Psychiatry:
An Evidence-Based Text

Psychiatry:
An Evidence-Based Text

Edited by

Professor Basant Puri
Honorary Consultant in Imaging and Psychiatry
Hammersmith Hospital and Imperial College, London, UK

Dr Ian Treasaden
Head of Forensic Neurosciences, Lipid Neuroscience Group
and Honorary Senior Lecturer in Psychiatry,
Imperial College London and Consultant Forensic Psychiatrist,
West London Mental Health NHS Trust, London, UK

HODDER
ARNOLD
AN HACHETTE UK COMPANY

First published in the UK in 2010 by
Hodder Arnold, an imprint of Hodder Education, an Hachette UK Company
338 Euston Road, London NW1 3BH

http://www.hodderarnold.com

British Library Cataloguing in Publication Data
A catalogue record for this book is available from the British Library

Library of Congress Cataloging-in-Publication Data
A catalog record for this book is available from the Library of Congress

ISBN 978 034 0950050

1 2 3 4 5 6 7 8 9 10

Commissioning Editor: Philip Shaw
Project Editors: Amy Mulick and Joanna Silman
Production Controller: Karen Dyer and Kate Harris
Cover Designer: Lynda King

Typeset in 9.5pt Rotis Serif by Phoenix Photosetting, Chatham, Kent
Printed in Italy

Contents

Contributors

Angela Attwood BSc PhD
Department of Experimental Psychology, University of Bristol, Bristol, UK

James Barrett MB BS(Hons) BSc MSc FRCPsych
Lead Clinician, National Gender Identity Clinic, London, UK

RH Belmaker MD
Hoffer-Vickar Professor of Psychiatry, Ben Gurion University of the Negev, Beer-Sheva, Israel

Boben Benjamin BSc (Hons) MD LRCP LRCS LMSSA MRCPsych
Specialist Registrar in Old Age Psychiatry, Wythenshawe Hospital, Manchester, UK

Dinesh Bhugra MA MSc MBBS FRCPsych MPhil Phd
Professor of Mental Health and Cultural Diversity, Institute of Psychiatry, Kings College London, London, UK

Jonathan Bird BSc MBChB FRCPsych
Consultant Neuropsychiatrist and Clinical Electro-encephalographer, The Burden Institute, Frenchay Hospital, Bristol, UK

Roger Bloor MD MPsyMed FRCPsych
Senior Lecturer and Consultant Psychiatrist, Keele University Medical School, Harplands Hospital, Staffordshire, UK

Mary Boulton BA PhD HonMFPH
Professor of Health Sociology, School of Health and Social Care, Oxford Brookes University, Oxford, UK

Andrew Brittlebank MA FRCPsych
Director of Medical Education, Northumberland Tyne and Wear NHS Trust, St Nicholas Hospital, Newcastle upon Tyne, UK

Ian Brockington MB B Chir MPhil MD FRCP FRCPsych
Professor Emeritus, University of Birmingham

Caroline Brown BSc PhD
Senior Lecturer, Department of Psychology, University of the West of England , Bristol, UK

Peter F Buckley MD
Professor and Chairman, Department of Psychiatry, Associate Dean for Leadership Development, Medical College of Georgia, Augusta, Georgia, USA

Alistair Burns MBChB FRCP FRCPsych MD MPhil DHMSA
Professor of Old Age Psychiatry, Deputy Dean (Clinical Affairs) University of Manchester, Manchester, UK

Stuart Carney MBChB MPH MRCPsych FAcadMed
Deputy National Director, UK Foundation Programme, Cardiff, UK

Charlotte Clark BSc (Hons) PhD
Lecturer in Environmental and Mental Health Epidemiology, Centre for Psychiatry, Wolfson Institute of Preventive Medicine, Barts and the London School of Medicine & Dentistry, Queen Mary, University of London, London, UK

Ilana Crome MA MD MPhil FRCPsych
Academic Director of Psychiatry and Professor of Addiction Psychiatry, Keele University Medical School, Harplands Hospital, Staffordshire, UK

Sean Cross BSc (Hons) MBChB MSt MRCPsych
SpR, Department of Liaison Psychiatry, St Thomas' Hospital, London, UK

Rudi Dallos BA MSc PhD Dip (Clin Psych)
Department of Clinical Psychology, University of Plymouth, UK

Mark Dickinson BSc MBBS MRCPsych
The Combined Learning Disability Team, Enfield, Middlesex, UK

Timothy G Dinan MD PhD FRCPsych
Department of Psychiatry, University College Cork, Ireland

Kedar Nath Dwivedi MBBS MD DPM FRCPsych
Director, International Institute of Child and Adolescent Mental Heath, Visiting Professor, London Metropolitan University, Formerly, Consultant Child and Adolescent Psychiatrist, Northampton, UK

Nicol Ferrier BSc MD FRCPsych FRCPed
Institute of Neuroscience, Newcastle University, Newcastle upon Tyne, UK

Peter Fitzgerald MB MRCPsych
Department of Psychiatry, University College Cork, Ireland

Peter Fonagy PhD FBA
Freud Memorial Professor of Psychoanalysis, University College London, Chief Executive, The Anna Freud Centre, London, UK

Bill (KWM) Fulford DPhil FRCP FRCPsych
Fellow of St Cross College, Member of the Philosophy Faculty and Honorary Consultant Psychiatrist, University of Oxford; Professor of Philosophy and Mental Health, University of Warwick; Co-Director, Institute for Philosophy, Diversity and Mental Health, University of Central Lancashire; and Special Adviser for Values-Based Practice, Department of Health, London, UK

Peter Garrard PhD FRCP
Reader in Neurology, University of Southampton School of Medicine Division of Clinical Neuroscience Southampton, UK

Steve Gentleman BSc PhD
Deputy Head of Division (Teaching), Reader in Experimental Neuropathology, Department of Clinical Neuroscience, Division of Neuroscience & Mental Health, Imperial College London, London, UK

Michael Gill MD MRCPsych FTCD
Professor of Psychiatry and Head of Department, Department of Psychiatry, Trinity Centre for Health Sciences, St. James' Hospital, Dublin, Ireland

Sandy Goldbeck-Wood MBChB MIPM MA (Psychoanalytic Studies) Dip (ERT)
Specialist Doctor in Obstetrics and Gynaecology, Ipswich Hospital, Suffolk, UK

John Gordon AB (Harvard)
Consultant Adult Psychotherapist, Forensic Psychotherapy Department and the Cassel Hospital, West London Mental Health NHS Trust; Psychoanalyst (British Psychoanalytic Association); Group Analyst (Institute of Group Analysis); Lecturer, Faculty of Continuing Education, Birkbeck College, University of London; and Honorary Senior Lecturer, Imperial College Medical School, London, UK

John Green BA MScClinPsych PhD
Chief Psychologist, CNW Department of Clinical Health Psychology, St. Mary's Hospital, London NHS Foundation Trust, UK; and Honorary Senior Lecturer in Behavioural Sciences, Imperial College, London

Richard Gross BA (Jt Hons) MA (Ed) Cert Ed
Full time academic author of many widely-used Psychology texts

Michael K Harte BSc PhD
Division of Pharmacology, School of Pharmacy, University of Bradford, Bradford, UK

Chris Hawley MB BS MRCPsych
Hertfordshire Partnership Foundation Trust, St Albans; and Bedfordshire and Hertfordshire Postgraduate Medical School, University of Hertfordshire, Hatfield, UK

David Hewison LLB PGDipSW CQSW MA ProfMbr SAP DipMarPsych FMbr SCPP DCplPsychPsych CertMgmt (Open)
Senior Couple Psychoanalytic Psychotherapist and Head of Research, Tavistock Centre for Couple Relationships, London, UK

Frank Holloway FRCPsych
Consultant Psychiatrist and Clinical Director, Croydon Integrated Adult Mental Health Service, South London and Maudsley NHS Foundation Trust, Bethlem Royal Hospital, Beckenham, UK

Malcolm Hooper PhD BPharm MRIC CChem
Emeritus Professor of Medicinal Chemistry, University of Sunderland, Sunderland, UK

Byron Hyde MD
Chairman, Nightingale Research Foundation, Ottawa, Canada

Borislav Iankov MBBS MRCPsych
Specialty Training Registrar – General Adult Psychiatry, Bedfordshire & Luton Mental Health and Social Care Partnership Trust, Luton, UK

Trisha A Jenkins BSc PhD
Department of Psychiatry, Queen's University Belfast, Belfast, UK

Peter B Jones MD PhD FRCIP FRCPsych FMedSci
Professor of Psychiatry and Head of Department, Department of Psychiatry, University of Cambridge, Cambridge, UK

Sridevi Kalidindi MRCPsych
Consultant Psychiatrist in Recovery and Rehabilitation Psychiatry, Croydon Integrated Adult Mental Health Service, South London and Maudsley Foundation NHS Trust, Bethlem Royal Hospital, Beckenham, UK

Gabriel Kirtchuk
Consultant Psychiatrist in Psychotherapy, Psychotherapy Training Department, West London Mental Health NHS Trust, Southall, Middlesex, UK

J Hubert Lacey MD MPhil FRCPsych
Professor of Psychiatry, St George's, University of London and Director of St George's Eating Disorders Service, London

Malcolm Lader OBE LLB DSc MD PhD FRCPsych FMed Sci
Emeritus Professor of Clinical Psychopharmacology, Institute of Psychiatry, King's College London, UK

Morven Leese MSc PhD
Health Service and Population Research Department, Institute of Psychiatry, Kings College London, London, UK

Pesach Lichtenberg MD
Department of Psychiatry, Herzog Hospital; and Clinical Senior Lecturer in Psychiatry, Hadassah Medical School of the Hebrew University of Jerusalem, Israel

Geoffrey G Lloyd FCC Psych MD MA
Visiting Consultant Psychiatrist, Priory Hospital North London, London, UK

Brian Lunn MB ChB FRCPsych
Honorary Clinical Senior Lecturer School of Medical Sciences Education Development, Newcastle University, Newcastle upon Tyne, UK

Chris Mace MD FRCPsych
Consultant Psychotherapist, Coventry and Warwickshire Partnership Trust, Honorary Associate Professor in Psychotherapy, University of Warwick, UK

Hameen Markar FRCP FRCPsych MPhil
Medical Director, Bedfordshire & Luton Mental Health and Social Care Partnership NHS Trust, Luton, UK

Rebecca Martinez DM MSc MRCEP MRCPsych
Clinical Lecturer in Psychiatry, Faculty of Medicine, University of Glasgow, Glasgow, UK

Jane McGrath MB MRCPsych
Department of Psychiatry, Trinity Centre for Health Sciences, St. James' Hospital, Dublin, Ireland

C Susan Mizen MBBS MRCPsych Memb SAP
Consultant Psychiatrist in Psychotherapy, Wonford House Hospital, Exeter, UK

David P Moore MD
Associate Clinical Professor, Department of Psychiatry and Department of Neurosurgery, University of Louisville School of Medicine, Louisville, Kentucky, USA

Ann Mortimer BSc MMedSc MD FRCPsych
Foundation chair in Psychiatry and Head of Department of Psychiatry, University of Hull, Hull, UK

Victoria Mountford BA Hons DClinPsych
Clinical Psychologist and Honorary Research Fellow, St George's Eating Disorders Service and St George's, University of London

Marcus R Munafò PhD
Reader in Biological Psychology, Department of Experimental Psychology, University of Bristol, Bristol, UK

Kingsley Norton MA (Cantab) MD FRCPsych
Consultant Psychotherapist, West London Mental Health Services, Southall, Middlesex, UK

Ash Padhi SpR
Specialist Trainee, Hertfordshire Partnership Foundation Trust, St Albans, UK

Hilary Pavis MA MRCGP
Consultant in Palliative Medicine, Nightingale Macmillan Unit, Royal Derby Hospital, Derby, UK

Raj Persaud FRCPsych
Consultant Psychiatrist, Emeritus Visiting Gresham Professor for the Public Understanding of Psychiatry, Gresham Collge, London, UK

Gavin P Reynolds BA PhD
Professor of Neuroscience, Department of Psychiatry, Queen's University Belfast, Belfast, UK

Allan Scott BSc MPhil MD MBA FRCPsych
Consultant Psychiatrist, Royal Edinburgh Hospital, Edinburgh, UK

John Shneerson MA DM MD FRCP FCCP
Sleep Disorders Unit, Papworth Hospital, Cambridge, UK

Iqbal Singh MB BS FRCPsych
Consultant Psychiatrist in Learning Disability, The Riverside Centre, Hillingdon Hospital, Uxbridge, Middlesex, UK

Georgina Smith
Department of Clinical Health Psychology, St. Mary's Hospital, London, UK

Paul St John Smith MA (Oxon) BM BCh FRCPsych
Consultant Psychiatrist, Hertfordshire Partnership Foundation Trust, St Albans, UK

Daniel Stahl Dipl Biol Dr rer nat
Lecturer in Biostatistics, Dept of Biostatistics & Computing, Institute of Psychiatry, Kings College London, London, UK

Stephen Stansfeld MB BS PhD MRCP FRCPsych
Chair & Centre Lead for Psychiatry, Centre for Psychiatry, Wolfson Institute of Preventive Medicine, Barts and the London School of Medicine & Dentistry, Queen Mary, University of London, London, UK

Maelie Swanwick FRCP
Consultant in Palliative Medicine, Nightingale Macmillan Unit, Royal Derby Hospital, Derby, UK

David Taylor BSc FFPH
Chief Pharmacist, South London and Maudsley NHS Foundation Trust, London, UK

Tim Thornton
Director of Philosophy and Professor of Philosophy and Mental Health, International School for Communities, Rights and Inclusion, University of Central Lancashire, Preston, UK

Sami Timimi MBChB MRCPsych
Consultant child and Adolescent Psychiatrist, Lincolnshire Partnership NHS Trust, Visiting Professor of Child and Adolescent Psychiatry, Faculty of Health and Social Sciences, Lincoln University

Lorna Torrens BA DClinPsych
Head of Clinical Psychology, Astley Ainslie Hospital, Edinburgh, UK

Trevor Turner DHMSA MD FRCPsych
Consultant Psychiatrist, East London Foundation Trust, Homerton University Hospital London; and Honorary Senior Clinical Lecturer, Barts and the London School of Medicine & Dentistry, Queen Mary, University of London, UK

Peter Tyrer FMedSci FRCPsych
Department of Psychological Medicine, Imperial College London, London, UK

Stephen Tyrer MB LMCC FRCPsych
Consultant in Psychiatry and Pain, Mental Health Unit, Southland Hospital, Invercargill, New Zealand

Fiona Warren MA PhD
Department of Psychology, Faculty of Arts and Human Sciences, University of Surrey, Guildford, UK

Kate Webb MRCPsych
Sp R and Honorary Research Assistant, St George's Eating Disorders Service and St George's, University of London, London, UK

Christopher J Williams BSc MBChB MMedSc MD FRCPsych
Senior Lecturer in Psychiatry, Faculty of Medicine, University of Glasgow, Glasgow, UK

Ewa Wisniewska Young MRCPsych
Specialist Registrar, Affective Disorders Unit, Royal Victoria Infirmary, Newcastle upon Tyne, UK

Ewa Zadeh MRCPsych
SpR and Honorary Research Assistant, St George's Eating Disorders Service and St George's, University of London, UK

Adam Zeman DM FRCP
Professor of Cognitive and Behavioural Neurology, Peninsula Medical School, Exeter, UK

Preface

Among the many demands on modern psychiatrists is keeping up to date with the ever-increasing pace of the development of psychiatric knowledge in recent years, both in the biological and psychosocial spheres. The basic sciences of psychology, neuroanatomy, neurophysiology, neuroendocrinology, neuroimaging, neuropathology, genetics, biochemistry, pharmacology, neuroscience, epidemiology and social sciences have now led to a better understanding of the basic mechanisms underlying clinical disorders. Sub-specialties of psychiatry have rapidly developed and the practice of psychiatry has increasingly moved from institutions to the community. Clinicians are now under pressure to deliver high quality cost-effective patient-focused care based upon the best evidence available.

The aim of this volume is to provide an up-to-date, solid, evidence-based text. Many of our contributors are acknowledged international leaders in their respective fields, have often been centrally involved at the forefront of shaping psychiatric research and practice and have, as a result, a first-hand feel of the evidence base of their contributions. The strength of the evidence base does still vary widely in different fields of psychiatry, but with the development of national guidelines, systematic reviews and meta-analyses, individual, sometimes idiosyncratic, clinical practices of the past are now no longer acceptable unless based on evidence. Thus, even if not entirely evidence based, psychiatry should always be evidence informed. Psychiatrists who increasingly work in multidisciplinary teams and whose practice is now increasingly challenged by other professionals, managers and, indeed, patients, now have to be able to defend the evidence base to their practice, if they are to maintain their medical leadership role in psychiatric practice.

In this book, we aim to comprehensively describe the basic sciences and clinical disorders and their treatments – using the UK and Ireland MRCPsych syllabus as a guide – while emphasising the evidence underlying theory and practice for the topics covered. However, we believe that this book will cater not only for trainee psychiatrists studying for the MRCPsych examinations, but also for trainees elsewhere and, indeed, will provide a valuable resource for psychiatrists who have completed their training and other professionals who work in psychiatry.

To facilitate the aim of this project, the book is divided into major sections and 79 chapters in a carefully considered order. Chapters have been standardised and cross referenced and include important and up to date references and generous use of tables, figures, boxes and pictures. At the end of each chapter major learning points are identified. While the book strives to provide an integrated overview of current knowledge through its sections and chapters, ,chapters have also been designed to stand alone, which inevitably implies some overlap in content between chapters which we hope has been kept to an acceptable minimum.

We hope this book will achieve wide acceptance through its succinct, user-friendly approach and its recognition of the importance of a solid evidence base for psychiatric practice. While a text book alone does not make a good psychiatrist, we hope this one will provide the sound foundation of evidence-based theoretical knowledge required for the competent practising clinician of today.

Basant K Puri
Ian Treasaden

Acknowledgements

We would like to warmly thank our contributors for their excellent contributions, delivered often on tight deadlines. We would also like to thank our publishers Hodder, including the Commissioning Editor, Philip Shaw, and the Project Editors, Amy Mulick and Joanna Silman, for their encouragement and always helpful assistance. We also wish to thank our Publisher, Caroline Makepeace. We would additionally like to thank Susan Oxlade for her administrative and secretarial assistance.

PART 1

The foundations of modern psychiatric practice

Chapter 1

History of psychiatry

Trevor Turner

INTRODUCTION

Psychiatric illness seems intrinsic to – and a necessary part of – being *Homo sapiens*, so it is not surprising that there are descriptions of abnormal behaviour, and even of symptoms resembling schizophrenia, in the earliest written fragments of Egypt, India and Babylon. Some evolutionary theorists consider psychosis to be inextricably linked to the genetic mutation(s) for our enlarged frontal lobe, with its unique capacity for memory and imagination. A history of psychiatry has to understand therefore how 'mental' symptoms – presentations of madness, sadness, foolishness, strangeness – were understood in all societies and accepted, or not, and what was done, or not, to help the sufferers.

There is thus a long history of mental illness consisting of 3000 years of random descriptions (in religious writings, legal documents, diaries, histories, romances and plays), and a shorter and more technical/medical history of practical psychiatry, in terms of professionalized attempts to understand, diagnose and treat mentally ill people. The long history precedes even the Bible and Classical Greece, while the short history starts some 200 years ago (at least in European terms), a product of the scientific advances of the Enlightenment, industrialization and city life. Supernatural 'apparitions' become secularized 'hallucinations', and psychopathology begins to erode the varieties of religious explanation.

HISTORIOGRAPHY – i.e. WHAT'S BEEN WRITTEN ABOUT IT

This chapter concentrates on the past two centuries as being essential to understanding what drives modern psychiatry. Just as taking a history is the key to psychiatric diagnosis, so knowing how and why we are at our present state of knowledge and organization helps us to make sense of our current work. In itself, the topic 'the history of psychiatry' has undergone a radical change in the past 30 years, from the obscure jottings of retired psychiatrists to a thriving subspecialty of modern historical research. It has its own quarterly journal, *History of Psychiatry* (first published in March 1990), its own European Association and a body of dedicated academic historians. The standard heavyweight tomes, such as *The History of Psychiatry* by Alexander and Selesnick (1966), have been replaced by more svelte versions, such as Edward Shorter's (1997) *A History of Psychiatry: From the Era of the Asylum to the Age of Prozac*, and diagnosis-based compilations such as *A History of Clinical Psychiatry: The Origin and History of Psychiatric Disorders* (Berrios and Porter, 1995). There has also been a series of reprints of core psychiatric textbooks and careful descriptions of whole eras of change, for example Andrew Scull's (1979) *Museums of Madness*, subtitled *The Social Organisation of Insanity in Nineteenth Century England*. Details of the most substantial histories of psychiatry, and the most influential secondary texts and textbooks (or versions thereof) are given in Tables 1.1–3.

Most importantly, there has been a prolonged, sometimes bitter but generally creative debate since the rise of the so-called 'anti-psychiatry movement' of the 1960s and 1970s as to what is even meant by a 'history of psychiatry' or a 'history of insanity' or of 'madness', and so on. Traditionally it had been the recording of notable forms of mental illness, whether in literature (e.g. Shakespeare's King Lear or Othello) or medical writings, accompanied by outlines of new diagnostic or treatment approaches, with admiring biographies of the leading doctors (not always medical) who had tried to help or even 'cure' the afflicted mad folk. This so-called 'meliorist' history – things getting better, in terms of more accurate diagnoses, more thoughtful doctors (and attendants/nurses) and more humane treatments – was challenged in the writings of social theorists such as Michel Foucault and Andrew Scull (see Table 1.2).

Foucault postulated a 'Great Confinement' in the seventeenth and eighteenth centuries, whereby the world of free-thinking and imaginative 'unreason' had been corralled by the mechanistic warriors of reason and social control. Psychiatrists and the psychiatric enterprise were even seen as a kind of thought police of this dark Enterprise. Mental illness was theorized as 'socially constructed', a means of rounding up the deviants and low life in society rather than a genuine part of medical practice dealing with real diseases. This debate goes on, has involved historians, psychologists, anthropologists, lawyers, sociologists and even a few psychiatrists, and has now swung back to some degree

Table 1.1 Ten histories of psychiatry

Reference	Comment
Tuke DH (1968; reprint of 1882 edn) *Chapters in the History of the Insane*, Amsterdam: Bonset	The original heroic nineteenth-century history, written as a celebration of Victorian achievement in building asylums and rescuing 'lunatics' from the neglect and abuse of whips, chains and supernatural beliefs
Zilboorg G, with Henry GW (1941) *A History of Medical Psychology*, New York: Norton & Co.	Zealously pro-Freudian ('the second psychiatric revolution'), this is written in the classic 'great men' style of history but has good details and nice photographs. Psychoanalysis is seen as the cure for all mental illness and more
Hunter R, Macalpine I (1963) *Three Hundred Years of Psychiatry 1535–1860*, Oxford: Oxford University Press	An extraordinary collection, over 1000 pages long, of extracts from several hundred original (primary) sources arranged chronologically and with a superb index. The ideal reference book for any facet of psychiatric diagnosis, language and treatment. Great for lecture introductions
Alexander FG, Selesnick ST (1966) *The History of Psychiatry*, New York: Harper & Row	The standard of its time but also in awe of Freud, more than half being devoted to the 'Freudian Age'. Much material from classical/medieval times, but unreliable in details. For example: 'It does not seem probable that ... pharmacological and biological methods will throw more light upon the complex phenomena of interpersonal relationships and replace psychological methods of treatment'
Jones K (1993) *Asylums and After: A Revised History of the Mental Health Services – From the Early Eighteenth Century to the 1990s*, London: Athlone Press	Describing how services developed, this is the best analysis of the rise and fall of the asylums, with special insight into the social, legal and political influences on psychiatry, including the deinstitutionalization of the past 50 years. Very critical of the weaknesses of 'care in the community'.
Scull A (1993) *The Most Solitary of Afflictions: Madness and Society in Britain 1700–1900*, New Haven, CT, and London: Yale University Press	An updated version of the author's groundbreaking *Museums of Madness* (1979), which introduced a radically new take on psychiatry as representing social power and social control, thus reinforcing the status quo via an often doubtful construct of 'mental illness'. A challenging way of looking at history, even if you disagree
Shorter E (1997) *A History of Psychiatry: From the Era of the Asylum to the Age of Prozac*, New York: John Wiley & Sons	The best modern history by far, though avowedly organicist in tone. Readable, beautifully detailed and with real narrative drive, concentrating on developments since *c.*1800. The author concludes that 'neurochem' and 'neurochat' augment each other as the optimum form of care
Andrews J, Briggs A, Porter R, Tucker P, Waddington K (1997) *The History of Bethlem*, London: Routledge	A highly detailed and extensively researched 750 pages of modern social history, published to celebrate Bethlem Hospital's 750th anniversary. A very technical text, for the specialist
Berrios G, Porter R (eds) (1995) *A History of Clinical Psychiatry: The Origin and History of Psychiatric Disorders*, London: Athlone	A multi-author volume reviewing the clinical and social history of our understanding of the major mental disorders (e.g. dementia, schizophrenia, anxiety), including neuropsychiatric conditions and the epilepsies. Not for reading through, but it is well referenced, and individual topic chapters (e.g. post-traumatic shock disorder, shell shock) are fascinating
Fuller Torrey E, Miller J (2001) *The Invisible Plague: The Rise of Mental Illness from 1750 to the Present*, Piscataway, NJ, and London: Rutgers University Press	A spirited and informative outline concentrating on the theory that severe schizophreniform mental illness represents a modern epidemic due to industrialization and urbanization. Diet, toxins, infectious agents (related to vaccination?) and even pet cats are among the postulated aetiological agents. Or is this retrospective history gone too far?

towards a general acceptance that there, probably, is such a thing as mental illness.

The key research has been into archival sources such as asylum records (going back to the mid-nineteenth century and sometimes earlier), the casebooks of individual doctors, for example the famed eighteenth-century 'mad-doctor' and physician to Bethlem ('Bedlam') Hospital, John Monro (1715–91), the writings of psychiatric patients themselves,

Table 1.2 Ten influential secondary texts

Foucault M (1965) *Madness and Civilization: A History of Insanity in the Age of Reason* (trans. R Howard), New York: Random House	The key work of the most celebrated cultural historian of the past 50 years, this posits a belief that mental illness is 'not a natural fact but a cultural construct', not a disease needing treatment but an issue of freedom, knowledge and power. Written in the impressionistic, deliberately indefinite style of much modern French philosophy, it is a real challenge, both to psychiatry as a reasonable profession and to the average empirical English reader
Hunter R, Macalpine I (1969) *George III and the Mad Business*, London: Penguin	Classic outline of good archival research into the much debated illness of King George III (1760–1820). Was it porphyria or just another routine manic disorder? More recently turned into a popular play and then a film, *The Madness of King George*, by the writer Alan Bennett
Ellenberger HF (1970) *The Discovery of the Unconscious: The History and Evolution of Dynamic Psychiatry*, New York: Basic Books	Over 900 pages on the development of psychological approaches to mental illness, and how Freud emerged successfully from numerous rivals. An absorbing matchless account of how theories come and go
Hunter R, Macalpine I (1974) *Psychiatry for the Poor: 1851 Colney Hatch Asylum–Friern Hospital 1973 – A Medical and Social History*, Folkestone: Dawson	Minutes, reports, photos, patients, medical and nursing staff – the archetypal asylum history, unvarnished but perfectly evocative of the practical management of an enormous institution (up to 2700 inmates) in a bygone era
Simon B (1978) *Mind and Madness in Ancient Greece: The Classical Roots of Modern Psychiatry*, Ithaca, NY: Cornell University Press	The classic exposition of Greek ideas, with chapters on 'tragedy and therapy' and 'Plato and Freud'
MacDonald M (1981) *Mystical Bedlam: Madness, Anxiety and Healing in Seventeenth Century England*, Cambridge: Cambridge University Press	A detailed analysis of the records of Richard Napier (1559–1634), a mystic and astrologer, much famed in his time, who treated over 2000 mentally disturbed patients who might be 'mopish', 'troubled in mind' or 'mad/lunatic'
Petersen D (ed.) (1982) *A Mad People's History of Madness*, Pittsburgh, PA: University of Pittsburgh Press	A collection of 27 accounts of being mentally ill, written by the patients, from the fifteenth to the twentieth century. A selective selection, but well edited historically. History from the patient's viewpoint, and so a unique version of common symptoms
Valenstein ES (1986) *Great and Desperate Cures: The Rise and Decline of Psychosurgery and Other Radical Treatments for Mental Illness*, New York: Basic Books	It will 'chill the marrow of naive readers' ran the blurb, and this is a well-researched account of lobotomy, its leading exponents (Moniz and Freeman) and its rationale. Imagine having your brain cut into as part of an out-patient procedure, and then being sent home to convalesce
Berrios GE, Freeman H (eds) (1991) *150 Years of British Psychiatry 1841–1991* London: Gaskell; and Berrios GE, Freeman H (eds) (1996) *Volume II: The Aftermath*, London: Athlone	A vivid collection of 28 essays, mainly by psychiatrists, covering the 'institutions', 'ideas' and 'people' dominating UK psychiatric development. Wonderfully, obsessionally(?) detailed. Much praised by professional historians
Porter R (2002) *Madness: A Brief History*, Oxford: Oxford University Press	A mere 230 or so pages. A brief, lively and easy-to-read historian's account of 'madness' – so not in fact confined to 'psychiatry'

and court records dealing with, for example, insane murderers. If you are prepared to hunt around in medieval documentation – and that is hard work, in terms of finding and even reading the material, which is often in Latin – and in dusty library records, a much more nuanced picture of how madness has been dealt with through the ages can be extracted, albeit often in bits and pieces, like the shards of pottery from an archaeological dig.

For example, if we consider how people deemed to be 'mad' or 'lunatic' were dealt with in Shakespeare's time (1564–1616), whether in his plays or in the plays of his contemporaries, it is not a lot different from today. Recognizing

Table 1.3 Ten interesting textbooks

Pinel P (1801) *A Treatise on Insanity* (trans. DD Davis), New York: Hafner Publishing	An outline of 'maniacal disorders', including an attempt at classification and numerous case histories. A humane, detailed and easy-to-read masterpiece – the first modern textbook with delightful descriptions of treatments, theatrical(s), and moral and physical approaches to managing very disordered people
Haslam J (1810) *Illustrations of Madness: Exhibiting a Singular Case of Insanity and a No Less Remarkable Difference in Medical Opinion*, London: Hayden; reprinted, Porter R (ed.) (1988) London: Tavistock Classics	A book-length account of a contended case, illustrating a 'first-rank' series of colourful symptoms typical of a florid paranoid schizophrenia, but that nevertheless generated considerable doubt and debate at that time
Bucknill J, Tuke DH (1858) *A Manual of Psychological Medicine*; facsimile edn (1968) New York: Hafner	The first proper English treatise of psychiatry, indicating the growing size of the specialty and the need for a student's textbook. Easy to read, quite sceptical, and with excellent clinical descriptions and references to the literature. Treatment is divided into 'hygienic', 'moral' and 'medical'
Maudsley H (1867) *The Physiology and Pathology of the Mind* London: Macmillan	A much admired textbook outlining the physical basis of mental disease as opposed to the 'metaphysical' theorizing that tended to dominate public discussion. Maudsley was a bluff Yorkshireman with a sarcastic tongue, but he was widely read in the French and German literature. Although much quoted, it was probably not practically used by working psychiatrists of his time
Von Krafft-Ebbing R (1886) *Psychopathia Sexualis: With Especial Reference to Contrary Sexual Instinct – A Medico-Legal Study* (trans. G Chaddock 1892), Philadelphia, PA: Davis & Co.	The first detailed description of abnormal sexual behaviours, including sadism, masochism, 'congenital inversion' (i.e. homosexuality) and fetishism. An entertaining collection of case histories, in great detail, bringing to light a wide range of sexual 'pathologies' usually suppressed even in the technical and medical literature of the time
Freud S (1900) *The Interpretation of Dreams* (trans. J Strachey 1976), London: Pelican Books	The classic Freud text on his theory of the unconscious, dreams being considered essential to understanding one's inner mental life. From this he moved on to developing his highly influential theories of childhood sexuality and the 'Oedipal complex' of character development. Lots of examples, but not 'scientific', although claimed as such
Kraepelin E (1904, 1905, 1912 – very popular) *Lectures on Clinical Psychiatry* (ed. T Johnston), London: Bailliere, Tindall and Cox	Summarizing the classic and groundbreaking textbook – Kraepelin in fact produced eight editions of his Lehrbuch from 1886 to 1924, which first described dementia praecox as a distinct psychotic disorder. His distinction between dementia praecox/schizophrenia and manic-depressive insanity continues to dominate diagnostic categories today
Bleuler E (1911) *Dementia Praecox or The Group of Schizophrenias* (trans. J Zinkin 1950), New York: International University Press	The book that introduced the term 'schizophrenia', fusing psychoanalytic theory derived from Freud with the clinical descriptions of Kraepelin. The Bleulerian outline of schizophrenia dominated psychiatry until the 1960s. His four 'A's (autism, affective impairment, ambivalence, impaired associations) made reliable diagnosis rather difficult
Sargant W, Slater E (1944) *An Introduction to Physical Methods of Treatment in Psychiatry*, Edinburgh: Livingstone	The (wartime) classic of biological psychiatry, trumpeting the use of insulin therapy, electroconvulsive therapy (ECT), chemical sedation, malaria treatment and prefrontal leucotomy, as opposed to psychotherapy, to which the authors barely paid lip service. Biology red in tooth and claw, claiming mental disorders as 'dependent on physiological changes'
Jung CG (1963) *Memories, Dreams, Reflections*; reprinted (1995) London: Fontana Press	The summation of the theories and work of Carl Jung (1875–1961), the long-lived alternative to Freud. Many 'Jungian analysts' are still influential today. His notion of archetypes and the collective unconscious are at the very edge of psychiatry, verging into spirituality, anthropology and religion. And he did actually try to psychoanalyse psychotics, unlike Freud, as outlined in his 1907 *The Psychology of Dementia Praecox*

mental illness was based on people's behaviours, what they said and what they perceived (e.g. Lady Macbeth's recurrent and obsessional hand-washing), doctors are called to attend them (e.g. Dr Caius in *The Comedy of Errors*), and disordered brains are seen as part of the problem ('canst thou not minister to a mind diseased ... raze out the written troubles of the brain ...', asks Macbeth of his physician). Confinement in madhouses, or 'dark houses' (e.g. Malvolio in *As You Like It*), or somewhere out of the way, is a common resort. We even have, in the character of Tom O'Bedlam in the play *King Lear* a vivid description of someone pretending to be mad. This is the eventual hero, Edgar, who in order to avoid entrapment and murder hides out half-naked, gibbering to himself and expressing a range of symptoms that today are entirely consistent with what we call 'schizophrenia'. If that is what early-seventeenth-century play-goers recognized as mental illness, then it seems reasonably indicative of the persistence of what we call schizophrenia, over some 400 years or more, rather than it being (as some have postulated) a relatively new disease of the industrial age of the nineteenth century and beyond (see especially Fuller Torrey, in Table 1.1).

TREATING MENTAL ILLNESS: WHERE, HOW, WHO?

The past 200 years have seen the rise and fall of a standard approach to mental illness – the asylum. Founded as a vehicle for delivery of what was essentially a structured psychosocial intervention, namely the 'moral treatment', the asylum has dominated psychiatric practice since the mid-nineteenth century – throughout the world – and only in the past 30 years has it became subservient to the notions of 'community care'. In fact the asylum arose because of the failures of community care – troubled souls wandering the countryside and dying of starvation, or being chained up in cellars or attics (à la Rochester's wife in the 1847 novel *Jane Eyre*) or unreliable private madhouses. The combination of Quaker concern, evangelical Christianity and the bricks-and-mortar solution of Victorian industrialization demanded that the 'pauper insane' be placed in large sanctuaries, i.e. the asylums, rather like medieval lepers in leprosaria. The rise of modern risk management and the medium-secure unit (MSU) are merely a replication of this process under a new guise. 'Normal' folk distrust (and exploit) 'mad' folk – thus the unique role of the psychiatrist in negotiating the relationship.

There is also during this period the development of a specialist profession, from a few scattered individuals, good-hearted clergymen looking after people in their houses, to the organization of medico-psychological associations and the first regular journals (e.g. *The Asylum Journal* in 1854, now the *British Journal of Psychiatry*). The troubled story of the development of psychiatry reflects another essential theme, namely stigma, the fear of the insane, and the difficulties their case has met in terms of resources, trained staff, research-based treatments and integration back into 'normal' society. Even today many doctors and nurses qualify, all over the world, without having partaken in any genuine psychiatric training or practice.

Yet psychiatry, one of the first true specializations in medicine, actually spawned the subspecialty of neurology and is the branch of medicine most outward-looking in terms of its relationship with sociology, psychology, criminology, the law, architecture, and social and working life. It has its heroes and its villains of course, more of the former than the latter, and has been cruelly mocked, not least in modern cinema (e.g. Hannibal Lecter in *The Silence of the Lambs* in 1991) and for indulging in what are termed 'desperate remedies' such as lobotomy and electroconvulsive therapy (ECT). But much retrospective criticism, which rarely comes from mainstream historians, often fails to understand how difficult it always has been to cope with chronic, unremitting, progressive psychosis.

The journey from essentially social and institutional treatments (e.g. asylums) to various psychological approaches (e.g. Sigmund Freud and friends), and on to the 1950s rise of psychopharmacology, is full of iconic stories. Philippe Pinel (1745–1826), the father of French psychiatry, unchaining the insane in 1792, in the middle of the chaos of the French Revolution (a battalion of soldiers hiding round the back of the hospital in case all hell broke loose); John Conolly (1794–1866) introducing, against mocking scepticism, non-restraint to the enormous Hanwell asylum (his monograph on non-restraint was published in 1856); the unravelling of 'general paralysis of the insane' (GPI) as in fact an infectious disease, tertiary syphilis, and its response to malaria therapy researched and developed by Julius Wagner-Jauregg (1857–1940), psychiatry's first Nobel Prize winner; the shell shock debate during and after the First World War (was it physical, a form of brain damage, or nervous, or cowardice even?), and the million or more war pensions generated; the transformed acute wards of the 1950s and the reported great interest of the nursing personnel when chlorpromazine, a 'neuroleptic', was introduced. These are mainly true, and some of the key historical themes are outlined in Table 1.4.

THE WORLD OF BEDLAM PRE-1800

Biblical and classical writings give many descriptions of people going mad, mainly kings and heroes such as Saul, Nebuchadnezzar and Ajax (who ran amok and slaughtered a herd of sheep). The long-influential Greco-Roman physician Galen (c.AD129–200) reinforced the Hippocratic doctrine of the humoral theory – the four humours (i.e. visible bodily secretions) being phlegm (tears or sweat), blood, yellow bile (choler) and black bile (= 'melancholia' in Greek), imbalances of which were seen as the basis of all

Table 1.4 Key historical themes

Language	From 'mania' and 'melancholia' to 'madness', 'insanity' and 'mental illness' – via 'neurosis' and 'psychosis' – there has been a constant and often confusing expansion of terms. Does this represent a changing pattern of illness or simply changing presentations? (Are mental illnesses cultural constructs or real diseases?) James Prichard's descriptions of cases of 'moral insanity', in 1835, would be diagnosed today as either personality disorder or bipolar illness. George Beard's 1869 outline of 'neurasthenia' is now covered by various forms of depression, anxiety and phobias. Modern 'schizophrenia' is relatively unique as a diagnostic term, surviving for over 100 years, unlike most of its contemporaries
Causation	Theories of humoral imbalance (i.e. some form of physical disorder) vied with supernatural beliefs (curses, witchcraft, secret sins) well into the eighteenth century. By the nineteenth century concerns about 'moral' causes (i.e. bad habits, sexual excess, cigar-smoking) vied with increasingly physical theories, as indicated by the practice of phrenology, with leading exponents being Drs Franz Gall (1758–1828) and JC Spurzheim (1776–1832). Phrenology considered the brain as the organ of the mind, different activities being located in different areas (the precursor of cerebral localization), demanding careful examination therefore of the shape of one's head (e.g. the notion of high-brow *v.* low-brow). This led on to the criminal anthropology of Cesare Lombroso (1836–1909) identifying criminality (and mental illness) via various physical stigmata. The ongoing debates as to nature *v.* nurture and organic *v.* psychological reflect this long-standing argument. The journey of the 'psychoses' from being disorders of the soul (i.e. psyche) to established diseases of the brain nicely illustrates this history
Treatment	Psychiatrists have always been asked to talk to patients in a special way ('fixing with the eye') in order to persuade them out of their delusions or into sober personal habits, voluntarily or by overt or covert enforcement. They have used 'behavioural' medications (e.g. to make one sweat or vomit), physical controls such as straitjackets or special chairs, locked wards and controlled diet and exercise, and social activities or even amusements, in a community context. Specific antipsychotics or monitored psychological therapies, as in the last half-century, are genuinely innovative. Putting mentally ill people into prisons is a reversion of Enlightenment principles
Law	When James Hadfield shot at King George III in a theatre on 15 May 1800 and was charged with 'high treason', he stated that he had been acting on God's instructions. Deemed not responsible, he was sent to Bethlem, and deciding on whether someone is 'mad' or 'bad' has subsequently dominated public attitudes to mental illness. The attempted murders of royalty (Queen Victoria endured at least seven failed assassinations), and murders by and of famous people, have always made excellent journalist copy. The McNaughton Rules, determining criminal insanity (e.g. 'knowing the nature of the act'), derive from the famous 1843 trial of Daniel McNaughton who murdered the then prime minister's private secretary, mistaking him for the prime minister. The 1863 founding of Broadmoor Hospital, for the reception of criminal lunatics, institutionalized the acceptance that capital punishment was not appropriate for people labouring under any 'defect of reason'. Henry Maudsley's 1874 *Responsibility in Mental Disease* was the first forensic psychiatric textbook, and the 'insanity defence' has been a key arbiter of psychiatry's public standing
Nervous disorders	Patients and practitioners have constantly wanted to distance themselves from 'raving and furious' madmen, even though they might seek help in dealing with chronic anxiety, tiredness, 'nerves', 'vapours', etc. The rise of a middle class generated a need for physicians specializing in 'office practice' (as opposed to asylum management). Mesmerism and hypnotism, spas and 'the water treatment', tonics and electric machines, and special dietary regimes such as Silas Weir Mitchell's 'Fat and Blood', a disgusting diet consisting of just those products while bed-bound for 6 weeks, could be fashionable and lucrative. The success of Sigmund Freud and other psychotherapists reflected this search for special, personal understanding. The ultimate mystique of the doctor therapist can be seen in TS Eliot's 1950 play *The Cocktail Party*

disease, physical or mental. Most of the latter came under the terms 'mania' and 'melancholia', people being overexcited by too much blood/choler or slowed down by too much phlegm or black bile. In the West the rise of Christianity led to the elaboration of supernatural and later witchcraft theories, mental illness even being seen as a punishment for wickedness, despite Jesus Christ 'casting out devils' from madmen, as regularly reported in the four Gospels.

From the fall of Rome to the Renaissance, such notions became a fixed part of approaches to treatment. The agrarian poor looked to holy shrines, magic potions, wise women or necessary beatings. The 'furious' mad were tied up in cellars or driven from parish to parish. Suicide was a sin – with a loss of possessions – and thus coroners' juries increasingly tried to establish a *non-compos mentis* verdict, medicalizing the deed in order to avoid penalizing the family. Physicians might be sought for the wealthy (Henry

VI, king of England from 1422 to 1461, when he heard 'voices' saw a learned doctor), with the use of laxatives ('purging') or bleeding as the standard approaches (to get rid of the excess humours).

With the Renaissance came a questioning of accepted ideas, with witchcraft trials (some 50 000 executions during the sixteenth and seventeenth centuries) providing one battleground. This European 'witch-craze' was fuelled by challenges to papal authority, for example by 'Protestant' preachers such as Martin Luther (1483–1546) or by scientists, such as Galileo Galilei (1564–1642) demonstrating that the earth went round the sun (not the other way round). Reactionary work appeared, famously *Malleus Maleficarum* (1486) written by two monks, Kraemer and Sprengler. A kind of handbook for witch-finding, this 'Hammer of Evil-Doing' was like a modern National Institute for Clinical Excellence (NICE) guideline, and it took a brave German physician, Johannes Weyer (1515–88), to produce the sceptical counterblast. His *De Praestigiis Daemonum* ('The Devil's Signs') of 1563 suggested that mental illness, with its ravings and imaginings, was often and easily mistaken for witchcraft.

Were these disordered women – and they were mainly women – dangerous witches, needing to be burnt at the stake, or brain-sick lunatics? Regular physicians such as William Harvey (1578–1657), discoverer of the circulation of the blood and physician to King Charles I, had another role as detectors of witchcraft, advising courts on what was illness and what was not. His contemporaries included Richard Burton, author of the *Anatomy of Melancholy* (1621), an enormous compendium of exemplary cases – troubled minds, not necessarily 'depressed', in all their different lifestyles and presentations – and Richard Napier (see Table 1.2), an astrologer-cum-psychotherapist who gained a reputation for helping mentally ill people and whose notebooks still survive.

By about 1700 most of Europe was over its witch beliefs, and during the seventeenth and eighteenth centuries a rising demand for sympathetic treatment rather than incarceration demonstrated the swing from religious supernaturalism to rationalist and early scientific explanations. Now come the first medical writings on mental illnesses and the beginnings of the 'mad-doctoring' business. William Battie (1703–76), with his *Treatise on Madness* (1758) and a famous debate with John Monro (1715–91) as to the real basis of mental illness (deluded imagination or impaired judgement?), and George Cheyne (1671–1743), with his 1733 description of *The English Malady*, were the most famous of their time, doing very well for themselves in a seemingly lucrative trade. The better-off English middle classes had discovered neurosis.

Apart from a 1744 Vagrancy Act, however, the first law passed 'for the better maintenance and care of Lunatics' was in 1808, fear of mental illness creating shame and family cover-ups. When George III went mad in 1788, putting the constitution itself at peril, psychiatry was represented by a self-made Lincolnshire reverend/therapist, Francis Willis. The king was 'knocked flat as a flounder' via a behavioural regime that eventually brought him back to his senses, and he was even 'cured'. Treatment of disease rather than punishment for sins gradually became the standard approach. Contemporary descriptions of Parkinson's disease (in 1817), delirium tremens (in 1813) and the brains of post-mortem syphilitics (in 1822) demonstrated the physical basis of some (but not most) disordered behaviours.

THE RISE OF THE ASYLUM 1800–1900

The early private madhouses have few records, as privacy was required, but business flourished in the rising prosperity and urbanization of the eighteenth century. There had always been St Mary Bethlem (founded in 1247) – home of the Tom-of-Bedlams, wandering madmen, of myth and Shakespeare – and from the 1750s new charitable institutions (e.g. St Luke's in London, the Bethel in Norwich) were set up. A flourishing area for private madhouses was around Shoreditch, Bethnal Green and Hackney in east London, some of them family businesses ('Mr Balme's House') with lurid reputations. Concerns about maltreatment (patients left tied up in filthy, faeces-coated cots), and especially the death of Hannah Mills, in the York Hospital, led the local Quakers to set up, for their 'brethren', 'the Retreat', which became a European model. Not least this reputation was thanks to the masterly public relations of the 1813 *Description of the Retreat* by Samuel Tuke, outlining a form of treatment called 'moral therapy' based on kindness, reason, behavioural limits, exercise and activities, a family atmosphere and setting a good example.

In the year of the Battle of Waterloo (1815), there was also a widely reported Inquiry into Bethlem Hospital, detailing abuses and negligence, for example keeping one notorious patient in a metal contraption and chains for over 7 years (Figure 1.1). Especially scapegoated was the apothecary John Haslam, whose case study (1810) of Bethlem inmate James Tilly Matthews, *Illustrations of Madness* (see Table 1.3), is often quoted as the first description of a full-blown schizophrenia-type illness, with delusions, hallucinations and a bizarre range of other symptoms, including the patient's belief in an infernal air loom machine, run by a dangerous gang, that could do things such as 'thigh-talking', 'thought-making' and 'cutting soul from sense'. The ignorance of such disorders among the medical profession was a particular target of Haslam, since two prominent society physicians actually tried to have Tilly Matthews released, on the grounds that he was perfectly sane.

The resultant evangelical reform movement, led by the long-lived Lord Ashley, seventh Earl of Shaftesbury (1801–84), based on the principles of moral therapy, unchaining the insane (as Philippe Pinel in revolutionary Paris) and the

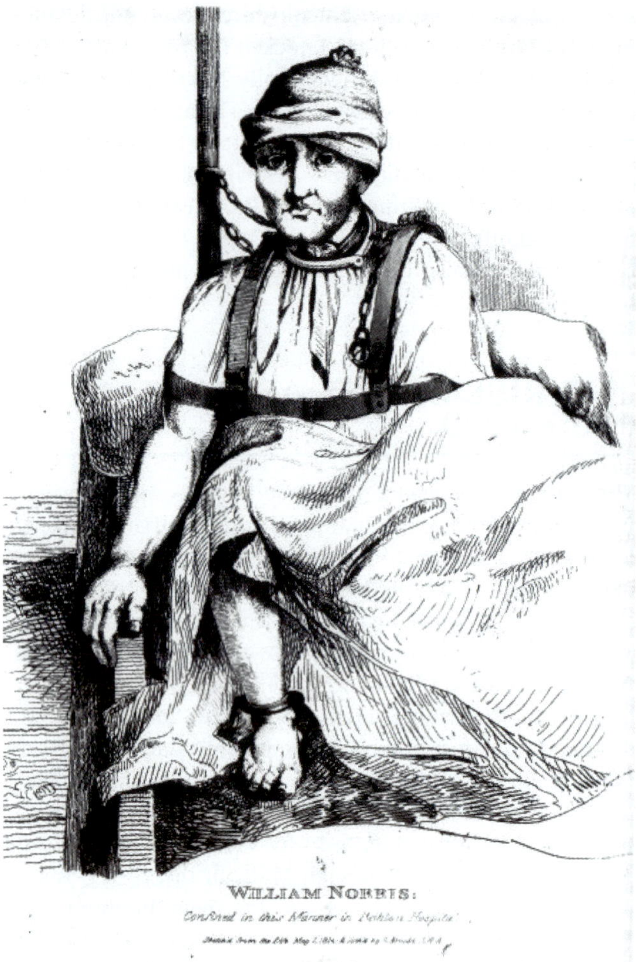

Figure 1.1 The iconic image of the Bethlem Inquiry: William Norris in the chained contraption in which he was kept in for 7 years

central role of the medical profession, created a specific therapeutic device for curing madness. This was the asylum, where 'lunatics' could be taken away from the hurly-burly of modern life (deemed to be driving them mad) and restored amidst fresh air, nice views, clean water and regular exercise. By 1845 every county in England had a statutory duty to build one (the Asylums Act). Such ring-fencing of money, for a particular specialty, has even been considered a kind of precursor to the start of the National Health Service (NHS), and over 120 asylums were eventually constructed in Britain (Figure 1.2), amidst a relentless rise in people deemed officially to be insane.

The psychiatric profession, throughout Europe, developed alongside the new asylums. Journals were founded, reports were published, posts were created and formal legal powers (certification) were introduced. Still readily stigmatized as 'mad-doctors' – hence the increasing fears about sane people being locked up for nefarious reasons (e.g. in novels such as *The Woman in White* by Wilkie Collins (1860) and *Hard Cash* by Charles Reade (1863)) – this new breed of 'alienists'-cum-'medical psychologists' wrote and held meetings and lobbied Parliament, but treatment approaches remained basic. Apart from the traditional purging, bleeding, confinement and exercise, they had to resort to devices such as whirling chairs, mustard baths (hot and cold), leeches and even early forms of electricity. Laying open the scalp, filling the wound with various herbs and ointments, and letting it suppurate for a week or two was practised by Dr Prichard, author of the much admired *A Treatise of Insanity*, published in 1835. For sedating medication they

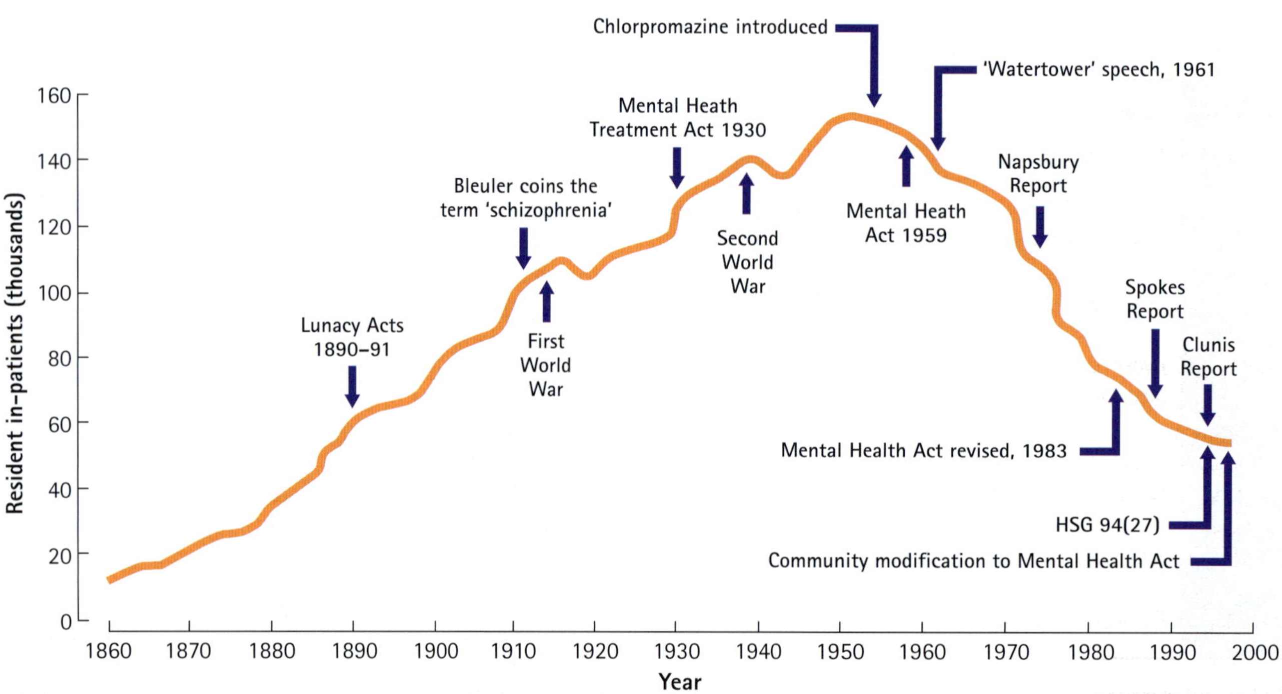

Figure 1.2 In-patients resident in mental illness hospitals, England and Wales, 1860–1995

had only opium/morphine, chloral hydrate and, of course, cannabis indica and brandy (Table 1.5).

But these first-generation psychiatrists and asylum superintendents did have one advantage. They could watch diseases evolve as the lunatic asylums grew larger and larger (see Figure 1.2), and they could start to classify the diseases more clearly. From the hordes of deranged, crippled, feeble-minded, epileptic and dementing inmates that filled up every new asylum, and each newly built asylum extension, doctors began to sort out different conditions, psychiatric, neurological, metabolic (e.g. hypothyroidism) and nutritional. Every leading alienist would publish his system, with new words, new diagnoses and new theories of causation. Abandoning the basics of 'mania' and 'melancholia', they created moral insanity, neurasthenia, catatonia, hebephrenia, lactational insanity and numerous others. By 1892 Daniel Hack Tuke, from the same family of Quaker Tukes that had founded the Retreat 100 years earlier, was able to publish his two-volume *Dictionary of Psychological Medicine*. This defined and discussed several thousand terms and phrases used by his zealous European-wide colleagues (including 200 legal cases).

But the asylums themselves, with their crowded 100-bed wards, their poorly paid and often untrained attendants, their handful of 'medical men' – perhaps four or five for two or three thousand patients – and their farms, drains and outbreaks of dysentery and typhoid, became less and less therapeutic and more and more just 'museums of madness'. Energetic superintendents burned themselves out trying to activate, morally treat, feed and semi-medicate their shuffling collections of 'chronic dements'. Paperwork and certificates dominated their days and nights, and ruthless magistrates imposed admissions and economies. Doctors could not refuse admissions, since all 'lunatics' were certified by the courts and simply sent in without warning. Formal inspections, unpleasant sounds and smells (incontinence was rife), and even random assaults dominated their day, although by the 1900s football matches and cricket leagues were well established. The good and bad of asylum life is summarized in Table 1.6.

Even worse news was that the numbers of insane people were rising faster than the population was growing, leading to fears of 'degeneration' – a theory first espoused by BA Morel (1809–73), a leading French asylum physician – and even a qualitative decline of the human race. Further classifying people as 'feeble-minded' led to more building (the Binet-Simon tests of intelligent quotient (IQ) appeared in 1905) of 'colonies' (i.e. very large asylums) of 'pauper imbeciles' designed to segregate the degenerate and to stop them overbreeding. In the early twentieth century some countries even sterilized large numbers of the 'mentally deficient', with certain American states such as California leading the way. The rise of eugenics (i.e. the theory of selective breeding of healthy genes) and the 1930s Nazis' attitudes to psychiatric patients, eliminating them as a precursor to the Holocaust, were the dark outcome of these developments.

The most positive effect of the asylums was the work of first-class researchers such as Emil Kraepelin (1856–1926). Using a computer-like system of library cards, he classified symptoms and followed their course, separating out dementia praecox (DP), a progressive, deteriorating psychotic disorder, from the better prognosis of manic-depressive illness, from which patients seemed to recover. This distinction, despite many attempts at redefinitions, remains at the heart

Table 1.5 Nineteenth-century medications

Traditional	Laxatives to 'purge' the bowel, e.g. croton oil
	Tonics, e.g. quinine, caffeine, strychnine
	Opium/morphine (hypodermic introduced 1855), cannabis, digitalis
1850s	Bromides
1870s	Hyoscyamus ⟶ hyoscine (from henbane plant) (also in combination with morphine/atropine)
1869	Chloral hydrate – widespread use in asylum, at home and as an addictive agent
1890s	Apomorphine – sedation and vomiting
1900s	Barbiturates

NB: By 1900, patent remedies were 72 per cent of pharmaceutical sales, often containing alcohol and stimulants (e.g. cocaine).

Table 1.6 Asylums: the good, bad (and ugly)

Positive	Negative
Sanctuary for 'lunatics'/ public safety	Stagnant, cut off from the 'normal' world
Food, shelter, clothes, 'attendants'	Internal abuses, neglect, scandals
Diagnostic research/ classification	Institutionalization*
Occupational activities (farm, laundry, woodwork)	Failure of moral therapy
Recognition of mental illness/ vulnerability	Distant, 'brooding', stigmatized
Financial/social commitment	Oversized, underfunded

*A twentieth-century term describing the effects on the individual of living in a controlled environment, with food, activities, contacts, clothes and time completely regimented by the needs of the institution.

of modern diagnosis, despite the term 'schizophrenia' replacing 'DP' as the standard terminology by the 1950s, probably because of its connotations of understandable treatability.

THE TWENTIETH CENTURY: I – THE BIOMEDICAL MODEL

Research advances in the late nineteenth century, especially in bacteriology, even started to pay dividends for psychiatry. Some 10 per cent of inmates of asylums had GPI, namely syphilis of the brain. When Noguchi and Moore discovered the syphilitic organism in 1913 (the brain abnormalities of syphilis had been known since the 1820s), it was the first clear connection of a mental illness to a disease process. Linked in with nineteenth-century knowledge of the effects of trauma to the brain, nutritional deficiencies, thyroid disease ('cretinism'), and the association between forms of epilepsy and types of hallucinations, a stronger line of research developed as to mental illness having a physical basis. Forget moral theories, 'religious excess' and the supernatural; here was cerebral disease generating crazy behaviours. Unfortunately this concentration on brain disorder did not generate much in the form of a biochemical marker or an effective treatment. Critics, often psychologists and psychotherapists, used the mocking term 'brain mythology'.

The pre-1950s asylums were full of chronic psychotics (schizophrenics and manic depressives), but the neuroses such as anxiety, depression, obsessionality and sexual perversions also had their proposed physical associations. A range of drugs, operations and shock therapies, of varying scientific reliability, ensued. Numerous records, photographic and written, graphically describe what happened. These unfortunately mainstream remedies may seem comic or gothic, for example excising colons or adenoids in search of 'focal infection', or giving injections of monkey gland cells to boost libido, but they reflect the desperation of patients, patients' families and physicians. The asylums had become enormous, crowded 'Private Worlds', as illustrated by Phyllis Bottome's 1932 novel of the same name and by the 1948 Warner Brothers movie *The Snake Pit*. In 1944, the textbook *Physical Methods of Treatment in Psychiatry* (Sargant and Slater) included insulin treatment, convulsion therapy (i.e. ECT), chemical sedation with drugs such as bromides and stimulation via Benzedrine (amphetamine), narcotherapy, malarial treatment (for GPI: give the patient malaria and a high fever and kill off the bugs before killing off the patient) and prefrontal leucotomy.

In the 1950s the discovery of chlorpromazine, other antipsychotics and a range of antidepressants led to the psychopharmacological revolution (Tables 1.7 and 1.8) and even new diagnoses to fit the new formulations available. The rise of the international drug companies in the 1970s and 1980s, pushing products such as Prozac, became a stock market phenomenon. Such approaches also enabled the gradual closure of the asylums, towards what has been called 'community care', and an increasing sense of neglect in that the sanctuary provided by the old asylums was no longer available. The continued failure, despite billions of dollars spent, to establish a clear biological marker for schizophrenia, depression or any other mental illnesses (although some brain imaging techniques are showing promise) has created a semi-mythical feeling about the need for 'counselling'. But the drugs do work, thus the now vociferous user movement and a rising anti-stigma campaign.

Table 1.7 Treatments for schizophrenia/psychosis

Pre-1950s	Sedative: chloral, hyoscine, opiates Physical: insulin coma, leucotomy, prolonged sleep Chemical/electrical shock Surgical excision (tonsils, colon, teeth) Psychological: psychoanalysis in various forms
1952	Deniken and Delay report on use of chlorpromazine in 38 patients treated at St Anne's Hospital, Paris
1952–1960	Widespread research/use worldwide; asylum numbers start to fall; term 'neuroleptic' coined
1958–1960	Haloperidol introduced
1960–1970s	Depot preparations of various dopamine-blocking antipsychotics
1969	Sulpiride
1974	Clozapine (reintroduced in the late 1980s)
1990s	'Atypical antipsychotics'

THE TWENTIETH CENTURY: II – PSYCHOLOGICAL APPROACHES

The asylums and classifications of the nineteenth century also led to a richer language of psychological description and a rising interest in psychological methods of treatment. Dominant personalities (among many) were Sigmund Freud (1856–1939) and Pierre Janet (1859–1947), the former's *Interpretation of Dreams* being published (but largely unsold) in 1900. For reasons that are hard to understand – although playing the sex card helped? – Freudian psychoanalysis swept aside many of its rivals. Like the Bolsheviks

Table 1.8 The road to modern psychopharmacology

1855	Von Bibra identified 17 different mind-altering plants (*Die Narkotischen Genusmittel unde der Mensch*)
1894	Adrenaline identified
1898	'Mezcal: a new artificial paradise' in *Contemporary Review* (a magazine of the time) by Havelock Ellis – 'an afternoon with peyote most educated gentleman should try once or twice'
1901	'Adrenalin' preparation marketed
1926	Acetylcholine identified in the synapse by Henry Dale
1929	Amphetamine (β-phenyl-isopropylamine) first used – 'feeling of wellbeing' noted 18 min after injection
1943	Lysergic acid diethylamide (LSD) discovered by Albert Hofmann – while cycling home, he found 'buildings yawned and rippled' and that his neighbour was wearing 'a lurid mask'
1950	Chlorpromazine (4560RP) and meprobamate synthesized
1955	Reserpine and meprobamate introduced for anxiety/depression
1956	Methylphenidate 'the happy medium in psychomotor stimulation' (marketed, and later targeted at childhood problems in 1961)
1957	Chlordiazepoxide, from a class of chemical dyes, 'causes a mouse to hang limply when held' (marketed in 1960 as Librium)
1957–1960	Imipramine, isoniazid and amitriptyline introduced as specific antidepressants
1959	Diazepam (marketed as Valium in 1963)
1974	Laboratory testing of fluoxetine (Lilly 110140)
1981	Zimelidine the first selective serotonin-reuptake inhibitor (SSRI) to be marketed (withdrawn in 1983 due to neurotoxic side effects)
1987	Fluoxetine (Prozac®) approved as an antidepressant
1994	Prozac had become the second best-selling drug in the world

in revolutionary Russia, the diehard commitment of Freud's followers created a new language of 'id', 'ego', 'transference' and 'Oedipus complex', loved by intellectuals and fitting the zeitgeist of post-First World War Europe. The shell shock of tens of thousands of previously 'normal' young men also helped to strengthen beliefs that mental illness was not due to heredity or degeneration, but rather was the understandable effects of a hellish environment, trench warfare. The treatment of the poet Siegfried Sassoon by the British psychoanalyst WHR Rivers (1864–1922), at Craiglockart Hospital, is especially well documented.

Although basing his theories upon some half a dozen famous cases, such as the Wolf Man (Sergei Pankaev, who died in 1979 having wandered around Europe, uncured, looking for help from many other therapists), Freud's approach to individual psychotherapy became the shibboleth of the cultured middle classes, especially in the USA. Despite schismatic alternatives developing under the leadership of Carl Jung (1875–1961) – the founder of analytical psychology and theories about archetypes – and Alfred Adler (1870–1937) – inventor of the inferiority complex, elaborated in *The Nervous Character* (1912) – the notion of the psychiatrist as a German Jewish professorial figure who put you on a couch while listening silently became the standard image. Even so, an undercurrent of – often misinformed – critical attitudes towards psychoanalysis persisted in mainstream medicine, not helped by some of the cruder approaches about childhood sexuality made by Freudian disciples such as Ernest Jones, who had to go off to Toronto to get away from the paedophilic taint. Scepticism also met the Freudians' beliefs that they could even 'cure' serious psychoses such as 'schizophrenia'. Given the looseness of that diagnostic term (i.e. the mistaken notion of a 'split' mind, like Dr Jekyll and Mr Hyde), this was not surprising. It took several decades of careful worldwide research to develop a reliable 'operational' system of diagnosing schizophrenia during the 1960s and 1970s, helped by the rise of effective antipsychotics, the need to counter the criticisms of anti-psychiatry and the new brain scanning techniques, such as magnetic resonance imaging (MRI).

In those same decades, however, radical psychology (e.g. RD Laing, Thomas Szasz), alongside alternative anti-establishment cultures, reached its pinnacle. This became the dominant mode of understanding the world, was critical of hidebound, asylum-bound, biology-bound 'straight' psychiatry, and scored notable victories. Diagnostic categories were seen as loose or corrupt (e.g. the Russian KGB's term 'latent schizophrenia' for political dissidents), and mental illness was seen as caused by parental impositions (e.g. the 1971 film *Family Life*; Table 1.9), social injustice and restrictive mores. Therapeutic drug experience using lysergic acid diethylamide (LSD) was even mooted as the real breakthrough. Increasingly influential, however, were the behavioural psychologists, developing sophisticated theories of – and treatments for – anxieties and phobias, and moving on to cognitive behavioural therapy (CBT) and cognitive analytical techniques. Linking the psychoanalytical and behavioural approaches were group therapies, family therapies and patient-centred approaches such as Alcoholics Anonymous (AA) and an increasingly vociferous user movement.

Psychiatrists, from being asylum keepers in the nineteenth century to being proto-neurologists in the first half of the twentieth century, were now trying to be eclectic – that is, doctors-cum-therapists-cum-psychopharmacologists, with sophisticated interpersonal and therapeutic skills and an enhanced awareness of social and legal constructions. The organizations, publications and legislation psychiatry in Britain are summarized in Tables 1.10 and 1.11.

Table 1.10 Psychiatry in Britain

	Organizations
1841	Association of Medical Officers of Asylums and Hospitals for the Insane
1865	Medico-Psychological Association (MPA)
1926	Royal Charter → R(oyal) MPA
1971	Royal College of Psychiatrists
	Publications
1843	*Annales Medico-Psychologiques*
1844	*American Journal of Insanity*
1848–1854	*Journal of Psychological Medicine and Mental Pathology*
1853	*Asylum Journal* (ed. JC Bucknill)
1858–1962	*Journal of Mental Science*
1963	*British Journal of Psychiatry*
1970	*Psychological Medicine*
1977	*Bulletin of the Royal College of Psychiatrists* (→ *Psychiatric Bulletin* 1988)

WHAT NOW?

By the 1990s, the 'talking therapies', although intellectually established in terms of art criticism and literature, had run into a series of debates as to effectiveness, cost–benefit and the nature of 'distress'. Why talk à la Woody Allen to a shrink three times a week for 15 years, when Prozac could make you feel alright within a month? Newly recognized,

Table 1.9 Psychiatry's history in the cinema

Witchfinder General (1968, dir. Michael Reeves)	'In 1645 a villainous lawyer finds it profitable to travel the country instigating witch hunts'. Hammer horror, colourful and savage, absorbs you in its world of supernatural belief and religious terror. The 'witchcraft delusion' as reality
Freud (1962, dir. John Huston)	Earnest and hagiographic biopic set in 1885 Vienna, when young Dr F uses hypnotism and discovers a boy who hates his father because he loves his mother; dream sequences and detailed discussions follow. A perfect outline of mid-century certainties as to the 'science' of psychoanalysis
The Snake Pit (1948, dir. Anatole Litvak)	Set in a 1940s' New York asylum, this film depicts electroconvulsive therapy (ECT) without anaesthesia, crowds of caged patients, chain-smoking psychiatrists and a heroic Freudian doctor/analyst. Warnings were posted that children were not allowed in the cinema and that conditions in British mental hospitals were 'unlike' those depicted
One Flew Over the Cuckoo's Nest (1975, dir. Milos Forman)	Set in a Californian state mental hospital, with staff and patients playing some roles, this reflects 1950s' rather than 1970s' in-patient treatments, but it is the classic 1970s' anti-psychiatry, patient-as-freedom-fighter (Jack Nicholson) movie, with 'Big Nurse', ECT and lobotomy used to enslave the inmates. A powerful reinforcement of the continuing stigmatization of psychiatry, and psychiatrists, in the movies and the media
Family Life (1971, dir. Ken Loach)	A small, TV-style, British take on a 'schizophrenogenic' family driving a young woman into psychosis via double-binds, excessive criticism and suburban life. Vividly redolent of the late 1960s and the predominant psychosocial theories

Table 1.11 Legislation (England and Wales)

1808	Act for 'better maintenance and care of Lunatics'
1844–5	Lunatics and Asylum Acts – statutory duty to provide asylums; lunacy commissioners appointed
1890	Lunacy Act – legalism triumphant, complex certification process
1913	Mental Deficiency Act – 'colonies' for mental defectives; 'Board of Control' to supervise asylums
1930	Mental Treatment Act – out-patients and involuntary admissions allowed
1959	Mental Health Act – ending of magistrates' courts and Board of Control; review tribunals introduced
1983	Mental Health Act – introduced consent, approved social workers (ASWs) and a Mental Health Act Commission
1995	Patients in the Community Act – Supervised Discharge and Supervision Register (abandoned later)
2007	Revised Mental Health Act – approved clinicians and approved mental health professionals

though still controversial (vis-à-vis their aetiological role), conditions such as child sex abuse and post-traumatic stress disorder were rife, but talking about them didn't necessarily help. 'Counselling' research in primary care showed limited evidence of making you feel better or even happier; CBT has become almost a panacea.

By the end of the twentieth century, therefore, psychiatric practice had become an embattled profession. Still enmeshed in stigma, and beset by homicide inquiries, risk management and a rising demand for public safety, psychiatrists are seen by many as poodles of corporate power (the drug companies) failing to deliver enough talking therapy or real understanding of user problems. Their own history has even been subverted by historical sociologists, who view its so-called 'advances' as nothing more than a cover-up for Orwellian social control and the medicalization of unhappiness. Ever the war zone of conflicting attitudes to the normal and the mad, psychiatry therefore continues to find itself fighting for the neglected Cinderellas of society, nowadays the prison-housed thousands yearning for understanding (asylum and prison populations tend to relate inversely, the one rising as the other falls, and vice versa). Key themes of this historical process are outlined in Table 1.4.

This 'history of psychiatry' is merely one version of a complex series of events, discoveries, social movements and intellectual developments. It has barely touched upon the philosophical basis to modern psychopathology, the numerous Parliamentary committees generating legislative change, the popular books and articles informing public attitudes, or even the individual case histories that have influenced clinical practice. There is a rich range of sources still awaiting thoughtful research, and some degree of cynicism as to, for example, why doctors became the agreed experts on managing mental illness. But one theme is constant: psychiatrists are in demand because of their unique combination of clinical and personal skills. History enables us to know what those mean and how they can work.

Chapter 2

Introduction to evidence-based medicine

Stuart Carney

INTRODUCTION

It is hard to argue with the principle that decisions should be informed by the best available evidence. However, since the early 1990s, evidence-based medicine (EBM) has evoked fierce debate. This debate has focused essentially on two questions: what is the best available evidence for clinical decision-making, and what role should this evidence play?

In this chapter, I use the term 'evidence-based medicine' to refer to decision-making in the care of an individual patient. Other terms in common use are 'evidence-based healthcare' (EBHC) and 'evidence-based practice' (EBP). EBHC relates to decision-making about groups of patients or populations. The generic descriptor EBP is often used to embrace both EBM and EBHC.[1]

EBM grew out of the need to improve the effectiveness and efficiency of medical education. It offers clinicians, mindful of their limitations, a strategy for recognizing and managing clinical uncertainty and information overload. With over two million articles published in 20 000 biomedical journals each year, it is impossible for busy clinicians to keep up to date without competence in EBM.

THE BEST AVAILABLE EVIDENCE

EBM proposes a paradigm shift in clinical decision-making. Instead of relying on reasoning from basic sciences, EBM demands that clinical decisions are informed by the best available clinical research data. In other words, evidence showing that a drug *does* work in clinical practice is valued above inferences from basic sciences that a drug *should* work.

Implicit in this paradigm shift is the principle of a hierarchy of evidence. Just as clinical trial data trump reasoning from basic sciences when considering what drug to prescribe, a systematic review of two or more randomized controlled trials (RCTs) will typically provide more convincing evidence than an individual RCT, which again provides more convincing evidence than an individual cohort or case–control study. Recognizing the inherent strengths and weaknesses of different study designs for different types of question is essential for the efficient identification of the best available evidence. The development of electronic databases has made searching for and retrieving research data much easier.

As a reader of the biomedical literature, you will be aware that publication in a scientific journal is no guarantee of study quality. The EBM revolution serves to equip all healthcare practitioners with the opportunity to question received wisdom and constructively, yet critically, appraise research findings in order to determine whether they are valid, important and applicable to the specific clinical situation. Critical appraisal requires a working knowledge of the possible pitfalls in scientific research.

Having identified the best available evidence, what role should it play in decision-making?

THE ROLE OF EVIDENCE IN CLINICAL DECISION-MAKING

Dave Sackett, one of the earliest advocates, defined EBM as 'the conscientious, explicit, and judicious use of best evidence in making decisions about the care of individual patients'.[2] Critics of EBM have drawn attention to the limitations of using research evidence alone when making clinical decisions. Approaches such as values-based medicine and 'the expert patient' have challenged traditional models for the doctor–patient relationship.[3,4] As these models have evolved, so has the philosophy of EBM. Perhaps EBM can be best understood as a component of clinical expertise that is 'the ability to integrate research evidence and patients' circumstances and preferences to help patients arrive at optimal decisions'.[5] This model for patient decision-making is illustrated in Figure 2.1.

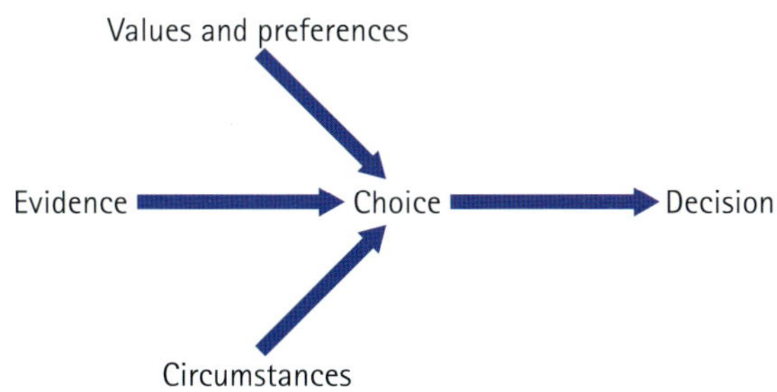

Figure 2.1 Role of evidence in patient decision-making

EVIDENCE-BASED PRACTICE AND CLINICAL EXPERTISE

Competence in EBM should help us empower patients to make optimal decisions. Helping patients to arrive at optimal decisions requires new and enhanced skills. These skills include the ability to use electronic databases, to critically appraise clinical research and data, and to communicate effectively with patients and other colleagues. Books and courses can help us develop our knowledge base, but the most effective way of developing competence in EBM is through reflective practice – that is, learning embedded in clinical practice.[6]

Drawing upon the public health disciplines of epidemiology and biostatistics, EBM seeks to simplify the process of accessing, appraising and applying research evidence. The EBM components of clinical expertise can be broken down into five steps:[7]

1. Translation of uncertainty to an answerable question.
2. Systematic retrieval of best available evidence.
3. Critical appraisal of evidence for validity, clinical relevance and applicability.
4. Application of results in practice (empowering patients to make clinical decisions).
5. Evaluation of performance.

The knowledge, skills and attitudes underpinning each of these five steps are summarized in Box 2.1.

It is clearly impractical to systematically retrieve and critically appraise the primary literature for every question that emerges in clinical practice. Meta-resources present pre-appraised summaries addressing some of the more common clinical questions, while evidence-based guidelines are becoming increasingly common. The art of EBM is judging, in partnership with patients, which questions are addressed adequately through guidelines, meta-resources and those that require appraisal of systematically retrieved primary evidence.[8]

Whatever the source of the evidence, the critical step in this process is the last one: the assessment of performance. This is easier to describe than to practise, but as we strive to improve patient safety and care we must not only evaluate our fidelity to the EBM process but also assess whether patients have been helped. The evaluation of performance remains the greatest challenge to truly practising EBM. Why? – because it requires a 'culture that is free of blame and encourages an open examination of error and failure'.[9]

Box 2.1 Knowledge, skills and attitudes underpinning the five steps of evidence-based medicine

To practise the five steps, clinicians should be able to:

- ***Translate their clinical uncertainty into answerable questions:***
  - Be able to assess patients and formulate a management plan.
  - Be aware of their own limitations and uncertainties.
  - Be motivated to seek guidance from published literature and colleagues.
  - Be able to translate these uncertainties into clinical questions.
- ***Systematically retrieve the best available evidence:***
  - Have knowledge and understanding of the resources available.
  - Have knowledge and understanding of how research is catalogued and strategies for efficient retrieval.
  - Have knowledge and understanding of the hierarchy of evidence.
  - Be able to effectively and efficiently access appropriate research evidence.
- ***Critically appraise the evidence:***
  - Have knowledge and understanding of basic epidemiology, basic biostatistics, basic qualitative methods, basic health economic methods and the principles of guideline/protocol development.
  - Be able to critically appraise primary research evidence and secondary sources, including guidelines.
  - Be able to determine whether the appraised evidence is applicable to this patient.
- ***Apply the results in practice:***
  - Be able to effectively communicate the strengths and weaknesses of the evidence, in a way that is respectful of the individual's circumstances and preferences, so that the patient is able to make an informed decision.
- ***Evaluate own performance:***
  - Have knowledge and understanding of the strategies to evaluate performance, including the importance of accurate, legible records, the role of electronic databases and the principles of audit.
  - Be able to evaluate their own performance and that of their team, and be actively engaged in developing strategies for quality improvement.
  - Be committed to monitoring performance (in a blame-free culture of learning).

REFERENCES

1. Gray J (2001) *Evidence-Based Healthcare*, 2nd edn. Edinburgh: Churchill Livingstone.
2. Sackett DL, Rosenberg WM, Gray JA, *et al.* (1996) Evidence based medicine: what it is and what it isn't. *British Medical Journal* **312**: 71–2.
3. Woodbridge K, Fulford K (2004) *Whose Values? A Workbook for Values-Based Practice in Mental Healthcare*. London: Sainsbury Centre for Mental Health.
4. Department of Health (2001) *The Expert Patient: A New Approach to Chronic Disease Management for the 21st Century*. London: Department of Health.
5. Guyatt G, Cook D, Haynes B (2004) Evidence based medicine has come a long way. *British Medical Journal* **329**: 990–1.
6. Coomarasamy A, Khan K (2004) What is the evidence that postgraduate teaching in evidence based medicine changes anything? A systematic review. *British Medical Journal* **329**: 1017–21.
7. Dawes M, Summerskill W, Glasziou P, *et al.* (2005) Sicily statement on evidence-based practice. *BMC Medical Education* **5**: 1.
8. Straus SE, Green ML, Bell DS, *et al.* (2004) Evaluating the teaching of evidence based medicine: conceptual framework. *British Medical Journal* **329**: 1029–32.
9. Halligan A, Donaldson L (2001) Implementing clinical governance: turning vision into reality. *British Medical Journal* **322**: 1413–17.

Chapter 3

History and philosophy of science

Bill (KWM) Fulford and Tim Thornton

INTRODUCTION

The psychiatrist and neuroscientist Nancy Andreasen has pointed out that a crucial characteristic of psychiatry as a research-led clinical discipline is the unique way in which it combines some of the most challenging scientific questions with equally challenging conceptual problems. Andreasen argues that the conceptual difficulties that we face have been driven increasingly to the top of psychiatry's practical agenda by the recent rapid pace of advances in the neurosciences.[1] These conceptual and empirical difficulties are evident in a wide range of contexts; examples include (i) disputes around the current revision processes for both the *International Classification of Diseases* (ICD) and the American Psychiatric Association's *Diagnostic and Statistical Manual*;[2] (ii) the contested shift in the UK and in many other countries in service delivery from psychiatry to a more multidisciplinary approach;[3] and (iii) growing pressure for a move away from professional-led mental health and social care services to a more equal partnership between professionals and service users and carers.[4]

In this chapter we set the conceptual difficulties surrounding current challenges of this kind in their historical context, with the aim of illustrating the extent to which the history and philosophy of science provide both context and direction for responding to the issues that we face today. It is natural to think of history and philosophy as perhaps subordinate to science as resources for improving service delivery in psychiatry. What we hope this chapter will illustrate is that the uniquely challenging nature of psychiatry, as a research-led clinical discipline, demands the resources of rigorous historical and philosophical work alongside, and as a full partner to, equally rigorous empirical methods.

Clearly, in a chapter of this length, we will not be able to cover the history and philosophy of science as it relates to psychiatry in any way comprehensively. Rather than giving an overview, therefore, we will adopt a case-study approach, exploring in some depth one particular strand in the history and philosophy of psychiatry that we believe is particularly relevant to current challenges. This strand concerns the role of both meanings and values as a complement to the brain sciences. The key protagonists that we will be considering are, respectively, one of the fathers of modern descriptive psychopathology, Karl Jaspers, and the Kantian philosopher of science Wilhelm Windelband, both writing around the start of the twentieth century.

The first section of this chapter focuses on Jaspers' work and in particular on his attempt to reconcile *meaningful* understanding with causal explanations in psychiatry. The second section examines Windelband's work, which focuses on the role of *values in understanding individuals*. Finally, we bring the story right up to date with recent developments in the counterparts of Jaspers' and Windelband's work, respectively phenomenology and what has become known as 'values-based practice'. This concluding section illustrates how these developments build on philosophical and empirical sources to provide practical approaches to decision-making in psychiatry that are directly complementary to the resources of the sciences.

JASPERS ON THE ROLE OF UNDERSTANDING MEANING IN PSYCHIATRY

Karl Jaspers was born in 1883. He studied first law and then medicine at university, graduating as a doctor in 1908 when he started to work as an assistant in the department of psychiatry in the University of Heidelberg. Kraepelin's influential textbook of psychiatry was in its eighth edition at this time. As a young man, Jaspers read widely, studying not only medicine but also psychology and philosophy, and it was the depth of his philosophical understanding that equipped him to make his unique contributions to psychiatry.

Jaspers and psychiatry's first biological phase

Jaspers was working at a time in the development of psychiatry very similar to our own, in that there were dramatic advances in the neurosciences of the day: the period has indeed become known as 'psychiatry's first biological phase'. Jaspers' professor in the Heidelberg department of psychiatry was Franz Nissl, a neurohistologist who discovered the dye that allowed the structure of nerve cells to be clearly seen for the first time. Using this technique, he had shown that the neurohistological changes in general paralysis were different from the changes described by Alois Alzheimer in dementia. General paralysis was a degenerative dementia that had swept Europe after the wars of the late nineteenth century. It was shortly to prove to be a form of neurosyphilis. These were dramatic discoveries, therefore, and the young Jaspers was impressed with Nissl as a scientist. But when it came to *clinical* work, however, Jaspers was considerably less impressed.

Psychiatry at the turn of the century in Germany had moved out of the large institutions into university clinics. There was considerable resentment among the institutional psychiatrists that their discipline had been taken over by academic neuroscientists, whose knowledge of clinical psychiatry was scant, and whom they perceived as being under the spell of a crudely natural scientific model, epitomized by the German psychiatrist Wilhelm Griesinger's famous aphorism 'Mental illnesses are brain illnesses'.[5] Psychiatric researchers at the time, such as Griesinger, Alzheimer, Nissl, Carl Meynert and Theodor Wernicke, were actively searching for the neuropathological changes by which they believed the major psychoses could be characterized. And, given their success with general paralysis, hopes were high. Jaspers shared these hopes. But he believed that the underlying biological approach had been pushed too far. 'These anatomical constructions, however, became quite fantastic (e.g. Meynert, Wernicke) and have rightly been called "Brain Mythologies"'.[5]

Jaspers and the *Methodenstreit*

Jaspers' reservations about what he perceived as the excessively natural-scientific approach to psychiatry were driven by his understanding of the philosophical debates about psychology in the late nineteenth century, the so-called *Methodenstreit*. This concerned whether the human sciences (*Geisteswissenschaften*) should try to emulate their far more successful cousins the natural sciences (*Naturwissenschaften*) or whether they should go their own methodological way. 'Positivists', including John Stuart Mill in England and both Auguste Comte and Emile Durkheim in France, argued that the human sciences were no different from the natural sciences. Others argued that the human or cultural sciences were different from the natural sciences, in terms of either the nature of their subject matter or their methodology, or both. The latter, in Germany, included Heinrich Rickert, Wilhelm Dilthey and Wilhelm Windelband, to whom we will return in the next section. Crucially for Jaspers, the German philosopher and sociologist Max Weber was among the latter camp.

Jaspers met Max Weber in 1909. He was invited to join Weber's elite intellectual circle, and he quickly became one of Weber's key intellectual antagonists. Jaspers thought of Weber as the 'Galileo of the human sciences'.[6] Although Weber believed that the human sciences involved a distinctive approach, he believed that sociology, his own discipline, was a hybrid subject, living partly within the natural and partly within the human sciences.

Jaspers and general psychopathology

Jaspers regarded psychopathology as Weber regarded sociology. It lay both within the natural sciences, pursuing abnormalities of brain functioning, and within the human sciences, pursuing the experiences, aims, intentions and subjective meanings of its patients. Of course, at a time when psychiatry was dominated by the 'brain mythologists', Jaspers' major aim was to bring psychiatry back within the ambit of the human sciences. He wanted to balance things up. In Weber's work, therefore, which in turn had drawn on the work of Dilthey, Windelband and Rickert, Jaspers saw things falling into place, and much of Weber's social theory – interpretation/understanding, *Evidenz*, ideal types and so forth – was to find its way into Jaspers' psychopathology. Some time later he wrote:

> My article of 1912 and this present book (1913) were greeted as something radically new, although all I had done was to link psychiatric reality with the traditional humanities. Looking back now, it seems astonishing that these had been so forgotten and grown so alien to psychiatry. In this way within the confines of psychopathology there grew a methodological comprehension of something which had always been present, but which was fading out of existence and which appeared in striking reverse, 'through the looking-glass' as it were, in Freud's psychoanalysis – a misunderstanding of itself. The way was clear for scientific consciousness to lay hold on human reality and on man's mental estate, his psychoses included, but there was an immediate need to differentiate the *various modes of understanding*, clarify them and embody them in all *the factual content* available to us.[5]

The period 1909–13 was a time of high output for Jaspers. He wrote papers on homesickness, hallucinations, pathological jealousy, phenomenology, and the need for both 'causal' (natural scientific) and 'understandable' (human scientific) connections in psychic life. We will discuss two papers published in this period below: 'The phenomenological approach in psychopathology'[7] and 'Causal and "meaningful" connections between life history and psychosis'.[8] But the culmination of this burst of output was that, in 1911, he was commissioned by the publisher Springer to write a textbook of psychopathology. It was thus that his *General Psychopathology* (*Allgemeine Psychopathologie*) appeared in its first edition in 1913.

Jaspers on subjective and objective

In 'The phenomenological approach in psychopathology',[7] Jaspers sets out his account of the role within psychopathology for a phenomenological approach. As we will explain shortly, phenomenology is, in Jaspers' view, a form of static understanding by contrast with what he calls genetic understanding (see below). But both forms of understanding have in common that they are attempts to explore subjective, as opposed to objective, symptoms. What is the distinction between subjective and objective? Jaspers describes objective symptoms as follows:

Objective symptoms include all concrete events that can be perceived by the sense, e.g. reflexes, registrable movements, an individual's physiognomy, his motor activity, verbal expression, written productions, actions and general conduct, etc.; all measurable performances... It is also usual to include under objective symptoms such features as delusional ideas, falsifications of memory, etc., in other words, the rational contents of what the patient tells us. These, it is true, are not perceived by the senses, but only understood; nevertheless, this 'understanding' is achieved through rational thought, without the help of any empathy into the patient's psyche.[7]

The distinction between what is available to rational thought and to empathy is important and one to which we will return. It helps to form a broader conception of what is objective than would generally be accepted today. But this in turn gives rise to a correspondingly narrower sense of 'subjective':

Objective symptoms can all be directly and convincingly demonstrated to anyone capable of sense-perception and logical thought; but subjective symptoms, if they are to be understood, must be referred to some process which, in contrast to sense perception and logical thought, is usually described by the same term 'subjective'. Subjective symptoms cannot be perceived by the sense-organs, but have to be grasped by transferring oneself, so to say, into the other individual's psyche; that is, by empathy. They can only become an inner reality for the observer by his participating in the other person's experiences, not by any intellectual effort.[7]

Jaspers complains that a purely objective psychology leads 'quite systematically to the elimination of everything that can be called mental or psychic'.[7] In order to illustrate what he means, Jaspers refers to the assessment of a patient's fatigue through measurable performances where 'It is not the feeling of fatigue but "objective fatigue" which is being investigated'.[7] This suggests a contrast between objective and measurable aspects of physiology and the subjective aspect of what it is like to be or to feel fatigued. Assessing such subjective symptoms requires a kind of imaginative transference or empathy, which, thus, lies at the heart of psychopathology.

Jaspers on phenomenological understanding

Having drawn this distinction between subjective and objective, Jaspers goes on to characterize the aims of phenomenological psychopathology in the following terms:

What then are the precise aims of this much-abused subjective psychology? ... It asks itself – speaking quite generally – what does mental experience depend on, what are its consequences, and what relationships can be discerned in it? The answers to these questions are its special aims... So before real inquiry can begin it is necessary to identify the specific psychic phenomena which are to be its subject, and form a clear picture of the resemblances and differences between them and other phenomena with which they must not be confused. This preliminary work of representing, defining, and classifying psychic phenomena, pursued as an independent activity, constitutes phenomenology.[7]

Thus, the key aim of phenomenology, or static understanding, is to identify the specific psychic phenomena that are to be its subject and to form a clear picture of the resemblances and differences between them and other phenomena. How does it set about this task?

We should picture only what is really present in the patient's consciousness; anything that has not really presented itself to his consciousness is outside our consideration. We must set aside all outmoded theories, psychological constructs or materialist mythologies of cerebral processes; we must turn our attention only to that which we can understand as having real existence, and which we can differentiate and describe. This, as experience has shown, is in itself a very difficult task. This particular freedom from preconception which phenomenology demands is not something one possesses from the beginning, but something that is laboriously acquired after prolonged and critical work and much effort – often fruitless – in framing constructs and mythologies.[7]

A key aspect of the task of getting a very clear picture of psychological phenomena is thus to attempt to strip away theoretical descriptions or constructs and to get back to the things themselves, to use a slogan of the philosophical phenomenologist Edmund Husserl (1859–1938) (the precise nature of whose influence on Jaspers is contested). Of course, from a modern perspective, the aim of a theory-free approach has echoes of the aetiological-theory-free approach of the glossary to ICD-8 and its successors in both the ICD and DSM series of classifications. Quite how successful a genuinely theory-free approach can be in the face of arguments as to the essential theory-ladenness of data is a matter of debate (see Fulford *et al.*[9]).

So far, Jaspers' discussion has presented the difficulties of the phenomenological method rather than offering specific guidance as to how it is to be achieved. The most concrete account offered of that in this essay runs as follows:

How then do we proceed when we isolate, characterise and give conceptual form to these psychic phenomena? We cannot portray them, or bring them before our eyes in any way that can be perceived by the senses. We can only guide ourselves by a multiple approach. We have to be led, starting *from the outside*, to a real appreciation of a particular psychic phenomenon by looking at its genesis, the conditions for its appearance, its configurations, its context and possible concrete contents; also by making use of intuitive comparison and symbolization, by directing our observations in whatever ways may suggest themselves (as artists do so penetratingly) ...

[T]he phenomenologist can indicate features and characteristics, and show how they can be distinguished and confusion avoided, all with a view to describing the qualitatively separate psychic data. But he must make sure that those to whom he addresses himself do not simply *think* along with him, but that they *see* along with him.[7]

Jaspers on genetic understanding

As remarked above, Jaspers distinguishes between two legitimate forms of understanding (of subjective phenomena): static understanding, which he also calls phenomenology, and genetic understanding. In 'The phenomenological approach in psychopathology', he characterizes the differences thus:

'Genetic understanding' [is] the understanding of the meaningful connections between one psychic experience and another, the 'emergence of the psychic from the psychic'. Now phenomenology itself has nothing to do with this 'genetic understanding' and must be treated as something entirely separate.[7]

What then *is* genetic understanding? A fuller discussion is given in another essay from this period, 'Causal and "meaningful" connections between life history and psychosis'.[8] Again, an important clue comes from the distinction mentioned above between rational connections and those that require empathy. Taking the case of understanding a speaker and understanding what the speaker has said, Jaspers comments:

The first important differentiation was made by Simnel, who showed the difference between the understanding of *what has been said* from understanding the *speaker*. When the contents of thoughts emerge one from another in accordance with the rules of logic, we understand the connections *rationally*. But if we understand the content of the thoughts as they have arisen out of the moods, wishes, and fears of the person who thought them, we understand the connections psychologically or empathetically. Only the latter can be called 'psychological understanding'. Rational understanding always only enables us to say that a certain rational complex, something which can be understood without any psychology whatever, was the content of a mind; empathic understanding, on the other hand, leads us into the psychic connections themselves. Whereas the rational understanding is only an *aid* to psychology, empathic understanding *is* psychology itself.[8]

This fits the earlier quotation in which the rational content of what a patient reports was characterized as an objective symptom. Equally, the rational interconnection between reports, their implications and so forth are also outside the domain of subjective psychology. But if empathy, in the service of genetic understanding, does not chart the logical or rational connection between one thought and another, then what is the basis of such psychological understanding? Jaspers' answer is not entirely clear. He says: 'We experience immediate evidence which we cannot reduce further nor base on any kind of other evidence... Meaningful connections are ideally typical connections. They are self-evident.'[8]

In other words, when there is a self-evident connection between one state and another, a connection that is typical although perhaps not always realized in practice, genetic understanding of it, through empathy, is possible. Realizing that one has won the lottery and thus solved all one's financial problems might lead, ideally and typically, to a state of happiness. Normally, to explain someone's sudden happiness, we might simply and sufficiently say that they have just heard that they have won the lottery. But, of course, in some unusual cases, that might not be a reason for happiness. The normal connection is basic – no more needs to be said – but it need not hold in all cases. It is ideally typical.

Thus, the relationship between static and genetic understanding is like this. The former articulates and vividly presents what it is like, for example, to have a sudden realization or what it is like to be in a state of happiness. It makes these kinds of state clear for further enquiry before the imposition of psychological theory. Genetic understanding adds to this the connection of how one state arises – ideally and typically – from the other. Such connections are shared empathically by psychological subjects, including psychiatrists and their patients.

Jaspers' characterization of static understanding has echoes in a more recent debate within the philosophy of mind between 'theory theory' and 'simulation theory' accounts of knowledge of other people's minds.[10] According to theory theory approaches, access to, and thus knowledge of, other people's minds is mediated by possession of a theory of mind. The theory is a body of deductively structured generalizations about the unseen causes of observable (speech and other) behaviour. This approach to the epistemological problem of how we can know about other minds thus dovetails with what are called 'functionalist' approaches to the ontological problem of what sort of things mental states are. Functionalism characterizes mental states in causal and functional terms, mediating between perceptual inputs and behavioural outputs. In other words, according to functionalism, mental states are akin to software states running on the brain as a computer. By characterizing types of mental state in second-order terms, functionalism aims to answer the problem of relating minds and bodies without simply reducing mental states to brain states. Theory theory approaches deploy broadly functionalist characterizations of what mental states are to explain, in addition, how we can have knowledge of them (in the case of other people).

Simulation theory, by contrast, explains knowledge of other minds not by possession of a theory of minds but merely by possession of a mind itself. The idea is that it is possible to have knowledge of another person's mental states by imaginatively putting oneself into his or her predicament. One 'runs' one's deliberative processes 'offline', as it were. Simulation theory is thus a form of empathy. But, unlike Jaspers' account, there is no restriction to non-rational patterns of thoughts emerging from one another. Indeed, one of the key arguments for simulation theory and against theory theory is that rational connections lie at the heart of mental phenomena but are not reducible to or codifiable in any set of principles of good thinking that could thus form part of a theory of mind.[11,12]

The limits of understanding

Despite its centrality in Jaspers' conception of psychopathology and thus psychiatry, understanding has limits. One kind of limit is quite general and concerns its scope by contrast with natural scientific explanation. In a section of 'Causal and "meaningful" connections between life history and psychosis' called 'The limits of understanding and the universal application of explaining', he says:

> The suggestive assumption that the psychic is the area of meaningful understanding and the physical that of causal explanation is wrong. There is no real event, be it physical or of psychic nature, which is not accessible to causal explanation ...
>
> The effect a psychic state may have could in principle lend itself to a causal explanation, while the psychic state itself of course must be phenomenologically (statically) understood. It is not absurd to think that it might one day be possible to have some rules which could causally explain the sequence of meaningfully connected thought processes without paying heed to the meaningful connections between them ...
>
> It is therefore in principle not at all absurd to try to understand as well as to explain one and the same real psychic event. These two established connections, however, are of entirely different kinds of validity.[8]

The thought here seems to be this: Understanding and explanation do not have two distinct subject matters. Rather, the difference between them is one of method or of the kind of intelligibility that they deploy. As applied in psychiatry, they share the same subject matter: 'real events' or 'thought processes', in Jaspers' terms. These can in principle be charted in either way: either by looking to the law-like causal relations between them or by looking to the meaningful relations between them.

The idea that neural events might be susceptible to two distinct patterns of intelligibility was articulated by the US philosopher of mind Donald Davidson (1917–2003). On his model of the mind, Anomalous Monism, the very same events that comprise mental events and that – according to Davidson – stand in essentially rational relations also comprise physical events and can be subsumed under nomological or law-like causal explanations.[13] When described in mental property terms, however, there are no laws that fit them. Hence – qua instantiations of mental properties – they are *anomalous*. But there are laws that fit them that use their physical or neurological properties.

Given this broad view of the relation between understanding and explanation, one might expect the following asymmetry between them. Although every mental event is also a physical event, not every physical event is a mental event. There were no mental properties in the event of comet Shoemaker Levy 9 colliding with Jupiter in 1994, for example. That collision was not a mental event. Thus, one might expect Jaspers to say that, although every event that can be understood can also be explained, not every event that can be explained can also be understood. It is rather curious, therefore, that he actually says: 'there is no event which cannot be understood as well as explained'.[8]

Although he does not recognize that plausible general limitation on understanding – that non-mental events can only be explained, not understood – Jaspers does suggest a more specific local limit in the case of psychopathology. He believes that 'primary delusions' cannot be understood. To unpack that claim, we will now outline his taxonomy of delusions.

Jaspers suggests that delusions fall into two kinds: primary and secondary, or delusions proper and delusion-like ideas. Primary delusions fall into four further kinds. The first is mentioned in *General Psychopathology* almost in passing: delusional atmosphere. He says:

> with this *delusional atmosphere* we always find an 'objective something' there, even though quite vague, a something which lays the seed of objective validity and meaning... Patients feel as if they have lost grip on things, they feel gross uncertainty...[5]

To a person with schizophrenia, the world as a whole can seem subtly altered, uncanny, portentous or sinister. This general transformation prompts Jaspers to say elsewhere: 'We observe that a new world has come into being'.[5] There are then three further forms of primary delusion:

> *Delusional perceptions.* These may range from an experience of some vague meaning to clear, delusional observation and express delusions of reference...
>
> *Delusional ideas.* These give new colour and meaning to memory or may appear in the form of a sudden *notion* – 'I could be King Ludwig's son' – which is then confirmed by a vivid memory of how when attending a parade the Kaiser rode by on his horse and looked straight at the patient...
>
> *Delusional awareness.* This constitutes a frequent element particularly in florid and acute psychoses. Patients possess a knowledge of immense and universal happenings, sometimes without any trace of clear perceptual experience of them...[5]

In each of these cases, there is a deep change in the experience of the significance of features of the world. In the case of delusional perceptions, an experience is transformed. In the case of delusional ideas, the significance of a memory is transformed. In delusional awareness, a delusional idea springs unbidden. But in all cases: 'All primary experience of delusion is an experience of meaning'.[5]

[T]he *experiences of primary delusion are analogous to this seeing of meaning*, but the awareness of meaning undergoes a radical transformation. There is an immediate, intrusive knowledge of the meaning and it is this which is itself the delusional experience.[5]

The key feature of primary delusions, however, is that they are un-understandable. While secondary delusions or delusion-like ideas are, in principle, understandable in the context of a person's life history, personality, mood state or presence of other psychopathology, primary delusions have a kind of basic status.

We can distinguish two large groups of delusion according to their *origin*: one group *emerges understandably* from preceding affects, from shattering, mortifying, guilt-provoking or other such experiences, from false perception or from the experience of derealisation in states of altered consciousness etc. The other group is for us *psychologically irreducible*; phenomenologically it is something final. We give the term '*delusion-like ideas*' to the first group; the latter we term '*delusions proper*'.[5]

As Andrew Sims says in a contemporary introduction to descriptive psychopathology:

[W]hen we consider the middle aged schizophrenic spinster who believes that men unlock the door of her flat, anaesthetize her and interfere with her sexually, we find an experience that is ultimately not understandable. We can understand, on obtaining more details of the history, how her disturbance centres on sexual experience; why she should be distrustful of men; her doubts about her femininity; and her feelings of social isolation. However, the *delusion*, her absolute conviction that these things are happening to her, that they are true, is not understandable. The best we can do is to try and understand externally, without really being able to feel ourselves into her position (*genetic empathy*), what she is thinking and how she experiences it [Sims 1988: 85].[14]

Thus, although Jaspers places empathic understanding (both static and genetic) at the heart of psychopathology and thus psychiatry, he also argues that some of the key phenomena that characterize psychopathology cannot be understood. They are un-understandable. If Jaspers is correct, then psychiatry has a fundamental limitation. We return to this point later, when we bring the story up to date with developments in modern phenomenology.

WINDELBAND ON THE ROLE OF UNDERSTANDING VALUES IN PSYCHIATRY

In this section, we consider a second strand of conceptual work from psychiatry's first biological phase, namely the role of values, which as a complement to the neurosciences has particular relevance to psychiatry today. As noted earlier, although Jaspers had important things to say about the role of meanings, he was less interested in the role of values. In the following passage, for example, he distances his conception of understanding meaning from forming or understanding value judgements:

It is a fact that when dealing with meaningful connexions as such we inevitably tend to value positively or negatively, while everything meaningless we merely value, if we do so at all, only in relation to something else. Thus the emergence of moral demands from resentment we may value as something despicable, whereas we value memory merely as a tool. In the *science* of psychology, however, we must strictly refrain from any such value judgement. Our task is merely to grasp the meaningful connexions as such and to recognize them.[8]

Thus, Jaspers separates understanding meanings from the kind of evaluation that properly involves the assessment of values. But another European philosopher of science, Wilhelm Windelband, did wish to stress the importance of values for a properly rounded scientific account. He did this via an account of idiographic understanding, which, as we will outline later, is itself at the forefront of contemporary thinking about psychiatry.[15]

Windelband and idiographic understanding

Wilhelm Windelband was a Kantian philosopher of science. He first introduced the distinction between 'idiographic' and 'nomothetic' in his rectorial address of 1894. Key components of the distinction between them are that it is a distinction of method not of subject matter, that it concerns treating events as unrepeated, and that it is a reaction against an overreliance on an essentially general conception of knowledge.

Windelband contrasts his own methodological distinction with one of substance, between natural sciences (*Naturwissenschaften*) and sciences of the mind (*Geisteswissenschaften*): 'I regard the dichotomy as unfortunate. Nature and mind is a substantive dichotomy ... not equivalent to a dichotomy based on modes of cognition.[16]

Such a distinction of substance is a hostage to the fortune of a metaphysical distinction of kind between mind and the rest of nature. In psychiatry, the interplay of both broadly psychological methods and neurology makes drawing such a distinction premature and unhelpful.

Windelband proposes, instead, a distinction that places psychology (as he understands it) and other natural sciences on one side and other disciplines, which in Germany at the time were called 'sciences of the mind' but which have a distinct method, on the other. This gives rise to a characterization of what he goes on to label 'idiographic', as follows:

[T]he majority of the disciplines that are usually called sciences of the mind have a distinctively different purpose: they provide a complete and exhaustive description of a single, more or less extensive process which is located within a unique, temporally defined domain of reality.[16]

Idiographic understanding and the uniqueness of individuals

As first introduced, idiographic understanding concerns individual or unique cases. But, given that the distinction is supposed to be at the level of method and not substance, this is fixed not by the subject matter so much as how that subject matter is approached. This is made clearer in the following passage, in which the term 'idiographic' is first introduced:

In their quest for knowledge of reality, the empirical sciences either seek the general in the form of the law of nature or the particular in the form of the historically defined structure. On the one hand, they are concerned with the form which invariably remains constant. On the other hand, they are concerned with the unique, immanently defined content of the real event. The former disciplines are nomological sciences. The latter disciplines are sciences of process or sciences of the event. The nomological sciences are concerned with what is invariably the case. The sciences of process are concerned with what was once the case. If I may be permitted to introduce some new technical terms, scientific thought is *nomothetic* in the former case and *idiographic* in the latter case.[16]

This suggests the following rough practical distinction: nomothetic approaches are those that chart law-like, or nomological, generalities. Their aim is to describe generalities. Idiographic understanding concerns individual cases described in non-general ways. Both are, however, forms of empirical enquiry.

Such a distinction fits modern psychological usage influenced by Gordon Allport (1897–1967), in which 'idiographic' is used to describe case-study-based qualitative research by contrast with quantitative cohort-based research (although whether Allport's use of nomothetic accords with Windelband's is a matter of dispute[17]). But although contemporary use in psychology suggests that idiographic and nomothetic forms of understanding are practically distinguishable but not fundamentally distinct, Windelband suggests that his distinction goes deeper. He relates it to a fundamental metaphysical divide:

[T]his distinction connects with the most important and crucial relationship in the human understanding, the relationship which Socrates recognized as the fundamental nexus of all scientific thought: the relationship of the general to the particular.[16]

What Windelband means is this. Scientific understanding has, since the Greeks, concentrated on generalities. It has concentrated on laws of nature that govern many objects and events. But in so doing it has neglected the importance of understanding individual objects, events or people not as instances of general kinds but in their individuality. He says:

The commitment to the generic is a bias of Greek thought, perpetuated from the Eleatics to Plato, who found not only real being but also real knowledge only in the general. From Plato this view passed to our day. Schopenhauer makes himself a spokesman for this prejudice when he denies history the value of a genuine science because its exclusive concern is always with grasping the specific, never with comprehending the general... But the more we strive for knowledge of the concept and the law, the more we are obliged to pass over, forget, and abandon the singular fact as such...[16]

Unique individuals and values

This raises a question – which arguably Windelband never answered satisfactorily – as to the nature of this individualistic understanding. What is it to understand an individual in essentially non-general terms? But he did give an important clue as to why he thought there was need for idiographic understanding. What we value when we value people or events is tied to their individuality, he argues.

In opposition to this [general, nomothetic] standpoint, it is necessary to insist upon the following: every interest and judgment, every ascription of human value is based upon the singular and the unique... Our sense of values and all of our axiological sentiments are grounded in the uniqueness and incomparability of their object.[16]

Examining value judgements helps to reveal the fundamental importance of particular cases as opposed to general kinds in judgements. It suggests that there is an important role for clinical judgement aimed at reflecting the nature of individuals and their experiences. Windelband himself seems to have taken this to imply the need for a particular kind of individualistic judgement in which there is no implicit comparison – as there is with any general concept – with other cases. Such a judgement would be essentially particular or individualized.

Windelband's fellow neo-Kantian Heinrich Rickert also argues that there can be essentially particular or individualized judgements and that these are exemplified by value judgements. Unlike nomothetic accounts of, for example, the forces acting on bodies, which are described and explained in general terms, judgements about the value of things are individualized judgements.

We are concerned here with the connection of objects with values; for a generalizing approach the objects are free of value-connection, they are exemplars, replaceable... This is what happens when we free the object of all connection with our interests – it becomes a mere exemplar of a general concept. An individualising approach is necessarily connected with the value-bound grasp of the object [*mit der wertverbindenen Auffassung der Objekte*]...[18]

But although Windelband's discussion supports the suspicion of subsuming individuals under categories and the role, instead, of a kind of individualized judgement, he does not offer a very clear account of what form such an idiographic judgement might have. How precisely is a judgement supposed to reject an historical overemphasis on the general? In fact, there is reason to be suspicious of the suggestion that reflecting individuals needs a special kind of individualistic judgement.[19,20]

Thus, the lasting importance of Windelband's discussion is this: he reminds us of the importance of the individual as well as the general. He suggests that judgement aimed at understanding individuals in their own terms rather than instances of generalities can be an important aspect of a scientific understanding, albeit one that contrasts with essentially general statistical or law-like explanation. And he suggests that understanding of individuals can be importantly connected to value judgements. In the final section of the chapter, we will outline a more recent approach to reflecting the values of individuals that avoids Windelband's reliance on the contested notion of 'individualising judgement'.

MEANING AND VALUES IN PSYCHIATRY TODAY

In this section we outline current developments in psychiatry as they reflect respectively meanings (phenomenology and related disciplines) and values (values-based practice), both of which are philosophically derived resources for clinical practice that are complementary to the resources of the sciences. Again, we are unable to cover either of these in detail, but we include a list of suggested further reading at the end of the chapter.

Phenomenology and related disciplines

Although not prominent in much of Anglo-American psychiatry, there was a strong continuing tradition of work in phenomenology and related disciplines in continental Europe through much of the twentieth century. This tradition was indeed one of a number of important sources of the remarkable resurgence of cross-disciplinary work between philosophy and psychiatry that began in the 1990s in parallel with the dramatic advances in the neurosciences of that period.[21]

As a rich theoretical discipline, phenomenology has continued to develop strongly along with other disciplines broadly within the 'philosophy of mind', very much in partnership with research in the neurosciences; see, for example, a number of papers in the double special issue of *Philosophy, Psychiatry, and Psychology*, edited by Christoph Hoerl.[22] As in Jaspers' day, it has been crucial in this respect that careful analysis of the subjective content of experience is available as a complement to the findings of empirical disciplines, such as functional neuroimaging and behavioural genetics. Equally important, though, has been the clinical impact of phenomenology, and related disciplines such as hermeneutics and existentialism, through improved understanding of the subjective experience of mental disorder. We return in a moment to a particular application of phenomenology to the problem of understanding as raised by Jaspers' work. Examples of other clinical applications of this area of philosophy include the work of the Dutch philosopher Guy Widdershoven on improved decision-making in old-age psychiatry;[23] of the American philosopher and psychologist Steven Sabat on interpretation of language difficulties in Alzheimer's disease;[24] and of the Oxford philosopher of mind Katherine Morris on body dysmorphic disorders.[25]

Returning, then, to the problem of understanding as raised by Jaspers, recent work by psychiatrists and philosophers alike has challenged the assumption that this rules out meaning-laden understanding as an aim, at least. The Italian psychiatrist and phenomenologist Giovanni Stanghellini, for example, treads a middle ground between explaining and understanding schizophrenia. In his book of essays *Disembodied Spirits and Deanimated Bodies*, he has argued that some understanding of the experiences of sufferers of schizophrenia is possible on the hypothesis that they experience a threefold breakdown of common sense.[26] This involves a breakdown of three distinct areas: the ability to synthesize different senses into a coherent perspective on the world (coenaesthia); the ability to share a common world view with other members of a community (sensus communis); and a basic pre-intellectual grasp of, or attunement to, social relations (attunement). Stanghellini says: 'The philosophical kernel of my proposal is to show how all these dimensions of the phenomenon of common sense (coenesthia, sensus communis, and attunement) *are related to each other*'.[26]

But Stanghellini does not attempt to use these ideas to step wholeheartedly inside the world view of subjects with schizophrenia. Rather, breakdowns of these are postulated as clues to interpret the strange things that people with schizophrenia report. But a basic phenomenon remains: the inaccessibility of experiences and thoughts:

> Listening to a person affected by schizophrenia is a puzzling experience for more than one reason. If I let his words actualize in me the experiences he reports, instead of merely taking them as symptoms of an illness, the rock of certainties on which my life is based may be shaken in its most fundamental features. The sense of being *me* the one who is now seeing this sheet, reading these lines and turning this page; the experience of perceptual unity between my seeing this book, touching its cover and smelling the scent of freshly printed pages; the feeling that it is me the one who agrees or disagrees with what I am reading; the sense of belonging to a community of people, of being attuned to the others and involved in my actions and future; the taken-for-granted of all these doubtless features of everyday life, may be put at jeopardy.
>
> Although my efforts to understand, by suspending all clinical judgement, allow me to see these person's self-reports as a pos-

sible configuration of human consciousness, I must admit that there is something incomprehensible and almost inhuman in these experiences, something that makes me feel radically different from the person I am listening to.[26]

This suggests that understanding is an ongoing and ultimately unfinishable task. The clinician has to make a series of interpretative judgements taking broad account of the life of the sufferer from, for example, schizophrenia. Such judgements can help towards at least a partial understanding of the person as a whole while at the same time taking account of the vividly alien quality of their psychopathological experiences.

On this approach, interpretative judgements presuppose that, as it were, the basic unit of meaning is the life of the whole person. Attempts at individual interpretation of specific delusions can be guided by a more general framework that takes schizophrenia, for example, to involve a breakdown of common sense. But such an approach goes only so far and, once they have given out, the interpretation of individual experiences has to be replaced by a sometimes partial and shifting understanding of the person as a whole based on contextual judgements. As in other areas of psychiatry, there is no quick route to bypass the need for good and sensitive judgement and hence to the irreducible role of the individual. It is the link between the general and the individual as mediated by values that is illustrated by recent developments in values-based practice outlined below.

Values and values-based practice

As described earlier, although Jaspers rather dismissed values, it was the particular contribution of Windelband during psychiatry's first biological phase to show their importance in relation to the uniqueness of individual people. As with phenomenology, then, so values have sprung back into prominence in recent years as part of the new philosophy of psychiatry, alongside and as a complement to developments in the neurosciences. The most familiar aspect of the new prominence of values is of course ethics; but other examples of emerging disciplines include health economics (e.g. Brown *et al.*[27]) and decision analysis (Hunink *et al.*[28]).

Values-based practice is distinctive theoretically in that it is derived from both philosophical and empirical sources. At a practical level, it is the closest to Windelband's work in providing a complement to the generalized sciences:

- in the emphasis it places on the importance of the *diversity of individual values*, including the values of clinicians, researchers and managers as well as those of patients and carers; and
- in relying on a number of elements of good *process*, in particular specific and learnable clinical skills, to support balanced decision-making where values conflict.

It is because it is process- rather than outcome-based that values-based practice is most directly complementary to the sciences as a resource for clinical decision-making. Values-based practice, as we describe further below, is indeed in this respect directly complementary to evidence-based practice.[29] In this section, we describe briefly (i) the theory and empirical base of values-based practice, including its philosophical roots, and (ii) illustrative examples of recent policy, training and service development initiatives in values-based practice in the UK and internationally.

The theory and empirical base of values-based practice

The theory underpinning values-based practice is based on work in linguistic analytical philosophy of the 'Oxford school' in the middle decades of the twentieth century, on the meanings of key value terms, such as 'good', 'ought' and 'right'. Exemplar work from this period includes RM Hare's *The Language of Morals*,[30] *Freedom and Reason*[31] and *Descriptivism*,[32] in which he explored the logic of value terms. Although not drawing directly on the work of Windelband and others in the *Methodenstreit*, Hare can be understood as being concerned with broadly the same issues, namely how factual terms are related to value terms. Hare's line on this was that there is always a logical distinction (i.e. a distinction of meaning) to be made between these two kinds of term: this is essentially because to evaluate something as good or bad always means something more than merely describing it. Thus, in one of Hare's examples, an eating apple that is (i.e. can be described as) red and crisp happens to be, for most people, a good eating apple; but to actually call such an apple a 'good eating apple' means more than merely describing it as red and crisp – it also commends it.

Hare's work did not go uncontested, of course: alternative views were put forward, for example by another Oxford philosopher, GJ Warnock, in his *The Object of Morality*.[33] The debate between Hare and Warnock was itself set in a tradition of analytical philosophy running through much of the twentieth century,[34] and also back to the work of the British empiricist philosopher David Hume.[35] The debate indeed continues to this day; see, for example, the 2002 collection by the American philosopher Hilary Putnam.[36]

Nonetheless, work in this tradition, and in particular Hare's disentangling of descriptive and evaluative meaning, provides a powerful set of insights that, although not developed originally with medicine in mind, can help us to understand the relationship between facts and values in healthcare. Fulford applied these insights to the meanings of medical terms such as 'illness', 'disease', 'disability', 'function' and 'dysfunction' in his *Moral Theory and Medical Practice* (Fulford, 1989).[37] As a contribution to the continuing debate about the meanings of these medical terms as they are used particularly in psychiatry, it is Fulford's work, in *Moral Theory and Medical Practice* together with a number of subsequent articles,[38–40] that provides the key theoretical underpinnings for values-based practice. We do not have space here to go into the theory of values-based practice in detail, but among the practical implications of the theory are clear ways of articulating the relationships between values-based practice and both ethics- and evidence-based practice.[29]

Values-based practice also builds on empirical work on values guided by the philosophical theory just outlined. Thus, a key prediction of the theory of values-based practice is that the implicit values driving medical decision-making are often far more diverse than is generally recognized. This prediction has been tested by the British social scientist Anthony Colombo in a major study of the models of disorder (including values and beliefs) guiding decisions in the management of people with long-term schizophrenia in the community.[41] The study combined empirical methods from the social sciences with the analytical philosophical theory just outlined and was innovative in a number of respects.[42] The results of the study were widely disseminated in both research and non-governmental organizations (NGO) journals (e.g. in the house journal of MIND), and the methods developed in this study became the basis for one of the main areas of skills training for values-based practice (see below).

Policy, training and service development initiatives in values-based practice

As noted above, values-based practice starts from the diversity of individual values and relies on good process to support balanced decision-making in practice. In its reliance on good process, rather than preconceived correct outcomes, values-based practice is very much a partner to evidence-based practice: evidence-based practice provides a process for effective healthcare decision-making where the relevant evidence is complex and possibly conflicting; values-based practice provides a different but complementary process for effective healthcare decision-making where the relevant values are complex and possibly conflicting.

Again, we do not have space here to describe the process of values-based practice in detail. Ten key principles of the process of values-based practice have been set out by Fulford, together with a detailed case history of a patient with manic–depressive disorder, showing how each of these principles interweaves in practice with evidence-based approaches.[29] The ten principles have been applied in mental health and social care as the basis of a series of policy, training and service development initiatives. This work has been carried out in partnership with both service users and service providers and with institutional support from NGOs, including the Sainsbury Centre for Mental Health (SCMH), the Mental Health Foundation (MHF) and Turning Point in London, and the World Psychiatric Association, and from government departments, in particular the UK Department of Health. Internationally, corresponding developments have been included in the World Psychiatric Association's Institutional Program on Psychiatry for the Person.[43,44] Examples of these developments are described below.

Policy

The National Institute for Mental Health in England (NIMHE), as the body responsible for mental health policy implementation in England and Wales, published a framework of values that was based explicitly on the approach of values-based practice (Box 3.1).[45] This in turn guided a range of subsequent policy developments, including a generic skills programme,[46] as the basis of moves towards more multidisciplinary and person-centred approaches to service delivery.[3] The approach has also been applied in a number of specific areas of policy development, including delivering race equality[47] and the introduction of community development workers.[48]

Training

The first training manual for values-based practice was developed in a partnership between the Sainsbury Centre for Mental Health and Warwick Medical School, with the support of NIMHE. Published as *Whose Values?*,[49] the training manual was launched at a conference in London by the minister Rosie Winterton and, together with the NIMHE values framework, supported the policy initiatives noted above. A further application of values-based practice has been in the training materials produced to support the amended Mental Health Act in England and Wales. These training materials combine evidence-based resources with an innovative values-based approach to using the guiding principles defined by the code of practice (Table 3.1) as a framework of values guiding the application of the general provisions of the Act to individual cases (Figure 3.1).[50] Outside the UK, training programmes in values-based

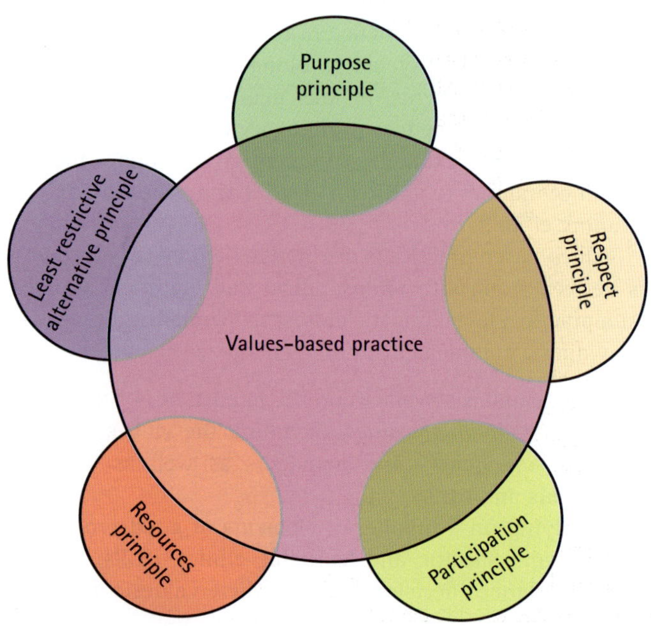

Figure 3.1 The guiding principles as a framework of values. Reproduced with permission from Ref. 50

> **Box 3.1 National framework of values for mental health**
>
> The work of the National Institute for Mental Health in England (NIMHE) on values in mental health care is guided by three principles of values-based practice:
>
> - *Recognition:* NIMHE recognizes the role of values alongside evidence in all areas of mental health policy and practice.
> - *Raising awareness:* NIMHE is committed to raising awareness of the values involved in different contexts, the role(s) they play and their impact on practice in mental health.
> - *Respect:* NIMHE respects diversity of values and will support ways of working with such diversity that makes the principle of service-user centrality a unifying focus for practice. This means that the values of each individual service user/client and their communities must be the starting point and key determinant for all actions by professionals.
>
> Respect for diversity of values encompasses a number of specific policies and principles concerned with equality of citizenship. In particular, it is anti-discriminatory because discrimination in all its forms is intolerant of diversity. Thus, respect for diversity of values has the consequence that it is unacceptable (and unlawful in some instances) to discriminate on grounds such as gender, sexual orientation, class, age, abilities, religion, race, culture or language.
>
> Respect for diversity within mental health is also:
>
> - *user-centred:* it puts respect for the values of individual users at the centre of policy and practice;
> - *recovery-oriented:* it recognizes that building on the personal strengths and resiliencies of individual users, and on their cultural and racial characteristics, there are many diverse routes to recovery;
> - *multidisciplinary:* it requires that respect be reciprocal, at a personal level (between service users, their family members, friends, communities and providers), between different provider disciplines (such as nursing, psychology, psychiatry, medicine, social work), and between different organizations (including health, social care, local authority housing, voluntary organizations, community groups, faith communities and other social support services);
> - *dynamic:* it is open and responsive to change;
> - *reflective:* it combines self-monitoring and self-management with positive self-regard;
> - *balanced:* it emphasizes positive as well as negative values;
> - *relational:* it puts positive working relationships supported by good communication skills at the heart of practice.
>
> NIMHE will encourage educational and research initiatives aimed at developing the capabilities (the awareness, attitudes, knowledge and skills) needed to deliver mental health services that will give effect to the principles of values-based practice.

practice have been developed in a number of European countries and in South Africa.[51]

Service developments

Many of the above policy and training initiatives have been associated with corresponding developments in service delivery. An example of a direct application of values-based practice to service development is a programme on diagnostic assessment in mental health and social care. This programme followed a series of international research seminars, initially in Dallas, USA,[52] and subsequently in London, supported by the Department of Health, exploring the role of values in psychiatric diagnosis. The last of these seminars, which was hosted jointly with the Mental Health and Substance Abuse section of the World Health Organization (WHO), led to the launch of a wide-ranging consultation on approaches to assessment that were considered best practice by all stakeholders – that is, by service providers from different disciplinary backgrounds, and also by service users and carers.

The programme on diagnostic assessment was distinctive in building on a specific prediction of the theory of values-based practice that, in psychiatry, values are as important in diagnosis – that is, in how we come to understand a problem – as they are in what we do about it – that is, in such areas as treatment and resource allocation. The programme has strongly practical outcomes, however, much of the publication itself comprising examples of innovative practice from the field. As with other work in values-based practice, these examples illustrate in a very practical way how the resources of generalized evidence-based science can be combined with an approach to assessment that is fully responsive to the needs, wishes, strengths and other values of the individual concerned (see Box 3.2).[53]

CONCLUSIONS

The period around the start of the twentieth century was one of great progress for biologically based neuroscience. It was a time of great promise for the science of psychiatry.

> **Box 3.2 Three keys to a shared approach to assessment in mental health and social care**
>
> - *Active participation* of the service user concerned in a shared understanding with service providers and, where appropriate, with their carers
> - Input from *different provider perspectives* within a multidisciplinary approach
> - A person-centred focus that builds on the *strengths, resiliencies and aspirations* of the individual service user and identifies his or her needs and challenges.

Table 3.1 Guiding principles in the code of practice for the new Mental Health Act (England and Wales)

Purpose	Decisions under the Act must be taken with a view to minimizing the undesirable effects of mental disorder, by maximizing the safety and wellbeing (mental and physical) of patients, promoting their recovery and protecting other people from harm
Least restrictive alternative	People taking action without a patient's consent must attempt to keep to a minimum the restrictions they impose on the patient's liberty, having regard to the purpose for which the restrictions are imposed
Respect	People taking decisions under the Act must recognize and respect the diverse needs, values and circumstances of each patient, including their race, religion, culture, gender, age, sexual orientation and any disability. They must consider the patient's views, wishes and feelings (whether expressed at the time or in advance), so far as they are reasonably ascertainable, and follow those wishes wherever practicable and consistent with the purpose of the decision. There must be no unlawful discrimination
Participation	Patients must be given the opportunity to be involved, as far as is practicable in the circumstances, in planning, developing and reviewing their own treatment and care in order to help ensure that it is delivered in a way that is as appropriate and effective for them as possible. The involvement of carers, family members and other people who have an interest in the patient's welfare should be encouraged (unless there are particular reasons to the contrary) and their views taken seriously
Resources (effectiveness, efficiency and equity)	People taking decisions under the Act must seek to use the resources available to them and to patients in the most effective, efficient and equitable way, to meet the needs of patients and achieve the purpose for which the decision was taken

Nevertheless, two figures of great importance for psychiatry realized that the science of natural laws and general mechanisms needed to be complemented by distinct approaches. As we have shown, Jaspers argued that the very nature of the subject matter of psychiatry called for an understanding of the meanings of and meaningful connections between subjects' experiences. Windelband argued that understanding the values that we place in and are held by individuals required a different approach from general nomological or nomothetic science.

As with any other area of research, their suggestions were not without problems, and there has been genuine progress in developing their key ideas. Jaspers' claim that key aspects of psychopathology are both genuinely mental phenomena and yet brutally 'un-understandable' has prompted attempts to explain simultaneously how there can be at least shifting and partial understanding of still difficult phenomena. We have mentioned work drawing on a phenomenological tradition, but equally the US psychologist Brendan Maher's suggestion that delusions are an understandable response to abnormal experiences[54] can be seen as a reaction to Jaspers' work. Similarly, Windelband's idea that value judgements require a special kind of individualistic judgement has been replaced by an approach, values-based practice, that is derived from analytical philosophy and relies on 'good process', in particular learnable clinical skills, as a basis for balanced decision-making where complex and conflicting values are in play.

Our aim in giving this brief outline of the work of Jaspers and Windelband, as two key figures in the history and philosophy of science, together with their modern counterparts, has been to indicate the extent to which resources derived from philosophy can contribute alongside the sciences to improving mental health care. Phenomenology and values-based practice, furthermore, it is important to add, are themselves set within a new and rapidly expanding international field of cross-disciplinary work between philosophy and psychiatry.[21] As Box 3.3 shows, this is a rapidly expanding field, and there are other potentially important practical developments, notably in relation to tacit knowledge (the basis of professional skills) and individual judgement (as in clinical judgement).[55]

It might seem surprising to some that there should have been this expansion of philosophy and psychiatry over the past two decades, in parallel with dramatic developments in the neurosciences underpinning psychiatry. The history of ideas outlined in the first two sections of this chapter not only makes sense of these parallel developments but also helps us to see their likely future direction. Then, as now, there were dramatic (actual or anticipated) advances in the sciences underpinning psychiatry; and these advances, far from reducing the need for careful conceptual work alongside empirical studies, actually increased it. There are several reasons for this: the challenge of applying generalized scientific knowledge to particular individual human beings, but also theoretical challenges

Box 3.3 Developments in the new philosophy of psychiatry

- 43 New academic and research groups around the world
- Special sections in the WPA and AEP
- Establishment of the International Network for Philosophy and Psychiatry (INPP), launched Cape Town, South Africa, 2002
- Annual international conferences in different parts of the world
- New professorial chairs in Italy, Netherlands, South Africa and the UK
- Training and research programmes, including a recently launched Oxford DPhil
- The international journal Philosophy, Psychiatry, and Psychology (PPP) now in its fourteenth year, from Johns Hopkins University Press
- Several book series, including International Perspectives in Philosophy and Psychiatry (IPPP) from Oxford University Press
- Establishment of the Institute for Philosophy, Diversity and Mental Health (IPDMH) at the University of Central Lancashire in the UK, with over £1 million funding
- Philosophy into practice, e.g. values-based practice (see text).

within the sciences themselves – we noted at the start of this chapter Nancy Andreasen's claim that advances in the neurosciences have driven many of the deepest problems of traditional philosophy to the top of our practical agenda.

Jaspers' work in the early twentieth century represented one clear response to these challenges. Naive models of empirical science, he believed, would reduce the sciences of the day to mere scientism (you will recall that he called such models 'brain mythologies'); and his response was to argue that we needed to find ways of working with meanings alongside and in parallel with scientific work on explanatory causes. Windelband's work on values represents a different response to scientism – one built on values in so far as these are distinct from meanings. What is shared by these approaches, then, is a recognition of the need to bring together in one way or another the findings of generalized science with the uniqueness of individual human beings.

The need to reconcile generalized science with individual human beings is perhaps particularly acute at the present time, with growing pressure to base service delivery on a narrow model of evidence-based practice that Jaspers would perhaps have characterized as scientistic. Yet, again as during psychiatry's first biological phase, the dangers of a scientistic use of evidence-based practice have been most evident to those who have been at the very forefront of developing this approach. As David Sackett puts it, in his seminal training manual on evidence-based practice, it is only when best research evidence is combined with clinical skills and, importantly, patient values that 'clinicians and patients form a diagnostic and therapeutic alliance which optimises clinical outcomes and quality of life'.[56] There is no better statement of the need for combining rigorous empirical methods with equally rigorous philosophical approaches in developing a psychiatry for the twenty-first century that is both fully science-based and genuinely patient-centred.

KEY POINTS

- Jaspers divides symptoms between subjective and objective. Another person's objective symptoms can either be detected by one's senses (such as by sight or hearing) or by merely rational understanding. To be sensitive to another's subjective symptoms requires that one imaginatively puts oneself into their predicament in a way that goes beyond merely rational understanding. The distinction between objective and subjective corresponds to a distinction between explanation and understanding.
- Jaspers distinguishes between two forms of (subjective) understanding. Static understanding, also called phenomenology, concerns what mental states feel like. Genetic understanding, also called empathy, concerns the way one mental state, ideally and typically, arises from another.
- Jaspers believes that some forms of apparently mental phenomena nevertheless cannot be understood. Primary delusions are, he claims, 'un-understandable'.
- Windelband distinguishes between idiographic and nomothetic sciences. Nomothetic sciences concern law-like and general phenomena. Idiographic sciences concern one-off events or processes. The most obvious need for an idiographic approach, according to Windelband, concerns judgements about values.
- Values-based practice is a new skills-based approach to working with complex and conflicting values that has been developed from philosophical value theory to stand alongside evidence-based practice as a support-tool for clinical decision-making in mental health.

WEBSITES AND FURTHER READING

Fulford and others have examined the links between values-based practice and a number of specific areas of medicine including Child and Adolescent Mental Health Services (CAMHS), management, spirituality and other aspects of the medical humanities, ethics, diagnosis and neuroscience. See Warwick Medical School website http://www2.warwick.ac.uk/fac/med/study/cpd/subject_index/pemh/vbp_introduction/.

Teaching and learning materials on values-based practice have now been published in a wide range of professional journals and textbooks. See the Warwick Medical School website noted above, and also the Royal College of General Practitioners' 2005 *Curriculum Statement: Ethics and Values Based Medicine* at www.rcgp.org.uk/gpcurriculum/pdfs/ethicsAndVBPsfRCGPCouncilDec2005.pdf.

Details of Jaspers' work and of other important figures in the early development of psychiatry are given in 'History of ideas' in *The Oxford Textbook of Philosophy and Psychiatry* (Fulford KWM, Thornton T, Graham G (2006) Oxford: Oxford University Press). Section 3 of this same book covers modern developments in the philosophy of science, Section 4 covers values-based practice and ethics, and Section 5 covers phenomenology and the philosophy of mind. *The Oxford Textbook* includes a series of readings (on a CD-ROM) and includes detailed guides to further reading and key learning points.

REFERENCES

1. Andreasen NC (2001) *Brave New Brain: Conquering Mental Illness in the Era of the Genome.* Oxford: Oxford University Press.
2. Kendler K, Appelbaum P, Bell C, *et al.* (2008) Issues for DSM-V: DSM-V should include a conceptual issues work group. *American Journal of Psychiatry* **165**: 1–2.
3. Department of Health (2005) *New Ways of Working for Psychiatrists: Enhancing Effective, Person-Centred Services through New Ways of Working in Multidisciplinary and Multi-Agency Contexts. (Final Report 'But Not the End of the Story'.)* London: Department of Health.
4. Department of Health (2008) *Putting People First: A Shared Vision and Commitment to the Transformation of Adult Social Care.* London: Department of Health.
5. Jaspers K ([1913] 1997) *General Psychopathology.* Baltimore, MD: Johns Hopkins University Press.
6. Ehrlich E, Ehrlich L, Pepper GB (eds) (1986) *Karl Jaspers: Basic Philosophical Writings.* Athens, OH: Ohio University Press.
7. Jaspers K ([1912] 1968) The phenomenological approach in psychopathology. *British Journal of Psychiatry* **114**: 1313–23.
8. Jaspers K ([1913] 1974) Causal and 'meaningful' connections between life history and psychosis (transl. J.Hoenig.) In SR Hirsch, M Shepherd (eds) *Themes and Variations in European Psychiatry.* Bristol: Wright: 80–93.
9. Fulford KWM, Thornton T, Graham G (2006) *Oxford Textbook of Philosophy and Psychiatry.* Oxford: Oxford University Press.
10. Carruthers P, Smith PK (eds) (1996) *Theories of Theories of Mind.* Cambridge: Cambridge University Press.
11. Heal J (1995) Replication and functionalism. In M Davies, T Stone (eds) *Folk Psychology.* Oxford: Blackwell.
12. McDowell J (1998) *Mind Value and Reality.* Cambridge, MA: Harvard University Press.
13. Davidson D (1980) *Essays on Actions and Events.* Oxford: Oxford University Press.
14. Sims, A. (1988) *Symptoms in the Mind: An Introduction to Descriptive Psychopathology.* London: Bailliere Tindall.
15. IDGA Workgroup, WPA (2003) IGDA 8: idiographic (personalised) diagnostic formulation. *British Journal of Psychiatry* **18** (suppl. 45): 55–7
16. Windelband W (1980) History and natural science. *History and Theory and Psychology* **19**: 169–85.
17. Lamiell JT (1997) Individuals and the differences between them. In R Hogan, J Johnson, S Briggs (eds) *Handbook of Personality Psychology.* New York: Academic Press.
18. Rickert H (1907) Geschichtsphilosophie. In W Windelband (ed.) *Die Philosophie im Beginn des zwanzigsten Jahrhunderts: Festschrift für Kuno Fischer.* Heidelberg: Carl Weinter.
19. Thornton T (2008) Does understanding individuals require idiographic judgement? *European Archives of Psychiatry and Clinical Neuroscience* **258** (suppl. 5): 104–9.
20. Thornton T (2008) Should comprehensive diagnosis include idiographic understanding? *Medicine, Healthcare and Philosophy* **11**: 293–302.
21. Fulford KWM, Morris KJ, Sadler JZ, Stanghellini G (2003) Past improbable, future possible: the renaissance in philosophy and psychiatry. In KWM Fulford, KJ Morris, JZ Sadler, G Stanghellini (eds) *Nature and Narrative: An Introduction to the New Philosophy of Psychiatry.* Oxford: Oxford University Press.
22. Hoerl C (2001) Introduction: understanding, explaining, and intersubjectivity in schizophrenia. *Philosophy, Psychiatry, and Psychology* **8**.
23. Widdershoven G, Widdershoven-Heerding I (2003) Understanding dementia: a hermeneutic perspective. In KWM Fulford, KJ Morris, JZ Sadler, G Stanghellini (eds) *Nature and Narrative: An Introduction to the New Philosophy of Psychiatry.* Oxford: Oxford University Press.
24. Sabat SR (2001) *The Experience of Alzheimer's Disease: Life Through a Tangled Veil.* Oxford: Blackwell.
25. Morris KJ (2003) The phenomenology of body dysmorphic disorder: a Sartrean analysis. In KWM Fulford, KJ Morris, JZ Sadler, G Stanghellini (eds) *Nature and Narrative: An Introduction to the New Philosophy of Psychiatry.* Oxford: Oxford University Press.
26. Stanghellini G (2004) *Disembodied Spirits and Deanimated Bodies.* Oxford: Oxford University Press.

27. Brown MM, Brown GC, Sharma S (2005) *Evidence-Based to Value-Based Medicine*. Chicago, IL: American Medical Association Press.
28. Hunink M, Glasziou P, Siegel J, *et al.* (2001) *Decision Making in Health and Medicine: Integrating Evidence and Values*. Cambridge: Cambridge University Press.
29. Fulford KWM (2004) Ten principles of values-based medicine. In J Radden (ed.) *The Philosophy of Psychiatry: A Companion*. New York: Oxford University Press.
30. Hare RM (1952) *The Language of Morals*. Oxford: Oxford University Press.
31. Hare RM (1963) *Freedom and Reason*. Oxford: Oxford University Press.
32. Hare RM (1963) Descriptivism. *Proceedings of the British Academy*, **49**: 115–34. Reprinted in Hare RM (1972) *Essays on the Moral Concepts*. London: Macmillan.
33. Warnock GJ (1971) *The Object of Morality*. London: Methuen.
34. Warnock GJ (1967) *Contemporary Moral Philosophy*. London: Macmillan.
35. Hume D (1972) *A Treatise of Human Nature: Book III*. London: Fontana/Collins.
36. Putnam H (2002) *The Collapse of the Fact/Value Dichotomy and other Essays*. Cambridge, MA: Harvard University Press.
37. Fulford, KWM (1989, reprinted 1995 and 1999) *Moral Theory and Medical Practice*. Cambridge: Cambridge University Press.
38. Fulford KWM (1998) Dissent and dissensus: the limits of consensus formation in psychiatry. In HAMJ ten Have, H-M Sass (eds) *Consensus Formation in Health Care Ethics*. Dordrecht: Kluwer.
39. Fulford KWM (1999) Nine variations and a coda on the theme of an evolutionary definition of dysfunction. *Journal of Abnormal Psychology* **108**: 412–20.
40. Fulford KWM (2000) Teleology without tears: naturalism, neo-naturalism and evaluationism in the analysis of function statements in biology (and a bet on the twenty-first century). *Philosophy, Psychiatry, and Psychology* **7**: 77–94.
41. Colombo A, Bendelow G, Fulford KWM, Williams S (2003) Evaluating the influence of implicit models of mental disorder on processes of shared decision making within community-based multi-disciplinary teams. *Social Science and Medicine* **56**: 1557–70.
42. Fulford KWM, Colombo A (2004) Six models of mental disorder: a study combining linguistic-analytic and empirical methods. *Philosophy, Psychiatry, and Psychology* **11**: 129–44.
43. Mezzich JE (2002) Comprehensive diagnosis: a conceptual basis for future diagnostic systems. *Psychopathology* **35**: 162–5.
44. Mezzich JE, Salloum IM (2007) Towards innovative international classification and diagnostic systems: ICD-11 and person-centered integrative diagnosis. *Acta Psychiatrica Scandinavica*, **116**: 1–5.
45. National Institute for Mental Health in England (2004) *The National Framework of Values for Mental Health*. London: National Institute for Mental Health in England.
46. Department of Health (2004) *The Ten Essential Shared Capabilities: A Framework for the Whole of the Mental Health Workforce*. London: Sainsbury Centre for Mental Health, National Health Service University (NHSU) and National Institute for Mental Health England (NIMHE).
47. Department of Health (2005) *Delivering Race Equality in Mental Health Care: An Action Plan for Reform Inside and Outside Services*. London: Department of Health.
48. Department of Health (2004) *Mental Health Policy Implementation Guide: Community Development Workers for Black and Minority Ethnic Communities*. London: Department of Health.
49. Woodbridge K, Fulford KWM (2004) *Whose Values? A Workbook for Values-Based Practice in Mental Health Care*. London: Sainsbury Centre for Mental Health.
50. Care Services Improvement Partnership (CSIP), National Institute for Mental Health in England (NIMHE) (2008) *Workbook to Support Implementation of the Mental Health Act 1983 as Amended by the Mental Health Act 2007*. London: Department of Health.
51. Van Staden CW, Fulford KWM (2007) Hypotheses, neuroscience and real persons: the theme of the 10th International Conference on Philosophy, Psychiatry and Psychology. *South African Journal of Psychiatry* **13**: 68–71.
52. Sadler JZ (ed.) (2002) *Descriptions and Prescriptions: Values, Mental Disorders, and the DSMs*. Baltimore, MD: Johns Hopkins University Press.
53. National Institute for Mental Health in England (NIMHE), Care Services Improvement Partnership (CSIP) (2008) *Three Keys to a Shared Approach in Mental Health Assessment*. London: Department of Health.
54. Maher BA (1999) Anomalous experience in everyday life: its significance for psychopathology. *Monist* **82**: 547–70.
55. Thornton T (2007) *Essential Philosophy of Psychiatry*. Oxford: Oxford University Press.
56. Sackett DL, Straus SE, Scott Richardson W, Rosenberg W, Haynes RB (2000) *Evidence-Based Medicine: How to Practice and Teach EBM*, 2nd edn. Edinburgh: Churchill Livingstone.

Chapter 4

Research methods and statistics

Daniel Stahl and Morven Leese

INTRODUCTION

In this chapter we review study designs and statistical techniques commonly used in psychiatry, focusing on the requirements of the MRCPsych examination. For reasons of space, we have not included details of all tests and definitions, but where appropriate we have given one or two key references. General texts that would be very useful to consult are: Bland (2000),[1] for a comprehensive guide to methods; Petrie and Sabin,[2] an excellent handbook covering all the standard statistical tests, including examples; and Everitt,[3] for concise definitions. Some useful articles can be found in the journals *Bandolier* and *BMJ Teaching*.

Psychiatric data: a typical scenario

We introduce here a typical scenario that will be used as an example throughout the rest of the chapter. A medication training package is offered to nurses, who each care for a caseload of patients. Each nurse willing to participate in a trial of this package is randomized to receive the training or be placed on a waiting list to receive training later, after the trial. Two patients are chosen at random from each nurse's caseload for assessment of patient outcomes. Outcomes are at two levels: a knowledge test for nurses, before and after the trial has taken place, and a global assessment of functioning (GAF) for patients. This is fairly typical of psychiatric data because it involves comparing groups at different levels within the same study, which leads to 'clustering' of data (because patients of a particular nurse are likely to be more similar to each other than patients of different nurses).

We shall use output from the package Stata to illustrate the results of analysing various types of data. Another package that is widely used is SPSS. Both programs are very comprehensive, but Stata has particularly good facilities for the types of data encountered in psychiatry. A good introduction to statistics using Stata is Dupont.[4] First we discuss some aspects of study design and general concepts such as precision and bias.

Classification of data types

The type of data being analysed determines which statistical methods are appropriate. In Table 4.1 we have given some examples of types of data that may be encountered in psychiatry and how they are classified.

Apart from the clustering feature mentioned above, psychiatric data have other characteristics that make them somewhat distinct from medical data in general. One of

Table 4.1 Data types encountered in psychiatry

Type of scale	Example	Data	Relation between values
Nominal	Gender, diagnostic group	Discrete (categorical, including binary)	No particular order; values are same/different
Ordinal	Age group, Likert scale, adjectival scale	Discrete (ordered categorical)	Categories are ranked – (ordered data); values are smaller/larger
Interval	Visual analogue pain score, functioning score	Discrete or continuous	Absolute difference; 0 has no real meaning
Ratio	Number of symptoms, cost of treatment	Discrete or continuous	Absolute difference and proportion; 0 has real meaning

these is the widespread assessment of patient outcomes from *questionnaires*. Establishing validity and reliability is particularly important for such data, as are issues concerned with combining responses to several individual questions (or *items*) into an aggregate score. Before describing the design and analysis of collected data, we first consider some aspects of scale development.

SCALE DEVELOPMENT

Measurement scales

Measurement involves the estimation of a quantity relative to some standard. Measurements usually need a *measuring instrument*, such as a measuring tape. The type of unit on which something is measured is called the *scale* (e.g. metre, second, kilogram) of the measuring instrument. In psychiatry, typical measurement problems involve identifying and assessing the severity of a disorder and evaluating the outcome of a treatment. However, many traits, such as abilities, attitudes, quality of life and personality, are difficult to measure, since they are unobservable and subjective. Psychometrics is concerned with the theory and technique of measuring such psychological phenomena, which are called *constructs*, *latent traits* or *attributes*. In psychometrics, unobservable and subjective phenomena are *inferred* from variables (items) that can be observed and measured, in the case of psychiatry through the use of questionnaires and structured interviews. Such questionnaires are sometimes called *instruments*. Adjectival, Likert and visual analogue scales (VAS) are often used in such situations. Figure 4.1 shows an example of each of these.

An example of a published adjectival scale is the Beck Depression Inventory (BDI).[5] This consists of a 21-question multiple-choice self-report inventory and asks questions about the feelings of the subject during the past couple of days. Each question (item) offers four possible answers, arranged in increasing severity. An example of statements for one item is:

0 – I do not feel like a failure.
1 – I feel I have failed more than the average person.
2 – As I look back on my life, all I can see is a lot of failure.
3 – I feel I am a complete failure as a person.

In Likert scales, a declarative sentence is given along with a number of response options. Respondents specify their level of agreement to this. While the descriptor of the adjectival scale is unipolar (from low to high), a Likert item is bipolar, with a neutral/undecided/no opinion term in the middle.

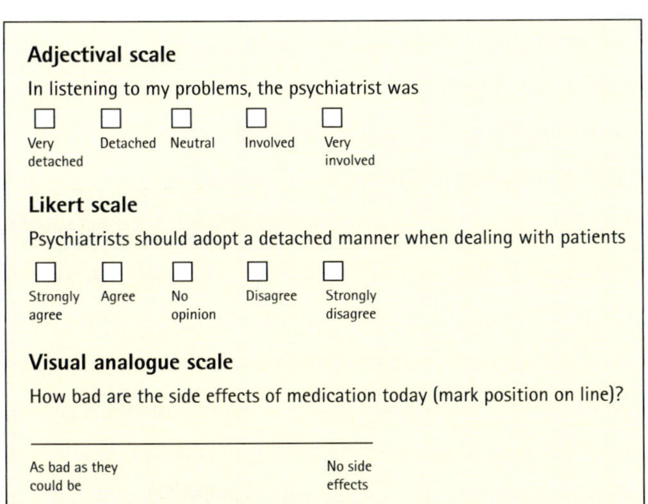

Figure 4.1 Examples of questionnaire data commonly used in psychiatry

Constructing a measuring instrument

The aim is to develop a scale that is *reliable* (i.e. measuring consistently) and *valid* (i.e. measuring what it is supposed to measure). The first step in the development of a questionnaire is to generate a pool of items, which is assumed to measure the latent construct(s).[6] From a statistical point of view, the choice of the scale (e.g. adjectival or Likert scale), the level (continuous, ordinal or categorical), the definition of the scaling responses (e.g. choice of adjective or the number of answer steps) and the wording of the question will influence the quality of the final scale. Particularly troublesome are floor and ceiling effects in short scales, where respondents tend to use a compressed interval at the top or bottom of the scale; this limits variability and hence the discriminatory power of the questionnaire.

To investigate how items might relate to latent constructs, it is common to perform a factor analysis, either exploratory (if little is known about how the items relate to factors) or confirmatory (if theory can predict this). Once the items that measure the construct(s) have been decided on, it is then common practice to add them up to make a scale total and/or subscale totals. In calculating totals, it is important that the response values (e.g. from 0 to 5) are in the same conceptual order to obtain a meaningful total score, so some items may need to be *reverse-coded* (e.g. 5 to 1, 4 to 2, 3 to 3, 2 to 4, 1 to 5). A summary of issues relating to health measurement scales in general is given in Streiner and Norman.[7]

Types of reliability

A reliable measure is measuring something consistently, in a reproducible fashion. In psychiatry, many questionnaires are self-administered and the reliability of the respondent needs to be evaluated by administering the scale on two or more occasions. This is called *test–retest reliability*. The choice of the time interval between two administrations is crucial. It must be sufficiently long that respondents do not remember their previous answers, but short enough that the underlying process (such as degree of depression) has not changed. Typical test–retest time intervals for health-related studies range between 2 days and 14 days. Often tests are administered through structured interviews. In this case, one needs to assess the degree to which different raters give consistent estimates of the same phenomenon when rating the same patients (*inter-rater reliability*). Finally, the individual items need to reliably estimate the latent construct. *Internal consistency reliability* assesses the consistency of items within a scale or subscale.

Indices of reliability

Classical test score theory assumes that each person has a true score that would be obtained if there were no errors in measurement. However, measuring instruments are imperfect and an observed score will be the sum of the true score and error. *Reliability* reflects the relative contributions of those two sources of variation. Reliability for continuous variables is usually based on the *intraclass correlation coefficient* (ICC).[8] It is the proportion of variance that reflects between-subject ('true') variability and ranges between 0 (no reliability) to 1 (perfect reliability). The most commonly used measure is the ICC for absolute agreement, which measures the absolute agreement between raters or between two observations at different time points and is the between-subject variance divided by the total variance. If we are interested only in relative agreement (i.e. ignoring constant bias between the raters or time points), then the between-rater or between-time-point variance would be removed from the model. The ICC for relative agreement would be estimated by the between-subject variance divided by the sum of between-subject variance and within-subject variance, and is consequently larger than the ICC for absolute agreement. Another statistic that can be used for pairs of observations (different occasions or two raters) is the so-called *concordance index* (see Bland and Altman[9]); this is numerically similar to the ICC for absolute agreement.

Although many software packages calculate ICCs, they can also be estimated through *random effects models* (see Multivariate and other more complex techniques, below), which can easily extend the ICC to account for more than two factors. It is, for example, possible to include therapist as another random factor in the model to estimate sources of errors due to therapist effects. This extension of reliability is known as *generalizability* theory and is a powerful tool to identify sources of error in a measurement process.[10]

The test–retest or inter-rater reliability of categorical variables is evaluated using *Cohen's kappa*, a measure of chance-adjusted agreement that takes a value of 1 when there is perfect agreement and of 0 when observed agreement is equal to chance. Ordinal categorical variables, such as symptom scores with possible scores of low, medium, high, can be assessed using *weighted kappa*, which penalizes according to the extent of disagreement. The kappa coefficient is dependent on the prevalence of the different response types. For example, if the prevalence of depression is low, we can obtain a good reliability for the diagnosis of depression between two raters, even if the raters disagree strongly about the classification of the few positive cases of depression. It is therefore advisable not to rely solely on the kappa but also to assess the percentage agreement within each class.

For internal consistency, a common approach is to calculate Cronbach's alpha for continuous data, which is the average of all possible split-half reliabilities (where the items are divided in half, e.g. odd versus even questions, and the reliabilities computed for the two halves). If the data are binary, the formula is the same but the index is known as the *Kuder–Richardson Formula 20* (KR20). Because reliability increases with the number of items, the index can be adjusted by the *Spearman–Brown formula*, so that the reliability of scales with different lengths can be compared directly.

Table 4.2 summarizes the various types of reliability discussed.

Intraclass correlations can be classified as 0.6 (fair), 0.7 (good), 0.8 (very good) and 0.9 (excellent), although note that these are all subjective terms; kappas and Cronbach's alphas are sometimes classified in a similar way.

Types of validity

Reliability does not say anything about what is being measured. A measure also requires validity – that is, finding

Table 4.2 Summary of reliability measures

Reliability	What it measures	Typical indices
Inter-observer	Agreement among interviewers, raters or coders who are rating the same information	Intraclass correlation (continuous data)
Test–retest (or intra-observer)	A measure at two different times with no treatment (or other changes) in between should yield the same results	Kappa (categorical data; possibly weighted if more than two categories)
Internal consistency (or item reliability)	Do the items measure the same construct/domain? Alternatively, do the scores of the items correlate with scores of all other items of the same construct/domain?	Cronbach's alpha (or Kuder–Richardson for binary data); possibly corrected using the Spearman–Brown formula

results that accurately reflect the concept being measured. Reliability is irrelevant without validity and validity implies reliability. Thus, reliability places the upper limit on validity. Some of the types of validity are summarized in Table 4.3.

The evaluation of validity is more of a scientific issue than a statistical one, since it depends on choosing appropriate scales for comparison. It is typically assessed through correlation or regression analysis, comparing the results of the scale of interest with results from other scales or designing experiments to reveal facets of the causal role of the construct. A common validity test involves comparing a screening test against a gold standard diagnosis that has established the true condition, for example as shown in the *contingency table* or cross-tabulation in Table 4.4.

Diagnostic test measures

In a diagnostic test (and other situations where one predicts the value of a binary variable), there are a number of measures of predictive accuracy. Sensitivity (specificity) is the proportion of those with (without) the true diagnosis who screen positive (negative). The (positive) likelihood ratio (LR) is the value of the screening test in predicting a positive result and is the ratio of the probability of a positive test from someone with the disorder to the probability of a positive test from someone without the disorder (and similarly for the negative LR). These measures are independent of prevalence and so are generalizable across samples. Positive (negative) predictive power is more useful in clinical situations and is the proportion of those who screen positive (negative) who do (do not) have the diagnosis. Positive predictive value (PPV) and negative predictive value (NPV) are specific to the particular clinical situation since they depend on prevalence. Table 4.5 summarizes these various quantities.

The post-test probability is a useful measure for clinicians in assessing a positive test result for individual patients. It takes account of known prevalence and combines it with the test result, through the intermediate step of computing odds from probabilities, using the following relationships:

$$\text{Odds} = \text{probability}/(1 - \text{probability})$$
$$\text{Probability} = \text{odds}/(1 + \text{odds})$$

The relevant prevalence is that for the specific population of interest or may be obtained from similar samples. The post-test odds, and hence the post-test probability, can be calculated as follows:

$$\text{Post-test odds} = \text{pre-test odds} \times \text{likelihood ratio}$$

If a patient undergoes a series of tests, the LRs can be multiplied together to obtain the post-test probability based on all the tests simultaneously.

For example, suppose the prevalence in the population of interest is 20 per cent, so the pre-test probability of the condition is 0.2 and odds is 0.2/0.8 = 0.25. A patient tests positive using a test that has sensitivity 0.8 and specificity 0.9, and that therefore has $LR_{+ve} = 0.8/0.1 = 8$. The post-test odds

Table 4.3 Types of validity

Type of validity	What it measures
Face	Subjective assessment that the instrument/item appears to measure the desired qualities
Content	Subjective assessment that the instrument samples all the important contents/domains of the attribute
Criterion	Is the measure consistent with what we already know and what we expect?
Concurrent	Does the new measure associate with a different scale that measures something similar?
Discriminate	The new measure should not associate with constructs that should not be related
Predictive	Does the measure predict outcome accurately?
Construct	Is the measure related to other variables as required by theory? Sensitivity to change, responsiveness

Table 4.4 Example of cross-tabulated data as used in a screening test

	True positive	True negative	Total
Screen positive	a	b	$a+b$
Screen negative	c	d	$c+d$
Total	$n_1 = a+c$	$n_2 = b+d$	$a+b+c+d$

Table 4.5 Diagnostic test measures

Measure	Formula
Sensitivity	$a/(a+c)$
Specificity	$d/(b+d)$
Likelihood ratio for a positive test	Sensitivity/(1 − specificity)
Likelihood ratio of a negative test	(1 − sensitivity)/specificity
Positive predictive power	$a/(a+b)$
Negative predictive power	$a/(c+d)$

is $8 \times 0.25 = 2$. Using the relationship above, the post-test probability is therefore $2/(1+2) = 0.667$ (67%).

Finally, we illustrate a receiver operator curve (ROC) in Figure 4.2. This is a plot of sensitivity versus 1 – specificity for situations where the screening tool produces a continuous score. In that case, by using different cut-offs, one can balance sensitivity and specificity. The area under the curve is an overall measure of the predictive success of the tool. The example in Figure 4.2 is not particularly good at 0.609: perfection would be 1, and 0.5, the diagonal line, no better than chance. The further the curve is towards the left-hand top corner, the better (high sensitivity and low specificity).

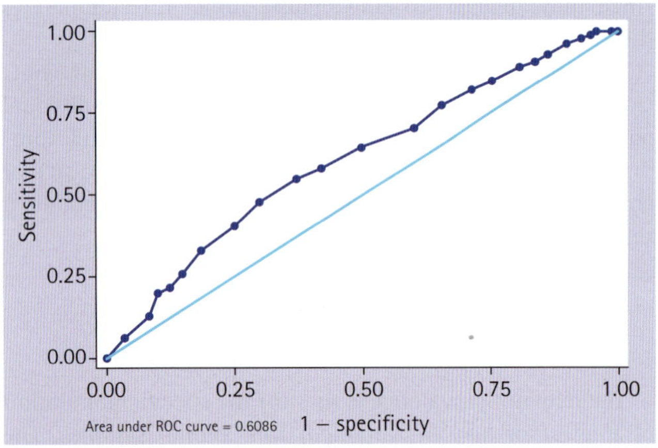

Figure 4.2 Example of a receiver operator curve (ROC)

STUDY DESIGNS

Although some psychiatric studies can be described as exploratory, most aim to answer specific questions such as: Does this new therapy work better than a standard therapy already in use? Can we identify factors that are risk or protective factors for developing certain diseases? Is it worth spending money on specific therapies or methods of delivering services? These three questions most often lead to intervention, observational and health economics studies, respectively. This classification is somewhat simplistic, as there are often going to be overlaps, but it provides a convenient way of thinking about study design. See Pocock[11] for an introduction to clinical trials.

Intervention studies

The main types of intervention (or 'experimental') study are now described.

In a *randomized controlled trial* (RCT), random allocation of patients to the treatments to be compared ensures fair comparisons. Any differences will be due to chance, and with large samples they will tend to be small. A *crossover* design involves giving the intervention and control to two randomized groups as usual but then, after a washout period, patients swap over, so that the controls have the intervention and vice versa. The advantage is that the difference between intervention and control is measured for each patient, so that patient differences are controlled for in the design. It is only possible for certain types of intervention (mainly drugs whose effect will become negligible during the washout period).

Randomization may be performed separately within strata (e.g. by centre in a multicentre trial, or by gender and/or age group). Methods of randomization include *permuted blocks* and *minimization*. The former produces sequences of codes (e.g. ABBA) that are generated at random and used to allocate patients to treatment arms A and B in small blocks, in this case four. Minimization is not a truly random method, but nevertheless it is generally acceptable and allows easy balance across several strata simultaneously. *Double blinding* means that neither the patient nor the therapist knows the group to which the patient has been assigned; a further protection is triple blinding, where the person analysing the data is also blind. The double-blind randomized, controlled trial is the gold standard of experimental designs since it minimizes most types of bias.

The interventions to be compared may include a *placebo* – that is, a dummy treatment that appears similar to patients but that has no medical effect. In *open-label studies*, both the patient and the therapist know the group to which the patient has been assigned. An example of the latter might be a comparison of cognitive-behaviour therapy (CBT) with drug treatment for anxiety; clearly neither the patient nor the therapist will be blind to the treatment arm and in this case a placebo is not feasible.

An ethical principal for RCTs is that there should be *equipoise* – a genuine uncertainty in the minds of the doctors concerned (whether specialists or the wider scientific community) about which arm would most benefit a subject. Another key issue is *intention-to-treat* (ITT): this refers to the recommended practice of analysing subjects as randomized, whether or not they are receiving the allocated treatment. This means that the benefits of randomization are retained, but it also means that it is the offer of treatment, rather than the receipt of treatment, that is being tested.

Trials are classified into phases depending on the stage of development of the intervention. The classification shown in Table 4.6 is most often used for drug trials. See also the Medical Research Council (MRC) Clinical Trial Unit definitions at www.ctu.mrc.ac.uk, from which some of these definitions were taken.

The reporting of trials is covered by the CONSORT guidelines,[12,13] which include a diagram showing the numbers recruited, randomized and followed up (Figure 4.3).

Loss to follow-up has traditionally been dealt with using *last observation carried forward* (LOCR), but this is now discredited and so-called *principled* methods of dealing with missing values are recommended, such as multiple imputation, model-based methods such as maximum likelihood with predictors of being missing, and probability weighting.

Table 4.6 Classification of phases in randomized controlled trials

Phase	Aim	Comment
I	Test the safety of a new treatment	Involve only a small number of people, who may be healthy volunteers
II	Test the new treatment in a larger group of people who usually have the disease for which the treatment is to be used, to see whether the treatment is effective	Usually a few hundred people are involved at this stage; phase II trials also look at safety
III	Test the new treatment in a larger group of people	Compares the new treatment with the treatment currently in use, or occasionally with a placebo; these trials look at how well the new treatment works and at any side effects it may cause
IV	Tests drugs that are already available for prescription (rather than new drugs under development)	Done after a drug has been tested in phases I–III and has been granted a licence

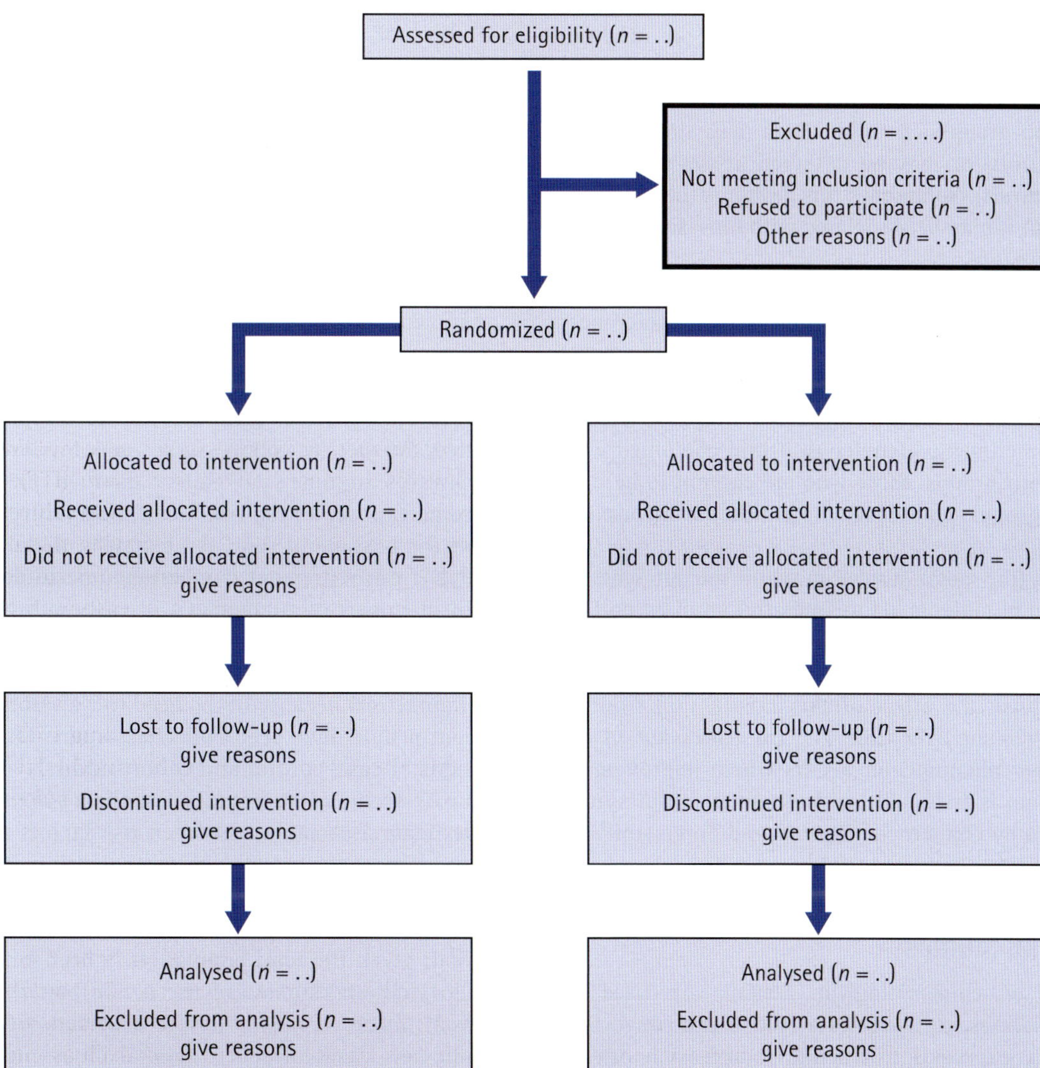

Figure 4.3 Example of a CONSORT diagram for an individually randomized trial

In a *cluster randomized trial*, a group of patients (e.g. those in a particular hospital ward) are randomized together; outcomes may be measured at the patient level (e.g. symptoms) or the group level (e.g. ward atmosphere), or both. This type of design is relatively common in psychiatry, since therapies are often administered to whole groups at a time. The phrase 'clustered data' should not be confused with 'cluster analysis' (see Multivariate and other more complex techniques, below). Although randomization can balance the characteristics of the groups across the arms of the trial, it may not be sufficient to balance those of patients. This is a disadvantage compared with individually randomized trials, although practical considerations or a need to avoid *dilution* may override this. Dilution refers to the possibility of patients randomized to the different arms interacting with one another and sharing some of the effect of therapy. A slightly different version of the CONSORT diagram would be used for clustered trials,[14] and sample sizes need to be increased to take account of the lack of independence within clusters.[15]

In *non-randomized controlled studies*, two groups are compared but individuals are not allocated at random; rather, the intervention is given to a group of patients and another group is chosen to be as similar in all respects to the intervention group as possible. Data may already exist (*historical controls*) or may be gathered at the same time (*concurrent controls*). Sometimes this design is the only feasible option, but it may be associated with bias (see Deeks *et al.*[16] for a discussion).

Patient preference trials allow patients or doctors to choose the arm of the trial according to their preference; clearly this design loses the bias-reduction advantages of randomization, and it tends to be used only where randomization is unethical or would lead to impossibly low recruitment rates. Sometimes preference trials are combined with RCTs to give four groups: those who are content to be randomized (two groups) and those who choose for themselves (two groups).

Before–after (pre–post) studies measure an outcome on the same group of patients before and after an intervention. Patients are sometimes described as being 'their own controls'. Major disadvantages of this approach are that one cannot distinguish the effect of the intervention from (i) natural improvement over time and (ii) *regression to the mean*. The latter phenomenon occurs where improvement of some patients is inevitable because their initial symptoms were high by chance. See Morton and Torgerson[17] for a discussion of this phenomenon.

Observational studies

Observational or epidemiological designs are used to describe populations, to investigate risk or protective factors, or to study interventions when it is not feasible or ethical to perform an RCT.[18]

In *case–control studies*, a group of cases is identified and then a comparison group of controls is assembled; if each case is matched individually with one or more controls, this is known as an *individually matched* case–control study. The important point is that a control would be a case *if* they had the outcome of interest. By comparing two groups with respect to hypothesized risk factors, one can infer something about the aetiology of the disease. If the control group is similar in general respects to the cases (e.g. they may be chosen to have a similar age range and to live in similar areas) without being individually matched, this is sometimes known as *group matching*. The analytical methods for an individually matched case–control study would be to estimate odds ratios (ORs) for the risk factor in relation to case–control status using, for example, conditional logistic regression (see Correlation and regression, below). Positive ORs indicate increased risk for those with the factor, but note that ORs can be numerically identified with risk ratios (RRs) only when the risk is small, say less than 5 per cent.

A typical scenario might be to identify cases of schizophrenia and find an individually matched control for each of them of the same age, within ±2 years, of the same ethnic group and born in the same postcode area. One might then look at birth records to determine whether birth trauma had occurred. Higher odds of birth trauma among those with schizophrenia compared with controls might imply that this was a risk factor.

Retrospective cohort studies compare outcomes in a group of people who have been exposed to a risk factor and another group who have not. An example would be a study of students in which previous neurotic symptoms in adolescence are self-reported. Current diagnosis of schizophrenia is made by a psychiatrist, and the association between the earlier self-reported symptoms and schizophrenia is estimated. *Prospective* cohort studies look forwards rather than backwards in time and collect data on patients as they become exposed to the risk factor, comparing the outcomes after the passage of time. An example might be a study of people from retirement comparing time to death for those with diagnosis of Alzheimer's disease with those without. Prospective studies are preferable scientifically because there is less danger of recall bias (see below), but they may be impractical because of the need to wait until data on sufficient people have been collected. Figure 4.4 contrasts the designs of case–control and cohort studies.

Cross-sectional studies take a snapshot in time in order to investigate associations between risk factors and outcomes or to estimate the prevalence of a condition. For example, a survey might seek to detect all people in contact with mental health services in a specific area over a 6-month period; given the total population figures for the area, this could yield an estimate of the *period prevalence* of severe mental illness. If health service providers were asked how many new cases of severe mental illness occurred in the period, this would yield an *incidence rate* per year. If patients' sociodemographic details were recorded, the

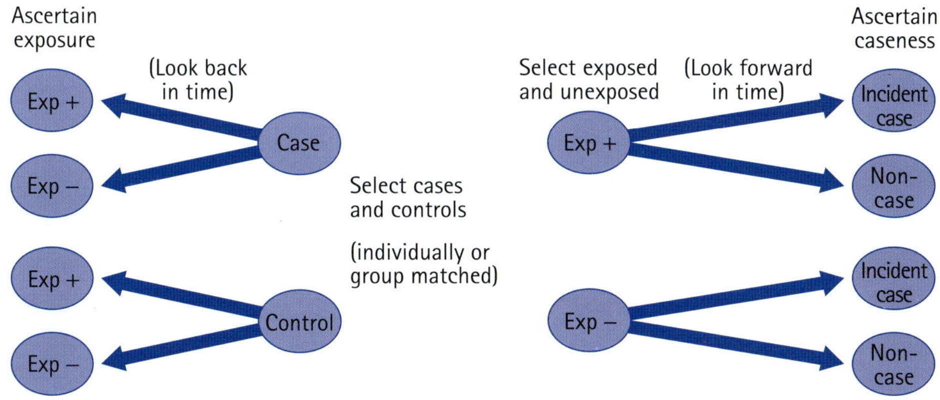

Figure 4.4 Contrast between the design of case–control (left) and cohort studies (right)

association between ethnic group and particular types of mental illness could be estimated (an *association* study).

Where the unit of observation is an area or group of people, such as a general practitioner's (GP) practice, rather than an individual, the study is termed *ecological*. Such studies are most useful for health service provision, where conclusions are sought at institutional level so that changes might be implemented at that level. The *ecological fallacy* refers to the incorrect attribution to individuals of findings at the group level. For example, the link between the levels of presentation with depression among adolescents might be studied at health authority level, with local information campaigns as a possible predictor. If a link were found, one could increase campaigns as a public health measure. The fallacy would be to assume that information campaigns affected individual adolescents when in fact their influence was more diffuse. Confounding is a particular problem for ecological studies, although they are convenient to perform because routinely collected administrative data can be used.

Health economic studies

Health economic studies are usually focused on comparing the costs and consequences of competing courses of action, such as the use of a new drug, or ways of providing health services, such as the use of assertive outreach teams. See Phelps[19] for a general introduction.

The consequences in a *cost-effectiveness analysis* might be, for example symptom reduction or social functioning. Cost-effectiveness analysis thus tends to be performed where there is a specific disease-related outcome. For example, if a new drug to lessen symptoms in schizophrenia were tested, the effectiveness might be the reduction in a symptom score. Typically, cost-effectiveness is measured as the average extra cost per unit increase in effectiveness – the incremental cost-effectiveness ratio (ICER). If this is less than a *maximum willingness to pay*, the therapy is considered cost-effective at that level. *Cost-utility analysis* is similar to cost-effectiveness analysis, except that, in order to place treatments for different diseases on a common basis, outcomes are measured in generalized units of utility. A commonly used utility is the *quality-adjusted life year* (QALY). One QALY is equivalent to 1 year of perfect health or 2 years in a health state valued at 0.5.

Typically, the results are displayed in a cost-effectiveness plane, as in Figure 4.5. Here, many samples consistent with the data have been *bootstrapped* to indicate the degree of uncertainty in the overall cost-effectiveness figure (the bold dot). Bootstrapping is a technique whereby many subsamples are taken from the observed data in which some cases are dropped and some replicated; each subsample supplies point estimates, the variation in which indicates the uncertainty in the data; it is used where distributional assumptions of standard statistics cannot be met – as is often the case for cost data. Two lines showing different values for willingness to pay are also shown. Points below these lines would be cost-effective using these criteria.

In *cost–benefit analysis*, clinical consequences are measured in monetary terms and can therefore be set directly against cost. It is used where different health technologies are to be compared with each other and/or with other types of expenditure. *Cost-minimization analysis* may also be a part of economic evaluation, where the health technologies to be compared have equal benefit, so that one requires only to compare costs. An increasingly widespread technique is the use of the *cost-effectiveness acceptability curve* (CEAC), a plot of the probability of cost-effectiveness against various choices of minimum willingness to pay.

IMPRECISION, BIAS AND CONFOUNDING

Psychiatrists want to know whether the observed advantages of a new therapy in comparison with one already existing can be generalized to all patients and need to be confident that the new therapy will work (on average) for all patients with the same diagnosis. A *population* in statistics represents all units of interests, such as all patients with a similar diagnosis or all nurses in the UK who care for patients with dual diagnosis. Usually we cannot study the entire population, and we have to draw a random sample

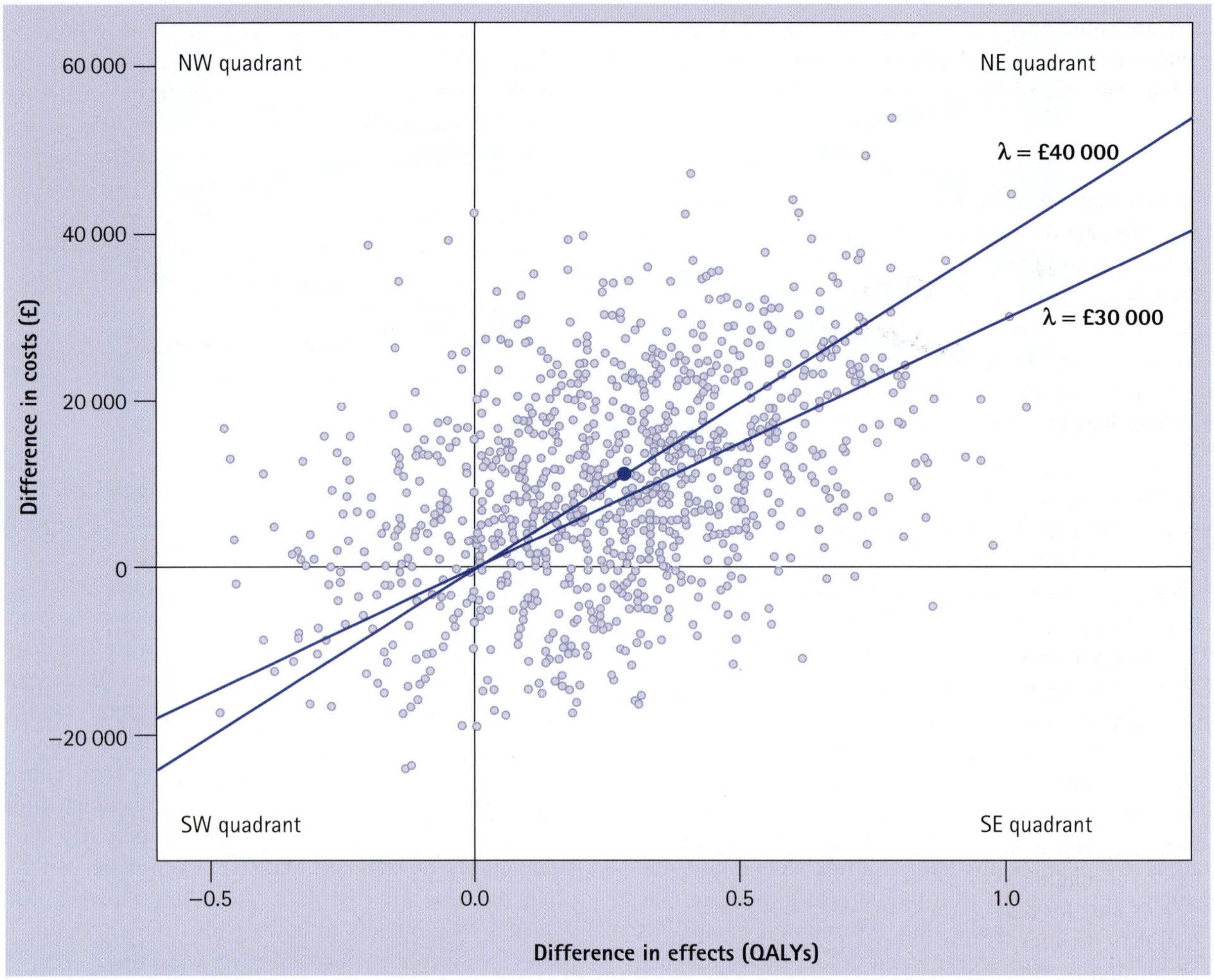

Figure 4.5 A cost-effectiveness plane showing bootstrapped samples

from a defined population, for example a sample of 30 nurses. Outcomes for the sample are assessed in relation to risk factors or interventions, and conclusions are assumed to be valid for the underlying population.

How far the conclusions can be justified depends on imprecision, bias and confounding. It is part of the job of the investigator to identify the sources of these errors and to control for them, as far as possible, either through an appropriate design or through the use of a particular type of analysis. On top of all of these factors is chance or random variation, which can affect results despite perfectly measured data, and the possibility of a conceptual error. An example of the latter might be reverse causality, when A is assumed to cause B because of an association between them, when in fact B causes A. Figure 4.6 shows a summary of these various factors.

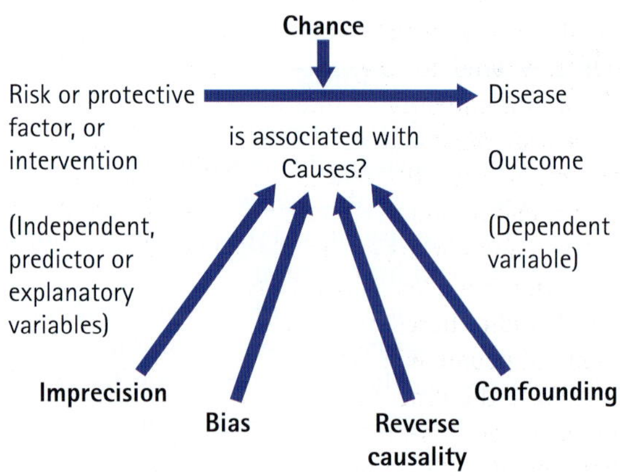

Figure 4.6 Factors that can affect inferences from data

Imprecision

Suppose we measure the mean knowledge before training for a random sample of nurses. This can be used to estimate the mean for the underlying population – that is, all nurses who care for similar patients. However, due to *sampling variation* (random fluctuations), parameter estimates differ from the true values in the population, and different studies will reveal different estimates. Precision can be increased by using larger sample sizes, since imprecision reflects the type of error that will be averaged out in summary statistics. Two measures are commonly reported to quantify the precision of parameter estimates: standard errors and 95 per cent confidence intervals (see Statistical inference, below).

Bias

Bias – a systematic error in results or inference – is potentially more serious than imprecision, since it will not average out. Often little can be done other than to recognize that bias may have occurred and to make due allowance in interpretation. Many sources of bias have been classified and given names. Some important ones are described below: see Sackett[20] for a more complete list and Lee *et al.*[21] for information about bias in case–control studies in psychiatry.

- *Attrition bias:* the loss to follow-up of subjects from a study (once the population to whom the study applies has been defined). Reasons for attrition include illness that prevents contact, death (unless this is the primary outcome), a move to another area, the patient becoming well and being less interested in participation, and some other personal reason for unwillingness to continue. Attrition is a common problem in long cohort studies, but it can also occur in randomized controlled trials.
- *Ascertainment bias:* occurs when the disease or risk factor is not perfectly identified. This would be a problem in the Alzheimer's cohort study mentioned above if it were designed as a prospective study, because of the difficulty of diagnosing Alzheimer's except postmortem.
- *Berkson's bias (or admission rate bias):* a spurious association may be inferred because the case data arise from a special source. This type of selection bias occurs especially in case–control studies based in hospitals; for example, if in-patients with schizophrenia are matched with controls, also in hospital, in order to investigate cannabis use as a risk factor. However, cannabis use in itself may tend to lead to admissions and therefore is seen more frequently among those in hospital.
- *Information bias:* a systematic difference in the information obtained for different groups of subjects. For example, risk factor data may be either easier or more difficult to obtain for controls than cases. *Recall bias* is a type of information bias particularly associated with case–control studies based on retrospective data. For example, parents of people with schizophrenia may be more likely to attribute the illness to childhood experiences because they have been searching for an explanation; on the other hand, they may be less likely to recall unfavourable circumstances such as poor nutrition if they felt themselves to be responsible. *Observer* or *interviewer bias* is another specific example of information bias, where the information gathered is affected by the views or experience of the observer.
- *Selection bias:* when those who are selected for a study are not representative of those to whom the conclusions are to apply. If each person in the population to whom results are to apply has an equal chance of being selected, then the sample is said to be representative. This is difficult to ensure, and representativeness is often tested after data collection by comparing characteristics of the sample obtained with the wider population. An example might be a study where advertisements are placed in the press for subjects. Only the section of society who read newspapers will be recruited. *Membership bias* is a subtype of this type of bias: people who choose to be a member of a group may tend to have particular characteristics, which differ from those people with the illness in general. For example, members of user groups may derive psychological advantage from campaigning on behalf of their fellow sufferers.

Causal inference and confounding

Causality can rarely be inferred directly from association with complete confidence. Some criteria for causal inferences have been suggested by a number of authors, including the famous epidemiologist Bradford Hill.[22] Table 4.7 lists Hill's criteria (the comments are from the useful discussion by Höfler).[23]

The applicability of the above needs to be judged in relation to each study, and those in Table 4.7 are perhaps common sense. However, confounding is a key issue that is ever present, although not always obvious. *Confounders* are variables associated with the outcome of interest and also with the risk factor or intervention. For example, keep-fit classes for patients with depression might be more attractive to young people than to middle-aged or older people. If young people were more likely to recover spontaneously from depression, then one might wrongly attribute a good outcome to the keep-fit classes rather than to youthfulness. Usually a confounding factor will produce a spurious positive finding, but in some cases confounding factors can mask a real association. Randomization (in intervention studies) and matching (in epidemiological studies) can average out unknown (or known but unmeasured) confounders to some degree. Analytical techniques such as regression can also deal with remaining confounding to some extent, by controlling for them. However, *residual confounding* can still occur when a particular factor has not been controlled for (perhaps because it was never measured or recognized or because it was measured inaccurately).

Sometimes intermediate variables are associated with both outcome and the explanatory factor of interest (e.g. intervention group or risk factor) but they lie on the *causal pathway*. Such variables are not considered as confounders and would not be controlled for in the analysis or design if the aim were to assess the increased risk associated directly with the factor of interest. For example, in a study of association between antipsychotics and bone fractures in elderly people, in order to predict who might need additional interventions, one would not control for bone density in assessing the risk of antipsychotics. This would control away the effect of interest. Finally, one would usually

Table 4.7 Bradford-Hill criteria for establishing a causal relationship

Criterion	Interpretation
Strength of association	A strong association is more likely to have a causal component than is a modest association
Consistency	A relationship is observed repeatedly
Specificity	A factor influences specifically a particular outcome or population
Temporality	The factor must precede the outcome it is assumed to affect
Biological gradient	The outcome increases monotonically with increasing dose of exposure or according to a function predicted by a substantive theory
Plausibility	The observed association can be plausibly explained by substantive matter, e.g. biological explanations
Coherence	A causal conclusion should not fundamentally contradict present substantive knowledge
Experiment	Causation is more likely if evidence is based on randomized experiments
Analogy	For analogous exposures and outcomes, an effect has already been shown

assume that, in a well-thought-out study, the exposure has the potential to cause the outcome. However, sometimes it is necessary to consider reversing the outcome and the exposure (*reverse causality*). An example might be a hypothesized causal relationship between cannabis and schizophrenia: does cannabis cause schizophrenia through a direct action on the brain, or are people with mental illness more likely to take cannabis because it helps with the side effects of medication?

DISTRIBUTIONS AND SUMMARY STATISTICS

In a clinical trial, the first table presented in a report might contain estimates of the means, standard deviations, frequencies and proportions for key variables for the randomised groups at baseline. (Contrary to some practice, there should be no significance tests here, because it can be assumed that any differences, even if large, are due to random fluctuation.) The second table might contain the estimates of the mean difference between the groups at follow-up (after the intervention), its 95 per cent confidence interval and an associated *P* value. The first table provides essentially descriptive information. The second provides information from which *inferences* can be made – because in that case we hope to come to some conclusion about the effectiveness of the intervention in the population at large. This is discussed later in the section Statistical inference; here, we give some information on summary statistics and distributions that describe data.

Distributions describing data

In many datasets encountered in psychiatry, the underlying population distribution from which such data arise is the bell-shaped *normal* or *Gaussian* distribution. An example is shown in Figure 4.7. It is fundamental to statistics because it underlies many standard summaries and test statistics. In the normal distribution, most of the cases are close to the centre and relatively few examples are at the extremes. It is characterized by the mean μ (the central value or average) and the standard deviation σ, a measure of variation in the same units as the data, and is denoted $N(\mu,\sigma)$. The variance is the square of the standard deviation. Conventionally, parameter values for the population (true but usually unknown) are denoted by Greek letters and estimates from samples by lower-case roman letters.

In a normally distributed population:

- 68 per cent of the cases in the population lie within $\pm\sigma$ from μ;
- 95 per cent of the cases in the population lie within $\pm 1.96\,\sigma$ from μ.

One reason why the normal distribution is so important is the *central limit theorem*, which states that under certain conditions the sum of a large number of independent and identically distributed random variables will be distributed approximately normally. Thus, the distribution of a mean tends to be normal, even when the distribution from which the means are derived is not, and it has the same mean as that of the original population. The theorem also explains why scores that reflect a diverse set of underlying additive biological or psychological influences emerge as approximately normal.

Two other distributions that are important in describing data are the Poisson and binomial distributions. The *Poisson distribution* describes counts that arise over time, in space or as rare events in a population. Examples might be the number of hospital admissions over a person's lifetime, the number of lesions in a particular volume of the brain, and the number of incident cases of schizophrenia in the population of a health authority. Although the counts observed over a fixed time period are the data to which the Poisson distribution applies, the interest is in estimating the rate that has produced them. The distribution underlies typical epidemiological methods used in incidence and prevalence studies such as Poisson regression. The distribution is characterized by the mean rate (with variance equal to the

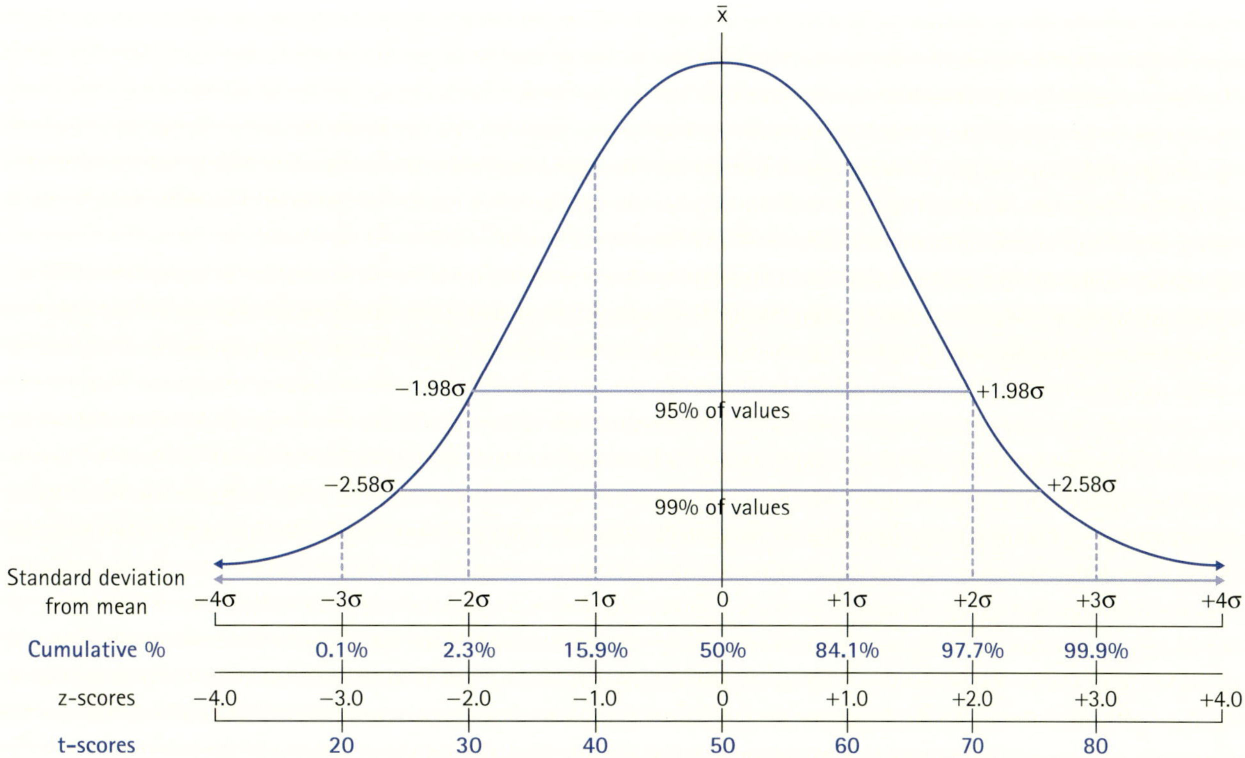

Figure 4.7 Normal or Gaussian distribution

mean), and it is approximated by the normal distribution as the rate increases (Figure 4.8).

A Bernoulli trial is a term describing a single event, for example admission of a patient to hospital within a given week. Given a fixed probability p that this event does or does not happen, the distribution of the number k of such events out of a fixed total n is described by the *binomial* distribution. The binomial distribution underlies the analysis of proportions (including logistic regression). The mean and variance of the binomial are np and $np(p-1)$. The observed proportion of events k/n estimates p. When p is small (say, < 0.05), $1 - p$ is close to 1 and $p(1 - p)$ is close to p. In this case, the binomial is close to a Poisson distribution with rate p. For example, if 1 person out of 10 000 dies over the course of a year, one could think of this either as a rate of 1 per 10 000 person-years or as a proportion of 1/10 000 (for a 1-year follow-up). The binomial distribution is approximated by a normal distribution in large samples unless p is very small. In both the Poisson and binomial distributions, the counts or events are assumed to be independent. In practice, this means that the probability of an event does not depend on what has happened before or, in the case of Poisson counts in a region, in the surrounding region.

Summary statistics calculated from data

For categorical data, the usual summary statistics are simply frequencies n and proportions p (expressed as a percentage) for each category. The odds $O = p/(1 - p)$, where p is a proportion, is a quantity used as an intermediate quantity in analysis, for example as illustrated above for diagnostic tests or via the odds ratio in epidemiology, but it is seldom presented as a simple summary statistic. Note that the mode may be used as a (not very useful) measure of the typical value in a categorical variable. For example, if ethnic group is recorded as white (70%), black Caribbean (15%), black African (5%) and other (10%), then the modal category is white.

For rates, it is usually important to give the number of events on which the rate is based and the exposure. The term 'exposure' is slightly confusing, because it can also mean exposure to a specific risk factor; in this context, it means the total population at risk or the total follow-up time accumulated over all those studied (e.g. in a cohort study). For example, the incidence rate of schizophrenia might be expressed as 25 cases over a follow-up period of 3567 person-years (e.g. 1000 people followed for an average of 3.567 years each), giving a rate of 0.007, or 7 per 1000 person-years. Standardized mortality ratios (SMRs) provide a way of comparing rates across different populations with different characteristics (e.g. age, gender). For example, one might be interested in the rate of schizophrenia among recent immigrants where a confounding factor might be their typically younger age distribution compared with other subgroups or the population at large. A standard population is chosen (e.g. that of the UK) and is divided up into bands (e.g. by age and gender). Rates of disease (e.g.

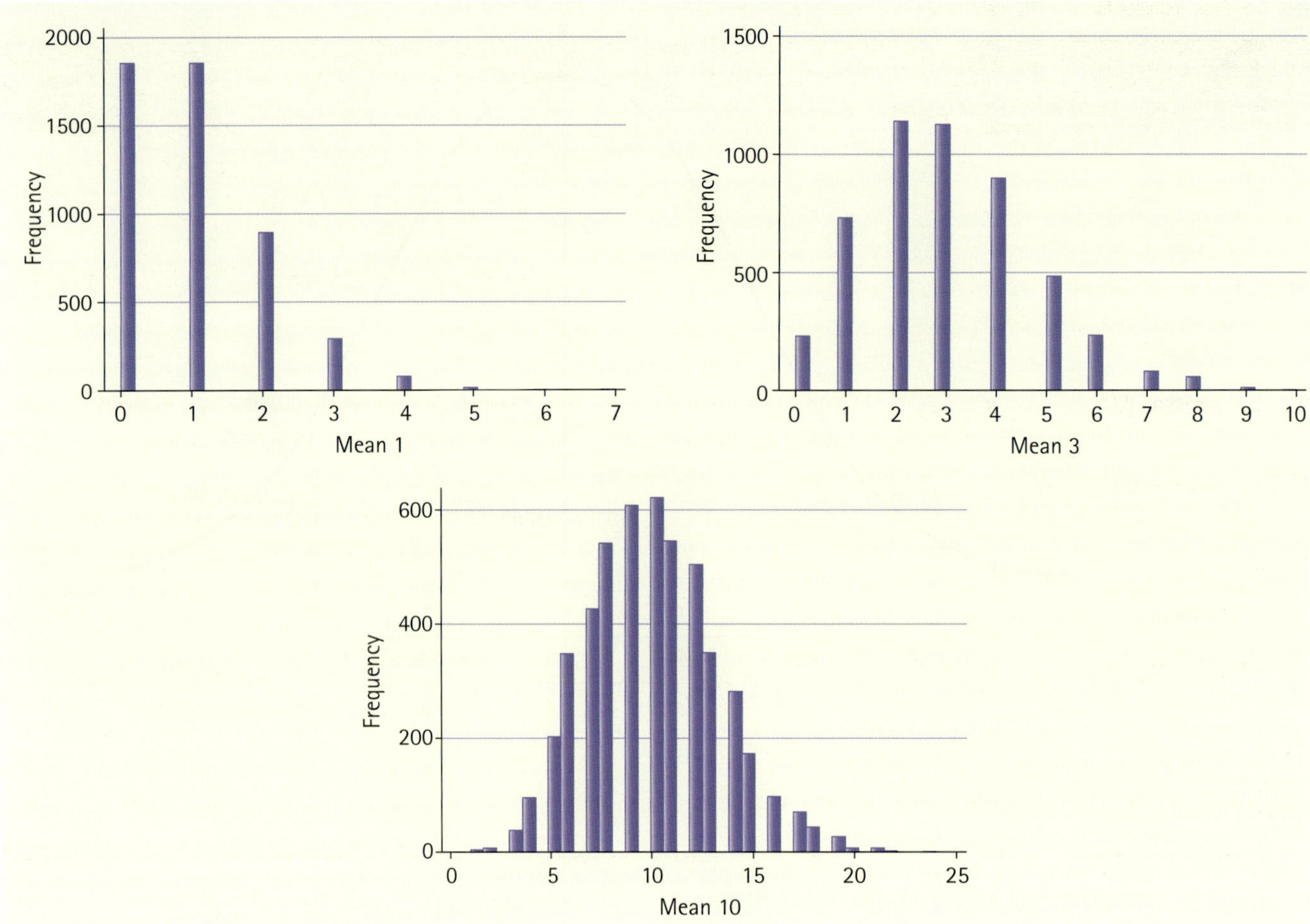

Figure 4.8 Examples of Poisson distributions (means 1, 3 and 10)

schizophrenia) in the population are found, for example from national records held by the Office for National Statistics, and are applied to the age and gender bands in the study sample. From this, the expected number of cases can be calculated for each band and accumulated to give the total expected, *E*. The ratio $O/E \times 100$ is the SMR, where *O* is the number actually observed.

For continuous data, there are a number of basic summary statistics, of which the mean, standard deviation and range, as shown in the Stata output for the change in knowledge scores for nurses in the scenario, are common:

```
Variable |   Obs      Mean    Std. Dev.     Min      Max
---------+------------------------------------------
  change |    30       2.8    2.483046      -2        8
```

Medians and percentiles are used to summarize skewed data (the median is equal to the mean in symmetrically distributed data but lower if the data are skewed with a tail to the right). The *mode* is the value corresponding to the peak of the distribution. Table 4.8 gives the formulae.

In papers, percentages should generally be quoted without decimal places, except in very large samples, and they are usually given in relation to the valid (non-missing) cases. The total sample size should be given with and without missing values. Means and standard deviations are usually given to a small number of decimal points (two or three). Note that confidence intervals or standard errors for means as descriptive data are usually not necessary. Rather, the important figure is the standard deviation, since this describes the variability of the data. (Confidence intervals are more useful for derived statistics from which inferences are to be made). Altman and Bland give some general guidelines on these issues.[1]

Graphical presentations

Plotting data should be the first step in any analysis. Categorical data can be displayed in bar charts and pie charts. Examples of box plots, histograms and QQ plots for two types of continuous data are illustrated in Figure 4.9. The box in a *box-and-whisker plot* (or box plot, for short) shows cases between the upper and lower quartiles. The *median* is indicated on the box plot as a bold line. It is often

Table 4.8 Basic formulae for summary statistics based on continuous data

Summary statistic	Formula (for a set of n data points $x_1, x_2 \ldots x_n$)	Notes
Mean	$\bar{x} = \frac{\sum_{i=1}^{n} x_i}{n}$	Most commonly used measure of the location of data for approximately normally distributed data
Variance	$v = \frac{\sum_{i=1}^{n} (x_i - \bar{x})^2}{n-1}$	Measure of the spread of the data around the mean
Standard deviation (SD)	$s = \sqrt{v}$	Expresses the variation in the same units as the data; the data deviate on average $\lvert s \rvert$ from the mean
95% reference range	$\bar{x} \pm 1.96 \times \text{SD}$	If data are distributed approximately normally, 95% of the individual observations lie within the reference range
Median	$\frac{(n+1)th}{2}$ value of the ordered observations	Midway value: half the data points lie below and half above the median; for an even number of cases, the average of the two middle values is used
Lower quartile (25th percentile)	$\frac{(n+1)th}{4}$ value of the ordered observations	The interquartile range is the range lying between the lower and upper quartiles; other percentiles can also be calculated
Upper quartile (75th percentile)	$\frac{3 \times (n+1)th}{4}$ value of the ordered observations	

taken as a 'typical' value, especially if the data are not distributed symmetrically. The whiskers on the plot (the thin lines) indicate the overall range of the data, after excluding very atypical values, which are known as *outliers*. The histograms show *frequency distributions*, where the range of the data are divided up into equal-sized 'bins' (usually 15–20) and the number on each bin counted and plotted. The y-axis scale here is frequency, but proportions can also be shown (in which case, it is important to give the total sample size). A theoretical normal probability distribution with the same mean and standard deviation is superimposed; here, the x-axis is continuous and the y-axis is a probability.

The QQ probability plots are shown on the right. They provide a way of visually estimating how close a distribution is to being normally distributed, as an alternative to formal tests such as the Kolmogorov-Smirnov test. If the data are normal, the points should lie on a straight line, as is the case for the first row of data. The second row of Figure 4.9 shows an example of a non-normal skewed distribution. (Duration of illness is often log-normally distributed.) *Skewness* refers to lack of symmetry and may be important to consider. (*Kurtosis* is another feature of non-normality, where the slope away from the peak is not so marked as for a normal distribution.) This latter feature of data is, however, rarely of any concern to data analysis. Here, the data have a tail to the right, with a few very high values, and the median is lower than the mean. Taking logs of such data sometimes produces a normal distribution (when the original distribution can be described as *log-normal*). Analysis can be carried out on the log-transformed values, and summaries such as the mean are then back-transformed.

Reference ranges and outliers

In medicine, the mean ± 1.96 standard deviations is sometimes known as the *reference range*, since it indicates where the vast majority of cases are expected to lie. It is not the same as the 95 per cent confidence interval (see Statistical inference, below). Values outside that range are not necessarily inconsistent with the distribution – they may be just at one end of a continuum. *Outliers*, on the other hand, are cases that are considered to be so extreme as to be unlikely to be part of the distribution, either because they derive from another underlying population that has been mixed in with the main population or because of a data measurement or transcription error.[24] The question of outliers is complex, but general advice would be to remove data only if there is definite evidence for a data error.

Dummy variables

In order to include the effects of categorical explanatory variables, many statistical models employ *dummy variables*

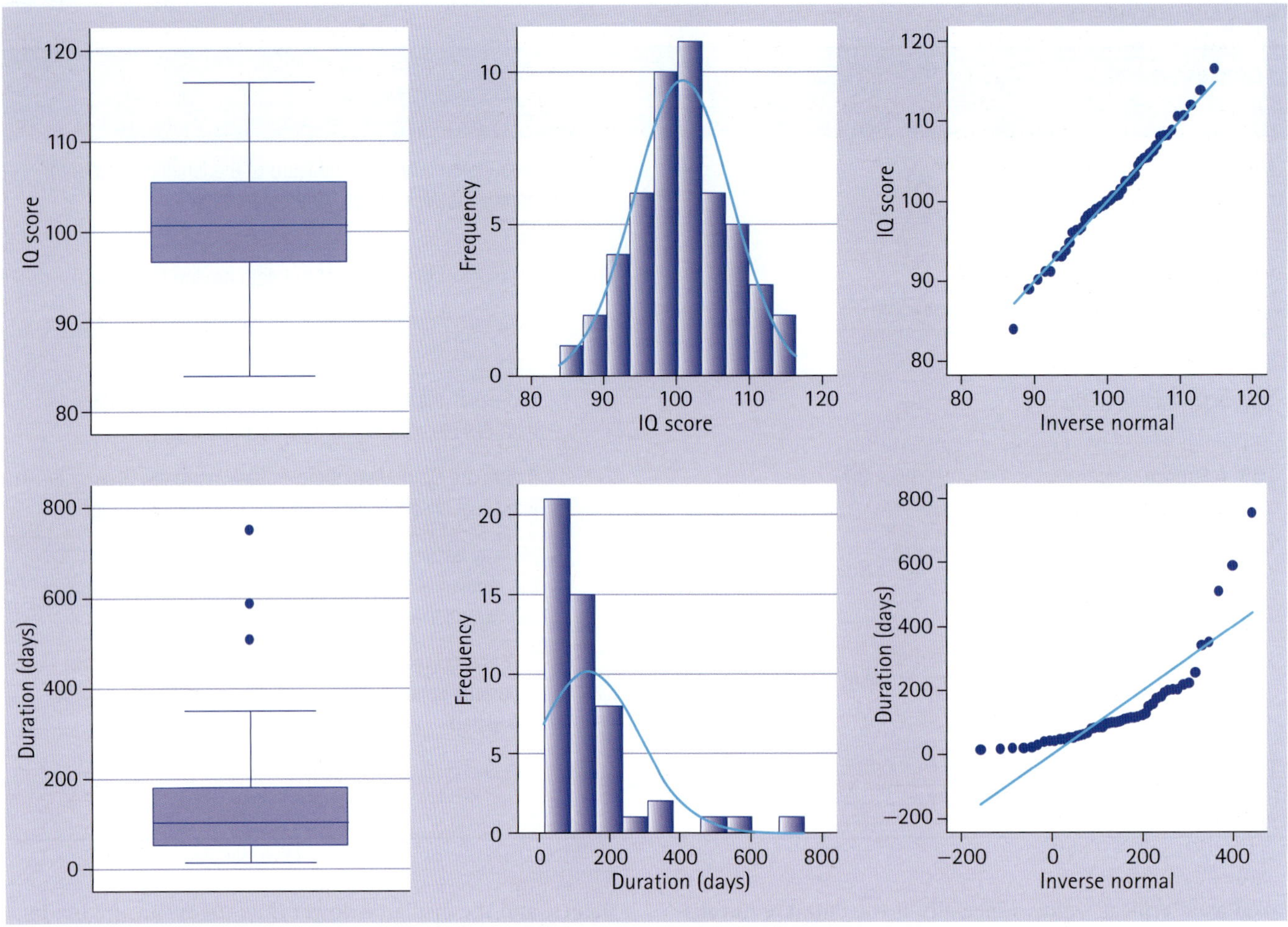

Figure 4.9 Box plots, histograms and QQ plots of a normally distributed variable (top row: intelligence quotient (IQ) of 50 patients) and a skewed, log-normally distributed variable (bottom row: days in hospital of 50 patients)

– binary indicator variables where the value 1 indicates that a subject falls into a specific category and the value 0 that it does not. Categorical variables with k categories can be represented by k dummy variables. Since the information provided by a factor with k categories is contained in k – 1 dummy variables (once you know the value of all but one, the value of the last one can be inferred), only k – 1 dummy variables are used in models. The category that has been left out then becomes the reference category.

Here is an example of dummy coding for a factor with three categories (the single variable Factor is replaced by three new variables Dum1, Dum2 and Dum3, only two of which would be included in an analysis).

Factor	Dum1	Dum2	Dum3
1	1	0	0
2	0	1	0
1	1	0	0
3	0	0	1
3	0	0	1
2	0	1	0

Effect sizes

The term 'effect size' often refers to the size of a mean difference or whatever quantity is the focus of interest. A measure of relative effect size can be presented to allow the scientific or clinical importance of the observed effects to be assessed on a common scale. The need for this arises because (i) a statistically significant difference in a large sample might be small and of no scientific importance; and (ii) different variables to be compared might be measured in different units. A widely used relative effect size is *Cohen's d*, which, for the comparison of two groups, is the mean difference between two groups divided by the pooled standard deviation.[25] The *standardized response mean* (SRM) may be more appropriate as a measure of responsiveness to change.[26] It is the mean of the change scores divided by the standard deviation of the change scores. Values for Cohen's d or SRMs between 0.2 and 0.5 would be regarded as small, between 0.5 and 0.8 as medium, and above 0.8 as large. It is important to explain how any such standardization has been performed and to be aware that using the standard deviation computed from a particular sample may limit the generalizability of the results. Because relative effect sizes can be compared across studies, they allow the accumulation of knowledge: a special statistical technique, meta-analysis, allows the combination of the results of several studies (see Multivariate and other more complex techniques, below).

STATISTICAL INFERENCE

Point estimates, standard errors and confidence intervals

Statistical inference is concerned with drawing conclusions from data and generalizing them to populations. It typically involves calculating point estimates and estimates of uncertainty such as confidence intervals, and performing hypothesis tests (e.g. comparing two or more groups, perhaps two arms in an RCT or those at risk and those not in a cohort study).

A *point estimate* is a single estimate such as a mean. In the Stata output for the nurse example below, the mean of the change from baseline to follow-up is 2.8 (point estimate). The standard error (SE) is an estimate of uncertainty in the point estimate and is the standard deviation of the distribution of the means (here, it is $0.453 = 2.483/\sqrt{30}$, 2.483 being the standard deviation (SD) of the raw data as shown earlier).

```
Variable |     Obs      Mean    Std. Err.        [95% Conf. Interval]
---------+-------------------------------------------------------------
  change |      30       2.8    .4533401          1.872815    3.727185
```

Confidence intervals (here, 1.87 to 3.73) are derived from standard errors (and they both give equivalent information), but the confidence interval is the preferred measure of the precision for a parameter estimate. In recent years, journals have increasingly recommended authors always to report confidence intervals, not least when results are inconclusive, because they indicate the largest and smallest estimates consistent with the data; these estimates are helpful in planning further research.[12,13]

What do confidence intervals show? If we repeat an experiment, trial or any other study involving a random sample many times and calculate each time a mean and its 95 per cent confidence interval, those intervals would contain the true population mean in 95 per cent of the repeats. An intuitive way of thinking about this is that it is the range within which we expect the true parameter to be with 95 per cent confidence.

The simulation illustrated in Figure 4.10 exemplifies this. We assumed that a distribution of a change score for the nurses was distributed normally with a true mean of 2 and a standard deviation of 2, and we drew 50 random numbers from this distribution, repeated 100 times. Each time, the sample mean and its 95 per cent confidence interval were calculated. Figure 4.10 shows the results. The average sample mean from the 100 simulations was 2.04, which is very close to the true mean. At no time was it estimated at the true population value of exactly 2, but 95 of the 100 95 per cent confidence intervals do include the true mean of 2. In only five simulations (filled circles) would we have made a wrong inference about the true population mean from the confidence interval.

Formulae for standard errors and confidence intervals

Tables 4.9–4.11 give formulae for standard errors and confidence intervals for a number of point estimates. It is not necessary to remember all of them but to remember rather the following key points, which relate to approximate standard errors and confidence intervals based on large samples ($n > 50$), unless otherwise stated:

- The 95 per cent confidence interval for a point estimate is given by estimate $\pm$ 1.96 $\times$ SE.
- Standard error for a mean of a normally distributed variable = $SD/\sqrt{n}$.
- In small samples, the 1.96 in the formula for the confidence interval of a mean is replaced by the corresponding value of a t distribution with $n-1$ degrees of freedom.
- Standard error for a proportion $p = \sqrt{p(1-p)/n}$.
- Standard error for a count $a = \sqrt{a}$.
- Standard error of A + B = standard error of A − B $= \sqrt{SE_A^2 + SE_B^2}$.
- Confidence limits for ratios of proportions, rates and odds are calculated on the log-transformed scale and then back-transformed.
- For samples smaller than 50, 'exact' methods using special tables or software are based on the underlying Poisson or binomial distributions.
- The larger the sample size n of a study, the smaller the standard error and 95 per cent confidence interval, and thus the more precise the estimate.

Table 4.9 gives formulae for summary statistics for a single proportion p based on k successes out of n trials or for a comparison of two proportions $p_1 = a/(a+c)$ and $p_2 = b/(b+d)$ (see Table 4.3 above for the layout of data assumed for these formulae). Ratios of proportions and odds, which are commonly used in case–control studies, are natural log-transformed before standard errors and confidence limits are calculated and are then back-transformed by exponentiation. For samples smaller than 50, 'exact' methods using special tables or software are based on the underlying binomial distribution.

Table 4.10 gives the formulae for a rate based on a events with a population or follow-up time (time at risk) in terms of person-years of N, or a comparison of two rates a/N_1 and b/N_2. For samples smaller than 50, 'exact' methods using

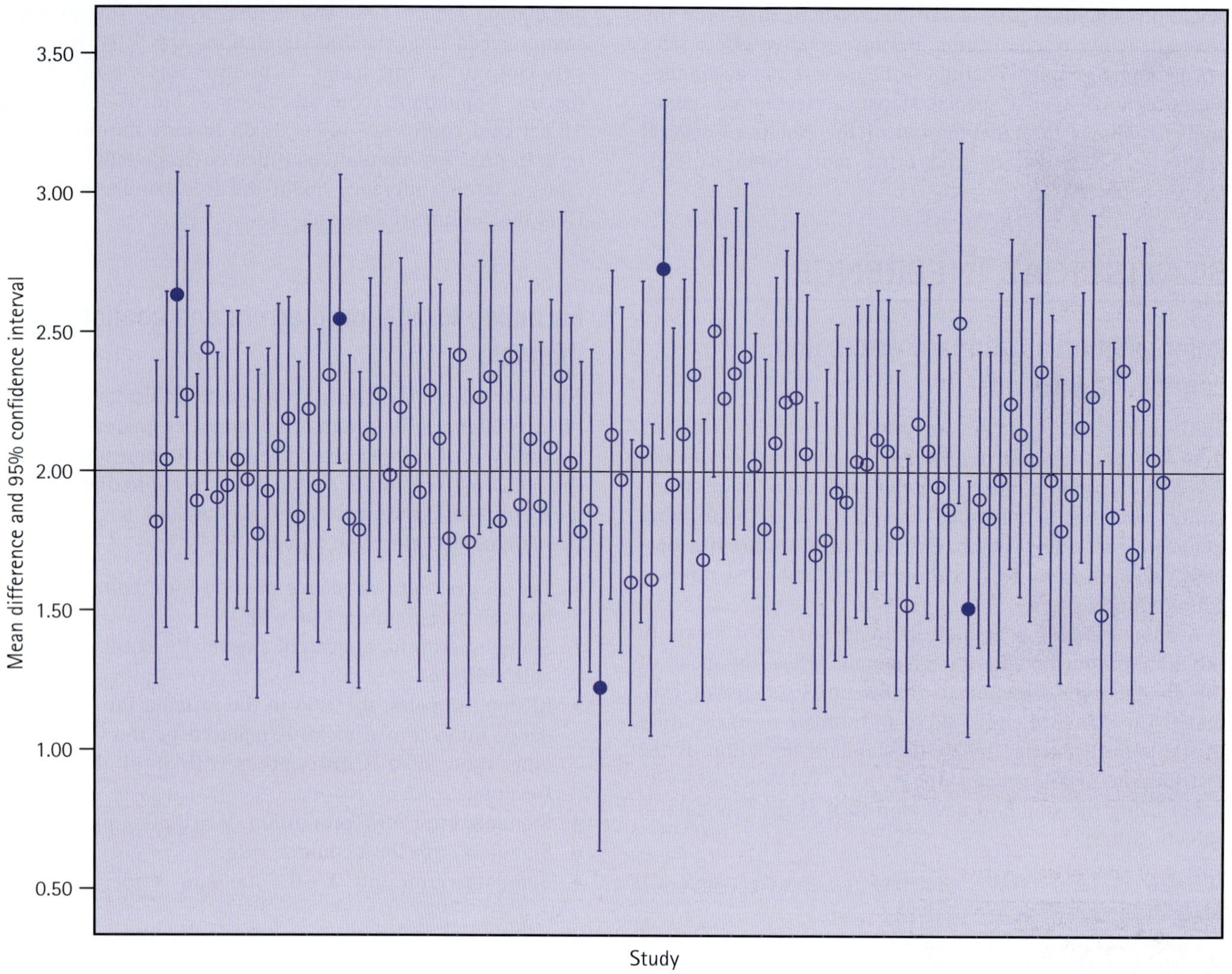

Figure 4.10 Results of 100 simulations from a distribution with mean 2 and standard deviation 2. Sample means and 95 per cent confidence intervals computed from 50 cases each time

special tables or software are based on the underlying Poisson distribution for counts.

The standard errors and confidence intervals for continuous data that can be assumed to be approximately normally distributed are shown in Table 4.11. For large samples (> 50), the 95 per cent confidence interval is given by estimate ± 1.96 × standard error; for small samples, the appropriate point of the T distribution should be used instead of 1.96.

Note that in the above formula for the variance, the denominator is $n - 1$ and is called the *degrees of freedom*. It can be shown that the estimate of the underlying population variance is unbiased if $n - 1$ is used as a denominator rather then n.

Hypothesis tests

In many studies there is a prediction of a difference between groups. This prediction is variously known as the experimental, research or *alternative hypothesis* (H1). The converse hypothesis is the *null hypothesis* (H0). We test H0 to see whether we can reject it beyond reasonable doubt in favour of H1. The procedure of classical hypothesis testing is to define a research and a null hypothesis, to collect sufficient data and to calculate a test statistic z^*; this is compared against a probability distribution, which is known if the null hypothesis is true. We reject H0 if the observed test statistic is very unlikely to occur if H0 is true, according to the probability that $Z > z^*$, where Z is a theoretical random variable with the known distribution. A null hypothesis is rejected if this probability – the P value – is below a *critical value*, α; thus, P is not the probability that H0 is true but the probability of an extreme value if it is true.

Typical values for α are 0.1, 0.05 and 0.01. They may be adjusted if multiple tests are to be performed using, for example, the Bonferroni correction: this would divide α by as many tests as are to be applied simultaneously (e.g. see Shaffer[27] for a discussion of multiple testing). In the vast majority of cases, one assumes that the null hypothesis

Table 4.9 Standard errors and confidence intervals for summary statistics based on binary data (proportions)

Standard error (SE) of proportion *p*	$\sqrt{\frac{p(1-p)}{n}}$	
Standard error for difference between two proportions	$\sqrt{\frac{p_1(1-p_1)}{n_1}+\frac{p_2(1-p_2)}{n_2}}$	When p_1 and p_2 are estimates of the same proportion (e.g. when two groups do not differ), the pooled estimate is used for both p_1 and p_2: $p=\frac{n_1p_1+n_2p_2}{n_1+n_2}$
Risk ratio (RR)	$\frac{p_1/n_1}{p_2/n_2}$	An alternative to risk difference
Standard error for ln(RR)	$\sqrt{(1/a+1/b+1/n_1+1/n_2)}$	Compute the CI for ln(RR), then exponentiate (anti-log) the limits for RR
Odds ratio (OR)	$\frac{p_1/(1-p_1)}{p_2/(1-p_2)}$ or equivalently $(a\times c)/(b\times d)$	An alternative to risk difference or ratio; produced by logistic regression
Standard error for ln(OR)	$\sqrt{(1/a+1/b+1/c+1/d)}$	Compute the CI for ln(OR), then exponentiate (anti-log) the limits for OR

CI, confidence interval, *a* and *b*, frequencies (see Table 4.3).

Table 4.10 Standard errors and confidence intervals for summary statistics based on count data (rates)

Standard error (SE) of rate	$\sqrt{\frac{a}{N_1}}$	Uses the variance = mean relationship for Poisson variables
Rate ratio	$\frac{a/N_1}{b/N_2}$	
Standard error for ln(ratio of counts *a* and *b*) to find confidence interval for rate ratio	$\sqrt{(1/a+1/b)}$	Compute the CI for ln(count ratio), then exponentiate (anti-log) the limits and multiply by N_2/N_1 to convert to rates

CI, confidence interval, *a* and *b*, counts N_1 and N_2, follow up times.

would be rejected with an extreme finding in either direction (i.e. large or very small), so a *double-sided test* is applied. Occasionally one knows in advance that deviations are impossible in one direction, so a *single-sided test* is applied.

In a single-sided test, α corresponds to the critical value z^*, such that:

$$\text{The probability that } Z > z^* = \alpha$$

For example, if the desired significance level is 0.05, testing a mean value assuming a normal distribution for Z, the corresponding value for z must be greater than or equal to 1.645 (or less than or equal to −1.645) for a single-sided test. For a double-sided test (where the extreme values can be at either end of the distribution), we are interested in:

$$\text{The probability that } Z > z^* = \alpha/2$$

Table 4.11 Standard errors and confidence intervals for summary statistics based on continuous data (assumed normally distributed)

Standard error for mean $\bar{x}$ (SE)	$\frac{s}{\sqrt{n}}$	s is SD; n is sample size
95% confidence interval for mean $\bar{x}$	$\bar{x} \pm 1.96 \times SE$ or $\bar{x} \pm t^* SE$	*If the total sample size is small (< 50), t^* is the 2.5% point of the t distribution with $n_1 - 1$ degrees of freedom
Standard error difference in two means $\bar{d}$	$\sqrt{\frac{s_1^2}{n_1} + \frac{s_2^2}{n_2}}$	$s = \sqrt{\frac{(n_1 - 1)s_1^2 + (n_2 - 1)s_2^2}{n_1^2 + n_2^2 - 2}}$ A pooled estimate of s can be used for s_1 and s_2 if they are not significantly different
95% confidence interval for difference between two means $\bar{d}$	$\bar{d} \pm 1.96 \times SE_d$ or $\bar{d} \pm t^* \times SE_d$	*If the total sample size is small (< 50), t^* is the 2.5% point of the t distribution with $n_1 + n_2 - 2$ degrees of freedom

so that probability is divided up between the two extremes of the distributions and the critical value z^* corresponds to the $\alpha/2$ significance level. To achieve a significance level of 0.05 for a double-sided test, the absolute value of the test statistic ($|z|$) must be greater than or equal to the critical value 1.96 (which corresponds to the level 0.025 for a single-sided test).

A 95 per cent confidence interval can also be used as a criterion to reject a null hypothesis: if it does not encompass the null hypothesis value, then the effect is statistically significant at $P = 0.05$. The null hypothesis value would be 0 (for a comparison of means in two groups) or 1 (for a comparison of proportions in two groups using ORs or RRs). A test based on P values and a test based on confidence intervals are closely related, and they will almost always result to the same conclusion about rejection of a null hypothesis.

Power and sample size calculations

When performing significance tests using $\alpha = 0.05$, over the long run the rejection of H0 will be mistaken in 5 per cent of occasions; this is a *type I error*. The probability of accepting the null hypothesis even though the alternative hypothesis is in reality true is denoted by β and $1 - \beta$ is known as the *power* of a test. The error is known as a *type II error*. The latter is more difficult to assess, but it is possible to control for it by doing a power analysis during the planning stage of a study. Here is a summary:

- *α-error:* probability of making a type I error (rejecting H0 although H0 is true).
- *β-error:* probability of making a type II error (accepting H0 although H1 is true).

A sample size calculation requires the following information:

- The power for the particular trial: $1 - \beta$, where β is the probability of a type II error – typically 80 per cent or 90 per cent
- The smallest difference (or 'effect') that is considered to be of clinical importance
- The significance level α, or probability of a type I error, to be used – typically 0.05
- The expected level of loss to follow-up.

For continuous data, one needs an estimate of the standard deviation within groups; if this is unknown, then Cohen's standard effect size (see above), which by definition has a standard deviation of 1, can be used as a generic solution. Sample sizes can be calculated using specialized computer software or using formulas and tables from standard textbooks (e.g. Cohen[25]). A rule of thumb for the sample size for a power of 80 per cent and a two-sided $\alpha = 0.05$ for independent t-tests or χ^2 tests is:

Sample size per group = $16/d$, where d = Cohen's d (the standardized difference)

Assumptions made by tests

Many statistical tests for continuous data depend on assumptions, for example that the data are distributed normally or that the variances of different groups are the same (*variance homogeneity*). Tests that depend on specific distributions are described as *parametric*. Before commencing with the main analysis, one may wish to investigate these assumptions. Some formal tests are available (e.g. Bartlett test for normality, Levene test for variance homogeneity), but they are often not helpful because datasets with small sample sizes will not reject the null hypothesis and datasets with large sample sizes may reject the null hypothesis even if the violations are minor and have little impact on the conclusions. Equality of variances can be evaluated by a rule of thumb: the larger standard deviation should be less than twice the smaller standard deviation.[28] Normality is best assessed visually by plotting box plots, histograms or QQ plots of the observed data for each group.

A further assumption that may be made is of independence of observations. This is often invalid for psychiatric data and then special methods are required, either robust methods or methods specially designed for non-independent or clustered data (see Multivariate and other more complex techniques, below). *Robust methods* include those that use standard models, such as regression, but with adapted variances for the parameter estimates (so-called *sandwich estimates*), with the aim of more realistic P values even when the distribution of the data is not as specified in the model. Bootstrapping is another robust method that works similarly to simulation (see section on health economics, where bootstrapping is commonly used).

Transformation

If the assumptions of a normal distribution and/or equal variances are not satisfied, then it may be advisable to transform the data. In psychiatric studies, data are often positively skewed, especially with essentially positive values such as service-use or cost data. Log-transformation is helpful both for producing normal distributions and also for unequal variances if the larger variance is associated with higher values. Note, however, that the back-transformed mean of a lognormal distribution is the geometric mean and is closer to the median of the original values rather than to the arithmetic mean. The arithmetic mean of the original untransformed data is estimated by $\exp(m + s^2/2)$, where m and s are the mean and standard deviation of the (natural) log-transformed values, respectively. Other transformations are the square transformation (x^2), which is used if the data are negatively skewed and the square root ($\sqrt{x}$), which is recommended for count data (although note that it is usually preferable to use methods based on the Poisson distribution rather than to transform and assume normality).

Non-parametric tests

An alternative to transformation is to use non-parametric tests, which do not assume particular distributions and are usually based on ranks. They do make other assumptions, however, depending on the test. A disadvantage of non-parametric tests is the difficulty of deciding on the appropriate summary statistic to illustrate group differences (instead of the mean and standard deviation). Another disadvantage is that it is difficult to extend analyses to take account of confounders (relatively easy with normally distributed data using regression). Siegel and Castellan[29] is a good basic text on non-parametric tests.

What do significant and non-significant results mean?

It is important to remember that statistical significance does not tell us anything about the importance of the effect. It reflects the amount of evidence that the effect exists. Small and clinically unimportant effects can become statistically significant if the sample size is large enough. Two quantities mentioned above are helpful in balancing statistical and clinical significance: the 95 per cent confidence interval for the point estimate, which quantifies the possible range of the effect, in original units, that is consistent with the data, and the standardized effect size, which places the point estimate on a scale measured in units of standard deviations.

As Altman and Bland discuss, 'absence of evidence is not "evidence of absence"'.[30] If the P value is above 0.05, this tells us that the observed effect is not large enough to exclude chance as an explanation. Thus, if there is no evidence to reject the null hypothesis, this does not mean that we have proved it to be true. Classical or *frequentist* hypothesis testing is thus fundamentally asymmetrical in that more weight is given to the null hypothesis, since it is accepted unless there is overwhelming evidence to reject it.

The Bayesian approach

The frequentist approach may seem not to address the aim of the study, which is to assess the probability that a hypothesis is true. Furthermore, this approach uses only information from the current study and does not integrate other available information, such as results of previous studies or opinions of psychiatrists. The *Bayesian* approach adopts a different viewpoint, more concerned with weighing the evidence both for and against a research hypothesis. It is based on the beliefs (about parameters and the hypothesis) as well as the data (see Bolstad[31] for an accessible introduction). In Bayesian statistics, population parameters are considered to be random variables and thus have probability distributions. In this context it is possible to express the belief or the probability that a research hypothesis is true. The belief in the hypothesis before the study starts is called the *prior probability*, which is converted to a *posterior probability* by the analysis of the data. This update is based on conditional probability through *Bayes' theorem*. A major criticism of Bayesian statistics is the subjectivity of describing prior belief and, in the past, the difficulty of the mathematics and computation involved. However, Bayesian methods have become increasingly popular, especially in decision-making analysis.[32]

ILLUSTRATIONS OF HYPOTHESIS TESTS

Summary of tests

Table 4.12 summarizes the most important parametric and non-parametric tests and when they are used. The most commonly used tests will be illustrated later in this section.

The statistical distributions used in the tests in Table 4.12 are the Student's t, χ^2 and F distributions. Their distributions depend on the *degrees of freedom*, which is generally

Table 4.12 Commonly used hypothesis tests

Comparison being made	Scale of measurement	Test
One group (one sample mean against population mean or distribution *v.* theoretical distribution)	Nominal	χ^2 goodness-of-fit test
	Ordinal	Mann–Whitney U test
	Interval/ratio	One sample *t*-test
Two groups (independent samples)	Nominal	χ^2 test, Fisher's exact test
	Ordinal	Mann–Whitney U test
	Interval/ratio	Two-samples *t*-test
Two groups (related samples)	Nominal	McNemar test
	Ordinal	Wilcoxon signed rank test
	Interval/ratio	Paired sample *t*-test
More than two groups (independent samples)	Nominal	χ^2 test for homogeneity
	Ordinal	Kruskal–Wallis test
	Interval/ratio	Analysis of variance (ANOVA)
	Survival	Log-rank test

the sample size minus the number of parameters that have been estimated (e.g. for the *t* distribution there are two parameters, the mean and standard deviation). Table 4.13 shows how these distributions are usually represented (the *d*s here are degrees of freedom, and some relationships that are worth remembering). The specific tests will be discussed later.

The independent samples *t*-test

Let us illustrate hypothesis testing with an example of the knowledge of nurses before and after a training programme. We are interested in whether nurses with training improved their knowledge more than nurses on the waiting list, on the basis of the change in knowledge test scores. What is the likely range of the true mean difference in change scores, and is there evidence that this difference is significantly different from the null hypothesis value of 0? The test statistic is the mean difference between the two groups divided by its standard error – the *t* statistic. The larger the difference between the two groups and the smaller the standard error, the larger the (absolute) value of *t*. The size of *t* is judged in relation to the theoretical *t* distribution; if it is above a critical value corresponding to $\alpha = 0.05$, it is deemed to be significant.

The output below presents the *P* value, which is 0.0018. The chance of obtaining a *t*-value greater than |3.45| if the null hypothesis is true is thus less than 0.05 and we can therefore reject the null hypothesis. Alternatively, we can say that the observed mean difference of improvement

Table 4.13 The main distributions used in statistical tests

Distribution	Used for	Equal to
χ^2_d	Comparing proportions, as a fit index and for some non-parametric test statistics	Distribution of sum of squares of $N(0,1)$ variables
t_d	Comparing means (one mean against a known value or two groups compared with each other)	$N(0,1)$ distribution, when n is large
$F_{d1,d2}$	Testing whether the ratio of variances is 1 and for comparing means (when there are more than two, in an analysis of variance)	t_{d2} distribution, when $d_1 = 1$

```
ttest   change, by(group)

Two-sample t test with equal variances
------------------------------------------------------------------------------
   Group |     Obs        Mean    Std. Err.   Std. Dev.   [95% Conf. Interval]
---------+--------------------------------------------------------------------
 Waiting |      15    1.466667    .4457916    1.726543    .5105388    2.422795
Training |      15    4.133333    .6314508    2.445599    2.779006    5.487661
---------+--------------------------------------------------------------------
combined |      30         2.8    .4533401    2.483046    1.872815    3.727185
---------+--------------------------------------------------------------------
    diff |           -2.666667    .7729556               -4.249994   -1.083339
------------------------------------------------------------------------------
    diff = mean(Waiting) - mean(Training)                         t =  -3.4500
Ho: diff = 0                                     degrees of freedom =       28

    Ha: diff < 0                 Ha: diff != 0                 Ha: diff > 0
 Pr(T < t) = 0.0009         Pr(|T| > |t|) = 0.0018          Pr(T > t) = 0.9991
```

between waiting list and training group nurses of −2.67 is too large to be explained by chance. The 95 per cent confidence interval of the difference in change score is −4.25 to −1.08 and does not include 0. It also informs us that the test can be rejected at 0.05. Additionally, it tells us that the possible mean difference ranges between −4.25 and −1.08 (see Stata output, above).

The *t*-test assumes that in the population the variable is distributed normally in each group, the variances are the same (variance homogeneity) and the observations are independent of each other. The *t*-test is fairly robust against some violations of the assumptions of normal distribution and variance homogeneity but not against violations of the independence of observations. As n increases, the t statistic approaches the z statistic, which has a $N(0,1)$ distribution. For large samples, therefore, any estimate of a mean difference from an approximately normal distribution whose absolute value is more than twice its standard error is significantly different from 0 at $P = 0.05$. This rule of thumb comes from the (rounded) double-sided 0.05 point of the normal distribution i.e. 1.96.

The Mann–Whitney U (Wilcoxon rank sum) test

A non-parametric test that can be used for comparing two independent groups when the data are not normally distributed is the Mann–Whitney U test (MWU; also known as the Wilcoxon rank sum test). The MWU test is based on the ranks of the data and does not have any distributional assumption. However, note that it tests equality of medians only if the distributions have the same shape. Figure 4.11 shows two types of non-normal data, illustrating how

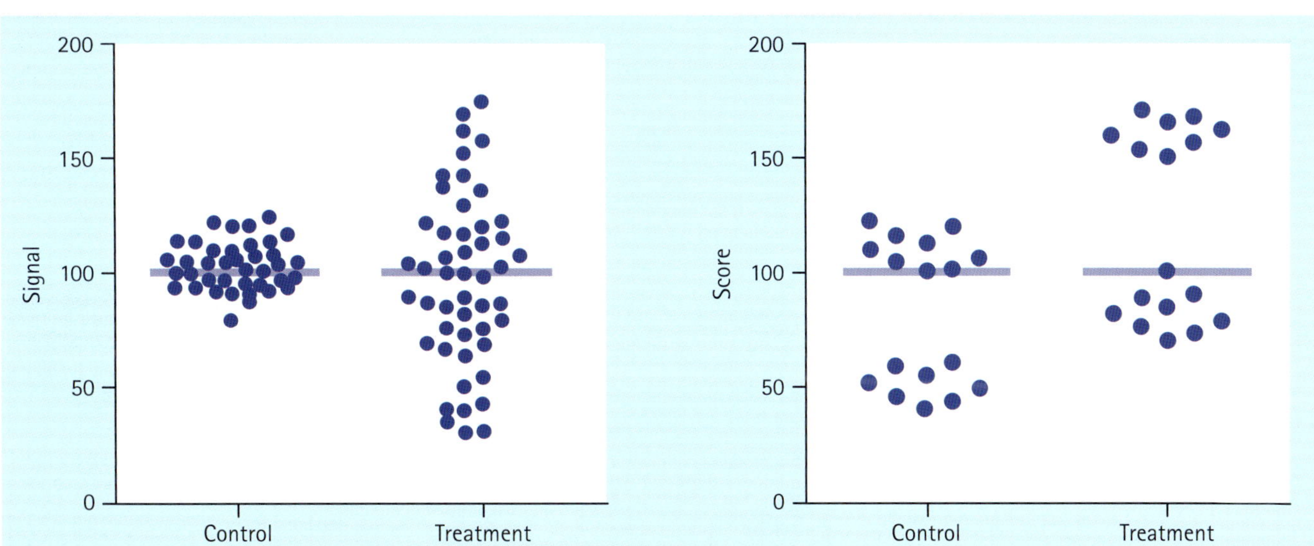

Figure 4.11 Examples showing medians that are the same but where the distributions differ and vice versa. The Mann–Whitney test would be significant in the first example but not the second

```
ranksum change, by(group)

Two-sample Wilcoxon rank-sum (Mann-Whitney) test

       group |      obs    rank sum    expected
-------------+---------------------------------
     Waiting |       15         157       232.5
    Training |       15         308       232.5
-------------+---------------------------------
    combined |       30         465         465

unadjusted variance       581.25
adjustment for ties       -18.36
                      ----------
adjusted variance         562.89

Ho: diff_k~e(group==Waiting) = diff_k~e(group==Training)
             z =  -3.182
    Prob > |z| =   0.0015
```

important it is to plot the data to decide whether the median interpretation is reasonable.

Using the MWU test for our example, we get the following output (see Stata output, above).

The test statistic is $z = -3.182$, $n_1 = 15$, $n_2 = 15$, $P = 0.0015$ (based on an approximation), so at the 0.05 level we can reject the null hypothesis that the two groups have the same distribution in the population. If the sample size is small (< 10), exact P values should be requested from the statistical software or the test statistics should be referred to statistical tables.[29]

Comparing more than two groups: analysis of variance

Analysis of variance (ANOVA) is used to test differences among two or more means. It is closely related to linear regression and can be analysed using regression techniques; the t-test is a special case. The F-test in an ANOVA compares the variability between means to that within means. Once an overall difference is established, post-hoc comparisons between groups can be applied using either specific predefined contrasts or all pair-wise comparisons with a suitable adjustment for multiple testing (e.g. Bonferroni adjustment or the Tukey test, which is less conservative). In the example below, the F-test indicates strong evidence for differences among the groups ($P = 0.0009$). The regression-style output below the F-test shows differences between dummy-coded variables (see Statistical inference, above) with the reference category, the highest-coded group in this case 3, denoted 'dropped'. Here, group 1 is not significantly different from group 3 but group 2 is (see Stata output, below).

Here is a contrast, that between groups 1 and 2, which

```
anova gaf  group3,regress

      Source |       SS       df       MS              Number of obs =      60
-------------+------------------------------           F(  2,    57) =    7.94
       Model |  1920.75756     2  960.378782           Prob > F      =  0.0009
    Residual |  6895.82577    57  120.979399           R-squared     =  0.2179
-------------+------------------------------           Adj R-squared =  0.1904
       Total |  8816.58333    59  149.433616           Root MSE      =  10.999

------------------------------------------------------------------------------
         gaf        Coef.   Std. Err.      t    P>|t|     [95% Conf. Interval]
------------------------------------------------------------------------------
_cons            61.86667   2.839946    21.78   0.000     56.17977    67.55356
group3
           1     4.061905   3.519373     1.15   0.253    -2.985518    11.10933
           2     14.66275   3.896374     3.76   0.000     6.860391     22.4651
           3    (dropped)
------------------------------------------------------------------------------
```

has not been produced by the regression output above: it has to be asked for specifically:

```
test _coef[group3[1]]=_coef[group3[2]]

 ( 1)  group3[1] - group3[2] = 0

       F(  1,     57) =     9.83
            Prob > F =    0.0027
```

In a *factorial design*, several factors are varied in the same experiment. For example, drugs A and B may be given at two levels, to give four combinations. This design allows two questions to be answered at the same time, and in particular it can test whether the combination of A and B is more effective than the additive effects of either (a phenomenon known as synergy). This design is easily analysed using the ANOVA framework. A synergistic effect would result in a significant interaction F-test between drug type and level. Figure 4.12 shows another example of an interaction between two factors, gender and time (pre- and post-drug treatment): the blood level of a certain hormone was measured in males and females before and after a drug treatment. The effect of the drug on hormone level depends on gender: only in females was an increase of the mean blood levels of a hormone after the drug treatment observed.

Where a continuous variable is controlled for (e.g. severity of illness), ANOVA is known as *analysis of covariance* (ANCOVA); and is usually analysed by regression. The Kruskal–Wallis test is a non-parametric version of ANOVA that compares medians in two or more groups.

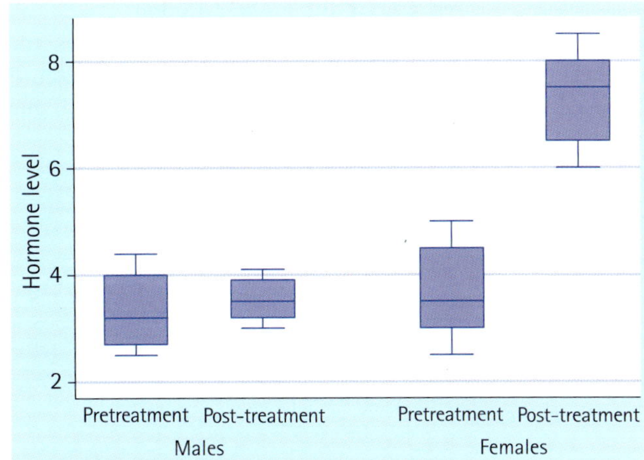

Figure 4.12 Example of an interaction between two categorical variables. The plot shows the blood levels of hormone before and after a drug treatment in males and females

Comparing two related samples: paired *t*-test and Wilcoxon signed rank test

Often we want to compare changes within a group, such as the pre- and post-training knowledge for those nurses who were trained. In this case, our two measurements are not independent. A nurse who scored above average in the knowledge test before the training started is more likely to score above average after the training programme than a nurse who scored poorly at the beginning. We need to consider the dependency of these repeated measurements, otherwise we will lose the advantage of the within-individual comparisons. This is done by the dependent samples *t*-test or its non-parametric equivalent, the Wilcoxon signed rank test. The null hypothesis here is that the mean change in the group with training is zero (see Stata output, below).

The mean difference between post- and pre-training knowledge is 4.13, with a 95 per cent confidence interval of 2.779 to 5.488. Because 0 is not included in the 95 per cent confidence interval, we can conclude that there is a significant increase in knowledge after the training. This conclusion is confirmed by the test statistic $t = 6.5458$.

A similar result is obtained if a non-parametric test is used. A Wilcoxon signed rank test shows that the pre- and

```
ttest   post_knowledge= preknowledge if group==1

Paired t test
------------------------------------------------------------------------------
Variable |     Obs        Mean    Std. Err.   Std. Dev.   [95% Conf. Interval]
---------+--------------------------------------------------------------------
post_k~e |      15        17.4     .623355    2.414243    16.06304    18.73696
prekno~e |      15    13.26667    .6723567    2.604026    11.82461    14.70873
---------+--------------------------------------------------------------------
    diff |      15    4.133333    .6314508    2.445599    2.779006    5.487661
------------------------------------------------------------------------------
     mean(diff) = mean(post_knowledge - preknowledge)              t =   6.5458
 Ho: mean(diff) = 0                               degrees of freedom =       14

 Ha: mean(diff) < 0           Ha: mean(diff) != 0           Ha: mean(diff) > 0
 Pr(T < t) = 1.0000       Pr(|T| > |t|) = 0.0000          Pr(T > t) = 0.0000
```

post-training scores are significantly different ($z = 3.358$, $N = 15$, $P < 0.001$). Here, N is the sample size minus the number of tied observations within a subject. Exact P values should be calculated from tables or software if the sample size is smaller than 10.

```
Wilcoxon signed-rank test

        sign |      obs   sum ranks    expected
-------------+---------------------------------
    positive |       14         119          60
    negative |        1           1          60
        zero |        0           0           0
-------------+---------------------------------
         all |       15         120         120

unadjusted variance          310.00
adjustment for ties           -1.38
adjustment for zeros           0.00
                         ----------
adjusted variance            308.63
Ho: post_knowledge = preknowledge
             z =    3.358
    Prob > |z| =    0.0008
```

The above paired tests are also used if the individuals of two groups are different but linked in some other way. In twin studies, twins with a psychiatric disorder are often compared with their respective unaffected sibling. Parent–child studies and comparison between the two halves of the brain are other examples.

Note that these paired tests look only at changes within a group; if a comparison between groups is the issue, one would use an independent t-test on the change scores as above: two separate within-group P values are not appropriate for comparing groups (e.g. a contrast between a significant P value in one group but not in the other). This is because, as already noted, the non-significant P value indicates not absence of an effect but lack of evidence for an effect.

A single group: one-sample *t*-test

The one-sample t-test assesses whether the mean value differs from a theoretical value, for example does the mean knowledge score of the nurses differ from 10? The comparison value is often called a *norm* (a value obtained from very large sample, perhaps over many years, and that becomes a standard; intelligent quotient (IQ) of 100 is one such norm). Again, the confidence interval of the estimated mean of 13.5 ranges between 12.58 and 14.49 and does not include 10. Therefore, we can conclude that the nurses score significantly better than 10. A formal one-sample t-test below shows that we can reject the null hypothesis that the knowledge score of the nurses before the treatment started is 10 at the 0.05 level and again conclude that nurses score significantly better than 10 (see Stata output, below).

If the data are seriously skewed, we can use the one-sample Wilcoxon test as a non-parametric alternative.

Chi-squared and Fisher's exact test, and McNemar's test for paired proportions

The chi-squared (χ^2) test can be used as a *goodness-of-fit* test to compare a theoretical and an observed distribution. More widely used is the χ^2 test for proportions in a two-way contingency table. It is based on a comparison of observed and expected frequencies in the cells of the table. The degrees of freedom are $(k_1 - 1) \times (k_2 - 1)$, where k_1 and k_2 are the number of categories in the rows and columns, respectively. An amendment to the basic χ^2 statistic, aimed at improving the fit to distributional assumption, is the *continuity correction* or *Yates' correction*. If any of the expected frequencies is less than 5, then the distributional approximation to the χ^2 test statistic is inaccurate and *Fisher's exact test* would be used. This test does not work with a test statistic as such but enumerates all possible tables with the same marginal totals to find the proportion as extreme as that observed and so produces only a P value. The example below illustrates a test of whether diagnostic groups differ according in the proportions above and below a functioning threshold as measured by the GAF.

```
  ttest pre_knowledge=10

One-sample t test
------------------------------------------------------------------------------
Variable |     Obs        Mean    Std. Err.   Std. Dev.   [95% Conf. Interval]
---------+--------------------------------------------------------------------
pre_kn~e |      30    13.53333    .4666667    2.556039    12.57889    14.48777
------------------------------------------------------------------------------
    mean = mean(pre_knowledge)                                    t =   7.5714
Ho: mean = 10                                    degrees of freedom =       29

    Ha: mean < 10               Ha: mean != 10               Ha: mean > 10
 Pr(T < t) = 1.0000         Pr(|T| > |t|) = 0.0000          Pr(T > t) = 0.0000
```

```
numerating sample-space combinations:
stage 3:  enumerations = 1
stage 2:  enumerations = 3
stage 1:  enumerations = 0

         |      primary diagnosis
         |
  gafbin | schizophr   bipolar   other | Total
         |                         psy |
---------+-----------------------------+------
       0 |        24        13      10 |    47
         |      24.3      14.1     8.6 |  47.0
---------+-----------------------------+------
       1 |         7         5       1 |    13
         |       6.7       3.9     2.4 |  13.0
---------+-----------------------------+------
   Total |        31        18      11 |    60
         |      31.0      18.0    11.0 |  60.0

     Pearson chi2(2) = 1.4363   Pr = 0.488
      Fisher's exact =               0.587
```

In the above table, the expected values E are given underneath the observed values O. These are the average values expected in tables with no association between rows and columns and hence are proportional to the row and column proportions. The E for the schizophrenia/gafbin = 0 cell is $47 \times 31/60 = 24.3$, very close to the observed value O of 24.

In anything more complicated than a 2×2 table, the aim would be to identify the proportions that were particularly high or low, once a significant overall difference had been established. One essentially exploratory approach appropriate for large tables is to scan the *Pearson residuals* in the cells ($|O - E|/\sqrt{E}$) (any of the latter above 2–3 being worth investigating). Correspondence analysis may also help (see Multivariate and other more complex techniques, below). In smaller tables, one can test for specific (preferably prespecified) comparisons using subsets of the cells, again using a χ^2 test but bearing in mind that, with k degrees of freedom, only k possible independent tests are possible (see Everitt[33]).

The *McNemar test* is used for paired proportions. For example, one might compare the proportion of nurses who passed an exam at baseline with the number passing at follow-up after training. If there were no effect of training, the proportion changing in either direction would be expected to be 50 per cent and so the test statistic compares this with the proportion who do change in one direction, for example from fail to pass. Those who pass or fail on both occasions do not enter into the calculation.

Kaplan–Meier analysis and log-rank test

Researchers are often interested in the time until participants in a study experience a specific event such as death or recovery or relapse (e.g. time until a relapse of a psychosis). The participants are followed from a starting point (which can be different for each participant) until the time when the event of interest occurs. If the participant withdraws or the study ends before the event occurs, the data are described as *censored*: we do know that the time to event (*survival time*) is longer than the measured follow-up, but we do not know the actual time. Simple statistics such as the standard χ^2 test or the mean time to the event are oversimplistic for censored data, which are preferably analysed with *survival analysis* methods.[34]

A popular non-parametric survival method is Kaplan–Meier analysis, which allows the estimation of a survival function (proportions of people at successive time intervals who survive without the event occurring). It is drawn as a plot with time on the x-axis and survival probability on the y-axis drawn as a step function, since only times when events actually happen are plotted. The time at which 50 per cent of people survive is the median survival time, and this is often used as a summary statistic, along with its 95 per cent confidence interval. Figure 4.13 shows the survival curve for patients with severe Alzheimer's disease in two different treatment groups. The difference in survival probability increases until about 50 months. Then the curves start to merge and after 12 months both curves approach 0.

Formal tests such as the *log-rank test* are used to compare the survival distributions for two or more groups. This is a χ_1^2 test that compares the observed numbers of events at each time point with the number expected if the survival curves were the same for the two groups. It does this by ordering the survival times of all participants and hence dividing up the follow-up time into intervals in which events occur. In each time interval, the number of events is recorded and the number of participants who remain at risk is reduced accordingly. The numbers observed and expected under the null hypothesis of no difference between the groups are accumulated over the whole time period. See Collet[35] for further details.

The distribution of the times to death for the two groups is significantly different according to the log-rank test. The median time to death of patients in the new treatment group is 40 months, while it is only 27 months in the old treatment group (see Stata output overleaf).

Other survival analysis methods such as Cox regression can allow for the effects of covariates (including covariates that change over time) on the survival time.

CORRELATION AND REGRESSION

So far, we have analysed measurements from different groups. Often, however, we want to assess the relationship between two variables in a single group. For example, using the nurse dataset, one might wish to assess the relationship between the knowledge score before and after the training program. Does a high score after training depend on a high score before training? Such an analysis should start with a scatter plot, in which one variable is plotted against a

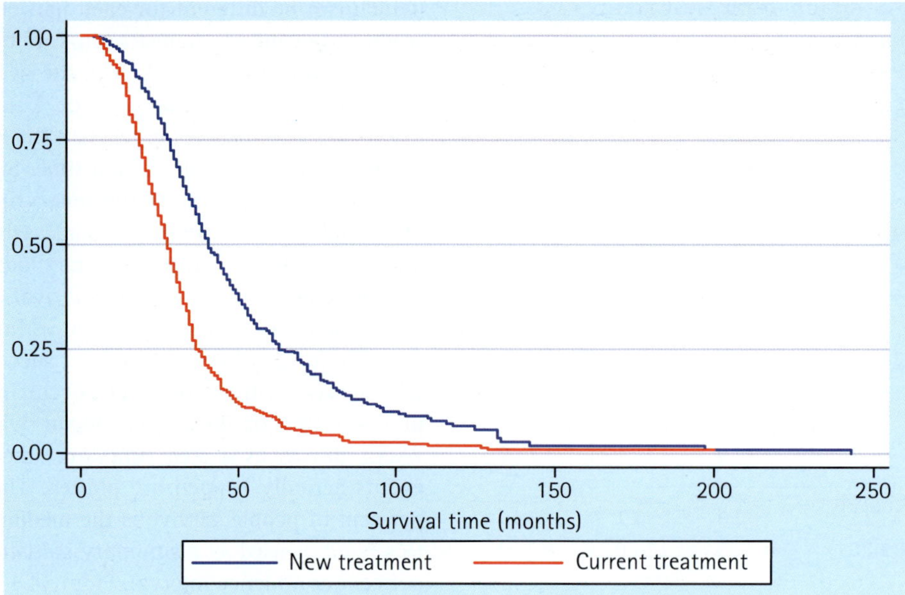

Figure 4.13 Example of Kaplan–Meier curve

```
        failure _d:  event == 1
  analysis time _t:  time

           |               incidence       no. of     |------ Survival time -----|
  treatm~t | time at risk     rate        subjects         25%        50%        75%
  ---------+---------------------------------------------------------------------
  new trea |        19695   .0181264           450          28         40         63
   current |        13437   .0305872           450          18         27         36
  ---------+---------------------------------------------------------------------
     total |        33132     .02318           900          21         32         50


  Log-rank test for equality of survivor functions

                           |   Events         Events
  treatment                |  observed       expected
  -------------------------+-------------------------
  new treatment method     |       357         486.23
  current treatment method |       411         281.77
  -------------------------+-------------------------
  Total                    |       768         768.00

                                 chi2(1) =     100.50
                                 Pr>chi2 =     0.0000
```

horizontal axis (x-axis) and another one against a vertical axis (y-axis). If one variable is considered to be dependent on the other (e.g. if one follows the other in time), then that variable should appear on the y-axis.

Figure 4.14 shows a scatter plot between pretreatment scores and post-treatment scores of the 30 nurses. Note that six cases have the same values and do not appear as separate points. The line is from a fitted straight-line regression of post-treatment on pretreatment score. This would differ from the regression the other way around, of pretreatment on post-treatment score, because it finds the line that minimizes the squared errors or *residuals*. These are measured by the vertical distances between the points and the line using a method of estimation known as *least squares*.

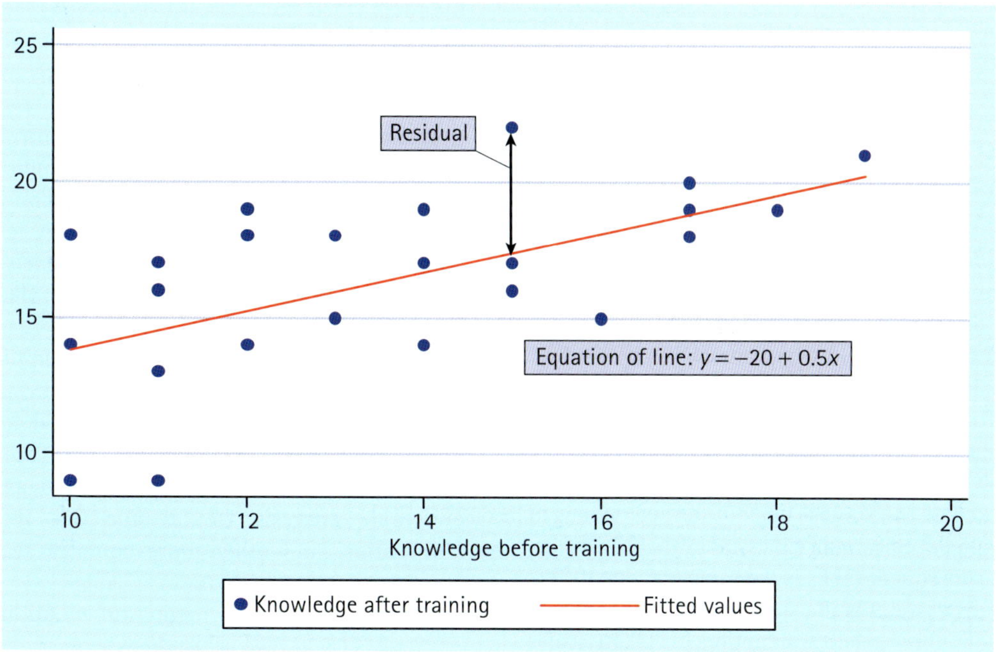

Figure 4.14 Scatter plot showing linear regression line

Regression assumes that one variable (the dependent variable on the *y*-axis) is a random variable whereas the other (the independent or explanatory variable) is a fixed error-free measurement. This is of course rarely the case and is not true of the nurse data. Errors of measurement in the independent variables attenuate the slope of the line (make it less steep), and it is worth bearing this in mind, although in practice this feature is usually ignored.

The difference between regression and correlation

Although mathematically (and in terms of the situations where they are used) correlation and regression are closely allied, there are conceptual differences between them. When one of the variables is thought to depend on or be predicted by the other, the natural approach is that of regression (see below). When the question is simply a matter of the degree of an association, then correlation analysis is more appropriate. Correlation is essentially symmetrical, and distributional assumptions about both variables are necessary for hypothesis tests, whereas in regression no distributional assumptions are made about the independent variables. In the above example, one could treat the data either way: correlation between the scores could be estimated, or a regression of knowledge after training could be fitted to that before training (the reverse relationship would probably not make much sense, indicating the importance of actively choosing what is to be the dependent variable and bearing in mind the criteria for causation, e.g. as in the Bradford-Hill criteria listed earlier).

Pearson's product moment correlation

The most commonly used measure of association is the Pearson *product moment correlation coefficient*, *r*, used to measure the strength of a linear relationship between two normally distributed variables with equal variances. It ranges between −1 (perfect negative relationship) and +1 (perfect positive relationship). The square of *r* is the percentage of variance in one variable explained by the other. In the nurse example, *r* for the relationship between pre- and post-training knowledge is 0.52. Pretraining scores explain therefore 0.52^2 or 27 per cent of the variance of the post-training scores. Hypothesis tests for the population correlation ρ can be based on the *Fisher transformation*:

$$z = 1/2 \ln((1 + r)/(1 - r))$$

which produces a test statistic *z* that is approximately *N*(0,1). A hypothesis test (single-sample *z*-test) of the null hypothesis that the population correlation is 0 shows that the observed *r* of 0.52 is significantly different from 0 ($P = 0.003$, 95 per cent confidence interval 0.20 to 0.74).

A correlation coefficient of 0 means that there is no linear relationship, but this does not mean that there is no relationship of any kind – it might be non-linear (hence the need to plot the data). It is important that there is no funnel shape in the data where the spread widens or narrows at different levels of the variables (indicating *heteroscedasticity*, i.e. a change in variance) and no outliers, to which Pearson's correlation is very vulnerable. *Partial correlations* are correlations between a pair of variables after adjusting for a third (and can be derived from the three pair-wise correlations).

Spearman and Kendall's tau correlation

Non-parametric alternatives are available, such as Spearman's rank correlation ρ. This is equivalent to the Pearson's correlation calculated on the ranked data and detects any monotonic (i.e. increasing or decreasing) relationship, such as an exponential relationship. Spearman's ρ ranges from −1 to 1 and is interpreted in a similar way to Pearson's *r*. However, ρ^2 cannot be interpreted as a percentage of variance explained in the same way as r^2. If there are tied observations in the data, a corrected version should be used. Furthermore, if the sample size is small (< 15) or if there are tied observations among the data, either exact *P* values should be computed or a statistical table for critical values of ρ should be consulted.[29] Spearman's ρ assumes that the difference between all subsequent ranks is the same (e.g. the difference between ranks 1 and 2 is the same as between ranks 10 and 11). This a commonly made assumption for Likert scales in psychiatric measurement scales. If the assumption of equidistance cannot be assumed, then Kendall's tau correlation coefficient is an alternative for ordinal-level variables.

Linear regression

Multiple linear regression is used for prediction of a variable from a set of other variables, or to control for confounders when the interest is in one particular variable (e.g. treatment arm). For example, one might use a *t*-test to compare the mean values of a continuous variable, such as symptom score, between two groups in a randomized controlled trial. Then one might wish to control for the baseline value and perhaps also sociodemographic variables using regression. This procedure is often known as ANCOVA. Regression and ANOVA, and ANCOVA (a mixture of the two), are examples of *general linear models* – not to be confused with the even more general *generalized linear models* (see below).

The example below shows typical output for a regression of functioning (GAF score) on days in hospital, randomization group of the patient's nurse and admission cohort (three categories, included as two dummy variables). (Because the patients are 'clustered' within the nurse, a preferable analysis would take this into account; see Multivariate and other more complex techniques, below) (see Stata output, below).

The linear regression prediction equation is (rounded):

GAF score = 59.39 + 7.470 (if randomization group = 1) + 2.844 (if admission group = 2) + 21.952 (if admission group = 3) + 0.00323 (days in hospital)

The coefficients are the estimates of the increase in the dependent variable for a one-unit increase in the independent variable, adjusted for all other variables. Thus, since *group* is coded 0 and 1, the coefficient for *group* in the

```
xi: regress gaf group i.admitgrp days
i.admitgrp        _Iadmitgrp_0-2       (naturally coded; _Iadmitgrp_0 omitted)

      Source |       SS       df       MS              Number of obs =      60
-------------+------------------------------           F(  4,     55) =   12.08
       Model |  4122.47021     4  1030.61755           Prob > F      =  0.0000
    Residual |  4694.11312    55  85.3475113           R-squared     =  0.4676
-------------+------------------------------           Adj R-squared =  0.4289
       Total |  8816.58333    59  149.433616           Root MSE      =  9.2384

------------------------------------------------------------------------------
         gaf |      Coef.   Std. Err.      t    P>|t|     [95% Conf. Interval]
-------------+----------------------------------------------------------------
       group |   7.470304   2.653043     2.82   0.007     2.153487    12.78712
 _Iadmitgrp_1 |   2.844533   2.652026     1.07   0.288    -2.470246    8.159311
 _Iadmitgrp_2 |   21.95218   3.820844     5.75   0.000     14.29504    29.60933
        days |   .0032465   .0086497     0.38   0.709    -.0140879    .0205808
       _cons |   59.39308   2.743692    21.65   0.000      53.8946    64.89156
------------------------------------------------------------------------------

. testparm  _Iadmitgrp_*

 ( 1)  _Iadmitgrp_1 = 0
 ( 2)  _Iadmitgrp_2 = 0

       F(  2,    55) =   17.15
            Prob > F =    0.0000
```

regression equation is the adjusted difference between groups. With no other variables in the equation, it would be the same as a *t*-test. The R^2 is the percentage of variance explained and is equal to the correlation between the predictions made by the above equation and the dependent variable. R^2 depends on the number of parameters; a value that is more comparable across different numbers of parameters is the adjusted R^2, which takes these into account. The F statistic in the top right corner reflects the significance of the group of explanatory variables taken together. The F statistic at the end reflects the significance of admission cohort as a categorical variable. Specific comparisons between the dummy-coded diagnostic groups 2 and 3 and the reference category appear in the main body of the result: $P = 0.288$ and $P < 0.001$, respectively.

Logistic regression

If one wished to compare the groups in terms of a binary variable, for example symptoms improved, then the approach would be a χ^2 test to compare proportions followed by logistic regression to control for other variables. Logistic regression analysis maximizes the *likelihood* (the probability *p* of the observed data given a particular statistical model) to estimate the parameters of a linear equation for the log of the odds – $\ln(p/(1-p))$ – also called the *logit*.

It does this through an iterative process to maximize the likelihood (*maximum likelihood estimation*). The output can be expressed in terms of the coefficients that apply to the logit through the linear predictor. An alternative formulation is in terms of exponentiated coefficients, which are the estimated adjusted ORs, and these are usually more useful for interpretation.

The example below shows the output in OR format for a logistic regression of binary (0/1) functioning category against randomization group (coded 0/1) and three-category diagnostic group for 30 of the patients (see Stata output ①, below).

Here, diagnosis 2 seems to be significant at about $P = 0.05$ compared with diagnosis 1. However, we need to test the whole variable, so we still need to perform a likelihood ratio test. We rerun the analysis without diagnosis to see whether the likelihood drops significantly, as illustrated below. Such tests can be validly applied when model A is *nested* in model B (i.e. A's parameters form a subset of B's) (see Stata output ②, below).

```
① Logistic regression                          Number of obs  =        30
                                               LR chi2(3)     =      7.76
                                               Prob > chi2    =    0.0512
  Log likelihood = -16.913369                  Pseudo R2      =    0.1866

  ------------------------------------------------------------------------------
       gaf_cat | Odds Ratio   Std. Err.      z    P>|z|     [95% Conf. Interval]
  -------------+----------------------------------------------------------------
         group |   4.444985   3.788074     1.75   0.080     .8364988    23.61975
  _Idiagnosi_2 |   7.141792   7.263598     1.93   0.053     .9729447    52.42353
  _Idiagnosi_3 |   1.903212   2.285294     0.54   0.592     .1808843    20.02503
  ------------------------------------------------------------------------------

② estimates store A

  logistic gaf_cat group

  Logistic regression                          Number of obs  =        30
                                               LR chi2(1)     =      3.40
                                               Prob > chi2    =    0.0653
  Log likelihood = -19.095425                  Pseudo R2      =    0.0817

  ------------------------------------------------------------------------------
       gaf_cat | Odds Ratio   Std. Err.      z    P>|z|     [95% Conf. Interval]
  -------------+----------------------------------------------------------------
         group |          4   3.098387     1.79   0.074     .8764398    18.25567
  ------------------------------------------------------------------------------

  . estimates store B

  . lrtest A B

  Likelihood-ratio test                             LR chi2(2)  =      4.36
  (Assumption: B nested in A)                       Prob > chi2 =    0.1128
```

The likelihood ratio test compares the likelihoods with and without diagnosis and shows that there is no significant reduction. Diagnosis as a whole is not significant and can be omitted from the model.

The output below illustrates the use of the linear predictor format as an alternative to the OR format to obtain logit (or log odds).

This linear predictor can be used to form predictions of the odds and hence the probabilities for individuals, as shown in the example for someone aged 20 years in group 1:

$$\text{Logit or } \ln(\text{odds}) = 3.466 + 2.132 - 20 \times 0.2783 = 0.0323$$
$$\text{Odds} = \exp(0.0323) = 1.0328$$
$$\text{Probability} = 1.0328/(1 + 1.0328) = 0.5081$$

The adjusted ORs for a positive outcome (gaf_cat = 1) in relation to a unit increase in the independent variables are found by exponentiating the coefficients, for example exp(2.131) = 4.

Logistic regression is commonly used in case–control studies: the case–control status is the binary dependent variable and the ORs measure the degree of association between the risk or protective factors and that status. In this situation the ORs are often interpreted as RRs, although this is numerically accurate only when the risk is very small (e.g. < 0.05). It is true, however, that, whatever the risk, a significant OR will indicate a significant RR, even if numerically they are not equivalent. Note that the calculation of probabilities as above cannot be performed: this is because the proportion of cases is determined by the design of the study (50% each in 1 : 1 matching), and so calculating a probability based on these proportions is meaningless.

Standardization of coefficients

In a regression analysis, either or both dependent and independent variables can be *standard scored* or *z*-scored – that is, the mean is subtracted and the value divided by the sample standard deviation (cf. standard effect sizes). The resulting coefficients are sometimes called 'beta coefficients'. If both dependent and independent variables are standardized, then the betas have a similar interpretation to partial correlation coefficients, although they are numerically slightly different. This is a useful way of comparing (within a given regression model) the relative sizes of coefficients for variables that are measured in different units. For logistic regression, one would only standardize the independent variables, because the dependent variable, being binary, does not need to be standardized.

Conditional logistic regression

One further type of regression that is especially important for individually matched case–control studies and other situations where the observations are not independent is *conditional logistic regression*. Here, the observations that are individually matched (e.g. in a case–control study) or connected in some other way (e.g. the two patients of each nurse in the example) are indicated by a 'link' variable or 'match group' (e.g. the nurse identification in the example). The likelihood that is maximized in estimating the parameters of a logistic model for case status is conditional on membership of the linked group and so effectively controls for characteristics that the members of the linked group have in common. This is the point of matching – to control for unmeasured confounders – and so it is important to make use of conditional logistic regression rather than standard logistic regression where appropriate, otherwise the benefits of matching may be wasted.

Other types of regression

Some other types of regression worth knowing about are *multinomial logistic regression*, where the dependent variable is categorical non-ordered, such as diagnosis; *ordered logistic regression*, where the dependent variable is ordered categorical, such as grade of illness; and *Poisson regression*, for count data, such as the number of admissions to hospital, or binary data, such as admitted or not where the time at risk is either measured or implied and one is interested in rates rather than proportions. Poisson regression is commonly used in cohort studies to estimate rate ratios over a follow-up period after controlling for confounders and produces *rate ratios*. *Cox regression* is appropriate where the outcome is time to an event, as in survival analysis. It produces *hazard ratios*, which are ratios of the risks of an event at any given point in time (rather than averaged over the follow-up time, as in Poisson regression). A more general model, which encompasses all of the above as well as linear and logistic regression and a number of others, is the *generalized linear model*.

Model-building in regression

The best way to include variables in a regression model of any type is on the basis of theoretical background in the subject matter of interest. However, sometimes investigators are faced with a large number of potential independent variables without much guidance as to which to use. A rule

gaf_cat	Coef.	Std. Err.	z	P>|z|	[95% Conf.	Interval]
group	2.13168	.9555024	2.23	0.026	.2589298	4.004431
age	-.2782977	.157653	-1.77	0.078	-.5872919	.0306965
_cons	3.466657	2.40287	1.44	0.149	-1.242881	8.176196

of thumb is to have at least ten cases per parameter to be estimated, so there is often a need to cut down the number of variables included. Some possible automatic methods are as follows:

- *Backward selection:* first include all variables, then omit variables one by one, starting with the least significant and refitting the model each time.
- *Forward selection:* start with the single most significant variable (having tested each separately), then progressively add in a variable at a time (again refitting the model each time).
- *Stepwise:* a mixture of the above procedures.

None of these is necessarily optimal, and they may give rise to different sets of variables. See Derksen and Keselman[36] for a discussion. An increasingly popular alternative to model selection based on significance testing is the use of information criteria, such as the Akaike information criterion (AIC).[37] This allows the comparison of the likelihood of a set of different candidate models, which need not be nested, as is the case with likelihood ratio tests.

MULTIVARIATE AND OTHER MORE COMPLEX TECHNIQUES

Principal components and factor analysis

Principal components analysis (PCA) transforms the data variables into components (linear combinations of original variables) that explain decreasing proportions of the variance in the data and that are uncorrelated.[38] It is essentially a data-reduction technique – often the first few components are plotted to illustrate the main features of multivariate data. The last few are useful for indicating any outliers. It is also used as the mathematical first step in a factor analysis. However, although factor and principal components analysis are often confused, they are conceptually distinct.

Exploratory factor analysis seeks underlying factors that explain the correlation or covariance between variables. The unmeasured variables are assumed to be linear functions of underlying unmeasured or latent variables, plus measurement errors (called residuals or *specific factors*). The analysis is often initiated by running a PCA to determine the number of factors. Factors are extracted using e.g. maximum likelihood methods, which can be rotated, either orthogonally (e.g. using the *varimax* method – axes are kept orthogonal/perpendicular) or obliquely (e.g. using the *oblimin* method – axes are allowed to form oblique patterns). The rotation often allows the coefficients that define the factors (factor loadings) to be interpreted more easily. It is common practice to set loadings to zero if they are below a cut-off (e.g. 0.40), with the aim of finding factors that are each associated with a mutually exclusive set of variables. (The others are not zero, but this presentation simplifies the results.) Costello and Osborne[39] provide some guidance on this method.

Table 4.14 shows typical factor solutions for hypothetical data from a quality-of-life scale. Interpretations of the factors are given along the top (these are the prerogative of the investigator). The percentage of the variance explained by each factor is given along the bottom. In this case the three-factor solution seems to be more interpretable because the variables load into different factors. Note that the negative coefficients do not matter for interpretation (so long as they are consistent within a factor). If scales were to be derived from the factors, then common practice would be to add up the values of the items within factors (i.e. set the factor loadings to 1). It is important that item response scores are in the same conceptual order.

In a *confirmatory factor analysis*, the researcher sets up

Table 4.14 Example of a factor analysis: oblimin-rotated factors based on principal components analysis of eight variables; factor loadings > 0.40 shown

Constituent scales of the SF-36	Two-factor solution		Three-factor solution		
	1 General health	2 Physical health	1 Mental health	2 Physical health	3 Roles
Physical functioning		0.85		0.78	
Role physical	0.41	0.40			−0.83
Bodily pain		0.85		0.82	
General health	0.64		0.70		
Vitality	0.78		0.82		
Social functioning	0.63		0.42		
Role emotional	0.74				−0.72
Mental health	0.91		0.90		
Percentage of variance explained	77%	10%	72%	15%	10%

in advance a hypothesis for the latent constructs and measures a number of variables that reflect different aspects of these constructs. The set of relationships between the observed variables and the constructs is called the *measurement model*, which is then tested for fit against real data. In more complicated models, the factors themselves will have a relationship with one another; this combination of factor analysis and regression analysis is called a *structural equation* and is analysed with specialist software. Figure 4.15 shows how such a theoretical model might be set up. Such diagrams are known as *path diagrams*.

Other multivariate methods

Principal components and factor analysis are widely used methods. Here, we mention some other methods that are much less popular but worth noting. *Discriminant analysis* is a method for classifying individuals into predefined groups by producing linear discriminant functions of the variables (if equal variances can be assumed) or quadratic functions (if not). It also provides a plot in a lower dimension than the original number of variables (analogous to principal components, except that the plot maximizes the variance between group means rather than between individual data points). It has a similar function to binary logistic regression (or multinomial logistic regression when there are more than two groups), but unlike those methods it assumes multivariate normality of the variables used and is hence somewhat more restrictive in application. The main advantage is the plot it produces. Another classification method is *classification and regression tree analysis* (CART); this focuses on finding interactive effects (i.e. combinations of variables) rather than linear functions, as in discriminant analysis or logistic regression analysis, and produces a tree-like diagram (e.g. see Thomas *et al.*[40]).

Correspondence analysis is a method for graphically displaying cross-tabulated data; although it is little used in psychiatry, it is potentially very useful for exploratory

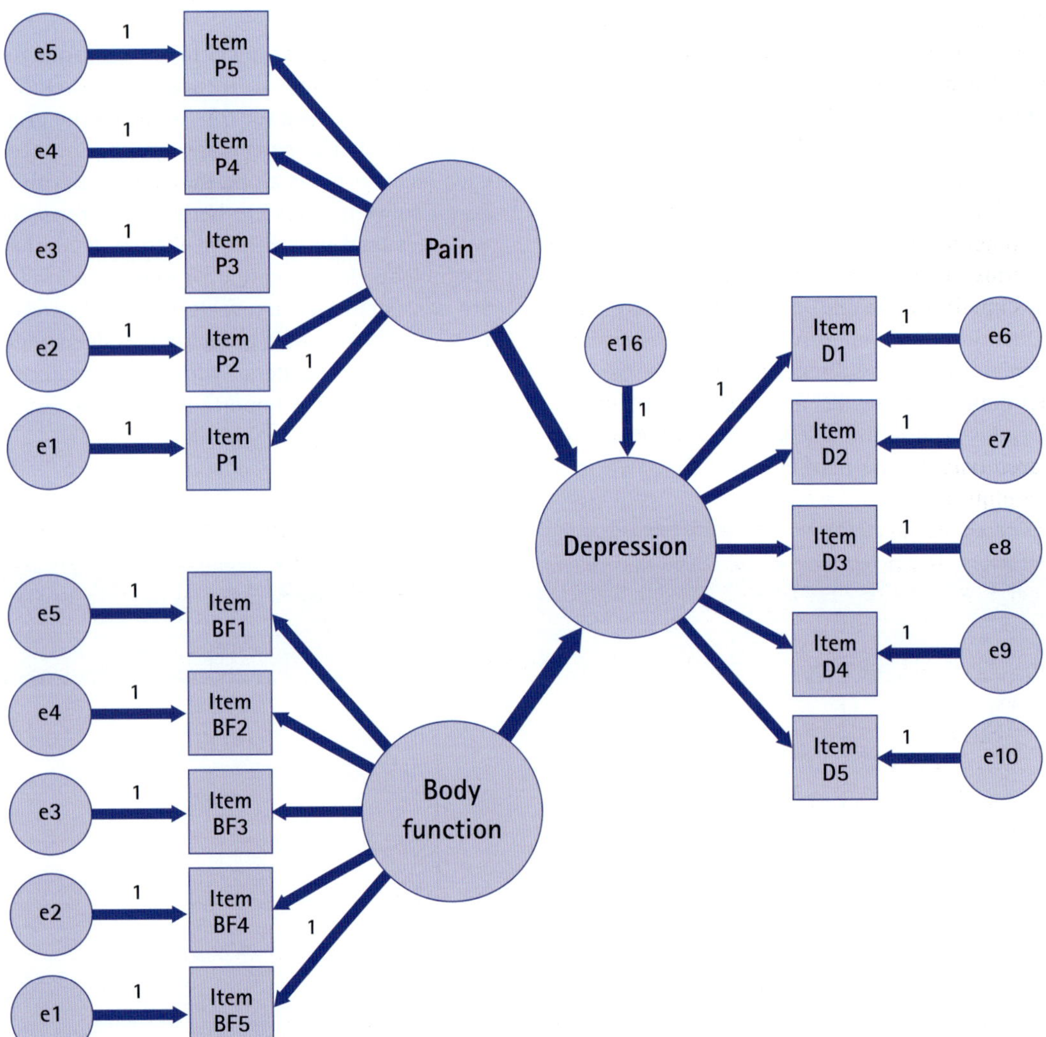

Figure 4.15 Example of a structural equation model. This relates the two latent traits 'Pain' and 'Body function' to the latent trait 'Depression'. Each latent trait is measured by five items (measurement model)

analysis of large cross-tabulations. *Canonical correlation analysis* again is little used, probably because the results are difficult to interpret; it is a method for investigating linear functions that maximize the correlation between the variables in one set with the variables in another set. *Cluster analysis* is a vast set of methods that seek subgroups within a dataset. It is a data-driven exploratory method, overlapping with data-mining, neural networks and pattern recognition. Everitt *et al.*[41] give an overview of the more standard methods. They differ from the classification methods mentioned above in that the groups are unknown a priori – the aim is to use the data to find the groups.

For an introduction to applied multivariate data analysis, see Everitt and Dunn[42] or Tabachnick and Fidell.[43]

Methods for non-independent data

Many standard statistical methods assume that each data point has been sampled independently of the others. However, in some situations this is not the case. Clustered trials and matched case–control studies have already been mentioned. Other examples are sampling of families where all members are interviewed, and of students within classes within schools. Repeated measurements for the same subject – sets of measurements of the same variable at different time points or sets of different variables that measure the same underlying within-subject factor – are also dependent.

In a *multivariate analysis of variance* (MANOVA), the purpose is to compare groups (e.g. gender or experimental condition) in terms of sets of dependent measures simultaneously. It is sometimes known as *profile analysis* when different variables are involved. It has been superseded to some extent by a number of specialized techniques appropriate for such data, such as *multilevel models* and *general estimation equation* (GEE) models. Other terms that will be encountered are *random effects* and *mixed models*. This collection of techniques is very flexible and can cope with within-subject repeated measures and multilevel sampling of different subjects. It can allow the inclusion of several levels of cluster (e.g. individuals clustered within families, families clustered within a therapist, and even cross-clustering, where individuals are clustered within families but family members do not have the same therapist). These modelling techniques allow the inclusion of both individual-level and cluster-level covariates.

To illustrate these, below is a simple regression of GAF score of the 60 patients on randomization group of the nurse in the training example. Because of the clustering of the pairs of patients within the nurses, this would not be correct and would underestimate the standard error for group and hence overestimate the significance.

Overleaf are the same data analysed as a *random effects regression*. Here, the effect of nurse that is common to his or her pair of patients has been explicitly modelled. The standard error increases and the estimate of the group effect is changed slightly, from 8.86 to 7.93 (see Stata output ①, overleaf).

Another approach is to use standard techniques such as linear regression but with specially adapted estimation methods that are *robust* to non-independence (such as the sandwich estimator mentioned earlier). Overleaf are the results for the above example: the point estimate for group is the same as the simple regression, but the standard error has been adjusted to take account of the clustering and is now called 'robust standard error' (see Stata output ②, overleaf).

A simple alternative approach for clustered data is to construct a *summary statistic* for each cluster and then analyse these summary values, for example with a weighted *t*-test using the numbers of subjects as a weight. However, this latter approach is not efficient and does not allow a more complex analysis including individual covariates.

Meta-analysis

Sample sizes in psychiatric studies are sometimes too small to detect clinically important effects. However, it is possible to combine the results of several similar studies by means of meta-analysis.[44,45] A typical meta-analysis starts with a

```
regress  gaf group

      Source |       SS       df       MS              Number of obs =      60
-------------+------------------------------           F(  1,     58) =    8.90
       Model |  1172.68601     1  1172.68601           Prob > F      =  0.0042
    Residual |  7643.89732    58  131.791333           R-squared     =  0.1330
-------------+------------------------------           Adj R-squared =  0.1181
       Total |  8816.58333    59  149.433616           Root MSE      =   11.48

------------------------------------------------------------------------------
         gaf |      Coef.   Std. Err.      t    P>|t|     [95% Conf. Interval]
-------------+----------------------------------------------------------------
       group |   8.861607   2.970743     2.98   0.004     2.915019    14.80819
       _cons |   63.78125   2.029404    31.43   0.000     59.71896    67.84354
------------------------------------------------------------------------------
```

```
① xtreg gaf group,i(nurse)

Random-effects GLS regression                   Number of obs      =        60
Group variable: nurse                           Number of groups   =        30

R-sq:  within  = 0.0154                         Obs per group: min =         2
       between = 0.1563                                        avg =       2.0
       overall = 0.1330                                        max =         2

Random effects u_i ~ Gaussian                   Wald chi2(1)       =      5.34
corr(u_i, X)       = 0 (assumed)                Prob > chi2        =    0.0208

------------------------------------------------------------------------------
         gaf |      Coef.   Std. Err.      z    P>|z|     [95% Conf. Interval]
-------------+----------------------------------------------------------------
       group |    7.92753   3.430114     2.31   0.021      1.20463    14.65043
       _cons |   64.21715   2.507726    25.61   0.000      59.3021    69.13221
-------------+----------------------------------------------------------------
     sigma_u |  9.5259075
     sigma_e |  6.6779359
         rho |   .6704923   (fraction of variance due to u_i)
------------------------------------------------------------------------------
```

```
② regress  gaf group, cluster(nurse)

Linear regression                                      Number of obs =      60
                                                       F(  1,    29) =    5.53
                                                       Prob > F      =  0.0257
                                                       R-squared     =  0.1330
                                                       Root MSE      =   11.48

                                  (Std. Err. adjusted for 30 clusters in nurse)
------------------------------------------------------------------------------
             |               Robust
         gaf |      Coef.   Std. Err.      t    P>|t|     [95% Conf. Interval]
-------------+----------------------------------------------------------------
       group |   8.861607   3.769132     2.35   0.026     1.152867    16.57035
       _cons |   63.78125   2.936454    21.72   0.000     57.77553    69.78697
------------------------------------------------------------------------------
```

systematic review: studies of the same or similar treatments of generally randomized controlled trials are collected in a formalized process.[46,47] Meta-analysis is a statistical technique that allows the combination of the effect sizes extracted from different studies into one overall estimate with an associated confidence interval and a hypothesis test of treatment effectiveness.

The statistical models used in meta-analysis weight the individual study results using either *fixed* or *random-effects* models, the choice between them depending on the degree of between-study variability, which can be tested in relation to pooled variation within studies with a χ^2 test for homogeneity (sometimes called the Q test). If they are homogeneous, then a fixed effects model should be used. In this case, the weights are proportional to the inverse of the within-study variation (e.g. as reported in the standard errors of the effects). If the studies are heterogeneous, then a random-effects model is more appropriate; here, the weight combines the studies' individual precisions with the between-study variation.

Figure 4.16 shows a so-called *forest* plot, a graphical summary of a meta-analysis. This shows the effect sizes obtained from the individual trials with their confidence intervals (the lengths of the lines); the size of the boxes is proportional to the sample sizes, and a vertical line indicates the overall effect.[48]

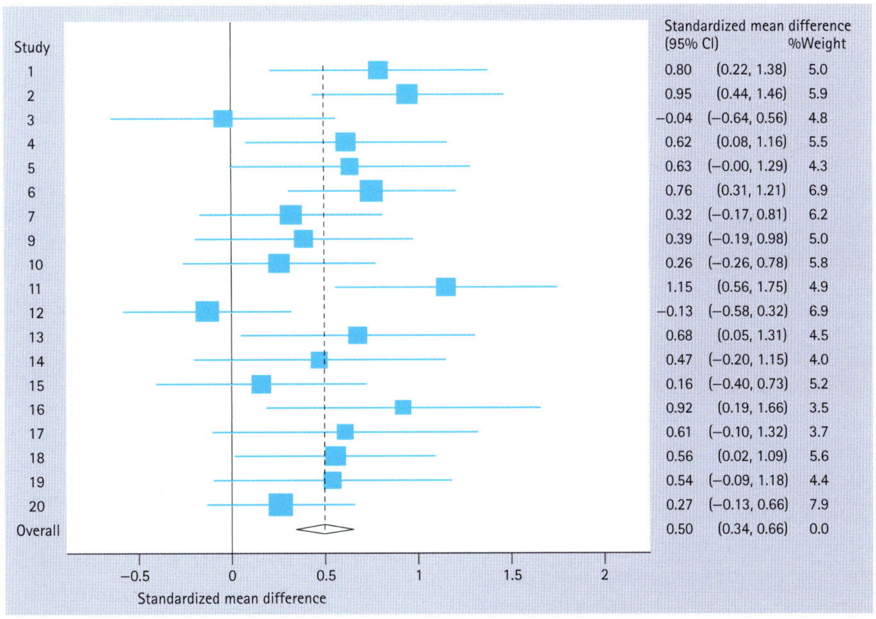

Figure 4.16 Forest plot of a random-effects meta-analysis of 20 studies of a particular type of group therapy. CI, confidence interval.

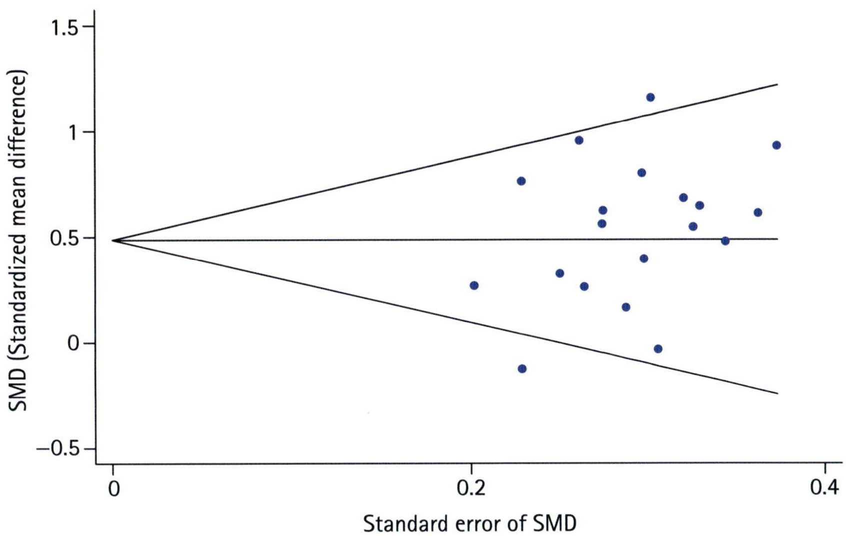

Figure 4.17 Funnel plot for the studies shown in Figure 4.16

A common problem is *publication bias*. Scientists tend to submit only studies with significant results, and editors of journals are more likely to publish such studies. Smaller studies without statistically significant effects or even contradictory effects are less likely to be published, so that the overall effect tends to be overestimated. The possibility of bias can be assessed informally by a *funnel plot* (Figure 4.17). This is a simple scatter plot of the sample sizes (or precision) of the studies against their estimated effect sizes.

The funnel plot in Figure 4.17 shows such a gap (bottom right), which suggests a publication bias although a formal test for bias (Begg's adjusted rank test) was not significant.

KEY POINTS

- Validity types include face; content; criterion; concurrent; discriminant; predictive; construct. Test–retest and inter-rater reliability are assessed by kappa coefficient (categorical data), intraclass correlation (continuous data), and item consistency by Cronbach's alpha.
- In diagnostic testing, post-test odds = pre-test odds × likelihood ratio where odds = probability/(1 − probability); receiver operator curves, sensitivity, specificity (both independent of base rate), PPV and NPV are also key concepts.
- The randomized controlled trial is the gold standard study design, and involves the following concepts: phases of development,

equipoise, placebo controls, blinding, intention-to-treat analysis, individual v. cluster randomization and the Consort diagram.

- Epidemiological designs include case–control studies (which are analysed using odds ratios, often via logistic regression), and cohort studies (which may use rates – or 'person-year analysis'– rate ratios and Poisson regression).
- Partly because of the central limit theorem, many statistical techniques are based on the bell-shaped normal or Gaussian distribution, characterized by the mean and standard deviation (square root of variance); the mean $\pm$ 1.96 $\times$ SD contains 95% of the observations.
- The approximate (large sample) 95% confidence interval for an estimate is the estimate $\pm$ 1.96 $\times$ its standard error, and indicates its uncertainty; the size of the estimate compared to its standard error produces the P value, the chance of obtaining so extreme a value under the null hypothesis (if P is below a critical value, alpha, it is said to be significant at that level, e.g. 0.05).
- Key basic techniques are: t-test (non-parametric Mann–Whitney or equivalently the Wilcoxon rank sum) and paired t-test (non-parametric Wilcoxon signed rank); chi-square test and McNemar test for proportions; analysis of variance, correlation (Pearson and non-parametric Spearman) and regression (linear for continuous and logistic for binary outcomes), and survival analysis (Kaplan–Meier, log-rank and Cox regression).
- Important multivariate techniques include principal components analysis, factor analysis (exploratory and confirmatory), discriminant analysis, cluster analysis, structural equation modelling and path analysis.
- Meta-analysis allows one to combine the results of several similar studies into one overall estimate with an associated confidence interval, and uses forest plots (to show the estimates) and funnel plots (to detect possible publication bias).

REFERENCES

1. Bland JM (2000) *An Introduction to Medical Statistics.* Oxford: Oxford University Press.
2. Petrie A, Sabin C (2005) *Medical Statistics at a Glance*, 2nd edn. Oxford: Blackwell.
3. Everitt BS (2006) *Medical Statistics from A to Z*, 2nd edn. Cambridge: Cambridge University Press.
4. Dupont WD (2002) *Statistical Modelling for Biomedical Research: A Simple Introduction to the Analysis of Complex Data.* Cambridge: Cambridge University Press.
5. Beck AT, Guth D, Steer RA, Ball R (1997) Screening for major depression disorders in medical inpatients with the Beck Depression Inventory for Primary Care. *Behavior Research and Therapy* **35**: 785–91.
6. Irvine SH, Kyllonen PC (eds) (2002) Mahwah, NJ: *Item Generation for Test Development.* Lawrence Erlbaum Associates.
7. Streiner DL, Norman GR (2003) *Health Measurement Scales: A Practical Guide to their Development and Use*, 3rd edn. Oxford: Oxford University Press.
8. Shrout P, Fleiss JL (1979) Intraclass correlation: uses in assessing rater reliability. *Psychological Bulletin* **86**: 420–28.
9. Bland J, Altman DG (1986) Statistical methods for assessing agreement between two methods of clinical measurement. *Lancet* **i**: 307–10.
10. Brennan RL (2001) *Generalizability Theory.* New York: Springer-Verlag.
11. Pocock SJ. (1994) *Clinical Trials: A Practical Approach.* Chichester: John Wiley & Sons.
12. Moher D, Schulz KF, Altman DG, CONSORT Group (2001) The CONSORT statement: revised recommendations for improving the quality of reports of parallel-group randomised trials. *Lancet* **357**: 1191–4.
13. Moher D, Schulz KF, Altman DG (2001) The CONSORT statement: revised recommendations for improving the quality of reports of parallel-group randomised trials. *Lancet* **357**: 1191–4.
14. Campbell MK, Elbourne DR, Altman DG, *et al.* (2004) CONSORT statement: extension to cluster randomised trials. *British Medical Journal* **328**: 702–8.
15. Donner A, Klar NS (2000) *Design and Analysis of Cluster Randomisation Trials in Health Research.* London: Arnold.
16. Deeks JJ, Dinnes J, D'Amico R, *et al.* (2003) Evaluating non-randomised intervention studies. *Health Technology Assessment* **7**: 1–173.
17. Morton V, Torgerson DJ (2003) Effect of regression to the mean on decision making in health care. *British Medical Journal* **326**: 1083–4.
18. Sackett D, Haynes RB, Tugwell P, Guyatt GH (1991) *Clinical Epidemiology: A Basic Science for Clinical Medicine*, 2nd edn. Boston, MA: Little Brown.
19. Phelps CE (2002) *Health Economics*, 3rd edn. Boston, MA: Addison-Wesley.
20. Sackett DL (1979) Bias in analytic research. *Journal of Chronic Diseases* **32**: 51–63.
21. Lee W, Bindman J, Ford T, *et al.* (2007) Bias in psychiatric case–control studies: a systematic review of current practice. *British Journal of Psychiatry* **190**: 204–9.
22. Hill AB (1965) The environment and disease: association or causation? *Proceedings of the Royal Society of Medicine* **58**: 295–300.
23. Höfler M (2005) The Bradford Hill considerations on causality: a counterfactual perspective. *Emerging Themes in Epidemiology* **2**: 11.
24. Miller JN (1993) Outliers in experimental data and their treatment. *Analyst* **118**: 455–61.
25. Cohen J (1988) *Statistical Power Analysis for the Behavioral Sciences*, 2nd edn. Hillsdale, NJ: Lawrence Erlbaum Associates.
26. Fitzpatrick R, Davey C, Buxton MJ, Jones DR (1998)

Evaluating patient-based outcome measures for use in clinical trials. *Health Technology Assessment* **2**: 1–74.
27. Shaffer JP (1995) Multiple hypothesis testing. *Annual Review of Psychology* **46**: 561–84.
28. Howell DC (1997) *Statistical Methods for Psychology*, 4th edn. Belmont, CA: Duxbury.
29. Siegel S, Castellan NJ (1988) *Nonparametric Statistics for the Behavioural Sciences*, 2nd edn. New York: McGraw-Hill.
30. Altman D, Bland NJ (2004) Confidence intervals illuminate absence of evidence. *British Medical Journal* **328**: 1016–17.
31. Bolstad WM (2007) *Introduction to Bayesian Statistics*, 2nd edn. New York: John Wiley & Sons.
32. Spiegelhalter DJ, Abrams KR, Myles JP (2003) *Bayesian Approaches to Clinical Trials and HealthCare Evaluation*. Chichester: John Wiley & Sons.
33. Everitt BS (1992) *The Analysis of Contingency Tables*. London: Chapman & Hall
34. Kleinbaum D, Klein M (2005) *Survival Analysis: A Self-Learning Text*. New York: Springer.
35. Collet D (1994) *Modelling Survival Data in Medical Research*. Boca Raton, FL: Chapman & Hall/CRC.
36. Derksen S, Keselman HJ (1992) Backward, forward and stepwise automated subset selection algorithms: frequency of obtaining authentic and noise variables. *British Journal of Mathematical and Statistical Psychology* **45**: 265–82.
37. Anderson DR (2008) *Model Based Inference in the Life Sciences: A Primer on Evidence*. New York: Springer.
38. Joliffe IT (1992) Principal component analysis and factor analysis. *Statistical Methods in Medical Research* **1**: 69–95.
39. Costello AB, Osborne JW (2005) Best practices in exploratory factor analysis: four recommendations for getting the most from your factor analysis. *Practical Assessment, Research and Evaluation* **5**: 1–9.
40. Thomas S, Leese M, Walsh E, *et al.* (2005) A comparison of statistical models in predicting violence in psychotic illness. *Comprehensive Psychiatry* **46**: 296–303.
41. Everrit B, Landau S, Leese M (2001) *Cluster Analysis*, 4th edn. London: Edward Arnold.
42. Everitt BS, Dunn G (2001) *Applied Multivariate Data Analysis*. London: Edward Arnold.
43. Tabachnick BG, Fidell LS (2007) *Using Multivariate Statistics*, 5th edn. Boston, MA: Allyn & Bacon.
44. Sutton AJ, Abrams KR, Jones DR, Sheldon TA, Song F (2002) *Methods for Meta-Analysis in Medical Research*. New York: John Wiley & Sons.
45. Rosenthal R (1991) *Meta-Analytic Procedures for Social Research*. Newbury Park, CA: Sage.
46. Davies HTO, Crombie IK (2001) What is a systematic review? *Bandolier* **1**: 1–6.
47. Egger M, Davey Smith G, Altman DG (2003) *Systematic Reviews in Health Care: Meta-Analysis in Context*. London: BMJ Books.
48. Lewis S, Clarke M (2001) Forest plots: trying to see the wood and the trees. *British Medical Journal* **322**: 1479–80.

Chapter 5

Epidemiology

Stephen Stansfeld and Charlotte Clark

INTRODUCTION

Epidemiology is the study of health in relation to populations. Succinctly, it has been described as the basic quantitative science of public health. It differs from clinical medicine in that the results of epidemiological research have relevance to public health with consequences for health at the level of the population rather than the individual. It has been described as the study of the distribution and determinants of health-related states or events in specified populations and the application of this to the control of health problems.

Epidemiological methods have a number of useful functions: to describe the burden of illness in a population; to elucidate the aetiology of disease and biological dysfunction; to test the effectiveness of health interventions; and to assess need for services.

Historically, psychiatric epidemiology began to develop from purely descriptive to analytical epidemiology, aimed at understanding the aetiology of disorders in the mid-1970s.[1] This began with empirical work on improving the reliability of psychiatric diagnoses, shown in the 1960s to be very unreliable. In the US/UK comparative diagnostic study, rates of schizophrenia in New York and London, which were thought to be very different, were found to be similar when standard methods of diagnosis were used in both settings. Operational criteria for a range of disorders were then developed and standardized psychiatric interviews were used to identify specific psychiatric disorders. Diagnoses such as schizophrenia were also strengthened by genetic adopted-away studies, which confirmed genetic rather than solely cultural transmission of disease between generations.[2] An important study of the time was the World Health Organization (WHO) International Pilot Study of Schizophrenia (IPSS), which found that a core syndrome of schizophrenia could be diagnosed reliably in different settings across the world by using a standardized psychiatric interview. More recent studies have questioned whether schizophrenic syndromes are equally frequent across cultures, but at the time this study greatly increased confidence in pursuing cross-cultural epidemiological research. This led to developing new diagnostic instruments that could be administered by interviewers without clinical training in large epidemiological field studies, such as the Epidemiologic Catchment Area Study (ECA) in the 1980s. This was followed in the 1990s by the National Co-morbidity Survey (NCS) and its replication study (NCS-R). Genetic epidemiology has progressed from family, twin and adoption designs to linkage including whole-genome studies. Analytical epidemiology has made substantial progress, for instance identifying, for schizophrenia, genetic inheritance, obstetric complications and, intriguingly, urban and winter birth as risk factors.

The advantages of studying an illness in a population rather than a clinical sample are several. Clinical samples, especially those seen in psychiatric out-patient and in-patient settings, are often the more severe or complex cases. Epidemiological samples give a better idea of distribution of the full range of illness severity, including milder cases, that may be helpful for understanding disease aetiology, and results found in epidemiological samples can be applied to the population from which they were taken. The type of bias observed through the choice of a sample of patients recruited from a health services source, to do with the selection processes involved in referral to health services, is called Berkson's bias.

Epidemiological studies are often used in determining causation of disease, where the potential aetiological or causal variables are referred to as the 'exposure', to be related to the dependent variable, the illness 'outcome'.

RATES OF DISEASE

The distribution of illness in a population is expressed in terms of rates of disease, which allow the frequency of diseases to be compared within and across populations (Box 5.1). There are two important rates: the prevalence rate and the incidence rate. Prevalence rate assesses the proportion of a specified illness or condition in a defined population. Point prevalence refers to the prevalence of illness at a specific point in time (e.g. on a census day), whereas period prevalence refers to the number of cases counted during a longer period (e.g. 6 months).

Prevalence is distinguished from incidence because incidence rates include the time dimension (see Box 5.1).

Box 5.1 Rates of disease

- *Rate of disease:* frequency of state or event/number of population at risk
- *Prevalence rate:* proportion of a defined population having a condition at any one time
- *Incidence rate:* proportion of a defined population developing a condition within a stated period.

Hence, incidence rates deal with the number of new cases or episodes of illness developing in a population over a unit time, usually a year. Strictly, for entirely new cases of an illness, the term 'inception rate' rather than 'incidence rate' is correct because incidence may include recurrent episodes.

Rates are always expressed in relation to the population at risk as the denominator. In other words, the denominator is specified as the population that is potentially at risk of developing the illness. For example, prevalence rates of Alzheimer's disease will be expressed as a proportion of the elderly population – it would make no sense to include children in the at-risk population.

Types of study in epidemiology

Epidemiological data can be collected either through new studies or by using routine statistical data. Useful routine data include statistics on mortality and cause of death drawn from death certificates, which can be accessed in the UK from the National Health Service (NHS Central) Registry and have nearly complete data on deaths. Other routine sources of data include the national cancer registry and birth certificates. In some areas, detailed systematic information is collected on health service attendees, including diagnoses, as a case register. When these data are complete and relate to a specific geographical area, they can be very useful for assessing burden of disease and trends in incidence of diagnosed disease. However, routine data sources should be treated cautiously, as there are often missing data. Usually, in order to understand the aetiology of a psychiatric disorder, it is necessary to carry out an epidemiological study. Broadly, studies may be either cross-sectional or longitudinal. Cross-sectional studies include straightforward prevalence studies and analytical case–control studies. Longitudinal studies include incidence and cohort studies.

Cross-sectional studies

A cross-sectional study is a study in which any association between two factors relates to a single point in time. Their uses include estimating needs for health services, providing statistics for health education, and screening for undiagnosed disease. Cross-sectional studies are quicker and cheaper than longitudinal studies, can be applied to the relevant population, and investigate hypotheses that are relevant at that point in time. Their disadvantages are that it is difficult to interpret associations in terms of causation, they are not suitable for rare or short-duration diseases, and they provide no estimate of incidence. They can, however, provide prevalence estimates, although these may be biased by movers in or out of the study area.

Case–control studies

In case–control studies, a type of cross-sectional study, a representative group of cases is compared with a group without disease that is representative of the population from which the cases derive. Unlike in observational cross-sectional studies, subjects are sampled on disease rather than exposure. All possible eligible cases should have an equal likelihood of selection; for example, patients with depression who undergo cognitive-behavioural therapy (CBT) could be matched to a control group of patients with depression who do not undergo CBT. Controls are then matched to cases either on an individual or a group basis. Matching is typically carried out for age, sex and sometimes social class, depending on the study. If subjects are inadvertently matched on a factor that is part of the study question, this is referred to as 'overmatching'.

As the selection of subjects is based on cases, this study design is useful for rare diseases, can involve screening for a wide range of possible risk factors and expensive or time-consuming tests, can test current hypotheses, and is not biased by dropout over time. This type of study is often seen as 'quick and dirty', as there is scope for bias in the selection of cases and controls, measurement bias and recall bias (see below for discussion of bias).

Longitudinal studies

In longitudinal studies, also referred to as prospective studies, a group of people are studied over a period of time. Certain characteristics are determined at the beginning of the study, and the incidence of disease in the group is then observed. This is a classical incidence study. Alternatively, in a cohort study, a group of subjects is studied at baseline and then followed up with recurrent waves of data collection, which collects data on new exposures and outcomes. Examples are the British Birth Cohort Studies that follow up a sample born in a week in 1946, 1958, 1970 and 2000.[3,4] A specialized form of cohort studies are occupational cohorts, where a group employed in the same organization is followed up over time (e.g. Whitehall II Study of civil servants[5]) or populations with special exposures are followed (e.g. victims of a disaster followed up for post-traumatic stress disorder[6]). The advantage of longitudinal studies over cross-sectional studies is that incidence rate can be measured, the longitudinal association of exposures and outcomes is more likely to indicate causation, and the longitudinal observation of cases gives a truer picture of severity, fatality, impact of therapy, and social class distribution of disease. Importantly, risk factor assessment at baseline is unbiased by presence of disease that develops by follow-up. Additionally, information about changing risk factor states may be obtained, and information given by subjects is not open to bias. However, these studies are expensive, gathering of results is slow, and refusals and dropouts may introduce bias. It is also difficult to maintain constant measurement techniques over time with changes in study researchers. In incidence studies, there is a need to test fixed hypotheses, and this design is not suitable for rare diseases.

Clinical trials

The intervention study or clinical trial can provide higher-quality data than observational studies because the investigator randomly allocates the exposure status (treatment) of the participants, thus ensuring greater validity to the results. Participants are randomly allocated to 'treatment' or 'control' groups. It is slightly more complex than that because intervention studies may be therapeutic (determining the ability of a treatment to diminish symptoms, prevent recurrence or decrease mortality) or preventive (testing whether a procedure can reduce the risk of developing a disease). Subjects are selected from an experimental population in which the trial is to be carried out; this will be a subset of the reference population to whom the results of the trial would be expected to apply. It is essential to select a large enough sample to give sufficient power to test the hypotheses and a sample that has enough outcomes (e.g. recovery from depression) to allow meaningful comparisons between the study groups within the study follow-up period.

Study subjects are invited to take part, having been informed of the nature of the study and the fact that they may be allocated to a control group without the active treatment. Potential participants are then screened to ensure they fit the inclusion criteria or may be ruled out on the basis of predefined exclusion criteria; such criteria control the population sampled in the study. Randomization of subjects to intervention or control group should be carried out in a double-blind fashion, so that neither the subject nor the investigator is aware of which group they are in. This reduces bias related to the subject's report and bias in the investigator's assessment of outcomes that could be influenced by knowledge of whether the subject was in the treatment or control groups (observation bias). This might also influence allocation to treatment or control group (e.g. investigators might tend to allocate more severe cases to the treatment rather than the control group). Another advantage of randomization is that groups will be similar in background and both known and unknown confounding variables.

A type of non-randomized intervention study uses a historical control group in which a group of patients allocated a new treatment is compared with a group that received an earlier, less advanced treatment. If the new treatment is much more effective than the old treatment, then a difference may be observed. However, if the difference between the groups is small, then it may be difficult to be certain whether the new treatment is more effective because of confounding by changes over time in patient populations, diagnoses or other treatments.

Compliance is an important issue, as non-compliance with, for example, a drug treatment will weaken the difference between treatment and control groups. Similarly, it is important to minimize dropout from the trial; frequent contact between investigators and participants can help to avoid this. To reduce bias in analysis, all subjects must be included (not excluding dropouts) in what is called 'intention to treat' analysis – 'once randomized, always analysed' – otherwise there may be a temptation to exclude subjects with less favourable outcomes.[7]

The progress of epidemiological knowledge is not straightforwardly linear. Often results of studies on the same topic are contradictory or show varying strengths of association between risk factors and outcomes. Observational studies may be subject to unmeasured confounding factors and may be contradicted by the results of randomized controlled trials (RCTs). How should the results of such a bewildering array of scientific knowledge be synthesized? Systematic reviews of the literature attempt to bring together all relevant studies on a topic by scanning the range of relevant databases (e.g. PubMed, PsycINFO, Web of Science), including those papers that fulfil predetermined quality criteria and then summarizing the results narratively or statistically. Where studies have comparable estimates of the magnitude of effects, these can be combined to give a summary measure of size of effect through a technique called meta-analysis. Pooled estimates of magnitude of effects are extremely useful as summary measures and are usually accompanied by measures of heterogeneity showing how consistent these effects are across studies and subgroups, such as by gender or age.

Selecting a sample

In epidemiological studies, it is important to select a sample that is representative of the population you are studying. The simplest method is to use random sampling to randomly select a sample from a defined population, so that all individuals within the population of interest should have an equal chance of being surveyed. This, however, is often difficult to achieve; the approach usually taken instead is to define a population that is thought to be representative of the population of interest and to sample from within this population. Bias can occur in the selection of the population fairly easily; for example, people who have an interest in the topic you are researching are more likely to participate in the study; alternatively, the use of a Web-based survey to collect data rules out the participation of people who do not have access to a computer. If you need greater numbers of one population group in your sample, then you may want to oversample in certain groups (e.g. women or elderly people) and you may use stratified sampling with a higher proportion or 'sampling fraction' from the specific groups. Samples are usually selected from a convenient source of names that covers the relevant population – a sampling frame – such as the electoral roll, general practice age–sex registers and postcode address files.

Bias

There are several important types of bias or potential error in epidemiological studies that you need to be aware of because they may lead to misleading results. In *selection bias*, errors arise from the initial identification of the study population – for instance, where the rate of response to the study is related to exposure status; this may be particularly an issue when control subjects are recruited from groups of students or staff or from newspaper advertisements.[8] *Observation (information) bias* results from a systematic difference in the way information on exposure or outcome is obtained from subjects. *Recall bias* refers to ill individuals recalling previous exposures differently from controls. A classic example of recall bias relates to studies of life events and depression, where individuals with depression tend to remember more negative life events, which non-depressed individuals forget or do not report. *Interview bias* involves bias in the interviewer's technique contingent on the interviewer knowing the disease status of subject; for example, if interviewers are aware of the case status of subjects, they may consciously or unconsciously put more or less effort into getting information on exposure variables. Control of bias may involve precautions taken in the study design, the choice of study population and the methods of data collection and can be addressed in the analysis of results.

Measurement in psychiatry

The easiest measuring instruments to use in psychiatry are self-report questionnaires, either as screening questionnaires for psychological distress, for example the General Health Questionnaire (GHQ) and the Malaise Scale, or for specific conditions, for example the Beck Depression Inventory (BDI), the Hospital Anxiety and Depression Scale (HADS) and the Center for Epidemiologic Studies Depression Scale (CES-D). The advantage of these scales is that they can be used as a continuous score for analysis, although they may not be normally distributed. The disadvantage is that they do not yield diagnoses.

Diagnostic agreement measured by kappa, intraclass correlations and Cronbach's alpha

It is important to ensure that such instruments are reliable. Reliability is of basically two types. One type of reliability refers to the internal consistency of the scale – whether the items on the scale are all measuring the same underlying dimension – assessed by high item–total score correlations, or *Cronbach's alpha*. The other type of reliability is retest reliability: does the test give the same score if it is repeated in the same individuals after a time interval? This is more relevant for dimensions that remain stable over time (e.g. neuroticism) rather than those that change (e.g. depressed mood).

Cronbach's alpha produces a value between 0 and 1. Typically, a value of 0.6 or higher is regarded as indicating adequate reliability, although ideally a value of 0.8 or higher should be sought. It is important to appreciate that the value of alpha will increase with the number of items in a scale.

Psychiatrists frequently measure various characteristics of individuals by the use of inventories, scales and measurements, making it necessary to measure the degree to which there is agreement between the raters undertaking the assessment. This is known as *inter-rater reliability*. The two most commonly used tests are described below.

The *kappa statistic* is used to assess agreement between two observers and an outcome. For example, if two psychiatrists both assess the same 30 patients for a diagnosis of schizophrenia, what is the extent of the agreement between them? Kappa assesses the reliability between the observers. Kappa can range from −1 to +1: −1 indicates no agreement at all between the two psychiatrists' diagnoses, 0 that there is agreement between the two psychiatrists but that this is not greater than the agreement we would expect by chance, and +1 that there is perfect agreement between the diagnoses for the psychiatrists. The significance of kappa is determined by a rule of thumb that states that agreement between observers should be at least 0.6 or higher if possible.

If there are more than two observers and with interval data, *intraclass correlation* (ICC) is used to assess agreement between observers. ICC compares the variability of different ratings of the same individual with the total variation in ratings across all the observers and individuals – that is, the variability of ratings for patient A are compared with the total variation across all the patients and all the observers. Like kappa, ICC produces an estimate that ranges from −1 to +1: it approaches +1 when there is little variability – that is, when the ratings for the individual patients are similar across observers. It is unusual to observe negative values in ICC.

In epidemiological research, case identification is important in counting the number of people with psychiatric disorders for assessing service need and changes in rates of illness. In most areas of psychiatry, there are no objective tests of psychiatric diagnosis such as raised blood sugar is for diabetes mellitus. Psychiatric diagnosis relies on clinical interview. In the past, different psychiatrists would have a range of diagnoses for the same patient. In other words, diagnoses had low reliability, where several assessors disagree in rating the same subjects; this is referred to as low inter-rater reliability. This has led to the development of internationally agreed systems of diagnosis based on symptoms such as the *International Classification of Diseases*, version 10 (ICD-10), championed by WHO, and the *Diagnostic and Statistical Manual of Mental Disorders*, 4th edition (DSM-IV), championed by the USA. Standardized interviews have been devised to gather data on symptoms in a systematic way in order to make diagnoses, such as the Present State Examination (PSE) and its successor Schedules for Clinical Assessment in Neuropsychiatry (SCAN), the Diagnostic Interview Schedule (DIS) and the Composite International Diagnostic Interview (CIDI). These interviews are often semi-structured, with screening questions that, if acknowledged, are followed up by additional probe questions. Such interviews require extensive training and are predicated on the interviewer being clinically trained. Increasingly, these interviews have been developed as fully structured, eliminating the need for interviewer discretion to enable their use by less expensive lay interviewers.

As well as reliability, an instrument needs to have validity – that is, does it measure accurately what it is supposed to measure? Face validity and content validity refer to whether the instrument appears to measure what you want to capture. Construct validity and discriminant validity relate to the instrument measuring the underlying construct but not other similar constructs. For instance, a valid measure of depression should not be measuring neuroticism or lack of social support. An important form of validity in psychiatry is criterion validity. In this, the sensitivity and specificity of a newly developed instrument are usually compared against a criterion, a so-called 'gold standard'. These gold-standard criteria are hard to find in psychiatry but often refer to a standardized psychiatric interview against which a simpler questionnaire is being assessed. Sensitivity of an instrument indicates the extent to which it identifies true positive cases of the illness. Those true cases of illness not identified by the test are false negatives and, together with true positives, comprise 100 per cent of cases. Specificity refers to the extent to which the instrument identifies true negatives, or non-cases of disease. Those who score positively on the screening instrument but who do not have the illness are false positives; this is often a fault of screening instruments for common mental disorders that tend to exaggerate the true prevalence of disorder. Together, true negatives and false positives comprise 100 per cent of non-cases. There are two other useful indices of the precision of an instrument. The positive predictive value (PPV) is the probability that a person actually has the illness given a positive test on the instrument. In contrast, the negative predictive value (NPV) is the probability that a person is free of the illness given an illness-free score on the instrument.

Increasingly, it is being recognized that psychiatric symptoms tend to fluctuate over time and may be transient indicators of more stable underlying latent traits or constructs. These underlying latent constructs may not be directly measurable and require sophisticated life-course analyses to identify them.[9] These underlying constructs may constitute endophenotypes that are linked more strongly to underlying genes than are symptoms or conventional psychiatric syndromes.

It is important to assess whether an association may be subject to bias. This may be due to *confounding*. A confounding factor is one that is associated with the exposure and also associated independently with the outcome and introduces a source of error that either diminishes or magnifies the true association. The association of the confounding factor with the outcome may not be causal, for example age and sex as confounding factors. It is important to adjust for confounding factors in analysis in order to see how much they may explain the association.

Descriptive and inferential statistics

Significance tests are used to evaluate numerical data, including categorical, ordinal and interval data, to test specific hypotheses between variables/measures. For example, imagine we are testing the hypothesis that, within a sample, females report higher rates of depression than males. Wherever there is a hypothesis, there is also a *null hypothesis* – which in this case would be that there are no differences between males and females in reports of depression.

Significance tests evaluate whether the results of a study are likely to have happened by chance. When epidemiological studies report the statistical significance of associations between variables, this is based on the P value. Levels of significance that are typically employed in epidemiological studies are 5 per cent ($P \leq 0.05$), 1 per cent ($P \leq 0.01$) and 0.1 per cent ($P \leq 0.001$), indicating, respectively, that the observed relationship between variables has a 5 in 100, 1 in 100 and 1 in 1000 probability of being due to chance. The lower the P value, the more certainty that the result is not due to chance. So, for example, if we found that females reported higher rates of depression than males and we found $P \leq 0.001$, we could be fairly certain that a gender difference did exist and we would accept our hypothesis that females report higher rates of depression than males. If the P value was greater than 0.05, this would indicate that there was no significant difference between males and females, and we would accept the null hypothesis. Note that the latter finding would be described as 'non-significant' in the text, not 'insignificant' – a frequently made lexical error.

In accepting and rejecting hypotheses, two types of error can be made. The first, known as a *type I error*, occurs when the null hypothesis is rejected even though it is true. In our example, this would mean that we would conclude that there was a gender difference in reports of depression, when actually there was not. The second, known as a *type II error*, occurs when we incorrectly reject the hypothesis and accept the null hypothesis. In our example, this would mean we would conclude that there was no gender difference, when there actually was. A type I error is most likely to occur when the P value that we are willing to accept is set high; type I errors can be avoided by setting a lower P value and thereby reducing the probability of chance findings. Conversely, type II errors are more likely when we set a very low P value. The standard approach to balance the chance of making type I and type II errors is to set $P \leq 0.05$.

When a population has been sampled randomly, results can be generalized reasonably accurately to the entire population from which the sample was drawn by the use of confidence intervals (CIs). Confidence intervals define the range of values within which the true estimate for the parameter must lie. Confidence intervals are expressed as percentages, so the commonly used metric of 95 per cent confidence intervals indicates that we can be 95 per cent sure that the estimate lies within the intervals. Epidemiological research often reports the 95 per cent confidence intervals for odds ratios, derived from logistic regressions. For example, a reported logistic regression analysis of the 1958 British Birth Cohort found that females were more likely to have a depressive episode at 45 years of age than males, with the odds ratio reported as 1.85 and the 95 per cent confidence intervals as 1.33 to 2.57.[4] Although the overall odds for the statistical analysis is 1.85, the confidence intervals indicate that we have 95 per cent certainty that the true odds lies between 1.33 and 2.57 – that is, there is a 5 per cent margin of error. The significance of logistic regression analyses is evaluated by assessing whether the confidence intervals include 1. In the example above, being female has a significant effect on depressive episode at 45 years of age, as the confidence intervals range from 1.33 to 2.57. If the odds ratios crossed 1, for example from 0.97 to 2.57, then there would be no significant effect of being female on reports of depressive episode. If the confidence intervals covered a range below 1, for example from 0.26 to 0.94, then this would indicate support for the hypothesis that males were more likely than females to report a depressive episode.

The width of a confidence interval is affected by the size of the sample under investigation. If confidence intervals become very wide, this suggests that the estimates are unreliable, which is usually associated with a small sample that lacks power. Ideally, confidence intervals should be fairly narrow in their range, indicating that the sample is large enough for reliable estimates to be produced. Confidence intervals can be derived for many different types of estimate, including odds ratios, relative risk, proportions, means and percentages.

The main advantage of confidence intervals over P values, which makes them particularly attractive to epidemiologists, is that they permit the range of true estimates to be derived, enabling the effect size of the relationship between variables to be identified: confidence intervals enable the highest and lowest true estimate to be identified. In the example above, from the P value analyses, we would know only that we were more likely to see more females than males with depression; from the confidence intervals, we would know that we were likely to see between 1.33 and 2.57 times more females than males, which may alter how resources are allocated.

Specific statistical tests

Different statistical tests are used to determine relationships between variables of different types of data, such as categorical/discrete, continuous and ordinal. *Descriptive statistics* are used to describe the data collected in a study or experiment, as opposed to inferential statistics, which use the data to draw inferences about the population. Epidemiological studies typically employ a *within-subject* approach to analyses, focusing on describing and assessing differences across the subjects within the study population. For example, a birth cohort study may make comparisons between males and females, or between people in employment and people not in employment. All the subjects are from the same population. Another commonly used approach is the *between-subject* approach, which is a more experimental method in which two or more populations are compared with each other. For example, an RCT compares subjects who receive the intervention with subjects who do not receive the intervention.

Tests exist for both of these types of study, ranging from tests that simply provide estimates that describe the data (e.g. means, measures of central tendency) to tests that compare differences in outcomes between groups, such as males versus females. Many tests describe the associations between variables (e.g. that depression is associated with life events) but are limited in terms of being able to draw conclusions about the strength of association or causality between variables. This section describes some commonly used and encountered statistical tests within epidemiology.

Descriptive statistics for categorical data

The chi-squared (χ^2) measure of association/goodness of fit is based on evaluating the *distribution of observed data*. The test is most often used to analyse data from independent samples, as in the contingency table in Table 5.1; the term 'independent' means that each individual in the sample can appear in only one of the four cells. The test assesses *goodness of fit*, which is the test of the null hypothesis that there is no significant difference between the observed frequencies in the cells. In this example, the null hypothesis would be that there is no difference between current rates of

Table 5.1 Example contingency table showing the frequency of reports of current depression by previous depression

	No current depression	Current depression	Total (N)
No previous depression	50	40	90
Previous depression	30	60	90

depression for people who have and people who have not experienced depression before.

The most commonly used test is Pearson's χ^2 test, which is applied to normally distributed data. If the P value for the test is above the level of significance, which is conventionally set as $P \leq 0.05$, then the null hypothesis is accepted. If $P \leq 0.05$, then the null hypothesis would be rejected and we would conclude that there was a significant association between previous and current depression. One disadvantage of the χ^2 test for epidemiologists is that it does not tell us where the difference lies between the different cells in the contingency table: the test simply identifies that there is a significant association.

Descriptive statistics for continuous data

Most inferential statistical tests (see Inferential statistics, below) require that data be *normally distributed*. This means that the mean, mode and median have the exact same value and are located in the centre of a symmetrical distribution.

Variance measures the degree to which the value for each individual in the sample differs from the mean for the whole sample, thus assessing variability within the data. Variance is always a positive number, as any negative numbers, which can result from an individual scoring lower than the mean, are squared. Calculating variance is the first step in calculating the *standard deviation*, which is the square root of the variance. Standard deviations are usually reported wherever mean scores are reported, as they indicate the spread of the scores from the mean value.

Confidence intervals have two further popular uses in epidemiology. The first is as a means of describing the range within which the true value of a mean, proportion or median lies for the sample. Confidence intervals can also be derived for assessing the difference between two estimates of means, proportions and medians. This test assumes that the two samples have the same variance and are independent and that the data are normally distributed. The test involves deriving the estimate for each group, for example males and females, calculating the standard error of the difference between the two groups, and then deriving the confidence intervals by computing the estimate for the group of interest (e.g.) females $\pm$ 1.96 $\times$ standard error. 1.96 is the value to use for 95 per cent confidence intervals and 2.58 the value to use for 99 per cent confidence intervals.

Inferential statistics

Inferential tests are applied to the data to enable researchers to draw inferences and make assumptions about the population under study.

t-Tests are applied to test the difference in mean scores between two samples. These can be independent samples, such as the difference in the mean score on a depression scale for males and females, or they can be dependent, such as the difference in a depression scale score for the same sample of people before and after an intervention such as CBT. The *t*-statistic relies upon knowing the mean, standard deviation and number in each of the samples and requires that the data be normally distributed. The P value is used to evaluate whether the hypothesis that there is a significant difference between the mean scores is supported or refuted.

Where the data are not normally distributed and are from independent samples, the *Mann–Whitney U test* may be used instead. This test assumes only that the distributions from the two independent samples be of a similar shape, not that they be normally distributed. The test produces a U-statistic and a P value.

t-Tests can be used only where there are two samples to be compared. Where there are more than two samples, analyses of variance (ANOVAs) can be used. Unlike *t*-tests, which assess mean scores, an ANOVA compares the variance of scores across the different samples. ANOVAs are appropriate where data are interval, ratio or ordinal; independent; and normally distributed. ANOVAs produce an F-statistic and a P value.

Epidemiologists frequently employ *regression* techniques to develop complex models that examine the role of a predictor variable or several predictor variables on an outcome variable. For example, air pollution levels near schools may be used to predict asthma in children, and smoking behaviour may be examined in relation to mortality or heart disease. Such techniques are extremely useful for analysis of longitudinal datasets, where predictors from earlier in life can be examined as predictors of later outcomes.

Regression techniques exist for a range of types of outcome data, including continuous and categorical data, and data that measure the time taken for an event measured as a binary outcome to occur, for example mortality or disease onset. Continuous-outcome data, such as a score on a test, are analysed using *linear regression*; categorical data are analysed using *logistic regression*; and time-to-event binary data are analysed using *Poisson* or *Cox regression*, the latter also being known as *survival analysis*.

One of the main advantages of regression techniques is that confounding factors can be included in the model, along with the predictor variables. This means that the association between the predictor and the outcome can be examined after taking into account other important factors. For example, if a researcher examines the association between smoking behaviour and heart disease, they may want to adjust for other lifestyle factors such as diet and socioeconomic factors, as well as gender and age.

Another attraction for epidemiologists of regression techniques is that regression techniques result in estimates of the size of the effect of the predictor on the outcome. Knowing the size of the influence of the predictor on the outcome is important for public health.

Factor analysis is a data-reduction technique that examines the underlying structure of a set of variables, using the variance between the variables. Factor analysis identifies traits from the intervariable correlation matrix between variables. Factor analysis requires that data are continuous: categorical data cannot be factor analysed, and typically this analysis is conducted on data that are collected using Likert scales.

Factor analysis is usually used to examine or identify unobserved latent traits or factors within datasets. For example, if the individual items on the Big 5 personality inventory were factor analysed, the result would be five different factors, or latent traits, of personality – neuroticism, conscientiousness, openness, extraversion and agreeableness. This is an example where the traits or factors are already known to the researcher. Factor analysis can also be used to identify factors where the researcher has not a priori identified the traits. For example, a number of continuous variables that measure attitudes towards antidepressant use could be factor analysed to identify the underlying structure of attitudes. It can be problematic to identify factors from the analysis; one approach, which has its critics and supporters, is to use *eigenvalues*, which identify the total variance that the factor accounts for in the analyses: factors with eigenvalues greater than 1 are typically thought to be worth examining. Factor scores can also be derived from the analysis, giving an estimate of each respondent's score for the factor, which can be used in further analysis.

Principal components analysis (PCA) is a similar data-reduction technique to factor analysis that also requires continuous data. PCA makes different mathematical assumptions about the nature of the relationship between the variables. PCA is usually used where the researcher wishes to reduce the number of variables in an analysis but to explain the same amount of variance, whereas factor analysis is used where underlying unobserved factors or latent constructs are of interest.

EPIDEMIOLOGY OF SPECIFIC PSYCHIATRIC DISORDERS

National surveys, such as the National Survey of Adults in Private Households carried out in the UK in 1993, 2000 and 2007, give useful estimates of the prevalence of psychiatric disorders (Table 5.2). In the USA, these include such surveys as the Epidemiologic Catchment Area (ECA) studies in the 1980s[10] and the National Comorbidity Survey (NCS) conducted in 1990–92 and its replication survey carried out in 2001–03 (Table 5.3). Rates of disorder differ between these studies, depending on the measuring instruments used, the study procedure, the choice of sample, and secular changes in rates of disorder. For instance, prevalence rates of psychiatric disorder were considerably higher in NCS than in

Table 5.2 Prevalence of psychiatric disorder in the UK general population: psychiatric morbidity among adults living in private households (2000)

	Total (%)	Women (%)	Men (%)
Neurotic disorder	16.4	19.4	13.5
Mixed anxiety and depression	8.8	10.8	6.8
Generalized anxiety disorder	4.4	4.6	4.3
Depressive episode	2.6	2.8	2.3
Psychotic disorder	0.5	0.5	0.6
Alcohol dependence	7.4	2.9	11.9

From Singleton *et al.*[13]

Table 5.3 Prevalence of psychiatric disorder in the National Comorbidity Survey Replication

Type of disorder	12-month prevalence*	Lifetime prevalence**
Panic disorder	2.7	4.7
Agoraphobia without panic	0.8	1.4
Specific phobia	8.7	12.5
Social phobia	6.8	12.1
Generalized anxiety disorder	3.1	5.7
Post-traumatic stress disorder	3.5	6.8
Obsessive–compulsive disorder	1.0	1.6
Major depressive disorder	6.7	16.6
Dysthymia	1.5	2.5
Bipolar I and II	1.5	3.9
Alcohol abuse	3.1	13.2
Alcohol dependence	1.3	5.4
Drug abuse	1.4	7.9
Drug dependence	0.4	3.0

*Kessler *et al.*;[14] **Kessler *et al.*[15]

the earlier ECA studies – it is unlikely that these changes represented a real increase in prevalence. More recent prevalence surveys include the WHO World Mental Health Survey using the CIDI across 28 countries and finding a broad range of prevalence estimates for mood disorders; the WHO Collaborative Study of Psychological Problems in Primary Care;[11] and the European Study of the Epidemiology of Mental Disorders project (ESEMED).[12]

A brief summary of epidemiological data for specific diagnoses follows.

Schizophrenia

The lifetime prevalence is 4.3 per cent, lifetime risk is 0.72 per cent and adult point prevalence is 4.5 per cent. Incidence of schizophrenia is 15.2 in 100 000. The male/female ratio is 1.4 : 1. Compared with native-born individuals, migrants have an increased incidence and prevalence of schizophrenia. Exposures related to urbanicity, less advantaged economic status and certain latitudes (increased in winter births) are associated with increased risk. People with schizophrenia have a two- to threefold increased risk of dying prematurely compared with the general population (median standardized mortality ratio = 2.6 for all-cause mortality).[16]

Manic–depressive psychosis (bipolar disorder)

Lifetime prevalence of bipolar I disorder in the NCS replication study is 1.0 per cent; 6-month prevalence is 0.6 per cent. Lifetime prevalence of bipolar II disorder is 1.1 per cent and 12-month prevalence is 0.8 per cent.[17] Onset is in late teens to late thirties. Regarding the co-morbidity of lifetime bipolar disorder, 63–87 per cent of patients have a lifetime anxiety disorder, and 35–60 per cent a lifetime substance use disorder. It is related inversely to age, educational level and previous marriage. It is unrelated to sex, ethnicity and income.

Major depression

Lifetime prevalence in the NCS replication study is 16.2 per cent (95% CI: 15.1% to 17.3%). The 6-month prevalence is 6.6 per cent (95% CI: 5.9% cent to 7.3%).[18] The male/female ratio is 2 : 1. Major depressive disorder (MDD) is highly co-morbid, with a 59 per cent risk of a lifetime anxiety disorder and 24 per cent risk of a substance use disorder. The median age of onset is 32 years (interquartile range 19–44 years). Risk factors include negative (loss) life events, low socioeconomic status, physical illness (e.g. coronary heart disease, cancer) and childhood adversities.

Suicide

The prevalence is 16.7/100 000 annually. Suicide makes up 1.5 per cent of all deaths and is the fourteenth leading cause of death.[19] The lifetime prevalence of suicide attempts is 0.4–5.1 per cent. The male/female ratio is between 3 : 1 and 7.5 : 1. There is an increase in non-fatal self-harm in people aged 12–20 years, peaking at age 16 years. Risk factors for completed suicide include male, adolescent, older adult, certain ethnic groups, unemployment, certain psychiatric disorders (depression, impulse-control disorders, alcohol/substance use disorders, psychotic disorders, personality disorder), hopelessness, stressful life events and certain occupations (e.g. military personnel, doctors, pharmacists).

Generalized anxiety disorder

The lifetime prevalence is 4.3, 5.9 per cent. The 12-month prevalence is 1.2–1.9 per cent. The male/female ratio is 1 : 2. Onset is usually before age 25 years. Some 66 per cent of patients have co-morbid major depression; a similar proportion have other anxiety disorders.[20]

Panic disorder

The adult prevalence of panic disorder with agoraphobia is 2–3 per cent; the prevalence is 1 per cent without agoraphobia. The lifetime prevalence is 1–2 per cent. The male/female ratio is 1 : 2. Onset is in late adolescence or early adulthood. Fifty per cent of patients develop depression during their lifetime, and there is an increased risk of suicide. Risk factors include heritability (40%), anxious temperament, anxiety sensitivity, neuroticism, early life trauma and recent life events.

Specific phobias

The adult prevalence is 2–5 per cent. The lifetime prevalence is 7–11 per cent. The male/female ratio is 1 : 2. Onset is usually at 5–8 years.

Agoraphobia

The adult prevalence is 2–3 per cent. The lifetime prevalence is 1.6 per cent. The male/female ratio is 1 : 4. Onset is usually around 18–35 years. It is associated with co-morbid major depression.

Social phobia

The adult prevalence is 4–6 per cent. The lifetime prevalence is 13 per cent. The male/female ratio is 1 : 1.5. Onset is usually in the teens (from 11 years) to early twenties (80% by 20 years). Risk factors include heritable components related to behavioural inhibition and neuroticism.[21]

Obsessive–compulsive disorder

The lifetime prevalence is 2.5 per cent. The 12-month prevalence is 0.7–2 per cent. The male/female ratio is between 1 : 1.5 and 1 : 1. There is increasing incidence with age from 15 years to 35 years; the mean age of onset is 19.5 years. The most common co-morbid conditions are anxiety disorders (75.8%), mood disorders (63.3%), impulse-control disorders (55.9%) and substance use disorders (38%). Sixty-five per cent of patients report severe role impairment.[22]

Post-traumatic stress disorder

The lifetime prevalence is 8 per cent. The 12-month prevalence is 1 per cent. The male/female ratio is 1 : 2.

Alcohol use disorders

The lifetime prevalence is 13.8, 23.5 per cent. The adult 12-month prevalence is 6.8, 7-7 per cent. The male/female ratio is 2 : 1. Alcohol use onset is usually in adolescence and peaks in late adolescence or early adulthood. Risk factors include alcohol-relieving negative affect, stimulating brain reward centres, pharmacological vulnerability, deviance proneness, heritability, parental substance abuse and peer influences. There is co-morbidity with all anxiety and mood disorders, particularly mania, antisocial behaviour disorders and drug use.

Drug dependence

The adult 12-month prevalence is 6.1, 7.5 per cent. The lifetime prevalence is 15 per cent. Eighteen per cent of people with a lifetime major depressive disorder have a substance use disorder. There is a higher risk for bipolar disorder.

Anorexia nervosa

The incidence rate is between 4.7 and 8.3 per 100 000. The lifetime prevalence is 1.2–2.2 per cent. The 12-month prevalence is 0.37 per cent. The 12-month prevalence of bulimia nervosa is 1.5 per cent. The male/female ratio is 1 : 8.[23]

Alzheimer's disease

The incidence rate is 1 per 1000 person-years in people aged 60–64 years, and 25 per 100 person-years in people over 85 years of age. The age-standardized prevalence rate is 4.4 per cent in people over 65 years and 22.2 per cent in people over 90 years. It is more frequent in people of advanced age, females, carriers of the apolipoprotein E4 gene, current smokers, people with a low education, income, and lower occupational status, and family history.

KEY POINTS

- Epidemiological methods can be used to describe the burden of illness in a population, to contribute to disease aetiology, to test the effectiveness of health interventions and to assess need for services.
- Epidemiological studies include cross-sectional (prevalence and case–control) studies and longitudinal (incidence and cohort) studies. Longitudinal studies are better than cross-sectional studies for assessing aetiology.
- Studies may be subject to bias. Observation bias occurs where there is a systematic difference in the way information on exposure or outcome is obtained from subjects. Selection bias relates to non-random selection of subjects. Recall bias refers to ill individuals recalling previous exposures differently from controls.
- The reliability of an instrument refers to the agreement between items making up a scale (internal consistency) and the stability of results over time in the same individuals, assuming no change in the construct measured (retest reliability).
- The criterion validity of an instrument measures how well it compares with an existing gold standard instrument. The sensitivity of an instrument is an index of how well it identifies true positive cases. The specificity of an instrument measures how well it identifies true negatives – that is, individuals without disease. The positive predictive value is the probability that a person actually has the illness given a positive test on the instrument. The negative predictive value is the probability that a person is free of the illness given an illness-free score on the instrument.
- A confounding factor is one that is associated with the exposure and also associated independently with the outcome and introduces a source of error, which either diminishes or magnifies the true association. Confounding can be dealt with either in the design or in the analysis of a study.
- A type I error occurs when the null hypothesis is rejected, even though it is true. A type II error occurs when we incorrectly reject the hypothesis and accept the null hypothesis.

REFERENCES

1. Eaton WW (1999) Psychiatric epidemiology. In H Freeman (ed.) *A Century of Psychiatry*. London: Mosby.
2. Kety SS, Rosenthal D, Wender PH, Schulsinger F, Jacobsen B (1975) Mental illness in the biological and adoptive families of adopted individuals who have become schizophrenic: a preliminary report based on psychiatric interviews. In RR Fieve, D Rosenthal, H Brill (eds) *Genetic Research in Baltimore Psychiatry*. Baltimore, MD: Johns Hopkins Press.
3. Wadsworth M, Kuh D, Richards M, Hardy R (2006) Cohort profile: the 1946 National Birth Cohort (MRC National Survey of Health and Development). *International Journal of Epidemiology* **35**: 49–54.
4. Clark C, Rodgers B, Caldwell T, Power C, Stansfeld S (2007) Childhood and adulthood psychological ill health as predictors of midlife affective and anxiety disorders: the 1958 British Birth Cohort. *Archives of General Psychiatry* **64**: 668–78.
5. Marmot MG, Smith GD, Stansfeld S, *et al.* (1991) Health inequalities among British civil servants: the Whitehall II study. *Lancet* **337**: 1387–93.

6. Van den Berg B, Grievink L, *et al.* (2008) Risk factors for physical symptoms after a disaster: a longitudinal study. *Psychological Medicine* **38**: 499–510.
7. Hennekens CH, Buring JE (1987) *Epidemiology in Medicine.* Philadelphia, PA: Lippincott Williams & Wilkins.
8. Lee W, Bindman J, Ford T, *et al.* (2007) Bias in psychiatric case-control studies: literature survey. *British Journal of Psychiatry* **190**: 204–9.
9. Colman I, Ploubidis GB, Wadsworth ME, Jones PB, Croudace TJ (2007) A longitudinal typology of symptoms of depression and anxiety over the life course. *Biological Psychiatry* **62**: 1265–71.
10. Regier DA, Boyd JH, Burke JD, Jr, *et al.* (1988) One-month prevalence of mental disorders in the United States: based on five Epidemiologic Catchment Area sites. *Archives of General Psychiatry* **45**: 977–86.
11. Ustun TB, Sartorius N (1995) *Mental Illness in General Health Care.* Chichester: John Wiley & Sons.
12. Alonso J, Angermeyer MC, Bernert S, *et al.* (2004) Prevalence of mental disorders in Europe: results from the European Study of the Epidemiology of Mental Disorders (ESEMeD) project. *Acta Psychiatrica Scandinavica* **109**: 21–7.
13. Singleton N, Bumpstead R, O'Brien M, Lee A, Meltzer H (2001) *Psychiatric Morbidity Among Adults Living in Private Households 2000.* London: Office for National Statistics.
14. Kessler RC, Chiu WT, Demler O, Merikangas KR, Walters EE (2005) Prevalence, severity, and comorbidity of 12-month DSM-IV disorders in the National Comorbidity Survey Replication. *Archives of General Psychiatry* **62**: 617–27.
15. Kessler RC, Berglund P, Demler O, *et al.* (2005) Lifetime prevalence and age-of-onset distributions of DSM-IV disorders in the National Comorbidity Survey Replication. *Archives of General Psychiatry* **62**: 593–602.
16. McGrath J, Saha S, Chant D, Welham J (2008) Schizophrenia: a concise overview of incidence, prevalence, and mortality. *Epidemiology Review* **30**: 67–76.
17. Merikangas KR, Akiskal HS, Angst J, *et al.* (2007) Lifetime and 12-month prevalence of bipolar spectrum disorder in the National Comorbidity Survey replication. *Archives of General Psychiatry* **64**: 543–52.
18. Kessler RC, Berglund P, Demler O, *et al.* (2003) National Comorbidity Survey Replication: the epidemiology of major depressive disorder – results from the National Comorbidity Survey Replication (NCS-R). *Journal of the American Medical Association* **289**: 3095–105.
19. Nock MK, Borges G, Bromet EJ, *et al.* (2008) Suicide and suicidal behavior. *Epidemiology Review* **30**: 133–54.
20. Tyrer P, Baldwin D (2006) Generalised anxiety disorder. *Lancet* **368**: 2156–66.
21. Stein MB, Stein DJ (2008) Social anxiety disorder. *Lancet* **371**: 1115–25.
22. Ruscio AM, Stein DJ, Chiu WT, Kessler RC (2008) The epidemiology of obsessive–compulsive disorder in the National Comorbidity Survey Replication. *Molecular Psychiatry* [forthcoming].
23. Hoek HW (2006) Incidence, prevalence and mortality of anorexia nervosa and other eating disorders. *Current Opinions in Psychiatry* **19**: 389–94.

Chapter 6

How to practise evidence-based medicine

Stuart Carney

INTRODUCTION

The practice of evidence-based medicine (EBM), which is the integration of the best available evidence of clinical experience and patient values in patient or clinical decision-making, can be broken down into five steps:[1]

1. Translation of uncertainty to an answerable question.
2. Systematic retrieval of the best available evidence.
3. Critical appraisal of the evidence.
4. Application of the results in practice.
5. Evaluation of performance.

Put another way, to practise EBM, you need to do the following:

1. Ask structured clinical questions.
2. Access the best available evidence.
3. Appraise the evidence.
4. Apply the evidence.
5. Assess performance and patient outcomes.

This chapter systematically considers each of these five steps. It builds upon the earlier chapters in this part on epidemiology and research methods and statistics.

STEP 1: ASK QUESTIONS

Many questions emerge in the course of clinical practice. One model for translating uncertainty into an answerable question is to break it down into four parts known by the acronym PICO:

- Patient
- Intervention (or E for exposure)
- Comparison
- Outcome.

For example, imagine you are faced with the following clinical situation:

Mrs B is a 31-year-old single mother with three primary school-aged children. She has suffered from recurrent episodes of depression since the age of 23 years. The latest depressive episode is severe, she is not eating and she is barely drinking. The treatment options include electroconvulsive therapy (ECT) and antidepressant medication.

We might ask: is ECT more effective and safer than antidepressants in the treatment of a woman with a severe depressive episode? Using the PICO model, we could break down this question into four parts:

- *Patient:* woman with a severe depressive episode
- *Intervention:* ECT
- *Comparison:* antidepressant treatment
- *Outcome:* remission of the depressive symptoms, side effects.

STEP 2: ACCESS THE EVIDENCE

Types of clinical question

Therapy questions, such as ECT versus antidepressants for the treatment of severe depression, are particularly common in clinical practice. However, clinical practice throws up other types of question: diagnosis, prognosis, aetiology and harm. Epidemiology, the study of the distribution and determinants of disease, provides a framework for addressing each type of question. Different types of study are best suited to answering specific types of question. It is essential to determine what type of question is being considered before searching the literature. The more common types of clinical question are described below.

Diagnostic questions (distribution of disease)

The medical paradigm is predicated on making a diagnosis. We seek to determine whether a patient is suffering from an illness and, if so, the exact nature of that illness. This decision-making process is informed by knowledge of the distribution of possible illnesses in the target population. Diagnostic instruments and tests are often used to assist in this process as the clinician seeks to confirm or refute hypotheses (differential diagnoses). As clinicians, we need to stay abreast of the evidence relating to prevalence and the accuracy of diagnostic tests. Cross-sectional studies are used to address these questions.

Prognosis questions

When patients ask what will happen to them, they are asking about their prognosis. Prognosis describes the likely course in a person with specific characteristics.

Aetiology, harm and therapy questions (determinants of disease)

What caused this disease? Is this drug an effective treatment for this disease? These are examples of aetiology, harm or therapy questions. Aetiology questions seek to ascertain what factor or factors caused a diagnosed disease, while therapy and harm questions focus on interventions that may change the course of the disease.

Hierarchy of evidence

The optimal study design to address a particular question depends on the type of question being asked. The pitfalls outlined in Chapter 4 can threaten the validity and importance of any clinical study, but certain designs are potentially better than others. The hierarchy of study architecture for each of the three groups of clinical questions is shown in Table 6.1.

It is also worth reflecting on two specific types of study, which are particularly important to the practice of EBM – systematic reviews and *N*-of-1 studies.

Systematic reviews

In 1979, Archie Cochrane, a British epidemiologist, lamented the failure of the medical profession to 'organise a critical summary, by specialty or subspecialty, adapted periodically, of all relevant randomised controlled trials'.[2] Thirteen years later, the Cochrane Collaboration was founded to 'Prepare, maintain and promote the accessibility of systematic reviews of the effects of health care interventions'. Although systematic review methodology is most advanced for the synthesis of randomized controlled trials (RCTs), the same principles can be applied to any study design. Consistent results from valid and important studies synthesized in a systematic review can provide the best available evidence for all clinical questions.

N-of-1 studies

Evidence-based medicine focuses on the care of the individual patient, while evidence-based healthcare relates to the effects of exposures in groups. It may not be appropriate or possible to apply population-based observations to the care of a particular patient. In certain circumstances, it may be possible to undertake research in partnership with an individual consenting patient. For conditions that are chronic

Table 6.1 Hierarchy of study designs

	Determinants of disease	Prognosis questions	Distribution of disease	
	Therapy, aetiology or harm questions		Diagnosis questions	
			Surveys (prevalence)	Evaluation of diagnostic instruments
1	*N*-of-1 study	Systematic review of cohort studies	Systematic review of cross-sectional surveys	Systematic review of cross-sectional diagnostic studies
2	Systematic review of RCTs	Individual cohort study	Single survey	Individual cross-sectional diagnostic study
3	Individual RCT	Follow-up of untreated control patients in an RCT	Expert opinion	Expert opinion
4	Controlled clinical trial	Case series		
5	Cohort study	Expert opinion		
6	Case–control study			
7	(Cross-sectional study)			
8	(Ecological survey)			
9	Case series			
10	Expert opinion			

RCT, randomized controlled trial.

and the effects of an intervention are transient, we could conduct an *N*-of-1 study.

By definition, the observations will be applicable to the patient under consideration. In an *N*-of-1 study, the patient is sequentially randomized to intervention and placebo and the outcomes assessed. Such a prospective design reduces the risk of performance and measurement bias and allows an assessment of the relative efficacy of an intervention. It is argued that the *N*-of-1 study design is primary for questions of therapeutic effect (therapy).[3]

Searching for the evidence

Having formulated a structured clinical question and determined the optimal study design, it should now be possible to search efficiently for the best available evidence. Developments in information technology, notably the development of electronic databases, have made the practice of EBM possible.

Table 6.2 lists some of the more common databases that may be of use when practising EBM. There are an increasing number of meta-resources, including clinical practice guidelines and evidence-based clinical decision support tools. These provide pre-appraised material addressing common clinical questions. To answer questions not covered by these resources, we must appraise systematic reviews or the original literature.

Electronic databases such as PubMed and Embase are useful resources for searching the scientific literature. PubMed is provided free by the US National Library of Medicine and is North American in focus, while Embase catalogues more European journals. The Cochrane Library includes the Cochrane Reviews, which are regarded as the gold standard for systematic reviews, and the Cochrane Controlled Trials Register (CCTR). The CCTR contains randomized and controlled trials drawn from sensitive searches of a number of databases, including Embase and PubMed.

Most electronic databases use Boolean logic to combine search terms. Table 6.3 provides some useful tips for searching. Returning to the clinical question about ECT, if we wish to find as many of the therapy studies as possible, then we could combine terms using the Boolean operator OR. As ECT is also known as electroshock therapy and electroconvulsive therapy, it would be sensible to search for these terms as well. A comprehensive search for papers on ECT could include the following search terms:

'electroconvuls*' or 'electro-convuls*' or 'electroshock*' or 'electro-shock*' or 'convuls*' or 'ECT'

As we are interested only in ECT for the treatment of a patient with depression, we could combine the ECT terms with search terms for depression. 'Depressive episode' is a synonym for 'depression', but both terms could be identified by truncating depression to 'depress*'. Similarly we could search for synonyms of 'antidepressants'. As we wish to restrict the search to these three criteria, we could use the Boolean operator AND.

Table 6.2 Databases useful in the practice of evidence-based medicine

Critically appraised databases/resources	Other electronic databases
Clinical Practice Guidelines	Cochrane Library
Clinical Evidence	PubMed
Evidence-based Medicine	Embase
Evidence-based Mental Health	PsycINFO
	Biological Abstracts
	Cinahl

Table 6.3 Electronic database search terms and tips

Search term	Notes
AND	Includes only those studies that contain both terms of interest, e.g. both 'depression' and 'ECT'
*	Can be used to search for all studies containing words beginning with the letters before the asterisk (*), e.g. 'depress*' will identify all studies with the words 'depression', 'depressive', etc. anywhere in the citation or abstract
OR	Includes all studies that contain term a, or term b, or both a and b
?	Can be used when various spellings are used for a term, e.g. '?etiology' will search for both 'aetiology' and 'etiology'
NOT	Includes all studies that contain term a, except for those that also contain term b
"..."	Can be used when a specific piece of text is to be searched for, e.g. 'University of Oxford' as a search term will identify only papers with this exact text and not those referring to 'Oxford University'

STEP 3: APPRAISE THE EVIDENCE

Critical appraisal addresses three questions: is the research applicable to my patient, is it valid, and is it important? Before considering the pitfalls in the design and execution of studies, it is worth pausing to consider how to efficiently extract the necessary data from papers.

Read a paper in less than 15 minutes

As busy clinicians, we often have to make rapid judgements. We do not have time to wade through piles and piles of research papers. With practice, it becomes easier to identify quickly which research papers are likely to address our clinical questions.

The title of the paper often gives clues as to whether it is likely to address the question of interest. More detail is given in the abstract. The title and the abstract help us to assess whether the paper is applicable to our patient – that is, whether it addresses our focused clinical question and uses an appropriate study design. Having spent no more than a minute looking at the paper, we should be able to make a judgement as to whether the paper is worth more detailed consideration.

The introduction rarely provides any useful information for critical appraisal, although the hypothesis under consideration or the aim of the study is usually described in the final paragraph. The methods and results sections should provide us with the data needed to critically appraise the paper. Having critically appraised the paper, there should be no need to read the discussion section, as we can draw our own conclusions. This whole process should take no more 15 min.

The GATE frame: critical appraisal with pictures[4]

Rod Jackson and colleagues have proposed a simplified approach to critical appraisal.[4] Inspired by the symbols on the Sony PlayStation®, they have created a frame (Graphic Appraisal Tool for Epidemiological studies, or GATE) comprising a triangle, circle, square and cross, upon which the key components of epidemiological studies can be hung (Figure 6.1).

The triangle represents the three levels of selecting participants for a study. For the ECT study, the source population would comprise patients with severe depression, the eligible population, those who satisfy the inclusion and exclusion criteria, and the sample those who agreed to take part. The circle is divided into two segments: those receiving the intervention (or exposure) and those receiving the

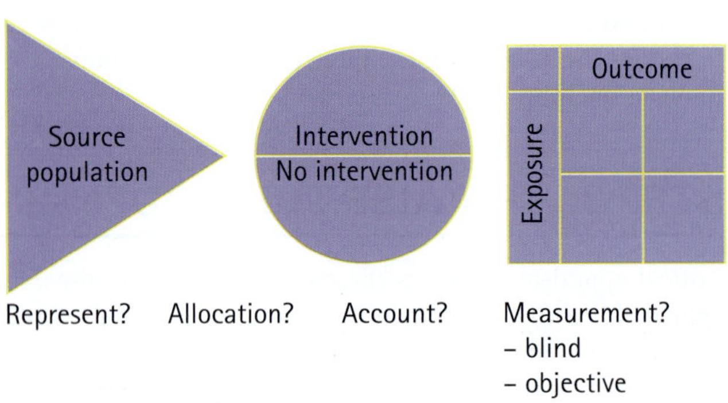

Figure 6.1 The GATE frame

comparison. The square can be broken down into a two-by-two table and is useful when we are interested in dichotomous outcomes (remission or no remission).

The triangle, circle and square serve as a template to guide the extraction of key data about where the participants came from and what happens to them during the course of the study. In parallel, we need to consider the potential pitfalls in the design and execution of the study. The GATE frame proposes that these can be summarized by the acronym RAAMbo.

- *Represent:* this asks the question 'Is my patient sufficiently similar to the participants in this study?' This is also known as generalizability, external validity or applicability.
- *Allocation:* for therapy studies, this considers how the participants were allocated to the intervention and comparison groups. Randomization with allocation concealment seeks to reduce the risk of selection bias, by achieving balance between the two groups with respect to known and unknown risk factors. Imbalance between the intervention and comparison group results in confounding. In prognostic studies, the cohorts are defined by whether or not they have a particular characteristic or exposure. Strategies may be employed to control for known prognostic factors when comparing the two groups in both the assembly (e.g. matching) of the groups and the analysis.
- *Accounted:* ideally, by the end of the study all participants should be accounted for, but this is rarely the case and typically some participants will drop out, switch treatment or be lost to follow-up. To maintain the integrity of the original allocation, attempts should be made to analyse all participants in the group to which they were allocated. This may require us to make judgements about how to handle dropouts (e.g. last observation carried forwards, best case/worst case scenario). Analysing all participants in the group to which they were originally allocated is known as 'intention-to-treat' analysis. Studies that experience a significant difference in dropouts across the two or more arms are prone to bias.
- *Measurement:* measuring outcomes typically requires some subjective judgement, and there is a risk that the outcome assessors may apply different thresholds, depending on whether the participant was allocated to a particular intervention. Blinding is a strategy to reduce the risk of measurement bias, and it is important that the study authors describe who was blinded and how blinding was achieved. There is less scope to make judgements if the outcome measures are objective (e.g. death).

The GATE frame provides a model for extracting data and making judgements about the applicability and validity of the study. If we are satisfied that any failings in the design or execution of the study are not catastrophic and that the study provides the best available evidence, we can turn our attention to the numbers or importance of the study. When dichotomous outcome measures are considered (event or no event), it is possible to calculate measures of effect such as absolute risk reduction (ARR), risk ratio (RR), relative risk reduction (RRR) and number needed to treat (NNT). These terms are described in Table 6.4. The terms ARR and RRR are used when the intervention reduces the risk of adverse events. Absolute benefit increase (ABI) and relative benefit increase (RBI) are more appropriate when considering positive outcomes.

Is it a poor-quality study or a poorly reported study?

There is a danger with critical appraisal that we become cynical about research. Most enterprises involving large numbers of people rarely go exactly to plan. Even the most perfectly designed study will encounter problems in its execution. It is common for participants to withdraw and no longer be available for follow-up.

Mindful that word limits and copy space present researchers and editors with challenges, even the most fundamental information about the conduct of the studies is often omitted. Therefore it is difficult to judge whether the study is of poor quality or just poorly reported.

In an attempt to ensure that readers of the scientific literature are equipped with all of the necessary information, editors and researchers have agreed standards for reporting research. The Consolidated Standards of Reporting Trials (CONSORT) statement recommends that authors and journal editors follow a 22-item checklist when reporting RCTs and use a flow diagram to describe the progress of study participants.[5] Although only 20 per cent of high-impact medical journals refer to the statement in their advice to authors, the quality of reporting of RCTs is improved in journals that have adopted it.[6,7]

Like the CONSORT statement, the Quality of Reporting of Meta-Analyses (QUORUM) statement describes the critical steps in a systematic review and meta-analysis of RCTs.[8] Guidance to authors and editors is not confined to RCTs and meta-analyses: there are also Standards for Reporting of Diagnostic Accuracy (STARD).[9]

STEP 4: APPLY THE EVIDENCE

The best available evidence is only one factor that should be taken into account for patient or clinical decision-making. There are clearly clinical considerations such as the severity of the illness and co-morbid risk factors. Patients, like clinicians, draw upon experience and have opinions and values. We make decisions in the context of healthcare policy, such as what is available in our particular health economy. There may be specific legal considerations that also need to be taken into account, such as the use of ECT when a patient refuses treatment or lacks capacity to give consent.

Clinical expertise is the ability to integrate research evidence and patients' circumstances and preferences in order to help patients arrive at optimal decisions.[1]. This is otherwise known as the X factor (Figure 6.2).[4]

Table 6.4 Effect measures

Term	Definition	How is it calculated?
Control event risk (CER)	Proportion with the event of interest in the control group	Number of events (controls)/total number in control group
Experimental event risk (EER)	Proportion with the event of interest in the intervention group	Number of events (intervention)/total number in intervention group
Absolute risk reduction (ARR)	Difference in risk between the control and experimental groups	ARR = CER – EER
Number needed to treat (NNT)	Number of patients that have to be treated with the intervention in order to prevent one additional person experiencing the adverse event; conventionally, NNT is rounded up	NNT = 1/ARR
Risk ratio (RR)	Risk of experiencing the event in the experimental group relative to the control group	RR = EER/CER
Relative risk reduction (RRR)	Proportion of events that would have been avoided in the control group had they been allocated the intervention	RRR = 1 – RR = ARR/CER

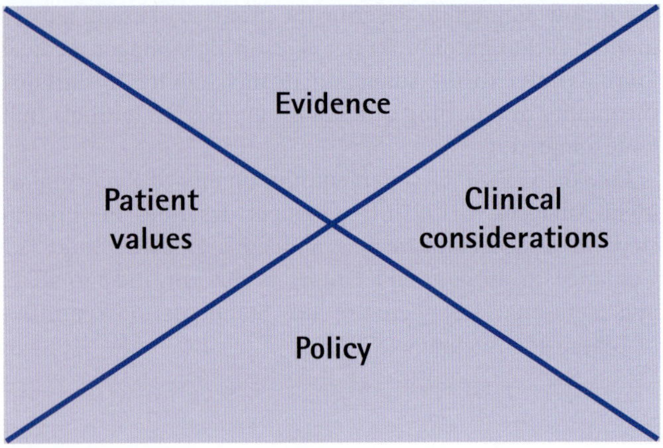

Figure 6.2 eXpertise

STEP 5: ASSESS PERFORMANCE AND PATIENT OUTCOMES

The most neglected step in the practice of EBM is the assessment of performance. As we strive to improve patient safety and care, we must assess whether patients have been helped and then consider what lessons can be learned from the care of individual patients. It may be the case that our review of the evidence focusing on the care of an individual patient highlights opportunities to improve the care of other patients.

REFERENCES

1. Straus S, Richardson W, Glasziou P, *et al.* (2005) *Evidence-Based Medicine: How to Practise and Teach*, 3rd edn. Edinburgh: Churchill Livingston.
2. Cochrane AL (1979) 1931–1971: a critical review, with particular reference to the medical profession. In Teeling-Smith G, Wells N, Office of Health Economics (eds) *Medicines for the Year 2000*. London: Office of Health Economics.
3. Guyatt GH, Haynes RB, Jaeschke RZ, *et al.* (2000) Users' guides to the medical literature XXV: evidence-based medicine – principles for applying the users' guide to patient care. *Journal of the American Medical Association* **284**: 1290–96.
4. Jackson R, Ameratunga S, Broad J, *et al.* (2006) The GATE frame: critical appraisal with pictures. *Evidence-Based Medicine* **11**: 35–8.
5. Moher D, Schulz KF, Altman DG, for the CONSORT Group (2001) The CONSORT statement: revisited recommendations for improving the quality of reports of parallel-group randomized trials. *Lancet* **357**: 1191–4.
6. Altman DG (2005) Endorsement of the CONSORT statement by high impact medical journals: survey of instructions for authors. *British Medical Journal* **330**: 1056–7.
7. Plint AC, Moher D, Morrison A, *et al.* (2006) Does the CONSORT checklist improve the quality of reports of randomised controlled trials? A systematic review. *Medical Journal of Australia* **185**: 263–7.
8. Moher D, Cook DJ, Eastwood S, *et al.* (1999) Improving the quality of reports of meta-analyses of randomized controlled trials: the Quorum statement. *Lancet* **354**: 1896–900.
9. Bossuyt PM, Reitsma JB, Bruns DE, *et al.* (2003) Towards complete and accurate reporting of studies of diagnostic accuracy: the STARD initiative. *British Medical Journal* **326**:41–4.
10. Guyatt G, Cook D, Haynes B (2004) Evidence based medicine has come a long way. *British Medical Journal* **329**: 990–91.

Chapter 7

Psychological assessment and psychometrics

Ann Mortimer

INTRODUCTION

The assessment of mental functions such as memory, concentration, language, intelligence, reasoning and judgement is a cornerstone of psychiatric practice. Impairment is germane to important disorders such as learning disability and the dementias, while there is some relevance to just about every other major diagnosis in psychiatry. It has been demonstrated repeatedly that poor cognitive ability is associated with both increased risk for mental disorder, and poorer personal and social function. A thorough understanding of cognitive function can, therefore, illuminate patient formulation to a surprising degree and may inform management in terms of how the patient can be expected to function in the future. This is particularly consequential for rehabilitation.

This chapter comprises an exposition of cognitive assessment beyond the usual few questions traditionally taught as part of mental state examination and the Mini-Mental State Examination (MMSE).[1] Comprehensive cognitive assessment starts with the taking of a history and examination of the rest of the mental state before formal screening for impairment. This in turn directs attention to more specific areas, or further psychometric tests may be indicated. The recognition of patterns of impairment informs diagnostic possibilities: common associations between specific profiles and the diagnoses which they imply will be given.

TAKING A HISTORY

Intelligence is a reasonable synonym for overall cognitive ability. Even without standard formal measures of intelligent quotient (IQ), a rough estimate can be made from the patient's history and general presentation. It should be possible to distinguish patients likely to be learning disabled (IQ 70, or IQ 75 where there is functional disability) with reasonable confidence.

IQ can be compromised by any significant insult to the brain, from gestation onwards. A history of adverse events in utero, birth complications, head injury, infections and systemic disorder in the preschool years or beyond may all be relevant here. The timescale of achievement of developmental milestones is useful information if available.

The patient's family background is also significant. Children brought up within very socially disadvantaged families or subjected to neglectful or abusive parenting are unlikely to learn as they should, through lack of appropriate stimulation and encouragement. There was previously a diagnosis, now obsolete, of 'subcultural subnormality', in which children assumed to be of ordinary intelligence were unable to manifest the intelligence because their parents were either very unintelligent or neglectful, or both.[2–4] These children could not learn from their parents, and they grew up with poor interest in and expectations of their achievement from family, schools and themselves. Presently, growing up with social and cultural deprivation potentially leads to a failure to access and benefit from learning opportunities, and a lack of interest in achieving potential in adulthood. Relevant enquiries about family poverty and disadvantage include the patient remembering being cold, hungry or in the dark, disconnection of utilities, the absence of a parent, separation from the parents, parenting from non-parents, family criminality, periods in foster care or on the Child Protection Register, and any kind of physical or emotional neglect and abuse.

These matters may impact equally, or more, on personality development in addition to compromising intellectual ability and potential. Although rather beyond the remit of this chapter, it is worth pointing out that deviance in cognition (as opposed to impairment) is one of the areas in which DSM-IV (*Diagnostic and Statistical Manual of Mental Disorders*, 4th edn) personality disorder manifests itself, cognition here defined qualitatively as ways of perceiving and thinking about oneself, other people and events.

School performance can be an important indicator of intelligence. Was the patient educated in remedial classes or in an educational facility for children with learning problems? Did the patient have a Statement of Special Educational Needs from the local education authority? If so, why, and what provision was made (e.g. one-to-one support)? Did the patient truant, or leave school early or without qualifications? What was the patient's attitude to leaning? Did the patient have a favourite subject? Again, this information has implications for a number of other issues apart from cognition, such as personality, cognitive style, attitudes and values.

It is unusual for patients with learning disability to be able to read, comprehend and write competently, and to be numerate. Establish everyday numeracy: the patient may be asked whether they can ensure that they pay the right amount for purchases and receive the correct change afterwards. Do they need help with filling in forms? Do they read regularly? If so, what can they read and understand (e.g. the tabloid press)?

Higher or further education, successfully completed, comprises additional evidence of cognitive ability. Even the patient who failed to complete secondary education may demonstrate the ability to learn new skills, such as driving a vehicle. Cognitive assessment naturally encompasses ability as well as deficit: what patients like to do and what they are good at. Such attributes are useful in addressing rehabilitative aspects of mental disorder. Interests, sports and hobbies may constitute evidence of intellectual aptitude or motor abilities, or both.

Apart from current intellectual capacity, psychiatric formulation is concerned with alterations in cognition, which may be related to or constitute illness: deterioration after traumatic or other insults to the brain, degenerative disorders such as dementia, and schizophrenia, in which there is evidence of cognitive decline in many patients. The patient's most senior position in employment can be a good indicator of what the patient was capable of, alongside an indication of what the patient actually had to do. The ubiquitous nature of euphemisms in job description may disguise an appointment that in reality required little skill, responsibility or motivation. An informant history may be extremely useful in mapping out what has changed since then: people living with or closely acquainted with the patient are in a good position to notice this. They may be asked about, or spontaneously describe, absent-mindedness, forgetfulness, lack of concentration, vacant spells, lack of understanding of what is said, loss of interest in intellectual pursuits such as reading and keeping up with current affairs, and carelessness in completion of tasks. The natural history of the change should not be omitted: when did it start, were there any clear precipitants, and was it acute, insidious, stepwise or fluctuating?

Enquiries should always be made regarding drug and alcohol abuse and dependence. Although alcohol-induced cognitive impairment is recognized in several guises (delirium, persistent dementia, amnesic syndrome), the literature on the cognitive impairment produced by illicit drug use is in its infancy. Alternatively, the possibility of exposure to environmental or industrial toxins should not be disregarded.

COGNITIVE ASSESSMENT IN MENTAL STATE EXAMINATION: NOT JUST AT THE END

In the author's experience, junior doctors prefer to keep things simple. The problem with this approach is that it can obscure the integration of relevant observations into a coherent whole, which is actually the purpose of the psychiatric history, examination and formulation. Otherwise, a series of disconnected comments is produced, tick-box fashion, which fails to inform diagnosis or management.

The patient's appearance may be relevant to cognition. A classic example is dressing apraxia, in which the patient puts their clothes on the wrong part of their body. An unkempt, dirty and malodorous appearance is non-specific but may be associated with learning disability, dementia or schizophrenia, where self-care skills are poorly developed or lost. Similarly, in the assessment of behaviour, there are classic phenomena related to organic disorder, such as perseverative *utilization behaviour* seen in patients with frontal lobe disorders, in which objects are used repeatedly, for instance wearing three pairs of glasses on top of each other. A more common example is the *catastrophic reaction*, also known as *emotional incontinence*, in which the dementing patient suddenly becomes very angry or upset for relatively minor reasons.

Facial expression can give some clues as to intellectual status: again, patients with dementia may have a fixed or vacant expression, while patients with learning disabilities may appear placid, child-like or restricted in their facial and general emotional expressions. Emotionally inert patients may present so for a variety of reasons, including cognitive compromise. There is a recognized association, for instance, between the negative syndrome in schizophrenia, with its poverty of emotional responsiveness, and intellectual decline.

Much may be inferred from the patient's manner of speaking. Indeed, formal cognitive assessment may be entirely unnecessary in the patient who gives an articulate, fluent, detailed and accurate account, who clearly understands all that is asked of them, and who demonstrates normal memory and concentration in their conversation. It makes little sense to ask such a patient if they know where they are, who they are and what time it is at the end of the interview. By contrast, patients with any kind of general intellectual impairment may speak little, and in simple concrete terms, betraying poor general knowledge and awareness of themselves and their environment. Even if the patient says a lot, they may impart very little information. They may struggle to understand and to answer more complex enquiries, look puzzled or perplexed, fail to come up with expected information, and demonstrate a surprisingly poor memory for fundamental facts about themselves and their families during their account. This may extend to the names and ages of their partner and children, for instance. A classic example is age disorientation in schizophrenia, when the patient says they are many years younger than their chronological age. This is considered cognitive rather than delusional.

Patients' language structure itself may be abnormal, as in expressive and receptive dysphasias, leaving aside formal thought disorder. Alternatively, poor educational standards are evinced by an overt ignorance of grammar (particularly the proper use of pronouns and verb conjugation in the author's experience) and correct pronunciation, although the vagaries of marked regional accents need to be taken into account to a certain degree.

Patients with delirium produce speech that is rambling, incoherent, disjointed and irrelevant. Acute intoxication with alcohol or other substances may present similarly. Such speech may be reminiscent of that of schizophrenic patients with marked thought disorder, but the latter should be fully conscious, alert and reasonably oriented, without the characteristic disturbance of sleep–wake cycle, fluctuation and worse presentation at night of the confused patient. Dysphasic patients produce characteristic speech anomalies: while the patient with receptive dysphasia may sound thought-disordered, with fluent but less than intelligible speech, expressive dysphasia manifests as very restricted speech and word-finding difficulties despite adequate comprehension.

Psychotic phenomena, by contrast, are linked less obviously to cognition. It is generally considered that the ability to experience and to express abnormal ideas and perceptions is related inversely to cognitive function: hence, the diagnosis of schizophrenia is difficult if not impossible to confirm in patients with moderate or severe learning disability. There are a handful of specific psychotic phenomena that may support diagnoses with cognitive impairment, such as visual hallucinations in Charles Bonnet syndrome and Lilliputian hallucinations in delirium tremens. Despite a great deal of research into the neuropsychological underpinnings of psychotic phenomena in schizophrenia throughout the 1990s, positive symptoms do not map easily on to the well recognized cognitive deficits manifest in more obviously organic brain disease, particularly deficits associated with circumscribed lesions.

Similarly, the relationship of insight to cognitive function is far from simple. Loss of insight is, like emotional inertia, a mental state anomaly that is possibly but not inevitably associated with cognitive impairment. In many patients, partial or absent insight may be understandably attributable to psychological defence mechanisms and personality factors. Do not forget to ask the patient whether they have noticed any problems with their memory or their ability to concentrate and pay attention. Can they take in a favourite TV programme, or read and remember a magazine or newspaper article? Are they absent-mindedly losing things, forgetting appointments, forgetting to switch off kitchen equipment, or becoming unaware of what people have said to them?

SPECIFIC COGNITIVE ASSESSMENT IN THE MENTAL STATE EXAMINATION

By the end of the mental state examination, it should be reasonably clear whether and what simple cognitive tests are appropriate. Essentially, these tests screen for clinically significant cognitive impairment in a variety of important intellectual functions. Language barriers should be taken into account in patients whose mother tongue is not English. The skill in appropriate cognitive assessment consists of deciding how much or how little to carry out, administering very simple bedside screening procedures for a reasonable spectrum of cognitive function where indicated, and adding further tasks if impairment is suggested by screening. Beyond this, the services of a clinical psychologist may be required.

As mentioned above, examination of orientation to place, person and time may be superfluous. Disorientation to time of day has the reputation of particular sensitivity, however. Ideally the patient should not have sight of a clock or a watch.

Use common sense in the interpretation of mistakes: patients living in a deprived environment may have little reason to know the exact date or even the day of the week – this is not the same as being presented with the date or day and then forgetting it. The patient should, however, know the month (except at the end or beginning of the month) and the year. If in doubt, ask additional questions such as what season it is, whether the patient has had breakfast today, and what sort of a job the patient does, in order to evaluate the patient's grasp and general awareness of their surroundings. Asking the patient to tell you what has been going on in the news can also be informative, particularly if momentous or highly publicized events have just taken place.

Memory should be divided into short-term or working memory (see below) and longer-term memory. Working memory can be tested by digit span – that is, repeating a series of digits after the doctor says them. The normal range is 5–9. Reversed digit span may also be tested and should normally extend to four or more digits. These and similar tests, such as saying the days of the week or the months of the year backwards, test attention and concentration as well as pure working memory. There is a good deal of overlap between the two. Mental arithmetic is another way of testing attention and concentration, plus the specific ability to calculate. Most patients find 'serial sevens' – subtracting seven repeatedly from 100 – rather challenging. Subtracting three from 20, or counting backwards from 20, is easier: again, take into account educational achievement.

Longer-term memory can be assessed by asking the patient to remember a name and an address comprising five or six elements. Use common sense: do not present something that is highly irregular or that you might not remember either. Make sure the patient has encoded the name and address by asking them to repeat it after you, correctly, at least once. Then ask the patient to perform other brief tasks for 2–5 minutes before asking them to repeat the name and address. The patient should be able to remember all of it, especially if it was only five items long.

Semantic memory may be assessed by asking the patient some general-knowledge questions, such as the name of the current monarch and prime minister, and the years during which the Second World War took place. Some questions may be so easy as to exclude the effects of incomplete education and disinterest in current affairs.

Frontal lobe function was classically assessed in terms of abstract conceptual ability – that is, asking patients to think beyond the concrete, by explaining the meaning of proverbs, or explaining the differences or similarities between objects. Proverb interpretation is in the author's experience performed very poorly, particularly by medical students asked the meaning of, 'It's an ill wind that blows nobody any good'. Again, take into account educational and cultural factors and keep it simple: 'Too many cooks spoil the broth' is probably OK to start with. Differences such as that between a fence and a wall, a child and a dwarf, and a table and a chair may be followed by an enquiry as to how the items are similar. More difficult abstract pairs include a poem and a statue, and praise and punishment. Reasoning and judgement can be examined by asking the patient to 'guesstimate' how fast racehorses gallop, the height of the average woman in the UK, the age of the oldest person in the UK, and the best paid occupation in the UK.

Frontal function is a somewhat overinclusive entity, unfortunately. What this means is that abstraction is not sufficient on its own. The best recognized frontal functions that lend themselves to bedside testing, apart from abstraction, are initiation (i.e. mental response to an external stimulus), maintenance of set (i.e. inhibition of inappropriate responses) and set-shifting (i.e. changing response as appropriate). To test initiation, ask the patient to generate as many animals as they can think of in one minute: ten or fewer indicates impairment, as does perseveration (repeating an answer). Similarly, ask the patient to say words beginning with the letter 's' (or 'f' or 'a') in one minute; again, fewer than ten per minute and perseveration indicate definite impairment.

Frontal lobe tasks tend to be performed poorly by people with learning disability, dementia or schizophrenia.

In the patient in whom dementia or other organic psychosyndrome is considered, it may be well worth carrying out tests of more localized dysfunction (see below). The tests from the MMSE comprise a useful screen: naming a watch and a pen (to which may be added naming the hands, winder, nib, clip, etc.), writing a sentence, repeating a phrase, following the written instruction 'Close your eyes', following a three-stage spoken instruction, and copying intersecting pentagrams. To this may be added basic praxis, for example, asking the patient to demonstrate how they would comb their hair, strike a match and wave goodbye.

WHY NOT JUST DO A MINI-MENTAL STATE EXAMINATION?

There is no doubt that the MMSE is a very well established screen for clinically significant cognitive impairment. However, it is based almost entirely on memory, with virtually no frontal testing. If the patient scores less than 24 on the MMSE, then this merely raises the question of definite deficit, which will not have been addressed in more specific cognitive or diagnostic terms. The MMSE does not constitute an end in itself.

More importantly for junior doctors, in the Royal College of Psychiatrists' clinical examinations that evaluate the candidate's ability to assess cognition, the MMSE test sheet is not available. It is of course possible to administer the MMSE from memory, and lots of candidates do, but it is highly likely that a more specific evaluation will be required. Candidates facing standardized clinical stations with role-players may be given instructions to examine any area of neuropsychological function and not just the presence of clinically significant cognitive impairment as per MMSE score. Outside formal examinations, however, the MMSE is clinically useful when there is a question-mark over whether the patient is cognitively impaired. Nonetheless, this circumstance should not be the rule, given the many other avenues of exploration possible. The other use of the MMSE is as repeated measure, to track emerging cognitive decline or response to treatment, particularly in dementing illness where memory deficit is to the fore.

CLINICAL PSYCHOLOGISTS AND PSYCHOMETRIC TESTING

Historically, clinical psychologists 'followed diagnosis with numbers' – that is, carried out IQ tests, memory tests, language tests, etc. at the behest of the psychiatrist, whose provisional diagnosis implied an impairment. Clinical psychology has now become a diffuse discipline in which psychometric testing is very much a minority interest. A vague non-specific referral is likely to lead to a 'full assessment' and 'formulation', which may prove completely free of any neurocognitive content whatsoever. It therefore behoves the referrer to know what they are talking about, to have carried out a range of bedside tests, to know the basics of more formal evaluation, and to demonstrate justification for what is asked for. The request should state what neuropsychological deficit is suspected and why, and should indicate what specific psychometric tests may be useful.

Psychologists sometimes return reports devoid of numbers, for instance describing current IQ as 'normal' or 'average'. This tendency should be discouraged and precision aimed for. After all, the investigation may need to be repeated in the future. The author would, furthermore, suggest that all psychiatrists should be capable of carrying out a premorbid IQ estimate, the National Adult Reading Test (NART)[5] and a current IQ estimate, the Quick Test.[6] The standard psychometric IQ evaluation, the Wechsler Adult Intelligence Scale (WAIS),[7] is a very lengthy test, onerous for both the patient and the clinical psychologist. Indeed, it is often 'pro-rated' – that is, a selection of sub-tests, rather than all of them, is administered and an IQ score derived from partial completion.

Finally, it is always well worth ordering all the patient's previous case notes. A summary of notes, although time-consuming, may generate much useful information about family history, development and previous personal function, which may not be available at initial interview. Occasionally there may have been a psychological assessment, even including an IQ score or other psychometric tests.

FROM THE CLINICAL TO THE THEORETICAL: STRUCTURAL–FUNCTIONAL RELATIONSHIPS

As a whole, cognitive function or the lack of it is as heterogeneous and variable as the spectrum of psychiatric disorder. Taking a hierarchical approach, the most gross cognitive impairments and anomalies are likely to be encountered in the dementias, learning disability and other organic psychosyndromes, produced by the usual range of neurodevelopmental, traumatic, neoplastic, metabolic, endocrine, vascular, infective, autoimmune, toxic and degenerative insults. An isolated area of cognitive dysfunction that can be attributed to a localized lesion, in the setting of preserved performance otherwise, is particularly likely to afford specific diagnostic implications. Moreover, 'functional' psychotic disorder, particularly schizophrenia, is increasingly recognized as including cognitive impairment in frontal function and long-term memory. These are disproportionate deficits considering overall intellectual ability. Even so, a fall in IQ from premorbid levels is extremely common in patients with schizophrenia. Similar chronic impairments are beginning to be described in bipolar affective disorder.

On the other hand, 'neurotic' disorder, personality disorder and substance (apart from alcohol) abuse were never of great interest in cognitive terms, although this is an emerging experimental field. Even so, it has long been recognized that depressed patients tend to complaints of absent-mindedness or inability to concentrate. On testing there can be a patchy impairment of memory and concentration owing to anxiety and difficulty in paying attention.

Occasionally, patients present with cognitive impairment that is more apparent than real, such as in dissociative amnesia and depressive pseudo-dementia. It pays to be aware of discrepancies between the pattern of impairment expected and that produced by the patient. Furthermore, there are particular issues with learning disability in the author's experience. Much subnormal IQ, whether original or recently acquired, goes undetected in psychiatric practice. Conversely, it is not rare to encounter patients thought to be learning disabled by other professions and who return a Quick Test estimate within one standard deviation of the mean.

Some important cognitive functions, principally attention, concentration, memory and executive function, are not localized to specific hemispheres or areas of the brain. These have a distributed neural basis and tend to be compromised by generalized cerebral dysfunction, by definition more than minor although not always permanent. Other functions such as verbal skills and visuospatial function are lateralized to the left and right hemispheres, respectively, depending on cerebral dominance. Discrete unilateral lesions, therefore, may have very different consequences compared with distributed compromise. Furthermore, the causes tend to differ: metabolic, electrolytic, infective, pharmaceutical and endocrine pathology is unlikely to target some parts of the brain more than others, as opposed to cerebrovascular, neoplastic and in some instances degenerative pathology.

The frontal lobes are something of an exception to the basic diffuse versus localized distinction, since they have a crucial integrative role across a number of important functions. Therefore, limited lesions of the frontal lobes can impact upon distributed functions. This is probably why 'frontal lobe function' is such an inherently overinclusive and unsatisfactory term.

DISTRIBUTED FUNCTIONS

Attention and concentration

The reticular activating system connects the brainstem to the thalamus and neocortex via ascending cholinergic, monoaminergic and serotonergic pathways. There is neocortical feedback, particularly from the prefrontal cortex and the posterior parietal and inferior temporal cortex, all of which receive afferent perceptual input. The result is conscious attention. Disruption of attention leads to confusion, termed delirium at the moment, at least when it comprises an acute presentation attributable to a new insult to the brain rather than a chronic degenerative picture.

Like any other disorder, there is a spectrum of severity applicable to attentional impairment. Clinically, it presents as poor orientation, an inability to sustain attention, distractibility by irrelevant stimuli, and inability to inhibit inappropriate responses. Such patients may perseverate, fail to repeat and reverse strings of digits, fail to reverse the days of the week, fail simple mental arithmetic, and fail to learn a name and address. There is obviously an overlap with compromise of working memory. Although usually the result of a diffuse insult, right-sided prefrontal lobe lesions are supposedly more likely to produce attentional impairment than the left-sided variety. Many delirious patients are quiet and lethargic, but some are actively agitated, deluded and hallucinated: this phenomenon is recognized in severely physically ill patients as 'ICU psychosis'. Some forms of delirium, the classic example being delirium tremens, are usually accompanied by hallucinosis.

Memory

The overall concept of memory is neuropsychologically quite complex and occasionally rather bewildering. The major subclassification into implicit and explicit memory has much more theoretical than clinical utility. Essentially, explicit (also known as declarative) memory subsumes what can be recalled by conscious (i.e. voluntary) recollection. Implicit memory is something of a 'rag-bag' and includes everything else. First, implicit memory includes what the patient has learned (i.e. not forgotten) but cannot voluntarily remember on demand. Such implicit memory material can be brought to consciousness by priming or cueing: if the patient is given a list of ten words to learn but can recollect only five of them, they may recall some of the others if given the initial letter or other clue. Second, implicit memory includes the learning and retention of motor skills, such as driving a car, typing, or playing a musical instrument. This is known as procedural memory. Third, implicit memory subsumes other non-verbal but entirely unconscious forms of learning such as conditioned reflexes.

Implicit memory tends to be relatively preserved, even in serious psychotic or degenerative disorder, and is not assessed routinely in psychiatry. However, loss of motor skills, if the patient had any, can be asked about in the history, particularly if an informant is available. It should not be forgotten that motor skills may deteriorate without regular practice, leaving aside the effects of mental disorder.

Explicit memory is divided into short-term memory (also known as working memory) and long-term memory. The working memory system serves to keep small amounts (five to nine items) of verbal, auditory or visual material present in conscious awareness for recall or manipulation, or both, for a brief period of up to 30 s. There is an obvious overlap with conscious attention. Working memory functions alongside long-term memory, but surprisingly the acquisition and retrieval of long-term memories can occur despite defective working memory.

Long-term memory is divided into episodic and semantic memory. Episodic memory is what most people would call memory – the recollection of personal experience – for instance, what one did yesterday. Semantic memory is what most people would call knowledge: the capital of France is Paris, and a dog is a four-legged domesticated animal that barks and wags its tail.

An added layer of complication in the understanding of memory is the processes through which the systems work. In other words, information of whatever kind must be encountered (consciously or otherwise), encoded, reinforced or consolidated, and then accessed for recall; otherwise, the information cannot become a memory. This may have practical clinical implications: for instance, the author was asked to complete a second opinion on a patient whom several 'assessments' had concluded was suffering from post-traumatic stress disorder. The flaw in the argument was that the traumatic incident comprised a blow to the head that produced unconsciousness accompanied by several minutes' amnesia both before and after the event. Logically, the patient could not suffer re-experiencing and avoidance symptoms related directly to an event of which he had no memory at all. This elementary error had understandably compromised the patient's management for the 3 years since presentation.

Another relevant process is forgetting: there are further theoretical distinctions between the functions of searching or accessing memories, and the existence of a store where representations are held. Recall is thought to be harder than recognition for these reasons: recall of material requires a search for and access to what is in the store, while recognition involves only a check for familiarity between the material presented and the content of the store.

Although memory is overall a distributed function, its subdivisions do have localized affiliations. Thus, the basal ganglia and cerebellum are thought to be of particular importance in conditioning and procedural memory. Regarding working memory, the substrates for verbal content (phonological loop) and non-verbal content (visuospatial sketch pad) devolve to the dominant and non-dominant hemisphere, respectively, while the frontal cortex includes a central executive function to operate them effectively. The circuit of Papez, a component of the limbic system comprising the medial temporal lobe, diencephalon, basal forebrain nuclei, fornix and cingulate gyrus, is essential for episodic memory. Semantic memory is lost with lesions of the dominant temporal neocortex.

Classic neuropsychological distinctions between these types of memory are of limited utility in psychiatry. Clinically, the ability to acquire, retain and recall new episodic material (i.e. anterograde memory) as opposed to the ability to recall old episodic material (retrograde amnesia) is much more relevant. Working memory and attention are usually compromised in anterograde amnesia, alongside this long-term episodic memory failure. The Rivermead Behavioural Memory Test (RBMT)[8] is the standard measure of episodic memory function in anterograde terms. The RBMT includes both non-verbal and verbal elements (words, drawings, faces) and tests of both recall and recognition. Interestingly, patients with schizophrenia perform very poorly on this test and on tests of semantic memory. The bedside test of verbal episodic memory recall, asking a name and address learned a few minutes previously, is a useful screen. Retrograde memory evaluation turns upon whether the autobiographical history given by the patient can be validated. In some patients it may be obviously confabulatory rather than missing. Formal tests exist, such as the Famous Faces Test, in which the patient is presented with photographs of famous people or events from different periods in the past.[9,10]

Amnesic syndrome is an important entity in psychiatry: anterograde or retrograde amnesia, or both, occur in the absence of other cognitive dysfunctions, including, surprisingly, implicit memory. Amnesic syndrome can be acute or chronic.

Acute amnesia occurs in delirium and in transient global amnesia: it may present with alcohol and drug intoxication, closed head injury and focal epilepsy. Anterograde amnesia is the rule, alongside some working memory/attentional impairment. Patients cannot remember anything for more than a few minutes: attentional impairment inevitably results in a degree of disorientation in place and time. Nonetheless, in transient global amnesia, the patient may have normal working memory and attention (i.e. normal digit span and reversal tests) and be acutely aware of their difficulty, repeatedly asking where they are, how they arrived at that location and what has happened. Furthermore, in transient global amnesia, there is a dense retrograde amnesia that may go back for decades. The patient may be unaware of the death of a relative or the achievements of their children, for instance.

Chronic amnesic syndrome indicates long-term bilateral damage to the medial temporal lobe, particularly the hippocampus, as in, for example, early Alzheimer's disease, herpes encephalitis and posterior cerebral artery stroke. It is also associated with closed head injury. Diencephalic damage is a classic complication of alcoholism in the form of Korsakoff psychosis. In chronic amnesic syndrome, there is a preserved intelligence quotient but severe anterograde amnesia accompanied by retrograde amnesia. This is much worse with diencephalic than hippocampal compromise. There is a temporal gradient that is counterintuitive, in that more distant memories are clearer than more recent memories. Working memory, attention and aspects of implicit memory are unaffected.

Semantic memory disorder occurs in Pick's disease, herpes encephalitis and severe schizophrenia. It also surfaces in progressive dementing disorder, particularly Alzheimer's disease. Bedside tests of semantic memory are not usually indicated, but there is some overlap with the 'frontal' category fluency test (i.e. naming as many items as possible, such as animals, or words beginning with a specific initial, in a brief period such as 1 minute). Asking about general knowledge (e.g. name of prime minister) is also useful. The patient may be asked to verify (or otherwise) statements such as 'Admirals are in charge of ships' and 'Beer is sold at a butcher's shop'. By far the best formal test of semantic memory is the Hodges semantic memory battery,[11] which has been used widely in formal neuropsychological assessment and research. The Graded Naming Test is much shorter: the patient is asked to look at a number of pictures of increasingly obscure items and say what they are.[12] The Silly Sentences Test consists of correct and nonsensical statements as above, the patient being asked to determined which is which.[13]

Frontal lobe function

Frontal lobe function, also known as executive function, is problematic in terms of its heterogeneity and ubiquity. In summary, frontal lobe function involves generating responses to stimuli, choosing the most appropriate, inhibiting inappropriate responses, planning and problem-solving, keeping a sequence of behaviours on course to achieve an overall goal, and yet changing response parameters when required by environmental variation. Bedside tests for frontal function have arisen from the study of patients with circumscribed frontal lobe lesions.

Frontal lobe compromise can be suggested by the history. Disinhibition in mood and behaviour and a lack of empathy for others are of course not specific to patients with frontal lobe disorders, but they can be of sufficient magnitude and difference compared with the normal personality and behaviour to be significant. Lack of suppression of inappropriate internal stimuli is thought to be responsible. On the other hand, the apathy and marked slowing also observed in frontal patients reflects that they may respond very poorly to internal and external stimuli. Adequate response to external stimuli enables patients to attempt testing, although this must be done carefully if cooperation is not to be lost. Category fluency for animals (or vehicles or household items, for instance) and words beginning with specific letters can be considered a frontal test. Perseveration occurs when items are repeated (the patient gets stuck rather than forgets they have said the item or word already), and irrelevant items or words may be offered owing to distractibility; one schizophrenic patient of the author's responded to a request to name sea creatures with the phrase 'men in aqualungs', for instance. Planning and strategy is compromised: most people when asked to name animals would use superordinate categorization to identify groups of animals, such as thinking of farm animals, domestic animals or jungle animals. Patients with frontal lobe disorders do not do this as effectively.

If frontal impairment is suspected, it may be useful to ask the patient to carry out non-verbal tasks as well as proverb, difference and similarity explanation, cognitive estimates and category fluency (see above). The patient may be asked to copy an alternating sequence of triangles and squares (Figure 7.1) or to tap on the desk twice when the examiner taps once (under the table), and vice versa (i.e. the patient should tap once when the examiner taps twice). This is repeated until the examiner is satisfied that the patient can or cannot do it. Further formal testing is within the remit of clinical psychologists. They may use a structured initiation task such as the formal FAS fluency test[14] (the patient is asked to say as many words as they can think of beginning with the letter F in 1 minute, then with the letter A, and then with the letter S) and 'dual tasks' of divided attention (since the working memory central executive is compromised), such as the Stroop Test[15] and the Trail Making Test.[16] Divided attention clearly overlaps with the ability to maintain and change set. The standard set maintenance and shifting task is, however, the Wisconsin Card Sorting Test, in which cards are sorted according to the different numbers of various shapes of separate colours that appear on each one.[17] The Tower of London (or Hanoi) test is used to assess planning and sequencing.[18] The Cognitive Estimates Test comprises ten 'guesstimate' questions (see above) and assesses reasoning and judgement.[19,20] The Behavioural Assessment of the Dysexecutive Syndrome (BADS)[21,22] is an ecologically valid test that covers functional aspects of frontal impairment.

Causes of frontal lobe syndrome include focal dementia such as Pick's disease, anterior cerebral artery stroke, head injury (closed or local trauma) and tumours. Frontal signs are eventually seen in degenerative disorders that have the effect of isolating the frontal lobes, for example subcortical dementias such as Huntingdon's and Parkinson's diseases, progressive supranuclear palsy, leucodystrophies and acquired immunodeficiency syndrome (AIDS) encephalopathy.

LOCALIZED COGNITIVE FUNCTIONS

The dominant hemisphere

The left hemisphere is dominant in right-handed people and about half of left-handed people: its functions include language, calculation and higher motor control (praxis).

Dysphasia (impairment of language function) should be distinguished from dysarthria (failure of articulation). Dysarthria has a variety of causes, the most common in psychiatric practice probably being antipsychotic drug treatment with extrapyramidal side effects. Cranial nerve palsies, cerebellar and basal ganglia pathology, and anterior left hemisphere lesions can also contribute to dysarthria.

Dysphasia presents in two forms, receptive and expressive. In receptive dysphasia there is a lesion affecting Wernicke's area in the dominant posterior superior temporal lobe. Language is not understood and speech output is fluent but unintelligible to varying degrees, including neologisms, grammatical and syntactical errors, and overinclusiveness. In expressive dysphasia there is a lesion affecting Broca's area in the dominant inferior frontal lobe, usually extending into the frontoparietal region served by the superior middle cerebral artery. Language is understood but the patient cannot find words and assemble phrases and sentences: speech output is simple, minimal and not entirely correct in structure, but it betrays better comprehension than the irrelevant speech output of patients with expressive dysphasia. Both types of dysphasia affect the ability to repeat and to name objects. The Graded Naming Test can be used to evaluate naming impairment and semantic memory. Repetition can be examined simply using the MMSE phrase 'No ifs, ands or buts'. Language comprehension can be evaluated with the Token Test: a number of tokens of different shapes and colours are assembled before the patient, who is then given standard verbal instructions of variable complexity, such as 'Put the small red circle on the big green square'.[23] Furthermore, most dysphasic patients are dyslexic, having difficulty in reading aloud or comprehension of text: they can be asked to read a short passage from a book, newspaper or magazine, and then describe its content. The distinction should be drawn between patients with learning disability and illiterate patients, however, and those who have lost a pre-existing ability. Similarly, there may be dysgraphia (difficulty in writing): the patient may fail to write a sentence or copy text. Dominant parietal lobe damage may be associated with dyspraxic dysgraphia, in which the motor control of writing is impaired. Both dysgraphia and dyslexia may present as neglect phenomena owing to non-dominant lesions (see below): the left (first) parts or words are not written or not read at all, or they are read or written incorrectly.

To the rear of Wernicke's area is the angular gyrus, which connects the temporal, parietal and occipital lobes. Lesions here produce Gerstmann syndrome: dysgraphia, dyscalculia, right–left disorientation and inability to name individual fingers according to convention (finger agnosia). The angular gyrus appears very important for numeracy in general. If a patient cannot carry out serial subtractions of three from 20, then simpler arithmetic function can be checked, for instance single-figure addition. If further examination is required, the patient may be asked to point to numbers on command, copy numbers, write numbers to dictation, and read aloud written numbers. Again, the context of overall intelligence quotient and educational and motivational factors should be considered.

Finally, apraxia, the loss of simple motor skills, can be a consequence of dominant hemisphere compromise. The patient may be asked to demonstrate buccofacial actions (how they would lick lips, cough, sip through a straw, blow out a match), limb actions (how they would wave goodbye, beckon 'come here', salute, hitch a lift) and object usage

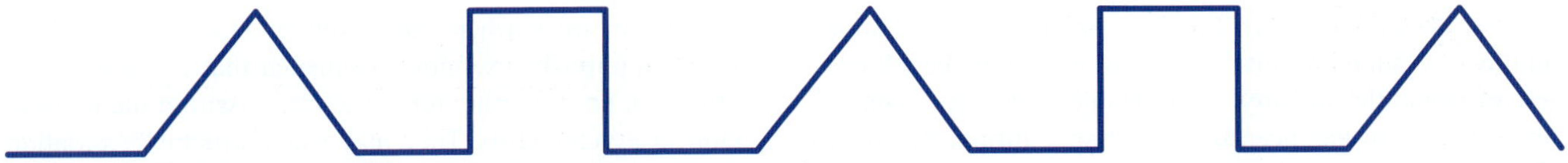

Figure 7.1 Ask the patient to copy the connected alternating shapes above

(how they would brush teeth, comb hair, strike a match, use scissors, hammer a nail). If there is difficulty, the action can be demonstrated by the examiner to see whether the patient can copy it.

The non-dominant hemisphere

Localized non-dominant hemisphere lesions result in neglect (lack of awareness) phenomena and visuospatial defect, particularly lack of visual recognition. Stroke-induced lesions can result in denial that the affected side exists, denial of hemiplegia (anosagnosia) or minimization (anosodiaphoria). Patients may ignore visual, auditory and tactile sensory input, usually from the left side of the body, since the right hemisphere is generally non-dominant. Extinction occurs when the patient is aware of such stimulation but, if the stimulus is presented bilaterally, ignores the stimulus on the neglected side. Neglect of space outside the body can occur after damage to either hemisphere but is persistent and severe following non-dominant insults. This can be determined by asking the patient to copy a clock face: half the numbers are left out or they are all squashed into one side. Other drawings are copied with the left half missing. Another aspect of visuospatial difficulty is manifest as dressing apraxia.

Visuospatial function can be tested at the bedside by asking the patient to copy simple line drawings such as the intersecting pentagons in the MMSE or a three-dimensional drawing of a cube. The Visual Object Space Perception Battery[24] is a very useful test for further evaluation of visuospatial function, although some of the more difficult tasks have a distinct executive element.

Visual agnosia (inability to name objects presented in pictorial form) may result from semantic memory impairment or deficits in visual processing (apperceptive agnosia). Patients with apperceptive agnosia cannot copy line drawings or match identical depictions. However, they may be able to identify an object by touch. The patient should be able to describe the attributes of an object named by the examiner, unlike patients with semantic memory disorder. Apperceptive agnosia may extend to an inability to recognize faces (prosopagnosia). Even so, patients with prosopagnosia may recognize people from their voice, gait or dress and can match the same face from portraits or photographs. They can describe facial features and expressions. The Recognition Memory Test[25] is a formal evaluation including faces presented singly and then in pairs, the patient needing to identify the face seen previously.

ESTIMATING PREMORBID AND CURRENT INTELLIGENCE QUOTIENT

Given the impact of current IQ upon personal and social function, it is important to judge the patient's general intellectual capacity to inform formulation and management. The population mean IQ score is 100: the range is between zero and 200. The standard deviation is 15. People with an IQ outwith two standard deviations of the mean are statistically abnormal: hence, learning disability is defined by an IQ below 70, while an IQ of over 130 denotes superiority. The measurement error is five points. For this reason, a person may be classed as having a learning disability with an IQ of 75 if there are sufficient impairments in (separately assessed) adaptive functioning. Conversely, if there is adequate adaptive functioning, then learning disability would not be diagnosed in the context of an IQ of 65. The low score would be attributed instead to measurement error. Because practice effects are observed in neuropsychological evaluation, and the WAIS does not include multiple versions, it can be misleading to repeat the evaluation particularly over a brief period of time.

WAIS assessment is, as mentioned above, rather lengthy and cumbersome, potentially presenting the individual with multiple experiences of failure, which can be demoralizing. Furthermore, IQ evaluation may be seen as undesirable for social reasons, undermining the value of people and constituting grounds for discrimination. IQ evaluation measures, it has been argued, no more than the ability to complete IQ tests successfully. Nonetheless, in cognitive terms, IQ tests load quite heavily on aspects of frontal and memory function, which are know to be crucial for independent living skills.

Availability of the WAIS equipment is limited by its publisher to properly qualified clinical psychologists. A good compromise is the Quick Test (Figure 7.2; Table 7.1).

Premorbid intelligence is of great interest where IQ decline is suspected, as in degenerative or other instances of permanent brain damage however caused. Estimation requires a test that accesses aspects of cognition at least relatively preserved subsequent to psychiatric or neurological disorder: scores on the test should correlate highly with current IQ in the normal population. The best established premorbid IQ evaluation is the NART (Table 7.2). This test asks the patient (whose first language should be English) to read 50 words whose spelling does not reflect their pronunciation. The implication is that because reading one's mother tongue is such a well established skill, acquired in childhood, it is resistant to the effects of cerebral pathology.

IQ decline can be assessed by comparing the NART score with the Quick Test score. Substantial discrepancies are manifest in dementia, after serious insults with permanent effects, and in some patients with chronic schizophrenia. Both the presence of decline and the current IQ estimate can be useful information in terms of diagnosis and prognosis.

CONCLUSION

Every competent psychiatrist must have an adequate working knowledge of cognition: the generality and specifics of

Table 7.1 Quick Test. Reproduced with permission from Ref. 6

Word	Difficulty/mental age (years)	Answer	Score out of 49	IQ estimate	Word	Difficulty/mental age (years)	Answer
Belt	Easy	4	49	135	Graceful	10	1
Dancing	Easy	1	48	130	Fluid	11	2
Traffic	Easy	4	47	120	Solution	11	2
Whistle	Easy	4	46	116	Discipline	12	4
Fence	Easy	3	45	110	Crystallised	13	2
Drink	Easy	2	44	108	Turntable	13	1
Wreck	Easy	3	43	104	Saccharin	14	2
Music	Easy	1	42	102	Immature	14	4
Medicine	Easy	2	41	100	Cordiality	15	1
Gun	Easy	4	40	98	Velocity	15	3
Pepper	Easy	2	39	96	Decisive	16	4
Racing	Easy	3	38	92	Laceration	16	3
Salt	Easy	2	36	90	Foliage	17	3
Woman	Easy	1	35	87	Imperative	17	4
Sugar	Easy	2	32	84	Intimacy	18	1
Track	Easy	3	30	80	Concoction	18	2
School	6	4	27	75	Conviviality	18	1
Partner	7	1	25	70	Chevrons	18+	4
Couples	7	1	22	65	Condiment	Hard	2
Rail	7	3	21	60	Cacophony	Hard	3
Respected	8	4	19	55	Miscible	Hard	2
Betting	8	3	18	50	Imbibe	Hard	2
Daring	9	3	16	45	Amicable	Hard	1
Stadium	9	3	15	40	Pungent	Hard	2
Pedestrian	10	4					

Table 7.2 The National Adult Reading Test (NART). Reproduced with permission from Ref. 5

Words			Number of errors	Premorbid IQ estimate	Number of errors	Premorbid IQ estimate	Number of errors	Premorbid IQ estimate
Chord	Placebo	Assignate	0	131	17	110	34	89
Depot	Detente	Subtle	1	129	18	108	35	87
Bouquet	Puerperal	Gist	2	128	19	107	36	86
Capon	Gauche	Superfluous	3	127	20	106	37	85
Nausea	Leviathan	Banal	4	126	21	105	38	84
Courteous	Prelate	Cellist	5	124	22	103	39	82
Equivocal	Demesne	Zealot	6	123	23	102	40	81
Catacomb	Labile	Aeon	7	122	24	101	41	80
Thyme	Ache	Abstemious	8	121	25	100	42	79
Radix	Aisle	Idyll	9	120	26	98	43	77
Hiatus	Psalm	Aver	10	118	27	97	44	76
Procreate	Deny	Topiary	11	117	28	96	45	75
Gouge	Debt	Beatify	12	116	29	95	46	74
Simile	Rarefy	Sidereal	13	115	30	94	47	73
Quadruped	Naive	Syncope	14	113	31	92	48	71
Façade	Gaoled	Campanile	15	112	32	91	49	70
Drachm	Heir		16	111	33	90		

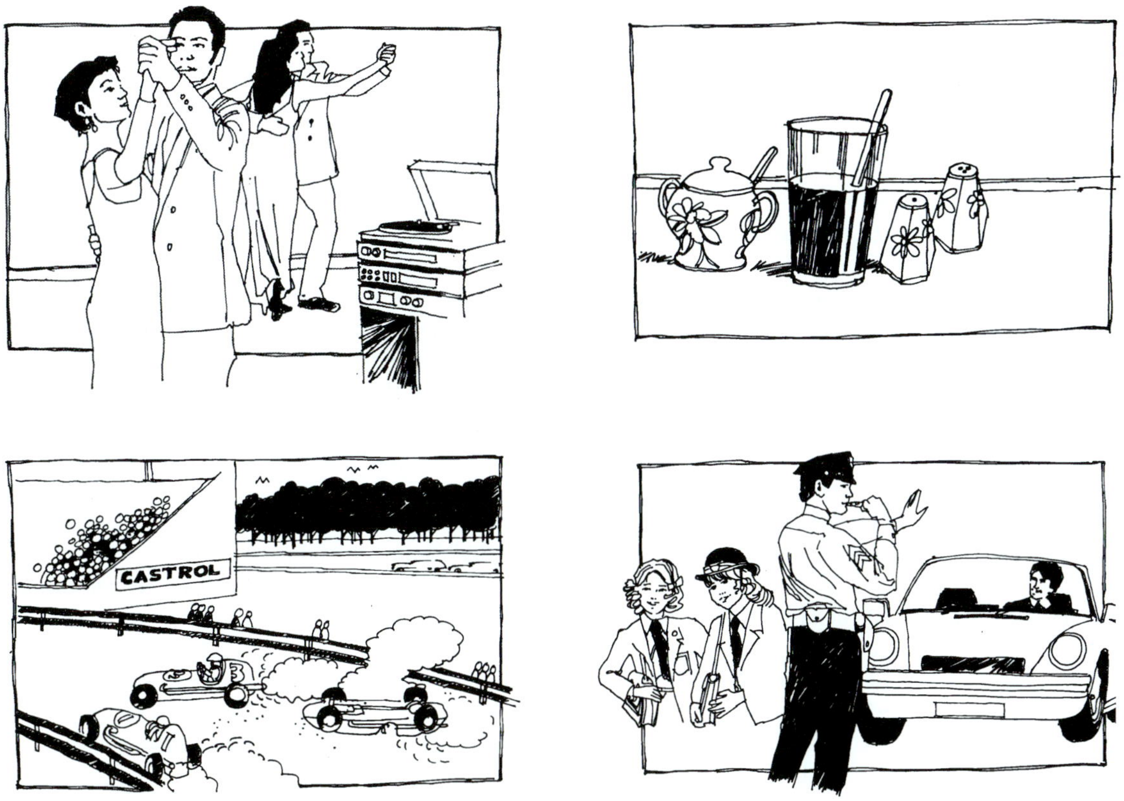

Figure 7.2 Quick Test. Place the cards in front of the patient on a table in a block of four. Leave a gap of about 15 cm between each card to make it easier for the patient to point at the picture they select in response to each test word. Reproduced with permission from Ref. 6

normal function, how it can go wrong, the clinical discovery of deficits, and their diagnostic and prognostic implications. Cognitive evaluation is, however, predicated not upon an afterthought of mental state examination but on foregoing referral information, and the patient's previous history, history at interview and mental state assessment. Only then can appropriate screening take place, followed up with further enquiry and referral to colleagues in clinical psychology when necessary.

Repeated and extensive practice with a broad spectrum of patients will illustrate how cognitive issues insinuate themselves into psychiatric formulation and so inform investigation, management and outcome. It is hoped that the material presented in this chapter constitutes a good starting point.

ACKNOWLEDGEMENT

The author is indebted to Professor John R Hodges, whose standard work, *Cognitive Assessment for Clinicians*,[26] very much informed a substantial minority of what is presented here. Professor Hodges' work is unreservedly recommended for further reading.

REFERENCES

1. Folstein M, Folstein S, McHugh P (1975) 'Mini-mental state': a practical method for grading the cognitive state of patients for the clinician. *Journal of Psychiatry Research* 12: 189–98.
2. Phillips C, Hon Y, Smith B, Sutton A (1986) Severe mental retardation in children from socially disadvantaged families. *Child: Care, Health and Development* 12: 69–91.
3. Rantakallio P (1987) Social class differences in mental retardation and subnormality. *Scandinavian Journal of Social Medicine* 15: 63–6.
4. Buchanan A, Oliver J (1977) Abuse and neglect as a cause of mental retardation: a study of 140 children admitted to subnormality hospitals in Wiltshire. *British Journal of Psychiatry* 131: 458–67.
5. Nelson H (1982) *The National Adult Reading Test (NART): Test Manual.* Windsor: NFER-Nelson.
6. Bowen K, Mortimer A, Rooke-Ley S (1999). Measuring IQ in schizophrenia: the 'Quick Test'. *Cognitive Neuropsychiatry* 4: 81–8.
7. Wechsler D. (1981) *Manual for the Wechsler Adult Intelligence Scale: Revised.* New York: Psychological Corporation.

8. Wilson B, Cockburn J, Baddeley A (1985) *The Rivermead Behavioural Memory Test*. Reading: Thames Valley Test Corporation.
9. Hodges J, Ward C (1989) Observations during transient global amnesia: a behavioural and neuropsychological study of five cases. *Brain* **112**: 595–620.
10. Estevez-Gonzalez A, Garcia-Sanchez C, Boltes A *et al.* (2004) Semantic knowledge of famous people in mild cognitive impairment and progression to Alzheimer's disease. *Dementia and Geriatric Cognitive Disorders* **17**: 188–95.
11. Hodges J, Salmon D, Butters N (1992) Semantic memory impairment in Alzheimer's disease: failure of access or degraded knowledge? *Neuropsychologia* **30**: 301–14.
12. McKenna P, Warrington E (1983) *The Graded Naming Test*. Oxford: Cambridge Cognition.
13. Collins A, Quillian M (1969) Retrieval time from semantic memory. *Journal of Verbal Learning and Verbal Behaviour* **8**: 240–47.
14. Benton A (1968) Differential behavioural effects in frontal lobe disease. *Neuropsychologia* **6**: 53–60.
15. Golden CJ (1978) *Stroop Color and Word Test: A Manual for Clinical and Experimental Uses*. Chicago, IL: Skoelting.
16. Reitan R (1958) Validity of the Trailmaking Test as an indication of organic brain damage. *Perceptual Motor Skills* **8**: 271–6.
17. Nelson H (1976) A modified card sorting test sensitive to frontal deficits. *Cortex* **12**: 313–24.
18. Shallice T (1982) Specific impairments of planning. In DE Broadbent, L Weiskrantz (eds) *The Neuropsychology of Cognitive Function*. London: The Royal Society.
19. Shallice T, Evans M (1978) The involvement of the frontal lobes in cognitive estimation. *Cortex* **14**: 294–303.
20. Nathan J, Wilkinson D, Stammers S, Low J (2001) The role of tests of frontal executive function in the detection of mild dementia. *International Journal of Geriatric Psychiatry* **16**: 18–26.
21. Wilson B, Evans J, Alderman N, Burgess P, Emslie H (1997) The Behavioural Assessment of the Dysexecutive Syndrome (BADS): behavioural assessment of the dysexecutive syndrome. In P Rabbit (ed.) *Theory and Methodology of Frontal and Executive Function*. Hove: Psychology Press.
22. Katz N, Tadmor I, Felzen B, Hartman-Maeir A (2007) The Behavioural Assessment of the Dysexecutive Syndrome (BADS) in schizophrenia and its relation to functional outcomes. *Neuropsychological Rehabilitation* **19**: 192–205.
23. McNeil A, Prescot T (2008) *The Revised Token Test*. Baltimore, MD: University Park Press.
24. Warrington E, James M (1991) *The Visual Object Space Perception Battery (VOSP)*. Bury St Edmunds: Thames Valley Test Company.
25. Warrington E (2008) *The Recognition Memory Test*. Windsor: NFER-Nelson.
26. Hodges J (2007) *Cognitive Assessment for Clinicians*, 2nd edn. Oxford: Oxford University Press.

PART 2

Developmental, behavioural and sociocultural psychiatry

Chapter 8

Human development

Marcus Munafò and Angela Attwood

CONCEPTUAL FRAMEWORKS

Nature and nurture

Are individual differences in behavioural and physical traits determined by genetic variation or by differences in environmental circumstances? Historically, theorists have tended to advocate extreme positions in this debate, but it is now widely accepted that genetic and environmental influences do not operate independently but are interactive. In most cases, genetic factors provide a set of parameters in which an infant can develop, with the exact nature of this development being determined by the environment. Thus, it seems that the important question is not *which* influence is most important, but rather *how* genetic and environmental factors interact to determine human development.

The heritability statistic used to express the relative contribution of genotype and environment to the observed behaviour or trait (i.e. phenotype) is widely misunderstood. This is a population statistic that provides information on the proportion of *variability* in the observed phenotype that may be accounted for by variability in the genotype (and, therefore, information on variability accounted for by the environment). The number of fingers on one hand, for example, although determined genetically, is not highly heritable, as any *variation* in this number is generally the result of environmental factors. Height, however, is highly heritable, since most diets – even relatively poor ones – are sufficient to promote growth, so that environmental variation plays a smaller role, with any residual variation being the result of genetic factors. The latter example also indicates that a heritability statistic for a given phenotype is specific to the time and population on which it was calculated: in populations where the diet is more variable, more of the variation in height in that population may be associated with this environmental factor, so that the heritability coefficient will be different even if the underlying distribution of genes is the same.

Stage theories

Many abilities and behaviours develop in a uniform way. The prerequisites for these behaviours, such as basic motor skills, are inherited, but through dynamic interaction with the environment children learn to develop these skills. Stage theories propose that development passes sequentially through qualitatively different phases. In most cases, accomplishment of one stage is necessary before development of the next can proceed. The rate of development is influenced by environmental factors, but some stage theories identify critical periods by which accomplishment of certain skills should be achieved.

Stage theories have been used to describe many aspects of development, including linguistic, moral and motor development. Piaget's theory of cognitive development is one of the best-known examples. The goal of stage theorists is to determine the distinct qualitative features of the developmental process and the important changes that characterize transition from one stage to the next.

Maturational tasks

Development of a skill or behaviour occurs when a child performs or practises tasks that strengthen, extend or consolidate current knowledge or abilities, so that higher levels of that skill or behaviour can be achieved. For example, a child will master the art of standing unaided before attempting his or her first steps, which will be unsteady at first, becoming more assured and steady over time. These tasks propel the child through the critical periods of development.

Maturation refers to a largely genetically determined 'blueprint' that sets out a child's critical periods of development (i.e. the sequential aspects of development that are under biological control). The concept of maturation is linked closely to the nature–nurture distinction, as it is the interaction between maturation and experience that shapes an individual's development.

Although it is relatively easy to understand maturation in the development of physical abilities, the applicability of this framework to psychological development is not accepted universally. It is also important to distinguish between simple maturation, which is the pure biological unfolding driven primarily by genetic factors, and development, which is the sequence of changes over the lifespan that results from the interaction of some behaviours and the environment.

Maturity

Maturity in a physical sense refers to the time in life when physical growth has ceased. From a psychological viewpoint, however, maturity is somewhat more difficult to define. Unlike growing in height, for example, there is no clear cessation in psychological growth. In fact, learning and development continue on an emotional, cognitive and intellectual level throughout an individual's lifetime. Therefore, it may be more relevant to think of maturity as the conclusion to a biologically predetermined pattern of development, or the culmination in the maturation process described above.

James Tanner devised a series of longitudinal charts to illustrate growth references on physical parameters, including height, weight, skin folds and puberty, ranging from birth to maturity. Their purpose was to provide a standardized tool for clinicians to assess whether a child's size and growth rate were within the normal limits for his or her age, sex, socioeconomic position and ethnic group, and to help diagnose growth disorders such as short stature and low growth velocity. Despite originally being designed for clinical use, the charts have also been used to predict adult physical characteristics such as height in adulthood. Questions have been raised regarding the validity of the charts, particularly due to trends of increasing size over time, which have been answered, to some extent, by revisions to the original work. There does, however, remain some confusion over the comparability of Tanner scales with other growth references. Tanner's charts are still in clinical use in the UK, often in combination with other growth references (Figure 8.1).

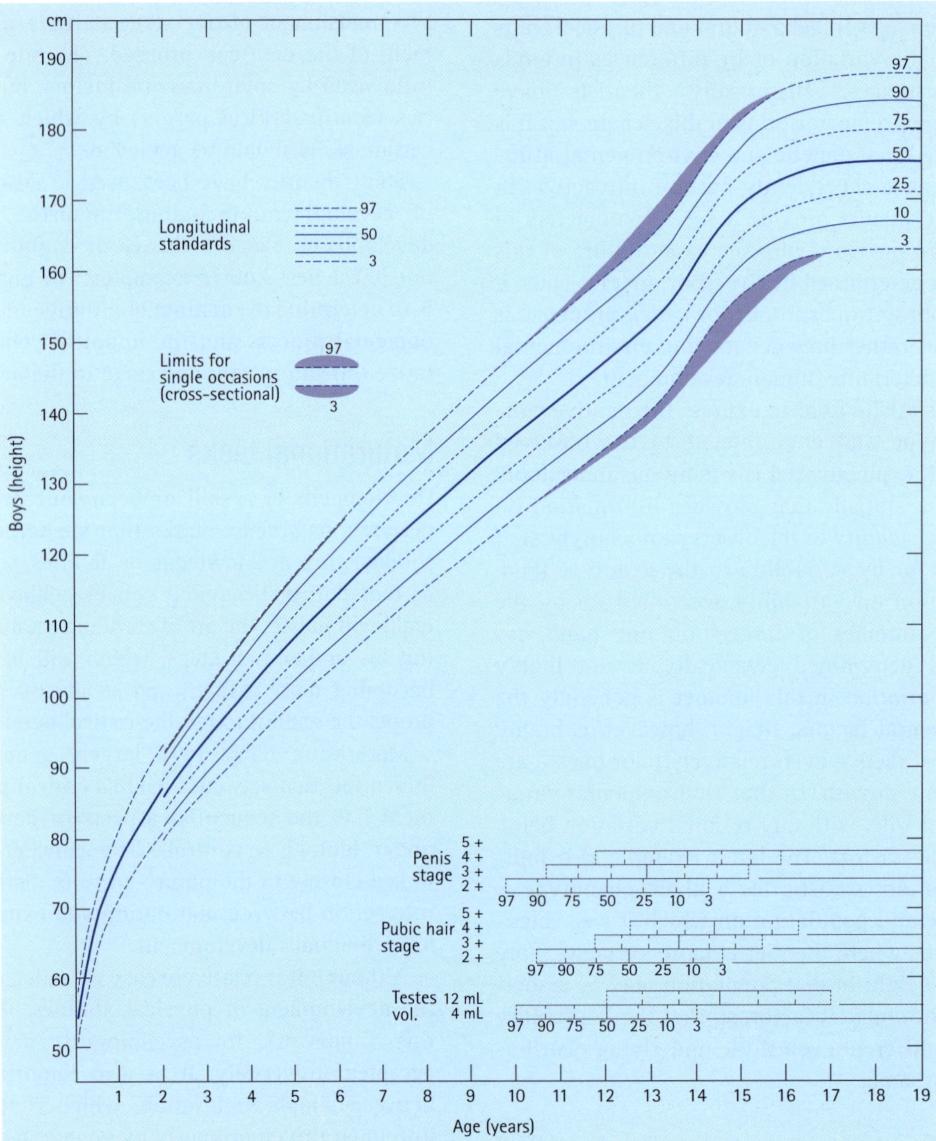

Figure 8.1 Example of Tanner growth chart for height. A series of charts of longitudinal growth standards for physical development (including parameters for height, weight, skin folds) were developed for children according to age, sex and sexual maturity. From Tanner JM, Whitehouse RH (1976) Clinical longitudinal standards for height, weight, height velocity, weight velocity, and stages of puberty. *Archives of Disease in Childhood* **51**: 170–79.

Gene–environment interactions

The broad implication of interactions between genetic and environmental influences has been described above. More recently, more specific findings have contributed to the debate concerning the nature and development of intelligence and personality, both of which have been claimed to be up to 80 per cent heritable, although most estimates range from 50 per cent to 60 per cent. Although twin studies and other methods have certainly suggested a genetic component to intellectual ability, the interpretation of these results is problematic, given the highly interactive nature of the factors in question and the complex nature of intelligence itself.

Early, simple additive genetic models of intelligence suggested that genotype and environment both contributed independently to the phenotypic expression of intelligence, so that the relative contribution could be determined by certain empirical means (e.g. the comparison of identical twins raised apart, or the comparison of monozygotic (MZ) versus dizygotic (DZ) twins). Notwithstanding the methodological limitations of many of these studies (and a few celebrated scientific frauds), the model of genetic influence guiding this research is potentially inappropriate. The model of genotype–phenotype interaction, proposed by Scarr and McCartney in 1983, highlights this (Figure 8.2).

Although genotype and environment will influence the phenotype of the individual, these relationships may not be

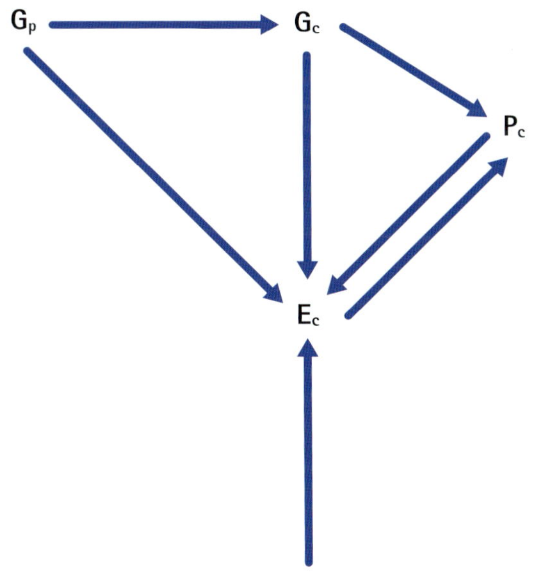

Figure 8.2 Scarr and McCartney's model of genotype–environment interaction in behavioural development. The child's observable behaviour (phenotype) will arise from an interaction between his or her genotype and rearing environment. The genotype of the parent will determine the genotype of the child and thus also indirectly influence the child's phenotype. Parental genotypes will have an additional influence over the child's rearing environment. The model also allows for a bidirectional influence between the child's behaviour and rearing environment, highlighting that the child actively contributes to their own behavioural development. E_c, child's rearing environment; G_c, child's genotype; G_p, parent's genotype; P_c, child's phenotype. From Scarr S, McCartney K (1983) How people make their own environments: a theory of genotype–environment effects. *Child Development* **54**: 424–35.

unidirectional. Most importantly, the phenotype of the individual will influence the environment, so that physically short individuals will be less likely to find themselves playing basketball, for example. In this sense, it would be possible to find a genetic component for basketball-playing, but this would not be interpreted as a gene 'for' basketball (whereas comparable findings in intelligence are so interpreted). Rather, the combined influence of a number of genes related to physical development, when expressed in a given context (i.e. a population where basketball is played) would influence the likelihood of an individual playing basketball. The various influences in this interactive model include the child's genotype on the child's phenotype, the child's environment on the child's phenotype, the child's phenotype on the child's environment, the parents' genotype on the child's genotype, the parents' genotype on the child's environment, and various external influences on the child's environment.

The influence of the parents' genotype on the child's environment may also, because of the obvious genetic relationship between parents and child, appear as a genetic influence rather than an environmental one. Finally, because of certain cultural norms, certain physical characteristics will result in the individual being treated in a certain way. Attractive children, for example, are likely to receive more stimulation in infancy, which may result in faster or improved cognitive development. This may appear as a genetic influence, even though the gene found is 'for' physical attractiveness, which, in a specific culture, results in certain treatment that may facilitate intellectual development, so that the genetic influence is mediated by a culturally determined environmental influence. In this case, it would be more proper to call the environmental mediating variable, rather than the genetic variable, causal.

Early versus late adversities

At various times in an individual's lifetime, they will encounter negative events or life stressors. A key question in developmental research is how the outcomes and coping strategies associated with these events differ as a function of when they occur. A young child may be particularly resilient to adversity; underdeveloped cognitive systems, for example, may restrict encoding of the event, such that its impact on future development is negligible. However, children are particularly vulnerable when the negative or traumatic event disrupts the normal course of development.

Over the last hundred years there have been several reports of children being rescued from severe adverse experiences, often involving considerable social and emotional neglect. Generally, the normal development of the child is severely compromised and, although improvements do occur with significant medical and psychiatric intervention, the child remains intellectually and socially impaired. These cases support the suggestion that children must attain specific developmental achievements within a critical age period.

These cases are, however, both extreme and rare. Many children experience some form of less severe adversity in childhood that may lead to behavioural disruption, but to what extent does this disruption persist – if at all? This will certainly depend on the nature of the negative event; a single short-lived adversity, such as a one-off hospitalization, while traumatic, may be less detrimental than sustained problems such as extreme poverty or an alcohol-dependent parent. However, individuals differ greatly in the extent to which they are vulnerable or resilient to the effects of negative events. Thus, it may be particularly important to consider why some individuals fare better than others following negative experience. Generally, events in early life will influence the development of risk factors such as self-concept, social skills and so on, while later events will act as causal factors given the existence of such risk or protective factors. This accounts for the apparent resilience found in some individuals where appropriate early experiences and subsequent emotional and cognitive development may act as protective factors.

Historical models and theories

Psychoanalytical theories

Psychoanalytical theories have common origins in the work of Sigmund Freud. They emphasize a role of unconscious as well as conscious processes in governing human behaviour. Early focus was on social and emotional characteristics of the adult and how these were shaped during early development. According to traditional theories, personality traits can be traced back to fixations held during various aspects of early development. An 'anal' personality type, for example, describes someone who is overly pedantic and compulsive, and would have had strong fixations in the anal stage of development. Parents and their methods of care are considered particularly important, with the infant playing a largely passive role in the outcome of their own development.

Social learning

A major component of social learning theory is learning through the observation and imitation of others, often termed 'observational learning' or 'modelling'. Although many imitated behaviours are reinforced in some way, studies by Albert Bandura in the 1960s and 1970s showed that children would mimic the behaviour of an observed model in the apparent absence of any positive or negative reinforcer. Imitation, however, does not occur spontaneously. Children appear to actively select the behaviours that they imitate. Contemporary social learning theorists are particularly interested in the factors that influence this selectivity, such as the personality or past experience of the child, or situational factors. More recently, social learning theory has been adapted to link closely with cognitive theories of development.

Jean Piaget's epistemological account of cognitive development is considered in more detail in other sections of this chapter. Based predominantly on the observations of his own children, Piaget developed a stage theory of cognitive development that emphasized the interaction between biological predispositions and environmental influence. His work also encompassed other aspects of development (e.g. moral development); however, it is his cognitive model of development that has been particularly influential. One of the most important contributions that Piaget made was to establish the child as playing a dynamic role in his or her own development, through interaction with physical and social worlds, that is driven by simple, inherited predispositions.

Summary

Understanding human development requires consideration of the relative influences of inherited biological dispositions and of environmental factors on phenotypic expression. This is referred to as the nature–nurture debate, and it is now accepted widely that genetic and environmental factors are not simply additive but interact in complex ways. Generally, it is believed that an individual may vary on any given characteristic within limits determined by their genotype, while the variation within these limits is determined by the environment.

Stage theories have been employed to explain many important aspects of human development. They describe qualitative changes that occur at various periods during development. Individuals pass through developmental stages in a fixed order, with attainment of the characteristic skills of one stage being required before the individual can pass on to the next. Although sometimes criticized for their rigidity, stage theories have been extremely influential and describe behaviours that are often readily observable in the developing child. A related concept is that of *maturational tasks*, which consolidate and expand current skills necessary for development on to higher levels of functioning.

It is important to be aware of several key theoretical frameworks, in particular psychoanalytical theory, social learning theory, and Piaget's stage theory of cognitive and intellectual development. These theories have been extremely influential in shaping understanding and research in human development.

METHODOLOGIES

Cross-sectional studies

Cross-sectional studies examine age-related differences in behaviour by comparing children of different age groups in the same situation and at the same point in time. This enables relatively quick and easy collection of large amounts of data. However, this method provides little information on how individual children develop or on the influence of past determinants on observed behaviour. It is possible to obtain self-reported retrospective accounts of past development, but this method is potentially flawed and has questionable reliability and validity. Furthermore, selection of different individuals means that comparison groups may differ on factors other than age. A 10-year-old child born in 1998, for example, may differ from a 5-year-old child born in 2003 due to different economic or social influences during their early development. Thus, there are limits on the conclusions that can be drawn from cross-sectional studies, and longitudinal or cohort methods are employed to tackle more complex questions such as individual stability over time.

Cohort studies

In cohort studies, individuals are chosen on the basis of one or more unifying characteristics. For example, studies examining the genetic and environmental risk factors for schizophrenia often enlist the children of schizophrenic patients, as the incidence of schizophrenia is elevated in these children compared with in the normal population. However, this presents problems relating to the generalizability of the findings. Longitudinal studies also require substantial resources to sustain them over the, often lengthy, study period. They also may achieve a less representative sample than a cross-sectional study, due to some people being unwilling to commit to repetitive testing over time. Furthermore, dropout rates are often high and such attrition may not be random.

Individual studies

On occasion it is beneficial to study an individual child in a detailed manner, which is not practical with larger groups of children. This method is particularly useful when studying unusual cases, such as rare diseases, where individual examples are uncommon. The fundamental limitation of such an idiographic approach, however, is an inability to generalize findings to the wider population; it is plausible that the observations are unique to the child being studied. Nevertheless, this method can provide useful insights that guide future research using more systematic techniques in a large number of individuals.

Identification and evaluation of influences

There is substantial interest in the relative influence of genetic and environmental factors on development. Methodologies for investigating this rely on comparison being made along certain phenotypic dimensions between individuals of varying genetic similarity. For example, identical (MZ) twins are genetically identical, while non-identical (DZ) twins share only, on average, one-half of their variegated genotype. As such, if a psychological characteristic is correlated more strongly in MZ twins compared with DZ twins, then this suggests a genetic influence. Several varying degrees of genetic and environmental similarity are possible: MZ twins reared together, MZ twins reared apart, DZ twins reared together, DZ twins reared apart, siblings reared together, siblings reared apart, cousins, and adopted (i.e. unrelated) children reared together. Other combinations are possible, but this demonstrates the variety of comparisons that may be made.

On a variety of phenotypic characteristics (e.g. personality and other psychological dimensions), the degree of similarity between individuals increases with genetic similarity (and also with environmental similarity). The interpretation of such results, however, is highly problematic, and it is becoming increasingly clear that accurate characterization and reliable measurement of the phenotypic characteristic of interest are of primary importance. Moreover, this basic methodology relies on a simple additive model of genetic and environmental influence that is probably incomplete, as it fails to take into account gene × environment interactions.

Summary

Three main methodologies have been employed to study human development, all of which have their own strengths and weaknesses. Cross-sectional studies are conducted at one point in time in groups of children of different ages. They provide a quick and easy method of collecting a large amount of data, but they do not enable deeper understanding of how individuals develop over time. Cohort studies recruit individuals based on a unifying characteristic; however, there are problems when generalizing these data to wider populations. Longitudinal studies involve the repeated testing of the same sample at various periods during their development, which allows analysis of individual development across time, but these studies are time-consuming and costly. Less commonly, a single child may be studied in depth, which is not possible with larger samples, although there are problems associated with the generalizability of the findings.

By studying individuals of varying genetic and environmental similarity, it is possible to examine the relative influence of these factors on phenotypic characteristics. However, interpretation of results from these studies can be problematic.

ATTACHMENT THEORY

Attachment theory attempts to describe the behaviour of infants (generally in primate species) and relate this to behaviour in adulthood, in particular focusing on the progression of these behaviours as they become focused on (usually) one primary caregiver, known as the attachment figure, through infancy, and the relationship between the resulting attachment style and interpersonal behaviour in adulthood. The main premise of attachment theory is that the need for physical proximity and emotional closeness is an innate behaviour and a necessary precursor to and stimulus of psychological, emotional and social development. The primary attachment figure (usually, but not necessarily, the mother) serves as the model for the development of future relationships in later childhood and through adulthood.

Attachment behaviours comprise relevant behaviours directed towards the primary attachment figure, who is the focus of these behaviours (Table 8.1). In early life (typically the first 6 months), the infant does not display selectivity in the direction of relevant behaviours (e.g. seeking closeness), but after this early period these become increasingly directed towards an attachment figure. This represents the formation of an attachment with this individual; interestingly, it depends primarily not on obtaining resources (e.g. food) from that individual but instead on proximity, affection and so on. Therefore, direct survival behaviours such as feeding appear to be distinct from attachment behaviours such as seeking affection.

For example, rhesus monkeys separated from their mother will spend the majority of time clinging to a wool doll rather than a wire doll, even when it is the latter that provides food. This suggests that attachment behaviours are related not to feeding but to proximity, nurturance and so on cued by other stimuli (such as the physical characteristics of the mother).

It has been suggested widely that the initial attachment forms a template for the development of subsequent social and emotional relationships, so that early behaviour may predict later social behaviour.

Table 8.1 Development of attachment behaviours

Evolutionary basis	Infant's best hope for survival lies in proximity to caretaker
Early weeks	Infant predisposed to achieve closeness
3rd month	Attachment remains indiscriminate and transient
6th month	A single (usually) attachment figure is established
12th month	Fear of strangers, attachment maintained over distance
24th month	Attachment figure (usually mother) of primary importance
36th month	Substitute attachment figures are accepted in absence of primary
Adulthood	Early attachment behaviour related to later emotional development

Emotional development

Attachment behaviours in early life appear to be highly correlated with subsequent development and behaviour. Secure attachment styles are related to initiative-taking, social competence and the ability to form friendships in later childhood. Insecure attachment styles, on the other hand, are related to subsequent social withdrawal and difficulty in forming friendships. Attachment behaviour seems to be relatively stable, once established, over the lifespan.

Affect regulation

Insecure attachment behaviours include inability to express affection with the attachment figure, either by being excessively dependent and at the same time irritated by the attachment figure, or by displaying avoidant behaviour, and this may be related to affect regulation in adult life. Generally, insecure attachments have been found to be related to emotional disturbance in adolescence and adulthood, although the strength of the relationship is modest.

Relationships

The primary attachment figure serves as the model for subsequent relationships, including friendships and romantic relationships. Patterns of adult romantic relationships appear similar to attachment behaviours, with the proportion of adults describing themselves as within each category roughly corresponding to the proportions found in infant attachment styles. Retrospective questionnaires suggest that these styles of romantic affection are related to the perceived or remembered behaviour of the mother towards the individual.

Secure attachment

Infants who display secure attachment behaviour use the attachment figure as a base from which to explore, occasionally returning to seek affection. Separation from the attachment figure induces anxiety and distress and interaction is sought when reunited, after which anxiety reduces and exploration resumes. This is most evident in the first 36 months of life, after which separation anxiety reduces and attachment substitutes may be accepted.

Secure attachment behaviour is related to early infant temperament, child-focused caring, nurturing behaviour from the attachment figure, encouragement for the child to explore independently, and provision of a secure base by the attachment figure.

Insecure attachment

Insecure attachment behaviours comprise two distinct categories:

Insecure-avoidant behaviours are characterized by muted distress in the absence of the attachment figure and a minimal response when reunited. What may appear to be secure attachment behaviour may in fact be insecure-avoidant behaviour, due to this apparent independence, and making the distinction may be difficult. The clearest difference lies in the fact that securely attached children still display closeness, balancing a desire for affection with independence, while insecure-avoidant children almost exclusively seek distance and self-sufficiency at the expense of closeness.

Insecure-ambivalent behaviours represent the least common attachment style and represent a mixture of excessively dependent behaviour towards the attachment figure with a lack of obvious affection. Separation results in excessive distress in the child but, when reunited, the child will then resist physical contact. Distress continues for some time after the return of the attachment figure.

There is evidence for a relationship between insecure attachment styles and future antisocial behaviour and affective disorders. If such attachment behaviours are identified in early life, then teaching parenting skills to the parents of the child, specifically to be more caring towards the child, may reduce this risk. However, it is simplistic to attribute attachment behaviours solely to the parenting style of the parents, and other factors such as early infant temperament appear relevant.

Early separation

Given the relationship between attachment behaviour and subsequent behaviour in adolescence and adulthood, separation from initial attachment figures is related to subsequent behavioural problems. This is related to the age at which such separation takes place. For example, selective attachments do not begin to form until 6 months of age, so that separation before this time may have relatively little effect, allowing the formation of attachment behaviours towards the adoptive caregiver. Similarly, after the first few years of life, the child will have developed a pattern of attachment behaviour, and therefore a model or template of relationships, so that separation will not result in excessive disturbance, as the child will be able to accept the adoptive caregiver as a substitute attachment figure.

The critical period appears to be between 6 and 36 months, when the greatest changes occur in the pattern of attachment behaviours. Separation during this period is likely to have the greatest impact on the child's subsequent behaviour, as it will disrupt the formation of normal attachment behaviour.

Failure to develop selective attachments

Autistic children are characterized by an unwillingness to seek physical contact with parents. This becomes most apparent between 12 and 36 months, when normal, selective attachments would otherwise typically form. This is highly correlated with similar behaviour in adult life and appears to be largely the result of physical and genetic factors rather than social or developmental processes.

The failure to develop selective attachments in autistic children as a result of internal factors should be distinguished from a breakdown of the normal attachment process because of environmental or rearing factors. In this case, the lack of a clear single caregiver results in incomplete development of attachment behaviours, so that strangers and parents are treated similarly, without any apparent stranger anxiety. At the same time, the behaviour towards such figures is superficial and any affection easily terminated, so that separation anxiety also does not occur. It is for this reason that early separation in the critical period is most detrimental to the child, in particular if the child is not placed in a caring adoptive or foster home.

Maternal bonding

The anxiety that results from separation of the child from the attachment figure is a necessary part of the development of secure attachments, since it is the eventual reunion that gives the child confidence in the attachment figure. This, in turn, gives the child confidence in relationships, understanding that they persist over time and distance. The term 'maternal bonding' is potentially inappropriate, however, in that, although usual in most Western cultures, it is not necessary that the primary attachment figure be the mother.

Summary

Attachment theory is a framework for understanding the behaviour of infant primates whereby proximity and affection are sought (attachment behaviours) and appear to act as primary drives, in a similar way to hunger and thirst. An attachment relationship develops between the infant and the care provider (attachment figure). This serves as the model for subsequent relationships of all kinds. Infant attachment behaviours appear to relate modestly to adolescent and adult friendships and romantic relationships. Selective attachments usually do not form before 6 months.

Attachment to an attachment figure may be either secure or insecure, with the latter further subdivided into avoidant and ambivalent. Secure attachment represents a relationship where the attachment figure provides a base for independent exploration, and, although separation from the attachment figure results in distress, this rapidly subsides on reunion. Insecure-avoidant attachment is characterized by a relative lack of distress on separation and a general tendency for affection to be muted. Apparent secureness masks an unwillingness to display closeness. Insecure-ambivalent behaviour is characterized by excessive dependence but an unwillingness to display affection towards the attachment figure. There is some evidence for a relationship between attachment style and subsequent antisocial behaviour and affective disturbance.

The development of attachment behaviours occurs between 6 and 36 months. This has implications for the separation of the child from the primary attachment figure (usually the mother), with this critical period being associated with the greatest impact on the child's behaviour if separation occurs.

A failure to develop selective factors may be the result of internal factors (e.g. autism) or external factors (e.g. disturbed family function). The latter situation may also be related to early separation of the child from the primary attachment figure during the critical period (i.e. the first 3 years of life).

FAMILY RELATIONSHIPS

Parental practices and attitudes

The behaviour of individuals towards their offspring is of primary importance in determining attachment behaviours in infants, with these factors further interacting with temperamental features of the infant. Parenting style is commonly characterized along two dimensions: restrictive-permissive and loving-hostile. Alternatively, three categories of parenting style have been suggested: permissive (warm and caring, while accepting unorthodox behaviour), authoritarian-restrictive (less emotionally close and highly controlling), and authoritative (enforce rules and demand achievement, yet warm and loving).

The development of the child depends greatly on the parenting style adopted by the child's parents. For example, authoritarian-restrictive parents tend to have highly submissive children, while authoritative parents tend to have independent children (largely as a result of the emphasis placed on expressiveness within set boundaries). The behaviour of the parents is most important in the early development of the child, and this establishes a pattern of behaviour in the child that is sustained over time. In particular, the *consistency* of the parents' behaviour towards the child, for example with reference to the rewards and punishments consequent on certain behaviour, is a strong predictor of subsequent emotional and social behaviour in the child. *Inconsistent* parenting behaviour is associated with negative outcomes along these dimensions, presumably because it inhibits the development of a clear social model to guide behaviour.

The extent to which specific attitudes of parents is mirrored in subsequent attitudes in their children is debatable: any relationship may be weak overall, and there are numerous examples of children adopting opposing attitudes and beliefs, in particular during adolescence.

Distorted family function

There are a variety of ways in which normal family function may be distorted. Such (dysfunctional) families are highly varied in the nature and extent of distorted function, so that care should be taken in making comparisons. Certainly there is no such thing as a 'typical' dysfunctional family. Distorted patterns of communication are often at the core of dysfunctional families; for example, positive or neutral remarks may be interpreted in a negative way, leading to potential discord. This situation may be self-sustaining, as individuals attempt to exert their influence in response to perceived insults by reacting in a similar way. Conversely, behaviour that would be useful in reducing discord (e.g. apology) is used rarely and is typically seen by those involved as an admission of defeat.

Overprotection may be the result of enmeshment within a family, in which case it is broadly applicable to all members of the family unit. It may also occur in specific cases; the central feature of overprotection is an unwillingness to allow a member of the family group to display individuality, especially outside of the family group. The characteristic feature of such family behaviour is an apparent excess of closeness that is selfishly motivated.

Rejection may be a specific individual effect, for example where a mother rejects closeness with her child, or a more general family effect. In this latter case, the family will not have a strong sense of collective identity, with individuals showing only weak attachment relationships to other members, often forming stronger attachments outside the family group. Isolation and loneliness commonly result.

Enmeshment refers to families where individual identity and individuality are lost to family status and role, in direct contrast to rejection. A high degree of homogeneity, especially of opinions and beliefs, results in little input in discussions regarding the family. Family structure is tightly defined, and any individual family member attempting to display independence is likely to have this suppressed.

Bereavement

Bereavement may involve the death of a loved one or relative, but more generally (and metaphorically) it can indicate loss of any kind (e.g. moving school, leaving home). This latter use is based on some evidence that the reaction to loss of any kind follows a similar pattern, although the intensity of these reactions will vary. Typical reactions to loss include: disbelief/denial, emotional blunting/numbness, and excessive rumination over the lost object or individual.

Considerable adjustment is required in any case of bereavement, and the effect on the child may be considerable. Behavioural problems are associated with the loss of a parent in children, and this is related to poor adjustment in the surviving parent, although the direction of causation may be complex. Subsequent development of the child may be influenced most by the subsequent behaviour of the surviving parent (e.g. change of parenting style, relative neglect due to increased time demands), rather than the loss of a parent specifically.

Divorce

The effects of divorce on child development are difficult to delineate, as parents who divorce have generally been in conflict for some time before the divorce. In general, in the first year following a divorce, the parents of the child become more permissive and less controlling, and communication between parents and child deteriorates. This behaviour occurs in both the parent without the child and the parent who cares for the child, but usually this change in parenting style resolves after the first year following the divorce. The effects of the divorce on the child depend on the age of the child, the degree of hostility resulting from the divorce, the use of the child by the conflicting parents to achieve their own aims, and the degree of adjustment of the parent who remains caring for the child.

In almost all cases there is a degree of distress in the child, allied to feelings of responsibility or guilt, and consequent depression or hostility. In most cases, however, this resolves relatively quickly (usually after the first year), provided that the parent with whom the child remains also adjusts over this period.

Intrafamilial abuse

Abuse of children is most dangerous in the early years of life (under 4 years), not least because this is when the child is physically most vulnerable. This is also the period when the antecedents of self-esteem and self-image are developing. Immediate effects of intrafamilial abuse (either physical or sexual) include sleep disturbance, eating disturbance, depression, phobias or anxiety, behavioural problems and social problems. Longer-term effects are more difficult to delineate, but there is some evidence that initial consequences may persist for several years if abuse continues. In particular, several problems appear to persist, including depression (especially in sexual abuse), self-harm, low self-esteem and impaired relationship formation.

These effects are greatest if the abuse comes from within the family group (which is the most common source), if the abuse is sustained over a substantial period, and if the abused is not believed when help is sought.

Non-orthodox family structures

The most common non-orthodox family structure is the single-parent family, a situation that has increased in prevalence recently. This may be the result of bereavement (uncommon), divorce (common) or single motherhood (also common). The consequences of living with only a mother (i.e. single-mother families) have been investigated extensively, since this is the most typical single-parent situation. Effects have been reported for self-identity (boys, in particular, may have problems achieving a clear sexual identity if the father is absent in early life), gratification (boys, again, are most affected and appear to show impaired ability to delay gratification and control impulses), and social skills (interaction with the opposite sex, in particular in girls, appears to be impaired).

There is also evidence that the relative difficulty in forming relationships with the opposite sex found in the children of single mothers persists into adulthood, although the effect is weak. The potential confound of differences in parenting behaviour existing in single-parent families is difficult to control for in studies that consider the impact of single-parent families on children, and it is difficult to conclude that behavioural and psychological correlates of a single parent upbringing are a consequence of the fact that only one parent was present. Similar consequences for child development have been found in other, rare family structures (e.g. children raised by grandparents).

Although the extended family structure found in some cultures and ethnic groups should not be regarded as unorthodox, it is not the common structure in Western cultures. In general, children raised in such families tend to develop high levels of self-esteem and the family structure seems to represent a protective factor (i.e. by providing high levels of social support).

Summary

Parenting style is an important determinant of child behaviour. The behaviour of the parents may be described as either dimensional (e.g. restrictive-permissive/loving-hostile) or categorical (e.g. permissive, restrictive, authoritative). Parenting style correlates with the behaviour of the child. For example, restrictive parents tend to have submissive children. This relationship is statistical, so that it is not possible to accurately predict behaviour in the child from the behaviour of the parents in specific cases.

The impact of bereavement and divorce on family function, in particular children's behaviour, may be regarded under the more general term of loss. There are certain similarities between bereavement and divorce, although there are also unique characteristics of each. Distress following loss of any kind is normal and only problematic if it becomes chronic in nature and extends beyond the normal time for adaptation and coping to take place.

Specific terms are used to describe different features of distorted family function, such as overprotection, rejection and enmeshment. Although there is no such thing as a typical dysfunctional family, and the causes of dysfunction may vary widely, certain characteristics appear repeatedly (e.g. distorted or impoverished communication between family members).

TEMPERAMENT

Temperament and parent–child relationships

From birth, infants display apparently innate differences in behaviour. They differ in their moods, activity levels, stability of sleeping and feeding patterns, sociability, and response to novel situations. These early biases are known as differences in temperament. Given that these differences are observed soon after birth, it is reasonable to suggest that differences in temperament are, at least in part, determined genetically.

Temperament also influences the relationship that forms between the child and the parent. A parent of a 'difficult' child may display irritability and frustration, which, in turn, increases the irritability of the child. In extreme cases, the stress of dealing with a difficult child may interfere with the natural attachment process, particularly in families where there is limited external support. Conversely, a parent is more likely to engage with a child who is sociable and quick to smile. Consequently, even within the same household, parents may encourage different patterns of development in their children, driven by differences in the children's temperament. Parenting style itself, however, is subject to change. Parents of a difficult child may learn to adapt and develop new and more fruitful ways of interacting with their offspring, so that even when bonding is initially compromised this can be rectified with appropriate parental adjustment.

Origins, typologies and stability of temperament

Early work on temperament identified several dimensions along which young children vary. The analysis of these dimensions resulted in three typologies of temperament: *easy children* (about 40%), characterized as having regular sleeping and feeding patterns, sociability, enjoyment of physical contact, and adaptability to new situations; *difficult children* (about 10%), characterized by irregular sleeping and feeding patterns, irritability, emotional lability and negative responding to new situations; and *slow-to-warm-up children* (about 15%), characterized by relatively low activity, slowness to adapt to new situations, and treating new situations with initial suspicion. A proportion cannot be reliably classified into one of these groups.

Around one-third of the original sample of children studied in this research did not clearly fall into any of these groups, but follow-up work suggested some degree of stability in temperament. Children identified as 'difficult' may not always be classified this way but are more likely to have problems in later life.

Temperament theory suggests that the nature and behaviour of a child is not simply a product of his or her environment (e.g. parenting style). Instead, the child interacts with the world and, in doing so, modifies behaviour directed towards them. The goodness-of-fit of the child's environment should be taken into account – a 'difficult' child may prompt negative responses in his or her parents. Alternatively, parents may work hard to overcome the challenges of dealing with a 'difficult' child, handling the child with emphasized patience and understanding. The latter case is more likely to result in healthy development of the child.

Temperament and personality

A critical question in developmental psychology is the extent to which personality in adulthood may be predicted by infant temperament. Although research has suggested links between early temperament and personality in later life, any continuity that does exist appears to be weak, presumably because of the strong environmental and societal influences on the development of personality. However, temperament does play an important role in the emerging personality of the individual; it sets a framework of behaviour, but personality will be a result of how this basic pattern of behaviour is affected by maturation and experience.

Temperament × environment interactions may serve to strengthen innate dispositions and mould personality. A sociable child, for example, will seek contact with others, in turn promoting sociability and social development. Furthermore, temperament is associated with various long-term outcomes, including the quality of familial and peer relationships, psychopathology and psychological adjustment.

There is some evidence to suggest that temperament of very young children is related to subsequent attachment behaviour (over a relatively short timespan): *easy* with secure attachment, *difficult* with anxious-avoidant attachment, and *slow-to-warm* up with anxious-ambivalent attachment. Attachment behaviour, in turn, has been shown to be weakly associated with adult behaviour. The greater the temporal distance between the temperament and current behaviour, the weaker the relationship.

Vulnerability and resilience

Psychosocial adversity and negative life events are associated with higher incidence of psychiatric disorder. However, individuals differ in the extent to which they are vulnerable or resilient to long-term negative impact following adverse experiences. Several factors have been identified that may increase vulnerability, such as family discord, intrafamilial abuse and early bereavement (particularly of the primary attachment figure).

Some children show great resilience to life stressors. Those that demonstrate secure attachment behaviour, for example, are likely to be able to form replacement attachments if the mother is lost (depending on the age at which the loss occurs). It is also possible that experience of early stress may result in resilience to stress in later life in some individuals but an increase in vulnerability in others.

The long-term impact of traumatic events will depend on the temperamental disposition of the child. Difficult and slow-to-warm-up children are more vulnerable to stressors and appear to be more at risk of subsequent deviant behaviours, including psychiatric problems such as depression, hysteria, neuroticism and psychosis.

Summary

From birth, infants display differences in behaviour that are referred to as individual *temperaments*. Children with 'difficult' temperaments are more irritable, less content and less sociable than children with 'easy' temperaments. An intermediate temperament, 'slow-to-warm-up', has been identified that describes children who may show initially negative emotional reactions that improve with time and experience. Development of temperament may be related to the development of attachment style in early infancy.

Some psychiatric disorders (e.g. unipolar depression) may develop as a result of certain environmental risk factors. However, individuals differ in the extent to which the presence of these risk factors is likely to result in the expression of psychiatric disturbance: some people seem particularly vulnerable, while others are resilient to these effects. The mechanisms underlying these differences are unclear but are likely to include the coping style of the individual.

COGNITIVE DEVELOPMENT

Jean Piaget developed an epistemological account of intellectual development that transformed our understanding of the way in which children think. He argued that the general pattern of cognitive growth was universal, and interaction with objects and people in the world forced children to follow comparable patterns of development. Piaget was particularly interested in *how* children think, the processes that underlie cognition, and how these processes change with age. An important feature of his theory, and one that is still largely accepted today, is that children's thought processes are qualitatively, not just quantitatively, different from adults'.

According to this model, children are not merely passive observers of the world. Cognitive development progresses via the interactive processes of *assimilation* and *accommodation*. At birth a child inherits relatively primitive mental structures, largely reflexive in nature, which enable basic interaction with the environment and which are modified with experience. First, the child interacts with the environment and interprets information in the context of existing mental structures (assimilation). Then, when presented with new information or objects that do not fit with existing cognitive schema, the child develops his or her repertoire of actions based on the environment (accommodation). Thus, in Piaget's view, cognitive development comprised a continuous interaction between the child and the environment, in which knowledge is repeatedly constructed and reconstructed in light of new experience.

Piaget argued that cognitive development was not a gradual process but advanced in a step-like fashion. He described specific, qualitatively distinct stages of development in which accomplishment of critical aspects of each stage was required before the child could advance to subsequent stages. These stages described a global process of cognitive development comprising the totality of cognitive growth from birth to maturity and are summarized in Table 8.2.

These transitions between stages suggest that, at critical periods, the child undergoes a comprehensive mental reorganization that encompasses all aspects of cognition. The ages described provide a guide to when these transitions occur, but children may vary considerably in the ages that they progress from one stage to another, with some individuals failing to achieve the final stage entirely.

Some key concepts should be noted that further characterize the different stages in development. *Object permanence* describes the acquired ability of the child to understand that objects in the environment exist even when

Table 8.2 Stages in Piaget's Model of Cognitive Epistemology

Stage	Description
Sensorimotor (birth–18 months)	Knowledge of the world is acquired primarily through sensory experience and basic motor actions (sucking, grasping, biting), which become more complex and coordinated over time. Only towards the end of this stage does the child begin to form internal mental representations of the world and begin to engage in intentional behaviour
Preoperational (18 months–7 years)	Characterized by the child beginning to engage in symbolic thought (imaginative play, drawing), where words/mental images stand for objects and people. Focus on static states rather than transformations
Concrete operations (7–11 years)	Logical thought and problem-solving ability emerges. Children acquire a number of cognitive operations that were not possible at earlier stages, including ability to see situations from the viewpoint of others, reversible thinking and ability to understand transformations. Abstract conceptualizations, however, are limited
Formal operational (11 years+)	Children can think in terms of abstract and hypothetical concepts. Logical and rational thought develop so that the child can conceive possible outcomes of actions and perform advanced problem-solving by constructing and testing hypotheses systematically. Complex self-identity develops

he or she can no longer see them. This ability is one of the most important developments during the sensorimotor stage. Preoperational children have a well-developed sense of object permanence but are largely *egocentric* – that is, they can only construe the world from their own viewpoint and lack understanding that alternative perspectives exist. Egocentrism is lost by the concrete operational stage, in which the most important acquired skill is *conservation.* This refers to an understanding that the fundamental nature of an object can remain constant despite changes in appearance. The classic example is that children in this stage understand that a set volume of liquid does not change when poured into different-shaped containers.

A particularly common criticism of Piaget's model is that he was overly pessimistic when describing the cognitive abilities of children. He believed that biological factors constrained the order and rate at which a child was able to develop. However, abilities such as object permanence have been observed in children much younger than Piaget would have predicted. Underdeveloped motor ability or difficulty in relaying task instructions to young children may have contributed to these underestimations in cognitive capability. In addition, the stage-like nature of development proposed by Piaget has been challenged. It appears that development may be more gradual and continuous than the model suggested. For example, children may show some aspects of object permanence or non-egocentric behaviour in some circumstances but not others, arguing against the abrupt changes in development associated with a stage theory.

Despite these limitations, Piaget's theory has been hugely influential due to its depth, testable hypotheses, and the observational and empirical basis of much of the theory. It provides a framework of global cognitive and intellectual development that explains the qualitative differences in thinking during development and also *how* changes occur. The assumption that children are not passive observers of the world has also had important implications for education.

Thought and communication

Piaget claimed that the acquisition of language progresses as part of the natural development of cognition, and therefore the way in which a child communicates with others depends on the developmental stage the child is at.

The first steps on the road to acquiring language occur with the emergence of symbolic thought towards the end of the sensorimotor stage. However, it is during the preoperational period that the child begins to display significant advances in linguistic skills, from single-word utterances, through short sentences, to competent, if unsophisticated, language. Towards the end of the preoperational stage, the child begins to learn and apply the *rules* of language (*language pragmatics*) as a means of more sophisticated communication. At this stage, children begin to show adult-like gestures associated with verbal communication and adapt their communication to the situation they are in or the person to whom they are talking. This social skill improves with the reduction of egocentrism, when children can appreciate the perspective of others and thus adapt communication appropriately. A noticeable change that occurs during the preoperational stage is the development of politeness in the linguistic competence of these children. More complex and subtle features of communication, such as indirect questions, hints and sarcasm, require a certain level of cognitive maturity before they can be learned.

The loss of egocentrism during the *concrete operational* stage characterizes a dynamic change in communication. Understanding the perspective of others means that, for the first time, the child appreciates that another person may not be interested in some topics of conversation and can identify what another person does or does not know. Persuasive communication marks another important development in linguistic ability; during earlier development, children tend to repeat crude requests, while concrete operational children form persuasive arguments that take into account the attitudes or desires of the person to whom the request is directed. During this stage, humour also develops, with children beginning to understand and tell rudimentary jokes.

Finally, the *formal operations* stage, in the context of communication, represents the final development of the social skills that must be allied to linguistic ability. An increasingly level of subtlety is evident in requests and persuasion, and sophistication in the use of humour (sarcasm, irony) and pragmatics appears. Children also acquire the ability to infer meaning of unfamiliar words by the context in which the word appears, without the need for explicit definition.

Therefore, the linguistic ability and communicative competence of children vary as a function of their level of cognitive development. As the capacity of abstraction develops, egocentrism declines and communicative social skills (pragmatics) develop, spoken language becomes more complex and goal-oriented, particularly in social situations.

Summary

Piaget's model of cognitive development proposes that children pass through step-like stages of cognitive development that are qualitatively different and proceed in an invariant order. These stages are the *sensorimotor, preoperational, concrete operational* and *formal operational.* To understand the model fully, one should be aware of the characteristics that define each stage and the approximate ages at which children move between them.

Although no longer accepted universally, Piaget's model remains influential. Key concepts include *assimilation, accommodation, operations* and *egocentricism.* These represent key mechanisms that allow the child to complete one stage of development and proceed on to the next.

As children progress through Piaget's stages, they acquire abilities necessary for communication and the development of linguistic ability. For example, with the loss of egocentricism, children develop social communicative skills, such as understanding that other people may not be interested in certain topics of conversation.

LANGUAGE DEVELOPMENT

Language develops as children learn to associate symbols with objects or people in the real world. However, language is not merely a collection of words but a coherent system comprising complex rules that the child must master if he or she is to become proficient in its use. Language comprises distinct elements that are achieved competently during different stages of development. Consequently, ascertaining the age at which a child develops language is difficult to determine and depends largely on how 'language' is defined. The main aspects of language are summarized in Table 8.3.

Despite the complexities of language, and the considerable cognitive capacity required to learn language, linguistic skills develop quickly. At birth, infants show a preference for the human voice and develop basic phonology during their first year of life. Vocabulary acquisition, although initially slow, increases rapidly between the ages of 18 months and 7 years. First words are universally similar across cultures and languages (including sign language) and are words of particular interest to the child ('doggie', 'mama', 'more'). Semantic understanding of newly learned words is initially minimal but becomes refined, with the child quickly learning multiple ways in which a single word can be used.

At around 2 years of age, early sentence structure appears. This is simplistic, comprising the combination of two or three words, and is often grammatically incorrect. However, by 3 years, children learn that simple grammatical manipulations such as changing word order (e.g. from 'cuddle Mummy' to 'Mummy cuddle') can alter the meaning of a sentence. In addition, children learn to alter sentence structure in order to ask questions and form negative sentences. They also learn to apply grammatical rules such as adding –ed to words in order to denote past tense (e.g. 'wash' becomes 'washed'). Once learned, these rules are often overapplied (e.g. 'drink' becomes 'drinked'), suggesting that children do not learn grammatical rules solely through imitation. At approximately 4 years of age children will also start to use future tense, and by 5 years language begins to resemble that of adults.

Contrasting theories of language development exist. Nativists (e.g. Chomsky) argue that language development is predominantly biologically determined, while behaviourists (e.g. Skinner) propose a learning account of language acquisition. Although simple learning accounts are insufficient to account fully for the complexity of language development, it is unquestionable that the learning of language is influenced strongly by the interaction with others.

Table 8.3 Components of language and linguistic competence

Phonology	Concerns the way in which basic units of sound (*phonemes*) are used to form words. This develops continuously through early childhood, from crying and cooing in infancy, through simple articulation (consonant sounds) and babbling (combining consonant and vowel sounds), to production of phonologically simple first words ('mama'). Phonological complexity increases with age, but full phonological competence takes time, and young children often have difficulty with the production of some sounds into school age despite good overall language competence
Semantics	Concerns the meaning of words. Early semantic development involves direct association of sounds with objects or people. Children may not, however, understand the meaning of a word in the same way that an adult does. They are prone to *overextensions* (e.g. the word 'cat' used to describe many different animals) and *underextensions* (e.g. the word 'cat' used only to identify black cats). At later ages, more sophisticated semantic understanding develops involving abstract meanings
Syntax	Concerns the structure and rules of language and how to combine words to form sentences, understanding grammatical structure of language including word order, use of pronouns, passive sentences, etc. Grammatical learning appears to develop spontaneously without explicit instruction. Furthermore, children show evidence of understanding grammatical rules when listening to the speech of others, even before they have begun to produce meaningful sentences themselves. This is a progressive skill that develops across the lifetime, with many adults never achieving a full understanding of syntax
Pragmatics	Concerns the social use of language. Children learn to use language in new ways to communicate effectively with others, e.g. use of tone to convey mood. Furthermore, language can be adapted to suit a particular situation or person (e.g. depending on familiarity or competence of listener)

Environmental influences

Whether children are born with innate mental structures that are specific to acquiring and using language is the subject of debate, but, given that language is used to communicate, it follows that successful language development requires significant exposure to interactions with others. Adults help the child to develop speech by adapting their own speech patterns. Speech is slowed and pauses between words are emphasized, so that words are separated clearly into individual 'chunks' of sound. Important words are also stressed and non-verbal gestures (e.g. pointing) often accompany the words to highlight meaning.

Traditional learning theories of language development claim that language is learned through the processes of operant conditioning. Parents will reinforce behaviour by praising the child when he or she produces phonetically (or grammatically) correct speech, which, in turn, shapes behaviour. A more popular approach is that of Albert Bandura, who suggested that children learn through imitation. In the case of language, children learn by listening to the speech of others and attempting to reproduce it. Learning theory accounts of language have been criticized, but nevertheless they identify important ways in which language development can be influenced by the child's environment.

The importance of environmental influence in language acquisition is also evident in cases of early isolation, where children have had little or no contact with humans during early development. Generally, these children develop elementary language skills, but complete communicative competence is rarely achieved. However, these cases involve a complete absence of social interaction, and the children often display a generally low level of cognitive competence. This has led some theorists to suggest that *critical periods* exist for language acquisition, referring to a set time period in which certain linguistic skills must be realized: if a child fails to learn these skills within this critical period, learning will never be achieved fully.

Communicative competence

The social conventions of language are known as *pragmatics*, described earlier. They develop throughout the lifespan and represent a shift from thinking about the meaning and grammatical structure of language to understanding how language is *used* to communicate. The art of being a good conversationalist requires the ability to engage the listener, to understand non-verbal gestures and to respond appropriately to feedback. By the age of 2 years, children begin to read facial expressions, offering more information, for example, if the listener looks confused. By 3–4 years, children develop a conversational structure more characteristic of adult speech by waiting their turn to speak, maintaining eye contact and adjusting speech to suit the listener. However, at this stage, children have difficulty keeping track of conversations involving two or more people and will often interrupt inappropriately. This may be judged as impolite to the casual observer, but this is a communicative skill that children need time to develop.

Communicative competence will naturally develop when important cognitive milestones are reached. The loss of egocentrism, for example, allows the child to understand that their listener may not know something they do or may have a different opinion to them. Children also learn communicative skills by the moral and cultural lessons of their parents. The use of 'please' and 'thank you', for example, is a first step towards effective cultural communication.

Although communicative competence, in the conventional sense, requires a substantial degree of linguistic skill and cognitive development, the distinction between language and communication is an important one. In truth, language itself is neither necessary nor sufficient for communication. Many species display communicative competence, but care should be taken when describing these as languages. Furthermore, non-verbal communication (body language) is a powerful means of communication. In sum, an individual may be highly skilled at constructing sentences but lack the social skills to be a good communicator, particularly with unfamiliar others. Although linguistic capability is good, communicative ability is impaired, illustrating the partial dissociation of the two concepts.

Summary

Language is a complex system that can be broken down into separate components – *phonetics*, *semantics*, *syntax* and *pragmatics* – which refer to the sounds, meanings, structure and social use of language. These components differ in complexity and the age at which they are understood and mastered. Ability in all of these components is required for the child to become a competent user of language.

It is important to distinguish between speaking and communicating. An individual may have relatively strong linguistic ability but be a poor communicator. Language is not necessary for communication, as seen in other animal species.

SOCIAL DEVELOPMENT

Development of social competence and relationships

Early attachment behaviours and styles correspond to the development of an internal model (or schema) of relationship formation. This provides the basis for the development of social competence, but this is by no means the endpoint. Children develop an understanding of their social world and the norms of social behaviour through interactions with peers, the nature of which will change as a function of age. In the first 6 months of life the child will display little interest in other infants, but after 6 months the child will begin to show specific emotional expressions and vocalizations in response to peers. Young children will initially engage in *solitary play*, but as time progresses the child will begin to play alongside other children, observing their actions but with little or no direct interaction (*parallel play*). As motor and cognitive skills develop (including language), he or she will engage in different forms of play that further develop his or her social skills and relationships with other children. Social interactions become more complex and reciprocal in nature, and the child coordinates with their play partner, taking turns in various aspects of play. The first explicit demonstrations of prosocial behaviour are also observed, such as sharing and helping, and the child develops the ability to understand and consider the viewpoint of others. Therefore, the goal of play is not only to have fun; it also enables children to practise the art of social interaction and to develop early peer relationships. In short, play provides the building blocks for the development of social competence. In mid- to late childhood there is a dramatic increase in the amount of time spent with peers, and peer groups grow in terms of both number and diversity. This change is influenced largely by the child's move into full-time schooling and participation in extracurricular group activities. In adolescence, the trend towards spending an increased amount of time with peers continues, and the child may perceive peer relationships as more influential and important than familial relationships.

Acceptance

There are several common determinants of acceptance within childhood peer groups. Children usually base their first impressions of others on surface characteristics such as names or physical appearance. Physically attractive children are typically accepted more readily by their peers and are more likely to be regarded as having more positive qualities. In some, but not all, cultures, children are most likely to interact and play with children of a similar age to themselves. More universally, children prefer same-sex playmates, particularly in mid- to late childhood, which may be a function of personality and interests, with boys more likely to engage in rough, physical games compared with girls. Generally, children prefer other children similar to themselves, and a child may not be accepted if they are seen to 'stand out' or be different from the norm.

Beyond these rather shallow determinants of acceptance, the personality of the child and their cognitive and social skills will also be influential in establishing whether they are viewed positively by their peers. Children who have a well-developed ability to cooperate and communicate will be particularly popular in favour of a child who demonstrates poor social skills.

Group formation

Children do not restrict their relationships to single-pair friendships. As their social skills develop, they forge multiple friendships that merge into friendship groups, within which a hierarchical structure forms. Members of the group assume different roles and form different relationships with other members, depending on their group status. Characteristics of group leaders change with age, with dominance being associated with 'toughness' in younger children, and with attractiveness, âthletic ability or popularity in older children. Hierarchies in groups develop quickly and serve to facilitate interaction and reduce intragroup conflict.

In adolescence, the development of social groupings or *cliques* becomes common. Cliques are cohesive, usually same-sex groups that share common interests, attitudes or goals. They play an important part in an individual's self-identity and psychological wellbeing. Although adolescents may continue to have strong attachment to their parents, they show extraordinarily high levels of conformity to the behaviours and attitudes of their peer group, which often exceeds familial influence. Cliques often combine to produce larger social groups or *crowds*, which may last a few years in adolescence, but generally disperse back to smaller groups, and then romantic relationships form as the individual advances into adulthood.

Cooperation

The development of social competence includes the emphasis placed on cooperation and competition. There appears to be a strong cultural influence here, with Western cultures being highly competitive and individualistic. In-group/out-group biases may be a result of the internalization of social norms that promote competition rather than cooperation. Nevertheless, cooperation is required in some cases and appears to be one of the major determinants of group behaviour. Cooperative behaviour appears in infants during the preoperational stage of cognitive development, when children will be seen to play together and achieve joint goals or take on individual roles in a broader game.

Friendships

The first experience of peer relationships occurs when children first engage in interactive play. Over repeated encounters with another child, a relationship will form (positive or negative), but the duration and frequency of contact at this stage in life will be dictated predominantly by the parent, and these early relationships do not equate to true friendships. Mutual liking is important for a friendship but not sufficient for its development or maintenance. A friendship additionally requires a level of commitment between individuals, which will not be achievable until a certain degree of cognitive development has been attained.

The function of friendships and conceptions of what constitutes a friendship change across childhood. For younger children friends are predominantly companions and playmates, but in mid-childhood friends begin to take on a supportive role and are more likely to be *chosen*, based on their personal characteristics. Friendships become more stable and long-lasting and are likely to be based on mutual liking. Thus, as children age, more intimate relationships are formed, and these friendships become important for emotional growth and wellbeing. There are also interesting differences in the quality of friendships between male and female children. Boys are more likely than girls to gather in groups, and these relationships are less intimate and more competitive. In contrast, friendships between young girls involve more agreement and self-disclosure.

Isolation and rejection

Children who are not readily accepted by their peer groups tend to report loneliness, social exclusion and low self-esteem. Rejected children also demonstrate poorer academic success and are more likely to play truant or drop out of school. However, recent evidence suggests that if a rejected child can secure one high-quality friendship, then the detrimental effects of poor social acceptance are reduced significantly. There is a well-supported association with rejection in childhood and negative outcome in later life. However, the direction of causality is ambiguous – it is unclear whether the rejection in childhood results in subsequent detriment or whether a negative disposition in the individual drives early rejection. Low self-esteem appears to be related closely to isolation and rejection. Children with low self-esteem often display reduced social skills, awkwardness when interacting with others, and general unwillingness to initiate friendships or join in group activities.

It may be important to distinguish between *rejected* children (who are explicitly ignored or disliked by their peers) and *neglected* children (who are reasonably well liked but lack individual friendships). Although less well studied, neglected children appear more likely than rejected children to establish friendships over time but will be more at risk of negative outcomes such as loneliness or depression than accepted children.

Popularity

In any group of children, there will be a few who stand out as being particularly well liked and popular among their peers, while others will find themselves on the periphery of the group, with little influence over other members of the group. Although the characteristics that define popularity may differ with age, in general, popular children are those who are physically attractive, friendly, sociable, intelligent and athletic (particularly in boys). For many of these positive traits, however, it is difficult to determine the direction of causation; for example, does extroversion lead to increased popularity, or does popularity result in extroversion?

There is also a strong relationship between popularity and *leadership*; indeed, popular children tend to be the informal leaders of group activities. One factor that is apparent in leaders rather than those who are simply popular is aggression, although this is highly controlled aggression, used primarily to reinforce the leader's position when required. Uncontrolled aggression, in contrast, is associated with unpopularity.

Summary

From 6 months, the infant will show interest in other babies and children. As they grow, children begin to play together, and the level of direct interaction that occurs during play increases with age. These interactions enhance social and communicative skills that become important for the formation and maintenance of friendships.

The nature and functions of friendships alter with age. In early to mid-childhood, friends serve as sources of fun (i.e. playmates); however, later friendships become a source of emotional support and acceptance, with greater levels of commitment and self-disclosure (particularly among females). Friendships are extremely important for emotional wellbeing and social fulfilment.

Certain traits are associated with popularity (e.g. physical attractiveness, extroversion, intelligence, sociability), while others are associated with rejection (e.g. social incompetence, excessive aggression). It is often difficult to ascertain the direction of causation – that is, does extroversion create popularity or does popularity create extroversion? Rejected children are more likely to have problems in school and are more at risk of psychiatric disturbance in later life.

MORAL DEVELOPMENT

Kohlberg's theory

Lawrence Kohlberg emphasized the need to understand how an individual *perceives* a morally challenging situation and to ascertain the moral reasoning underlying a response. As such, he rejected response-oriented approaches that focused on overt behavioural responding. Instead, he conducted a series of interviews in which subjects were presented with moral dilemmas and were asked to justify what they believed to be the 'right' course of action. As a result of this work, Kohlberg proposed a stage theory of moral development comprising three levels of moral reasoning, which each comprised two qualitatively distinct stages:

- *Level 1:* pre-conventional moral reasoning
  Stage 1: obedience and avoidance of punishment
  Stage 2: acquisition of rewards (for self or others)
- *Level 2:* conventional moral reasoning
  Stage 3: acquisition of social reward (approval)/avoidance of disapproval
  Stage 4: maintaining social rules, laws, etc.
- *Level 3:* post-conventional moral reasoning
  Stage 5: defined by the 'public good', a social contract
  Stage 6: conscience, individual moral code, abstract personal ethics.

Although ages were not associated explicitly with Kohlberg's stages of moral reasoning, varying degrees of cognitive competence are necessary to achieve transition through the stages. The first two stages of pre-conventional morality require representational ability and therefore are unlikely to emerge until the child reaches Piaget's preoperational stage of cognitive development. During early to mid-childhood, moral judgements are made predominantly in reference to punishment and rewards. In this context, the notion of physical punishment will gradually make way for social punishment as social skills develop. However, the concept of the 'public good' requires higher-level operational thought and therefore will generally not be realized until adolescence or adulthood. However, Kohlberg himself noted that the highest level of moral reasoning will be achieved by very few people in their lifetime and would be evident only in those regarded as paradigms of morality.

Unfortunately, the correlation between moral development as assessed by Kohlberg's model and actual behaviour is quite weak. This is probably due to the emphasis that the model places on abstract reasoning and the description of moral behaviour, as opposed to its actual performance. In addition, the reliability of the interview process, on which the model was based, has been questioned, due to a lack of standardization in both the administration and the scoring of the interview. Moreover, the interviews were conducted only with male subjects, and the imaginary moral dilemmas presented during the interviews were culturally oriented to North America, limiting the generalizability of the findings. Progression through the levels of morality with age may simply result from increased awareness of and ability to describe moral rules, without necessarily being related to any desire to follow these.

Social perspective-taking

The ability to form a detached opinion from another person's perspective, or from a general 'social' perspective, represents a significant advance in the cognitive and moral development of the individual. This requires a strong sense of personal identity, an understanding of the independence of the thoughts and actions of others, and an understanding that morality is not defined simply by one's own desires and corresponding rewards and punishments. Consequently, it is unsurprising that Kohlberg's level at which an understanding of social norms for moral behaviour becomes apparent corresponds (roughly) with the development of concrete operational thought and a corresponding decline in egocentrism.

The ability to reason from a perspective other than one's own, however, is distinct from the desire to act in a moral way. Social perspective-taking is a largely cognitive ability that may be applied to moral dilemmas, so that the stages of Kohlberg's theory may represent only an increasing ability to reason from perspectives other than one's own (rather than any actual development of personal morality).

Summary

Kohlberg's stage theory of moral development comprises three distinct levels, each comprising two stages. It is not as rigid as some stage theories (e.g. Piaget's cognitive model), and not all individuals accomplish all of the developmental stages fully.

There is some correspondence between moral development and cognitive development, with some level of cognitive capacity being required before specific aspects of morality can be achieved.

DEVELOPMENT OF FEARS

Childhood and adolescence

From around 6 months, an infant will display fear or anxiety in some situations, for example during maternal separation or in the presence of strangers. However, with a few exceptions (e.g. darkness, heights), younger infants are characterized by a general lack of fear, leading to the assumption that the majority of fear responses are learned, particularly in younger children.

There is, however, individual variability in physiological and psychological reactions to a potentially fearful event. For example, some introverted children may display relatively high levels of stress in response to mild environmental stressors. That is not to say that the fear response is consistent across all situations or inevitable in all individuals. For example, fear in response to the presence of a stranger is reduced markedly if the meeting occurs in the infant's home.

As children grow, their understanding of reality changes, so that fears relating to imaginary figures or unlikely threats to personal safety diminish. Instead, as the child enters late childhood and adolescence, new fears develop, often relating to social concerns, and that begin to resemble the profile of adulthood fears.

Aetiological and maintenance mechanisms

Very young infants show relatively low levels of fear, so that learning models of fear development have proved popular. In particular, associative models of learning have been used to describe how fears are learned and maintained, and have suggested therapeutic interventions that have been successful if also controversial.

Fears are suggested to be the result of the association of neutral objects with fear-evoking objects. For example, when a neutral object is paired with an aversive or frightening stimulus (e.g. shock), that object will acquire the ability to elicit fear through the processes of classical conditioning. Individuals appear to develop fears of certain objects more readily than others (e.g. snakes), and it is suggested that there may be a genetic component to this readiness.

Although valuable in understanding the development and maintenance of phobias, this model is also appropriate in understanding normal fear. In particular, infants appear to learn fearful behaviour from the observation of attachment figures, in particular the mother. This may be described as a form of vicarious classical conditioning or as social learning theory. Note that the two models are not exclusive.

Although classical conditioning models are particularly relevant to the understanding of development of fears, operant conditioning models provide some insight into how these fears (or fear responses) are *maintained*. Operant conditioning concerns the association of behaviour with either positive or negative reinforcement. In the context of fear, avoidance of fear (i.e. the behavioural response) will be reinforced by reduction in the feelings of fear and anxiety. Thus, once a fear has been established, the fear response serves to maintain the fear, which, in turn, has implications of the treatment of fears.

All learning processes are more powerful in childhood, and this corresponds with the fact that most fears develop early in life and are sustained through it. Adults rarely develop new fears, except in extreme circumstances (e.g. post-traumatic stress disorder).

Summary

Certain fears seem to be innate (e.g. the dark, heights), and there may be an evolutionary component to this. However, the relative lack of fear in infants suggests a strong learning component in the development of fears. The most common fears in babies are separation anxiety and fear of strangers, although the expression of these fears may be affected by factors such as attachment style, temperament and context.

Models of learning, particularly associative learning, have been used to describe how fears develop and are maintained. All also have implications for the treatment of fears.

SEXUAL DEVELOPMENT

Physical sexual development takes place primarily over a 3- to 5-year period, characterized by rapid physical growth and more gradual development of sexual characteristics (e.g. facial hair and deeper voice in males). There is substantial variation in the time of onset of puberty and the rate of development, although in the majority of cases this is complete by the age of 16–17 years.

Physical development is accompanied by increases in emotionality and, importantly, changes in self-identity, self-esteem and social relationships. This is related in part to the hormonal changes associated with sexual development, although this relationship is weak. In particular, sexual development significantly earlier or later than one's peers can be distressing. Late-maturing boys show greatest distress compared with early-maturing boys, while the reverse pattern is true of girls. Behavioural and emotional problems that exist during puberty and adolescence usually disappear with age.

Sexual identity

The development of personal identity is the central feature of adolescence. A significant component, most closely related to sexual development, is the development of sexual identity. Specifically, sexual identity refers to the elements of self-identity and self-perception that pertain to sexual preference. It is more general than simply the delineation of sexual preference, in that it also encompasses the extent to and way in which an individual's sexuality is expressed and portrayed to others. Certain behavioural and psychological characteristics may be described as masculine or feminine, with any individual (regardless of sex) displaying both masculine and feminine features. Several theories have suggested ways in which sexual identity develops.

Psychoanalytical theories argue that the sex drive is initially directed towards the father (in females) and blocked by the mother, so that the child identifies with the mother in order to achieve the father (or substitute), leading to appropriate gender roles. The basic mechanism of Freudian theory is identification; incestuous love or sex drive is repressed, resulting in the Oedipus or Electra complex, which culminates around the age of 5 years, with identification leading to the adoption of a gender role.

Social learning theory argues that cultural and societal forces model the behaviour of the child from birth, as well as the behaviour of others towards the child (e.g. girls play with dolls and are dressed in pink), leading to the development of sexual and gender identity. Behaviour, and therefore self-identity, is socially learned, and learning proceeds through reward, punishment and observation, while physical development and sexual characteristics are of minor importance. The child gradually learns appropriate social behaviour, which is internalized, and part of this includes the internalization of appropriate gender behaviour.

Cognitive developmental theories argue that, as the cognitive development of the child progresses, there is an increasing awareness of the self, including important elements of the self-concept such as 'she' or 'he', which is gradually incorporated into the child's understanding. Sex and gender concepts are poorly understood in young children, and before the age of about 5 years sex is identified by clothing, hair length and other external characteristics; changing a simple characteristic is enough (e.g. a zebra without stripes becomes 'a horse'). Around 5 years of age, clearer understanding of concepts develops, and this results in awareness of own sex and corresponding sexual identity and role.

These alternative explanations are not exclusive. Furthermore, similar processes (especially social learning) may account for the development of other elements of personal identity, self-image and self-concept, such as socio-economic status and ethnic group.

Sexual preference

Sexual preference is the preferred sex of one's partner and is a behavioural index defined by the usual sex of the partner. It is a relatively recent term, used to distinguish between subjective sexuality, which may not be polarized as either heterosexual or homosexual, and actual sexual behaviour, which usually is. Sexual orientation comprises several components, including attraction, behaviour, affection, and so on. As a result, the classification of individuals as heterosexual, homosexual or bisexual is simplistic. There is substantial current interest in the extent to which sexual orientation and sexual preference are innate or learned.

Evidence to date is equivocal – such research has been more successful at disconfirming hypotheses, so that the following conclusions have been supported to some degree (disconfirming some common hypotheses and popular beliefs). Sexual preference appears to be established relatively early, usually before puberty and adolescence, even if the individual is uncomfortable with this identity, and precedes sexual activity. The nature of the first sexual encounter appears unimportant, with homosexuals being as likely as heterosexuals to have had a first sexual encounter with a partner of the opposite sex. Homosexuals appear to have participated in less sexually stereotyped behaviour as children, so that a lack of conformity appears to be associated with subsequent homosexuality. Parental relationships appear to be of little importance, undermining psychoanalytical theories of the development of sexual preference.

There may be a genetic component to sexuality; for example, increasing genetic similarity is related to an increasing correspondence of sexual behaviour. However, as in the case of intelligence or personality, care must be taken in interpreting these results, given the complex nature of genotype–phenotype correlations. It is possible that certain genetically determined characteristics result in certain behaviour being more or less likely, which, in specific societies, is likely to result in a certain self-identity being developed (i.e. more or less stereotypically masculine), which is likely to be reinforced externally.

Summary

Physical and psychological sexual development are distinct. While the former, to a large extent, drives the latter, it is the latter where there is greater scope for individual variation, and a description of the causal factors is more difficult. Psychological sexual development corresponds broadly to the development of a distinct sexual identity.

Three broad theoretical positions exist for understanding the development of sexual identity and preference: psychoanalytical theories emphasize the role of basic drives and desires; social learning theories focus on the role of social and cultural norms; and cognitive developmental theories suggest that cognitive development results in an increasing awareness of the self, including sexual identity.

The development of sexual identity includes the development of sexual preferences. Preference appears to be established in early life, with parental influence being minimal. Such research is clearly controversial, and care must be taken in interpreting results.

ADOLESCENCE

Pubertal changes

Pubertal changes are those associated with development of the sex organs such that these enable reproduction. These changes are more obvious in females at menarche, while in males the changes are more gradual. Certain physical changes are apparent, in particular in males, such as the development of facial hair and deepening of the voice. The point at which puberty ends is difficult to define, and there is no clear value in attempting to set a period for this, in particular given the wide variation across individuals in onset and rate of development. Primary sexual changes (of the sex organs) are distinct from secondary sexual changes (of other physical characteristics, e.g. facial hair).

It is secondary sexual changes that are most noticeable: males grow significantly in size and body proportions also change, while in females breasts develop. Cognitive differences between males and females also emerge at puberty, with males being more likely to take spatial and mathematical subjects at school and females being more likely to take verbal and literary subjects. Evidence for these differences is somewhat controversial, and the effect may be determined largely by social pressures. Nevertheless, it has been suggested that there are sex-related differences in brain organization.

These physical changes are accompanied by important developments in self-image. For example, drawings of the self change noticeably over the first menstrual period in females, even though this is a short period of time, incorporating far more stereotypically feminine characteristics (not necessarily reflecting actual physical changes).

Task mastery

Physical and cognitive changes associated with puberty and adolescence allow for the development of new abilities. This period is also associated with a high degree of social development, in particular the development of sexual relationships. Social development is also accelerated as a result of the stronger peer relationships that develop, providing a set of group and attitude norms that become internalized. Self-esteem and personal achievements are also highly correlated. This physical, cognitive and social development results in the achievement of autonomy, including behavioural autonomy (the ability to select activities and friends independently), emotional autonomy (increasing independence from family members) and value autonomy (value and beliefs determined more by peers than by family).

Adolescence therefore requires mastery of two developmental tasks: development and acceptance of adult sexuality, and development and acceptance of social identity (and autonomy).

Conflict

It is a common stereotype that adolescence and puberty are associated with conflict with authority figures, in particular parents and teachers. Although there is some support for this, it appears that such behaviour is also culturally determined. For example, in Western cultures childhood is regarded as unique and the transition to adulthood an important one, while at the same time parental control is high. This results in the characteristic desire of adolescent children to assert their individuality and achieve independence. In contrast, there is evidence that the distinction between childhood and adulthood is less clear in some cultures (e.g. in east Asian), and the degree of parental control sought is less, and that this corresponds to a relatively conflict-free adolescence.

Conflict appears to be not only largely generated by social norms (rather than, say, excessive emotionality related to hormonal changes) but also a function of changes in self-image and self-esteem. Development into an adult is associated with increased self-esteem and confidence and a greater ability to assert oneself. Finally, the stereotype of adolescent conflict is too general, and a large proportion of individuals pass through adolescence without any major conflict or turmoil.

Affective stability

The hormonal and other physiological changes associated with adolescence may result in some degree of emotional instability. Although there is some evidence that emotionality is higher during adolescence, this effect is weak. Moreover, the effect is likely to be the result of social conflict as well as physiological factors. The notion of adolescent affective lability has existed in literature at least as far back as the eighteenth century, suggesting a role for social construction. Although there is certainly a degree of conflict associated with adolescence, this is likely to be primarily the result of changing self-image and self-esteem rather than affective instability. Moreover, those adolescents who do experience a high degree of emotional instability are likely to continue to display this in adulthood.

Normal and abnormal development

Adolescence should be regarded as a developmental stage characterized by significant physical and psychosocial changes, and these changes require a degree of adaptation on the part of the adolescent. The majority of these changes, while initiated by physical changes and the psychological and social consequences of these, are related to self-image and self-expression. Normal development will be associated with changes in a variety of areas, including values and beliefs, social behaviour, sexual behaviour, cognitive abilities, physical abilities, self-esteem, self-image and self-concept.

Although there is evidence that some adolescents do experience distress and turmoil, this appears to be abnormal and is associated with similar affective instability in later life. Adequate adjustment to the demands of adolescence is a very strong predictor of successful adaptation in adulthood. Adolescent conduct and behavioural problems are associated strongly with criminal behaviour, both in adolescence and later in adulthood. This is in part influenced culturally: the incidence of adolescent criminality is far higher in cultures where pubertal and adolescent turmoil is regarded as normal than in cultures where the emphasis on adolescence is far less.

Summary

Physical change in adolescence is marked, and there are correspondingly marked psychological changes, in particular in social and sexual identity. There is an important distinction between primary and secondary sexual changes.

Physical, cognitive and social development results in the accomplishment of specific tasks (task mastery). In particular, the adolescent must develop sexually and socially and, most importantly, be comfortable with and accept these changes.

Changes in self-image, social identity and so on may result in a degree of conflict between the adolescent and, usually, authority figures. This, however, is less common than popularly believed. Although some have suggested that emotionality is elevated during adolescence as a result of hormonal fluctuations, the evidence for this is weak.

Abnormal adolescent development is usually characterized by an inability to accept sexual and social changes associated with this period or by development in this area being impaired in some way.

ADAPTATIONS IN ADULT LIFE

Adulthood is not the endpoint of development, and adaptation proceeds throughout life. Certain specific adaptations are common to most individuals, each representing a significant change in lifestyle and an attendant change in self-identity and responsibility. These may include the decision to choose a partner for life, whether or not to have children, and choosing an occupation.

Pairing

It is likely that the first significant change in the lifestyle of an adult will be the formation of a romantic relationship that is intended to be permanent. Although an increasing number of couples do not marry, most still do. Regardless of the exact nature of the relationship with the partner, certain features are common. Several factors appear to be important in the development of romantic relationships, including attractiveness, common attitudes and emotional stability.

There is an association between marriage and health, both physical and mental. A happy and stable relationship is a protective factor, while unhappy relationships have been associated with poorer immune function, depression and other negative health outcomes.

Parenting

The transition to parenthood affects the behaviour of both the mother and the father and may change the quality of the marital relationship. Mothers tend to become more sexually stereotyped, engaging in more feminine behaviours and fewer masculine behaviours. In contrast, fathers become less sexually stereotyped, showing a relative increase in feminine behaviour. Several factors may influence the quality of the marital relationship, including relative reduction in income, potential absolute reduction in income, sleep disturbance and reduction in privacy.

Although these factors suggest that the transition to parenthood should have negative consequences for the marriage, there is also contrasting evidence that intimacy and affection increase between the marital partners, so that the stress of parenthood is reduced. In general, parenthood is likely to be more stressful if the parents are young, the birth takes place before marriage, and the relationship has existed for a long period before the birth (possibly due to greater lifestyle change). The temperament of the child will also have an impact on how stressful the transition to parenthood is, with difficult children representing a greater challenge.

Illness

Illness may be regarded as a relatively common but nevertheless serious source of stress in individuals. Beyond the physical effects of the illness, the individual will be required to appraise their condition and, in adults, typically include both current concerns (e.g. loss of income) and concerns about the future.

The nature of illness that individuals have to cope with and adapt to changes with age. With increasing age, illness becomes more common and chronic illness more likely. Illnesses suffered also become more serious and debilitating (e.g. stroke). In the case of chronic illness, individuals may pass through several stages of adjustment: shock (bewilderment and a sense of detachment), encounter (grief, despair and depression), retreat (denial, either of the illness or its implications) and intrusion (the individual comes to terms with the illness and adapts). This model has been criticized for being excessively rigid and prescriptive, but there is some evidence that at least a large proportion of individuals react to the diagnosis of chronic illness in roughly the way described above, although not necessarily as a linear progression through these stages.

Bereavement and loss

Bereaved individuals are likely to see their doctor more often, become preoccupied with the object or individual that has been lost, show loss of appetite and general apathy, and exhibit signs of denial. These responses to bereavement are common and should be regarded as normal, provided the individual eventually adjusts to the loss. Mortality also increases in the 6 months following bereavement, in particular among married men who have lost their wife. Several factors have been associated with poor adjustment, including lower socioeconomic status, several concurrent stressful life events, self-blame, severe depression, and lack of forewarning and preparation. Although in some cases adjustment to the loss may be difficult and lengthy, the majority of individuals eventually do adapt effectively.

Although the term 'bereavement' is generally used to refer to the loss of a relative, close friend or loved one, it may also be used metaphorically to refer to other forms of loss, such as limb amputation or loss of a job. The common feature of these cases is that a considerable degree of adjustment is required after the loss, although there will be variation in severity and reaction across individuals.

Summary

Adaptations in adult life are characterized by the requirement to interact in specific socially defined ways with others. One example is the search for a partner and subsequent parenting. It is common, although not universal, to follow a fairly clearly defined path through life, punctuated by periods of adaptation (e.g. marriage, parenthood, bereavement, death).

No definitive list of the adaptations required in adulthood exists, but in general these include major events that require a significant change in lifestyle. In such cases there will be a role played by self-image, self-esteem and so on, and also by others (e.g. social support).

PREGNANCY AND CHILDBIRTH

The 9 months of pregnancy represent a gradual build-up to the stresses of childbirth and parenthood, while also representing a stressful episode itself.

Physiological stresses

The physical changes associated with pregnancy are (perhaps paradoxically) not regarded as particularly feminine, in particular by women themselves. The increase in weight, and the hormonal and dietary changes that result from pregnancy, represent a significant source of physiological stress, with consequent problems such as low back pain and morning sickness. The physiological consequences also contribute to a great extent to the feeling of unattractiveness common in many pregnant women.

At the time of birth, the most important consideration of the mother is the pain associated with childbirth. Relaxation and focused-attention techniques do allow significantly improved tolerance of pain, while other methods of childbirth have broader objectives such as the maintenance of contact between the mother and child.

Psychological stresses

The onset of pregnancy will have consequences not only for the mother but also for the father. For example, the preoccupation of the mother with the fetus may result in feelings of alienation and separation in the father. Although there is no reason why sexual contact should be reduced during pregnancy, it commonly is. There is some evidence that sexual behaviour during pregnancy is related to the ease of labour. Several stereotypes and attitudes exist towards pregnancy: pregnancy as illness (the substantial medical intervention in births may result in a conception that the birth is a medical rather than a natural process), pregnancy as crisis (the professional consequences of pregnancy for employed women may be substantial, in particular if the pregnancy is unplanned or unexpected), and pregnancy as a task (there is substantial pressure, in some cases, from other family members for a couple to begin a family, which may not correspond to the couple's wishes).

These stereotypes and attitudes tend to be strongest during the first pregnancy; contact with the realities of pregnancy and childbirth tend to modify the attitudes of mothers having a second child. However, this may also have negative consequences if the events during pregnancy are particular distressing, such as prolonged labour, so that the mother may expect a difficult labour again, even if this is relatively unlikely.

Anxiety is a common feature of pregnant women and may be focused on several potential risks or outcomes, such as possible handicap of the child, preoccupation with cleanliness, one's own abilities as a mother, the financial consequences of a child, and the risk of miscarriage. Although some degree of anxiety is perhaps to be expected, there is evidence that excessive stress during pregnancy may influence fetal development in several ways and has also been shown to be related to the risk of miscarriage and low birth weight. The incidence of miscarriage is significant and results in very strong grief reactions from both parents, especially the mother, being associated with subsequent depression for several weeks or months following the event.

Summary

The physiological and psychological stresses of pregnancy and childbirth are distinct, although they interact. Postnatal depression, for example, is likely to include a strong physiological (i.e. hormonal) component.

Specific social stereotypes contribute to the stress of pregnancy and childbirth (e.g. the pathologization of pregnancy).

A degree of anxiety is normal in pregnant women (and in their partner), generated by a variety of potential negative outcomes or consequences (e.g. financial burden, doubt in one's ability to act as a good parent).

DEVELOPMENT OF PERSONAL IDENTITY

Erik Erikson suggests a stage model of psychosocial and personal development, with each stage being characterized by a particular crisis that the individual must overcome in order to develop (Table 8.4).

Although Erikson specifies favourable outcomes, the result of each psychosocial crisis may not in fact be favourable (e.g. anxiety, insecurity, loneliness). The ability to face each crisis depends to a large extent on the outcome

Table 8.4 Stages in Erikson's model of psychosocial development

Stage	Crisis	Favourable outcome
1st year	Trust/mistrust	Trust and sense of security (attachment)
2nd–3rd years	Autonomy/self-doubt	Self-control and self-efficacy
3rd–5th years	Initiative/guilt	Confidence in own ability to act/initiate
6th–13th years	Competence/inferiority	Competence in social and intellectual skills
Adolescence	Identity/confusion	Development of self-identity
Adulthood	Intimacy/isolation	Commitment to others, career, etc.
Middle age	Generativity/stagnation	Concern beyond self to family, society, future
Later life	Integrity/despair	Sense of satisfaction, completion

of the previous crisis, so that a child who develops secure attachments and a strong sense of self-control in early life will be well prepared to face future challenges and crises.

Various social identities

Social identities derive largely from the membership of groups, although these groups need not be explicit (e.g. football team) and may be more implicit (e.g. recognition of occupying a certain socioeconomic position). Individuals will possess a number of social identities that may overlap and, in some cases, conflict.

Group membership appears to be a fundamental need. Individuals will very rapidly regard themselves as belonging to a group, even on the basis of random and meaningless criteria, and display a preference for other members of the group. Individual identity (self-concept) depends to a large extent on social identities, intergroup comparisons contribute to self-esteem, and the need for a positive self-concept results in intergroup prejudice and bias.

The question 'Who am I?', asked of subjects and repeated several times, results in an interesting and insightful hierarchy of self-descriptions, many of which are related to social identities and group membership. This is influenced by cultural factors also, so that in Western cultures there is a bias towards individual characteristics while in Eastern cultures there is more emphasis on group membership.

Social identities need not necessarily be related to group membership (although the majority are) and may instead relate to perceived relationships and interactions with other (e.g. a strong component of self-concept may be 'father').

Adaptations in adult life

Typical adaptations in adult life include the development of permanent romantic relationships, the birth of the first child, the onset of serious illness and bereavement. Nevertheless, the development of the individual, in particular social support, self-esteem and self-efficacy beliefs, will influence the degree to which the individual adapts to various life crises. Therefore, factors that influence the extent to which adaptations in adult life will be successful include self-esteem, self-efficacy, locus of control, attributional style and social support.

Erikson's model of the development of personal identity makes it clear that developmental experiences, in particular those in early and middle childhood, will influence these factors and directly influence coping responses to stressful events. An individual with a strong, coherent and positive sense of self will be better prepared to cope with major life events requiring adaptation.

The 'mid-life crisis' represents the generativity versus stagnation crisis of middle adulthood suggested by Erikson. The proposal is that adults at this stage question their achievements to date and what they will achieve in the remainder of their life. Priorities tend to be restructured and greater emphasis is placed on the development of children rather than the self. Nevertheless, the term 'crisis' is debatable, as the evidence that individuals in middle adulthood are particularly distressed is weak. As such, it is perhaps more valuable to examine specific crises (i.e., adaptations) separately, with middle adulthood simply representing a period when several of these are likely to occur close together (e.g. illness, children leaving home, etc.).

Summary

The basic structure of Erikson's model of personal development is important, in particular the crises that characterize different stages of the model. For each of these there is a generally favourable (or unfavourable) outcome. These outcomes are appropriate at different stages in the lifespan, and the model is therefore distinct in that it covers the entire lifespan, from birth to death. Concern for the future and society in general, for example, is appropriate by this model in middle age but inappropriate in adolescence, where personal development and self-identity are paramount.

The stages of Erikson's model correspond to an extent to the different social roles adopted by individuals over the lifespan. Parenthood in adult life corresponds to the development, in Erikson's model, of a commitment to others.

AGEING

Individual functioning and ageing

The physical, physiological and cognitive changes related to ageing result in corresponding changes in functioning. For example, speed of performance generally becomes slower, although this is not uniform across tasks, and corresponds to a decline of less than 10 per cent between 20 years and 70 years of age for aimed movement, a roughly 25 per cent decline for simple sensorimotor decision tasks, and approximately a 50 per cent decline for complex sensorimotor decision tasks. Sensory function, in particular vision and hearing, also declines. The most significant changes begin after 40 years of age, when decline in function becomes more rapid.

Memory and learning

Learning of new skills declines, while longer explicit recall also declines with age. Some memory tasks show improvement (possibly due to greater use of memory aids, such as diaries and notes).

Personality

Erikson regards development through the lifespan as continual (see above), and norms for psychometric personality questionnaires (e.g. measures of extraversion and neuroticism) change with age. Individuals generally become less extroverted and less neurotic, and emotionality is often more stable and easily controlled in older adults.

Sexuality

The nature of sexual function changes greatly, although pleasure derived from intercourse commonly remains. It has been argued that sexuality in the elderly is often not socially accepted, and there is a common misconception that elderly people cannot (or should not) remain sexually active.

Social functioning and ageing

Social contact generally reduces with age. Although this is in part due to a reduction in the number of friends, the changes in individual functioning associated with age also lead to a reluctance or inability to maintain social contact. Social situations may be frightening if hearing or vision is impaired (e.g. on busy streets), for example, while difficulties in performing certain tasks may reduce social contact (e.g. walking to a bus stop). In particular, society may not allow for the differences in individual functioning found in elderly people (objects are designed by young and healthy people, usually without consideration for elderly people).

Nevertheless, there are certain gains associated with age, such as reduced emotional lability, which may allow certain losses to be compensated for. Selective optimization with compensation refers to the ability of individuals to select appropriate and realistic goals, focus on goals of primary importance, and use alternative strategies to compensate for declining abilities (e.g. memory aids). This conceptualization is universal, although clearly the pattern of behaviour and compensation will vary widely across individuals.

Summary

The normal ageing process has both physical and psychological consequences. The physical consequences are relatively straightforward, including a gradual decline in sensorimotor ability, memory and so on. Apparent improvements in certain types of memory with age may be ascribed to increasing use of memory aids.

Psychological consequences of ageing include changes in the sexual behaviour of individuals. This is due primarily to social norms rather than to any decline in the desire for or pleasure derived from intercourse. Social contact also changes, as a consequence of a declining social network and an inability to perform certain social tasks as a result of physical changes.

KEY POINTS

- Development is the result of the interaction between innate behaviours and the environment and may entail progression through a series of stages. It is distinct from maturation, where less emphasis is placed on this interaction.
- Key models of the development of cognitive (e.g. Piaget), social (e.g. attachment theory) and moral (e.g. Kohlberg) abilities exist, which are separate but may be mutually compatible (e.g. a certain degree of development may be necessary to understand certain moral concepts).
- Attachment theory describes the need for proximity and nurturance as separate from the need for sustenance, and suggests distinct types of attachment behaviour (secure, insecure-avoidant, insecure-ambivalent), which may relate to behaviour in adult life.
- The development of personal identity accelerates in adolescence, as personal autonomy increases and puberty brings results in important physical and psychological changes. This results in changes in self-image and self-identity.
- Although most developmental theories focus on infancy, childhood and adolescence, there are developmental changes throughout the lifespan, and these are sometimes characterized by challenges that need to be met (c.f. Erikson).
- Other developmental models exist for linguistic and sexual development and for the development of fears. Many of these share core features, such as the role of cognitive development, learning processes and social learning theory.

Chapter 9

Introduction to basic psychology

Richard Gross

IS PSYCHOLOGY A SCIENCE?

Throughout psychology's history as a separate discipline and field of study, psychologists, as well as philosophers of science and other interested parties, have continued to ask this question. One feature of psychology that makes it special is that its scientific status is part of its subject matter: it's as though we need to know what kind of discipline it is before we can evaluate and apply the research findings that are published under the name of psychology.

Behind the question 'Is psychology a science?' is the fundamental assumption of *scientism*:

> ... the borrowing of methods and a characteristic vocabulary from the natural sciences in order to discover causal mechanisms that explain psychological phenomena.[1]

For much of its history, psychology has taken physics and chemistry as the 'model' it aspired to; this perhaps suggests that we might rephrase the original question and ask: 'How successful is psychology in identifying causal mechanisms that explain psychological phenomena?' This, in turn, begs all sorts of questions about the aims or goals of psychology, how psychology has changed during its near-130-year history, and the appropriateness and viability of studying human beings using the methods of natural science.

The scope of this chapter doesn't allow for discussion of these issues, but for a detailed account, see Gross[2,3] and Gross *et al.*[4]

A BRIEF HISTORY

The word 'psychology' is derived from the Greek *psyche* (= mind, soul, spirit) and *logos* (= knowledge, discourse, study). Literally, then, psychology is the 'study of the mind'.

The emergence of psychology as a separate discipline is generally dated at 1879, when Wilhelm Wundt, a German physiologist, opened the first psychology laboratory at the University of Leipzig. Wundt and his co-workers were attempting to investigate 'the mind' through *introspection* (observing and analysing the structure of their own conscious mental processes). The aim of introspection was to analyse conscious thought into its basic elements and perception into its constituent sensations, much as chemists analyse compounds into elements. This attempt to identify the structure of conscious thought is called *structuralism*.

Wundt and his fellow researchers recorded and measured the results of their introspections under controlled conditions, using the same physical surroundings, the same stimulus (such as a clicking metronome), the same verbal instructions to each participant, and so on. This emphasis on measurement and control marked the separation of the 'new psychology' from its parent discipline of philosophy.

Philosophers had discussed 'the mind' for thousands of years. For the first time, scientists applied some of the basic methods of scientific investigation to the study of mental processes. This was reflected in James's definition of psychology as

> ... the Science of Mental Life, both of its phenomena and of their conditions... The Phenomena are such things as we call feelings, desires, cognitions, reasoning, decisions and the like.[5]

However, by the early twentieth century, the validity and usefulness of introspection were being seriously questioned, particularly by the American psychologist John B Watson. Watson believed that the results of introspection could never be proved or disproved, since, if one person's introspection produced different results from another's, then how could we ever decide which was correct? Objectively, of course, we cannot, since it is impossible to 'get behind' an introspective report to check its accuracy. Introspection is subjective, and only the individual can observe his or her own mental processes.

Consequently, Watson proposed that psychologists should confine themselves to studying behaviour, since only this is measurable and observable by more than one person.[6] Watson's form of psychology was known as *behaviourism*. It largely replaced introspectionism and advocated that people should be regarded as complex animals to be studied using the same scientific methods as those used in chemistry and physics. For Watson, the only way psychology could make any claim to being scientific was to emulate the natural sciences and adopt its own objective methods (i.e. scientism). He defined psychology as:

> ... that division of Natural Science which takes human behaviour – the doings and sayings, both learned and unlearned – as its subject matter.[7]

The study of inaccessible, private, mental processes was to have no place in a truly scientific psychology.

Especially in the USA, behaviourism in one form or another remained the dominant force within psychology for the next 40 years or so. The emphasis on the role of learning (in the form of conditioning) was to make that topic one of the central areas of psychological research as a whole (see Chapter 14). Box 9.1 outlines psychoanalytic theory and Gestalt psychology, two major European alternatives to American behaviourism.

In the late 1950s, many British and American psychologists began looking to the work of computer scientists to try to understand more complex behaviours, which, they felt, had either been greatly oversimplified or neglected altogether by learning theory (conditioning). These complex behaviours were what Wundt, James and other early scientific psychologists had called 'mind' or mental processes. They were now referred to as *cognition* or *cognitive processes* and denote all the ways in which we come to know the world around us – how we attain, retain and regain information through the processes of attention, perception, memory, problem-solving, language and thinking in general.

Box 9.1 Psychoanalytic theory and Gestalt psychology

In 1900, Sigmund Freud, an Austrian neurologist living in Vienna, first published his *psychoanalytic theory* of personality, in which the *unconscious* mind plays a crucial role. In parallel with this theory, he developed a form of psychotherapy called *psychoanalysis*. Freud's theory (which forms the basis of the *psychodynamic* approach) represented a challenge and a major alternative to behaviourism (see Gross[2] and Chapter 8).

A reaction against both structuralism and behaviourism came from the *Gestalt* school of psychology, which emerged in the 1920s in Austria and Germany. Gestalt psychologists were interested mainly in perception and believed that perceptions could not be broken down in the way that Wundt advocated. They identified several 'laws' or *principles of perceptual organization* (such as 'the whole is greater than the sum of its parts'), which have made a lasting contribution to our understanding of the perceptual process (see Chapter 10).

Cognitive psychologists see people as information-processors, and cognitive psychology has been heavily influenced by computer science, with human cognitive processes being compared to the operation of computer programs (the *computer analogy*). Cognitive psychology now forms part of cognitive science, which emerged in the late 1970s (Figure 9.1). The events that together constitute the 'cognitive revolution' are described in Box 9.2.

Box 9.2 The 1956 'cognitive revolution'

At a meeting at the Massachusetts Institute of Technology (MIT), Noam Chomsky presented his theory of language (see Gross[2]), George Miller presented a paper on the 'magical number seven' in short-term memory (see Chapter 5), and Newell and Simon presented a paper on the logical theory machine (or logic theorist), with a further paper by Newell *et al.*[8], which Newell and Simon extended into the general problem-solver (GPS)[9] (see Gross[2]).

The first systematic attempt to investigate concept formation (in adults) from a cognitive psychological perspective was reported.[10]

At Dartmouth College, New Hampshire (the 'Dartmouth Conference'), ten academics met to discuss the possibility of producing computer programs that could 'behave' or 'think' intelligently. These academics included McCarthy (generally attributed with having coined the term 'artificial intelligence'), Marvin Minsky, Simon, Newell, Chomsky and Miller.

Based on Eysenck and Keane.[11]

Although mental or cognitive processes can only be inferred from what a person does (i.e. they cannot be literally or directly observed), they are now accepted as being valid subject matter for psychology, provided that they can be made 'public' (as in memory tests or problem-solving tasks). Consequently, what people say and do are perfectly acceptable sources of information about their cognitive processes, although the processes themselves remain inaccessible to the observer, who can study them only indirectly.

The influence of both behaviourism and cognitive psychology is reflected in Clark and Miller's definition of psychology as:

> ... the scientific study of behaviour. Its subject matter includes behavioural processes that are observable, such as gestures, speech and physiological changes, and processes that can only be inferred, such as thoughts and dreams.[12]

Similarly, Zimbardo states:

> Psychology is formally defined as the scientific study of the behaviour of individuals and their mental processes.[13]

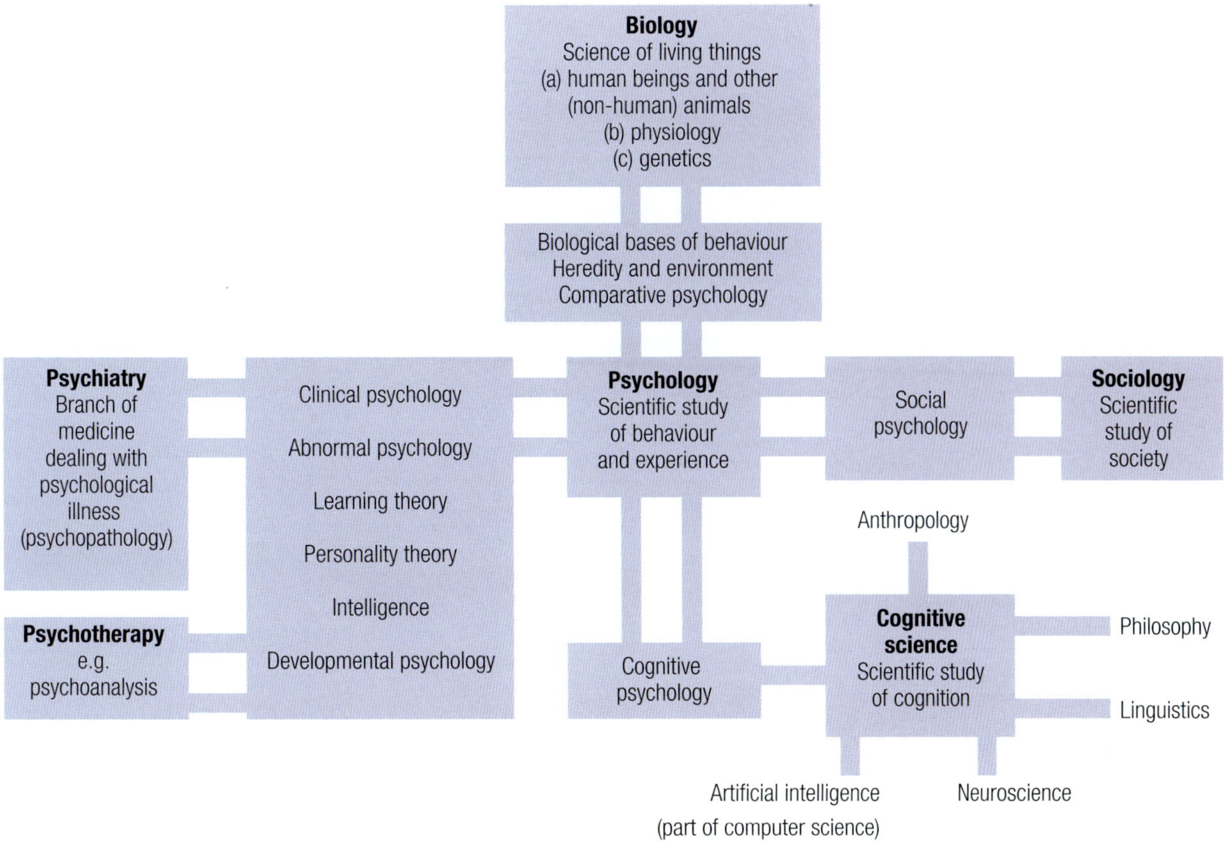

Figure 9.1 Relationship between psychology and other scientific disciplines

CLASSIFYING THE WORK OF PSYCHOLOGISTS

Despite behaviourist and cognitive psychology's influence on psychology's general direction during the past 90 years or so, much more goes on within the discipline than has been outlined so far. There are other theoretical approaches or orientations (such as the humanistic, social constructionist and evolutionary), other aspects of human (and non-human) activity that constitute the special focus of study, and different kinds of work that different psychologists do.

A useful, although not hard and fast, distinction can be made between the *academic* and *applied* branches of psychology (Figure 9.2). Academic psychologists conduct research and are attached to a university or research establishment, where they also teach undergraduates and supervise the research of postgraduates. Research may be *pure* (done for its own sake and intended, primarily, to increase our knowledge and understanding) or *applied* (aimed at solving a particular problem). Applied research is usually funded by a government institution, such as the Home Office, National Health Service (NHS) or Department for Education and Skills (DfES), or by a commercial or industrial institution. The range of topics that may be investigated is as wide as psychology itself, but they can be classified as focusing either on the processes or mechanisms underlying various aspects of behaviour, or more directly on the person.[14]

The process approach

This is divided into three main areas: physiological, cognitive and comparative psychology.

Physiological (or bio-) psychology

Physiological (or bio-) psychologists are interested in the physical basis of behaviour, how the functions of the nervous system (in particular, the brain) and the endocrine (hormonal) system are related to and influence behaviour and mental processes. For example, are there parts of the brain concerned specifically with particular behaviours and abilities (localization of brain function)? What role do hormones play in the experience of emotion, and how are these linked to brain processes? What is the relationship between brain activity and different states/levels of consciousness/awareness (including sleep)?

A fundamentally important biological process with important implications for psychology is genetic transmis-

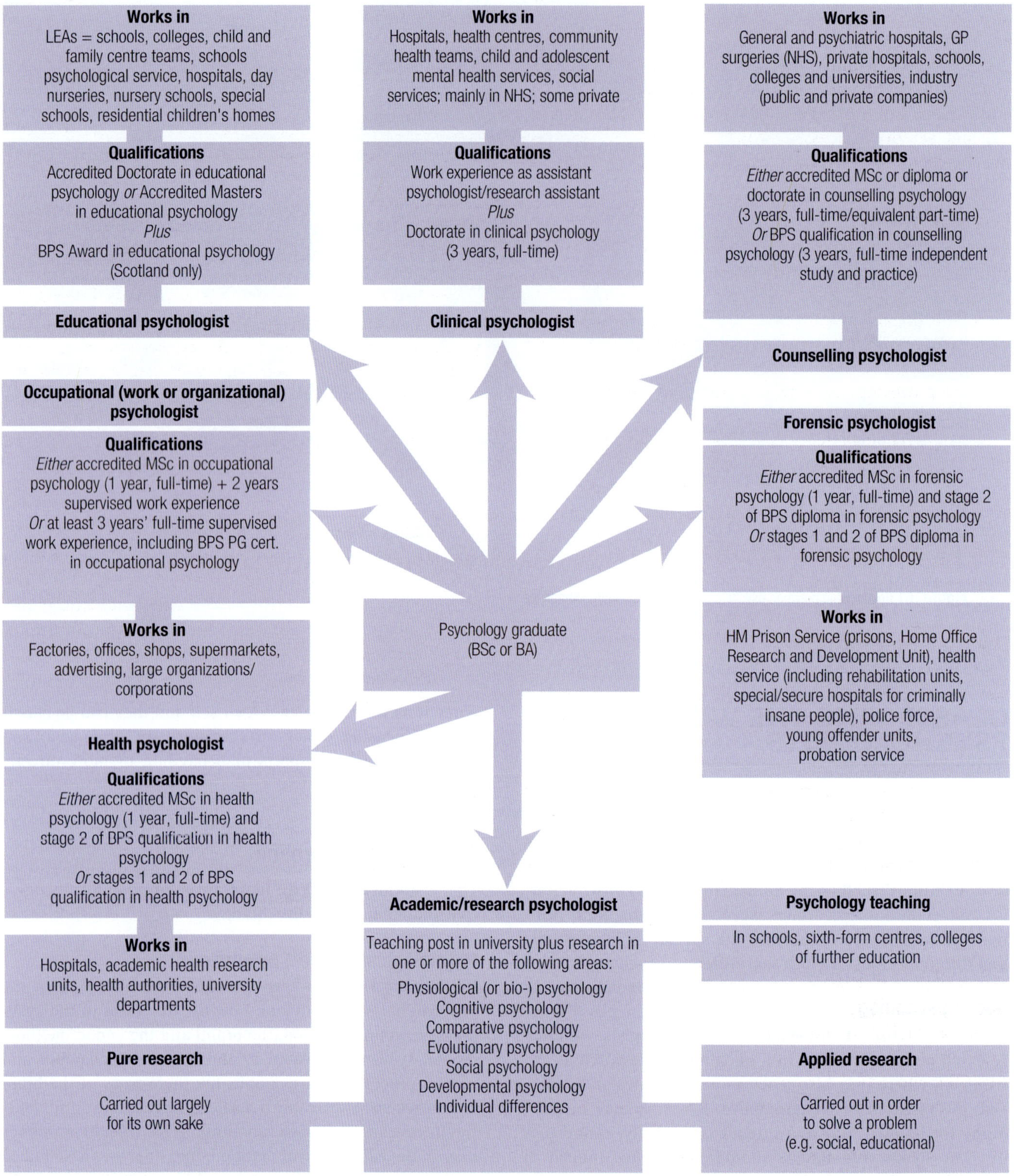

Figure 9.2 Some of the main areas of academic and applied psychology open to psychology graduates

sion. The *heredity–environment* (or *nature–nurture*) issue draws on what geneticists have discovered about the characteristics that can be passed from parents to offspring, how this takes place, and how genetic factors interact with environmental ones (see Gross[2,3]).

Other topics within physiological psychology include motivation (see Chapter 11), stress (which is commonly discussed as part of health psychology; see below and Chapter 13) and sensory processes, which are connected closely with perception (see Chapter 16).

Cognitive psychology

As we saw earlier, cognitive (or mental) processes include attention, perception, memory, language, thinking, problem-solving, decision-making, reasoning and concept-formation (*higher-order* mental activities). Although these are often studied for their own sake, they may also have important practical implications, such as understanding the memory processes involved in eyewitness testimony (see Gross[2]).

Social psychology (classified here as belonging to the person approach) is heavily cognitive in flavour: for example, many social psychologists study the mental processes that we use when trying to explain people's behaviour (*social cognition*). Also belonging to the person approach is the Swiss psychologist Jean Piaget's influential theory of cognitive development (see Gross[2]).

Comparative psychology

Comparative psychology is the study of the behaviour of non-human animals, aimed at identifying similarities and differences between species. It also involves studying non-human animal behaviour in order to gain a better understanding of human behaviour.

The basis of comparative psychology is *evolutionary theory*. Areas of research include classical and operant conditioning (see Chapter 14), animal communication, language and memory (see Gross *et al.*[15]), and evolutionary explanations of human behaviour (see Clamp[16] and Gross[2]).

The person approach

Social psychology

Some psychologists would claim that all psychology is social psychology, because all behaviour takes place within a social context and, even when we're alone, our behaviour continues to be influenced by others. However, other people usually have a more immediate and direct influence upon us when we are actually in their presence (as in *conformity* and *obedience*).

Social psychology is also concerned with *interpersonal perception* (forming impressions of others) and *interpersonal attraction* (why we like some people more than others, both friends and romantic partners), which forms a part of *interpersonal relationships*. Other areas of research interest include *prejudice* and *discrimination*, and *pro-* and *antisocial behaviour* (especially altruism and aggression, respectively).

Developmental psychology

Developmental psychologists study the biological, cognitive, social and emotional changes that take place in people over time. One significant change within developmental psychology during the past 40 years or so is the recognition that development is not confined to childhood and adolescence but is a lifelong process (the *lifespan approach*). It is now generally accepted that development continues beyond childhood and adolescence into adulthood and old age.

Developmental psychology is not an isolated or independent field, and advances in it depend on progress within psychology as a whole (such as behaviour genetics, (neuro)physiological psychology, learning, perception and motivation). Although Piaget's theory of cognitive development was meant to map the changes that take place up to about 15 years of age, he is considered to have made a major contribution to psychology as a whole.

Individual differences

This is concerned with the ways in which people can differ from one another, including personality, intelligence and psychological abnormality. Other examples are age, gender and cultural/ethnic background. Another source of individual differences is criminal behaviour. Major mental/psychological disorders include schizophrenia, depression, anxiety disorders, sexual and eating disorders, and addictive behaviours.

Abnormal psychology is linked closely with clinical psychology, one of the major applied areas of psychology (see below). Clinical psychologists and psychologists who study abnormality are also concerned with the effectiveness of different forms of treatment and therapy. Each major theoretical approach (such as the behavioural, psychodynamic and cognitive-behavioural) has contributed to both the explanation and the treatment of mental disorders.

Comparing the process and person approaches

In practice, it is very difficult to separate the two approaches, even if it can be done theoretically. However, there are important relative differences between them (Box 9.3).

Areas of applied psychology

Discussion of the process/person approaches has been concerned largely with the academic branch of psychology. Since the various areas of applied psychology are all concerned with people, they can be thought of as the applied aspects of the person approach.

Box 9.3 Some important differences between the process and person approaches

- The *process approach* is typically confined to the laboratory (where experiments are the 'method of choice'). It makes far greater experimental use of non-human animals and assumes that psychological processes (particularly learning) are essentially the same in all species; any differences between species are only quantitative (differences of degree).
- The *person approach* makes much greater use of field studies (such as observing behaviour in its natural environment) and of non-experimental methods (such as correlation studies; see Coolican[17]). Typically, human participants are studied, and it is assumed that there are qualitative differences (differences in kind) between humans and non-humans.

According to Hartley and Branthwaite,[18] most applied psychologists work in four main areas: clinical, educational and occupational psychology, and government service (such as forensic psychology). In addition, Coolican and colleagues identify forensic (or criminological), sport and exercise, health, and environmental psychology.[19,20] Hartley and Branthwaite argue that the work psychologists do in these different areas has much in common: it is the subject matter of their jobs that differs, rather than the skills they employ. Consequently, they consider an applied psychologist to be a person who can deploy specialized skills appropriately in different situations (Box 9.4).

Clinical psychology

Clinical psychologists are the largest single group of psychologists, in both the UK and the USA.[21] Clinical psychology represents the largest single division within the British Psychological Society (BPS) and probably the largest number of Chartered Psychologists holding a Practising Certificate within the UK (see below). In 2005, those belonging to the Division of Clinical Psychology (DCP) constituted approximately 52 per cent of the entire register of Chartered Psychologists.[19]

According to Coolican, clinical psychology can be defined as:

> ... the application of psychological theory to human distress, manifested as psychological problems. Therefore, clinical psychology is a profession primarily concerned with the alleviation of psychological problems ...[19]

Even within psychology, clinical psychologists cannot claim to be the only practitioners concerned with the alleviation of psychological problems. Counselling and health psychologists also play a vital role in the application of psychological therapy. Outside psychology, psychotherapists, counsellors, specialist nurses and psychiatrists are all

Box 9.4 Seven major skills (or roles) used by applied psychologists

- *The psychologist as counsellor:* helping people to talk openly, express their feelings, explore problems more deeply, and see these problems from different perspectives. Problems include school phobia, marriage crises and traumatic experiences (such as being the victim of a hijacking). The counsellor can adopt a more or less directive approach.
- *The psychologist as colleague:* working as a member of a team and bringing a particular perspective to a task, namely drawing attention to the human issues, such as the point of view of the individual end user (be it a product or a service of some kind).
- *The psychologist as expert:* drawing upon psychologists' specialized knowledge, ideas, theories, and practical knowledge to advise on issues ranging from incentive schemes in industry to appealing to an 'expert witness' in a court case.
- *The psychologist as toolmaker:* using and developing appropriate measures and techniques to help in the analysis and assessment of problems. These include questionnaire and interview schedules, computer-based ability and aptitude tests and other *psychometric tests* (tests of mental measurement, such as intelligence quotient (IQ) tests and personality tests).
- *The psychologist as detached investigator:* many applied psychologists carry out evaluation studies to assess the evidence for and against a particular point of view. This reflects the view of psychology as an objective science, which should use controlled experimentation whenever possible. The validity of this view is a recurrent theme throughout psychology.
- *The psychologist as theoretician:* theories try to explain observed phenomena, suggesting possible underlying mechanisms or processes. They can suggest where to look for causes and how to design specific studies that will produce evidence for or against a particular point of view. Results from applied psychology can influence theoretical psychology, and vice versa.
- *The psychologist as agent for change:* applied psychologists are involved in helping people, institutions and organizations, based on the belief that their work will change people and society for the better. However, some changes are much more controversial than others, such as the use of psychometric tests to determine educational and occupational opportunities, and the use of behaviour therapy and modification techniques to change abnormal behaviour.

involved in the same overall aim; the main difference between these professional groups lies in the methods and techniques used to achieve it (as well as the theories and research on which they are based).

Clinical psychologists work largely in health and social care settings, including hospitals, health centres, community mental health teams, child and adolescent mental health services, and social services (Box 9.5). They usually work as part of a team, with, for example, social workers, medical practitioners and other health professionals. In the UK, most clinical psychologists work in the NHS, but some work in private practice.

Box 9.5 Major functions of the clinical psychologist

A clinical psychologist has had work experience as an assistant psychologist/research assistant, plus 3 years' postgraduate training (doctorate in clinical psychology).[22] The clinical psychologist's functions include:

- assessing people with learning difficulties, administering psychological tests to brain-damaged patients, devising rehabilitation programmes for long-term psychiatric patients, and assessing elderly people for their fitness to live independently;
- planning and carrying out programmes of therapy, usually behaviour therapy/modification or psychotherapy (group or individual) in preference to, or in addition to, behavioural techniques;
- conducting research into abnormal psychology, including the effectiveness of different treatment methods ('outcome studies'); patients are usually adults, many of whom are elderly, or in psychiatric hospitals, psychiatric wards in general hospitals or psychiatric clinics;
- involvement in community care, as psychiatric care in general moves out of the large psychiatric hospitals ('asylums');
- teaching other groups of professionals, such as nurses, social workers and psychiatrists.

Counselling psychology

Counselling psychology as an applied field of psychology

> ... aims to facilitate personal and interpersonal functioning across the life span with a focus on *emotional, social, educational, health-related, developmental* and *organizational* concerns. Through the integration of psychological theory, research and practice, counselling psychology includes a broad range of practices that help people improve their well-being, alleviate distress, resolve crises, and increase their ability to live more fulfilling lives.[19]

Counselling psychology is a relatively new division within the BPS. Counselling psychologists work within the NHS (in general and psychiatric hospitals and primary care settings), in private hospitals and in private practice, in schools, colleges and universities, in public and private corporate institutions, and, most recently, within the prison service.

Forensic (or criminological) psychology

Forensic psychology is a branch of applied psychology that applies psychological principles to the criminal and civil justice system. It is very much rooted in empirical research, theory and practice, and it is one of the fastest-growing areas of applied psychology, following a funded expansion of psychologists working with offenders in prison in 1996.[19]

Drawing on cognitive, developmental, social and clinical psychology, a major focus of forensic psychology is the study of criminal behaviour and its management, but in recent years research interests have expanded to include other areas, most notably those with a high media profile (such as stalking) (Box 9.6).

The largest single employer of forensic psychologists in the UK is HM Prison Service (which includes the Home Office Research and Development Unit as well as prisons). Forensic psychologists also work in the health service (including rehabilitation units and special/secure hospitals for criminally insane people, such as Broadmoor and Rampton), the police service, young offender units and the probation service. Some work in university departments or in private consultancy.

Educational psychology

According to Coolican, educational psychology is an

> ... area of applied psychology, linking knowledge about the development of children and young people to education. It is concerned with how children feel, interact, learn and behave. It involves the application to education of psychological theories, research and techniques, with the aim of establishing a body of

Box 9.6 Recent areas of research interest among forensic psychologists

- Jury selection
- Presentation of evidence
- Eyewitness testimony (see Chapter 17 and Gross[2])
- Improving the recall of child witnesses
- False memory syndrome and recovered memory (see Chapter 17)
- Offender profiling
- Crime prevention
- Devising treatment programmes, such as anger management
- Assessing the risk of releasing prisoners
- Falling convictions for rape.

From Coolican[19] and Coolican *et al.*[20]

knowledge about the psychological and educational development of children within the context of home, school and the community.[19]

Educational psychologists in England, Wales and Northern Ireland must have a first degree, followed by 3 years' full-time professional training leading to a doctorate in educational psychology.[23]

Educational psychologists are mostly employed by local education authorities (LEAs), working in schools, colleges, child and family centres (previously called 'child guidance'), the Schools Psychological Service, hospitals, day nurseries, nursery schools, special schools (day and residential) and residential children's homes). Clients are aged up to 18 years, but most fall into the 5–16 years age group. Educational psychologists regularly liaise with other professionals from the departments of education, health and social services. A growing number work as independent or private consultants.[22] Box 9.7 lists some of the responsibilities of educational psychologists.

Box 9.7 Some of the responsibilities of the educational psychologist

- Administering psychometric tests, particularly intelligence quotient (IQ) tests, as part of the assessment of learning difficulties (LDs)
- Planning and supervising remedial teaching; research into teaching methods, the curriculum, interviewing, and counselling methods and techniques
- Planning educational programmes for people with mental and physical impairments (including visual impairment and autism), and other groups of children and adolescents not attending mainstream schools (special educational needs)
- Advising parents and teachers on how to deal with children and adolescents with physical impairments, behaviour problems and LDs
- Teacher training.

Health psychology

Health psychology is one of the newer fields of applied psychology, having become a separate division in 1997.

Health psychologists work in a variety of settings, such as hospitals, academic health research units, health authorities and university departments (Box 9.8). They may deal with the problems identified by healthcare agencies, including NHS trusts and health authorities, health professionals (such as general practitioners (GPs), nurses and rehabilitation therapists), and employers outside the healthcare system.

Chartered psychologists

Calling yourself a 'psychologist' even if you have never formally studied psychology is not illegal (unlike calling yourself a 'doctor' or a 'psychiatrist'), and the BPS has long sought some kind of statutory status for practising psychologists of the type that doctors and nurses enjoy.[19]

Since 1987, the BPS, the only professional body for British psychologists incorporated by Royal Charter, has been authorized under its charter to keep a register of chartered psychologists. Entry to the register is restricted to members of the BPS who have applied for registration and who have the necessary qualifications or experience to have reached a standard sufficient for professional practice in psychology without supervision.[24]

All of the applied areas described above (as well as occupational) lead to chartered status, entitling the individual to take the title CPsychol. As yet, sport psychology and psychotherapy do not grant chartered status.[18] Now, not just anyone can call themselves a 'chartered psychologist' without facing prosecution: chartered status is a form of Kitemark for psychologists that should reassure members of the public that they are consulting a competent, experienced and professional practitioner.[19]

In spring 2005, the UK government issued a consultation document on statutory regulation, which proposed that psychologists should be regulated by the Health Professions

Box 9.8 Breadth of health psychology

Health psychology involves the use of psychological principles to promote changes in people's attitudes, behaviour and thinking about health and illness. This may involve:

- the use of psychological theories and interventions to prevent damaging behaviours (e.g. smoking, drug abuse, poor diet), and to change health-related behaviour in community and workplace settings;
- promoting and protecting health by encouraging behaviours such as exercise, healthy diet, teeth-brushing, health checks and self-examination;
- health-related cognitions – investigating the processes that can explain, predict and change health and illness behaviours;
- processes influencing healthcare delivery – the nature and effects of communication between healthcare practitioners and patients, including interventions to improve communication, facilitate adherence (such as taking medication) and prepare for stressful medical procedures;
- psychological aspects of illness – looking at the psychological impact of acute and chronic illness on individual families and carers.

Based on British Psychological Society.[22]

Council (HPC). The BPS raised several serious objections, not least being the fact that most psychologists work outside the NHS. The BPS continues to argue for a new, more appropriate, regulatory body.

Psychology and common sense

In a sense we are all psychologists (see Gross[3]). This is a theme explored at length by Joynson in *Psychology and Common Sense.*[25] He begins by stating that human beings are not like the objects of natural science – we understand ourselves and can already predict and control our behaviour to a remarkable extent. This creates for the psychologist a paradoxical task: what kind of understanding can we seek of a creature that already understands itself?

For Joynson, the fundamental question is: 'If the psychologist did not exist, would it be necessary to invent him?' Conversely, for Skinner, 'it is science or nothing',[26] while Broadbent also rejects the validity of our everyday understanding of ourselves and others (what Joynson calls 'the behaviourists' prejudice').[27] But given our cognitive abilities, and the nature of social interaction, we cannot help but try to make sense of our own and other people's behaviour, and, to this extent, we are all psychologists. Heather points to ordinary language as embodying our 'natural' understanding of human behaviour: as long as human beings have lived, they have been psychologists, and language provides us with an 'elaborate and highly refined conceptual tool, developed over thousands of years of talking to each other'.[28]

Formal versus informal psychology

Legge and others resolve this dilemma by distinguishing between formal and informal psychology (or professional versus amateur/scientific versus non-scientific).[14]

Our common-sense, intuitive or 'natural' understanding is unsystematic and does not constitute a body of knowledge. This makes it very difficult to 'check' an individual's 'theory' about human nature, as does the fact that each individual has to learn from his or her own experience. So, part of the aim of formal psychology (or 'Psychology' – the scientific discipline – as opposed to 'psychology' – every individual's cognitive, emotional, behavioural make-up[29]) is to provide such a systematic body of knowledge, which represents the unobservable basis of our 'gut reactions'.

Yet it could be argued that informal psychology *does* provide a 'body of knowledge' in the form of proverbs or sayings or folk wisdom, handed down from generation to generation, for example 'birds of a feather stick together', 'too many cooks spoil the broth' and 'don't count your chickens until they're hatched'. Although each of these may contain at least a grain of truth, for each one there's another proverb that states the opposite: 'opposites attract', 'many hands make light work' or 'two heads are better than one', and 'time and tide wait for no man' or 'nothing ventured, nothing gained'.

However, formal psychology may help us to reconcile these apparently contradictory statements. For example, there is evidence to support both proverbs in the first pair. Formal psychology tries to identify the conditions under which each statement applies; they appear to be contradictory only because we assume that only one or the other can be true. In this way, scientific psychology throws light on our everyday informal understanding, rather than negating or invalidating it (see Gross[2] and Rolls[30]).

Legge believes that most psychological research should indeed be aimed at demonstrations of 'what we know already', but that it should also aim to go one step further. Only the methods of science, he argues, can provide us with the public, communicable body of knowledge that we're seeking. According to Allport, the aim of science is 'Understanding, prediction and control above the levels achieved by unaided common sense', and this is meant to apply to psychology as much as to the natural sciences.[31]

CONCLUSIONS

Psychology is a diverse discipline. Psychologists investigate a huge range of behaviours and mental or cognitive processes. There is a growing number of applied areas, in which theory and research findings are brought to bear in trying to improve people's lives in various ways.

During the course of its life as a separate discipline, definitions of psychology have changed quite fundamentally, reflecting the influence of different theoretical approaches. Rather than having to choose between our common-sense understanding of people and the 'scientific' version, psychology as a scientific discipline can be seen as complementing and illuminating our 'everyday' psychological knowledge.

KEY POINTS

- The question as to whether psychology is a science has been part of its subject matter throughout its history as a separate discipline.
- Early psychologists, such as Wundt, attempted to study the mind through introspection under controlled conditions, aiming to analyse conscious thought into its basic elements (structuralism).
- Watson rejected introspectionism's subjectivity and replaced it with behaviourism. Only by regarding people as complex animals, using the methods of natural science, and studying observable behaviour could psychology become a true science.
- Gestalt psychologists criticized both structuralism and behaviourism, advocating that 'the whole is greater than the sun of its parts'. Freud's psychoanalytic theory offered another major alternative to behaviourism, stressing the role of the unconscious mind.

- Following the cognitive revolution, people came to be seen as information-processors, based on the computer analogy. Cognitive processes, such as perception and memory, became an acceptable part of psychology's subject matter.
- Academic psychologists are concerned mainly with conducting research (pure or applied), which may focus on underlying processes/mechanisms or on the person.
- The process approach comprises physiological (bio-), cognitive and comparative psychology, while the person approach covers developmental and social psychology, and individual differences.
- The process approach is confined largely to laboratory experiments using non-humans; the person approach makes greater use of field studies and non-experimental methods involving humans. The two approaches see species differences as quantitative and qualitative respectively.
- Most applied psychologists work in clinical, counselling, forensic (criminological) and educational psychology. Newer fields include health psychology.
- In a sense we are all psychologists, creating a dilemma for psychologists: are they necessary? One solution is to distinguish between informal/common-sense and formal/scientific psychology. The latter aims to go beyond common-sense understanding and to provide a public, communicable body of knowledge.

REFERENCES

1. Van Langenhove L (1995) The theoretical foundations of experimental psychology and its alternatives. In JA Smith, R Harré, L Van Langenhove (eds) *Rethinking Psychology*. London: Sage.
2. Gross R (2005) *Psychology: The Science of Mind and Behaviour*, 5th edn. London: Hodder Arnold.
3. Gross R (2009) *Themes, Issues and Debates in Psychology*, 3rd edn. London: Hodder Education.
4. Gross R, Humphreys P, Petkova B (1997) *Challenges in Psychology*. London: Hodder & Stoughton.
5. James W (1890) *The Principles of Psychology*. New York: Henry Holt & Company.
6. Watson JB (1913) Psychology as the behaviourist views it. *Psychological Review* **20**: 158–77.
7. Watson JB (1919) *Psychology from the Standpoint of a Behaviourist*. Philadelphia, PA: J.B. Lippincott.
8. Newell A, Shaw JC, Simon HA (1958) Elements of a theory of human problem-solving. *Psychological Review* **65**: 151–66.
9. Newell A, Simon HA (1972) *Human Problem Solving*. Englewood Cliffs, NJ: Prentice-Hall.
10. Bruner JS, Goodnow JJ, Austin GA (1956) *A Study of Thinking*, New York: John Wiley & Sons.
11. Eysenck MW, Keane MJ (1995) *Cognitive Psychology: A Student's Handbook*, 3rd edn. Hove: Lawrence Erlbaum Associates.
12. Clark KE, Miller GA (eds) (1970) *Psychology: Behavioural and Social Sciences Survey Committee*. Englewood Cliffs, NJ: Prentice-Hall.
13. Zimbardo PG (1992) *Psychology and Life*, 13th edn. New York: HarperCollins.
14. Legge D (1975) *An Introduction to Psychological Science*. London: Methuen.
15. Gross R, McIlveen R, Coolican H, Clamp A, Russell J (2000) *Psychology: A New Introduction*, 2nd edn. London: Hodder & Stoughton.
16. Clamp A (2001) *Evolutionary Psychology*. London: Hodder & Stoughton.
17. Coolican H (2004) *Research Methods and Statistics in Psychology*. London: Hodder & Stoughton.
18. Hartley J, Branthwaite A (1997) Earning a crust. *Psychology Review* **3**: 24–6.
19. Coolican H (ed.) (2007) *Applied Psychology*, 2nd edn. London: Hodder Arnold.
20. Coolican H, Cassidy T, Chercher A, *et al.* (1996) *Applied Psychology*. London: Hodder & Stoughton.
21. Atkinson RL, Atkinson RC, Smith EE, Bem DJ (1990) *Introduction to Psychology*, 10th edn. New York: Harcourt Brace Jovanovich.
22. British Psychological Society (2004) *So You Want To Be a Psychologist?* Leicester: British Psychological Society.
23. Dunsmuir S, Turner J (2004) MPs debate future of educational psychology. *Psychologist* **17**: 429.
24. Gale A (1990) *Thinking about Psychology?*, 2nd edn. Leicester: British Psychological Society.
25. Joynson RB (1974) *Psychology and Common Sense*. London: Routledge & Kegan Paul.
26. Skinner BF (1971) *Beyond Freedom and Dignity*. New York: Knopf.
27. Broadbent DE (1961) *Behaviour*. London: Eyre & Spottiswoode.
28. Heather N (1976) *Radical Perspectives in Psychology*. London: Methuen.
29. Richards G (2002) *Putting Psychology in its Place: A Critical Historical Overview*, 2nd edn. Hove: Routledge.
30. Rolls G (2007) *Taking the Proverbial: The Psychology of Proverbs and Sayings*. Edinburgh: Chambers.
31. Allport GW (1947) *The Use of Personal Documents in Psychological Science*. London: Holt, Rinehart and Winston.

Chapter 10

Awareness

Richard Gross

INTRODUCTION

For the first 30 years or so of its life as a separate discipline, pioneered by figures such as William James and Wilhelm Wundt, psychology took conscious human experience as its subject matter. As described in Chapter 9, introspection – the observation of one's own mind – was the primary method used to study it. This interest in consciousness should not come as a surprise, given how fundamental it is to everything we do.[1]

And yet it is the very subjectivity of our experience that led Watson to reject introspectionism in favour of a truly scientific (i.e. objective) approach to the study of psychology, namely behaviourism. Writing from the perspective of a modern neuroscientist, Greenfield states:

> Any scientific explanation of consciousness must be objective and embrace physical properties of the brain: but at the same time it must, nonetheless, somehow take account of the subjective. This is why consciousness has been such an anathema to scientists, because the whole essence of science is objectivity. And yet we are going to deal with a phenomenon that is subjective ...[2]

However, as part of the 'cognitive revolution' in the 1950s (which removed behaviourism from its dominant position within psychology), 'the mind' once more became an acceptable, respectable focus of psychological research. Reflecting the current interest in consciousness among neuroscientists, philosophers and psychologists, one of the questions we will ask is: how might the brain generate consciousness?

There has been a considerable amount of research since the 1950s into sleep as a state of consciousness, much of which involves trying to find correlations between objective measures of physiological activity and subjective experience, in particular dreaming. Sleep is increasingly discussed in relation to bodily rhythms; disruption of these through our modern lifestyle is increasingly seen as a risk to health. According to Hobson, the rhythm of rest and activity, '... the primordia of sleeping and waking ...', represents one of the most universal and basic features of life.[3] So, the study of sleep is of interest to biologists as well as to psychologists.

WHAT IS 'CONSCIOUSNESS'?

Are only human beings 'conscious'?

In Edelman's terms, non-humans possess *primary consciousness*;[4] this comprises sensory awareness, attention, perception, memory (or learning), emotion and action. What makes human beings distinct is their additional possession of *secondary consciousness*; that is, *self*-consciousness or awareness. This, according to Singer, is the experience of one's own individuality, the ability to experience oneself as an autonomous individual with subjective feelings.[5] It is considered to be '... the result of social interactions, and hence of cultural evolution'. This suggests that it is a rather human thing to have.

Singer also claims that when we say we are conscious, we usually mean that we perceive and remember in a way that makes it possible to report about the perceived and remembered content, or to make it the object of intentional deliberations. As Hobson puts it:

> Consciousness may be defined as our awareness of our environment, our bodies, and ourselves. Awareness of ourselves implies an awareness of awareness, that is, the conscious recognition that we are conscious beings.[6]

Given the crucial role of language in these processes, and given that language is regarded by many as unique to humans, the rest of this chapter focuses on consciousness as a characteristic of human beings.

Some other definitions

- When we are awake, we are *conscious*; but when we are asleep, are in a coma or have been 'knocked out' by a punch to the head, we are *unconscious*. The term 'unconscious' is often reserved for the latter two examples, but, as we shall see, when we fall asleep we do 'lose consciousness'.
- When we do something *consciously*, we do it deliberately or knowingly; but to do something *unconsciously* means doing it automatically or without having to think about it (e.g. an experienced driver or typist; see Chapter 13).

- Public-health campaigns (such as those promoting safe sex) are aimed at increasing *public consciousness* or awareness of the dangers of certain types of behaviour.

Freud's theory of consciousness

Freud saw consciousness as a whole comprising three levels:

- *The conscious:* what we are fully aware of at any one time.
- *The preconscious:* what we could become aware of quite easily if we switched our attention to it.
- *The unconscious:* what we have pushed out of our conscious minds, through repression, making it extremely inaccessible, although it continues to exert an influence on our thoughts, feelings and behaviour (see Chapters 15, 17 and 61).

Most psychologists agree that thoughts, feelings, memories and so on differ in their degree of accessibility. But most would not accept Freud's formulation of the unconscious (based on repression). Indeed, other psychodynamic theorists, in particular Jung, disagreed fundamentally with Freud's view of the unconscious.

CONSCIOUSNESS, AROUSAL AND ALERTNESS

Objective physiological measures, such as the electroencephalogram (EEG), electromyogram (EMG), electrooculogram (EOG) (see below), breathing and heart rates, and other correlates of consciousness, are often described as measures of level of *arousal* or *alertness*. Both subjectively and in terms of overt behaviour, there is an obvious difference between being sleepy and being wide awake regarding the degree of arousal or alertness. Less obvious are the smaller changes that occur during normal wakefulness and that are of two kinds – *tonic* and *phasic*. These are mediated by different brain systems.[7]

Tonic alertness

Changes in tonic alertness reflect intrinsic (and usually quite slow) changes of the basic level of arousal throughout a 24-hour period (or even across a lifetime). They are related closely to various biological rhythms, in particular the circadian rhythm (see below). It was originally thought that the reticular formation (RF)/reticular activating system (RAS) was solely responsible for arousing and maintaining consciousness (it has been called a 'consciousness switch'). For instance, if the brainstem is severed below the RAS, then the animal is paralysed but remains fully alert when awake and shows normal sleep–wake EEG patterns. However, if the brainstem is sectioned above the RAS, then the animal falls into a state of continuous slow-wave sleep (see below).

It is known that other brain structures (in both the thalamus and the hypothalamus) are involved in the sleep–wake cycle, and the coordination of all these systems is necessary for the initiation and maintenance of conscious awareness. Both during wakefulness and sleep, there are periodic, fairly predictable changes in the degree of alertness: the daytime changes are governed by a diurnal rhythm and the sleep (night-time) changes by an ultradian rhythm.

Phasic alertness

Changes in phasic alertness involve short-term, temporary variations in arousal, over a period of seconds, initiated by novel and important environmental events. An important component of these changes is the orienting response to arousing stimuli. It involves a decrease in heart rate and breathing rate, pupil dilation, tensing of the muscles and characteristic changes in the EEG, which becomes desynchronized.

If the stimuli are continuously presented, then the orienting response is replaced by *habituation*: the person or animal stops responding to the stimuli. Habituation is, in fact, a form of *adaptation*. It is more important from a survival point of view to respond to novel stimuli rather than constant stimuli, and, since most stimuli are relatively constant, we need to be able to attend selectively to those that are different or unexpected. It is the changing aspects of the environment that demand, and usually receive, our attention, and the nervous systems of animals and humans have evolved so as to make them especially responsive to change.

CONSCIOUSNESS AND ATTENTION

Although consciousness is difficult to describe because it is fundamental to everything we do,[1] one way of trying to 'pin down' consciousness is to study what we are paying attention to – that is, what is in the forefront of our consciousness. According to Allport, 'attention is the experimental psychologist's code name for consciousness'.[8]

Focal attention

Focal attention/awareness is what we are currently paying deliberate attention to and what is in the centre of our awareness (this corresponds to Freud's conscious). All those other aspects of our environment, or our own thoughts and feelings, that are on the fringes of our awareness but that could easily become the object of our focal attention are within our peripheral attention/awareness (corresponding to Freud's preconscious).

We seem to be capable of doing many things quite unconsciously or automatically, without having to think about what we are doing. A good illustration of this is perception. It is difficult to imagine what it would be like if we were aware of how we perceive (Box 10.1).

> **Box 10.1 Perception as an automatic process: doing what comes naturally**
>
> If you haven't seen the picture shown in Figure 10.1 before, what do you see? If you have seen it before, try to explain how you saw what you saw when you first saw it.
>
> 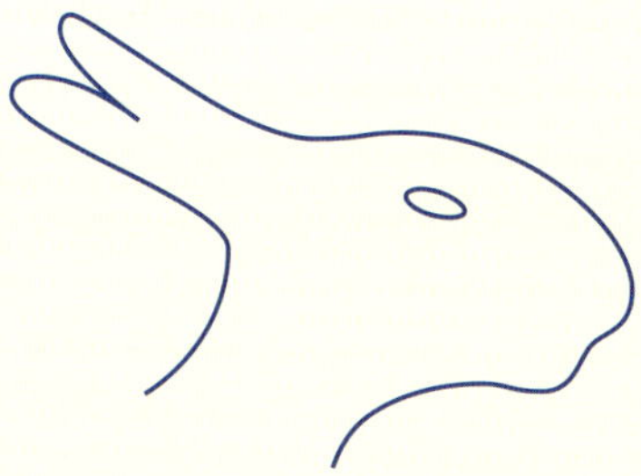
>
> **Figure 10.1** Duck or rabbit?
>
> - To consciously select one version of the ambiguous duck/rabbit figure, we must either know that there is a duck and a rabbit in the picture, or we must have already perceived both versions (in which case, how did the original perception come about?).
> - You may have had difficulty perceiving the duck if your immediate perception was of the rabbit, even though you consciously searched for, and tried to see, the alternative version.
> - This illustrates the very important difference between *conception* and *perception*: most of the time, perception is something that we 'just do' (see Chapter 16).

Conversely, something we normally do quite automatically, such as walking down stairs, might be disrupted if we try to bring it into focal awareness (e.g. thinking about each step as we take it – but don't try this at home!). In general, being able to do things automatically makes sense in terms of freeing us to attend to those environmental events that are unfamiliar or threatening in some way. If we had to think about our bodily movements when walking, this would add to the long list of sources of stimulation competing for our attention (see Chapter 13).

Even with skills that definitely do require focal attention when first acquired, such as driving or playing the piano, once they have been mastered, they become automatic. As Lloyd and colleagues put it, unconscious processes seem to be 'precipitates' of earlier conscious processes.[7]

Nisbett and Wilson go so far as to claim that all psychological activities (including social behaviour) are governed by processes *of which we are unaware*.[9] If people are asked about what they think governed their behaviour after participating in a social psychology experiment, then the answers they give do not usually correspond very well with the explanations that psychologists offer for the same behaviour (and that they believe are the real reasons).

Nisbett and Wilson argue that our belief that we can account for our own behaviour ('common-sense' or intuitive explanations) is illusory, because what really guides our behaviour is not available to consciousness. We do not have direct or privileged access to our cognitive processes, only to the products/outputs of those processes. Joynson,[10] Heather[11] and other psychologists present an opposing view, arguing that people are psychologists and that common-sense explanations may be as valid as theoretical, scientific explanations (see Gross[12]).

CONSCIOUSNESS AND BRAIN ACTIVITY

Passingham at Oxford University and his colleagues from the Institute of Neurology in London (see McCrone[13]) conducted a finger-tapping experiment, which may have revolutionary implications for our understanding of what it means to consciously experience something (Box 10.2).

McCrone believes that Passingham and colleagues' results are not especially surprising. After all, we would expect the brain to be capable of automating motor tasks such as typing or riding a bike. However, McCrone refers to other imaging studies that have shown that a similar

> **Box 10.2 Could finger-tapping be the key to conscious experience?**
>
> - Participants positioned their head into the centre of a brain scanner and rested one hand on a keypad. Then, by trial and error, they started to work out an unknown sequence of eight finger-taps.
> - A tick flashed up on a screen whenever they pressed the correct key. Once they knew the sequence, their instruction was to keep drumming out the pattern until it became an unthinking rhythm. After an hour, their fingers were skipping through the complex routine almost of their own accord and they were barely conscious of what they were doing.
> - In the learning phase, having to remember what they had just discovered while groping for the next step, regions all over the brain were clearly very active. These regions included a range of high-level cognitive areas in the forebrain (such as those involved with planning and memory), as well as other, lower brain areas that regulate movements (such as the basal ganglia and the cerebellum).
> - Yet, within minutes of 'getting' the sequence, this wash of activity began to fade. The job of moving the fingers became confined to a small set of motor areas:
>
> **... It seems, having used the whole brain consciously to establish the individual finger movements, just the bare bones of the routine are left. The brain now has a template or habit that can produce the same behaviour 'as if' it were still going through all the hoops of being consciously aware.**[13]

process occurs when we learn more cognitive skills, such as matching verbs to nouns (e.g. 'hammer' and 'hit'), learning to play a computer game, and learning a path through a drawn maze. Studies using these various tasks show that

> ... paying focal, effortful attention to something calls large regions of the brain into action. The brain does not behave like a collection of isolated pathways, each doing their own thing, but as a coherent system.[13]

There seem to be general-purpose planning centres that come into play whenever the brain is dealing with any kind of novel or difficult mental situation. These planning centres guide the more specialist language and motor centres to an appropriate output. Once the brain has found an optimal way to respond to a certain situation, the 'wider scaffolding' quickly falls away. It is not a case of practice making more efficient use of the pathways that were active during conscious learning, but rather the response can be reduced to its bare essentials. When Passingham and colleagues asked their participants to pay close attention to their finger-tapping rhythm (after this had become automatic), the participants' prefrontal cortex immediately became active again. Just as significantly, their actual performance became more ragged, as if the brain were being put back into exploratory mode.

How might the brain generate consciousness?

Greenfield suggests that consciousness may have three properties:[2]

- Where might a 'consciousness centre' in the brain be? She claims that a recurring problem in neuroscience in general is the difficulty of 'location of function'. Vision, memory, movement and other brain/mind functions seem almost certainly *not* to be related in a modular way to single respective brain regions. Many different regions play parallel roles, analysing the outside world in various ways and reintegrating it into a connected whole. This is likely to be true of consciousness: it could be spatially multiple but also temporally unitary (i.e. we are usually conscious of only any one state at a time). This view is consistent with Passingham and colleagues' research discussed above.
- Rather than being all or nothing (either you are conscious or you are not), a more plausible scenario is that consciousness is more like the light on a dimmer switch that grows as the brain does. The more complex the brain, the greater the consciousness, with a continuum running from minimal to profound. This view can accommodate non-human animal consciousness, children's consciousness, and differences between the same individuals on different occasions (e.g. changes in consciousness induced by drugs (see Chapters 58 and 70), religious experience and listening to music).
- We are always conscious *of something*: there is always some kind of focus, epicentre or trigger (Box 10.3).

Box 10.3 Epicentres and neuronal connectivity

The circuitry of the brain changes with learning and development. It is connections between neurons, rather than neurons themselves, that are established as a result of postnatal experience.

This *plasticity* is especially marked in humans, and the brain remains adaptable and sensitive to life experiences even in adults (e.g. as in the phantom limb phenomenon). Experience changes the connectivity of neurons according to which circuits are most stimulated and hence the most active.

The *epicentre* is like a stone thrown into a pond, causing ripples to spread out over the surface of the water. The extent of these neuronal 'ripples' would affect the degree of consciousness at any one time. The epicentre that is going to trigger consciousness at any one moment is mediated by a group of neurons with relatively long-lasting connections between them. The activated hub of neurons generates the ripples in the brain that constitute consciousness.

From Greenfield.[2]

How might this happen? Greenfield cites an experiment by Libet, in which he pricked participants' skin and recorded the activity of large parts of the brain surface using the EEG. There was a huge amount of activity in the somatosensory cortex, but participants reported no conscious experience of tingling or any other sensations. They felt nothing, although their brain was registering signals of the touch to the skin, via the spinal cord. In Greenfield's model, it is this early component in the response that is equivalent to the 'epicentre'. But then, after about 500 ms, the activity evoked by the skin-prick spread away from the somatosensory cortex to a much larger area of the brain. Only at this stage did participants report feeling a tingle.

Because we never have the same conscious experience on two separate occasions, the same number of neurons will never be stimulated to exactly the same extent or in exactly the same way more than once. Greenfield's model, therefore, needs a neuronal mechanism that can bias a large number of neurons to become activated simultaneously, and she believes that *neuromodulators* fit the bill. These chemicals 'prime' (*bias* or *modulate*) neurons for stimulation by neurotransmitters.

THE FUNCTIONS OF CONSCIOUSNESS: WHAT IS IT FOR?

Like perception, many cases of problem-solving seem to involve processes that are 'out of consciousness'. For example, answers often seem to 'pop into our head', but we do not know how we reached them. If what is important is the solution (as opposed to the process involved in reaching it), then consciousness may be seen as incidental to information-processing (consistent with Nisbett and Wilson's view: see above). But although perception and other basic cognitive and behavioural processes may not *require* consciousness, they are at least usually accompanied by consciousness. Assuming that most other species lack our kind of consciousness, we can infer that consciousness evolved in human beings for some purpose.

The complexity of our nervous system, which makes our consciousness possible, provided our ancestors with the flexibility of behaviour that helped them to survive. However, it is less obvious whether consciousness was itself adaptive or simply a side effect or by-product of a complex nervous system. Some psychologists and biologists believe that consciousness is a powerful agent for controlling behaviour, which has evolved in its own right. Accordingly, non-conscious problem-solving systems are seen as the 'servants of consciousness' (Box 10.4).[14]

Box 10.4 Evolution of the 'inner eye'

Humphrey argues that if consciousness (what he calls the 'inner eye'; Figure 10.2) is the answer to anything at all, then it must be to a biological challenge that human beings have had to meet, namely the human need to understand, respond to and manipulate the behaviour of other human beings:[15,16] '... The first use of human consciousness was – and is – to enable each human being to understand what it feels like to be human and so to make sense of himself and other people from the inside'.[16]

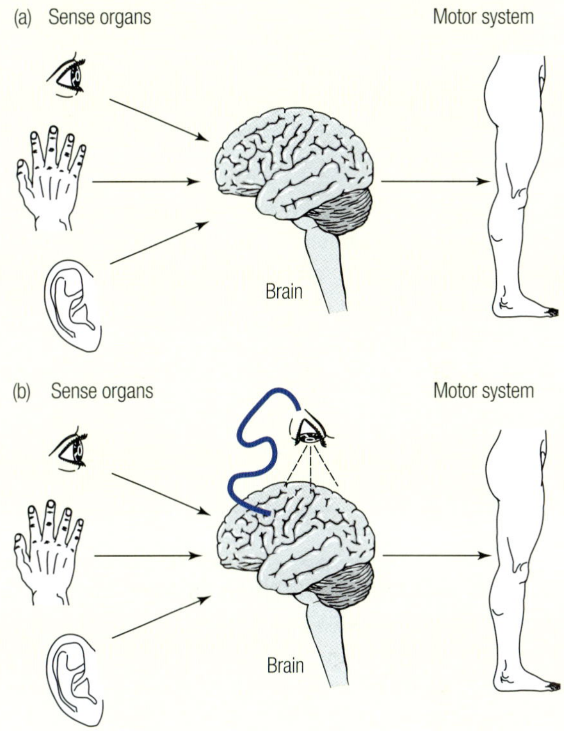

Figure 10.2 (a) How an animal without insight works; (b) how the addition of an 'inner eye' affects the animal

This inner eye allowed our ancestors to raise social life to a new level, so that consciousness is essential for human social activity. We are natural psychologists in a way that species lacking consciousness cannot be.

TWO KINDS OF CONSCIOUSNESS

According to Hilgard's 'neo-dissociation' theory of hypnosis (see Gross[17]), the consciousness that solves a problem may be different from the consciousness that reports the solution: neither is 'higher' or 'lower' than the other, they're simply different.[18] This is consistent with the work on *split-brain patients* (e.g. see Sperry[19]) – that is, people who have undergone surgery (usually for intractable epilepsy) that involves cutting the corpus callosum linking the two hemispheres.

Some psychologists believe that the two cerebral hemispheres are specialized (although they share the potential for many functions and both participate in most psychological activities), so that each is dominant with respect to particular functions. The most common way of distinguishing between them has been the claim that the left is specialized for verbal processes, while the right is specialized for visuo-spatial processes. But this is rather oversimplified, and the distinction is most accurate in relation to higher-order cognitive processes within these domains. For example, although the basic processes of language may be present in both hemispheres, only the left has the specialized neural processes needed to carry out the complex linguistic functions of everyday life.[20] In the vast majority of intact brains, only the left hemisphere retains the person's ability to speak, enabling verbal report of conscious experience.[21]

Ornstein believes that these two modes of operation represent two distinct modes of consciousness.[22] In daily life, we normally just alternate between them and, although they might complement each other, they do not readily substitute for one another (as when you try to describe a spiral staircase or how you tie a shoelace). Is there any evidence to support these claims (Box 10.5)?

CONSCIOUSNESS AND THE ELECTROENCEPHALOGRAM

A major method (since the 1930s) of studying the working of the brain is to monitor its electrical activity. Exactly the same information can be used to throw light on consciousness, because particular patterns of electrical activity are correlated with other measures of arousal and alertness (Box 10.6).

Electroencephalography (literally, 'electric-in-head writing') detects the output of minute electrical 'ripples' caused

Box 10.5 Alpha rhythms and hemispheric lateralization

Galin and Ornstein (1972; see Ornstein[22]) recorded changes in participants' electroencephalograms (EEGs) when presented with either verbal or spatial tasks.

On verbal tasks, alpha rhythms (associated with a waking adult with the eyes closed) in the right hemisphere increased relative to the left; on spatial tasks, the reverse was true (see Box 10.6).

The appearance of alpha rhythms indicates a 'turning off' of information-processing in the area of the brain involved. So, on verbal tasks, information-processing is turned off in the right hemisphere. This is the side of the brain not being used (as if to reduce the interference between the two conflicting modes of operation of the two hemispheres).

Similarly, people with damage to the left hemisphere have greater problems with consciously executed writing, while those with right hemisphere damage have greater problems with more automatic writing, such as signing their name.

This suggests that the left hemisphere may be more involved in highly conscious processes that require intentional behaviour and the focusing of attention. The right hemisphere may be more involved with automatic or unconscious actions, and may be more sensitive to material outside the conscious focus of attention.

Box 10.6 The four major types of brain wave (measured in frequency)

- *Delta (1–2 Hz):* found mainly in infants, sleeping adults and adults with brain tumours.
- *Theta (3–7 Hz):* found mainly in children aged 2–5 years and in psychopaths. May be induced by frustration.
- *Alpha (8–12 Hz):* found mainly in adults who are awake and relaxed, and whose eyes are closed. Most reliably recorded from the back of the scalp.
- *Beta (≥ 13 Hz):* found mainly in adults who are awake and alert, whose eyes are open, and who may be concentrating on some task or other. Most reliably recorded from the middle of the scalp and related to activity in the somatosensory and motor cortex.

See also Box 10.8.

by changes in the electrical charges in different parts of the brain (usually the synchronized activity of large groups of neurons). Although there are characteristic patterns common to all individuals of a particular age or developmental stage, an individual's brain activity is as unique and distinctive as their fingerprints.

Computerized electroencephalography has recently been used to detect evoked potentials (EPs), minute voltage changes induced in the brain by fairly specific visual and auditory stimuli. Often the average of a number of responses to similar kinds of stimuli is used (the average evoked potential – AEP) in order to amplify the signal-to-noise ratio. AEPs are used to study newborns, some children with learning difficulties, people in coma, people who have had a stroke, people with tumours and people with multiple sclerosis. However, for certain brain conditions, brain scanning has largely replaced the EEG (see Chapter 32).[23]

SLEEP

Sleep and the circadian rhythm

According to Blakemore:

> For all the advances of modern society, we cannot afford to ignore the rhythms of the animal brain within us, any more than we can neglect our need to breathe or eat. Without the biological clocks in our brains, our lives would be chaotic, our actions disorganized. The brain has internalized the rhythms of Nature, but can tick on for months without sight of the sun ...[24]

Most animals display a circadian (from the Latin *circa dies* = about one day) rhythm. This is a periodicity or rhythmical alternation of various physiological and behavioural functions, synchronized to the 24-hour cycle of light and dark. So, during a 24-hour period, there is a cycle of several physiological functions (heart rate, metabolic rate, breathing rate, body temperature, hormonal secretion, urine excretion, immune function, alertness and so on), which all tend to reach maximum values during the late afternoon and early evening and to reach minimum values in the early hours of the morning. (The disruption of circadian rhythms is discussed in Box 10.7 and in Chapter 11 as a source of stress.)

Box 10.7 Siffre and the 25-hour day

In 1972, Michel Siffre, a young French cave explorer, spent 7 months underground with no cues as to the time of day. He had adequate food, water, books and exercise equipment. His only contact with the outside world was via a telephone, which was staffed permanently. He was linked up to a computer and video camera, by which scientists on the surface could monitor his physiological functions and state of mind. He organized his life into a fairly normal pattern of alternating periods of activity and sleep, and his 'day' was broken up by a normal meal pattern. The remarkable finding was that he chose to live a 25-hour (rather than 24) day. For every real day that passed, he rose an hour later – the clock in his brain was running a little slow.

From Blakemore.[24]

The internal or biological clock

Rats, like humans, have an inherent rhythm of about 25 hours, which dictates their cycle of sleep and waking if they are put in the dark. This internal clock is as reliable and regular as most manufactured ones – the rhythm deviates by no more than a few minutes over several months. So how is the internal (biological) clock reset each day to the cycle of the real world, and where is the clock to be found?

The internal clock is thought to be a tiny cluster of neurons, the *suprachiasmatic nucleus* (SCN), situated in the medial hypothalamus. For example, damage to the SCN in rats produces complete disappearance of the circadian rhythm: the sleep–wake cycle, eating and drinking, hormone secretion and so on become completely random during the course of the 24-hour period. Most of what is known about the SCN is based on experiments with non-human animals, and we cannot make direct electrophysiological recordings from the human brain. But anatomical studies show that humans have an SCN.[25] The function of the SCN is to synchronize all the bodily functions that are governed by the circadian rhythm.

The SCN is situated directly above the optic chiasma (the junction of the two optic nerves en route to the brain). A tuft of thin nerve fibres branches off from the main nerve and penetrates the hypothalamus above, forming synaptic connections with cells in the SCN. This anatomically insignificant pathway is the link between the outside world and the brain's own clock.[24] So, the retina projects directly onto the SCN, which ensures that the sleep–wake cycle is tuned to the rhythm of night and day. If this connection with the retina is severed, then the cycle goes 'haywire'.

The effects of disrupting the biological clock

In human adults at least, it appears that the circadian rhythm does not depend primarily on external cues, although it is surprisingly easy to outsmart our body clock by external means such as alarm clocks.

According to Melton, scientists are warning that we ignore our natural bodily rhythms at our peril:

> ... Fighting our natural sleep tendencies ... may be grinding away at our health, triggering a string of maladies... Giving up the late nights and weekend lie-ins in favour of a strict daily routine and a regular bedtime might be as important to our health as quitting smoking or cutting back on saturated fat.[26]

How much sleep do we need?

We are biologically ill-prepared to function on minimal sleep: our prehistoric genetic blueprint for sleep has not evolved fast enough to keep up with the pace of twenty-first-century life. Humans are more likely to need an average of 10 hours of sleep a night than the 4 hours that Margaret Thatcher famously claimed to get by on. In the sleep laboratory, people who average 8 hours of sleep a night and maintain that they are fully alert during the day, and who then get an extra hour's sleep at night, find their productivity levels increase by 25 per cent.

It has been suggested that each of us maintains a personal sleep bank account. We need enough sleep in the account in order to be able to function properly during the day. This means at least 8 hours of sleep for most people, in order to cancel out the sleep debt incurred by 16 hours of continuous alertness. Similarly, Dement, one of the pioneers of sleep research and the founder of the world's first sleep disorders centre (see below), proposes a rough rule of thumb: most people require about an hour's sleep for every two waking hours.[27]

We live in a sleep-deprived society.[28,29] For example, in the past 20 years, we've added about 158 hours to our annual working and commuting time – equal to a full month of working hours. (The British work longer hours compared with any other nation in Europe). Young mothers with children have added an astonishing 241 hours since the 1960s. According to the National Sleep Survey, we have just 6.5 hours' sleep per night (rather than 8 hours), although the almost 2000 respondents were mainly younger than in other surveys.[30] This is more than 2 hours less every night than our grandparents slept. In our 24-hour society, the pace of life is becoming faster and harder, and the stresses and pressures of work are leading to longer working hours and disrupted sleep. But, as Griffey says: '... sleep isn't a social inconvenience, it's a physical necessity and more and more studies are showing that sleep deprivation is a growing problem'.[29]

How does sleep deprivation produce negative effects on health?

Dement believes that most of us carry a heavy 'sleep debt', a deficit of sleep built up over days, weeks and months.[27] Sleep debt is dangerous, and it is potentially lethal. Examples are drivers who fall asleep at the wheel, pilots who are too sleepy to land planes safely, and surgeons who botch surgical procedures because they are exhausted. Both the *Exxon Valdez* and the *Challenger* space shuttle disasters were attributed to human error caused by extreme sleep deprivation. Dement also links high blood pressure, heart attacks and strokes to sleep apnoea, a chronic failure to sleep well because of problems breathing during sleep (see Chapter 54).

According to Melton, reduced sleep can interfere with the regulation of the immune system (see Chapter 11).[26] Griffey reports on the findings of several studies showing why sleep deprivation is so harmful.[29] The metabolic and endocrine changes resulting from a significant sleep debt mimic many of the hallmarks of ageing. Chronic sleep loss could not only speed up the onset but also increase the severity of age-related diseases such as diabetes, hypertension, obesity and memory loss. This might happen through chronic increases in the level of cortisol, a stress-related hormone, which in large quantities acts as a neurotoxin, killing billions of brain cells. Cortisol is also associated with increased risk of heart disease (see Chapter 11). Shift workers are especially at risk.

The physiology of sleep

When darkness falls, the eyes indirectly inform the pineal gland (the 'third eye'). This is a tiny structure at the top of the brainstem, which keeps track of the body's natural cycles and registers external factors such as light and darkness. The pineal gland secretes melatonin in response to darkness, making us drowsy. Downing calls melatonin 'nature's sleeping draught'.[31] Melatonin is a hormone that affects brain cells that produce serotonin, concentrated in the raphe nuclei (situated near the pons), which secrete a substance that acts on the RAS to induce light sleep. Jouvet found that lesions of the raphe nuclei in cats produced severe insomnia, and naturally occurring lesions in humans seem to have a very similar effect.[32]

Another important sleep centre is the locus coeruleus (LC), a tiny structure on each side of the brainstem whose cells are rich in noradrenaline, thought to be involved in inducing active (rapid eye movement – REM) sleep (see below). The LC may well serve many of the functions previously attributed to the RAS. Studies with rats suggest that the LC regulates the animal's level of vigilance to environmental stimuli.[25]

There is also evidence that a substance called *factor S* accumulates gradually in the brain of animals when they are awake. If this factor is removed from the fluid surrounding the brain and transferred into another animal, then sleep is induced. It is likely that factor S contributes to our feelings of sleepiness.[23]

Varieties of sleep and the ultradian rhythm

In the typical sleep laboratory, a volunteer settles down for the night with not only EEG wires attached, but also with wires from an EOG ('oculo' = eye) and an EMG ('myo' = muscle) (Figure 10.3).

A typical night's sleep comprises a number of ultradian cycles (lasting approximately 90 min), and each cycle consists of a number of stages (Box 10.8).

The cycle then goes into reverse, so we re-enter stage 3 and then stage 2. Instead of re-entering stage 1, however, a different kind of sleep (*active sleep*) appears. Pulse and respiration rates increase, as does blood pressure, and all three processes become less regular. The EEG begins to resemble that of the waking state, showing that the brain is active, supported by increases in oxygen consumption, blood flow and neural firing in many brain structures. But it is even more difficult to wake us from this kind of sleep than from the deep stage 4 sleep, hence the term *paradoxical sleep*.[33]

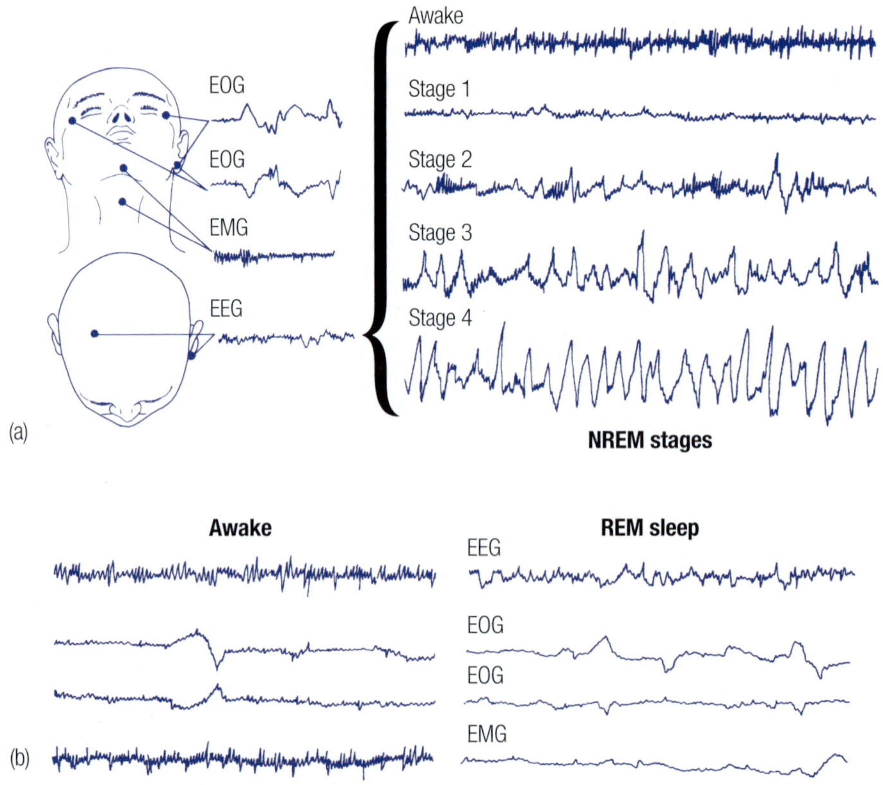

Figure 10.3 Comparison of physiological measures for different types of sleep. (a) The non-rapid eye movement (NREM) stages are represented in typical order of appearance; in reality, each one gradually blends into the next. (b) Rapid eye movement (REM) sleep is in some ways similar to waking, but in other ways it is quite different; the electroencephalogram (EEG) is more similar to waking than to that in any NREM stage, and REMs are present, but the body muscles are deeply inhibited. EMG, electromyogram; EOG, electro-oculogram.

Box 10.8 Typical night's sleep: the four stages of non-rapid eye movement (NREM) sleep

After we shut our eyes and prepare to sleep, *alpha waves* begin to punctuate the high-frequency *beta waves* of active wakefulness. The transition from being awake to entering stage 1 sleep is called the *hypnagogic period*, and is sometimes included in stage 1.

- *Stage 1:* When we first fall asleep, the electroencephalogram (EEG) is irregular and lacks the pattern of alpha waves that characterizes the relaxed waking state. At first, there is a reduction in frequency of alpha waves, which are then replaced by low-voltage, slow theta waves, accompanied by slow rolling eye movements. The heart rate begins to slow down and the muscles relax, but we can still be woken up easily.
- *Stage 2:* This is a deeper state of sleep, but it is still fairly easy to wake the person. The EEG shows bursts of activity called *sleep spindles* (1- to 2-second waxing and waning bursts of 12- to 14-Hz waves). There are also occasional sharp rises and falls in amplitude of the whole EEG (*K complexes*), which last for up to 2 seconds.
- *Stage 3:* Sleep is becoming deeper, and the spindles disappear and are replaced by long, slow *delta waves* for up to 50 per cent of the EEG record. We are now quite unresponsive to external stimuli, and so it is difficult to wake us up. Heart rate, blood pressure and body temperature continue to drop.
- *Stage 4:* We now enter *delta sleep* (deep or 'quiet' sleep: 50% or more of the record consists of delta waves) and will spend up to 30 minutes in this stage. About an hour has elapsed since stage 1 began. As in stage 3, it is difficult to wake us unless something happens of great personal significance, such as our baby crying.

Stages 2–4 collectively are called *slow-wave sleep* (SWS). As we pass through stages 1–4, the frequency of the waves decreases, and the amplitude and voltage increase. Also, muscle tone steadily declines.

Another characteristic of active sleep are the rapid eye movements (the eyeballs moving back and forth, and up and down, together) under the closed lids (hence the term 'rapid eye movement sleep'). Finally, although the brain may be very active, the body is not. REM sleep is characterized by muscular paralysis (especially of the muscles of the arms and legs), so that all the tossing and turning and other typical movements associated with sleep occur only during stages 1–4 (non-rapid eye movement (NREM) sleep). The distinction between REM and NREM sleep was originally made by Dement and Kleitman.[34]

Another feature of REM sleep is the appearance of *pontine-geniculo-occipital* (PGO) *spikes/waves*, which are generated in the pons and travel through the lateral geniculate nucleus (LGN). These were discovered by Jouvet working with cats in the 1960s. PGO spikes typically occur in bursts, often preceding individual eve movements. According to the activation-synthesis model of dreaming (see below), PGO activity is the prime source of dreaming experience.[25]

After 15 minutes or so in REM sleep, we re-enter NREM sleep (stages 2–4), and so another ultradian cycle begins (Figure 10.4). However, with each 90-minute cycle (of which

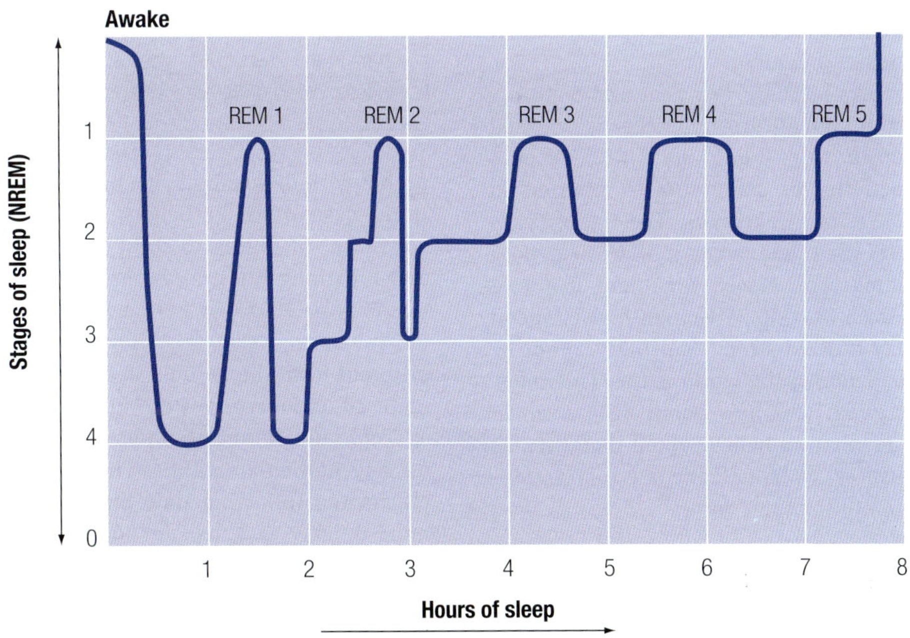

Figure 10.4 Typical night's sleep stages. NREM, non-rapid eye movement; REM, rapid eye movement.

there are four to five on average per night), the duration of the REM sleep increases and that of NREM sleep decreases. The first cycle normally provides the deepest sleep and the shortest REM period. As the night goes on, we spend relatively more time in REM and less in NREM sleep. In later cycles, it is quite common to go from REM to stage 2, and then straight back into REM sleep (bypassing stages 3 and 4). Natural waking usually occurs during a period of REM sleep.

According to Empson:

> While most all-night recording experiments are over brief periods (of up to a week), some very extended studies have been done and there is no evidence that the patterns of sleep we observe over short periods (after the first night) are in any way peculiar to the unfamiliarity of the laboratory environment.[25]

Sleep and dreaming

People woken from REM sleep commonly report that they have been dreaming,[35] and dreaming is associated primarily with REM sleep.[36] Rapid eye movements seem to be a very reliable indicator that a person is dreaming (especially in combination with the fairly high-frequency and low-amplitude brain waves). However, it is now generally agreed that there is no one-to-one correspondence between dream action and eye movement, although cues about the general nature of the dream can often be gleaned from the REM record.[37] Faraday notes that research has shown that movements of the inner ear also occur during sleep and may be correlated with the auditory content of dreams.

REM sleep has been called 'dream sleep' or the 'D-state', and some writers have gone so far as to call it the 'third state of existence', because it is in many ways as different from NREM sleep (the 'S-state') as it is from waking. Since brain activation is most intense in REM, dreaming is most highly correlated with that brain state,[6] and dream reports from REM sleep have remained the principal focus of empirical investigations of dreaming.[38]

Blackmore gives figures of 70–95 per cent and 5–10 per cent, respectively, for the (vivid) dreaming that is reported when people are woken from REM and NREM sleep.[39] Mentation (mental activity) of some sort is reported in about 50 per cent of NREM awakenings. The figures vary according to the criteria used.[40] So, being in REM sleep does not guarantee dreaming; conversely, dreaming can and does occur in NREM sleep (Box 10.9). Human fetuses spend about 15 hours per day in REM sleep – but they cannot be 'dreaming', since experience of the world is the 'raw material' of dreams. From what we know about REM sleep in other species, and from what we believe about their dreams and state of consciousness, we must conclude that dreaming and REM sleep are not the same thing.[39]

Box 10.9 There's more to dreaming than rapid eye movement sleep

Is it possible that the difference between dreams in rapid eye movement (REM) and non-rapid eye movement (NREM) sleep is actually an artefact of the ability to recall dreams following the 'rude awakening'?

Beaumont argues that being awoken from NREM sleep may lead to the dream being forgotten before the participant is sufficiently awake to report it (since this is a deeper kind of sleep, in which the brain is much less active).[41] By contrast, being woken from REM sleep may allow the ongoing dream to be remembered and then reported (as the brain is much more active).

Clearly, if this is so, then we have stumbled upon a major confounding variable that challenges the very basis of much of the sleep/dream research. An appreciable amount of mental activity occurs during NREM sleep, and there are no completely consistent differences between dream reports obtained when participants are woken from either kind of sleep.

Research in the 1990s indicated that REM sleep may not be the driving force behind dreams. Dreaming seemed to be more of a continuous process, not confined to periods of REM sleep. Rather than seeing NREM sleep as 'dream-free', research suggested that NREM dreams are relatively short and rationally constructed in terms of facts and logic, compared with the more visual, emotional and detailed REM dreams.[42]

Participants woken from NREM sleep tend to report dreams that are shorter, less vivid and less visual than REM dreams and, in fact, they often describe themselves as having been 'thinking' rather than dreaming. NREM sleep is also associated with sleepwalking (somnambulism), sleeptalking and some types of nightmare.

However, evidence from studies of sleep deprivation seems to support the view of REM sleep as a dream-state sleep quite independently of the sleeper's report of having dreamed (or not).

The effects of sleep deprivation

As far as rats are concerned, long-term sleep deprivation is definitely not good for their health: it causes impaired thermoregulation, metabolic dysfunction and eventually death.[3] In the case of human beings, studies have been remarkably consistent in failing to show any marked changes in heart and breathing rates, blood pressure, skin conduction, body temperature, EMG or EEG, even when deprivation continues for up to 200 hours.[43] But as we have seen, this is very different form the *chronic* sleep deprivation that is symptomatic of a modern Western lifestyle.

Webb and Bonnet limited participants to 2 hours' sleep on one particular night.[44] The participants suffered no ill effects the following day, but that night they fell asleep more quickly and slept for longer than usual. Longer periods of sleep deprivation may result in some unpleasant psychological effects, but people are remarkably able to do without sleep. Webb and Bonnet gradually reduced the length of sleep in a group of volunteers from 8 hours to 4 hours per night over a 2-month period, with no detectable effect. Box 10.10 describes the sleep rebound.

Theories of sleep

According to Blakemore:

> Our planet is a dangerous place; there is ruthless competition for limited resources and only the fittest survive. And yet all the most advanced animals, normally alert, shrewd, watchful, drop their defences to sleep. Even human beings, the most spectacularly successful species, spend one-third of their lives more or less paralysed and senseless. If sleep is so risky, it must bestow a huge benefit on animals that indulge in it, or it would have been eliminated by the powerful forces of natural selection. Animals that did not need sleep would surely have evolved and prevailed over their sleepy competitors ... sleep must surely be valuable ...[24]

Empson maintains that, even though physiologists have made great strides in understanding sleep mechanisms, this has not helped greatly in understanding what sleep is for.[25] Sleep has the features of a primary drive (such as hunger and sex), but what makes it unique as a primary biological drive is that the need for sleep is reflected in decreased levels of arousal, and its satisfaction is associated with further decreases. Sleep, therefore, represents a serious exception to the view that organisms seek a single optimal level of (non-specific) arousal (see Chapter 11).[7]

Box 10.10 The rapid eye movement rebound

When sleep is reduced *abruptly* (e.g. in the case of hospital doctors, who may be on duty for 50 hours at a stretch), the effects may be serious and may include irritability, intellectual inefficiency, and an intense fatigue and need for sleep.

These effects mirror those produced by depriving participants of approximately 2 hours of rapid eye movement (REM) sleep (but otherwise allowing them to sleep normally). The following night, there is an increase in REM sleep (to compensate for the previous night's loss). This is called the *REM rebound*.

When volunteers are able to get by on greatly (but gradually) reduced amounts of sleep, it is apparently because they pack their 2 hours of REM sleep tightly into their sleeping time (thus reducing the amount of non-rapid eye movement (NREM) sleep in between their dreams). When sleep is reduced abruptly, there is no time to adopt this alternative dreaming-sleep pattern.

Dement woke participants from their REM sleep on five successive nights (a control group were woken only during NREM sleep periods).[45] When the participants were allowed to sleep uninterruptedly, they did 60 per cent more dreaming until they had made up their lost REM time. For as many as five nights following their REM deprivation, they spent more time in REM sleep than usual, and on some nights they doubled their REM time.

The restoration theory

Oswald maintains that both REM and NREM sleep serve a restorative, replenishing function.[46] NREM restores bodily processes that have deteriorated during the day, while REM sleep is a time for replenishing and renewing brain processes, through the stimulation of protein synthesis (Box 10.11).

Box 10.11 Rapid eye movement sleep and the developing brain

Restoration theory helps to explain the large proportion of babies' sleeping time spent in rapid eye movement (REM) sleep.

During much of their first year, babies sleep for about 18/24 hours. By about 12 months old, they have two periods of sleep every 24 hours (one daytime and one night-time). Not until the age of about 5 years has an 'adult' pattern become established, probably as a result of both environmental and maturational factors.

Within these changing patterns, the relative proportions of REM and non-rapid eye movement (NREM) sleep change quite dramatically. Whereas newborns spend half their 18 hours in REM sleep, adults usually spend only one-quarter of their 8 hours in REM sleep.

The developing brain needs a great deal of protein synthesis for cell manufacture and growth, and REM sleep helps to achieve this.

An evaluation of restoration theory

- Patients who survive drug overdoses and withdrawal, and other brain 'insults', such as intensive electroconvulsive therapy (ECT) (see Chapter 59), experience prolonged increases in REM sleep. These increases are consistent with the estimated time for the half-life of proteins in the brain; that is, in a 6-week period, about half the brain's total protein is replaced, and this is the approximate length of the increased REM period.
- Nocturnal secretion of growth hormone (which produces bodily protein synthesis) depends on uninterrupted stage 4 sleep. In adults, a chronic lack of normal stage 4 is found in people with fibrositis, whose EEG during sleep is characterized by 'alpha-delta' patterns, a mixture of sleeping and waking EEG (typically experienced as fitful, unrestorative sleep). The disturbance of stage 4 in healthy volunteers produces the symptoms of fibrositis.
- According to Empson, all this evidence is consistent with a general anabolic function for sleep: REM sleep underlies brain growth, repair and memory functions, and slow-wave (stage 4) sleep promotes bodily growth and repair.[25] However, cell repair goes on 24 hours a day (even though it reaches a peak at night).
- A more serious objection is that REM sleep is an active

state (at least as far as the brain is concerned) and probably burns up a substantial amount of energy. Indeed, blood flow to the brain *increases* during REM sleep, and this would actually prevent high levels of protein synthesis. In view of this kind of evidence, Oswald maintains that both types of sleep are involved in the process of restoring bodily tissue.[47]

- However, Oswald may have been a little premature. According to Siegel, although most brain cells are at least as active during REM sleep as in waking, there is a specific group of cells that goes against this trend.[48] These are the cells that produce the monoamine neurotransmitters (noradrenaline, serotonin, histamine). These key neurotransmitters inhibit body movement and reduce awareness of the environment, and the cells that produce them stop discharging completely during REM sleep. This cessation of neurotransmitter release is vital for the functioning of these neurons and their receptors on recipient neurons. This interruption may allow the receptor systems to 'rest' and regain full sensitivity, which may be crucial during waking for mood regulation. The monoamines also play a part in rewiring the brain to respond to new experiences. So, turning them off during REM may help to prevent changes in brain connections that might otherwise be 'accidentally' created as a consequence of the activation of other neurons during REM sleep. The REM rebound might result from the need to rest monoamine systems and other 'off' systems.[48]

Evolutionary theory

Different species characteristically sleep for different periods. Those at risk from predators, that cannot find a safe place to sleep or that spend large parts of each day searching for and consuming food and water (such as herd animals) sleep very little (e.g. zebras sleep for only 2–3 hours per day). Predators that sleep in safe places and can satisfy their food and water needs fairly quickly sleep for much of the day (e.g. lions often sleep more or less continuously for 2–3 days after gorging themselves on a kill).

According to Meddis, sleep is an advantage because it keeps the animal immobilized for long periods, making it less conspicuous to would-be predators and, therefore, safer.[49,50] The safer the animal from predators, the longer it is likely to sleep. Meddis also argues that the long sleep periods of babies have evolved to prevent exhaustion in their mothers and, in this sense, sleep is still functional – at least for mothers of babies and young children. As to the need for immobilization, this no longer seems viable as an explanation of sleep in humans, and so it may be regarded as a remnant of our evolutionary past.

An evaluation of evolutionary theory

- According to the theory, a preyed-upon species may sleep for both *shorter* periods (because of the constant need to stay on guard against predators) and *longer* periods (because this makes it safer from predators). In other words, whatever sleep pattern a species has, it can be explained in 'evolutionary' terms – an example of *non-falsifiability*. This represents a serious limitation of evolutionary theory.
- Empson characterizes Meddis's theory as a 'waste of time' theory.[25] Empson believes that the fact that sleep is universal among animals contradicts the theory, as does the finding that sleep deprivation can be fatal (at least in rats: see above).
- A weaker version of the 'waste of time' theory was proposed by Horne, who distinguishes between *core sleep* (which is necessary) and *optional sleep* (which is not).[51] Evidence from sleep-deprivation experiments (both partial and total) shows that accumulated sleep 'debts' are made up to some extent on recovery nights, but never entirely. For example, REM rebound accounts for approximately 50 per cent of the REM sleep lost during selective awakenings. This suggests that only the first 3 hours of sleep are truly necessary (core sleep), and the rest is optional (having no physiological function).
- But most of us eat more than we absolutely need to in order to keep body and soul together, and yet no biologist would say that, because a proportion of feeding was optional, feeding was only partly functional.[25]

Empson concludes by saying:

> ... sleep appears to be ubiquitous and necessary; it is a complex function of the brain involving far-reaching changes in body physiology as well as brain physiology. It is difficult to believe that it does not have an important function and the restorative theories provide a coherent account of what this might be.[25]

Hobson's levels

Although not a discrete theory, Hobson proposes that the function of sleep can be analysed at different levels:[3]

- At the *behavioural level*, sleep suppresses activity at a time (night-time/darkness) when the chances of finding food or a mate are relatively low. Also, such activities have a high energy cost in warm-blooded animals when the temperature is low. This makes sleep behaviourally very efficient. In addition, the enforced nature of sleep and its relation to resting activity serves to unite animals in a family or pair-bonded situation, which may encourage sexual behaviour and promote care and development of the young.
- At the *developmental level*, a function of REM sleep for developing organisms could be the guaranteed activation of neural circuits underlying crucial, survival behaviours (see Box 10.11). From an evolutionary point of view, there would be great advantages gained from ensuring the organized activation of the complex systems of the brain before the organism has developed the ability to test them in the real world. In both the developing and the adult animal, REM sleep could constitute a form of *behavioural rehearsal*.

- At the *metabolic level*, the recurring cycles of NREM/REM sleep are accompanied by major changes in all the body's physiological systems. NREM sleep involves decreased blood pressure, heart rate and breathing rate, as well as the release of growth and sex hormones from the pituitary (consistent with the restoration theory), while REM sleep involves increased blood pressure, heart rate and breathing rate, as well as penile erection and clitoral engorgement.

DREAMING

Although dreaming and REM sleep are not the same thing, dreaming is associated with REM sleep, and psychologists have developed reliable techniques for establishing when a person is likely to be dreaming. But there has been no equivalent progress in understanding the nature of dreams. According to Empson,[25] a starting point must be to establish clearly how dreaming differs from waking consciousness. Empson identifies four such differences:

- Dreams *happen to us* as opposed to being a product of our conscious control: 'When dreaming we are the spectators of an unfolding drama, and only rarely does one have the impression of being in control ...'[25]
- *Lucid dreaming*, in which the dreamer 'knows' that he or she is dreaming and decides how the dream plot should develop, is very rare.
- The *logic* of waking consciousness is suspended (see Freud's theory in Chapter 61).
- Dreams reported in the laboratory tend to be mundane and lack the *bizarre quality* of 'normal' dreams, probably because only the strangest experiences are remembered when we wake normally after a night's sleep.

Dreams have a single-mindedness: the imagery of the dream totally dominates the dreamer's consciousness. But when we are awake, we normally reflect on the stream of consciousness as it goes on, and we can be aware of one thing but simultaneously imagine something else. (Recall that Greenfield claims that waking consciousness is single-minded:[2] see above).

Hobson describes dreams as typically including:[3]

- *hallucinations* (predominantly visual, although auditory, tactile and movement sensations are also prominent, with taste and smell underrepresented and pain extremely rare);
- *delusions* (believing that the events are real);
- *cognitive abnormalities* (such as the occurrence of events that would be physically impossible in the real world);
- *emotional intensification* and *amnesia* (we forget over 95 per cent of our dreams).

These characteristics have led to a comparison between dreams and abnormal states of mind, as in schizophrenia and organic mental disorders, in particular delirium (see Chapters 37 and 38).

Theories of dreaming

Reorganization of mental structures

According to Ornstein, REM sleep and dreaming may be involved in the reorganization of our *schemas* (mental structures), so as to accommodate new information.[22] People placed in a 'disturbing and perplexing' (asked to perform difficult tasks with no explanation) atmosphere for 4 hours just before sleep spend longer in REM sleep than normal. REM time also increases after people have had to learn complex tasks.

This may explain why REM sleep decreases with age. As we have seen, newborns spend 50 per cent of their (approximately) 18 hours of sleep in REM sleep, compared with 25 per cent spent by adults in their (approximately) 8 hours of sleep. Oswald suggested that babies' brains need to process and assimilate the flood of new stimuli pouring in from the outside world (as part of the very construction of the brain), and that this is achieved (partly) through REM sleep (see above). However, we go on throughout our lives needing to reconstruct our brains and our minds.[52]

Activation-synthesis model[53,54]

The cortex is highly active during REM sleep (*activation*), although it receives little external stimulation. While the motor cortex is highly active (generating activity that would normally produce bodily movement), these commands do not reach the muscles of the limbs but are 'switched off' at a relay station at the top of the spinal column: we are effectively paralysed (*output blockade*).

Not only is the cortex isolated (unable to control muscles), but also there is inhibition of incoming signals produced by the sensory systems. Consequently, perceptions of the 'real' world are selectively attenuated (*input blockade*). Hindbrain and midbrain structures, normally associated with relaying sensory information to the cortex, spontaneously generate signals (PGO waves; see above) responsible for cortical activation. These are indistinguishable from signals that would normally have been relayed from the eyes and ears. This activity is under the control of a periodic triggering mechanism in the pontine brainstem (the top of the spinal column, at the base of the brain).

What we call a dream is the simplest way of interpreting these internally produced signals, by combining them into some meaningful whole (i.e. *synthesis*). The cognitive system, which organizes sensory information into the simplest meaningful interpretation when we are awake, processes all the internally generated signals as if they came from the outside world. In combination with oculomotor activity, PGO waves are sent to the visual and association cortex and the thalamus.

It is the unusual intensity and rapidity of brain stimulation (often involving simultaneous activation of areas not usually activated together during waking) that account for the highly changeable and sometimes bizarre content of dreams. According to Hobson: '... the now autoactivated and autostimulated brain processes these signals and interprets them in terms of information stored in memory'.[3]

Many dream experiences do seem to reflect the brain's and body's state, and so they can be thought of as interpretations of these physical states. For example, being chased, locked up or frozen with fear may well reflect the blocked motor commands to the muscles; floating, flying and falling experiences may reflect vestibular activation; and the sexual content of dreams may reflect vaginal engorgement and penile erection.[22]

Evaluation of the activation-synthesis model

- In a sense, we dream instead of acting (perhaps suggesting the need for rest and restoration for the body). Cats with brainstem injury act out their dreams by, for example, chasing the mouse of their dreams while ignoring the real mouse in their cage: they are not paralysed in the normal way during REM sleep.
- Crick and Mitchison proposed a modified version of the model, which they called *reverse learning*.[55] The basic idea is that we dream in order to forget. The cortex (unlike other parts of the brain) is composed of richly interconnected neuronal networks. The problem with such a network system is that it malfunctions when there is overload of incoming information. To deal with such overload, the brain needs a mechanism to 'debug' or 'clean up' the network, and REM sleep is that mechanism. In this way, we awake with a cleaned up network, and the brain is ready for new input. According to Crick and Mitchison, trying to remember our dreams may not be a good idea: they are the very patterns of thought that the system is trying to tune out.
- For others, especially psychoanalysts and other psychodynamic psychologists, it is essential that we do remember our dreams, so that we can try to understand their meaning. For example, Freud saw dreams as wish fulfilments. Both he and Jung saw symbolism as being of central importance in dreams, which put the dreamer in touch with parts of the self usually inaccessible during waking life (see Chapter 61). Hall saw dreams as 'a personal document, a letter to oneself' and, like Jung, advocated the study of dream series rather than single isolated dreams.[56]

CONCLUSIONS: INTEGRATING NEUROBIOLOGICAL, EVOLUTIONARY AND PSYCHOLOGICAL ACCOUNTS OF DREAMING

Winson, a neuroscientist, argues that neural and psychological theories of dreams are not mutually exclusive.[57] While Crick and Mitchison argue that we need to forget our dreams, Winson claims that:

> ... dreams may reflect a memory-processing mechanism inherited from lower species, in which information important for survival is reprocessed during REM sleep. This information may constitute the core of the unconscious.[57]

To maintain sleep, locomotion had to be suppressed by inhibiting motor neurons. But suppressing eye movements was not necessary, because this does not disturb sleep. With the evolution of REM sleep, each species could process the information most needed for its survival (such as the location of food and the means of predation or escape). In REM sleep, this information may be re-accessed and integrated with past experience to provide an ongoing strategy for behaviour. Similarly, threat simulation theory claims that dreaming evolved to simulate the very real threats to individuals' physical survival (and hence to reproductive success) during human evolution.[58] Ways of dealing with these threats could be 'practised' in dreams.

According to Humphrey, dreams are also about practising all sorts of physical, intellectual and social skills ('dreaming as play').[15,16] But dreams may just be an evolutionary 'epiphenomenon', without any adaptive function,[59] and it may also be true that many people function perfectly well without remembering their dreams.[52] Nevertheless:

> ... studying our own dreams can be valuable in all sorts of ways. They can reveal our inner motivations and hopes, help us face our fears, encourage growing awareness, and even be a source of creativity and insight.[39]

KEY POINTS

- Since the cognitive revolution dislodged behaviourism from its dominant position in psychology, cognitive processes and consciousness have once more become important areas of psychological research.
- Freud distinguished three levels of consciousness: conscious, preconscious and unconscious. Most psychologists do not accept Freud's view of the unconscious as based on repression, but they would accept that there is a continuum of consciousness.
- Arousal/alertness can be defined objectively in terms of various physiological measures, such as EEGs, EOGs, EMGs, breathing rate and heart rate. These are correlates of consciousness.
- Changes in tonic alertness are linked closely to various biological rhythms, especially the circadian rhythm. The RF/RAS plays an important role in arousing/maintaining consciousness. Alertness changes in fairly predictable ways both during wakefulness (controlled by a diurnal rhythm) and sleep (ultradian rhythm).
- Changes in phasic alertness involve changes in the orienting response to arousing stimuli. This is complemented by habituation, a form of adaptation. Human and non-human nervous systems have evolved such that they are especially responsive to change.
- Consciousness can be experimentally pinned down by studying attention (focal or peripheral). Perception seems to take place largely unconsciously, and many behaviours are carried out quite

automatically, allowing us to consciously attend to the unfamiliar or threatening aspects of our environment.

- Most animals display a circadian rhythm that is synchronized to the 24-hour cycle of light and dark, involving a rhythmical alternation of various physiological and behavioural functions.
- The internal/biological clock is thought to be the SCN, part of the hypothalamus. The retina projects directly on to the SCN, ensuring that the sleep–wake cycle is tuned to the rhythm of night and day.
- When darkness falls, the pineal gland begins to secrete melatonin, making us drowsy. It affects the brain cells that produce serotonin concentrated in the raphe nuclei; these secrete a substance that acts on the RAS to induce light sleep. The LC is rich in noradrenaline, which induces REM sleep.
- Modern living increases the likelihood that the circadian rhythm will be disrupted, and people are sleeping less than human beings are designed for by evolution. This has harmful effects on people's mental and physical health.
- Sleep is measured in the laboratory using an EEG, EOG and EMG. A typical night's sleep comprises four to five ultradian cycles, each consisting of several stages. Stages 2–4 are collectively called SWS or 'deep' sleep; stages 1–4 are collectively called NREM sleep.
- REM or active sleep replaces stage 1 at the beginning of the next cycle. Physiological processes increase and EEGs begin to resemble those of the waking state, and yet it is more difficult to wake someone than from stage 4 sleep (making it paradoxical). With each ultradian cycle, the duration of REM sleep increases.
- Depriving people of REM sleep produces the REM rebound, suggesting that dreaming associated with REM sleep is perhaps the most important function of sleep. But psychologists are still very unclear about the functions of sleep. It is unique as a primary biological drive in that the need for sleep is reflected in decreased levels of arousal.
- According to Oswald's restoration theory, REM and NREM sleep help to replenish bodily and brain processes, respectively. However, the fact that cell repair goes on 24 hours a day, and that the brain is highly active during REM sleep, led Oswald to claim that both REM and NREM sleep are involved in restoration of bodily tissue.
- Meddis's evolutionary theory claims that both longer and shorter periods of sleep are associated with greater safety from predators, and that longer sleep is also characteristic of certain predators such as lions. This makes the theory unfalsifiable. Hibernation theory is a variant of evolutionary theory.
- According to the activation-synthesis model, dreams are the simplest way of interpreting all the internal, brain-produced signals that occur during REM sleep. This activation of the brain is consciously interpreted (synthesis) in the form of a dream. Psychological theories of dreams, such as those of Freud, Jung and Hall, focus on the synthesis component, stressing their significance for the dreamer.
- According to Crick and Mitchison's reverse learning theory, dreams are a way of 'cleaning up' the cortex's neural networks and preparing them for new input – so, we need to forget our dreams. Psychological theories, on the other hand, stress the need to remember our dreams.
- Different theories of dreaming are not mutually exclusive. REM sleep may have evolved in order to help animals' biological survival, but dreams continue to serve a vital function for individuals, helping them to survive psychologically.

REFERENCES

1. Rubin Z, McNeil EB (1983) *The Psychology of Being Human*, 3rd edn. London: Harper & Row.
2. Greenfield S (1998) How might the brain generate consciousness? In S. Rose (ed.) *From Brain to Consciousness?: Essays on the New Sciences of the Mind.* Harmondsworth: Penguin.
3. Hobson JA (1995) Sleeping and dreaming. In D Kimble, AM Colman (eds) *Biological Aspects of Behaviour.* London: Longman.
4. Edelman G (1992) *Bright Air, Brilliant Fire: On the Matter of the Mind.* Harmondsworth: Penguin.
5. Singer W. (1998) Consciousness from a neurobiological perspective. In S Rose (ed.) *From Brains to Consciousness? Essay on the New Sciences of the Mind.* Harmondsworth: Penguin.
6. Hobson JA (2007) Normal and abnormal states of consciousness. In M Velmans, S Schneider (eds) *The Blackwell Companion to Consciousness.* Oxford: Blackwell.
7. Lloyd P, Mayes A, Manstead ASR, Meudell PR, Wagner HL (1984) *Introduction to Psychology: An Integrated Approach.* London: Fontana.
8. Allport DA (1980) Patterns and actions: cognitive mechanisms are content specific. In G Claxton (ed.) *Cognitive Psychology: New Directions.* London: Routledge & Kegan Paul.
9. Nisbett RE, Wilson T (1977) Telling more than we can know: verbal reports on mental processes. *Psychological Review* **84**: 231–59.
10. Joynson RB (1974) *Psychology and Common Sense.* London: Routledge & Kegan Paul.
11. Heather N (1976) *Radical Perspectives in Psychology.* London: Methuen.
12. Gross R (2009) *Themes, Issues and Debates in Psychology*, 3rd edn. London: Hodder Education.
13. McCrone J (1999) Left brain, right brain. *New Scientist* **163**: 26–30.
14. Ruch JC (1984) *Psychology: The Personal Science.* Belmont, CA: Wadsworth Publishing Co.
15. Humphrey N (1986) *The Inner Eye.* London: Faber & Faber.
16. Humphrey, N. (1993) Introduction. In N. Humphrey (1986) *The Inner Eye.* London: Vintage.
17. Gross R (2008) *Key Studies in Psychology*, 5th edn. London: Hodder Education.
18. Hilgard ER (1977) *Divided Consciousness: Multiple Controls in Human Thought and Action.* New York: John Wiley & Sons.
19. Sperry RW (1968) Hemisphere deconnection and unity in conscious awareness. *American Psychologist* **23**: 723–33.
20. Gazzaniga MS (2000) Cerebral specialization and interhemispheric communication: does the corpus callosum enable the human condition? *Brain* **123**: 1293–326.

21. Colvin MK, Gazzaniga MS (2007) Split-brain cases. In M Velmans, S Schneider (eds) *The Blackwell Companion to Consciousness*. Oxford: Blackwell.
22. Ornstein R (1986) *The Psychology of Consciousness*, 2nd end (revised). Harmondsworth: Penguin.
23. Diagram Group (1982) *The Brain: A User's Manual*. New York: Putnam.
24. Blakemore C (1988) *The Mind Machine*. London: BBC.
25. Empson J (1993) *Sleep and Dreaming*, 2nd revised edn. Hemel Hempstead: Harvester Wheatsheaf.
26. Melton L (2000) Rhythm and blues. *New Scientist* **166**: 28–31.
27. Dement W (2000) Tired of counting sheep? The world's greatest sleep expert on how to hit the snooze button. *Independent on Sunday, Real Life*, 16 January: 1–2.
28. Williams A (1998) *Doctor, I Can't Sleep*. East Horsley: Amberwood Publishing.
29. Griffey H (2004) Are you dead on your feet? *Independent Review*, 26 April: 8–9.
30. Channel 4 (2004) National Sleep Survey: Initial Results. www.channel4.com/entertainment/tv/microsites/S/shattered/index.html.
31. Downing D (1988) *Day Light Robbery*. London: Arrow Books.
32. Jouvet M (1967) Mechanisms of the states of sleep: a neuropharmacological approach. *Research Publications of the Association for the Research in Nervous and Mental Diseases* **45**: 86–126.
33. Aserinsky E, Kleitman N (1953) Regularly occurring periods of eye motility and concomitant phenomena during sleep. *Science* **118**: 273–4.
34. Dement W, Kleitman N (1957) The relation of eye movements during sleep to dream activity: an objective method for the study of dreaming. *Journal of Experimental Psychology* **53**: 339–46.
35. Hobson JA (1999) *Dreaming as Delirium: How the Brain Goes Out of Its Mind*. Cambridge, MA: MIT Press.
36. McCarley RW (1995) Sleep, dreams and states of consciousness. In PM Conn (ed.) *Neuroscience and Medicine*. Philadelphia, PA: J.B. Lippincott.
37. Faraday A (1972) *Dream Power*. London: Pan Books.
38. Mueller A, Roberts R (2001) Dreams. In R Roberts, D Groome (eds) *Parapsychology: The Science of Unusual Experience*. London: Hodder Arnold.
39. Blackmore S (2003) *Consciousness: An Introduction*. London: Hodder & Stoughton.
40. Empson J (2001) *Sleep and Dreaming*, 3rd edn. New York: Palgrave Macmillan.
41. Beaumont JG (1988) *Understanding Neuropsychology*. Oxford: Blackwell.
42. Klosch G, Kraft U (2005) Sweet dreams are made of this. *Scientific American Mind* **16**: 38–45.
43. Pinel JPJ (1993) *Biopsychology*, 2nd edn. Boston, MA: Allyn & Bacon.
44. Webb WB, Bonnett MH (1979) Sleep and dreams. In ME Meyer (ed.) *Foundations of Contemporary Psychology*. New York: Oxford University Press.
45. Dement W (1960) The effects of dream deprivation. *Science* **131**: 1705–7.
46. Oswald I (1966) *Sleep*. Harmondsworth: Penguin.
47. Oswald I (1974) *Sleep*, 2nd edn. Harmondsworth: Penguin.
48. Siegel JM (2003) Why we sleep. *Scientific American* **289**: 72–7.
49. Meddis R (1975) On the function of sleep. *Animal Behaviour* **23**: 676–91.
50. Meddis R (1977) *The Sleep Instinct*. London: Routledge & Kegan Paul.
51. Horne J (1988) *Why We Sleep: The Functions of Sleep in Humans and Other Mammals*. Oxford: Oxford University Press.
52. Hobson JA (2002) *Dreaming: A Very Short Introduction*. Oxford: Oxford University Press.
53. Hobson JA, McCarley RW (1977) The brain as a dream state generator: an activation-synthesis hypothesis of the dream process. *American Journal of Psychiatry* **134**: 1335–48.
54. McCarley RW (1983) REM dreams, REM sleep and their isomorphism. In MH Chase, ED Weitzman (eds) *Sleep Disorders: Basic and Clinical Research*, Vol. 8. New York: Spectrum.
55. Crick F, Mitchison G (1983) The function of dream sleep. *Nature* **304**: 111–14.
56. Hall CS (1966) *The Meaning of Dreams*. New York: McGraw-Hill.
57. Winson J (1997) The meaning of dreams. *Scientific American Mysteries of the Mind* **791**: 58–67.
58. Revonso A (2000) The reinterpretation of dreams: an evolutionary hypothesis of the function of dreaming. *Behavioural and Brain Sciences* **23**: 877–901, 904–1018, 1083–121.
59. Flanagan OJ (2000) *Dreaming Souls: Sleep, Dreams, and the Evolution of the Conscious Mind*. New York: Oxford University Press.

Chapter 11

Stress

Richard Gross

INTRODUCTION

According to Bartlett:

> ... the notion that stress is bad for you and can make you ill has become a modern cultural truism. However, there is also a significant body of research evidence which lends support to this idea... The study of stress must ... be central to ... health psychology which concerns, at its most basic level, the role of psychosocial processes in health and disease.[1]

Definitions of stress fall into three categories:[1,2]

- Stress as a *stimulus*
- Stress as a *response*
- Stress as *interaction* between an organism and its environment.

In turn, this classification corresponds very closely to three models of stress identified by Cox: the *engineering model* (which is concerned mainly with the question 'what causes stress?'), the *physiological model* ('what are the effects of stress?') and the *transactional model* (both of these questions, plus 'how do we cope with stress?).[3]

Although stressors are faced by everyone (especially, perhaps, people living in constantly changing Western cultures), some people face greater demands than others. As a group, patients (both in and out of hospital) face sources of stress that they did not have to deal with before becoming ill. Similarly, although all occupations are stressful, some occupations are more stressful than others. Several studies have suggested that health workers experience more stress than comparable groups of non-health workers.[4] In terms of Warr's *vitamin model*, which identifies several environmental factors that affect mental health, nurses and other health professionals are likely to suffer from organizational stressors that are common to many other occupations (e.g. lack of clarity, conflicting roles, work overload, lack of control).[5] However, doctors and nurses often suffer additional stressors that are intrinsic to the job (e.g. providing terminal care, counselling bereaved parents, dealing with disturbed and violent patients).

MODELS OF STRESS

The *engineering model* sees external stresses giving rise to a stress reaction, or strain, in the individual.[3] The stress is located in the stimulus characteristics of the environment: stress is what happens *to* a person, and not what happens within a person. Up to a point, stress is inevitable and can be tolerated; moderate levels may even be beneficial (*eustress*[6]).

The *physiological model* is concerned primarily with what happens *within* the person as a result of stress (the 'response' aspects of the engineering model), in particular the physiological changes. The impetus for this view was Selye's definition of stress as '... the individual's psychophysiological response, mediated largely by the autonomic nervous system and the endocrine system, to any demands made on the individual'.[6]

As a medical student, Selye noticed a general malaise or syndrome associated with 'being ill', regardless of the particular illness. The syndrome was characterized by (i) a loss of appetite, (ii) an associated loss of weight and strength, (iii) loss of ambition and (iv) a typical facial expression associated with illness. Further examination of extreme cases revealed major physiological changes (confirmed by Cox[3]). This non-specific response to illness reflected a distinct phenomenon, which Selye called the *general adaptation syndrome* (GAS; see below).

The *transactional model* represents a kind of blend of the first two models. It sees stress as arising from an interaction between people and their environment, in particular when there is an imbalance between the person's perception of the demands being made of them by the situation and their ability to meet those demands. Because it is the person's *perception* of this mismatch between demand and ability that causes stress, the model allows for important individual differences in what produces stress and how much stress is experienced. There are also wide differences in how people attempt to cope with stress, psychologically and behaviourally.

WHAT CAUSES STRESS?

The causes of stress do not exist objectively, and individuals differ in what they see as a stressor in the first place.[7] In this section we identify potential stressors – the kinds of event or experience that most people are likely to find exceed their capacity to handle the demands that are involved.

Disruption of circadian rhythms

The word 'circadian' ('about 1 day') describes a particular periodicity or rhythm of a number of physiological and behavioural functions that can be seen in almost all living creatures (see Chapter 10). Many studies have shown that these rhythms persist if we suddenly reverse our activity pattern and sleep during the day and are active during the night. This indicates that these rhythms are controlled internally (endogenous).

However, our circadian rhythms are kept on their once-every-24-hours schedule by regular daily environmental (exogenous) cues called *zeitgebers* (German = 'time-givers'). The most important zeitgeber is the daily cycle of light and dark. If we persist with our reversal of sleep and activity, then the body's circadian rhythms reverse (after a period of acclimatization) and become synchronized to the new set of exogenous cues.

Individual differences and the effects of shift work

Some people take 5–7 days to adjust, while others take up to 14 days and some never achieve a complete reversal. Not all physiological functions reverse at the same time: body temperature usually reverses within a week for most people, while the rhythms of adrenocortical hormone take much longer to reverse. During the changeover period, the body is in a state of *internal desynchronization*.[8] This is very stressful, and shift workers often report experiencing insomnia, digestive problems, irritability, fatigue and even depression when changing work shifts. In shift work, the zeitgebers stay the same, but workers are forced to adjust their natural sleep–wake cycles in order to meet the demands of changing work schedules (Box 11.1).[10]

Coffey *et al.* examined the influence of day, afternoon, night and rotating shifts on the job performance and job-related stress of 463 female nurses at five US hospitals.[11] Using a structured questionnaire, they found that job performance was highest for nurses on the day shift, followed by the night, afternoon and rotating shifts. Rotating-shift nurses reported the highest job-related stress, followed by afternoon-, day- and night-shift nurses. These results contrast with those of mainly male factory workers, where individuals are doing essentially the same type of work regardless of the shift. The type of work carried out by nurses differs considerably depending on their particular shift, and so performance by shift may be affected by both the social organization of hospital work and circadian rhythm synchronization.

Box 11.1 Night nurses aren't all the same

Hawkins and Armstrong-Esther studied 11 nurses during the first seven nights of a period of night duty:[9]

- They found that performance was significantly impaired on the first night but improved progressively on successive nights. However, body temperature had not adjusted fully to night working after seven nights.
- There were significant differences between individual nurses, with some appearing relatively undisturbed by working nights and others never adjusting.

Rotating-shift nurses may suffer the most stress and have the least successful job performance due to both the disturbance of circadian rhythms and the fact that they often work with different colleagues and patients on each shift. This may make it more difficult to establish working relationships. Although day-shift nurses suffer the least from circadian rhythm disruption, they are responsible for the instrumental activities of supervising patient preparation for diagnostic testing, treatment and therapy. The pace is rapid and the nurse is interacting with a maximum number of colleagues, both nursing and non-nursing. This can be very stressful (see below).

Conversely, the pace is slower and interaction with others considerably reduced on night shift, helping to reduce stress levels. Concentration is on the expressive activities of making patients comfortable and ensuring rest and sleep.

In the afternoon shift, circadian rhythm disruption is moderate, but nurses face the stress of both instrumental and expressive functions. The nurses are responsible for continuing and monitoring the medical treatment initiated during the day shift, while at the same time dealing with the social and psychological aftermath of the medical regimen. This may account for their high stress levels.[11]

According to Singer (see Brown[12]), who compared rota systems in different countries, there is a very high error and accident rate among people working an early-morning shift that follows a late-afternoon/evening shift. This combination should be avoided at all costs. However, a late shift followed by an early shift is the staple diet of the internal rotation duty pattern in the UK.[12]

Jet lag

Other occupational groups affected by disruption to their circadian rhythms are airline pilots and cabin crew, who experience jet lag because they cross time zones during the course of a flight. If you have travelled across a time zone, you will know what it is like to have your biological rhythms 'out of sync' with your surroundings. If you arrive in Washington, DC, at 7 p.m., after an 8-hour flight from London, you may want to start your evening's entertainment – but as far as your body is concerned, it is time to sleep, because back in London it is 1 a.m.

Most people suffer much less jet lag when travelling in an east–west direction compared with a west–east direction. When going west ('chasing the sun'), the day is temporarily lengthened. Because the natural circadian rhythm cycle is 25 hours (see Chapter 10), an increase in day length is much easier to deal with than a decrease. Secretion of melatonin reaches a peak during the night, helping to make us sleepy. After a long flight, the cyclical release of melatonin stays locked into the day/night pattern of the home country for some days. This could account for the fatigue felt during the day and the insomnia experienced at night. If jet-lagged volunteers are given melatonin during the evening, far fewer report feeling jet-lagged than controls who receive only a placebo.[13]

Cabin crew flying across time zones had significantly raised salivary cortisol (one of the glucocorticoid stress hormones; see Figure 11.1) compared with when the same cabin crew flew short distances, and compared with ground crew. In a response-time test, the jet-lagged crew performed more poorly when there was a 25-second delay between presentation of the target symbol and having to recognize the symbol (but not when the delay was only 1 or 5 seconds).[14] De Quervain *et al.* found poorer recognition memory among non-flight crew participants given cortisone (another glucocorticoid).[15] The researchers believe that raised glucocorticoid levels may cause impairments in memory retrieval in stressful situations such as exams, job interviews, combat and courtroom testimony (see Chapter 17).

Life changes: the Social Readjustment Rating Scale

Holmes and Rahe examined 5000 patient records and made a list of 43 life events, of varying seriousness, that seemed to cluster in the months preceding the onset of the patients' illnesses.[16] Out of this study grew the Social Readjustment Rating Scale (SRRS). Several studies have shown that people who experience many significant life changes (a score of 300 or more life change units – LCUs) are more susceptible to physical and mental illness than people with lower scores. The range of health problems includes sudden cardiac death, heart attacks (non-fatal), tuberculosis (TB), diabetes, leukaemia, accidents and athletics injuries (Table 11.1).

Evaluation of the Social Readjustment Rating Scale

The SRRS assumes that *any* change, by definition, is stressful; that is, certain events are inherently stressful, but the undesirable aspects of events are at least as important as the fact that they change people's lives.[17] A quick glance at Table 11.1 suggests that life changes have a largely negative feel, especially those in the top ten, which receive the highest LCU scores; so, the scale may be confusing 'change' and 'negativity'.

Similarly, life changes may be stressful only if they are unexpected and, in this sense, uncontrollable. In other words, it may not be change as such that is stressful, but rather change that we cannot prevent or reverse. Studies have shown that if people are asked to classify the undesirable life events on the SRRS as either 'controllable' or

Table 11.1 Selected items from the Social Readjustment Rating Scale (SSRS)

Rank	Life event	Mean value
1	Death of spouse	100
2	Divorce	73
3	Marital separation	65
4	Jail term	63
5	Death of close family member	63
6	Personal injury or illness	53
7	Marriage	50
8	Fired at work	47
9	Marital reconciliation	45
10	Retirement	45
11	Change in health of family member	44
12	Pregnancy	40
13	Sex difficulties	39
16	Change in financial state	38
17	Death of close friend	37
18	Change to different line of work	36
22	Change in responsibilities at work	29
23	Son or daughter leaving home	29
28	Change in living conditions	25
30	Trouble with boss	23
31	Change in work hours or conditions	20
32	Change in residence	20
38	Change in sleeping habits	16
41	Going on holiday	13
42	Christmas	12
43	Minor violations of the law	11

The amount of stress a person has experienced in a given period of time, say 1 year, is measured by the total number of life change units (LCUs). These units result from the addition of the values (shown in the right-hand column) associated with events that the person has experienced during the target time period. The mean values (item weightings) were obtained empirically by telling 100 judges that 'marriage' had been assigned an arbitrary value of 500 and asking them to assign a number to each of the other events in terms of 'the intensity and length of time necessary to accommodate ... regardless of the desirability of the event relative to marriage'. The average of the numbers assigned to each event was divided by 10 and the resulting value became the weighting of each life event.

Adapted from Holmes TH, Rahe RH (1967) The social readjustment rating scale. *Journal of Psychosomatic Research* **11**: 213–18, with permission from Elsevier.

'uncontrollable', then only the latter are correlated significantly with subsequent onset of illness.[18]

Some of the items are ambiguous (e.g. those that refer to 'changes in' could be positive or negative changes). Others (e.g. items 6 and 12) refer to states of health, and so the total LCU score is already contaminated with the individual's current health status.[19]

The list of events is incomplete. For example, the list does not include death of a child, there is no reference to the problems of old age, and there is no mention of natural or 'man-made' disasters.[20] The list also fails to take into account individual circumstances. For example, the impact of the death of a spouse is generally affected by the partner's age at the time, the nature of their relationship and the cause of death.[21] The SRRS was developed over 40 years ago. This makes some of the original LCU scores associated with particular life events potentially out of date.

Evaluation of studies using the Social Readjustment Rating Scale

Although many studies have found statistically significant correlations between LCUs and subsequent illness, the correlations are typically too low to be of any practical value.[20] Since the data produced by these studies are correlational, it is possible that, instead of life events causing illness, some life events (e.g. being fired from work, sexual difficulties, trouble with in-laws, change in sleeping habits) are themselves early manifestations of an illness that is already developing.[18,19,22]

Many of these studies are also retrospective: people are asked to recall both the illnesses and the stressful life events that occurred during the specified period, which is likely to produce distorted, unreliable data (see Chapter 17). For example, what people say about a past illness may be different from what the illness was actually like.[22]

The need for control

According to Parkes, the psychosocial transitions that are most dangerous to health are those that are sudden and allow little time for preparation.[23] The sudden death of a relative from a heart attack, in an accident or as a result of crime are examples of the most stressful kind of life changes (see Chapter 57).

Using Rotter's Locus of Control Scale,[24] and devising a new scale – the Life Events Scale – Johnson and Sarason found that life events stress was related more closely to psychiatric symptoms (in particular, depression and anxiety) among people rated as high on external locus of control than among those rated as high on internal locus of control.[25] In other words, people who believe that they do not have control over what happens to them are more vulnerable to the harmful effects of change than those who believe they do. This is related to Seligman's concept of *learned helplessness* (see Chapter 14).[26]

The hassles and uplifts of everyday life

By definition, most of the 43 changes included in the SRRS are not everyday occurrences. Kanner *et al.* designed a hassles scale comprising 117 items, and an uplifts scale containing 135 items.[27] They define 'hassles' as:

> ... the irritating, frustrating, distressing demands that to some degree characterize everyday transactions with the environment. They include annoying practical problems, such as losing things or traffic jams and fortuitous occurrences such as inclement weather, as well as arguments, disappointments, and financial and family concerns.[27]

Daily uplifts are:

> ... positive experiences such as the joy derived from manifestations of love, relief at hearing good news, the pleasure of a good night's rest, and so on.[27]

In a study of 100 men and women aged 45–64 years over a 12-month period, Kanner *et al.* confirmed the prediction that hassles are related positively to undesirable psychological symptoms; but the effect of uplifts was unclear, and research interest waned.[1] Kanner and colleagues also found that hassles are a more powerful predictor of symptoms than life events (as measured by the SRRS). 'Divorce', for example, may exert stress by any number of component hassles, such as cooking for oneself, handling money matters and having to tell people about the situation. So, daily hassles may intervene between major life events and health: it is the cumulative impact of these day-to-day problems that may prove detrimental to health.

An evaluation of the hassles and uplifts scales

According to Lazarus, life events (as measured by the SSRS) are *distal* (remote) causes of stress.[20] We need to know the psychological meaning that a person attaches to an environmental event – the personal significance of what is happening (the *proximal* cause). This is what makes Kanner and colleagues' scales a more valid approach. According to Lazarus:

> Although daily hassles are far less dramatic than major life changes ... and what constitutes a hassle varies greatly from person to person, our research has suggested that, especially when they pile up or touch on special areas of *vulnerability* ... they can be very stressful for some people and very important for their subjective well-being and physical health ...[20]

Bartlett claims that implicit in the concept of hassles is a stimulus-based definition of stress.[1] This is inconsistent with the transactional approach advocated by Lazarus (see above). This apparent contradiction stems from focusing on the hassles themselves while simultaneously believing that it is their psychological meaning that causes stress.

Occupation-linked stressors

Along with social work, teaching and the police force, nursing is identified as a high-stress occupation. A study by

Borrill *et al.* (see Carson *et al.*[28]) of 11 000 National Health Service (NHS) staff found that nurses had the second-highest stress score among seven staff groups. We have already seen how shift work, although not unique to nurses, is an inherently stressful aspect of the job; this is common to doctors and to all people working in the emergency services (e.g. police, fire, ambulance, emergency medical teams, mountain rescue). These staff groups share routine encounters with death, tragedy and horror, are required to deal with people in pain and distress and to handle dead bodies, and may face personal danger and injury.

Mental health nurses

O'Donnell reported the findings of a survey in which nurses were asked about 16 different stressors.[29] Overall, most of these stressors were perceived as being more extensive in mental health nursing (MHN) than in nursing as a whole. Violence was found to be substantially more extensive than average, as were job insecurity, not being involved in decision-making and career uncertainty.

According to Sullivan (see Nolan *et al.*[30]), a growing body of research evidence suggests that nursing in general, and MHN in particular, is a stressful occupation. All those professionals working in mental health may be at greater risk of stress than their colleagues working in physical healthcare; for example, psychiatrists have the highest suicide rate among doctors. As MHN is often carried out against a background of risk-taking and uncertainty because of the volatile and potentially aggressive nature of some psychiatric patients, nurses inevitably experience stress.[30]

According to Burnard *et al.*, psychological distress, emotional exhaustion and increased alcohol consumption are just some of the consequences of increased workplace stressors among community mental health nurses (CMHNs).[31] These nurses see themselves as overworked, struggling with too much paperwork and administration, having too many clients, and having serious concerns about their client groups. As many as 20 per cent feel they have no job security. These are among the key findings of a survey into stress among CMHNs in Wales, the largest of its kind in the UK. The survey included nurses working in a wide range of urban and rural settings. The findings describe *burnout*, which Cherniss (see Firth *et al.*[32]) defines simply as 'negative changes in work-related attitudes and behaviour in response to job stress'. Burnout is an 'occupational hazard' in a variety of healthcare professionals, especially those caring for terminally ill patients.[33]

WHAT ARE THE EFFECTS OF STRESS?

The general adaptation syndrome

According to Selye, GAS represents the body's defence against stress.[6] The body responds in the same way to any stressor, whether the stressor is environmental or arises from within the body itself. The GAS comprises three stages: the *alarm reaction*, *resistance* and *exhaustion*.

Alarm reaction

When a stimulus is perceived as a stressor, there is a brief, initial *shock phase*. Resistance to the stressor is lowered. This is followed quickly by a *countershock* phase. The sympathetic branch of the autonomic nervous system (ANS) is activated, which, in turn, stimulates the adrenal medulla to secrete increased levels of adrenaline and noradrenaline (catecholamines). These are associated with sympathetic changes, collectively referred to as the *fight-or-flight syndrome* (the individual's instinctive, biological preparation for confronting or escaping danger). The catecholamines mimic sympathetic arousal (*sympathomimetics*), and noradrenaline is the transmitter at the synapses of the sympathetic branch of the ANS. Consequently, noradrenaline from the adrenals prolongs the action of noradrenaline released at synapses in the ANS. This prolongs sympathetic arousal after the stressor's removal. This is referred to as the ANS–adrenal medulla system or sympatho-adrenomedullary axis.

Resistance

If the stressor is not removed, there is a decrease in sympathetic activity but an increase in output from the other part of the adrenal gland, the *adrenal cortex*. This is controlled by the amount of adrenocorticotrophic hormone (ACTH) in the blood. ACTH is released from the anterior pituitary (the 'master' endocrine gland) upon instructions from the hypothalamus. The adrenal cortex is essential for the maintenance of life and its removal results in death.

The effect of ACTH is to stimulate the adrenal cortex to release corticosteroids (or adrenocorticoid hormones), one group of which are the glucocorticoid hormones (chiefly, corticosterone, cortisol and hydrocortisone). These control and conserve the amount of glucose in the blood (glucogenesis), which helps to resist stress of all kinds. The glucocorticoids convert protein into glucose, make fats available for energy, increase blood flow and generally stimulate behavioural responsiveness. In this way, the anterior pituitary–adrenal cortex system (or hypothalamic-pituitary-adrenal axis) contributes to the fight-or-flight syndrome.

Exhaustion

Once ACTH and corticosteroids are circulating in the bloodstream, they tend to inhibit the further release of ACTH from the pituitary. If the stressor is removed during the resistance stage, then blood sugar levels will gradually return to normal. But if the stress situation continues, the pituitary–adrenal excitation continues. The body's resources are now becoming depleted, the adrenals can no longer function properly, blood glucose levels drop and, in extreme cases, hypoglycaemia could result in death.

At this stage psychophysiological disorders develop, including hypertension, coronary artery disease (CAD), coronary heart disease (CHD), asthma and peptic ulcers. Selye calls these 'diseases of adaptation' (Figures 11.1 and 11.2).

Evaluation of the general adaptation syndrome

Lazarus cites a study of patients dying from injury or disease.[20] Postmortem examination showed that those patients

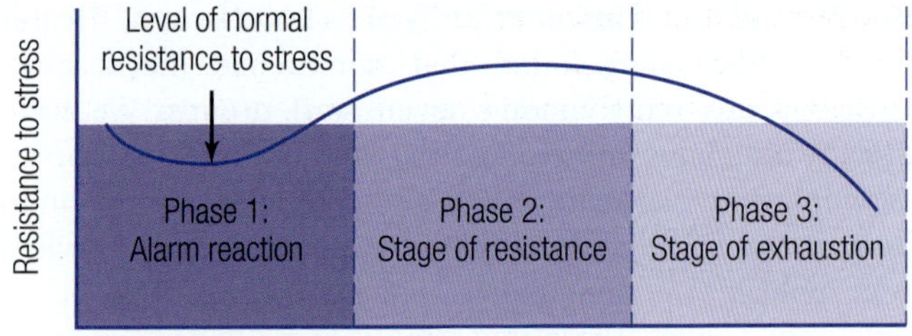

Figure 11.2 Three stages of the general adaptation syndrome

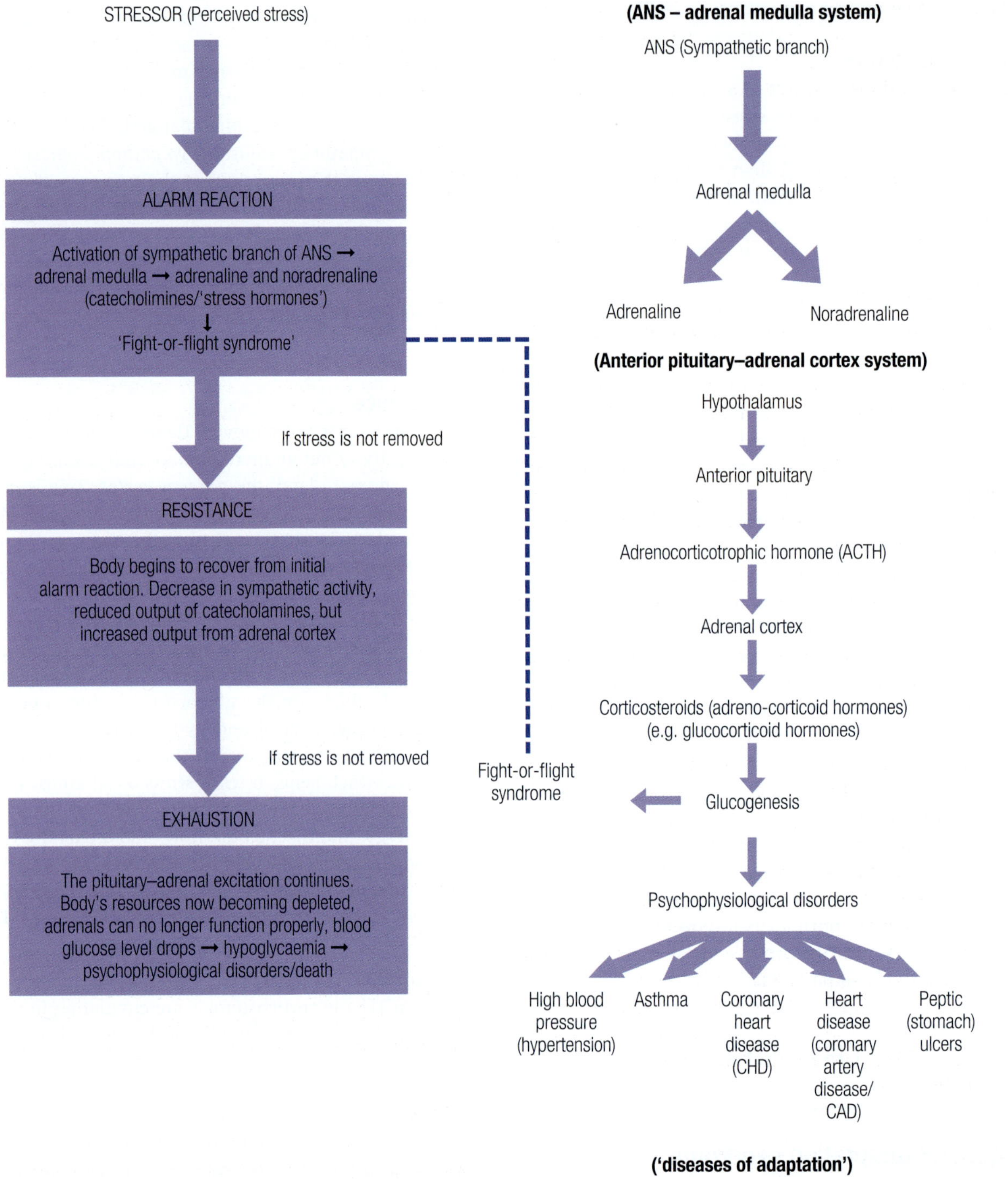

Figure 11.1 Summary diagram of the three stages of the general adaptation syndrome (GAS) and their relationship with the physiological changes associated with (i) the autonomic nervous system (ANS)-adrenal medulla and (ii) the anterior pituitary-adrenal cortex systems

who remained unconscious had normal levels of corticosteroids, while the opposite was true for those who were conscious, presumably aware that they were dying. Lazarus infers from this that:

> ... some psychological awareness – akin to a conscious perception or appraisal – of the psychological significance of what is happening may be necessary to produce the adrenal cortical changes of the GAS.[20]

Although Selye helped us to understand how stressors affect the body, in order to understand what makes a psychological event stressful, we must put the person into the equation. In effect, says Lazarus: '... it takes both the stressful stimulus conditions and a *vulnerable person* to generate a stress reaction ...'

HOW DOES STRESS MAKE US ILL?

An evolutionary perspective

The sympathetic branch of the ANS responds as a unit, causing a state of generalized, undifferentiated arousal. This was probably of crucial importance in our evolutionary past, when our ancestors were frequently confronted by life-threatening dangers. This is precisely what the fight-or-flight syndrome is for. But although an increase in heart rate may be necessary to supply more blood to the muscles when facing a hungry-looking bear, it may be quite irrelevant to most of the stressors we face in modern life, which involve a far higher psychological element.

Most stressors do not pose a physical threat, but our nervous and endocrine systems have evolved in such a way that we typically react to stressors as if they did. What may have been adaptive responses for our ancestors have become maladaptive today. So, what happens to all that internal activity?

In the case of heart rate and blood pressure, chronic stress involves repeated episodes of increases in heart rate and blood pressure, which in turn produces increases in plaque formation within the cardiovascular system. Stress also produces an increase in blood cholesterol levels, through the action of adrenaline and noradrenaline on the release of free fatty acids. This produces a clumping together of cholesterol particles, leading to clots in the blood and in the artery walls, and occlusion of the arteries. In turn, raised heart rate is related to a more rapid build-up of cholesterol on artery walls. High blood pressure results in small lesions on the artery walls, and cholesterol tends to get trapped in these lesions.[34]

Stress and the immune system

The immune system (Figure 11.3) is a collection of billions of cells that travel through the bloodstream and move in and out of tissues and organs, defending the body against invasion by foreign agents such as bacteria, viruses and cancerous cells. The immune cells are produced mainly in the spleen, lymph nodes, thymus and bone marrow. The study of the effect of psychological factors on the immune system is called *psychoneuroimmunology* (PNI; see Ogden[35]).

Many people catch a cold soon after a period of stress because stress seems to reduce the immune system's ability to fight off cold viruses (we become 'run down'). Goetsch and Fuller[2] refer to studies that show decreases in the activity of lymphocytes among medical students during their final exams (e.g. Kiecolt-Glaser *et al.*[36]). Lymphocytes (natural killer cells) are a particular type of white blood cell that normally fight off viruses and cancer cells. Levels of immunoglobulin A (IgA) increase immediately after an oral exam (if it appeared to go well) but not after a written exam, suggesting that the stress is not relieved until much later, when the exam results are known.[37]

Of course, none of these findings means that stress actually *causes* infections. Stress makes us more susceptible to infectious agents by temporarily suppressing immune function (the immunosuppressive effects of stress). Stressors that seem to have this effect include exams (see above) and the death of a spouse (see Chapter 57). For example, Schliefer *et al.* found that the immune systems of men whose wives had died from breast cancer functioned less well than before their wife's death.[38]

Interleukin-b (see Figure 11.3) is produced soon after tissue damage, helping to remodel connective tissue in wounds and to form collagen (scar tissue). Kiecolt-Glaser *et al.* compared the rate of wound healing in two groups: (i) a group of 13 'high-stress' women, caring for relatives with Alzheimer's disease and (ii) a 'stress-free' matched control group.[39] All the women underwent a 3.5-mm full-thickness punch biopsy on their non-dominant forearm. Healing took significantly longer in the caregivers than in the controls (48.7 days *v.* 39.3 days). Box 11.2 describes another study investigating psychological techniques to boost the immune system.

Moderators and mediators of stress

Moderator variables are antecedent conditions (e.g. personality, ethnic background, gender) that interact with exposure to stress to affect health outcome. *Mediator variables* intervene in the link between stress exposure and health outcome (e.g. appraisal[41]). If a mediator variable reduces the impact of a stressful event, then it is a 'protective' or 'buffering' variable (it softens or cushions the impact[1]).

Personality

What is now referred to as *type A behaviour pattern* (TABP) was originally called 'type A personality' (a stable personality trait[42]). TABP is now conceptualized as a stereotypical set of behavioural responses, including:

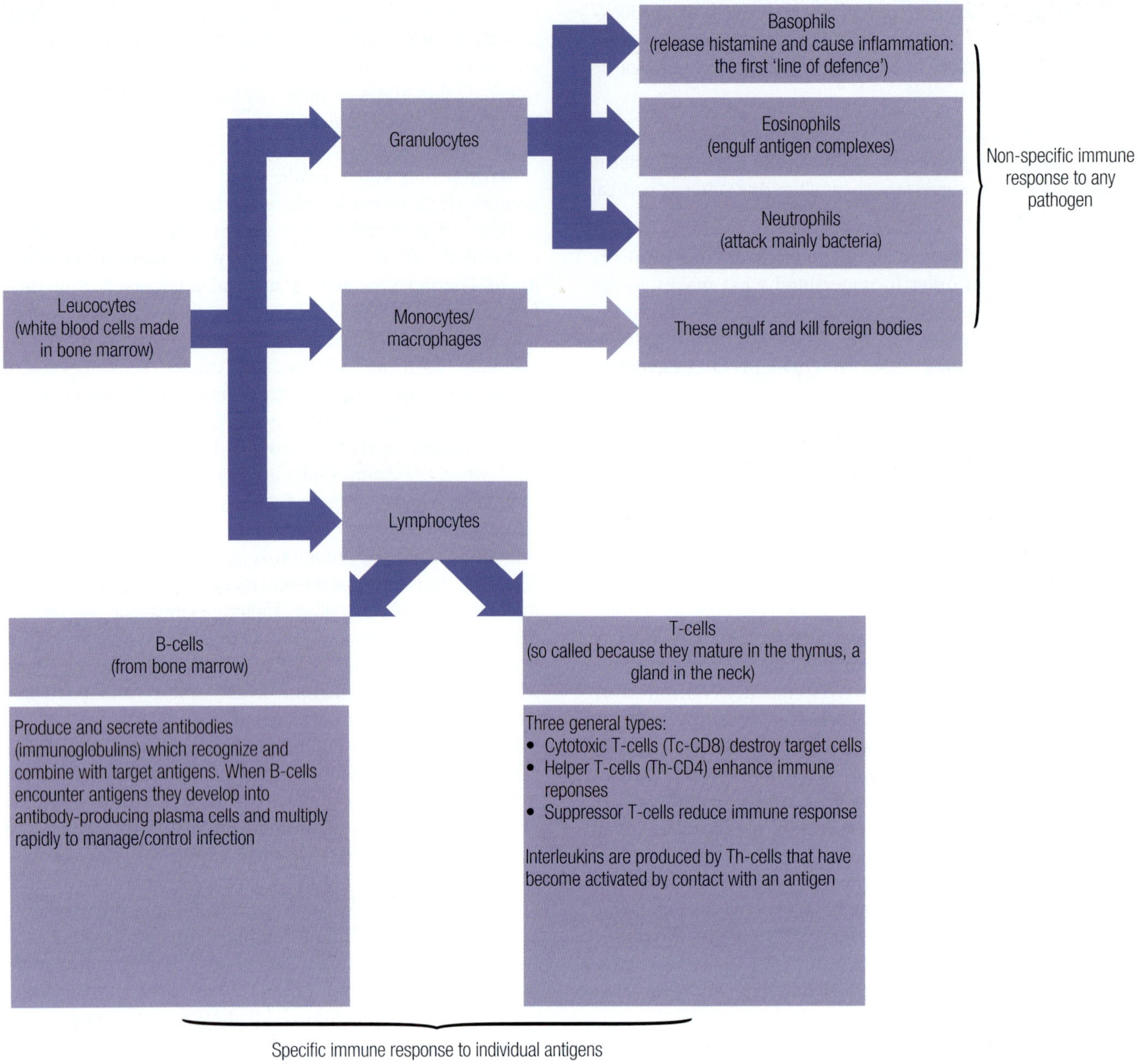

Figure 11.3 The immune system

- competitiveness and achievement orientation;
- aggressiveness and hostility;
- sense of time urgency.

Many early studies showed that people who display TABP were at much greater risk of high blood pressure and CHD, compared with type B people. However, these risks are only *relative*: the vast majority of type A people do not develop CHD, and many type B people *do* develop CHD.[17] Also, most studies have found that TAPB assessed immediately following a heart attack does not predict future attacks. This suggests that TAPB is not a distinct risk for CHD in people already at risk for the disorder.[19]

However, there seem to be clear physiological differences between type A people and type B people in response to stress, even when the person is not conscious.[43] Krantz *et al.* (see Fletcher[43]) found that, compared with type B patients, type A patients undergoing coronary bypass surgery showed greater blood-pressure changes while anaesthetized (by as much as 30 mmHg) and were much more likely to have complications during surgery, which could be attributed to enhanced sympathetic nervous system activity.

According to Temoshok, people with type C personalities are cancer-prone.[44] People with the type C personality have difficulty expressing emotion and tend to suppress or inhibit emotions, particularly negative emotions such as

Box 11.2 Using psychological techniques to boost the immune system

Norton reports on a study in which women with breast cancer were encouraged to visualize their white blood cells waging war against the cancer cells.[40] This was intended to boost the immune system in a way that could help the women fight the disease. This guided imagery was combined with progressive muscle relaxation, as well as standard surgery, chemotherapy and radiotherapy.

Compared with women in a control group (given only the medical treatment), those who used the psychological techniques had higher numbers of mature T-cells, activated T-cells and cells carrying T-cell receptors. These are important for attacking malignant cells.

At the end of the 9-month study, the women who used the psychological techniques also had higher levels of lymphokines (activated killer cells), which help prevent the disease from spreading. The women reported a better quality of life and fewer side effects from medical treatments.

anger. Although there is no clear-cut evidence to show that these personality characteristics can actually cause cancer, it does seem likely that they influence the progression of cancer and, hence, the survival time of people with cancer.[45]

Greer and Morris found that women diagnosed with breast cancer showed significantly more emotional suppression than women with benign breast disease (especially among those aged under 50 years).[46] This emotional suppression had been a characteristic for most of their life. Cooper and Faragher reported that experiencing a major stressful event is a significant predictor of breast cancer.[47] This was especially so in women who did not express anger but who used denial as a form of coping (Box 11.3).

Self-esteem

This is an important factor in moderating stress (see Burnard *et al.*[31]). The study of CMHNs in Wales described above found that those with high self-esteem/self-worth used a wide range of coping skills to deal with work stress. However, 40 per cent of respondents reported low self-esteem and felt that others had little respect for them. Low self-esteem scores were associated with higher levels of psychological distress, greater emotional exhaustion, lower use of coping skills and increased alcohol consumption.

A positive and resilient self-esteem is a crucial resource in combating the negative implications for an individual that often accompany stressful events (see Carson *et al.*[28]). Research has shown a significant inverse relationship between self-esteem and symptoms of depression (the lower the self-esteem, the greater the symptoms of depression; see Carson *et al.*[28]). Although self-esteem has not featured much in the literature on nursing stress, Carson *et al.* believe that it is reasonable to predict that nurses with high

Box 11.3 Beating breast cancer

Greer *et al.* studied women who had had a mastectomy after being diagnosed with breast cancer.[48] Those women who reacted either by denying what had happened ('I'm being treated for a lump, but it's not serious') or by showing a 'fighting spirit' ('This is not going to get me') were significantly more likely to be free of cancer 5 years later than women who stoically accepted it ('I feel an illness is God's will ...') or were described as 'giving up' ('Well, there's no hope with cancer, is there?').

A follow-up at 15 years confirmed the improved prognosis.[49,50] Survival was almost three times lower in the stoical or 'giving up' women. This difference obtained independently of factors such as age, menopausal status, clinical stage, type of surgery, tumour size and postoperative radiotherapy.

According to Hegarty:

> **Such research ... appears to give scientific support to the advice ... 'to think positive' in the face of a diagnosis of cancer. It suggests the value of having psychological resources which will allow individuals to adapt to, rather than succumb to, a severe threat to their well-being. It might even be possible to teach such strategies to people who neither have nor use them.[51]**

self-esteem will have lower levels of stress and burnout, and better coping skills, than those with low self-esteem.

The Claybury community psychiatric nurse (CPN) study was a survey of stress, coping and burnout in 245 MHNs and 323 ward-based nurses in five large mental hospitals and two district hospital psychiatric units.[28] A range of standardized measures were used, including the modified Rosenberg Self-Esteem Scale, the General Health Questionnaire (a well-validated measure of psychological distress) and the Maslach Burn-Out Scale.[52] Overall, the results confirmed the prediction that levels of stress, burnout and use of coping skills are related to levels of self-esteem in MHNs.

COPING WITH STRESS

What do we mean by 'coping'?

Lazarus and Folkman define coping as '... constantly changing cognitive and behavioural efforts to manage external and/or internal demands that are appraised as taxing or exceeding the resources of the person'.[53]

This mirrors the definition of stress as the individual's belief that his or her available biological, psychological and social resources are not sufficient to meet the demands of the situation.

Different kinds of coping

According to Roger and Nash, the term 'coping' conjures up ideas about being able to handle any situation that comes our way.[54] But in relation to stress, they distinguish between *maladaptive* and *adaptive* coping styles:

- *Maladaptive* styles involve failing to adjust appropriately to our environment and experiencing misery and unhappiness as a result. They can take the form of *emotional* and *avoidance* coping styles.
- *Adaptive* styles involve an appropriate adjustment to the environment and gaining from the experience. These can be either *detached* or *rational.*

In fact, the term 'maladaptive coping' is a contradiction in terms (Table 11.2).

Cohen and Lazarus classified all the coping strategies that a person might use into five general categories:[55]

- *Direct action response:* the individual tries to directly change or manipulate his or her relationship to the stressful situation, such as escaping from or removing it.
- *Information-seeking:* the individual tries to understand the situation better and to predict future events related to the stressor.
- *Inhibition of action:* doing nothing. This may be the best course of action if the situation is seen as short-term.
- *Intrapsychic or palliative coping:* the individual reappraises the situation (e.g. through the use of psychological defence mechanisms; see Chapter 19) or changes the internal environment (e.g. through drugs, alcohol, relaxation, meditation).
- *Turning to others:* for help and emotional support.

These five categories of coping overlap with the distinction between problem-focused coping (PFC) and emotion-focused coping (EFC) (Box 11.4).[53]

An evaluation of different methods of coping

- Many researchers simply assume that EFC and avoidant coping are a less adaptive way of dealing with stress.[56] But, as Lazarus and Folkman state, the effectiveness of coping depends on the situation. For example, a situa-

Table 11.2 Maladaptive and adaptive coping and their short- and long-term consequences

Maladaptive coping		Adaptive coping	
Emotional	Feeling overpowered and helpless	Detached	Not seeing the problem or situation as a threat
	Becoming miserable, depressed, angry		Keeping a sense of humour
	Taking out frustrations on other people		Taking nothing personally and seeing the problem as separate from yourself
	Preparing for the worst possible outcome and seeking sympathy from others		Resolving the issue by getting things into proportion
	Short-term benefits: expression of emotion		*Short-term benefits:* able to stand back and take stock of problem
	Long-term consequences: increasingly overwhelmed by problem		*Long-term consequences:* prevents overidentification with problem
Avoidance	Sitting tight and hoping it all goes away	Rational	Using past experience to work out how to deal with the situation
	Pretending there is nothing the matter if people ask		Taking action to change things
	Thinking about something else and talking about it as little as possible		Taking one step at a time and approaching the problem with logic
	Trusting in fate and believing things will sort themselves out		Giving the situation full attention and treating it as a challenge to be met
	Short-term benefits: temporary relief as problem blocked out		*Short-term benefits:* logic determines resolution of problem
	Long-term consequences: blocking out cannot be sustained		*Long-term consequences:* problems put into perspective

Adapted from Roger and Nash.[54]

> **Box 11.4 Problem-focused and emotion-focused coping**
>
> - *Problem-focused coping* (PFC) involves taking direct action in order to solve the problem, or seeking information that is relevant to a solution.
> - *Emotion-focused coping* (EFC) involves trying to reduce the negative emotions that are part of the experience of stress.
>
> Lazaraus and Folkman claim that effective coping depends on the situation; sometimes using both kinds of coping might offer the best solution.[53]

tion that is controllable calls for more problem-focused efforts because the individual is in a position to do something about it. In contrast, situations that do not allow for control require management of the emotions triggered by such situations.

- Effectiveness must also take into account how long the stressor lasts. With short-term stressors, avoidant strategies are preferable, while long-term stressors require more focused attention. This implies (i) that men would be better at coping with short-term problems (because of their predominant use of avoidant coping) and (ii) women would adjust better to less frequent but more extreme events (e.g. death of a spouse; see Stroebe[57] and Chapter 57) because of their more frequent use of attentional strategies, which provides them with timely warning signs to take action.
- Although many studies report that women engage more often than men in EFC, the majority of female coping is PFC: the observation that women are emotion-oriented copers is a relative one and does not support the stereotype of all women as emotional copers.[56]
- Stanton *et al.* have questioned the very concept of EFC.[58] They found that women worked through their emotions more often than men and that this greater effort to understand and express their emotions was more adaptive for them. Similarly, Stroebe has suggested that widowers may be more vulnerable to physical illness and depression compared with widows because widowers find it easier to avoid confrontation with feelings and to deal with the problems that are created by their wife's death, rather than dealing with their grief.[57] Widows can access their emotions and express them more easily.

Stress management

Much of what we have said about coping with stress refers to what people do in a largely spontaneous way. In this informal sense, we all 'manage' our stress more or less effectively. More formally, the term 'stress management' refers to a range of physiological and psychological techniques used in a quite deliberate way, in a professional setting, to help people reduce their stress. These techniques may be used singly or in combination.

Psychotherapeutic drugs act directly on the ANS, and anxiolytic drugs are commonly used in cases of chronic stress. The benzodiazepines (a group of anxiolytic drugs) usually succeed in reducing the physiological effects of stress, but they may produce side effects, tolerance and physical dependence (see Chapter 58).

With *biofeedback* (see Chapter 14), the focus is on treating the symptoms of stress rather than the stressor itself. Biofeedback is based on the principle that stress can be reduced by gaining control over autonomic functions about which we normally have little knowledge, let alone control. The same is true for a number of procedures used to bring about a state of relaxation, in particular progressive muscle relaxation, meditation and hypnosis.

Cognitive restructuring refers to a number of specific methods aimed at trying to change the way the individual thinks about their life situation and self, in order to change their emotional responses and behaviour. This approach is based largely on the work of Beck (treatment of automatic thoughts) and Ellis (rational emotive therapy), two major forms of cognitive-behaviour therapy (CBT; see Chapter 66). This approach provides information to reduce uncertainty and to enhance the individual's sense of control.

KEY POINTS

- Stress has been defined as a stimulus (corresponding to the engineering model), a response (corresponding to the physiological model) and an interaction between an organism and its environment (corresponding to the transactional model).
- The physiological model is based on Selye's GAS, which comprises the alarm reaction, resistance and exhaustion.
- The alarm reaction involves changes in the sympathetic branch of the ANS, which are collectively called the fight-or-flight syndrome. This is associated with the ANS-adrenal-medulla system/sympatho-adrenomedullary axis.
- Resistance is associated with the anterior pituitary-adrenal cortex system/hypothalamic-pituitary-adrenal axis.
- Exhaustion is related to psychophysiological disorders ('diseases of adaptation').
- Potential causes of stress (stressors) include disruption of circadian rhythms (e.g. shift work, jet lag), life changes (as measured by the SRRS) and occupation-linked stressors.
- Burnout is an occupational hazard for a variety of healthcare professionals, especially those working with terminally ill people.
- Chronic stress makes us ill through repeated increases in heart rate and blood pressure, increased blood cholesterol, and suppression of the functioning of the immune system (the immunosuppressive effects of stress).
- Personality and self-esteem represent moderators of the effects of stress.

- Type A behaviour is associated with an increased risk of high blood pressure and CHD, while people with type C personalities may be cancer-prone.
- So-called coping with stress can be both adaptive and maladaptive.
- All coping strategies can be classified as direct action response, information-seeking, inhibition of action, intrapsychic/palliative coping, or turning to others for emotional support. These overlap with the distinction between problem-focused and emotion-focused coping.
- Formal stress management refers to physiological and psychological techniques used by professionals to reduce people's stress.
- Physiological techniques include the use of anxiolytic drugs and biofeedback.
- Many psychological techniques involve cognitive restructuring, which forms the basis of various types of CBT.

REFERENCES

1. Bartlett D (1998) *Stress: Perspectives and Processes*. Buckingham: Open University Press.
2. Goetsch VL, Fuller MG (1995) Stress and stress management. In D Wedding (ed.) *Behavior and Medicine*, 2nd edn. St Louis, MO: Mosby.
3. Cox T (1978) *Stress*. London: Macmillan.
4. Jones F (1995) Managing stress in health care: issues for staff and patient care. In D Messer, C Meldrum (eds) *Psychology for Nurses and Health Care Professionals*. Hemel Hempstead: Prentice Hall/Harvester Wheatsheaf.
5. Warr PB (1987) Job characteristics and mental health. In PB Warr (ed.) *Psychology as Work*. Harmondsworth: Penguin.
6. Selye H (1956) *The Stress of Life*. New York: McGraw-Hill.
7. Lazarus RS (1966) *Psychological Stress and the Coping Process*. New York: McGraw-Hill.
8. Aschoff J (1979) Circadian rhythms: general features and endocrinological aspects. In DT Krieger (ed.) *Endocrine Rhythms*. New York: Raven Press.
9. Hawkins LH, Armstrong-Esther CA (1978) Circadian rhythms and night shift working in nurses. *Nursing Times* 4 May: 49–52.
10. Pinel JPJ (1993) *Biopsychology*, 2nd edn. Boston, MA: Allyn & Bacon.
11. Coffey L, Skipper K, Jung F (1988) Nurses and shift work: effects on job performance and job related stress. *Journal of Advanced Nursing* **13**: 245–54.
12. Brown P (1988) Punching the body clock. *Nursing Times* **84**: 26–8.
13. Blakemore C (1988) *The Mind Machine*. London: BBC.
14. Cho K, Ennaceur A, Cole JC, Suh CK (2000) Chronic jet-lag produces core defects. *Journal of Neuroscience* **20**: 1–5.
15. De Quervain DJF, Roozendaal B, Nitsch RM, McGaugh JL, Hoch C (2000) Acute cortisone administration impairs retrieval of long-term declarative memory in humans. *Nature Neuroscience* **3**: 313–14.
16. Holmes TH, Rahe RH (1967) The social readjustment rating scale. *Journal of Psychosomatic Research* **11**: 213–18.
17. Davison G, Neale JM (1994) *Abnormal Psychology*, 6th edn. New York: John Wiley & Sons.
18. Brown R (1986) *Social Psychology*, 2nd edn. New York: Free Press.
19. Penny G (1996) Health psychology. In H Coolican (ed.) *Applied Psychology*. London: Hodder & Stoughton.
20. Lazarus RS (1999) *Stress and Emotion: A New Synthesis*. London: Free Association Books.
21. Forshaw M (2002) *Essential Health Psychology*. London: Arnold.
22. Davison G, Neale JM, Kring AM (2004) *Abnormal Psychology*, 9th edn. New York: John Wiley & Sons.
23. Parkes CM (1993) Bereavement as a psychosocial transition: processes in adaptation to change. In MS Stroebe, W Stroebe, RO Hansson (eds) *Handbook of Bereavement: Theory, Research and Intervention*. New York: Cambridge University Press.
24. Rotter J (1966) Generalized expectancies for internal versus external control of reinforcement. *Psychological Monographs* **30**: 1–26.
25. Johnson JH, Sarason IG (1978) Life stress, depression, and anxiety: internal/external controls as a moderator variable. *Journal of Psychosomatic Research* **22**: 205–8.
26. Seligman MEP (1975) *Helplessness: On Depression, Development and Death*. San Francisco, CA: W.H. Freeman.
27. Kanner AD, Coyne JC, Schaefer C, Lazarus RS (1981) Comparison of two modes of stress measurement: daily hassles and uplifts versus major life events. *Journal of Behavioural Measurement* **4**: 1–39.
28. Carson J, Fagin L, Brown D, Leary J, Bartlett H (1997) Self-esteem and stress in mental health nurses. *Nursing Times* **93**: 55–8.
29. O'Donnell E (1996) Stressing the point. *Nursing Standard* **10**: 22–3.
30. Nolan P, Cushway D, Tyler P (1995) A measurement tool for assessing stress among mental health nurses. *Nursing Standard* **9**: 36–9.
31. Burnard P, Edwards D, Fothergill A, Hannigan B, Coyle D (2000) When the pressure's too much. *Nursing Times* **96**: 28–30.
32. Firth H, McKeown P, McIntee J, Britton P (1987) Burn-out, personality and support in long-stay nursing. *Nursing Times* **83**: 55–7.
33. Hedge B (1995) Psychological implications of HIV infection. In D Messer, C Meldrum (eds) *Psychology for Nurses and Health Care Professionals*. Hemel Hempstead: Prentice-Hall/Harvester Wheatsheaf.

34. Holmes DS (1994) *Abnormal Psychology*, 2nd edn. New York: HarperCollins.
35. Ogden J (2004) *Health Psychology: A Textbook*, 3rd edn. Maidenhead: Open University Press/McGraw-Hill Education.
36. Kiecolt-Glaser JK, Garner W, Speicher CE, *et al.* (1984) Psychosocial modifiers of immunocompetence in medical students. *Psychosomatic Medicine* **46**: 7–14.
37. Petit-Zeman S (2000) Mmm, guilt-free chocolate. *The Times*, 18 July: 10.
38. Schliefer SJ, Keller SE, Camerino M, Thornton JC, Stein M (1983) Suppression of lymphocyte stimulation following bereavement. *Journal of the American Medical Association* **250**: 374–7.
39. Kiecolt-Glaser JK, Marucha PT, Malalrkey WB, Mercado AM, Glaser R (1995) Slowing of wound healing by psychological stress. *Lancet* **346**: 1194–6.
40. Norton C (2000) Brains can fight breast cancer. *Independent on Sunday*, 16 April: 12.
41. Folkman S, Lazarus RS (1988) *Manual for the Ways of Coping Questionnaire*. Palo Alto, CA: Consulting Psychologists Press.
42. Friedman M, Rosenman RH (1974) *Type A Behaviour and Your Heart*. New York: Harper & Row.
43. Fletcher BC (1995) The consequences of stress. In D Messer, C Meldrum (eds) *Psychology for Nurses and Health Care Professionals*. Hemel Hempstead: Prentice-Hall/Harvester Wheatsheaf.
44. Temoshok L (1987) Personality, coping style, emotions and cancer: towards an integrative model. *Cancer Surveys* **6** (suppl.): 545–67.
45. Weinman J (1995) Health psychology. In AM Colman (ed.) *Controversies in Psychology*. London: Longman.
46. Greer S, Morris T (1975) Psychological attributes of women who develop breast cancer: a controlled study. *Journal of Psychosomatic Research* **19**: 147–53.
47. Cooper C, Faragher B (1993) Psychological stress and breast cancer: the interrelationship between stress events, coping strategies and personality. *Psychological Medicine* **23**: 653–62.
48. Greer A, Morris T, Pettingale KW (1979) Psychological response to breast cancer: effect on outcome. *Lancet* **13**: 785–7.
49. Greer S (1991) Psychological response to cancer and survival. *Psychological Medicine* **21**: 43–9.
50. Greer S, Morris T, Pettingale KW, Haybittle JL (1990) Psychological responses to breast cancer and fifteen year outcome. *Lancet* **335**: 49–50.
51. Hegarty J (2000) Psychologists, doctors, and cancer patients. In J Hartley, A Branthwaite (eds) *The Applied Psychologist*, 2nd edn. Buckingham: Open University Press.
52. Maslach C, Jackson SE (1986) *Maslach Burn-Out Inventory*. San Francisco, CA: Consulting Psychologists Press.
53. Lazarus RS, Folkman S (1984) *Stress, Appraisal and Coping*. New York: Springer.
54. Roger D, Nash P (1995) Coping. *Nursing Times* **91**: 42–3.
55. Cohen F, Lazarus RS (1979) Coping with the stress of illness. In GC Stone, Adler NE, Cohen F (eds) *Health Psychology: A Handbook*. Washington, DC: Jossey-Bass.
56. De Ridder DTD (2000) Gender, stress and coping: do women handle stressful situations differently from men? In L Sherr, JS St Lawrence (eds) *Women, Health and the Mind*. Chichester: John Wiley & Sons.
57. Stroebe MS (1998) New directions on bereavement research: explorations of gender differences. *Palliative Medicine* **12**: 5–12.
58. Stanton AL, Danoff-Berg S, Cameron CL, Ellis AP (1994) Coping through emotional approach: problems of conceptualization and confounding. *Journal of Personality and Social Psychology* **66**: 350–62.

Chapter 12

Emotion

Richard Gross

INTRODUCTION

Mr Spock in *Star Trek* often points out to Captain Kirk how much energy human beings waste through reacting emotionally to things, when a more logical and rational approach would be more productive. But would we be human if we did not react in this way? This is not to advocate 'being emotional' in the sense of losing control of our feelings, or being unable to consider things in a calm and detached way; but it is the richness of our emotions, and our capacity to both have feelings and think things through and reason that makes us unique as a species. Emotions set the tone of our experience and give life its vitality. Emotions are internal factors that can energize, direct and sustain behaviour.[1]

At the same time, we often respond emotionally to events and situations that we believe make demands on us that we cannot meet, either because we do not have the necessary abilities or resources or because they force us to make very difficult choices and decisions. We describe these negative kinds of events as 'stressful' and our emotional responses to them as the experience of 'stress' (see Chapter 11).

One of the key issues running through research into the nature of emotional experience is to what extent it is a physiological phenomenon. Related to this is the question of whether different subjective emotions (feeling angry, afraid and so on) are also physiologically distinct. More recent theories have emphasized the role of cognitive factors in our experience of emotion and are collectively referred to as *cognitive appraisal theories.*

WHAT IS EMOTION?

Wundt, one of the founders of scientific psychology (see Chapter 9), believed that emotional experience can be described in terms of combinations of three dimensions – pleasantness/unpleasantness, calm/excitement and relaxation/tension (based on introspection). Schlosberg[2] also identified pleasantness/unpleasantness, together with acceptance/rejection and sleep/tension, based on photographs of posed facial expressions.

Ekman *et al.*[3] and Ekman and Friesen[4] identified six primary emotions: surprise, fear, disgust, anger, happiness and sadness, based on photos of posed facial expressions (Figure 12.1). These primary emotions are taken to be universal; that is, they are expressed facially in the same way, and are recognized as such, by members of diverse cultures. This suggests very strongly that the emotions are *innate.*

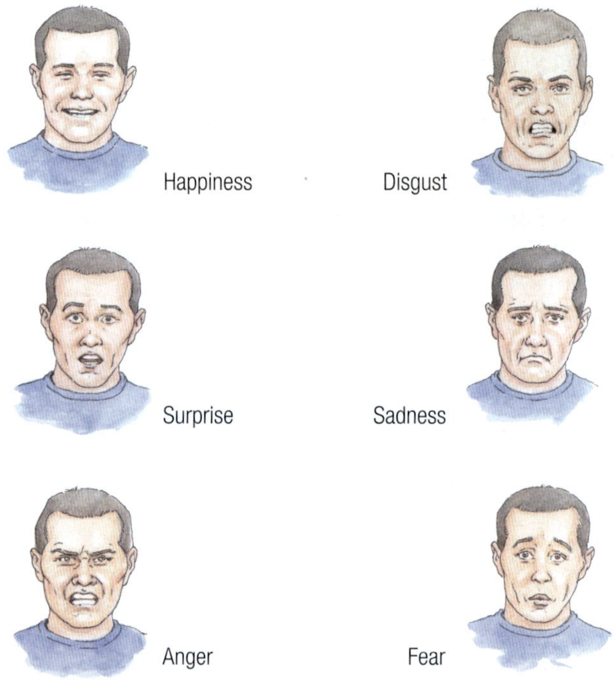

Figure 12.1 Six universal facial expressions

Plutchik proposed an 'emotion wheel' (Figure 12.2), in which eight basic or primary emotions (composed of four pairs of opposites) are shown inside the circle, with a further eight complex emotions on the outside.[5] The primary emotions correspond to Ekman and Friesen's six emotions, except that the terms 'joy' and 'sorrow' are used instead of 'happiness' and 'sadness', respectively, plus 'acceptance' and 'expectancy' are also included. Plutchik believes that the primary emotions are both biologically and subjectively distinct.

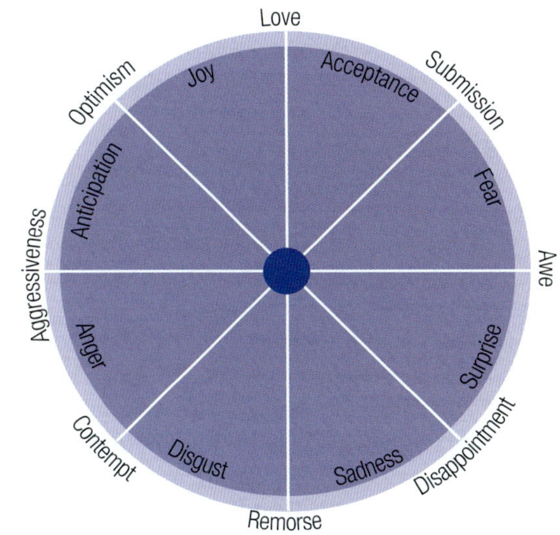

Figure 12.2 The emotion wheel

Basic or primary emotions

Ekman uses the term 'basic' to emphasize the role that evolution has played in shaping both the unique and the common features that emotions display, as well as their current function.[6] Emotions evolved for their adaptive value in dealing with fundamental life tasks: they helped species to survive. Three major characteristics of emotions follow from this adaptive function:

- There are certain common elements in the contexts in which emotions are found to occur, despite individual and cultural differences in social learning.
- The emotions are likely to be observable in other primates (although it is possible that there are certain emotions that are unique to humans, there is no convincing evidence that this is so).
- The emotions can be aroused so quickly that they start to happen before we are even aware of them:

Quick onset is central to the adaptive value of emotions, mobilizing us quickly to respond to important events.[6]

Emotions can occur with very rapid onset, through automatic appraisal (see below), with little awareness, and with involuntary changes in expression and physiology. Indeed, we often experience emotions as happening *to* us rather than chosen by us.

Evidence exists of distinctive patterns of autonomic nervous system (ANS) activity for different emotions (see below). Ekman believes that these patterns are likely to have evolved because they support patterns of motor behaviour that were adaptive for each of these emotions, preparing the organism for quite different actions.[6] For example, fighting may have been the adaptive action in anger (which is consistent with the finding that blood flow increases to the hands when we are angry). There may also be unique patterns of central nervous system (CNS) activity for each emotion, which is not found in other mental activity.

Averill also recognizes the influence that an evolutionary approach has had in the study of emotions, defining basic emotions as those 'that fulfil vital [to the survival of the species] biological functions'.[7] Like Ekman, Averill believes that basic emotions should be universal, be seen (at least in rudimentary form) in non-human primates and be heritable.

However, what is considered 'basic' varies between cultures and within the same culture over time. For example, in the Middle Ages, hope was classified as a basic emotion, but today hope is regarded as a secondary emotion (if it is considered an emotion at all) by most emotion theorists (Box 12.1).[7]

Box 12.1 The social construction of emotions

According to *social constructionism* (see Gross[8]), emotions are the products of culture. Human cultures influence the emotions by influencing their members' beliefs, values, and social environments.

Emotions may be understood as enmeshed within an entire system of beliefs and values, so they cannot exist independently of the culture. For example, *accida* is an emotion that existed in Western cultures in medieval times but seems to have become extinct by about 1400. It involved a mixture of boredom with one's religious duties, attempting to put off carrying them out, sadness about one's religious failings, and a sense of loss of one's former religious enthusiasm. It disappeared during the Renaissance, when values started to change.[9] Today, someone facing the same religious 'crisis' is likely to feel guilt, an emotion related to a culture based on individual responsibility rather than spiritual duty.[10]

According to Markus and Kitayama, 'ego-focused' emotions (e.g. anger, frustration, pride) are experienced more by people in individualist cultures with more independent selves.[11] 'Other-focused' emotions (e.g. shame, belongingness, sympathy) are more common in collectivist cultures with more interdependent selves.

Most basic of all are emotions that are psychologically basic: when people are asked to recount emotional episodes that evoked their 'true feelings', they typically describe incidents that reinforce or transform or enhance their sense of self.[12]

Components of emotion

For each distinct emotion, there are three components:

- The *subjective experience* of happiness, sadness, anger and so on

- *Physiological changes*, involving the ANS and the endocrine system, over which we have little if any conscious control; however, we may become aware of some of their effects (e.g. 'butterflies in the stomach', gooseflesh, sweating)
- *Associated behaviour* such as smiling, crying, frowning, running away or being 'frozen to the spot'.

The latter two components are sometimes categorized together as 'bodily reactions', with the physiological changes being described as 'visceral' and the associated behaviour 'skeletal'. This distinction relates to the ANS and CNS, respectively. However, although running away is largely under voluntary (CNS) control, crying and sweating definitely are not: and yet in all three cases, we infer another person's emotional state from this observable behaviour.

Different theories of emotion are distinguished by:

- how they see the relationship between three components;
- the relative emphasis given to each component;
- how they see the relationship between the components and our cognitive appraisal or interpretation of the emotion-producing stimulus or situation.

Consistent with this is Parrott's definition of an emotion as:

> ... a reaction to personally significant events, where 'reaction' is taken to include biological, cognitive and behavioural reactions, as well as subjective feelings of pleasure or displeasure ...[9]

THEORIES OF EMOTION

The James–Lange theory

If there is a common-sense theory of emotion, it is that something happens that produces in us a subjective emotional experience and, as a result of this, certain bodily and/or behavioural changes occur. James (originally in 1878 and then in 1890) and Lange (at first quite independently of James) turned this common-sense view on its head. They argued that our emotional experience is the result, not the cause, of perceived bodily changes.

To give an example used by James, the common-sense view says that we meet a bear, are frightened and run. The James–Lange theory maintains that we are frightened *because* we run. Similarly, 'We feel sorry because we cry, angry because we strike, afraid because we tremble ...' According to James: '... the bodily changes follow directly the perception of the exciting fact, and ... our feeling of the same changes as they occur is the emotion'.[13]

The crucial factor in the James–Lange theory is feedback from the bodily changes (Figure 12.3). We label our subjective state by inferring how we feel based on perception of our own bodily changes ('I'm trembling, so I must be afraid').

You may be able to think of situations in which you have reacted in a fairly automatic way. For example, if you slip while walking down stairs, only after you've grabbed the banister do you become aware of feeling frightened and a little shaken. It is almost as if the sudden change in your behaviour – rather than your reason for grabbing the banister in the first place – has caused the fear.

Evaluation of the James–Lange theory

The theory implies that by deliberately altering our behaviour, we can control our emotional experiences. Try smiling – do you feel any happier? A crucial test (which James admitted would be very difficult to perform) would be to examine the emotional experience of a completely anaesthetized, but not intellectually or motor impaired, individual.

In the examples that James gives of inferring emotion from bodily changes, such as running away from the bear, he clearly attaches much more importance to skeletal rather than visceral changes. Parrott calls this the 'peripheral' approach.[9] In this respect, the James–Lange theory probably differs from other theories, which usually mean 'visceral' when they say 'physiological'. Given this emphasis on skeletal changes, there are two important studies that support the James–Lange theory (Box 12.2).

The Valins[14] and Laird[15] studies suggest that overt behaviour may cause subjective feelings without there being any

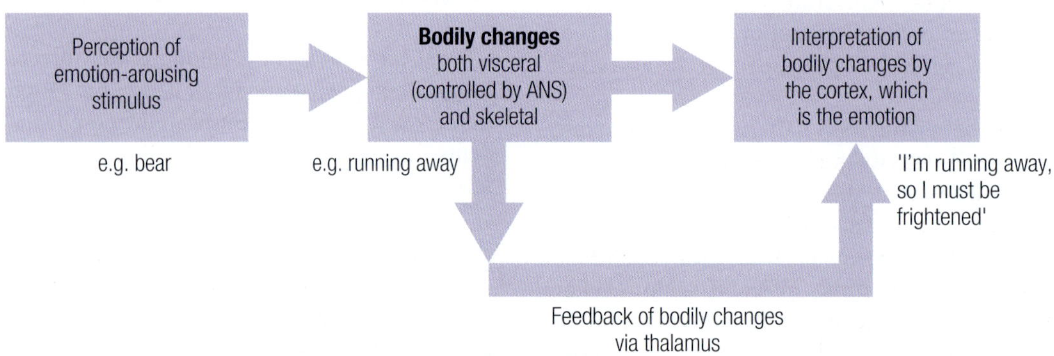

Figure 12.3 James–Lange theory of emotion. (ANS: autonomic nervous system).

> **Box 12.2 Listen to your heart and smile if you want to be happy**
>
> Valins provided male participants with feedback of their heart rate while watching slides of semi-nude *Playboy* pin-ups.[14] The heart rate was in fact pre-recorded and programmed to increase in response to presentation of half the slides; but the participants *believed* the feedback was an indication of their true response. This is the *false feedback paradigm*. The models in the slides associated with the apparent heart-rate increase were judged to be more attractive than those associated with unchanged heart rate.
>
> Laird tested the *facial feedback hypothesis* by falsely informing 32 students that they were participating in an experiment to measure activity in facial muscles.[15] Bogus electrodes were attached to the face, as if to measure physiological response, and the participants were instructed to raise their eyebrows, contract the muscles in their forehead and make other facial expressions. They did not realize the emotional significance of what they were being asked to do.
>
> While this was going on, cartoon slides were projected on to a screen. Regardless of the content of the cartoons, participants rated the slides they had seen while 'smiling' as funnier. They also described themselves as happier when 'smiling', angrier when 'frowning' and so on.

obvious physiological arousal taking place: visceral changes may not be necessary. But neither Valins nor Laird attempted to measure any accompanying visceral changes. What if smiling triggers certain physiological changes? Might these changes, rather than the change in our facial muscles, be the real cause of our feeling happy? And, if so, is this quite damaging to the James–Lange theory, which places so much stress on behavioural (skeletal) changes?

Levenson *et al.* asked participants to move particular facial muscles, in order to simulate the emotional expression of fear, anger, surprise, disgust, sadness and happiness.[16] The authors also monitored several physiological responses controlled by the ANS while this was going on. They found that the simulated expressions did alter ANS activity; for example, anger increased heart rate and skin temperature, fear increased heart rate but decreased skin temperature, and happiness decreased heart rate without affecting skin temperature.

In the James–Lange theory, these bodily changes occur spontaneously, rather than consciously and deliberately. This makes it difficult to draw any firm conclusions from experiments like those of Valins and Laird. However, both studies strongly suggest that physiological arousal is not sufficient to account for emotional experience. The fact that participants in the Valins study were prepared to infer emotion on the basis of (false) information about their reactions to stimuli suggests that physiological arousal may not even be necessary, and that cognitive factors may be sufficient.[17]

According to Parrott, for the body to 'know' how to respond appropriately, more than simply 'perception of the exciting fact' must be involved.[9] The event (e.g. the bear) must be interpreted or evaluated (or appraised) as a threat. The James–Lange theory fails to account for why the bear is seen as frightening in the first place. (We shall return to this issue below.)

Cannon's crtique of the James–Lange theory

According to Cannon, there are four major faults with the James–Lange theory:[18]

- The theory assumes that for each subjectively distinct emotion there is a corresponding set of physiological changes enabling us to label the emotion that we are experiencing.
- Even if this assumption were true, physiological arousal would still not be sufficient.
- Physiological arousal may not even be necessary.
- The speed with which we often experience emotions seems to exceed the speed of response of the viscera, so how could the physiological changes be the source of sudden emotion?

Cannon argued that 'the same visceral changes occur in very different emotional states and in non-emotional states'. In other words, the James–Lange theory was built on the assumption that different emotional stimuli induce different patterns of ANS activity, and that perception of these different patterns results in different emotional experiences.

According to the Cannon–Bard theory, the ANS responds in the same way to all emotional stimuli: the sympathetic branch prepares the organism for flight or fight, through increased heart rate and blood pressure, pupil dilation, increased blood flow to the muscles, increased respiration and increased release of adrenaline and noradrenaline from the adrenal medulla. This means that there must be more to our emotional experience than simply physiological arousal, otherwise we would not be able to tell one emotional state from another.

Evidence for physiological specificity

According to LeDoux, this represents 'one of the most pesky problems in emotion research'.[19] He points out that the emphasis of research has been on ANS activity, and this emphasis is due partly to Cannon's criticism of the James–Lange theory.

The methods of Ax (Box 12.3) would be ethically unacceptable today, but his findings have been confirmed by others (e.g. Frankenhaeuser[21]). Schachter confirmed Ax's original findings that fear is influenced largely by adrenaline;[22] but he also found that anger produces a mixed adrenaline–noradrenaline response and that pain produces a noradrenaline-like pattern. Schachter and Singer concluded:

Whether or not there are physiological distinctions among the various emotional states must be considered an open question. Any differences which do exist are at best rather subtle and the variety of emotion, mood and feeling states do not appear to be matched by an equal variety of visceral patterns.[23]

This conclusion is consistent with Schachter's *cognitive labelling theory*, which sees physiological arousal as necessary for emotional experience,[24] but the nature of the arousal is irrelevant (see below).

Less extreme and controversial methods than Ax's include:

- the *directed facial action method*, in which participants are instructed to make the facial expressions characteristic of various emotions while ANS activity is recorded;
- the *relived emotion method*, in which participants are asked to think about previous emotional experiences while these measures are being made.

Levenson carried out a series of experiments using both methods. He maintains that it is a 'myth' that every emotion is autonomically different (Box 12.4). It seems far more likely that reliable differences will be found only between emotions for which there are different associated typical behaviours, and even among this smaller set it is quite unlikely that they will not share some features.

Even if there were identifiable patterns of physiological response associated with different subjective emotions, Cannon argued that such physiological changes themselves do not necessarily produce emotional states. In other words, physiological arousal is not sufficient. This was demonstrated by Marañon (Box 12.5).[26] However, the study by Hohmann suggests that, although physiological changes are not sufficient for the experience of 'full-blooded' emotions, they may still be necessary (Box 12.6).[27]

Box 12.3 Be afraid: the Ax man's coming

In a famous, but ethically highly dubious, experiment, Ax measured various aspects of electrodermal (skin conductance), electromyographic (muscle action potential), cardiovascular and respiratory activity in participants who were deliberately frightened and made angry.[20]

The participants were told that they were participating in a study of hypertension and were asked to lie quietly on a couch while physiological measures were taken.

As the electrodes were attached, it was casually mentioned that the technician who usually operated the technical equipment in an adjacent room was sick, and a man who had recently been fired for incompetence and arrogance was filling in for him. A few minutes later, after baseline measures had been recorded, either the 'anger condition' followed by the 'fear condition' occurred, or vice versa.

In the fear condition, a continuous mild shock was administered to one finger, without any warning or explanation. The intensity increased gradually, until the participant complained. Then sparks were made to jump.

In the anger condition, the technician (an actor) entered the room and spent 5 minutes checking the wiring. During this time, he jostled the participant, criticised the attending nurse, and blamed the participant for causing a fault in the equipment.

Of 14 different measures taken, Ax found that seven were significantly different between the two conditions. For example, fear was associated with increased heart rate, skin conduction level, muscle action potential frequency and breathing rate (reflecting the effects of adrenaline). Anger was accompanied by increased diastolic blood pressure, frequency of spontaneous skin conduction responses and action potential size (reflecting the greater influence of noradrenaline).

Box 12.4 The physiology of positive and negative emotions

Levenson *et al.* compared anger, disgust, fear and sadness (negative emotions), and happiness (positive emotion) and surprise.[16] They identified a small number of fairly reliable differences in patterns of autonomic nervous system (ANS) activity, both between the negative emotions, and between the negative emotions as a group and happiness.

For example, anger, fear and sadness all produce larger increases in heart rate than disgust does, while anger produces a larger increase in finger temperature than fear does.

These differences have been found consistently across populations differing in occupation, age (from young people to 71- to 90-year-olds), culture (Americans and Minangkabau males living in western Sumatra, Indonesia) and gender, and across the directed facial action and relived emotion methods.

Levenson believes that positive emotions might not be associated with any particular pattern of behaviour, or, if they are, it would be characterized by low activity, making little metabolic demand on the ANS:

> **Instead of having distinctive autonomic signatures ... positive emotions might be associated with a state of physiological quiescence ... their primary function might be to 'undo' the autonomic activation produced by negative emotions ... to restore the organism to its pre-arousal state in a more efficient and rapid manner than would be the case if the negative emotions were allowed to run their natural course.[25]**

This implies that, at least in our present state of knowledge, we cannot draw general conclusions about the specificity of the body's response to emotional stimuli – it depends partly on which emotion (positive or negative) we are talking about.

Box 12.5 As if emotion were just adrenaline

Marañon injected 210 people with adrenaline.[26] Seventy-one per cent said they experienced only physical symptoms, with no emotional overtones at all. Most of the rest reported 'as if' emotions.

The few who experienced genuine emotion had to imagine – or remember – a highly emotional event.

Box 12.6 Real emotions need an intact autonomic nervous system

Hohmann studied 25 adult males with spinal cord injuries who suffered corresponding ANS damage.[27] The participants reported significant changes in the nature and intensity of certain emotional experiences, especially anger, fear and sexual feelings. Generally, the higher the lesion in the spinal cord, the greater the disruption of visceral responses, and the greater the disturbance of normal emotional experiences.

Like Marañon's participants, Hohmann's participants reported 'as if' emotions, a 'mental kind of anger' for example.

According to Schachter, what Marañon's and Hohmann's participants reported is precisely what would be expected from his cognitive labelling theory, which sees emotional experience as a joint function of cognitive and physiological factors (see below).[24]

The Cannon–Bard theory

Cannon removed the sympathetic nervous system in cats,[28] and Sherrington severed the spinal cord and vagus nerve in dogs.[29] In both cases, feedback from the viscera to the brain was prevented, but the animals showed apparently normal emotional reactions. Cannon took these findings to mean that physiological changes may not even be necessary for emotional experience. In addition, Dana studied a patient with a spinal-cord lesion: despite having no sympathetic functioning and only extremely limited muscular movement, the patient showed a range of emotions, including grief, joy, displeasure and affection.[30] Similarly, Chwalisz *et al.* found that people with spinal-cord injuries experience emotion as intensely as before the injury, as intensely as 'normal' people, and as intensely as people with spinal-cord injuries that do not block bodily sensations.[31] These findings seem to support Cannon's view.

As Figure 12.4 shows, the subjective emotion is quite independent of the physiological changes involved. The emotion-producing stimulus is processed by the thalamus. This sends impulses to the cortex, where the emotion is consciously experienced, and to the hypothalamus, which sets in motion certain autonomic physiological changes.

An evaluation of the Cannon–Bard theory

Cannon also questioned how, because we often feel emotions quite rapidly and yet the viscera are quite slow to react, the physiological changes could be the source of such sudden emotion (as required by the James–Lange theory). However, although the viscera are not sensitive to certain kinds of stimulation (e.g. burning, cutting), they provide much better feedback than Cannon suspected. Many visceral changes can occur sufficiently quickly that they could be the causes of feelings of emotion.[32]

Pinel advocates a position falling between the extreme views represented by the Cannon–Bard and James–Lange theories.[33] On the one hand, the Cannon–Bard view that the ANS responds in the same way to all emotional stimuli is clearly incorrect: several differences have been well documented. On the other hand, there is insufficient evidence to make a strong case for the James–Lange view that each emotion is characterized by a different pattern of ANS activity.

Schachter's cognitive labelling theory

According to Schachter, Cannon was wrong in thinking that bodily changes and the experience of emotion are independent, and the James–Lange theory was mistaken in claiming that physiological changes cause the feeling of emotion.[24] Although sharing the James–Lange belief that physiological changes precede the experience of emotion,

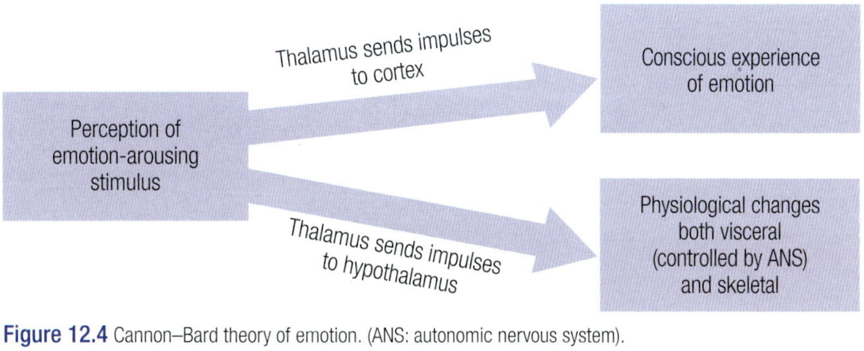

Figure 12.4 Cannon–Bard theory of emotion. (ANS: autonomic nervous system).

Schachter argues that we have to decide which particular emotion we are feeling. The label we attach to our arousal depends on what we attribute that arousal to (Figure 12.5).

Schachter is saying that physiological arousal (factor 1) is necessary for the experience of emotion, but the nature of arousal is immaterial: what is important is how we interpret that arousal (factor 2). Hence, the theory is also known as the *two-factor theory of emotion.* The classic experiment that demonstrates this cognitive theory of emotion is Schachter and Singer's 'adrenaline experiment' (Box 12.7).[23]

Schachter and Singer were testing three interrelated hypotheses regarding the interaction between physiological and cognitive factors in the experience of emotion:

- If we experience a state of physiological arousal for which we have no immediate explanation, we will label this state and describe it in terms of the cognitions available. So, precisely the same state of arousal could receive different labels (e.g. 'euphoria'/'anger' – groups B and C). (Physiological arousal and cognitive labelling are necessary.)
- If we experience a state of physiological arousal for which we have a completely appropriate explanation (e.g. 'I've just been given an injection of adrenaline'), we will label this state accordingly (group A).
- Given the same circumstances, we will react emotionally or describe our feelings as emotions only to the extent

Box 12.7 Schachter and Singer's adrenaline experiment[23]

Participants were given an injection of adrenaline but told that they were given a vitamin injection in order to see its effect on vision. The participants were then tested under one of four conditions:

- *Group A* participants were given accurate information about the side effects of the injection (palpitations, tightness in the throat, tremor, sweating).
- *Group B* participants were given false information about the side effects (itching, headache).
- *Group C* participants were given no information about the side effects.
- *Group D* (control group) participants were given a saline injection but otherwise treated like group C participants.

Before being given a 'vision test', each participant (one at a time) sat in a waiting room with another 'participant' (a stooge of the experimenters). For half the participants in each condition, the stooge acted either in a happy, frivolous way (making paper aeroplanes, laughing out loud, playing with a hula-hoop: *euphoria condition*), or very angrily (eventually tearing up the questionnaire that he and every participant was asked to complete: *anger condition*). (The group B condition was run only with a euphoric stooge.)

Participants' emotional experience was assessed in two ways:

- Observers' ratings of the degree to which they joined in with the stooge's behaviour.
- Self-report scales.

As predicted:

- participants in groups A and D were much less likely to join in with the stooge or to report feeling euphoric or angry;
- participants in groups B and C were much more likely to assume the stooge's behaviour and emotional state.

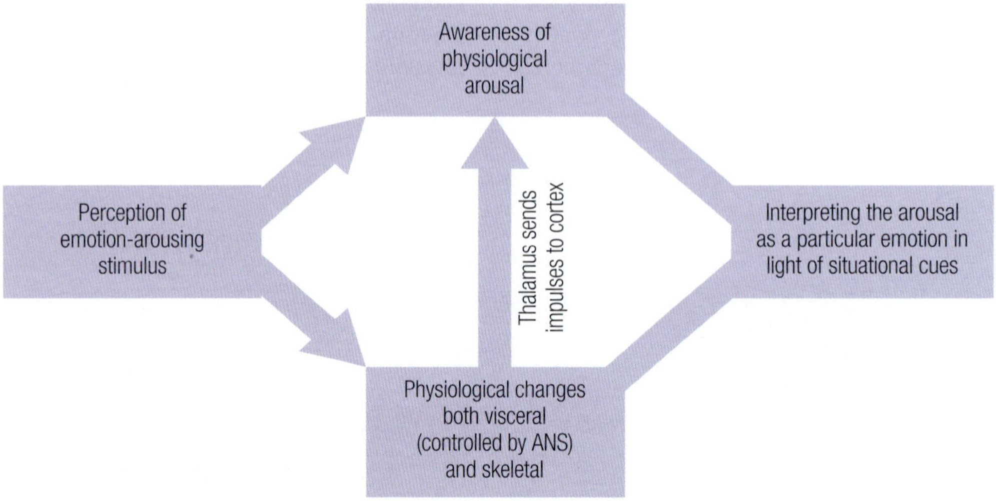

Figure 12.5 Schachter's cognitive labelling (or two-factor) theory. (ANS: autonomic nervous system).

that we experience a state of physiological arousal (groups A–C). (Physiological arousal is necessary.)

An evaluation of cognitive labelling theory

- Schachter and Wheeler confirmed these results by injecting participants with either adrenaline or chlorpromazine (which inhibits arousal); controls were injected with a placebo.[34] While watching a slapstick comedy, the adrenaline participants laughed more, and the chlorpromazine participants less, than the controls.
- Dutton and Aron's study (Box 12.8) confirms Schachter's claim that the autonomic arousal that accompanies all emotions is similar and that it is our interpretation of that arousal that matters – even though sometimes this results in our misidentifying our emotions. Dutton and Aron's suspension-bridge participants seemed to be mislabelling their fear as sexual attraction to the interviewer.
- The focus of Schachter's model is an atypical state of affairs, where the participant is unsure about the cause of arousal (groups B and C). But Schachter admitted that usually we *are* aware of a precipitating situation before the onset of arousal (which usually takes 1–2 seconds to reach consciousness).[24] Therefore, it is normally perfectly obvious to us what aspects of the situation have provoked the emotion. However, even here the meaning of the emotion-inducing circumstances requires some cognitive analysis before the emotion can be labelled.
- Schachter claims that the *quantitative* aspect of emotion can arise without cognitive mediation ('Am I in a state of emotional arousal?' – as in Valins' study). But the *qualitative* aspect requires prior cognition ('What emotion is it that I am experiencing?' – as in Laird's study). Mandler has called Schachter's theory the 'jukebox theory' – arousal is like the coin that gets the machine going, and cognition is the button we push to select the emotional tune.[36]
- According to Parkinson, the view that affect (emotion) is post-cognitive is now probably the most popular attitude among emotion theorists.[17] But even if we accept the important role of cognitive factors, is our emotional experience really as labile or malleable as Schachter claims? Are environmental cues really as easily accepted as the basis for inferences about our own feelings?[37]
- Using the original Schachter and Singer paradigm, several studies have concluded that when we try to explain a state of arousal, we do not merely use others' behaviour as a guide to what we are feeling.[38–40] We call on many other sources of information as well, particularly our own past history: we search for previous occasions on which we felt this arousal state to explain why it is occurring now. Although other people's behaviour might suggest – or even dictate (through conformity) – how we should behave in that situation, it does not tell us how we're feeling. At the very least, others' behaviour must in some way be appropriate.[41]
- These later studies also found that people who do not have a ready-made explanation for their adrenaline-produced arousal are more likely to attach a negative emotional label to it, such as unease or nervousness, similar to 'free-floating anxiety'. This suggests that emotional lability is not as great as Schachter maintains: unexplained arousal has a negative, unpleasant quality about it.

Box 12.8 Falling in love on a suspension bridge[35]

The study participants were unsuspecting males, aged 18–35 years, visiting the Capilano Canyon in British Columbia, Canada.

An attractive female interviewer approached the men and asked them questions as part of a survey on the effects of scenery on creativity. One of the things the men were asked to do was invent a short story about an ambiguous picture of a woman (a picture from the Thematic Apperception Test (TAT); see Chapter 15). This was later scored for sexual content, taken to reflect the men's sexual attraction towards the interviewer.

Some men were interviewed on an extremely unstable suspension bridge, less than 2 metres wide and 150 metres long, composed of wooden boards attached to wire cables, running from one side of the canyon to the other. This bridge, about 75 metres above the canyon, tends to sway, tilt and wobble, giving the impression that one is about to fall over the side. There are only very low handrails of wire cable for support (*high arousal condition*).

Other men were interviewed on a solid wooden bridge upstream, about 3 metres above a shallow rivulet, with high handrails and without any swaying or tilting (*low arousal condition*).

As predicted, the stories of the men in the high arousal condition contained significantly more sexual imagery.

The interviewer also invited the men to contact her if they wanted more information about the research. Again in line with predictions, four times as many men from the high arousal condition contacted the researcher compared with men in the low arousal condition.

To show that arousal was the independent variable, Dutton and Aron also arranged for another group of men to be interviewed at least 10 minutes after crossing the suspension bridge. By this time, the symptoms of their physical arousal should have been declining. These non-aroused men did not show the signs of sexual arousal shown by those in the high arousal condition.

The role of attribution

According to Schachter, group A participants in the adrenaline experiment could attribute their arousal to the injection (they had a ready-made explanation and so did not need an emotional explanation). For those in groups B and C, however, no such ready-made explanation was available, and so the stooge's behaviour was used as a cue for explaining their own state of arousal (as either euphoria or anger).

Taking one of James's original examples (running away from the bear), the original cause of the bodily reactions (the bear) is irrelevant. This is because our emotional experience is based on feedback from our bodily reactions (running away). But for Schachter, it is what we attribute our arousal to that determines the label we give to it. In the adrenaline experiment, the initially unexplained arousal is attributed to the (rather extreme) behaviour of the confederate and so is labelled euphoria or anger accordingly.

Similarly, the men in Dutton and Aron's experiment who were tested on the swaying suspension bridge were unaware of the 'real' cause of their arousal. They attributed it instead to the female interviewer. We know that arousal was the independent variable, and it is highly likely that, if the attractive interviewer had not approached the men, they would have labelled their arousal 'fear', because it would have been attributed to a frightening stimulus (the bridge).

What all these examples show is that the cognitive labelling theory is essentially based on *attributional principles* (see Gross[8]). This represents a major form of influence that Schachter's theory has had on cognitive theories of emotion in general.

According to Weiner, certain kinds of attribution produce specific emotions.[41,42] For example, success produces a very general positive feeling (e.g. happiness), while failure produces a very general negative feeling (e.g. sadness). But if the outcome (either success or failure) either is very different from what is expected or has very important consequences, then we try to figure out the reasons for or causes of the outcome. These reasons will take the form of internal or external attributions, which in turn can be broken down into controllable or uncontrollable. It is the combination of internal/external and controllable/uncontrollable that will determine specific emotional responses (Figure 12.6).

The misattribution effect

The adrenaline and suspension-bridge experiments show that people can make mistakes in how they attribute their arousal. This mislabelling of our feelings, and drawing mistaken conclusions about the causes of those feelings, is called the *misattribution effect*.[43]

As part of their suspension-bridge experiment, and in a later experiment, Dutton and Aron invited male students to participate in a learning experiment.[35,44] After meeting an attractive female partner, half the students were frightened with the news that they would be suffering some 'quite painful' electric shocks. Before the experiment was due to begin, they were given a short questionnaire 'to get some information on your present feelings and reactions, since these often influence people on the learning task'. Asked how much they would like to date and kiss their partner, the aroused (frightened) men expressed more intense attraction than the non-frightened men.

By definition, the female partner was sexually attractive, and so it was far easier for the men to transfer their arousal to her and to mislabel their arousal as sexual. In this way, the female partner represented a salient or credible source of arousal.[45] (She also represents a clear, unambiguous source of arousal.) Similarly, if female participants are

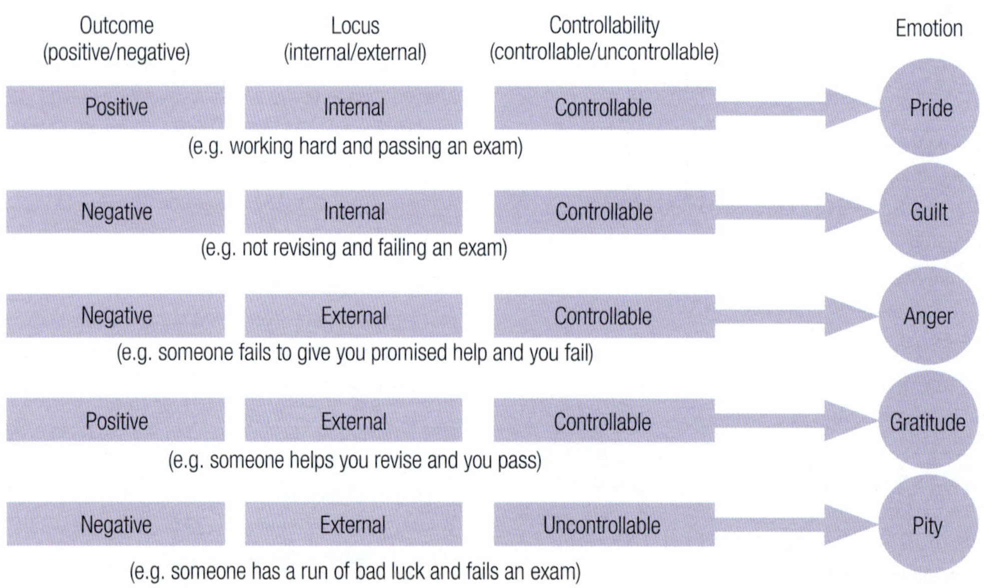

Figure 12.6 Examples of how particular kinds of attribution can produce particular emotions

shown slides of attractive nude males, it may be easy to alter their preferences among the pictures based on false heart-rate feedback, whereas this would be very difficult to achieve if the nude males were replaced by slides of naked hippos. (This is a deliberately modified version of an example given by Taylor *et al.*[46])

Cognitive appraisal or affective primacy?

When evaluating the James–Lange theory earlier, we noted that it fails to account for why a bear, say, should make us run away. In other words, it fails to take into account our appraisal of the emotional 'stimulus' (Box 12.9). Appraisal is the thinking that leads to emotion,[9] and appraisal theory is a development of Schachter's cognitive labelling theory.

According to Lazarus, some degree of cognitive processing is an essential prerequisite for an affective reaction to a stimulus to occur and is an integral feature of all emotional states. For Lazarus, '... emotion results from evaluative perception of a relationship (actual, imagined or anticipated) between a person (or animal) and the environment'.[47]

Lazarus proposes that cognitive appraisal invariably precedes any affective reaction, although it does not have to involve any conscious processing. Zajonc argues that there is generally little direct evidence of either the existence or nature of such preconscious cognitive processing[49] (although the study of subliminal perception suggests otherwise; see Gross[50]). Zajonc argues that cognition and affect operate as independent systems, and an emotional response may precede cognitive processes under certain circumstances. For example, we may meet someone very briefly and form a positive or negative impression, despite not being able to remember any detailed information about them later, such as hair or eye colour.[51]

Parrott asks how it is possible to describe certain emotions as 'irrational' if emotions do not intrinsically entail beliefs.[9] Also, most emotions are 'about' something – and this is cognitive. The most important problem for Zajonc is that how we think about a situation influences how we feel (e.g. *why* we think someone behaved as they did determines whether we feel angry or sympathetic; see Figure 12.6).

Zajonc seems to overestimate the amount of cognitive processing that Lazarus and other cognitive appraisal theorists are claiming. For example, Lazarus simply argues that some minimal cognitive analysis at some level always precedes emotional experience. But this can be quite automatic, and so 'cognitive appraisal' is quite consistent with the sense of 'immediacy' that so much emotional experience has (and which Frijda sees as a characteristic of emotion[52]).

Box 12.9 Subincision in the Arunta[48]

Participants were shown a film (*Subincision in the Arunta*) that depicts aboriginal boys undergoing circumcision as part of a puberty rite. The boys are shown having their penis cut with a jagged flint knife. This usually causes high levels of stress in viewers of the film (and probably in the boys too). The sound track was manipulated, so that:

- the pain, jaggedness of the knife and so on were emphasized (*trauma*);
- the boys' anticipation of entering manhood was stressed (*denial*);
- the emotional elements were ignored and the traditions of the aboriginal people were emphasized (*intellectualization*);
- there was no commentary (*silent control*).

As predicted, arousal (measured by galvanic skin response (GSR) and heart rate) was highest in the trauma condition, next highest in the control condition, and lowest in the other two conditions.

What we tell ourselves about external situations (*cognitive appraisal*) influences our level of arousal.

What is 'an emotion'?

Clore defines emotions as *mental states*.[53] Neither physiological arousal nor feeling states provide the best way of trying to capture the nature of an emotion. Emotions are special kinds of feeling, namely those that we judge to have an emotional cause. This is why feelings that are generated artificially by electrical stimulation or hormone injection (or some other non-cognitive means) are not emotions (see Box 12.5). For Clore, emotion terms seem to refer to something beyond feelings, to psychological states of which feelings are perhaps a necessary but not a sufficient condition.

Many of the examples Zajonc gives of emotion without cognition (*affective primacy* or 'preferences need no inferences') do not seem to describe emotional states at all. For example, when someone leaps out in front of you and shouts 'Boo!', your physiological and bodily response (including your facial expression) would be described more accurately as a startle reflex than as fear.

According to Scherer, the classic debate between Lazarus and Zajonc, which had a major impact on the psychology of emotion during the 1980s, was concerned mostly with the level of processing involved – and not with whether any processing took place.[54] This, in turn, revolved around the definition of 'cognition'.

What is cognition?

If 'cognition' means or includes basic sensory processing, then most, if not all, emotions will have some cognitive component. However, LeDoux[19] and Panksepp,[55] both biologists, suggest that the brain circuitry underlying emotion and cognition is different. Cognition is seen as depending on the neocortex and hippocampus. If 'cognition' is restricted to processes involving these brain areas, then emotion can occur without cognition, since non-humans with extensive lesions in these structures still display emotional responses.

CONCLUSIONS

According to Davidson and Ekman, most theorists now acknowledge that emotion can be elicited in the absence of conscious cognitive mediation.[56] If a broad view of cognition is taken, then most would also agree that some cognitive processing is required for most emotion. Dalgleish maintains that the view that cognition is an integral part of emotion is predominant within the psychology of emotion.[57] The challenge is to specify more precisely the types of cognitive processing that may be critical to the emotion generation process, and to identify the neural circuitries that underlie emotion and cognition respectively. We also need to study the interactions between emotion and cognition.

KEY POINTS

- Ekman and Friesen identify six primary universal emotions, which are probably innate. Plutchik's emotion wheel also incorporates primary emotions, but distinguishes these from complex emotions.
- An evolutionary approach to understanding primary or basic emotions includes considering their current function. But 'basic' emotions differ between cultures and over time within the same culture. They may be psychologically or culturally basic – rather than biologically basic.
- According to social constructionism, emotions are culturally and historically relative. They exist within a system of beliefs and values, which differ between cultures and change over time.
- For each distinct emotion, there is the subjective experience, physiological changes, associated behaviour and cognitive appraisal of the emotion-producing stimulus/situation.
- The James–Lange theory turns the common-sense theory of emotion on its head, by claiming that our emotional experience is the result of perceived bodily changes, in particular skeletal changes.
- Studies by Valins (using the false feedback paradigm) and Laird (testing the facial feedback hypothesis) support the James–Lange theory, although they fail to take into account any visceral changes that may be taking place. They both suggest that physiological arousal is not sufficient to account for emotional experience.
- Cannon criticized the James–Lange theory for assuming that different emotional states are associated with different patterns of ANS activity. The Cannon–Bard theory claims that the ANS responds in the same way to all emotional stimuli.
- Using the directed facial action and the relived emotion methods, Levenson reports physiological differences between anger, disgust, fear and sadness. Both the James–Lange and the Cannon–Bard theories take too extreme a view regarding physiological specificity, and the truth lies somewhere in between.
- Marañon's and Hohmann's studies support Cannon's claim that physiological arousal is not sufficient for emotional experience, although they indicate that it is necessary. However, Cannon's own study of cats, plus those of Sherrington and Dana, suggest that it might not even be necessary.
- According to Schachter's cognitive labelling theory, the experience of emotion depends on both physiological changes and the interpretation of those changes. Cannon was, therefore, mistaken in claiming that emotional experience and bodily changes are independent.
- Schachter and Singer's 'adrenaline experiment' demonstrates that, although physiological arousal is necessary, the nature of the arousal is irrelevant. What is crucial is the cognitive label that we give that arousal.
- Dutton and Aron's suspension-bridge experiment supports Schachter's theory, but it also shows that our labelling of our arousal can be mistaken (the misattribution effect).
- Failure to replicate the adrenaline experiment suggests that emotional experience is much less malleable than Schachter claims, and that unexplained arousal is likely to be interpreted negatively.
- Lazarus's cognitive appraisal theory clams that some minimal cognitive analysis always precedes emotional experience, although this can be unconscious and automatic. Zajonc's affective primacy theory claims that emotional responses can occur without any cognition being involved.
- The basic disagreement between Lazarus and Zajonc seems to be about the level of processing involved, rather than whether or not any cognitive processing takes place. This, in turn, centres around the definition of 'cognition'.

REFERENCES

1. Rubin Z, McNeil EB (1983) *The Psychology of Being Human*, 3rd edn. London: Harper & Row.
2. Schlosberg HS (1941) A scale for the judgement of facial expression. *Journal of Experimental Psychology* 29: 497–510.
3. Ekman P, Friesen WV, Ellsworth P (1972) *Emotion in the Human Face: Guidelines for Research and an Integration of Findings*. New York: Pergamon.
4. Ekman P, Friesen WV (1975) *Unmasking the Face*. Englewood Cliffs, NJ: Prentice-Hall.
5. Plutchik R (1980) *Emotion: A Psychobioevolutionary Synthesis*. New York: Harper & Row.
6. Ekman P (1994) All emotions are basic. In P Ekman, RJ Davison (eds) *The Nature of Emotion: Fundamental Questions*. New York: Oxford University Press.
7. Averill JR (1994) In the eyes of the beholder. In P Ekman, RJ Davidson (eds) *The Nature of Emotion: Fundamental Questions*. New York: Oxford University Press.
8. Gross R (2005) *Psychology: The Science of Mind and Behaviour*, 5th edn. London: Hodder Arnold.
9. Parrott WG (2004) The nature of emotion. In MB Brewer, M Hewstone (eds) *Emotion and Motivation*. Oxford: Blackwell.
10. Harré R, Finlay-Jones R (1986) Emotion talk across times. In R Harre, R Finlay-Jones (eds) *The Social Construction of Emotion*. Oxford: Blackwell.

11. Markus HR, Kitayama S (1991) Culture and the self: implications for cognition, emotion, and motivation. *Psychological Review* **98**: 224–53.
12. Morgan C, Averill JR (1992) True feelings, the self, and authenticity: a psychological perspective. In DD Franks, V Gecas (eds.) *Social Perspectives on Emotion*, Vol. 1. Greenwich, CT: JAI Press.
13. James W (1890) *The Principles of Psychology*. New York: Henry Holt & Company.
14. Valins S (1966) Cognitive effects of false heart-rate feedback. *Journal of Personality and Social Psychology* 4: 400–408.
15. Laird JD (1974) Self-attribution of emotion: the effects of facial expression on the quality of emotional experience. *Journal of Personality and Social Psychology* **29**: 475–86.
16. Levenson RW, Ekman P, Friesen WV (1990) Voluntary facial action generates emotion-specific autonomic nervous system activity. *Psychophysiology* **27**: 363–84.
17. Parkinson B (1987) Emotion: cognitive approaches. In H Beloff, AM Colman (eds) *Psychology Survey 6*. Leicester: British Psychological Society.
18. Cannon WB (1929) *Bodily Changes in Pain, Hunger, Fear, and Rage*. New York: Appleton.
19. LeDoux JE (1994) Emotion-specific physiological activity: don't forget about CNS physiology. In P Ekman, RJ Davidson (eds) *The Nature of Emotion: Fundamental Questions*. New York: Oxford University Press.
20. Ax AF (1953) The physiological differentiation of fear and anger in humans. *Psychosomatic Medicine* **15**: 422–33.
21. Frankenhaeuser F (1975) Experimental approaches to the study of catecholamines and emotion. In L Levi (ed.) *Emotions: The Parameters and Measurement*. New York: Raven Press.
22. Schachter S (1957) Pain, fear and anger in hypertensives and normotensives: a psychophysiologic study. *Psychosomatic Medicine* **19**: 17–29.
23. Schachter S, Singer JE (1962) Cognitive, social, and physiological determinants of emotional state. *Psychological Review* **69**: 379–99.
24. Schachter S (1964) The interaction of cognitive and physiological determinants of emotional state. In L Berkowitz (ed.) *Advances in Experimental Social Psychology*, Vol. 1. New York: Academic Press.
25. Levenson RW (1994) The search for autonomic specificity. In P Ekman, RJ Davidson (eds) *The Nature of Emotion: Fundamental Questions*. New York: Oxford University Press.
26. Marañon G (1924) Contribution a l'etude de l'action emotive de l'adrenaline. *Revue Francaise d'Endocrinologie* 2: 301–25.
27. Hohmann GW (1966) Some effects of spinal cord lesions on experienced emotional feelings. *Psychophysiology* 3: 143–56.
28. Cannon WB (1927) The James–Lange theory of emotions: a critical re-examination and an alternative theory. *American Journal of Psychology* **39**: 106–24.
29. Sherrington CS (1900) Experiments on the value of vascular and visceral factors for the genesis of emotion. *Proceedings of the Royal Society* **66**: 390–403.
30. Dana CL (1921) The anatomic seat of the emotions: a discussion of the James–Lange theory. *Archives of Neurology and Psychiatry* **6**: 634.
31. Chwalisz K, Diener E, Gallagher D (1988) Autonomic arousal feedback and emotional experience: evidence from the spinal cord injured. *Journal of Personality and Social Psychology* **54**: 820–28.
32. Carlson NR (1992) *Foundations of Physiological Psychology*, 2nd edn. Boston, MA: Allyn & Bacon.
33. Pinel JPJ (1993) *Biopsychology*, 2nd edn. Boston, MA: Allyn & Bacon.
34. Schachter S, Wheeler L (1962) Epinephrine, chlorpromazine and amusement. *Journal of Abnormal and Social Psychology* **65**: 121–8.
35. Dutton DC, Aron AP (1974) Some evidence for heightened sexual attraction under conditions of high anxiety. *Journal of Personality and Social Psychology* **30**: 510–17.
36. Mandler G (1967) Organization and memory. In KW Spence, JT Spence (eds) *The Psychology of Learning and Motivation*, Vol. 1. New York: Academic Press.
37. Fiske ST, Taylor SE (1991) *Social Cognition*, 2nd edn. New York: McGraw-Hill.
38. Plutchik R, Ax AF (1967) A critique of determinants of emotional state by Schachter and Singer (1962). *Psychophysiology* **4**: 79–82.
39. Marshall G, Zimbardo P (1979) Affective consequences of inadequately explaining physiological arousal. *Journal of Personality and Social Psychology* **37**: 970–88.
40. Maslach C (1979) Negative emotional biasing of unexplained arousal. *Journal of Personality and Social Psychology* **37**: 953–69.
41. Weiner B (1986) *An Attributional Theory of Motivation and Emotion*. New York: Springer-Verlag.
42. Weiner B (1992) *Human Motivation: Metaphors, Theories and Research*, Newbury Park, CA: Sage.
43. Ross L, Nisbett RE (1991) *The Person and the Situation: Perspectives of Social Psychology*. New York: McGraw-Hill.
44. Dutton DC, Aron AP (1989) Romantic attraction and generalized liking for others who are sources of conflict-based arousal. *Canadian Journal of Behavioural Science* **21**: 246–57.
45. Olson JM, Ross M (1988) False feedback about placebo effectiveness: consequences for the misattribution of speech activity. *Journal of Experimental Social Psychology* **24**: 275–91.
46. Taylor SE, Peplau LA, Sears DO (1994) *Social Psychology*, 8th edn. Englewood Cliffs, NJ: Prentice-Hall.

47. Lazarus RS (1982) Thoughts on the relations between emotion and cognition. *American Psychologist* **37**: 1019–24.
48. Speisman JC, Lazarus RS, Mordkoff AM, Davidson LA (1964) The experimental reduction of stress based on ego defence theory. *Journal of Abnormal and Social Psychology* **68**: 397–8.
49. Zajonc RB (1984) On the primacy of affect. *American Psychologist* **39**: 117–23.
50. Gross R (2008) *Key Studies in Psychology*, 5th edn. London: Hodder Education.
51. Eysenck MW, Keane MJ (1990) *Cognitive Psychology: A Student's Handbook*. Hove: Lawrence Erlbaum Associates.
52. Frijda NH (1994) Varieties of affect: emotions and episodes, moods and sentiments. In P Ekman, RJ Davidson (eds) *The Nature of Emotion: Fundamental Questions*. New York: Oxford University Press.
53. Clore GL (1994) Why emotions require cognition. In P Ekman, RJ Davidson (eds) *The Nature of Emotion: Fundamental Questions*. New York: Oxford University Press.
54. Scherer KR (1994) Toward a concept of 'modal emotions'. In P Ekman, RJ Davidson (eds) *The Nature of Emotions: Fundamental Questions*. New York: Oxford University Press.
55. Panksepp J (1994) The basics of basic emotion. In P Ekman, RJ Davidson (eds) *The Nature of Emotion: Fundamental Questions*. New York: Oxford University Press.
56. Davidson RJ, Ekman (1994) Afterword: what are the minimal cognitive prerequisites for emotion? In P Ekman, RJ Davidson (eds) *The Nature of Emotion: Fundamental Questions*. New York: Oxford University Press.
57. Dalgleish T (1998) Emotion. In M Eysenck (ed.) *Psychology: An Integrated Approach*. Harlow: Longman.

Chapter 13

Information-processing and attention

Richard Gross

INTRODUCTION

According to Titchener, a student of Wundt: 'The doctrine of attention is the nerve of the whole psychological system'.[1] However, the Gestalt psychologists (see Box 9.1 in Chapter 9) believed that the concept of attention was unnecessary (a stimulus array's properties were sufficient to predict the perceptual response to it: see Chapter 16). The behaviourists argued that, since 'attention' was unobservable, it was not worthy of experimental study (see Chapters 10 and 14).

Interest in the study of attention re-emerged following the publication of Broadbent's *Perception and Communication*, which also had a great impact on the development of cognitive psychology overall.[2] Broadbent argued that the world is composed of many more sensations than can be handled by the perceptual and cognitive capabilities of the human observer. To cope with the flood of available information, humans must selectively attend to only some information and somehow 'tune out' the rest. Attention, therefore, is the result of a limited-capacity information-processing system. Solso calls this a 'pipeline' theory.[3] To understand our ability to selectively attend to things, researchers study focused (or selective) attention.

Central to the information-processing approach is the computer analogy. This is arguably most evident in explanations of memory (see Chapter 17) and attention. Concepts such as buffer store and limited-capacity processor are drawn from information technology (IT) and built into the models of attention that we discuss in this chapter.

Almost all the early models of attention assumed *serial processing*, a step-by-step process in which each operation is carried out in turn. The first of these was Broadbent's *filter model*,[2] followed by Treisman's *attenuation model*[4] and the *pertinence model*.[5,6] These are all single-channel models of selective attention. But early attempts to explain *divided attention*, such as Kahneman's *central capacity theory*,[7] also assumed serial processing. In *parallel processing*, two or more operations are carried out at the same time. This is the view taken in Allport's *multi-channel theory* of divided attention (doing more than one thing at a time).[8]

Assumptions about serial and parallel processing reflect changes in the underlying computer analogy, which in turn reflect developments in computer technology. For much of the 1950s and 1960s, computers were capable only of serial processing. During the 1980s and 1990s, machines capable of massive parallel processing were built, and theorists have returned to an earlier belief that cognitive theories should be based more closely on the brain's neural networks.[9,10] The human brain is the parallel processing machine par excellence.

WHAT IS ATTENTION?

One famous definition of attention is that of William James, according to whom:

> It is the taking possession by the mind, in clear and vivid form, of one out of what seem several simultaneously possible objects or trains of thought. Focalization, concentration of consciousness are of its essence. It implies withdrawal from some things in order to deal effectively with others.[11]

Although we cannot necessarily equate attention with consciousness (see below), James's definition underlines the selective nature of attention. This is echoed in Solso's definition: '... the concentration of mental effort on sensory or mental events'.[3] However, this is only one of two major ways in which attention has been defined and investigated. A crucial distinction is made between the following:

- The mechanisms by which certain information is registered and other information is rejected, whether or not the latter enters conscious awareness (*selective* or *focused attention*).
- Some upper limit to the amount of processing that can be performed on incoming information at any one time (*capacity* or *divided attention*).

As we saw in Chapter 10, the term 'attention' has also been used to refer to arousal level, vigilance, and the ability to stay alert and concentrate.

METHODS OF STUDYING ATTENTION

Selective attention

People are presented with two or more simultaneous 'messages' and are instructed to process and respond to only one of them. The most popular way of doing this is to use *shadowing*, in which one message is fed into the left ear and a different message into the right ear (through headphones). Participants have to repeat one of these messages aloud as they hear it.

The shadowing technique is a particular form of *dichotic listening*.[12] This is the simultaneous reception of two different stimulus inputs, one to each ear. Shadowing was first used by Cherry, who wanted to study the *cocktail party phenomenon*, in which we manage to select one or two voices to listen to from the hubbub of conversations taking place at the same time and in the same room.[13] The participant is asked to select, which can tell us something about the selection process and what happens to unattended stimuli. Most studies have looked at auditory attention.

Divided attention

In the *dual-task technique*, people are asked to attend and respond to both or all of the messages. Whereas shadowing focuses attention on a particular message, the dual-task method deliberately divides the participant's attention. This provides useful information about a person's processing limitations, attention mechanisms and their capacity.

SELECTIVE (OR FOCUSED) AUDITORY ATTENTION

Cherry's dichotic listening and shadowing research

In his initial experiments, Cherry's participants wore headphones through which pairs of spoken prose messages were presented to both ears simultaneously (*binaural listening*). Cherry found that various physical differences affected a person's ability to select one of the messages to attend to, in particular voice intensity, the speaker's location and the speaker's gender. Cherry also found that, when these differences were controlled for in the two messages (so that each message was, say, spoken in an equally intense female voice), their meaning was extremely difficult to separate. In later experiments, Cherry used dichotic listening and shadowing. Although participants were able to shadow the specified message, little of the non-shadowed message was remembered. Box 13.1 lists other research findings from shadowing.

Box 13.1 Other research findings using shadowing

- Little of the non-shadowed message was remembered, even when the same word was presented 35 times to the non-shadowed ear.[14]
- Participants did not notice whether the message was spoken in a foreign language or changed from English to a different language.
- Although speech played backwards was reported as having 'something queer about it', most participants believed it to be normal speech.
- A pure tone of 400 cycles/s was nearly always noticed, as was a change of voice from male to female or from female to male.

These data suggested that, although the physical properties of the message in the non-shadowed ear were 'heard', semantic content (its meaning) was completely lost.

Researchers quickly moved on from Cherry's original question about how we can attend to one conversation, and began asking why so little seemed to be remembered about the other conversations.[15]

Broadbent's split-span studies

Broadbent reported the results of a series of studies using the *split-span procedure*.[12] In this study, three digits (e.g. 8, 2, 1) are presented via headphones to one ear at the rate of one digit every half-second. Simultaneously, three different digits (e.g. 7, 3, 4) are presented to the other ear. The task is to listen to the two sets of numbers and then write down as much as can be remembered.

The digits can be recalled either:

- according to the ear of presentation – *ear-by-ear recall*: the numbers above could be recalled as either 8, 2, 1, 7, 3, 4 or 7, 3, 4, 8, 2, 1; or
- according to their chronological order of presentation – *pair-by-pair recall*. Since the digits have been presented in pairs, this would involve recalling the first pair (8, 7 or 7, 8), followed by the second pair (2, 3 or 3, 2) and finally the third pair (1, 4 or 4, 1).

When subjects are simply given a list of six digits at a rate of one every half-second, serial recall is typically 95 per cent accurate. However, Broadbent found that the split-span procedure produced accurate recall only 65 per cent of the time. Moreover, pair-by-pair recall was considerably poorer than ear-by-ear recall. If given a choice, people preferred ear-by-ear recall.

SINGLE-CHANNEL THEORIES OF FOCUSED AUDITORY ATTENTION

Single-channel theories propose that somewhere in information processing is a 'bottleneck' or filter that allows some information to be passed on for further analysis, while the other information is either discarded or processed to only a limited degree. The three theories that have been proposed differ mainly over whether the filtering takes place early or late in information-processing. This means that they differ in terms of the nature and extent of processing of the non-attended material.

Broadbent's early-selection filter theory

Broadbent's theory was the first systematic attempt to explain both Cherry's findings and the findings of split-span experiments.[2] Broadbent assumes that our ability to process information is capacity-limited. Information from the senses passes 'in parallel' to a short-term store. This is a temporary 'buffer system', which holds information until it can be processed further and, effectively, extends the duration of a stimulus (see Chapter 17). The various types of information (e.g. two or more voices) are preserved in their original form and then passed to a selective filter. This operates on the basis of the information's physical characteristics, selecting one source for further analysis and rejecting all others.

Information allowed through the filter reaches a limited-capacity channel (the filter is necessary precisely because the channel is capacity-limited). This corresponds to the 'span of consciousness',[11] or what we experience as happening now. The information allowed through the filter is analysed in that it is recognized, possibly rehearsed and then transferred to the motor effectors (muscles), producing an appropriate response (Figure 13.1).

Broadbent considered the short-term store to be capable of holding information for a period of time before it decayed. So, two simultaneous stimuli can be processed, provided that the processor can get back to the store before the information in it has disappeared. Consequently, attending to one thing does not necessarily mean that everything else is lost. However, Broadbent maintained that processing two different pieces of information from two channels would always take longer, and be less efficient, than processing the same information from one channel. This is because switching attention between channels takes a substantial period of time.

Tests of Broadbent's theory

According to the filter theory, (i) the non-shadowed message is not allowed to pass through the filter and (ii) the input to the relevant ear is the physical property on which the information is selected.

However, the theory assumes that, because the non-shadowed message is filtered out according to its physical characteristics, its meaning should not be subject to any sort of higher-level analysis. But when we are at a party, our attention sometimes switches from the person with whom we are conversing to another part of the room (e.g. if we hear our name mentioned). This was demonstrated

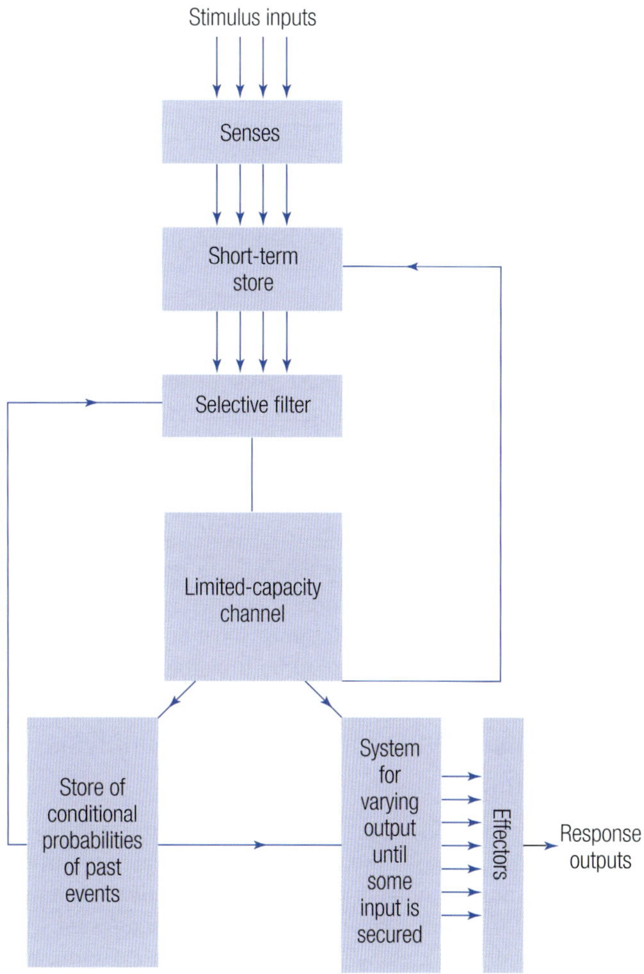

Figure 13.1 Broadbent's theory of the flow of information between stimulus and response

experimentally by Moray, who found that when the participant's name was presented to the non-attended (non-shadowed) ear, attention switched to that ear about one-third of the time.[14]

An evaluation of Broadbent's theory

- Treisman found that if meaningful material presented to the attended ear was switched in mid-sentence to the non-attended ear, participants would occasionally change the focus of their attention to the non-attended ear and then shadow that material before changing back to the attended ear.[16]
- Treisman discovered that if a French translation of the shadowed material was presented as non-shadowed material, some bilingual participants realized that the shadowed and non-shadowed material had the same meaning.[4]
- Corteen and Wood conditioned participants to produce a galvanic skin response (GSR) whenever they heard a particular target word.[17] A small electric shock was delivered immediately after the target word was heard.

The target word produced a GSR when presented to the non-attended ear, as did synonyms. However, GSRs did not occur every time the conditioned words were presented.

- Mackay presented the word 'bank' in a sentence, and participants subsequently had to recognize the sentence they had heard. Recognition was influenced by whether the word 'river' or 'money' had been presented to the non-attended ear.[18]

These studies, and that of Gray and Wedderburn (Box 13.2),[19] suggest that the meaning of the input to the non-attended ear is processed at least some of the time. Further, Underwood found that participants trained at shadowing can detect two-thirds of the material presented to the non-attended ear.[20] This throws doubt on Broadbent's claim that the non-shadowed message is always rejected at an early stage of processing. Also, when the material used is sufficiently different (such as one being auditory and the other visual), then memory for the non-shadowed message is good. This indicates that the material must have been processed at a higher level than that proposed by Broadbent.[21]

Treisman's attenuation (or stimulus-analysis system) model

According to Treisman,[4,16] competing information is analysed for things other than its physical properties, including sounds, syllable patterns, grammatical structure and the information's meaning.[15] Treisman suggested that the non-shadowed message is not filtered out early on, but that the selective filter *attenuates* it (Figure 13.2). So, a message that is not selected on the basis of its physical properties would not be rejected completely, but its 'volume' would be 'turned down'.

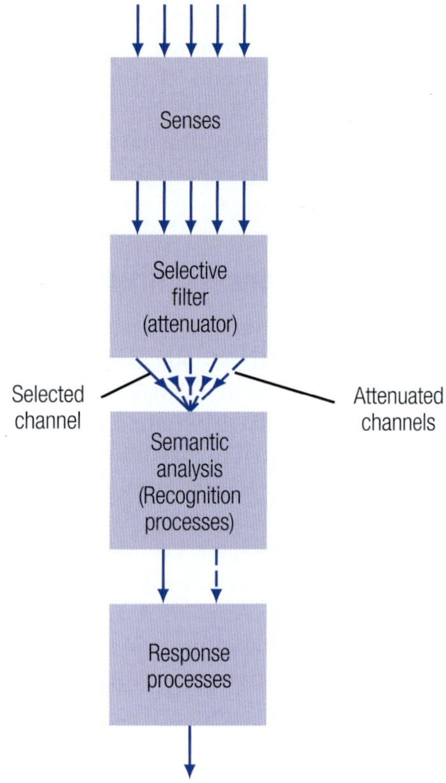

Figure 13.2 Treisman's attenuation model

Both non-attenuated and attenuated information undergoes these further analyses. This may result in an attenuated message being attended to, depending on its features. Treisman suggested that biologically relevant and emotionally important stimuli may be 'pre-sets' to which attention is switched, irrespective of the content of the attenuated message. This accounts for our ability to switch attention to a different conversation when our name is mentioned. Since it is the features of a stimulus that determine whether or not the stimulus is attended to, the concept of *probabilistic filtering* is perhaps a better way of appreciating Treisman's theory than that of attenuation.[22]

Box 13.2 Why use one ear when two will do?[19]

Gray and Wedderburn presented, to each ear alternately, the syllables composing a word, plus random digits. Thus, when one ear 'heard' a syllable, the other 'heard' a digit. For example, in one experiment, participants heard the following:

- *Left ear:* OB 2 TIVE
- *Right ear:* 6 JEC 9

In other experiments, phrases were used in place of words, such as 'Dear Aunt Jane', 'Mice eat cheese' and 'What the hell'.

According to Broadbent, participants should have reported 'ob-two-tive', or 'six-jec-nine'. This, of course, is nonsense. But the filter model maintains that it is the physical nature of the auditory signal (which ear receives which input), and not meaning, that determines what is attended to and, hence, what is recalled.

What participants actually reported was 'objective' or 'Dear Aunt Jane', etc. In other words, they acted 'intelligently'. The ears do not always function as different information channels, and switching between channels is fairly easy to do.

The Deutsch–Norman late-selection filter model

Deutsch and Deutsch[5] and Norman[23,24] completely rejected Broadbent's claim that information is filtered out early on. According to the Deutsch–Norman model, filtering or selection occurs only after all inputs have been analysed at a high level, for example after each word has been recognized by the memory system and analysed for meaning (Figure 13.3).

The filter is placed nearer the response end of the processing system; hence, it is a 'late' selection filter. Because processing will have already been undertaken on the infor-

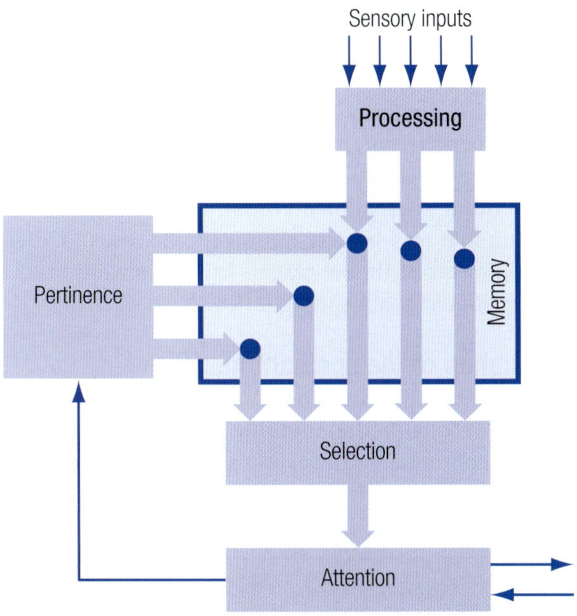

Figure 13.3 The Deutsch–Norman theory of focused attention. All sensory inputs receive perceptual processing and are recognized in the sense that they excite their representations (●) in memory. The information selected is that which has the greatest pertinence[23]

mation that has been presented, some information will have been established as pertinent (most relevant) and will have activated particular memory representations; this is why the model is sometimes called the *pertinence model*. When one memory representation is selected for further processing, attention becomes selective. The model implies that we perceive everything we encounter but are consciously aware of only some of it.[15]

Tests of the Treisman and Deutsch–Norman models

Both the Treisman and the Deutsch–Norman model can account for the processing of non-shadowed material (whereas Broadbent's theory cannot). If the Deutsch–Norman model is correct, then participants should be able to identify as many target words in the non-shadowed message as in the shadowed message, since both are allegedly completely analysed for meaning. Treisman and Geffen, however, found that target words were much better detected in the shadowed message (87%) than in the non-shadowed message (8%).[25] This is consistent with Treisman's view that the non-shadowed message is attenuated.

However, Treisman and Geffen's findings assume that the shadowed and non-shadowed messages are equally important. Deutsch and Deutsch argued that this assumption wasn't met, because participants had to indicate when they heard a target word by tapping.[26] In other words, participants had to shadow and tap in one message, but only tap in the other. This made the target words in the shadowed message more important than those in the non-shadowed message. Treisman and Riley overcame this problem by requiring participants to stop shadowing and to tap as soon as they detected a target word in either ear.[27] Under such conditions, performance was still better for the shadowed message (76%) than for the non-shadowed message (33%).

This finding is consistent with Treisman's model, but inconsistent with the Deutsch–Norman claim that performance should not differ (since the targets were equally pertinent, irrespective of the ear to which they were presented). However, the detection rate for the non-attended ear in Treisman and Riley's study (33%) was much higher than that in Treisman and Geffen's study (8%). This provides some support for the Deutsch–Norman model.

The Deutsch–Norman model predicts that participants asked immediately afterwards should be able to repeat back the words presented to the non-shadowed ear. However, the non-shadowed message gets into short-term memory for only a brief period and is then forgotten very quickly. Norman found that participants could remember the last couple of words presented to the non-attended ear if tested immediately, but not after a short continuation of the shadowing task.[6] This finding was replicated by Glucksberg and Cowan.[28]

An evaluation of single-channel models

- Despite some support for the Deutsch–Norman model, Wilding believes that less is known about non-attended messages than the model claims.[29] However, more is known than can be explained by either Broadbent's or Treisman's models.
- The major criticism of single-channel theories is their lack of flexibility, and several more 'flexible' theories have been advanced. According to Johnston and Heinz, attentional selectivity can occur at several different stages of processing, depending on the demands made by the experimental task.[30] In order to minimize demands on capacity, selection is made as early as possible.
- Johnston and Heinz[31] and Johnston and Wilson[32] presented findings consistent with their view that processing is more flexible than predicted by single-channel theories. For example, Johnston and Wilson showed that participants processed words presented to both ears, but only when they did not know to which ear particular target words would be presented. These data suggest that non-target words are processed only to the extent necessary to perform a task.
- Many researchers question whether any single, general-purpose, limited-capacity central processor can, in principle, account for the complexities of selective attention.[8,33,34] Much of the relevant evidence comes from dual-task studies, which are concerned more directly with processing capacity – that is, divided attention (see below).

FOCUSED VISUAL ATTENTION

According to Driver:

The cluttered scenes of everyday life present more objects than we can respond towards simultaneously, and often more than we can perceive fully at any one time. Accordingly, mechanisms of attention are required to select objects of interest for further processing. In the case of vision, one such mechanism is provided by eye movements, which allow us to fixate particular regions so that they benefit from the greater acuity of the fovea.[35]

The fovea provides maximum acuity for visual stimuli. So, when we fixate on an object, maximum visual processing is carried out on the object whose image is projected on to the fovea. The resources given to the other parts of the visual field are 'attenuated'.[36]

Posner and colleagues found that when individuals are told to fixate on one part of the visual field, it is still possible to attend to stimuli about 7 degrees either side of the fixation point.[37,38] Also, attention can be shifted more quickly when a stimulus is presented in an expected rather than an unexpected location. Thus, visual attention is not confined to the part of the visual field that is processed by the fovea but can be shifted without corresponding changes in eye movements. Indeed, such shifts in attention frequently precede the corresponding eye movement.[36] Posner calls this 'covert attention'.[39]

The internal mental spotlight and the zoom lens

Posner likened covert attention to an internal mental spotlight that 'illuminates' any stimulus in the attended region, so that it is perceived in greater detail. It essentially duplicates the functions of eye movements internally, by allowing a particular region of space to be perceptually enhanced.[35]

LaBerge required participants to judge whether the middle letter of five letters (e.g. L A C I E) came from the beginning or end of the alphabet (*directed attention condition*).[40] But on some occasions, a stimulus such as – 7 – – – was presented, and the task was to determine whether the 7 was one of two letters (T or Z). LaBerge found that the speed of judgement was a function of the distance from the centre of attention. Thus, reaction times were fastest for items at the centre of the stimulus and slower for those at its periphery, even though all items were within the fovea's region.

LaBerge concluded that visual attention is most concentrated at the centre of the internal spotlight and least at its periphery. When information beyond its centre needs to be processed, the spotlight must be shifted to ensure maximal processing. Because this takes time, participants in Posner and colleagues' experiments took longer to judge a stimulus when it appeared in an unexpected location.[41]

LaBerge also found that when participants were required to attend to the whole five-letter word string (*global attention condition*), the 'width' of the spotlight's 'beam' increased (based on the similarity of reaction times for items at the centre and periphery). These findings led Eriksen to propose the *zoom-lens model* of visual attention.[42] This accepts the existence of an internal mental spotlight but suggests that it has a beam that may be very narrow (in the case of LaBerge's letter task) or broad (in the case of LaBerge's word task). It is simply a variable-beam spotlight.[43]

An evaluation of the spotlight model

Despite evidence that little or no processing occurs beyond the spotlight,[44] both the spotlight and zoom-lens models have been contradicted in several studies (Box 13.3).

Box 13.3 Neisser and Becklen's study of selective visual attention[45]

Visual selective attention was studied by superimposing a film of three people playing a ball game on a film that showed two people's hands clapping (Figure 13.4).

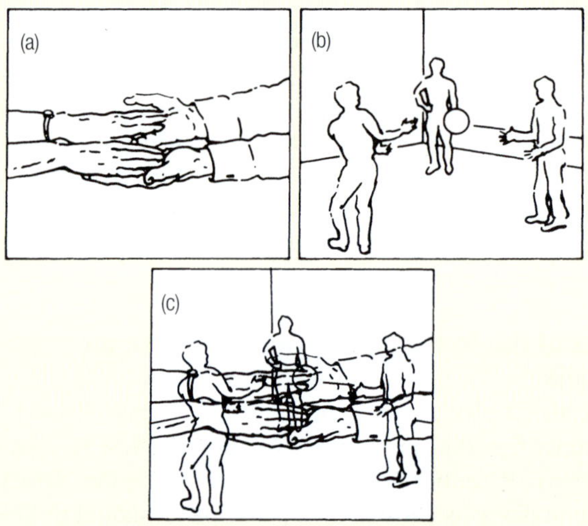

Figure 13.4 A film of two people clapping hands (a) and a film of three people playing a ball game (b) have been superimposed (c)

The task was to follow one of the films and press a key to indicate that a critical event, such as the ball being thrown, had occurred.

Adults found it difficult to follow both films simultaneously, but they were able to attend selectively to one or other of the films easily. This is difficult for the zoom-lens model to explain, since the model proposes that the focus of attention is a given area in visual space, rather than objects within that area.[9]

Using Neisser and Becklen's methodology, it has been shown that infants as young as 4 months can selectively follow one of the two films. This suggests that selective visual attention is innate rather than learned.

The fate of unattended visual stimuli

For Johnston and Dark, stimuli beyond the focus of visual attention are subject to no, or virtually no, semantic processing.[44] Any such processing is limited to mainly simple physical features. However, Driver disagrees.[35] For example, when a picture is shown as the unattended stimulus on one trial, it slows the processing of an attended word with an identical or similar meaning on the next trial (*negative priming*). The fact that processing of the attended stimulus is reduced suggests that the meaning of the unattended stimulus must have been subject to some sort of processing.[46]

Treisman's feature-integration theory

Treisman's theory was developed on the basis of findings using the visual search procedure.[47] Participants are presented with an array of visual material (Figure 13.5) in which a target item is embedded on some trials but absent on others, and the 'distractor' items can be varied so that they are similar to or different from the target letter. The participant's task is to decide whether the target is present or absent.

X P T L A B N T

A R H N J I F R

E W R N P A Z X

A H Y 5 Y T E S

A N H C E S T I

G D T K D Y U I

Figure 13.5 Visual search array. The task is to find the number 5 among the letters

Neisser argued that when people perform a visual search task, they process many items simultaneously, without being fully aware of the exact nature of the distractor items.[48] Visual information-processing might occur pre-attentively, depending on the nature of the stimuli (such as whether they have angular or curved features when the task is to detect a particular letter).

However, Treisman argues that attention must be focused on a stimulus before its features can be synthesized into a pattern. In one of Treisman and Gelade's experiments, participants were required to detect the presence of the letter T among an array of Is and Ys.[49] Because the horizontal bar at the top of a T distinguishes it from an I and a Y, this could be done fairly easily just by looking for the horizontal bar. Participants took around 800 ms to detect the T, and the detection time was not affected by the size of the array (i.e. the number of Is and Ys). In another experiment, the T was embedded in an array of Is and Zs. Here, looking for a horizontal bar on its own does not aid detection, since the letter Z also has a horizontal bar at the top. To detect a T, participants needed to look for the conjunction of a horizontal and vertical line. This took around 1200 ms. Moreover, detection time was longer when the size of the array was increased. On the basis of these (and other) findings, Treisman proposed her *feature-integration theory* (Box 13.4).

An evaluation of Treisman's theory

- Treisman has claimed evidence for the occurrence of illusory conjunctions in her visual search experiments. Treisman and Schmidt, for example, required participants to identify two black digits flashed in one part of the visual field.[50] In another part, letters in various colours were presented (e.g. a blue T or a red S). After reporting the digits, participants were asked what letters they had seen and their colour. Most participants reported seeing illusory conjunctions (e.g. a blue S) almost as frequently as correct conjunctions. This supports the view that accurate perception occurs only when attention is focused on an object. When it is not, the features of objects are processed but not always combined accurately.
- However, results from experiments in which moving items are intermingled with static items challenge Treisman's theory (Box 13.5).

Visual attention and brain damage

Many researchers are interested in the brain regions involved in attention (e.g. Driver,[35] Halligan[52]). People who have had a right-hemisphere stroke involving the parietal

Box 13.4 Treisman's feature-integration theory

According to Treisman, it is possible to distinguish between objects (e.g. a strawberry) and their features (e.g. being red, possessing curves, being of a particular size).

In the first stage of visual processing, we process the features of stimuli in the visual environment rapidly and in parallel, without attention being required. Next, the features are combined to form objects (e.g. a small, red, curved object). This second stage of processing is a slow and serial process.

Focusing attention on an object's location provides the 'glue' that allows meaningless features to be formed into objects. But features can also be combined on the basis of knowledge stored in memory (e.g. the knowledge that strawberries are typically red).

When relevant stored knowledge is not available or focused attention is absent, feature combination occurs in a random way. This can produce illusory conjunctions (e.g. a blue banana) or odd combinations of features.

Based on Anderson[36] and Eysenck and Keane.[9]

Box 13.5 The moving target experiment[51]

Participants were asked to search for the presence or absence of a single moving X among static Xs and moving Os (Figure 13.6). The target is defined only by its specific conjunction of form and movement, since its shape is shared with the static Xs and its movement with the Os.

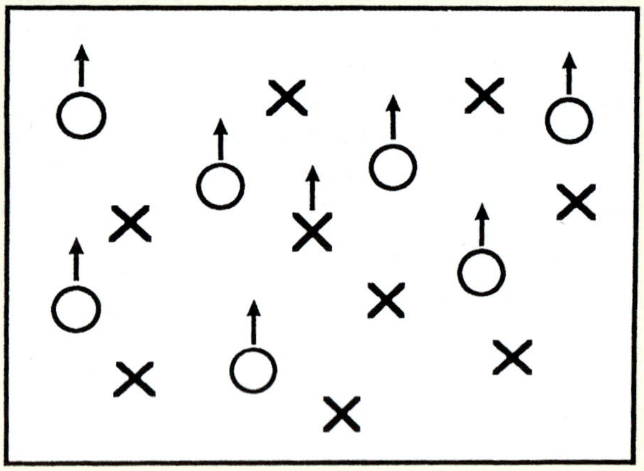

Figure 13.6 Schematic representation of the display used by McLeod *et al.*[51] The arrows indicate motion, and the task is to search for a single moving X among moving Os and intermingled static Xs

Treisman's theory would predict that serial attention was necessary for each item when searching for the target, so that decision times would increase with an increasing number of distractors.

In fact, the target was found easily, regardless of the display's size. This implies a *parallel process*, and in other experiments McLeod *et al.* showed that the parallel search arose because attention could be restricted to just the group of items with common motion to the exclusion of the static items. Because the target has a unique shape, it can be detected in parallel.

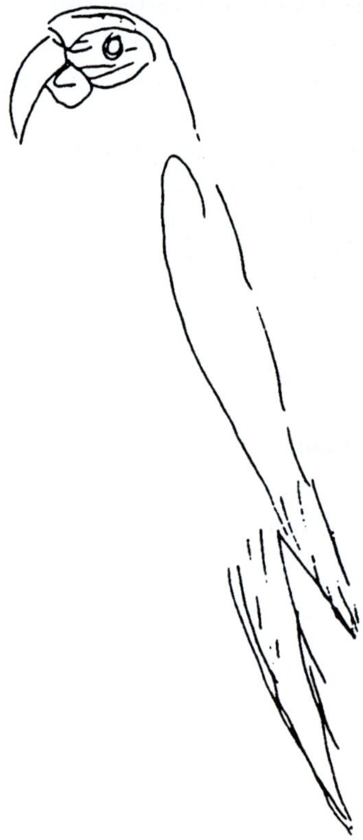

Figure 13.7 Drawing of a parrot by a person with left-side neglect

lobe may completely ignore stimuli occurring on the left side; for example, they may fail to eat food from the left side of their plate and be unaware of their body on that side (Figure 13.7). The fascinating thing about this *unilateral visual neglect* is that these effects occur even though the pathways from the receptors to the central nervous system (CNS) for the neglected information remain intact.

According to Posner and Petersen, the parietal lobe is responsible for disengaging attention from its present focus,[53] and patients with damage to the pulvinar nucleus (part of the thalami) have difficulty in shifting attention to a new target.[54]

Interestingly, among 4- to 10-year-old children, those who took less time to switch attention in a specially devised computer game were more likely to show awareness of traffic as they approached a busy road.[55]

DIVIDED ATTENTION

Some demonstrations of dual-task performance

Allport *et al.* showed that skilled pianists were able to read music successfully while shadowing speech.[21] Later, Shaffer reported the case of an expert typist who could type accurately from sight while shadowing speech.[56] Perhaps the most striking example of dual-task performance comes from Spelke *et al.*, who had two students spend 5 hours a week training at performing two tasks simultaneously.[57] Initially, the students were required to read short stories while writing down dictated words. At first they found this difficult, and both their comprehension and writing suffered. But after 6 weeks of training, the students could read as quickly, and comprehend as much of what they read, when reading with dictation as when reading without it. Interestingly, though, they could remember very little of what they had written down, even though thousands of words had been dictated to them over the course of the experiment.

At this point, the task was altered and the students had to write down the category to which a word belonged (requiring more processing of the words), while simultaneously reading the short stories. Although again the task was difficult initially, they eventually performed it without any reduction in their comprehension of the stories.

Factors affecting dual-task performance

According to Hampson, factors that make one task easier also tend to make the other easier because 'Anything which minimises interference between processes or keeps them "further apart" will allow them to be dealt with more readily either selectively or together'.[58]

Eysenck and Keane identify three factors that affect our ability to perform two tasks at once: difficulty, practice and similarity (Box 13.6).[9]

Theories of divided attention

As we noted earlier, models of selective attention assume the existence of a limited-capacity filter capable of dealing with one information channel at a time. As Hampson and Morris have observed, these theories

> ... imply a series of stages of processing, starting with superficial, physical analysis, and working 'upwards' towards the 'higher' cognitive analyses for meaning.[15]

> **Box 13.6 Effects of difficulty, practice and similarity on dual-task performance**
>
> - *Difficulty:* generally, the more difficult the task, the less successful is dual-task performance. However, it is hard to define task difficulty objectively, since a task that is difficult for one person might not be difficult for another (this relates to practice: see below). Also, the demands made by two tasks individually are not necessarily the same as when the tasks are performed concurrently. Thus, performing two tasks together may introduce fresh demands and the risk of interference.
> - *Practice:* as we have seen, practice improves dual-task performance. This could be because people develop new strategies for performing each task, minimizing interference between them. Another possibility is that practice reduces a task's attentional demands. Finally, practice may produce a more economical way of functioning that uses fewer resources.
> - *Similarity:* Allport *et al.* showed that when people are required to shadow one message and learn pictorial information, both tasks can be performed successfully.[21] This is, presumably, because they do not involve the same stimulus modality. Two tasks also disrupt performance when both rely on related memory codes (e.g. visual memory), make use of the same stages of processing (e.g. the input stage) or require similar responses to be made.
>
> Based on Eysenck and Keane.[9]

In Hampson and Morris's view, these processes are better thought of as an integrated mechanism, with the high and low levels interacting and combining in the recognition of stimuli. Accordingly, it is better to look at the system's overall processing.

Limited-capacity theories

Kahneman's theory

According to Kahneman, humans have a limited amount of processing capacity, and whether or not tasks can be performed successfully depends on how much demand they make on the limited-capacity processor.[7] Some tasks require little processing capacity, leaving plenty available for performing another task simultaneously. Others require much more, leaving little 'spare'.

The process of determining how much capacity is available ('effort') is related to the allocation of that capacity. How much capacity a task requires depends on things such as its difficulty and a person's experience of it. How capacity is allocated depends on *enduring dispositions*, *momentary intentions* and the *evaluation of the attentional demands* (Figure 13.8). The central processor is responsible for the allocation policy and constantly evaluates the level of demand. When demand is too high, the central processor must decide how available attention should be allocated.

Kahneman sees arousal as playing an important part in determining how much capacity is available. Generally,

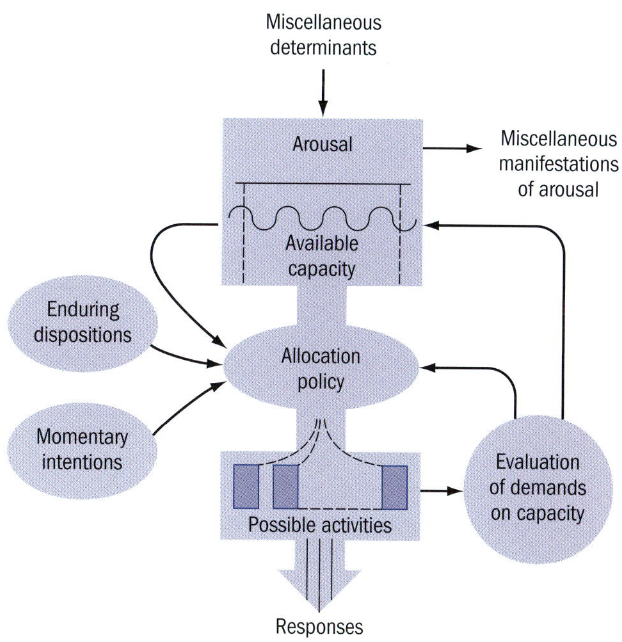

Figure 13.8 Kahneman's theory of attention. Enduring dispositions are the rules for allocating capacity that are outside voluntary control. These include allocating capacity to novel stimuli and hearing one's own name used in a different conversation. Momentary intentions are voluntary shifts in attention such as listening to a message in a dichotic listening task. Evaluation of demands on capacity include rules for overload on the system, such as deciding to complete one task rather than failing to complete two tasks

more attentional resources are available when we are aroused and alert than when we are tired and lethargic. Attention can be divided between tasks, provided that the total available capacity is not exceeded. This explains the findings of the dichotic listening tasks discussed earlier: shadowing requires almost all of the capacity available, leaving the non-shadowed message insufficient capacity. Kahneman's theory also predicts that, as skill at carrying out a task increases, so less capacity is needed for it and more becomes available for other tasks. Thus, when people are trained at shadowing, they become able to shadow and to attend to the non-shadowed message.[20]

Evaluation of Kahneman's theory

Kahneman's theory portrays attention as a much more flexible and dynamic system than do the models of focused attention. However, it does not address the issue of how decisions to channel attention are made. The difficulty in defining the general limits of capacity has led some researchers to suggest that the concept of limited capacity should be abandoned.[15]

Norman and Bobrow's theory

Following on from Kahneman, Norman and Bobrow have offered a *central capacity interference* account of attentional phenomena (Box 13.7).[33]

Evaluation of Norman and Bobrow's theory

This distinction between resource- and data-limited processes can explain findings from both focused and divided attention research. For example, Treisman and Geffen found that participants shadowing words in one ear had difficulty recognizing target words presented simultaneously to the other ear.[25] Lawson, however, found that under similar conditions, participants could detect target tones presented in the non-attended ear.[59] This finding can be explained by proposing that the tone-detection process becomes data-limited much sooner than the word-recognition process.

Box 13.7 Norman and Bobrow's central capacity interference theory[33]

This theory's central feature is its distinction between *resource-limited* and *data-limited* processes. On a complex task, performance is related to the amount of resources devoted to it. As more resources are allocated, so task performance improves up to some point. Performance is thus resource-limited.

But on some tasks, applying more resources does not lead to improved performance because of external influences (e.g. when participants are required to identify a quiet tone among loud, masking 'white' noise). This sort of task is data-limited, because performance can be improved only by altering the stimuli (e.g. by making the tone louder or the masking noise quieter).

However, the theory's biggest weakness is its inability to predict beforehand the results that an experiment is likely to produce. Because it allows for differential allocation of resources to tasks, an experimenter can never know the level of resources allocated to a particular task. Any results can therefore be interpreted in a way consistent with the theory, and no results can ever be taken as negative evidence.

Multi-channel theories

Supporters of limited-capacity models defend their approach by pointing out that the attentional system breaks down as more and more is demanded of it. Also, if data from divided-attention studies are considered carefully, it is not true that two tasks can be performed together with no disruption at all.[60] Nevertheless, several researchers have rejected the concept of a general-purpose, limited-capacity processor completely. For Allport, the concept of attention is often used synonymously with 'consciousness', with no specification of how it operates.[8,61,62] This has done little to increase our understanding of the very problems that it is meant to explain.

Modules and multiple resources

According to Allport, it is difficult to see how the neurology of the brain could produce a system of processing capacity that was completely open to any of the tasks that might be presented to it.[15] It is much more profitable to view the data in terms of tasks competing for the same specialized processing mechanisms or modules, each of which has a limited capacity but none of which is uniquely 'central'.

When two tasks are highly similar, they compete for the same modules, and this leads to performance impairments. However, because dissimilar tasks use different modules, both can be performed simultaneously. A virtually identical theoretical account has been proposed by Navon and Gopher[63] and Wickens[64] in their *multiple-resource theory*. Certainly, the findings of dual-task studies (e.g. Allport *et al.*[21]) are consistent with the idea of different processing mechanisms handling the requirements of different tasks.

However, this approach is also non-falsifiable, since any pattern of data can be explained by proposing the existence of a particular pattern of modules.[65] If multiple resources do operate in parallel, then they must do so in a highly integrated way, since our behaviour is typically coherent.[9]

Attempts at synthesizing capacity and module accounts

According to Eysenck[66–68] and Baddeley,[69] a much better way of accommodating the data from divided-attention studies is to see capacity and module accounts as being complementary rather than competitive. *Synthesis models* propose the existence of a *modality-free central capacity processor*, which is involved in the coordination and control of behaviour, and *specific processing systems*. In Baddeley's *working memory model*, for example, there are two independently operating and specific systems – an *articulatory/phonological loop* and a *visuospatial scratch-*

pad.[69] These systems can explain why overt repetition of an overlearned sequence of digits does not interfere with verbal reasoning, since the former uses an articulatory loop and the latter a central processor (see Chapter 17).

Automatic *v.* controlled processing

As we have seen, both laboratory evidence and everyday experience indicate that we can learn to perform two tasks simultaneously and highly efficiently. For some researchers, this is because many processes become automatic; that is, they make no attentional demands if they are used or practised often enough. Two important theoretical contributions are those of Schneider and Shiffrin[70] and Norman and Shallice.[71]

Schneider and Shiffrin's automaticity model

Schneider and Shiffrin distinguish between controlled and automatic attentional processing:[70]

- *Controlled processing* makes heavy demands on attentional resources, is slow, is capacity-limited and involves consciously directing attention towards a task.
- *Automatic processing* makes no demands on attentional resources, is fast, is unaffected by capacity limitations, is unavoidable and difficult to modify (it always occurs in the presence of an appropriate stimulus), and is not subject to conscious awareness.

The results of several studies (e.g. Schneider and Fisk[72]) are consistent with Schneider and Shiffrin's view. If people are given practice at a task, then they can perform it quickly and accurately, but their performance is resistant to change. An example of apparent automaticity in real life occurs when we learn to drive a car. At first, focused attention is required for each component of driving, and any distraction can disrupt performance. Once we have learned to drive, and as we become more experienced, our ability to attend simultaneously to other things increases.

Logan suggests that automaticity develops through practice, because automatic responses involve an almost effortless retrieval of an appropriate and well-learned response from memory.[73] This does not involve conscious memory, because no thought processes intervene between the presentation of a stimulus and the production of an appropriate response. In Logan's view, then, automaticity occurs when stored information about the sequence of responses necessary to perform a task can be accessed and retrieved rapidly.

An evaluation of Schneider and Shiffrin's model

Despite its intuitive appeal, it is unclear whether automaticity results from a speeding up of the processes involved in a task or from a change in the nature of the processes themselves. Also, the view that automatic processing makes no demands on attention has been challenged by findings indicating that allegedly automatic tasks do influence the performance of simultaneously performed tasks (e.g. Hampson[58]). Additional problems occur with the Stroop effect (Box 13.8).

Box 13.8 The Stroop effect

Stroop showed that if a colour word (e.g. 'blue') is written in a conflicting colour (e.g. the word 'blue' written in red ink), then participants find it difficult to name the colour in which the word is written.[74]

Because reading is such a well-learned, unavoidable and automatic activity, the word interferes with the requirement to name the colour.

An analogue of the Stroop effect can be tried here. Say as quickly as you can the number of characters in each of the rows below.

5 5 5
1 1 1 1
2
3 3 3 3 3
4 4
5 5 5
4 4 4 4 4
5 5 5 5
3
4 4 4
2 2 2 2
3 3
4 4 4
1 1 1 1
3
2 2 2

Flowers *et al.* found that people have difficulty resisting saying the numbers that make up each row rather than counting the numbers, because number recognition is much more automatic compared with number counting.[75] But automatic responses are not always unavoidable.[76]

Norman and Shallice's supervisory attentional system model

To overcome what Eysenck calls the 'unavoidability criterion',[76] Norman and Shallice proposed that processing involves two separate control systems: *contention scheduling* and the *supervisory attentional system* (SAS).[71] Some behaviours involve fully automatic processing, which occurs with little conscious awareness of the processes involved and is controlled by *schemas* (organized plans for behaviour; see below and Chapter 17).

However, such processes are capable of disrupting behaviour, and so contention scheduling occurs as a way of resolving conflicts among schemas. This produces partially automatic processing, which generally involves more conscious awareness than fully automatic processing but does not require deliberate direction or conscious control. Deliberate control involves the SAS and occurs in decision-making and trouble-shooting, allowing flexible responding to occur in novel situations. Baddeley claims that SAS is like the operation of free will, while contention scheduling leaves no place for free will.[77]

An evaluation of Norman and Shallice's model

According to Eysenck and Keane, Norman and Shallice's model is superior to Schneider and Shiffrin's because it '... provides a more natural explanation for the fact that some processes are fully automatic whereas others are only partially automatic'.[9]

Their SAS model is not worked out in the same degree of detail, or empirically tested as extensively, as Schneider and Shiffrin's automaticity model. However, it does provide a very useful basis for conceptualizing the central executive of Baddeley and Hitch's[78] working-memory model (Box 13.9; see also Chapter 17).[77]

Box 13.9 Is working memory's central executive just an attentional system?

As we have noted, Baddeley and Hitch identified the central executive with Norman and Shallice's supervisory attentional system (SAS), agreeing that the SAS was often disrupted in patients with frontal lobe damage. Such patients sometimes show paradoxical behaviour, such as perseveration (becoming locked into a specific activity) or its opposite (being unable to resist the temptation to respond inappropriately to features in the immediate environment). An example of the latter is *utilization behaviour*, in which the patient responds automatically to surrounding objects (e.g. drinking someone else's coffee, or, on one occasion, seizing a hypodermic needle and injecting the examining doctor).[79]

According to Baddeley, there has been an explosion of research into how behaviour is controlled, with an emphasis on how the frontal lobes are related to the ability to focus, divide and switch attention. Although the first two appear to be separable functions of the central executive, switching seems to be more complex. Baddeley's own research has pointed to the important role of the phonological loop in controlling behaviour via sub-vocal speech.

If the central executive is a purely attentional system, which could not itself store information, how did the phonological loop and the visuospatial sketchpad (the other 'slave' system) work together in the absence of a common code or language? And how could the whole system interface with long-term memory (LTM)?

Baddeley's solution to these critical problems is to propose a fourth slave (or sub-) system, namely the *episodic buffer*. This sits between the central executive and LTM, accepting information from any part of the system and holding it in a multidimensional code. It is taken to be of limited capacity (about four episodes or chunks; see Chapter 17) and accessible through conscious awareness. It is an essentially passive store – a television screen rather than a stage: the hard work goes on elsewhere but depends on the episodic buffer for its display.[79]

Action slips

Action slips have been defined as the performance of unintended actions, or actions that deviate from the actor's intentions, and have been researched extensively by Reason.[80,81] Reason originally asked 36 participants to keep a diary record of the action slips they made over a 4-week period. The participants recorded 433 action slips between them. Reason was able to place 94 per cent of these action slips into one of five categories (Box 13.10).

Explaining action slips

Closed- and open-loop control

Paradoxically, action slips seem to occur with highly practised and overlearned actions, which should, therefore, be least subject to errors. Reason[81] proposes that, when we first learn to perform a behaviour, our actions are subject to *closed-loop control*.[83] In this, a central processor or attentional system guides and controls a behaviour from start to finish. When we are skilled at a behaviour, it is under *open-loop control*, controlled by motor programmes or other automatic processes.

Closed-loop control is slow and effortful, whereas open-loop control is fast and allows attentional resources to be given over to other activities. However, closed-loop control is less prone to error and responds more flexibly to environmental demands compared with open-loop control. As a result, action slips occur because of an overreliance on

Box 13.10 Reason's five categories of action slips

- *Storage failures (40%):* repeating an action that has already been completed; for example, pouring a second kettle of boiling water into a teapot of freshly made tea without any recognition of having made the tea already.
- *Test failures (20%):* forgetting the goal of a particular sequence of actions and switching to a different goal; for example, intending to turn on the radio but walking past it and picking up the telephone instead. These slips occur, presumably, because a planned sequence of actions is not monitored sufficiently at some crucial point in the sequence.
- *Sub-routine failures (18%):* either omitting or reordering the stages in a sequence of behaviour; for example, making a pot of 'tea' but failing to put any tea in it.
- *Discrimination failures (11%):* failing to discriminate between two objects involved in different actions; for example, mistaking toothpaste for shaving cream.
- *Programme assembly failures (5%):* incorrectly combining actions; for example, unwrapping a sweet, putting the paper in your mouth and throwing the sweet in the bin.

Based on Eysenck[82] and Reason.[81]

open-loop control when closed-loop control (selectively attending to the task) should be occurring.

As shown in studies of focused attention, material not attended to is typically poorly remembered because it is not stored in long-term memory (LTM). So, the most common type of action slip, storage failures, can be explained in terms of open-loop induced attentional failures leading to a failure to store (and hence recall) previous actions. As a result, an action may be repeated. Other slips also seem amenable to explanation in terms of open-loop control.[82]

Schema theory

An alternative theoretical account has been advanced by Norman[84] and elaborated by Sellen and Norman (Box 13.11).[85] Their theory is based on the concept of the schema, first proposed by Bartlett (see Chapter 17).[86] Briefly, a schema is an organized mental representation of everything we understand by a given object, concept or event, based on past experience.

Box 13.11 Sellen and Norman's schema theory of action slips[85]

Parent schemas are the highest-level schemas, corresponding to an overall intention or goal (e.g. going to a football match). At a lower level are *child schemas*, which correspond to the actions involved in accomplishing the overall intention or goal (e.g. driving the car to the football ground and buying a ticket).

Each schema has a particular activation level, and a behaviour occurs when the activation level is reached (which depends on the current situation and current intentions) and when appropriate 'triggering' conditions exist. An action slip occurs if:

- there is an error in the formation of an intention; or
- an incorrect schema is activated; or
- activation of the correct schema is lost; or
- there is faulty triggering of an active schema.

Reason and Mycielska believe that a thorough understanding of the nature of action slips is necessary in order to avoid potential disaster occurring in the real world.[87] Eysenck maintains that action slips would be eliminated if we were to use closed-loop control for all behaviours, but this would be a waste of valuable attentional resources.[88] The frequency of action slips reported by Reason's participants (an average of about one action slip per day) suggests that people alternate between closed-loop and open-loop control as circumstances dictate.[80] For Eysenck:

> The very occasional action slip is a price which is generally worth paying in order to free the attentional system from the task of constant monitoring of our habitual actions.[88]

Action slips represent the minor errors of an action system that typically functions very well indeed.[82] Similarly, 'Absent-minded errors demonstrate misapplied competence rather than incompetence'.[89]

Each type of action slip might require its own explanation. Although the mechanisms underlying them may appear similar, they might actually be very different.[9] Consider Box 13.12.

Box 13.12 Reason's 'oak–yolk effect' experiment[81]

Answer the following series of questions as quickly as possible:

- *Q:* What do we call the tree that grows from acorns?
- *A:* Oak

- *Q:* What do we call a funny story?
- *A:* Joke

- *Q:* What sound does a frog make?
- *A:* Croak

- *Q:* What is Pepsi's major competitor?
- *A:* Coke

- *Q:* What's another word for cape?
- *A:* Cloak

- *Q:* What do you call the white of an egg?
- *A:* Yolk

'Yolk' is, in fact, the *wrong* answer (correct answer = albumen). Reason found that 85 per cent of his participants made this error, compared with only 5 per cent of a control group given just the final question. However, are such trick-induced action slips comparable to those that occur spontaneously in everyday life? According to Sellen and Norman, the laboratory environment is the least likely place to see truly spontaneous absent-minded errors.[85] In Eysenck & Keane's words:

> The number of occurrences of any particular kind of action slip is meaningful only when we know the number of occasions on which the slip might have occurred but did not. Thus, the small number of discrimination failures [reported by Reason] may reflect either good discrimination or a relative lack of situations requiring anything approaching a fine discrimination.[9]

CONCLUSIONS

It is possible sometimes to divide attention between two different tasks, although how this is achieved has not been explained satisfactorily. Two broad types of explanation are those that propose a general-purpose limited-capacity processor, and those that identify modules, each with a limited capacity but none of which is central. The idea that many processes become automatic and make no demands on attention has some support and helps to explain why we sometimes perform behaviours that we did not intend. Action slips involve behaviours that are highly practised and are the price we pay for not having to monitor our actions continuously.

KEY POINTS

- According to Broadbent, who was trying to account for Cherry's cocktail party phenomenon, humans must selectively attend to some information and tune out the rest.
- Using binaural listening, Cherry identified several physical differences affecting selective attention to one of two messages. He also used dichotic listening, in which participants had to shadow one of the messages. They could do this, but they remembered little, if anything, of the non-shadowed message, whose meaning was lost completely.
- Three single-channel models share the belief in a 'bottleneck' or filter that allows some information to be passed on for further processing, either discarding the rest or processing it to only a limited degree. The models differ mainly in terms of how early or late the filtering takes place.
- Broadbent's early-selection filter theory accounts for Cherry's findings and his own split-span data. But people's ability to switch attention to the non-attended ear when their name is spoken, together with other research findings relating to the processing of meaning, are inconsistent with Broadbent's theory.
- According to Treisman's attenuation model, competing information is analysed for its physical properties, and for sounds, syllable patterns, grammatical structures and meaning. The selective filter 'turns down' the non-shadowed message. If this includes biological 'pre-sets', our attention will switch to the non-shadowed message.
- The Deutsch–Norman late-selection filter theory/pertinence model sees selection as occurring only after all inputs have been analysed at a high level. The filter is nearer the response end of the processing system.
- Mechanisms involved in focused visual attention include eye movements that allow us to fixate specific regions of the visual field. But visual attention is not confined to the part of the visual field processed by the fovea, as demonstrated by covert attention. This is like an internal mental spotlight.
- According to Eriksen's zoom-lens model, the internal spotlight has a beam that may be very narrow or very broad.
- According to Treisman's feature-integration theory, focusing attention on their location allows unitary features to be formed into their various objects. Illusory conjunctions can arise in the absence of relevant stored knowledge or focused attention.
- Researchers interested in divided attention typically measure dual-task performance. Three factors affecting dual-task performance are task difficulty, practice and similarity.
- According to Kahneman, humans have only a limited processing capacity. Different tasks require different amounts of processing capacity, leaving more or less available for performing other tasks. Arousal is important for determining the amount of available capacity.
- Norman and Bobrow's central capacity interference theory distinguishes between resource-limited and data-limited performance.
- Several researchers have rejected the concept of a general-purpose limited-capacity processor. The most useful way of interpreting the data is in terms of tasks competing for the same modules, each of which has a limited capacity but none of which is uniquely 'central'.
- Two highly similar tasks compete for the same modules, leading to performance deficits, while dissimilar tasks use different modules and thus do not compete. This view is also taken by multiple-resource theory.
- Synthesis models propose the existence of a modality-free central capacity processor, plus specific independent processing systems, such as Baddeley's articulatory/phonological loop and visuospatial scratchpad. More recently, the episodic buffer has been identified.
- Schneider and Shiffrin distinguish between controlled and automatic processing. The Stroop effect shows that well-learned, unavoidable and automatic skills (e.g. reading) can interfere with other tasks (e.g. naming the colour of a written word).
- Contention scheduling is used to resolve conflicts among schemas that control fully automatic processing and produces partially automatic processing. The SAS is involved in deliberate control, which allows flexible responses in novel situations.
- The most common action slips are storage failures. Other categories include test, sub-routine, discrimination and programme assembly failures.
- Action slips seem to involve actions that are highly practised or overlearned. They reflect an overreliance on open-loop control when closed-loop control (focused attention) is needed.

REFERENCES

1. Titchener EB (1903) *Lectures on the Elementary Psychology of Feeling and Attention.* New York: Macmillan.
2. Broadbent DE (1958) *Perception and Communication.* Oxford: Pergamon.
3. Solso RL (1995) *Cognitive Psychology*, 4th edn. Boston, MA: Allyn & Bacon.
4. Treisman AM (1964) Verbal cues, language and meaning in selective attention. *American Journal of Psychology* **77**: 206–19.
5. Deutsch JA, Deutsch D (1963) Attention: some theoretical considerations. *Psychological Review* **70**: 80–90.
6. Norman DA (1969) Memory while shadowing. *Quarterly Journal of Experimental Psychology* **21**: 85–93.
7. Kahneman D (1973) *Attention and Effort.* Englewood Cliffs, NJ: Prentice-Hall.
8. Allport DA (1980) Attention and performance. In G Claxton (ed.) *Cognitive Psychology: New Directions.* London: Routledge & Kegan Paul.
9. Eysenck MW, Keane MJ (1995) *Cognitive Psychology: A Student's Handbook*, 3rd edn. Hove: Erlbaum.

10. Jarvis M (1994) Attention and the information processing approach. *Psychology Teaching* December: 12–22.
11. James W (1890) *The Principles of Psychology*. New York: Henry Holt & Company.
12. Broadbent DE (1954) The role of auditory localization and attention in memory span. *Journal of Experimental Psychology* **47**: 191–6.
13. Cherry EC (1953) Some experiments on the recognition of speech with one and two ears. *Journal of the Acoustical Society of America* **25**: 975–9.
14. Moray N (1959) Attention in dichotic listening: affective cues and the influence of instructions. *Quarterly Journal of Experimental Psychology* **11**: 56–60.
15. Hampson PJ, Morris PE (1996) *Understanding Cognition*. Oxford: Blackwell.
16. Treisman AM (1960) Contextual cues in selective listening. *Quarterly Journal of Experimental Psychology* **12**: 242–8.
17. Corteen RS, Wood B (1972) Autonomic responses to shock-associated words in an unattended channel. *Journal of Experimental Psychology* **94**: 308–13.
18. Mackay DG (1973) Aspects of the theory of comprehension, memory and attention. *Quarterly Journal of Experimental Psychology* **25**: 22–40.
19. Gray JA, Wedderburn AA (1960) Grouping strategies with simultaneous stimuli. *Quarterly Journal of Experimental Psychology* **12**: 180–84.
20. Underwood G (1974) Moray vs the rest: the effects of extended shadowing practice. *Quarterly Journal of Experimental Psychology* **26**: 368–72.
21. Allport DA, Antonis B, Reynolds P (1972) On the division of attention: a disproof of the single-channel hypothesis. *Quarterly Journal of Experimental Psychology* **24**: 225–35.
22. Massaro DW (1989) *Experimental Psychology: An Information Processing Approach*. New York: Harcourt Brace Jovanovich.
23. Norman DA (1968) Toward a theory of memory and attention. *Psychological Review* **75**: 522–36.
24. Norman DA (1976) *Memory and Attention*, 2nd edn. Chichester: John Wiley & Sons.
25. Treisman AM, Geffen G (1967) Selective attention: perception or response? *Quarterly Journal of Experimental Psychology* **19**: 1–18.
26. Deutsch JA, Deutsch D (1967) Comments on 'Selective attention: Perception or response?'. *Quarterly Journal of Experimental Psychology* **19**: 362–3.
27. Treisman AM, Riley JGA (1969) Is selective attention selective perception or selective response? A further test. *Journal of Experimental Psychology* **79**: 27–34.
28. Glucksberg S, Cowan N (1970) Memory for non-attended auditory material. *Cognitive Psychology* **1**: 149–56.
29. Wilding JM (1982) *Perception: From Sense to Object*. London: Hutchinson.
30. Johnston WA, Heinz SP (1978) Flexibility and capacity demands of attention. *Journal of Experimental Psychology: General* **107**: 420–35.
31. Johnston WA, Heinz SP (1979) Depth of non-target processing in an attention task. *Journal of Experimental Psychology* **5**: 168–75.
32. Johnston WA, Wilson J (1980) Perceptual processing of non-targets in an attention task. *Memory and Cognition* **8**: 372–7.
33. Norman DA, Bobrow DG (1975) On data-limited and resource-limited processes. *Cognitive Psychology* **7**: 44–64.
34. Neisser U (1976) *Cognition and Reality*. San Francisco, CA: W.H. Freeman.
35. Driver J (1996) Attention and segmentation. *Psychologist* **9**: 119–23.
36. Anderson JR (1995) *Cognitive Psychology and Its Implications*. New York: W.H. Freeman.
37. Posner MI, Nissen MJ, Ogden WC (1978) Attended and unattended processing modes: the role of set form spatial location. In HL Pick, IJ Saltzman (eds) *Modes of Perceiving and Processing Information*. Hillsdale, NJ: Lawrence Erlbaum Associates.
38. Posner MI, Snyder CRR, Davidson BJ (1980) Attention and the detection of signals. *Journal of Experimental Psychology: General* **109**: 160–74.
39. Posner MI (1980) Orienting of attention: the VII Sir Frederic Bartlett lecture. *Quarterly Journal of Experimental Psychology* **32A**: 3–25.
40. LaBerge D (1983) Spatial extent of attention to letters and words. *Journal of Experimental Psychology: Human Perception and Performance* **9**: 371–9.
41. Eriksen CW, Yeh YY (1987) Allocation of attention in the visual field. *Journal of Experimental Psychology: Human Perception and Performance* **11**: 583–97.
42. Eriksen CW (1990) Attentional search of the visual field. In D Brogan (ed.) *Visual Search*. London: Taylor & Francis.
43. Groome D, Dewart H, Esgate E, *et al.* (1999) *An Introduction to Cognitive Psychology: Processes and Disorders*. London: Psychology Press.
44. Johnston WA, Dark VJ (1986) Selective attention. *Annual Review of Psychology* **37**: 43–75.
45. Neisser U, Becklen R (1975) Selective looking: attending to visually specified events. *Cognitive Psychology* **7**: 480–94.
46. Tipper SP, Driver J (1988) Negative priming between pictures and words: evidence for semantic analysis of ignored stimuli. *Memory and Cognition* **16**: 64–70.
47. Treisman AM (1988) Features and objects: the fourteenth Bartlett memorial lecture. *Quarterly Journal of Experimental Psychology* **40A**: 201–37.
48. Neisser U (1967) *Cognitive Psychology*. New York: Appleton Century Crofts.
49. Treisman AM, Gelade G (1980) A feature-integration theory of attention. *Cognitive Psychology* **12**: 97–136.
50. Treisman AM, Schmidt H (1982) Illusory conjunctions

in the perception of objects. *Cognitive Psychology* **14**: 107–41.

51. McLeod P, Driver J, Dienes Z, Crisp J (1991) Filtering by movement in visual search. *Journal of Experimental Psychology: Human Perception and Performance* **17**: 55–64.
52. Halligan PW (1995) Drawing attention to neglect: the contribution of line bisection. *Psychologist* **8**: 257–64.
53. Posner MI, Petersen SE (1990) The attention system of the human brain. *Annual Review of Neuroscience* **13**: 25–42.
54. Rafal RD, Posner MI (1987) Deficits in human visual spatial attention following thalamic lesions. *Proceedings of the National Academy of Sciences* **84**: 7349–53.
55. Dunbar G, Lewis V, Hill R (1999) Control processes and road-crossing skills. *Psychologist* **12**: 398–9.
56. Shaffer LH (1975) Multiple attention in continuous verbal tasks. In PMA Rabbitt, S Dornic (eds) *Attention and Performance*, Vol. V. London: Academic Press.
57. Spelke ES, Hirst WC, Neisser U (1976) Skills of divided attention. *Cognition* **4**: 215–30.
58. Hampson PJ (1989) Aspects of attention and cognitive science. *Irish Journal of Psychology* **10**: 261–75.
59. Lawson EA (1966) Decisions concerning the rejected channel. *Journal of Experimental Psychology* **18**: 260–65.
60. Broadbent DE (1982) Task combination and selective intake of information. *Acta Psychologica* **50**: 253–90.
61. Allport DA (1989) Visual attention. In M Posner (ed.) *Foundations of Cognitive Science*. Cambridge, MA: MIT Press.
62. Allport DA (1993) Attention and control: have we been asking the wrong questions? A critical review of twenty-five years. In DE Meyer, SM Kornblum (eds) *Attention and Performance*, Vol. XIV. London: MIT Press.
63. Navon D, Gopher D (1979) On the economy of the human processing system. *Psychological Review* **86**: 214–55.
64. Wickens CD (1992) *Engineering Psychology and Human Performance*, 2nd edn. New York: HarperCollins.
65. Navon D (1984) Resources: a theoretical soup stone? *Psychological Review* **91**: 216–34.
66. Eysenck MW (1982) *Attention and Arousal: Cognition and Performance*. Berlin: Springer.
67. Eysenck MW (1984) *A Handbook of Cognitive Psychology*. London: Lawrence Erlbaum Associates.
68. Eysenck MW (1997) Doing two things at once. *Psychology Review* **4**: 10–12.
69. Baddeley AD (1986) *Working Memory*. Oxford: Oxford University Press.
70. Schneider W, Shiffrin RM (1977) Controlled and automatic human information. *Psychosomatic Medicine* **19**: 17–29.
71. Norman DA, Shallice T (1986) Attention to action: willed and automatic control of behaviour. In RJ Davidson, GE Schwartz, D Shapiro (eds) *The Design of Everyday Things*. New York: Doubleday.
72. Schneider W, Fisk AD (1982) Degree of consistent training: improvements in search performance and automatic process development. *Perception and Psychophysics* **31**: 160–68.
73. Logan GD (1988) Toward an instance theory of automatization. *Psychological Review* **95**: 492–527.
74. Stroop JR (1935) Studies of interference in serial verbal reactions. *Journal of Experimental Psychology* **18**: 643–62.
75. Flowers JH, Warner JL, Polansky ML (1979) Response and encoding factors in ignoring irrelevant information. *Memory and Cognition* **7**: 86–94.
76. Eysenck MW (1993) *Principles of Cognitive Psychology*. Hove: Lawrence Erlbaum Associates.
77. Baddeley AD (1997) *Human Memory: Theory and Practice*, revised edn. Hove: Psychology Press.
78. Baddeley AD, Hitch G (1974) Working memory. In GH Bower (ed.) *Recent Advances in Learning and Motivation*, Vol. 8. New York: Academic Press.
79. Baddeley AD (2008) What's new in working memory? *Psychology Review* **13**: 2–5.
80. Reason J (1979) Actions not as planned: the price of automatization. In G Underwood, R Stevens (eds) *Aspects of Consciousness*, Vol 1: Psychological Issues. London: Academic Press.
81. Reason J (1992) Cognitive underspecification: its variety and consequences. In BJ Baars (ed.) *Experimental Slips and Human Error: Exploring the Architecture of Volition*. New York: Plenum Press.
82. Eysenck MW (1997) Absent-mindedness. *Psychology Review* **3**: 16–18.
83. Adams JA (1976) Issues for a closed-loop theory of motor learning. In GE Stelmach (ed.) *Motor Control: Issues and Trends*. London: Academic Press.
84. Norman DA (1981) Categorization of action slips. *Psychological Review* **88**: 1–15.
85. Sellen AJ, Norman DA (1992) The psychology of slips. In BJ Baars (ed.) *Experimental Slips and Human Error: Exploring the Architecture of Volition*. New York: Plenum Press.
86. Bartlett FC (1932) *Remembering*. Cambridge: Cambridge University Press.
87. Reason J, Mycielska K (1982) *Absentmindedness: The Psychology of Mental Lapses and Everyday Errors*. Englewood Cliffs, NJ: Prentice-Hall.
88. Eysenck MW (1995) Attention. In CC French, AM Colman (eds) *Cognitive Psychology*. London: Longman.
89. Reason J (1984) Absent-mindedness. In J Nicholson, H Beloff (eds) *Psychology Survey 5*. Leicester: British Psychological Society.

Chapter 14

Learning theory

Richard Gross

INTRODUCTION

As we note in Chapter 9, psychology comprises a number of different theoretical perspectives or approaches. Each approach makes different assumptions about the particular aspects of a person that are worthy of study, which helps to determine an underlying model or image of what people are like. In turn, this model or image determines a view of the nature of development, the preferred methods of study, the nature of psychological normality, the major cause(s) of abnormality, and the preferred methods and goals of treatment.

Learning theory is associated with the *behaviourist* approach, which dominated American psychology in particular for much of the first half of the twentieth century. Given the central role of learning in philosophical behaviourism, it is hardly surprising that the topic of learning itself should be central within psychology as a whole.

WHAT DO WE MEAN BY 'LEARNING'?

The concept of learning is a good example of the discrepancy between the everyday, common-sense use of a term and its technical, scientific use (see Chapter 9). In everyday conversation, the emphasis is usually on *what* is learned (the end product), such as learning to drive a car, use the Internet or speak French. But when psychologists use the term, their focus is on *how* the learning takes place (the learning process).

Learning is a *hypothetical construct*: it cannot be observed directly; instead, it can only be inferred from observable behaviour. So, for example, if a person's performance on a task at time 1 differs from performance on the task at time 2, then we might infer that learning has taken place. But if that change is observed just once, then we may be much more hesitant about making such an inference. Learning, therefore, normally implies a fairly permanent change in a person's behavioural performance. Again, temporary fluctuations in behaviour can occur as a result of fatigue, drugs, temperature changes and so on, and this is another reason for taking permanence as a minimum requirement for saying that learning has taken place.

However, permanent changes in behaviour can also result from things that have nothing to do with learning, such as the effects of brain damage on behaviour, and the changes associated with puberty and other maturational processes. So, if a change in behaviour is to be counted as learning, then the change must be linked to some kind of past experience (regardless of whether there was any attempt to bring about that change). For these reasons, psychologists usually define learning as '... a relatively permanent change in behaviour due to past experience'[1] or '... the process by which relatively permanent changes occur in behavioural potential as a result of experience'.[2]

Learning versus performance

The second definition has one major advantage over the first; namely, it implies a distinction between learning (*behavioural potential*) and performance (*actual behaviour*).

If you can swim, you are almost certainly not doing so as you read this chapter – but you could readily do so if faced with a pool full of water. So what you could do (potential behaviour based on learning) and what you are actually doing (current performance) are two different things. Ultimately, of course, the only proof of learning is a particular kind of performance (e.g. exams). Performance can fluctuate due to fatigue, use of drugs and emotional factors, and so it is much more variable than learning, which is more permanent. (Exams come to mind again – many students have left an exam knowing what they could not demonstrate during the exam itself.)

Some basic questions about learning

Although it is generally agreed by psychologists that learning is relatively permanent and due to past experience, there is much less agreement about exactly what changes when learning takes place and what kinds of past experience are involved. Put another way, how do the changes occur? And what mechanisms are involved? One important issue that divides psychologists is the extent to which they focus on the overt, behavioural changes as opposed to the covert, cognitive changes.

THE BEHAVIOURIST APPROACH

Basic principles and assumptions

According to Skinner:

The first explicit behaviourist was John B. Watson, who in 1913 issued a kind of manifesto called *Psychology as the Behaviourist Views It*. As the title shows, he was not proposing a new science but arguing that psychology should be redefined as the study of behaviour... Most of the psychologists at the time believed they were studying mental processes in a mental world of consciousness, and they were naturally not inclined to agree with Watson. Early behaviourists wasted a good deal of time, and confused an important issue, by attacking the introspective study of mental life.[3]

Watson claimed that only by modelling itself on the natural sciences could psychology legitimately call itself a science (see Chapter 9).[4] He argued for a certain type of behaviourism, namely *methodological behaviourism*: only events/phenomena that can be verified intersubjectively (i.e. agreed upon by two or more people) are suitable for scientific investigation. Cognition, thinking, believing, feeling, pain and so on are private events, and so they are not accessible to anyone else. Therefore, they should be excluded from a science of psychology.

In this sense, what was revolutionary about Watson's behaviourist manifesto has become almost taken-for-granted, 'orthodox' psychology. It could be argued that all psychologists are methodological behaviourists.[5] Belief in the importance of empirical methods, especially the experiment, as a way of collecting data about humans (and non-humans), which can be quantified and statistically analysed, is a major feature of mainstream psychology.

Skinner's radical behaviourism

Skinner, generally regarded as the arch-behaviourist, rejected Watson's insistence on 'truth by agreement'. According to his radical behaviourism, cognitions are covert behaviours ('within the skin') that should be studied by psychologists along with overt behaviours (capable of being observed by two or more people). He was not 'against cognitions', but he said that 'so-called mental activities are metaphors or explanatory fictions and ... behaviour attributed to them can be more effectively explained in other ways'.

For Skinner, these more effective explanations of behaviour come in the form of the principles of reinforcement derived from his experimental work with rats and pigeons (see below). What is 'radical' about Skinner's radical behaviourism is the claim that feelings, sensations and other private events cannot be used to explain behaviour but are to be explained in an analysis of behaviour (*behaviour analysis*). Since private events cannot be manipulated, they cannot serve as independent variables; but they can serve as dependent variables. Some recent studies of consciousness seem to support Skinner's claim that our common-sense belief that we will our actions is an illusion (see Chapter 10 and Gross[6]).

Although methodological behaviourism proposes to ignore such inner states (they are inaccessible), Skinner ignores them only as variables used for explaining behaviour (they are irrelevant) and argues that they can be translated into the language of reinforcement theory.[7] According to Nye, Skinner's ideas are also radical because he applied the same type of analysis to both covert and overt behaviour.[8]

Skinner stressed the importance of identifying functional relations between environmental conditions and behaviours. According to Leslie:

... the psychology of an individual consists primarily of an account of those functionally defined behavioural characteristics that occur in the environments typically encountered by that individual. A person, if you like, is primarily to be understood as 'what he or she does' and that account of their behaviour cannot ... be described without also describing the location or occasion of those behaviours and the important consequences of those behaviours ...[9]

From the perspective of behaviour analysis, the key process of psychological change is operant conditioning:

... whereby those behaviours that are functionally effective for the individual become more frequent (in the corresponding environment) while other behaviours decline in frequency ...[9]

The behaviour is not caused by either the individual or the environment. Rather:

... it is the history of interaction between the behavioural repertoire of the individual (that is, the whole range of behaviours shown by the person) and the environment that selects, and in a sense causes, the behaviour ...[9]

Skinner also saw his brand of behaviourism as a thoroughgoing, 'deep' behaviourism.[10] According to Skinner, radical behaviourism is not a scientific law or set of empirical findings. It is meta-scientific; that is, it attempts to define what a science of behaviour should look like.[3] The questions that Skinner asks are essentially philosophical. According to O'Donohue and Ferguson:

... radical behaviourism is a philosophy of science, or more exactly, a philosophy of psychology. Skinner calls the science based on this philosophy the experimental analysis of behaviour or behaviour analysis.[10]

Given this important distinction between methodological and radical behaviourism, we need to consider some principles and assumptions that apply to behaviourism in general (Box 14.1).

Skinner made the crucial distinction between *respondents* (or respondent behaviour), which are triggered automatically by particular environmental stimuli, and *operants* (or operant behaviour), which are essentially voluntary (Figure 14.1). A related distinction is that between classical or

Box 14.1 Basic principles and assumptions made by the behaviourist approach

- Behaviourists emphasize the role of *environmental factors* in influencing behaviour, often to the (apparent) exclusion of innate or inherited factors. This amounts essentially to a focus on *learning*, the key form of which is *conditioning* – either *classical* (the basis of Watson's research) or *operant* (the basis of Skinner's).
- Classical and operant conditioning are often referred to collectively as *learning theory*, as opposed to 'theories of learning', which usually imply theories other than conditioning theories (i.e. non-behaviourist theories; see text).
- Skinner saw psychology as a branch of biology and was influenced heavily by Darwin's theory of evolution. The environment selects certain behaviours over others, and this determines their frequency in future generations. Operant conditioning is itself an evolutionary adaptation: the ability to learn from the consequences of behaviour is an evolutionary development that proved advantageous. Classical conditioning is another learning mechanism that evolution has produced.[10]
- Behaviourism is often referred to as 'S–R' (stimulus–response) psychology. However, the stimulus and response relationship can be defined in fundamentally different ways. Only in classical conditioning is the stimulus seen as triggering a response in a predictable, automatic way, and this is what is conveyed by S–R psychology. It is, therefore, a mistake to describe operant conditioning as an S–R approach (see text).
- The mechanisms proposed by a theory should be as simple as possible. Behaviourists stress the use of *operational definitions* (defining concepts in terms of observable, measurable events).
- The aim of a science of behaviour is to predict and control behaviour. This raises both conceptual questions (about the nature of science, in particular the role of theory) and ethical questions (e.g. about power and the role of psychologists as agents of change; see Gross[6]).

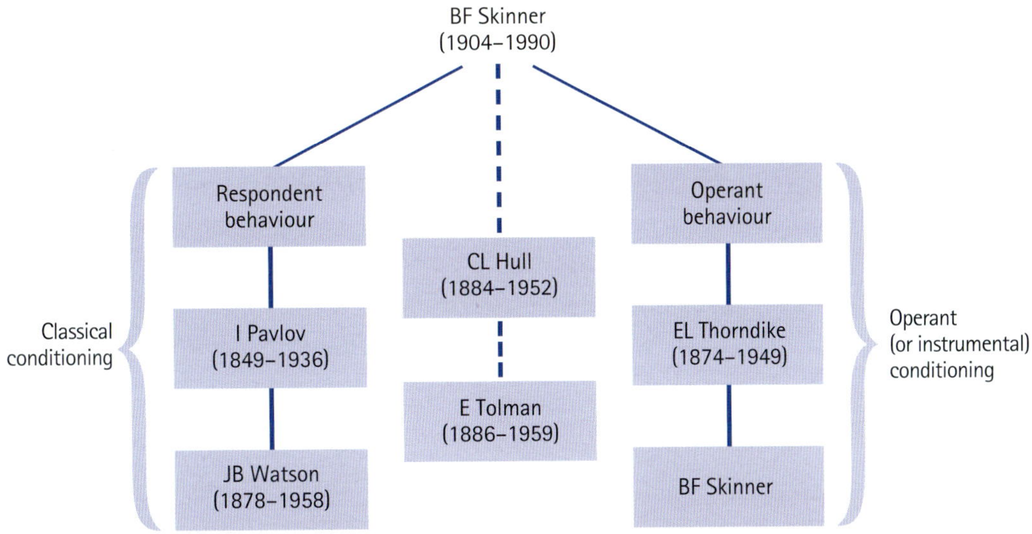

Figure 14.1 Major figures in the behaviourist (learning theory) tradition

respondent (*Pavlovian*) conditioning and operant or instrumental (*Skinnerian*) conditioning.

Classical conditioning: why do dogs drool over bells?

Ivan Pavlov was a physiologist interested in the process of digestion in dogs. He was awarded the Nobel Prize in 1904 (the year Skinner was born). He developed a surgical technique for collecting a dog's salivary secretions. A tube was attached to the outside of its cheek, so the drops of saliva could be measured easily (Figure 14.2).

Pavlov noticed that the dogs would often start salivating before they were given any food, such as when they looked at the food or saw the feeding bucket, or even when they heard the footsteps of the laboratory assistant who was coming to feed them.[11] These observations led to the study of what is now called classical (or Pavlovian) conditioning: a stimulus (e.g. a bell) that would not normally produce a particular response (e.g. salivation) eventually comes to do

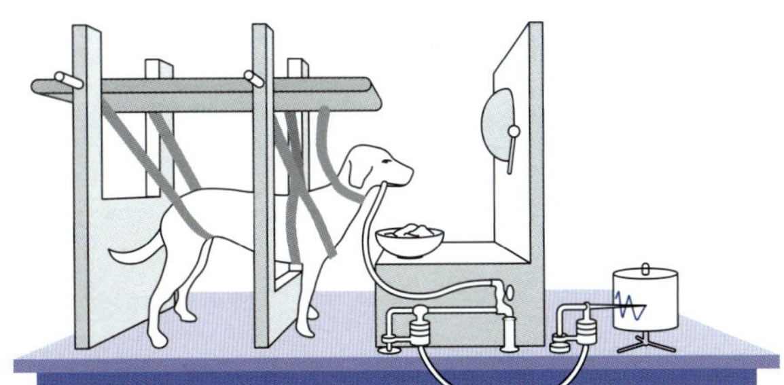

Figure 14.2 Apparatus used by Pavlov in his experiments on conditioned reflexes

so by being paired with another stimulus (e.g. food) that does normally produce the response (Figure 14.3).

Before conditioning, the taste of food will naturally and automatically make the dog salivate, but the sound of a bell will not. The food is thus referred to as an *unconditioned stimulus* (UCS), and the salivation is an *unconditioned response* (UCR): an automatic, reflex, biologically built-in response. The dog does not have to learn to salivate in response to food, because it does so naturally.

During conditioning, the bell is paired with the food. Because the bell does not naturally produce salivation, it is called a *conditioned stimulus* (CS): it produces salivation only on the condition that it is paired with the UCS. It is also neutral with regard to salivation before conditioning.

If the bell and food are paired often enough, the dog starts to salivate as soon as it hears the bell and before the food is presented. When this occurs, conditioning has taken place. The salivation is now referred to as a *conditioned response* (CR), because it is produced by a conditioned stimulus (CS) – the bell.

This basic procedure can be used with a variety of conditioned stimuli, such as buzzers, metronomes, lights and geometric figures. The exact relationship between the CS and the UCS can also be varied to give different kinds of conditioning. What is described above involves *delayed/forward* conditioning (Table 14.1).

Higher-order conditioning

Pavlov demonstrated that a strong CS could be used instead of food to produce salivation in response to a new stimulus that had never been paired with food. For example, a buzzer (previously paired with food) is paired with a black square. After ten pairings (using delayed conditioning), the dog will salivate a small but significant amount at the sight of the black square before the buzzer is sounded. The black square has never been associated with food directly, but only indirectly through association with the buzzer. It is as if the CS were functioning as a UCS.

The buzzer–food combination is referred to as *first-order conditioning*, and the black square–buzzer pairing as

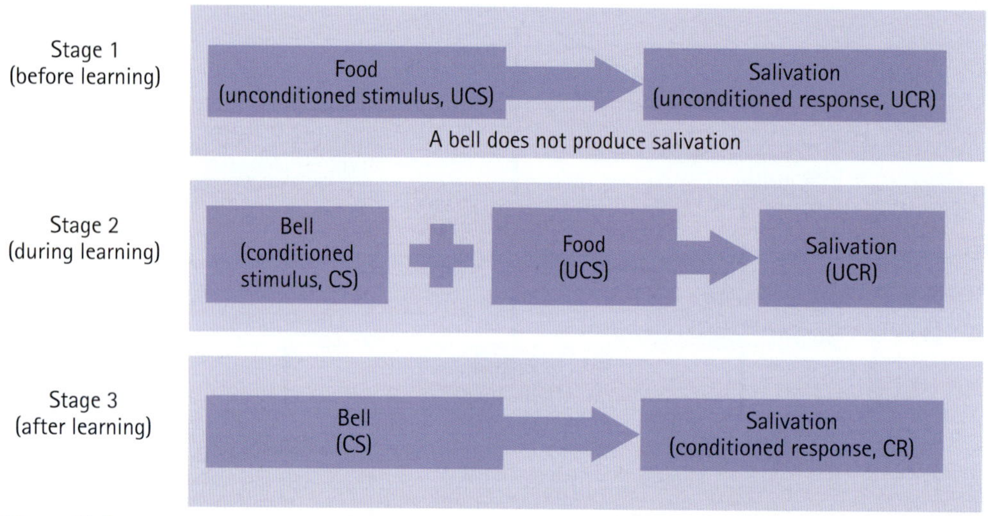

Figure 14.3 Basic procedure involved in classical conditioning

Table 14.1 Four types of classical conditioning based on different conditioned stimulus (CS)–unconditioned stimulus (UCS) relationships

Delayed or forward	The CS is presented before the UCS, and remains 'on' while the UCS is presented and until the unconditioned response (UCR) appears. Conditioning has occurred when the conditioned response (CR) appears before the UCS is presented. A half-second interval produces the strongest learning. As the interval increases, learning becomes poorer. This type of conditioning is typically used in the laboratory, especially with non-humans.
Backward	The CS is presented after the UCS. Generally this produces very little, if any, learning in laboratory animals. However, much advertising uses backward conditioning (e.g. the idyllic tropical scene is set, and then the coconut bar is introduced).
Simultaneous	The CS and UCS are presented *together*. Conditioning has occurred when the CS on its own produces the CR. This type of conditioning often occurs in real-life situations (e.g. the sound of the dentist's drill accompanies the contact of the drill with your tooth).
Trace	The CS is presented and removed before the UCS is presented, so that only a 'memory trace' of the CS remains to be conditioned. The CR is usually weaker than in delayed or simultaneous conditioning.

second-order conditioning. Pavlov found with dogs that learning could not go beyond third- or fourth-order conditioning. Even so, conditioning is beginning to look a rather more complex process.

Generalization and discrimination

In *generalization*, the CR transfers spontaneously to stimuli similar to, but different from, the original CS. For example, if a dog is trained using a bell of a particular pitch and is then presented with a bell a little higher or lower in pitch, the dog will still salivate, although only one bell (the original CS) was actually paired with food. However, if the dog is presented with bells that are increasingly different from the original, the CR will gradually weaken and eventually stop altogether – the dog is showing *discrimination* (Figure 14.4).

Pavlov also trained dogs to discriminate in the original conditioning procedure. For example, if a high-pitched bell is paired with food but a low-pitched bell is not, the dog will start salivating in response to the former but not to the latter (*discrimination training*). An interesting phenomenon related to discrimination is what Pavlov called *experimental neurosis* (Box 14.2).

Extinction and spontaneous recovery

If dogs have been conditioned to salivate to a bell, and the bell is repeatedly presented without food, the CR of salivation gradually becomes weaker and eventually stops altogether (*extinction*). However, if a dog that has undergone extinction is removed from the experimental situation and then put back a couple of hours or so later, it will start salivating again. Although no further pairing of the bell and food has occurred, the CR of salivation reappears in response to the bell (*spontaneous recovery*). This shows that extinction involves not an 'erasing' of the original learning but rather a learning to *inhibit* or *suppress* the CR when the CS is continually presented without a UCS.

CS1 (The bell used in the original conditioning procedure) → CR (salivation)

Bells CS2, CS3 and CS4 are of increasingly lower pitch but still produce salivation through **Generalization**

CS2 → CR
CS3 → CR
CS4 → CR

Salivation is gradually becoming weaker as the pitch becomes lower compared with CS1

Bells CS5, CS6 and CS7 fail to produce salivation because they are sufficiently different from CS1 The dog is showing **Discrimination**

CS5 ↛ CR
CS6 ↛ CR
CS7 ↛ CR

No salivation occurs

Figure 14.4 Example of discrimination occurring spontaneously as a result of generalization stopping

Box 14.2 Experimental neurosis: how to drive a dog mad

Pavlov trained dogs to salivate to a circle but not to an ellipse, and then gradually changed the shape of the ellipse until it became almost circular. As this happened, the dogs started behaving in 'neurotic' ways – whining, trembling, urinating and defecating, refusing to eat and so on. It was as if the dogs did not know how to respond: was the stimulus a circle (in which case, through generalization, they 'ought' to salivate), or was it an ellipse (in which case, through discrimination, they 'should not' salivate)?

Classical conditioning and human behaviour

There have been many laboratory demonstrations involving human participants. It is relatively easy to classically condition and extinguish CRs, such as the eye-blink and galvanic skin response (GSR). But what relevance does this have for understanding human learning and memory, let alone thinking, reasoning or problem-solving?

In normal adults, the conditioning process can apparently be overridden by instructions: simply telling participants that the UCS will not occur causes instant loss of the CR, which would otherwise extinguish only slowly.[12] Most participants in a conditioning experiment are aware of the experimenter's *contingencies* (the relationship between stimuli and responses) and, in the absence of such awareness, often fail to show evidence of conditioning.[13]

There are also important differences between very young children, and those with severe learning difficulties, and older children and adults, regarding their behaviour in a variety of operant conditioning and discrimination learning experiments. These seem largely attributable to language development (see below).[14]

All this suggests that people have rather more efficient, language- (or rule-) based forms of learning at their disposal than the laborious formation of associations between a CS and UCS. Even behaviour therapy, one of the apparently more successful applications of conditioning principles to human behaviour, has given way to cognitive-behaviour therapy (see Chapter 66).[15]

Classical conditioning and phobias

Watson was the first psychologist to apply the principles of classical conditioning to human behaviour. He did this in what is considered to be one of the most ethically dubious psychology experiments ever conducted (Box 14.3).

It is unclear whether Watson and Rayner intended to remove Little Albert's phobia. What is certain is that Albert's mother removed him from the hospital before this could happen. They might have attempted to remove the phobia through the method of *direct unconditioning* as used by Jones (Box 14.4).[17] This is an early example of what Wolpe called *systematic desensitization* (see Chapter 67).[18]

Behaviour therapists, such as Eysenck, regard the Little Albert experiment as demonstrating how all phobias are acquired in everyday life. A fear of the dentist, for example, could be learned in the following way:

Box 14.3 The case of Little Albert[16]

Albert B's mother was a wet-nurse in a children's hospital. Albert was described as 'healthy form birth', and 'on the whole stolid and unemotional'. When he was about 9 months old, his reactions to various stimuli were tested – a white rat, a rabbit, a dog, a monkey, masks with and without hair, cotton-wool, burning newspapers, and a hammer striking a steel 4-foot steel bar just behind his head. Only the last of these frightened him, so this was designated the unconditioned stimulus (UCS; the fear was the unconditioned response, UCR). The other stimuli were neutral because they did not produce fear.

When Albert was just over 11 months old, the rat and the UCS were presented together: as Albert reached out to stroke the animal, Watson crept up behind the baby and brought the hammer crashing down on the steel bar.

This occurred seven times in total over the next 7 weeks. By this time, the rat (the conditioned stimulus, CS) on its own frightened Albert, and the fear was now a conditioned response (CR). Watson and Rayner had succeeded in deliberately producing in a baby a phobia of rats.

The CR transferred spontaneously to the rabbit, the dog, a sealskin fur coat, cotton-wool, Watson's hair and a Santa Claus mask. But it did not generalize to Albert's building blocks or to the hair of two observers (so Albert was showing discrimination).

Five days after conditioning, the CR produced by the rat persisted. After 10 days it was 'much less marked', but it was still evident a month later.

Box 14.4 The case of Little Peter[17]

Peter was a 2-year-old living in a charitable institution. Jones was interested mainly in those children who cried and trembled when shown an animal (e.g. a frog, rat or rabbit). Peter showed an extreme fear of rats, rabbits, feathers, cotton-wool, fur coats, frogs and fish, although in other respects he was regarded as well adjusted. It was not known how these phobias had arisen.

Jones, supervised by Watson, put a rabbit in a wire cage in front of Peter while the child ate his lunch. After 40 such sessions, Peter ate his lunch with one hand and stroked the rabbit (now on his lap) with the other hand.

In a series of 17 steps, the rabbit (still in the cage) had been brought a little closer each day, and then let free in the room. Eventually the rabbit sat on Peter's lunch tray.

- Drill hitting a nerve (UCS) → pain/fear (UCR).
- Sound of drill (CS) + drill hitting nerve (UCS) → pain/fear (UCR).
- Sound of drill (CS) → fear (CR).

If you are looking at the dentist peering into your mouth, you may become afraid of upside-down faces. If the dentist is wearing a mask, you may acquire a fear of masks too. Also, through generalization, you can come to fear all drill-like noises or all white coats worn by medical personnel and laboratory technicians.

Human phobias may be perpetuated through avoiding the object of our fears. In other words, we do not give the fear a chance to undergo extinction (see Chapter 67). This occurs in conjunction with operant conditioning, whereby the avoidance behaviour becomes strengthened through negative reinforcement.

Operant conditioning: why do rats press levers?

When Skinner drew the distinction between respondent and operant behaviour, he was not rejecting the discoveries of Pavlov and Watson. Rather, he was arguing that most animal and human behaviour is not triggered or elicited by specific stimuli. He was interested in how animals operate on their environment, and how this operant behaviour is instrumental in bringing about certain consequences, which then determine the probability of that behaviour being repeated. Skinner saw the learner as much more active than Pavlov or Watson did (Box 14.5).

Just as Watson's ideas were based on the earlier work of Pavlov, so Skinner's study of operant conditioning grew out of the earlier work of another American, Edward Thorndike.

Thorndike's law of effect

Thorndike built puzzle-boxes for use with cats, whose task was to operate a latch that would automatically cause the door to spring open (Figure 14.5).[19] Each time they managed to escape, there was a piece of fish, visible from inside the puzzle-box, waiting for them. The cats were deprived of food for a considerable time before the experiments began and so were highly motivated. After eating the fish, the cats

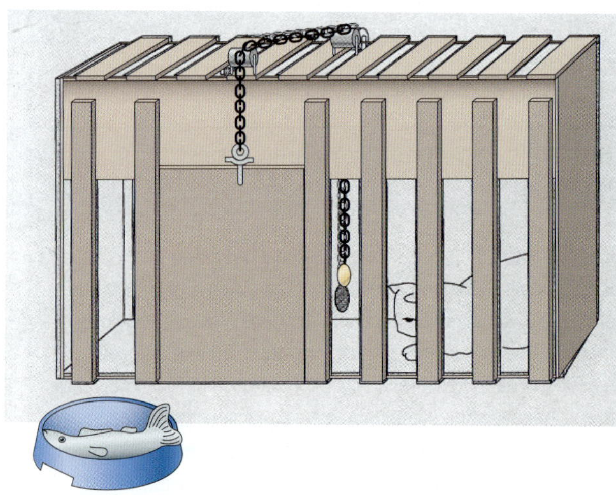

Figure 14.5 Thorndike's puzzle-box

Box 14.5 Major similarities and differences between classical and operant conditioning

SIMILARITIES

- They are both types of associative learning.
- Generalization, discrimination, extinction and spontaneous recovery occur in both.

DIFFERENCES

- In classical conditioning, the unconditioned response (UCR) or conditioned response (CR) is elicited (triggered automatically) by the unconditioned stimulus (UCS) or conditioned stimulus (CS) (it is essentially a reflex, involuntary response). In operant conditioning, behaviour is emitted by the organism and is essentially voluntary.
- In classical conditioning, the stimulus is guaranteed to produce the response, while the likelihood of a particular operant response being emitted is a function of the past consequences of such behaviour (it is more or less probable, but never certain).
- In classical conditioning, the UCS works in basically the same way regardless of whether it is pleasurable (e.g. food) or aversive (e.g. electric shock). In operant conditioning, responses that result in pleasurable outcomes are likely to be repeated, while those that result in aversive outcomes are not.
- In classical conditioning, completely new stimulus–response (S–R) connections are formed; operant conditioning, however, involves the strengthening or weakening of response tendencies already present in the animal's behavioural repertoire.
- In classical conditioning, the reinforcer (UCS) is presented regardless of what the animal does, and is presented before the response. In operant conditioning, the reinforcer is presented only if the animal emits some specified, preselected behaviour and is presented after the behaviour.
- In classical conditioning, the strength of conditioning is typically measured in terms of response magnitude (e.g. how many drops of saliva) and/or latency (how quickly a response is produced by a stimulus). In operant, strength is measured mainly as response rate (Table 14.2).

were put straight back in the box, and the whole process was repeated.

At first the cats struggled to get out, behaving in a purely random way, and it was only by chance that the first escape was made. But every time the cats were returned to the puzzle-box, it took them less time to operate the latch and escape again. For instance, with one of the boxes, the average time for the first escape was 5 min, but after 10–20 trials this was reduced to about 5 s.

Thorndike accounted for this by claiming that the learning was essentially random or trial-and-error. There was no sudden flash of insight into how the releasing mechanism worked, but rather there was a gradual reduction in the number of errors made and hence the escape time. What was being learned was a connection between the stimulus (the manipulative components of the box) and the response (the behaviour that allowed the cat to escape). Further, the stimulus–response (S–R) connection is 'stamped in when pleasure results from the act, and stamped out when it doesn't' (law of effect). This is crucially important as a way of distinguishing classical and operant conditioning, which Skinner did 40 years later.

Skinner's 'analysis of behaviour'

Skinner used a form of puzzle-box known as a 'Skinner box'. This was designed for a rat or pigeon to do things in, rather than escape from. The box has either a lever (in the case of rats) or illuminated discs (in the case of pigeons), under which is a food tray. The experimenter decides exactly what the relationship shall be between pressing the lever and the delivery of a food pellet, providing total control of the animal's environment. But it is the animal that has to do the work.

Skinner used the term 'strengthen' in place of Thorndike's 'stamping in', and 'weaken' in place of 'stamping out'. He regarded Thorndike's terms as too mentalistic, and his own as more objective and descriptive (Box 14.6).

Box 14.6 Skinner's analysis of behaviour (or the ABC of operant conditioning)

The analysis of behaviour requires an accurate but neutral representation of the relationship (or *contingencies*) between the following:

- *Antecedents:* the stimulus conditions, e.g. the lever, the click of the food dispenser, a light that may go on when the lever is pressed
- *Behaviours or operants:* e.g. pressing the lever
- *Consequences:* what happens as a result of the operant behaviour – i.e. reinforcement or punishment.

Table 14.2 Common reinforcement schedules and associated patterns of response and resistance to extinction

Reinforcement schedule	Example	Pattern and rate of responding	Resistance to extinction	Example of human behaviour
Continuous reinforcement (CRF)	Every single response is reinforced	Response rate is low but steady	Very low; the quickest way to bring about extinction	Receiving a high grade for every assignment Receiving a tip for every customer served
Fixed interval (FI)	A reinforcement is given every 30 s (FI 30), provided the response occurs at least once during that time	Response rate speeds up as the next reinforcement becomes available; a pause after each reinforcement; overall response rate fairly low	Fairly low; extinction occurs quite quickly	Being paid regularly (every week or month) Giving yourself a 15-min break for every hour's studying done
Variable interval (VI)	A reinforcement is given on average every 30 s (VI 30), but the interval varies from trial to trial, so the interval on any one occasion is unpredictable	Response rate is very stable over long periods of time; still some tendency to increase response rate as time elapses since the last reinforcement	Very high; extinction occurs very slowly and gradually	Many self-employed people receive payment irregularly, depending on when the customer pays for the product or service
Fixed ratio (FR)	A reinforcement is given for a fixed number of responses, however long this may take, e.g. 1 reinforcement in every 10 responses (FR 10)	There is a pronounced pause after each reinforcement, and then a very high rate of responding leading up to the next reinforcement	As in FI	Piece work (the more work done, the more money earned) Commission (extra money for so many goods made or sales completed)
Variable ratio (VR)	A reinforcement is given on average every 10 responses (VR 10), but the number varies from trial to trial, so the number of responses required on any one occasion is unpredictable	Very high response rate; very steady	Very high; the most resistant of all the schedules	Gambling

According to Skinner's version of the law of effect, 'behaviour is shaped and maintained by its consequences'. The consequences of operants can be positive reinforcement, negative reinforcement or punishment (Figure 14.6).

Although both positive and negative reinforcement strengthen behaviour (making it more probable), each works in a different way. Positive reinforcement involves presenting something pleasurable (e.g. food), while negative reinforcement involves the removal or avoidance of some 'aversive' (literally 'painful') state of affairs (e.g. electric shock). Punishment weakens behaviour (making it less probable), through the presentation of an aversive stimulus (Figure 14.7).

Reinforcers and reinforcement

Food is a reinforcer, and electric shock a punisher. The process whereby food is presented as a result of, say, lever-pressing is (positive) reinforcement; when electric shock is presented, it is called punishment. Skinner argues that deciding whether something is a reinforcer or a punisher can be done only after it has been made contingent on a specific behaviour on a number of occasions. Thus, if the behaviour is strengthened when followed by food, then the food is a reinforcer; if the shock weakens the behaviour, then the shock is a punisher. Reinforcers and punishers cannot be defined independently of the effects they have on behaviour.

Skinner's definition could be accused of circularity ('a

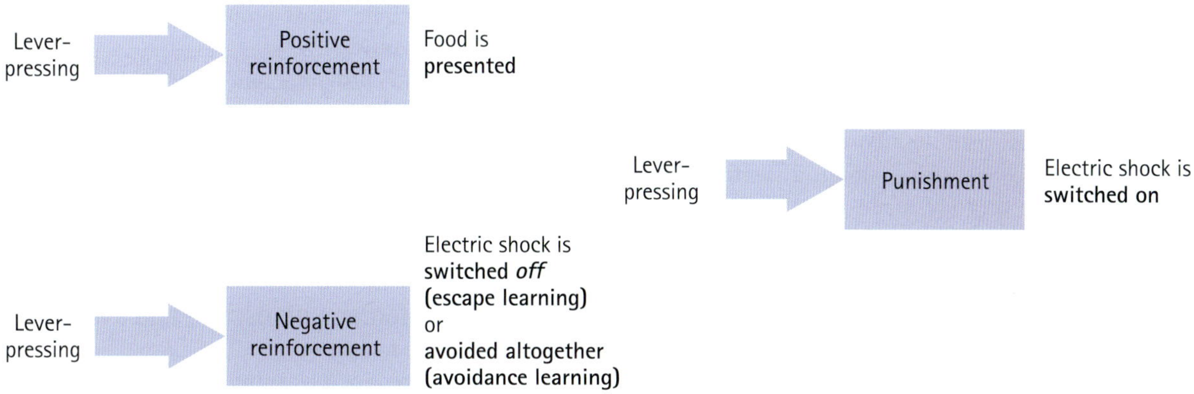

Figure 14.6 Three possible consequences of lever-pressing in a Skinner box

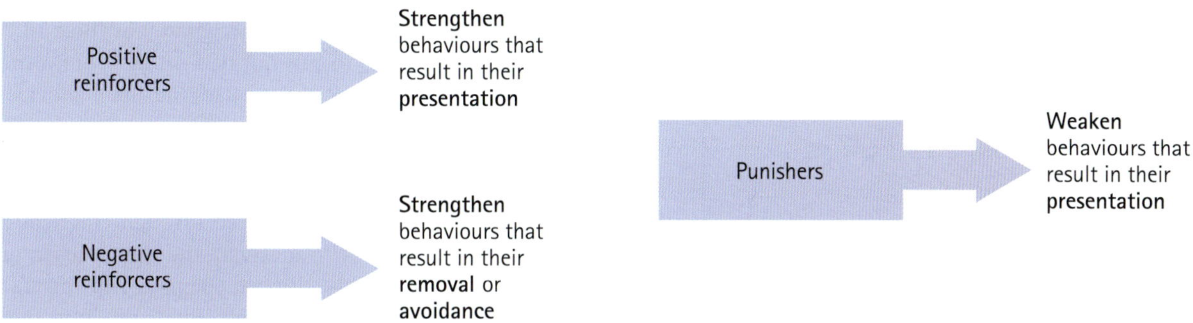

Figure 14.7 Consequences of behaviour and their effects

reinforcer is whatever strengthens behaviour' and 'whatever strengthens behaviour is a reinforcer'). In practice, animals are starved for several hours before the experiments begin, in order to ensure that they will be motivated and find food reinforcing.

Skinner argues that his approach is more scientific, since the intended effect may not always coincide with the actual effect. For example, if a child who feels deprived of his or her parents' attention is smacked and shouted at when misbehaving, the child is more likely to carry on being naughty. For a child who feels ignored, any attention is better than no attention at all. So, what is 'punishment' as far as the parents are concerned may be a positive reinforcement for the child. Similarly, a positive reinforcement can be called a reward only loosely, since the term 'reward' implies that the rewarder expects to strengthen some behaviour, whereas 'positive reinforcement' refers to what has been shown to strengthen it.

Primary and secondary reinforcers

Primary reinforcers (e.g. food, water, sex) are natural reinforcers (reinforcing in themselves). Secondary reinforcers acquire their reinforcing properties through association with primary reinforcers; that is, we have to learn (through classical conditioning) to find them reinforcing. Examples of human secondary (or conditioned) reinforcers are money, trading stamps, cheques and tokens (see Chapter 67).

In a Skinner box, if a click accompanies the presentation of each pellet of food, then the rat will eventually come to find the click on its own reinforcing. The click can then be used as a reinforcer for getting the rat to learn some new response. (Clickers are used in dog training, at first in conjunction with a primary reinforcer, such as a food treat, and then on their own). Secondary reinforcers are important because they bridge the gap between the response and the primary reinforcer, which may not be presented immediately.

Schedules of reinforcement

Another important aspect of Skinner's work is concerned with the effects on behaviour of how frequently and how regularly (or predictably) reinforcements are presented. Ferster and Skinner identified five major schedules, each of which is associated with a characteristic pattern of responding.[20] This part of Skinner's research is largely counter-intuitive.[21]

Rats and pigeons (and probably most mammals and birds) typically 'work harder' (press the lever/peck the disc at a faster rate) for scant reward: when reinforcements are relatively infrequent and irregular or unpredictable, they will go on working long after the reinforcement has been withdrawn. So, each schedule can be analysed in terms of pattern and rate of response and resistance to extinction (see Table 14.2).

The rate of response can be represented by plotting responses cumulatively as steps along a vertical axis, against the time when they are made along the horizontal axis (Figure 14.8). Skinner called this a 'cumulative record'.

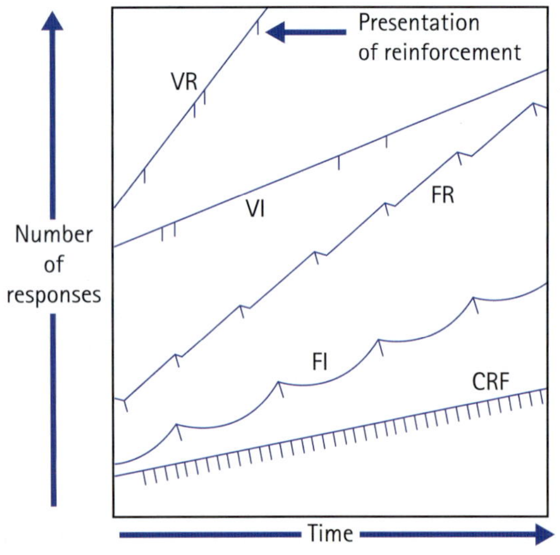

Figure 14.8 Typical cumulative records for a response (e.g. ever pressing) reinforced using fives schedules of reinforcement. CRF, continuous reinforcement; FR, fixed ratio; FI, fixed interval; VI, variable interval; VR, variable ratio.

A continuous schedule is usually used only when some new response is being learned. Once it has being emitted regularly and reliably, it can be maintained by using one of the four partial or intermittent schedules, but this change must be gradual. If the animal is switched from a continuous schedule to, say, a reinforcement given on average every 50 responses (VR 50), it will soon stop responding. Skinner originally used an interval schedule, because a reinforcer is guaranteed, sooner or later, so long as one response is made during the interval.

Shaping: the reinforcement of successive approximations

Reinforcement can be used to build up relatively complex behaviour (not part of the animal's natural repertoire) by reinforcing closer and closer approximations to the desired behaviour (*shaping*). First, the behaviour must be broken down into a number of small steps, each of which is reinforced in sequence. Gradually, what the animal can do is much more like what the experimenter is trying to teach it. This is what animal trainers have been doing for hundreds of years, and it is the method of reinforcement that Skinner used to teach pigeons to play ping-pong or to turn a full anticlockwise circle. Most human skills are learned in this step-by-step manner.

Shaping also provides an important foundation for behaviour modification. This is used to teach children and adults with learning difficulties to use the toilet, feed and dress themselves, and other social skills. It has also been used to develop speech in children with autism and adults with schizophrenia (see Chapter 67).

Negative reinforcement: escape and avoidance learning

Escape and avoidance learning are the two major ways in which negative reinforcement has been studied in the laboratory. Escape learning is relatively simple. For example, rats can learn to press a lever in order to turn off electric shock. Avoidance learning is more complex and more relevant to certain aspects of human behaviour (Box 14.7).

Miller trained rats to run out of a white room, through a small door, into a black room by giving them shocks in the white room.[24] After pretraining, the door was closed and could be opened only by the rat turning a wheel. Even though no further shocks were given, the residual 'aversiveness' of the white room (acquired through classical conditioning) was sufficient to motivate the rats to learn quickly to turn the wheel. This allowed them to run through into the 'safe' room, thus relieving their anxiety (negative reinforcement).

This illustrates an important difference between positive and negative reinforcement in relation to extinction. If we try to teach a rat a new response in order to get it into a black box that used to contain food, the rat will soon stop responding (it soon 'discovers' that the food is no longer

Box 14.7 Avoidance learning through negative reinforcement

Most laboratory studies use a *shuttle box*, a box divided into two compartments, sometimes with a barrier or door between them. Electric shocks can be delivered through the floor of either compartment independently of the other. Neither side is permanently safe, but only one is electrified at any one time.

The animal's task is to find which is the safe side on any one occasion. A *warning signal* (a light or buzzer) is given whenever the electrified side is to be changed, so the animal can always avoid being shocked if it switches sides when it hears or sees the signal.

According to the *two-factor theory*[22] or the *two-process theory*,[23] the animal first learns to be afraid (the warning signal elicits an anticipatory emotional response of fear/anxiety through classical conditioning). It then learns a response to reduce the fear (jumping the barrier is negatively reinforced by avoiding the shock before it is switched on).

available). But if a rat successfully escapes from a white room that used to be dangerous, the rat may go on escaping indefinitely (it does not stay around long enough to 'discover' that the shock is no longer happening).

So, responses motivated by conditioned fear/anxiety should take longer to extinguish than those motivated by positive incentives. Avoidance learning prevents the learner from testing reality, and this has been found in dogs and humans.[25,26] This can explain both the persistence of human phobias and the use of methods to remove them based on the principle of *forced reality testing* (see Chapter 67).

Punishment

Skinner maintained that, with both humans and non-humans, positive (and, to a lesser extent, negative) reinforcement is a much more potent influence on behaviour than is punishment. This is largely because punishment can only make certain responses less likely: you cannot teach anything new by punishment alone.

However, Campbell and Church argue that punishments are, if anything, *a stronger influence* on behaviour than the incentive effects of reinforcements (at least as far as laboratory animals are concerned).[27] But punishment produces unpleasant side effects, such as stress, anxiety, withdrawal and aggression.

Estes concluded that punishment merely *suppresses* lever-pressing in the short term but does not weaken it.[28] Other experiments have shown that the strength and duration of the suppression effect depend on the intensity of the punishment and the degree of deprivation. However, the response is still suppressed rather than unlearned.

When alternative ways of obtaining reinforcers are available, punishment has a more powerful suppressive effect on the punished behaviour.[29] For example, Azrin and Holz combined punishment and reinforcement, so that response A was punished while response B (incompatible with A) was positively reinforced.[30] Skinner advocates this with human beings.

The antecedents of behaviour: stimulus control

In operant conditioning, the stimulus indicates the likely consequence of emitting a particular response: the operant behaviour is more likely to occur in the presence of some stimuli than others. If a rat has been reinforced for pressing the lever, then it is more likely to go on emitting that response as the lever becomes associated with both reinforcement and the action of pressing (probably through classical conditioning). Technically, lever-pressing has now come under the stimulus control of the lever. But there is still no inevitability about pressing it, only an increased probability. (This is why the term 'S–R psychology' strictly applies only to classical conditioning.)

Similarly, drivers' behaviour is brought under the stimulus control of traffic signals, road signs, other vehicles, pedestrians and so on. Much of our everyday behaviour can be seen in this way. Sitting on a chair, answering the telephone, turning on the television and so on are all operants that are more likely to occur in the presence of those stimuli because of the past consequences of doing so.

A special case of stimulus control is a *discriminative stimulus*. If a rat in the Skinner box is reinforced for lever-pressing only when a light is on, then the light soon becomes a discriminative stimulus (the rat presses the lever only when the light is on).

Does conditioning work in the same way for all species?

The fact that many experiments involving a variety of species can all be described as classical conditioning does not in itself mean that there is only one mechanism involved, or only one explanation that applies equally to all species and all cases.[21] Although *conditionability* seems to be an almost universal property of nervous systems (including those of sea snails, flatworms and fruit flies), many psychologists have argued that there can be no general laws of learning.[31]

If such laws do exist, then one of them is likely to be the *law of contiguity*: events (or stimuli) that occur close together in time and space are likely to become associated with each other. Most of the examples of conditioning that we have considered so far would appear to 'obey' the law of contiguity. Box 14.8 describes some very important exceptions to this law.

Although rats can also be conditioned to novel smells, auditory, visual and tactile stimuli are not associated so readily with internal illness. As for pigeons, it is impossible to deter them from water and, for other species, taste aversions are very difficult to establish, even if the animal is made very ill. In almost all species, aversions to new

Box 14.8 Learning to feel as sick as a rat[32,33]

In Garcia *et al.*'s study, rats were given a novel-tasting solution, such as saccharine-flavoured water (the conditioned stimulus, CS), before the drug apomorphine (the unconditioned stimulus, UCS), which has a delayed action, inducing severe intestinal illness (the unconditioned response, UCR).[33]

In two separate experiments, the precise time-lapse between tasting the solution and onset of the drug-induced nausea was either (i) 5, 6, 7, 8, 9, 10, 11, 12, 15, 16, 17, 18, 19, 20, 21 and 22 min, or (ii) 30, 45, 75, 120 and 180 min.

In (i), the rats received just four treatments (one every third day). In all cases, there was a conditioned aversive response to the solution: intestinal illness became a conditioned response (CR) (a response to the solution alone). In some replications, just a single treatment was required.

flavours are learned more easily than aversions to familiar flavours (saccharine solution is a novel taste for the rat).

Biological constraints on conditioning

It seems, then, that there are definite biological limitations on the ability of animals to develop a conditioned aversion. Similarly, rats typically learn very quickly to avoid shock in a shuttle box and to press a lever for food. However, they do not learn very readily to press a lever in order to avoid shock. Pigeons can be trained quickly to fly from one perch to another in order to avoid shock, but it is almost impossible to train them to peck a disc in order to avoid shock.

Findings such as these have led Bolles and others to conclude that we cannot regard the basic principles of learning as applying equally to all species in all situations.[34] We must take into account the evolutionary history of the species, as well as the individual organism's learning history. An important idea in this context is Seligman's concept of *preparedness*.[31] Animals are biologically prepared to learn actions that are related closely to the survival of their species (e.g. learned water or food aversions), and these prepared behaviours are learned with very little training. Equally, *contra-prepared* behaviours are contrary to an animal's natural tendencies and so are learned with great difficulty, if at all. Seligman believes that most of the behaviour studied in the laboratory falls somewhere in between these two extremes.

As far as human behaviour is concerned, much of the relevant data relate to how easily certain conditioned fear responses can be induced in the laboratory or how common certain naturally occurring phobias are compared with others. For example, Ohman *et al.* paired slides of snakes and spiders with a strong electric shock and quickly established conditioned emotional responses to these slides – but not to slides of flowers, houses or berries.[35,36]

Seligman observed that human phobias tend to fall into certain narrow categories – mostly animals and dangerous places.[37] Most common of all were fears of snakes, spiders, the dark, high places and closed-in places; often there is no previous evidence for the fear actually having been conditioned (see Chapter 40). Also, classically conditioned responses extinguish faster in humans than animals. This is because the CRs are modulated by more complex human memories.[38]

The role of cognition in conditioning

According to Mackintosh, conditioning cannot be reduced to the strengthening of S–R associations by the automatic action of a process called reinforcement.[39] It is more appropriate to think of it as a matter of detecting and learning about relations between events. Animals typically discover what signals or causes events that are important to them, such as food, water, danger or safety. Salivation and lever-pressing are simply a convenient index of what the subject has learned, namely that certain relationships exist in its environment.

Classical conditioning

Pavlov described the CS as a 'signal' for the UCS, the relationship between CS and the UCS as one of 'stimulus substitution', and the CR as an 'anticipatory' response (or 'psychic secretions'), suggesting that his dogs were expecting the food to follow the bell. Consistent with this interpretation, Rescorla presented two groups of animals with the same number of CS–UCS pairings, but the second group also received additional presentations of the UCS on its own without the CS.[40] The first group showed much stronger conditioning than the second group, indicating that the most important factor (at least in classical conditioning) is how predictably the UCS follows the CS, rather than how often the CS and UCS are paired.

Blocking also supports a more cognitive interpretation.[41] For example, if an animal is shown a light, quickly followed by an electric shock, then the light soon comes to elicit fear as a CR. If a noise is then added (noise + light + shock), then the noise should also soon become a CS, because it too is being paired with shock. However, this is not what happens. If the noise is later presented alone, it fails to produce a CR. It seems that the noise has somehow been 'blocked' from becoming a CS because of the previous conditioning to the light. In cognitive terms, since the light already predicts shock, the noise is irrelevant. It provides no additional information – the animal already 'knows' that shock will follow the light.

Operant conditioning

Seligman's study of learned helplessness is described in Box 14.9.[42] According to Seligman, the dogs learned that no behaviour on their part had any effect on the occurrence (or non-occurrence) of a particular event (the shock). This has

Box 14.9 Learned helplessness[42]

Dogs were strapped into a harness and given a series of shocks from which they could not escape. The dogs were later required to jump a barrier in a shuttle box within 10 s of a warning signal, or suffer 50 s of painful shock.

Control dogs (which had not been subjected to the inescapable shocks) learned the avoidance response very quickly, but about two-thirds of the experimental dogs seemed unable to do so. The experimental dogs seemed passively resigned to suffering the shock. Even if they did successfully avoid the shock on one trial, they were unlikely to do so on the next trial. Some dogs had to be pushed over the barrier 200 times or more before this learned helplessness wore off.

been demonstrated by Miller and Norman using human participants.[43] Maier and Seligman have tried to explain depression in humans in terms of learned helplessness (see Chapter 39).[44]

Skinner's claim that reinforcements and punishments automatically strengthen and weaken behaviour has been challenged by Bandura: 'Reinforcements serve principally as an informative and motivational operation rather than as a mechanical response strengthener.'[45,46]

Reinforcement provides the learner with information about the likely consequences of certain behaviour under certain conditions; that is, it improves our prediction of whether a given action will lead to pleasant (reinforcement) or unpleasant (punishment) outcomes in the future. It also motivates us by causing us to anticipate future outcomes. Our present behaviours are governed largely by the outcomes that we expect them to have, and we are more likely to learn behaviour if we value its consequences.

Social learning theory

This cognitive reinterpretation of reinforcement forms part of Bandura's *social learning theory* (SLT),[45,46] which has been applied to a variety of behaviours, including aggression, moral and gender development, and personality (see Gross[47] and Chapter 19). SLT represents an attempt to reinterpret certain aspects of Freud's psychoanalytical theory in terms of classical and operant conditioning.

As well as focusing on human social behaviour, Bandura and other social learning theorists believe that there are important *cognitive mediating variables* between stimulus and response without which we cannot explain human behaviour adequately. Some of the most important cognitive variables include *self-concept*, *self-monitoring* (or self-regulation) and *self-efficacy* (our belief that we can act effectively and exercise control over events that influence our lives.[45,48] Self-efficacy is crucially important for motivation: how we judge our own capabilities is likely to affect our expectations about future behaviour (see Chapter 15). The central importance of cognitive factors is reflected in Bandura's renaming of SLT as *social cognitive theory*.[48,49]

Social learning theorists also emphasize the role of *observational learning* (or modelling); that is, learning through the behaviour of others – models). This occurs spontaneously, with no deliberate effort by the learner, or any intention by the model to teach anything. Observational learning takes place without any reinforcement: mere exposure to the model is sufficient for learning to occur.[50]

Tolman's cognitive behaviourism

Although working within the behaviourist tradition in the 1920s, 1930s and 1940s, Tolman would be regarded today as a cognitive psychologist. He explained the learning of rats in terms of inferred cognitive processes, in particular cognitive or mental maps.

In Box 14.10, clearly the rats in group 3 had been learning their way through the maze during the first 10 days, but the learning was *latent* (hidden or 'behaviourally silent'). In other words, the learning did not show up in their actual behaviour until they received the incentive of the reinforcement on day 11. Tolman and Honzik concluded that reinforcement may be important in relation to performance of learned behaviour, but that it is not necessary for the learning itself.[51]

Box 14.10 Latent learning: who needs reinforcement?[51]

- *Group 1* rats were reinforced every time they found their way through a maze to the food box.
- *Group 2* rats were never reinforced.
- *Group 3* rats received no reinforcement for the first 10 days of the experiment, but did so from day 11.

Not surprisingly, the rats in group 1 learned the maze quickly and made fewer and fewer mistakes, while the rats in group 2 never reduced the time it took to find the food, and moved around aimlessly much of the time.

The rats in group 3 made no apparent progress during the first 10 days, but they then showed a sudden decrease in the time it took to reach the goal box on day 11, when they received their first reinforcement. They caught up almost immediately with the rats in group 1 (Figure 14.9).

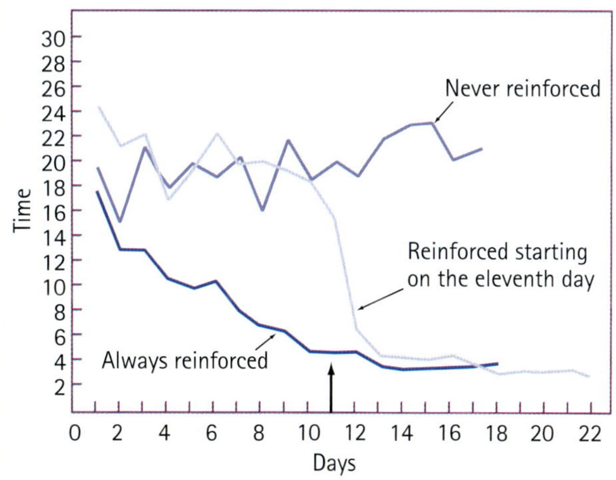

Figure 14.9 Results of Tolman and Honzik's study of latent learning in rats

Tolman's *place learning* (or *sign learning*) theory maintains that rats learn expectations as to which part of the maze will be followed by which other part of the maze.[52] Tolman called these expectations *cognitive maps*, a primitive kind of perceptual map of the maze, an understanding of its spatial relationships (much like the mental map you have of familiar streets leading to places you know well).

Although a cognitive map can only be inferred from actual behaviour, it is difficult to know how else to explain the findings that rats will take shortcuts to the food box if the old path is blocked. Similarly, if the maze were rotated, the rats could find the usual food location from several different starting points.[53] Restle flooded a maze immediately after a group of rats had learned to run it, and they were able to swim to the goal box with no more errors than when they had walked.[54] This clearly supports Tolman's interpretation.

Practical applications of learning theory

As we have seen, methodological behaviourism's emphasis on experimentation, operational definitions and the measurement of observable events has had a major influence on the practice of scientific psychology in general, quite unrelated to any views about the nature and role of mental events. Other, more tangible, contributions include the following:

- *Behaviour therapy* and *behaviour modification* (based on classical and operant conditioning, respectively) are major approaches to the treatment of abnormal behaviour (see Chapter 67) and one of the main tools in the clinical psychologist's kit bag (see Chapter 9). Specific examples of behaviour modification in particular have been given above.
- *Behavioural neuroscience* is an interdisciplinary field of study, using behavioural techniques to understand brain function and neuroscientific techniques to elucidate behavioural processes. Although many researchers believe that behaviour can be reduced to, or explained by, brain processes, the evidence shows that each is dependent on the other.[9]
- *Behavioural pharmacology* involves the use of schedules of reinforcement to assess the behavioural effects of new drugs that modify brain activity. Most importantly, the research has illustrated how many behavioural effects of drugs are determined as much by the current behaviour and reinforcement contingencies as by the effects of the drug on the brain.[9]
- *Environmental enrichment studies* have produced evidence for neuronal plasticity; that is, the brain's capacity for change and adapting to changing environmental conditions. These findings have exciting implications for the treatment of strokes and other conditions involving brain damage.

According to Leslie:

> The life-long interaction between the behaviour of the individual and the environment produces changes in the brain. This in turn changes behaviour, and so the interaction goes on. Any attempt to deal with a human behavioural problem can involve changes to the nervous system, behaviour or the environment.[9]

Learning theory and addiction

Classical conditioning

According to Claridge and Davis, the common reward pathway in the brain is also involved in *associative learning*; that is, in establishing the conditioned reinforcement of environmental cues that signal the approach or onset of the natural reward state.[55] They are referring to *classical conditioning*.

As applied to addiction, classical conditioning might be able to explain how a stimulus associated with a drug (e.g. drug paraphernalia) can come to produce a similar response to the response produced by the drug itself (as well as a similar reaction in the brain), but it cannot explain how or why the drug is taken in the first place. Unless the drug is forced upon the individual in some way, we need to account for how addiction is initiated, and classical conditioning (on its own) cannot do this because it can account only for involuntary behaviour.

Because of the powerful nature of the response produced by most drugs, classical conditioning can better explain the maintenance of addictive behaviours (e.g. through the process of *stimulus generalization*). However, what about addictive activities that do not involve such powerful, biologically determined UCRs? For example, by definition, gamblers win only some of the time (they usually lose more often than they win); so why does gambling not stop through extinction? The answer seems to rely on operant conditioning (see below).

As we have seen, when experimental animals are presented with the CS without the UCS, the CR gradually weakens and eventually stops altogether (*experimental extinction*); this is equivalent to the addict being denied access to the substance or activity of their addiction and abstaining. However, when the UCS is later reintroduced, experimental animals will display the CS again (through *spontaneous recovery*). This corresponds to the addict's relapse and shows that in extinction the CS is merely suppressed rather than destroyed.

From an evolutionary perspective, the ability of environmental cues to signal the approach or onset of the natural reward state is clearly a very adaptive function: the organism will fare much better if it can discriminate between stimuli that predict when a rewarding event is likely to happen, and those that do not.[55] A relatively large body of research supports the role of the amygdala in this process, because it maintains a representation of the affective (emotional) value of the CS (see Claridge and Davis[55]).This is a good example of how the function of brain structures complements, and is correlated with, psychological processes (here, acquiring conditioned responses through classical conditioning).

The strength of conditioned reinforcement is greatly enhanced when the CS is paired with certain kinds of UCS (in particular, pharmacological rewards, e.g. cocaine) than others (e.g. food). This demonstrates that classical conditioning is a more complex learning process than it might at first appear: its effects are mediated by which particular UCS is used (which suggests the role of biological factors). Other research has demonstrated the role of cognitive factors (see above).

Operant (instrumental or Skinnerian) conditioning

One of the best-known explanations of gambling behaviour is that it illustrates very well the process of operant conditioning, specifically, a *variable ratio reinforcement schedule* (see Table 14.2). As in all cases of operant conditioning, the organism must perform some specified action in order to receive a particular positive reinforcement.

In general terms, applying this framework to drug dependence is straightforward if we define dependence operationally as an excessive tendency to engage in drug-taking behaviour. According to Powell:

> ... This implies that the rewards to the addict are so salient, and sufficiently reliable, that he or she has become motivated to take the drug progressively more often in order to achieve these effects, eventually reaching a point where the desire overwhelms all else ...[56]

If a gambler is used to winning only on a certain proportion of occasions, then not winning on any particular occasion will come as no surprise and will not cause the behaviour to extinguish (as might happen if the gambler wins every time). Tied to this irregularity of success is the unpredictability (the gambler does not know when the next success will come): not winning will not 'throw' the gambler. However, wins and losses average out over a large number of bets. (Of course, if the gambler never won again, the behaviour would, eventually, cease).

This account relates to maintenance of behaviour: the gambling will persist in the absence of reinforcement because the gambler is used to receiving only intermittent, irregular reinforcements. However, as with classical conditioning, its ability to explain initiation is very limited. Unlike classical conditioning, a VR schedule describes a situation where the reinforcer is presented a specific proportion of times the response is made. As we have seen, the behaviour persists for much longer than it would if the reinforcement occurred every time (i.e. abstinence is more difficult to achieve); relapse (which occurs only after a period of abstinence) is, therefore, less likely to occur in the first place, but if it does occur, it can be also be explained in terms of spontaneous recovery.

However, just because gambling is commonly given as the classic example of human behaviour controlled by a VR schedule does not mean that other addictive behaviours can necessarily be explained in similar terms. The equivalent for the drug addict would be that only sometimes does snorting cocaine produce a high; although some highs may be higher than others, this is hardly equivalent to winning or not winning on, say, a fruit machine. Also, different classes of drug exert very different pharmacological effects, so that the rewards that have contributed to the development of the addiction will vary from drug to drug.[56]

As well as accounting for maintenance/persistence of certain addictive behaviours, operant conditioning also offers an explanation of how difficult it might be for someone to break their habit. For example, the decision to try to break a habit can be seen as reflecting the strength of its punishing outcomes: since most habits produce mixed effects, some pleasant and others aversive, addicts may find themselves in an *approach-avoidance conflict*, where motivation fluctuates between wanting to use and wanting to stop.[56]

In the context of gambling, Sharpe (cited in Bennett[57]) claims that, although VR schedules undoubtedly contribute to high levels of social gambling, they do not fully explain pathological gambling, where consistent and significant losses do not cause the individual to stop gambling. Sharpe suggests that large payouts and, in particular, a 'big win' early in a gambling career establish and sustain pathological gambling. These presumably distort expectations of the outcomes of gambling and support losses in the expectation of future 'big wins'.

Social learning theory

As we saw above, neither classical nor operant conditioning can easily explain how addictive behaviours occur in the first place. But SLT, through its emphasis on observational learning/modelling, together with its claim that mere exposure to the model is sufficient for learning to take place, can quite easily explain why someone would begin engaging in behaviour that leads to addiction. Although reinforcement of some kind might be necessary for the learned behaviour to actually show, this may only require the model to be rewarded.[50] So, for example, observing a model win at a fruit machine might be enough for a child to begin developing the habit.

KEY POINTS

- Learning has played a major part in the development of psychology as a scientific discipline and is central to the behaviourist approach. Psychologists are interested in learning as a process.
- It is generally agreed that learning involves a relatively permanent change in behaviour due to past experience.

- Watson's methodological behaviourism focuses on what can be observed and quantified by different observers. Skinner's radical behaviourism regards mental processes as both inaccessible and irrelevant to explaining behaviour.
- The distinction between respondent and operant behaviour corresponds to classical (respondent or Pavlovian) and operant (instrumental or Skinnerian) conditioning, respectively.
- In classical conditioning, the pairing of a conditioned and an unconditioned stimulus results in the former eliciting a response that formerly was produced only by the latter.
- Delayed/forward, backward, simultaneous and trace conditioning differ according to the relationships between the conditioned and the unconditioned stimuli.
- Generalization, discrimination, extinction and spontaneous recovery represent conditioning phenomena that make it more complex and versatile. Spontaneous recovery demonstrates that extinction involves a learning to inhibit/suppress the conditioned response.
- Watson applied classical conditioning to human behaviour for the first time by inducing fear of a rat in Little Albert. Jones removed animal phobias from Little Peter using an early form of systematic desensitization.
- Compared with classical conditioning, operant conditioning considers learning to be a much more active process. Skinner was interested in how animals operate on their environment, and how their activity is instrumental in producing certain consequences.
- Skinner's work was based on Thorndike's law of effect. He designed a form of puzzle-box (a Skinner box), and called the consequences of behaviour positive reinforcement, negative reinforcement and punishment.
- Reinforcement (both positive and negative) strengthens behaviour, while punishment weakens it.
- Primary reinforcers are naturally reinforcing, while secondary/conditioned reinforcers come to be reinforcing through association with primary reinforcers.
- Different schedules of reinforcement can be analysed in terms of pattern/rate of response and resistance to extinction. Variable schedules involve high, steady rates of response and high resistance to extinction, compared with fixed and continuous schedules.
- Shaping involves the reinforcement of successive approximations to the desired behaviour.
- Escape and avoidance learning are two forms of negative reinforcement. They have been explained by the two-factor theory, according to which both classical and operant conditioning are involved. The persistence of human phobias can be understood in terms of avoidance learning.
- Punishment seems to involve a suppression of behaviour and is most effective when combined with the reinforcement of an incompatible response.
- Taste-aversion experiments contribute to the view that the basic principles of conditioning do not apply equally to all species in all situations.
- Preparedness helps to explain experimental findings showing that different species acquire certain conditioned responses more or less easily, and why certain human phobias are more common than others.
- Classical conditioning involves learning about relations between environmental events, rather than a simple strengthening of S–R associations. Seligman's concept of learned helplessness illustrates the complexity of operant conditioning and has been used to explain human depression.
- Tolman's studies of latent learning show that learning can take place in the absence of reinforcement. Rats learn a cognitive map of the maze rather than the individual movements of walking or running that take them to the food box.
- Methodological behaviourism has influenced the practice of scientific psychology in general. Other applications of learning theory include behaviour therapy and modification, behavioural neuroscience and pharmacology, and environmental-enrichment studies.
- Although classical and operant conditioning can both explain the maintenance of various addictions, only social learning theory can account for their initiation.

REFERENCES

1. Coon D (1983) *Introduction to Psychology*, 3rd edn. St Paul, MN: West Publishing Co.
2. Anderson JR (1995a) *Learning and Memory: An Integrated Approach*. Chichester: John Wiley & Sons.
3. Skinner BF (1974) *About Behaviorism*. New York: Alfred Knopf.
4. Watson JB (1913) Psychology as the behaviourist views it. *Psychological Review* **20**: 158–77.
5. Blackman DE (1980) Images of man in contemporary behaviourism. In AJ Chapman, DM Jones (eds) *Models of Man*. Leicester: British Psychological Society.
6. Gross R (2009) *Themes, Issues and Debates in Psychology*, 3rd edn. London: Hodder Education.
7. Garrett, R (1996) Skinner's case for radical behaviourism. In W O'Donohue, RE Kitchener (eds) *The Philosophy of Psychology*. London: Sage.
8. Nye RD (2000) *Three Psychologies: Perspectives from Freud, Skinner and Rogers*, 6th edn. Belmont, CA: Wadsworth/Thomson Learning.
9. Leslie JC (2002) *Essential Behaviour Analysis*. London: Arnold.
10. O'Donohue W, Ferguson KE (2001) *The Psychology of BF Skinner*. Thousand Oaks, CA: Sage.
11. Pavlov IP (1927) *Conditioned Reflexes*. Oxford: Oxford University Press.
12. Davey GCL (1983) An associative view of human classical conditioning. In GCL Davey (ed.) *Animal Models of Human Behaviour: Conceptual, Evolutionary, and Neurobiological Perspectives*. Chichester: John Wiley & Sons.

13. Brewer WF (1974) There is no convincing evidence for operant or classical conditioning in adult humans. In WB Weimar, DS Palermo (eds) *Cognition and the Symbolic Processes.* Hillsdale, NJ: Lawrence Erlbaum Associates.
14. Dugdale N, Lowe CF (1990) Naming and stimulus equivalence. In DE Blackman, H Lejeune (eds) *Behaviour Analysis in Theory and Practice: Contributions and Controversies.* Hillsdale, NJ: Lawrence Erlbaum Associates.
15. Mackintosh NJ (1995) Classical and operant conditioning. In NJ Mackintosh, AM Colman (eds) *Learning and Skills.* London: Longman.
16. Watson JB, Rayner R (1920) Conditioned emotional reactions. *Journal of Experimental Psychology* **3**: 1–14.
17. Jones MC (1924) The elimination of children's fears. *Journal of Experimental Psychology* **7**: 382–90.
18. Wolpe J (1958) *Psychotherapy by Reciprocal Inhibition.* Stanford, CA: Stanford University Press.
19. Thorndike EL (1898) Animal intelligence: an experimental study of the associative processes in animals. *Psychological Review Monograph* **8** (suppl. 2).
20. Ferster CB, Skinner BF (1957) *Schedules of Reinforcement.* New York: Appleton-Century-Crofts.
21. Walker S (1984) *Learning Theory and Behaviour Modification.* London: Methuen.
22. Mowrer OH (1960) *Learning Theory and Behaviour.* New York: John Wiley & Sons.
23. Gray JA (1975) *Elements of a Two-Process Theory of Learning.* London: Academic Press.
24. Miller NE (1948) Theory and experiment relating psychoanalytic displacement to stimulus–response generalization. *Journal of Abnormal Psychology* **43**: 155–78.
25. Solomon RL, Wynne LC (1953) Traumatic avoidance learning: the outcomes of several extinction procedures with dogs. *Psychological Monographs* **4**: 66–7.
26. Turner LH, Solomon RL (1962) Human traumatic avoidance learning. *Psychological Monographs* **76**: 40.
27. Campbell BA, Church RM (1969) (eds) *Punishment and Aversive Behaviour.* New York: Appleton-Century-Crofts.
28. Estes WK (1970) *Learning Theory and Mental Development.* New York: Academic Press.
29. Howe M (1980) *The Psychology of Human Learning.* London: Harper & Row.
30. Azrin NH, Holz WC (1966) Punishment. In WK Honig (ed.) *Operant Behavior: Areas of Research and Application.* New York: Appleton-Century-Crofts.
31. Seligman MEP (1970) On the generality of the laws of learning. *Psychology Review* **77**: 406–18.
32. Garcia J, Koelling RA (1966) The relation of cue to consequence in avoidance learning. *Psychonomic Science* **4**: 123–4.
33. Garcia J, Ervin FR, Koelling RA (1966) Learning with prolonged delay of reinforcement. *Psychonomic Science* **5**: 121–2.
34. Bolles RC (1980) Ethological learning theory. In GM Gazda, RJ Corsini (eds) *Theories of Learning: A Comparative Approach.* Itaska, IL: Free Press.
35. Ohman A, Erikkson A, Olofsson C (1975) One-trial learning and superior resistance to extinction of autonomic responses conditioned to potentially phobic stimuli. *Journal of Comparative and Physiological Psychology* **88**: 619–27.
36. Ohman A, Erixson G, Loftberg L (1975) Phobias and preparedness: phobic and neutral pictures as conditioned stimuli for human autonomic responses. *Journal of Abnormal Psychology* **84**: 41–5.
37. Seligman MEP (1972) *Biological Boundaries of Learning.* New York: Academic Press.
38. Weiskrantz L (1982) Comparative aspects of studies of amnesia. *Philosophical Transactions of the Royal Society, London B* **298**: 97–109.
39. Mackintosh NJ (1978) Cognitive or associative theories of conditioning: implications of an analysis of blocking. In SH Hulse, M Fowler, WK Honig (eds) *Cognitive Processes in Animal Behaviour.* Hillsdale, NJ: Lawrence Erlbaum Associates.
40. Rescorla RA (1968) Probability of shock in the presence and absence of CS in fear conditioning. *Journal of Comparative and Physiological Psychology* **66**: 1–5.
41. Kamin L J. (1969) Predictability, surprise, attention, and conditioning. In BA Campbell, RM Church (eds) *Punishment and Aversive Behaviour.* New York: Appleton-Century-Crofts.
42. Seligman MEP (1975) *Helplessness: On Depression, Development and Death.* San Francisco, CA: W.H. Freeman.
43. Miller I, Norman W (1979) Learned helplessness in humans: A review and attribution theory model. *Psychological Bulletin* **86**: 93–118.
44. Maier SF, Seligman MEP (1976) Learned helplessness: theory and evidence. *Journal of Experimental Psychology: General* **105**: 3–46.
45. Bandura A (1977) Self-efficacy: toward a unifying theory of behaviour change. *Psychological Review* **84**: 191–215.
46. Bandura A (1977) *Social Learning Theory,* 2nd edn. Englewood Cliffs, NJ: Prentice-Hall.
47. Gross R (2005) *Psychology: The Science of Mind and Behaviour,* 5th edn. London: Hodder Arnold.
48. Bandura A (1986) *Social Foundations of Thought and Action.* Englewood Cliffs, NJ: Prentice-Hall.
49. Bandura A (1989) Social cognitive theory. In R Vasta (ed.) *Six Theories of Child Development.* Greenwich, CT: JAI Press.
50. Bandura A (1965) Influence of model's reinforcement contingencies on the acquisition of imitative responses. *Journal of Personality and Social Psychology* **1**: 589–95.
51. Tolman EC, Honzik CH (1930) Introduction and removal of reward and maze-learning in rats. *University of California Publications in Psychology* **4**: 257–75.

52. Tolman EC (1948) Cognitive maps in rats and man. *Psychological Review* **55**: 189–208.
53. Tolman EC, Ritchie BF, Kalish D (1946) Studies in spatial learning: 1 – orientation and the short-cut. *Journal of Experimental Psychology* **36**: 13–25.
54. Restle F (1957) Discrimination of cues in mazes: a resolution of the 'place versus response' question. *Psychological Review* **64**: 217–28.
55. Claridge G, Davis C (2003) *Personality and Psychological Disorders*. London: Arnold.
56. Powell J (2000) Drug and alcohol dependence. In L Champion, M Power (eds) *Adult Psychological Problems: An Introduction*, 2nd edn. Hove: Psychology Press.
57. Bennett P (2006) *Abnormal and Clinical Psychology: An Introductory Textbook*, 2nd edn. Maidenhead: Open University Press.

Chapter 15

Motivation

Richard Gross

INTRODUCTION

Trying to define motivation is a little like trying to define psychology itself. Taking as a starting point the layperson's view of psychology as the study of 'what makes people tick', motivation is concerned with why people act and think the way they do. 'Why' questions – and related 'how' questions – usually imply causes and underlying mechanisms or processes.

Each of the major theoretical approaches within psychology (behaviourist, psychodynamic, humanistic, neurobiological/biogenic, cognitive, evolutionary, social constructionist: see Gross[1]) tries to identify the key processes and mechanisms. This is also true of the neurobiological/biogenic approach. At the heart of each approach lies an image of human beings that, in essence, is a theory of the causes of human behaviour.

Motivated behaviour is goal-directed, purposeful behaviour. It is difficult to think of any behaviour, human or non-human, that is not motivated in this sense. However, just how the underlying motives are conceptualized and investigated depends very much on the persuasion of the psychologist. For example:

- A *psychodynamic* psychologist will try to discover internal, unconscious drives and motives (see Chapter 19 for a discussion of Freud's psychoanalytical theory).
- A *behaviourist* psychologist will look for environmental schedules of reinforcement, which can explain the behaviour of rats and pigeons as effectively as that of human beings (see Chapter 14). As a radical behaviourist, Skinner rejects the claim that mental or other internal events or processes – conscious or unconscious – can influence behaviour in any way. For him, 'motivation' and other mentalistic terms are 'explanatory fictions'.
- A *humanistic* psychologist, such as Maslow, will try to understand a person's behaviour in terms of a hierarchy of motives, with self-actualization at the top of the hierarchy.
- For a *biopsychologist*, what is crucial are bodily events and processes taking place in the central nervous system (CNS), the autonomic nervous system (ANS) and the endocrine system, or interactions between these different systems. These events and processes are related to the biological survival of the person or animal.

Although we shall consider a range of different motives, this chapter has a very 'biological' flavour. Maslow's *hierarchy of needs* is useful as a general framework for examining other approaches. *Homeostatic drive theories* try to explain hunger and thirst. But even in the case of such basic biological motives as these, cognitive and other individual factors, as well as social, cultural and other environmental factors, play a crucial role.

We shall also consider non-homeostatic needs and drives, including electrical self-stimulation of the brain (ES-SB), competence and cognitive motives, and some important social motives.

WHAT IS MOTIVATION?

According to Rubin and McNeil, motives are a special kind of cause that '... energize, direct and sustain a person's behaviour (including hunger, thirst, sex and curiosity)'.[2] Similarly, 'Motivation refers, in a general sense, to processes involved in the initiation, direction, and energization of individual behaviour ...'[3]

The word 'motive' comes from the Latin *movere* (= move), and this is captured in Miller's definition:

> The study of motivation is the study of all those pushes and prods – biological, social and psychological – that defeat our laziness and move us, either eagerly or reluctantly, to action.[4]

As we noted in the introduction to this chapter, different schools of thought within psychology look for the causes of behaviour in very different places. These differences indicate that motives may vary with regard to a number of features or dimensions, including:

- internal or external;
- innate or learned;
- mechanistic or cognitive;
- conscious or unconscious.

Several attempts have been made to classify different kinds of motive. For example, Rubin and McNeil classify motives into (i) survival or physiological motives and (ii) competence or cognitive motives.[2] Social motives represent a third category. Clearly, humans share survival motives with all other species, as well as certain competence motives (see below). But other motives are peculiarly and uniquely human, notably *self-actualization*, which lies at the peak of a 'hierarchy of needs' in Maslow's humanistic theory.[5]

Maslow's hierarchy of needs

Although Maslow's theory is commonly discussed in relation to personality (see Chapter 19), its focus on needs makes it equally relevant to motivation (Figure 15.1). (The book in which Maslow first proposed his hierarchy was called *Motivation and Personality*.[6]) According to Maslow, we are subject to two quite different sets of motivational states or forces:

- those that ensure survival by satisfying basic physical and psychological needs (physiological, safety, love and belongingness, esteem); and
- those that promote the person's self-actualization; that is, realizing one's full potential, 'becoming everything that one is capable of becoming',[6] especially in the intellectual and creative domains.

As Maslow states, 'We share the need for food with all living things, the need for love with (perhaps) the higher apes, [and] the need for Self-Actualization with [no other species].'

Behaviours that relate to survival or deficiency needs (*deficiency* or *D-motives*) are engaged in because they satisfy those needs (a means to an end). But behaviours that relate to self-actualization are engaged in for their own sake, because they are intrinsically satisfying (*growth*, *being* or *B-motives*). The latter include the fulfilment of ambitions; the acquisition of admired skills; the steady increase of understanding about people, the universe and oneself; the development of creativeness in whatever field; and, most importantly, simply the ambition to be a good human being. It is simply inaccurate to speak in such instances of tension reduction, which implies the overcoming of an

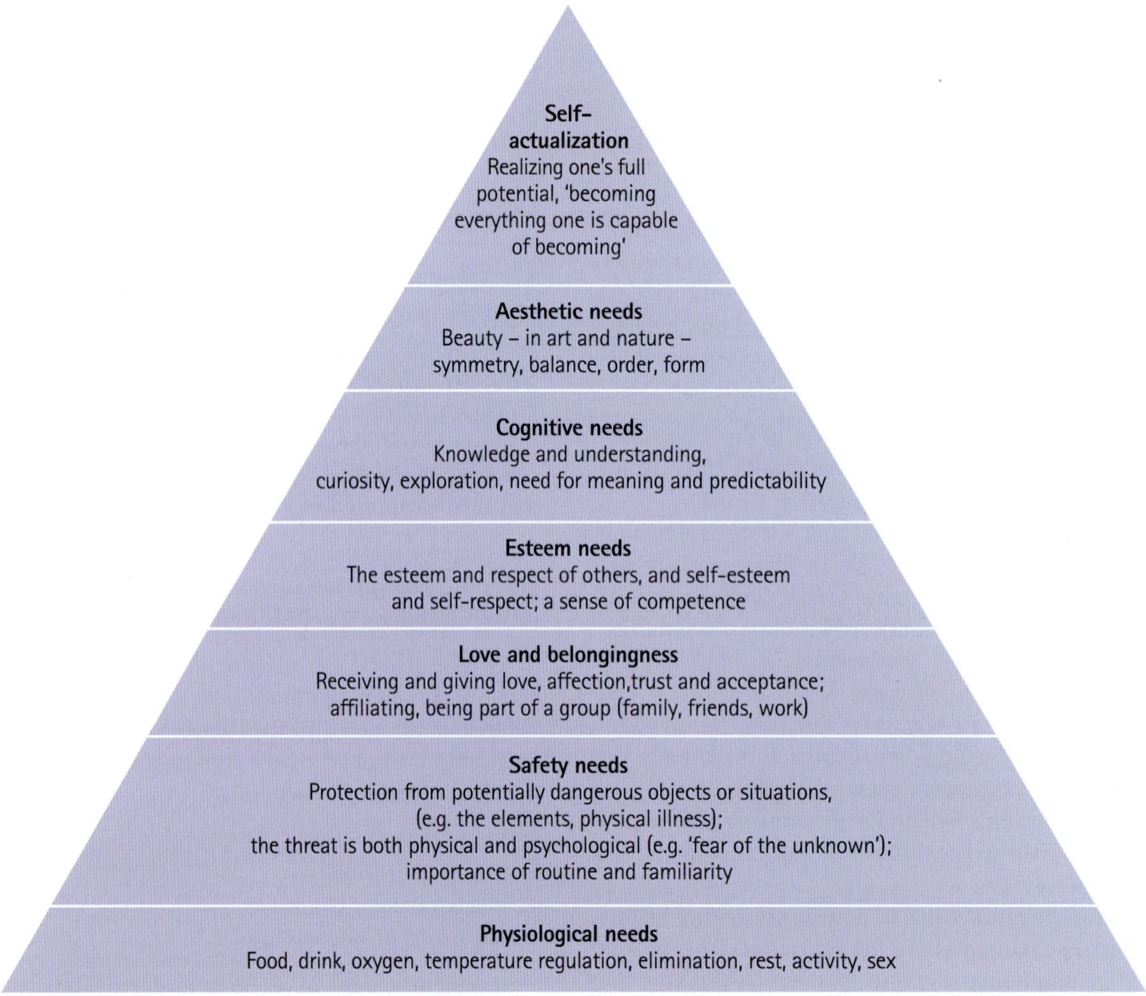

Figure 15.1 Maslow's hierarchy of needs. Based on Maslow.[5]

annoying state, for these states are not annoying.[7] (Another term for 'tension reduction' is 'drive reduction', which is discussed below). Maslow's argument is that to reduce the full range of human motives to drives that must be satisfied or removed is simply mistaken.

The hierarchical nature of Maslow's theory is intended to highlight the following points:

- Needs lower down in the hierarchy must be satisfied before we can attend to needs higher up. For example, if you are reading this while your stomach is trying to tell you that it is lunchtime, you probably won't absorb much about Maslow (pun intended!). Similarly if you are tired or in pain. Yet you can probably think of exceptions, such as the starving artist who finds inspiration despite hunger, or the mountain climber who risks his or her life for the sake of adventure (what Maslow would call a 'peak' experience – an unintended pun!).
- Higher-level needs are a later evolutionary development: in the development of the human species (phylogenesis), self-actualization is a fairly recent need. This applies equally to the development of individuals (ontogenesis): babies are concerned much more with their bellies than with their brains. But it is always a case of one need *predominating* at any one time rather than excluding all other needs.
- The higher up the hierarchy we go, the more the need becomes linked to life experience and the less 'biological' it becomes. Individuals achieve self-actualization in different ways, through different activities and by different routes. This is related to experience, not biology: 'A musician must make music, an artist must paint, a poet must write, if he is to be ultimately at peace with himself. What a man can be, he must be.'[7] This quote from Maslow captures nicely the idiographic nature of Maslow's theory – that is, the view that every individual is unique (see Chapter 19).
- The higher up the hierarchy we go, the more difficult it becomes to achieve the need. Many human goals are remote and long-term and can be achieved only in a series of steps. This pursuit of aims and goals that lie very much in the future is unique to human beings, although individuals differ in their ability to set and realize such goals.

THE EARLY STUDY OF MOTIVATION

As with many other aspects of psychology, the study of motivation has its roots in philosophy (see Chapter 9 and Gross[8]). Rationalists saw human beings as free to choose between different courses of action. This makes the concept of motivation almost unnecessary: it is our reason that determines our behaviour. This idea of freedom and responsibility is a basic premise of both humanistic and cognitive approaches (but see Chapter 10).

The seventeenth-century British philosopher Hobbes proposed the theory of hedonism. This maintains that all behaviour is determined by the seeking of pleasure and the avoidance of pain. These are the 'real' motives (whatever we may believe), and this idea is central to Freud's psychoanalytical theory, captured in the concept of the *pleasure principle*. Similarly, the basic principles of positive and negative reinforcement can be seen as corresponding to the seeking of pleasure and the avoidance of pain, respectively, and these are central to Skinner's operant conditioning (see Chapter 14).

During the 1920s, the concept of instinct (Box 15.1) was largely replaced by the concept of drive. The term 'drive' was first used by Woodworth, who compared human behaviour with the operation of a machine: the mechanism of a machine is relatively passive and drive is the power applied to make it 'go'. The concept of drive has taken two major forms: *homeostatic drive theory*,[12] which is a physiological theory, and *drive-reduction theory*,[13] which is primarily a theory of learning.

Box 15.1 Motives as instincts

The concept of instinct played a major role in early psychological approaches to motivation. Many psychologists, inspired by Darwin's theory of evolution, which argued that humans and animals differ only quantitatively,[9] identified human instincts that would explain human behaviour.

For example, McDougall originally proposed 12, and by 1924 over 800, separate instincts.[10] But to explain behaviour by labelling it explains nothing (e.g. 'We behave aggressively because of our aggressive instinct' is a circular statement). This, combined with the sheer proliferation of instincts, seriously undermined the whole approach.

However, the concept of instinct – with certain important modifications – remains a central feature of the ethological approach to behaviour, in particular non-human animal behaviour (see Gross *et al.*[11]).

HOMEOSTATIC DRIVE THEORY

The term 'homeostasis' is derived from the Greek *homos* (= same), and *stasis* (= stoppage). The term was coined by Cannon to refer to the process by which an organism maintains a fairly constant internal (bodily) environment; that is, how body temperature, blood sugar level, salt concentration in the blood, and so on are kept in a state of relative balance or equilibrium.[12]

The basic idea is that when a state of imbalance arises (e.g. through a substantial rise in body temperature), something must happen to correct the imbalance and restore equilibrium (sweating). In this case, the animal does not have to 'do' anything, because sweating is completely automatic and purely physiological. However, if the imbalance is caused by the body's need for food or drink (*tissue need*), then the hungry or thirsty animal has to do something in order to obtain food or water. This is where the concept of a homeostatic drive becomes important. Tissue need leads to internal imbalance, which leads to homeostatic drive, which leads to appropriate behaviour, which leads to restoration of internal balance, which leads to drive reduction.

The internal environment requires a regular supply of raw materials from the external world.[14] Although oxygen intake, for example, is involuntary and continuous, eating and drinking are voluntary and discontinuous (or spaced). We talk about a hunger and thirst drive, but we do not talk about an oxygen drive. Because of the voluntary nature of eating and drinking, hunger and thirst are the homeostatic drives that biopsychologists have been most interested in.

Hunger and eating

Does hunger cause eating?

If there is a common-sense theory of eating, it is that we eat because – and when – we are hungry. What could be simpler? If asked why we get hungry, most people would probably say that 'our bodies get hungry'; that is, certain events take place in our bodies when we have not eaten for a certain period of time, and these events act as the signal to eat. We experience that signal as hunger.

This fits neatly with the hunger drive outlined above. If we place the experience of hunger in between internal imbalance and homeostatic drive, we get a blend of the common-sense and drive-reduction theories, with hunger towards the end of a chain of causation that results in eating.

But is hunger either a necessary or sufficient condition for eating to occur? Can eating occur in the absence of hunger, and is it possible that we might not eat despite being hungry? We have all been tempted by the look or the smell of food when not feeling hungry, and we are not usually still hungry by the time the dessert trolley comes along. In other words, we often eat simply because we like it. This suggests that hunger is not necessary for eating. Conversely, people who go on weight-loss diets or hunger strike choose to not eat (or to eat less than they might otherwise do) despite being very hungry, suggesting that hunger is not sufficient.

So, there seems to be no biological inevitability about the hunger–eating relationship. However, as Blundell and Hill point out, under many circumstances there is a close relationship between the pattern of food intake and the rhythmic fluctuation of hunger.[15] For example, many experimental studies confirm a strong link between the intensity of experienced hunger sensations and the amount of food eaten. This fairly consistent finding has been interpreted as showing that there is a causal connection between hunger and the size of a following meal. But in reality, certain physiological mechanisms are probably producing both the sensations of hunger and the eating behaviour.

Blundell and Hill propose an *appetite-control system*, in which hunger, eating and physiological mechanisms are coupled together, but the coupling is not perfect. There will be circumstances where uncoupling can occur, as in the hunger strike example and in cases of eating disorders (e.g. obesity, anorexia nervosa; see Chapter 42). So, what might some of these physiological mechanisms be? Assuming that, normally, these are coupled (or correlated) with hunger, what happens when the 'body gets hungry'?

What prompts us to eat?

Carlson points out that the physiological signals that cause eating to begin are not necessarily the same signals that cause it to end.[16] There is considerable delay between the act of eating (the *correctional mechanism*) and a change in the state of the body. So, although we may start eating because the level of nutrients has fallen below a certain point, we certainly do not stop because that level has been restored to normal. In fact, we usually stop eating long before this, since digestion takes several hours to complete. Therefore, the signals for hunger and for satiety (the state of no longer being hungry) are sure to be different. Probably the earliest formal theory of hunger was proposed by Cannon (Box 15.2).

An evaluation of Cannon's 'hunger pangs' theory

Sometimes patients have their stomach removed because of disease and the oesophagus is 'hooked up' directly to the duodenum or small intestine. The patients continue to report feeling hungry and satiated. Even though their stomachs are bypassed, they maintain normal body weight by eating more frequent, smaller meals.[18]

Similarly, cutting the neural connections between the gastrointestinal tract (comprising mainly the stomach and intestine) and the brain (i.e. cutting the vagus nerve) has little effect on food intake either in experimental animals or in human patients.

These findings suggest that Cannon exaggerated the importance of stomach contractions in causing hunger. But this does not mean that the stomach and the gastrointestinal tract play no part in hunger and satiety. If the vagus nerve is cut, then signals arising from the gut can still be communicated to the brain via the circulatory system. These signals convey information about the components of the food that has been absorbed. Some of the nutrients whose depletion acts as a signal to start eating are fats (lipids), carbohydrates (including glucose), vitamins/mineral salts and proteins/amino acids. Fats and carbohydrates are burned up in cellular reactions and provide the energy to fuel metabolic processes.

Also, the presence of food in the stomach (*stomach load-*

Box 15.2 'Swallow a balloon if you're hungry'[17]

Cannon originally believed that the hunger drive is caused by stomach contractions ('hunger pangs') and that food reduces the drive by stopping the contractions.

Washburn swallowed an empty balloon tied to the end of a thin tube. Then Cannon pumped some air into the balloon and connected the end of the tube to a water-filled glass U-tube, so that Washburn's stomach contractions would cause an increase in the level of water at the other end of the U-tube (Figure 15.2). He reported a 'pang' of hunger each time a large stomach contraction was recorded.

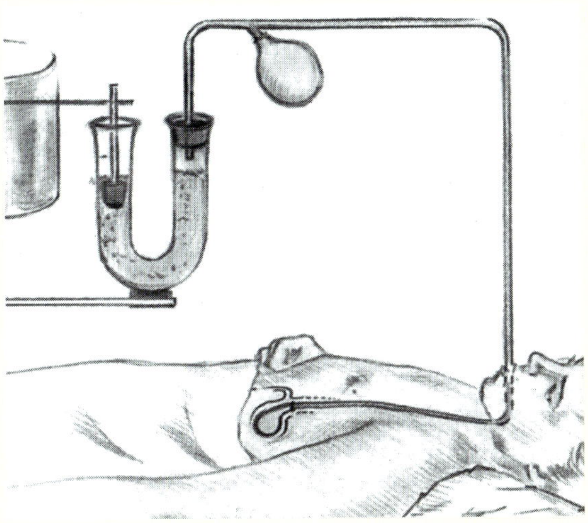

Figure 15.2 System developed by Cannon and Washburn in 1912 for measuring stomach contractions

These results were soon confirmed by a case study (cited in Carlson[16]) of a patient with a tube implanted through his stomach wall, just above the navel. He had accidentally swallowed some acid, which caused the walls of his oesophagus to fuse shut. The tube allowed him to feed himself and provided a means of observing his stomach activities.

When there was food in his stomach, small rhythmic contractions (subsequently named peristaltic contractions/peristalsis) mixed the food and moved it along the digestive tract. When it was empty, the contractions were large and associated with the patient's reports of hunger.

ing) is important in the regulation of feeding: if the exit from the stomach to the duodenum is blocked, rats will still eat normal-sized meals. It seems that information about the stretching of the stomach wall caused by the presence of food is passed to the brain (via the vagus nerve), allowing the brain's feeding centres to control meal size.

When we engage in vigorous physical activity, the muscles are fuelled by fats and carbohydrates, which are stored as energy reserves. The cells that store our fat reserves are called adipocytes, which clump together as adipose tissue (or simply 'fat'). Carbohydrates are stored as glycogen. Two major accounts of why we start eating are the glucostatic and the lipostatic theories.

Glucostatic theory

According to the glucostatic theory (GT), the primary stimulus for hunger is a decrease in the level of blood glucose below a certain set-point. Glucose is the body's (especially the brain's) primary fuel. The 'glucostat' was assumed to be a neuron (probably in the hypothalamus) that detects the level of blood glucose in much the same way as a thermostat measures temperature.

According to Pinel,[18] Mayer's version of GT was particularly influential, because it dealt with a serious problem associated with earlier versions.[19] He proposed that it was glucose utilization (the rate at which glucose is used), rather than absolute blood glucose level, that was regulated by feeding. Although these are usually highly correlated, Mayer's version could account for those few occasions where high levels are associated with hyperphagia (overeating). For example, people with diabetes mellitus overeat despite having high blood glucose levels. This is because, in diabetes mellitus, the pancreas fails to produce sufficient quantities of insulin (needed for glucose to enter most body cells and to be utilized by them).

Mayer's hypothesis was supported by experiments with mice, which appeared to identify the location of the glucoreceptors in the ventromedial hypothalamus (VMH).[20] Mayer and Marshall concluded that the VMH is a satiety centre.[20] However, although a fall in blood glucose may be the most important physiological signal for hunger, it is not the only one. If animals eat a meal that is low in carbohydrate but high in fats or proteins, they still manage to eat a relatively constant amount of calories, even though their blood glucose is reduced slightly. If eating were controlled exclusively by blood glucose, we would expect the animals to overeat and become fat.[16]

Lipostatic theory

According to Green, the lipostatic theory (LT) focuses on the end product of glucose metabolism, namely the storage of fats (lipids) in adipocytes.[21] Body fat is normally maintained at a relatively constant level. Similarly, fluctuations in the amount of stored fats largely determine variations in body weight. According to Nisbett's version of LT, we all have a body-weight set-point around which our weight fluctuates within quite narrow limits; this is determined by the level of fats in the adipocytes.[22]

The most frequently cited evidence in support of LT is the failure of short-term dieting programmes to produce long-term weight loss: as soon as dieting stops, the person regains the weight that has been lost. Other evidence comes from animal experiments in which lesions are made in the hypothalamus. When the lateral hypothalamus is damaged, rats stop eating, even when food is readily available, to the point of death from starvation. This failure to feed is called *aphagia*. It was originally taken to indicate that the lateral hypothalamus normally functions to stimulate eating and so represents another partial answer to the question 'Why do we start eating?' (Box 15.3).

Box 15.3 Lowering body weight before the lesion[23]

Keesey and Powley deprived rats of food so that the rats' body weight was substantially lowered. When lesions were then made in the lateral hypothalamus, the rats started eating more rather than less food.

In normal rats, the lesion lowers the body-weight set-point, and the resulting failure to eat occurs because the animal is trying to adjust to this lower target weight.

However, if the weight is reduced before the lesion is made to below the lesion-produced target, the rat increases feeding (following the lesion) in order to reach the new (higher) set-point.

Keesey and Powley's findings mean that damage to the lateral hypothalamus affects feeding only indirectly (as Nisbett suggests), by altering the body-weight set-point.[23] Feeding is aimed at attaining this new target.

Set-point or settling point?

According to Pinel, the GT and LT are complementary rather than mutually exclusive.[18] The GT was meant to account for the initiation and termination of eating (relatively short-term processes), while the LT was proposed to explain long-term feeding habits and the regulation of body weight. Both theories assume the existence of mechanisms within the CNS that are sensitive to deviations from one or more hypothetical set-points. This assumption is itself based on another, namely that homeostasis implies the existence of set-point mechanisms.

Many current biopsychological theories of eating reject these assumptions in favour of the view that body weight tends to drift around a natural *settling point* – that is, the level at which the various factors that influence it achieve balance or equilibrium. Pinel believes that earlier theorists were seduced by the analogy with the thermostat, which is a compelling set-point model.[18] His analogy for a settling-point theory is the *leaky barrel model*: the level of fat in the body, like the water level in a leaky barrel, is regulated around a natural settling point rather than a predetermined set-point.

Other factors that influence eating

A settling-point theory is more compatible with research findings that implicate factors other than internal energy deficits as causes of eating. As we noted earlier, hunger is neither a necessary nor a sufficient condition for eating to take place. For example, even if it were possible to explain hunger purely in terms of lowered levels of glucose and fat, we would still need to identify other influences on eating. According to Pinel:

> The modern era of feeding research has been characterized by an increasing awareness of the major role played by learning in determining when we eat, what we eat, how much we eat, and even how the food that we eat is digested and metabolised. The concept of the feeding system has changed from that of an immutable system that maintains glucose and fat levels at pre-determined set points, to that of a flexible system that operates within certain general guidelines but is 'fine-tuned' by experience ...[18]

Eating for pleasure

Both humans and other animals are drawn to eat (rather than driven to eat) by food's *incentive properties* – that is, its anticipated pleasure-producing effects (or palatability). According to incentive theories, both internal and external factors influence eating in the same way, namely by changing the incentive value of available foods. Signals from the taste receptors seem to produce an immediate decline in the incentive value of similar-tasting food, and signals associated with increased energy supply from a meal produce a general decrease in the incentive properties of all foods.

Support for this view comes from the discovery of lateral hypothalamus neurons that respond to the incentive properties of food rather than to food itself.[24] When monkeys were repeatedly allowed to eat one palatable food, the response of lateral hypothalamus neurons to the food declined (a form of habituation?), but the response to other palatable foods did not decline. Neurons that responded to the animal's sight of food would begin to respond to a neutral stimulus that reliably predicted the presentation of food. These findings explain very neatly the common experience of the mouth watering (salivating) at the mere mention of, or even seeing a picture of, a favourite food (Box 15.4).

Box 15.4 Learning to salivate[25]

The smell of food, and the dinner bell, are food-predicting cues (or classically conditioned stimuli). They trigger digestive and metabolic events such as salivation, insulin secretion and gastric secretions (classically conditioned responses). These digestive/metabolic events are also called *cephalic phase responses*.

Pavlov was the first to demonstrate that a cephalic phase response can be conditioned: the sight or smell of milk produced abundant salivation in puppies raised on a milk diet, but not in those raised on a solid diet.

Feeling hungry at the times of the day when we usually eat (whether or not we are experiencing an energy deficit) is another example of a classically conditioned response (see Chapter 14).

Knowing what to eat

If learning is involved in the way that humans and other animals respond to foods that are already palatable, could learning be involved in what is found palatable in the first place?

We have innate preferences for tastes that are associated in nature with vital nutrients. For example, sweetness detectors on the tongue are probably there because they helped our ancestors identify food that is safe to eat. Even when we are not particularly hungry, we tend to find a sweet taste pleasant, and eating something sweet tends to increase our appetite.[16]

Both humans and other animals also have the ability to learn the relationship between taste and the post-ingestion consequences of eating certain food. In taste-aversion studies, rats learn to avoid novel tastes that are followed by illness (see Chapter 14).[26] Rats are also able to learn to prefer tastes that are followed by the infusion of nutrients and flavours that they smell on the breath of other rats.

Rats and human beings have in common a metabolism that requires them to eat a variety of different foods: no single food provides all essential nutrients. We generally find a meal that consists of moderate amounts of several different foods more interesting than a huge plate of only one food, however palatable that food might be. If we have access to only one particular food, we soon become tired of it (*sensory-specific satiety*). This encourages the consumption of a varied diet.

Cultural evolution helps the selection of balanced diets. For example, Mexicans increased the calcium in their diet by mixing small amounts of mineral lime into their tortillas. But in the industrialized societies of Europe and North America, we seem to prefer diets that are fundamentally detrimental to our health. Manufacturers tend to sell foods that are highly palatable and energy-dense but that often have little nutritional value. This encourages us to overeat and, as a result, to increase fat deposits and body weight. Blundell and Hill maintain that in evolutionary terms, overeating makes good sense:

> ... For human beings it can be supposed that during most of the tens of thousands of years of human evolution the biggest problem facing human-kind was the scarcity of food ... the existence of an abundance of food, highly palatable and easily available, is a very recent development in evolutionary terms. Accordingly, it is unlikely that evolutionary pressure has ever led to the development of mechanisms to prevent overconsumption ...[15]

What stops a meal?

According to Blundell and Hill (1995), satiety (feeling 'full up' or satisfied) is, by definition, not instantaneous but something that occurs over a considerable period of time.[15] It is useful, therefore, to distinguish different phases of satiety associated with different mechanisms, which, together, comprise the satiety cascade. Most important for understanding the suppression and subsequent control of hunger are:

- *post-ingestive effects*, including gastric distension, the rate of gastric emptying, the release of hormones (e.g. cholecystokinin (CCK); Box 15.5), and the stimulation of certain receptors along the gastrointestinal tract;
- *post-absorptive effects* – that is, mechanisms arising from the action of glucose, fats, amino acids and other metabolites after absorption across the intestine into the bloodstream.

> **Box 15.5 Cholecystokinin**
>
> After food reaches the stomach, the protein is broken down into its constituent amino acids. As digestion proceeds, food gradually passes into the duodenum (small intestine). This controls the rate of stomach emptying by secreting a peptide hormone (short chains of amino acids) called cholecystokinin (CCK). CCK is secreted in response to the presence of fats, detected by receptors in the walls of the duodenum.
>
> Many studies have found that injecting CCK into hungry rats causes them to eat smaller meals. Wolkowitz *et al.* gave people injections of a drug that blocks CCK receptors in the peripheral nervous system (but not in the brain): they reported feeling more hungry and less full after a meal than controls given a placebo.[27]
>
> Based on Carlson.[16]

There is currently considerable research interest in whether protein, fat and carbohydrate differ in their satiating efficiency and their capacity to reduce hunger. One clear finding is that carbohydrates are efficient appetite suppressants. Also, the fat content of food influences its texture and palatability, but it has a disproportionately weak effect on satiety.[15]

Although the stomach may not be very important in causing hunger (see Box 15.2), it does seem to be important in satiety. For example, we noted that stomach-loading and stretching of the stomach wall play a part in reducing hunger. The gastric branch of the vagus nerve carries emergency signals from the stretch receptors in the stomach wall, preventing us from overeating and damaging the stomach.

The brain's control of eating

It has been known since the early 1800s that tumours of the hypothalamus can cause *hyperphagia* (excessive overeating) and obesity in humans.[18] But not until the advent of *stereotaxic surgery* in the late 1930s were experimenters able to assess the effects of damage to particular areas of the hypothalamus on the eating behaviour of experimental animals (Box 15.6).

Ventromedial hypothalamus syndrome

Paradoxically, ventromedial hypothalamus (VMH)-lesioned rats are not 'hell-bent' on eating – they will not simply eat anything and everything. The taste of food seems to be

Box 15.6 Hyperphagia in rats[28]

Hetherington and Ranson found that large bilateral lesions in the lower central portion of the hypothalamus (the ventromedial nucleus, VMN) cause hyperphagia: the rat will carry on eating until it becomes grotesquely fat, doubling or even trebling its normal body weight.

Although several structures were damaged by such lesions, it was generally assumed that the ventromedial hypothalamus (VMH) was the crucial structure.

The resulting hyperphagia was taken to indicate that the normal function of the VMH is to inhibit feeding when the animal is 'full'. Hence, the VMH became known as the *satiety centre*. The centre has been found in rats, cats, dogs, chickens and monkeys.[29]

especially important in hyperphagic rats. Most animals will eat even bad-tasting food ('you'll eat anything if you're hungry enough'), but hyperphagic rats are very fussy and will refuse their regular food if quinine is added, even if this means that they become underweight.[30]

What about people?

One possible explanation for the finicky eating of VMH-lesioned rats is that they become less sensitive to internal cues of satiation (e.g. blood glucose level, body fat content) and more responsive to external cues (e.g. taste). Schachter claims that this may also apply to overweight people.[31] Schachter *et al.* found that normal-weight people responded to the internal cue of stomach distension ('feeling bloated') by refusing any more food, but obese people tended to go on eating.[32] The obese people seemed to be responding to the availability of food, although they are less willing than normal-weight people to make an effort to find food; normal-weight people will search for food, but only if they are genuinely hungry.[31]

Overweight people tend to report that they feel hungry at prescribed eating times, even if they have eaten only a short time before. Normal-weight people tend to eat only when they feel hungry, and this is relatively independent of clock time. However, this increased sensitivity to external cues is not necessarily what causes some people to become obese – it could just as easily be an *effect* of obesity.

Although people with hypothalamic tumours tend towards obesity, there is no evidence that the hypothalamus does not function properly in overweight people generally.

Differences in basal metabolic rate largely determine our body weight and are probably hereditary. There is very little evidence to suggest that lack of impulse control, poor ability to delay gratification and eating too quickly contribute to overweight.[16] However, the role of complex psychological variables has been studied much more extensively in relation to anorexia nervosa and bulimia nervosa (see Chapter 42).

Lateral hypothalamus syndrome

If the VMH has traditionally been regarded as a 'brake' on eating, then the lateral hypothalamus has been seen as the 'accelerator'. Bilateral lesions to the lateral hypothalamus cause aphagia, a refusal to eat, even to the point of death from starvation.[33,34] Even rats made hyperphagic by VMH lesions will become aphagic by the addition of lateral hypothalamus lesions. These findings suggest very strongly that the lateral hypothalamus is a feeding centre.

However, the lateral hypothalamus syndrome also includes *adipsia* (complete cessation of drinking). Both aphagia and adipsia are, in turn, part of a more general lack of responsiveness to sensory input. The lateral hypothalamus itself is a relatively large, complex and ill-defined area, with many nuclei and several major nerve tracts running through it. Although electrical stimulation of the lateral hypothalamus produces eating, it also triggers drinking, gnawing, temperature changes and sexual activity. Conversely, eating can also be elicited by stimulation of other areas of the hypothalamus, the amygdala, hippocampus, thalamus and frontal cortex. For all these reasons, Pinel believes that to call the lateral hypothalamus a 'hunger centre' is a misnomer.[18]

THIRST AND DRINKING

What starts us drinking?

It was thought until recently that drinking is motivated by a deficit in the body's water resources – that is, by deviation from set-points, as part of a homeostatic drive mechanism. However, most drinking (like most eating) occurs in the absence of deficits. This suggests that the motivation to drink comes from anticipating its pleasurable effects (positive incentive properties). We tend to prefer drinks that have a pleasant taste (e.g. fruit juice) or pleasant pharmacological effects (e.g. alcoholic drinks, coffee, tea).

Positive incentive theory

Water deprivation increases the positive incentive value of almost all salt-free drinks. After 24 h without a drink, people report that even plain water has a pleasant taste.[35] If you add a little saccharine to the water of non-deprived rats, their water intake rockets. Like people, rats with unlimited access to water or other palatable fluids drink far more than they actually need.

As with food, sensory-specific satiety has a major effect on drinking. As fond as rats are of saccharine, if saccharine solution is available constantly ('on tap'), they begin to prefer it less than when it is available only periodically.

Dry-mouth theory

A dry mouth and throat are obvious cues to thirst (the counterpart of the stomach contraction cues to hunger; see

Box 15.2). Although a dry mouth is one consequence of water deficiency, it is not the primary factor in thirst. For example, producing a chronic dry mouth by removal of the salivary glands does not substantially increase water intake, unless rats are fed dry food or kept in a very hot environment. Conversely, blocking the sensation of a dry mouth fails to decrease water intake.

The most convincing evidence against the dry-mouth theory comes from *sham drinking*, in which water flows down the oesophagus and then out through a fistula before it can be absorbed. Despite the lack of a dry mouth, animals sham-drink continuously.[18]

What makes us stop drinking?

According to set-point theories, drinking brings about a return to an internal water resource set-point. When this has been achieved, drinking stops. But, like hunger, thirst and drinking seem to stop long before enough time has elapsed for the body to have absorbed the water from the stomach, and for the water–salt balance in the blood to have been restored.

Stomach distension probably contributes to satiety. Cold water is more thirst-quenching because it moves out of the stomach much more slowly and so provides a clearer stomach-distension signal to the brain. The *mouth-metering mechanism* also plays a part; this gauges the amount of water being ingested and compares the amount needed to restore the water balance.

If set-point theories were correct, we would expect that delivering water directly to where it is needed would eliminate thirst and deprivation-induced drinking. However, if water is injected directly into a rat's stomach or bloodstream, drinking is reduced by only 30 per cent of the amount injected. Even total replenishment of an animal's water resources has only a modest inhibitory effect on deprivation-induced drinking (about 30 per cent). These findings pose difficulties for any set-point theory.[18]

HULL'S DRIVE-REDUCTION THEORY

As we noted earlier, Hull's motivational theory must be considered in the context of his theory of learning. The drive-reduction theory was intended to explain the fundamental principle of reinforcement, both positive (reduction of a drive by the presentation of a stimulus) and negative (reduction of a drive by the removal or avoidance of a stimulus).

Hull was interested in the primary (physiological) homeostatic needs and drives of hunger, thirst, air, avoiding injury, maintaining an optimum temperature, defecation and urination, rest, sleep, activity and propagation (reproduction). He believed that all behaviour (human and animal) originates in the satisfaction of these drives (Figure 15.3).

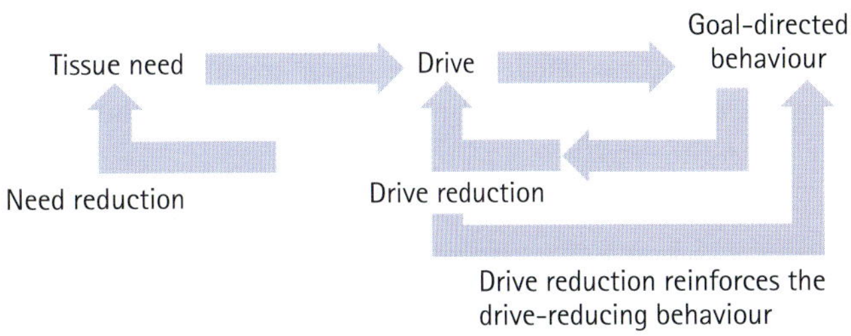

Figure 15.3 Summary of drive-reduction theory

Needs versus drives

Although the terms 'need' and 'drive' are often used interchangeably, they are fundamentally different:

- *Needs* are physiological and can be defined objectively, such as in terms of hours without food or blood sugar level.
- *Drives* are psychological (behavioural) and are hypothetical constructs – that is, abstract concepts that refer to processes/events believed to be taking place inside the person/animal but that cannot be directly observed or measured.

However, Hull operationalized drives as hours of deprivation. He proposed a number of equations, which were meant to be testable in laboratory experiments.[36] Perhaps the most important of these was:

$$sEr = D \times V \times K \times sHr$$

where *sEr* is the intensity or likelihood of any learned behaviour, which can be calculated if four other factors are known, namely:

- *D:* the *drive or motivation*, measured by some indicator of physical need, such as hours of deprivation;
- *V:* the *intensity* of the signal for the behaviour;
- *K:* the *degree of incentive*, measured by the size of the reward or some other measure of its desirability;
- *SHr:* the *habit strength*, measured as the amount of practice given, usually in terms of the number of reinforcements.

Evaluation of drive-reduction theory

Hull's basic premise is that animals (and, by implication, people) *always* and *only* learn through primary drive reduction. But the relationship between primary drives and needs is very unclear, as we saw earlier when discussing the eating behaviour of obese people.

At its simplest, needs can arise without specific drives, as in learning what and how much to eat (see above). For example, we need vitamin C, but we would not normally talk of a 'vitamin C drive' in the same way that we talk about a general hunger drive.

Conversely, drives can occur in the absence of any obvious physiological need. An important example of a non-homeostatic drive in rats is electrical (self)-stimulation of the brain (ES-SB) (Box 15.7).

Box 15.7 What a rat wouldn't do for a shock[37]

Olds and Milner implanted an electrode near a rat's septum (part of the limbic system), so that every time the rat pressed a lever it received an electric shock (Figure 15.4).

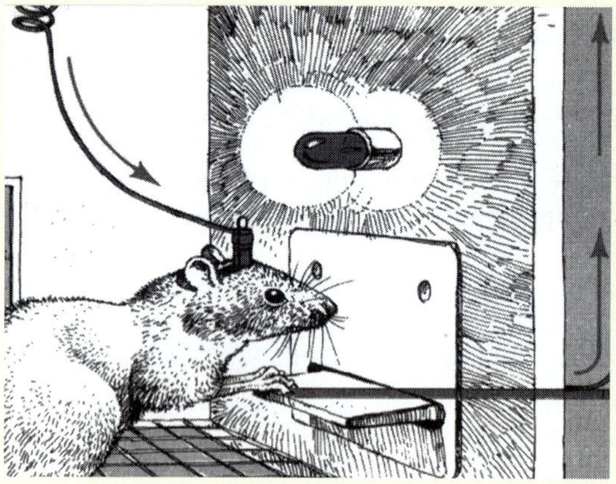

Figure 15.4 Olds implanted electrodes in the hypothalamus of rats.[38] The rats could trigger an electrical stimulus by depressing a lever. The region where the electrode was implanted constitutes some kind of pleasure centre

Rats made between 3000 and 7500 lever-pressing responses in a 12-h period. Olds reported that one rat stimulated itself more than 2000 times/h for 24 consecutive hours.[38]

Olds reported that rats that normally press a lever 25 times/h for food reward will press 100 times/min for a reward of electrical (self)-stimulation of the brain (ES-SB).[39]

Box 15.8 The 'addicted brain'[41]

Neurobiologists have known for a long time that drugs have their effects because they ultimately boost the activity of the brain's reward system: a complex circuit of neurons that evolved to make us feel flush after eating or having sex. At least initially, stimulating this system makes us feel good, which encourages us to repeat whatever induced the pleasure (the feeling is a powerful reinforcer). But research has indicated that chronic drug use can actually produce structural and functional changes in the system's neurons that can last for weeks, months or years after the fix.

A key part of the circuit is the pathway extending from dopamine-producing neurons of the ventral tegmental area (VTA) to dopamine-sensitive neurons in the nucleus accumbens (NA), situated deep beneath the frontal cortex. Changes to these neurons contribute significantly to the tolerance, dependence and craving that fuel repeated drug use and lead to relapses, even after long periods of abstinence.

There are also pathways linking the NA and VTA with other brain regions that can help make addicted people highly sensitive to reminders of past highs – such as drug paraphernalia (the equipment used in drug-taking) and places where they have scored – vulnerable to relapse when stressed, and unable to control the urge to seek drugs.

Functional magnetic resonance imaging (fMRI) and positron-emission tomography (PET) scans have revealed that the NA in the brains of people addicted to cocaine 'lights up' when they are offered a snort or when shown a video of someone using cocaine or even a photograph of white lines on a mirror. The amygdala and NA influence both the cocaine-induced rush and the craving for more of the drug, which becomes stronger as the euphoria wears off (see Chapter 70).

Brain stimulation is such a powerful reinforcer that a male rat with an electrode in its lateral hypothalamus will self-stimulate in preference to eating if hungry, drinking when thirsty or having access to a sexually receptive female. This effect has been found in rats, cats, monkeys and pigeons (and humans, occasionally). The main reward site for ES-SB is the median forebrain bundle (MFB), a fibre tract that runs from the brainstem up to the forebrain through the lateral hypothalamus.[16,40] The effect seems to depend on the presence of dopamine and noradrenaline. These reward centres are generally thought of as the neural substrate of 'pleasure', so that any behaviour defined as pleasurable involves their activation. ES-SB is seen as a shortcut to pleasure, eliminating the need for natural drives and reinforcers (Box 15.8).

Tolman's cognitive behaviourism challenged Skinner's theory of operant conditioning, because it showed that learning could take place in the absence of reinforcement (*latent learning*; see Chapter 14). By implication, Tolman showed that learning could take place in the absence of drive reduction.

Hull's theory emphasized primary (homeostatic) drives to the exclusion of secondary (non-homeostatic) drives. Primary drives are based on primary (innate) needs, but much human (and, to a lesser extent, non-human) behaviour can be understood only in terms of secondary (acquired) drives. Several behaviourist psychologists, notably Miller,[42] Mowrer[43] and Dollard and Miller,[44] modified Hull's theory to include acquired drives (in particular, anxiety), which led to a great deal of research on avoidance learning in the 1950s (see Chapter 14).

In Maslow's terms, drive-reduction theory deals only with survival needs, completely ignoring the self-actualization (or 'growth') needs that make human motivation distinctively different from that of non-humans.

NON-HOMEOSTATIC NEEDS AND DRIVES

Just as ES-SB cannot be accommodated by drive reduction when considering only non-human motivation, so non-humans seem to have other non-homeostatic drives that they share, to some degree, with humans.

Competence motives: motives without specific primary needs

According to White, the 'master reinforcer' that keeps most of us motivated over long periods of time is the need to confirm our sense of personal competence: our capacity to deal effectively with the environment.[45] It is intrinsically rewarding and satisfying to feel that we are capable human beings, to be able to understand, predict and control our world.

Unlike hunger, which comes and goes, competence seems to be a continuous, ongoing motive. We cannot satisfy it and then do without it until it next appears, because it is not rooted in any specific physiological need. This is why it is not very helpful to think of the competence motive as a drive that pushes us into seeking its reduction. While homeostatic drives involve an attempt to reduce something (tissue need), competence motives often involve the search for stimulation.

Seeking stimulation

If rats are allowed to become thoroughly familiar with a maze, and then the maze is changed in some way, they spend more time exploring the altered maze. This occurs even in the absence of any obvious extrinsic reward, such as food. The rats are displaying a curiosity drive.[46] Butler[46] and Harlow *et al.*[47] gave monkeys mechanical puzzles to solve, such as undoing a chain, lifting a hook and opening a clasp. The monkeys did these puzzles over and over again, for hours at a time, with no other reward: they were displaying their *manipulative drive*.[47]

Play and motivation

Much of the behaviour normally described as play can be thought of in terms of the drives for curiosity, exploration and manipulation. The purpose of play from the child's point of view is simple enjoyment. The child does not consciously play in order to find out how things work, or to exercise the imagination; instead, the child plays simply because playing is fun and intrinsically satisfying. Any learning that does result is quite incidental. However, for the young child, there is no real distinction between 'work' and 'play' in an adult sense.

Piaget distinguishes between *play*, which is performed for its own sake, and *intellectual activity* or *learning*, which has an external aim or purpose.[48] This distinction is meant to apply to all three major types of play that he describes: mastery, symbolic/make-believe and play with rules (see Chapter 8). Nor is play confined to humans. The young of many species engage in activities that seem to have little to do with homeostatic or survival needs. However, the higher up the evolutionary scale the species is, the more apparent and purposeful the play becomes, and the more the nature of play changes as the young animal develops.[49]

Motivation and adaptation

Piaget saw play as essentially an adaptive activity. Throughout development, play helps to consolidate recently acquired abilities and to aid the development of additional cognitive and social skills. In the same way, the competence motives of curiosity, exploration and manipulation undoubtedly have adaptive significance for an individual and, ultimately, for the species. Investigating and exploring the environment equips an animal with 'knowledge' that can be used in times of stress or danger.[50]

Optimum-level (or arousal) theories

According to Berlyne, investigation and exploration are based on an inbuilt tendency to seek a certain 'optimum' level of stimulation or activity.[51] Exploring the unfamiliar increases arousal, but if it is very different from what we are used to, arousal will be too high (we feel anxious and tense). If it is not different enough, then arousal is too low (we soon become bored).

Optimum-level theories are supported by sensory-deprivation experiments. In classic experiments carried out by Hebb and colleagues at McGill University in the 1950s, participants were almost completely cut off from their normal sensory stimulation by wearing blindfolds, earmuffs, cardboard tubes on their arms and legs, and so on (Figure 15.5).[52,53] They soon began to experience extreme psychological discomfort, reported hallucinations (Figure 15.6), and could not tolerate their confinement for usually more than 3 days.

Cohen and Taylor studied the psychological effects of long-term imprisonment.[54] They found that sensory deprivation and monotony are experiences that prisoners share with explorers, space travellers and round-the-world sailors. Conversely, excessive stimulation ('sensory overload') is also debilitating and may be responsible for some kinds of psychological disorders in highly urbanized societies (see Chapter 11).

The need for control

Another major kind of competence motive is the need to be in control of our own destiny and not at the mercy of external forces.[2] This is linked closely to the need to be free from the controls and restrictions of others, to dictate our own actions and not to be dictated to. According to Brehm, when our freedom is threatened, we tend to react by reasserting our freedom (*psychological reactance*).[55]

When people initially expect to have control over the outcomes of their actions, the first experience of not being

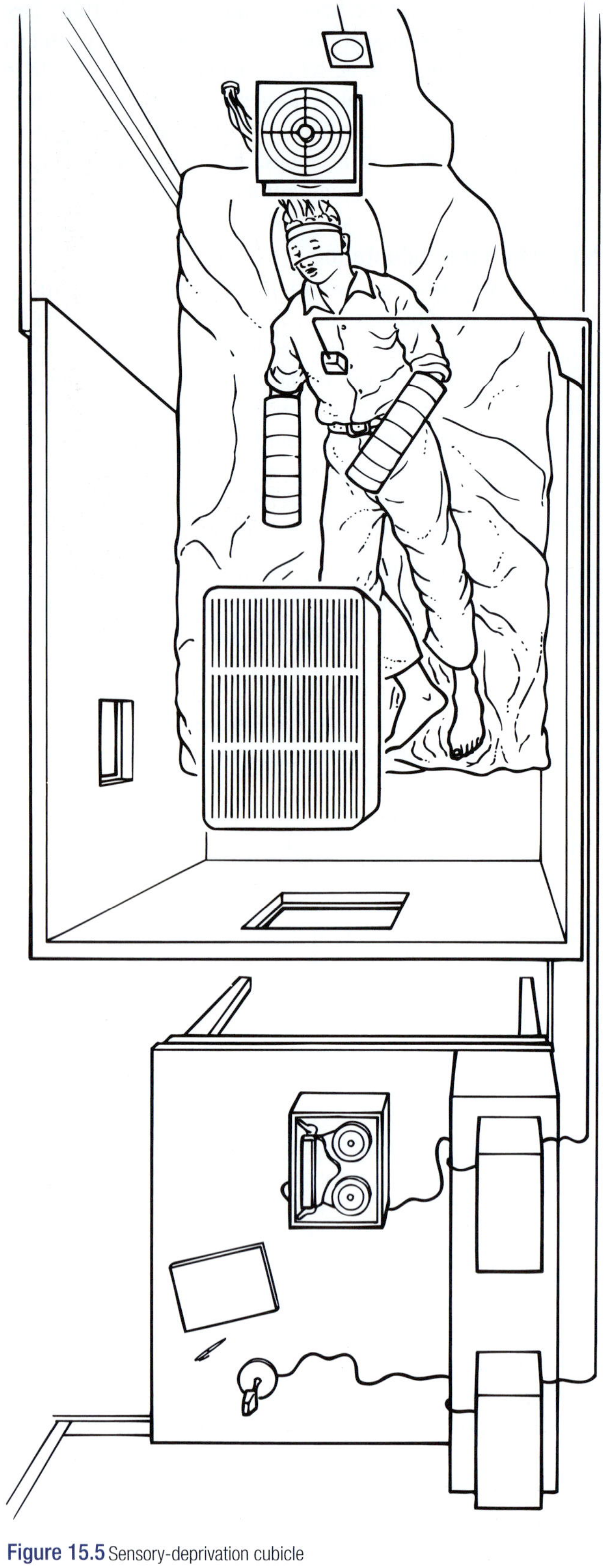

Figure 15.5 Sensory-deprivation cubicle

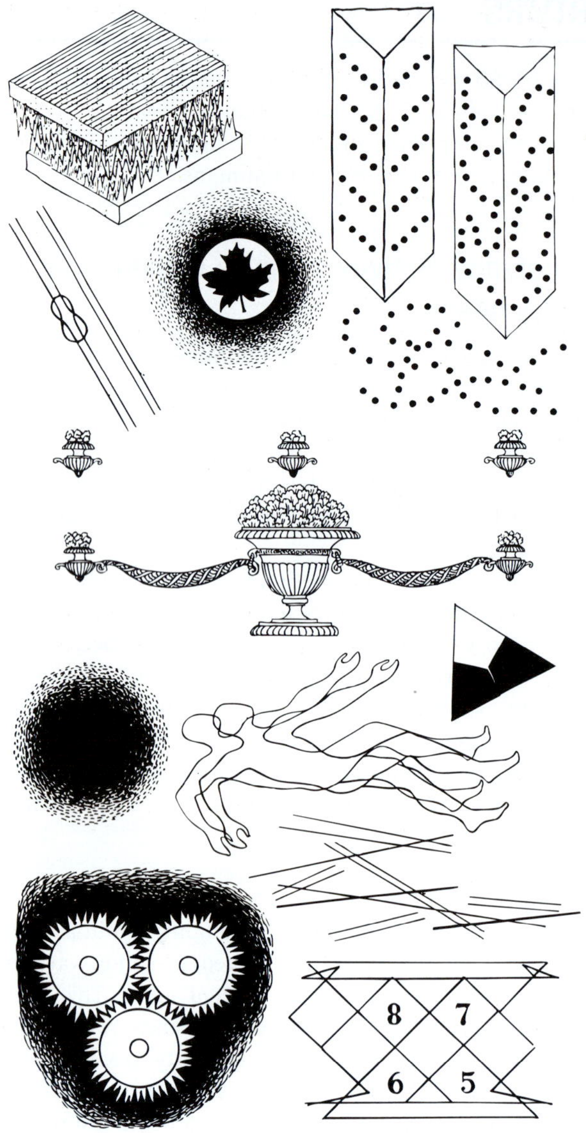

Figure 15.6 Hallucinations of sensory-deprived participants

so is likely to produce reactance. Further bad experiences, however, are likely to result in *learned helplessness*.[56] Rotter's concept of *locus of control* refers to individual differences in people's beliefs about what controls events in their everyday lives (see Chapter 11).[57]

Cognitive motives

Consistency and achievement

One of the most researched cognitive motives is the need for *cognitive consistency*, which is central to Festinger's cognitive dissonance theory[58] (see also Gross[1]). Another cognitive motive that has generated an enormous amount of research and theorizing is *achievement motivation/need for achievement* (*nAch*). This was one of the 20 human motives identified by Murray in 1938.[59] Murray drew a sharp distinction between 'psychogenic' (or psychological) needs, which are learned, and 'viscerogenic' (or physiological) needs, which are innate.

Murray agreed with Freud that people express their true motives more clearly in free association than in direct self-reports (or questionnaire-type personality tests). Based on this belief, Murray devised the Thematic Apperception Test (TAT). This test consists of a series of 20 pictures (Figure 15.7), presented one at a time, 10 in each of two sessions separated by at least 1 day. Slightly different versions are used for men and women, and for boys and girls. The participant is told that the TAT is a test of imagination and asked to make up a story that describes:

- what is happening and who the people are;
- what has led up to the situation;
- what is being thought and what is wanted and by whom;
- what will happen and what will be done.

The pictures are sufficiently ambiguous with regard to the events depicted and the emotions of the characters to allow a wide range of interpretations. How a person interprets the pictures reveals their unconscious motives. Hence, the TAT is a major projective test used in motivation and personality research (see Chapter 19). A person who scores high on nAch is concerned with standards of excellence, high levels of performance, recognition of others and the pursuit of long-term goals (the person is ambitious).

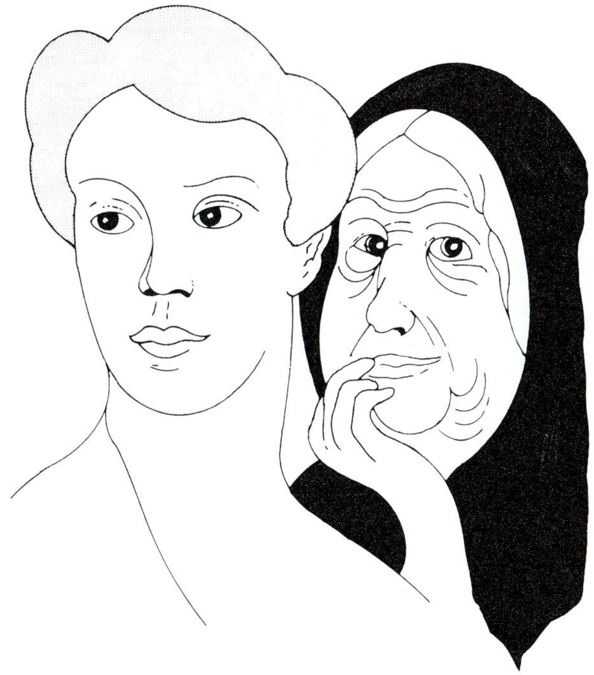

Figure 15.7 Sample Thematic Apperception Test (TAT) picture

Social motives

According to Geen, social motivation refers to the activation of processes involved in the initiation, direction and energization of individual behaviour '... by situations in which other people are in close contact with the individual ...'[3] It is usually assumed that these situations do not provide specific cues for individual behaviour (they are 'weak'). Geen contrasts 'weak' situations with 'strong' situations, such as those in which there is direct social influence (e.g. Milgram's famous obedience experiments: see Chapter 20). Geen gives three main examples:

- *Social facilitation:* the enhancing effect on behaviour of the mere presence of others.
- *Social presentation:* behaving in ways that attempt to present a desirable impression to others.
- *Social loafing:* the tendency for individual effort to diminish in group task situations, partly as a result of diffusion of responsibility.

Each of these may be thought of as a manifestation of the more general influence of *social anxiety*, a state created when a person who wishes to make a certain impression on others doubts that this impression can actually be made. But why should the fear of making a bad impression be such a powerful motive for individual behaviour?

One answer can be found at quite a low level of Maslow's hierarchy, namely love and belongingness. This includes the need for affiliation, the company of other people, especially family, friends and work colleagues, and the need to be accepted by, and included within, society. Certain kinds of conformity can be understood in terms of this basic need (a survival need in Maslow's terms). But does this need itself stem from some other, even more fundamental need?

According to Greenberg *et al.* (cited in Geen[3]), human culture, which society represents, provides a buffer against facing one's own vulnerability and mortality. Society provides a 'cultural drama' that gives meaning to life and without which the individual would experience a dread of being alive. We are, therefore, motivated to play an approved role in that drama: by meeting cultural standards, the individual achieves the approval and acceptance of others and avoids rejection and isolation. This can be seen in relation to safety needs, the second level of Maslow's hierarchy, and includes 'fear of the unknown'. The ultimate example of this is the fear of death (see Chapter 57).

Fiske argues that, from the idea that we need other people for our basic survival, it follows that over time we would have developed some core social motives that interact with the social situation in order to help us survive in groups.[60] We are motivated to get along with other people, because it is adaptive to do so. Fiske defines core social motives as '... fundamental, underlying psychological processes that impel people's thinking, feeling, and behaving in situations involving other people ...'[60]

Fiske identifies five core social motives: *belonging* (see above), *understanding*, *controlling*, *self-enhancing* and *trusting*. Belonging underlies the others.

KEY POINTS

- The study of motivation is the study of the causes of behaviour. Although there is general agreement that motivated behaviour is purposeful, goal-directed behaviour, different theoretical approaches see the underlying causes in very different ways.
- Motives have been classified in various ways, but the most comprehensive classification is Maslow's hierarchy of needs, which distinguishes survival, deficiency or D-motives, and growth, being or B-motives.
- Hedonism can be seen as a central theme in both Freud's psychoanalytic theory and Skinner's operant conditioning.
- Influenced by Darwin's theory of evolution, many early psychologists tried to explain human behaviour in terms of large numbers of instincts. This approach was replaced by Woodworth's concept of drive.
- Two major forms of drive theory are Cannon's homeostatic drive theory and Hull's drive-reduction theory.
- Hunger and thirst are the homeostatic drives that have been most researched by biopsychologists. The earliest formal theory of hunger was Cannon's theory of stomach contractions.
- According to the glucostatic theory, the primary stimulus for hunger is a decrease in the level of blood glucose below a certain set-point. The glucostat (probably a neuron in the hypothalamus) detects the level of blood glucose in the way a thermostat measures temperature.
- The other major set-point theory is the lipostatic theory, which focuses on the storage of lipids (fats) in the adipose tissue. It is supported by several observations, including the finding that damage to the lateral hypothalamus affects feeding indirectly by altering the body-weight set-point.
- The glucostatic theory was meant to account for the relatively short-term processes of eating initiation (and termination), while the lipostatic theory was meant to explain long-term feeding habits and regulation of body weight. They share the belief in predetermined set-points.
- Eating, in both humans and other animals, is determined partly by food's palatability. Food-predicting cues elicit cephalic phase responses, such as salivation, through classical conditioning.
- Sensory-specific satiety encourages the consumption of a varied diet. Although humans are capable of learning which diets best meet their biological needs, people in industrialized societies seem to prefer diets that are fundamentally harmful to health, with obesity becoming increasingly common.
- Lesions in the VMN of the rat's hypothalamus cause hyperphagia, and the VMH became known as the 'satiety centre'. However, the VMH syndrome also involves increased sensitivity to external cues of satiation. This also seems to be true of obese humans.
- Lesions to the lateral hypothalamus cause aphagia, which suggests that it is a feeding centre. However, the effects of lateral hypothalamus lesions are much more diffuse than originally thought.
- Drinking has traditionally been seen as motivated by deviation from set-points induced by water deprivation. Although there is some support for the dry-mouth theory, this is not the primary factor in thirst.
- It is difficult for set-point theories to explain why drinking stops, whether this is water-deprived drinking or not. Both stomach distension and the mouth-metering mechanism play a part in satiety.
- Hull's drive-reduction theory was intended to explain the principle of reinforcement. However, needs can arise without specific drives and drives can occur in the absence of any obvious tissue need, as in ES-SB. Brain stimulation is a very powerful reinforcer that can override the primary drives of hunger, thirst and sex.
- Latent learning shows that learning can take place in the absence of reinforcement. Much behaviour can be understood only in terms of secondary (non-homeostatic) drives, such as anxiety and its avoidance.
- Humans and non-humans share certain non-homeostatic needs and drives, such as curiosity, manipulation and play. These are linked to the search for stimulation and the need for competence, important for adaptation to our environment.
- Optimum-level theories can help to explain why both sensory deprivation and sensory overload can be stressful and disturbing.
- Cognitive consistency and nAch are two very important cognitive motives.
- Many kinds of social behaviour can be seen as a manifestation of social anxiety, which in turn may reflect the more fundamental need for safety and protection from our fear of death.
- Core social motives include belonging, understanding, controlling, self-enhancing and trusting.

REFERENCES

1. Gross R (2005) *Psychology: The Science of Mind and Behaviour*, 5th edn. London: Hodder Arnold.
2. Rubin Z, McNeil EB (1983) *The Psychology of Being Human*, 3rd edn. London: Harper & Row.
3. Geen RG (1995) Social motivation. In B Parkinson, AM Colman (eds) *Emotion and Motivation*. London: Longman.
4. Miller GA (1962) *Psychology: The Science of Mental Life*. Harmondsworth: Penguin.
5. Maslow A (1954) *Motivation and Personality*. New York: Harper & Row.
6. Maslow A (1970) *Motivation and Personality*, 2nd edn. New York: Harper & Row.
7. Maslow A (1968) *Towards a Psychology of Being*, 2nd edn. New York: Van Nostrand.
8. Gross R (2009) *Themes, Issues and Debates in Psychology*, 3rd edn. London: Hodder Education.
9. Darwin C (1859) *The Origin of Species by Means of Natural Selection*. London: John Murray.
10. McDougall W (1908) *An Introduction to Social Psychology*. London: Methuen.

11. Gross R, McIlveen R, Coolican H, Clamp A, Russell J (2000) *Psychology: A New Introduction*, 2nd edn. London: Hodder & Stoughton.
12. Cannon WB (1929) *Bodily Changes in Pain, Hunger, Fear, and Rage*. New York: Appleton.
13. Hull CL (1943) *Principles of Behaviour*. New York: Appleton-Century-Crofts.
14. Green S (1980) Physiological Studies I and II. In J Radford, E. Govier (eds) *A Textbook of Psychology*. London: Sheldon Press.
15. Blundell JE, Hill AJ (1995) Hunger and appetite. In B Parkinson, AM Colman (eds) *Emotion and Motivation*. London: Longman.
16. Carlson NR (1992) *Foundations of Physiological Psychology*, 2nd edn. Boston, MA: Allyn & Bacon.
17. Cannon WB, Washburn AI (1912) An explanation of hunger. *American Journal of Physiology* **29**: 441–54.
18. Pinel JPJ (1993) *Biopsychology*, 2nd edn. Boston, MA: Allyn & Bacon.
19. Mayer J (1955) Regulation of energy intake and the body weight: the glucostatic theory and the lipostatic hypothesis. *Annals of the New York Academy of Sciences* **63**: 15–43.
20. Mayer J, Marshall NB (1956) Specificity of gold thioglucose for ventromedial hypothalamic lesions and obesity. *Nature* **178**: 1399–400.
21. Green S (1994) *Principles of Biopsychology*. Hove: Lawrence Erlbaum Associates.
22. Nisbett RE (1972) Hunger, obesity and the ventromedial hypothalamus. *Psychological Review* **79**: 433–53.
23. Keesey RE, Powley TL (1975) Hypothalamic regulation of body weight. *American Scientist* **63**: 558–65.
24. Rolls ET, Rolls BJ (1982) Brain mechanisms involved in feeding. In LM Barker (ed.) *The Psychobiology of Human Food Selection*. Westport, CT: AVI Publishing Co.
25. Pavlov IP (1927) *Conditioned Reflexes*. Oxford: Oxford University Press.
26. Garcia J, Ervin FR, Koelling RA (1966) Learning with prolonged delay of reinforcement. *Psychonomic Science* **5**: 121–2.
27. Wolkowitz OM, Bertz B, Weingartner H, *et al.* (1990) Hunger in humans induced by MK-329: a specific peripheral-type cholecystokinin receptor antagonist. *Biological Psychiatry* **28**: 169–73.
28. Hetherington AW, Ranson SW (1942) The relation of various hypothalamic lesions to adiposity in the rat. *Journal of Comparative Neurology* **76**: 475–99.
29. Teitelbaum P (1967) Motivation and control of food intake. In CF Code (ed.) *Handbook of Physiology: Alimentary Canal*, Vol. 1. Washington, DC: American Physiological Society.
30. Teitelbaum P. (1955) Sensory control of hypothalamic hyperphagia. *Journal of Comparative and Physiological Psychology* **48**: 156–63.
31. Schachter S (1971) *Emotion, Obesity and Crime*. New York: Academic Press.
32. Schachter S, Goldman R, Gordon A (1968) The effects of fear, food deprivation, and obesity on eating. *Journal of Personality and Social Psychology* **10**: 107–16.
33. Anand BK, Brobeck JR (1951) Hypothalamic control of food intake in rats and cats. *Yale Journal of Biological Medicine* **24**: 123–40.
34. Teitelbaum P, Stellar E (1954) Recovery from the failure to eat produced by hypothalamic lesions. *Science* **120**: 894–5.
35. Rolls BJ, Wood R, Rolls ET, Lind H, Ledingham JG (1980) Thirst following water deprivation in humans. *American Journal of Physiology* **239**: 476–82.
36. Walker S (1984) *Learning Theory and Behaviour Modification*. London: Methuen.
37. Olds J, Milner P (1954) Positive reinforcement produced by the electrical stimulation of the septal area and other regions of the rat brain. *Journal of Comparative and Physiological Psychology* **47**: 419–27.
38. Olds J (1956) Pleasure centres in the brain. *Scientific American* **October**: 105–6.
39. Olds J (1958) Self-stimulation of the brain. *Science* **127**: 315–23.
40. Beaumont JG (1988) *Understanding Neuropsychology*. Oxford: Blackwell.
41. Nestler EJ, Malenka RC (2004) The addicted brain. *Scientific American* **290**: 50–57.
42. Miller NE (1948) Theory and experiment relating psychoanalytic displacement to stimulus–response generalization. *Journal of Abnormal Social Psychology* **43**: 155–78.
43. Mowrer OH (1950) *Learning Theory and Personality Dynamics*. New York: Ronald Press.
44. Dollard J, Miller NE (1950) *Personality and Psychotherapy*. New York: McGraw-Hill.
45. White RW (1959) Motivation reconsidered: the concept of competence. *Psychological Review* **66**: 297–333.
46. Butler RA (1954) Curiosity in monkeys. *Scientific American* **February**: 70–75.
47. Harlow HF, Harlow MK, Meyer DR (1950) Learning motivated by a manipulation drive. *Journal of Experimental Psychology* **40**: 228–34.
48. Piaget J (1951) *Play, Dreams, and Imitation in Children*. London: Routledge & Kegan Paul.
49. Fontana D (1981) Play. In D Fontana (ed.) *Psychology for Teachers*. London: British Psychological Society/Macmillan.
50. Bolles RC (1967) *Theory of Motivation*. New York: Harper & Row.
51. Berlyne DE (1960) *Conflict, Arousal and Curiosity*. London: McGraw-Hill.
52. Bexton WH, Heron W, Scott TH (1954) Effects of decreased variation in the sensory environment. *Canadian Journal of Psychology* **8**: 70.
53. Heron W (1957) The pathology of boredom. *Scientific American* **196**: 52–69.

54. Cohen S, Taylor L (1972) *Psychological Survival: The Experience of Long-Term Imprisonment.* Harmondsworth: Penguin.
55. Brehm JW (1966) *A Theory of Psychological Reactance.* New York: Academic Press.
56. Seligman MEP (1975) *Helplessness: On Depression, Development and Death.* San Francisco, CA: W.H. Freeman.
57. Rotter J (1966) Generalized expectancies for internal versus external control of reinforcement. *Psychological Monographs* 30: 1–26.
58. Festinger L (1957) *A Theory of Cognitive Dissonance.* New York: Harper & Row.
59. Murray HA (1938) *Explorations in Personality.* New York: Oxford University Press.
60. Fiske ST (2004) *Social Beings: A Core Motives Approach to Social Psychology.* New York: John Wiley & Sons.

Chapter 16

Perception

Richard Gross

INTRODUCTION

When we compare our experience of the world (in which objects remain stable and constant) with what our sense organs receive in the form of physical stimulation (a state of near-continuous flux), it is almost as if there are two entirely different 'worlds'. Psychologists call these 'worlds' *sensation* and *perception*, respectively. Sensations are the experiences that physical stimuli elicit in the sense organs. Perception is the organization and interpretation of incoming sensory information to form inner representations of the external world.

This chapter begins by looking at some basic visual perceptual phenomena, namely form and depth perception, perceptual constancy and visual illusions. Many of the principles that govern human visual perception were first identified by the German school of Gestalt psychology. As Dodwell has observed, 'To perceive seems effortless. To understand perception is nevertheless a great challenge.'[1]

One response to this challenge claims that our perception of the world is the end result of a process that also involves making inferences about what things are like. Those who subscribe to this end-result view, such as Bruner,[2] Neisser[3] and Gregory,[4,5] are called *top-down* (or *conceptually driven*) *perceptual processing* theorists. Making inferences about what things are like means that we perceive them indirectly, drawing on our knowledge and expectations of the world. Others argue that our perception of the world is essentially determined by the information presented to the sensory receptors, so that things are perceived in a fairly direct way. The most influential of these *bottom-up* (or *data-driven*) *perceptual processing* theorists is Gibson.[6,7] Others still, notably Marr,[8] display elements of both approaches (see Gross[9]).

GESTALT PSYCHOLOGY AND PERCEPTUAL ORGANIZATION

Von Ehrenfels claimed that many groups of stimuli acquire a pattern quality that is greater than the sum of their parts.[10] A square, for example, is more than a simple assembly of lines – it has 'squareness'. Von Ehrenfels called this 'emergent property' *Gestalt qualität* (= form quality). In the early 1900s, Gestalt psychologists (notably Wertheimer, Koffka and Köhler) attempted to discover the principles through which sensory information is interpreted. They argued that, as well as creating a coherent perceptual experience that is more than the sum of its parts, the brain does this in regular and predictable ways. They believed that these organizational principles are largely *innate* (see Gross[9]).

Form perception

In order to structure incoming sensory information, we must perceive objects as being separate from other stimuli and as having meaningful form.

Figure and ground

The first perceptual task when confronted with an object (or *figure*) is to recognize it. To do this, we must perceive the figure as being distinct from its surroundings (or *ground*). A figure's familiarity can help determine whether it is perceived as figure or ground, but unfamiliar and even meaningless 'blobs' are also seen as figures. One of the strongest determinants of figure and ground is *surroundedness*. Areas enclosed by a contour are generally seen as figures, whereas the surrounding area is generally seen as ground. Size, orientation and symmetry also play a role in figure–ground separation.

Sometimes, though, there may not be enough information in a pattern to allow us to distinguish easily between figure and ground. A good example of this is shown in Figure 16.1, which illustrates the principle underlying camouflage.

In *figure–ground reversal*, a figure may have clear contours, but it is capable of being perceived in two very different ways: it is unclear which part of it is the figure and which the ground. A famous example is shown in Figure 16.2, usually called Rubin's vase.[11] Here, the figure–ground relationship continually reverses, so that it is perceived as either a white vase with a black background, or two black profiles on a white background. However, the stimulus is always organized into a figure seen against a ground, and

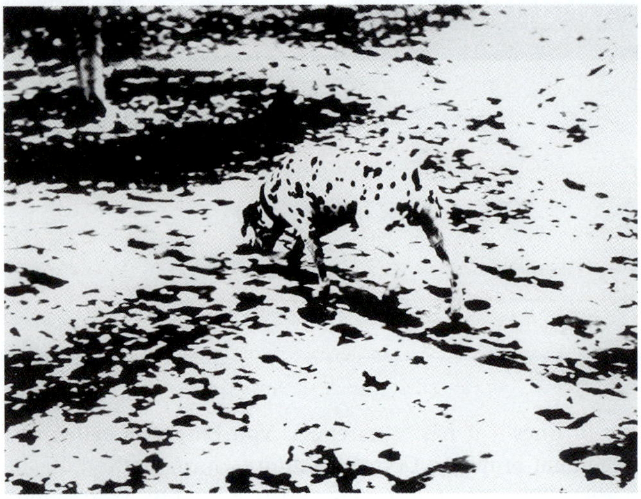

Figure 16.1 The Dalmatian dog (the figure) is difficult to distinguish from the ground because the dog has few visible contours of its own

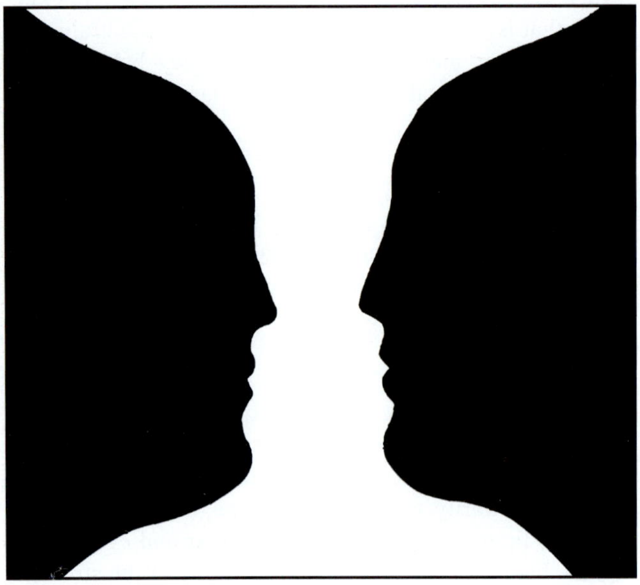

Figure 16.2 Rubin's vase. What else can you see?

the reversal indicates that the same stimulus can trigger more than one perception.

The artist Escher used figure–ground reversal in many of his paintings.

A map is another example of figure–ground reversal. We normally see the land as figure and the sea as (back)ground, because we are more familiar with the shape of Africa, say, than with the shape of the Atlantic ocean. An auditory example is the *cocktail party phenomenon* (see Chapter 13). Here is another example: try repeating 'over-run' out loud and you'll find the two words alternating as figure and ground.

Grouping

Once we have discriminated figure from ground, the figure can be organized into a meaningful form. Gestalt psychologists believed that objects are perceived as *Gestalten* (= organized wholes, configurations, patterns) rather than combinations of isolated sensations. They identified several laws of perceptual organization or grouping, which illustrate their view that the perceived whole of an object is more than the sum of its parts.

These laws can be summarized under one heading, the *law of prägnanz* (= precision), according to which, 'Psychological organisation will always be as good as the prevailing conditions allow. In this definition, "good" is undefined'.[12]

In practice, the 'best' way of perceiving is to see things as symmetrical, uniform and stable, and this is achieved by following the laws of *prägnanz* (Box 16.1).

An evaluation of the Gestalt contribution

A major philosophical influence on Gestalt psychology was *phenomenology*. This sees the world as we ordinarily experience it as being of central concern. Koffka, for example, believed that the most important question for perceptual psychologists was 'Why do things look as they do?' For Köhler, 'There seems to be a single starting point for psychology, exactly as for all the other sciences: the world as we find it, naïvely and uncritically.'[13]

The most comprehensive account of perceptual grouping is still that provided by the Gestalt psychologists,[14] and, in Gordon's view, Gestalt psychology's discoveries 'are now part of our permanent knowledge of perception'.[15]

However, many contemporary researchers (e.g. Greene[16]) have argued that, as originally expressed, the various Gestalt 'laws' are at best only descriptive and at worst extremely imprecise and difficult to measure. Several studies have attempted to address the various criticisms made of the Gestalt laws. For example, Navon tested the idea that the whole is perceived before the parts that make it up by presenting participants with various stimuli, as shown in Figure 16.8 opposite.[17]

Navon distinguished between the global (or 'whole-like' features of a stimulus) and the local (or more specific and 'part-like' features). Each stimulus consisted of a large (global) letter made up of many small (local) letters. In some cases, the global and local letters matched (as shown in the stimulus on the left in Figure 16.8), and in some cases they did not match (as shown on the right).

Participants had to identify either the large or the small letter as quickly as possible. Navon found that the time taken to identify the large letter was unaffected by whether the small letters matched or not. However, the time taken to identify the small letters was affected by whether the large letter matched or not: when the large and small letters were different, response times were longer (Table 16.1). This suggests that it is difficult to avoid processing the whole, and that global processing necessarily occurs before any more detailed perceptual analysis.

Box 16.1 Gestalt laws of perception

PROXIMITY

Elements appearing close together in space or time tend to be perceived together, so that different spacings of dots produce four vertical lines or four horizontal lines (Figure 16.3).

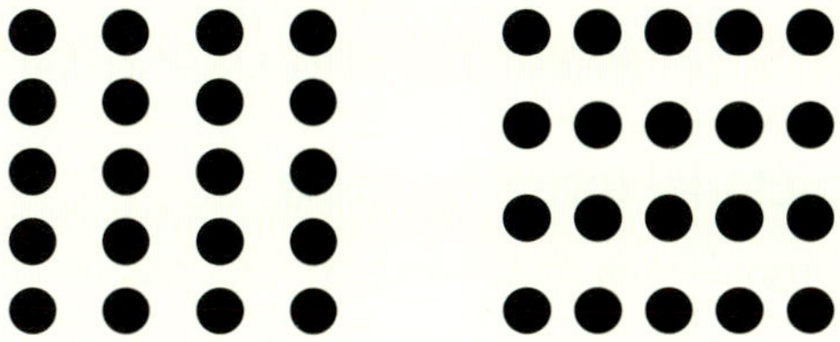

Figure 16.3 Proximity

An auditory example would be the perception of a series of musical notes as a melody, because they occur soon after one another in time.

SIMILARITY

Similar figures tend to be grouped together. So, the triangles and circles in Figure 16.4 are seen as columns of similar shapes rather than rows of dissimilar shapes.

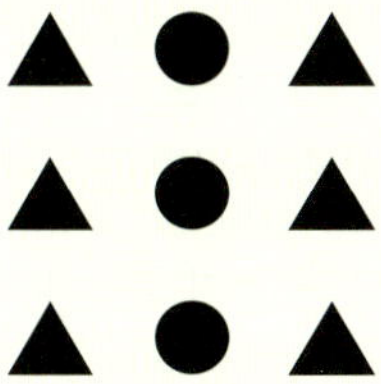

Figure 16.4 Similarity

Hearing all the separate voices in a choir as an entity illustrates the principle of similarity.

CONTINUITY

We tend to perceive smooth, continuous patterns rather than discontinuous ones. The pattern in Figure 16.5 could be seen as a series of alternating semicircles, but it tends to be perceived as a wavy line and a straight line.

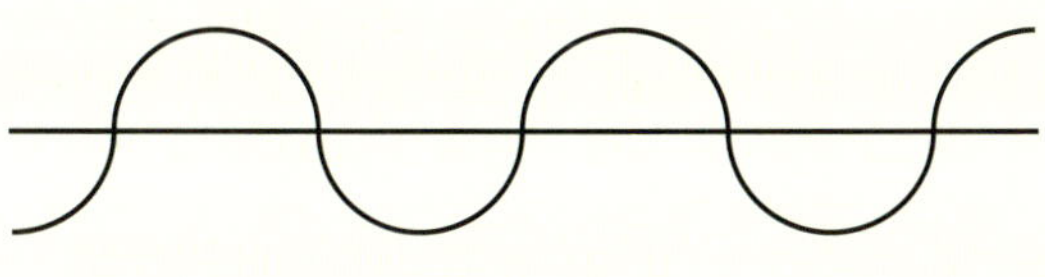

Figure 16.5 Continuity

Music and speech are perceived as continuous, rather than as a series of separate sounds.

CLOSURE

Closed figures are perceived more easily than open/incomplete ones. So, we often supply missing information in order to close a figure and separate it from its background. By filling in the gaps, the illustrations in Figure 16.6 are seen as a triangle and a seashell.

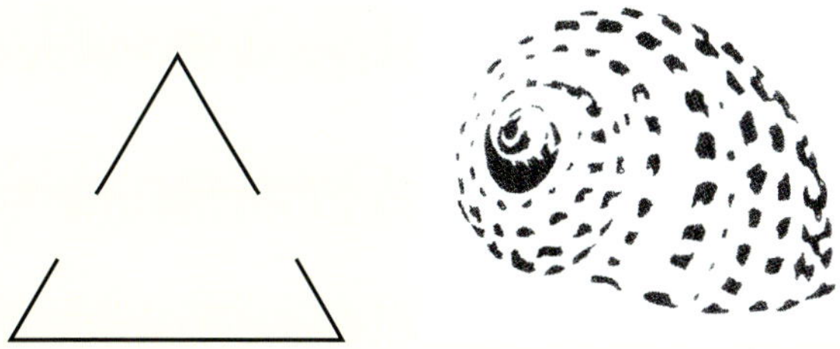

Figure 16.6 Closure

PART–WHOLE RELATIONSHIP

As well as illustrating continuity and proximity, the three images in Figure 16.7 illustrate the principle that the whole is greater than the sum of its parts. Despite the similarity of the parts (each pattern is composed of 12 crosses), the Gestalten are different.

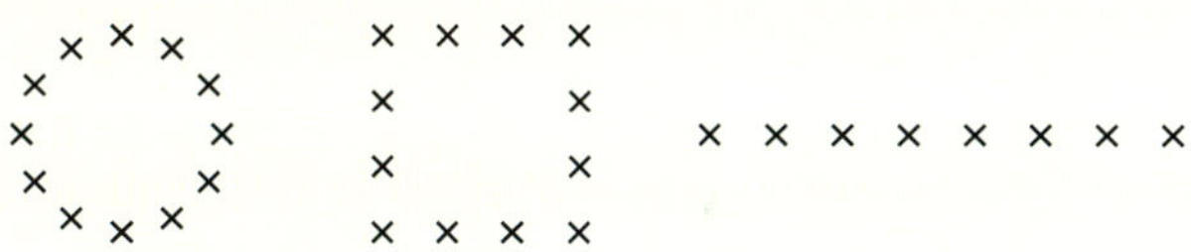

Figure 16.7 Part–whole relationship

The same melody can be recognized when hummed, whistled or played with different instruments and in different keys.

COMMON FATE

Elements seen moving together are perceived as belonging together. This is why a group of people running in the same direction appear to be unified in their purpose.

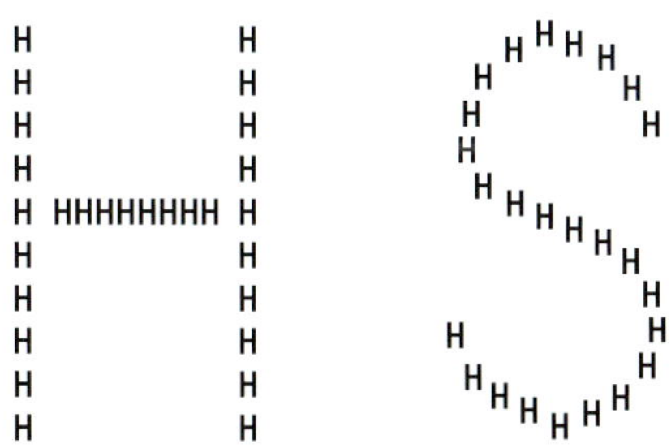

Figure 16.8 The whole is perceived before the constituent parts

Table 16.1 Decision time for global and local letters under match and mismatch conditions

Condition	Response time (ms)	
	Match	Mismatch
Global	471	477
Local	581	664

Based on Navon.[17]

Does the global always predominate?

The findings from Navon's (and others') experiments clearly support Gestalt laws. But the Gestalt laws are difficult to apply to the perception of solid (three-dimensional, 3D) objects as opposed to two-dimensional (2D) drawings. Our eyes evolved to see 3D objects, and when 3D arrays have been studied, Gestalt laws have not been consistently upheld.[18] The world around us comprises 'whole' scenes, in which single objects are but 'parts'.[19] Because many of the Gestalt displays involve single objects, they have very low ecological validity' that is, they are not representative of 'the objects and events which organisms must deal with in order to survive'.[15]

Factors such as the sizes of the local and global features, the viewing conditions and the nature of the observer's task are all likely to play a part in determining the role played by individual features in pattern recognition.[20] In everyday life, it is easier sometimes to process 'forests' and sometimes easier to process 'trees'.[14]

Some theorists (e.g. Palmer[21]) have suggested that, under most circumstances, the interpretation of parts and wholes takes place in top-down and bottom-up directions simultaneously, such as in the recognition of parts of a face with and without context. As shown in Figure 16.9, the features that can be recognized easily in context are somewhat ambiguous when seen alone (out of context), but they are recognizable when more detail is provided. (Compare Palmer's approach with that of Neisser's analysis-by-synthesis model.)

Marr found the Gestalt principles useful in achieving accurate *segmentation* – that is, how visual information is used to decide which regions of a visual scene belong together and form coherent structures.[22] Marr devised a computer program aimed at achieving segmentation (e.g. of a teddy bear) using the Gestalt principles. He succeeded in obtaining appropriate segmentation of the teddy's outline, eyes and nose. But some scenes are ambiguous and require using knowledge about objects in order to achieve segmentation (such as two leaves overlapping substantially in a bowl of flowers[8]).

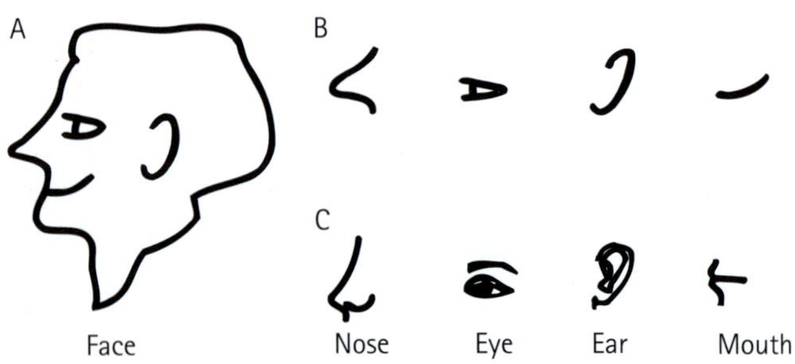

Figure 16.9 The features that can be recognized easily in context (a) are rather ambiguous when see alone – that is, out of context (b) – although they become more recognizable when more detail is provided (c). Based on Palmer.[21]

DEPTH PERCEPTION

From the 2D images that fall on our retinas, we manage to organize 3D perceptions. This ability is called *depth perception*, and it allows us to estimate an object's distance from us. Some of the cues used to transform 2D retinal images into 3D perceptions involve both eyes and rely on their working together. These are called *binocular cues*. *Monocular cues* are available to each eye separately.

Non-pictorial (primary) cues

Most preyed-upon non-humans (e.g. rabbits) have their eyes on the side of the head, allowing them to see danger approaching over a wide area. Most predators (e.g. lions) have their eyes set close together on the front of the head, equipping them with binocular vision, which helps in hunting prey. Like non-human predators, humans have predatory vision, which influences the way we perceive the world. Four important non-pictorial cues are retinal disparity, stereopsis, accommodation and convergence. These are all binocular, except for accommodation.

Because our eyes are nearly 8 cm apart, each retina receives a slightly different image of the world. The amount of *retinal disparity* (the difference between the two images) detected by the brain provides an important cue to distance.

Hold your finger directly in front of your nose. The difference between the two retinal images is large, and this can be shown by looking at your finger first with the left eye closed and then with the right eye closed. When the finger is held at arm's length, retinal disparity is much smaller.

Ordinarily, we do not see double images because the brain combines the two images in a process called *stereopsis* (literally, 'solid vision'[23]). This allows us to experience one 3D sensation rather than two different images.

In *accommodation*, which is a muscular cue, the lens of the eye changes shape when we focus on an object, thickening for nearby objects and flattening for distant objects.

Convergence, another muscular cue to distance, is the process by which the eyes point more and more inward as an object gets closer. By noting the angle of convergence, the brain provides us with depth information over distances from about 180 cm to 610 cm.[24]

Pictorial (secondary) cues

Except with relatively near objects, each eye receives a very similar retinal image when looking ahead. At greater distances, we depend on pictorial cues. These refer to features of the visual field itself (rather than to the eyes) and are all also monocular (Table 16.2).

PERCEPTUAL CONSTANCY

Having perceived an object as a coherent form and located it in space, we must next recognize the object without being

Table 16.2 Some pictorial depth cues

Depth cue	Description
Relative size	In an array of objects of different sizes, smaller objects are usually seen as more distant (especially if they are known to have a constant size)
Relative brightness	Brighter objects normally appear to be nearer
Superimposition (or overlap)	An object that blocks the view of another is seen as being nearer
Linear perspective	Parallel lines (e.g. railway tracks) appear to converge as they recede into the distance
Aerial perspective	Objects at a great distance appear to have a different colour (e.g. the hazy bluish tint of distant mountains)
Height in the horizontal plane	When looking across a flat expanse (e.g. the sea), objects that are more distant seem higher (closer to the horizon) than nearer objects, which seem lower (closer to the ground)
Light and shadow	Three-dimensional objects produce variations in light and shade (e.g. we normally assume that light comes from above)
Texture gradient	Textured surfaces (e.g. sand) look rougher close up than from a distance; a stretch of beach looks more smooth and uniform
Motion parallax	This is the major dynamic depth cue (pictorial/non-pictorial); objects nearer to us seem to move faster than more distant objects (e.g. telegraph poles seen from a (moving) train window flash by when close to the track)

'fooled' by changes in its size, shape, location, brightness and colour. The ability to perceive an object as unchanging, despite changes in the sensory information that reaches our eyes, is called *perceptual constancy*.

Size constancy

The image on the retina of an average-height person would be the same size for a dwarf seen from close up or a giant viewed from a distance.[25] Size constancy occurs because the perceptual system takes into account an object's distance from the perceiver. So, perceived size is equal to retinal image size taking distance into account.

The perception of an *after-image* demonstrates how distance can be varied without changing the retinal image's size.

Stare at a bright light for a few seconds and then look away. You'll experience an after-image. This has a fixed size, shape and position on the retina. Now quickly look at a nearby object and then at an object further away. The after-image seems to shrink and swell, appearing to be largest when you look at a more distant object.

Real objects cast smaller images the further away they are. To maintain perceptual constancy, the brain 'scales up' the image (*constancy scaling*). The same constancy scaling is applied to an after-image, producing changes in its apparent size.

Shape constancy

We often view objects from angles at which their 'true' shape is not reflected in the retinal image they project. For example, rectangular doors often project trapezoid shapes (Figure 16.10), and round cups often project elliptical-shaped images. Just as with size constancy, the perceptual system maintains constancy in terms of shape.

However, shape and size constancy do not always work. When we look down at people from the top of a very tall building, they look more like ants to us, even though we know they are people.

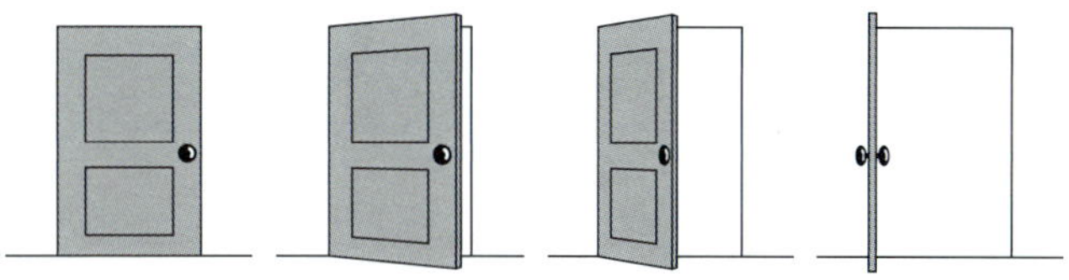

Figure 16.10 No matter what angle a door is viewed from, it remains a door

Location constancy

Moving our head around produces a constantly changing pattern of retinal images. However, we do not perceive the world to be spinning around. This is because *kinaesthetic feedback* from the muscles and balance organs in the ear is integrated with the changing retinal stimulation in the brain in order to inhibit perception of movement. To keep the world from moving crazily each time we move our eyes, the brain subtracts the eye-movement commands from the resulting changes on the retina. This helps to keep objects in a constant location.

Brightness constancy

We see objects as having a more or less constant brightness, even though the amount of light they reflect changes according to the level of illumination. For example, white paper reflects 90 per cent of light falling on it, whereas black paper reflects only 10 per cent of light. But in bright sunlight black paper still looks black, even though it may reflect 100 times more light than does white paper indoors. Perceived brightness depends on how much light an object reflects relative to its surroundings (*relative luminance*).

Colour constancy

Familiar objects retain their colour (or, more correctly, their *hue*) under a variety of lighting conditions (including night light), provided there is sufficient contrast and shadow. However, when we do not already know an object's colour, colour constancy is less effective. If you have ever bought new clothes under fluorescent light without viewing them in ordinary lighting conditions, you may well agree.

ILLUSIONS

Although perception is usually reliable, our perceptions sometimes misrepresent the world. When our perception of an object does not match its true physical characteristics, we have experienced an illusion. Some illusions are due to the physical distortion of stimuli, whereas others are due to our misperception of stimuli.[26] An example of a physical illusion is the bent appearance of a stick when placed in water. Gregory identifies four types of perceptual illusion:[27]

- Distortions (or geometric illusions)
- Ambiguous (or reversible) figures
- Paradoxical figures (or impossible objects)
- Fictions.

Distortions

Figure 16.11 shows several examples of distortions. The Poggendorf illusion (Figure 16.11b) is accentuated when the diagonal line is slanted more steeply and when the parallel bars are more separated. As the line is brought closer to the horizontal, the illusion disappears.[28] The horizontal–vertical illusion (Figure 16.11d) illustrates our tendency to overestimate the size of vertical objects. This helps to explain why a small tree that we have chopped down looks shorter than it did when it was standing.[26]

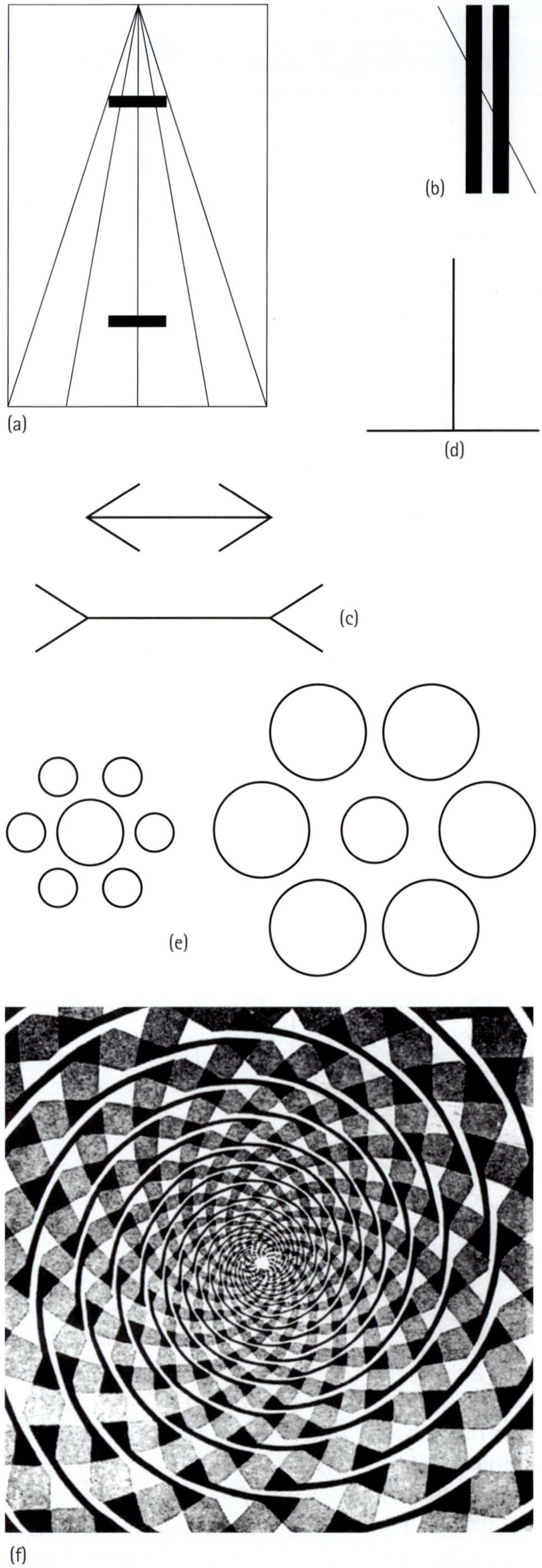

Figure 16.11 Distortions, or geometric illusions. In the Ponzo illusion (a), the horizontal bar at the top is seen as being longer than the horizontal line at the bottom, even though both lines are the same length. The Poggendorf illusion (b) suggests that the segments of the diagonal line are offset, even though they are not. The line with the outgoing fins in the Müller–Lyer illusion (c) appears to be longer than the line with the ingoing fins, but in fact the lines are the same length. In the horizontal–vertical illusion (d), the vertical line is seen as being longer, although it is the same length as the horizontal line. In Titchener's circles (e), the central circle in the left-hand group is seen as being larger than the central circle of the right-hand group, but both circles are the same size. Finally, in the twisted card illusion (f), the twisted cards appear to form a spiral pattern, but in fact the circles are concentric

Ambiguous figures

In addition to Rubin's vase (see above), two other well-known reversible figures are shown in Figure 16.12. In the Necker cube (Figure 16.12a), the figure undergoes a *depth reversal*. The cube can be perceived with the crosses being drawn either on the back side of the cube or on the top side looking down. Although our perceptual system interprets this 2D line drawing as a 3D object, it seems unsure as to which of the two orientations should be perceived. Hence, the cube spontaneously reverses in depth orientation if looked at for about 30 s.

Figure 16.12b shows Boring's 'old/young woman'. These two are examples of reversible figures in which the change in perception illustrates object reversal. The figure can be perceived as the profile of a young woman's face with the tip of her nose just visible, or the young woman's chin can be perceived as the (very large) nose of a much older woman (who also has a very long chin).

Paradoxical figures

Although paradoxical figures look ordinary enough at first, on closer inspection we realize that they cannot exist in reality (hence 'paradoxical'). Figure 16.13 illustrates three such paradoxical figures.

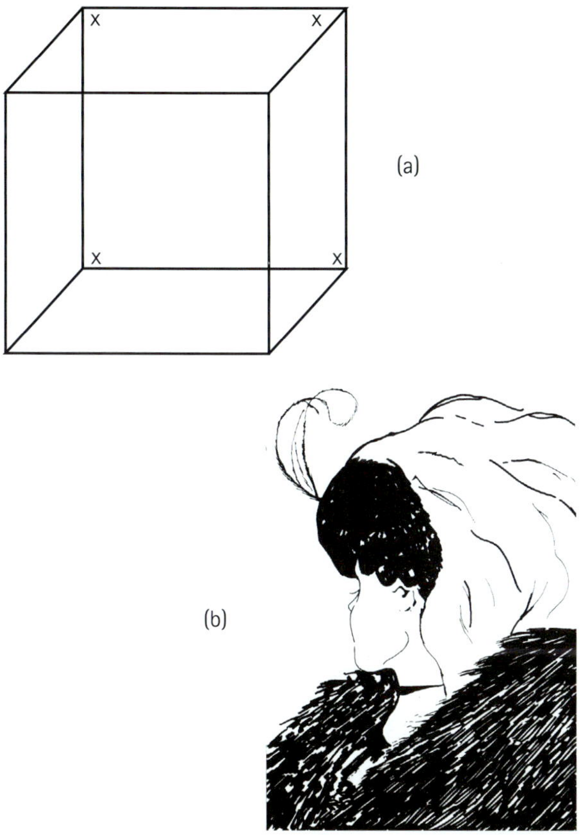

Figure 16.12 Two ambiguous/reversible figures: (a) the Necker cube; (b) Boring's 'old/young woman'

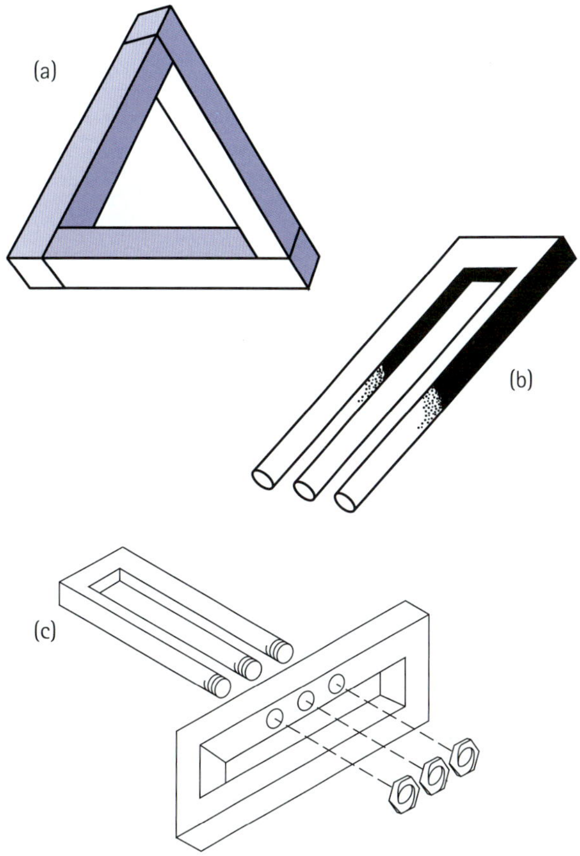

Figure 16.13 Three paradoxical objects: (a) the Penrose impossible triangle; (b) variously known as 'trident' and the 'devil's pitchfork'. (c) Trident has been combined with another impossible object

According to Hochberg, it takes us a few seconds to realize that a figure is impossible.[24] This is because we need time to examine the figure fully or to scan it and organize its parts into a meaningful whole. When we look at a figure, our eyes move from place to place at the rate of about three changes per second.[29] So, when we look at an impossible figure, it takes time for us to scan it and perceive its form; only after this scanning can we appreciate its impossible nature.

Fictions

Fictions help us to explain how we perceive that objects possess specific shapes. The idea that shape is determined by the physical contours of an object (causing edge-detectors in the cells of the visual system to fire) has been challenged by the existence of *subjective contours*. These are the boundaries of a shape perceived in the absence of physical contours.[30]

In Figure 16.14a, there is no white triangular contour physically present. But we perceive the shape of a white triangle, which appears to be opaque and lighter than the background. There are some contours that are physically present (the overlap of the triangle and the disc), and these

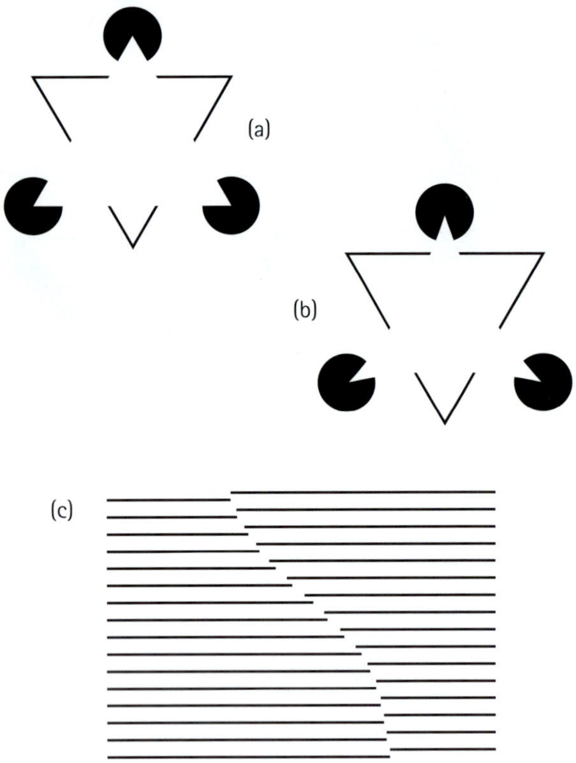

Figure 16.14 Three fictions: (a) the 'white triangle' is banded by a subjective contour, rather than a continuous physical one; (b) the subjective contours are curved; (c) lines of different orientation produce a subjective contour

might cause enough edge-detector cells to fire. However, this explanation cannot account for the fact that, in Figure 16.14b, the partial and straight physical contours give rise to a curved triangle. Nor can it explain the subjective contour in Figure 16.14c, which is marked by lines in a totally different orientation.[31]

It is the relationship between its parts that defines a shape, rather than its physical contours.[32] Physical contours are, of course, usually indicative of the location of an object's parts, but the location of the parts can also be determined by subjective contours. As a result, the perception of shape must involve more than simply detecting the elements of a pattern.[31]

Illusions of movement

We are surrounded by illusions in our everyday life. The use of perspective cues by artists leads us to infer depth and distance; that is, we add something to a picture that is not physically present, just as we do to the images projected on our television screens. Television pictures also use the illusion of movement. Just as it is possible for changes in patterns of retinal stimulation not to be accompanied by the perception of movement, so it is possible to perceive movement without a successive pattern of retinal stimulation.[33] This is called *apparent movement* (Box 16.2).

Box 16.2 Some examples of apparent movement

AUTOKINETIC EFFECT

If you look at a stationary spot of light in an otherwise completely dark room, the light will appear to move. According to Gregory, this illusion is produced by small and uncontrollable eye movements.[34] Another explanation suggests that it is caused by the absence of a stimulating background to provide a frame of reference for measuring movement. This is supported by the fact that the autokinetic effect disappears if other lights are introduced.

STROBOSCOPIC MOTION

The illusion of movement is created by the rapid succession of slightly different stationary images. If these are presented sufficiently quickly (around 16–22 frames/s), an illusory impression of continuous movement is produced. This is the mechanism by which moving pictures operate. With fewer than 16 frames/s, the moving picture looks jumpy and unnatural. Smooth slow motion is achieved by filming at a rate of 100+ frames/s and then playing back at about 20 frames/s.

PHI PHENOMENON

This is a simpler form of stroboscopic motion, in which a number of separate lights are turned on and off in quick succession. This gives the impression of a single light moving from one position to another. Both stroboscopic motion and the phi phenomenon can be explained by the law of continuity (see Box 16.1).

INDUCED MOVEMENT

This occurs when we perceive an object to be moving, although in reality the object is stationary and the surroundings are moving. Movie stars, for example, are often filmed in a stationary car with a projection of a moving background behind them. Similarly, when the moon is seen through a thin cover of moving clouds, we sometimes perceive it to be moving very quickly. Another example is the experience of sitting in a car at traffic lights and noticing that we are 'moving backwards', when in fact the car at our side is moving forwards.

MOTION AFTER-EFFECTS

People who work on inspection belts in factories experience movement after-effects when the belt suddenly stops but is then perceived as moving backwards. Similarly, if you stare at a waterfall and then switch your gaze to the ground surrounding the water, the ground appears to be moving in the opposite direction.

Illusions of shading

According to Ramachandran and Rogers-Rachamandran, the visual image is inherently ambiguous.[25] Perception is partly a matter of using certain assumptions about the world in order to resolve such ambiguities, and illusions can help to uncover the brain's hidden rules and assumptions.

- How would you describe the group of disks on the left in Figure 16.15?
- How would you describe those on the right?
- Can you try to explain the different perceptions?

The disks on the left in Figure 16.15 are usually seen as eggs, while those on the right are seen as cavities. The eggs are light on the top, and the cavities are light on the bottom. According to Ramachandran and Rogers-Ramachandran, this reveals an assumption made by the visual system, namely that it expects light to shine from above.[25]

Now turn the page upside down and look at Figure 16.15 again. All the eggs and cavities instantly switch places.

Ask a friend to hold the page right side up for you. Then bend down and look between your legs at the page (which is now behind you). Again, the switch occurs '... as if the sun is stuck to your head and shining upward from the floor'.[25]

PERCEPTION OF REAL MOVEMENT

The importance of eye movements

To perceive real (actual) movement, there must be changes in the retinal image. Indeed, it seems that the receptors only respond to changes in the environment. The eyes are constantly making minute, oscillatory movements, which keep the receptors stimulated. A device for stabilizing the retinal image shows that these movements are necessary for seeing things at all.[35] A tiny slide projector, mounted on a contact lens, is attached to the cornea and a slide projected on to a screen. Since the lens and the projector move with the eye, the retinal image is stabilized. In other words, eye movements and the movement of the image on the screen cancel each other out, so the retinal image stays in the same place. After initially seeing the picture with normal acuity, the image begins to fade within a few seconds and after a minute disappears altogether.

If you turn your head slowly around with your eyes open, or you scan a stationary scene, you create a succession of different retinal images, but you will not perceive movement (location constancy kicks in). So, changes in the retinal image cannot be a sufficient basis for the perception of movement. Conversely, when an object moves across your visual field and you follow the object with your eyes, the retinal image remains the same but you do perceive movement.

Configurational change

Objects moving in the environment usually do so against a background of stationary or differently moving objects. Also, the nose and other anatomical borders to the visual field provide stationary reference points against which to judge movement. This causes a *configuration change*, or change in the overall pattern and interrelationship between objects. However, although in practice this is often an important source of information, it may not be a necessary one. If a lighted cigarette is moved about in a dark room, the cigarette will be perceived as moving, even though there are no background cues or frames of reference.[34] (This should not be confused with the autokinetic effect; see Box 16.2.)

How does the brain do it?

It seems that the brain is capable of distinguishing between eye movements that signal movement of objects (real movement) and those eye movements (and head movements) that do not signal movement. Probably the superior colliculus plays an important role in making this distinction. Gregory describes two systems:[34]

- The *image–retina system*, which responds to changes in the visual field that produce changes in the retinal image
- The *eye–head system*, which responds to movements of the head and eyes.

The perception of movement is the product of an interplay between the two systems.

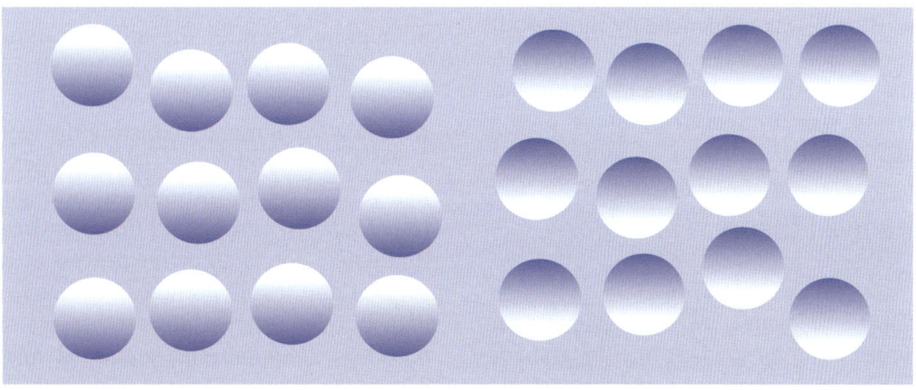

Figure 16.15 Illusions of shading. From Ramachandran and Rogers-Ramachandran.[25]

According to Braddick, the human visual system seems to have two separate systems for measuring the speed and direction of individual features moving in the retinal image:[36]

- A long-range, *feature-tracking* system seems to infer motion from one instant to the next, which underpins our conscious impression of motion in films and television.
- A short-range, *motion-sensing* system seems to measure motion more directly by signalling changes in the image content over time.

Although neither system is fully understood, the basic requirements are in place even at the retina. P-type ganglion cells respond to abrupt spatial changes in the image, while M-type ganglion cells may respond to abrupt temporal (time-related) changes. Additionally, the temporal cortex contains many cells selective for different types of motion, and most visual cortical cells prefer moving to stationary stimuli.[23]

THEORIES OF VISUAL PERCEPTION

Classifying theories

As we noted above, one way in which theories of perception differ is in terms of whether they regard perception as a direct (bottom-up, data-driven) or indirect (top-down, conceptually driven) process. Bruce and Green describe these as 'ecological' and 'traditional', respectively.[37] The term 'ecological' was used by Gibson, the major bottom-up theorist, to imply that visual information from the whole physical environment is available for analysis by retinal receptor cells.

Another issue that divides theories relates to the nature–nurture debate (see Gross[9]). *Empiricists* regard perception as primarily the result of learning and experience, while *nativists* believe that perception is essentially an innate ability, requiring little, if any, learning. All the top-down theorists are also empiricists, and the major nativists are the Gestalt psychologists. Gibson was influenced by the Gestalt school, but he is generally regarded as an empiricist. Finally, Marr's theory has both top-down and bottom-up components, and he too was influenced by some of the Gestalt laws (Table 16.3).

Table 16.3 Classification of theories of perception

	Direct (bottom-up/ecological)	Indirect (top-down/traditional)
Empiricist	Gibson[6,7]	Gregory[4,5] Bruner[2] Neisser[3] Marr[8]
Nativist	Gestalt	

Gregory's constructivist theory

According to Gregory:

> Perception is not determined simply by stimulus patterns. Rather, it is a dynamic searching for the best interpretation of the available data ... [which] involves going beyond the immediately given evidence of the senses.[38]

To avoid sensory overload, we need to select from all the sensory stimulation that surrounds us. Also, we often need to supplement sensory information, because the total information that we need might not be directly available to the senses. This is what Gregory means by 'going beyond the immediately given evidence of the senses', and it is why his theory is described as *constructivist*. For Gregory, we make inferences about the information that the senses receive (based on Helmholtz's nineteenth-century view of perception as consisting of *unconscious inferences*).

Gregory's theory and perceptual constancies

Perceptual constancies tell us that visual information from the retinal image is sketchy and incomplete, and that the visual system has to 'go beyond' the retinal image in order to test hypotheses that fill in the 'gaps'.[16] To make sense of the various sensory inputs to the retina (*low-level information*), the visual system must draw on all kinds of evidence, including distance cues, information from other senses and expectations based on past experience (*high-level knowledge*). For all these reasons, Gregory argues that perception must be an indirect process involving a construction based on physical sources of energy.

Gregory's theory and illusions

Gregory argues that, when we experience a visual illusion, what we perceive may not be physically present in the stimulus (and hence not present in the retinal image). Essentially, an illusion can be explained in terms of a perceptual hypothesis that is not confirmed by the data: our attempt to interpret the stimulus figure turns out to be inappropriate. In other words, an illusion occurs when we attempt unsuccessfully to construe the stimulus in keeping with how we normally construe the world (Box 16.3).

All illusions illustrate how the perceptual system normally operates by forming a 'best guess', which is then tested against sensory inputs. For Gregory, illusions show that perception is an active process of using information to suggest and test hypotheses.[38] What we perceive is not the data but an interpretation of them, so that 'A perceived object is a hypothesis, suggested and tested by sensory data.'[38] As Gregory has noted, '... this makes the basis of knowledge indirect and inherently doubtful.'[38]

Box 16.3 Explaining the Ponzo illusion

In the Ponzo illusion (see Figure 16.11a), our system can either:

- accept the equal lengths of the two central bars as drawn on a flat two-dimensional surface (which would involve assuming that the bars are equidistant from us); or
- 'read' the whole figure as a railway track converging into the distance, so that the two horizontal bars represent sleepers, the top one of which would be further away from us but appears longer, since it 'must' be longer in order to produce the same-length image on the retina.

The second interpretation is clearly inappropriate, since the figure is drawn on a flat piece of paper and there are no actual distance differences. As a result, we experience an illusion.

Gregory argues that when we view a 3D scene with many distance cues, the perceptual system can quickly select the hypothesis that best interprets the sensory data. However, reversible figures supply few distance cues to guide the system. For example, the spontaneous reversal of the Necker cube (see Figure 16.12) occurs because the perceptual system continually tests two equally plausible hypotheses about the nature of the object represented in the drawing.

With the impossible triangle (see Figure 16.13a), our perceptual system makes reasonable, but incorrect, judgements about the distance of different parts of the triangle.

Misapplied size constancy theory

According to Gregory, the Müller–Lyer illusion can be explained as follows (Figure 16.16):

- The arrow with the ingoing fins provides linear perspective cues, suggesting that it could be the outside corner of a building. Hence, the fins are seen as walls receding away from us, making the shaft look closer to us.
- In the arrow with the outgoing fins, the cues suggest that it could be the inside corner of a room, and the outgoing fins as walls coming towards us. This would make the shaft appear 'distant'.
- The retinal images produced by the arrows are actually equal. According to size constancy, if equally sized images are produced by two lines, one of which is further away from us than the other, then the line that is furthest from us must be longer. Because this interpretation is taking place unconsciously and quickly, we immediately perceive the illusion.
- However, if the perspective cues are removed, the illusion remains, suggesting that the misapplied size constancy theory is itself misapplied (Figure 16.17). Alternatively, the apparent distance of the arrow could be caused by the apparent size of the arrows rather than, as Gregory claims, the other way around.[39]

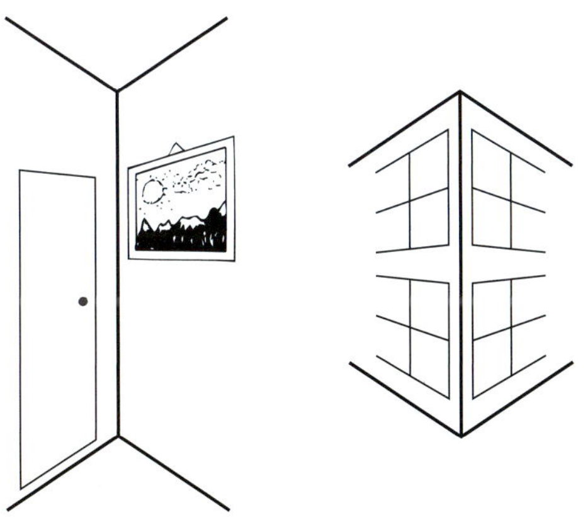

Figure 16.16 Representation of the Müller–Lyer illusion as suggested by Gregory's misapplied size constancy theory

In the Müller–Lyer illusion, we know the arrows are the same length, and yet we still experience the illusion. Our knowledge should enable us to modify our hypotheses in an adaptive way. Although some illusions can be explained in terms of the same unconscious processes occurring (an example being size constancy), not all illusions are amenable to explanation in the way Gregory proposes.[39]

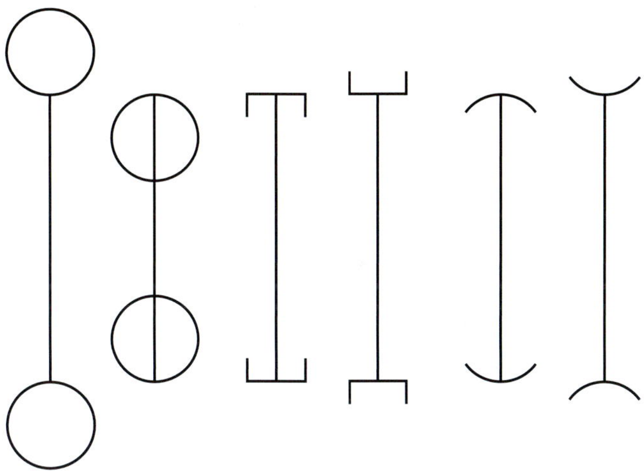

Figure 16.17 Müller–Lyer illusion with the depth cues removed

Gregory's theory and perceptual set

Perceptual set is directly relevant to Gregory's view that perception is an active process involving selection, inference and interpretation. Allport describes perceptual set as '... a perceptual bias or predisposition or readiness to perceive particular features of a stimulus'.[40]

It refers to the tendency to perceive or notice some aspects of available sense data and ignore others. According to Vernon, set acts as:[41]

- a *selector* (the perceiver has certain expectations that help to focus attention on particular aspects of the incoming sensory information);
- an *interpreter* (the perceiver knows how to deal with the

selected data, how to classify, understand and name them, and what inferences to draw from them).

Several factors can influence or induce set, most of them being *perceiver* (or *organismic*) variables. But some relate to the nature of the stimulus or the conditions under which it is perceived (*stimulus* or *situational variables*). Both types of variable influence perception indirectly, through directly influencing set, which, as such, is a perceiver variable or characteristic (Figure 16.18, Box 16.4).

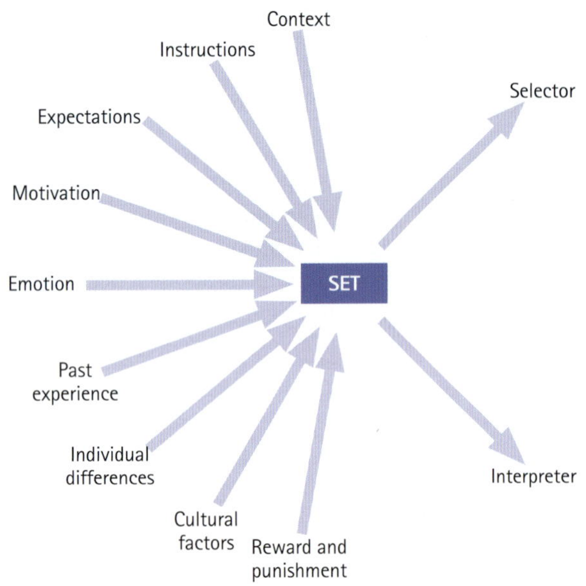

Figure 16.18 Indirect influence of perceiver and stimulus variables on perception through their direct influence on set

An evaluation of Gregory's theory of perception

- Gregory's theory raises many important questions that have yet to be answered satisfactorily.[15] For example, if perception is essentially constructive, then we need to know how it gets started and why there is such common experience among different people, all of whom have had to construct their own idiosyncratic perceptual worlds. Also, given that perception is typically accurate (and our hypotheses are usually correct), it seems unlikely that our retinal images are really as ambiguous and lacking in detail as Gregory suggests.
- Gregory has been much more successful in explaining at least some types of illusion than in explaining perception as a whole.[51] His theory may be most relevant when stimuli are ambiguous, incomplete or presented very briefly, or their processing is interrupted.[52] In Gordon's view, constructivist theories have underestimated the richness of sensory evidence in the real world.[15] For Gordon:

It is possible that we perceive constructively only at certain times and in certain situations. Whenever we move under our

Box 16.4 Some findings relating to perceptual set

MOTIVATION

People with some particular need (e.g. hunger) are more likely to perceive vague or ambiguous pictures as relating to that need.[42,43]

EMOTION

The term 'perceptual defence' refers to the findings from laboratory experiments that subliminally perceived words (below the threshold of conscious awareness) that evoke unpleasant emotions take longer to be perceived at a conscious level than neutral words.[44]

VALUES

Lambert *et al.* found that when children were taught to value something more highly than they had done previously, they perceived the valued thing as being larger (*perceptual accentuation*).[45]

BELIEFS

The beliefs we hold about the world can affect our interpretation of ambiguous sensory signals. A person who believes in UFOs is likely to perceive an ambiguous object in the sky differently from a person who does not share that belief.[46]

COGNITIVE STYLE

The way we deal with our environment appears to affect our perception of it. Some people perceive the environment as a whole and do not clearly differentiate the shape, colour and other aspects of individual items. Others perceive the elements of the environment as separate and distinct.[47]

CONTEXT AND EXPECTATIONS

The interaction between context and expectations was demonstrated by Bruner and Postman[48] and Bruner *et al.*[49] When participants are asked to copy a briefly presented stimulus such as:

PARIS IN THE THE SPRING	ONCE IN A A LIFETIME	A BIRD IN THE THE HAND

it is typically copied as PARIS IN THE SPRING/ONCE IN A LIFETIME/A BIRD IN THE HAND. One reason eyewitness testimony is so unreliable is that our general expectation of people is that they will be of 'average' height and weight, and this is what almost all eyewitness accounts describe people as being (see Chapter 17 and Gross[9]).[50]

own power on the surface of the natural world and in good light, the necessary perceptions of size, texture, distance, continuity, motion and so on, may all occur directly and reflexively.[15]

Gibson's theory of direct perception

Constructivists use the retinal image as their starting point for explaining perception. According to Gibson, this approach mistakenly describes the input for a perceiver in the same terms as that for a single photoreceptor, namely a stream of photons.[6] For Gibson, it is better to begin by considering the input as a pattern of light extended over time and space (an *optic array* containing all the visual information from the environment striking the eye of a stationary perceiver).

The optic array provides unambiguous, invariant information about the layout and relevant properties of objects in space. This information takes three main forms: *optic flow patterns*, *texture gradient* and *affordances*. Perception essentially involves picking up the rich information provided by the optic array in a direct way, which involves little or no (unconscious) information processing, computations or internal representations.[23]

Optic flow patterns

During the Second World War, Gibson prepared training films describing the problems that pilots experience when taking off and landing. He called the information available to pilots 'optic flow patterns' (OFPs). As shown in Figure 16.19, the point to which a pilot moves appears motionless, with the rest of the visual environment apparently moving away from that point. Thus, all around the point there is an apparent radial expansion of textures flowing around the pilot's head.

The lack of apparent movement of the point towards which the pilot moves is an invariant, unchanging feature of the optic array. Such OFPs provide unambiguous information about direction, speed and altitude. OFPs in general refer to changes in the optic array as the perceiver moves about.

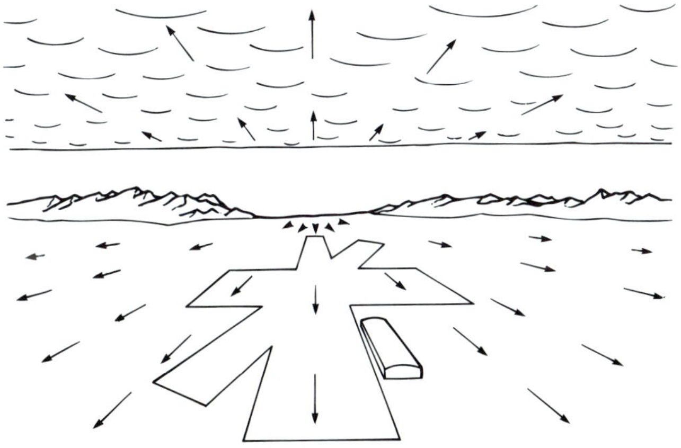

Figure 16.19 Optic flow patterns as a pilot approaches the landing strip. From Gibson.[53]

Texture gradients

Textures expand as we approach them and contract as they pass beyond our head. This happens whenever we move toward something, so that over and above the behaviour of each texture element there is a higher-order pattern or structure available as a source of information about the environment (and so the flow of the texture is invariant). Texture gradients (or *gradients of texture density*) are important depth cues perceived directly without the need for any inferences. The depth cues described in Table 16.2 are all examples of directly perceived, invariant, higher-order features of the optic array. For Gibson, then, the third dimension (depth) is available to the senses as directly as the other two dimensions, automatically processed by the sense receptors, and automatically producing the perceptual experience of depth.

Affordances

The environment contains invariant information, the detection of which has survival value for the perceiver. Affordances are directly perceivable, potential uses of objects, such as surfaces that are stand-on-able or sit-on-able, objects that are graspable or throwable, and things that afford eating (are 'edible'). In other words, affordances are the meanings that an environment has for an animal, and the relationship between perceiver and environment is vitally important.

An evaluation of Gibson's theory

- Gibson was concerned with the problem of how we obtain constant perception in everyday life, based on continually changing sensations. According to Marr, this indicated that Gibson correctly regarded the problem of perception as that of recovering from sensory information 'valid properties of the external world'.[8]
- However, as Marr points out, Gibson failed to recognize two equally critical things: 'First, the detection of physical invariants, like image surfaces, is exactly and precisely an information-processing problem... Second, he vastly underrated the sheer difficulty of such detection.'[8]
- An interesting study by Lee and Lishman tends to support Gibson's belief in the importance of movement in perception, and the artificiality of separating sensory and motor aspects of behaviour (Box 16.5).[54]
- Gibson's concept of affordances is part of his attempt to show that all the information needed to make sense of the visual environment is directly available in the visual input (a purely bottom-up approach to perception). Bruce and Green argue that this concept is most powerful and useful in the context of visually guided behaviour, as in insects.[37] Here, it makes sense to speak of an organism detecting information available in the light needed to organize its activities, and the idea of it needing a conceptual representation of its environment seems redundant.

Box 16.5 If the room sways, there may be an experiment going on[54]

Lee and Lishman used a specially built swaying room (suspended above the floor), designed to bring texture flow under experimental control. As the room sways (so changing the texture flow), adults typically make slight unconscious adjustments and children tend to fall over. Normally, the brain is very skilled at establishing correlations between changes in the optic flow, signals to the muscles and staying upright.

Arguably, the most important reason for having a visual system is to be able to anticipate when contact with an approaching object is going to be made. Lee and Lishman believe that estimating 'time to contact' is crucial for actions such as avoidance of objects and grasping them, and thus represents extremely important ecological information. This can be expressed as a formula:

$$\text{Time to contact} = \frac{\text{size of retinal image}}{\text{rate of expansion of retinal image}}$$

This is a property shared by all objects and so is another invariant, demonstrating the unambiguous nature of the retinal image.

Measures of optic flow have also provided some understanding of how skilled long-jumpers control their approaches to the take-off position.[15]

- However, humans act in both a cultural and a physical environment. It is inconceivable that we do not need any knowledge of writing or the postal system in order to detect that a pen affords writing or a post-box affords posting a letter, and that these are directly perceived invariants. People see objects and events as what they are in terms of a culturally given conceptual representation of the world, and Gibson's theory says much more about 'seeing' than about 'seeing as'.

'Seeing' and 'seeing as'

According to Fodor and Pylyshyn:

> What you see when you see a thing depends upon what the thing you see is. But what you see the thing as depends upon what you know about what you are seeing.[55]

This view of perception as 'seeing as' is the fundamental principle of *transactionalism*. Transactionalists (such as Ames, cited in Ittelson[56]) argue that, because sensory input is always ambiguous, the interpretation selected is the one most likely to be true given what has been perceived in the past.

Ames experimented with a distorted room, constructed in such a way that, when viewed with one eye through a peephole, a person at one end may appear very small and the person at the other end very tall. When the people cross the room, they appear to change size. The observer has to choose between two different beliefs about the world built up through past experience. The first is that rooms are rectangular, consist of right-angles and so on. The second is that people are usually of 'average' height. Most observers choose the first and so judge the people to be an odd size. However, a woman who saw her husband in the room and judged the room to be odd shows that particularly salient past experiences can override more generalized beliefs about the world.

The Ames room is another example of a visual illusion, and the inability of Gibson's theory to explain mistaken perception is perhaps its greatest single weakness. Gibson argues that most 'mistaken perceptions' occur in situations very different from those that prevail in the natural environment. However, to suggest that illusions are nothing but laboratory tricks designed to baffle ordinary people is not true, since at least some illusions produce effects similar to those found in normal perception.

A possible synthesis of Gregory's and Gibson's theories

Despite the important differences between Gibson's and Gregory's theories, they also agree on certain points:

Similarities

- Visual perception is mediated by light reflected from surfaces and objects.
- Some kind of physiological system is needed in order to perceive.
- Perception is an active process. (In Gibson's view, 'a perceiving organism is more like a map-reader than a camera'.[6])
- Perceptual experience can be influenced by learning.

Differences

- Gregory believes that meaningless sensory cues must be supplemented by memory, habit, experience and so on in order to construct a meaningful world. Gibson argues that the environment (initially the optic array) provides us with all the information we need for living in the world. Perceptual learning consists not of 'gluing' together sensory 'atoms' but of coming to differentiate and discriminate between the features of the environment as presented in the optic array.
- To the extent that Gibson acknowledges the role of learning (albeit a different kind of learning from Gregory), he may be considered an empiricist (see above), together with his emphasis on what is provided by the physical world. In other respects, though, Gibson can be considered a nativist. As we noted earlier, he was very much influenced by the Gestalt psychologists, stressing the organized quality of perception. However, although for Gibson this organized quality is part of the physical structure of the light impinging on the observer's eye, for Gestaltists it is a function of how the brain is organized.

Eysenck and Keane argue that the relative importance of bottom-up and top-down processes is affected by several factors.[51] When viewing conditions are good, bottom-up processing may be crucial. However, with brief or ambiguous stimuli, top-down processing becomes increasingly important. Gibson seems to have been concerned more with optimal viewing conditions, while Gregory and other constructivists have tended to concentrate on suboptimal conditions.[18] In most circumstances, both bottom-up and top-down processes are probably needed, as claimed by Neisser (Box 16.6).[57]

Box 16.6 Neisser's analysis-by-synthesis model[58]

Neisser assumes the existence of a perceptual cycle involving schemata, perceptual exploration and stimulus environment. *Schemata* contain collections of knowledge based on past experience (see Chapter 17), and these direct perceptual exploration towards relevant environmental stimulation. Such exploration often involves moving around the environment, leading the perceiver to actively sample the available stimulus information. If this fails to match the information in the relevant schema, then the hypothesis is modified accordingly.

An initial analysis of the sensory cues and features (a bottom-up process) might suggest the hypothesis that the object being viewed is, say, a chair.

This initiates a search for the expected features (e.g. four legs and a back), which is based on our schema of a chair (this synthesis is a top-down process).

But if the environmental features disconfirm the original hypothesis (the 'chair' has only three legs and no back), then a new hypothesis must be generated and tested (it might be a stool), and the appropriate schema activated.

Neisser argues that perception never occurs in a vacuum: our sampling of sensory features of the environment is always guided by our knowledge and past experience. Perception is an interactive process, involving both bottom-up feature analysis and top-down expectations (Figure 16.20).

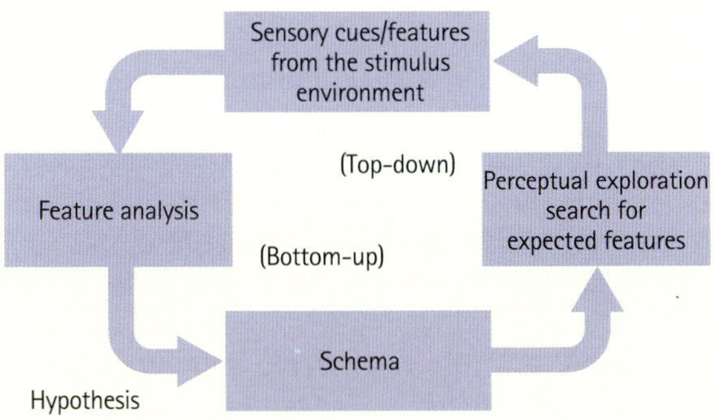

Figure 16.20 Neisser's analysis-by-synthesis model of perception

CONCLUSIONS

Form and depth perception, perceptual constancy and visual illusions are all concerned with perceptual organization, and many of the principles governing perceptual organization are commonly referred to as Gestalt laws.

Although Gregory's constructivist ('top-down') and Gibson's direct ('bottom-up') approaches may appear to contradict each other, it is possible to see them as complementary. According to Harris:

> Perception is not just a single task but ... contributes in many different ways to everyday life... Some of these ... are obviously more difficult than others and it seems likely that some can be accomplished directly, as Gibson maintained, whilst others may require sophisticated internal knowledge and are thus better described by the indirect approach.[23]

KEY POINTS

- Sensation involves physical stimulation of the sense organs, while perception is the organization and interpretation of incoming sensory information.
- Gestalt psychologists identified innately determined principles through which sensory information is interpreted and organized. The most basic of these is form perception, which organizes incoming sensory information into figure and ground.
- Laws for grouping stimuli together rest on the belief that the whole is greater than the sum of its parts. These laws can be summarized under Koffka's law of *prägnanz*. Major Gestalt laws of perception include proximity, similarity, continuity, closure, part–whole relationship and common fate.
- Despite empirical support, Gestalt laws are difficult to apply to 3D perception and to whole scenes (they lack ecological validity).
- Depth perception allows us to estimate the distance of objects from us. Pictorial cues refer to aspects of the visual field and are monocular. Non-pictorial cues include convergence and retinal disparity, which are binocular.
- Perceptual constancy refers to the ability to recognize an object as unchanging despite changes in its size, shape, location, brightness and colour.
- Four main kinds of perceptual illusion are distortions/geometric illusions, ambiguous/reversible figures, paradoxical figures and fictions. Other illusions include those involving apparent movement and shading.
- According to top-down (conceptually driven) perceptual processing theorists, perception is the end result of an indirect process that involves making inferences about the world, based on knowledge and expectations. Bottom-up (data-driven) theorists argue that perception is a direct process, determined by the information presented to the sensory receptors.
- According to Gregory's constructivist theory, we often supplement perception with unconscious inferences. His misapplied size constancy theory claims that we interpret the ingoing and outgoing fins

of the arrows in the Müller–Lyer illusion as providing perspective cues to distance.

- Perceptual set acts as a selector and interpreter and can be induced by perceiver/organismic and stimulus/situational variables. Perceiver variables include expectations, which often interact with context.
- According to Gibson, the optic array provides information about the layout and properties of objects in space requiring little or no (unconscious) information-processing, computations or internal representations. Optic flow patterns, texture gradients and affordances are all invariant, unchanging and higher-order features of the optic array.
- Gibson overlooked the role of culturally determined knowledge in perception. He also failed to distinguish between 'seeing' and 'seeing as', the latter forming the basic principle of transactionalism.
- Both Gibson and Gregory agree that perception is an active process, influenced by learning (making them empiricists), although they propose different kinds of learning. Gibson is also a nativist in certain respects and was influenced by the Gestalt psychologists.
- Bottom-up processing (Gibson) may be crucial under optimal viewing conditions, but under suboptimal conditions top-down processing (Gregory) becomes increasingly important.
- According to Neisser's analysis-by-synthesis model, perception is an interactive process, involving both bottom-up feature analysis and top-down expectations (appearing at different stages of a perceptual cycle).

REFERENCES

1. Dodwell PC (1995) Fundamental processes in vision. In RL Gregory, AM Colman (eds) *Sensation and Perception.* London: Longman.
2. Bruner JS (1957) On perceptual readiness. *Psychological Review* **64**: 123–52.
3. Neisser U (1967) *Cognitive Psychology.* New York: Appleton-Century-Crofts.
4. Gregory RL (1972) Visual illusions. In BM Foss (ed.) *New Horizons in Psychology 1.* Harmondsworth: Penguin.
5. Gregory RL (1980) Perception as hypotheses. *Philosophical Transactions of the Royal Society of London, Series B* **290**: 181–97.
6. Gibson JJ (1966) *The Senses Considered as Perceptual Systems.* Boston, MA: Houghton Mifflin.
7. Gibson JJ (1979) *The Ecological Approach to Visual Perception.* Boston, MA: Houghton Mifflin.
8. Marr D (1982) *Vision: A Computational Investigation into the Human Representation and Processing of Visual Information.* San Francisco, CA: W.H. Freeman.
9. Gross R (2005) *Psychology: The Science of Mind and Behaviour*, 5th edn. London: Hodder Arnold.
10. Von Ehrenfels C (1890) Uber Gestaltqualitaten Vierteljahrschrift fur wissenschaftliche. *Philosophie und Soziologie* **14**: 249–92.
11. Rubin E (1915) *Synsoplevde Figurer.* Copenhagen: Gyldendalaske Boghandel.
12. Koffka K (1935) *The Principles of Gestalt Psychology.* New York: Harcourt Brace.
13. Köhler W (1925) *The Mentality of Apes.* New York: Harcourt Brace.
14. Roth I (1986) An introduction to object perception. In I Roth, JP Frisby (eds) *Perception and Representation.* Milton Keynes: Open University Press.
15. Gordon IE (1989) *Theories of Visual Perception.* Chichester: John Wiley & Sons.
16. Greene J (1990) Perception. In I Roth (ed.) *Introduction to Psychology*, Vol. 2. Milton Keynes: Open University Press.
17. Navon D (1977) Forest before trees: the precedence of global features in visual perception. *Cognitive Psychology* **9**: 353–83.
18. Eysenck MW (1993) *Principles of Cognitive Psychology.* Hove: Lawrence Erlbaum Associates.
19. Humphreys GW, Riddoch MJ (1987) *To See But Not To See: A Case Study of Visual Agnosia.* London: Lawrence Erlbaum Associates.
20. Eysenck MW, Keane MJ (1990) *Cognitive Psychology: A Student's Handbook.* Hove: Lawrence Erlbaum Associates.
21. Palmer SE (1975) The effects of contextual scenes on the identification of objects. *Memory and Cognition* **3**: 519–26.
22. Marr D (1976) Early processing of visual information. *Philosophical Transactions of the Royal Society of London, B* **275**: 483–524.
23. Harris M (1998) Perception. In P Scott, C Spencer (eds) *Psychology: A Contemporary Introduction.* Oxford: Blackwell.
24. Hochberg JE (1971) Perception. In JW Kling, LA Riggs (eds) *Experimental Psychology.* New York: Holt.
25. Ramachandran VS, Rogers-Ramachandran D (2004) Illusions. *Scientific American Special: Mind* **14**: 100-C3.
26. Coren S, Girgus JS (1978) *Seeing is Deceiving: The Psychology of Visual Illusions.* Hillsdale, NJ: Lawrence Erlbaum Associates.
27. Gregory RL (1983) Visual illusions. In J Miller (ed.) *States of Mind.* London: BBC.
28. Mackay DC, Newbigging PL (1977) The Poggendorf and its variants do arouse the same perceptual processes. *Perception and Psychophysics* **21**: 26–32.
29. Yarbus AL (1967) *Eye Movements and Vision* (transl. B Haigh). New York: Plenum.
30. Kanizsa A (1976) Subjective contours. *Scientific American* **234**: 48–52.
31. Krebs D, Blackman R (1988) *Psychology: A First Encounter.* New York: Harcourt Brace Jovanovich.

32. Rock I (1984) *Perception*. New York: W.H. Freeman.
33. Ramachandran VS, Anstis SM (1986) The perception of apparent motion. *Scientific American* **254**: 80–87.
34. Gregory RL (1973) *Eye and Brain*, 2nd edn. New York: World Universities Library.
35. Cornsweet TN (1970) *Visual Perception*. New York: Academic Press.
36. Braddick OJ (1974) A short-range process in apparent motion. *Vision Research* **14**: 519–27.
37. Bruce V, Green PR (1990) *Visual Perception*, 2nd edn. Hove: Lawrence Erlbaum Associates.
38. Gregory RL (1966) *Eye and Brain*. London: Weidenfeld & Nicolson.
39. Robinson JO (1972) *The Psychology of Visual Illusions*. London: Hutchinson.
40. Allport GW (1955) *Theories of Perception and the Concept of Structure*. New York: John Wiley & Sons.
41. Vernon MD (1955) The function of schemata in perceiving. *Psychological Review* **62**: 180–92.
42. Sanford RN (1937) The effects of abstinence from food upon imaginal processes: a further experiment. *Journal of Psychology* **3**: 145–59.
43. McClelland DC, Atkinson JW (1948) The projective expression of need: I. The effect of different intensities of the hunger drive on perception. *Journal of Psychology* **25**: 205–22.
44. McGinnies E (1949) Emotionality and perceptual defence. *Psychological Review* **56**: 244–51.
45. Lambert WW, Solomon RM, Watson PD (1949) Reinforcement and extinction as factors in size estimation. *Journal of Experimental Psychology* **39**: 637–41.
46. Wade C, Tavris C (1999) *Invitation to Psychology*. New York: Longman.
47. Witkin HA, Dyk RB, Faterson HF, Goodenough DR, Karp SA (1962) *Psychological Differentiation*. London: John Wiley & Sons.
48. Bruner JS, Postman L (1949) On the perception of incongruity. *Journal of Personality* **18**: 206–23.
49. Bruner JS, Busiek RD, Minturn AL (1952) Assimilation in the immediate reproduction of visually perceived figures. *Journal of Experimental Psychology* **44**: 151–5.
50. Loftus EF (1980) *Memory*. Reading, MA: Addison-Wesley.
51. Eysenck MW, Keane MJ (1995) *Cognitive Psychology: A Student's Handbook*, 3rd edn. Hove: Lawrence Erlbaum Associates.
52. Groome D, Dewart H, Esgate E, *et al.* (1999) *An Introduction to Cognitive Psychology: Processes and Disorders*. London: Psychology Press.
53. Gibson JJ (1950) *The Perception of the Visual World*. Boston, MA: Houghton Mifflin.
54. Lee DN, Lishman JR (1975) Visual proprioceptive control of stance. *Journal of Human Movement Studies* **1**: 87–95.
55. Fodor JA, Pylyshyn ZW (1981) How direct is visual perception? Some reflections on Gibson's 'ecological approach'. *Cognition* **9**: 139–96.
56. Ittelson WH (1952) *The Ames Demonstrations in Perception*. Princeton, NJ: Princeton University Press.
57. Neisser U (1976) *Cognition and Reality*. San Francisco, CA: W.H. Freeman.

Chapter 17

Memory

Richard Gross

INTRODUCTION

Learning and memory represent two sides of the same coin: learning depends on memory for its 'permanence', and memory would have no 'content' without learning. Hence, we could define memory as the retention of learning and experience. As Blakemore says, 'In the broadest sense, learning is the acquisition of knowledge and memory is the storage of an internal representation of that knowledge ...'[1]

Both learning and memory featured prominently in the early years of psychology as a science (see Chapter 9). William James, one of the pioneers of psychology, was arguably the first to make a formal distinction between primary and secondary memory, which correspond to short-term and long-term memory, respectively. This distinction is central to Atkinson and Shiffrin's very influential *multi-store model* (MSM).[2,3]

As with other cognitive processes, memory remained a largely unacceptable area for psychological research until the cognitive revolution of the mid-1950s, reflecting the dominance of behaviourism until this time. However, some behaviourists, especially in the USA, studied verbal behaviour using paired-associate learning. This associationist approach was (and remains) most apparent in *interference theory*, an attempt to explain forgetting. Other theories of forgetting include *trace decay*, *displacement*, *cue-dependent forgetting* and *repression*.

Several major accounts of memory have emerged from criticisms of the MSM. These include Craik and Lockhart's *levels-of-processing approach*,[4] Baddeley and Hitch's *working-memory model*[5] and attempts to identify different types of long-term memory (e.g. Tulving[6]). Psychologists are increasingly interested in everyday memory rather than studying it merely as a laboratory phenomenon.

THE MEANINGS OF 'MEMORY'

Memory, like learning, is a hypothetical construct denoting three distinguishable but interrelated processes (Figure 17.1):

- *Registration (or encoding):* the transformation of sensory input (e.g. a sound or visual image) into a form that allows it to be entered into (or registered in) memory. With a computer, for example, information can be encoded only if it is presented in a format that the computer recognizes.
- *Storage:* the operation of holding or retaining information in memory. Computers store information by means

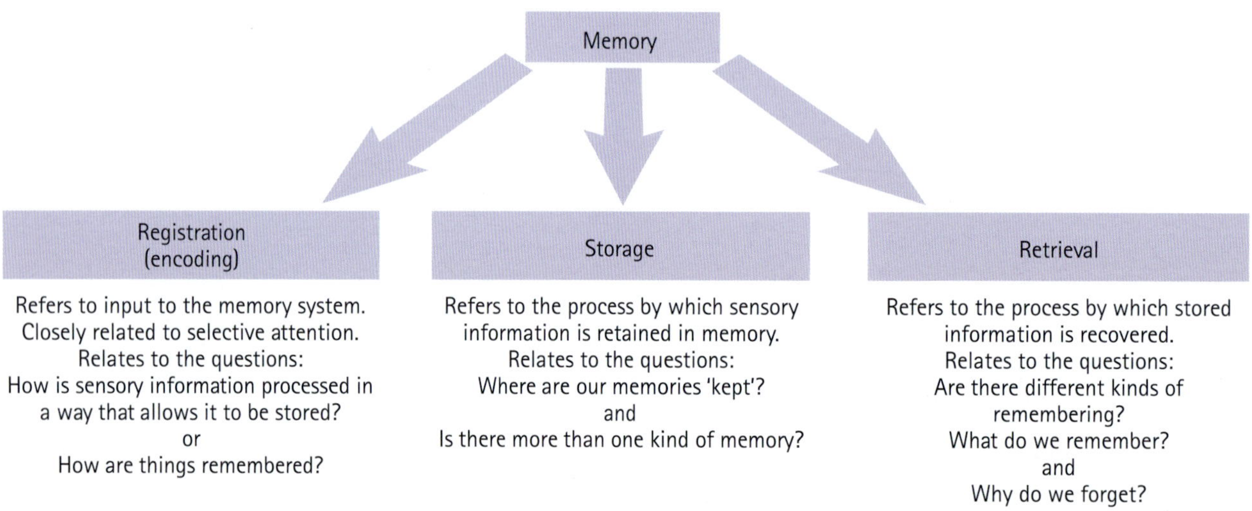

Figure 17.1 The three processes of memory

of changes in the system's electrical circuitry. In humans, the changes occurring in the brain allow information to be stored, though exactly what these changes involve is unclear.

- *Retrieval:* the process by which stored information is extracted from memory.

Registration can be thought of as a necessary condition for storage to take place, but not everything that registers on the senses is stored. Similarly, storage is a necessary, but not sufficient, condition for retrieval: we cannot recover information that has not been stored, but the fact that we know the information is no guarantee that we will remember it on any particular occasion. This is the crucial distinction between *availability* (whether or not the information has been stored) and *accessibility* (whether or not the information can be retrieved), which is especially relevant to theories of forgetting.

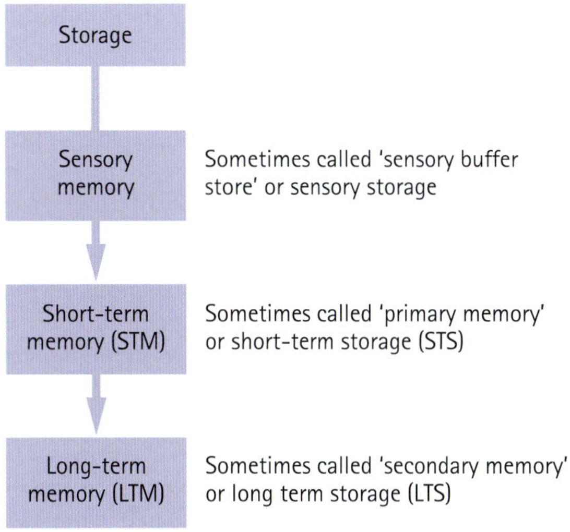

Figure 17.2 The three forms of storage

STORAGE

In practice, storage is studied through testing people's ability to retrieve. This is equivalent to the distinction between learning and performance: learning corresponds to storage, while performance corresponds to retrieval. But there are several kinds of retrieval (see below). So, if we are tested by recall, it may look as though we have not learned something, but a test of recognition may show that we have. For these reasons, it is useful to distinguish between memory as storage and memory as retrieval. When people complain about having a 'poor memory', they might mean storage or retrieval, but they are unlikely to make the distinction (they would simply say 'I can't remember').

As we noted earlier, it was James who first distinguished between primary and secondary memory. Ebbinghaus, the pioneer of memory research, would have accepted it.[7] Many psychologists since James have also made the distinction, including Hebb,[8] Broadbent[9] and Waugh and Norman.[10] In Atkinson and Shiffrin's MSM, primary and secondary memory are called short-term memory (STM) and long-term memory (LTM), respectively (Figure 17.2).[2,3] Strictly, STM and LTM refer to experimental procedures for investigating short-term and long-term storage, respectively.

Sensory memory

Sensory memory gives us an accurate account of the environment as experienced by the sensory system. We retain a literal copy of the stimulus long enough for us to decide whether it is worthy of further processing. Any information that we do not attend to or process further is forgotten. It is probably more useful to think of sensory memory as an aspect of perception and as a necessary requirement for storage proper (i.e. STM).

The storage (such as it is) occurs within the sensory system that received the information (it is *modality-specific*). Additional information entering the same sensory channel immediately disrupts the storage. For example, if two visual stimuli are presented within quick succession, memory of the first stimulus may be lost; but if the second stimulus is a sound or smell, it will not interfere with memory of the visual stimulus. Although it is likely that a sensory memory exists for each of our sensory systems, most research has concentrated on:

- *iconic memory* (an icon is an image), which stores visual images for about half a second;
- *echoic memory*, which stores sounds for up to two seconds.

We are usually unaware of sensory memory, but if you watch someone wave a lighted cigarette in a darkened room you see a streak rather than a series of points.[11] If we had no iconic memory, we would perceive a film as a series of still images interspersed with blank intervals, rather than as a continuously moving scene. Without echoic memory, instead of hearing speech as such, we would hear a series of unrelated sounds.[12]

Short-term memory

Probably less than one-hundredth of all the sensory information that impinges on the human senses every second reaches consciousness. Of this, only about 5 per cent is stored permanently.[13] Clearly, if we possessed only sensory memory, then our capacity for retaining information about the world would be extremely limited. However, according to models of memory such as Atkinson and Shiffrin's MSM,[2,3] some information from sensory memory is successfully passed on to STM.

Short-term (and long-term) memory can be analysed in terms of the following:

- *Capacity:* how much information can be stored

- *Duration:* how long the information can be held in storage
- *Coding:* how sensory input is represented by the memory system.

Capacity

Ebbinghaus[7] and Wundt in the 1860s were two of the first psychologists to maintain that STM is limited to six or seven bits of information. But the most famous account is given by Miller in his article 'The magical number seven, plus or minus two'.[14] Miller showed how *chunking* can be used to expand the limited capacity of STM by using already established memory stores to categorize or encode new information. If we think of STM's capacity as seven slots, with each slot being able to accommodate one bit, or unit, of information, then seven individual letters would each fill a slot and there would be no room left for any additional letters. But if the letters are chunked into a word, then the word would constitute one unit of information, leaving six free slots. In the example below, the 25 bits of information can be chunked into (or reduced to) six words, which could quite easily be reduced further to one bit (or chunk) based on prior familiarity with the words:

S	A	V	A	O
R	E	E	E	G
U	R	S	Y	A
O	O	D	N	S
F	C	N	E	R

To be able to chunk, you have to know the rule or code, which in this case is: starting with F in the bottom left-hand corner, read upwards until you get to S; then drop down to C and read upwards until you get to A; then go to N and read upwards; and so on. This should give you 'four score and seven years ago'.

Chunking is involved whenever we reduce a larger amount of information to a smaller amount. This (i) increases the capacity of STM and (ii) represents a form of encoding information, by imposing a meaning on otherwise meaningless material. For example:

- arranging letters into words, words into phrases and phrases into sentences;
- converting 1066 (four bits of information) into a date (one chunk), so a string of 28 numbers could be reduced to seven dates;
- using a rule to organize information: the series 149162536496481100121 (21 bits) is generated by the rule by which $1^2 = 1$, $2^2 = 4$, $3^2 = 9$ and so on. The rule represents a single chunk, and that's all that has to be remembered.

These examples demonstrate how chunking allows us to bypass the seven-bit bottleneck. Although the amount of information contained in any one chunk may be unlimited (e.g. the rule above can generate an infinitely long set of digits), the number of chunks that can be held in STM is still limited to seven plus or minus two.

Duration

A way of studying pure STM was devised by Brown[15] and Peterson and Peterson[16] – the *Brown–Peterson technique.* By repeating something that has to be remembered (maintenance rehearsal), information can be held in STM almost indefinitely. The Brown–Peterson technique overcomes this problem (Box 17.1).

Box 17.1 The Brown–Peterson technique[16]

In the Brown–Peterson technique, participants hear various trigrams, such as 'XPJ'. Only one trigram is presented on each trial.

Immediately afterwards, the participants are instructed to recall what they heard or to count backwards, in threes, out loud, from some specified number for 3, 6, 9, 12, 15 or 18 s (the retention interval). The function of this distractor task is to prevent rehearsal.

At the end of the time period, participants try to recall the trigram.

Peterson and Peterson found that the average percentage of correctly recalled trigrams was high with short delays, but decreased as the delay interval increased. Nearly 70 per cent were forgotten after only a 9-s delay, and 90 per cent after 18 s (Figure 17.3).

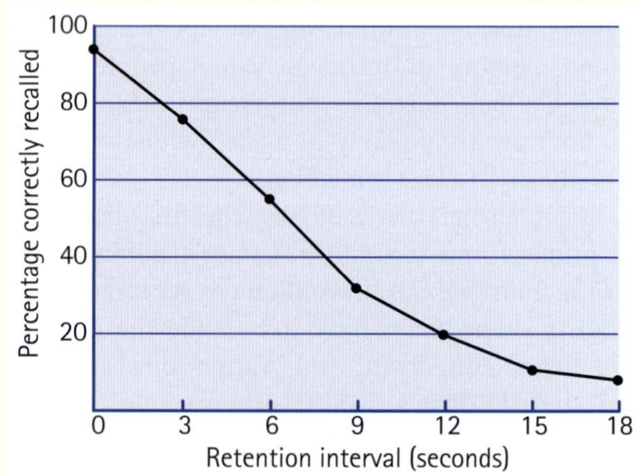

Figure 17.3 Data reported by Peterson and Peterson in their experiment on the duration of short-term memory[16]

In the absence of rehearsal, then, the duration of short-term memory is very short, even with very small amounts of information. If a more difficult distractor task is used, the duration can be made even shorter.

Coding

Conrad presented participants visually with a list of six consonants (e.g. BKSJLR), each of which was seen for about three-quarters of a second.[17] Participants were instructed to write down the consonants. Mistakes tended to be related to a letter's sound. For example, there were 62 instances of 'B' being mistaken for 'P' and 83 instances of 'V' being mistaken for 'P', but only two instances of 'S' being mistaken for 'P'. These *acoustic confusion errors* suggested to Conrad that STM must code information according to its sound. Even when information is presented visually, it must somehow be transformed into its acoustic code (see also Baddeley's study[18]).

Other forms of coding in short-term memory

Shulman showed participants lists of ten words.[19] Recognition of the words was then tested using a visually presented 'probe word', which was:

- a homonym of one of the words on the list (e.g. 'bawl' for 'ball'); or
- a synonym of one of the words on the list (e.g. 'talk' for 'speak'); or
- identical to one of the words on the list.

Shulman found that homonym and synonym probes produced similar error rates. These results imply that some *semantic coding* (coding for meaning) had taken place in STM. If an error was made on a synonym probe, then some matching for meaning must have taken place.

Visual images (e.g. abstract pictures, which would be difficult to store using an acoustic code) can also be maintained in STM, if only briefly.

Long-term memory

Capacity and duration

It is generally accepted that LTM has unlimited capacity. It can be thought of as a vast storehouse of all the information, skills, abilities and so on that are not currently being used but that are potentially retrievable. According to Bower, some of the kinds of information contained in LTM include:[20]

- a spatial model of the world around us;
- knowledge of the physical world, physical laws and properties of objects;
- beliefs about people, ourselves, social norms, values and goals;
- motor skills, problem-solving skills, and plans for achieving various things;
- perceptual skills in understanding language, interpreting music and so on.

Many of these are included in what Tulving calls *semantic memory* (see below).[6] Information can be held for between a few minutes and several years (and may in fact span the individual's entire lifetime).

Coding

With verbal material, coding in LTM appears to be mainly semantic. For example, Baddeley presented participants with words that were:

- *acoustically similar* (e.g. 'caught', 'short', 'taut', 'nought'); or
- *semantically similar* (e.g. 'huge', 'great', 'big', 'wide'); or
- *acoustically dissimilar* (e.g. 'foul', 'old', 'deep'); or
- *semantically dissimilar* (e.g. 'pen', 'day', 'ring').[18]

When recall from STM was tested, acoustically similar words were recalled less well than acoustically dissimilar words. This supports the claim that acoustic coding occurs in STM. There was a small difference between the number of semantically similar and semantically dissimilar words recalled (64% and 71%, respectively). This suggests that although some semantic coding occurs in STM, it is not dominant. When an equivalent study was conducted on LTM, fewer semantically similar words were recalled, while acoustically similar words had no effect on LTM recall. This suggests that the dominant code of LTM is semantic. Similarly, Baddeley found that immediate recall of the order of short lists of unrelated words was seriously impeded if the words were acoustically similar, but not if they were semantically similar.[18] After a delay, however, exactly the opposite effect occurred.

Does long-term memory use only semantic coding?

Findings such as Baddeley's do not imply that LTM uses only a semantic code.[21] Our ability to picture a place we visited on holiday indicates that at least some information is stored or coded visually. Also, some types of information in LTM (e.g. songs) are coded acoustically. Smells and tastes are also stored in LTM, suggesting that LTM is a very flexible system, as well as being large and long-lasting.

Table 17.1 shows the main differences between STM and LTM.

RETRIEVAL

There are many different ways of recovering or locating information that has been stored; that is, 'remembering' can

Table 17.1 Summary of main differences between short-term memory (STM) and long-term memory (LTM)

	Capacity	Duration	Coding
STM	Seven bits of (unrelated) information; can be increased through *chunking*	15–30 s (unaided); can be increased by (maintenance) *rehearsal*	Mainly acoustic; some semantic; visual also possible
LTM	Unlimited	From a few seconds to several years (perhaps permanently)	Semantic, visual, acoustic; also olfactory and gustatory; very flexible

take many different forms. Likewise, there are also different ways of measuring memory in the laboratory.

How is memory measured?

The systematic scientific investigation of memory began with Ebbinghaus (Box 17.2).[7]

Other techniques for measuring memory include the following:

- *Recognition:* this involves deciding whether or not a particular piece of information has been encountered before (e.g. in a multiple-choice test, where the correct answer is presented along with incorrect answers). Recognition is a very sensitive form of retrieval.
- *Recall:* this involves participants actively searching their memory stores in order to retrieve particular information (e.g. in timed essays). Retrieval cues are missing or very sparse. The material can be recalled either in the order in which it was presented (*serial recall*) or in any order at all (*free recall*).
- *Memory-span procedure:* this is a version of serial recall, in which a person is given a list of unrelated digits or letters, and then required to repeat them back immediately in the order in which they were heard. The number of items on the list is increased successively until an error is made. The maximum number of items that can be consistently recalled correctly is a measure of *immediate memory span.*
- *Paired-associates recall:* participants are required to learn a list of paired items (e.g. 'chair' and 'elephant'). When one of the words (e.g. 'chair') is re-presented, the participant must recall the paired word ('elephant').

Box 17.2 Pure memory[7]

To study memory in its purest form, Ebbinghaus invented three-letter nonsense syllables – a consonant followed by a vowel followed by another consonant, such as XUT and JEQ.

Ebbinghaus spent several years using only himself as the subject of his research. He read lists of nonsense syllables out loud; when he felt he had recited a list sufficiently to retain it, he tested himself.

If Ebbinghaus could recite a list correctly twice in succession, he considered the list to have been learned. After recording the time taken to learn a list, he then began learning another list.

After specific periods of time, he returned to a particular list and tried to memorize it again. He calculated the number of attempts (or trials) it took him to relearn the list, as a percentage of the number of trials it had originally taken to learn it (a *savings score*).

Ebbinghaus found that memory declines sharply at first, but then levels off. For example, in one set of experiments involving a series of eight different lists of 13 nonsense syllables, he found the following savings scores:

- 58% 20 min after training.
- 44% 60 min after training.
- 34% 24 h after training.
- 21% 31 days after training.

> **'... Thus, most of the memory loss occurred within the first minutes after training; once the memory had survived this hurdle it seemed much more stable...'**[22]

This finding has subsequently been replicated many times.

THE MULTI-STORE MODEL

Atkinson and Shiffrin's MSM (sometimes called the *dual-memory model* because of the emphasis on STM and LTM) was an attempt to explain how information flows from one storage system to another (Figure 17.4).[2,3] The model sees sensory memory, STM and LTM as permanent structural components of the memory system (built-in features of the human information-processing system). In addition to these structural components, the memory system comprises more transient control processes. Rehearsal is a key control process serving two main functions:

- to act as a *buffer* between sensory memory and LTM by maintaining incoming information within STM;
- to transfer information to LTM.

Information from sensory memory is scanned and matched with information in LTM. If a match (i.e. pattern

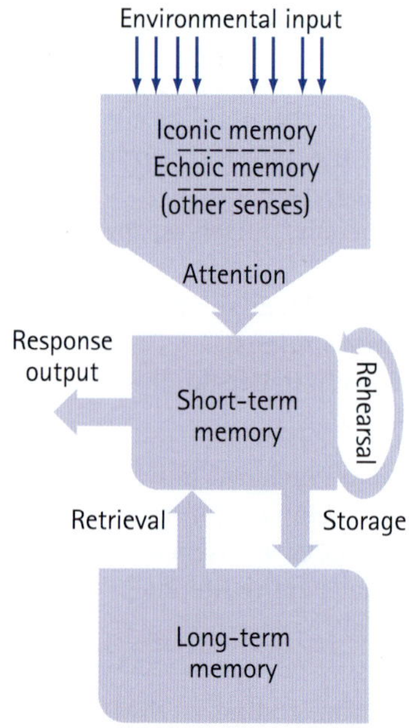

Figure 17.4 Multi-store (dual-memory) model of memory proposed by Atkinson and Shiffrin

recognition) occurs, then it might be fed into STM along with a verbal label from LTM.

Evidence for the multi-store model

Three kinds of evidence are relevant here:

- Experimental studies of STM and LTM (sometimes referred to as *two-component tasks*)
- Studies of *coding*
- Studies of patients with brain damage.

Experimental studies of short- and long-term memory

The serial position effect

Murdock presented participants with a list of words at a rate of about one word per second.[23] Participants were asked to free-recall as many of these words as they could. Murdock found that the probability of recalling any word depended on its position in the list (its *serial position*; the graph shown in Figure 17.5 is a *serial position curve*). Participants typically recalled those items from the end of the list first and got more of these correct than earlier items (the *recency effect*). Items from the beginning of the list were recalled quite well relative to those in the middle (the *primacy effect*), but not as well as those at the end. Poorest recall is for items in the middle. The serial position effect holds, regardless of the length of the list.[23]

The primacy effect occurs because the items at the beginning of the list have (presumably) been rehearsed and transferred to LTM, from where they are recalled. The recency effect occurs presumably because items currently in STM are recalled from there. Because the capacity of STM is limited and can hold items for only a brief period of time, words in the middle are either lost from the system completely or otherwise unavailable for recall. The last items are remembered only if recalled first and tested immediately, as demonstrated by Glanzer and Cunitz in a variation of Murdock's study (Box 17.3).[24]

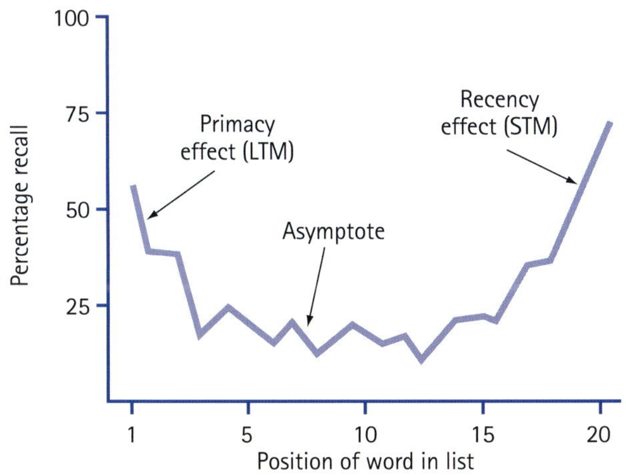

Figure 17.5 Typical serial position curve

Box 17.3 Removing the recency effect[24]

Glanzer and Cunitz presented two groups of participants with the same list of words.

One group recalled the material immediately after presentation, while the other group recalled the material after 30 s. The participants had to count backwards in threes (the Brown–Peterson technique), which prevented rehearsal and caused the recency effect to disappear (Figure 17.6).

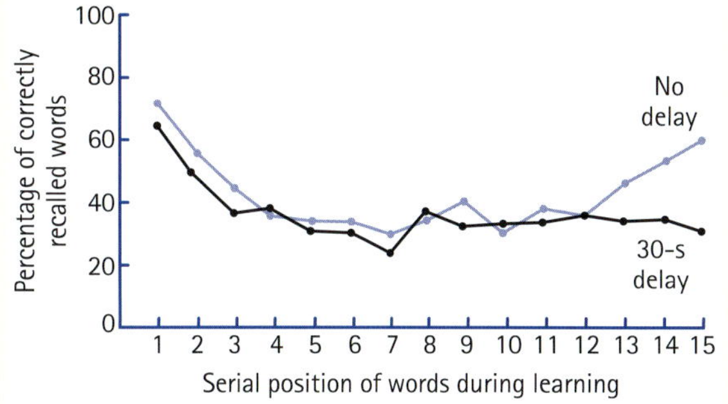

Figure 17.6 Data from Glanzer and Cunitz's study[24] showing serial position curves after no delay and after a delay of 30 s

The primacy effect was largely unaffected.

In Glanzer and Cunitz's study, it is likely that the earlier words had been transferred to LTM (from where they were recalled), while the most recent words were vulnerable to the counting task.[25]

Brown–Peterson technique and rehearsal

When discussing the characteristics of STM earlier, we noted the rapid loss of information from memory when rehearsal is prevented using the Brown–Peterson technique. This is usually taken as evidence for the existence of a STM with rapid forgetting (see below). But the concept of rehearsal itself has been criticized as both unnecessary and too general (Box 17.4).

An earlier study by Glanzer and Meinzer found that participants who were asked to repeat items aloud recalled fewer items than participants given an equal period of silent rehearsal.[27] Perhaps in silent rehearsal the material is not merely being repeated but is recoded into a different form that enhances recall.

Rehearsal and the levels-of-processing approach

It seems, then, that what is important is the kind of rehearsal or processing, rather than how much. This has been investigated in particular by Craik and Lockhart,[4] in the form of the *levels-of-processing approach* (LOP) (see Gross[28]). Maintenance rehearsal may not even be necessary for storage. Jenkins found that participants could remember material even though they were not expecting to be tested and so were unlikely to have rehearsed the material.[29] This is called *incidental learning*.

Box 17.4 Maintenance *v.* elaborative rehearsal[26]

Craik and Watkins asked participants to remember only certain 'critical' words (those beginning with a particular letter) from lists presented either rapidly or slowly.

The position of the critical words relative to the others determined the amount of time a particular word spent in short-term memory (STM) and the number of potential rehearsals it could receive.

Craik and Watkins found that long-term remembering was unrelated to either how long a word had spent in STM or the number of explicit or implicit rehearsals it received.

Based on this and later findings, Craik and Watkins distinguished between:

- *maintenance rehearsal*, in which material is rehearsed in the form in which it was presented ('rote');
- *elaborative rehearsal* (or elaboration of encoding), which elaborates the material in some way (e.g. by giving it a meaning or linking it with pre-existing knowledge stored in long-term memory).

Craik and Lockhart also considered that the MSM view of the relationship between structural components and control processes was, essentially, the wrong way round. According to the MSM, the structural components (sensory memory, STM, LTM) are fixed, while control processes (e.g. rehearsal) are less permanent. The LOP model begins with the proposed control processes. The structural components (the memory system) are what results from the operation of these processes. In other words, memory is a by-product of perceptual analysis. This is controlled by the central processor, which can analyse a stimulus (e.g. a word) on various levels:

- At a superficial (*shallow*) level, the surface features of a stimulus (e.g. whether the word is in lower- or upper-case letters) are processed.
- At an intermediate (*phonemic* or *phonetic*) level, the word is analysed for its sound.
- At a deep (or *semantic*) level, the word's meaning is analysed.

The level at which a stimulus is processed depends on both its nature and the processing time available. The more deeply information is processed, the more likely it is to be retained.

Studies of coding

Table 17.1 indicates that the major form of coding used in STM is acoustic, while LTM is much more flexible and varied in how it encodes information. It also suggests that semantic coding is used primarily by LTM. This is usually taken to support the MSM. However, not everyone accepts this view.

Chunking and short- and long-term memory

When discussing the characteristics of STM, we saw that chunking increases the capacity of STM by imposing meaning on otherwise meaningless material. According to Miller, chunking represents a *linguistic recoding* that seems to be the 'very lifeblood of the thought process'.[14] But this cannot occur until certain information in LTM is activated and a match is made between the incoming items and their representation in LTM.

Miller and Selfridge gave participants 'sentences' of varying lengths, which resembled true English to different degrees, and asked the participants to recall the words in the correct order.[30] The closer a 'sentence' approximated normal English, the better it was recalled. This suggests that knowledge of semantic and grammatical structure (presumably stored in LTM) is used to aid recall from STM.

In a similar study, Bower and Springston presented one group of American college students with letters that formed familiar acronyms (e.g. fbi, phd, twa, ibm).[31] A second group was presented with the same letters, but in a way that did not form those acronyms (e.g. fb, iph, dtw, aib, m). The first group recalled many more letters than the second group. The pause after 'fbi' and so on allowed the students to 'look up' the material in their mental dictionaries and so encode the letters in one chunk.

The study of patients with brain damage

Anterograde amnesia and the amnesic syndrome

If STM and LTM really are distinct, then there should be certain kinds of brain damage that impair one without affecting the other. One such form of brain damage is *anterograde amnesia* (Box 17.5).

An equally dramatic but in many ways more tragic case is that of Clive Wearing (Box 17.6).

Atkinson and Shiffrin regard the kind of memory deficits displayed by HM and Clive Wearing as 'perhaps the single most convincing demonstration of a dichotomy in the memory system'. According to Parkin, the *amnesic syndrome* is not a general deterioration of memory function but is a selective impairment in which some functions, such as learning novel information, are severely impaired, while others, including memory span and language, remain intact.[34]

If amnesic patients do have an intact STM, then they should show a similar recency effect (based on STM) but a poorer primacy effect (based on LTM) compared with normal controls. This is exactly what is found (e.g. Baddeley and Warrington[35]). These results have led most psychologists to accept that, in the amnesic syndrome, STM function is preserved but LTM function is impaired.

However, this difference in STM and LTM functioning could mean that:

- the problem for amnesic patients is one of transfer from STM to LTM, which is perfectly consistent with the MSM; or

Box 17.5 HM[32]

HM is probably the most studied amnesic patient in the history of neuropsychology.[22] HM had had epileptic fits of devastating frequency since the age of 16 years. In 1953, aged 27 years, he underwent surgery aimed at alleviating his epilepsy. The anterior two-thirds of his hippocampus and amygdala, plus part of the temporal lobe (on both sides of the brain), were removed.

Although the surgery was fairly successful in curing his epilepsy, at the time the role of these brain structures in memory was unknown and he was left with severe anterograde amnesia; that is, he has near-normal memory for anything learned before the surgery, but he has severe memory deficits for events that occurred afterwards.

His short-term memory is generally normal. He can retain verbal information for about 15 s without rehearsal, and for much longer with rehearsal. But he cannot transfer information into long-term memory or, if he can, he is unable to retrieve it. He seems entirely incapable of remembering any new fact or event.

He has almost no knowledge of current affairs because he forgets all the news almost as soon as he has read about it. He has no idea what time of day it is unless he has just looked at the clock, he cannot remember that his father has died or that his family has moved house, and he rereads the same magazine without realizing he has already read it.

People he has met after the operation remain, in effect, total strangers to him, and he has to 'get to know them' afresh each time they come into his house. Brenda Milner has known him for 25 years, and yet she is a stranger to him each time they meet.

He is able to learn and remember perceptual and motor skills, although he has to be reminded each day just what skills he has. However:

> **... new events, faces, phone numbers, places, now settle in his mind for just a few seconds or minutes before they slip, like water through a sieve, and are lost from his consciousness.[1]**

Box 17.6 Clive Wearing

Clive Wearing was the chorus master of the London Sinfonietta, a world expert on Renaissance music and a BBC radio producer.

In March 1985 he suffered a rare brain infection caused by the cold sore virus (Herpes simplex). The virus attacked and destroyed his hippocampus, along with parts of his cortex.

Like HM, Clive lives in a snapshot of time, constantly believing that he has just awoken from years of unconsciousness. For example, when his wife, Deborah, enters his hospital room for the third time in a single morning, he embraces her as if they have been parted for years, saying, 'I'm conscious for the first time' and 'It's the first time I've seen anybody at all'.

At first his confusion was total and very frightening to him. Once he held a chocolate in the palm of one hand, and covered it with the other hand for a few seconds until its image disappeared from his memory. When he uncovered the chocolate, he thought he had performed a magic trick, conjuring it up from nowhere. He repeated it again and again, with total astonishment and growing fear each time.

Like HM, Clive can still speak and walk. He can also still read music, play the organ and conduct. In fact, his musical ability is remarkably well preserved.

Also like HM, Clive can learn new skills (e.g. mirror-reading). Over the course of a few days of testing, the speed of reading such words doubles, and it can be done just as well 3 months later. Yet for Clive, it is new every time.

Unlike HM, however, Clive's capacity for remembering his earlier life is extremely patchy. For example, when shown pictures of Cambridge (where he spent 4 years as an undergraduate and had often visited subsequently) he recognized only King's College Chapel – the most distinctive Cambridge building – but not his own college. He could not remember who wrote *Romeo and Juliet*, and he thought the Queen and the Duke of Edinburgh were singers he had once known from a Catholic church.

According to Deborah, 'Without consciousness he's in many senses dead'. In his own words, his life is 'Hell on earth – it's like being dead – all the bloody time'.

Based on Blakemore[1] and Baddeley.[33]

- amnesic patients have difficulties in retrieval from LTM.[36,37]

The latter interpretation is more consistent with Craik and Lockhart's LOP approach.[4]

Another major implication of cases such as those of HM and Clive Wearing is that the 'unitary' LTM of the MSM is a gross oversimplification (see below).

Retrograde amnesia

In retrograde amnesia, the patient fails to remember what happened before the surgery or accident that caused it. Retrograde amnesia can be caused by head injuries, electroconvulsive therapy (ECT; see Chapter 59), carbon monoxide poisoning and extreme stress. As in anterograde amnesia, there is typically little or no disruption of STM, and the period of time for which the person has no memories may be minutes, days or even years. When retrograde amnesia is caused by brain damage, it is usually accompanied by anterograde amnesia. Similarly, patients with Korsakoff's syndrome (caused by severe, chronic alcoholism involving damage to the hippocampus) usually experience both kinds of amnesia.

Retrograde amnesia seems to involve a disruption of consolidation, whereby, once new information has entered

LTM, time is needed for it to become firmly established physically in the brain.

ALTERNATIVES TO THE MULTI-STORE MODEL

Multiple forms of long-term memory

Episodic and semantic memory

Despite their brain damage, HM and Clive Wearing retained many skills, both general and specific (e.g. talking, reading, walking, playing the organ). They were also capable of acquiring and retaining new skills, although they did not know that they had them. This suggests very strongly that there are different kinds of LTM. But as far as the MSM is concerned, there is only 'LTM' (i.e. LTM is unitary).

Box 17.7 differentiates episodic memory (EM) and semantic memory (SM). Our general knowledge about, say, computers (part of our SM) is built up from past experiences with particular computers (part of EM), through abstraction and generalization. This suggests that, instead of regarding EM and SM as two quite distinct systems within the brain (which is what Tulving originally intended[6]), it might be more valid to see SM as made up from multiple EMs.[12]

Autobiographical *v.* experimental episodic memory

Tulving maintained that EM is synonymous with *autobiographical memory* (AM). For example, the forgetting of words in a free-recall task can be thought of as a failure in our EM. Clearly, we already know the words as part of our SM, but we fail to remember that they appeared in that particular list just presented to us. However, Cohen argues that learning word lists is not what most people understand by AM.[38] Instead, AM is a special kind of EM, concerned with specific life events that have personal significance. Accordingly, she distinguishes between autobiographical EM and experimental EM; taking part in an experiment in which we are required to learn lists of words is an example of the latter.

Box 17.7 Episodic and semantic memory[6]

Episodic memory (EM) is an autobiographical memory responsible for storing a record of our past experiences – the events, people, objects and so on that we have personally encountered. EM usually includes details about the particular time and place in which objects and events were experienced (they have a spatiotemporal context, e.g. 'Where did you go on your holiday last year?' and 'What did you have for breakfast this morning?'). They have a subjective (self-focused) reality, but most could, in principle, be verified by others.

Semantic memory (SM) is our store of general, factual knowledge about the world, including concepts, rules and language. It is '... a mental thesaurus, organised knowledge a person possesses about words and other verbal symbols, their meanings and referents ...'[6] SM can be used without reference to where and when that knowledge was originally acquired. For example, we do not remember 'learning to speak' – we just 'know English' (or whatever our native language happens to be). But SM can also store information about ourselves. For example, if we are asked how many siblings we have, we do not have to remember specific past experiences in order to answer the question.

Flashbulb memories

Flashbulb memories are a special kind of EM, in which we can give vivid and detailed recollections of where we were and what we were doing when we first heard about some major public national or international event.[39]

According to Brown and Kulik, a neural mechanism is triggered by events that are emotionally arousing, unexpected or extremely important, with the result that the whole scene becomes 'printed' on the memory.[40] However, Neisser argued that the durability of flashbulb memories stems from their frequent rehearsal and reconsideration after the event.[41] Also, the detail and vividness of people's memories are not necessarily signs of their accuracy – we can be very confident about something and still be mistaken.

Procedural *v.* declarative memory

Procedural memory (PM) refers to information from LTM that cannot be inspected consciously.[42,43] For example, riding a bike is a complex skill that is even more difficult to describe. In the same way, native speakers of a language cannot usually describe the complex grammatical rules by which they speak correctly (perhaps because the skills were not learned consciously in the first place). By contrast, EM and SM are both amenable to being inspected consciously, and the content of both can be described to another person.

Cohen and Squire distinguish between PM and declarative memory,[44] which correspond to Ryle's distinction between *knowing how* and *knowing that*, respectively (Table 17.2).[45] Anderson argues that, when we initially learn something, it is learned and encoded declaratively, but with

Table 17.2 Distinctions between different kinds of long-term memory

Tulving[43]	Example	Cohen and Squire[44]
Episodic	'I rode my first two-wheeler when I was 7'	Declarative ('knowing that')
Semantic	'I know that bicycles have two wheels'	
Procedural	'I know how to ride a bike'	Procedural ('knowing how')

practice it becomes compiled into a procedural form of knowledge.[46]

Regarding the LTM of HM and Clive Wearing, most aspects of their PM seemed to be intact, but both their EM and SM were partially impaired. For instance, HM was given extensive training by Gabrieli *et al.* in the task of learning the meaning of unfamiliar words that had come into popular use since his operation.[47] He made very little progress, despite extensive practice every day for 10 days.

Most other amnesic patients similarly fail to update their SM in order to take account of changes in the world since onset of their dysfunction.[48] For example, many such patients do not know the name of the current leader of their country, and they have very poor recognition for faces of people who have become famous only quite recently.[49]

The major problem seems to involve recent declarative memory. We saw earlier that Clive Wearing denied all knowledge of having learned to mirror-read. Similarly, HM was trained to solve the Tower of Hanoi problem-solving task (see Gross[28]) over several days, but each time he was presented with the task he denied ever having seen it before. Yet their performance on these two tasks steadily improved. As Rose puts it, '... procedural memory continued to testify to the truth of what declarative memory denied'.[22]

Procedural memory involves more automatic processes and allows patients to demonstrate learning without the need for conscious recollection of the learning process. But declarative learning/memory involves conscious recollection of the past. Damage to a number of cortical and subcortical areas (including the temporal lobes, hippocampus and mamillary bodies) seriously impairs declarative memory in patients with amnesia. PM does not appear to be impaired by damage to these areas.[12]

The working-memory model: rethinking short-term memory

In their MSM, Atkinson and Shiffrin saw STM as a system for temporarily holding and manipulating information. However, Baddeley and Hitch criticized the model's concept of a unitary STM.[5] Although accepting that STM rehearses incoming information for transfer to LTM, they argued that it was much more complex and versatile than a mere 'stopping-off station' for information.

Short-term memory is an active store used to hold information that is being manipulated. According to Groome *et al.*, working memory (WM) is like the computer screen, a kind of mental workspace where various operations are performed on current data.[50] By contrast, LTM resembles the computer's memory ('storage memory'), which holds large amounts of information in a fairly passive state for possible future retrieval. Working memory is a cognitive function that:

- helps us to keep track of what we are doing or where we are from moment to moment;
- holds information long enough to allow us to make a decision, dial a telephone number or repeat a strange foreign word that we have just heard.

Instead of a single, simple STM, Baddeley and Hitch proposed a more complex, multicomponent WM.[5] This comprises a *central executive*, which is in overall charge, plus sub- or *slave systems*, whose activities are controlled by the central executive. These are the *articulatory* (or *phonological*) loop (the *inner voice*) and the *visuospatial scratchpad* (or *sketchpad*; the *inner eye*) (for a more detailed discussion, see Gross[28]).

An evaluation of the working-memory model

- It is generally accepted that (i) STM is better seen as a number of relatively independent processing mechanisms than as the single unitary store of the MSM; and (ii) attentional processes and STM are part of the same system (they are probably used together much of the time in everyday life).
- The idea that any one slave system (such as the phonological loop) may be involved in the performance of apparently very different tasks (e.g. memory span, mental arithmetic, verbal reasoning, reading) is a valuable insight.
- It has practical applications that extend beyond its theoretical importance,[51,52] such as explaining children's problems in learning to read.
- One weakness of the WM model is that least is known about the most important component, namely the central executive.[53] This can, apparently, carry out an enormous variety of processing activities in different conditions. This makes it difficult to describe its precise function, and the idea of a single central executive might be as inappropriate as that of a unitary STM.[54]

MEMORY AND THE REPRESENTATION OF KNOWLEDGE

What psychologists have traditionally called knowledge is information that is represented mentally in a particular format and is structured or organized in some way.[48] This leads to two interrelated questions about the nature of knowledge:

- What format do mental representations take?
- How are these mental representations organized?

This subject area was neglected until quite recently, when attempts to provide a knowledge base for computer systems stimulated an interest in how '... this enormously important but complex facility operates in people'.[33]

The organized nature of memory

As we have seen, chunking is a way of increasing the limited capacity of STM by imposing a meaning on unrelated items of information. We do this by organizing it, giving it a structure that it does not otherwise have. As Baddeley says:

> The secret of a good memory, as of a good library, is that of organisation; good learning typically goes with the systematic encoding of incoming material, integrating and relating it to what is already known.[12]

Organization can be imposed either by the experimenter (experimenter organization, EO) or spontaneously by the participant (subjective organization, SO).[55] Mandler found that instructions to organize will facilitate learning, even though the participant is not trying to remember the material.[56]

Schemas and reconstructive memory

As we saw above, Ebbinghaus was the first to study memory systematically, using nonsense syllables. Although this tradition is still popular with today's memory researchers, Bartlett argued that:[57]

- Ebbinghaus's use of nonsense syllables excluded 'all that is most central to human memory';
- the study of 'repetition habits' had very little to do with memory in everyday life;
- research should examine people's active search for meaning, rather than their passive responses to meaningless stimuli presented by an experimenter.

Although meaningful material is more complex than meaningless material, Bartlett argued that it too could be studied experimentally. Bartlett's concept of a schema is central to theories that attempt to explain the structure and organization of knowledge in SM (a major part of LTM). Because of the large amount of work on the organizational aspects of memory, and because of the growing recognition of the need to study meaningful material (as opposed to lists of unrelated words, numbers and so on), there has been a rediscovery of Bartlett's research into reconstructive memory.

Bartlett concluded from his research findings that interpretation plays a major role in the remembering of stories and past events. Learning and remembering are both active processes involving 'effort after meaning' – that is, trying to make the past more logical, coherent and generally 'sensible'. This involves making inferences or deductions about what could or should have happened. We reconstruct the past by trying to fit it into our existing understanding of the world. Unlike a computer's memory, where the output matches the input exactly, human memory is an 'imaginative reconstruction' of experience.

Bartlett called this existing understanding of the world a schema. Schemas (or schemata):

- provide us with ready-made expectations that help us to interpret the flow of information reaching the senses;
- help us to make the world more predictable;
- allow us to 'fill in the gaps' when our memories are incomplete;
- can produce significant distortions in memory processes, because they have a powerful effect on the way in which memories for events are encoded. This happens when new information conflicts with existing schemas (or schemata).

THEORIES OF FORGETTING

In order to understand why we forget, we must recall the distinction between availability (whether or not material has been stored) and accessibility (being able to retrieve what has been stored). In terms of the MSM, since information must be transferred from STM to LTM for permanent storage:

- availability concerns mainly STM and the transfer of information from STM into LTM;
- accessibility is concerned mainly with LTM.

Forgetting can occur at the encoding, storage or retrieval stages (Figure 17.7).

One way of looking at forgetting is to ask what prevents information staying in STM long enough to be transferred to LTM (some answers are provided by the *decay* and *dis-*

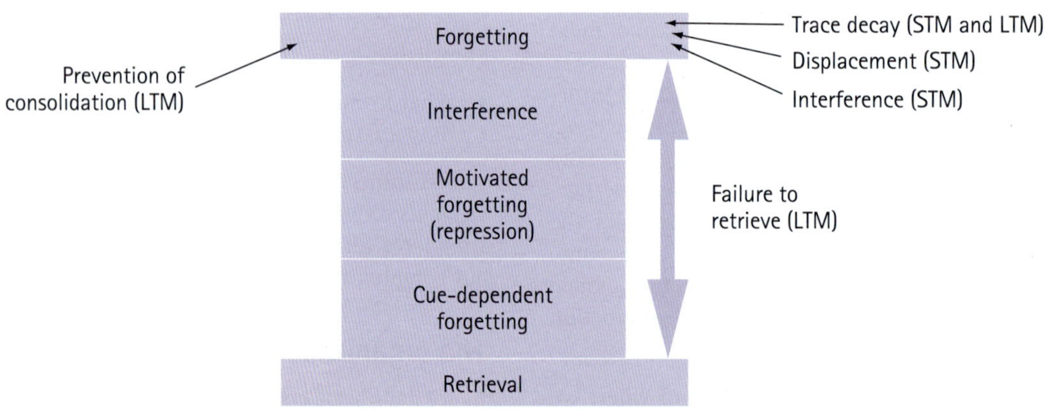

Figure 17.7 Different theories of forgetting, including retrieval failure. LTM, long-term memory; STM, short-term memory.

placement theories). Some answers to the question about what prevents us from locating the information that is already in LTM include those offered by *interference theory*, *cue-dependent forgetting* and *motivated forgetting* (or *repression*).

Decay theory

Decay (or trace decay) theory tries to explain why forgetting increases with time. Clearly, memories must be stored somewhere, the most obvious place being the brain. Presumably, some sort of structural change (the *engram*) occurs when learning takes place. According to decay theory, metabolic processes occur over time that cause the engram to degrade (break down), unless it is maintained by repetition and rehearsal. This results in the memory contained within it becoming unavailable.

Hebb argued that while learning is taking place, the engram that will eventually be formed is very delicate and liable to disruption (the *active trace*).[8] With learning, the engram grows stronger, until a permanent engram is formed (the *structural trace*) through neurochemical and neuroanatomical changes.

Decay in short- and long-term memory

The active trace corresponds roughly to STM, and, according to decay theory, forgetting from STM is due to disruption of the active trace. Although Hebb did not apply the idea of decay to LTM, other researchers have argued that it can explain LTM forgetting if it is assumed that decay occurs through disuse (hence, *decay-through-disuse theory*). So, if certain knowledge or skills are not used or practised for long periods of time, the corresponding engram will eventually decay away.[58]

Is forgetting just a matter of time?

Peterson and Peterson's experiment (see Box 17.1) has been taken as evidence for the role of decay in STM forgetting.[16] If decay did occur, then we would expect poorer recall of information with the passage of time, which is exactly what the Petersons reported.

The difficulty with the Petersons' study in particular, and decay theory in general, is that other possible effects need to be excluded before a decay-based account can be accepted. The ideal way to study the role of decay in forgetting would be to have people receive information and then do nothing, physical or mental, for a period of time. If recall was poorer with the passage of time, then it would be reasonable to suggest that decay had occurred. Such an experiment is, of course, impossible. However, Jenkins and Dallenbach were the first to attempt an approximation to it (Box 17.8).[59]

Although some data exist suggesting that neurological breakdown occurs with age and disease (e.g. in Alzheimer's disease), there is no evidence that the major cause of forgetting from LTM is neurological decay.[60]

Box 17.8 If you want to remember, sleep on it[59]

Participants learned a list of ten nonsense syllables. Some participants then went to sleep immediately (approximating the ideal 'do nothing' state), while the others continued with their normal activities.

After intervals of 1, 2, 4 or 8 h, all participants were tested for their recall of the syllables.

Although there was a fairly steady increase in forgetting as the retention interval increased for the 'waking' participants, this was not true for the sleeping participants (Figure 17.8).

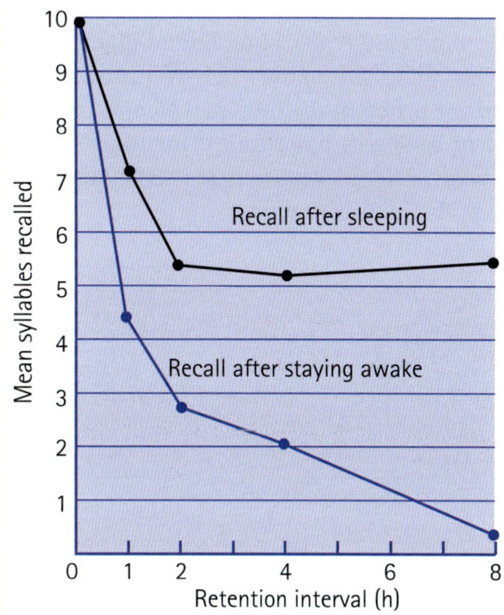

Figure 17.8 Mean number of syllables recalled by participants in Jenkins and Dallenbach's experiment[59]

If decay is a natural result of the passage of time alone, then we should have expected equal forgetting in both groups. The results suggest that it is what happens in between learning and recall that determines forgetting, not time as such. This led Jenkins and Dallenbach to conclude:

> **Forgetting is not so much a matter of decay of old impressions and associations as it is a matter of interference, inhibition or obliteration of the old by the new.**

Interference theory is discussed in the text.

Displacement theory

In a limited-capacity STM system, forgetting might occur through displacement. When the system is 'full', the oldest material in it would be displaced ('pushed out') by incoming new material. This possibility was explored by Waugh and Norman using the serial probe task.[10] Participants were presented with 16 digits at the rate of either one or four per second. One of the digits (the 'probe') was then repeated, and participants had to say which digit followed the probe. Presumably:

- if the probe was one of the digits at the beginning of the list, then the probability of recalling the digit that followed would be small, because later digits would have displaced earlier digits from the system;
- if the probe was presented towards the end of the list, then the probability of recalling the digit that followed would be high, since the last digits to be presented would still be available in STM.

When the number of digits following the probe was small, recall was good; but when the number of digits was large, recall was poor. This is consistent with the idea that the earlier digits are replaced by later digits (Figure 17.9).

Since less time had elapsed between presentation of the digits and the probe in the four-per-second condition, there would have been less opportunity for those digits to have decayed away. This makes it unclear whether displacement is a process distinct from decay.

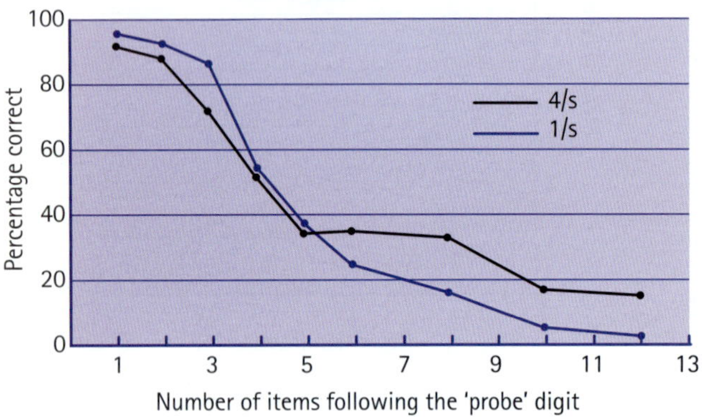

Figure 17.9 Data from Waugh and Norman's serial probe experiment[10]

Retrieval-failure theory and cue-dependent forgetting

According to retrieval-failure theory, memories cannot be recalled because the correct retrieval cues are not being used. The role of retrieval cues is demonstrated by the *tip-of-the-tongue phenomenon* (TOT), in which we know that we know something but cannot retrieve it at that particular moment in time (Box 17.9).[61]

Tulving and Pearlstone read participants lists of varying numbers of words (12, 24 or 48) consisting of categories (e.g. animals) of one, two or four exemplars (e.g. dog) per list, plus the category name.[62] Participants were asked to try to remember only the exemplars. Half the participants (group 2) free-recalled the words and wrote them down on blank pieces of paper. The other half (group 1) were given the category names. Group 1 recalled significantly more words, especially on the 48-item list. However, when the participants in group 2 were given the category names, recall improved (Figure 17.10).

Box 17.9 It's on the tip of my tongue[61]

Brown and McNeill gave participants dictionary definitions of unfamiliar words and asked them to provide the words themselves. Most participants either knew the word or knew that they did not know it.

Some participants, however, were sure that they knew the word but could not recall it (it was 'on the tip of the tongue'). About half could give the word's first letter and the number of syllables and often offered words that sounded like the word or had a similar meaning. This suggests that the required words were in memory, but the absence of a correct retrieval cue prevented them from being recalled.

Examples of definitions used by Brown and McNeill include the following:

1. 'A small boat used in the harbours and rivers of Japan and China, rowed with a scull from the stern, and often having a sail.'
2. 'Favouritism, especially governmental patronage extended to relatives.'
3. 'The common cavity into which the various ducts of the body open in certain fish, reptiles, birds and mammals.'

Answers:

1 Sampan
2 Nepotism
3 Cloaca.

This illustrates very well the availability/accessibility distinction. The category name acted as a contextual cue, helping to make accessible what was available. Group 2 participants knew more than they could actually retrieve under the cue-less conditions.

According to Tulving's *encoding-specificity principle* (ESP), recall improves if the same cues are present during

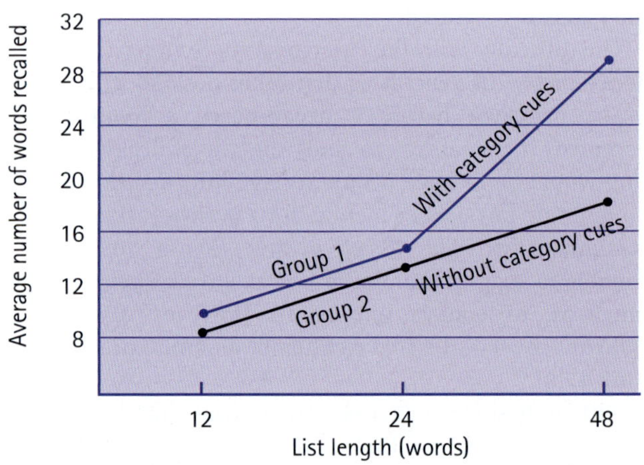

Figure 17.10 Average number of words recalled with and without cues in Tulving and Pearlstone's experiment[62]

recall as during the original learning.[63] In Tulving and Pearlstone's experiment, the category names were presented together with the exemplars for group 1. Presumably, they were encoded at the time of learning. The ESP explains why recall is sometimes superior to recognition (even though recognition is generally considered to be easier than recall).

Tulving used the term 'cue-dependent forgetting' to refer jointly to context-dependent and state-dependent forgetting (Table 17.3).[64]

Interference theory

According to interference theory, forgetting is influenced more by what we do before or after learning than by the mere passage of time (see Box 17.8):

- In *retroactive interference/inhibition* (RI), later learning interferes with the recall of earlier learning.
- In *proactive interference/inhibition* (PI), earlier learning interferes with the recall of later learning.

Interference theory has been studied extensively in the laboratory using paired-associate lists. The usual procedure for studying interference effects is shown in Figure 17.11.

Usually, the first member of each pair in list A is the same as in list B, but the second member of each pair is different in the two lists:

- In RI, the learning of the second list interferes with recall of the first list (the interference works backwards in time).
- In PI, the learning of the first list interferes with recall of the second list (the interference works forwards in time).

Wickens found that participants became increasingly poor at retaining information in STM on successive trials.[69] However, when the category of information was changed, they performed just as well as on the first list. So, performance with lists of numbers became poorer over trials, but if the task was changed to lists of letters, it improved. This is known as *release from proactive inhibition.*

Limitations of laboratory studies of interference theory

The strongest support for interference theory comes from laboratory studies. However:

- Learning in such studies does not occur in the same way as it does in the real world, where learning of potentially interfering material is spaced out over time. In the laboratory, learning is artificially compressed in time, which maximizes the likelihood that interference will occur.[33] Such studies therefore lack ecological validity.
- Laboratory studies tend to use nonsense syllables as the stimulus material. When meaningful material is used, interference is more difficult to demonstrate.[60]

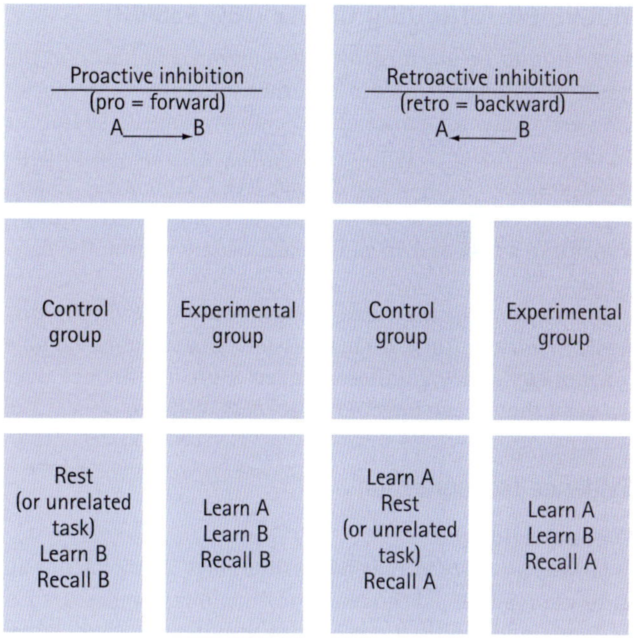

Figure 17.11 Experimental procedure for investigating retroactive and proactive interference

Table 17.3 Cue-dependent forgetting

Context-dependent forgetting	State-dependent forgetting
Occurs in absence of relevant environmental or contextual variables; these represent external cues	Occurs in absence of relevant psychological or physiological variables; these represent internal cues
Abernathy:[65] one group had to learn and then recall material in the same room, while a second group learned and recalled in different rooms; the first group's recall was superior	Clark *et al.*:[66] victims' inabilities to recall details of a violent crime may be due at least partly to the fact that recall occurs in a less emotionally aroused state (see Gross[28])
Godden and Baddeley:[67] divers learned lists of words either on land or 15 feet under water; recall was then tested in the same or a different context; those who learned and recalled in different contexts showed a 30% deficit compared with those who learned and recalled in the same context	McCormick and Mayer:[68] the important link may be between mood and the sort of material being remembered; so, we are more likely to remember happy events when we are feeling happy rather than when we are feeling sad

- When people have to learn, for example, the response 'bell' to the stimulus 'woj', the word 'bell' is not actually learned in the laboratory, since it is already part of SM. What is being learned (a specific response to a specific stimulus in a specific laboratory situation) is stored in EM. SM is much more stable and structured than EM and so is much more resistant to interference effects. No amount of new information will cause someone to forget the things they know that are stored in their SM.[60]

However, in support of interference theory, it is generally agreed that, if students have to study more than one subject in the same timeframe, then the subjects should be as dissimilar as possible.

Motivated-forgetting theory (repression)

According to Freud, forgetting is motivated rather than the result of a failure to learn or other processes.[70] Memories that are likely to induce guilt, embarrassment, shame or anxiety are actively, but unconsciously, pushed out of consciousness as a form of *ego defence* (see Chapters 15, 19 and 61): 'The essence of repression lies simply in turning something away, and keeping it at a distance, from the conscious ...'[71]

Unconscious or repressed memories are exceedingly difficult to retrieve (they are inaccessible) but remain available ('in storage'). They continue to exert a great influence over us, even though we have no awareness of them.

Evidence for repression

Clinical evidence

It is widely accepted that repression plays a crucial role in different types of psychogenic (or functional) amnesia, such as fugue and multiple personality disorder (or dissociative identity disorder) (see Chapter 40 and Gross[72]). These disorders involve a loss of memory associated with a traumatic experience (as opposed to brain injury or surgery). A relatively common form of psychogenic amnesia is *event-specific amnesia*: loss of memory for a fairly specific period of time. For instance, some violent criminals claim they cannot remember carrying out their crimes. Even when we have ruled out both malingering and the effects of intoxication at the time the crime was committed, there is still a substantial number of criminals whose memories of their crimes seem to have been repressed.[73] This is especially likely when the victim is a close relative or lover of the murderer and killed in a 'crime of passion'.[74]

Ian Brady, convicted along with Myra Hindley of the 'Moors Murders', repressed memories of his hideous crimes for many years before finally remembering where he had buried his victims.[75] However, in a study of children who had seen a parent killed, none showed evidence of repression; on the contrary, the experience tended to be recalled all too frequently.[76] This, and the observation that psychogenic amnesia can disappear as suddenly as it appeared, are difficult for motivated-forgetting theory to explain.

Parkin also cites evidence that repressive mechanisms may play a beneficial role in enabling people with post-traumatic stress disorder to adjust.[73] For example, survivors of the Holocaust who were judged to be better adjusted were significantly less able to recall their dreams when woken from rapid eye movement (REM) (dream) sleep (see Chapter 10) than less well-adjusted survivors.[77]

However, 'repression' does not necessarily imply a strictly Freudian interpretation. When the concept is considered more broadly than Freud intended – that is, in the general sense that our memory systems can in some way block particular forms of memory – it deserves to be taken seriously.[75] This is also the view taken by the British Psychological Survey on 'recovered memories'.[78] Similarly, although traumatic experiences can undoubtedly produce memory disturbances, there is greater doubt as to whether Freud's explanation is the best one.[79]

Experimental evidence

Levinger and Clark tested Freud's repression hypothesis (Box 17.10).[80]

However, other studies show that, although highly arousing words tend to be recalled poorly when tested immediately, the effect reverses after a delay.[81] If the words are being repressed, this should not happen (they should stay repressed), suggesting that arousal was the crucial factor.

Parkin *et al.* replicated the original study but added a delayed recall condition: participants were asked to recall their associations 7 days after the original test.[82] The results supported Eysenck and Wilson's interpretation[81] – higher arousal levels inhibit immediate recall but increase longer-term recall. In a later replication, Bradley and Baddeley

Box 17.10 Testing Freud's repression hypothesis[80]

Levinger and Clark looked at the retention of associations to negatively charged words (e.g. 'quarrel', 'angry', 'fear') compared with those for neutral words (e.g. 'window', 'cow', 'tree').

When participants were asked to give immediate free associations to the words (to say exactly what came into their minds), it took them longer to respond to the emotional words. These words also produced higher galvanic skin responses (GSR; a measure of emotional arousal).

Immediately after the word-association tests had been completed, participants were given the cue words again and asked to try to recall their associations. They had particular trouble remembering the associations to the emotionally charged words.

This is exactly what Freud's repression hypothesis predicted, and for some years the study stood as the best experimental demonstration of repression.[73]

used an immediate and a 28-day delayed condition.[83] They found clear support for the arousal hypothesis. But later research has not always supported the arousal interpretation, and the question of emotional inhibition remains open.[73]

Recovered memories and the false-memory debate

Since the early 1990s, considerable publicity has been given to court cases in the USA, where parents are being sued for damages by their teenage or adult children who accuse them of child sexual abuse (CSA). Such abuse has been remembered during the course of psychotherapy. It is assumed that these recovered memories (RMs) had been repressed since the alleged CSA happened and that the safety and support provided by the therapist allows the memories to become conscious many years later.

However, accused parents, and retractors (people who had recovered memories of CSA, accused their parents and then later withdrew the accusations) have also sued therapists and hospitals for implanting false memories (FMs) in their clients' minds. The False Memory Syndrome Foundation was set up in the USA in 1992, and in 1993 the British False Memory Society was founded, with 1000 families currently on its books.[84] Freud is regarded by many to be at least partly responsible for the phenomenon of false-memory syndrome (FMS).

This brief account of the FM debate raises several, interrelated issues, spanning the psychology of memory and forgetting, the nature of psychotherapy (in particular, Freudian psychoanalysis) and the ethics of psychotherapy in general. The FM debate has caused division among psychologists, as well as between psychologists and psychiatrists. Two key questions are: (i) do RMs exist and (ii) do FMs exist?

Do recovered memories exist?

The answer to this question depends very largely on how the concept of repression is understood. If these memories have been repressed, and are now retrieved from the unconscious during the course of therapy, then there must first be sound evidence for the existence of repression. This is the process that is supposed to keep recollections of the CSA hidden from the abused person in the first place, until many years later, as an adult in therapy, the unconscious is 'unlocked'.

When discussing repression above, we saw that the strongest evidence is clinical but that this is far from conclusive. We also need to take a closer look at Freud's view of memory (Box 17.11).

If Freud is right, then RMs can no longer be memories of actual CSA but fantasies of abuse. This reflects Freud's rejection of the *seduction theory* in favour of the Oedipal theory (see Gross[28]). According to Esterson (2000, personal communication), Freud's theory of repression and his therapeutic methods are the basic tools of RM therapists, which makes Freud the arch-enemy of accused parents and the BFMS. But if it is pointed out that RM therapists have misunderstood Freud's theory of repression and the nature of childhood memories, then this also seems to play into the hands of Freud's accusers. In other words, if memories are essentially constructed rather than 'discovered' or 'recovered' (or 'unearthed', to use an archaeological analogy that Freud himself used), it becomes easier to understand how FMS occurs: vulnerable patients can easily be 'persuaded' that a constructed memory (a fantasy that CSA took place) is, in fact, an objectively true, historically verifiable event (the CSA actually happened).

In defence of Freud, Ofshe (cited in Jaroff[87]) contends that RM therapists have invented a mental mechanism ('robust' repression) that supposedly causes a child's awareness of sexual abuse to be driven entirely from consciousness. According to Loftus:

If repression is the avoidance in your conscious awareness of unpleasant experiences that come back to you, yes, I believe in

Box 17.11 Freud and screen memories

According to Mollon, it is sometimes asserted that Freud believed that the events of a person's life are all recorded accurately somewhere in the mind, like video-recordings.[85] They are supposedly preserved in their original form, available but made inaccessible by repression.

However, in a paper on 'screen memories', Freud argued that memories, especially of events of long ago, may be constructed like dreams.[86] A screen memory is a memory that is apparently emotionally insignificant but is actually a substitute for a more troubling memory with which it has become associated. But he argued that the distinction between screen memories and other memories from childhood is unclear:

> **It may indeed be questioned whether we have any memories at all from our childhood: memories relating to our childhood may be all that we possess. Our childhood memories show us our earliest years not as they were but as they appeared at the later periods when the memories were aroused. In these periods of arousal, the childhood memories did not, as people are accustomed to say, emerge; they were found at that time. And a number of motives, with no concern for historical accuracy, had a part in forming them, as well as in the selection of the memories themselves.[86]**

Thus, Freud argued that memories of childhood may not be what they seem. The subjective sense of remembering does not mean that the memory is literally true. Memories are like dreams or works of fiction, constructed out of psychodynamic conflict, serving wish-fulfilment and self-deception. True memories of childhood may simply be unobtainable. Our apparent memories may be fabrications created later.[85]

repression. But if it is a blocking out of an endless stream of traumas that occur over and over that leave a person with absolutely no awareness that these things happen ... and re-emerge decades later in some reliable form, I don't see any evidence for it. It flies in the face of everything we know about memory.[89]

Many practising psychotherapists would agree with Loftus.

A report published in the *British Journal of Psychiatry* distinguishes between (i) CSA that is reported in childhood or kept secret although unforgotten and (ii) RMs of CSA, previously completely forgotten, that emerge in adulthood during therapy, usually in women in their thirties or forties.[88] For some patients, RMs can escalate into FMS, in which a person's identity comes to centre around the:

... memory of a traumatic experience which is objectively false but in which the person strongly believes... The individual avoids confrontation with any evidence that might challenge the memory ...[88]

Brandon *et al.* summarize the findings of studies that have compared these two kinds of CSA:

- About 90 per cent of patients with RM are women, while in documented abuse cases the sex ratio is close to 50:50.
- Although only 3 per cent of accusations of RM are made against stepfathers, stepfathers are much more likely to be involved in documented childhood cases.
- Although documented abuse usually involves older children and adolescents, people with RM recall abuse before the age of 4 years or even in infancy.

Do false memories exist?

According to the 1995 British Psychological Society (BPS) report on RMs, CSA that is alleged to have occurred before 4 years of age and that does not continue beyond that age might not be retrievable in adulthood in a narrative form (describable in words).[78] Very early memories are implicit rather than explicit, and are reflected in behaviour, outside conscious awareness. This means that we do not need the concept of repression in order to explain the 'forgetting' of childhood experiences, but it also implies that some RMs could be false (or at the very least inaccurate).

In a survey of 810 chartered psychologists, about 90 per cent believed that RMs are sometimes or usually 'essentially correct', a negligible number believed they are always correct, about 66 per cent believed they are possible, and over 14 per cent believed that one of their own clients had experienced FMs.[78]

CONCLUSIONS

The fact that FMs can be created does not mean that all RMs are false.[89] The BPS has published a draft set of new guidelines for psychologists working with clients in contexts in which issues related to RMs may arise. The preamble states that:

... there can be no doubt for psychologists of the existence of ... [CSA] as a serious social and individual problem with long-lasting effects. In addition, there can be little doubt that at least some recovered memories of CSA are recollections of historical events. However, there is a genuine cause for concern that some interventions may foster in clients false beliefs concerning CSA or can lead them to develop illusory memories.[90]

KEY POINTS

- Memory can be defined as the retention of learning or experience. Learning and memory are interdependent processes.
- Ebbinghaus began the systematic study of memory, using nonsense syllables. He showed that memory declined very rapidly at first and then levelled off.
- Memory is now studied largely from an information-processing approach, which focuses on registration/encoding, storage and retrieval. Storage corresponds to availability, retrieval to accessibility.
- Techniques for measuring memory include testing recognition, recall (serial or free), paired-associates recall and the memory-span procedure.
- James's distinction between primary and secondary memory corresponds to that between STM and LTM. Sensory memory is modality-specific.
- The limited capacity of STM can be increased by chunking, which draws on LTM to encode new information in a meaningful way. Rehearsal is a way of holding information in STM almost indefinitely, and the primary code used by STM is acoustic. But semantic and visual coding are also used.
- LTM probably has an unlimited capacity, and information is stored in a relatively permanent way. Coding is mainly semantic, but information may also be coded visually, acoustically and in other ways.
- Atkinson and Shiffrin's MSM sees sensory memory, STM and LTM as permanent structural components of the memory system. Rehearsal is a control process that acts as a buffer between sensory memory and LTM, and helps the transfer of information to LTM.
- Craik and Watkins' distinction between maintenance and elaborative rehearsal implies that it is not the amount but the kind of rehearsal or processing that matters.
- According to Craik and Lockhart's LOP model, memory is a by-product of perceptual analysis, such that STM and LTM are the consequences of the operation of control processes. The more deeply information is processed, the more likely it is to be retained
- The primacy effect reflects recall from LTM, while the recency effect reflects recall from STM. Together they comprise the serial position effect.
- Studies of brain-damaged patients with amnesia appear to support the STM–LTM distinction. While STM continues to function fairly normally, certain aspects of LTM functioning are impaired.
- LTM is not unitary but comprises semantic, episodic and procedural memory. Autobiographical memory and flashbulb memories are two

kinds of episodic memory. An overlapping distinction is that between procedural and declarative memory/learning.

- Baddeley and Hitch's working-memory (WM) model rejected the MSM view of STM as unitary. Instead, STM is seen as comprising a central executive, which controls the activities of the phonological loop (inner voice) and visuospatial scratchpad (inner eye).
- Chunking is a means of organizing information, making it easier both to store and to retrieve.
- Bartlett introduced the concept of schema to help explain how we remember meaningful material, such as stories. Reconstructive memory uses schemas (schemata) to interpret new information, making the world more predictable.
- Decay/trace decay theory attempts to explain why forgetting increases over time. STM forgetting is due to disruption of the active trace, and decay-through-disuse explains LTM forgetting.
- Displacement theory is supported by data from Waugh and Norman's serial probe task. However, displacement may not be distinct from decay.
- According to retrieval-failure theory, memories cannot be recalled because the correct retrieval cues are missing. This is demonstrated by the tip-of-the-tongue phenomenon and the provision of category names. Unlike decay theory, retrieval-failure theory can explain our ability to recall different items on different occasions.
- Cue-dependent forgetting comprises context-dependent and state-dependent forgetting, which refer to external and internal cues, respectively.
- According to interference theory, forgetting is influenced more by what we do before/after learning than by the mere passage of time. Retroactive interference/inhibition works backwards in time, while proactive interference/inhibition works forwards in time.
- According to Freud's motivated-forgetting theory, unacceptable memories are made inaccessible through repression.
- Although cases of psychogenic amnesia are consistent with Freud's theory, a strictly Freudian interpretation may not be necessary and experimental support for the repression hypothesis is inconclusive.
- There is currently great controversy over recovered memories (RMs) of CSA and false-memory syndrome (FMS). Some RM therapists are accused of implanting false memories of CSA into clients, while some clients accuse their parents of the abuse.
- Most psychologists and psychiatrists seem to accept the possibility of FMs, but this does not mean that all RMs of CSA are false.

REFERENCES

1. Blakemore C (1988) *The Mind Machine*. London: BBC.
2. Atkinson RC, Shiffrin RM (1968) Human memory: a proposed system and its control processes. In KW Spence, JT Spence (eds) *The Psychology of Learning and Motivation*, Vol. 2. London: Academic Press.
3. Atkinson RC, Shiffrin RM (1971) The control of short-term memory. *Scientific American* **224**: 82–90.
4. Craik FIM, Lockhart R (1972) Levels of processing. *Journal of Verbal Learning and Verbal Behaviour* **11**: 671–84.
5. Baddeley AD, Hitch G (1974) Working memory. In GH Bower (ed.) *Recent Advances in Learning and Motivation*, Vol. 8. New York: Academic Press.
6. Tulving E (1972) Episodic and semantic memory. In E Tulving, W Donaldson (eds) *Organization of Memory*. London: Academic Press.
7. Ebbinghaus H (1885) *On Memory*. Leipzig: Duncker.
8. Hebb DO (1949) *The Organization of Behaviour*. New York: John Wiley & Sons.
9. Broadbent DE (1958) *Perception and Communication*. Oxford: Pergamon.
10. Waugh NC, Norman DA (1965) Primary memory. *Psychological Review* **72**: 89–104.
11. Woodworth RS (1938) *Experiment Psychology*. New York: Holt.
12. Baddeley AD (1995) Memory. In CC French, AM Colman (eds) *Cognitive Psychology*. London: Longman.
13. Lloyd P,Mayes A, Manstead ASR, Meudell PR, Wagner HL (1984) *Introduction to Psychology: An Integrated Approach*. London: Fontana.
14. Miller GA (1956) The magical number seven, plus or minus two: some limits on our capacity for processing information. *Psychological Review* **63**: 81–97.
15. Brown JA (1958) Some tests of the decay theory of immediate memory. *Quarterly Journal of Experimental Psychology* **10**: 12–21.
16. Peterson LR, Peterson MJ (1959) Short-term retention of individual items. *Journal of Experimental Psychology* **58**: 193–8.
17. Conrad R (1964) Acoustic confusion in immediate memory. *British Journal of Psychology* **55**: 75–84.
18. Baddeley AD (1966) The influence of acoustic and semantic similarity on long-term memory for word sequences. *Quarterly Journal of Experimental Psychology* **18**: 302–9.
19. Shulman HG (1970) Encoding and retention of semantic and phonemic information in short-term memory. *Journal of Verbal Learning and Verbal Behaviour* **9**: 499–508.
20. Bower GH (1975) Cognitive psychology: an introduction. In W Estes (ed.) *Handbook of Learning and Cognitive Processes*, Vol. 1. Hillsdale, NJ: Lawrence Erlbaum Associates.
21. Baddeley AD (1976) *The Psychology of Memory*. New York: Basic Books.
22. Rose S (2003) *The Making of Memory: From Molecules to Mind*, revised edn. London: Vintage.
23. Murdock BB (1962) The serial position effect in free recall. *Journal of Experimental Psychology* **64**: 482–8.
24. Glanzer M, Cunitz AR (1966) Two storage mechanisms in free recall. *Journal of Verbal Learning and Verbal Behaviour* **5**: 928–35.
25. Eysenck MW (1993) *Principles of Cognitive Psychology*. Hove: Lawrence Erlbaum Associates.
26. Craik FIM, Watkins MJ (1973) The role of rehearsal in short-term memory. *Journal of Verbal Learning and Verbal Behaviour* **12**: 599–607.

27. Glanzer M, Meinzer A (1967) The effects of intra-list activity on free recall. *Journal of Verbal Learning and Verbal Behaviour* **6**: 928–35.
28. Gross R (2005) *Psychology: The Science of Mind and Behaviour*, 5th edn. London: Hodder Arnold.
29. Jenkins JJ (1974) Remember that old theory of memory? Well, forget it! *American Psychologist* **29**: 785–95.
30. Miller GA, Selfridge JA (1950) Verbal context and the recall of meaningful material. *American Journal of Psychology* **63**: 176–85.
31. Bower GH, Springston F (1970) Pauses as recoding points in letter series. *Journal of Experimental Psychology* **83**: 421–30.
32. Milner B, Corkin S, Teuber HL (1968) Further analysis of the hippocampal amnesic syndrome: 14-year follow-up study of H.M. *Neuropsychologica* **6**: 215–34.
33. Baddeley AD (1990) *Human Memory*, Hove: Lawrence Erlbaum Associates.
34. Parkin AJ (1987) *Memory and Amnesia: An Introduction*. Oxford: Blackwell.
35. Baddeley AD, Warrington EH (1970) Amnesia and the distinction between long- and short-term memory. *Journal of Verbal Learning and Verbal Behaviour* **9**: 176–89.
36. Warrington EH, Weiskrantz L (1968) New method of testing long-term retention with special reference to amnesic patients. *Nature* **217**: 972–4.
37. Warrington, EH, Weiskrantz L (1970) Amnesic syndrome: consolidation or retrieval? *Nature* **228**: 628–30.
38. Cohen G (1993) Everyday memory and memory systems: the experimental approach. In G Cohen, G Kiss, M Levoi (eds) *Memory: Current Issues*, 2nd edn. Buckingham: Open University Press.
39. Brown R, Kulik J (1977) Flashbulb memories. *Cognition* **5**: 73–99.
40. Brown R, Kulik J (1982) Flashbulb memories. In U Neisser (ed.) *Memory Observed*. San Francisco, CA: W.H. Freeman.
41. Neisser U (1982) (ed.) *Memory Observed*. San Francisco, CA: W.H. Freeman.
42. Anderson JR (1985) *Cognitive Psychology and Its Implications*. New York: W.H. Freeman.
43. Tulving E (1985) How many memory systems are there? *American Psychologist* **40**: 385–98.
44. Cohen NJ, Squire LR (1980) Preserved learning and retention of pattern-analyzing skills in amnesia: dissociation of knowing how from knowing that. *Science* **210**: 207–10.
45. Ryle G (1949) *The Concept of Mind*. London: Hutchinson.
46. Anderson JR (1983) *The Architecture of Cognition*, 2nd edn. Cambridge, MA: Harvard University Press.
47. Gabrieli JDE, Cohen NJ, Corkin S (1983) The acquisition of lexical and semantic knowledge in amnesia. *Society for Neuroscience Abstracts* **9**: 238.
48. Eysenck MW, Keane MJ (1990) *Cognitive Psychology: A Student's Handbook*. Hove: Lawrence Erlbaum Associates.
49. Baddeley AD (1984) Neuropsychological evidence and the semantic/episodic distinction. *Behavioral and Brain Sciences* **7**: 238–9.
50. Groome D, Dewart H, Esgate E, *et al.* (1999) *An Introduction to Cognitive Psychology: Processes and Disorders*. London: Psychology Press.
51. Gilhooly K (1996) Working memory and thinking. *Psychologist* **9**: 82.
52. Logie RH (1999) Working memory. *Psychologist* **12**: 174–8.
53. Hampson PJ, Morris PE (1996) *Understanding Cognition*. Oxford: Blackwell.
54. Eysenck MW (1986) Working memory. In G Cohen, MW Eysenck, MA Le Voi (eds) *Memory: A Cognitive Approach*. Milton Keynes: Open University Press.
55. Tulving E (1962) Subjective organization in free recall of unrelated words. *Psychological Review* **69**: 344–54.
56. Mandler G (1967) Organization and memory. In KW Spence, JT Spence (eds) *The Psychology of Learning and Motivation*, Vol. 1. New York: Academic Press.
57. Bartlett FC (1932) *Remembering*. Cambridge: Cambridge University Press.
58. Loftus EF (1980) *Memory*. Reading, MA: Addison-Wesley.
59. Jenkins JG, Dallenbach KM (1924) Oblivescence during sleep and waking. *American Journal of Psychology* **35**: 605–12.
60. Solso RL (1995) *Cognitive Psychology*, 4th edn. Boston, MA: Allyn & Bacon.
61. Brown R, McNeill D (1966) The 'tip-of-the-tongue' phenomenon. *Journal of Verbal Learning and Verbal Behaviour* **5**: 325–337.
62. Tulving E, Pearlstone Z (1966) Availability versus accessibility of information in memory for words. *Journal of Verbal Learning and Verbal Behaviour* **5**: 389–91.
63. Tulving E (1983) *Elements of Episodic Memory*. London: Clarendon Press/Oxford University Press.
64. Tulving E (1974) Cue-dependent forgetting. *American Scientist* **62**: 74–82.
65. Abernathy EM (1940) The effect of changed environmental conditions upon the results of college examinations. *Journal of Psychology* **10**: 293–301.
66. Clark MS, Millberg S, Erber R (1987) Arousal and state dependent memory: evidence and some implications for understanding social judgements and social behaviour. In K Fiedler, JP Forgas (eds) *Affect, Cognition and Social Behaviour*. Toronto: Hogrefe.
67. Godden D, Baddeley AD (1975) Context-dependent memory in two natural environments: on land and under water. *British Journal of Psychology* **66**: 325–31.
68. McCormick LJ, Mayer JD (1991) Mood-congruent recall and natural mood. Poster presented at the annual meeting of the New England Psychological Association, Portland, ME.

69. Wickens CD (1972) Characteristics of word encoding. In A Melton, E Martin (eds) *Coding Processes in Human Memory*. Washington, DC: Winston.
70. Freud S (1901 [1976b]) *The Psychopathology of Everyday Life*. Harmondsworth: Penguin.
71. Freud S (1915) *Repression: Standard Edition of the Complete Psychological Works of Sigmund Freud*, Vol. 14. London: Hogarth Press.
72. Gross R (2008) *Key Studies in Psychology*, 5th edn. London: Hodder Education.
73. Parkin AJ (1993) *Memory: Phenomena, Experiment and Theory*. Oxford: Blackwell.
74. Taylor PF, Kopelman MD (1984) Amnesia for criminal offences. *Psychological Medicine* **14**: 581–8.
75. Parkin AJ (2000) *Essential Cognitive Psychology*. Hove: Psychology Press.
76. Baddeley AD (1999) *Essentials of Human Memory*. Hove: Psychology Press.
77. Kaminer H, Lavie P (1991) Sleep and dreaming in Holocaust survivors: dramatic decrease in dream recall in well-adjusted survivors. *Journal of Nervous and Mental Diseases* **179**: 664–9.
78. British Psychological Society (1995) *Recovered Memories: The Report of the Working Party of the British Psychological Society*. Leicester: British Psychological Society.
79. Anderson JR (1995) *Cognitive Psychology, Its Implications*. New York: W.H. Freeman.
80. Levinger G, Clark J (1961) Emotional factors in the forgetting of word associations. *Journal of Abnormal Psychology* **62**: 99–105.
81. Eysenck HJ, Wilson GD (1973) (eds) *The Experimental Study of Freudian Theories*. London: Methuen.
82. Parkin AJ, Lewinson J, Folkard S (1982) The influence of emotion on immediate and delayed retention: Levinger and Clark reconsidered. *British Journal of Psychology* **73**: 389–93.
83. Bradley BP, Baddeley AD (1990) Emotional factors in forgetting. *Psychological Medicine* **20**: 351–5.
84. Showalter E (1998) Sex, lies, and therapy. *Independent on Sunday, Section 2*, 5 April: 5.
85. Mollon P (2000) *Freud and False Memory Syndrome*. Cambridge: Icon Books.
86. Freud S (1899) *Screen Memories*: *Standard Edition of the Complete Psychological Works of Sigmund Freud*, Vol. III. London: Hogarth Press.
87. Jaroff L (1993) Lies of the mind. *Time* **143**: 56–61.
88. Brandon S, Boakes J, Glaser D, Green R (1998) Recovered memories of childhood sexual abuse: implications for clinical practice. *British Journal of Psychiatry* **172**: 293–307.
89. Loftus EF (1997) Creating false memories. *Scientific American* **September**: 50–55.
90. Frankland A, Cohen L (1999) Working with recovered memories. *Psychologist* **12**: 82–3.

Chapter 18

Language and thought

Richard Gross

INTRODUCTION

The relationship between language and thought is one of the most fascinating and complex issues within psychology and has been debated by philosophers for over 2000 years. Our thinking often takes the form of imagery, and our thoughts and feelings are often expressed unconsciously through gestures and facial expressions. Artists 'think' non-linguistically. Knowing what we want to say but being unable to 'put it into words' is one of several examples of thought taking place without language.[1]

However, the exact relationship between language and thought has been the subject of much debate among philosophers and psychologists. Views fall into four main categories:

- *Thought is dependent on, or caused by, language:* this view is taken by people working in a variety of disciplines, including psychology, sociology, linguistics and anthropology. Sapir (a linguist and anthropologist) and Whorf (a linguist) were both interested in comparing languages, which they saw as a major feature of a culture. Language is shared by all members of a culture, or sub-cultures within it, and this makes it a determining influence on how individuals think. Bernstein (a sociologist) focused on subcultural (social class) differences in language codes, which he saw as a major influence on intelligence and educational attainment. *Social constructionists* (e.g. Gergen) regard language as providing a basis for all our thought, a system of categories for dividing up experience and giving it meaning (see Gross[2]).
- *Language is dependent on, and reflects, thought:* probably the most extreme version of this view is Piaget's, according to whom language reflects the individual's level of cognitive development (see Chapter 8).
- *Thought and language are initially quite separate activities:* they then come together and interact at a later point in development (about age 2 years). This view is associated with the Russian psychologist Vygotsky (see Chapter 8).
- *Language and thought are one and the same:* this rather extreme view is associated mainly with Watson, the founder of behaviourism.

The focus of this chapter is the various versions of the first of these viewpoints.

LANGUAGE AND THOUGHT ARE THE SAME

Watson's 'peripheralist' approach

The earliest psychological theory of the relationship between language and thought was proposed by Watson.[3] In his view, thought processes are really no more than the sensations produced by tiny movements of the speech organs too small to produce audible sounds. Essentially, then, thought is talking to oneself very quietly. Part of Watson's rejection of 'mind' was his denial of mentalistic concepts such as 'thought' (see Chapters 9 and 14) and hence his reduction of it to 'silent speech'.

Watson's theory is called *peripheralism*, because he regards 'thinking' as occurring peripherally in the larynx rather than centrally in the brain. Movements of the larynx do occur when 'thought' is taking place, but this indicates only that such movements may accompany thinking, not that the movements are thoughts or are necessary for thinking to occur.

Smith *et al.* attempted to test Watson's theory by injecting Smith himself with curare, a drug that causes total paralysis of the skeletal muscles without affecting consciousness.[4] The muscles of the speech organs and the respiratory system are paralysed, and Smith's breathing had to be maintained artificially. When the drug's effects had worn off, Smith was able to report on his thoughts and perceptions during the paralysis.

Additionally, Furth has shown that people who are born deaf and mute and who do not learn sign language can think in much the same way as hearing and speaking people.[5] For Watson, deaf and mute individuals should be incapable of thought, because of the absence of movement in the speech organs.

THOUGHT IS DEPENDENT ON, OR CAUSED BY, LANGUAGE

Bruner has argued that language is essential if thought and knowledge are not to be limited to what can be learned through our actions (the *enactive mode of representation*) or images (the *iconic mode*).[6] If the *symbolic mode* (going beyond the immediate context) is to develop, then language is crucial (see Gross[7]).

Social constructionists (e.g. Gergen[8]) have argued that our ways of understanding the world derive from other people (past and present), rather than from objective reality. We are born into a world where the conceptual frameworks and categories used by people in our culture already exist. Indeed, these frameworks and categories are an essential part of our culture, since they provide meaning, a way of structuring experience of both ourselves and the world of other people. Language is of fundamental importance in this process. This view has much in common with the 'strong' version of the *linguistic relativity hypothesis* (LRH), the most extensively researched of the theories arguing that thought is dependent on, or caused by, language.

The linguistic relativity hypothesis

According to the philosopher Wittgenstein, 'The limits of my language mean the limits of my world'.[9] By this, he meant that people can think about and understand the world only through language; and if a particular language does not possess certain ideas or concepts, then these ideas and conceps could not exist for the native speakers of that language.

The view that language determines how we think about objects and events, or even what we think (our ideas, thoughts and perceptions), can be traced to the writings of Sapir[10] and Whorf,[11] a student of Sapir. Their perspective is often called the *Sapir–Whorf linguistic relativity hypothesis* (LRH) or, in acknowledgement of the greater contribution made by Whorf, the *Whorfian hypothesis*. For Whorf:

> We dissect nature along the lines laid down by our native languages. The categories and types that we isolate from the world of phenomena we do not find there because they stare every observer in the face; on the contrary, the world is presented in a kaleidoscopic flux of impressions that has to be organised by our minds – and this means largely by the linguistic systems in our minds. We cut nature up, organise it into concepts and ascribe significance as we do, largely because we are parties to an agreement to organise it this way – an agreement that holds throughout our speech community and is codified in patterns of our language.[11]

According to Whorf's *linguistic determinism*, language determines our concepts, and we can think only through the use of concepts. So, acquiring a language involves acquiring a 'world view' (or *Weltanschauung*). People who speak different languages have different world views (hence linguistic 'relativity').

Whorf's evidence

Whorf compared standard average European (SAE) languages, such as English, French and Italian (Indo-European), with Native American languages, particularly Hopi. While in English we have a single word for snow, the Inuit Eskimos have approximately 20 words (including one for 'fluffy snow', one for 'drifting snow', another for 'packed snow' and so on). The Hopi Indians have only one word for 'insect', 'aeroplane' and 'pilot', and the Zuni Indians do not distinguish verbally between yellow and orange.

Whorf also saw a language's grammar as determining an individual's thought and perception. In the Hopi language, for example, no distinction is made between past, present and future, which, compared with English, makes it a 'timeless language'. In European languages, 'time' is treated as an objective entity, with a clear demarcation between past, present and future. Although the Hopi language recognizes duration, Hopis talk about time only as it appears subjectively to the observer. For example, rather than saying 'I stayed for ten days', Hopis say 'I stayed until the tenth day' or 'I left on the tenth day'.

In English, nouns denote objects and events, and verbs denote actions. But in the Hopi language, 'lightning', 'wave', 'flame', 'meteor', 'puff of smoke' and 'pulsation' are all verbs, since events of necessarily brief duration must be verbs. As a result, a Hopi would say 'it lightninged', 'it smoked' and 'it flamed'.

Greene asks us to imagine a Hopi linguist applying a Whorfian analysis to English.[12] Would the linguist think that English speakers have 'primitive' beliefs, that ships are really female or that mountains have feet, or that 'driving a car', 'driving off in golf' and 'driving a hard bargain' all involve the same activity? Of course not. (See 'An evaluation of the linguistic relativity hypothesis' below.)

Testing the linguistic relativity hypothesis

Miller and McNeill distinguish between three different versions of the LRH, all of which are consistent with the hypothesis but vary in the strength of claim they make:[13]

- The strong version claims that language determines thought.
- The weak version claims that language affects perception.
- The weakest version claims that language influences memory: information that is described more easily in a particular language will be better remembered than information that is more difficult to describe.

The questions and criticisms that we considered above relate mainly to the strong version of the hypothesis, but almost all the research has focused on the weak and weakest versions. One of the few attempts to test the strong version was a study by Carroll and Casagrande (Box 18.1).[14]

Attempts at testing the 'weak' and 'weakest' versions of the LRH have typically involved the perception and memory of colour. The Jalé from New Guinea have terms

Box 18.1 How Navaho children shape up on cognitive development[14]

Carroll and Casagrande compared Navaho Indian children who spoke either only Navaho (Navaho–Navaho) or both English and Navaho (English–Navaho) with American children of European descent who spoke only English.

The children were tested on the development of form or shape recognition.

The Navaho language stresses the importance of form, such that 'handling' verbs involve different words depending on what is being handled. For example, long and flexible objects (e.g. string) have one word form, whereas long and rigid objects (e.g. sticks) have another.

American children of European descent develop object recognition in the following order: size, colour, form or shape.

If, as the strong version of the linguistic relativity hypothesis (LRH) claims, language influences cognitive development, then the developmental sequence of the Navaho children should differ from the English-only American children, and their form or shape recognition abilities should be superior.

This is what Carroll and Casagrande found, thus supporting the strong version of the LRH.

However, they also found that the English–Navaho group showed form recognition later than the English-only American children, which does not support the strong version of the LRH.

Carroll and Casagrande attributed the superior performance of the English-only children to the fact that they had had a great deal of experience of shape classification at nursery school. This made them an atypical sample.

only for black and white, while the Dani from New Guinea use the word 'mola' for bright, warm hues and 'mili' for dark, cold hues. The Shona people of Zimbabwe have three colour words, and members of the Ibibio culture from Nigeria have terms for black, white, red and green.

According to the weaker versions of the LRH, tests of colour perception and memory should be more difficult for the Jalé than the Ibibio. Since the Ibibio word for green encompasses the English green, blue and yellow, the Ibibio should find colour perception and memory tasks more difficult than English speakers. Taking a previous example, since the Zuni language does not distinguish between yellow and orange, Zuni speakers should be unable to discriminate them (they should be 'blind' for these two colours).

Brown and Lenneberg found that Zuni Indians did make more mistakes than English speakers in recognizing these colours.[15] But Lenneberg and Roberts found that the number of errors made by bilingual Zuni–English speakers in distinguishing orange and yellow fell midway between that of monolingual Zuni and monolingual English speakers.[16] This suggests that the two languages do not determine two different sets of conflicting perceptions but rather determine two sets of labels for essentially the same colour perceptions. Language serves to draw attention to differences in the environment and acts as a label to help store these differences in memory. Sometimes the label we apply to what we see may distort our recall of what was seen, since the label determines how we code our experiences into memory storage (Box 18.2; see also Chapter 17).

So, although there is very little direct evidence to support the strong form of the LRH, there is rather more support for the weaker versions. Language merely predisposes people to think or perceive in certain ways or about certain things.[18] However, Brown and Lenneberg's results,[15] and those of other researchers using a similar methodology, have been challenged in a way that throws doubt even on the weaker versions.

Perceiving focal colours

Berlin and Kay used a chart with an array of 329 small coloured chips, comprising almost all the hues that the human eye can discriminate.[19] They asked native speakers of 20 languages other than English (i) to trace the boundaries of each of their native language's basic colour terms and (ii) to point to the chip that was the best example of each basic colour term. A basic or focal colour was defined by a list of linguistic criteria, including the following:

- A term should consist of only a single unit of meaning (e.g. 'red' rather than 'dark red').
- A term should name only colours and not objects (e.g. 'purple' rather than 'wine').

As expected from anthropological research, there was considerable variation in the placement of boundaries; but the choice of best examples was surprisingly similar. The largest clusters were for black and white and red, for which all the 20 languages have colour terms, followed by 19 for green, 18 for yellow, 16 for blue, 15 for brown and purple, 14 for grey, and 11 for pink and orange. Berlin and Kay concluded that 'colour categorization is not random and the foci of basic colour terms are similar in all languages'.[19]

So, although cultures may differ in the number of basic colour terms they use, all cultures draw their focal terms from only 11 colours: black, white, red, green, yellow, blue, brown, purple, pink, orange and grey. Moreover, the colour terms emerge in a particular sequence in the history of languages (Figure 18.2).

For cultures with only two colours, these will always be black and white, whereas in cultures with three colours, these will always be black, white and red.[20] As Newstead has observed:

> This, then, gives a rather different perspective on the use of colour terms. It had been assumed that verbal labels were chosen more or less arbitrarily, and that those chosen influenced

Box 18.2 Drawing different conclusions[17]

Two separate groups of participants were given identical stimulus figures but two different sets of labels. After a period of time, both groups were asked to reproduce the figures.

The drawings of both groups were distorted in comparison with the original stimulus according to which label had been presented (Figure 18.1).

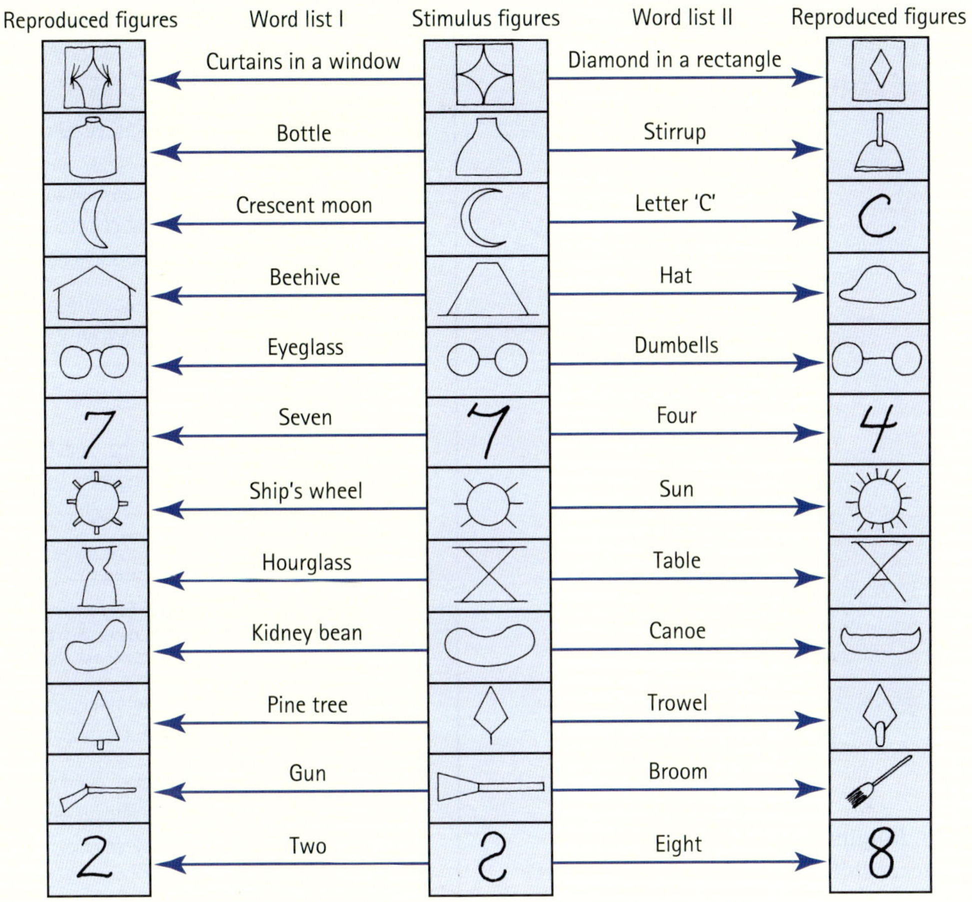

Figure 18.1 Stimulus figures, word lists and reproduced figures from the experiment by Carmichael *et al.*[17]

the way in which colour was perceived. Berlin and Kay's findings suggest that there are certain focal colours which will always be labelled if colour terms are used at all. This suggests an alternative explanation for Brown and Lenneberg's findings: that the colours which participants in their study had found easier to learn were the focal colours and these were easy to remember not because they had verbal labels but because they were the most basic colours.[20]

A study that supports Berlin and Kay's findings was conducted by Heider and Oliver (Box 18.3).[21]

Heider concluded:

> Far from being a domain well suited to the study of the effects of language on thought, the colour-space would seem a prime example of the influence of underlying perceptual-cognitive factors on the formation and reference of linguistic categories.[22]

By this, Heider (sometimes referred to as Rosch, her married name) means that her data are explained better in terms of physiological factors underlying colour vision than in terms of linguistic factors. Thus, people are sensitive to focal colours because the human visual system processes reality in a certain way.[23] Indeed, evidence suggests that focal colours can be discriminated before any verbal labels for them have been learned. Bornstein, for example, has argued that preverbal infants categorize the visible spectrum in a similar way to adults, namely on the basis of the relatively discrete hues of blue, green, yellow and red.[24]

However, Kay (cited in Ross[25]) denies that there is any evidence to support a physiological explanation. In addition, a study of another New Guinea people, the Berinmo, casts doubt on Heider's interpretation and seems to support the weakest and weak versions of the LRH (Box 18.4).

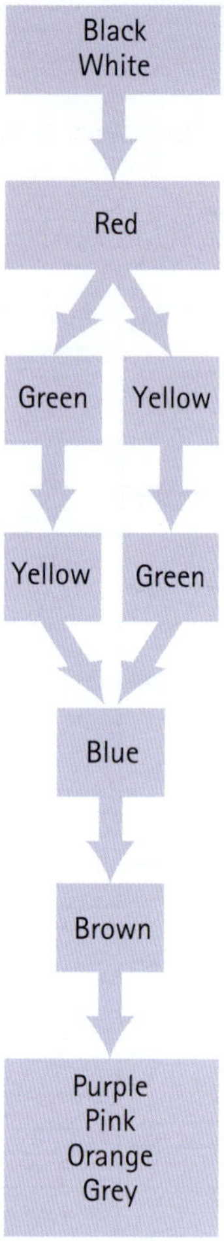

Figure 18.2 Sequence in which focal colours emerge[19]

An evaluation of the linguistic relativity hypothesis

Berry *et al.*[28] and Jackendoff[29] have argued that Whorf's evidence was anecdotal rather than empirical and that he exaggerated the differences between Hopi and other languages. Moreover, far from having 'over 20' words for 'snow', the Inuit Eskimos have relatively few such words[20] and no more than do English speakers.[30] According to Pagel, Whorf simply got his facts wrong.[31]

There is an important difference between a language's grammar and our perceptual experience. The fact that Hopi can be translated into English (and vice versa) implies a universally shared knowledge of the world that is independent of the particular language in which it is expressed.[31]

A crucial question that Whorf seems to have overlooked is *why* Eskimos have so many names for snow (if, indeed, they do) and SAE languages so few. One answer is that the more significant an experience or some feature of our environment is for us, the greater the number of ways of expressing it in the language. In other words, while Whorf argued that language structures the Eskimo's world, it could equally well be argued that the Eskimos' language develops as a result of their different perception of the world.[32] According to Solso:

Box 18.3 Colour-naming among the Dani[21]

The Dani, a 'Stone Age' agricultural people of Indonesian New Guinea, have only two words for colours, whereas native English speakers have words for 11 basic colours.

Heider and Oliver gave both Dani- and English-speaking participants a coloured chip, which they were allowed to look at for 5 s. After a 30-s delay, participants were asked to pick out a chip of the same colour among a set of 40 different-coloured chips.

On the weakest version of the linguistic relativity hypothesis (LRH) the Dani's colour vocabulary should have influenced their memory for colours, and on the weak version they should have had difficulty discriminating similar colours of a slightly different hue that they had labelled with the same name.

Both the Dani-speaking and the English-speaking participants made many mistakes. But there were no significant differences between them in their rate of confusion of similar colours, despite the differences in their colour vocabularies.

In other research, Heider showed that both Dani and English speakers were better at recognizing focal colours than non-focal colours, and that the Dani found it much easier to learn labels for focal than non-focal colours.

Box 18.4 Colour-naming among the Berinmo

Robertson *et al.*[26,27] studied the Berinmo people of New Guinea, who live a simple hunter–gatherer lifestyle in remote forests.

The Berinmo have five colour names: one for green, blue and purple, another for yellow, orange and brown, a third for all dark colours, a fourth for white and all light colours, and a fifth for all shades of red and pink.

Using a procedure similar to that of Heider and Oliver,[21] Robertson *et al.* found that the Berinmo could remember only those colours that matched their colour names, and that they were unable to discriminate between colours that their language did not discriminate, such as green and blue.

Although all the focal colours were represented by the Berinmos' five colour names, the fact that green, blue and purple were lumped together, as were yellow, orange and brown, and red and pink, seems inconsistent with the claim that colour terms emerge in a particular order in the history of languages (see Figure 18.2).

> The development of specific language codes ... is dependent on cultural needs; the learning of these codes by members of a language group also involves the learning of significant values of the culture, some of which must be related to survival ...[33]

Solso's view is supported by the fact that English-speaking skiers learn to discriminate between varied snow conditions and invent a vocabulary to describe these differences. Such terms include 'sticky snow', 'powder', 'corn' and 'boilerplate' (or ice).[34] Similarly, the Hanunoo people of the Philippines have modified their language in response to environmental conditions. For example, women have developed a more complex vocabulary for shades of blue to distinguish the colours of dyed textiles that have been introduced into their society.[35]

It is now widely accepted that Whorf overestimated the importance of language differences. As Berry *et al.* have observed:

> Language as an instrument for thinking has many cross-culturally variant properties. As humans, we may not all be sharing the same thoughts, but our respective languages do not seem to predestine us to different kinds of thinking.[28]

What language may do, however, is affect the ease of information processing. Newstead,[20] for example, describes research conducted by Hunt and Agnoli that supports this view.[36] The English word 'seven' has two syllables, whereas the equivalent French word ('sept') has only one. The English word 'eleven' has three syllables, whereas the French word 'onze' has one. Hunt and Agnoli argue that, when a name is shorter, information is processed more quickly, and so French speakers would have an advantage over English speakers when performing mental arithmetic involving these numbers, at least in processing terms.

According to Price and Crapo, the study of semantic domains (e.g. colour naming) helps us to discover what is important in the daily lives of different cultural groups and demonstrates the changing cultural history of a society.[35] Similarly, Kay (cited in Ross[25]) argues that the degree to which the world is man-made seems to explain the variation in the number of colour words. Hunter–gatherers need fewer colour words, because colour data rarely provide much crucially distinguishing information about a natural scene or object; but industrialized societies get a bigger 'information payoff' for colour words.

Kay (cited in Ross[25]) claims that his research into focal colours has been interpreted by some as undermining the LRH as a whole. But he and Berlin were concerned with one restricted domain, namely colour. Even if it is accepted that the colour perception research does not support the LRH, there is no reason to rule it out in relation to other domains (Box 18.5).

Although this shows that the LRH may be correct:

> ... it is unlikely that the various languages of the world are so different from one another, in underlying conceptual structure, that the ways their speakers think are incommensurable.[25]

The linguistic relativity hypothesis, social class and race

Social-class differences in language and thought

Stones gives examples of imaginary conversations on a bus between a mother and child:[37]

- *Mother:* Hold on tight.
- *Child:* Why?
- *Mother:* Hold on tight.
- *Child:* Why?
- *Mother:* You'll fall.
- *Child:* Why?
- *Mother:* I told you to hold on tight, didn't I?

- *Mother:* Hold on tight, darling.
- *Child:* Why?
- *Mother:* If you don't you'll be thrown forward and you'll fall.
- *Child:* Why?
- *Mother:* Because if the bus suddenly stops, you'll jerk forward on to the seat in front.
- *Child:* Why?
- *Mother:* Now, darling, hold on tightly and don't make such a fuss.

Box 18.5 'There's a fly to the north of your nose'

Ross cites a study of speakers of Guugu Yimithirr (a language of Australia).[25] Like several world languages, Guugu Yimithirr lacks subjective terms equivalent to 'left' and 'right' and instead uses absolute directions akin to 'north' and 'south'. In such a language, you might say 'There's a fly to the north of your nose.'

If Guugu speakers are presented with an arrow pointing to their left, they will later draw it pointing to the left only if they are still facing in the direction in which they saw the arrow originally. If they turn round, they will draw the arrow pointing to the right – that is, in the same absolute direction as the original arrow.

This illustrates strikingly how linguistic categories can mould thought and behaviour.[25]

Restricted and elaborated codes

Bernstein was interested in language's role as a social, rather than an individual, phenomenon, especially its relation to cultural deprivation.[38] He showed that there were generally no differences between the verbal and non-verbal intelligence test performance of boys from public schools and boys from lower-working-class homes. But the latter often showed considerable differences, with non-verbal performance sometimes being as much as 26 points better than verbal performance. Bernstein argued that working-class and middle-class children speak two different kinds (or *codes*) of language, which he called *restricted code* and *elaborated code*, respectively (Table 18.1).

Bernstein saw the relationship between potential and actual intelligence as being mediated through language; consequently, the lack of an elaborated code would prevent working-class children from developing their full intellectual potential. The different language codes underlie the whole pattern of relationships (to objects and people) experienced

Table 18.1 Characteristics of restricted and elaborated codes[38]

Restricted code	Elaborated code
Grammatically crude, repetitive and rigid; limited use of adjectives and adverbs; greater use of pronouns than nouns; sentences often short, grammatically simple and incomplete	Grammatically more complex and flexible; uses a range of subordinate clauses, conjunctions, prepositions, adjectives and adverbs; uses more nouns than pronouns; sentences longer and more complex
Context-bound: meaning is not made explicit but assumes listener's familiarity with the situation being described, e.g. 'He gave me it'; listener cannot be expected to know what 'he' or 'it' refers to	Context-independent: meaning is made explicit, e.g. 'John gave me this book'
'I' used very rarely; much of the meaning conveyed non-verbally	'I' used often, making clear speaker's intentions and emphasizing precise description of experiences and feelings
Frequent use of uninformative but emotionally reinforcing phrases, e.g. 'you know' and 'don't I?'	Relatively little use of emotionally reinforcing phrases
Tends to stress the present, the here-and-now	Tends to stress the past and future
Does not allow expression of abstract and hypothetical thought	Allows expression of abstract and hypothetical thought

by members of different classes, as well as the patterns of learning that their children bring with them to school.

In support of Bernstein's views, Hess and Shipman found that social-class differences influence children's intellectual development.[39] In particular, there was a lack of meaning in the mother–child communication system for low-status families. Language was used much less to convey meaning (to describe, explain, express and so on), and much more to give orders and commands to the child (see the two mother–child conversations above).

However, instead of seeing 'restricted' and 'elaborated' as distinct types of language code, they are better thought of as two ends of a continuum. Also, the terms 'restricted' and 'elaborated' imply a value judgement of middle-class speech as being superior to working-class speech (closer to 'standard' or 'the Queen's' English). The lack of objectivity makes this judgement difficult to defend.

Black English

A version of English spoken by segments of the African-American community is called 'black English'. When asked to repeat the sentence 'I asked him if he did it, and he said he didn't do it', one 5-year-old girl repeated the sentence like this: 'I asks him if he did it, and he says he didn't did it, but I knows he did'.[40] Bernstein argued that black English is a restricted code and that this makes the thinking of black English speakers less logical than that of their white elaborated-code counterparts.

One major difference between black English and standard English relates to the use of verbs.[41] In particular, black English speakers often omit the present tense copula (the verb 'to be'). So, 'He be gone' indicates the standard English 'He's been gone for a long time', and 'He gone' signifies 'He's just gone'. Black English is often described as 'sub-standard' and regarded as illogical rather than 'non-standard'.[42] According to Labov, black English is just one dialect of English, and speakers of both dialects are expressing the same ideas equally well.[43]

Black English and prejudice

Although the grammatical rules of black English differ from those of standard English, black English possesses consistent rules that allow the expression of thoughts as complex as those permitted by standard English.[40] Several other languages, such as Russian and Arabic, also omit the present-tense verb 'to be', and yet we do not describe those languages as 'illogical'. This suggests that black dialects are considered substandard as a matter of convention or prejudice rather than because they are poorer vehicles for expressing meaning and logical thinking. However, because the structure of black English does differ in important ways from standard English, and since intelligence tests are written in standard English, black English speakers are at a linguistic disadvantage (as, indeed, are white working-class children: see Gross[7]).

Language in context

Labov also showed that the social situation can be a powerful determinant of verbal behaviour. A young boy called Leon was shown a toy by a white interviewer and asked to tell him everything he could about it. Leon said very little and was silent for much of the time, including when a black interviewer took over. However, when Leon sat on the floor and shared a packet of crisps with his best friend and with the same black interviewer introducing topics in a local black dialect, Leon became a lively conversationalist. Had he been assessed with the white or black interviewers on their own, Leon might have been labelled 'non-verbal' or 'linguistically retarded'.

Black children may actually be bilingual. In their home environments, the school playground and their neighbourhoods, they speak the accepted vernacular. In the classroom, however, and when talking to people in authority, they may adopt standard English, with which they are unfamiliar; this results in short sentences, simple grammar and strange intonation. Out of school, their natural language is easy, fluent, creative and often gifted. So, although black English is certainly non-standard, it is another language with its own grammar, which is certainly not substandard (Box 18.6).

Box 18.6 'Ebonics': an ongoing debate

'Ebonics' is a fusion of the words 'ebony' and 'phonics' and was coined in 1975 as an alternative for the term 'black English'. In 1996, Ebonics (or African–American vernacular English, AAVE) was officially recognized by the Oakland public school board in California, and schools were ordered to teach 28 000 black children in their 'own tongue'. The board claimed that Ebonics was a separate language, genetically rooted in the West African and Niger–Congo language system, rather than a dialect of standard American English.[44,45]

In early 1997, the school board edited its statement so that the word 'genetically' referred to linguists' use of the word for the roots of a language rather than to a gene pool. They also indicated that it was not the intent to teach in Ebonics, but rather to have teachers use the vernacular to be able to understand their children.[46]

Both conservatives and liberals in America claim that the decision to require Ebonics to be taught would be 'political correctness run amok'.[47] Educationalists such as Zinberg disagree. In her view, many students are '... bewildered, then angered and finally alienated from the schools where their language and self-esteem are belittled by a seemingly insensitive system'.

Although regional dialects in the USA are diverging, there is no evidence of convergence between black and white vernaculars.[48] By contrast, black and white British people still speak the same language, partly because there is no segregation in housing in Britain as there is in the USA (Labov, cited in Hawkes[48]).

LANGUAGE IS DEPENDENT ON, AND REFLECTS, THOUGHT

According to Piaget, children begin life with some understanding of the world and try to find linguistic ways of expressing their knowledge.[49] As language develops, it 'maps' on to previously acquired cognitive structures, and so language is dependent upon thought.[50] For example, a child should begin talking about objects that are not present in his or her immediate surroundings only after *object permanence* has developed (i.e. understanding that things continue to exist even when they are not being perceived). Similarly, children who could *conserve* liquid quantity (understanding that, when liquid is poured from one container into a taller, thinner container, the quantity of liquid remains the same) understood the meaning of phrases and words such as 'as much as', 'bigger' and 'more'. However, children who could not conserve did not improve their performance of the correct use of these words after receiving linguistic training.[51]

In Piaget's view, children can be taught words but they will not understand them until they have mastered certain intellectual skills during the process of cognitive growth. So, language can exist without thought, but only in the sense that a parrot can 'speak'. Thought, then, is a necessary forerunner to language if language is to be used properly.

Contrary to Piaget's view that thought structures language, Luria and Yudovich suggest that language plays a central role in cognitive development (Box 18.7).[52]

Box 18.7 The Russian twins[52]

Luria and Yudovich studied 5-year-old twin boys whose home environment was unstimulating. They played almost exclusively together and had only a very primitive level of speech. The boys received little adult encouragement to speak and made little progress towards the symbolic use of words. Essentially, their speech was *synpraxic*, a primitive form in which words cannot be detached from the action or object they denote.

The twins hardly ever used speech to describe objects or events or to help them plan their actions. They could not understand other people's speech, and their own speech constituted a kind of signalling rather than a symbolic system.

Although the boys never played with other children, and they played with each other in only a primitive and repetitive way, they were otherwise normal.

After the twins were separated, one twin was given special remedial treatment for his language deficiency, but the other was not. The former made rapid progress and, 10 months later, was ahead of his brother. However, both twins made progress and their synpraxic speech died away. For Luria and Yudovich:

> **The whole structure of the mental life of both twins was simultaneously and sharply changed. Once they acquired an objective language system, [they] were able to formulate the aims of their activity verbally, and after only three months we observed the beginnings of meaningful play.**

THOUGHT AND LANGUAGE AS INITIALLY SEPARATE ACTIVITIES

For Vygotsky, language is by far the most important psychological tool the human species possesses, capable of transforming how we think about the world and altering 'the entire flow and structure of mental functions'.[53] So, while for Piaget thought is prior to language (the development of representational thinking enables the child to use words), Vygotsky sees language as prior to thought (developing the ability to use words makes representational thought possible).[54]

According to Vygotsky, language and thought begin as separate and independent activities.[55] Early on, thinking occurs without language (consisting primarily of images) and language occurs without thought (as when babies cry or make other sounds to express feelings, attract attention or fulfil some other social aim). But at about age 2 years, *prelinguistic thought* and *pre-intellectual language* '... meet and join to initiate a new kind of behaviour [in which] thought becomes verbal and speech rational' (Figure 18.3).[55]

Vygotsky believed that between the ages of 2 years and 7 years, language performs two functions:

- An *internal* function, which enables internal thought to be monitored and directed
- An *external* function, which enables the results of thinking to be communicated to others.

However, children cannot distinguish between the two functions and, as a result, their speech is *egocentric* (Box 18.8): they talk out loud about their plans and actions, and they can neither think privately nor communicate publicly to others. Instead, they are caught somewhere between the two and cannot distinguish between 'speech for self' (what Piaget calls *autistic speech*) and 'speech for others' (*socialized speech*).

Vygotsky believed that around age 7 years (when children typically enter Piaget's *concrete operational stage* of cognitive development: see Chapter 8), overt language begins to be restricted to communication, while the thought function of language becomes internalized as *internal speech* (*verbal thought*). For Piaget, egocentric speech is a kind of 'running commentary' on the child's behaviour. At about age 7 years, it simply fades away and is replaced by socialized (or communicative) speech.

Box 18.8 The function of egocentric speech

When 6- and 7-year-olds are trying to solve a problem and something goes wrong (e.g. a pencil breaking, which requires them to revise their thinking), they often revert to overt verbalization.[55] Adults sometimes do the same in similar situations, especially when they believe no one can hear them. For example, we often retrace our steps out loud (e.g. 'Now, I know I didn't have it when I went in the room, so what did I do before that?').

Vygotsky concluded that the function of egocentric speech was similar to that of inner speech. It does not merely accompany the child's activity but

> **'... serves mental orientation, conscious understanding; it helps in overcoming difficulties, it is speech for oneself, intimately and usefully connected with the child's thinking. In the end it becomes inner speech ...' [Figure 18.4].[55]**

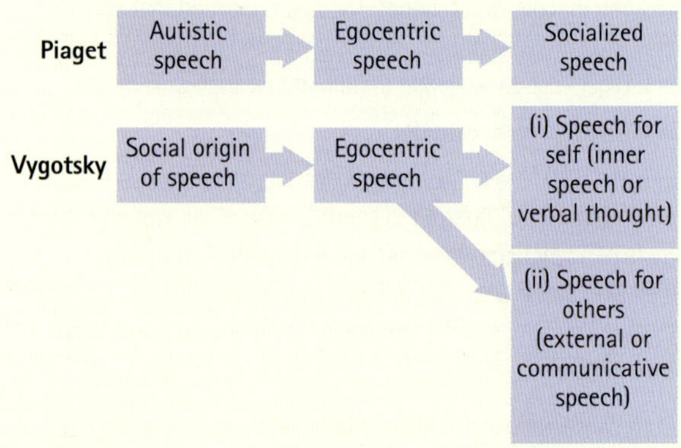

Figure 18.4 Difference between Piaget and Vygotsky with respect to egocentric speech

An evaluation of Vygotsky's position

A considerable body of research into inner speech has largely supported Vygotsky's account, demonstrating how closely language and thought become intertwined during development.[54]

Egocentric speech commonly accompanies problem-solving, even in young children. But with increasing age, egocentric speech becomes less and less audible, eventually becoming silent. For example, Bivens and Berk observed 6- and 7-year-olds as they worked on maths problems.[56] This was repeated 1 and 2 years later. The overall incidence of egocentric speech was extremely high and remained high over the 3 years of observation, but task-relevant speech increased greatly and the nature of the speech changed: there was more inaudible muttering and lip movements. These changes were paralleled by the children's greater ability to inhibit extraneous movements and restlessness and to pay closer attention to the task. This is consistent with Vygotsky's belief that inner speech is used increasingly to aid the child's self-regulation/self-control (Box 18.9).[54]

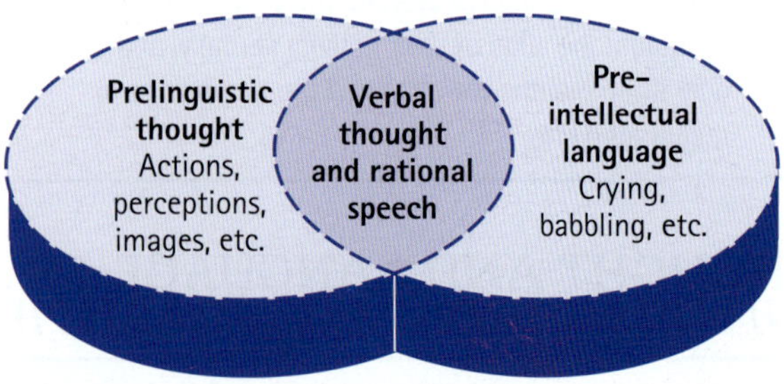

Figure 18.3 Diagrammatic representation of Vygotsky's views on the relationship between language and thought

Box 18.9 Language and self-regulation

According to Luria, a colleague and supporter of Vygotsky, there are three stages in children's ability to use language for directing their behaviour:[57]

1 Up to about age 3 years, another person's verbal instructions can trigger but not inhibit an action. For example, given a rubber bulb to squeeze, children will correctly squeeze in response to 'Squeeze!', but 'Stop!' will simply make them squeeze again.

2 Around 4–5 years, the child responds to instructions in an impulsive way: told to squeeze when a light comes on, the child squeezes repeatedly. The child is responding more to the energizing quality of speech than to its content (the louder the instructions, the more often the child squeezes).

3 After about 5 years, the child responds to the contents of speech and becomes capable of using it to inhibit or activate their behaviour.

Both inner speech and egocentric speech differ from speech for others in that they do not have to satisfy grammatical conventions. Thus, both are abbreviated, incomplete, and concerned more with the essential meaning rather than how the meaning is expressed. For Vygotsky, inner speech is a 'dynamic, shifting and unstable thing which "flutters" between word and thought' (see Figure 18.3).

Overt speech can sometimes resemble inner speech in its abbreviated nature, long after egocentric speech has been replaced. For example, people who know each other well may talk in an abbreviated form that they would not use with strangers. Understanding occurs because, the more familiar we are with others, and the more experiences we have in common, the less explicit our speech has to be. 'Coffee?', for example, asked with a rising inflection and in a particular context, would be interpreted as 'Would you like a cup of coffee?' This is similar to how adults interpret the holophrastic speech of young children. In Bernstein's terms, we use restricted code when talking in familiar surroundings to familiar others, whose view of the world we assume is similar to our own.

CONCLUSIONS

Although there are many examples indicating that thought can occur without language, the exact relationship between thought and language remains unclear. What is certain, however, is that no one account of this relationship is true, with all others being false; several theoretical perspectives can claim some support from the experimental literature. However, since language represents such a central feature of culture, both shaping it and being shaped by it, any theory that fails to take account of cultural factors is likely to be inadequate.

KEY POINTS`

- According to Watson's peripheralism, thought is no more than sensations produced by tiny movements of the larynx, too small to produce audible sounds. Although these movements accompany thought, they are not necessary for thinking to occur.
- Contrary to Watson's view, thinking can occur despite complete paralysis, and people who are born deaf and mute are also capable of thinking.
- Bruner argues that language is essential for thought and knowledge to progress beyond the enactive and iconic modes of representation to the symbolic mode.
- Social constructionists claim that conceptual frameworks and categories provide meaning within a culture, a way of structuring our experience of ourselves and the world.
- According to the Sapir–Whorf LRH, language determines how we think about objects and events, and even what we think. This is related to linguistic determinism.
- The 'weak' and 'weakest' versions of the LRH have typically been tested through perception and memory of colour. The fewer colour words there are in a language, the more difficult native speakers should find tests of colour perception and memory.
- Early studies seemed to support these two versions. But although cultures may differ in the number of basic colour terms they use, all cultures draw their colour terms from only 11 focal colours, which emerge in a particular sequence in the history of languages.
- Whorf's evidence was anecdotal rather than empirical, and he exaggerated the differences between Hopi and other languages. Also, he mistakenly equated language's grammar with perceptual experience. Translation between languages implies a universally shared knowledge of the world independent of any particular language.
- Bernstein claimed that working-class children speak a restricted code and middle-class children an elaborated code. The relationship between actual and potential intelligence is mediated through language, so working-class children are prevented from developing their full intellectual potential.
- Differences between standard and Black English have resulted in the latter being called substandard rather than non-standard. According to Labov, this is an expression of prejudice.
- Black children may be bilingual, using the accepted register fluently at home and with their peers, but adopting unfamiliar standard English in the classroom.
- According to Piaget, language 'maps' on to previously acquired cognitive structures, so that language is dependent on thought. Words can be understood only if certain intellectual skills (e.g. object permanence, conservation) have already been mastered.
- For Vygotsky, language and thought are initially separate and independent activities. At around age 2 years, prelinguistic thought and pre-intellectual language begin to interact to form verbal thought and rational speech.

- Between the ages of 2 years and 7 years, language performs both internal and external functions. The child's failure to distinguish between them results in egocentric speech. For Vygotsky, this indicates the separation of the two functions.
- According to both Vygotsky and Luria, language plays a vital role in self-regulation and self-control.

REFERENCES

1. Weiskrantz L (1988) *Thought Without Language*. Oxford: Oxford University Press.
2. Gross R (2009) *Themes, Issues and Debates in Psychology*, 3rd edn. London: Hodder Education.
3. Watson JB (1913) Psychology as the behaviourist views it. *Psychological Review* **20**: 158–77.
4. Smith EM, Brown HO, Torman JEP, Goodman LS (1947) The lack of cerebral effects of D-tubo-curarine. *Anaesthesiology* **8**: 1–14.
5. Furth HG (1966) *Thinking Without Language*. New York: Free Press.
6. Bruner JS (1983) *Child's Talk: Learning to Use Language*. Oxford: Oxford University Press.
7. Gross R (2005) *Psychology: The Science of Mind and Behaviour*, 5th edn. London: Hodder Arnold.
8. Gergen KJ (1973) Social psychology as history. *Journal of Personality and Social Psychology* **26**: 309–20.
9. Wittgenstein L (1921) *Tractatus Logico-Philosophicus*. London: Routledge.
10. Sapir E (1929) The study of linguistics as a science. *Language*, **5**: 207–14.
11. Whorf BL (1956) *Language, Thought and Reality*. Cambridge, MA: MIT Press.
12. Greene J (1975) *Thinking and Language*. London: Methuen.
13. Miller GA, McNeill D (1969) Psycholinguistics. In G Lindzey, E Aronson (eds) *The Handbook of Social Psychology*, Vol. 3. Reading, MA: Addison-Wesley.
14. Carroll JB, Casagrande JB (1958) The function of language classifications in behaviour. In EE Maccoby, TM Newcombe, EL Hartley (eds) *Readings in Social Psychology*, 3rd edn. New York: Holt, Rinehart and Winston.
15. Brown R, Lenneberg EH (1954) A study in language and cognition. *Journal of Abnormal Psychology* **49**: 454–462.
16. Lenneberg EH, Roberts JM (1956) *The Language of Experience, Memoir 13*. Bloomington, IN: University of Indiana, Publications in Anthropology and Linguistics.
17. Carmichael L, Hogan P, Walter A (1932) An experimental study of the effect of language on the reproduction of visually perceived forms. *Journal of Experimental Psychology* **15**: 1–22.
18. Brown JA (1958) Some tests of the decay theory of immediate memory. *Quarterly Journal of Experimental Psychology* **10**: 12–21.
19. Berlin B, Kay P (1969) *Basic Colour Terms: Their Universality and Evolution*. Berkeley, CA: University of California Press.
20. Newstead S (1995) Language and thought: the Whorfian hypothesis. *Psychology Review* **1**: 5–7.
21. Heider E, Oliver D (1972) The structure of the colour space in naming and memory for two languages. *Cognitive Psychology* **3**: 337–54.
22. Heider E (1972) Universals in colour naming and memory. *Journal of Experimental Psychology* **93**: 10–20.
23. Lakoff G (1987) *Women, Fire and Dangerous Things: What Categories Reveal about the Mind*. Chicago, IL: University of Chicago Press.
24. Bornstein MH (1988) Perceptual development across the life-cycle. In MH Bornstein, ME Lamb (eds) *Perceptual, Cognitive and Linguistic Development*. Hove: Lawrence Erlbaum Associates.
25. Ross PE (2004) Draining the language out of colour. *Scientific American* **290**: 24–5.
26. Robertson D, Davidoff J, Davies IRL, Shapiro LR (2005) Colour categories: evidence for the cultural relativity hypothesis. *Cognitive Psychology* **50**: 378–411.
27. Robertson D, Davies IRL, Davidoff J (2000) Colour categories are not universal: replications and new evidence from a Stone-age culture. *Journal of Experimental Psychology, General* **129**: 369–398.
28. Berry JW, Poortinga YH, Segall MH, Dasen PR (1992) *Cross-Cultural Psychology*. Cambridge: Cambridge University Press.
29. Jackendoff R (1993) *Patterns in the Mind: Language and Human Nature*. Hemel Hempstead: Harvester Wheatsheaf.
30. Pinker S (1997) *How the Mind Works*. New York: Norton.
31. Pagel M (1995) Speaking your mind. *Times Higher Educational Supplement*, 7 July: 17–18.
32. Baddeley AD (1999) *Essentials of Human Memory*. Hove: Psychology Press.
33. Solso RL (1995) *Cognitive Psychology*, 4th edn. Boston, MA: Allyn & Bacon.
34. Crooks RL, Stein J (1991) *Psychology: Science, Behaviour and Life*, 2nd edn. London: Holt, Rinehart and Winston.
35. Price WF, Crapo RH (1999) *Cross-Cultural Perspectives in Introductory Psychology*, 3rd edn. Belmont, CA: Wadsworth Publishing Co.
36. Hunt E, Agnoli A (1991) The Whorfian hypothesis: a cognitive psychological perspective. *Psychological Review* **98**: 377–89.
37. Stones E (1971) *Educational Psychology*. London: Methuen.
38. Bernstein B (1961) Social class and linguistic development: a theory of social learning. In AH Halsey J Floyd, CA Anderson (eds) *Education, Economy and Society*. London: Collier-Macmillan.
39. Hess RD, Shipman V (1965) Early experience and the

socialization of cognitive modes in children. *Child Development* **36**: 860–86.
40. Labov W (1973) The boundaries of words and their meanings. In CJN Bailey, RW Shuy (eds) *New Ways of Analyzing Variations in English*. Washington, DC: Georgetown University Press.
41. Rebok GW (1987) *Life Span Cognitive Development*. New York: Holt, Rinehart and Winston.
42. Bereiter C, Engelman S (1966) *Teaching Disadvantaged Children in the Pre-School*. Englewood Cliffs, NJ: Prentice-Hall.
43. Labov W (1970) The logic of non-standard English. In F Williams (ed.) *Language and Poverty*. Chicago, IL: Markham.
44. Hiscock J (1996) Schools recognize 'Black English'. *Daily Telegraph*, 21 December: 12.
45. Whittel G (1996) Black American slang wins place in classroom. *The Times*, 21 December: 11.
46. Zinberg DS (1997) Ebonics unleashed tongues. *Times Higher Education Supplement*, 14 February: 14.
47. Cornwell T (1997) Board tones down Ebonics policy. *Times Educational Supplement*, 31 January: 14.
48. Hawkes N (1998) Tongue-twisters. *The Times*, 23 February: 15.
49. Piaget J (1950) *The Psychology of Intelligence*. London: Routledge & Kegan Paul.
50. Piaget J, Inhelder B (1969) *The Psychology of the Child*. London: Routledge & Kegan Paul.
51. Sinclair-de-Zwart H (1969) Developmental psycholinguistics. In D Elkind, J Flavell (eds) *Handbook of Learning and Cognitive Processes*, Vol. 5. Hillsdale, NJ: Lawrence Erlbaum Associates.
52. Luria AR, Yudovich FI (1971) *Speech and the Development of Mental Processes in the Child*. Harmondsworth: Penguin.
53. Vygotsky LS (1981) The genesis of higher mental functions. In JV Wertsch (ed.) *The Concept of Activity in Soviet Psychology*. Armonk, NY: Sharpe.
54. Schaffer HR (2004) *Introducing Child Psychology*. Oxford: Blackwell.
55. Vygotsky LS (1962 [1934]) *Thought and Language*. Cambridge, MA: MIT Press.
56. Bivens JA, Berk LA (1990) A longitudinal study of the development of elementary school children's private speech. *Merrill-Palmer Quarterly* **36**: 443–63.
57. Luria AR (1961) *The Role of Speech in the Regulation of Normal and Abnormal Behaviour*. New York: Liveright.

Chapter 19

Personality

John Green and Georgina Smith

INTRODUCTION

The concept of personality is an everyday one. People seem to have distinct ways of behaving towards the world that are characteristic of them. Some people appear cheerful, others morose; some seem warm, others cold and distant. The concept of personality disorder is an important one in clinical practice. However, it has proved remarkably difficult for personality researchers to reach a consensus on how personality is structured, how important it is in everyday life and even what it is.

Various attempts have been made to define personality. Carver and Scheier suggested: 'Personality is a dynamic organization, inside the person, of psychophysical systems that create a person's characteristic patterns of behaviour, thoughts, and feelings.[1] The *Diagnostic and Statistical Manual of Mental Disorders*, 4th edition (DSM-IV) states that personality is 'enduring patterns of perceiving, relating to, and thinking about the environment and oneself that are exhibited in a wide range of social and personal contexts'.[2] The central idea is that an individual's behaviour is not driven solely by their environment but is influenced across situations by something characteristic of them personally.

There are some immediate difficulties with the idea of personality. First, there is huge disagreement about what personality is, with a range of startlingly different theories and explanations as to how it arises. Disturbingly, it is known that our subjective belief in personality is, at least in part, misleading. If we see you at a party telling jokes and ask you why, then you are likely to respond with a reason such as 'To make people laugh', 'To break the ice' or 'Because it is a good way to get to know people'. If, on the other hand, we point out someone else at the party who is telling jokes and ask you why they are doing that, then you are much more likely to respond with a description that calls on their personality, such as 'He's a funny man', 'He's a real extrovert' or 'He's always like that'. In other words, we tend to explain our own behaviour as reasoned but attribute that of others to enduring personal characteristics consistent across situations – that, is to their personality. This effect has been called the 'fundamental attribution error' and, more recently, the 'correspondence bias'; it arises, in large part at least, because we have access to our own thoughts and motives but not to those of others.[3,4] The tendency to see people in terms of personality is compounded by an erroneous tendency to believe that certain characteristics cluster together (e.g. warm and generous, old and wise) and our tendency to use these 'representations' in our dealings with others.[5,6]

Approaches to the study of personality have tended to take one of two approaches, which Allport called the nomothetic approach and the idiographic approach.[7]

Nomothetic approaches assume that everyone has the same basic elements to their personality but that they differ from each other in how strongly each of those elements are represented. So, if we believe that every human being has a sense of humour but that some people have a strong sense of humour while others have a weak sense of humour, then we are taking a nomothetic approach to personality. However, many theories of personality are not primarily nomothetic. If we believe that a person can have unique characteristics or that some people have characteristics that many others do not have, then that is an idiographic theory. It is possible to believe that some people are greedy and some are not: they are not just low on greediness – rather, they lack greediness altogether. For the latter category, measuring the greed level makes as much sense as measuring the colour of water. What makes the distinction particularly important is in our assumptions about measuring personality. Under a nomothetic approach, it is possible, at least in theory, to identify the key personality dimensions common to every person, and to measure where an individual lies on each of these dimensions using a standardized questionnaire or observation system; the information obtained will allow us to completely describe a person's personality. With an idiographic approach, we cannot specify in advance which dimensions will be important to any individual. With a nomothetic approach to personality, each person is unique in the combination of amounts of particular personality elements they happen to have; with an idiographic approach, people differ in personality because they have different elements to their personality.

In areas where personality is an important concept, for instance in personnel selection and in clinical practice, people tend to act as though personality is made up of a mixture of nomothetic and idiographic elements. Many personality theorists, including Allport, accept that personality is made up of both elements. Nonetheless, the distinction is a useful and helpful one in thinking about personality.

In order to illustrate some of these issues, we will first look at three different personality models and then look at some of the overall issues in personality theory. The three types of model we will look at are *trait models*, *humanistic approaches* and *cognitive approaches*. There are other theories that merit attention, particularly the psychoanalytical model, but we have chosen these three models because they illustrate key general issues. For the reader who wishes to look more widely at the area, there are a number of excellent textbooks that provide overviews of the field (e.g. Larsen and Buss[8] and Ryckman[9]).

TRAIT MODELS

Trait models are perhaps the personality models that most closely resemble what might be called 'natural' theories of personality – the way that we see others in everyday life. They are nomothetic theories par excellence seeking to identify traits, enduring dimensions of personality shared by everyone, and then distinguishing between individuals by measuring the amounts of each of these traits that an individual has. Trait theorists make a number of general assumptions: that traits are relatively stable over time, that their levels differ among individuals, and that they influence behaviour. People are expected to have unique combinations of scores on the different dimensions. Critical to understanding trait theories is to understand that they are based on a particular statistical technique, factor analysis. The strengths and weaknesses of trait theory are ultimately derived from the strengths and weaknesses of factor analysis.

Trait theories have a long history. Hippocrates (460–377BC) was an early trait theorist. He suggested that humans have four basic humors and that the amount of each determines an individual's personality.

One of the best known modern trait models is that of Cattell.[10] Cattell assembled a very large number of questionnaire items thought to measure aspects of personality. He then administered these to large numbers of respondents. The problem was to identify common elements within this large body of items. Some items were clearly measuring the same underlying concept, so that if an individual scored highly on item A, then they would be very likely to score highly on item B – that is, their scores would be strongly correlated. Cattell used factor analysis to reduce a large number of items to a small number of overall dimensions and to identify which items best measured those overall dimensions.

Cattell came up with 16 factors. A widely used questionnaire derived from his factor analyses is called the 16PF (PF = personality factor). He also looked at personality by using ratings by observers of actual behaviour using a similar approach, and got a good overlap on 12 of the 16 factors with the questionnaire approach. He tried to use specially designed tasks as a third check, but with rather less satisfactory results.[10]

However, factor analysis is a modelling technique. Unlike statistical tests of significance, there is no single correct answer. In fact, there are, in theory, an almost infinite number of possible answers to the question 'What factors underlie this dataset?' The answer will also differ according to whether one assumes that different personality dimensions must be wholly uncorrelated or whether some degree of correlation occurs between different underlying traits.

By making different assumptions, Cattell was able to derive a smaller number of second-order factors. These can be regarded as higher-level classifications. The easiest way to understand this is by analogy. The cat *Felis silvestris catus* can be classified as a member of the species *F. sylvestris*, as a member of the genus *Felis*, as a Felid, as a carnivore, and so on. Each of these levels is correct, but they all address somewhat different questions.

The most studied alternative model is that of Eysenck.[11,12] Eysenck also used a pool of questionnaire items. He derived two independent uncorrelated main dimensions, introversion–extroversion and neuroticism. High neuroticism scorers tend to be high in anxiety and depression (e.g. Weinstock and Whisman[13]) rather than necessarily attracting a neurotic-spectrum diagnosis. Later, Eysenck added a third factor, psychoticism. The name of the latter factor is unfortunate: high scorers seem to be eccentric or unsocialized rather than psychotic per se, and the label generated some controversy.[8]

Eysenck produced a questionnaire called the Eysenck Personality Questionnaire (EPQ),[14] which measured all three items as well as including a 'lie scale'. This was originally intended to identify people who were trying to 'fake good' on the questionnaire – in other words, to appear 'better' than they were in reality. In fact, it seems to measure social acceptability, the tendency of some respondents to questionnaires to give socially acceptable answers rather than seeking to deliberately mislead. Eysenck also viewed intelligence as a key characteristic of the individual. There have been differences of opinion among personality theorists about whether intelligence should be viewed as a personality dimension or something separate.

Eysenck's personality dimensions match up rather well with Cattell's second-order factors, the two most important of which are exvia–invia, roughly introversion–extroversion, and anxiety. It is possible to argue that they are tapping similar key underlying dimensions. However, the exact structure of personality suggested by the two workers remains markedly different at lower levels of their models.

Eysenck believed that his main factors would reflect underlying biological differences between individuals. For instance, he believed that extroverts would differ from introverts in their degree of brain arousal, specifically differing in the balance of inhibition and excitation of the brain by the ascending reticular activating system. In order to test this hypothesis, a number of studies compared introverts with extroverts on physiological measures gathered under conditions of various degrees of stimulation (e.g. Gale[15]). In addition, neuroticism, Eysenck thought, was related to autonomic nervous system lability, and he tentatively suggested that psychoticism might be related to hormone levels, particularly androgens. The evidence in favour of these various propositions has been very mixed, and most modern researchers would take the view that these hypotheses are, at best, oversimplifications.

More recently, there has been an emerging consensus on a five-factor personality model often nicknamed 'the big five model' (e.g. John,[16] McCrae and John,[17] Saucier and Goldberg[18]). This includes the higher-order factors from both Eysenck and Cattell. The factors are extroversion, agreeableness (warmth *v.* cold), conscientiousness, emotional stability (Eysenck's neuroticism) and intellect/openness to experience (a mix of intelligence and imaginativeness). The convergence of different models at higher levels on these factors, particularly extroversion, emotional stability and intelligence, does suggest that there are underlying measurable traits, but it does not tell us how important these are in absolute terms as determinants of behaviour.

Trait theories have more or less replaced the older type theories. Trait theories assume, for instance, that extroversion and introversion are points on a continuum, while type theories (e.g. Jung and Hull[19]) take the view that some people are one and some the other. Although type theories attract little attention these days, they form the basis for some standardized measures, for instance the Myers–Briggs type indicator still sometimes used in personnel selection and similar applications. Perhaps the most recent type theory to reach prominence was in the 1950s, when Friedman and colleagues suggested that a particular personality type, 'type A', was associated with a higher risk of coronary heart disease than 'type B'.[20] Although subsequent research has not always upheld this proposition, the concept has passed into popular speech.

COGNITIVE MODELS – KELLY'S CONSTRUCT THEORY

Many people thinking about personality take a different perspective from trait theorists. Perhaps the strongest alternative approach is that emphasizing cognition. Instead of people's behaviour being determined by underlying traits, it is determined by how they construe particular situations, their characteristic ways of thinking about the world and how they interpret particular situations. Many therapists favour cognitive models. They do not necessarily deny the existence of traits, but they are less interested in them because they see them as being difficult to change. Cognitions, however, are theoretically and practically changeable. Cognitive-behavioural therapy (CBT) is based on a model that emphasizes the importance of thoughts, perceptions and feelings as determinants of behaviour.

Unfortunately, there is no single model of cognition underlying CBT, partly because CBT therapists tend to be more interested in changing behaviour and symptoms than in personality per se. Static personality factors – those less susceptible to change – are of little interest to most therapists. CBT therapists have also tended to concentrate narrowly on particular aspects of cognition relevant to the condition they are treating, such as anxious thoughts, rather than trying to derive some overall model of personality.

Kelly's personal construct theory[21] is included here mainly because it shows the characteristics of a fully formed cognitive model (see Fransella[22] for a more recent summary). Although this theory enjoyed considerable attention in the past as a basis for therapy, the rise of CBT and the somewhat weak therapeutic results[23] have led to its relative eclipse. A technique for measuring personality derived from it, the repertory grid,[21,24] attracted a great deal of interest, but again its utility, consistency and reliability proved disappointing in practice. Nonetheless, it illustrates how such models work and their potential limitations.

Kelly's view was that the way we behave is fundamentally determined by how we perceive the world and how we have learnt to react to it. In fact, most of our cognitive structures are learnt. It is not a necessary tenet of trait theories that traits are innate or biologically determined; however, they are usually assumed to be so. Kelly, however, was clear not only that our perceptions of the world and our responses to it could change but also that we were constantly monitoring the effectiveness of our view of the world by predicting and then seeing whether those predictions come true. The model is that of 'humans as scientists', and Kelly suggested that we are all, to an extent, scientists acting on the world and getting feedback from it, on the basis of which we change our cognitive structures. Kelly believed that one source of psychopathology was a situation where cognitive structures did not fit the needs of particular situations or where they were positively harmful. Specifically, for Kelly, these were where a person's constructs were such that they could not adequately monitor feedback from the world or where the structures were in such a mess or so rigid that they could not be changed easily in response to feedback that they were inadequate. These are propositions that most modern CBT therapists would have no difficulty with, although they might disagree greatly with the details of his theory.

Kelly envisaged cognitive structures as being hierarchical bipolar constructs, such as warm–cold. If we have this construct, he said, then we see people as either warm or cold. There are no degrees of constructs, only either/or. However, constructs such as warm–cold do not exist in isolation but are linked hierarchically and laterally to other constructs and, taken together, we are able to utilize structures made out of constructs to see gradations in the world, even though the constructs themselves are categorical.

One of the difficulties of this sort of theory is that it is very difficult to fit emotion into it. Kelly himself struggled with the issue and made a number of propositions about how it might be dealt with. However, none of these was very satisfactory. More recently, research has managed to integrate cognition, perception and emotion in a much more effective manner (e.g. investigations into the neural systems underlying human behaviour demonstrate that the mechanisms of emotion and cognition are intertwined from early perception to reasoning[25,26]). At the same time, we understand much more about how perceptions of the world are organized within the brain and how they are turned into action, and it may be that the time is right for another attempt to formulate a cognitive theory of personality.

HUMANISTIC THEORIES

It is exceedingly difficult to pigeonhole humanistic theories of personality or to define exactly what makes a humanistic theory, but they do have a number of features in common. One thing they share is the idea that every person has a unique experience of the world and that to understand their personality it is necessary to understand their experience. Humanistic theories are, thus, idiographic theories par excellence. There is also a strong undercurrent of the idea of the importance of people reaching their full potential. Growth is a key concept, and hence these ideas are represented strongly in areas such as life coaching and self-help organizations. They are also very important in many counselling approaches.

The apotheosis of this view of personality probably comes in Maslow's theory of self-actualization (see Maslow and Hoffman[27]). Life for Maslow was a process of striving to reach the highest level of functioning one can. He viewed humankind as individuals seeking to climb a pyramid of levels of personal integration. The theory concentrates on this process of self-actualization, and people can be located according to their degree of progress towards this fulfilment of human potential.

Probably the most important humanistic theorist, however, was Carl Rogers because his ideas formed the basis of client-centred counselling, a particularly important strand in the counselling movement. For Rogers, personality was about how a person sees themselves, their self-image, and their interactions with others and the world. He saw these things as being unique to the person and, although he had little or no interest in traits, he would probably have regarded these as artificial externally imposed structures. People could grow and change by reflecting on their experiences and, if they were having difficulties, seeing opportunities for alternative ways of looking at things and of living. In order to do this, the therapist had to create an environment in which the client felt able to look at these issues. This environment was best created through 'unconditional positive regard', and the therapist needed to react to the client with empathy, warmth and genuineness. Perhaps the most familiar therapeutic technique was reflecting back to the client important things that they said in order to facilitate their thinking about them and moving forward. This is not simply parroting, but rather the therapist and the client seek to identify and explore important themes in the client's experience. Thus, Rogers' theory is based around therapy and its importance and, essentially, around the idea that the client can heal themselves; it is the main job of the therapist to facilitate this rather than to offer advice.

GENETICS

In recent years, there has been an increasing tendency to try to link traits to underlying genetic factors, whether directly to specific alleles or more generally through twin studies (e.g. Birley *et al.*[28]). While one could imagine an idiographic model of personality being partly determined by genes, in practice most genetic theorists are concerned with the explanation of traits, particularly with the 'big five' traits, although some researchers have sought to identify genetic linkages to other characteristics of the individual such as fearlessness, impulsive non-conformity[29] and even sexual orientation.[30]

Twin studies are the main tool for estimating the probable size of behavioural genetic effects. Summaries of the behavioural genetic data for many of the major personality traits – extroversion, agreeableness, conscientiousness, neuroticism, openness to experiences – yield heritability estimates of around 50 per cent.[31] Studies have also yielded surprisingly large values for genetic components for other traits such as emotionality, sociability, persistence, fear and distractibility.[32] Most studies have found surprisingly low values for familial influences. In twin studies, monozygotic (MZ) twins are compared against dizygotic (DZ) twins and, ideally, non-twin siblings. MZ twins share all their genes and their intrauterine environment, DZ twins share half their genes (if they are the same sex) and their intrauterine environment, and non-twin siblings share half their genes but do not share an intrauterine environment. Most of the information is contained within the MZ–DZ twin contrast. A comparison between the degree of agreement for MZ twins and the degree of agreement for DZ twins allows a calculation of the proportions of the variance in a particular behaviour attributable to genes, shared environment (particularly family and intrauterine environments), and individual developmental history and experience. Furthermore, it is the proposed heritability of personality that is believed to be responsible for the fact that personality traits remain fairly stable over time.[31,33–35]

However, although these studies suggest a genetic influence on personality, possibly a sizeable one, the estimates of the size of such an effect are subject to several possible errors. Twin models make important assumptions about the underlying genes, particularly no dominance effects (interactions between alleles at a single locus), no epistasis (interactions between alleles at different loci), and, ideally, many genes of small effect. These assumptions are very unlikely to be true for every trait. There are also assumptions about the statistical distributions of behaviour and genes. It is assumed that the environment experienced by MZ twins is no more similar than that of DZ twins and, although some evidence is put forward that there are few differences in, for instance, sharing rooms or property, it is not clear how relevant some of these data are to the underlying issue. The difficulty is that if these assumptions are not met, then the effect is, in the main, to inflate the apparent size of the genetic component. The apparent size of familial influences will be reduced.[36]

Much effort has gone into identifying candidate alleles and measuring their association with personality. Unfortunately, to date the outcomes of these studies have often been inconsistent. A good example is the proposed linkage between alleles of the *DRD4* dopamine receptor gene and novelty-seeking behaviour. Early reports were positive, but a more recent meta-analysis was negative.[37] Nonetheless, this approach would seem to be the most promising avenue of research into the impact of genes on personality.

Many researchers hope that genetic studies will cast new light on the underlying structure of personality. Although one would hope that this is true, there is something of a circularity here. In order to accurately identify allelic influences on personality, we have to be able to identify and delineate the aspect of personality that we expect those alleles to affect. If the boundaries of a trait are defined poorly, or we cannot measure it accurately, or we identify a single underlying trait as several traits, or incorrectly combine several underlying traits into a single trait, then we make identifying allelic influences much more difficult. Thus, our uncertainties about the nature of personality are likely to weaken behavioural genetic studies.

PERSONALITY DISORDER

Personality disorder per se is dealt with in Chapter 43. Here we are concerned with the extent to which the idea of personality disorder overlaps with ideas about personality. Personality disorders are treated in DSM-IV and the *International Classification of Diseases*, 10th revision (ICD-10), as typological and idiographic – some people have one, and others do not. It is not possible to have 'a bit of a personality disorder'. However, this may owe more to the need to classify and pigeonhole for diagnostic purposes than to any underlying assumed structure to personality disorder. Research is complicated by our poor understanding of the structure of personality disorder, particularly at the level of the individual disorder, with many patients meeting the criteria for more than one diagnosis. Unlike with axis I disorders, DSM-IV more or less encourages mix-and-match multiple diagnoses. Indeed, the relationship between axis I and axis 2 disorders remains an area of some uncertainty, with many patients at least effectively having both.

It has always been difficult to link personality disorder on to the sorts of theory discussed in this chapter. It would be possible in practice to describe personality disorders in terms of any of the sorts of theory, or none, and it is possible to find just that in the literature. However, most researchers have concentrated on trait approaches, the idea that people with personality disorders might have extreme scores on particular traits or, more likely, some combination of trait scores that account for their condition. Widiger and colleagues describe how extremes on either end of specific trait dimensions can be associated with personality disorders.[38] For example, someone with a combination of high levels of hostility and a lack of trust in others might be disposed to paranoid personality disorder. According to Ball, 'the application of personality trait models to the conceptualization of personality disorders has forged a much needed integration of what were separate areas of study for most of the 20th century'.[39]

A considerable amount of effort has gone into carrying out personality profiling of people with personality disorders over many years, with generally rather disappointing results. However, more recent applications of the 'big five' framework have been more successful, with several studies reporting fair predictive values for 'big five' factors (see Saulsman and Page[40] for a meta-analytical review of the empirical literature). Unfortunately, there has not always been good agreement about what trait patterns predict particular personality disorders, which may owe as much to the weaknesses of diagnostic criteria as to the weaknesses of personality theory.

Existing research is incomplete, and where it will end up is open to speculation. However, the picture does not, to our eye, suggest that personality disorder can be wholly ascribed to some combination of 'big five' traits. Either there is an idiographic component, something that people with personality disorder have or lack that others do not, or some trait or traits outside the 'big five' are important, or it may be impossible to adequately describe personality disorder within a trait framework at all and we may need to look at other possible ways to describe personality.

SUMMARY

Personality has been studied systematically by psychologists for almost 100 years. It is hard not to feel disappointed at the lack of consensus on crucial issues such as what it is and how it is structured. Personality tests were, at one time, used quite widely in clinical practice. They have gradually fallen into disuse in most areas of clinical work (although not in areas such as personnel selection) because they proved of very limited value in determining treatment and in understanding patients' problems. There is now speculation that a five-factor model (FFM) diagnosis would prove to have considerable clinical utility,[38] but, at the time of writing, there have been only four published studies on the use of the FFM by practising clinicians.[41–44] Estimates of the percentage of variance in behaviour accounted for by personality measures are usually low, although there is evidence that interaction between personality and situation may be more important. At one level this is hardly surprising: the behaviour of an individual at a funeral would be likely to be very different from their behaviour at a party, regardless of personality. Weaknesses in current models and measures of personality obviously weaken the ability of personality theorists to predict behaviour. Nonetheless, the acid test of the value of future research into personality will be precisely the extent to which new approaches and new measures are able to predict real-life behaviour.

KEY POINTS

- There is no agreement about what personality is and how it is structured.
- Different theorists have taken radically different approaches to personality.
- In recent years, there has been a growing consensus around a five-factor model of personality.
- Personality usually explains only a small part of the variance of human behaviour.
- Although there has been much interest in possible genetic influences on personality, this is an area with more promise than hard data.
- The link between 'personality' and 'personality disorder' is unclear; the two fields of enquiry have developed more or less separately.

REFERENCES

1. Carver CS, Scheier MF (2000). *Perspectives on Personality*, 4th edn. Boston, MA: Allyn & Bacon.
2. American Psychiatric Association (1994) *Diagnostic and Statistical Manual of Mental Disorders*, 4th edn. Washington, DC: American Psychiatric Association.
3. Ross L (1977) The intuitive psychologist and his shortcomings: distortions in the attribution process. In L Berkowitz (ed.) *Advances in Experimental Social Psychology*. New York: Academic Press.
4. Gilbert DT (1998) Speeding with Ned: a personal view of the correspondence bias. In JM Darley, J Cooper (eds) *Attribution and Social Interaction: The Legacy of E. E. Jones*. Washington, DC: APA Press.
5. Tversky A, Kahneman D (1974). Judgment under uncertainty: heuristics and biases. *Science* **185**: 1124–31.
6. Tversky A (2003) *Preference, Belief and Similarity*. Cambridge, MA: MIT Press.
7. Allport G W (1937) *Personality: A Psychological Interpretation*. New York: Holt, Rinehart and Winston.
8. Larsen RJ, Buss DM (2005) *Personality Psychology: Domains of Knowledge about Human Nature*, 2nd edn. Boston, MA: McGraw-Hill.
9. Ryckman R (2004) *Theories of Personality*. Belmont, CA: Thomson/Wadsworth.
10. Cattell RB (1965) *The Scientific Analysis of Personality*. London: Penguin.
11. Eysenck HJ (1970) *The Structure of Human Personality*. London: Methuen.
12. Eysenck HJ (1981) *A Model for Personality*. Berlin: Springer-Verlag.
13. Weinstock LM, Whisman MA (2006) Neuroticism as a common feature of the depressive and anxiety disorders: a test of the revised integrative hierarchical model in a national sample. *Journal of Abnormal Psychology* **115**: 68–74.
14. Eysenck HJ, Eysenck SB (1972) *Manual of the Eysenck Personality Questionnaire*. San Diego, CA: Educational and Industrial Testing Service.
15. Gale A (1986) Extraversion–introversion and spontaneous rhythms of the brain: retrospect and prospect. In J Strelau, F Farley, A Gale (eds) *The Biological Basis of Personality and Behavior*, Vol. 2. Washington, DC: Hemisphere.
16. John OP (1990) The 'big five' factor taxonomy: dimensions of personality in the natural language and questionnaires. In LA Pervin (ed.) *Handbook of Personality*. New York: Guilford Press.
17. McCrae RR, John OP (1992) An introduction to the five-factor model and its applications. *Journal of Personality* **60**: 175–215.
18. Saucier G, Goldberg LR (1998) What is beyond the big five? *Journal of Personality* **66**: 495–524.
19. Jung CG, Hull RFC (1992) *Psychological Types* (rev. edn). London: Routlege.
20. Friedman HS, Booth-Kewley S (1987) Personality, type A behavior, and coronary heart disease: the role of emotional expression. *Journal of Personality and Social Psychology* **53**: 783–92.
21. Kelly GA (1955) *The Psychology of Personal Constructs*. London: Routledge.
22. Fransella F (2003). *International Handbook of Personal Construct Psychology*. New York: John Wiley & Sons.
23. Holland JS, Neimeyer RA, Currier J, Berman JS (2007) The efficacy of personal construct therapy: a comprehensive review. *Journal of Clinical Psychology* **63**: 93–107.
24. Fransella F, Bannister D (1977). *A Manual for Repertory Grid Technique*. London: Academic Press.
25. Phelps EA (2005) Emotion and cognition: insights from studies of the human amygdala. *Annual Review of Psychology* **57**: 27–53.
26. Rolls ET (2007) *Emotion Explained*. Oxford: Oxford University Press.

27. Maslow AH, Hoffman E (1996) *Future Visions: The Unpublished Papers of Abraham Maslow*. Thousand Oaks, CA: Sage Publications.
28. Birley AJ, Gillespie NA, Heath AC, *et al.* (2006) Heritability and nineteen-year stability of long and short EPQ-R Neuroticism scales. *Personality and Individual Differences* **40**: 737–47.
29. Blonigen DM, Carlson SR, Krueger RF, Patrick CJ (2003) A twin study of self-reported psychopathic personality traits. *Personality and Individual Differences* **35**: 179–97.
30. Bailey JM, Kirk KM, Zhu G, Dunne MP, Martin NG (2000) Do individual differences in sociosexuality represent genetic or environmentally contingent strategies? Evidence from the Australian twin registry. *Journal of Personality and Social Psychology* **78**: 537–45.
31. Caspi A, Roberts BW, Shiner RL (2005). Personality development: stability and change. *Annual Review of Psychology* **56**: 453–8.
32. Oniszczenko W, Zawadzki B, Strelau J, *et al.* (2003) Genetic and environmental determinants of temperament: a comprehensive study based on Polish and German samples. *European Journal of Personality* **17**: 207–20.
33. Blonigen DM, Hicks BM, Krueger RF, Patrick CJ, Iacono WG (2006) Continuity and change in psychopathic traits measures via normal-range personality: a longitudinal-biometric study. *Journal of Abnormal Psychology* **115**: 85–95.
34. Johnson W, McGue M, Krueger RF (2005) Personality stability in late adulthood: a behaviour genetic analysis. *Journal of Personality* **73**: 523–51.
35. Van Beijsterveldt CEM, Bartels M, Hudziak JJ, Boomsma DI (2003) Causes of stability of aggression from early childhood to adolescence: a longitudinal genetic analysis of Dutch twins. *Behavior Genetics* **33**: 591–605.
36. Plomin R, DeFries JC, McClearn GE, McGuffin P (2000) *Behavioural Genetics*, 4th edn. New York: W.H. Freeman.
37. Kluger AN, Siegfried Z, Ebstein RP (2002) A meta-analysis of the association between DRD4 polymorphism and novelty seeking. *Molecular Psychiatry* **7**: 712–17.
38. Widiger TA, Trull TJ, Clarkin JF, Sanderson C, Costa PT, Jr (2002) A description of the DSM-IV personality disorders with the five-factor model of personality. In PT Costa, Jr, TA Widiger (eds) *Handbook of Personality Psychology*. Washington, DC: American Psychological Association.
39. Ball SA (2001) Reconceptualizing personality disorder categories using personality trait dimensions: introduction to special section. *Journal of Personality* **69**: 147–53.
40. Saulsman LM, Page AC (2004) The five-factor model and personality disorder empirical literature: a meta-analytic review. *Clinical Psychology Review* **23**: 1055–85.
41. Blais MA (1997) Clinician ratings of the five-factor model of personality and the DSM-IV personality disorders. *Journal of Nervous and Mental Disease* **185**: 388–93.
42. Samuel DB, Widiger TA (2004) Clinicians' personality descriptions of prototypic personality disorders. *Journal of Personality Disorders* **18**: 286–308.
43. Sprock J (2002) A comparative study of the dimensions and facets of the five-factor model in the diagnosis of cases of personality disorder. *Journal of Personality Disorders* **16**: 402–23.
44. Sprock J (2003) Dimension versus categorical classification of prototypic and nonprototypic cases of personality disorder. *Journal of Clinical Psychology* **59**: 991–1014.

Chapter 20

Social psychology

Raj Persaud

INTRODUCTION: WHY PSYCHIATRISTS ARE SOCIAL PSYCHOLOGISTS TOO

'No man is an island' might be said to be the catchphrase and guiding philosophy of social psychologists. This is the branch of psychology that focuses on how what we do, feel and think is influenced by others. Oftentimes those outside the field find it difficult to discern the precise difference between social psychology and sociology, but as a general rule, although the areas of interest of the two fields often overlap, social psychologists tend to be more quantitative and to deploy more experimental methods.[1]

Since medicine frequently involves interactions between people, perhaps most notably between doctors and patients, social psychological theory and findings have much to offer in understanding the outcomes that occur when doctors and patients encounter each other.

As we will see, social psychology has made important contributions to understanding many of the behavioural phenomena with which psychiatrists must grapple daily, such as aggression. It has also been influential in the introduction of new treatment approaches, such as cognitive-behavioural therapy (CBT).

SOCIAL PSYCHOLOGY AND AGGRESSION

Social psychology has been seen as productive in understanding many of the phenomena that psychiatrists must deal with clinically. Perhaps one of the most famous examples is aggression.

The traditional Freudian view of aggression is that this arises out of inner drives. For example, a child's unconscious desire to possess the opposite-sex parent sexually inevitably elicits aggression to the other, same-sex parent, who is now perceived as a threat.

A later theory was the frustration–aggression hypothesis produced by John Dollard, an anthropologist/sociologist based at Yale who suggested that it is not only the inner drive that needs to be studied but also the idea that aggression occurs when that drive is frustrated by an environmental obstacle, which then generates exasperation. Wherever you saw aggression, if you dug deeper you would find a frustrated goal. Simplistic though this theory is now perceived as being, it is still more sophisticated than many lay views of aggression. Consider, for example, modern media theorizing about the causes of terrorism.

The frustration–aggression theory was more complex than even this simplistic summary, because the two elements in the system appeared to act synergistically. Frustration generated aggression, while the aggressive drive was also more likely to be frustrated.

However, the proposal suffered from the neglect that many people are frustrated but not all turn to aggression, and so inhibition mechanisms combined with individual variability were relatively ignored aspects of the whole aggression story.

At least with the development of the frustration–aggression hypothesis, the environment entered academic thinking about the causes of aggression as opposed to the more inner-world theorizing of the psychoanalytical view.

Albert Bandura, a social psychologist based at Stanford University, pioneered one of the ultimate developments of inputting the environment into the genesis of aggression, and moving away from purely internal mechanisms, with his famous 'social learning' theory.

Hostility, like most other behaviours, is viewed as learned from the environment. This theory posits that, for learning to occur, suitable opportunities for witnessing similar behaviours must pertain, and reinforcing conditions must also be involved, so allowing the behaviour to be mimicked and produced again and again.

Social learning would be the background theory on which ideas that television, film and video games contribute to increased aggression in viewers are based. This is because the theory emphasizes just how easily we are influenced by others. Reinforcement might be subtle, in the form of identification with role models and admired others, leading to the expectation of increased status amongst peers if aggression is exhibited.

Social learning is not a pure behaviourist theory, which would instead rely on the environment as the sole shaper of behaviour. Instead, Bandura's view was that 'reciprocal determinism' occurred. Others' as well as your own behaviour becomes an environmental influence. You shape the environment, which in turn moulds you. Behaviourism tends to see us as passive recipients of influence rather than active contributors to the transforming effect of our world.

SOCIAL PSYCHOLOGICAL THEORIES ABOUT RELATIONSHIPS

Social learning theory appears to be a modern link between behaviourist and contemporary cognitive learning theories, because it invokes cognitive routes such as attention, memory and motivation in order to explain the chain of internal or mental processes that mediate between an environmental stimulus and its ability to influence a person's eventual behaviour.

Similar theories in social psychology that appear to have their roots in stimulus–reward behaviourism include social exchange theory. This posits that one key way of thinking about relationships and why they occur, as well as why they end or how long they endure, is that relationships are sources of rewards and costs. Tangible benefits of relationships include material compensations, such as a father extending a loan to his son, as well as less tangible compensations, such as attention, approval and status.

According to social exchange theory, we engage in relationships very much with a sense of this exchange. Some people give much of themselves and make sacrifices in their relationships, but they do so in order to obtain something from others. The theory suggests that the benefits we gain from, and the sacrifices we make for, relationships must evolve into some kind of equilibrium in terms of the value we place on what we gain and invest for relationships to endure. The theory could be criticized as relying on people to constantly and rationally self-interestedly determine the cost–benefit pros and cons of all their relationships.

This perspective appears to be based on a view that we see others as means to our ends as opposed to being reinforced just by having relationships in themselves. Also, it does not appear to leave much room for altruism.

Social psychologists might be forgiven for being somewhat cynical about concepts such as altruism following their intensive investigation of why a large crowd of people can witness another person being criminally attacked and yet not intervene to help. The research literature began after a famous case where numerous bystanders failed to assist a victim of serious crime – Kitty Genovese – who was supposedly stabbed to death in 1964 in front of numerous witnesses who failed to offer her assistance. Since then, the phenomenon has been referred to as the 'bystander effect'.

The social psychological research finds that, paradoxically, the larger a group witnessing a crime or a person needing assistance, the less likely any one individual within that group is to take it upon themselves to intervene. The most popular theory to explain this finding is the 'diffusion of responsibility' effect, whereby if you are alone witnessing a crime you tend to feel more personally responsible if nothing is done, in comparison with how you feel if others are around and similarly doing nothing.

Another social psychological factor could be group influence. We view the inertia or otherwise of others as determining our assessment of what is going on. Perhaps if no one else is doing anything, then we have misread the predicament and the serious injury that we appear to be witnessing is not really occurring.

The bystander effect is a good example of social psychology in action – it reveals that our behaviour is governed by complex processes involving the impact of others combined with how we are thinking about other people and what they would think about us.

SOCIAL PSYCHOLOGY OF PERSUASION AND INFLUENCE

Another example of social psychology in action would be in the area of persuasion. Much of the work of healthcare professionals, and perhaps particularly psychiatrists, centres on the art of persuasion. Psychiatrists need to persuade patients to accept treatment or a medical understanding of their experiences, for example hallucinations.

One technique developed from a famous strand of social psychological research is referred to as the 'foot-in-the-door' technique.[2] The experiments follow a particular strand whereby subjects are asked for a small favour, followed later by a much bigger favour. The second request involves much more trouble or sacrifice for the subject. The intriguing finding from social psychology is that you are much more likely to secure agreement to the bigger request if you have presaged it with a smaller one.[3]

So, for example, psychologists might venture into a suburban neighbourhood and ask residents if they would allow a large and ugly poster in support of a local charity or good cause to be displayed at home. Not surprisingly, only a small number of residents might say yes to this request.

In the second condition of the experiment, the psychologists go to a similar neighbourhood but this time ask the residents to sign a petition or wear a small innocuous badge in support of the same charity or good cause. This is such a small task, and therefore a small yes for most people, that they agree to this apparently inconsequential request readily.

Later, the psychologists return to the same neighbourhood and now ask for the large poster, which was usually rejected in the first condition of the experiment, to be hung in the home. However, on this occasion many more people agree to put up the poster, compared with when they were asked without a presaging minor request. The theoretical reasons for why so many more people agree to the large poster after first agreeing to the small badge or favour are many and varied.

One theory is about the idea that, once you start saying yes, it is much more difficult to say no. Another theory is that, having accepted the badge or signed the petition, it does not seem to make sense to reject the poster. People like to be consistent and accepting wearing the badge means that you agreed with the principle of supporting the charity, so why now reject the poster? This is an important social psychological principle, which is that apparent consistency seems to be extremely important to most people. We shall come back to this principle shortly when we explore the issue of cognitive dissonance.

Another interesting idea is that, having said yes to the badge, you identified yourself as a supporter of the charity or good cause and therefore your identity was now tied up with the cause. To reject the large poster was now in conflict with this newly established identity.

By starting with small yeses and building to a bigger one, you are using powerful social psychology that makes it much more likely that you will secure the big yes at the end. Controversy remains in the field about how effective the foot-in-the-door technique would be when dealing with more strongly held opposing views.[3]

An almost opposite social psychological principle appears to be in play in another famous series of experiments, which lead to what is termed the 'door-in-the-face' technique.[4] Here, in marked contrast to the foot-in-the-door approach, the key idea is to elicit a 'no' with your first request. This sets up a situation where paradoxically you appear much more likely to get a 'yes' with the real request that you have been storing up and building up to all along.

These experiments follow a pattern that would be something along the lines of psychological experimenters going into the high street to ask passers-by to donate blood or make a commitment to help with a blood-transfusion drive. In the first condition, the experimenters stop people and ask them, but as usual they get a limited response.

In another condition, the experimenters stop people and ask for big donations or large personal commitments to assist with the blood-transfusion drive. Unsurprisingly, given the large scale of the 'ask', very few people indeed volunteer.

In a third condition of the experiment, they indeed start similarly to the second condition by asking for a large personal commitment to a massive blood-donation drive. But, after this 'big ask' was tried first, upon hearing the refusal, the experimenter says something like: 'OK, we understand this is a big ask but as the blood transfusion truck is just round the corner why not just donate one pint today and we'll forget the other rather demanding scheme?'

Many more people end up giving a pint of blood after they were first asked to give much more than if they were just asked for the pint up front.

Why is this?

One theory is that, in asking for so much more and then scaling down the request, it appeared that the blood transfusion people had made a concession – they had conceded that the first request was too much and were now asking for much less. There is a natural human tendency to reciprocate – that is, once one person has made a concession in a negotiation, it seems only natural to reciprocate with a concession yourself, in this case agreeing to giving a small amount of blood.[4]

Another explanation relies on a 'perceptual contrast' effect, which is that donating a pint of blood does not now seem that big an ask if it were preceded by a much bigger request. The contrast between the two renders the final request appearing much smaller in size.[5]

COGNITIVE DISSONANCE

Returning to the foot-in-the-door technique and the theory that consistency is extremely important to people, this argument has been one of the most productive in social psychology. It has opened up a field referred to as 'cognitive dissonance'.[6]

Cognitive dissonance theory has become one of the most dominant ways of accounting for many otherwise puzzling behavioural phenomena. The key idea behind cognitive dissonance is that we like to think of ourselves as rational, reasonable and consistent beings; therefore, if we come to notice that our performance is at variance with consistency, we will tend to modify our attitudes or behaviour, in order to bring consistency back into the frame. This drive for consistency is so powerful that it can have a massive effect, although an often unconscious one, on our attitudes and behaviour.

The theory is largely the brain child of one of the most famous social psychologists of the twentieth century, Leon Festinger, who came up with the idea following what appeared to him to be a puzzling incident involving rumours following an infamous Indian earthquake of 1934. Festinger noticed that rumours of a worse earthquake to come did not appear to be based on hard evidence or logic but could instead be explained by an idea: that people at an unconscious level needed to consistently account for their high levels of anxiety.[7]

Cognitive dissonance theory has a wide range of applications. For example, as argued by Robert Oxoby,[8] it effectively accounts for the puzzling tendency of people who work in hazardous industries to ignore safety regulations more than people who do not work in such dangerous predicaments. The argument from cognitive dissonance theorists goes something like this: those who toil in a dangerous occupation must experience dissonance between their choice to work in such a perilous area and their understandable fear of injury. Oxoby contends that it is impossible to keep turning up to work with such high anxiety and also to reconcile the idea that you are a rational intelligent person and yet you are making such a decision to put yourself in such danger.[8]

Reducing dissonance in this context takes the form of mentally minimizing the probability of injury in your own mind. Because you resolve the inner conflict by deciding that it is not that dangerous, it is inevitable according to cognitive dissonance theory that people exposed to daily danger will come to reduce the assessment of the risk in their own minds, compared with people who are not so exposed.

Indeed, cognitive dissonance works the other way for people outside the industry.[8] If the industry is well paid, then we who are not working there will reason to ourselves that it makes sense that we do not take these big rewards because it is just too dangerous.

One key flaw with cognitive dissonance theory is that individual variability may not be properly taken account of over the need for consistency, and indeed this drive may often be subsumed under other more pressing needs. Thus, it may be an effect that emerges in the rarefied atmosphere of controlled laboratory conditions but not so much usefully in the more messy real world.

MEASUREMENT OF ATTITUDE

Cognitive dissonance theory hinges not only on the experimental demonstration of behaviour change but also on the ability to measure attitude reliably. Attitudes and their measurement are a cornerstone of social psychological research and have been influential on psychiatric journals as well.

The scientific approach to an attitude and its formal measurement derives from social psychology, where an attitude is measured as a psychological tendency that is expressed by evaluating a particular entity with some degree of favour or disfavour. So, patients prefer a nice waiting room and charming nurses, and this contributes to their 'attitude' to the hospital, clinic or treatment.

Thurstone scales, first developed by Louis Leon Thurstone in 1928, were the first attempt to scientifically measure attitudes, and this derived from first finding a large number of attitudinal statements towards the object being measured, such as attitudes to religion.[9]

One statement might be that 'belief in religion is irrational'. Independent judges are asked to rate the statements in terms of degree of negativity or positivity towards religion. Once there is a convergence in the judges' ratings of these statements in terms of their ranking along a spectrum of positivity and negativity (e.g. the above statement is rated as an extremely negative view), they are put to the population to be tested. Anyone who endorses the above statement is measured as having a very negative attitude to religion.

Several problems arise out of this technique: it is complex statistically and procedurally, and it crucially hinges on the assumption that the judges used for scale construction are similar in outlook to the population intended to be tested.

In contrast to Thurstone scales, the most popular method for measuring attitudes today uses Likert scales.[10] Likert scales involve measuring a person's level of agreement with a statement, so the format of a typical five-level Likert item is: Strongly disagree, Disagree, Neither agree nor disagree, Agree, Strongly agree.

Likert scales suffer from statistical problems when differences between groups are analysed, as not only means but also variances might contrast. There are also problems over recurring patterns of responding, such as central tendency bias, which is a tendency for responses to cluster around the middle of the rating scale offered, and acquiescence bias, which is about the general tendency to agree rather than disagree.

When social psychologists look for correlations between attitudes or possible descriptions, they uncover three basic factors. A factor is a term derived from social statistics and is a hypothetical construct that is supposed to explain real-world outcomes.

So, intelligence quotient (IQ) was a factor that first emerged when statistically examining correlations across a wide range of examination results in school students. It was noticed that some students tended to do well across all subjects, while others tended to do, roughly speaking, equally badly across all subjects.

If your score in mathematics bore no relationship whatsoever to your score in anything else, then a factor could not emerge. But if those students who scored high in maths tended to score high in other subjects, then perhaps something more is going on underneath the data, such as a general cognitive ability factor.

Across attitudes, three general factors appear to emerge: evaluation, potency and activity. Evaluation as a factor loads highest on adjective pairs that are most similar to 'good–bad'. The 'strong–weak' adjective pair defines the potency factor. The adjective pair 'active–passive' defines the activity factor. This factorial structure makes intuitive sense from an evolutionary standpoint.

Osgood's semantic differential technique measures these three factors.[11] It contains sets of adjective pairs such as warm–cold, bright–dark, beautiful–ugly, sweet–bitter, fair–unfair, brave–cowardly and meaningful–meaningless. In questionnaires, these are generally seven steps apart so you can record how close your attitude is to fair or unfair when, for example, your attitude to the National Health Service (NHS) is measured. For example, a scale for rating how a person feels about smoking may include the following:

FOOLISH	−3	−2	−1	0	+1	+2	+3	WISE
PLEASANT	−3	−2	−1	0	+1	+2	+3	UNPLEASANT

Semantic differential scales do not have individualized questions as Likert scales do, and they do not specify mathematically the levels of agreement or disagreement.

There appears to be an evolutionary underpinning to the factors that emerge from attitude scaling. In ancient times, when personal safety was the paramount issue in our minds, when we met someone we did not already know well, and therefore could be sure we knew their personality disposition, there was possibly survival value in a rapid summary analysis of all their readily apparent characteristics.

The most efficient approach would be along the lines of determining instinctively and primarily whether this stranger represented a danger. This translates into modern attitude measurement of the strongly emergent factor of: is the person good or bad? The next: is the person strong or weak? If the stranger is strong and bad, then this is a much more hazardous encounter than if they are weak and bad.

The evaluation, potency and activity factors are key according to Osgood's system to understanding how people's attitudes to another person or a phenomenon are likely to translate into real-world action. If your attitude to a third runway at Heathrow Airport is measured and no difference can be found along the evaluation, potency and activity factors from another person, then, although you may have answered some attitude questions differently, is there an *essential* contrast in your attitude to the third runway that is in any way meaningful in terms of what you might do about it? Factor analysis is a statistical technique that originated in psychometrics.

There are many problems with all these different essentially mathematical and statistical approaches to methods of measuring attitudes, but the generic issue is the relatively low correlations that stubbornly persist between attitude and actual real-world behaviour.

Possible reasons for this include the conundrum that most attitude measurement does not properly consider two crucial social psychological issues. Subjects may be loath to tell you directly what they really think; for example, they may not own up to racist attitudes or stigmatizing attitudes to mental illness, because these are not opinions that are socially acceptable.

Attitudes also make sense only in terms of an appreciation of the implicit trade-offs involved. Charming nurses who have a lot of time to spend with you may not, for example, turn out to be quite so vital to patients when attitudes to this are rated if they understood that this benefit could be bought only at the expense of numbers of nurses.

This more realistic concept of preferences comes from economics, where preferences are defined as individuals' 'utility' for consuming healthcare goods and services. The assumption is that we aim to maximize our utility. Economic theory argues that utilities or benefits can be measured in money-equivalence terms. In other words, the real strength of preferences is the monetary compensation that would leave people indifferent between having a given utility change and not having the change (i.e. willingness to pay or willingness to accept).

If you could be given a money substitute for charming nurses, then how much would compensate you for their absence? This figure in comparison with the monetary value for what you would accept to forgo clean waiting rooms tells us which you really prefer.

The technique currently popular in social psychology that takes this point on board is called 'conjoint analysis'. This assumes that individuals make trade-offs within a resource constraint.[12]

Attitude researchers have also long been sceptical of assuming that our reports of our own attitudes are not tempered by concerns over impression management. So, attitudes towards immoral or illegal behaviour need to be probed in a more sophisticated manner other than just eliciting attitudes on simple scales that measure intensity of evaluation.

Response latency measures are one of the currently favoured approaches. These yield evaluations that are unlikely to be consciously controlled or censored, as pointed out by Laurie Rudman, a social psychologist based at Rutgers University in the USA in a review of attitude measurement.[13] This is because they are taken from reaction time tasks that measure people's attitudes or beliefs indirectly (i.e. without asking people how they feel or think).

That is, people's attention is focused not on the attitude object but on performing an objective task, and attitudes are then inferred from systematic variations in task performance.

For example, in the Implicit Association Test, automatic pro-white bias is indicated when people show faster performance categorizing pleasant words and white people (and unpleasant words and black people) together, compared with categorizing unpleasant words and white people (and pleasant words and black people) together. Thus, implicit attitudes can be characterized as the automatic association people have between an object and evaluation (whether it is good or bad).

IMPRESSION MANAGEMENT

Susan Fiske, Amy Cuddy and Peter Glick based at Princeton University, Northwestern University and Lawrence University, respectively, all in the USA, have published an intriguing outline as to how the key factors that emerge in attitude research are linked with impressions that we create in others and therefore what the most effective way of creating a good impression might be, based on evolutionary theory.[14]

In our evolutionary past, we often met strangers and had to make some key decisions that would determine our future survival. At the heart of these quandaries was the basic issue: does this stranger intend to harm me? A subsidiary question then became: if they do intend to harm me, how likely are they to inflict significant damage?

Another way of thinking about these crucial social decisions that we are probably making at an unconscious level all the time, whenever we encounter someone, is that we are constantly evaluating how 'warm' or otherwise another person is and how 'competent' they are.

Warmth as a quality has particularly vital evolutionary significance, as it translates into an assessment of whether another intends to harm or help us. Competence may seem a slightly strange quality to place so high up on the scale of fundamental assessments that we make of others, but again this has huge evolutionary significance because it relates to the question of whether another has the ability to enact their intentions. There is little real point to a helpful but incompetent person – you would not find them of positive survival value in the jungle.

Fiske and colleagues point out that psychology first got a hint that this assessment of warmth lay at the foundations of our assessments of others with one of the most famous experiments in social psychology.[14] In 1946, Solomon Asch, perhaps the most famous social psychologist of all time, examined how impressions of others are formed using a list of adjectives – for example, 'determined', 'practical', 'industrious', 'intelligent' and 'skilful'; the list of adjectives also included either 'warm' or 'cold', depending on the experimental condition.[15] The power that was uncovered of the term 'warm' versus 'cold' as primary to our assessment of another's personality, and its ability to profoundly alter impressions, continues to surprise to this day.

Asch found that a 'warm' intelligent person is perceived to be wise, whereas a 'cold' yet intelligent person is viewed as 'sly'. No other personality attribute has been found in the half-century since Asch's experiment to profoundly alter our view of another.

How warm someone is, is linked profoundly to our sense of their fundamental intent, including linked issues such as friendliness, helpfulness, sincerity, trustworthiness, morality, fairness, generosity, sincerity, tolerance and understanding, so all of these overlap with the warmth–trustworthiness dimension. The competence dimension, on the other hand, reflects personality attributes that are related to perceived ability, including intelligence, skill, creativity, efficiency, foresightedness and ingeniousness.

Other research confirms that our sense of another's warmth and competence accounts for over 80 per cent of our perceptions of everyday social life.[14] When we try to interpret the behaviour or form impressions of others, warmth and competence account almost entirely for how we characterize them.

Fiske and colleagues point out that the evidence suggests that warmth judgements are primary: warmth is judged before competence, and warmth judgements carry more weight in affective and behavioural reactions. From an evolutionary perspective, the primacy of warmth is fitting because another person's intent for good or ill is more important to survival than whether the other person can act on those intentions.

So, social psychology has developed an understanding of person perception – how we perceive others founded on measurement of attitude, otherwise known more colloquially as impression formation and impression management.[16]

We are all involved in impression management, trying to influence others' perception of ourselves. For example, wearing a smart suit at an interview is an attempt to create a certain impression. This deploys a branch of person perception known as the 'halo effect'. The halo effect is about the recurrent finding that we seem to assume that characteristics cluster, for example that attractive people are more intelligent and outgoing. This may explain why attractive people attract more lenient sentences from juries. Somehow, we assume that attractive people are less guilty.[17]

In wearing a smart suit at an interview, we are deploying the psychology that the person who looks intelligent and organized is indeed this way when it comes to doing the job. This is a major assumption, but the halo effect demonstrates a huge number of assumptions we make when it comes to person perception. Indeed, it is theorized that, as we often have to make snap judgements in social interaction, it makes sense to jump to conclusions and to stereotype. For example, we automatically assume that an elderly person will have a cluster of personality characteristics that differ from a younger individual, without bothering to actually check that this is so.[18]

The problem with using person perception findings too readily is that there is also individual variation in perceptions. Some people are more skilled than others in working out intentions behind impression-management techniques such as wearing a smart suit.

THEORY OF MIND

A branch of social psychology comes into play here that is referred to as 'theory of mind'.[19] First-order theory of mind is the theory or account you have of what is going on in your own mind. Second-order theory of mind is the theory you have of what is going on in another's mind. So, you might theorize that a smartly dressed person is intelligent, organized and cooperative. However, third-order theory of mind is thinking what the other person is thinking about what you are thinking. So, as an interviewer, you might realize that the person is wearing a smart suit merely in order to impress you superficially, and therefore you may discount this behaviour.

Theory of mind is gathering influence in understanding the psychological deficits that may be at the heart of disorders such as autism and schizophrenia.[20]

It might be that much puzzling behaviour becomes more explicable once it is understood from a theory-of-mind perspective. It might be, for example, that, with delusion formation, the key issue becomes not that people believe they are the next coming of the messiah but that theory-of-mind deficits mean that they do not grasp the personal repercussions of openly venturing these beliefs to the mental health services. Theory of mind hinges on the issue of ability to take perspectives other than one's own as lying at the heart of communication, social skill and discourse.

Theory of mind underpins relationships because, in order to conduct relationships successfully, we need to be able to theorize at a lay level about what is going on in others' minds.

IMPROVING YOUR RELATIONSHIPS

This naturally leads on to another favourite topic of social psychology – relationship formation. This is founded on the question: how does how we perceive others guide us in forming affiliations with them?

Part of the answer comes from research by a team of psychologists led by Rachael Potter from Southwest Minnesota State University in the USA, who examined a key issue, our fear of rejection from others.[21]

The authors point out the need to be accepted by others is one of the most profound of all human motivations, and therefore it follows that rejection is frequently extremely painful. Their argument is that, because this is such a dreadful outcome, a group of us start to over-monitor our environment – the faces and behaviour of those we are talking to – on the lookout for early signs of rejection.

Psychologists such as Potter use the buzz term 'interpersonal rejection sensitivity' to describe this phenomenon. It is basically a tendency to anxiously expect, readily perceive and overreact to rejection. 'Rejection sensitivity' is now thought to lie at the heart of poor social skills and unease, because a state of social hypervigilance associated with anxious expectations of rejection naturally tends to distort perceptions of others' behaviour. This in turn produces an often defensive reaction in the perceiver, which in itself undermines relationships.

So, these psychologists are arguing that the tragic irony of interpersonal rejection sensitivity is that it creates a vicious cycle of self-fulfilling prophecies in the form of actual rejection following from the imagined rejection.

For example, another group of psychologists, led by Geraldine Downey at Columbia University in New York, found that people who enter romantic relationships with anxious expectations of rejection tend to too readily perceive intentional rejection in the 'insensitive' behaviour of their new partner.[22] Lo and behold – what then happened was that these 'rejection-sensitive' people and their romantic partners became dissatisfied with their relationships. The rejection sensitivity led to jealousy and hostility in those who were rejection-sensitive, and it was this diminished supportiveness that subsequently produced their partners' dissatisfaction.

Given that being too sensitive to interpersonal rejection produces such terrible social outcomes – either you avoid social encounters altogether and therefore do not learn how to become more socially skilled, or when you enter relationships you are too needy or anxious and this messes things up – why are people some so interpersonally sensitive in the first place?

A collaboration between psychologists based in the USA and Australia, led by Nathan Gillespie at the Queensland Institute of Medical Research, found that just under a third of how sensitive you were to rejection was the proportion accounted for by genes. This is good news for those of us who are not the most socially assured in the world, because it suggests that there is quite a lot we can still do about the problem, even if dealt a poor social skills hand in the game of life.[23]

Rachael Potter's group found that bullying and teasing during childhood seemed to account for a large part of the story as to why some of us are more sensitive to rejection than others.[21] If bullying and teasing lead to low self-esteem and feelings of inadequacy, then perhaps the direct antidote is acceptance by others – the problem is if you expect to be rejected, then you tend not to be so socially competent.

Social psychology has a lot to say on the issues of self-concept and related matters such as self-esteem and personal identity. Social psychology argues that these apparently 'self' concepts are in fact very social. The views we develop on ourselves might appear intensely private and personal, but ultimately they tend to derive from what we understand others think of us. If you were bullied at school and you deduced that you were viewed with contempt by others, then this will contribute to low self-esteem because you internalize others' views of you.

Getting on with and managing others' views of you – impression management being a cornerstone of this project – then appears a way to boost self-esteem. Through greater social skills, we derive more social rewards from others in the form of rewards and praise, and so we enter a positive feedback loop whereby self-esteem is raised.

In order to learn how to be more socially assured, it is useful to break down the skill into its component parts. These are described by social skills specialists as abilities in the areas of initiating relationships, self-disclosure, asserting displeasure with others' actions, providing emotional support, and managing interpersonal conflicts.[21]

People who expect rejection tend not to self-disclose about themselves because they are embarrassed about themselves, and yet it is only through self-disclosure that others come to know us and feel closer to us. Asserting displeasure is oddly enough a vital social skill, as otherwise we find ourselves in relationships that irritate us and lead to gradual building resentment.[21]

Social skills rely on some other deeper psychological abilities. These are described by Nathan Gillespie's team as including 'need for approval' and 'fragile inner self'. Need for approval is the extent to which we subjugate our personal needs in order to keep others happy, so as to avoid rejection, and this will tend naturally to produce low ability to assert displeasure with others' actions. Fragile inner self refers to our fear of being rejected or ridiculed.

It would seem that the needier you are of others, the less you are able to be a socially rewarding person to be with. You have to give first in order to get.

But what about those people apparently at the other end of the scale of social skill, the socially powerful among us – how do they achieve this? A group of psychologists at the University of Illinois using personality testing examined the link between personality and the attainment of leadership or higher-status positions in student organizations at universities.[24] The research has made an important contribution to our understanding of what the secret ingredient is to the personality type who climbs the greasy pole of power in organizations.

The pursuit of power appears to be a fundamental determinant in eventual success in status attainment. Status, and in particular relative status between people, appears to be a key influence on how relationships are conducted and how much influence we have over others. Status-seeking, argue the researchers in this study, could be considered a primary and universal human motive, although this appears to have been surprisingly relatively neglected by psychological researchers.[24]

A large part of the strain of working in medicine as a doctor or nurse could be said to centre on issues linked to frustrations over a lack of personal influence over others, including colleagues and patients.

This research found that some essential personality characteristics were linked strongly to how much influence you attained over others. These characteristics included extroversion (being sociable and socially confident) and conscientiousness (fulfilling obligations). The authors argue that extroversion facilitates getting noticed and conscientiousness enables potential leaders or seekers after higher status to present themselves as role models.

Although many people are often extremely conscientious, they may not realize that 'getting noticed' is key to achieving higher status and may need to draw more attention to themselves or the valuable role they play in the organizations in which they work.

Interestingly, this research found that extroversion and conscientious were not sufficient key predictors of who attained formal executive power or genuine high formal status, which was instead linked most closely with having an 'ambitious power orientation'.

Also particularly notable was that the attainment of prestigious offices in democratic organizations where you needed to court the favour of an electorate was associated with high 'agreeableness'. Agreeableness, argue the authors of this study, provides the necessary social skills to offset the negative impressions that colleagues often have of overtly ambitious individuals.

So, the art of attaining higher status or power appears to revolve around a delicate combination of both ambition and likeability. Perhaps many of us try too hard to be liked and therefore lose power that way. Most power in the social world is deployed most effectively by getting people to think the way you want them to – so they end up agreeing to your plan without feeling coerced. This is wielding power through cooperation rather than conflict.

One famous social psychology technique used to explore cooperation between people is to use experiments that take the form of inviting subjects to participate in a game called the 'ultimatum' game, which is basically a way of exploring and measuring cooperation between two people.[25] Classically, the game is played between a 'proposer' and a 'responder', whereby the proposer is given by the experimenter a sum of money to divide with the responder. The proposer must suggest a way of dividing the funds, and the responder can decide whether or not to accept the offer. The key twist in the game is that, if the responder accepts the offer made by the proposer, then the two are allowed to split the money accordingly and therefore keep the bounty. However, if the responder rejects the offer made by the proposer, then neither party gets to retain any cash.

Theoretically, since the responder had no capital at all given to them in the first place, then any offer at all made by the proposer, no matter how inequitable (e.g. 'I keep £95 and offer you £5' rather than the equitable 50/50 split), makes logical sense to accept. Accepting £5 means that you are still £5 better off than having nothing at all. Accepting a low offer is rational, given that the key alternative is no money at all, but it is also in the responder's self-interest to accept any offer, no matter how low, because it is not self-interested to make oneself poorer by refusing an offer, particularly when no work had to be done for the money in the first place.

Yet, the astonishing result found repeatedly when both psychologists and economists play this ultimatum game in their laboratories is that offers below 20 per cent are usually rejected by responders, even when this amounts to a substantial amount, such as the equivalent of half a day's pay.

The other intriguing finding is that offers by proposers tend to be near the 50 per cent mark, so many are making much more generous offers than they theoretically really need to.

What is going on? The answer is important because these findings run counter to current prevalent wisdom that our behaviour is motivated by and largely accounted for by self-interested attitudes.

A relatively new theory proposed by Terence Burnham, an economist based at Harvard University who has published a novel take on the ultimatum game experiments, is that what the experiment demonstrates is that we are quite willing to suffer a personal loss if that stops someone else getting ahead – particularly if it looks like they are doing better than us.[26]

In other words, it is not that we seek money, but more that we seek to have more money relative to others. So, if everyone else does better than us – even if we have more as well – then we end up more upset than if we had not gained at all.

It is this relativity of success that Burnham's work emphasizes. To put it another way, all doing well turns on social comparison – more money is not the problem, even if it does buy us wonderful things such as greater freedom and more control over our own lives. The key issue instead becomes how we compare what we have with what others have.

Burnham came to this conclusion because his twist on the ultimatum game experiments was to obtain saliva samples from the participants in order to investigate whether the testosterone levels of the male players affected their strategy. The results described in *Proceedings of the Royal Society* are quite startling: responders who reject a low offer had an average testosterone level more than 50 per cent higher than the average of those who accept. Five of the seven men with the highest testosterone levels in the study rejected a $5 ultimate offer from a starting stake of $50, but only one of the 19 others made the same decision.

High testosterone in men is associated with greater competitiveness, risk-taking and a drive for greater social dominance. Those who win at games appear to have consistently higher testosterone than losers. It would appear that those who are keenest to win at social comparison are most likely to reject low derisory offers – they in particular can not stand others getting on and moving past them, even if they are benefiting as well.

Burnham's results ask a startling question about the whole point of money – which is in fact to produce a sense of social superiority. Money has meaning in terms of a social universe only because what we really want is relative rather than absolute prosperity – we would actually much prefer to be absolutely poorer if we at the same time became the richest people (in comparison to others) in the village or on the desert island.

There is absolutely no point in being a multimillionaire on a desert island if no one knows about it, and similarly there is little benefit in being a multimillionaire if everyone else is one as well.

But there are other interpretations of this kind of ultimatum game result. For example, Darine Zaatari and Robert Trivers from the Center for Human Evolutionary Studies at Rutgers University in the USA found that more physically symmetrical men are also more likely to make small initial offers (and, in turn, reject relatively larger ones).[27]

Psychologists have found that how symmetrical your body and face are appears to be a profound measure of not only physical attractiveness but also your body's ability to cope with a wide range of environmental stressors during development, ie resistance to parasites, immunological strength, ability to escape predators, speed, strength, and mental acuity.

Zaatari and Trivers argue that this superior genetic quality, as displayed by people with more body symmetry, increases their ability to gain access to resources without cooperation, for example by physical aggression.[27] Zaatari and Trivers point out that previous research confirms that symmetrical men are more likely to be aggressive and to start and participate in fights, and have a high opinion of their ability to win when it comes to violence. This bias makes sense if their physical symmetry is a measure of general physical and genetic fitness. The interesting thing about aggression as a strategy is that it could be said to be the negotiating opposite of cooperation.[27]

Zaatari and Trivers contend that aggression permits the seizing of another's resources without having to bother offering any cooperative benefit in return. Weaker men are more likely therefore to seek to try a cooperative strategy, as they have most to lose from a confrontational strategy. Sure enough, Zaatari and Trivers found that more asymmetrical men (and therefore the less genetically fit) were more likely to make more generous offers in ultimatum games, supposedly in order to induce a more cooperative relationship with the other party. Symmetrical males made significantly lower offers than asymmetrical males. For the stronger man, why bother to offer to cooperate when you can take aggressively anyway?[27]

Sometimes players adopt an aggressive strategy in order to create an intimidating impression – we may readily accept a low offer if we feel the alternative is having our head bitten off. How much of the low offer strategy is a bluff, though, as opposed to comprising an iron fist in a relatively velvet glove?

One reason those offered low sums in the ultimatum game might decline such offers is that they are thinking of what happens in the future of this relationship – if you accept a lower offer now, maybe that means the person making the offer will continue to make low offers in the future. If you refuse the low offer, then it means that the person making offers in the future may be more inclined to up the offer. This way of thinking about relationships puts the issue of power at their heart.

Dacher Keltner and colleagues at the University of California at Berkeley documented some of the surprising personal psychological benefits of being a 'high-power' individual and demonstrated that suffering from 'low power' was accompanied by profound emotional burdens.[28] They found that because elevated power is associated with increased rewards and freedom, it was associated strongly with 'approach-related' tendencies – in other words, high-power individuals tend to be more assertive and exploratory in human affairs, take more risks and try out more novel activities. Reduced power, on the other hand, was inevitably accompanied by a constant sense of increased 'threat, punishment, and social constraint', and thereby this activated what the psychologists referred to as 'inhibition-related tendencies'. Low-power individuals will tend to be less assertive and constantly living in a climate of fear and anxiety about what higher-power people around them will do to them.[28]

As a result of this research, Keltner and colleagues conclude that power is associated with more positive mood and a tendency to focus on any potential rewards in the environment. They also conclude, perhaps more surprisingly, that certain cognitive skills such as thinking for oneself and more lucidly are likely to be associated with higher power. Perhaps most intriguingly for the various sex and financial scandals in which our leaders tend to be trapped so commonly, they also conclude that high power is linked with more 'disinhibited behaviour' – in other words, people higher up the power tree tend to take more risks and indulge their fantasies, while the rest of us cowering below tend to restrain ourselves more, perhaps cognizant of what the higher-power authorities might do to us.[28]

The authors of this study argue that reduced power is associated with more negative mood and constant vigilance for threat and punishment, which, among other consequences, is likely to lead to lower creativity. There is also a tendency to be preoccupied with others' interests and those features of the self that are relevant to others' goals, in other words trying to please others by modifying the self to fit in. All of this naturally leads to more inhibited social behaviour and less assertiveness.

The bottom line that Keltner and colleagues are making is that suffering from low power when it comes to your impact on others at work or at home has massive psychological consequences in terms of your mood and behaviour and the whole way you think about the world. This in turn probably has surprising implications for your general physical health. Keltner and colleagues paint a picture of the relatively powerless being under chronic strain, which in turn probably has a negative impact on their health.[28]

OBEDIENCE

People of low power tend to obey others – indeed, that is one of the signals of their low power. But social psychologists have been interested to see whether, when people perform actions, we should consider the drivers of their actions as lying within them or within their situation. When Nazis brought to trial after the Second World War claimed to be 'just following orders', was this an adequate account of why they committed atrocities, or was the reason to be found in their personalities?

The personality theory produced a literature devoted to the 'authoritarian personality type' primarily ignited by Theodore Adorno and colleagues in the 1950s. They argued that early childhood experiences, based on Freudian theory, could be linked to adult tendencies to prefer conservative conventional political views and to favour obedience to strong leaders.[29]

In contrast to this trait or personality basis for behaviour, an alternative tradition developed in the 1960s; this was a situationist school, which preferred to contend that we do what we do because of the predicament in which we find ourselves. We need to refer more to the situation than to the personality.

Stanley Milgram's 'obedience to authority' experiments conducted at Yale University in the early 1960s are perhaps the most famous empirical counter to the authoritarian personality type theory.[30] Milgram found that 65 per cent of ordinary members of the public were willing to administer apparently deadly electric shocks to a clearly distraught victim simply because an authority figure commanded them to. Not all of these ordinary subjects surely could score high on Adorno's F scale measuring authoritarianism?

Actually, the 'shock box' from which the electric shocks were apparently administered was in fact a home-constructed prop, and the 'learner' who was being punished for failing to learn was an actor who did not actually get shocked.

But it was not only the result of the experiment that was groundbreaking. That a clear majority of the subjects administered what they believed to be life-threatening 450-V shocks simply because a white-coated authority figure commanded them to was shocking. However, Milgram had pioneered a new experimental paradigm that invoked aspects of theatre in social psychology experiments. It was key to his work that, although the subjects were debriefed afterwards, the experience felt profoundly real and impactful during their time in the laboratory.

However, the field has since been plagued with controversy over the ethics involved in the use of deception and stressful stimuli, and as a result the experimental paradigm that Milgram initiated has not been clearly developed since.

Controversy also remains over the interpretation of Milgram's results. Are people really as passive in the face of authority as his results indicated? Milgram's own data revealed that if just one other subject was witnessed rebelling and refusing to obey the experimenter, then compliance rates dropped dramatically in those subjects waiting in line to take part. In the real world, is it not the case that some disobedience to authority is a regular feature of everyday life?[31]

The practical implication is that the key to disobeying authority appears to be to find collaborators, band together and disobey as a group.

Exactly why the passive compliers obey remains controversial to this day. The latest incarnation of a social psychological account is that the subjects who obey do so because they accept definitions of action provided by the apparently legitimate authority figures governing them. So, although it is the subject who indeed performs the final action, they do so only because they have allowed someone else, an authority, to define its meaning.

In Abu Ghraib, for example, the soldiers abusing and torturing prisoners did not define their actions in that way. Instead, they probably saw themselves as defensively trying to save their own country by using legitimate methods to extract information or attain compliance.

The attempt to lay the blame of causation at the door of the situation or the inner drives of the individual relates to a broader field referred to as attribution theory.[32] This is a branch of social psychology that focuses on the nature of explanation for events, particularly human behaviours.

It has been determined that, although there are myriad possible attributions or explanations for behaviours, these different explanations can be classified most usefully into three key dimensions in terms of their own impact on our behaviour and attitudes. These dimensions are whether the causes for a behaviour are internal (i.e. you are an aggressive impatient person) or external (the traffic warden was being particularly provocative). Another dimension is stability – will the causes change over time or not? The final dimension is controllability – can you or someone else affect them over time?

CBT for depression is founded partly on the finding that people with low mood tend to make a particular constellation of attributions about the causes of negative life events that may have befallen them recently. These are that the bad thing that happened is down to the individual – 'It's my fault, there is nothing I can do about it because I am just that way, and this will continue for ever more.' Exploring and shifting attributions is theorized to be a key part of producing change in psychotherapies such as CBT.

So, we can see that social psychology has important contributions to make in all branches of psychiatry, from theorizing about aetiology, to pioneering new treatments.

KEY POINTS

- Social psychology theories of aggression include the following:
- Frustration–aggression hypothesis – note the contrast with strict Freudian ideas.
- Social learning theory – note the contrast with simple behaviourism.
- Social psychology theories of relationships include social exchange theory.
- The bystander effect predicts some counterintuitive and surprising human behaviour.
- Theories of persuasion include foot-in-the door and door-in-the face techniques.
- Cognitive dissonance invokes the drive for consistency as important and predicts some counterintuitive outcomes in attitude change.
- Contrasting approaches to measurement of attitudes include techniques subsumed under the names of Osgood, Likert and Thurstone.
- Response latency and the implicit association test are newer approaches to get past the problem of people telling us what they think we want to hear when we probe their attitudes.
- The halo effect is important in impression management and may derive from evolutionary antecedents.
- Theory of mind has vital influence on sophisticated impression management techniques.
- Interpersonal rejection sensitivity can lead to self-fulfilling prophecy.
- People who tend to be successful in relationships display predictable social psychological personality characteristics and strategies.
- The attainment of interpersonal power can be charted from a social psychological perspective.
- Personal sense of power in the social world produces profound mental health implications.
- Worrying and surprising levels of obedience have been predicted by a variety of social psychological theories.

REFERENCES

1. Alcock JE, Garment DW, Sadava S (2001) *A Textbook of Social Psychology*, 5th edn. Toronto: Prentice Hall.
2. Freedman JL, Fraser SC (1966) Compliance without pressure: the foot-in-the-door technique. *Journal of Personality and Social Psychology* **4**: 195–202.
3. Burger JM (1999) The foot-in-the-door compliance procedure: a multiple-process analysis and review. *Personality and Social Psychology Review* **3**: 303–25.
4. Cialdini RB, Vincent JE, Lewis SK, *et al.* (1975) Reciprocal concessions procedure for inducing compliance: the door-in-the-face technique. *Journal of Personality and Social Psychology* **31**: 206–15.
5. Cialdini RB (2000) *Persuasion: Influence and Practice*, 4th edn. New York: Allyn & Bacon.
6. Festinger L (1957) *A Theory of Cognitive Dissonance*. Stanford, CA: Stanford University Press.
7. Festinger L, Carlsmith JM (1959) Cognitive consequences of forces compliance. *Journal of Abnormal and Social Psychology* **58**: 203–10.
8. Oxoby RJ (2004) Cognitive dissonance, status and growth of the underclass. *Economic Journal* **114**: 727–49.
9. Thurstone LL (1928) Attitudes can be measured. *American Journal of Sociology* **33**: 529–54.
10. Likert RA (1932) Technique for the measurement of attitudes. *Archives of Psychology* **140**: 1–55.
11. Osgood C, Suci G, Tannenbaum P (1957) *The Measurement of Meaning*. Chicago, IL: University of Illinois Press.
12. Green P, Srinivasan V (1978) Conjoint analysis in consumer research: issues and outlook. *Journal of Consumer Research* **5**: 103–23.
13. Rudman LA (2004) Sources of implicit attitudes. *Current Directions in Psychological Science* **13**: 279–82.
14. Fiske ST, Cuddy AJE, Glick P (2007) Universal dimensions of social cognition: warmth and competence. *Trends in Cognitive Sciences* **11**: 77–83.
15. Asch SE (1946) Forming impressions of personality. *Journal of Abnormal and Social Psychology* **41**: 258–90.
16. Leary MR, Kowalski RM (1990) Impression management: a literature review and two-component model. *Psychological Bulletin* **107**: 34–47.
17. Kaplan RM (1978) Is beauty talent? Sex interaction in the attractiveness halo effect. *Sex Roles* **4**: 195–204.
18. Macrae CN, Stangor C, Hewstone M (1996) *Stereotypes and Stereotyping*. New York: Guilford Press.
19. Brüne M, Brüne-Cohrs U (2006) Theory of mind: evolution, ontogeny, brain mechanisms and psychopathology. *Neuroscience and Biobehavioral Reviews* **30**: 437–55.
20. Chung YS, Kang DH, Shin NY, Yoo SY, Kwon JS (2008) Deficit of theory of mind in individuals at ultra-high-risk for schizophrenia. *Schizophrenia Research* **99**: 111–18.

21. Butler JC, Doherty MS, Potter RM (2007) Social antecedents and consequences of interpersonal rejection sensitivity. *Personality and Individual Differences* **43**: 1376–85.
22. Downey G, Feldman SI (1996) Implications of rejection sensitivity for intimate relationships. *Journal of Personality and Social Psychology* **70**: 1327–43.
23. Gillespie NA, Johnstone SJ, Boyce P, Heath AC, Martin NG (2001) The genetic and environmental relationship between the interpersonal sensitivity measure (IPSM) and the personality dimensions of Eysenck and Cloninger. *Personality and Individual Differences* **31**: 1039–51.
24. Harms PD, Roberts BW, Wood D (2007) Who shall lead? An integrative personality approach to the study of the antecedents of status in informal social organizations. *Journal of Research in Personality* **41**: 689–99.
25. Rotemberg JJ (2008) Minimally acceptable altruism and the ultimatum game. *Journal of Economic Behavior and Organization* **66**: 457–76.
26. Burnham TC (2007) High-testosterone men reject low ultimatum game offers. *Proceedings: Biological Sciences* **274**: 2327–30.
27. Zaatari D, Trivers R (2007) Fluctuating asymmetry and behavior in the ultimatum game in Jamaica. *Evolution and Human Behavior* **28**: 223–7.
28. Keltner D, Gruenfeld DH, Anderson C (2003) Power, approach and inhibition. *Psychological Review* **110**: 265–84.
29. Adorno TW, Frenkel-Brunswik E, Levinson DJ, Sanford RN (1950) *The Authoritarian Personality*. New York: Harper & Row.
30. Blass T (1999) The Milgram paradigm after 35 years: some things we now know about obedience to authority. *Journal of Applied Social Psychology* **29**: 955–78.
31. Blass T (ed.) (2000) *Obedience to Authority: Current Perspectives on the Milgram Paradigm*. New York: Lawrence Erlbaum Associates.
32. Moore MT, Fresco DM (2007) Depressive realism and attributional style: implications for individuals at risk for depression. *Behavior Therapy* **38**: 144–54.

Chapter 21

Social science and sociocultural psychiatry

Mary Boulton

INTRODUCTION

Social science is a generic term for a range of disciplines that are concerned with structural level processes of a social system and their impact on social organization, social groups and individuals. It includes sociology, anthropology, economics and political science.

SOCIAL DIVISIONS AND THE SOCIAL PATTERNING OF MENTAL HEALTH

The main divisions in British society, as in other advanced industrial nations, are based on social class, gender and ethnicity. These divisions are associated with social inequalities and, to varying degrees, social stratification. *Social stratification* is the arrangement of individuals into social strata, or layers, in a hierarchy of advantage reflecting their relative power in society. An individual's location within the social structure affects her or his *life chances* – the chances of sharing in society's cultural and material rewards such as education, employment, income and health.

Social class

Social classes may be defined as 'segments of the population sharing broadly similar types and levels of resources, with broadly similar styles of living and (for some sociologists) some shared perception of their common condition'.[1] In the UK, the most common measure of social class is based on occupation. *Socioeconomic status* (SES) is a term for a comparable concept commonly used in North America. The National Statistics Socio-economic Classification (NS-SEC),[2] introduced for the analysis of the 2001 Census, groups occupations into 14 operational categories (based on their market positions), which can be combined into eight classes for analytical purposes. These in turn can be collapsed into a five-class version – managerial and professional; intermediate; small employers and own-account workers; lower supervisory and technical; and semi-routine and routine – or a three-class version – managerial and professional; intermediate; and routine and manual.

There are marked social class differences in diagnosed psychiatric disorders, including schizophrenia, alcoholism, drug addiction and organic psychoses, and common mental disorders, with highest rates in the lower social classes.[3,4] Types of treatment are also related to social class and poverty. People from lower social classes are more likely to be admitted to hospital, to remain hospitalized for longer and to receive physical forms of care such as electroconvulsive therapy (ECT), while people from higher social classes are more likely to be treated on an out-patient basis and to receive treatments such as psychotherapy.[5]

The higher rates of psychiatric disorders among individuals in the lowest social classes are generally seen as the product of the adverse life situations they experience, deriving from economic hardships and the range of negative life events associated with poverty and social disorganization.[6–8] The consequences of material deprivation include higher stress from crime, traffic, pollution and poor housing. Manual jobs entail little control and satisfaction and are more subject to redundancies, all of which contribute to lower levels of self-esteem.

Class differences in psychiatric morbidity may also arise as a consequence of processes associated with mental illness itself. Individuals who become mentally ill may find it difficult to perform adequately in more skilled and demanding jobs and over time may drift down the occupational hierarchy.[1] This has been noted particularly in relation to individuals suffering from schizophrenia, where downward social mobility has made the class gradient even more marked.

Gender

Gender refers to differences in social characteristics assigned to males and females. *Gender roles* refer to roles in society typically assigned to men (breadwinner, fighter) or women (homemaker, carer). *Gender stereotypes* are preconceived ideas about appropriate styles of behaviour for men (active, aggressive) and women (passive, compliant). The system of male dominance over women is called *patriarchy*.

In industrialized societies, women generally have lower mortality rates than men but higher rates of morbidity. This is particularly noticeable in relation to psychiatric illness, where women have almost twice the rates of neurotic disorders, affective psychoses and dementia.[9] One set of explanations for these differences relates to women's disadvantaged position within society generally and the particular nature of their domestic roles.[10] Women have fewer resources and less influence in society and are more likely to be in subordinate and dependent positions. Their domestic roles are characterized by boring, repetitive and non-productive activities, social isolation, and little social recognition or prestige. This produces low levels of chronic stress, the effects of which are exacerbated by the lack of structure in their work, which allows women time to brood over their problems. An increasing proportion of women work outside the home and may benefit from this additional source of rewards, but they may also suffer from the *double burden* of employment and domestic roles, which generates stress as a result of both *role accumulation* and *role conflict*.[11,12]

Other explanations point to the importance of gender stereotypes in producing higher rates of psychiatric illness among women. One version of this argument suggests that gender role socialization, which emphasizes passivity, helplessness and dependence as appropriate feminine behaviour, produces *learned helplessness*. This means that women are less able to cope with stressful situations and hence are at greater risk of depression. The other version suggests that higher rates of minor psychiatric morbidity may also be an artefact of women's illness behaviour.[9] Gender stereotypes may make it easier for women to acknowledge their emotions and to seek professional help when in difficulty, while their roles as mothers and carers may themselves bring them into contact with doctors.[5] Cultural stereotypes may also predispose doctors to diagnose mental illness more readily in women.

'Race' and ethnicity

Ethnicity denotes membership of a social group with a distinct culture – expressed in a common language, religion, dress, diet and other symbols – and some sense of a common origin or homeland. It needs to be distinguished from '*race*', which is a classification system based on visible physical characteristics, and *immigrant status*, which refers to place of residence. Discrimination based on race or ethnicity is racial prejudice or racism. *Institutional racism* is the systematic disadvantage of people from ethnic minorities built in to the way institutions operate, which may be unintentional and go unrecognized.

In the 2001 census, 7.9 per cent of the population of England and Wales described themselves as belonging to a non-white ethnic group, and one in 12 of the population was born overseas. Although immigration has occurred throughout British history, since the middle of the twentieth century immigration has involved migrants from further away and with different languages, religions and skin colours. Public policies and attitudes were initially based on assumptions of *acculturation* – the adoption by people from minority groups of the norms, values and traditions of the host population – and *assimilation* – the decline of distinct ethnic identities and their social significance. Subsequently there has been greater recognition of *multiculturalism* – the valuing of the distinctiveness and diversity of ethnic minority cultures – although this in turn is being questioned on the grounds of its perceived consequences for social cohesion.

Compared with people from the white population, people from non-white ethnic minorities have been disadvantaged in a number of ways, for example in relation to education, policing, housing and healthcare. However, there is considerable diversity among ethnic minorities, and this is also reflected in differences in their life experiences. In terms of labour market participation and occupational attainment, for example, Chinese and Indian minorities are doing as well as the white majority, while Pakistani and Bangladeshi minorities are doing significantly worse.

There are striking differences in rates of diagnosed psychiatric disorder between different ethnic groups,[13] with higher rates of schizophrenia among the Afro-Caribbean and Irish populations and lower rates of mental illness generally among the Asian populations.[14–18] Early explanations for these patterns emphasized the effects of migration, as either selecting for emigration individuals with schizophrenia or a predisposition for schizophrenia or as creating stress among immigrants, which precipitated schizophrenia among those people predisposed to it. With the end of large-scale immigration to Britain in the 1970s and the observation of increased rates of schizophrenia among second-generation British-born Afro-Caribbean people, research has focused more on the responses of the host population, in terms of hostility and discrimination, and the material deprivation, frustrated ambitions and social stress they produce.

Alternative approaches point to the way social and cultural factors affect both the expression and the recognition of mental illness. For example, noisy, antisocial behaviour in public is likely to attract the attention of the authorities, as is black skin colour. Young male Afro-Caribbeans in Britain are much more likely than their white counterparts to come into contact with psychiatric services through the police and more than twice as likely to be admitted as a result of a compulsory detention order and to be detained in locked wards.[5,16,17] For a doctor who does not understand the person's cultural beliefs or practices, it may be difficult to determine whether problematic behaviour is evidence of schizophrenia or any of the other possibilities (e.g. religious fervour, youthful rebelliousness, criminal intentions).

Similarly, doctors, particularly inexperienced general practitioners (GPs), may find it difficult to understand the significance of symptoms presented by Asian patients from cultures where depression and anxiety are somatized and much morbidity may go unrecognized. In addition, mental illness carries a particularly high degree of stigma in some cultures, which discourages seeking help from the health services and means that, especially among women, minor psychiatric morbidity may be contained within the nuclear or extended family. These considerations taken together have led some authors to argue that misdiagnosis is common and that the pattern of mental illness among ethnic groups presented by official statistics is a distorted and unhelpful representation of psychiatric need.[5,19]

ILLNESS IN SOCIETY AND THE SOCIAL ROLE OF MEDICINE

The sick role and the doctor–patient relationship

Illness may be regarded as a form of deviance in as much as it inhibits an individual's ability to perform his or her usual social roles and hence disrupts the smooth functioning of society.[20] In order to cope with this threat to social order, society must develop mechanisms of social control to keep the deviance within manageable bounds and to return the individual to normal social roles. This it does by creating an approved social role for the deviant – which Parsons called the 'sick role' – and by recruiting others to a reciprocal social role – that of the doctor – to help the deviant return to normality. The doctor and patient may thus be seen as occupying a pair of reciprocal and complementary roles that share the same aim of returning the patient to normal social functioning.

Parsons went on to specify the reciprocal rights and obligations of doctors and patients. He saw the sick role as an essentially undesirable, temporary role that imposes on the individual entering it the obligation to leave it as soon as possible. To this end, patients are accorded two privileges: they are allowed to shed normal roles and responsibilities (e.g. work roles or household responsibilities), and they are regarded as being not responsible for the illness (relieving the individual of any sense of moral culpability and allowing the disavowal of inferiority) and as being in need of care in order to return to health. These privileges confer considerable benefits on patients and are thus conditional on them accepting other obligations: they must want to get well as soon as possible and must seek help from the doctor to achieve this; and they must then cooperate with the doctor in his or her investigations, accept the doctor's advice and follow the doctor's recommended treatment. Failure to fulfil these obligations may lead to the label of 'malingerer' and the withdrawal of the benefits of the sick role.

Parsons viewed the doctor as society's gatekeeper, determining the official labelling of conditions as 'health' or 'sickness' and thus controlling access to the sick role. The medical profession alone has the authority to legitimate an individual's claim to illness or, conversely, to impose on an individual the diagnosis of illness. This may be particularly important in relation to psychiatric disorders, where conditions may be ill-defined, ambiguous or contentious.

Parsons described the doctor's role as complementary, but not equal, to that of the patient. Whereas the patient is expected to cooperate with the doctor, the doctor occupies a position of authority in relation to the patient. The doctor is given the right to examine the patient physically, to enquire into intimate areas of the patient's life, and to exercise considerably autonomy in their professional practice. In return for these rights, the doctor is expected to apply their specialist knowledge and skills for the benefit of the patient and community and to follow the rules of professional practice. The potential tensions arising from the personal nature of medical practice are reduced by the further obligations on the doctor to remain objective and emotionally detached and to use their privileged position for the benefit of the patient and not for personal or professional advantage.

Although Parson's analysis has proved extremely useful to understanding the social role of medicine, it has been widely criticized for placing too much emphasis on the consensus between doctors and patients. Friedson, by contrast, emphasized the differences in knowledge, interests and expectations that can lead to tensions and conflict between doctors and patients.[21] Conflicts may arise, for example, between the competing interests of individual patients (e.g. for the doctor's time and attention); between the interests of a patient now and in the future (e.g. between the immediate relief provided by tranquillizers and the long-term potential for dependency); between the interests of the patient and the interests of the patient's family (e.g. in deciding on whether to hospitalize a depressed patient); and between the doctor's duties to the patient and the doctor's duties as an agent of the state (e.g. in deciding whether a stressed patient's request for a sick note for time off work is warranted or not). This model suggests that the face-to-face consultation between doctor and patient may be understood as a process of negotiation, with both the doctor and the patient having their own agenda and using interaction strategies in an attempt to achieve their objectives.[22]

Illness behaviour and the clinical iceberg

Parson's formulation of the sick role assumes that individuals who experience illness seek professional help as soon as possible. A number of empirical studies, however, have shown that patients are much more likely to deal with their symptoms themselves, either ignoring the symptoms or using non-prescribed medicines, alternative practitioners or self-help groups, and only rarely consult a doctor. The vast amount of illness in the community, unseen by the medical profession, is known as the *clinical iceberg*. Much mental illness, because it is highly stigmatizing, is likely to remain unrecognized and untreated in the community.

Whether and when individuals seek help from a doctor depends on a number of factors, both in their social environment and in the organization and provision of healthcare services. Mechanic used the term 'illness behaviour' to describe the way individuals perceive, evaluate and act upon pain, discomfort or other signals of organic malfunction.[23] Illness behaviour is influenced fundamentally by the social meanings attributed to symptoms, often by friends or colleagues, who may constitute a *lay referral network*, which suggest appropriate ways of dealing with them. Most symptoms tend to be *normalized* – that is, seen as the expected consequences of everyday life – and adjustments made to accommodate them. For example, families of schizophrenic patients have been found to tolerate symptoms for considerable periods, defining the symptoms as signs of malice or religious zeal and compensating for them by altering their own behaviour and expectations. Help may be sought only when something happens to disrupt this pattern of accommodation. The kinds of thing that happen to cause this are known as *triggers to action*. Zola identified five such triggers – interference with work; interference with personal relationships; sanctioning; interpersonal crisis and temporalizing of symptomatology – and argued that doctors need to understand and address these contextual issues as much as the symptoms themselves.[24]

The way healthcare services are organized and provided can also influence illness behaviour by altering the balance of perceived costs and benefits of seeking medical help. A range of social and psychological costs to patients may be reduced by changing the times and locations of clinics – for example, siting them in health centres rather than in hospitals – or by altering the attitudes and responses of clinic staff.

Mental hospitals and the sociology of residential institutions

Goffman used the term 'total institution' to describe places such as large mental hospitals where inmates are segregated from the wider society and live in a social world of their own.[25] In total institutions, all aspects of life are conducted in the same place and under a single authority. Daily life is characterized by *batch living*, with activities carried out as part of a group and the usual distinction between work, leisure and home life removed. A clear differentiation is made between the managers and the managed (binary management) and the behaviour of inmates is highly regulated. There is an institutional perspective and hence the assumption of an overall rational plan.

Institutionalization is the process whereby individuals admitted to large institutions gradually withdraw from normal life and become dependent on the structures of the institution. It starts with admission procedures and continues with the establishment of deference patterns and assimilation into the subculture of the institution. The result is gradual changes in perception of individuals about themselves and others, which Goffman terms the 'moral career' of the patient.

Goffman described a number of processes designed to ensure the smooth operation of total institutions but that contribute to *depersonalization* and have adverse psychological effects. *Degradation rituals* remove the individual's 'normal' identity and strip away their usual sense of self. Patients may be discouraged from maintaining contacts outside the institution and information about what is going on both within the institution and in relation to their own care may be kept from them. Their freedom of movement may also be controlled.

Patients may initially respond to these processes in a number of ways, including rebelling, withdrawing or pretending to accept them (conforming in the hope of speedy discharge) but, in the long term, most succumb to institutional pressures. Acceptance means a loss of personal identity, its replacement by the identity of a mental patient, and a growing dependence on the institution for all decisions.

Strauss introduced the concept of the hospital as a *negotiated order*, where those people with limited power (patients, lower-level staff) were able to make life more comfortable for themselves by negotiating around the formal rules of the institution, for example through a series of bargains and informal agreements between staff and patients.[26] The constant negotiation and renegotiation of the way roles and responsibilities are fulfilled is crucial to the smooth functioning of long-stay residential institutions and points to the importance of the informal structures that develop within them.

Wing provided empirical evidence for the relationship between the social withdrawal and passivity of hospitalized patients and their length of stay and the poverty of their hospital environment (measured in terms of ward restrictiveness and lack of occupation, personal possessions and contact with the outside world).[27] This relationship was independent of clinical conditions and was shown to be reversible if chronic patients were placed in a stimulating social environment.

Care or control?

As well as being a body of knowledge and skills, medicine is also a system of power and control. Doctors have power over patients because of their specialized knowledge and because they define what is, or what is not, illness. Doctors control the work of other occupational groups through their monopoly over decisions about patient diagnosis and treatment. The medical profession has also been able to determine what is acceptable as treatment and to exclude alternative therapies from state recognition.

It has been argued that the power and control of the medical profession has increased. The term 'medicalization' refers to the process of expansion by which more and more areas of life become subject to medical definitions and management. Aspects of daily life become defined as illnesses (e.g. anorexia, alcoholism) to be treated and cured and individuals turn to their doctors for solutions (e.g. tranquillizers, diet pills) to their problems of living. Medicalization increases the remit of the medical profession and, through the sick role, diminishes the responsibility of the individual. Public morality in areas of personal behaviour is maintained, but under the auspices of medicine rather than religion or the law.

Psychiatry has been a particular target for critics of medicine, who see psychiatry as an institution of social control. In his historical analysis of the origins of mental hospitals, Foucault saw asylums as representing a new age of incarceration and the new medical discourses – which presented 'reason' as the source of healthy civilization and 'madness' as a sickness to be cured – as part of the process of normalization and self-discipline.[28] Foucault rejected the notion that asylums arose from a desire to provide more humane care for 'mad' people and instead saw them as a way of persecuting those people who did not act rationally and as reinforcing social control. They served the interests not of the patients but of the professions and bureaucracies whose authority was grounded in the dominant discourses of an increasingly rational world.

Kennedy developed a somewhat different argument in relation to twentieth-century practices, making the case that, by defining deviant behaviour as illness and offering to cure it, the psychiatric profession helps to reinforce accepted ways of thinking and legitimates the punitive treatment of people who do not conform.[29] The fact that many people are being treated in hospital not because they want to be there but because others such as relatives, neighbours or the police want them there has been taken to indicate that psychiatric legislation and psychiatry are much more about the social control of people whose behaviour is causing problems for others than they are about caring for sick people themselves. According to Szasz, the *myth of mental illness* persists in modern societies not because of its scientific validity but because it is such an effective means of social control.[30]

FAMILIES, FAMILY LIFE AND EXPRESSED EMOTION

There is a growing diversity in the forms of family and household arrangements in contemporary Britain, with increases in the proportion of people living in households comprising single people, cohabiting couples, lone parents and dependent children, and step- or reconstituted families (a couple living together with children from one or more previous relationships). This diversity is the result of a number of current demographic trends, most notably the decline in marriage and increase in cohabitation, the rising rates of birth outside marriage, and the increase in divorce and remarriage. These trends in turn can be seen as reflecting the effects of an increasing individualism or *individualization* of society – the breakdown in normal social constraints and fixed guidelines for living, and the opening up of greater individual choice in the way individuals can lead their lives. Although this widens the scope for individuals to pursue personally fulfilling goals, greater choice also creates greater uncertainty and the potential for conflict within relationships. These changes have significant implications for mental health: lone-parent and reconstituted families have been shown to experience more life events in their own lives and in the lives of friends and relatives, while two-parent families provide greater protection from economic hardship and two- (birth) parent families provide greater family support.[31]

Family relationships and environment have also been shown to affect mental health, most notably in relation to *expressed emotion* (EE). Expressed emotion is a construct encompassing critical, hostile or emotionally overinvolved attitudes on the part of a family member towards a relative with a disorder or impairment. Although EE is now a well-validated predictor of poor clinical outcome for a wide range of psychiatric disorders, it was originally developed as a measure of the emotional climate of families of schizophrenic patients who had been discharged from hospital,[32] demonstrating that high levels of EE were related significantly to higher rates of relapse. Early conceptualizations of EE focused on the contrasting styles of low-EE families (tolerant, non-intrusive, sensitive to patient needs) and high-EE families (intolerant, intrusive, adopting inappropriate and inflexible strategies in dealing with difficulties).[33] More recent work has focused on the role of *attributions* in understanding differences in the way families respond to patients, and evidence is accumulating that critical relatives are more likely than non-critical relatives to hold patients responsible for their difficulties.[34]

SOCIAL FACTORS AND MENTAL ILLNESS

Social factors are aspects of the social environment that elicit recurrent stressful experience and increase risk of physical and mental illness.[35] Social factors commonly associated with the onset of a broad range of psychiatric disorders include low educational attainment, unemployment, poverty, poor housing, family breakdown, family dysfunction (e.g. childhood abuse, neglect, domestic violence, substance misuse) and neighbourhood disorganization (e.g. drugs, crime, urban decay).

An important mediating factor is *social support* – the ties that an individual has with other people or groups that provide a sense of self-worth (of being loved and valued) and other resources. Social support includes instrumental, informational, appraisal and emotional dimensions. It acts to buffer the negative effects of social adversity and to reduce the likelihood of subsequent psychiatric disorder by enhancing *adaptive coping. Social capital* is a related concept at a neighbourhood level that refers to aspects of social organization, such as trust among neighbours, norms of reciprocity and group membership, that facilitate collective action.

Depression

Research on social factors and depression has focused on *life events* and *social support.* Life events are sudden changes, positive or negative, which disrupt the normal course of an individual's life. By disrupting social life to the point where previous norms and values are no longer appropriate, severe events may give rise to *anomie* or a sense of *normlessness.* Brown and Harris initially argued that it is only this type of event – life events that involve long-term threat – that is important in the onset of depression in women.[36] This points to the importance of the meaning of events, which can be determined only by considering them in the context of individual lives. For example, the birth of a baby has different meanings for a middle-class couple with a house and a garden and for a woman living in bed-and-breakfast accommodation with two other children and whose partner is in jail. In recent refinements of their work, Brown and Harris have identified losses involving humiliation or entrapment as particularly important in the onset of depression and 'fresh start' experiences (which promise new hope) as important in remission.[37]

Brown and Harris also argue that the influence of life events depends on the existence of *vulnerability factors,* which increase susceptibility to depression. These include loss of mother before 11 years of age; absence of a confiding relationship with a partner; lack of employment outside the home; and three or more children under 15 years of age living at home. Vulnerability factors contribute to low self-esteem, which reduces the ability to cope with life events and reflects low social support. Working-class women are likely to experience higher rates of both severe life events and vulnerability factors than middle-class women.

Schizophrenia

The most convincing evidence for the role of social factors in schizophrenia comes from research in a number of European countries that found high rates among first- and second-generation immigrants from a wide range of ethnic and geographical backgrounds.[38] According to Cantor-Graae and Selten, the most likely explanation for markedly raised rates of schizophrenia in such disparate groups as Africans and Greenlanders is chronic experience of discrimination or long-term exposure to *social defeat.*[39] These authors base their argument on the observation that the relative risk of schizophrenia is especially high in groups with black skin colour and originating in a developing country or of second-generation immigrant status (for whom being treated as an 'outsider' in their country of birth may be particularly distressing). Incidence rates in this population are lower in neighbourhoods with higher proportions of ethnic minority residents, most likely because of the protection they offer against discrimination and isolation. The social defeat hypothesis also proposes that stress related to social rank may be particularly harmful.

In non-immigrant populations, urban birth or upbringing, social and material deprivation, childhood victimization, substance misuse (most notably cannabis use in adolescence) and 'psychotogenic' neighbourhoods have been shown to be related to raised incidence of schizophrenia.

Alcohol and illicit drug addiction

Although growing medicalization of everyday life is reflected in the range of behaviours that are now regarded as addictive, including shopping, computer games, the Internet and sex, addiction to or dependence on alcohol and illicit drugs remains the main focus of public concern.[40]

Alcohol consumption and drug-taking are most likely to start in adolescence, but progression to dependence or addiction is less common.[41] Men are more likely than women to have illicit drug and alcohol problems, possibly because they are exposed to heavier alcohol use and more drug-taking, although this may be changing.

Problematic substance misuse is more likely to take root in deprived neighbourhoods where local people feel cut off from mainstream society and powerless to change their environment; where selling illegal drugs can appear to be an efficient way of earning a living; and where law-breaking and violence associated with drug-dealing and drug-using may seem glamorous and attractive.[42,43] Substance misuse is also associated with poor attachment to or communication with parents; childhood conduct disorder; and low school grades, truancy and exclusion from school. Many illegal substances are expensive and need to be acquired through illegal means, resulting in high rates of criminality and periods in prison among problematic substance users. Substance misuse is also associated with increased levels of violence and the risk of danger to self and others.[44]

Social exclusion

Mental illness also has social consequences: people with mental health problems are more likely to become and remain unemployed, to have poor accommodation or become homeless, to live in socially disorganized and poor localities, and to experience hostility and discrimination from the public and mass media. They also experience difficulties in accessing statutory services, including financial services and healthcare. These problems interact and persist over time, with the consequence that the people are no longer integrated into society and are excluded from adequate social participation. This is known as *social exclusion*, a concept that conveys the multiple, complex and interlocking social problems experienced by people with mental health problems.[45]

DEVIANCE, STIGMA AND PREJUDICE

The process of socialization means that members of a social group are likely to share similar conceptions of appropriate attitudes and behaviour, but it does not mean that all think or act in a way that is acceptable to the group. Behaviour that contravenes the norms of the group is considered *deviant behaviour*. Deviance can be defined only in relation to some notion of normality, and one of the functions of identifying deviant behaviour is to clarify norms and values and to reinforce definitions of normal behaviour. However, in the context of late modernity – where established ways of doing, thinking and being are constantly questioned and social life is characterized by ambivalence, insecurity and disorder – distinctions between normal and deviant behaviour may be increasingly difficult to make.

Deviance that contravenes fundamental social values attracts particular social disapproval and may be stigmatizing. Goffman defined *stigma* as an attribute, trait or behaviour that is considered shameful or disgraceful and that symbolically marks the possessor as unacceptable, inferior or dangerous.[46] In a society that values rationality, control and achievement, psychiatric disorders carry strong negative meanings and are highly stigmatized.

Deviance that is immediately visible to others, such as psychotic behaviour, is *discredited* and creates problems for the stigma bearer in 'the management of tensions' generated during social interaction. Deviance that is not immediately visible, such as a diagnosis of schizophrenia, is *discreditable* and requires the stigma bearer to 'manage information' about the stigmatized attribute (e.g. through 'passing' as normal, 'covering' or withdrawal). *Enacted stigma* refers to a stigma bearer's experience of discrimination; *felt stigma* refers to the fear of discrimination and is more prevalent, and hence more disabling, than enacted stigma.

Individuals who are stigmatized are perceived in terms of a *stereotype* – as an example of a 'type' of individual – that has negative connotations. The stereotype evokes emotional reactions in others, such as fear, contempt and disgust, and a social response of distancing, rejection or withdrawal. As a result, the stigmatized person is set apart and may feel depersonalized, rejected and disempowered. Pilgrim suggests that the basis of the prejudice against people with mental health problems is a cultural stereotype that incorporates a lack of intelligibility, a lack of social competence and the presence of violence.[47]

PRINCIPLES OF CRIMINOLOGY AND PENOLOGY

Criminology and understanding crime

Criminology is concerned with the causes, consequences, forms and incidence of a particular category of deviance – crime. Crime is difficult to define as it is impossible to identify activities that would be regarded as criminal in all societies at all times.[48,49]

Although early criminological research attempted to identify what distinguished criminals from non-criminals in terms of biological or personality characteristics or psychopathology, more recent research has been concerned with explaining the causes of criminal behaviour.

Functionalist theories see deviance and crime as an inevitable and integral part of society and look to explain excessive levels of crime. Merton's *strain theory* suggests that, in any particular society, the scope and character of deviance will depend on how well society makes cultural goals (e.g. financial success) accessible to its population by providing institutionalized means (e.g. schooling, job opportunities) to achieve those goals.[50] The disparity between what society expects individuals to achieve and what individuals come to realize they will actually achieve creates strain (which Merton called anomie). Where structural inequalities prevent individuals from achieving their goals through legitimate means, some individuals will turn to illegitimate means – crime – in order to achieve them; others will reject society's goals and the conventional means of achieving them and retreat into deviant or unconventional subcultures; and others will go further, rebelling against both the goals and the conventional means of achieving them and advocating radical alternatives to the social order.

The theory of *deviant subcultures* suggests that delinquency among working-class youths is a consequence of *status frustration* and a reaction against the norms of middle-class society. Cohen suggested that working-class boys are alienated and frustrated at school and so seek self-respect by building a deviant subculture.[51] Others have argued that an individual's tendency towards conformity or deviance depends on the relative frequency of association with other people who encourage conventional or deviant behaviour (peer pressure) and that criminal deviance results in part from the availability of opportunities for illegal behaviour.

Interactionist theories focus on the complex process of becoming a deviant or criminal. *Labelling theory* draws attention to the importance of reactions of other people to deviant behaviour in 'creating' deviance.[52] Most deviant behaviour is normalized and accommodated (cf. illness behaviour) until something happens to make it intolerable to others (e.g. it becomes more visible or threatening). At this point, it may be labelled as one of a number of types of behaviour, including criminal behaviour and mental illness.

Labelling refers to the process whereby individual characteristics are identified and given a particular meaning by other people. Both convicting an individual and giving a diagnosis are acts of labelling *primary deviance. Secondary deviance* (or deviance amplification) refers to the change in behaviour that occurs as a consequence of labelling. Once an individual has been convicted of a crime or diagnosed as mentally ill, social expectations promote behaviour that conforms to this label. In this sense, agencies of social control (e.g. law, medicine) act as amplifiers or even manufacturers of deviance. Labelling individuals in this way has a profound effect because deviance is a master status that overshadows other aspects of identity. It also creates outsiders and may provoke individuals to adopt a deviant lifestyle and begin a deviant career.

Critical criminology and *conflict theorists* see crime not as a problem of individual offenders or strains in society but as a process related to wider economic and political structures of power. They are concerned with exploring why and how the activities of some groups – for example, black working-class youths – come to be subjected to criminal law and question the way in which mechanisms of social control are used.[48] Theories based on *classical Marxism* focus on the way in which social norms and laws support the interests of the rich and powerful, while the *new criminology* focuses on the various ways in which capitalism itself produces crime and criminals.[53]

A further development is *left realism*, which takes seriously the impact of crime on victims and seeks to produce realistic ways of dealing with crime.[54] It sees deep structural inequalities as the root cause of crime and focuses on the 'square of crime' – the state, society, offenders and victims – each element of which, and their interrelationships, must be explored and addressed.

Penology and the principles of punishment

Penology is the study of punishment imposed by the judiciary in accordance with penal law and administered by penal institutions. In liberal democratic societies, such punishment generally equates to some form of deprivation, which may entail the loss of liberty (curfew, imprisonment), time (community service), money (fines, compensation orders) or reputation ('naming and shaming').

There are four types of justification for judicial punishment.[55] Three are concerned with preventing future crimes and reflect utilitarian and consequentialist philosophies and reductivist aims:

- *Deterrence* aims to prevent criminal activity through the development and application of effective and efficient sanctions. It is based on the assumption that criminal behaviour is rational, self-interested and freely chosen, and that the wellbeing of the community can be protected by providing rational individuals with good reasons not to commit crimes. Critics point to the limited conception of human action and the lack of attention to social and material context. In addition, punishment may be a deterrent only when apprehension and conviction are certain, punishment is severe and the link between the crime and its punishment is clear to the offender.
- *Rehabilitation* has the aim of reintegrating the offender into society after a period of punishment and so requires that the content of the punishment is designed to achieve this end. It is based on the belief that change and improvement are possible (through a range of interventions, including individual and group therapy, education and training) and that crime is best prevented by addressing directly the social, economic and personal factors that are the causes of crime. Critics point to limited evidence of its effectiveness or object on moral grounds to the deterministic view of human behaviour and the social engineering approaches to behaviour change that it implies.
- *Incapacitation* has the aim of protecting potential victims, and the community more generally, by removing the offender's ability to commit further crimes through some form of incarceration or, at the extreme, capital punishment. Selective incapacitation is based on the view that a small number of offenders commit a relatively large amount of crime and involves identifying those offenders likely to re-offend and giving them long prison sentences. Critics point to the difficulty in predicting who will re-offend (and hence how much crime will be prevented) and question the justice of punishing someone not for what they have done but for what it is thought they might do if left at liberty.

The fourth type of justification for judicial punishment – *retribution* – is concerned solely with punishing crimes that have already been committed. It is based on the view that, in committing a crime, the offender has disturbed the moral equilibrium of the community and that, in order to restore that equilibrium, the offender must be identified and punished. In other words, society has a moral obligation to punish wrongdoers, and wrongdoers deserve their punishment. The punishment should always fit the crime and should be proportionate to the harm done rather than adjusted to the circumstances of the offender. Critics argue that it is, in essence, simply a primitive demand for vengeance and that it is not morally justifiable to inflict punishment for its own sake when no positive good can be achieved.

Rather than trying to define a good justification for punishment, some penologists question its necessity or desirability as the usual response to crime. *Abolitionists* have advocated the abolition of the death penalty or of imprisonment as a response to all but exceptional crime. The *restorative justice* movement aims to abolish not only imprisonment but punishment generally, seeking to shift the focus from the offender to the victim, with the intention of securing recompense and reconciliation between offender and victim.

KEY POINTS

- There are marked differences in rates of mental illness by social class and, for particular conditions, by gender and ethnicity.
- Type of treatment differs between social classes, with higher rates of hospitalization and physical treatments among people from lower classes.
- Social factors play a significant role in the onset of a wide range of mental health problems.
- Mental illness and criminal behaviour are forms of deviance. Medicine and the law are key social institutions for controlling deviance.
- Stigma is an attribute that is considered shameful and marks the possessor as inferior or unacceptable.
- The stigma of mental illness contributes to discrimination, social and material disadvantage, and social exclusion.

REFERENCES

1. Townsend P, Davidson N, Whitehead M (1988) *Inequalities in Health: The Black Report/The Health Divide.* Harmondsworth: Penguin.
2. Office for National Statistics (2004) *The National Statistics Socio-economic Classification User Manual (NS-SEC).* London: Office for National Statistics. www.statistics.gov.uk/methods_quality/ns_sec/default.asp.
3. Goldberg D, Morrison S (1963) Schizophrenia and social class. *British Journal of Psychiatry* **109**: 785–802.
4. Fryers T, Melzer D, Jenkins R (2003) Social inequalities and the common mental disorders: a systematic review of the evidence. *Social Psychiatry and Psychiatric Epidemiology* **38**: 229–37.
5. Pilgrim D, Rogers A (2005) *A Sociology of Mental Health and Illness*, 3rd edn. Buckingham: Open University Press.
6. Hauk K, Rice N (2004) A longitudinal analysis of mental health mobility in Britain. *Health Economics* **13**: 981–1001.
7. Wiggins R, Scholfiled P, Sacjer A, Head J, Bartley M (2004) Social position and minor psychiatric morbidity over time in the British Household Panel Survey 1991–1998. *Journal of Epidemiology and Community Health* **58**: 779–87.
8. Fone D, Dunstan F, Williams G, Lloyd K, Palmer S (2007) Places, people and mental health: a multilevel analysis of economic inactivity. *Social Science and Medicine* **64**: 633–45.
9. Piccinelli M, Wilkinson G (2000) Gender differences in depression. *British Journal of Psychiatry* **177**: 486–92.
10. Gove W (1984) Gender differences in mental and physical illness: the effects of fixed roles and nurturant roles. *Social Science and Medicine* **19**: 77–91.
11. Arber S, Gilbert G, Dale A (1985) Paid employment and women's health: a benefit or a source of role strain? *Sociology of Health and Illness* **7**: 375–400.
12. Chandola T, Martikainen P, Bartley M, *et al.* (2004) Does conflict between home and work explain the effect of multiple roles on mental health? A comparative study of Finland, Japan and the UK. *International Journal of Epidemiology* **33**: 884–93.
13. Smaje C (1996) The ethnic patterning of health: new directions for theory and research. *Sociology of Health and Illness* **18**: 139–71.
14. Cochrane R, Bal S (1989) Mental hospital admission rates of immigrants to England: a comparison of 1971 and 1981. *Social Psychiatry* **24**: 2–11.
15. Carpenter I, Brockington I (1980) A study of mental illness in Asians, West Indians and Africans living in Manchester. *British Journal of Psychiatry* **137**: 201–5.
16. McGovern D, Cope R (1987) The compulsory detention of males of different ethnic groups with special reference to offender patients. *British Journal of Psychiatry* **150**: 505–12.
17. Koffman J, Fulop N, Pashley D, Coleman K (1997) Ethnicity and the use of psychiatric beds: a one day survey in North and South Thames Regions. *British Journal of Psychiatry* **171**: 238–41.
18. Bracken P, Greenslade L, Griffen B, Smyth M (1998) Mental health and ethnicity: an Irish dimension. *British Journal of Psychiatry* **172**: 103–5.
19. Littlewood R, Lipsedge M (1982) *Aliens and Alienists.* Harmondsworth: Penguin.
20. Parsons T (1951) *The Social System.* Glencoe, IL: Free Press.
21. Friedson E (1970) *The Profession of Medicine.* New York: Harper & Row.
22. Tuckett D, Boulton M, Olson C, Williams A (1985) *Meetings Between Experts: An Approach to Sharing Ideas in Medical Consultations.* London: Tavistock.
23. Mechanic D (1978) *Medical Sociology*, 2nd edn. New York: Free Press.
24. Zola I (1973) Pathways to the doctor: from person to patient. *Social Science and Medicine* **7**: 677–89.
25. Goffman E (1961) *Asylums: Essays on the Social Situation of Mental Patients and Other Inmates.* Harmondsworth: Penguin.
26. Strauss A (1963) The hospital and its negotiated order. In E Freidson (ed.) *The Hospital in Modern Society.* New York: Free Press.
27. Wing J (1962) Institutionalism in mental hospitals. *British Journal of Social and Clinical Psychology* **1**: 38–51.
28. Foucault M (1965) *Madness and Civilization.* New York: Random House.
29. Kennedy I (1981) *The Unmasking of Medicine.* London: Paladin.
30. Szasz T (1970) *The Manufacture of Madness.* New York: Harper & Row.

31. Barrett A, Turner RJ (2006) Family structure and substance use problems in adolescence and early adulthood: examining explanations for the relationship. *Addiction* **101**: 109–20.
32. Brown G, Birley J, Wing J (1972) Influences of family life on the course of schizophrenic disorders: a replication. *British Journal of Psychiatry* **121**: 241–8.
33. Leff J, Vaughn C (1985) *Expressed Emotion in Families*. New York: Guilford Press.
34. Barrowclough C, Hooley J (2003) Attributions and expressed emotion: a review. *Clinical Psychology Review* **23**: 849–80.
35. Gabe J, Bury M, Elston MA (2004) *Key Concepts in Medical Sociology*. London: Sage.
36. Brown G, Harris T (1978) *The Social Origins of Depression*. London: Tavistock.
37. Harris T (2001) Recent developments in understanding the psychosocial aspects of depression. *British Medical Bulletin* **57**: 17–32.
38. Cantor-Graae E (2007) The contribution of social factors to the development of schizophrenia: a review of recent findings. *Canadian Journal of Psychiatry* **52**: 277–86.
39. Cantor-Graae E, Selten J (2005) Schizophrenia and migration: a meta-analysis and review. *American Journal of Psychiatry* **162**: 12–24.
40. Adrian M (2003) How can sociological theory help our understanding of addictions? *Substance Use and Misuse* **38**: 1385–423.
41. McIntosh J, MacDonald F, McKeganey N (2005) The reasons why children in their pre- and early teenage years do or do not use illegal drugs. *International Journal of Drug Policy* **16**: 254–61.
42. Advisory Council on the Misuse of Drugs (ACMD) (1998) *Drug Misuse and the Environment*. London: The Stationery Office.
43. Johnston L, MacDonald R, Mason P, Ridley L, Webster C (2000) *Snakes and Ladders: Young People, Transition and Social Exclusion*. Bristol: Policy Press/Joseph Rowntree Foundation.
44. Neale J (2002) *Drug Users in Society*. Basingstoke: Palgrave.
45. Bradshaw J, Kemp P, Baldwin S, Rowe A (2003) *The Drivers of Social Exclusion: A Review of the Literature for the Social Exclusion Unit*. London: Social Exclusion Unit.
46. Goffman E (1963) *Stigma: Notes on the Management of Spoiled Identity*. Englewood Cliffs, NJ: Prentice-Hall.
47. Pilgrim D (2005) *Key Concepts in Mental Health*. London: Sage.
48. Croall H (1998) *Crime and Society in Britain*. London: Longman.
49. Doherty M (2003) *Criminology*, 4th edn. London: Old Bailey Press.
50. Merton R (1938) Social structure and anomie. *American Sociological Review*, **3**: 672–82.
51. Cohen A (1955) *Delinquent Boys*. Glencoe, IL: Free Press.
52. Becker H (1963) *Outsiders: Studies in the Sociology of Deviance*. New York: Free Press.
53. Taylor I, Walton P, Young J (1973) *The New Criminology*. London: Routledge & Kegan Paul.
54. Young J (1997) Left realist criminology: radical in its analysis, realist in its policy. In M Maguire, R Morgan, R Reiner (eds) *The Oxford Handbook of Criminology*, 2nd edn. Oxford: Clarendon Press.
55. Hudson B (2003) *Understanding Justice: An Introduction to Ideas, Perspectives and Controversies in Modern Penal Theory*. Buckingham: Open University Press.

Chapter 22

Cultural psychiatry

Dinesh Bhugra and Sean Cross

INTRODUCTION

Culture plays a significant role in people's lives. The way people dress, behave, eat, drink and generally deal with emotional distress and idioms to express their distress are all influenced by culture. Culture and society define what is deviant and what is normal and where and how people seek help. In this chapter we propose to define culture and to describe its impact on mental illness and its management.

THEORETICAL BACKGROUND

What is culture?

The word 'culture; has been described as 'one of the two or three most complicated words in the English language',[1] and as a result many misunderstandings ensue. It has been described as being used in three main ways:[2]

- Culture as a supposed 'civilizing' process, from migratory to agrarian to urban societies, which have become more cultivated in a historical sense, or contemporaneously of an artistic or rarefied existence. Both imply that a higher or better level has evolved.
- Culture as collective identity with the setting apart of one group of people from another on the basis of historical lineage, language, religion, gender or ethnicity.[3]
- Culture as it is currently used in anthropology, as a 'way of life', with all the norms, values, customs, beliefs and practices that form a complex system.[4]

We all carry different cultures with us, such as cultures related to gender, specialties and work-related milieu. Conflation of these different ways of looking at culture can lead to problems. The first definition is often associated with notions of class and superiority. However, the other definitions also use different sources of identities to create complex levels of influence. Cultural identity is fluid and changes with exposure to other cultures and different components work at different levels. For example, an Indian person may well behave differently in an Indian formal setting than in a formal British setting.

An individual's culture consists of different elements, including age, gender, nationality, ethnicity, language, religion, politics, sexual orientation and career. Some elements may have stronger meanings than others. The term 'subculture' is also used without an exact definition. There are important components in the construction (Table 22.1).

Table 22.1 Summary of important components in cultural identity construction

Time	Not only a question of ageing but also the fluidity of different priorities at different times in identity construction
Place	The Internet has challenged the need for definitive boundaries in identity construction, but nationality and ethnicity are still largely geographically based
Other	An 'other' is required to define against and becomes integral to the identity construct

Variations in presentation of any health issue can be influenced by a variety of different forces in an individual's identity, as represented in Figure 22.1.

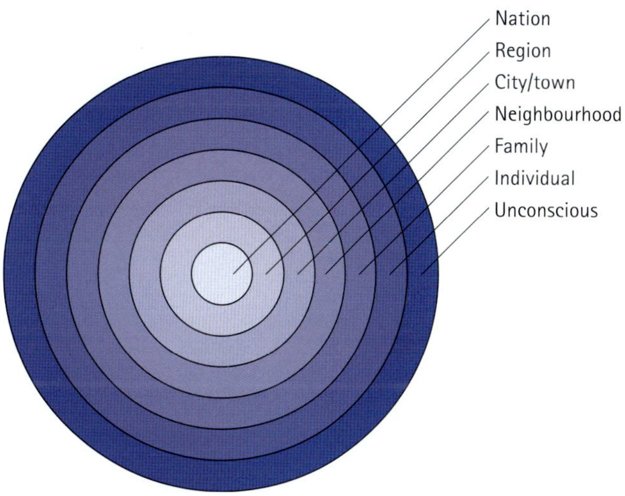

Figure 22.1 Where is culture located, and how is it to be measured? Reproduced with permission from Kohn R and Bhui K (2007) Psychiatric epidemiology and its contributions to cultural psychiatry. In D Bhugra and K Bhui (eds) *Textbook of Cultural Psychiatry*. Cambridge: CUP

We will argue that culture, made up of many aspects of these, forms a strong mediating role in the presentation, identification and management of mental health problems.

Key concepts in cultural psychiatry

In the history of cultural psychiatry, the argument between universalism and relativism across cultures is relevant in our understanding of the role of culture in the genesis and presentation of symptoms.

Universalist position

This is often taken by psychiatrists and argues that people are primarily of one type, i.e. one species. It is at this level of 'sameness' that most of the aetiological factors influencing mental disorders act. All members of the species are potentially affected by these genetic or environmental pressures, which result in variation. The symptoms of a disorder, its course and its outcome are taken to have a 'normal expected' path, with deviation from it explainable by the lesser effects such as social pressures.

Relativist position

This is the position espoused by many anthropologists, who argue that people are one species but are also members of many other groupings. It is at these lower-than-species level groupings that aetiological factors influencing mental disorders can act. Variation may be due to cultural pressures against which different individuals or different groups may react differently. As such, the symptoms of a disorder and its course can have many different understandable outcomes, with any attempt at creating a 'normal' outcome resisted. Attempts at understanding the process can be done only by also recognizing the relative position of the observer.

Psychiatry is affected by the contemporaneous sociopolitical context. Many of the early works on phenomenology were influenced by the colonial activities of European nations of the time. Imposition of European-style management of psychotic mental disorders occurred globally, and asylums for the custodial care of the long-term mentally ill were built. Orientalist understanding of the presentations of mental disorders also occurred and in various forms remains today. Kraeplin concluded that his basic forms of *dementia praecox* existed in Javanese people, 'though racial characteristics, religion and customs' might modify their clinical manifestations.[5] It was assumed that there was a fully explainable biological causative pathway for mental disorders, with culture playing a peripheral pathoplastic effect. Now this is viewed as naive.

Cultural psychiatric studies, along with many others, spent much of the latter part of the twentieth century adjusting to this legacy. The civil rights movement in the USA successfully challenged the notion of racial supremacy within the West, even if its impact is still ongoing today. Various guises of sociopolitical accommodation of immigrant groups across Western Europe and the USA have also resulted in the advancement of concepts that help to explain aetiology of mental disorders. In particular, the concept of acculturation is important and defined as 'the process of cultural and psychological change that takes place as a result of contact between cultural groups and their members'.[6]

This contact can be brief, such as a holiday, be the result of a war, conquest or colonization, or be the result of immigration processes. A relationship between assimilation and integration between different groups is represented in Figure 22.2.

From the 1960s onwards, large cross-national epidemiological studies were undertaken under the auspices of the

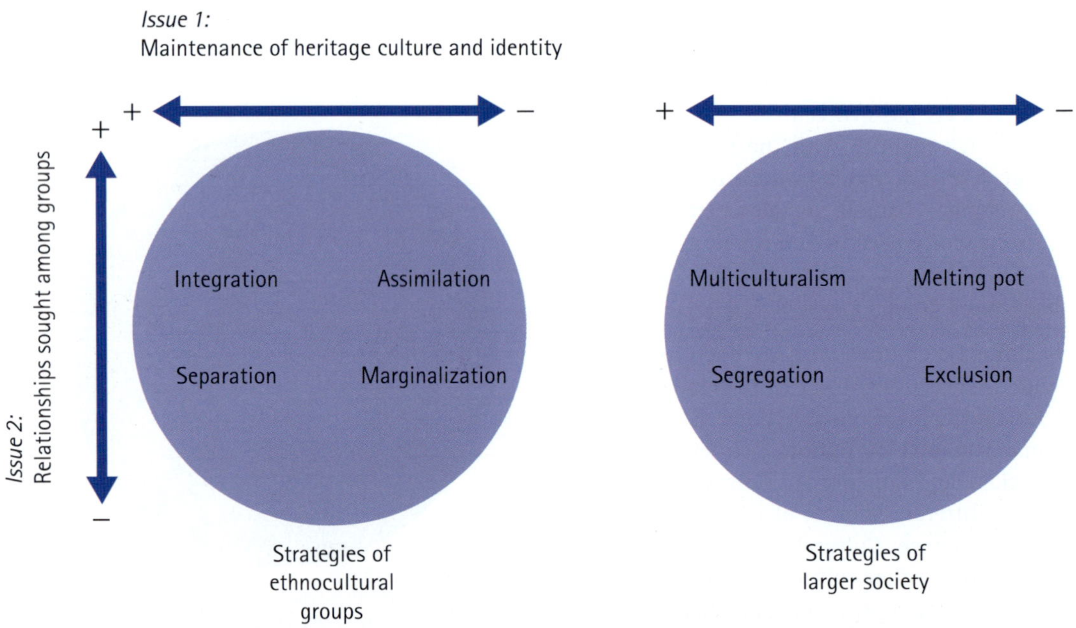

Figure 22.2 Acculturation strategies in ethnocultural groups and in the larger society. Based on John Berry's model of acculturation. Berry J (1997) Immigration, Acculturation and Adaptation. *Applied Psychology: An International Review* **46:** 5–68

World Health Organization (WHO). Such universalist ventures occurred while anthropological concepts were influencing psychiatric practice.

Etic

This description accounts for culturally neutral observations, in which the same entities can be identified across different cultures. The term is derived from linguistics and is short for phonetic, i.e. 'sounds like'. The WHO's multi-country studies on a number of psychiatric conditions are more etic in origin. They are useful in understanding the application of epidemiological methods. They have significant face validity because, in every culture that has been studied, clusters of symptoms such as feeling bad or hearing voices have been described.

Emic

This description accounts for culturally meaningful observations, which grow out of the culture and vary between cultures. This is derived from linguistics too and is short form for phonemic. More emic traditions also exist. The advocacy by Kleinman of a philosophical category fallacy in psychiatry is the most famous relativist critique.[7] It argues against the presumption that psychiatric categorization has the same meaning between cultures.

Tseng highlights differences in various roles that culture plays in relationship to psychiatric disorders. The impact of culture on psychopathology has also been classified in a further way, depending on how causative or associative it is seen to be (Table 22.2).[8]

Table 22.2 Summary of Tseng's description of effects on psychopathology

Effects	Description
Pathogenic	Culture is directly causative of psychopathology, e.g. through heightened stress of cultural expectation or necessity
Pathoselective	Tendency to select certain culturally influenced reactions, e.g. culturally sanctioned suicide
Pathoplastic	Culture influences or models the manifestation, e.g. types of delusional beliefs such as 'I am Christ' or 'I am Buddha'
Pathoelaborating	Universal behaviour reactions that may become exaggerated through reinforcement, e.g. types of suicidal act
Pathofacilitative	Culture does not affect the actual universalism of the disorder, but it does affect the frequency of onset, e.g. excessive concern with body weight and association with onset of eating disorders
Pathoreactive	Although not directly affecting the disorder, it does affect how the disorder is viewed and dealt with within the culture

CULTURE AND MENTAL DISORDERS

In this section we illustrate some of the cultural factors in major psychiatric disorders.

Schizophrenia and psychoses

Because of the perceived importance and striking pathology, schizophrenia was the first of the mental disorders to be studied across cultures. Determining the homogeneity of the pathophysiological process is a major difficultly due to the lack of an objective test. There is little doubt that a relapsing and remitting psychotic condition occurs in all human cultures of a sufficient size that have so far been studied. Positive symptom constellations are similar across cultures, namely hallucinatory voices in the third person, thought withdrawal or broadcast, and the sense of surroundings being imbued with special meaning. Negative symptoms also display commonalities across cultures, including psychomotor poverty, social withdrawal and amotivation. Age and sex distribution also appear similar.

Two major large-scale studies occurred in the 1960s – the International Pilot Study of Schizophrenia (IPSS)[9–11] and the Determinants of Outcome of Severe Mental Disorders, a WHO ten-country study.[12–14] These were some of the first key studies to gather information in an epidemiologically valid way, reducing but not eradicating observer bias through the use of standardized assessment tools. They looked for and found commonalities but ignored differences in their discussion of the implications of their findings. However, it is in those differences that greater understanding of the actual disorder process may occur.

Comparison of rates of schizophrenia

It is important to stress that the rates show variation according to methodologies. The following rates are summarized in greater detail in other work.[15]

Prevalence

- *Developed country studies:* 2.4–7.0 per 1000.
- *Developing country studies:* 1.4–7.3 per 1000.

Incidence

The time at which symptoms reach a threshold of recognition is prone to significant national and cultural variance. Based on *International Classification of Diseases*, version 8 (ICD-8) or version 9 (ICD-9) 'broad' definitions of schizophrenia, the incidence is between 0.17 and 0.54 per 1000 population per year. Using the more restrictive *Diagnostic and Statistical Manual*, 3rd edition (DSM-III), 3rd edition revised (DSM-IIIR) or fourth edition (DSM-IV) or ICD-10 criteria, it is two to three times lower.

Two systematic reviews of the literature highlight considerable variation in schizophrenia rates across countries,[16,17] but less variance is demonstrated than in other medical conditions such as insulin-dependent diabetes mellitus and multiple sclerosis. Causative or protective influences in the development of schizophrenia may be hypothesized following identification of characteristics of groups with high or low rates.

Low rates of schizophrenia

The Hutterites in South Dakota are a close-knit Protestant community of 35000 people originally descended from about 90 forebears. A lifetime prevalence rate for schizophrenia of 1.1 per 1000 was recorded[18] and replicated.[19,20] Several causes have been suggested:

- Genetic, due to a low frequency of psychosis-predisposing alleles
- Social/cultural, due to protective community support factors
- Social/cultural, due to a negative selection of individuals with schizoid traits unable to tolerate the communal lifestyle leaving the group.

Low rates have also been recorded in aboriginal Taiwanese people compared with mainland Chinese people who migrated to the island after the Second World War. Two studies show rates of 2.1 and 1.4 per 1000 population, respectively.[21,22]

High rates of schizophrenia

Two to three times the national rate have been found in certain population isolates in northern Sweden[23] and several areas of Finland.[24,25] High estimated lifetime risks for schizophrenia – recorded as 2.77 per cent for males and 1.99 per cent for females – were reported from the Palau islands in Micronesia.[26] The highest lifetime risk estimate for schizophrenia at 4.95 per cent was recorded in a community in Daghestan, in the Russian Federation.[27]

There are also data showing high rates of schizophrenia in both immigrant and subsequent minority ethnic communities (Table 22.3).

Table 22.3 Summary of increased rates of schizophrenia symptoms in different groups

Rate variations	Group and country
Increased rates of psychotic symptoms	Norwegian immigrants in the USA[28]
Increased rates of psychosis	Afro-Caribbean immigrants to the UK[29]
Higher rates of incidence of schizophrenia – 0.6 per 1000	Afro-Caribbean population in the UK[30,31]
Four-fold increase in rates of psychosis	Dutch Antillean and Surinamese immigrants in the Netherlands[32]
Increased rates of psychosis	Moroccan and other non-Western immigrants in the Netherlands[33]

Migration stress as a direct cause has been advanced, as several studies have shown lower rates of schizophrenia in the home countries of the Caribbean.[34,35] However, simple migratory stress is not the whole answer. There is an additional explanation that needs to be explored. From Odegaard's work onwards, the rates have been higher in migrants, but after they have been in the new country for long periods rather than an immediate development of illness, indicating that migratory stress may not work in isolation. There is no evidence that these psychotic events are somehow different from the normal course of a psychotic disorder.[36,37] No other links with other biological explanations – such as increased obstetric complications or increased maternal influenza rates – have been found.[38,39] A further complicating factor against a pure migration stress theory is that increased rates of schizophrenia occur in siblings of second-generation Afro-Caribbean individuals with schizophrenia when compared with white British individuals with schizophrenia.[40] Of further concern remains the distinct possibility of continuing observer bias difficulties demonstrated in one study showing significant diagnostic disagreement between a Jamaican and a British psychiatrist.[41]

The Aetiology and Ethnicity in Schizophrenia and Other Psychoses (AESOP) study is a large, ongoing, first-presentation study based in London, Nottingham and Bristol in the UK and has revealed similar findings (Table 22.4).

Given these data, a variety of explanations have been advanced, including lack of supportive community structures, lack of stable family structures, lower social capital (the concept that social networks have value and give advantage in some way to individuals possessing them), acculturation stresses, trans-generational acculturation processes, demoralization due to racial discrimination, institutional racism, and blocked opportunity for upward social mobility.

Table 22.4 Summary of major Aetiology and Ethnicity in Schizophrenia and Other Psychoses (AESOP) study findings

- Two-fold increase in rate of psychosis in London compared with in Nottingham and Bristol, adding an extra dimension to urbanization hypotheses[42]
- Nine-fold increase in rates of psychosis in Afro-Caribbean people and six-fold increase in black African compared with white British counterparts[42]
- Afro-Caribbean and black African individuals are far more likely to be detained at first presentation and more likely to access care via police rather than GP[43]
- Detection of an association between early separation, parental loss and social isolation and development of psychosis[44]

GP, general practitioner.

Comparison of the content of symptoms of schizophrenia

The WHO ten-country study noted that variations in the type of the disorder occur in different cultural settings (Table 22.5).[13]

Table 22.5 Percentage of patients with different forms of schizophrenia

	Developing countries	Developed countries
Acute-onset schizophrenia	40.3	10.9
Catatonic schizophrenia	10.3	1.2

The pathoplastic influence of culture on specific psychotic symptoms is undoubted. However, for both delusions and hallucinations, further influences have been identified. A developing/developed nation dichotomous split is an oversimplification, with religion playing a strong cultural mediating role.

Delusions

Religious delusions and delusional guilt are common in Christian culture but less frequent in Hindu, Buddhist and Islamic societies.[45] The same study demonstrated that delusions of grandeur were rarer in village communities, where it was postulated as wrong to strive for a higher level.[45] In the IPSS study, persecution was the most common delusional theme, but Pakistan (the only Islamic country in the study noted above) showed far fewer religious, grandeur and guilt themes. The religious delusions centred on Djinn possession. Prophet-type delusions, common in Africa, were virtually absent from Pakistan, where they are far less culturally sanctioned.[45]

Hallucinations

Visual and tactile hallucinations appeared more frequently in individuals from Africa and the Middle East than in those from Europe.[46] Higher rates of auditory and visual hallucinations were also recorded in non-European patients compared with English and other European patients in a study in London.[47] Furthermore, Pakistanis in Pakistan reported higher rates of visual and lower rates of auditory hallucinations than British Pakistani or white British people in the UK.[48]

Comparison of the outcome of schizophrenia

Since the early twentieth century, it has been proposed that a less disabling course of the disorder played out in developing nations. The WHO multicentre studies appeared to confirm this, with the IPSS showing better outcomes for patients from India, Colombia and Nigeria in a range of measures.[9,10] The WHO ten-country study confirmed these findings with the data shown in Table 22.6.[13]

Table 22.6 Percentage of patients with different outcome measures

	Developing countries	Developed countries
Remitting/complete remission	62.7	36.8
Impaired social functioning	15.7	41.6

However, developing nation status may simply be an artefact to some other aspect of culture. It may reflect changing culture in response to urbanization and industrialization, and it may well also indicate changing social mores, with changes in socioeconomic and educational status.

Although genetic variations may account for some of the differences, psychosocial and cultural factors have been proposed to play a role in the outcome, such as close-knit family/communities in sociocentric non-Western countries where the social expectations are from the kinship rather than from the individuals; family set-ups where less able individuals may be looked after; higher rates of marriage and resulting support in developing nations; acute onset in developing nations, with possibility of organic and infectious agents playing a part; higher individual–environment fits that minimize social isolation and withdrawal in developing nations; and lower incidences of chronic stressors associated with developed market economies.

The influence of expressed emotion (EE) as a predictor of psychotic relapse was investigated in the WHO ten country study.[49] It was noted that EE was as effective at predicting a relapse in Indian as European or North American families, but that it was in itself a much rarer phenomenon in India, thus demonstrating a potentially strong candidate for a cultural precipitant.

Affective disorders

Affective disorders are common in all cultures, but their presentation is likely to be affected by cultural factors too, in that mania or depression will carry with them different cultural symbolism. The majority of this section is devoted to depression, although some evidence is also available on mania and bipolar disorders across different cultures. A contemporaneous study to the IPSS found that rates of mania occurred at similar rates across countries.[50]

Early theories held the opinion that depression was rare in non-Western cultures. An argument has been advanced that this came from an alliance between colonial-era psychiatrists and cultural anthropologists, with the former believing racist assumptions in the capacity of people to experience depression and the latter believing in different culturally specific ways of displaying distress.[51]

Comparison of rates of depression

Cross-community comparative psychiatric surveys demonstrate significant variation, from 2.6 per cent in Nagasaki to 29.5 per cent in Santiago.[52] However, the conclusion that

Chileans are ten times more depressive than Japanese people is untenable. Variations are likely to measure health systems, pathways to care and attitudes to health. However, comparisons of rates between countries using the same tools have occurred, and several of these are presented in Table 22.7.[51]

Several studies have also attempted to detect differences in rates between different ethnic groups within countries (Table 22.8).[51]

Variations in rates of depression occur within culturally homogenous groups in relation to basic demographic factors such as age, gender and socioeconomic status, as well as more complex factors such as the pressures of urban living, all of which may be interwoven in minority ethnic communities. The presence of extreme political events such as war or genocide can often result in the diagnosis of high levels of depression, such as the Lebanon study below. To look for explanatory cultural factors on the meanings of dysphoria in such a universally miserable setting may be inappropriate. However, culturally relevant coping strategies may also play a role in understanding how distress is experienced and expressed.

Comparison of the content of depressive symptoms

The WHO Collaborative Study on Standardised Assessment of Depressive Disorder studied 583 patients in five urban centres in four countries (Basle, Montreal, Tehran, Nagasaki, Tokyo) using the Schedule for Standardised Assessment of Depressive Disorder.[67] The results highlighted quantitative rather than qualitative differences. There was similarity in core symptoms such as sadness, joylessness, anxiety, tension, lack of energy, loss of interest, loss of concentration, and ideas of inadequacy, insufficiency and worthlessness. Feelings of guilt, often associated with a

Table 22.7 Summary of depression rates using different tools

Tool used	Prevalence rates
Diagnostic Interview Schedule	Lifetime low: 1.5% – Taiwan[53]
	Lifetime: 9.6% – Canada[54]
	Lifetime: 9.2% – West Germany[55]
	Lifetime: 3.7% – Hong Kong[56]
	Lifetime high: 41.9% – Lebanon[57]
Composite International Diagnostic Interview	Lifetime low: 2.3% – Nigeria[58]
	Lifetime: 10.5% – Spain[59]
	Lifetime: 14.6% – Ukraine[60]
	Lifetime high: 21.4% – France[61]

Table 22.8 Summary of rates of depression in different ethnic groups

Study	Group	Prevalence (%)
Riolo *et al.* (2005)[62]	USA – white	10.4 – lifetime
	USA – African-American	7.5 – lifetime
	USA – Mexican-American	8.0 – lifetime
Weich *et al.* (2004)[63]	UK – Irish	1.8
	UK – black Caribbean	2.2
	UK – Bangladeshi	2.1
	UK – Indian	1.7
	UK – Pakistani	2.4
	UK – white	2.4
Takeuchi *et al.* (1998)[64]	Los Angeles Chinese Americans	6.9 – lifetime
Beals *et al.* (2005)[65]	American Indian tribes	5.5 – lifetime
Hicks (2002)[66]	Chinese American women	21 – lifetime

Judeo-Christian tradition, were most common in Basle and Montreal and least common in Tehran, where suicidal ideation was also least common. Somatic symptoms were more common in Tehran than in Basle or Montreal.

Other studies have also highlighted further differences. Although guilt remains a ubiquitous symptom, its focus can vary. Guilt directed towards ancestors, parents and fellow workers is common in Japan compared with guilt directed towards children and God in Germany.[68] Attempts at subdividing types of guilt into different culturally specific components have not succeeded so far.[69] Other symptoms such as poor libido, loss of energy and hypochondriasis occur at different rates in different groups, such as one study where they were related more commonly by people with depression in southern than northern India.[70]

In China it is more socially acceptable to receive the diagnosis of neurasthenia than depression, and neurasthenia is a commoner diagnosis there than anywhere else.[71] However, in 100 patients with neurasthenia in Taiwan who were examined using standardized tools, 93 were found to have clinical depression and 87 major depressive disorder according to DSM-III. On being treated with tricyclic antidepressants, a majority experienced mood lift but social function deterioration. The diagnosis of neurasthenia was viewed as important in maintaining or sanctioning this higher level of functioning.

The low rates in certain populations from the studies above, such as Taiwnanese people, may be explained in Kleinmanian terms. However, this is challenged when looking at levels of diagnosed depression in Chinese groups outside China when the importance of acculturation is taken into account. Australian Chinese immigrants are able to recognize and ascribe depressive symptoms more easily. Their likelihood of gaining a diagnosis of depression is increased in line with the level of acculturation.[72] East Asian immigrants to the USA were found to have increased attention to the affective component and less to the somatic component of self with increased acculturation.[73] In a further study, the overall level of somatic symptoms in presentation of dysphoria in Chinese-Americans was also unaffected, suggesting that acculturation regarding dysphoria in Western culture works primarily at an affective-cognitive level.[74]

Abandonment of notions of earlier culture has been suggested to be a depressogenic factor, with Korean Americans who abandon their identity seen as likelier to become depressed.[75] The study also found that learning the new language and increasing social contacts were protective against developing depression, although in another, larger study, bilingualism in itself was found not to be a protective factor.[76]

Once again, migration has been suggested as a precipitating factor in depression. However, it is a complex model when considering other influences such as culture clash and general chronic stressors encountered by most immigrants, including poor housing, lower incomes and urban living.[77] Understandably, significantly higher levels of depression have been measured in groups of refugees and asylum seekers,[78] and clear differences in levels of depression have been measured in different Hispanic groups in the USA, with higher levels linked to illegality of presence.[79]

Anxiety and the stress disorders

There is much less evidence on cross-cultural comparisons of anxiety disorders. Data are presented on several different disorders collected loosely as 'anxiety and stress disorders'. It is within this milieu that the culture-bound syndromes will be addressed. Although not all are anxiety-related, they are discussed here in an attempt to normalize them as human experiences and purposefully move away from the orientalist view of them as some kind of peculiar exotic behaviour or other.

Panic disorder

The somatic experiences that hyperventilation can bring leave open many different interpretations influenced by the individual's cultural beliefs. *Ode-ori* has been postulated to be a cultural variation of panic that is described in some Nigerian cultures with symptoms such as heat in the head or parasites crawling in the head at times of heightened fear.[80]

Social phobia

Fear of scrutiny or criticism by others, together with somatic symptoms of blushing, sweating and other symptoms of anxiety, can lead to significant avoidance behaviour. *Taijinkyofusho* from Japan has a core symptom of a fear of offending others through inappropriate behaviour or presentation. These symptoms were found to correlate strongly with social phobia in Japanese-Americans in Hawaii, but with more symptoms specific to *taijinkyofusho* associated with lower levels of acculturation.[80]

Obsessive–compulsive disorder

Religious and superstitious themes have a major impact on obsessive–compulsive disorder (OCD) symptoms, as do widely culturally differing approaches to cleanliness, contamination and purification, which often lie at the heart of ritualistic behaviour.[81] Conflicting information exists on rates of OCD. The Cross National Collaborative Study described similar lifetime prevalence rates of approximately 2.3 per cent in many countries, with the exceptions of South Korea at 1.9 per cent and Taiwan at 0.7 per cent.[82] Lower rates for minority ethnic populations have been recorded in the UK[83] and for Australian Aborigines.[84]

Dissociative disorders

Of central importance to these diagnoses is loss of integrative function between different aspects of the self – from mind or memories to body parts or bodily functions. The symptoms are classified as affecting specific body parts (conversion disorders), the memory (dissociative amnesia or fugue) and the personality (dissociative identity disorder or even trance or possession disorders). It is unsurprising that this area has considerable history in the field of cross-cultural psychiatry, but epidemiological data are sadly lacking.

The precipitous decline of the use of the term 'hysteria' as a diagnosis across the twentieth century in the West has been mirrored by an increase in the use of the terms 'depression' and 'anxiety'. Distress has become more readily communicable verbally in a way that previous hysterical symptoms were an expressed conversion. The pejorative inference of the term 'hysterical', challenged within the West not least by feminist theory, means it has to all intents and purposes been abandoned. However, it is still a commonly asserted view that hysterical symptoms are more common within the developing world.

It is within this context that other culture-bound disorders are described, such as *latah*, in which echolalia in dissociative states has been described in North Africa, and *amok* in South-East Asia, in which these states are seen as associated with severe episodes of violence and amnesia. The danger once again with such classification is that they are seen as entities that 'they' are prone to and 'we' are not. It is more valid to view these as cultural variations on a theme of symptom complexes in response to stressors, rather than as separate entities themselves. A wider discussion on the re-evaluation of culture-bound syndromes is available.[85] Figure 22.3 attempts to show a probable relationship between culture-bound syndromes and psychiatric disorders.

Somatization disorder

Associated with some form of conversion process, somatization disorder has strict criteria according to ICD-10 and DSM-IV. Variations within different cultural contexts have, however, been postulated, such as *ataque de nervios* among Hispanic people and *hwa byung* in Korea.

Hypochondriacal disorder

No recognizable disease pattern is described, but repeated investigation of symptoms is requested without reassurance. Variations on the type of presentation will depend on the cultural context, but several anxiety states based on irrational fears of sexual function are very common globally. Within certain parts of South-East Asia this has been described as *koro*, in which death is seen as possible due to retraction of the penis into the body.

Post-traumatic stress disorder

Perhaps more than any other contemporary diagnosis, post-traumatic stress disorder (PTSD) has led to vociferous arguments among psychiatrists over the cross-cultural validity of the construct since its use describing American soldiers' psychopathology after the Vietnam War. The cluster of symptoms includes a triad of flashbacks to the prior traumatic event, hypervigilance and avoidance behaviour.

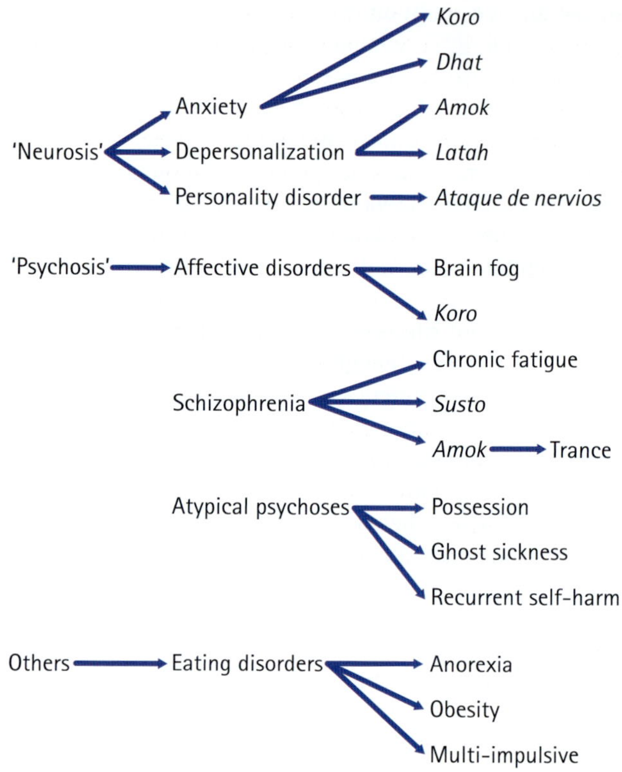

Figure 22.3 Interaction between psychiatric disorders and culture-bound syndromes. Modified from Bhugra D and Jacob KS (1997) Culture bound syndromes. In *Troublesome disguises: Undiagnosed Psychiatric Syndromes*. Oxford: Blackwell science

All humans can experience traumatic events. There are a variety of ways that people from different cultures use to adapt to these events. There are multiple examples of studies from across the globe in which high rates of PTSD have been recorded in many different cultures with culturally validated tools.[86,87] However, the use of a medicalized framework for this process has been critiqued as being imperialistic due to the etic imposition of such a framework.[88] In the contemporary world, this has specific and growing cross-cultural relevance within the field of conflict psychiatry, reactions to war and natural disasters and refugee health. The use of 'traumascape' theories attempts to build consensus around the need to see the individual as part of a wider cultural and historical setting in which different ways, rituals and processes can be drawn upon in order to heighten resilience and lower vulnerability.[89]

Substance misuse

Most cultures around the world have a history of use of different mind-altering substances for social or religious practices. The cultural influences in assessment of these practices tend to be complex. In the context of a substance, use, misuse and dependence may be seen as a continuum.[90] There is significant agreement between ICD-10 and DSM-IV on the classification of dependence syndromes, with both influenced by research on alcohol.[91] There is also evidence for the validity of the dependence syndromes for alcohol, opioids and cannabis across different countries according to the WHO, but not for other substances.[92]

In the absence of a dependence syndrome, there is less unanimity in how to classify, due to misuse or problematic use being subjective and inextricably judged against cultural norms. There are examples throughout history of widely differing attitudes to different substance usage, which is often linked with legality. These include the criminalization of substances such as opium across time,[93] and the medicalization of khat, which has occurred in Europe following its use within a new social and cultural context.[90]

Despite the difficulties, some studies have tried to measure the levels of substance misuse across cultures.[94] It has been estimated that globally 1 billion people smoke tobacco, 76 million people suffer from alcohol use disorders and 15 million people have a drug use disorder.[95] Further studies suggest the influence of migration and acculturation processes, with evidence that substance misuse in ethnic minorities in the UK is lower than for the indigenous population.[96] However, potentially contradictory evidence also exists – depending on levels of use in originator countries – for substance misuse being higher in immigrants to the UK than in their equivalents in countries of origin.[97]

The manner in which culture interacts with the socioeconomic consequences of poverty is also important. Making causal links between particular cultures and increased susceptibility to substance misuse may be misleading. Several studies from a number of different cultures have identified a pattern of behaviour most loosely described as a 'poverty trap', which encourages ongoing substance misuse. It has been argued that poverty itself gives rise to a culture that promotes and maintains substance misuse in Sri Lanka.[98] Similar themes exist in evidence of higher rates of substance misuse in indigenous communities such as Australia and New Zealand[99] and the USA.[100]

Eating disorders

The relationship between individuals and their food is heavily influenced by the culture to which they belong.[101] Food is often used as a means of welcoming guests and is used as an important and significant symbol in relationships. Sociocultural pressures have been advanced as causative to the development of eating disorders. The 10 : 1 ratio of women to men may be a reflection of their higher associated target status for such notions as thinness. This is reinforced by high rates in certain subcultural groupings, such as dancers and models, in which a demand for thinness is even more marked than in society at large.[102–104] In addition, higher rates have been recorded in urban settings in all societies, with explanations varying from the changes in family structure and social mobility,[105,106] to easier availability of food, marked changes in meal timings, increased obesity and higher weight consciousness.[107]

Eating disorders have been considered as a culture-bound phenomenon, due to a low prevalence rate within many non-Western cultures.[108] However, this has been challenged with evidence including significant variation within the West, between the USA and central Europe,[109] and between different areas of a single country, in north and south Italy.[110]

There are reports of significant increases in certain areas of the world such as in black South African girls post Apartheid,[111] and in developing nations generally since 1990,[112] leading to an argument that eating disorders should be seen as markers of a 'westernization' process[107] or more latterly as 'markers of cultural transition' in general.[101]

Personality disorders

Disorders based on personality raise problematic cross-cultural issues due to the normative understanding of what personality means and how it fits within a wider societal framework. Classification of personality traits or types dates back to ancient Greece, but it was Pinel in the nineteenth century who first attempted to separate out psychopathological processes and behaviours that were not illnesses. The subsequent development of ICD-10 and DSM-IV has seen an evolution in the way in which these have been classified to the current ten categories.

Diagnostic reliability between psychiatrists is low even when working within a culturally homogenous setting,[113] perhaps due to pejorative connotations[114] or the inherent discrimination of the psychiatric profession.[115] In addition, the notion of culturally acceptable or unacceptable behaviour arises as an important marker in diagnosis. The overlap between the legal system and people with personality disorders is therefore unsurprising, with up to 80 per cent of people on remand in UK found to have an antisocial personality disorder.[116]

It is therefore important to consider how the concept of the self varies across cultures. It has been argued that, in the West, the self is individuated, detached, self-sufficient and separate – an egocentric position.[117] A corollary of this is the notion of a more sociocentric individual, whose conception of self is linked inextricably with a role in which individual choice is not absent but is subsumed within wider responsibilities. The importance of early formative years and subsequent experiences are seen as highly influential in the development of personality disorders, particularly to cluster B. The very different approaches to societal structure in which individuals develop would, unsurprisingly, result in different views of the self, different personal expectations, and different measures of failure to conform to societal norms and values.

Attempts at measuring personality disorders across cultures have occurred. The International Personality Disorder Examination (IPDE) was used in a study of 716 individuals in 14 centres in 11 countries, which showed a two-fold higher rate of diagnosis of personality disorder using DSM-IIIR as opposed to ICD-10.[118] Antisocial personality disorder is the only type to have been studied in cross-national community surveys of morbidity. Rates ranged from 0.14 per cent in Taiwan to 3.7 per cent in Canada.[119] However, the cause of such differences may be a true high prevalence or a reflection on how antisocial behaviour is defined in both societies.

Disorders of childhood and adolescence

Differences in the way childhood is experienced add a level of complexity when evaluating mental health problems cross-culturally. Children are at the forefront of the mechanisms of cultural continuation and absorb the norms and values of a particular way of life readily. Two important basic epidemiological factors are important (Table 22.9).[120]

Table 22.9 Summary of the importance of age and gender

Age	At 7, 14 or even 21 years old, different relationships with schooling, employment, marriage and psychoactive substances occur in different cultures
Gender	In much of the world, being female results in a different childhood experience than being male

A range of different international studies have estimated prevalence rates of 'child mental health problems' of 20–25 per cent and more specific 'child psychiatric disorders' of 9–12 per cent in several countries.[83,121,122] Increased rates are associated with lower socioeconomic status and with urban living.

Data on the attention spectrum disorders do reveal some cultural differences. In the USA, rates range from 3 per cent to 7 per cent of the general population. However, use of psychostimulant medication has been found to be associated strongly with the type of insurance policy held, meaning that white children are far more likely to be treated this way.[123]

Disorders of ageing

Although all humans age, not all experience old age in a similar way – if at all.[124] However, in both high- and low-income countries, the elderly population is increasing. It is estimated that the number of people over age 65 years will increase from 50 million in 1990 to 1 billion by 2025.[125] However, there is a paucity of epidemiological and clinical information on elderly people from low-income countries as well as minority ethnic populations in high-income countries.[126,127]

The different roles experienced by elderly people in different cultures towards employment, family and social responsibilities all potentially mediate mental health problems. The concept of multiple disadvantages is also pertinent for elderly people, who may experience problems associated not only with ageism but also with racism, class problems and restricted access to health and social care.[128]

Prevalence rates for dementia are influenced by several factors, including that individuals in lower-income countries have a shorter lifespan generally and that mortality rates once dementia has been diagnosed are worse in low-income countries.[129] There are many problems with cross-cultural comparisons, including difficulties in exact age identification, associations with pre-existing physical impairment confounders such as visual and hearing difficulties, high rates of illiteracy and innumeracy, and translational artefacts. However, some comparative prevalence studies of dementia are available and reveal rates between zero and 13.2 per cent, with a median of 4 per cent.[127] Universally the prevalence increases with age and is higher in women, with a rough rule of a doubling every 5 years after the age of 60 years.[130,131] In addition, prevalence of Alzheimer's disease is lower and of vascular dementia higher in Asian than Western countries.[132]

Intra-country cross-cultural studies reveal significant similarities in prevalence rates across groups in the UK.[133–135] However, a population-based study in the UK revealed that having an African or Caribbean origin increased the risk of dementia.[136] This matches data on higher prevalence rates in African-American and Hispanic people in the USA.[137] Higher rates of stroke and hypertension in African-American people have been recorded, suggesting a link with higher rates of vascular dementia.[138,139]

Deliberate self-harm and suicide

Comparative studies in this field are difficult due to a number of factors, as deliberate self-harm (DSH) and suicide rates are not recorded accurately in many places. It is suggested that a recent rise in youth suicide in Ireland is explained in part by a reduction in the number of coroner's verdicts of 'open' or 'accidental' deaths as a result of changing attitudes towards matters formerly taboo.[140]

Some attempt at comparative work is available.[141] In general global terms, European nations record the highest rates of suicide and Central and South American countries the lowest.[142] Most risk factor studies have occurred in high-income nations. Gender, rural communities, alcohol misuse, life events and a history of DSH increase risks globally. Being single, divorced or widowed, all of which increase risks in the West, do not appear to do so in China or India.[143] More 'religious' countries appear to have lower rates of suicide.[144] Although the meaning of self-harm and suicide varies across cultures, it appears that the attitudes to intentions when self-harming are actually consistent across many countries.[145] Variation in method of self-harming occurs, with firearm use an obvious cause of increased mortality in the USA. The same method but different agent can also reveal marked rate differences in suicide, for example with the use of pesticides as opposed to analgesics in China and Sri Lanka compared with Europe.[146] Accessibility to primary and secondary healthcare can also have a significant impact on survival rates post-incident. Some specific regional and country data are available.

Russia and Eastern Europe

High rates of suicide and DSH were recorded in Russia in the 1990s following the break-up of the USSR and all the social changes that came with it.[147] Of the former 15 Soviet states, 10 experienced a rise in suicide rates post-1991.[148] The Russian minority in Estonia were found to have higher suicide rates after that republic's independence.[149]

India

It has been estimated that 300 000 people die by suicide in India – three times the official figure.[150] Gender ratios are more equal than other nations, making cultural factors seemingly important.[151] There are even figures showing higher rates of young females in India to young males, with one study showing 50–75 per cent of all deaths of women aged 10–19 years in Vellore, southern India, as opposed to 25 per cent of equivalent males.[152] These higher rates for young women were replicated in New Delhi, but by a lesser margin of 1.2 : 1. Hanging was a more common method with young women and poisoning with young males, in a reversal of most other places.[153]

Japan

Traditionally this country has a high rate of suicide, with more complex cultural sanctioning of the behaviour in certain circumstances. In 2002 the rate was 23.8 per 100 000, but when broken down it is much higher in men aged 50–59 years at 71 per 100 000 and accounted for 24 per cent of all older person's deaths.[154] In middle-aged men, economic pressures and *inseki-jisatu*, or responsibility-driven suicides to demonstrate remorse for untoward events, are thought to be culpable factors.[155]

China

Overall more females than males die by suicide – the only country for which such rates are available.[156] Rural women are found to have a greater risk than urban women, in a reversal of Western risks.[157] Organophosphate usage is the most common method used by women, with impulsivity in the presence of family conflict noted as important.[158]

There are also data on suicide and DSH within different minority ethnic groupings.

The UK

Rates of DSH have been measured as 2.5 times higher in Asian women than white women and seven times higher in Asian women than in Asian men. Black men had much lower rates of DSH presentation than white men in one London study.[159] Additionally, Asian women were found to be more likely to report they wanted to die during DSH, more likely not to regret the incident, likely to take fewer tablets and less likely to use alcohol.[160]

Suicide data reveal further evidence of cultural differences, with high rates detected in men in general and in Indian women as a subgroup, mirroring the country data above. One study showed that Indian women were more likely to use hanging and burning as methods of suicide than white women, for whom self-poisoning was the main method.[161]

A further study revealed the age-specific rates of suicide for 20- to 44-year-olds in London (Table 22.10) and presented evidence that coroners appear less likely to return a verdict of suicide in ethnic minority groups.[162]

The USA

Data are also available on differences in DSH and suicide rates for different ethnic groupings within the USA (Table 22.11).[163]

Historically, the rate of suicide by African-Americans has been lower than by their white counterparts.[164] The black/white split in the USA also differs in a couple of epidemiologically important ways: (i) the rate of male to female suicides is higher, and (ii) the rates increase in early adulthood, follow a mid-life plateau and then decrease in later life. With the white population, the increase continues across life. Explanations about the protective nature of better social support networks and single motherhood among African-American women have been advanced.[165]

DSH data are more inconsistent, but several important themes have emerged, including that more DSH occurs

Table 22.10 Summary of suicide rates from one London study, 1997

Group	Rate per 100 000 people
Indian women	23.2
White women	9.5
African-Caribbean women	0.5
White men	27.0
African-Caribbean men	26.5
African origin men	15.0
Indian origin men	18.1

Table 22.11 Summary of US suicide rates, 2002

Group	Male rates per 100 000	Female rates per 100 000
White	20.0	4.7
American Indian/Alaskan native	16.4	4.1
African-American	9.8	1.6
Hispanic	8.3	1.8

among women in all groups and more African-American adolescents engage in self-harm than do their white counterparts.[166] African-American males are also more likely to require medical attention.[79]

Indigenous groups

Several additional countries with significant indigenous populations have data suggesting an overrepresentation of their populations in death by suicide, including First Nations People/Canadian Metis and Inuit,[167] and Australian Aborigines.[168] The impact of social marginalization, unemployment and increased alcohol and substance misuse are all advanced as causative.

Refugees

Refugees and asylum seekers show high rates of anxiety, depression and PTSD, all of which are risk factors for DSH behaviour and suicide, even though there are few studies demonstrating elevated risk for completed suicide, suggesting resilience is an important factor.[169,170]

CULTURE IN ASSESSMENT AND MANAGEMENT

This section focuses on cultural factors in the assessment process and management, including medication and psychotherapies.

Conducting a culturally aware assessment

As clinicians, we all must be aware of our cultural inheritance and prejudices so that we can understand how our response to patients is seen by patients and their carers. The assessment needs to gain an accurate and relevant amount of information quickly. It is easier to gain that information with someone similar to oneself, as various verbal and non-verbal communication mechanisms are used within a context of shared knowledge and are generally understood in the context of culture. Difficulties may arise as differences grow, whether these are related to language, religious values or broader cultural factors – but communicating across these differences is an essential skill for any psychiatrist to learn.

Any of the differences in Table 22.12 may result in a lack of shared knowledge. Into that vacuum assumptions may arise, from which prejudice may spring. Building shared knowledge requires you to have an awareness of relevant issues, which, even if somewhat alien, are accepted as valid. In a culturally aware assessment process, there are three important strands, as shown in Table 22.13.

Table 22.12 Some of the many ways in which cultural difference may occur

- Age
- Ethnicity
- Sexual orientation
- Gender
- Religion
- Nationality
- Class
- Language
- Political persuasion

Management with medication

The influence of culture in pharmacological management has been succinctly detailed, a summary of which now follows.[171] Culture can be thought of as influencing at three different levels, as shown in Table 22.14.

The first is a resource issue, but the latter two provide a basis for genuine variation. Many drug trial data, in particular on antidepressants, demonstrate significant placebo effects, which have a significant culturally mediated component. In addition, most trial data have also been generated from testing in the Caucasian populations of North America and Europe.

There is also evidence for the biological basis to variation. Absorption, distribution, metabolism and excretion of any given drug will vary across individuals and to some extent across ethnocultural groups. There are very few examples of full ethnocultural homogeneity, which means that stereotyping can lead to inaccuracies, but there are many examples of cross ethnocultural variances. An early study demonstrated a higher serum haloperidol level 7 h after dosing in Asian people versus Caucasian people, even taking into account body surface area. This was thought most likely due to differential hepatic first-pass rates.[172,173] More widely, there are two main ways in which this variation might act – through pharmacokinetic processes (variation in the amount of the drug that is present) and pharmacodynamic processes (variation in organism response to the drug).

Pharmacokinetics

The P450 enzyme system is important in metabolism. A highly studied part of this system is CYP2D6, which is responsible for about 25 per cent of metabolism of many drugs, including tricyclic antidepressants, selective serotonin reuptake inhibitors (SSRIs) and antipsychotics. Depending on a large number of allelic variants, enzyme activity has been measured and grouped according to the following types:[174,175]

- *UM:* ultra-rapid metabolizer (gene duplication or multiplication)
- *EM:* extensive metabolizer (gene duplication or multiplication)
- *IM:* intermediate metabolizer (one defective gene or two less effective genes)
- *PM:* poor metabolizer (two defective genes).

Table 22.13 Important ideas in a culturally aware interview

Be aware of oneself	Be aware of other	Be aware of circumstance
Beliefs about how certain problems should present according to one's own cultural norms	Variations in presentation of the same problem, e.g. different idioms of distress	Wider sociopolitical context within which you are working
How one's own cultural norms affect the formulation process	Variety of symptom cluster profiles that may occur, e.g. different emphases on the somatic	Acceptance of the reality of institutionalized prejudice processes
Any general assumptions and prejudices held by one's own culture about others	Basic norms and values of other cultures without assuming they are automatically held	Understanding that acculturation can result in hybrid responses becoming common
The way one has previously accepted or challenged these assumptions and prejudices differently	Avoidance of both negative and positive assumptions of others	Multiculturalism may mean different groups access and use the same services
Knowledge of the assumptions and prejudices made by other cultures about one's own	Assessment of the impact of assumptions or prejudices directed at your culture	
One's own non-verbal communication methods	Other kinds of non-verbal communication method	

Table 22.14 Three levels of cultural influence on pharmacology

Basic funding level	Globally, there are financial restrictions within many cultures on availability of medicines
Biological level	Variation in enzyme phenotypes resulting in different rates of metabolism
Non-biological level	'Expectation effect' of medications mediated by cultural norms and values; factors such as religious or dietary taboos

Table 22.15 Frequency of poor metabolizer (PM) variation in different groups

Group	PM variable frequency (%)	Study
Caucasians	5–10	177, 178
Black Africans	0–8	179
African-Americans	3.7	180, 181
Chinese	1	182

A study of 100 consecutively phenotyped hospital patients revealed that the number of adverse drug effects was highest in PMs, then IMs, and then EMs or UMs.[176] The cost of treating PMs and UMs was highest, and the total hospital duration was highest in PMs, which may have relevance due to the ethnocultural linkages (Table 22.15).

In addition to genetics, external factors, such as drugs and diet, and internal factors, such as hormones, may influence the activity of P450 enzymes. It has been postulated that diet as a cultural mediator is an important factor in the differential expression of CYP1A2, which may explain why significantly longer antipyrine half-life occurs in Sudanese people living in home villages compared with Sudanese people in the UK and white UK citizens.[183] Additionally, in clomipramine and antipyrine trials, significantly faster rates of metabolism have been demonstrated in South Asian subjects who switched to a 'British' diet, comparable with white British, than South Asians who followed 'Indian' vegetarian diets and South Asians in South Asia.[184,185]

CYP3A4 is a further enzyme in the P450 series and is involved in metabolism of many antipsychotics, including clozapine and benzodiazepines. Inhibition of this enzyme results in significant accumulation of certain drugs and a prolonged period of their action. A number of different potent inhibitors are readily available that will heighten the drug availability. Increased drowsiness in people who drank grapefruit juice after taking midazolam and triazolam has been described,[186,187] and black pepper from South Asia and piper cubeba from Indonesia are also both known to be potent inhibitors of CYP3A4.[188,189]

Pharmacodynamics

These processes, mediated by the transporters, receptors and enzyme systems, result in differential activities in response to pharmacological agents. The two most studied systems around which ethnocultural variation has been detected are the serotonin transporter (*5-HTT*) gene and the catecholamine-O-methyltrasferase (*COMT*) gene.

A serotonin transporter gene-linked polymorphism has been studied in its effects on the psychopathology of depression[190] and alcoholism.[191] In addition, it has been studied for its treatment effects on antidepressants in OCD[192] and depression.[193–196] Two alleles, *l* and *s*, demonstrate differential treatment responses, with *l* having a significantly better treatment response to SSRIs than the *s* variant. Results of further analysis in different groups have still revealed inconclusive findings but could be of importance because there have been ethnocultural variations in the preponderance of *l* alleles – people with African ancestry have the highest rates at 70 per cent, and people of East Asian origin the lowest at 17 per cent.[197]

The *COMT* gene mediates one of the pathways for metabolizing catecholamines, including dopamine and noradrenaline. Variant alleles that have been studied include the H and L varieties, with the latter demonstrating a three to four times lower rate of activity.[198]

Again, although findings have yet to be replicated robustly, there have been studies investigating the impact of such variation in panic disorder;[199,200] schizophrenia and Parkinson's disease;[201] treatment-resistant schizophrenia;[202] aggressive and violent behaviour;[198,203] and L-dopa therapy, with H/H genotype individuals suffering more dyskinesia than L/L genotype individuals.[204] One of the spurs to ongoing research in this area is due to the ethnocultural variations in L allele frequency that have been detected, with rates in Caucasians the highest at 50 per cent and East Asians the lowest at 18 per cent.[205]

Management with psychotherapies

The focus of psychotherapy aims to aid an individual's greater understanding of self, thereby eliminating or reducing the impact of psychopathological processes. Over the course of the twentieth century, many variations of talking therapies emerged from different intellectual traditions. These have been viewed as being most relevant to Western cultures. Although there are variations that focused on processes involving greater-than-self work such as family or systems therapy, the basis for much of the work is the concept of the self. Therefore, at the very core of the one-to-one psychotherapeutic alliance is the fundamentally important cross-cultural question of what it means to be an individual.

There is a dearth of empirical studies with psychotherapies, even without addressing cross-cultural complexities. Psychotherapies do not form the basis of services to people in most parts of the globe. The effective use of psychotherapies in a multicultural setting is still little studied.[206] However, smaller proportions of individuals from ethnic minority groups take up psychotherapy than do their white counterparts in both the USA and the UK, and more patients from ethnic minority groups drop out of psychotherapy. It appears that most people prefer a therapist from the same culture.

CONCLUSION

This chapter has presented evidence on the importance of cultural concepts in many aspects of psychiatric practice, from classification and identification of disorders to assessment and management of them. It is a complex field of endeavour, and there is still much to be discovered. However, in an age of increasing globalization in which the boundaries between cultures are transcended, it is vital to be aware of how different cultural norms and values may lead to a greater understanding of mental disorders and wider psychiatric practice.

REFERENCES

1. Williams R (1983) *Keywords: A Vocabulary of Culture and Society* (rev. and expanded edn). London: Fontana.
2. Kirmayer L (2007) Cultural psychiatry in historical perspective. In D Bhugra, K Bhui (eds) *Textbook of Cultural Psychiatry*. Cambridge: Cambridge University Press.
3. Banks M (1996) *Ethnicity: Anthropological Constructions*. London: Routledge.
4. Kuper A (1999) *Culture: The Anthropologists' Account*. Cambridge, MA, London: Harvard University Press.
5. Kraepelin E (1904) Vergleichende Psychiatrie. *Ztbl Nervenheilk Psychiat* 27: 433–7.
6. Redfield R, Linton R, Herkovits M (1936) Memorandum on the study of acculturation. *American Anthropologist* 38: 149–52.
7. Kleinman AM (1977) Depression, somatization and the 'new cross-cultural psychiatry'. *Social Science and Medicine* 11: 3–10.
8. Tseng W (2007) Culture and psychopathology: general view. In D Bhugra, K Bhui (eds) *Textbook of Cultural Psychiatry*. Cambridge: Cambridge University Press.
9. World Health Organization (1973) *Report of the International Pilot Study of Schizophrenia*. Geneva: World Health Organization.
10. World Health Organization (1979). *Schizophrenia: An International Follow-Up Study*. Geneva: World Health Organization.
11. Leff J, Sartorius N, Jablensky A, Korten A, Ernberg G (1992) The International Pilot Study of Schizophrenia: five-year follow-up findings. *Psychological Medicine* 22: 131–45.
12. Sartorius N, Jablensky A, Korten A, *et al.* (1986) Early manifestations and first-contact incidence of schizophrenia in different cultures: a preliminary report on the initial evaluation phase of the WHO Collaborative Study on determinants of outcome of severe mental disorders. *Psychological Medicine* 16: 909–28.
13. Jablensky A, Sartorius N, Ernberg G, *et al.* (1992) Schizophrenia: manifestations, incidence and course

in different cultures – a World Health Organization ten-country study. *Psychological Medicine Monograph Supplement* **20**: 1–97.
14. Jablensky A (2000) Epidemiology of schizophrenia: the global burden of disease and disability. *European Archives of Psychiatry and Clinical Neuroscience* **250**: 274–85.
15. Jablensky A (2007) Schizophrenia and related psychoses. In D Bhugra, K Bhui (eds) *Textbook of Cultural Psychiatry*. Cambridge: Cambridge University Press.
16. Goldner EM, Hsu L, Waraich P, Somers JM (2002) Prevalence and incidence studies of schizophrenic disorders: a systematic review of the literature. *Canadian Journal of Psychiatry* **47**: 833–43.
17. McGrath J, Saha S, Welham J, *et al.* (2004) Systematic review of the incidence of schizophrenia: the distribution of rates and the influence of sex, urbanicity, migrant status and methodology. *BMC Medicine* **2**: 13.
18. Eaton JW, Weil RJ (1955) *Culture and Mental Disorders: A Comparative Study of the Hutterites and Other Populations*. Glencoe, IL: Free Press.
19. Torrey EF (1995) Prevalence of psychosis among the Hutterites: a reanalysis of the 1950–53 study. *Schizophrenia Research* **16**: 167–70.
20. Nimgaonkar VL, Fujiwara TM, Dutta M, *et al.* (2000) Low prevalence of psychoses among the Hutterites, an isolated religious community. *American Journal of Psychiatry* **157**: 1065–70.
21. Rin H, Lin TY (1962) Mental illness among Formosan aborigines as compared with the Chinese in Taiwan. *Journal of Mental Science* **108**: 134–46.
22. Lin TY, Chu HM, Rin H, *et al.* (1989) Effects of social change on mental disorders in Taiwan: observations based on a 15-year follow-up survey of general populations in three communities. *Acta Psychiatrica Scandinavica Supplement* **348**: 11–33, discussion 167–78.
23. Book JA, Wetterberg L, Modrzewska K (1978) Schizophrenia in a north Swedish geographical isolate, 1900–1977: epidemiology, genetics and biochemistry. *Clinical Genetics* **14**: 373–94.
24. Hovatta I, Terwilliger JD, Lichtermann D, *et al.* (1997) Schizophrenia in the genetic isolate of Finland. *American Journal of Medical Genetics* **74**: 353–60.
25. Arajarvi R, Suvisaari J, Suokas J, *et al.* (2005) Prevalence and diagnosis of schizophrenia based on register, case record and interview data in an isolated Finnish birth cohort born 1940–1969. *Social Psychiatry and Psychiatric Epidemiology* **40**: 808–16.
26. Myles-Worsley M, Coon H, Tiobech J, *et al.* (1999) Genetic epidemiological study of schizophrenia in Palau, Micronesia: prevalence and familiality. *American Journal of Medical Genetics* **88**: 4–10.
27. Bulayeva KB, Leal SM, Pavlova TA, *et al.* (2005) Mapping genes of complex psychiatric diseases in Daghestan genetic isolates. *American Journal of Medical Genetics. Part B, Neuropsychiatric Genetics* **132B**: 76–84.
28. Odegaard O (1932) Emigration and insanity: a study of mental disease among Norwegian born population in Minnesota. *Acta Psychiatrica Neurologica Scandinavica* **7** (suppl. 4): 1–206.
29. Hemsi L (1967) Psychiatric morbidity of West Indian Immigrants. *Social Psychiatry* **2**: 95–100.
30. Bhugra D, Leff J, Mallett R, *et al.* (1997) Incidence and outcome of schizophrenia in whites, African-Caribbeans and Asians in London. *Psychological Medicine* **27**: 791–8.
31. Harrison G, Glazebrook C, Brewin J, *et al.* (1997) Increased incidence of psychotic disorders in migrants from the Caribbean to the United Kingdom. *Psychological Medicine* **27**: 799–806.
32. Selten JP, Slaets JP, Kahn RS (1997) Schizophrenia in Surinamese and Dutch Antillean immigrants to the Netherlands: evidence of an increased incidence. *Psychological Medicine* **27**: 807–11.
33. Veling W, Selten JP, Veen N, *et al.* (2006) Incidence of schizophrenia among ethnic minorities in the Netherlands: a four-year first-contact study. *Schizophrenia Research* **86**: 189–93.
34. Hickling FW, Rodgers-Johnson P (1995) The incidence of first contact schizophrenia in Jamaica. *British Journal of Psychiatry* **167**: 193–6.
35. Selten JP, Zeyl C, Dwarkasing R, *et al.* (2005) First-contact incidence of schizophrenia in Surinam. *British Journal of Psychiatry* **186**: 74–5.
36. Harrison G, Amin S, Singh SP, Croudace T, Jones P (1999) Outcome of psychosis in people of African-Caribbean family origin: population-based first-episode study. *British Journal of Psychiatry* **175**: 43–9.
37. Hutchinson G, Takei N, Sham P, Harvey I, Murray RM (1999) Factor analysis of symptoms in schizophrenia: differences between white and Caribbean patients in Camberwell. *Psychological Medicine* **29**: 607–12.
38. Hutchinson G, Takei N, Bhugra D, *et al.* (1997) Increased rate of psychosis among African-Caribbeans in Britain is not due to an excess of pregnancy and birth complications. *British Journal of Psychiatry* **171**: 145–7.
39. Selten JP, Slaets J, Kahn R (1998) Prenatal exposure to influenza and schizophrenia in Surinamese and Dutch Antillean immigrants to the Netherlands. *Schizophrenia Research* **30**: 101–3.
40. Hutchinson G, Takei N, Fahy TA, *et al.* (1996) Morbid risk of schizophrenia in first-degree relatives of white and African-Caribbean patients with psychosis. *British Journal of Psychiatry* **169**: 776–80.
41. Hickling FW, McKenzie K, Mullen R, Murray R (1999) A Jamaican psychiatrist evaluates diagnoses at a London psychiatric hospital. *British Journal of Psychiatry* **175**: 283–5.
42. Kirkbride JB, Fearon P, Morgan C, *et al.* (2006)

Heterogeneity in incidence rates of schizophrenia and other psychotic syndromes: findings from the 3-center AeSOP study. *Archives of General Psychiatry* **63**: 250–58.

43. Morgan C, Fearon P, Hutchinson G, *et al.* (2006) Duration of untreated psychosis and ethnicity in the AESOP first-onset psychosis study. *Psychological Medicine* **36**: 239–47.
44. Morgan C, Fisher H, Fearon P (2006) Child abuse and psychosis. *Acta Psychiatrica Scandinavica* **113**: 238, author reply 238–9.
45. Stompe T, Friedman A, Ortwein G, *et al.* (1999) Comparison of delusions among schizophrenics in Austria and in Pakistan. *Psychopathology* **32**: 225–34.
46. Murphy HB, Wittkower ED, Fried J, Ellenberger H (1963) A cross-cultural survey of schizophrenic symptomatology. *International Journal of Social Psychiatry* **9**: 237–49.
47. Ndetei DM, Vadher A (1984) A comparative cross-cultural study of the frequencies of hallucination in schizophrenia. *Acta Psychiatrica Scandinavica* **70**: 545–9.
48. Suhail K, Cochrane R (2002) Effect of culture and environment on the phenomenology of delusions and hallucinations. *International Journal of Social Psychiatry* **48**: 126–38.
49. Wing JK (1987) Has the outcome of schizophrenia changed? *British Medical Bulletin* **43**: 741–53.
50. Leff JP, Fischer M, Bertelsen A (1976) A cross-national epidemiological study of mania. *British Journal of Psychiatry* **129**: 428–42.
51. Bebbington P, Cooper C (2007) Affective disorders. In D Bhugra, K Bhui (eds) *Textbook of Cultural Psychiatry*. Cambridge: Cambridge University Press.
52. Üstürn TB, Sartorius N (1995) *Mental Illness in General Health Care: An International Study*. Chichester: John Wiley & Sons.
53. Hwu HG, Yeh EK, Chang LY (1989) Prevalence of psychiatric disorders in Taiwan defined by the Chinese Diagnostic Interview Schedule. *Acta Psychiatrica Scandinavica* **79**: 136–47.
54. Bland RC, Newman SC, Orn H (1988) Period prevalence of psychiatric disorders in Edmonton. *Acta Psychiatrica Scandinavica Supplement* **338**: 33–42.
55. Wittchen HU, Essau CA, von Zerssen D, Krieg JC, Zaudig M (1992) Lifetime and six-month prevalence of mental disorders in the Munich Follow-Up Study. *European Archives of Psychiatry and Clinical Neuroscience* **241**: 247–58.
56. Chen CN, Wong J, Lee N, *et al.* (1993) The Shatin community mental health survey in Hong Kong: II. Major findings. *Archives of General Psychiatry* **50**: 125–33.
57. Karam EG, Howard DB, Karam AN, *et al.* (1998) Major depression and external stressors: the Lebanon wars. *European Archives of Psychiatry and Clinical Neuroscience* **248**: 225–30.
58. Gureje O, Lasebikan VO, Kola L, Makanjuola VA (2006) Lifetime and 12-month prevalence of mental disorders in the Nigerian Survey of Mental Health and Well-Being. *British Journal of Psychiatry* **188**: 465–71.
59. Haro JM, Palacin C, Vilagut G, *et al.* (2006) [Prevalence of mental disorders and associated factors: results from the ESEMeD-Spain study.] *Medicina Clinica (Barcelona)* **126**: 445–51.
60. Bromet EJ, Gluzman SF, Paniotto VI, *et al.* (2005) Epidemiology of psychiatric and alcohol disorders in Ukraine: findings from the Ukraine World Mental Health survey. *Social Psychiatry and Psychiatric Epidemiology* **40**: 681–90.
61. Lepine JP, Gasquet I, Kovess V, *et al.* (2005) [Prevalence and comorbidity of psychiatric disorders in the French general population]. *Encephale* **31**: 182–94.
62. Riolo SA, Nguyen TA, Greden JF, King CA (2005) Prevalence of depression by race/ethnicity: findings from the National Health and Nutrition Examination Survey III. *American Journal of Public Health* **95**: 998–1000.
63. Weich S, Nazroo J, Sproston K, *et al.* (2004) Common mental disorders and ethnicity in England: the EMPIRIC study. *Psychological Medicine* **34**: 1543–51.
64. Takeuchi DT, Chung RC, Lin KM, *et al.* (1998) Lifetime and twelve-month prevalence rates of major depressive episodes and dysthymia among Chinese Americans in Los Angeles. *American Journal of Psychiatry* **155**: 1407–14.
65. Beals J, Manson SM, Whitesell NR, *et al.* (2005) Prevalence of major depressive episode in two American Indian reservation populations: unexpected findings with a structured interview. *American Journal of Psychiatry* **162**: 1713–22.
66. Hicks M (2002) Validity of the CIDI probe flow chart for depression in Chinese American women. *Transcultural Psychiatry* **39**: 434–51.
67. World Health Organization (1983) *Depressive Disorders in Different Cultures*. Geneva: World Health Organization.
68. Kimura B (1965) Vergleichende untersuchungen uber depressive erkrankungen im Japan und im Deutschland. *Fortscritte de Neurologie-Psychiatrie* **33**: 202–15.
69. Stompe T, Ortwein-Swoboda G, Chaudhry HR, *et al.* (2001) Guilt and depression: a cross-cultural comparative study. *Psychopathology* **34**: 289–98.
70. Campion J, Bhugra D (1997) Experiences of religious healing in psychiatric patients in south India. *Social Psychiatry and Psychiatric Epidemiology* **32**: 215–21.
71. Kleinman A (1988) *Social Origins of Distress and Disease: Depression, Neurasthesia and Pain in Modern China*. New Haven, CT: Yale University Press.
72. Parker G, Chan B, Tully L, Eisenbruch M (2005)

Depression in the Chinese: the impact of acculturation. *Psychological Medicine* **35**: 1475–83.

73. Chen H, Guarnaccia, PJ, Chung H (2003) Self-attention as a mediator of cultural influences on depression. *International Journal of Social Psychiatry* **49**: 192–203.
74. Mak WW, Zane NW (2004) The phenomenon of somatization among community Chinese Americans. *Social Psychiatry and Psychiatric Epidemiology* **39**: 967–74.
75. Oh Y, Koeske GF, Sales E (2002) Acculturation, stress, and depressive symptoms among Korean immigrants in the United States. *Journal of Social Psychology* **142**: 511–26.
76. Hwang WC, Myers HF, Takeuchi DT (2000) Psychosocial predictors of first-onset depression in Chinese Americans. *Social Psychiatry and Psychiatric Epidemiology* **35**: 133–45.
77. Bhugra D (2003) Migration and depression. *Acta Psychiatrica Scandinavica Supplement* (418): 67–72.
78. Burnett A, Peel M (2001) Health needs of asylum seekers and refugees. *British Medical Journal* **322**: 544–7.
79. Oquendo MA, Lizardi D, Greenwald S, Weissman MM, Mann JJ (2004) Rates of lifetime suicide attempt and rates of lifetime major depression in different ethnic groups in the United States. *Acta Psychiatrica Scandinavica* **110**: 446–51.
80. Chaturvedi S, Desai G (2007) Neurosis. In D Bhugra, K Bhui (eds) *Textbook of Cultural Psychiatry*. Cambridge: Cambridge University Press.
81. De Silva P, Bhugra D (2007) Culture and obsessive complusive disorder. In D Bhugra, K Bhui (eds) *Textbook of Cultural Psychiatry*. Cambridge: Cambridge University Press.
82. Weissman MM, Bland RC, Canino GJ, *et al.* (1994) The cross national epidemiology of obsessive compulsive disorder. The Cross National Collaborative Group. *Journal of Clinical Psychiatry* **55** (suppl.): 5–10.
83. Meltzer H, Gatward R (2000) *The Mental Health of Children and Adolescents in Great Britain: The Report of a Survey Carried Out in 1999 by Social Survey Division of the Office for National Statistics on Behalf of the Department of Health, the Scottish Health Executive and the National Assembly for Wales*. London: The Stationery Office.
84. Jones IH, Horne DJ (1973) Psychiatric disorders among aborigines of the Australian western desert: further data and discussion. *Social Science and Medicine* **7**: 219–28.
85. Bhugra D, Sumathipala A, Siribaddanna S (2007) Culture-bound syndromes: a re-evaluation. In D Bhugra, K Bhui (eds) *Textbook of Cultural Psychiatry*. Cambridge: Cambridge University Press.
86. Mollica RF, Caspi-Yavin Y, Bollini P, *et al.* (1992) The Harvard Trauma Questionnaire: validating a cross-cultural instrument for measuring torture, trauma, and posttraumatic stress disorder in Indochinese refugees. *Journal of Nervous and Mental Disease* **180**: 111–16.
87. Silove D, Manicavasagar V, Mollica R, *et al.* (2007) Screening for depression and PTSD in a Cambodian population unaffected by war: comparing the Hopkins Symptom Checklist and Harvard Trauma Questionnaire with the structured clinical interview. *Journal of Nervous and Mental Disease* **195**: 152–7.
88. Summerfield D (1998) Trauma, post-traumatic stress disorder, and war. *Lancet* **352**: 911.
89. De Jong JTVM (2007) *Traumascape: An Ecological-Cultural-Historical Model of Extreme Stress*. Cambridge: Cambridge University Press.
90. Wanigaratne S, Sala S, Strang J (2007) *Substance Misuse*. Cambridge: Cambridge University Press.
91. Edwards G, Gross MM (1976) Alcohol dependence: provisional description of a clinical syndrome. *British Medical Journal* **1**: 1058–61.
92. Nelson CB, Rehm J, Ustun TB, Grant B, Chatterji S (1999) Factor structures for DSM-IV substance disorder criteria endorsed by alcohol, cannabis, cocaine and opiate users: results from the WHO reliability and validity study. *Addiction* **94**: 843–55.
93. Berridge V, Edwards G (1987) *Opium and the People: Opiate Use in Nineteenth-Century England*. New Haven, CT: Yale University Press.
94. Vega WA, Aguilar-Gaxiola S, Andrade L, *et al.* (2002) Prevalence and age of onset for drug use in seven international sites: results from the international consortium of psychiatric epidemiology. *Drug and Alcohol Dependence* **68**: 285–97.
95. West R, Hardy A (2006) *Theory of Addiction*. Oxford: Blackwell.
96. McCambridge J, Strang J (2005) Age of first use and ongoing patterns of legal and illegal drug use in a sample of young Londoners. *Substance Use and Misuse* **40**: 313–19.
97. Wanigaratne S, Unninthan S, Strang J (2001) Substance misuse and ethnic minorities: issues for the UK. In D Bhugra, R Cochrane (eds) *Psychiatry in Multi-Cultural Britain*. London: Gaskell.
98. Baklien B, Samarasinghe D (2003) *Alcohol and Poverty*. Colombo: Forut.
99. Saggers S, Gray D (1998) *Dealing With Alcohol: Indigenous Usage in Australia, New Zealand and Canada*. Cambridge: Cambridge University Press.
100. O'Connell J, Novins DK, Beals J, *et al.* (2006) The relationship between patterns of alcohol use and mental and physical health disorders in two American Indian populations. *Addiction* **101**: 69–83.
101. Nasser M (2007) Culture and eating disorders. In D Bhugra, K Bhui (eds) *Textbook of Cultural Psychiatry*. Cambridge: Cambridge University Press.
102. Garner DM, Garfinkel PE (1980) Socio-cultural factors in the development of anorexia nervosa. *Psychological Medicine* **10**: 647–56.

103. King MB, Mezey G (1987) Eating behaviour of male racing jockeys. *Psychological Medicine* **17**: 249–53.
104. Weight LM, Noakes TD (1987) Is running an analog of anorexia? A survey of the incidence of eating disorders in female distance runners. *Medicine and Science in Sports and Exercise* **19**: 213–17.
105. Rathner G, Messner K (1993) Detection of eating disorders in a small rural town: an epidemiological study. *Psychological Medicine* **23**: 175–84.
106. Hoek HW, Bartelds AI, Bosveld JJ, *et al.* (1995) Impact of urbanization on detection rates of eating disorders. *American Journal of Psychiatry* **152**: 1272–8.
107. Nasser M, Katzman MA (1999) Transcultural perspectives inform prevention. In N Piran, MP Levine, C Steiner-Adair (eds) *Preventing Eating Disorders: A Handbook of Interventions and Special Challenges.* Philadelphia, PA: Brunner/Mazel.
108. Prince R (1983) Is anorexia nervosa a culture bound syndrome? *Transcultural Psychiatry Research and Review* **20**: 299.
109. Neumarker U, Dudeck U, Voltrath M, Neumarker K, Steinhausen H (1992) Eating attitudes among adolescent anorexia nervosa patients and normal subjects in former West and East Berlin: a transcultural comparison. *International Journal of Eating Disorders* **12**: 281–9.
110. Ruggiero GM, Hannower W, Mantero M, Papa R (2000) Body acceptance and culture: a study in Northern and Southern Italy. *European Eating Disorders Review* **8**: 40–50.
111. Le Grange D, Telch CF, Tibbs J (1998) Eating attitudes and behaviors in 1,435 South African Caucasian and non-Caucasian college students. *American Journal of Psychiatry* **155**: 250–54.
112. Gordon RA (2001) Eating disorders east and west: a culture bound syndrome unbound. In M Nasser, M Katzman, RA Gordon (eds) *Eating Disorders and Cultures in Transition.* Hove: Brunner-Routledge.
113. Mellsop G, Varghese F, Joshua S, Hicks A (1982) The reliability of axis II of DSM-III. *American Journal of Psychiatry* **139**: 1360–61.
114. Tyrer P, Casey P, Ferguson B (1991) Personality disorder in perspective. *British Journal of Psychiatry* **159**: 463–71.
115. Lewis G, Appleby L (1988) Personality disorder: the patients psychiatrists dislike. *British Journal of Psychiatry* **153**: 44–9.
116. Singleton N, Gatward R, Meltzer H (1998) *Psychiatric Morbidity Among Prisoners in England and Wales.* London: The Stationery Office.
117. Morris B (1994) *Anthropology of the Self: The Individual in Cultural Perspective.* London: Pluto.
118. Loranger AW, Sartorius N, Andreoli A, *et al.* (1994) The International Personality Disorder Examination. The World Health Organization/Alcohol, Drug Abuse, and Mental Health Administration international pilot study of personality disorders. *Archives of General Psychiatry* **51**: 215–24.
119. De Girolamo G, Reich JH (1993) *Personality Disorders.* Geneva: World Health Organization.
120. Dogra N, Vostanis P, Karnik N (2007) Child and adolescent psychiatric disorders. In D Bhugra, K Bhui (eds) *Textbook of Cultural Psychiatry.* Cambridge: Cambridge University Press.
121. Eapen V, al-Gazali L, Bin-Othman S, Abou-Saleh M (1998) Mental health problems among schoolchildren in United Arab Emirates: prevalence and risk factors. *Journal of the American Academy of Child and Adolescent Psychiatry* **37**: 880–86.
122. Fleitlich-Bilyk B, Goodman R (2004) Prevalence of child and adolescent psychiatric disorders in southeast Brazil. *Journal of the American Academy of Child and Adolescent Psychiatry* **43**: 727–34.
123. Zito JM, Safer DJ, Zuckerman IH, Gardner JF, Soeken K (2005) Effect of Medicaid eligibility category on racial disparities in the use of psychotropic medications among youths. *Psychiatric Services* **56**: 157–63.
124. Shah A, Mackenzie S (2007) Disorders of ageing across cultures. In D Bhugra, K Bhui (eds) *Textbook of Cultural Psychiatry.* Cambridge: Cambridge University Press.
125. Desjarlais RR (1995) *World Mental Health: Problems, and Priorities in Low-Income Countries.* New York: Oxford University Press.
126. Subedi S, Tausig M, Subedi J, Broughton CL, Williams-Blangero S (2004) Mental illness and disability among elders in developing countries: the case of Nepal. *Journal of Aging and Health* **16**: 71–87.
127. Shah A, Lindesay J, Nnatu I (2005) Cross cultural issues in the assessment of cognitive impairment. In AS Burns, JDM O'Brien, D Ames (eds) *Dementia*, 3rd edn. London: Hodder Arnold.
128. Boneham M (1989) Ageing and ethnicity in Britain: the case of elderly Sikh women in a Midlands town. *New Community* **15**: 447–459.
129. Suh GH, Shah A (2001) A review of the epidemiological transition in dementia: cross-national comparisons of the indices related to Alzheimer's disease and vascular dementia. *Acta Psychiatrica Scandinavica* **104**: 4–11.
130. Jorm AF, Korten AE, Henderson AS (1987) The prevalence of dementia: a quantitative integration of the literature. *Acta Psychiatrica Scandinavica* **76**: 465–79.
131. Hofman A, Rocca WA, Brayne C, *et al.* (1991) The prevalence of dementia in Europe: a collaborative study of 1980–1990 findings. Eurodem Prevalence Research Group. *International Journal of Epidemiology* **20**: 736–48.
132. Li G, Shen YC, Chen CH, *et al.* (1989) An epidemiological survey of age-related dementia in an urban area of Beijing. *Acta Psychiatrica Scandinavica* **79**: 557–63.

133. Bhatnagar K, Frank J (1997) Psychiatric disorders in elderly from the Indian sub-continent living in Bradford. *International Journal of Geriatric Psychiatry* **12**: 907–12.
134. Lindesay J, Jagger C, Mlynik-Szmid A, *et al.* (1997) The Mini-Mental State Examination (MMSE) in an elderly immigrant Gujarati population in the United Kingdom. *International Journal of Geriatric Psychiatry* **12**: 1155–67.
135. McCracken CF, Boneham MA, Copeland JR, *et al.* (1997) Prevalence of dementia and depression among elderly people in black and ethnic minorities. *British Journal of Psychiatry* **171**: 269–73.
136. Livingston G, Leavey G, Kitchen G, *et al.* (2001) Mental health of migrant elders: the Islington study. *British Journal of Psychiatry* **179**: 361–6.
137. Gurland BJ, Wilder DE, Lantigua R, *et al.* (1999) Rates of dementia in three ethnoracial groups. *International Journal of Geriatric Psychiatry* **14**: 481–93.
138. Heyman A, Fillenbaum G, Prosnitz B, *et al.* (1991) Estimated prevalence of dementia among elderly black and white community residents. *Archives of Neurology* **48**: 594–8.
139. Perkins P, Annegers JF, Doody RS, *et al.* (1997) Incidence and prevalence of dementia in a multiethnic cohort of municipal retirees. *Neurology* **49**: 44–50.
140. Cantor C, Leenaars, AA, Lester D (1997) Underreporting of suicide in Ireland 1960–1989. *Archives of Suicide Research* **3**: 5–12.
141. Fortune S, Hawton K (2007) Culture and mental disorders: suicidal behaviour. In D Bhugra, K Bhui (eds) *Textbook of Cultural Psychiatry.* Cambridge: Cambridge University Press.
142. Lester D, Yang B (2005) Regional and time-series studies of suicide in nations of the world. *Arch Suicide Res* **9**: 123–33.
143. Vijayakumar L, John S, Pirkis J, Whiteford H (2005) Suicide in developing countries (2): risk factors. *Crisis* **26**: 112–9.
144. Vijayakumar L, Nagaraj K, Pirkis J, Whiteford H (2005) Suicide in developing countries (1): frequency, distribution, and association with socioeconomic indicators. *Crisis* **26**: 104–11.
145. Hjelmeland H, Hawton K, Nordvik H, *et al.* (2002) Why people engage in parasuicide: a cross-cultural study of intentions. *Suicide and Life-Threatening Behavior* **32**: 380–93.
146. Eddleston M, Gunnell D, Karunaratne A, *et al.* (2005) Epidemiology of intentional self-poisoning in rural Sri Lanka. *British Journal of Psychiatry* **187**: 583–4.
147. Pridemore WA, Spivak AL (2003) Patterns of suicide mortality in Russia. *Suicide and Life-Threatening Behavior* **33**: 132–50.
148. Lester D (1998) Suicide and homicide after the fall of communist regimes. *European Psychiatry* **13**: 98–100.
149. Varnik A, Kolves K, Wasserman D (2005) Suicide among Russians in Estonia: database study before and after independence. *British Medical Journal* **330**: 176–7.
150. Joseph A, Abraham S, Muliyil JP, *et al.* (2003) Evaluation of suicide rates in rural India using verbal autopsies, 1994–9. *British Medical Journal* **326**: 1121–2.
151. Steen DM, Meyer P (2004) Modernization and the male–female suicide ratio in India 1967–1997: divergence or convergence? *Suicide and Life-Threatening Behavior* **34**: 147–59.
152. Aaron R, Joseph A, Abraham S, *et al.* (2004) Suicides in young people in rural southern India. *Lancet* **363**: 1117–18.
153. Lalwani S, Sharma GA, Kabra SK, Girdhar S, Dogra TD (2004) Suicide among children and adolescents in South Delhi (1991–2000). *Indian Journal of Pediatrics* **71**: 701–3.
154. Shiho Y, Tohru T, Shinji S, *et al.* (2005) Suicide in Japan: present condition and prevention measures. *Crisis* **26**: 12–19.
155. Takei N, Nakamura K (2004) Is inseki-jisatsu, responsibility-driven suicide, culture-bound? *Lancet* **363**: 1400.
156. Cantor C, Neulinger K (2000) The epidemiology of suicide and attempted suicide among young Australians. *Australian and New Zealand Journal of Psychiatry* **34**: 370–87.
157. Pearson V, Liu M (2002) Ling's death: an ethnography of a Chinese woman's suicide. *Suicide and Life-Threatening Behavior* **32**: 347–58.
158. Pearson V, Phillips MR, He F, Ji H (2002) Attempted suicide among young rural women in the People's Republic of China: possibilities for prevention. *Suicide and Life-Threatening Behavior* **32**: 359–69.
159. Bhugra D, Desai M, Baldwin DS (1999) Attempted suicide in west London: I. Rates across ethnic communities. *Psychological Medicine* **29**: 1125–30.
160. Bhugra D, Baldwin DS, Desai M, Jacob KS (1999) Attempted suicide in west London: II. Inter-group comparisons. *Psychological Medicine* **29**: 1131–9.
161. Soni Raleigh V, Bulusu L, Balarajan R (1990) Suicides among immigrants from the Indian subcontinent. *British Journal of Psychiatry* **156**: 46–50.
162. Neeleman J, Mak V, Wessely S (1997) Suicide by age, ethnic group, coroners' verdicts and country of birth: a three-year survey in inner London. *British Journal of Psychiatry* **171**: 463–7.
163. US Department of Health and Human Services, Centers for Disease Control and Prevention, National Center for Health Statistics (2004) *Health, United States, 2004.* Washington, DC: US Department of Health and Human Services, Centers for Disease Control and Prevention, and National Center for Health Statistics.
164. Castle K, Duberstein PR, Meldrum S, Conner KR, Conwell Y (2004) Risk factors for suicide in blacks and

whites: an analysis of data from the 1993 National Mortality Followback Survey. *American Journal of Psychiatry* **161**: 452–8.

165. Fernquist RM (2004) Does single motherhood protect against Black female suicide? *Archives of Suicide Research* **8**: 163–71.
166. Joe S, Kaplan MS (2001) Suicide among African American men. *Suicide and Life-Threatening Behavior* **31** (suppl.): 106–21.
167. Kirmayer LJ, Malus M, Boothroyd LJ (1996) Suicide attempts among Inuit youth: a community survey of prevalence and risk factors. *Acta Psychiatrica Scandinavica* **94**: 8–17.
168. Tatz CM (2001) *Aboriginal Suicide Is Different: A Portrait of Life and Self-Destruction.* Canberra: Aboriginal Studies Press.
169. Keller AS, Rosenfeld B, Trinh-Shevrin C, *et al.* (2003) Mental health of detained asylum seekers. *Lancet* **362**: 1721–3.
170. Fazel M, Wheeler J, Danesh J (2005) Prevalence of serious mental disorder in 7000 refugees resettled in western countries: a systematic review. *Lancet* **365**: 1309–14.
171. Yu S, Liu S, Lin K (2007) Psychopharmacology across cultures. In D Bhugra, K Bhui (eds) *Textbook of Cultural Psychiatry.* Cambridge: Cambridge University Press.
172. Lin KM, Poland RE, Lau JK, Rubin RT (1988) Haloperidol and prolactin concentrations in Asians and Caucasians. *Journal of Clinical Psychopharmacology* **8**: 195–201.
173. Lin K-M, Poland RE, Nakasaki G (1993) *Psychopharmacology and Psychobiology of Ethnicity.* Washington, DC: American Psychiatric Press.
174. Aitchison KJ, Jordan BD, Sharma T (2000) The relevance of ethnic influences on pharmacogenetics to the treatment of psychosis. *Drug Metabolism and Drug Interactactions* **16**: 15–38.
175. Kinnear CJ, Niehaus DJ, Moolman-Smook JC, *et al.* (2000) Obsessive-compulsive disorder and the promoter region polymorphism (5-HTTLPR) in the serotonin transporter gene (SLC6A4): a negative association study in the Afrikaner population. *International Journal of Neuropsychopharmacology* **3**: 327–31.
176. Chou WH, Yan FX, de Leon J, *et al.* (2000) Extension of a pilot study: impact from the cytochrome P450 2D6 polymorphism on outcome and costs associated with severe mental illness. *Journal of Clinical Psychopharmacology* **20**: 246–51.
177. Steiner E, Bertilsson L, Sawe J, Bertling I, Sjoqvist F (1988) Polymorphic debrisoquin hydroxylation in 757 Swedish subjects. *Clinical Pharmacology and Therapeutics* **44**: 431–5.
178. Carrillo JA, Herraiz AG, Ramos SI, *et al.* (2003) Role of the smoking-induced cytochrome P450 (CYP)1A2 and polymorphic CYP2D6 in steady-state concentration of olanzapine. *Journal of Clinical Psychopharmacology* **23**: 119–27.
179. Masimirembwa C, Persson I, Bertilsson L, Hasler J, Ingelman-Sundberg M (1996) A novel mutant variant of the CYP2D6 gene (CYP2D6*17) common in a black African population: association with diminished debrisoquine hydroxylase activity. *British Journal of Clinical Pharmacology* **42**: 713–19.
180. Leathart JB, London SJ, Steward A, *et al.* (1998) CYP2D6 phenotype-genotype relationships in African-Americans and Caucasians in Los Angeles. *Pharmacogenetics* **8**: 529–41.
181. Wan YJ, Poland RE, Han G, *et al.* (2001) Analysis of the CYP2D6 gene polymorphism and enzyme activity in African-Americans in southern California. *Pharmacogenetics* **11**: 489–99.
182. Loub WD, Wattenberg LW, Davis DW (1975) Aryl hydrocarbon hydroxylase induction in rat tissues by naturally occurring indoles of cruciferous plants. *Journal of the National Cancer Instituge* **54**: 985–8.
183. Branch RA, Salih SY, Homeida M (1978) Racial differences in drug metabolizing ability: a study with antipyrine in the Sudan. *Clinical Pharmacology and Therapeutics* **24**: 283–6.
184. Allen JJ, Rack PH, Vaddadi KS (1977) Differences in the effects of clomipramine on English and Asian volunteers: preliminary report on a pilot study. *Postgraduate Medical Journal* **53** (suppl. 4): 79–86.
185. Fraser HS, Mucklow JC, Bulpitt CJ, *et al.* (1979) Environmental factors affecting antipyrine metabolism in London factory and office workers. *British Journal of Clinical Pharmacology* **7**: 237–43.
186. Hukkinen SK, Varhe A, Olkkola KT, Neuvonen PJ (1995) Plasma concentrations of triazolam are increased by concomitant ingestion of grapefruit juice. *Clinical Pharmacology and Therapeutics* **58**: 127–31.
187. Kupferschmidt HH, Ha HR, Ziegler WH, Meier PJ, Krahenbuhl S (1995) Interaction between grapefruit juice and midazolam in humans. *Clinical Pharmacology and Therapeutics* **58**: 20–28.
188. Bhardwaj RK, Glaeser H, Becquemont L, *et al.* (2002) Piperine, a major constituent of black pepper, inhibits human P-glycoprotein and CYP3A4. *Journal of Pharmacology and Experimental Therapeutics* **302**: 645–50.
189. Usia T, Watabe T, Kadota S, Tezuka Y (2005) Potent CYP3A4 inhibitory constituents of *Piper cubeba. Journal of Natural Products* **68**: 64–8.
190. Rosenthal NE, Mazzanti CM, Barnett RL, *et al.* (1998) Role of serotonin transporter promoter repeat length polymorphism (5-HTTLPR) in seasonality and seasonal affective disorder. *Molecular Psychiatry* **3**: 175–7.
191. Konishi T, Luo HR, Calvillo M, *et al.* (2004) ADH1B*1, ADH1C*2, DRD2 (-141C Ins), and 5-HTTLPR are associated with alcoholism in Mexican American men

living in Los Angeles. *Alcoholism, Clinical and Experimental Research* **28**: 1145–52.

192. Di Bella D, Erzegovesi S, Cavallini MC, Bellodi L (2002) Obsessive-compulsive disorder, 5-HTTLPR polymorphism and treatment response. *Pharmacogenomics Journal* **2**: 176–81.
193. Kim DK, Lim SW, Lee S, *et al.* (2000) Serotonin transporter gene polymorphism and antidepressant response. *Neuroreport* **11**: 215–19.
194. Pollock BG, Ferrell RE, Mulsant BH, *et al.* (2000) Allelic variation in the serotonin transporter promoter affects onset of paroxetine treatment response in late-life depression. *Neuropsychopharmacology* **23**: 587–90.
195. Zanardi R, Serretti A, Rossini D, *et al.* (2001) Factors affecting fluvoxamine antidepressant activity: influence of pindolol and 5-HTTLPR in delusional and non-delusional depression. *Biological Psychiatry* **50**: 323–30.
196. Arias B, Catalan R, Gasto C, Gutierrez B, Fananas L (2003) 5-HTTLPR polymorphism of the serotonin transporter gene predicts non-remission in major depression patients treated with citalopram in a 12-weeks follow up study. *Journal of Clinical Psychopharmacology* **23**: 563–7.
197. Gelernter J, Kranzler H, Cubells JF (1997) Serotonin transporter protein (SLC6A4) allele and haplotype frequencies and linkage disequilibria in African- and European-American and Japanese populations and in alcohol-dependent subjects. *Human Genetics* **101**: 243–6.
198. Lachman HM, Papolos DF, Saito T, *et al.* (1996) Human catechol-O-methyltransferase pharmacogenetics: description of a functional polymorphism and its potential application to neuropsychiatric disorders. *Pharmacogenetics* **6**: 243–50.
199. Woo JM, Yoon KS, Yu BH (2002) Catechol O-methyltransferase genetic polymorphism in panic disorder. *American Journal of Psychiatry* **159**: 1785–7.
200. Domschke K, Freitag CM, Kuhlenbaumer G, *et al.* (2004) Association of the functional V158M catechol-O-methyl-transferase polymorphism with panic disorder in women. *International Journal of Neuropsychopharmacology* **7**: 183–8.
201. Kunugi H, Nanko S, Ueki A, *et al.* (1997) High and low activity alleles of catechol-O-methyltransferase gene: ethnic difference and possible association with Parkinson's disease. *Neuroscience Letters* **221**: 202–4.
202. Inada T, Nakamura A, Iijima Y (2003) Relationship between catechol-O-methyltransferase polymorphism and treatment-resistant schizophrenia. *American Journal of Medical Genetics. Part B, Neuropsychiatric Genetics* **120B**: 35–9.
203. Jones G, Zammit S, Norton N, *et al.* (2001) Aggressive behaviour in patients with schizophrenia is associated with catechol-O-methyltransferase genotype. *British Journal of Psychiatry* **179**: 351–5.
204. Rivera-Calimlim L, Reilly DK (1984) Difference in erythrocyte catechol-O-methyltransferase activity between Orientals and Caucasians: difference in levodopa tolerance. *Clinical Pharmacology and Therapeutics* **35**: 804–9.
205. Ameyaw MM, Syvanen AC, Ulmanen I, Ofori-Adjei D, McLeod HL (2000) Pharmacogenetics of catechol-O-methyltransferase: frequency of low activity allele in a Ghanaian population. *Human Mutation* **16**: 445–6.
206. Bhui K, Morgan N (2007) Effective psychotherapy in a racially and culturally diverse society. *Advances in Psychiatric Treatment* **13**: 187–93.

PART 3

Neuroscience

Chapter 23

Neuroanatomy

Basant K Puri and Bari M Logan

INTRODUCTION

Neuroanatomy is one of the fundamental basic neurosciences that underpin the practice of clinical psychiatry. In this chapter the following aspects are covered, with an emphasis on those aspects that are of particular importance to psychiatry: the general anatomy of the brain and spinal cord, including the lobes, the major gyri, the limbic system and the cranial nerves; the basal ganglia; the internal anatomy of the temporal lobes; the major white-matter tracts of the brain; the types of cells found in the central nervous system; and the major neurochemical pathways. In our experience, the study of neuroanatomy is made easier by dissecting the brain, or at the very least by examining specimens; the reader is strongly encouraged to do so.

THE SKULL

Bones

The skull includes the mandible, whereas the term 'cranium' is without it. Excluding the six auditory ossicles, a normal adult human skull is formed from 22 bones.

Single bones

These are the:

- frontal bone;
- ethmoid bone;
- sphenoid bone;
- vomer;
- occipital bone;
- mandible.

Paired bones

The paired bones of the skull (left and right) are the:

- maxilla (the maxillae);
- nasal bone;
- lacrimal bone;
- inferior nasal concha;
- palatine bone;
- temporal bone;
- zygomatic bone;
- parietal bone.

Auditory ossicles

In addition, the paired auditory ossicles within the middle cavities of the temporal bones are (left and right) the:

- incus;
- malleus;
- stapes.

Dura mater

The cranial cavity, within the upper part of the skull, which encloses the brain, is lined with a covering of double-layered dura mater, which forms:

- the falx cerebri in the midsagittal plane, separating the two cerebral hemispheres;
- the tentorium cerebelli, which forms a roof over the cerebellum, in an almost axial plane, and separates it from the posterior under-surface of the occipital lobes of the brain.

Cranial fossae

The base of the skull (floor of the cranial cavity) is divided into three areas: the anterior, middle and posterior cranial fossae. Some key important structures to note with these are given below.

Anterior cranial fossa

- The cribriform plate of the ethmoid bone through the multi-perforations of which pass olfactory (I) nerve filaments connecting to the under surface of the olfactory bulbs
- The foramen caecum, through which passes an emissary vein.

Middle cranial fossa

- The pituitary fossa (sella turcica) containing the pituitary gland, which has a posterior lobe (neurohypophysis) and an anterior lobe (adenohypophysis)

- The optic canal, through which passes the optic (II) nerve
- The superior orbital fissure transmits the ophthalmic (V1), oculomotor (III), trochlear (IV) and abducent (VI) nerves and ophthalmic veins
- The foramen spinosum transmits the middle meningeal artery
- The foramen ovale transmits the mandibular division of the trigeminal (V3) nerve
- The foramen lacerum, upper aspect, opening of the carotid canal
- The trigeminal ganglion in a recess near the apex of the petrous temporal bone.

Posterior cranial fossa

- The internal acoustic meatus transmits the facial (VII) and vestibulocochlear (VIII) nerves
- The jugular foramen transmits the glossopharyngeal (IX), vagus (X) and accessory (XI) nerves
- The foramen magnum, through which passes the medulla oblongata, vertebral arteries and spinal root of the accessory nerves.

CERVICAL VERTEBRAE

There are seven cervical vertebrae. The first is the atlas, on which the skull articulates. The second is the axis; fracture of its odontoid peg (dens) can cause spinal cord damage or severance. The third to sixth (inclusive) cervical vertebrae have bifid spinous processes. The seventh (the vertebra prominens) has a single, palpable spinous process.

All seven cervical vertebrae have a foramen in each of their transverse processes (foramen transversarium). It is important to note that on each side, the vertebral artery, ascending from the subclavian artery, passes only through the foramina transversaria of the first to sixth cervical vertebrae, entering at the sixth. The vertebral vein emerges from the sixth cervical foramen transversarium. A variable, companion vein may emerge from the foramen transversarium of the seventh cervical vertebra.

GENERAL ANATOMY OF THE BRAIN AND SPINAL CORD

Lobes and major gyri

The four major lobes of the brain (the frontal lobe, parietal lobe, temporal lobe and occipital lobe) are named after the approximately adjacent skull bones.

The frontal lobe extends rostrally from the central sulcus (formerly known as the fissure of Rolando) and superiorly from the lateral fissure (formerly known as the Sylvian fissure). It contains the primary motor cortex (M1 or MI; Brodmann area 4) just anterior to the central sulcus, occupying the precentral gyrus (Figure 23.1). Electrical stimulation of M1 leads to contralateral muscular contraction. The somatotopic representation in M1, as the motor homunculus, was described by Penfield and Boldry.[1] The premotor cortex (Brodmann area 6) lies rostral to M1 (see Figure 23.1). It is divided functionally into the dorsal (PMd) and ventral (PMv) areas; the PMd receives input from the dorsolateral prefrontal cortex (DLPFC), while the PMv receives input from the ventrolateral prefrontal cortex (VLPFC). The premotor cortex has important functions in both motor activity and preparing for motor activity. In addition, the PMd may also be involved in decision circuits activated by free choice.[2] The frontal eye field (FEF; mainly Brodmann area 8 – see Figure 23.1) receives afferent connections via the thalamus from the cerebellum (the dentate nucleus), substantia nigra and superior colliculus, and from ipsilateral regions, including V5 (medial temporal cortex; visual), Brodmann area 7a (see Figure 23.1; parietal cortex) and the superior temporal gyrus (auditory/language). The FEF is particularly important in controlling ocular movements; spatial selection for locating behaviourally relevant stimuli for guiding attention and eye movements appears to be computed locally in the FEF from spatially non-selective inputs.[3] The prefrontal cortex (PFC) contains Brodmann areas 9, 10, 11, 12, 45 and 46; in the dominant (usually left)

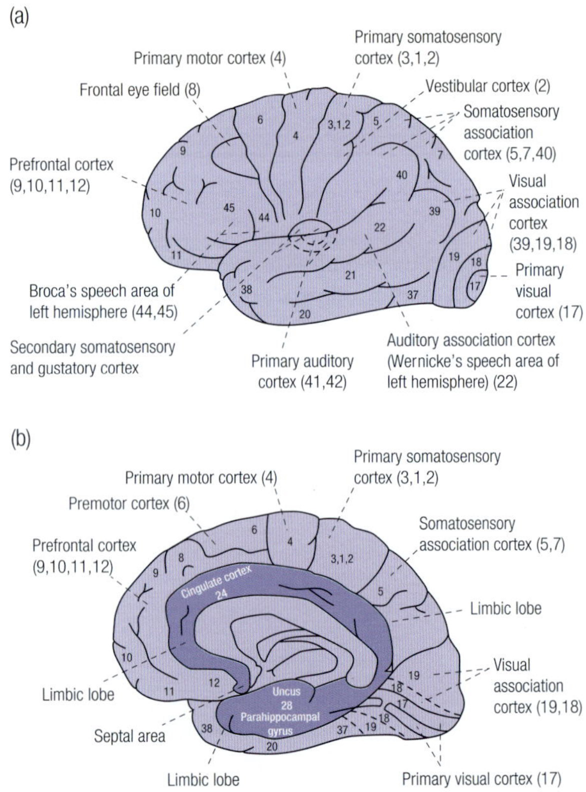

Figure 23.1 (a) Lateral and (b) medial aspects of the cerebral hemisphere, showing important Brodmann areas (numbered)

Reproduced with permission from Graham *et al.*, *Adams & Graham's Introduction to Neuropathology*, 3rd edn. Hodder, London. (2006).

hemisphere, areas 44 and 45 comprise Broca's area (see Figure 23.1), which is the motor speech area. The DLPFC has been much studied in psychiatric disorders such as schizophrenia and in psychological experiments. It appears to be involved particularly in self-ordered working memory, monitoring and the action of the central executive.[4–7] The VLPFC, on the other hand, appears to be involved in mnemonic processing and rule representation.[8] The supplementary motor cortex (SMA; M2 or MII) is on the superolateral border and medial side of the hemisphere, rostral to M1, and appears to be involved in the assembly of central motor programming of sequential movements.[9] The orbitofrontal cortex occupies the orbital gyri on the inferior surface of the frontal lobe and appears to be involved in processes involving the motivational or emotional value of incoming information, including the representation of primary reinforcers, the representation of learned relationships between arbitrary neutral stimuli and rewards or punishments, and the integration of this information to guide response selection, suppression and decision-making.[10]

The parietal lobe extends between the central sulcus (fissure of Rolando) and the parieto-occipital fissure, and laterally as far as the lateral (Sylvian) fissure. It contains the primary somatosensory cortex (S1 or SI; Brodmann areas 3, 1 and 2) just posterior to the central sulcus, occupying the postcentral gyrus and the posterior wall of the central sulcus (see Figure 23.1), which receives medial lemniscal, spinothalamic and trigeminothalamic input via the thalamic ventral posterior nucleus. The location of the somatosensory association cortex (Brodmann areas 5, 7a, 7b and 40) in the superior and inferior parietal lobules is also shown in Figure 23.1.

The temporal lobe lies inferior to the lateral (Sylvian) fissure and extends posteriorly to the parieto-occipital fissure. It contains the primary auditory cortex (A1 or AI; Brodmann areas 41 ± 42; see Figure 23.1), which receives auditory sensory input from the medial geniculate nucleus and has a tonotopic cochlear representation (low auditory frequencies anterior and high frequencies posterior). As shown in Figure 23.1, the dominant temporal lobe also contains Wernicke's (sensory speech) area, which is variously designated as Brodmann area 22 ± 39 ± 40 and may include part of the parietal cortex. The middle temporal cortex, Brodmann area 21 (see Figure 23.1), has connections with different sensory modality pathways, including those related to vision, somatosensory input and auditory input. In contrast, the inferior temporal cortex, Brodmann area 20 (see Figure 23.1), is particularly related to the higher processing of visual stimuli. The internal anatomy of the temporal lobes is considered later in this chapter.

The occipital lobe lies behind the parieto-occipital fissure and contains Brodmann areas 17, 18 and 19. Brodmann area 17 is the primary visual cortex (V1 or VI; see Figure 23.1), also known as the striate cortex, and receives visual sensory input from the lateral geniculate nucleus by means of the branches (lower and upper fields) of the optic radiation, as shown in Figure 23.2. The calcarine sulcus is shown

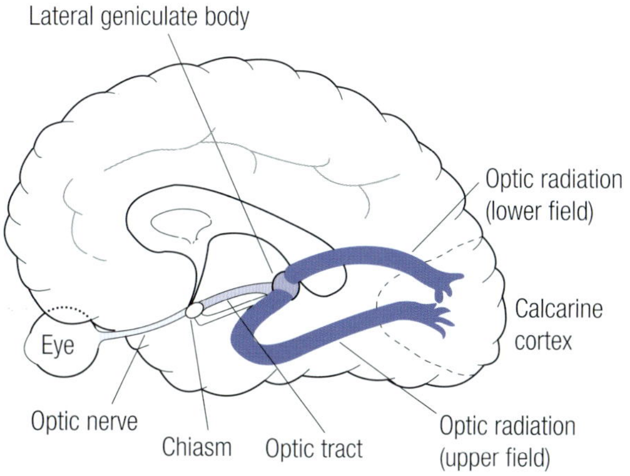

Figure 23.2 Medial sagittal view of the brain, showing the visual pathways that traverse the brain from the front to the back

Reproduced with permission from Fowler and Scadding, *Clinical Neurology*, 3rd edn. Hodder, London. (2003).

in Figure 23.3; the part of V1 above this sulcus receives a retinotopic visual input (macular to a large posterior part of V1 and peripheral to anterior V1) from the contralateral inferior visual hemifields (superior retinal quadrants), while the part of V1 below the sulcus receives a similar retinotopic input from the contralateral superior visual hemifields (inferior retinal quadrants). V2, the second visual area, is found in much of Brodmann area 18 (see Figure 23.1), just concentric to area 17, and also contains a retinotopic mapping of the contralateral visual hemifield. V3, the third visual area, is also mainly found in Brodmann area 18 and is divided into dorsal (V3d or V3), ventral (V3v or VP) and anterior (V3a) parts. V4, the fourth visual area, is found in Brodmann area 19 (see Figure 23.1). Cells in V2 and V3 tend to be orientation-selective but not selective for stimulus colour or direction or movement, whereas V4 appears to be particularly involved in the discrimination of colour, orientation, form and movement.[11]

The major gyri are shown in Figures 23.3–5.

Figure 23.6 summarizes some of the key linguistic and visual parts of the cerebral cortex of the left hemisphere, together with some of the disorders that occur when there is damage to these areas.

Limbic system

Papez put forward the notion of a neural network theory of emotion, suggesting that

> The central emotive process of cortical origin may ... be conceived as being built up in the hippocampal formation and as being transferred to the mamillary body and thence through the anterior thalamic nuclei to the cortex of the gyrus cinguli. The cortex of the [cingulate] gyrus may be looked on as the receptive region for the experiencing of emotion... Radiation of the emotive process from the gyrus cinguli to other regions in the cerebral cortex would add emotional colouring to psychic processes.[12]

1 Superior frontal gyrus
2 Cingulate sulcus
3 Cingulate gyrus
4 Callosal sulcus
5 Corpus callosum – body
6 Corpus callosum – genu
7 Corpus callosum – splenium
8 Fornix
9 Caudate nucleus (head) in wall of lateral ventricle
10 Choroid plexus, third ventricle
11 Interventricular foramen (Monro)
12 Thalamus
13 Massa intermedia
14 Anterior commissure
15 Pineal body
16 Posterior commissure
17 Superior colliculus
18 Aqueduct (of Sylvius)
19 Inferior colliculus
20 Mesencephalon
21 Hypothalamus
22 Mamillary body
23 Infundibulum
24 Uncus
25 Optic nerve (II)
26 Oculomotor nerve (III)
27 Trochlear nerve (IV)
28 Parahippocampal gyrus
29 Rhinal sulcus
30 Pons
31 Pontine tegmentum
32 Fourth ventricle
33 Nodulus
34 Anterior lobe of cerebellum
35 Parieto-occipital fissure
36 Calcarine sulcus
37 Cerebellar hemisphere
38 Tonsil of cerebellum
39 Inferior cerebellar peduncle
40 Pyramid
41 Medulla oblongata

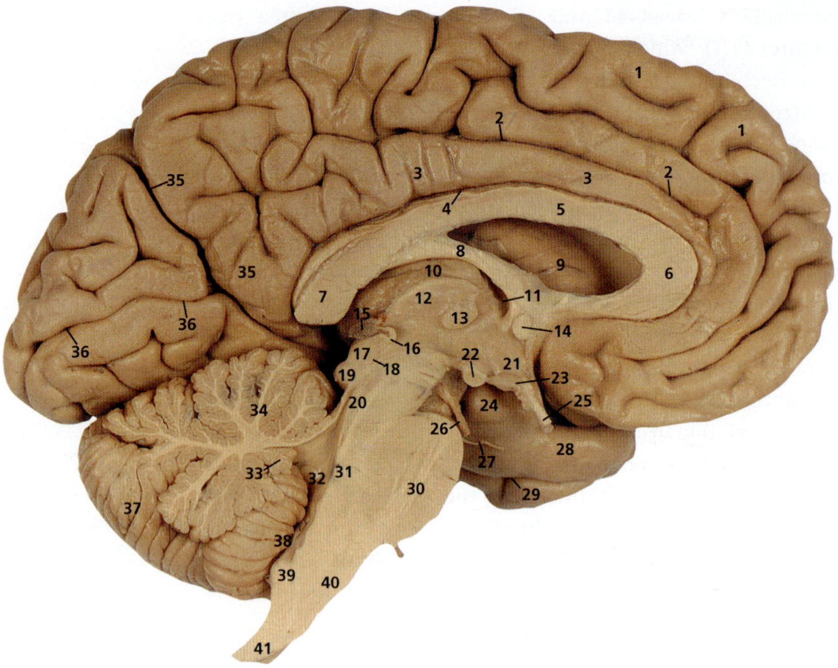

Figure 23.3 Median sagittal section of the left hemisphere

Reproduced with permission from Ellis, Logan and Dixon, *Human Sectional Anatomy*, 3rd edn. Hodder, London. (2007).

A Left cerebral hemisphere. From above, with the arachnoid mater and blood vessels removed
1 Longitudinal cerebral fissure (arrowed)
2 Frontal pole
3 Middle frontal gyrus
4 Superior frontal sulcus
5 Precentral gyrus
6 Central sulcus
7 Postcentral gyrus
8 Postcentral sulcus
9 Inferior parietal lobe
10 Parieto-occipital fissure
11 Occipital gyri

B Right cerebral hemisphere. From above, with the arachnoid mater and blood vessels intact
12 Arachnoid granulations
13 Superior cerebral veins

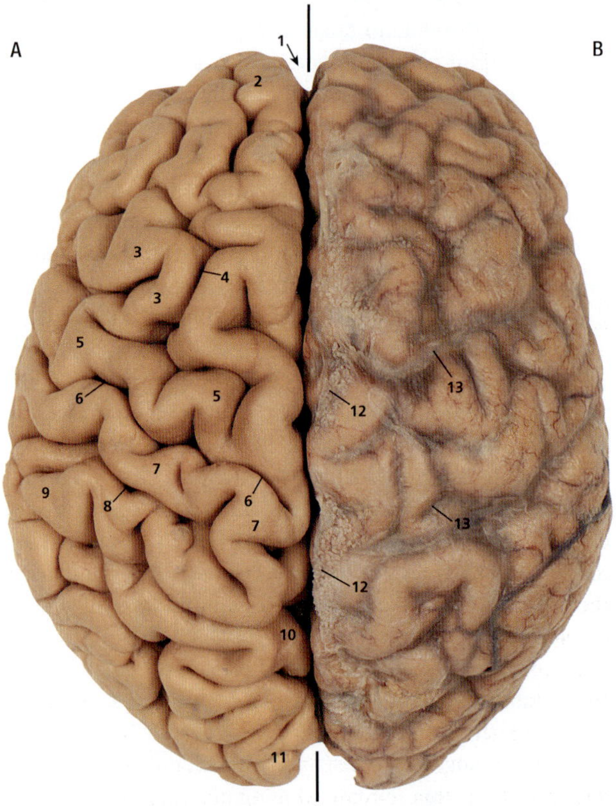

Figure 23.4 Superficial dissection of the brain viewed from above

Reproduced with permission from Ellis, Logan and Dixon, *Human Sectional Anatomy*, 3rd edn. Hodder, London. (2007).

1 Central sulcus
2 Precentral gyrus
3 Postcentral gyrus
4 Precentral sulcus
5 Inferior frontal sulcus
6 Superior frontal gyrus
7 Inferior frontal gyrus
8 Orbital gyri
9 Postcentral sulcus
10 Lateral fissure
11 Superior temporal gyrus
12 Superior temporal sulcus
13 Middle temporal gyrus
14 Inferior temporal sulcus
15 Inferior temporal gyrus
16 Parieto-occipital fissure (arrowed)
17 Lunate sulcus
18 Anterior occipital sulcus
19 Pons
20 Flocculus
21 Cerebellar hemisphere
22 Medulla oblongata

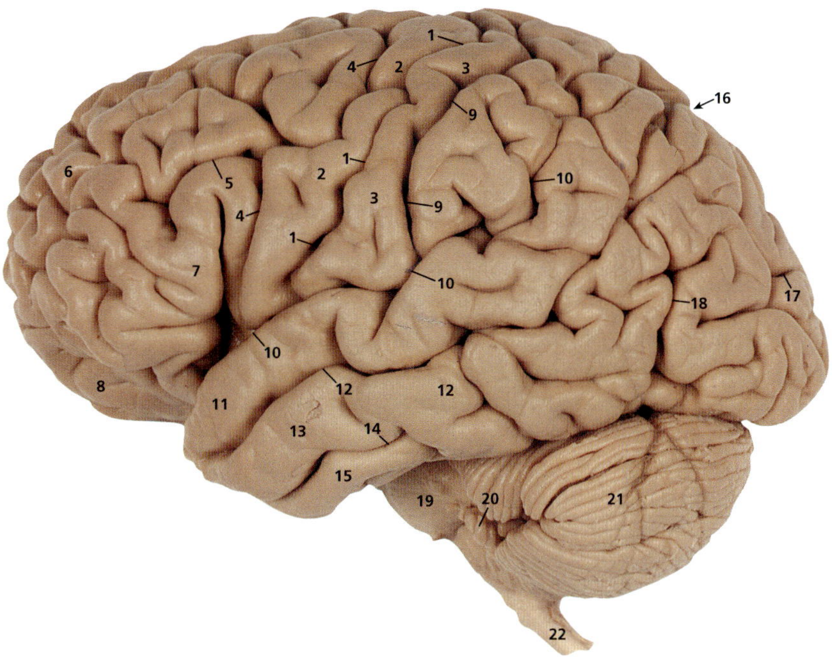

Figure 23.5 Superficial dissection of the brain viewed from the left side

Reproduced with permission from Ellis, Logan and Dixon, *Human Sectional Anatomy*, 3rd edn. Hodder, London. (2007).

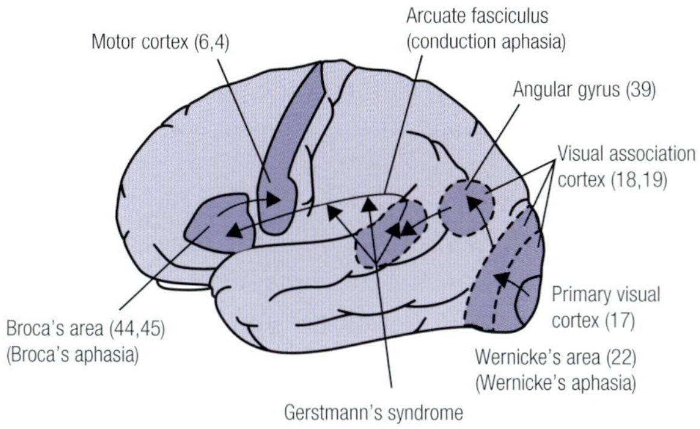

Figure 23.6 Left hemisphere: language, vision and Gerstmann syndrome

Reproduced with permission from Graham *et al.*, *Adams & Graham's Introduction to Neuropathology*, 3rd edn. Hodder, London. (2006).

Papez also included parts of the brain involved in olfaction in his circuit. Many of these regions are shown as the shaded limbic lobe in Figure 23.1b. Papez argued that lesions directly involving or impinging on this anatomical circuit (the Papez circuit) caused symptoms largely confined to the person's affective behaviour. Thus, in rabies affecting the hippocampus and cerebellum, Papez noted that patients are subject to anxiety, apprehension and paroxysms of rage and terror.[12,13] He pointed out that intact neural pathways from the mamillary bodies to the cingulate gyrus, via the anterior nuclei of the thalamus, appeared to be required for a state of vigilance and wakefulness, from which he deduced that this circuit was concerned with affective behaviour.[12,13] In respect of the possible emotional function of the cingulate gyrus, Papez noted that corpus colossal tumours impinging on this gyrus are often associated with personality change, loss of affect, and a degree of somnolence and stupor.[12,13]

The Papez circuit was further elaborated upon by MacLean, who included the following structures (in approximately this sequence) in his version of the limbic system: olfactory bulb, olfactory tubercle, lateral olfactory stria, amygdala, stria terminalis, septal nuclei, stria medullaris, interpeduncular nucleus, medial forebrain bundle and mamillary body; and also a pathway from the septal nuclei via the supracallosal striae, dentate gyrus, hippocampus and fornix back to the mamillary body. Other components of this version of the limbic system included the anterior nuclear group of the thalamus, the diagonal band of Broca and the habenula (part of the epithalamus).[13]

There is no consistent agreed set of components of the limbic system. Most modern definitions tend to include the cingulate gyrus, the rest of the hypothalamus and, at least partly, the basal ganglia (described later in this chapter). The cingulate gyrus is shown in Figure 23.3; the anterior cingulate cortex in particular appears to be implicated in a number of psychiatric disorders.

It has been argued that attributing emotional functions primarily to the limbic system may be inherently incorrect. For example, Pessoa stated:

> In attempting to localize affect in the brain, an appealing approach has been to separate the 'emotional brain' from the 'cognitive brain' ... parcelling the brain into cognitive and affective regions is inherently problematic, and ultimately untenable for at least three reasons: first, brain regions viewed as 'affec-

tive' are also involved in cognition; second, brain regions viewed as 'cognitive' are also involved in emotion; and critically, third, cognition and emotion are integrated in the brain.[14]

Cranial nerves

At the base of the brain the cranial nerves are attached to the brainstem.

The fibres of cranial nerve I, the olfactory nerve, which subserves the function of olfaction, originate from the olfactory mucosa and pass to the olfactory bulb. The fibres of cranial nerve II, the optic nerve, which subserves the function of vision, originate from the retinal ganglion layer. The blind spot is caused by the lack of photoreceptors in the part of the retina from which this cranial nerve exits the eye. The optic nerve is ensheathed in the three meningeal layers of, from internal to external, the pia mater, arachnoid mater and dura mater. It passes backwards to form the optic chiasma with the optic nerve from the other eye.

Cranial nerve III, the oculomotor nerve, which subserves the function of eye movement and also carries a parasympathetic innervation to the ciliary ganglion, emerges between the cerebral peduncles in the brainstem. The superior division of the nerve supplies the superior rectus and levator palpebrae superioris muscles, while the inferior division supplies the inferior oblique, inferior rectus and medial rectus, and carries the parasympathetic innervation.

Cranial nerve IV, the trochlear nerve, which subserves the function of eye movement, emerges from the midbrain (mesencephalon) and supplies the superior oblique.

Cranial nerve V, the trigeminal nerve, which subserves the functions of general sensory input from the head and motor output to the muscles of mastication, originates from the pons. The sensory (larger) and motor roots that leave the brainstem at the middle cerebellar peduncle eventually reach the trigeminal ganglion from which the following three divisions take form: the ophthalmic division, the maxillary division and the mandibular division. Their main branches are given in Table 23.1; the only motor branches are those to the muscles of mastication and the mylohyoid branch of the inferior alveolar nerve to the mylohyoid muscle and the anterior belly of the digastric muscle.

Cranial nerve VI, the abducens (abducent) nerve, which subserves the function of eye movement, emerges from between the pons and the medulla oblongata and supplies the lateral rectus.

Cranial nerve VII, the facial nerve, which subserves the functions of facial movement, taste and lacrimal and salivary gland parasympathetic innervation, has the following major branches: greater petrosal nerve (secretomotor to the pterygopalatine ganglion); the nerve to the stapedius; chorda tympani (taste from anterior two-thirds of the tongue and parasympathetic supply to the submandibular ganglion); posterior auricular nerve (to the occipital belly of occipitofrontalis and auricular muscles); nerves to the posterior belly of the digastric and stylohyoid; and five terminal motor branches from the parotid plexus (pes anserinus), namely the temporal, zygomatic, buccal, mandibular and cervical branches, which supply the muscles of facial expression and the platysma and buccinator muscles.

Cranial nerve VIII, the vestibulocochlear nerve, has two components: the vestibular nerve, which subserves sensory functions related to balance and posture; and the cochlear nerve, which is concerned with the sensation of hearing. This cranial nerve emerges from the pontocerebellar angle and eventually, upon entry into the petrous temporal bone (through the internal acoustic meatus), it splits into its two main components. The spiral organ of the cochlea is supplied by the cochlear nerve.

Cranial nerve IX, the glossopharyngeal nerve, has several functions: taste; pharyngeal sensory and motor innervation; a parasympathetic supply to the parotid gland; carotid body and sinus innervation; and a motor supply to the stylopharyngeus muscle. This cranial nerve leaves the skull through the jugular foramen. Its main branches include the carotid, carrying afferents from carotid body chemoreceptors and carotid sinus baroreceptors; the lingual branch to the pharyngeal (postsulcal) part of the tongue and to the circumvallate papillae of the oral (presulcal) part of the tongue; the muscular branch, which supplies the stylopharyngeus muscle; pharyngeal branches supplying pharyngeal sensory mucosal fibres; tonsillar branches, which, with the lesser palatine nerves, form the circulus tonsillaris from which occurs innervation of the palatine tonsil region, soft palate and oropharyngeal isthmus; and the tympanic nerve.

Cranial nerve X, the vagus nerve, has widespread functions that include sensory and motor innervation of the pharynx, larynx, palate and oesophagus; a parasympathetic supply to the viscera of the thorax and the alimentary tract as far as the splenic fissure; and sensory innervation of thoracic and abdominal viscera and the external acoustic meatus and tympanic membrane. The vagus nerve leaves the skull through the jugular foramen. Its branches in the neck include meningeal branches to the posterior cranial fossa dura mater; the auricular branch, which, after supplying a branch to the facial nerve, ultimately ends in two branches, one of which combines with the posterior auricular nerve and the other of which supplies the external acoustic meatus and part of the skin of the external ear; the pharyngeal branch, which supplies motor innervation to the pharynx; branches to the carotid body; the superior laryngeal nerve, which gives rise to the internal and external laryngeal nerves; and the recurrent laryngeal nerve.

Cranial nerve XI, the accessory nerve, which enables the head and shoulders to move and supplies muscles of the pharynx and larynx, comprises a smaller cranial root and a spinal root. The cranial root emerges from the skull through the jugular foramen whence it is joined briefly with the larger spinal root. After separating from the latter, the cranial root joins the tenth cranial nerve and supplies the pharyngeal and laryngeal muscles (with the exception of tensor

Table 23.1 Divisions and main branches of the trigeminal nerve (simplified)

Division	Branches	Structures supplied (sensory unless otherwise stated)
Ophthalmic	Tentorial	Tentorium cerebelli and supratentorial falx cerebri
	Lacrimal	Skin and conjunctiva of lateral upper eyelid and adjacent conjunctiva
	Communicating branch with zygomatic (see below)	
	Frontal	
	Supraorbital	Upper eyelid, frontal sinuses and scalp (to vertex)
	Supratrochlear	Skin of upper eyelid and medial forehead
	Nasociliary	
	Anterior ethmoidal	Anterior cranial fossa dura, ethmoidal air cells, upper anterior nasal cavity and, via the terminal branch (external nasal nerve), the skin at the tip of the nose
	Communicating branch with ciliary ganglion	Ethmoidal air cells, sphenoidal air sinuses
	Posterior ethmoidal	
	Infratrochlear	Medial upper eyelid, conjunctiva, adjacent nose
	Long ciliary nerves	Cornea, sclera and pass sympathetic supply to dilator pupillae
Maxillary	Meningeal	Dura mater
	Ganglionic branches to the pterygopalatine ganglion	
	Orbital	Orbital periosteum and sphenoidal and ethmoidal sinuses
	Nasal branches	Nasal septal mucosa
	Pharyngeal	Nasopharyngeal mucosa
	Greater palatine	Gingivae, mucosa and glands of hard palate
	Posterior inferior nasal	Posterior inferior lateral wall of nasal cavity
	Lesser palatine	Uvula, tonsil and soft palate
	Zygomatic	
	Zygomaticotemporal	Skin of temple
	Zygomaticofacial	Skin of cheek prominence
	Infraorbital	
	Superior alveolar	
	Branches of the superior alveolar: posterior, middle and anterior superior alveolar; sub-branches: superior dental plexus (superior dental and superior gingival)	Upper teeth and gingiva, nasal septum, side of nose and maxillary air sinus
	Inferior palpebral	Skin and conjunctiva of lower eyelid
	Nasal branches (external nasal and internal nasal)	Skin of side of nose and of movable part of nasal septum
	Superior labial	Skin of anterior cheek and upper lip
Mandibular	Motor branches	Muscles of mastication (motor)
	Meningeal branch	Middle cranial fossa dura
	Buccal	Cheek skin over anterior buccinator and mucous membrane of cheek
	Auriculotemporal	Auricle, external acoustic meatus, tympanic membrane, temporomandibular joint, posterior temple; parasympathetic supply to parotid gland
	Inferior alveolar	
	Mylohyoid	Motor supply to mylohyoid and anterior belly of digastric muscles
	Dental branches	Teeth and gingiva adjacent to the mandibular canal
	Incisor	Incisor and canine teeth
	Mental	Skin and mucous membrane of lower lip and of chin
	Lingual	Lingual gum, anterior two-thirds of tongue, floor of mouth; parasympathetic supply to sublingual and submandibular glands

veli palatine). The spinal root supplies the sternocleidomastoid and trapezius muscles.

Cranial nerve XII, the hypoglossal nerve, enables tongue movement. It supplies all the muscles of the tongue, with the exception of palatoglossus.

Spinal cord

Housed in the vertebral canal, the spinal cord is continuous with the brain, extending caudally from the medulla oblongata of the brain, just inferior to the foramen magnum of the skull, to the conus medullaris, which has a bony anchoring connection via the filum terminale to the dorsal aspect of the sacrococcygeal region. It has meningeal coverings that are continuous with those of the brain. There is a small central canal in the central grey matter of the spinal cord, which contains cerebrospinal fluid; this is continuous with the cerebrospinal fluid of the fourth ventricle of the brain.

Figure 23.7 shows the ascending sensory pathways that lie in the white matter of the spinal cord and include the following:

- The posterior or dorsal columns or fasciculi – the fasciculus cuneatus and the more medial fasciculus gracilis, which carry proprioceptive, vibratory and exteroceptive (i.e. relating to touch and pressure) information to higher levels of the central nervous system
- The lateral spinothalamic tract, which carries pain and temperature sensations to the somatosensory part of the thalamus
- The anterior or ventral spinothalamic tract, which carries sensations of pressure and coarse touch to the somatosensory part of the thalamus
- The posterior (dorsal) and anterior (ventral) spinocerebellar tracts, which carry proprioceptive and cutaneous sensations to the cerebellum
- The spinoreticular pathway, within the spinothalamic tracts, which appear to carry cutaneous and deep pain sensations to the pontomedullary reticular formation
- The spinocervicothalamic pathway, which carries sensations of pressure, pinching, hair movement and temperature to the contralateral thalamus via the lateral cervical nucleus and medial lemniscus.

Descending spinal cord pathways also lie in spinal cord white matter and have important motor control functions relating to movement, muscle tone and posture. They also influence spinal reflexes. Descending pathways include the following:

- The lateral and anterior (ventral) corticospinal tracts: fibres originate mainly in the cerebral cortex (with the corticobulbar tracts), including the motor cortex (Brodmann area 4) and premotor cortex (Brodmann area 6). The course of the corticospinal tracts is shown in Figure 23.8
- The rubrospinal tract: fibres originate in the magnocellular part of the red nucleus

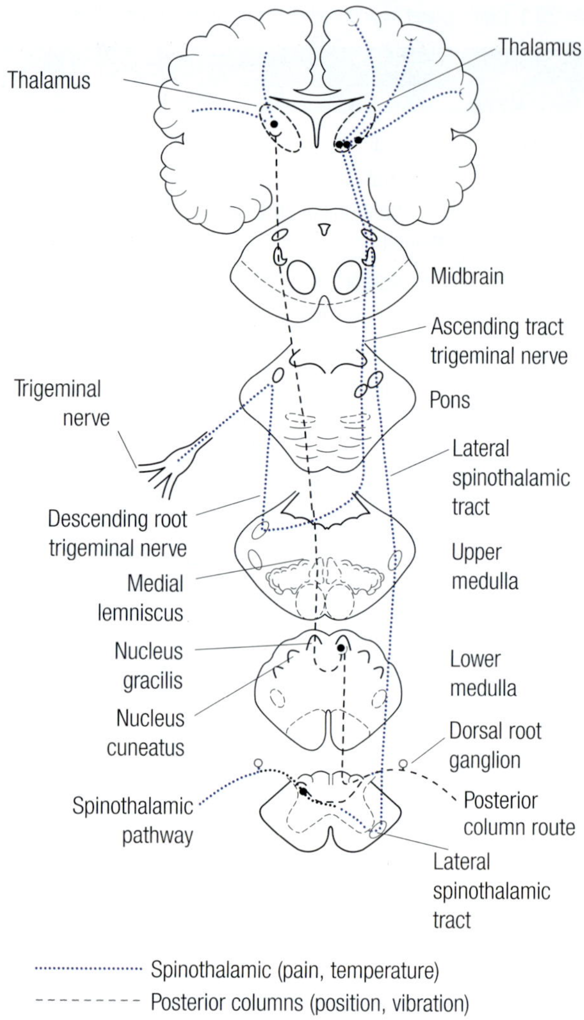

Figure 23.7 Ascending sensory pathways

Reproduced with permission from Fowler and Scadding, *Clinical Neurology*, 3rd edn. Hodder, London. (2003).

- The tectospinal tract: fibres originate in the superior colliculus
- The lateral and medial reticulospinal tracts: fibres originate in the reticular formation
- The interstitiospinal tract: fibres originate in the interstitial nucleus of Cajal
- The lateral and medial vestibulospinal tracts: fibres originate in the vestibular nuclear complex (in the floor of the fourth ventricle)
- The solitariospinal tract: fibres originate in the nucleus solitarius
- Spinal pathways using monoamines for neurotransmission: these originate from brain regions that are part of these neurochemical pathways (vide infra). For example, noradrenergic coeruleospinal spinal pathways project from the locus coeruleus.

The grey matter forms a central butterfly-shaped core of the spinal cord and contains multipolar neurons. The grey

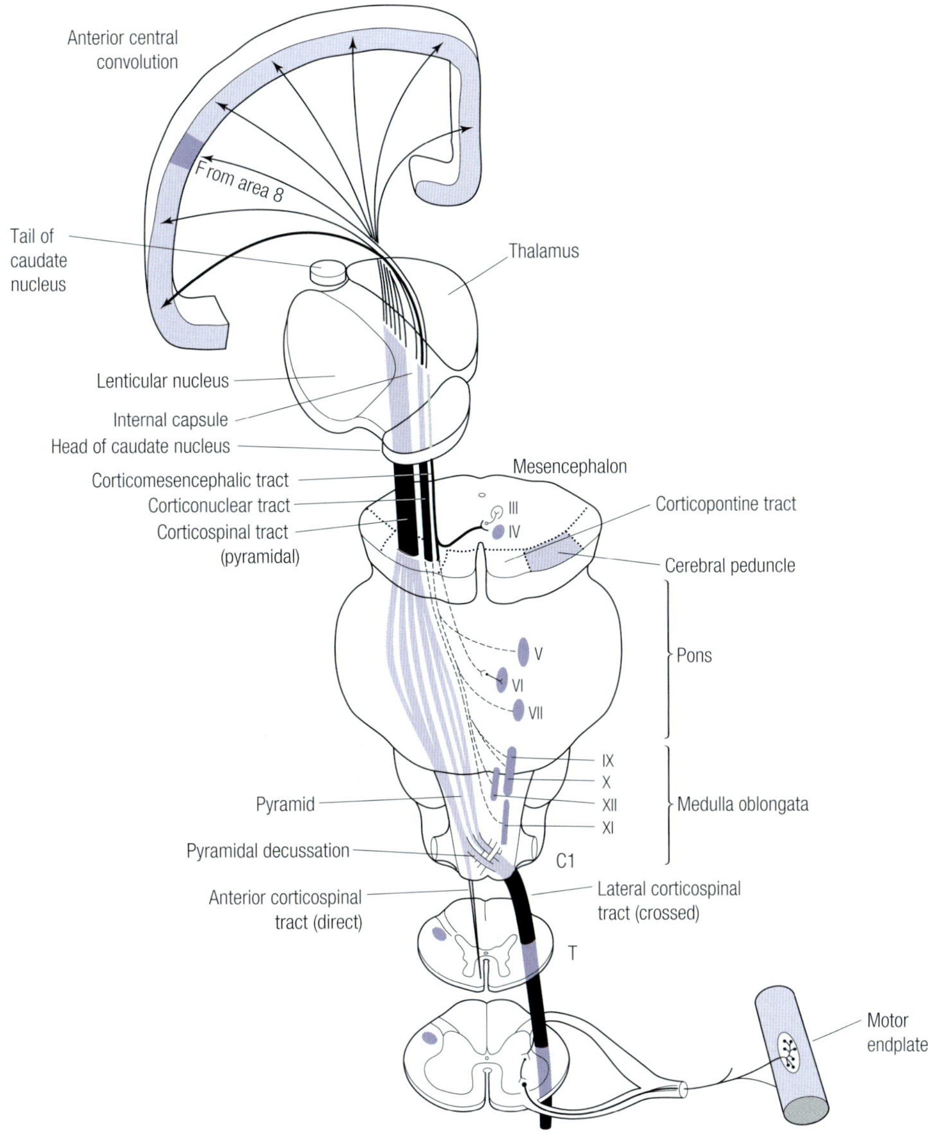

Figure 23.8 Course of the corticospinal tracts

Reproduced with permission from Fowler and Scadding, *Clinical Neurology*, 3rd edn. Hodder, London. (2003).

matter is related to the spinal nerves. Primary afferents from spinal nerve sensory dorsal rootlets terminate in the dorsal horn of grey matter (Figure 23.9). Efferents from the ventral horn of grey matter give rise to ventral motor rootlets, which join to form a ventral motor root. Figure 23.9 also shows the formation of the mixed spinal nerve, its division into dorsal and ventral primary rami, and the connection to the latter of sympathetic ganglia via white (myelinated) afferent rami communicantes and grey (unmyelinated) efferent rami communicantes.

BASAL GANGLIA

The basal ganglia have important functions in respect of the control of movement and posture.

Components

The basal ganglia refer to deep subcortical paired nuclear masses that lie close to the internal capsule. A modern definition of the basal ganglia is shown in Box 23.1. Note that, although the putamen and globus pallidus have traditionally been grouped together as the lentiform nucleus, in practice it is the caudate nucleus rather than the globus pallidus with which the putamen should be paired, based on cytoarchitectural and connectivity similarities; this pairing of the caudate nucleus with the putamen is relatively recent in phylogenetic terms and is known as the striatum (or neostriatum), in contrast to the older palaeostriatum consisting of the globus pallidus.

Box 23.1 Components of the basal ganglia

- Corpus striatum:
  - (Neo)striatum
    - Caudate nucleus
    - Putamen
  - Paleostriatum = globus pallidus
- Amygdala ± claustrum.

Anatomical relationships

A three-dimensional diagram showing the striatum (caudate nucleus and putamen) and its relationship to nearby structures is shown in Figure 23.10.

Connections

The basal ganglia interact with the cerebral cortex through a complex series of loop circuits; there is a functional division into connections with different parts of the cerebral cortex (such as motor and associative areas) and the limbic system.[15] In particular, functionally defined regions of the frontal cortex (the orbital and medial prefrontal cortex (OMPFC), involved in emotions and motivation; the DLPFC, involved in higher cognitive processes or executive functions; the premotor and motor areas, involved in motor planning and the execution of those plans) project topographically through the basal ganglia, to the thalamus, and back to the cortex.[16] The concept of the ventral striatum refers to a ventral extension of the striatum that includes the nucleus accumbens, the medial and ventral portions of the caudate nucleus and putamen, and the striatal cells of the olfactory tubercle.[16–18] Using this definition, projections from frontal cortex may be considered to form a functional gradient of inputs from the ventromedial sector through the dorsolateral striatum, with the medial and orbital prefrontal cortex terminating in the ventromedial part, and the motor cortex terminating in the dorsolateral region; furthermore, afferents from interconnected and functionally associated thalamic and cortical regions terminate in the same striatal area, resulting in a tight, anatomical and functional organization to the striatum.[16] These connections are illustrated in Figure 23.11. The cortical functional topography maintained through cortical connections to the striatum is likely to be continued from the striatum to the pallidum (relating predominantly to the globus pallidus) and pars reticulata of the substantia nigra, from these output structures to the thalamus, and finally, back to cortex.[16]

Alexander and colleagues put forward a model of five functionally segregated circuits linking the basal ganglia with the cortex in a parallel organization.[19] Evidence supporting this model has been forthcoming from non-human primate studies, such as that of Middleton and Strick.[20] The five circuits are designated the motor, oculomotor, dorsolateral prefrontal, lateral orbitofrontal and anterior cingulate

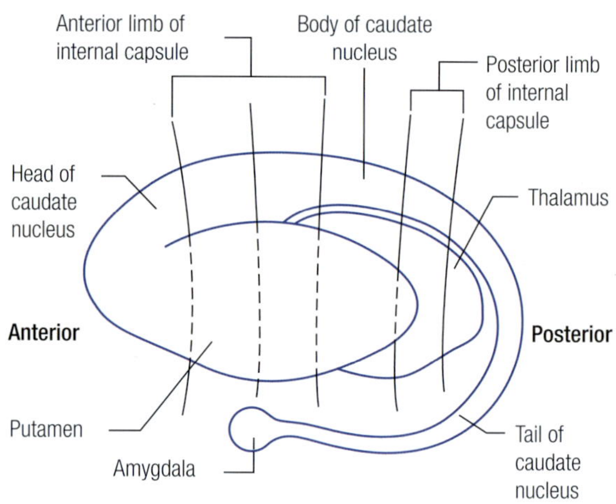

Figure 23.10 Three-dimensional view of the striatum of the left cerebral hemisphere

Reproduced with permission from Crossman and Neary, *Neuroanatomy*, 3rd edn. Churchill Livingstone, Edinburgh. (2000).

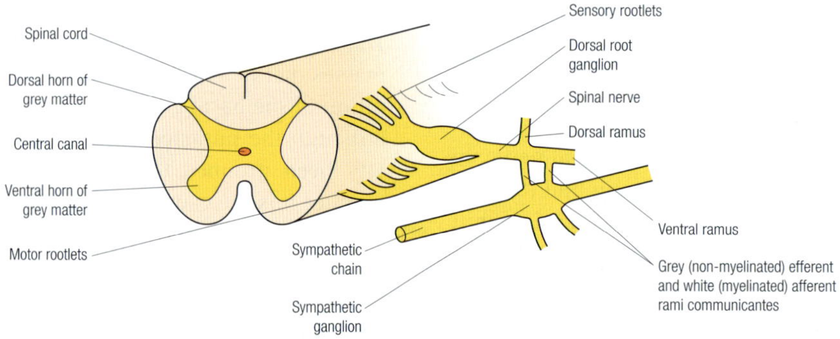

Figure 23.9 Typical spinal nerve formation and connections to the sympathetic ganglia and chains. The ventral motor rootlets unite to form a ventral motor root, joining with the dorsal sensory root, which comes from the sensory rootlets and dorsal root ganglion of each spinal segment. The mixed spinal nerve then divides into a dorsal and a ventral primary ramus. The dorsal rami supply the back, whereas the ventral rami supply all the limbs and trunk. The sympathetic ganglia are connected to the ventral rami via white (presynaptic) rami communicantes and grey (postsynaptic) rami communicantes.

Reproduced with permission from Abrahams *et al. Illustrated Clinical Anatomy.* Hodder, London. (2005).

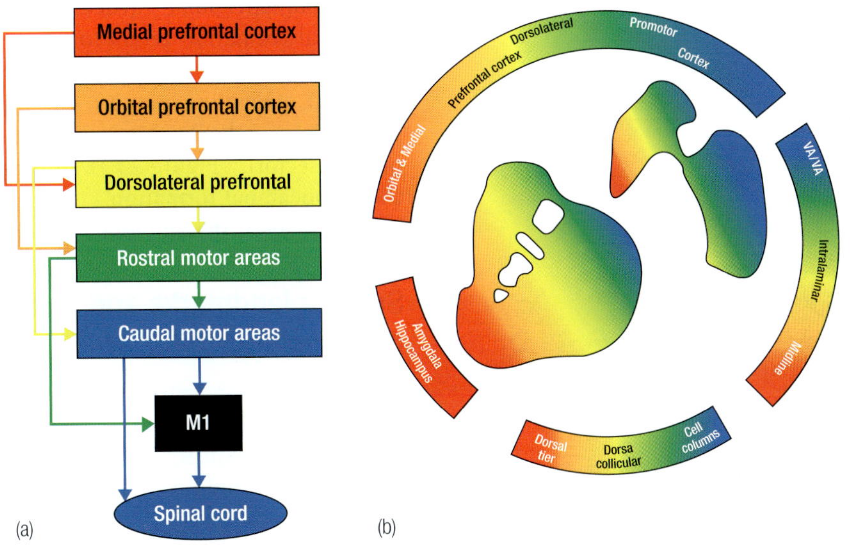

Figure 23.11 (a) Schematic illustration of the functional connections linking frontal cortical brain regions. (b) Organization of cortical and subcortical inputs to the striatum. In both (a) and (b), the colours denote functional distinctions. Blue: motor cortex, execution of motor actions; green: premotor cortex, planning of movements; yellow: dorsal and lateral prefrontal cortex, cognitive and executive functions; orange: orbital prefrontal cortex, goal-directed behaviours and motivation; red: medial prefrontal cortex, goal-directed behaviours and emotional processing

Reproduced with permission from ref. 16

circuits; each is centred on a different part of the frontal lobe, as shown in Figure 23.12. The circuits consist of partially overlapping corticostriate inputs, which are progressively funnelled via the pallidum (globus pallidus) and substantia nigra to the thalamus and thence back to the cortex, as shown in Figure 23.13. Details of the five proposed circuits are shown in Figure 23.14.

Figure 23.15 depicts the organization of thalamocorticothalamic projections that relate to the basal ganglia; nuclei appear to mediate information flow from higher cortical association areas of the prefrontal cortex to rostral motor areas involved in cognitive or integrative aspects of motor control to primary motor areas that direct movement execution.[16]

Within each area of connected corticobasal ganglia structures, there are reciprocal connections linking up regions associated with similar functions (maintaining parallel networks); in addition, there exist non-reciprocal connections linking up regions that are associated with different cortical–basal ganglia circuits.[16]

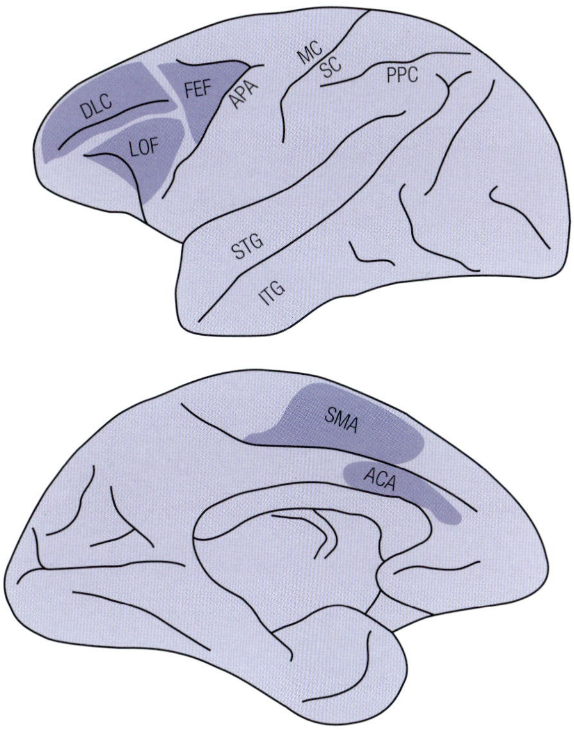

Figure 23.12 Frontal cortical targets of basal ganglia output. Schematic illustration of the five cortical areas that contribute to the closed loop portions of the Alexander basal ganglia–thalamocortical circuits

ACA, anterior cingulate area; APA, arcuate premotor area; DLC, dorsolateral prefrontal cortex; FEF, frontal eye fields; ITG, inferior temporal gyrus; LOF, lateral orbitofrontal cortex; MC, motor cortex; PPC, posterior parietal cortex; SC, somatosensory cortex; SMA, supplementary motor area; STG, superior temporal gyrus.

Reproduced with permission from ref. 19.

INTERNAL ANATOMY OF THE TEMPORAL LOBES

Components

In this section, particular consideration is given to the anatomy of the hippocampal formation and the amygdala. There are essentially three components to the medial temporal lobe: the hippocampal formation, the amygdala and the parahippocampal cortices that cover them; the hippocampal formation refers to a constellation of structures including the subicular cortices (parasubiculum, presubiculum and subiculum proper), the hippocampus (CA1–CA3 pyramids) and the dentate gyrus (including its hilar neurons or CA4 sector).[21] Figure 23.16 illustrates the components of the hippocampal formation.

The nuclei of the amygdala are described below.

Surface landmarks and anatomical relationships

Figure 23.17 is a coronal section through the brain of a human female, showing the relationship of the hippocampi to nearby structures in addition to the parahippocampal gyrus and the fimbria of the hippocampus.

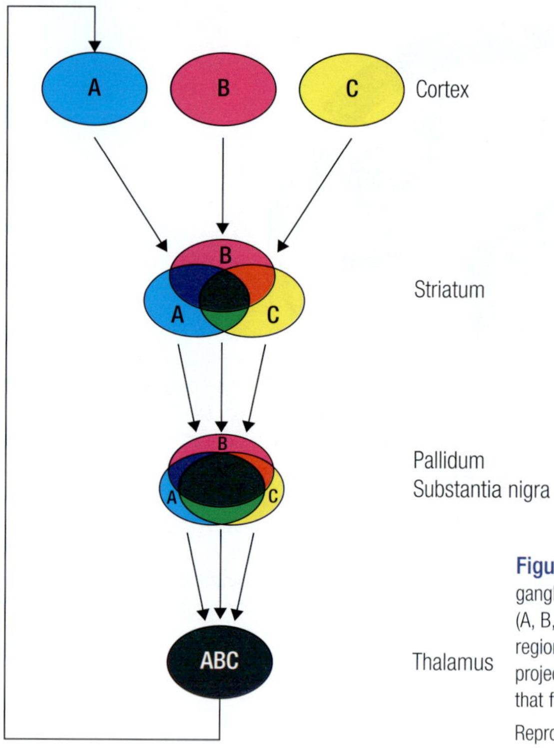

Figure 23.13 Generalized basal ganglia–thalamocortical circuit. Skeleton diagram of the basal ganglia–thalamocortical circuits. Each circuit receives output from several functionally related cortical areas (A, B, C), which send partially overlapping projections to a restricted portion of the striatum. These striatal regions send further converging projections to the globus pallidus and substantia nigra, which in turn project to a specific region of the thalamus. Each thalamic region projects back to one of the cortical areas that feeds into the circuit, thereby completing the closed-loop portion of the circuit

Reproduced with permission from ref. 19.

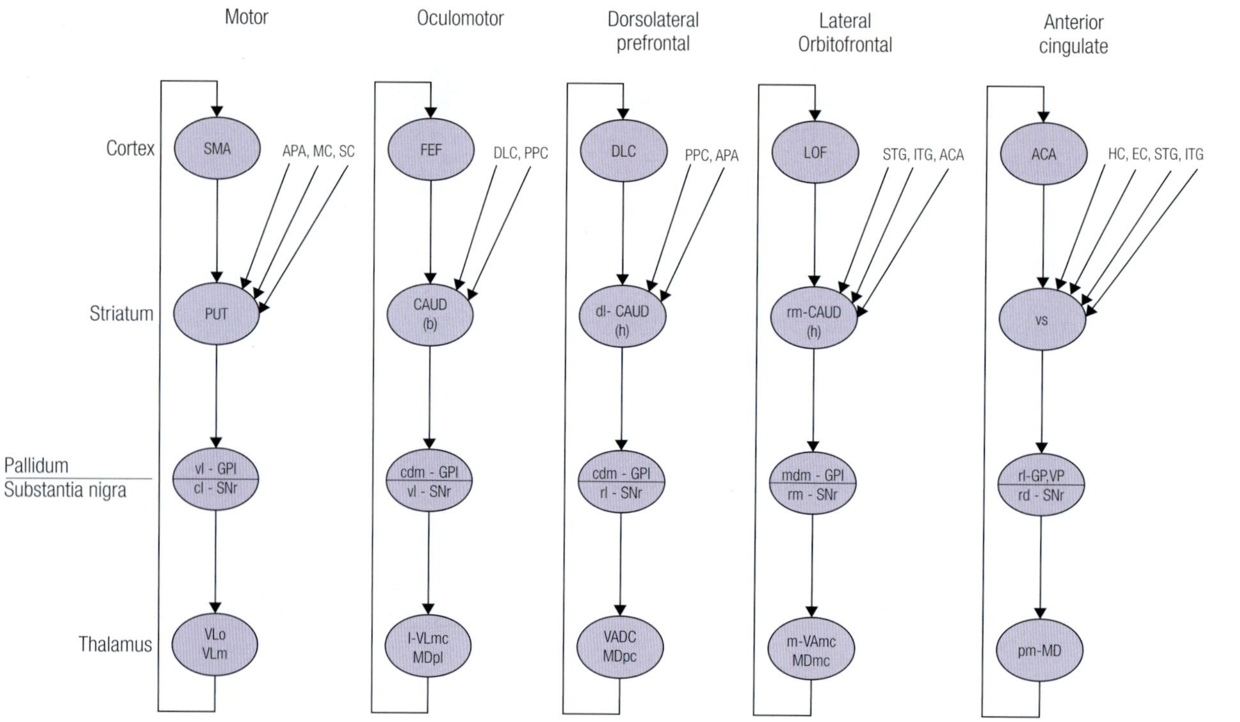

Figure 23.14 Proposed basal ganglia–thalamocortical circuits

ACA, anterior cingulate area; APA, arcuate premotor area; CAUD, caudate, (b) body, (h) head; cdm-, caudal dorsomedial; cl-,caudolateral; dl-, dorsolateral; DLC, dorsolateral prefrontal cortex; EC, entorhinal cortex; FEF, frontal eye fields; GPi, internal segment of globus pallidus; HC, hippocampal cortex; ITG, inferior temporal gyrus; l-, lateral; ldm-, lateral dorsomedial; LOF, lateral orbitofrontal cortex; m-, medial; MC, motor cortex; mdm-, medial dorsomedial; MDpl, medialis dorsalis pars paralamellaris; MDmc, medialis dorsalis pars magnocellularis; MDpc, medialis dorsalis pars parvocellularis; pm-, posteromedial; PPC, posterior parietal cortex; PUT, putamen; rd-, rostrodorsal; rl-, rostrolateral; rm-, rostromedial; SC, somatosensory cortex; SMA, supplementary motor cortex; SNr, substantia nigra pars reticulata; STG, superior temporal gyrus; VAmc, ventralis anterior pars magnocellularis; VApc, ventralis anterior pars parvocellularis; vl-, ventrolateral; VLm, ventralis lateralis pars medialis; VLo, ventralis lateralis pars oralis; vm-, ventromedial; VP, ventral pallidum; VS, ventral striatum.

Reproduced with permission from ref. 19.

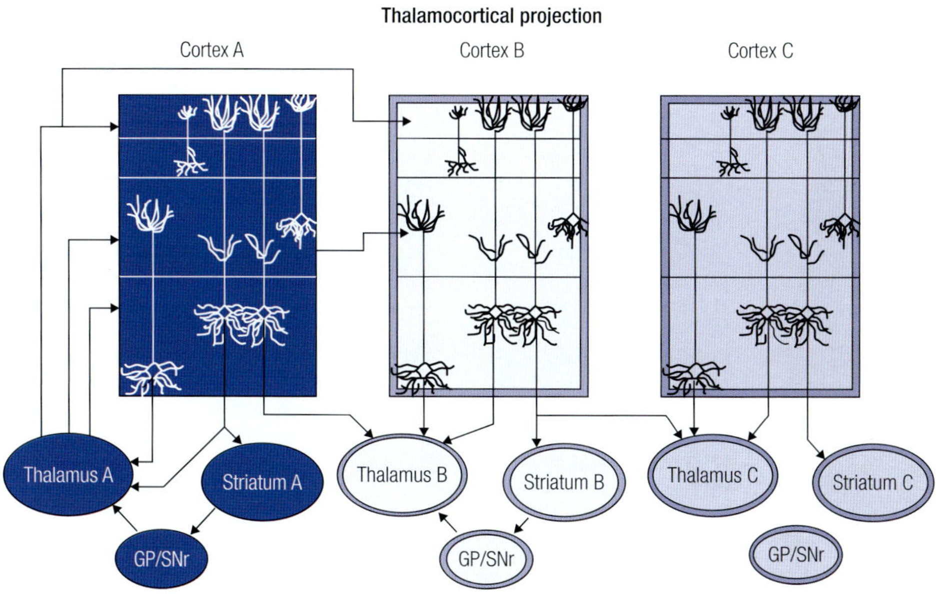

Figure 23.15 Diagram of the organization of thalamocorticothalamic projections. Through the non-reciprocal corticothalamic projection, cells in layer V may also interface with other corticobasal ganglia circuits by projecting to a thalamic region that is part of another circuit system

GP, globus pallidus; SNr, substantia nigra pars reticulata.

Reproduced with permission from ref. 16.

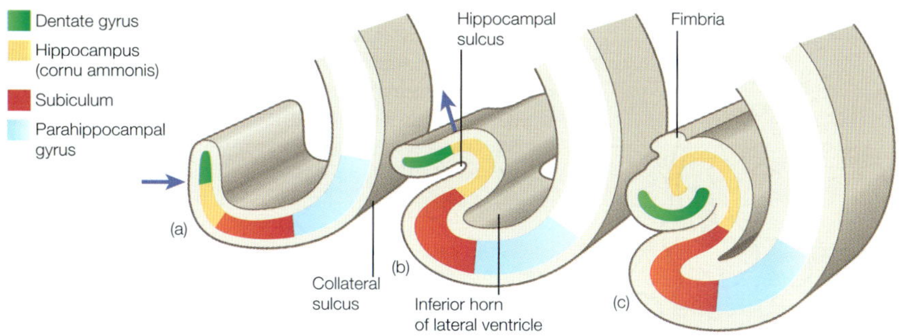

Figure 23.16 Series of coronal sections of the temporal lobe and inferior horn of the lateral ventricle, illustrating the relationships between the components of the hippocampal formation

Reproduced with permission from Standring, *Gray's Anatomy,* 40th edn. Churchill Livingstone, Edinburgh. (2008).

The following sulci may be seen on the surface of the medial temporal lobe: the rhinal sulcus, which passes anteriorly and laterally and is often more prominent in great apes than in humans; the collateral sulcus, which passes posteriorly and laterally; the uncal sulcus, which separates the uncus (uncal hippocampal formation) from the parahippocampal gyrus; the hippocampal sulcus or fissure, which separates the rolled up main body of the hippocampal formation from the posterior parahippocampal gyrus; and the sulcus semianularis, which separates the entorhinal cortex from the cortical nuclei of the amygdala.[21] The position of the amygdala is shown in Figure 23.10. Interestingly, the surface of the entorhinal cortex often has a corrugated appearance, which is probably the result of the presence of cytochrome oxidase-reactive islands (in layer II).[21,22]

Connections

In Figure 23.18 the disposition of the cell fields CA1–CA4 in the hippocampal formation, and its different strata, are illustrated. Different cell fields are probably involved in different connections. For example, CA2 pyramidal cells appear to receive the hypothalamic input (from the supramamillary region of the hypothalamus). Cortical and subcortical connections of the hippocampal formation are shown in Figure 23.19, with further details being given in the legend.

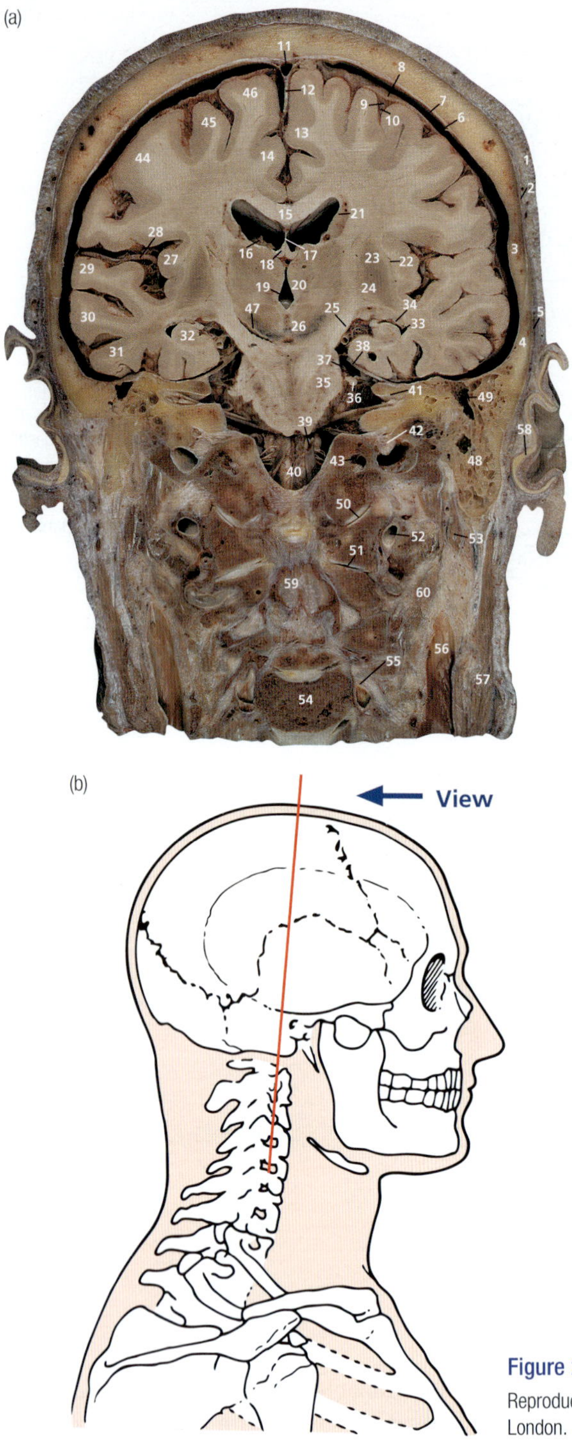

1 Skin and dense subcutaneous tissue
2 Epicranial aponeurosis (galea aponeurotica)
3 Parietal bone
4 Temporal bone
5 Temporalis
6 Dura mater
7 Subdural space
8 Arachnoid mater
9 Subarachnoid space
10 Pia mater
11 Superior sagittal sinus
12 Falx cerebri
13 Medial frontal gyrus
14 Cingulate gyrus
15 Body of corpus callosum
16 Choroid plexus within lateral ventricle
17 Septum pellucidum
18 Fornix
19 Third ventricle
20 Thalamus
21 Caudate nucleus
22 Claustrum
23 Putamen
24 Globus pallidus
25 Posterior limb of internal capsule
26 Mamillary body
27 Insula
28 Lateral cerebral fissure and branches of middle cerebral artery
29 Superior temporal gyrus
30 Middle temporal gyrus
31 Inferior temporal gyrus
32 Hippocampus
33 Inferior horn of lateral ventricle
34 Tail of caudate nucleus
35 Pons
36 Trigeminal nerve (V)
37 Trochlear nerve (IV)
38 Free margin of tentorium cerebelli
39 Vertebral artery (see 52)
40 Medulla oblongata
41 Facial nerve (VII) and vestibulocochlear nerve (VIII) entering internal auditory meatus within petrous part of temporal bone
42 Glossopharyngeal nerve (IX), vagus nerve (X) and cranial part of accessory nerve (XI) entering jugular foramen within petrous part of temporal bone
43 Hypoglossal nerve (XII) entering hypoglossal canal within petrous part of temporal bone
44 Postcentral gyrus
45 Precentral gyrus
46 Superior frontal gyrus
47 Substantia nigra
48 Mastoid air cells within mastoid process of the petrous part of temporal bone
49 Mastoid antrum within petrous part of temporal bone
50 Atlanto-occipital joint
51 Atlanto-axial joint
52 Vertebral artery within foramen transversarium of axis (see 39)
53 Posterior belly of digastric
54 Body of C4 vertebra
55 C4 dorsal root ganglion
56 Internal jugular vein
57 Sternocleidomastoid
58 Auricular cartilage of ear
59 Dura of spinal canal
60 Levator scapulae

Figure 23.17 (a) Coronal section of the brain at the level shown in (b)
Reproduced with permission from Ellis, Logan and Dixon, *Human Sectional Anatomy*, 3rd edn. Hodder, London. (2007).

To understand the connections of the amygdala (or amygdaloid complex), it is useful first to have an overview of its many nuclei. These are shown in Figure 23.20 for the rat amygdala. These nuclei may be divided into groups (in Figure 23.20 by different colours): the deep or basolateral group, which includes the lateral nucleus (LA), the basal nucleus (B) and the accessory basal nucleus (AB); the superficial or cortical-like group, which includes the nucleus of the lateral olfactory tract (NLOT), the bed nucleus of the accessory olfactory tract (BAOT), the anterior and posterior cortical nucleus (CoA and CoP, respectively) and the periamygdaloid cortex (PAC); the centromedial group composed of the central (CeA) and medial (M) nuclei and the amygdaloid part of the bed nucleus of stria terminalis (BNST); and a separate set of nuclei that do not easily fall into any of these three previous groups and include the intercalated cell

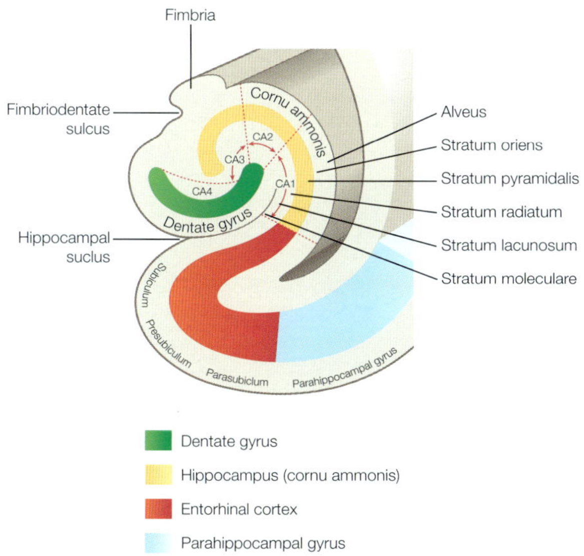

Figure 23.18 Hippocampal formation, showing the disposition of the various cell fields

masses and the amygdalohippocampal area.[23,24,25] The CeA has four divisions: the capsular subdivision (CeC), lateral subdivision (CeL), intermediate subdivision (CeI) and medial subdivision (CeM).[24,26,27] Figure 23.21 summarizes the main afferents to the nuclei of the amygdala, while Figure 23.22 summarizes the main efferents from the nuclei. Intra-amygdaloid connections are summarized in Figure 23.23.

MAJOR WHITE-MATTER PATHWAYS

In this section, two major white-matter pathways of relevance to psychiatry are considered, namely the corpus callosum and the fornix. Papez' circuit and its relationship to the limbic system were described earlier in this chapter.

Corpus callosum

This constitutes the largest white-matter pathway in the brain and is a set of commissural fibres providing both

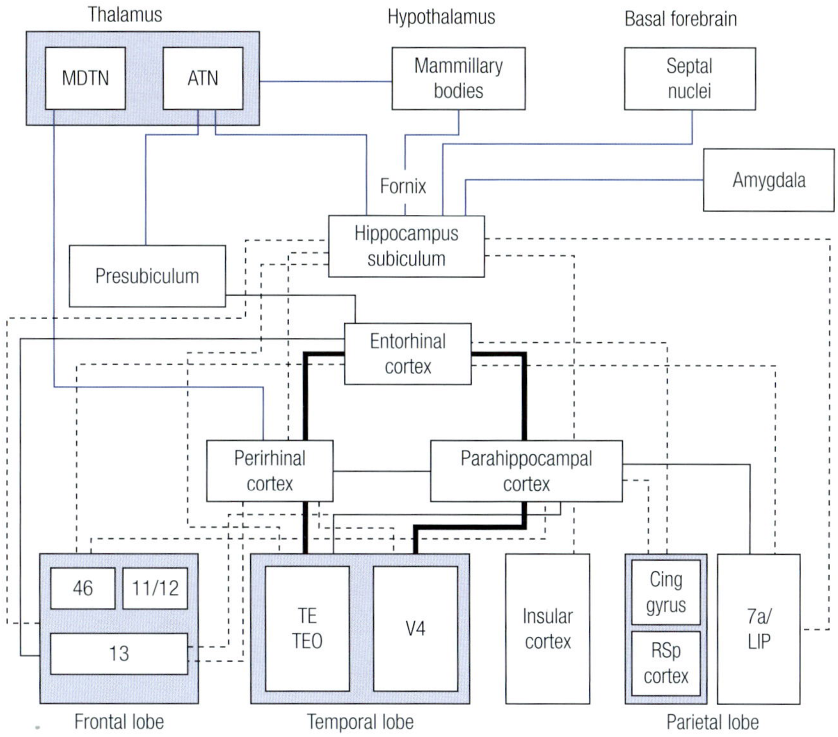

Figure 23.19 Cortical and subcortical connections of the hippocampal formation. Subcortical connections are indicated by blue lines; cortical connections are indicated by black lines. The thickness of the black lines approximates to the strength of the connections. Most of the hippocampus's neocortical inputs come from the perirhinal and parahippocampal cortices, through the entorhinal cortex, and most of its neocortical output is through the subiculum, which also projects back to the entorhinal cortex. Both the perirhinal cortex and the parahippocampal cortex lie at the end of the ventral visual processing ('what') stream. The perirhinal cortex is crucial for the representation of complex objects, whereas the parahippocampal cortex, with its strong connections to the posterior parietal (7a/lateral intraparietal area, LIP) and retrosplenial (RSp) cortices, has a greater role in the processing of visuospatial information (from the dorsal visual processing ('where') stream). Head-direction cells are found in the mamillary bodies, the anterior thalamic nuclei (ATN), the presubiculum and the entorhinal cortex. Some researchers have proposed that recollection is dependent on the hippocampus and its links with the ATN, whereas familiarity can be mediated by direct connections between the perirhinal cortex and the medial dorsal thalamic nuclei (MDTN)

Cing gyrus, cingulate gyrus; TE and TEO, inferior temporal areas TE and TEO.

Reproduced with permission from ref. 23.

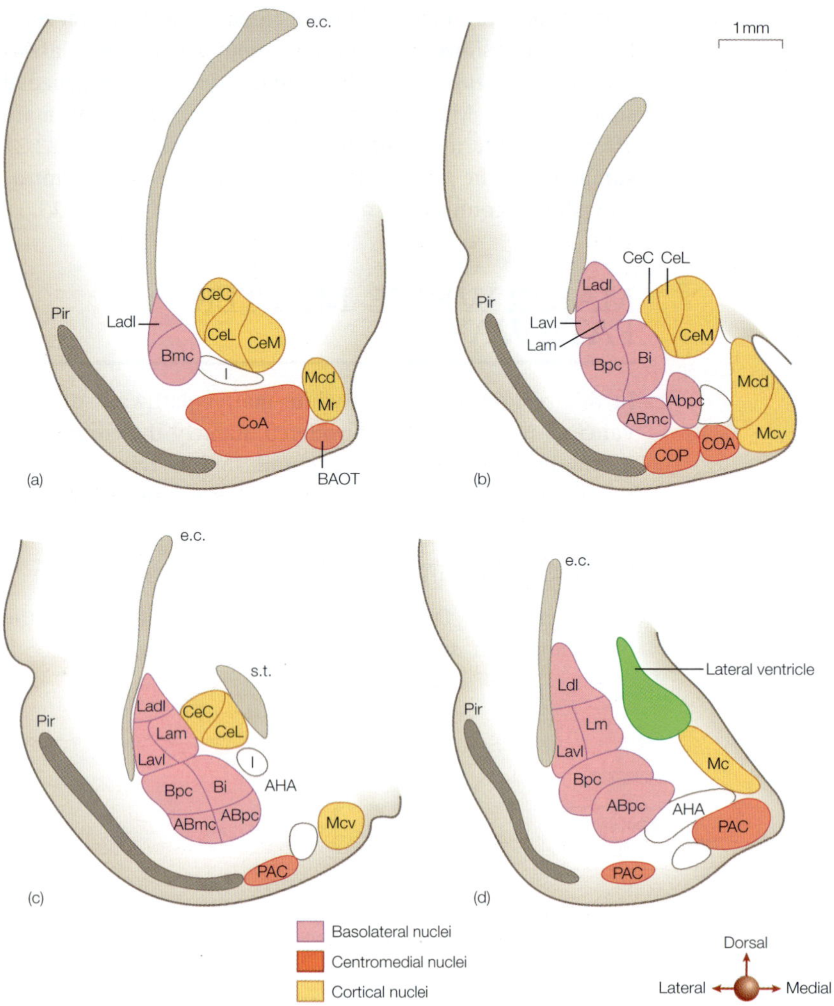

Figure 23.20 Nuclei of the rat amygdaloid complex. Coronal sections are drawn from rostral (a) to caudal (d). The different nuclei are divided into three groups, as described in text. Areas in blue form part of the basolateral group, areas in yellow are the cortical group, and areas in green form the centromedial group

ABmc, accessory basal magnocellular subdivision; ABpc, accessory basal parvicellular subdivision; Bpc, basal nucleus magnocellular subdivision; e.c., external capsule; Ladl, lateral amygdala medial subdivision; Lam, lateral amygdala medial subdivision; Lavl, lateral amygdala ventrolateral subdivision; Mcd, medial amygdala dorsal subdivision; Mcv, medial amygdala ventral subdivision; Mr, medial amygdala rostral subdivision; Pir, piriform cortex; s.t., stria terminalis.

Reproduced with permission from ref. 24.

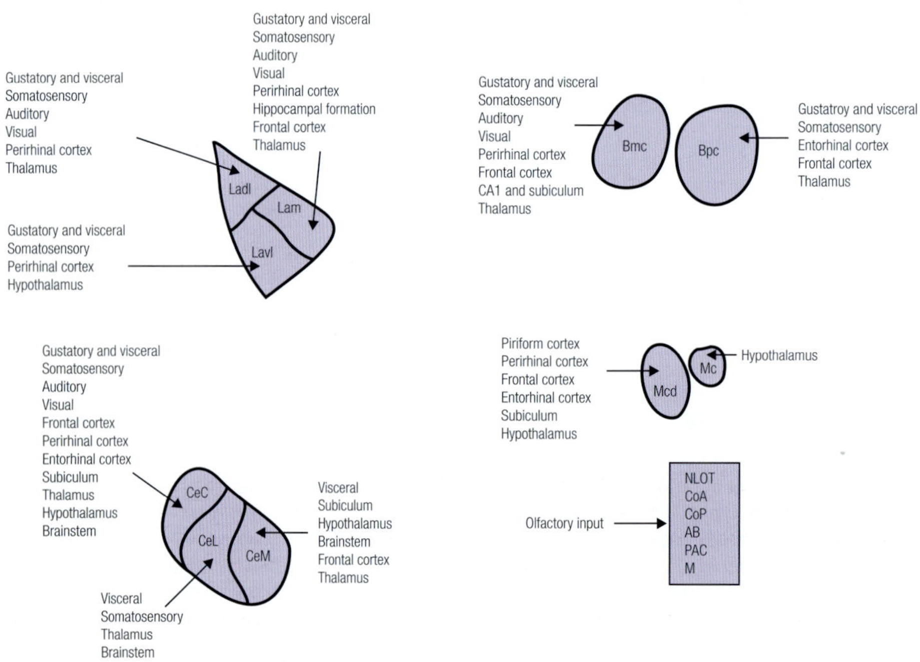

Figure 23.21 Summary of the inputs to the amygdaloid nuclei. Neuromodulatory inputs (e.g. acetylcholine, serotonin) have been omitted for clarity. See Figure 23.22 and text for definitions

Reproduced with permission from ref. 24.

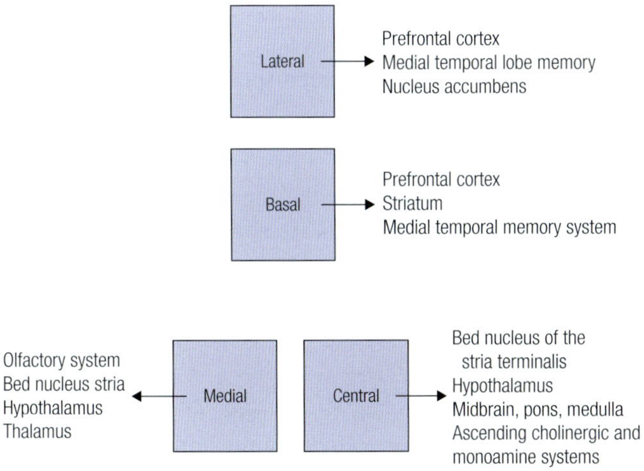

Figure 23.22 Summary of the main outputs from the nuclei of the amygdala. See Figure 23.20 and text for definitions

Reproduced with permission from ref. 24.

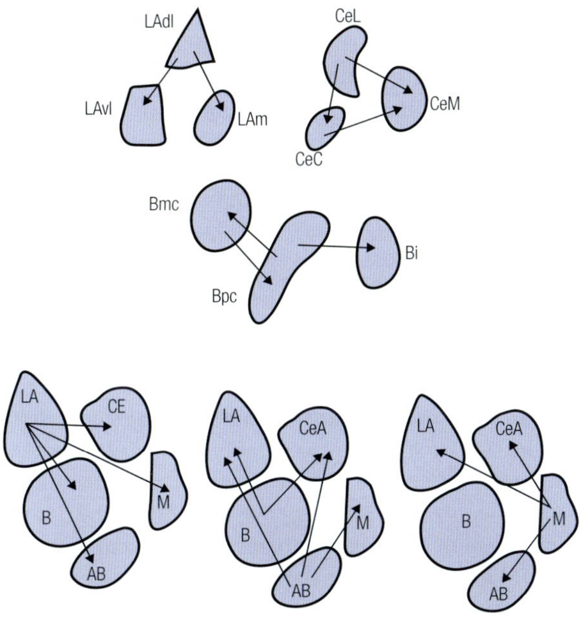

Figure 23.23 Intra-amygdaloid connections as described by anatomical tract tracing studies. Most of the connections between nuclei within the amygdala are glutamatergic. See Figure 23.20 and text for definitions

Reproduced with permission from ref. 24.

homotopic and heterotopic connections between the right and left cerebral hemispheres. The corpus callosum in the sectional anatomy views of Figures 23.3 and 23.18, from which it can be seen that it extends rostrally from the splenium, via its body, to the genu, just inferior to the callosal sulcus (see Figure 23.3). Its relationship to close structures is evident from these three figures. A summary of the destinations of fibres that pass through different parts of the corpus callosum is given in Table 23.2.

Fornix

The course of the fornix is shown in Figure 23.3. As the fornix passes ventrally towards the anterior commissure (labelled 14 in Figure 23.3), it divides into two parts, the precommissural part and the post-commissural part. As can be seen from Figure 23.19, fibres of the fornix connect the hippocampal formation with the hypothalamus, septal nuclei of the basal forebrain and anterior thalamic nuclei.

TYPES OF CELL FOUND WITHIN THE CENTRAL NERVOUS SYSTEM

Neurons

Neurons, or nerve cells, have a variety of different sizes and shapes, but all have one axon emerging from the axon hillock and at least one dendrite; some neurons possess many dozens of dendrites. The axon can vary in length, from a few millimetres to almost a metre. In larger neurons, it can be seen that the nucleus is round and centrally placed and contains a prominent nucleolus, in which ribosomal RNA (rRNA) is transcribed (by RNA pol I), while the cytoplasm of the neuronal soma contains large numbers of basophilic granular Nissl bodies extending into the dendrites (although typically not in the axon hillock), which are the site of protein biosynthesis, consisting of rough endoplasmic reticulum and polyribosomes. Neuronal cytoplasm also contains mitochondria, which are the sites of oxidative phosphorylation; Golgi apparatus, which carries out glycosylation and phosphorylation, synthesizes proteoglycans and carbohydrates, transports lipids and creates lysosomes (from endosomes by the addition of hydrolytic

Table 23.2 Corpus callosal fibre destinations

Part of corpus callosum	Name of fibres (if applicable)	Destinations
Splenium	Forceps major	Occipital lobes
Splenium and posterior body	Tapetum	Temporal lobes
Body		Widespread neocortical areas
Genu	Forceps minor	Frontal lobes

enzymes); and lipofuscin granules, which are membrane-bound yellow–brown organelles containing non-metabolizable remnants of lysosomal digestion.

Synaptic vesicles are the organelles of the boutons terminaux, which store neurotransmitters. Details of synaptic function are given in Chapter 24.

The dark tyrosine-derived pigment neuromelanin is normally found in granules in the neuronal cytoplasm of the central nervous system in the following locations: substantia nigra; pars compacta; locus coeruleus, from which arises the ascending noradrenergic pathway (see below); dorsal motor nucleus of the vagus nerve; and the pontine median raphe nucleus.

Macroglia

Astrocytes

Astrocytes, or astroglia, are classified as being either protoplasmic or fibrous/fibrillary. Protoplasmic astrocytes are found mainly in grey matter and tend to have short processes with numerous branches. In contrast, fibrous or fibrillary astrocytes are found mainly in white matter and tend to have long processes; they form a thick feltwork beneath the pia mater. Their cytoplasm tends to contain glial fibrillary acidic protein (GFAP), an intermediate filament protein.

Variants of astrocytes include Bergmann glia in the granule layer of the cerebellar cortex; and the round laminate PAS-positive corpora amylacea found in subpial and periventricular white matter and in the spinal cord, particularly in subjects of advanced age.

Astrocytes have numerous functions, which may include structural functions: central nervous system repair, astrocytes having been considered to be functionally homologous to fibroblasts in the central nervous system and helping to form scar tissue (astrocytic gliosis); the nourishment of neurons; their end-feet may play a role in the formation of the blood–brain barrier; aiding in neurotransmission; vasomodulation; ion-concentration regulation; and promoting myelination by oligodendrocytes.

Oligodendrocytes

Oligodendrocytes, or oligodendroglia, possess few cell processes (hence their name) and do not have cytoplasmic filaments. Those in grey matter tend to cluster around neuronal cell bodies and are known as perineuronal satellite cells. They probably play an important role in sustaining these neurons. Those in white matter are arranged in rows between myelinated fibres and are known as interfascicular glia. These white-matter oligodendrocytes are responsible for the formation of the myelin sheaths.

Ependymal cells

Ependymal cells, ependyma, are ciliated cuboidal cells that usually form a continuous lining of the ventricular system of the brain (including its foramina and the cerebral aqueduct) and the central canal of the spinal cord (with which the ventricles are continuous). Ependymal cells may play a role in fluid homeostasis (between cerebrospinal fluid and brain parenchyma) and in cerebrospinal fluid circulation.

Choroid plexus cells

The cuboidal cells that cover the fibrovascular cores of the choroid plexi of the ventricles are non-ciliated. The choroid plexi are mainly responsible for the production of cerebrospinal fluid.

Microglia

Microglia are now known to be resident central nervous system immune cells that provide surveillance in the normal brain and spinal cord and become activated following tissue insult to perform a number of functions, including proliferation, migration, phagocytosis, and secretion of cytokines, chemokines, trophic factors, nitric oxide and other bioactive molecules and reactive species. Detailed mechanisms by which they detect and respond to their environment are not fully understood, but it is known that microglia express a number of surface receptors and ion channels, including voltage-gated sodium channels, that participate in transduction of external stimuli to intracellular responses.[28–32] When activated, microglia usually become rod-shaped.

Stem cells

Stem cells are multipotent cells that can give rise to a differentiated progeny and self-renewed progeny; the balanced coordination of these two stem cell fates is essential for embryonic development and tissue homeostasis in the adult.[33,34] Stem cells are aided by their environment, which provides support and regulatory signals; this microenvironment is the stem cell niche and is the sum of all factors, cellular and molecular, that interact with and regulate the stem cell.[35] At the time of writing, the following two stem cell niches have been established as existing in the adult mammalian brain: the subventricular zone (SVZ) of the lateral wall of the lateral ventricle, and the subgranular zone (SGZ) of the dentate gyrus of the hippocampal formation.[34,35] Progenitor cells of the SVZ continually migrate rostrally to the olfactory bulb and differentiate into interneurons, which integrate into the granule cell layer and olfactory glomerular layer and serve important olfactory functions.[35,36] Postnatal neurogenesis in the dentate gyrus plays a critical role in normal cognitive development, specifically in learning and memory functions associated with the hippocampus.[35]

MAJOR NEUROCHEMICAL PATHWAYS

Dopaminergic pathways

Major dopaminergic pathways of the human brain are detailed in Figure 23.24. Note that the nigrostriatal dopamin-

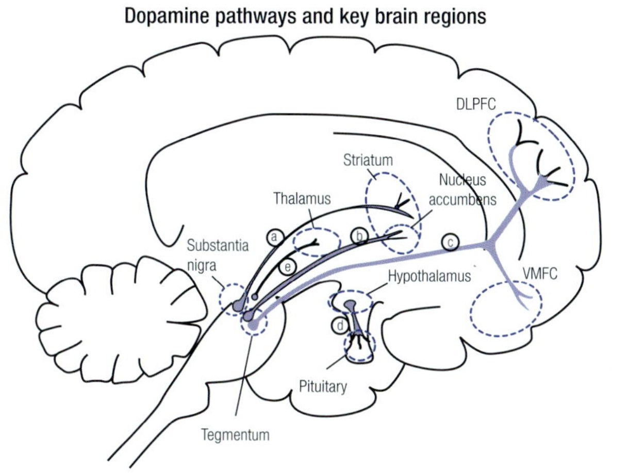

Figure 23.24 Major dopamine pathways in the brain. (a) The nigrostriatal dopamine pathway, which projects from the substantia nigra to the corpus striatum of the basal ganglia, is part of the extrapyramidal system and controls motor function and movement. (b) The mesolimbic dopamine pathway projects from the midbrain ventral tegmental area to the nucleus accumbens, a part of the limbic system thought to be involved in many behaviours such as pleasurable sensations, the powerful euphoria of drugs of abuse, and delusions and hallucinations of psychosis. (c) The mesocortical dopamine pathway is related to the mesolimbic pathway and also projects from the ventral tegmental area but sends its axons to areas of the prefrontal cortex, where they may have a role in mediating cognitive symptomatology (dorsolateral prefrontal cortex) and affective symptomatology (ventromedial prefrontal cortex) of schizophrenia. (d) The tuberoinfundibular dopamine pathway projects from the hypothalamus to the anterior pituitary gland and controls prolactin secretion. (e) A fifth dopamine pathway arises from multiple sites, including the periaqueductal grey, ventral mesencephalon, hypothalamic nuclei and lateral parabrachial nucleus, and projects to the thalamus. Its function is not currently well known

Reproduced with permission from *Stahl's Essential Psychopharmacology,* 3rd edn. Cambridge University Press. (2008).

ergic pathway has its origin in the pars compacta of the substantia nigra of the mesencephalon (midbrain) and projects to the corpus striatum of the basal ganglia; the pars compacta is part of dopaminergic cell group A9. The nigrostriatal pathway is sometimes referred to as the mesostriatal pathway. The origin of the mesolimbic and mesocortical dopaminergic pathways is also in the mesencephalon, in the ventral tegmental area (dopaminergic cell group A10). In addition to the prefrontal cortex, the mesocortical pathway probably also projects to the cingulate and entorhinal cortices.

Noradrenergic pathways

Major ascending noradrenergic (norepinephrinergic) projections from the locus coeruleus of the pons are detailed in Figure 23.25. Most of these tracts ascend in the medial forebrain bundle, an exception being the tract supplying the cerebellum, which does so via the superior cerebellar peduncle. The major descending noradrenergic projection to the spinal cord (coeruleospinal pathway) is also illustrated in Figure 23.25.

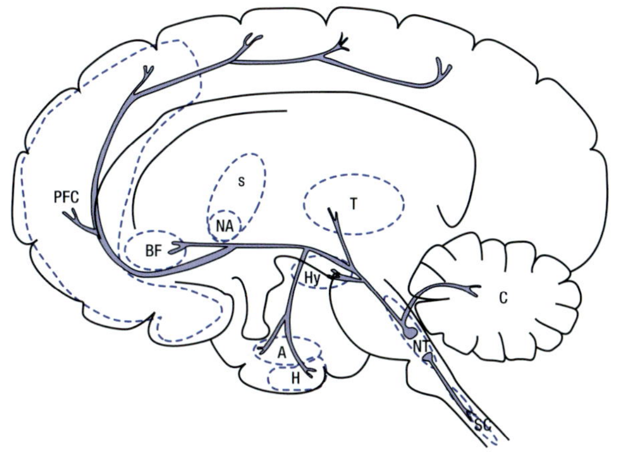

Figure 23.25 Major noradrenergic projections. Ascending noradrenergic projections originate mainly in the locus coeruleus of the brainstem; they extend to multiple brain regions, as shown here, and regulate mood, arousal, cognition and other functions. Descending noradrenergic projections extend down the spinal cord and regulate pain pathways

A, amygdala; BF, basal forebrain; C, cerebellum; H, hippocampus; Hy, hypothalamus; NA, nucleus accumbens; NT, brainstem neurotransmitter centres; PFC, prefrontal cortex; S, striatum; SC, spinal cord; T, thalamus.

Reproduced with permission from *Stahl's Essential Psychopharmacology,* 3rd edn. Cambridge University Press. (2008).

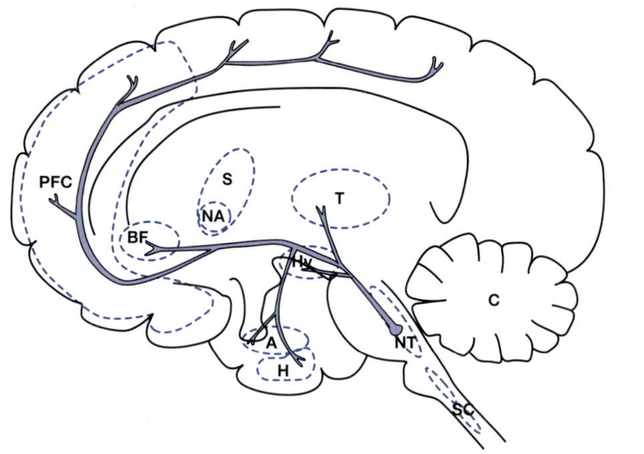

Figure 23.26 Brainstem cholinergic pathway. Acetylcholine projections originating in the brainstem extend to many regions, including the prefrontal cortex, basal forebrain, thalamus, hypothalamus, amygdala and hippocampus. These projections regulate arousal, cognition and other functions

A, amygdala; BF, basal forebrain; C, cerebellum; H, hippocampus; Hy, hypothalamus; NA, nucleus accumbens; NT, brainstem neurotransmitter centres; PFC, prefrontal cortex; S, striatum; SC, spinal cord; T, thalamus.

Reproduced with permission from *Stahl's Essential Psychopharmacology,* 3rd edn. Cambridge University Press. (2008).

Cholinergic pathways

Two major brain cholinergic (acetylcholine) pathways are of importance in psychiatry. One is the brainstem cholinergic pathway, which takes its origin in the brainstem and is detailed in Figure 23.26. The second is the basal forebrain cholinergic pathway, which originates in the basal forebrain and projects widely to the prefrontal cortex, amygdala and hippocampus, as illustrated in Figure 23.27.

Cholinergic projections from basal forebrain

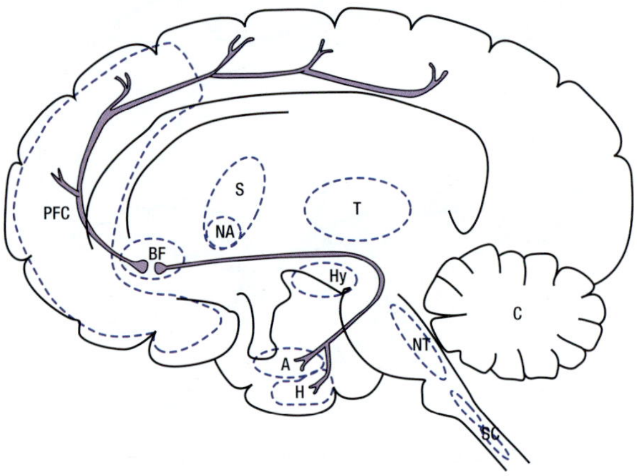

Important cholinergic neurons in the basal forebrain project to the cortex, hippocampus, and amygdala.

Figure 23.27 Basal forebrain cholinergic pathway. Cholinergic neurons originating in the basal forebrain project to the prefrontal cortex, hippocampus and amygdala; they are believed to be involved in memory

A, amygdala; BF, basal forebrain; C, cerebellum; H, hippocampus; Hy, hypothalamus; NA, nucleus accumbens; NT, brainstem neurotransmitter centres; PFC, prefrontal cortex; S, striatum; SC, spinal cord; T, thalamus.

Reproduced with permission from *Stahl's Essential Psychopharmacology*, 3rd edn. Cambridge University Press. (2008).

Corticofugal glutamate system

Corticofugal fibres project from the cerebral cortex to subcortical structures, including the basal ganglia and thalamus. These fibres form a fan-shaped arrangement of white matter known as the corona radiata (Figure 23.28a). Since the corona radiata appears as a curved linear area of low attenuation on computed tomography (CT) scans of the

(a)

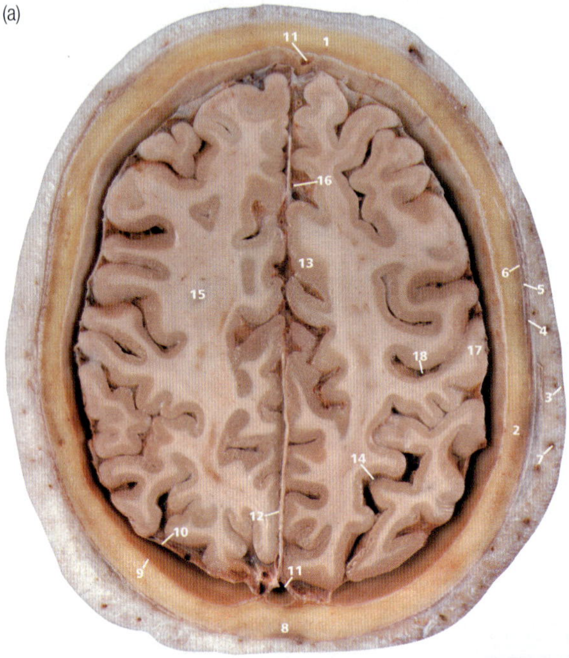

1 Frontal bone
2 Parietal bone
3 Skin and dense subcutaneous tissue
4 Epicranial aponeurosis (galea aponeurotica)
5 Temporalis
6 Pericranium
7 Branch of superficial temporal artery
8 Sagittal suture
9 Dura mater
10 Arachnoid mater
11 Superior sagittal sinus
12 Falx cerebri
13 Cingulate gyrus
14 Parieto-occipital sulcus
15 Corona radiata
16 Anterior cerebral artery (branches)
17 Postcentral gyrus
18 Central sulcus

(b)

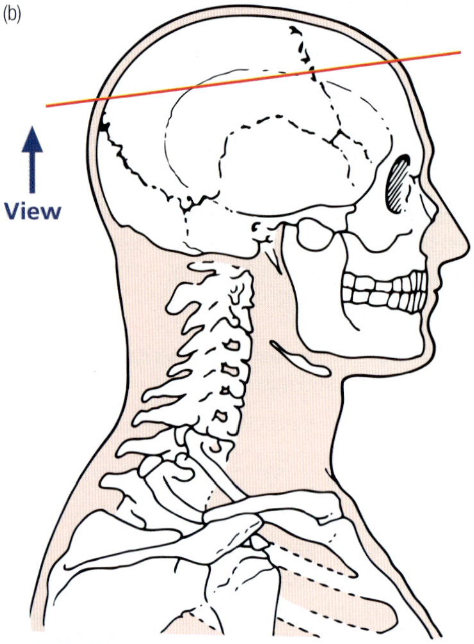

(c)

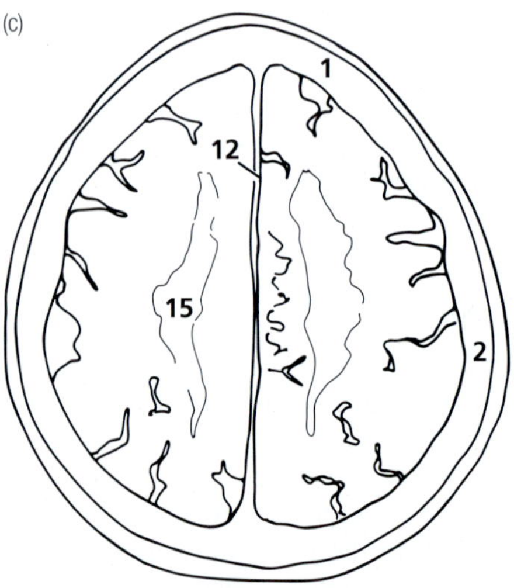

(d)

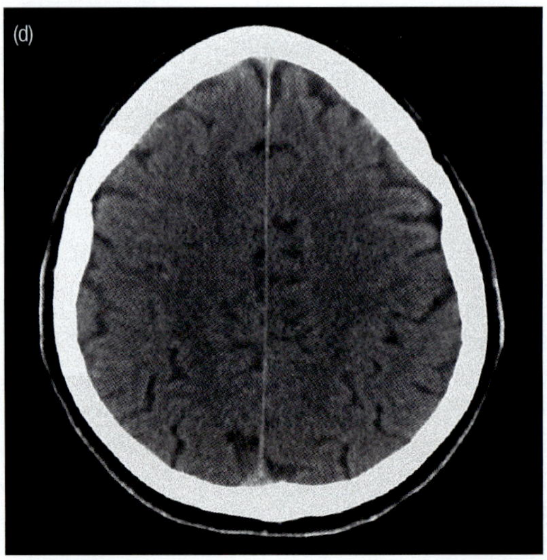

Figure 23.28 (a) Transverse section of the brain at the level shown in (b). (c) Features seen in the transverse (axial) computed tomography (CT) brain scan (d). Note the prominent appearance of the corona radiata or centrum semiovale

Reproduced with permission from Ellis, Logan and Dixon, *Human Sectional Anatomy*, 3rd edn. Hodder, London. (2007).

brain (Figure 23.28d), it is also known as the centrum semi-ovale, particularly in the field of structural neuroimaging. As mentioned in the section on the basal ganglia (vide supra), cortical-striatal-thalamic-cortical loops are likely to subserve many important functions (see Figures 23.13–15). These and similar loops of importance in psychiatry include the DLPFC-striatal-thalamic-DLPFC loop for executive functions, the anterior cingulate cortex-striatal-thalamic-anterior cingulate cortex loop for attention, the orbitofrontal cortex-caudate-thalamic-orbitofrontal cortex loop for impulsivity, and possibly an anterior cingulate cortex-nucleus accumbens-thalamic-anterior cingulate cortex loop for some aspects of emotion. The output from the cortical pyramidal neurons that begin and end these loops is illustrated in Figure 23.29. As the neurotransmitter output is the amino acid glutamate, this whole arrangement is referred to as the corticofugal glutamate system.

Serotonergic pathways

Major ascending and descending serotonergic projections from the brainstem are detailed in Figure 23.30. The origins are from three groups of midline brainstem raphe nuclei: the medullary raphe group, comprising the nucleus raphe pallidus, nucleus raphe obscurus and nucleus raphe magnus, from which project the descending bulbospinal tract into the spinal cord and the propriobulbar tract to the inferior olivary complex; the mesencephalic raphe group, comprising the nucleus raphe dorsalis, from which project ascending tracts; and the pontine raphe group, comprising the nucleus raphe pontis and nucleus centralis superior, from which project ascending tracts, the pontocerebellar tract to the cerebellum, and propriobulbar tracts to the locus coeruleus and reticular formation.

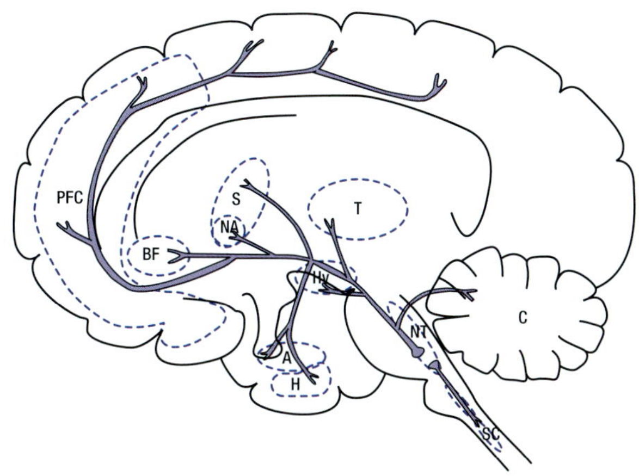

Figure 23.30 Major serotonergic projections. Like noradrenaline, serotonin has both ascending and descending projections. Ascending serotonergic projections originate in the brainstem and extend to many of the same regions as noradrenergic projections, with additional projections to the striatum and nucleus accumbens. These ascending projections may regulate mood, anxiety, sleep and other functions. Descending serotonergic projections extend down the brainstem and through the spinal cord; they may regulate pain

A, amygdala; BF, basal forebrain; C, cerebellum; H, hippocampus; Hy, hypothalamus; NA, nucleus accumbens; NT, brainstem neurotransmitter centres; PFC, prefrontal cortex; S, striatum; SC, spinal cord; T, thalamus.

Reproduced with permission from *Stahl's Essential Psychopharmacology,* 3rd edn. Cambridge University Press. (2008).

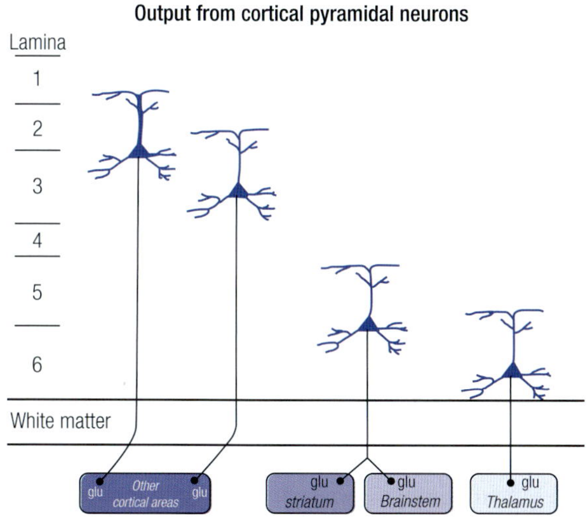

Figure 23.29 Output from cortical pyramidal neurons. Corticostriatal-thalamic-cortical loops begin and end with a pyramidal neuron in the cortex. These pyramidal cells are located in various laminae of the cortex, which influence the direction in which they send their outputs. Cortical pyramidal neurons located in laminae 2 and 3 send output to other cortical areas; those located in lamina 5 send output to the striatum and brainstem; and those in lamina 6 send output to the thalamus. The neurotransmitter output of all cortical pyramidal neurons is glutamate (glu)

Reproduced with permission from *Stahl's Essential Psychopharmacology,* 3rd edn. Cambridge University Press. (2008).

KEY POINTS

- The frontal cortex contains M1, PMd, PMv, FEF, DLPFC, VLPFC, SMA and the orbitofrontal cortex; the parietal cortex contains S1 and S2; the temporal cortex contains A1 and, on the dominant side, Wernicke's area; the occipital cortex contains V1, V2, V3d, V3v, V3a and V4.
- The limbic system is based on the Papez circuit, which was further elaborated upon by MacLean to include the following structures: olfactory bulb, olfactory tubercle, lateral olfactory stria, amygdala, stria terminalis, septal nuclei, stria medullaris, interpeduncular nucleus, medial forebrain bundle and mamillary body; and also a pathway from the septal nuclei via the supracallosal striae, dentate gyrus, hippocampus and fornix back to the mamillary body. Other components of this version included the anterior nuclear group of the thalamus, the diagonal band of Broca and the habenula (part of the epithalamus).
- The cranial nerves are I olfactory (smell), II optic (vision), III oculomotor (motor/parasympathetic), IV trochlear (motor), V trigeminal (sensory/motor), VI abducent (motor), VII facial (motor/sensory/parasympathetic), VIII vestibulocochlear (motor/sensory), IX glossopharyngeal (sensory/parasympathetic), X vagus (motor/sensory/parasympathetic), XI accessory (motor) and XII hypoglossal (motor).

- Each of the basal ganglia consists of the corpus striatum and amygdala and interacts with the cerebral cortex through a complex series of loop circuits; there is a functional division into connections with different parts of the cerebral cortex (such as motor and associative areas) and the limbic system.
- There are essentially three components to the medial temporal lobe: the hippocampal formation, the amygdala and the parahippocampal cortices that cover them; the hippocampal formation refers to a constellation of structures including the subicular cortices (parasubiculum, presubiculum and subiculum proper), the hippocampus (CA1–CA3 pyramids) and the dentate gyrus (including its hilar neurons or CA4 sector).
- The corpus callosum constitutes the largest white-matter pathway in the brain and is a set of commissural fibres providing both homotopic and heterotopic connections between the right and left cerebral hemispheres.
- Fibres of another important white-matter pathway, the fornix, connect the hippocampal formation with the hypothalamus, septal nuclei of the basal forebrain and anterior thalamic nuclei.
- Types of cell found within the central nervous system include neurons, macroglia (astrocytes and oligodendrocytes), ependymal cells, choroid plexus cells, microglia and stem cells.
- Major neurochemical pathways in the brain include the nigrostriatal, mesolimbic and mesocortical dopaminergic pathways; the ascending noradrenergic (norepinephrinergic) projections from the locus coeruleus; the coeruleospinal pathway; the brainstem cholinergic pathway; the basal forebrain cholinergic pathway; the corticofugal glutamate system; and major ascending and descending serotonergic projections from the brainstem.

REFERENCES

1. Penfield W, Boldrey E (1937) Somatic motor and sensory representation in the cerebral cortex of man as studied by electrical stimulation. *Brain* **60**: 389–433.
2. Pesaran B, Nelson MJ, Andersen RA (2008) Free choice activates a decision circuit between frontal and parietal cortex. *Nature* **453**: 406–9.
3. Monosov IE, Trageser JC, Thompson KG (2008) Measurements of simultaneously recorded spiking activity and local field potentials suggest that spatial selection emerges in the frontal eye field. *Neuron* **57**: 614–25.
4. Baddeley AD, Hitch G (1974) Working memory. In GA Bower (ed.) *The Psychology of Learning and Motivation.* New York: Academic Press.
5. D'Esposito M, Postle BR, Rypma B (2000) Prefrontal cortical contributions to working memory: evidence from event-related fMRI studies. *Experimental Brain Research* **133**: 3–11.
6. Champod AS, Petrides M (2007) Dissociable roles of the posterior parietal and the prefrontal cortex in manipulation and monitoring processes. *Proceedings of the National Academy of Sciences USA* **104**: 14837–42.
7. Chase HW, Clark L, Sahakian BJ, Bullmore ET, Robbins TW (2008) Dissociable roles of prefrontal subregions in self-ordered working memory performance. *Neuropsychologia* **46**: 2650–61.
8. Donohue SE, Wendelken C, Bunge SA (2008) Neural correlates of preparation for action selection as a function of specific task demands. *Journal of Cognitive Neuroscience* **20**: 694–706.
9. Roland PE, Larsen B, Lassen NA, Skinhøj E (1980) Supplementary motor area and other cortical areas in organization of voluntary movements in man. *Journal of Neurophysiology* **43**: 118–36.
10. Ramnani N, Owen AM (2004) Anterior prefrontal cortex: insights into function from anatomy and neuroimaging. *Nature Reviews Neuroscience* **5**: 184–94.
11. Essen DC, Zeki SM (1978) The topographic organization of rhesus monkey prestriate cortex. *Journal of Physiology* **277**: 193–226.
12. Papez JW (1937) A proposed mechanism of emotion. *Archives of Neurology and Psychiatry* **38**: 725–43.
13. MacLean PD (1949) Psychosomatic disease and the visceral brain: recent developments bearing on the Papez theory of emotion. *Psychosomatic Medicine* **11**: 338–53.
14. Pessoa L (2004) On the relationship between emotion and cognition. *Nature Reviews Neuroscience* **9**: 148–58.
15. Yelnik J (2008) Modeling the organization of the basal ganglia. *Revue Neurolique* **164**: 969–76.
16. Haber SN (2003) The primate basal ganglia: parallel and integrative networks. *Journal of Chemical Neuroanatomy* **26**: 317–30.
17. Heimer L (1978) The olfactory cortex and the ventral striatum. In KE Livingston, O Hornykiewicz (eds) *Limbic Mechanisms.* New York: Plenum Press.
18. Heimer L, Switzer RD, Van Hoesen GW (1982) Ventral striatum and ventral pallidum: components of the motor system? *Trends in Neuroscience* **5**: 83–7.
19. Alexander GE, DeLong MR, Strick PL (1986) Parallel organization of functionally segregated circuits linking basal ganglia and cortex. *Annual Review of Neuroscience* **9**: 357–81.
20. Middleton FA, Strick PL (2002) Basal ganglia 'projections' to the prefrontal cortex of the primate. *Cerebral Cortex* **12**: 926–35.
21. Van Hoesen GW (1995) Anatomy of the medial temporal lobe. *Magnetic Resonance Imaging* **13**: 1047–55.
22. Hevner RF, Wong-Riley MT (1992) Entorhinal cortex of the human, monkey, and rat: metabolic map as revealed by cytochrome oxidase. *Journal of Comparative Neurology* **326**: 451–69.
23. Bird CM, Burgess N (2008) The hippocampus and memory: insights from spatial processing. *Nature Reviews Neuroscience* **9**: 182–94.
24. Sah P, Faber ES, Lopez De Armentia M, Power J (2003) The amygdaloid complex: anatomy and physiology. *Physiological Reviews* **83**: 803–34.
25. Price JL, Russchen FT, Amaral DG (1987) *The Limbic*

Region: II. The Amygdaloid Complex. New York: Elsevier Science.

26. Jolkkonen E, Pitkänen A (1998) Intrinsic connections of the rat amygdaloid complex: projections originating in the central nucleus. *Journal of Comparative Neurology* **395**: 53–72.
27. McDonald AJ (1982) Cytoarchitecture of the central amygdaloid nucleus of the rat. *Journal of Comparative Neurology* **208**: 401–18.
28. Black JA, Liu S, Waxman SG (2009) Sodium channel activity modulates multiple functions in microglia. *Glia* **57**: 1072–81.
29. Garden GA, Moller T (2006) Microglia biology in health and disease. *Journal of Neuroimmune Pharmacology* **1**: 127–37.
30. Hanisch U-K, Kettenmann H (2007) Microglia: active sensor and versatile effector cells in the normal and pathologic brain. *Nature Neuroscience* **10**: 1387–94.
31. Van Rossum D, Hanisch U-K (2004) Microglia. *Metabolic Brain Disease* **19**: 393–411.
32. Korotzer AR, Cotman CW (1992) Voltage-gated currents expressed by rat microglia in culture. *Glia* **6**: 81–8.
33. Yadirgi G, Marino S (2009) Adult neural stem cells and their role in brain pathology. *Journal of Pathology* **217**: 242–53.
34. Walker MR, Patel KK, Stappenbeck TS (2009) The stem cell niche. *Journal of Pathology* **217**: 169–80.
35. Hellström NA, Björk-Eriksson T, Blomgren K, Kuhn HG (2009) Differential recovery of neural stem cells in the subventricular zone and dentate gyrus after ionizing radiation. *Stem Cells* **27**: 634–41.
36. Gheusi G, Lledo PM (2007) Control of early events in olfactory processing by adult neurogenesis. *Chemical Senses* **32**: 397–409.

Chapter 24

Basic concepts in neurophysiology

Paul Strutton

INTRODUCTION

This chapter covers the basic concepts in neurophysiology: ion flux and channels, membrane potential, graded potential, action potential, synapses, and neurotransmission (neurotransmitter synthesis, release and reuptake).

It is estimated that the human brain contains of the order of 100 billion (10^{11}) nerve cells, or neurons. Neurons are excitable cells that are capable of converting various stimuli into electrical impulses. A typical neuron is composed of a cell body and a number of elongated projections. One of these projections (an axon) joins the cell body at an elongated cylindrical point called the axon hillock and forms the output pathway for the neuron, and a network of other projections (dendrites) forms the input pathway to the neuron (Figure 24.1). There are exceptions to this somewhat simplified morphological description, with some neurons having no dendrites and other neurons using dendrites as the output in addition to the input pathway. Neurons can be classified on the basis of their structural characteristics (Figure 24.2). A neuron may make connections with as many as 1000–2000 other neurons by way of synapses, specialized junctions between neurons. Communication between neurons takes place using chemical transmitters, which are released at the presynaptic terminal of the axon, cross the synaptic cleft and bind to receptors on the postsynaptic membrane. The electrical signals of the neurons are action potentials; these can cover quite considerable dis-

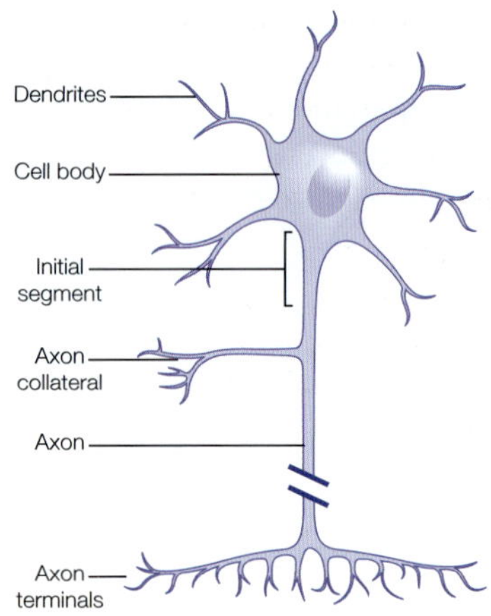

Figure 24.1 Diagrammatic representation of a neuron. The break in the axon indicates that axons may extend for long distances; in fact, they may be 5000–10 000 times longer than the cell body is wide. This neuron is a common type, but there are a wide variety of neuronal morphologies, one of which has no axon. Redrawn with permission from Widmaier, Raff and Strang (2008) *Vander's Human Physiology* 11th edn. Maidenhead: McGraw Hill.

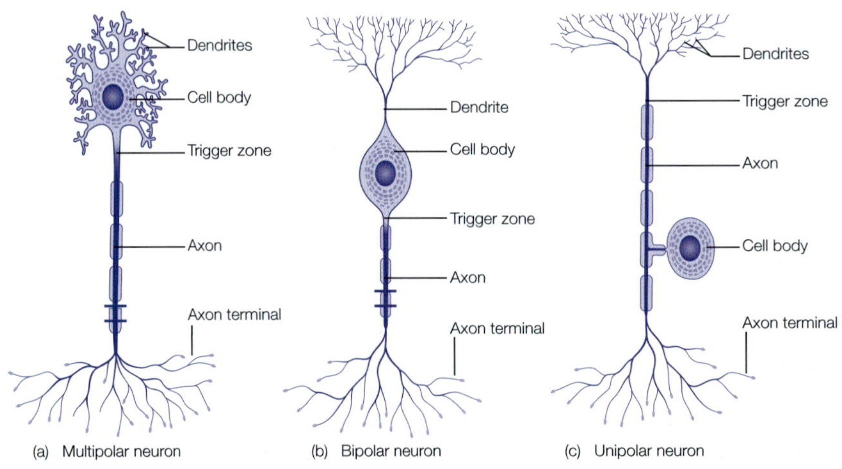

Figure 24.2 Structural classification of neurons. Breaks indicate that axons are longer than shown. A multipolar neuron has many processes extending from the cell body (a), a bipolar neuron has two (b), and a unipolar neuron has one (c). Redrawn with permission from Tortora and Derrickson (2006) *Principles of Anatomy and Physiology* 11th edn. Oxford: Wiley Blackwell.

tances along the length of an axon (up to 1 m in humans). Some larger axons are surrounded by layers of myelin, a lipid substance that improves the speed with which axons can conduct action potentials. The generation of action potentials by the neuron relies on two features of the cell membrane: the resting potential and the presence of channels through which ions can flow. The resting potential is the separation of electrical charge across the membrane, with the outside being more positive by approximately 70 mV. This potential difference is altered by the opening and closing of ion channels located in the membrane itself and the flow of ions from the outside of the cell through the membrane to the inside, and vice versa. When the potential difference reaches a threshold level, an action potential is produced. The action potential is propagated along the length of the axon until it reaches the presynaptic terminal, where it causes the release of a chemical transmitter. This diffuses across the synaptic cleft and binds to receptors located on the postsynaptic membrane. The result is an increase in the likelihood of the postsynaptic neuron being brought to threshold and continuing with the propagation of the action potential (excitation), or a decrease in the likelihood of the postsynaptic neuron being brought to threshold and continuing with the propagation of the action potential (inhibition).

ION FLUX AND CHANNELS

The basis for the generation of action potentials is the movement of ions across the plasma membrane through ion channels, altering the separation of electrical charge that exists under resting conditions. The molecules contained within a liquid move continuously, and equilibrium is reached when they are distributed uniformly throughout. If there is an initial region of higher concentration, then the molecules will move away from this area towards the area of lower concentration, down their concentration gradient, until equilibrium is reached. If two compartments containing equal volumes of a solution of differing concentrations are separated by a barrier permeable to the molecules in that solution, then there will be diffusion across this membrane from the compartment containing the solution of higher concentration to that containing the lower concentration. At the same time, there will be random movement of molecules in the opposite direction. The movement of substance across a surface in a unit of time is called flux, and the net flux is the difference between two one-way fluxes. Eventually the concentrations become equal and the net flux is zero.

Charged particles (ions) such as sodium (Na^+), potassium (K^+), chloride (Cl^-) and calcium (Ca^{2+}) move across the plasma membrane due not only to concentration gradients but also, since they are charged, electrical gradients. Positively charged ions (cations) move towards negatively charged areas, and negatively charged ions (anions) move towards areas of positive charge. Since an electrical gradient exists across the plasma membrane of neurons (the membrane potential; see below), which exerts a driving force on the ions present on either side of the membrane, there are two driving forces at work across the neuronal membrane. These two driving forces (chemical and electrical) are collectively known as the electrochemical gradient.

Ions traverse the plasma membrane from the extracellular fluid to the intracellular fluid, and vice versa, by way of ion channels, protein structures within the plasma membrane that selectively allow ions to pass through. The channels are closed by the movement of a part of the protein called a gate and are opened when this gate moves out of the way. The opening and closing of ion channels is a process called gating, a rapid process that can occur many times per second. The channels open and close in response to a range of stimuli and are described as 'leakage', 'voltage-gated', 'ligand-gated' and 'mechanically gated'. Leakage channels open and close randomly and allow ions to pass through. There are more leakage channels for potassium in the plasma membrane than for sodium, and as a result the plasma membrane is more permeable to potassium than it is for sodium. Voltage-gated channels open in response to a change in the membrane potential (see below); movement of sodium and potassium ions through these channels is critical for the generation and propagation of action potentials, and movement of calcium ions through these plays a role in the release of neurotransmitters at the presynaptic terminal. A ligand-gated channel opens or closes in response to a chemical stimulus, such as a neurotransmitter. This type of channel can be opened or closed in one of two ways: the chemical can bind directly to a portion of the protein of the channel itself (as in the case of the neurotransmitter acetylcholine) or it can activate a specialized protein (G-protein) in the membrane, which activates an additional second-messenger protein in the intracellular fluid, which in turn operates the channel's gate. A mechanically gated channel opens or closes in response to a mechanical stimulus, such as vibration, which physically distorts the membrane and as a result alters the physical properties of the channel in order to activate its gate. An example of this type of gate is found in the inner ear. The structure of the voltage-gated sodium channels and potassium channels is shown in Figure 24.3. It can be seen that sodium channels can be closed, open or inactivated whereas potassium channels can be closed or open.

In addition to these ion channels, the plasma membrane contains sodium/potassium pumps that move sodium and potassium ions across the membrane. These pumps move sodium ions out of the cell into the extracellular fluid and potassium ions into the intracellular fluid against their electrochemical gradients; this active transport process requires a constant input of energy. Three sodium ions are moved out through the membrane and two potassium ions are moved in. This process contributes to the maintenance of the membrane potential by maintaining a separation of

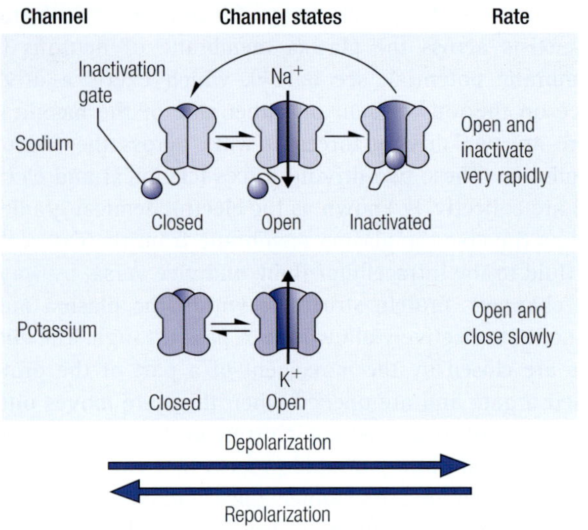

Figure 24.3 Behaviour of voltage-gated sodium and potassium channels. Depolarization of the membrane causes sodium channels to rapidly open and then undergo inactivation, followed by the opening of potassium channels. When the membrane repolarizes to negative voltages, both channels return to the closed state. Redrawn with permission from Widmaier, Raff and Strang (2008) *Vander's Human Physiology* 11th edn. Maidenhead: McGraw Hill.

electrical charge and is therefore described as 'electrogenic'. Its contribution to the resting membrane potential of –70 mV is small, in the region of –3 mV.

RESTING MEMBRANE POTENTIAL

Under resting conditions, the plasma membrane of a neuron has a separation of charge across it and is therefore polarized. This charge separation is a form of potential energy and is measured in millivolts (mV), or thousandths of volts. Conventionally, the extracellular fluid is designated as zero voltage, such that when it is measured using an intracellular electrode and an extracellular electrode as the reference, if the potential difference across the membrane is measured to be 70 mV, then the resting membrane potential is said to be –70 mV. This potential ranges from –40 mV to –75 mV in different neurons and is steady unless electrical current changes occur across the membrane. When alterations occur to this separation of charge due to the movement of ions across the cell membrane (see above), the membrane is said to *hyperpolarize* if the inside becomes more negative with respect to the outside (e.g. the potential changes from –70 mV to –80 mV) and to *depolarize* if the potential reduces (e.g. the potential changes from –70 mV to –60 mV). As will be discussed later, hyperpolarization of the membrane decreases the neuron's ability to generate an action potential and is therefore inhibitory, while depolarization increases the neuron's ability to generate an action potential and is therefore excitatory.

The separation of charge is due to the differential distribution of various ions outside and inside the cell.

Table 24.1 Concentrations of ions across the plasma membrane of a typical neuron

Ion	Extracellular concentration (mmol/L)	Intracellular concentration (mmol/L)
Sodium (Na^+)	145	15
Chloride (Cl^-)	100	7
Potassium (K^+)	5	150

Extracellular fluid has a high concentration of positively charged sodium ions (Na^+) and negatively charged chloride ions (Cl^-). The intracellular fluid is rich in positively charged potassium ions (K^+) and negatively charged molecules such as phosphates and amino acids (Table 24.1). The positively charged ions (cations) in the extracellular fluid are attracted to the negatively charged ions (anions) in the intracellular fluid, and they congregate closely to the outer and inner surfaces of the plasma membrane, respectively. In reality, these excess ions represent only a tiny fraction of the total number of ions present inside and outside the cell. In addition to these ions, there are a number of other ions present in both the intracellular and extracellular fluid, such as Mg^{2+}, Ca^{2+}, H^+, HCO_3^-, HPO_4^{2-} and SO_4^{2-}.

The membrane potential is maintained by a combination of the sodium/potassium pump and the differential permeability of the membrane to sodium and potassium ions and their movements. The membrane is more permeable to potassium than to sodium. Consequently, as the sodium/potassium pump moves sodium out of and potassium into the cell in unequal proportions, the inside becomes more negative with respect to the outside. The sodium that is accumulating outside the cell is prevented from moving down its concentration gradient by the membrane's low permeability to sodium. Potassium, however, moves more readily down its concentration gradient and therefore does not continuously build up in the intracellular fluid, since it leaks out through the leakage channels. However, potassium does not equilibrate with respect to its concentration, due to the electrical gradient. As sodium is pumped out of the cell, the inside of the cell is left negative with respect to the outside, and this attracts the positively charged potassium ions and repels the negatively charged chloride ions.

GRADED POTENTIALS AND ACTION POTENTIALS

Changes in the membrane potentials of neurons underlie the basis of neuronal processing and transmission of electrical impulses. These alterations in membrane potential can take one of two forms: graded potentials and action potentials. Graded potentials arise when a stimulus causes activation of ligand-gated or mechanically gated channels. This potential is a small deviation of the membrane potential; its size is related to the intensity of the stimulus (hence the term 'graded') and its polarity is related to the nature of the stimulus. If the stimulus induces a reduction in the membrane potential (i.e. a decrease in the difference in charge between the inside and the outside of the cell), then it is called a 'depolarizing graded potential'. Conversely, if the stimulus induces an increase in the membrane potential (i.e. an increase in the difference in charge between the inside and the outside of the cell), then it is called a 'hyperpolarizing graded potential'. If the stimulus is small, only a few channels will be activated and a small graded potential will occur. These potentials are usually confined to small regions of the membrane and usually occur in the dendrites and the cell body of the neuron; they are named in relation to the location or their function, for example 'synaptic potential' or 'receptor potential'. They also decrease in size within a short distance from the site from which they were initiated and are therefore useful as signal generators over a short distance. Many stimuli arriving in quick succession, however, can cause graded potentials to summate, and this has importance in the initiation of larger potentials, called action potentials.

An action potential is a large brief alteration in the membrane potential that occurs mainly in the axon plasma membrane and the axon terminals. The alteration may be as large as 100 mV, taking the membrane potential from its resting value of −70 mV to +30 mV (thus depolarizing it), and last up to 4 ms. The action potential is comprised of two phases, a depolarizing phase in which the membrane potential becomes less negative, followed by a repolarizing phase in which the potential is restored to its resting level of −70 mV. An action potential is initiated by a depolarizing stimulus (e.g. a neurotransmitter binding to a receptor), and this causes voltage-gated sodium channels to open. Sodium ions move rapidly across the membrane, down their concentration and electrical gradients, into the intracellular fluid. This influx causes depolarization of the membrane potential; when the membrane potential reaches a critical level, the threshold potential (about −55 mV in many neurons, or approximately 15 mV less negative than the resting membrane potential for that cell), depolarization becomes a positive-feedback loop. Influx of sodium causes further depolarization, which in turn causes opening of more sodium channels and further depolarization. When the membrane potential reaches a peak at about +30 mV (the inside now being more positive than the outside), sodium influx declines rapidly as sodium channels are inactivated by closure of the inactivation gate (this is in contrast to the gate being closed; see Figure 24.3). At this peak, voltage-gated potassium channels open, permeability to potassium increases, and potassium moves down its concentration and electrical gradients from the intracellular fluid to the extracellular fluid; depolarization halts and repolarization of the membrane potential starts to occur. Potassium channels are slower to close than sodium channels; as a result, there is a brief period following repolarization in which the membrane is transiently more permeable to potassium than it is in the resting state, and the membrane potential drops below that seen at rest (Figure 24.4). This is the hyperpolarization phase, when the membrane potential becomes more negative than the resting potential, at about −90 mV. During this period, another stimulus (however large) cannot produce further action potentials; this is due to sodium channels being open already or having been inactivated. This period is known as the absolute refractory period. Following this refractory period, and after some of the sodium channels have returned to their resting state and some of the potassium channels are still open, it is possible for a second stimulus to evoke another action potential, but only if this is of a sufficient size. This period of up to 15 ms coincides with the hyperpolarization period and is known as the 'relative refractory period'.

If a stimulus is not of a sufficiently high intensity to cause the membrane potential to depolarize to the critical

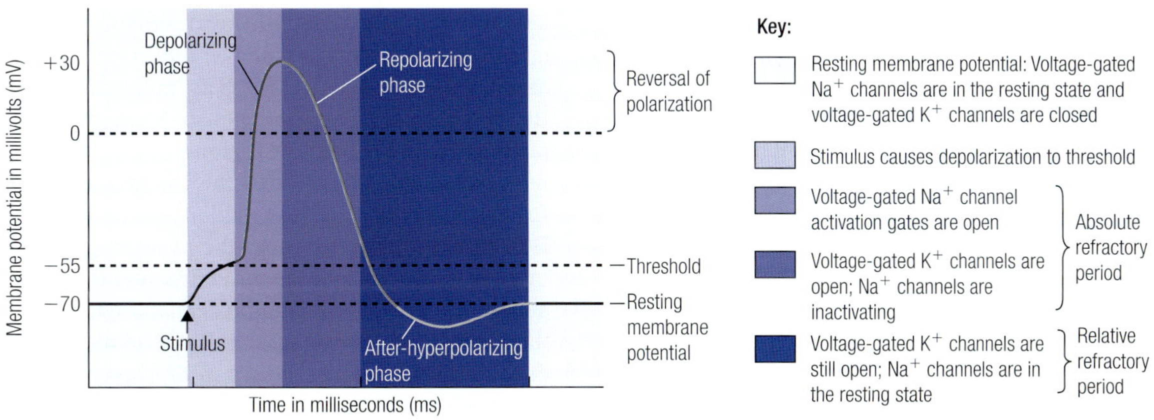

Figure 24.4 Action potential (AP) or impulse. When a stimulus depolarizes the membrane to threshold −55 mV, an AP is generated. The AP arises at the trigger zone (at the junction of the axon hillock and the initial segment) and then propagates along the axon to the axon terminals. Redrawn with permission from Tortora and Derrickson (2006) *Principles of Anatomy and Physiology* 11th edn. Oxford: Wiley Blackwell.

threshold, then an action potential will not be produced. Such potentials are termed 'subthreshold potentials'. An action potential is therefore an all-or-none phenomenon – there cannot be fractions of action potentials.

For an action potential to have an effect distant from its origin, it needs to be transmitted along the length of the axon, sometimes a considerable distance. This requires the membrane potential at each segment of the axon along the way to be brought to the threshold potential. Local currents are produced in adjacent segments of the axon distal to the point of the action potential, but the refractoriness of the membrane in the trailing segment of axon means that the action potential is propagated in one direction only (an exception to this is following artificial stimulation in the middle of an axon). Since the generation of an action potential is dependent upon the positive feedback cycle of voltage-gated sodium channels further along the axon, the size of the action potential is not diminished in size at the axon terminals. This type of propagation of action potentials due to depolarization and repolarization of adjacent segments occurs in unmyelinated axons and in muscle fibres; since it is continuous along the length of the cell, it is known as 'continuous conduction'. In myelinated axons, action potentials can be transmitted at much greater speeds. The myelin sheath (see Chapter 23) is a multilayered sheath of lipid wrapped around the axon. This highly resistant sheath effectively insulates the axon and prevents electrical conduction. This sheath, however, is not wrapped in a continuous fashion along the entirety of the axon but is periodically interrupted at the nodes of Ranvier (approximately 1 μm in length, or 1×10^{-6} m). At these nodes there is no covering of myelin sheath, and it is here that there are large numbers of voltage-gated channels (in contrast to the few voltage-gated channels found in the membrane covered by myelin). The flow of local currents that occurs across the plasma membrane occurs mainly at these nodes. The nerve impulses carried along the myelinated axon effectively jump from one node to the next as current is carried in the intracellular fluid between the nodes and across the plasma membrane at the nodes. This type of nerve conduction is known as 'saltatory conduction' (from the Latin *saltare*, meaning 'to leap'). The propagation of action potentials by saltatory conduction in myelinated axons is much faster than the continuous conduction of unmyelinated axons. In addition to the speed of nerve conduction in myelinated axons being faster, this type of conduction is also more energy-effective, since fewer sodium/potassium pumps are required to restore the resting membrane potential due to the presence of the nodes.

The diameter of an axon also affects the speed with which it conducts axon potentials, since a larger-diameter axon offers less resistance to the production of local currents. Conduction velocities range from 0.5 m/s for small-diameter unmyelinated axons up to approximately 100 m/s for large-diameter myelinated axons.

All cell membranes are capable of transmitting graded potentials, but only excitable cells such as nerve and muscle cells can propagate action potentials; this forms the basis for communication over large distances.

SYNAPSES

Neurons within the central nervous system are driven by communication with other neurons via specialized regions called synapses (named by Sherrington, from the Greek – *syn*, meaning 'with', and *-aptein*, meaning 'to join'), of which there are, according to latest estimates, approximately 100 trillion (10^{14}) within the central nervous system. Their presence is therefore fundamental to the functioning of the nervous system. The neuron from which the impulses are being transmitted is termed the 'presynaptic neuron' and the neuron that receives the impulses is known as the 'postsynaptic neuron'. The majority of synapses occur between axon and dendrite (axodendritic), between axon and cell body (axosomatic) and between axon and axon (axoaxonic). Based on their morphology, two classes of synapse exist: those in which the cytoplasms of the pre- and postsynaptic cells are bridged by tubular structures called connexons, and those in which they are not, with the cells being separated by a synaptic cleft measuring 20–50 nm (10^{-9} m). These morphological differences account for the functional differences of these synapses, with the bridged (gap) junctions mediating electrical transmission and the unbridged junctions mediating chemical transmission. Electrical synapses are found in cardiac muscle and in the visceral smooth muscle but are present in much lower numbers in the human nervous system (in the cerebral and cerebellar cortices) compared with chemical synapses.

The activity of the postsynaptic neuron can be increased by the membrane potential being brought closer to its firing threshold (i.e. depolarizing it); this is an excitatory synapse. Alternatively, the activity of the postsynaptic neuron can be decreased by moving the membrane potential further way from its threshold (i.e. hyperpolarizing it); this is an inhibitory synapse. At an excitatory chemical synapse, the action potential arriving at the presynaptic terminal causes a sequence of events (see above) that result in the release of an excitatory transmitter (such as glutamate), which crosses the synaptic cleft and induces an excitatory postsynaptic potential (EPSP). One EPSP alone (of the order of 0.5 mV) may not be enough to bring the postsynaptic neuron to its firing threshold, and no action potential is generated. However, for a brief period, the postsynaptic membrane is more receptive to subsequent EPSPs, and the likelihood of it generating an action potential is increased; this is known as 'facilitation'. If a presynaptic cell is stimulated in quick succession, it may induce EPSPs in a postsynaptic cell before the previous EPSPs have died away; this is known as 'temporal summation' (EPSPs generated at about the same time). If many presynaptic cells induce EPSPs in the postsynaptic cell, spatial summation may occur (Figure 24.5).

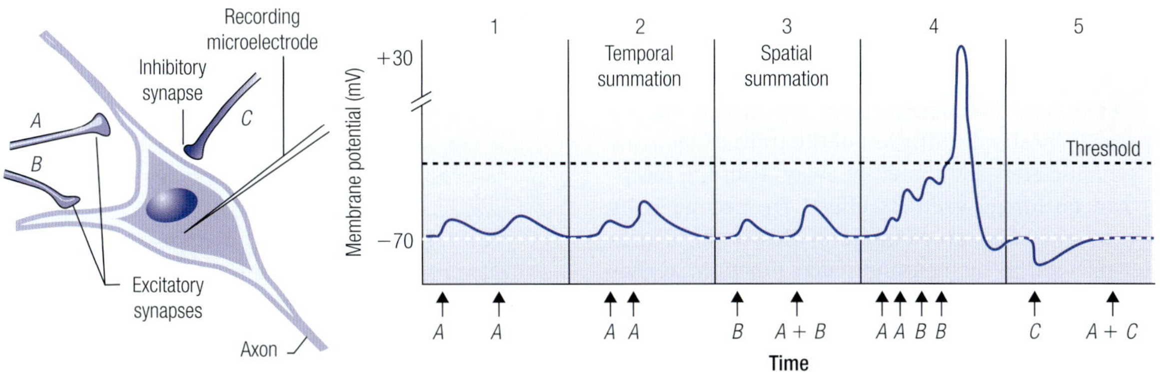

Figure 24.5 Interaction of excitatory postsynaptic potentials (EPSPs) and inhibitory postsynaptic potentials (IPSPs) at the postsynaptic neuron. Presynaptic neurons (A–C) were stimulated at times indicated by the arrows, and the resulting membrane potential was recorded in the postsynaptic cell by a recording microelectrode. Redrawn with permission from Widmaier, Raff and Strang (2008) *Vander's Human Physiology* 11th edn. Maidenhead: McGraw Hill.

At an inhibitory chemical synapse, the action potential arriving at the presynaptic terminal causes release of an inhibitory transmitter, such as γ-aminobutyric acid (GABA), which induces an inhibitory postsynaptic potential (IPSP) in the postsynaptic cell. This IPSP is generated by the opening of chloride or potassium channels. Once open, these channels allow Cl^- ions into the cell and K^+ ions out of the cell, causing the inside of the cell to become more negative (i.e. hyperpolarized). An additional type of inhibition is presynaptic inhibition, in which small presynaptic cells terminate on other presynaptic cells; these later cells normally produce EPSPs. However, the functioning of the inhibitory presynaptic cells is to reduce the size of these EPSPs, and in this way the postsynaptic cell is less likely to be brought to firing threshold. Many thousands of presynaptic neurons can exert influence over a single postsynaptic cell (convergence), or many branches of a single presynaptic neuron can influence many postsynaptic neurons (divergence).

NEUROTRANSMISSION

At chemical synapses, neurotransmitters are the signal carrier by which action potentials are propagated from one neuron to another. These transmitters can be broadly classified by their size into small-molecule transmitters and larger neuropeptides. Small-molecule transmitters are synthesized from precursor molecules located in the nerve terminals using enzymes that have been synthesized in the soma of the neuron. These transmitters are transported down the axon using a slow axonal transport (0.5–5 mm/day) to the nerve terminal. Larger peptide transmitters (neuropeptides) are synthesized in the neuronal cell body and transported down the length of the axon via a cytoplasmic scaffold of microtubules at a much faster rate of up to 400 mm/day (fast axonal transport). In each case, the transmitters are packaged into vesicles before release. Thousands of neurotransmitter molecules are stored in these vesicles, which are either anchored to the presynaptic membrane at active zones or freely located within the terminal. When an action potential arrives at the presynaptic terminal, it causes calcium channels to open in the membrane, leading to calcium influx into the presynaptic terminal. This influx of calcium into the cell causes the vesicles containing the neurotransmitter to fuse with the plasma membrane, releasing the neurotransmitter into the synaptic cleft. A small fraction of the neurotransmitter released into the synaptic cleft binds to receptors located in the plasma membrane of the postsynaptic cell. Even under conditions of no stimulation (i.e. no action potential has arrived at the presynaptic terminal), these vesicles can release their contents into the synaptic cleft spontaneously and at a very low rate; this in turn causes small membrane potential changes in the postsynaptic neuron. These potentials have been studied extensively in the neuromuscular junction, where they are called 'miniature end-plate potentials' (mEPPs). The size of these mEPPs is not altered by altering degrees of depolarization, which implies that the release of neurotransmitter from the vesicle is an all-or-none phenomenon with a fixed amount, or quantum, of neurotransmitter released.

In order for the neurotransmitter to propagate the action potentials to the postsynaptic cell, it has to activate receptors. These can have a central opening that allows the movement of ions across the membrane (ionotropic), or they may activate other ion channels through a second-messenger system (metabotropic).

It is important to note that the term 'receptor' has two distinct meanings in neurophysiology. One relates to the type of sensory receptor that is a transducer (converts different forms of stimuli into electrical signals) for various sensory stimuli. These receptors can be classified as mechanoreceptors (detect physical pressure or deformation), thermoreceptors (detect changes in temperature), photoreceptors (detect changes in light levels), nociceptors (detect noxious or painful stimuli) and chemoreceptors (detect various chemical stimuli). However, the type of receptor referred to in this chapter is a protein embedded in the plasma membrane that binds a neurotransmitter and propagates action potentials.

Once the neurotransmitter has exerted its effect at the receptors, it needs to be removed from the synaptic cleft. This removal is essential for the normal functioning of the synapse. There are three main ways by which this is achieved. One is by simple diffusion of the transmitter away from the synaptic cleft and therefore away from the receptors so it can no longer exert its effect. The second is by breakdown by enzymes; an example of this is the neurotransmitter released at the neuromuscular junction, acetylcholine. This is degraded by acetylcholinesterase into choline and acetate. The third way by which neurotransmitters are removed is by reuptake. This can be back into the neurons that released it (for repackaging into new vesicles, ready for release) or into adjacent cells such as glia. An important action of many pharmacological agents is to prolong the activity of the neurotransmitter by blocking its breakdown by the enzyme or by preventing its reuptake.

KEY POINTS

- A membrane potential exists due to the separation of charged particles across the neuronal membrane.
- At rest, the inside of the neuron is negative with respect to the outside. The flow of ions can change this membrane potential in either direction – hyperpolarize it or depolarize it.
- If the threshold is reached, an action potential is generated, which is propagated to the synaptic terminal.
- The speed of propagation of the action potential is increased by a larger-diameter axon and the presence of a myelin sheath.
- Calcium influx at the presynaptic terminal causes neurotransmitter release, binding of the neurotransmitter to a postsynaptic receptor and a postsynaptic potential (excitatory – EPSP, or inhibitory – IPSP).
- The neurotransmitter is broken down or taken up by nerve terminals, and its action terminated.

FURTHER READING

Carpenter R (2002) *Neurophysiology.* London: Hodder Arnold.

Kandel ER, Schwartz JH, Jessell TM, Siegelbaum SA, Hudspeth AJ (2009) *Principles of Neural Science.* New York: McGraw-Hill Medical.

Schmidt RF (1985) *The Fundamentals of Neurophysiology.* Berlin: Springer-Verlag.

Tortora GJ (2005) *Principles of Anatomy and Physiology.* New York: John Wiley & Sons.

Widmaier EP, Raff H, Strang KT (2007) *Vander's Human Physiology.* Boston, MA: McGraw-Hill Higher Education.

Chapter 25

Neurophysiology of integrated behaviour

Basant K Puri

INTRODUCTION

This chapter covers the physiology and anatomical pathways of the neural and endocrine systems involved in integrated behaviour, including perception, pain, memory, motor function and drives. The pathways concerned with arousal are described in Chapter 28. Motivation and emotions are described in Chapters 15 and 12, respectively.

PERCEPTION

Visual pathway

The visual pathway from the retina to V1, with the projection of retinal ganglion cell axons to the lateral geniculate nucleus (LGN) (via the optic nerve, the optic chiasma and the optic tract) and the projection from here to V1 (via the optic radiation), is shown in Figure 25.1. This figure also illustrates the visual field defects that can result from lesions at different parts of this pathway. From the details on the right-hand side of Figure 25.2, it can be seen that in V1 the LGN axons terminate primarily in layer 4 and form ocular dominance columns, with the termination site depending on the layer in which the LGN neuron is found: parvocellular cells project mainly to layer 4Cβ, magnocellular cells to layer 4Cα and koniocellular cells to layer 4A and lower layer 3.[1]

The construction of visual experiences is dependent on attention. According to a comprehensive review by Kanwisher and Wojciulik, attention affects processing at the first stage of cortical information processing, in V1; attention not only modulates the gain on incoming visual information but can also add a pure top-down signal that increases baseline activity in striate and extrastriate cortex; attention can, under different conditions, select locations, features, objects or a combination thereof; and large regions within the frontoparietal network, which apparently provide the source of top-down bias signals in visual areas, support a very heterogeneous set of attention tasks.[2] In other words:

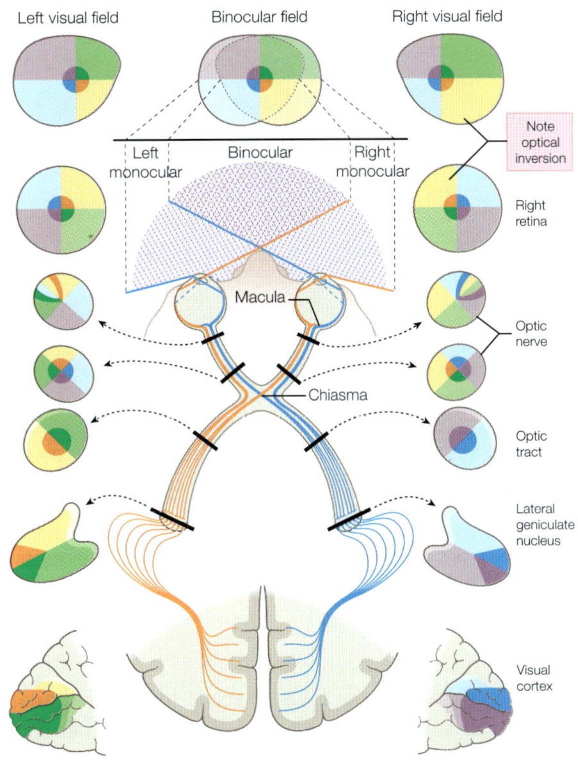

Figure 25.1 Visual pathway, showing the spatial arrangement of neurons and their fibres in relation to the quadrants of the retinae and visual fields. The proportions at various levels are not exactly to scale. In particular, the macula is exaggerated in size in the visual fields and retinae. In each quadrant of the visual field, and in the parts of the visual pathway subserving it, two shades of each respective colour are used: the paler shade denotes the peripheral field and the darker shade the macular part of the quadrant. From the optic tract onwards, these two shades are both made more saturated to denote intermixture of neurons from both retinae, the palest shade being reserved for parts of the visual pathway concerned with monocular vision

Reproduced with permission from Standing, *Gray's Anatomy*. 40th edn. Churchill Livingstone, Edinburgh. 2008.

We are not passive recipients of the information that impinges on our retinae, but active participants in our own perceptual processes. Visual experience depends critically on attention. We

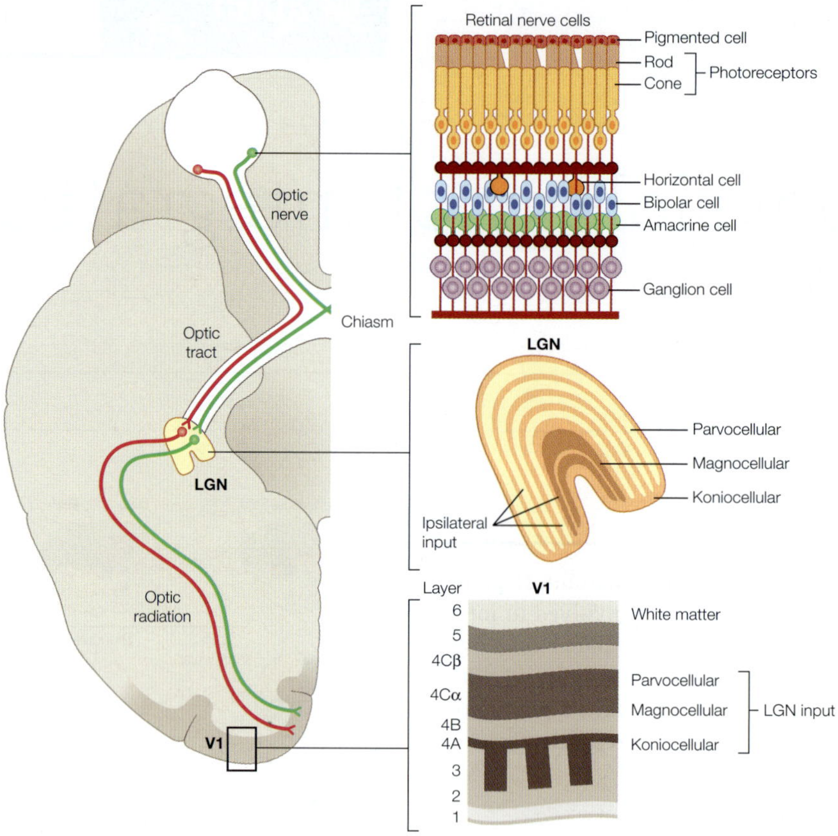

Figure 25.2 The left panel shows a schematic drawing of the pathway from the retina to the primary visual cortex (V1) through the dorsal lateral geniculate nucleus (LGN) of the thalamus. The right panels highlight the important anatomical structures. Light entering the eye passes through the ganglion cells and is imaged on the photoreceptor layer. Signals from photoreceptors pass through bipolar cells to ganglion cells, the axons of which form the optic nerve, which projects principally to the LGN. The horizontal and amacrine cell pathways within the retina allow spatial comparisons of cone signals. Ganglion cells from the temporal retina project to the ipsilateral LGN (red lines) and those from the nasal retina project to the contralateral LGN (green lines). Within the LGN, the projections from the two eyes are aligned, so the same topographic map (of the contralateral half of the visual field) is found in all layers. The axons of LGN neurons project almost exclusively to V1, where they terminate primarily in layer 4 and form ocular dominance columns (a small fraction of LGN cells project to extrastriate areas). The termination site within layer 4 depends on the layer in which the LGN neuron is found. The shading depicts the distinct pattern that emerges when slices through V1 are stained for cytochrome oxidase activity. Reactivity is particularly high in layer 4 and in patches that dot the superficial layers 2 and 3.

Reproduced with permission from ref. 1.

select particular aspects of a visual scene for detailed analysis and control of subsequent behaviour, but ignore other aspects so completely that moments after they disappear from view we cannot report anything about them.[2]

Further aspects of the psychology of vision are covered in Chapter 16.

Auditory pathway

The anatomical pathways of the ascending auditory pathway, from the cochlear nerve to the auditory cortex, are shown in Figure 25.3a. Figure 25.3b illustrates the key stations in this pathway, from the cochlear hair cells to the inferior colliculus and thence to the primary auditory cortex via the medial geniculate body; there is also an output from the inferior colliculus to the superior colliculus, thereby allowing auditory stimuli to have an input into ocular movements (including reflex movements).

Griffiths and Warren have argued that it is meaningful to consider auditory objects as fundamental elements of the auditory world; operationally, an auditory object might be defined as an acoustic experience that produces a two-dimensional image with frequency and time dimensions.[3] Figure 25.4 illustrates their consideration of models of auditory-object analysis, presented schematically as a hierarchy of operational processing stages, together with plausible neuroanatomical substrates for these operations.[3]

PAIN

Chapter 52 details psychological and psychiatric aspects of pain. Here, neurophysiological aspects of pain are considered.

Peripheral pain mechanisms

Nociceptors

Nociceptors (pain receptors) may be dichotomized into C-polymodal nociceptors (C-PMNs) and A-mechanoheat

Figure 25.3 Main features of the human ascending auditory pathway. (a) Series of sections showing that ipsilateral and commissural connections occur at most levels in this system. The major connections are shown by the red and blue arrows; other arrows denote less heavy projections. (b) Main stations of the auditory pathway.

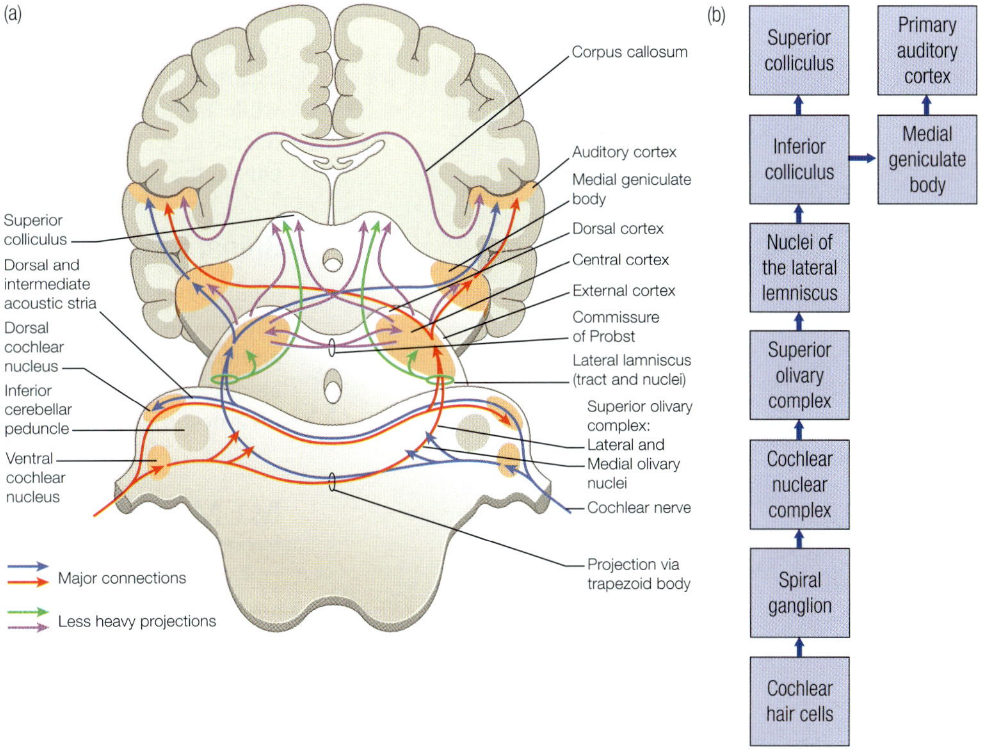

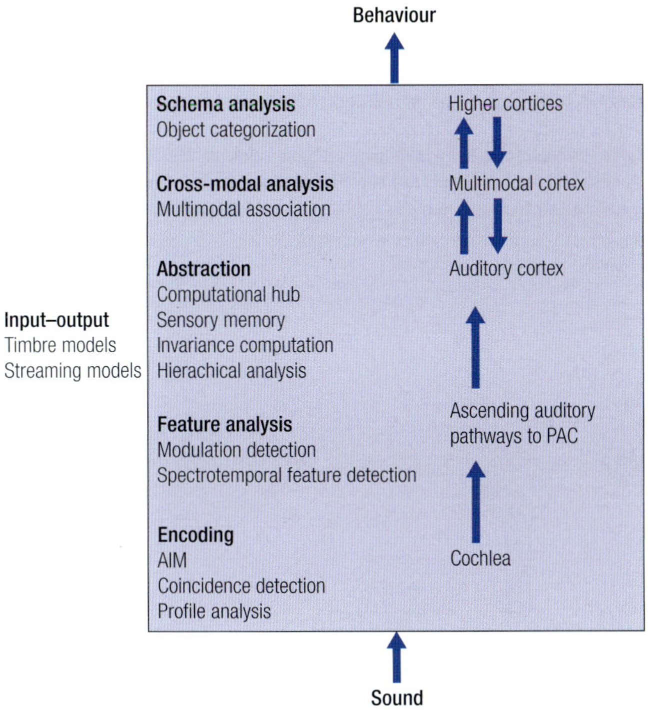

Figure 25.4 Models of auditory-object analysis presented schematically as a hierarchy of operational processing stages (left). Plausible neuroanatomical substrates for these operations are shown (right); however, these require further experimental validation. The putative flow of auditory information is indicated (blue arrows); the exchange of information with higher-order cortices and other sensory modalities is probably reciprocal (bidirectional arrows). The precise order of processing stages (e.g. cross-modal analysis and schema analysis) probably depends on task demands

AIM, auditory-image model; PAC, primary auditory cortex.

Reproduced with permission from ref. 3.

(AMH) nociceptors. As their names imply, AMN receptors respond primarily to mechanical and thermal stimuli. C-PMNs respond not only to mechanical and thermal stimuli but also to chemical stimuli.

Peripheral inflammation

Tissue damage leads to direct stimulation of nociceptors and also the release of inflammatory mediators, including eicosanoids, cytokines, neurotransmitters, neuropeptides and adenosine triphosphate (ATP), which in turn reduce the nociceptor stimulation threshold and sensitize and stimulate the nociceptors further. Further details of the events that occur during peripheral activation and sensitization, as part of the inflammatory response, and spread of this sensitization, are shown in Figure 25.5. Peripheral inflammation leads to the production of opioid receptors by the dorsal root ganglion and their transport towards the peripheral terminal (Figure 25.6), which also depicts the fact that these peripheral opioid receptors may be activated by endogenous opioid peptides released by monocytes, T-cells, B-cells and macrophages.

Peripheral trauma

Figure 25.7 summarizes the neural mechanisms underlying the generation of pain and other symptoms associated with complex regional pain syndromes following peripheral trauma.

Dorsal horn mechanisms

Endogenous ligands that act in the dorsal horn of the spinal cord in respect of nociception include glutamate, which is an

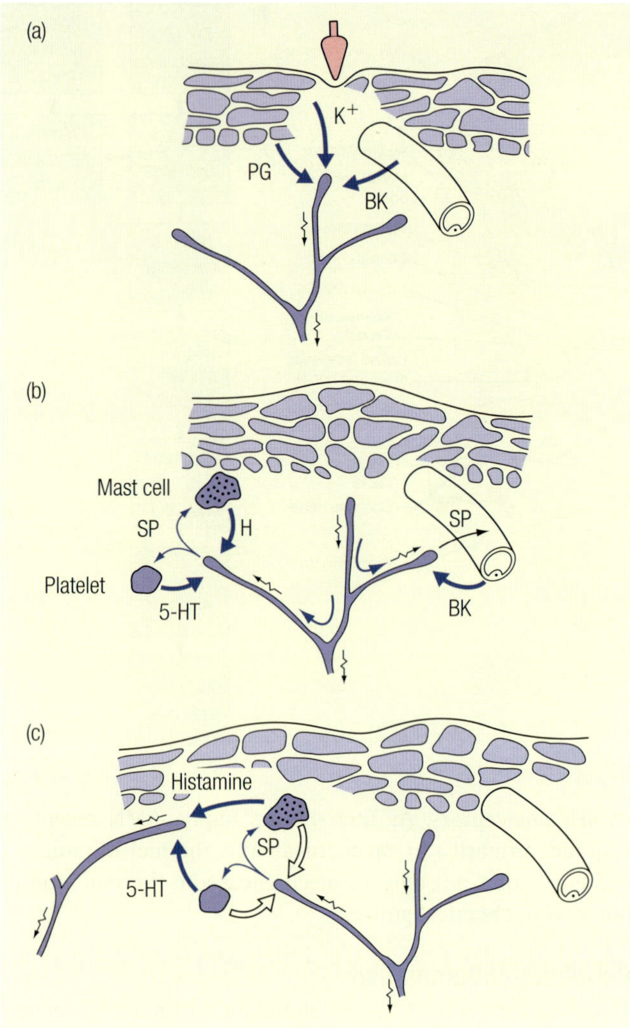

excitatory amino acid, and substance P (Figure 25.8).[4] The cascade of intracellular events activated by *N*-methyl-D-aspartate (NMDA) receptor activation is shown in Figure 25.9, while Figure 25.10 illustrates postsynaptic events following release of glutamate from central terminals of primary afferents in the spinal cord, including the role of nitric oxide.

Spinal cord and brain pathways

Figure 25.11 illustrates the main ascending nociceptive pathway in the spinal cord and descending modulatory pathways arising from the mesencephalon and medulla oblongata. Further details of the ascending pathways and their destination in the brain are given in Chapter 23.

MEMORY

The neuroanatomy of the limbic system and the medial temporal lobe is considered in Chapter 23. Figure 25.12 is a

Figure 25.5 Events leading to activation, sensitization and spread of sensitization of primary afferent nociceptor terminals. (a) Direct activation by intense pressure and consequent cell damage, leading to release of K^+ and biosynthesis of prostaglandins (PGs) and bradykinin (BK). PGs increase the sensitivity of the terminal to BK and other pain-producing substances. (b) Secondary activation. Impulses generated in the stimulated terminal propagate not only to the spinal cord but also into other terminal branches, where they induce the release of peptides such as substance P (SP), which in turn causes vasodilation and neurogenic oedema, with further accumulation of BK and also the release of histamine (H) from mast cells and serotonin (5-HT) from platelets. (c) Histamine and serotonin levels rise in the extracellular space, secondarily sensitizing nearby nociceptors, leading to a gradual spread of hyperalgesia and/or tenderness

Reproduced with permission from Power and Kam, *Principles of Physiology for the Anaesthetist*. Hodder, London. (2007).

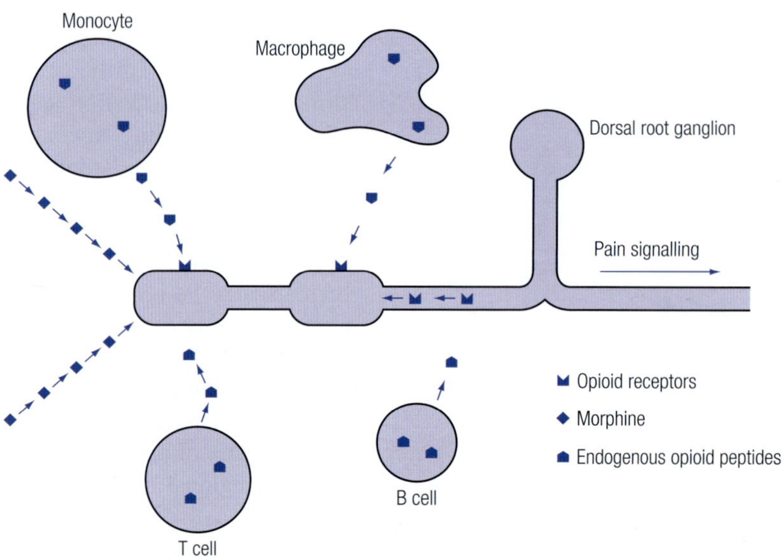

Figure 25.6 Peripheral inflammation leads to the production of opioid receptors by the dorsal root ganglion. These opioid receptors are transported towards the peripheral terminal. Peripheral opioid receptors may be activated by endogenous opioid peptides released by monocytes, T-cells, B-cells and macrophages, and by exogenous application of morphine

Reproduced with permission from Power and Kam, *Principles of Physiology for the Anaesthetist*. Hodder, London. (2007).

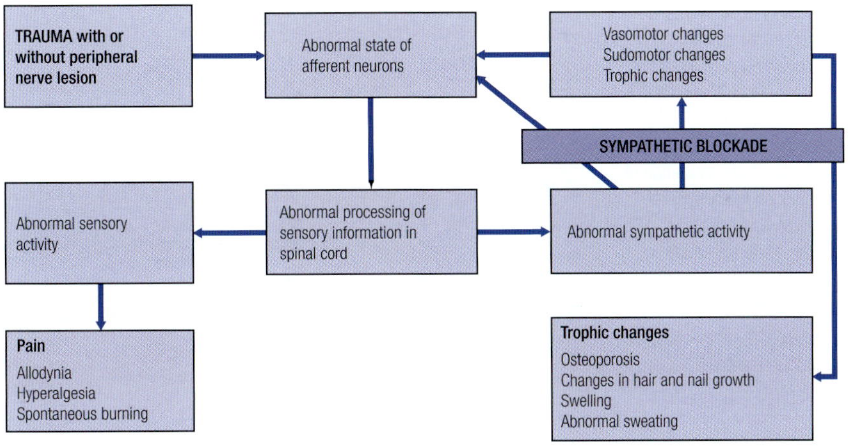

Figure 25.7 General hypothesis about the neural mechanisms underlying the generation of pain and other symptoms associated with complex regional pain syndromes following peripheral trauma with and without nerve lesions

Reproduced with permission from Power and Kam, *Principles of Physiology for the Anaesthetist*. Hodder, London. (2007).

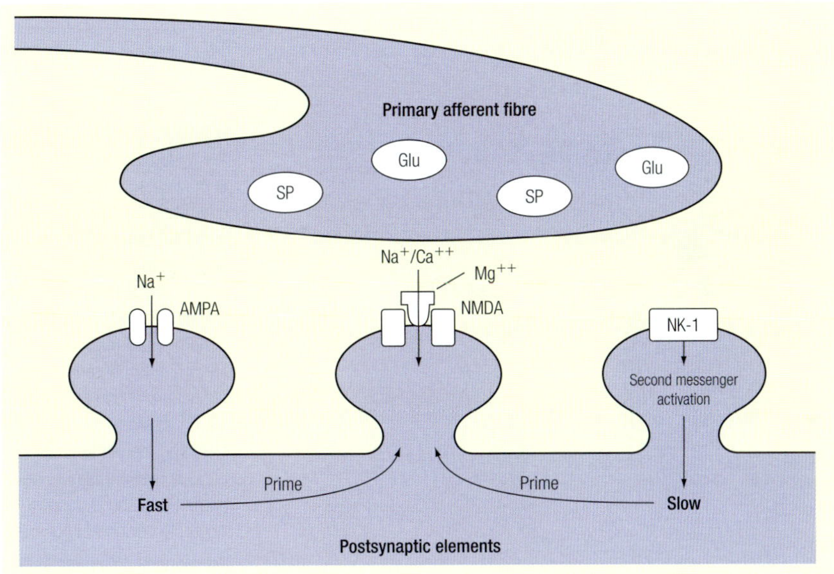

Figure 25.8 Release of glutamate (Glu) and substance P (SP) from the terminals of nociceptive primary afferents activates α-amino-3-hydroxy-5-methyl-4-isoxazole-propionate (AMPA) and neurokinin-1 (NK-1) receptors, respectively, on the postsynaptic membrane. Activation of these receptors leads to Na^+ influx at the AMPA receptor and activation of second messengers. These processes prime the *N*-methyl-D-aspartate (NMDA) receptor with removal of the Mg^{2+} plug and Na^+ and Ca^{2+} influx

Reproduced with permission from Power and Kam, *Principles of Physiology for the Anaesthetist*. Hodder, London. (2007).

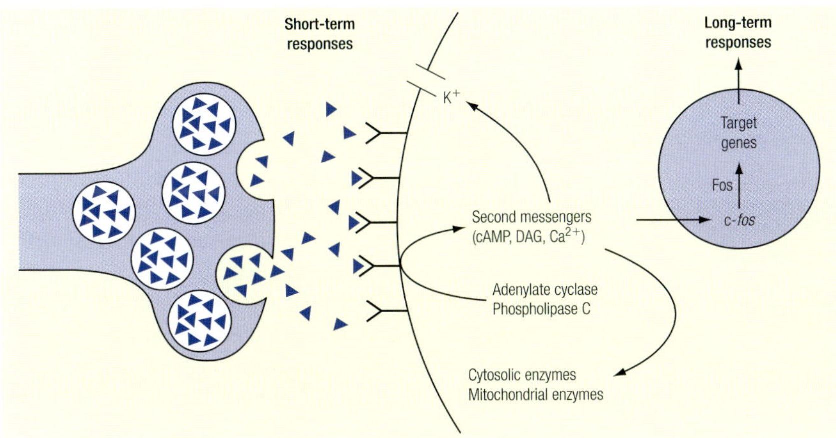

Figure 25.9 Neurotransmitter release from the central terminal of peripheral afferents leads to activation of postsynaptic membrane receptor sites. Activation of phospholipase C (PLC) and adenylate cyclase leads to the biosynthesis of the second messengers cyclic adenosine monophosphate (cAMP) and diacylglycerol (DAG), mobilization of which may result in decreased K^+ efflux and elevated intracellular Ca^{2+}. The latter results in induction of the proto-oncogene *c-fos*, production of Fos protein and a presumed action on target genes to alter cellular long-term responses to further stimuli

Reproduced with permission from Power and Kam, *Principles of Physiology for the Anaesthetist*. Hodder, London. (2007).

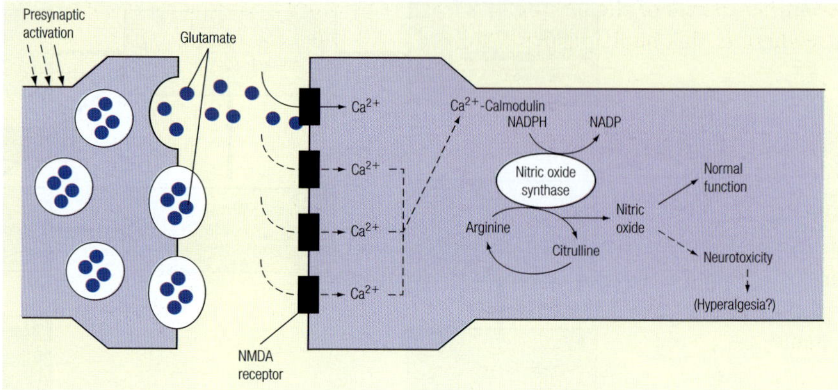

Figure 25.10 Diagram illustrating postsynaptic events following release of glutamate from central terminals of primary afferents in the spinal cord. Following priming of the *N*-methyl-D-aspartate (NMDA) receptor, glutamate release results in NMDA receptor activation with subsequent Ca^{2+} influx. Intracellular Ca^{2+} then acts on a calmodulin-sensitive site to activate nitric oxide synthase (NOS). In the presence of the cofactor nicotinamide adenine dinucleotide phosphate (reduced) (NADPH), NOS uses arginine as a substrate to produce nitric oxide and citrulline. Nitric oxide has a role in normal cellular function, but increased production may be involved in hyperalgesia and may lead to neurotoxicity

Reproduced with permission from Power and Kam, *Principles of Physiology for the Anaesthetist*. Hodder, London. (2007).

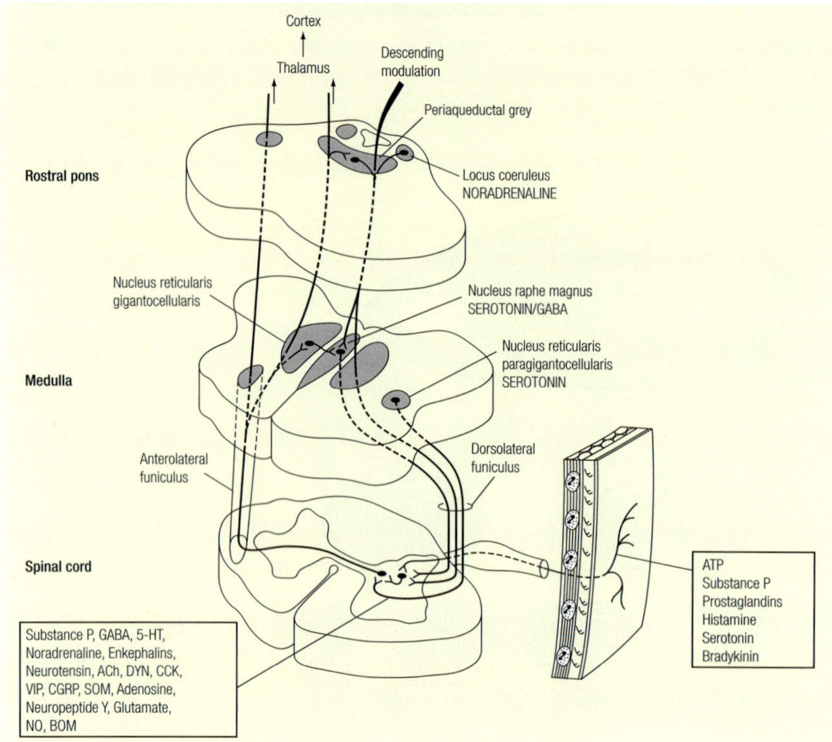

Figure 25.11 Simplified schema of afferent sensory pathways and descending modulatory pathways arising from the midbrain and medulla. Note the various sites for enhancement or reduction in pain signalling. Release of chemicals from peripheral terminals of primary afferents results in peripheral sensitization. The main ascending nociceptive pathway travels primarily via the anterolateral funiculus and terminates in the thalamus (spinothalamic) and reticular formation (spinoreticular). Incoming signals from the periphery are then modulated at the spinal dorsal horn by intrinsic interneurons and descending influences from the brainstem. These descending influences travel primarily via the dorsolateral funiculus and arise from several regions, including the periaqueductal grey matter, locus coeruleus and nucleus raphe magnus. Neurotransmitters released from the terminals of these descending pathways then act to inhibit incoming peripheral nociceptive input

Reproduced with permission from Power and Kam, *Principles of Physiology for the Anaesthetist*. Hodder, London. (2007).

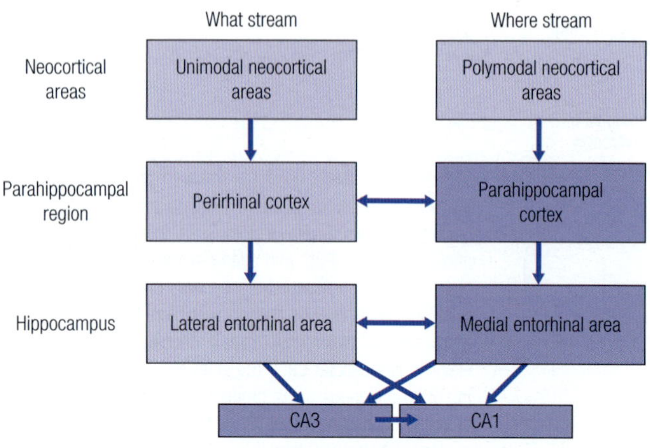

Figure 25.12 Schematic representation of anatomical connections between neocortex, parahippocampal region and hippocampus

Reproduced with permission from ref. 3.

schematic representation of anatomical connections between the neocortex, parahippocampal region and hippocampus. According to Eichenbaum and Lipton:

Information flows between areas of the cerebral cortex and components of the parahippocampal region and between the parahippocampal region and areas of the hippocampus through two partially distinct channels. The perirhinal cortex receives inputs from areas that identify the nonspatial identity of stimuli. In contrast, parahippocampal/postrhinal cortex receives inputs from many areas that appear to be involved in processing the spatial content of sensory information. Thus, in the monkey, whereas the perirhinal cortex receives more inputs from areas along the ventral visual pathway considered important for object recognition, the parahippocampal cortex receives more inputs from areas along the dorsal visual stream considered important for spatial attention and visuospatially guided actions.[5]

Further details of the neurophysiology of memory appear elsewhere in this book, particularly in Chapter 17.

MOTOR FUNCTION

The course of the corticospinal tract is shown in Figure 23.8 in Chapter 23. Further details of the various parts of the brain and spinal cord concerned with motor function appear in Chapter 23, and there are clinical details in Chapter 36.

DRIVES

Sexual behaviour

Sexual behaviour is a non-regulatory form of behaviour; that is, it is not under the control of a homeostatic mechanism.

Sex hormones are clearly of importance in sexual behaviour and have effects on both the developing brain and the adult brain. Testosterone masculinizes the brain in the male fetus, with particular effects in the preoptic area of the hypothalamus, which is much larger in males than females following testosterone exposure. Prenatal exposure to testosterone is of importance in the development of gender-related behaviour. Hines has reviewed this area:

> In neural regions with appropriate receptors testosterone, or its metabolites, influences patterns of cell death and survival, neural connectivity and neurochemical characterization. Consequently, testosterone exposure during critical periods of early development produces permanent behavioural changes. In humans, affected behaviours include childhood play behaviour, sexual orientation, core gender identity and other characteristics that show sex differences (i.e. differ on average between males and females).[6]

Sex hormones have an activating effect on the adult brain. Higher levels of circulating testosterone are associated with increased sexual activity in both men and women.[7] In the latter, testosterone activity increases at around the time of ovulation and is associated with increased sexual desire.[8] In adult male primates, testosterone acts on the amygdala to stimulate the sexual drive, while its action on the hypothalamus stimulates copulatory behaviour; in adult female primates, ovarian hormones also act on the amygdala to stimulate sexual drive.

There are clearly important cognitive influences on sexual behaviour. Beauregard and colleagues studied the neural substrate underlying emotional self-regulation by measuring brain activation in ten normal male subjects while they either responded in a normal manner to erotic film excerpts (oral or vaginal intercourse, etc., between one woman and two or three men, between two women and one man, and between two or more women) or voluntarily attempted to inhibit the sexual arousal induced by viewing the erotic stimuli.[9] Their results demonstrated that the sexual arousal experienced in response to the erotic film excerpts was associated with activation in the limbic and paralimbic structures, such as the right amygdala, right anterior temporal pole and hypothalamus (Figure 25.13):

> In addition, the attempted inhibition of the sexual arousal generated by viewing the erotic stimuli was associated with activation of the right superior frontal gyrus and right anterior cingulate gyrus. No activation was found in limbic areas. These findings reinforce the view that emotional self-regulation is normally implemented by a neural circuit comprising various prefrontal regions and subcortical limbic structures. They also suggest that humans have the capacity to influence the electrochemical dynamics of their brains, by voluntarily changing the nature of the mind processes unfolding in the psychological space.[9]

The same group have also compared sexual arousal and brain activation in men and women, using erotic film segments depicting sexual interactions, including vaginal intercourse in some of the scenes, between a man and a woman, using those scenes with the lowest disgust scores among the women.[10] Key differences in relation to brain activation related to the hypothalamus and thalamus:

> In male subjects only, processing of the erotic film segment was also associated with significant activation in the hypothalamus and thalamus. Furthermore, a regression analysis revealed the existence of a positive correlation between the intensity of the SA [sexual arousal] experienced by male subjects and the mag-

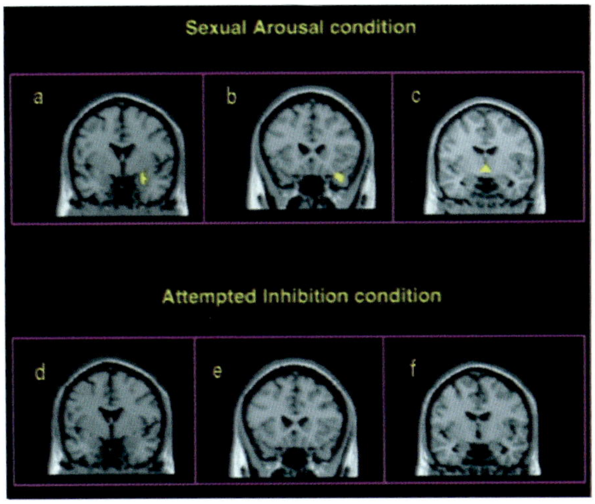

Figure 25.13 Statistical activation maps for limbic-paralimbic structures defined a priori. Images are coronal sections for the data averaged across subjects. The right hemisphere of the brain corresponds to the right side of the image. In the sexual arousal condition, greater activation during the viewing of erotic film excerpts relative to the viewing of emotionally neutral film excerpts was noted in the right amygdala (a), right anterior temporal pole (b) and hypothalamus (c). In the attempted inhibition condition, no significant loci of activation were seen in the amygdalae (d), anterior temporal polar region (e) or hypothalamus (f)
Reproduced with permission from ref. 9.

nitude of hypothalamic activation. No such correlation was noted in female subjects.[10]

Other important aspects of sexual behaviour are detailed in Chapter 45.

Hunger

In terms of the neuroanatomical pathways related to the hunger drive, it is noteworthy that many descending afferent fibres from forebrain structures converge in the rostral division of the nucleus tractus solitarius (rNTS) of the medulla, including dense projections from the central nucleus of the amygdala, the lateral hypothalamus and the gustatory cortex.[11] A neuroanatomical overview of the central taste pathways is given in Figure 25.14.

Hunger is a regulatory behaviour – that is, controlled by homeostatic mechanisms – and the endocrine system plays a very important role. According to Coll and colleagues, the hormonal control of food intake may be summarized as follows:

> We now know a number of circulating peptides and steroids that are produced in the body can have significant influence on appetitive behavior through their actions on the hypothalamus, the brain stem or afferent autonomic nerves. These hormones come from at least three sites: fat cells, the gastrointestinal tract and the endocrine pancreas.[12]

Details of the control of food intake by the hypothalamus are shown in Figure 25.15. The peptide leptin is produced in adipose tissue, and circulating levels rise with overfeeding and fall with starvation.

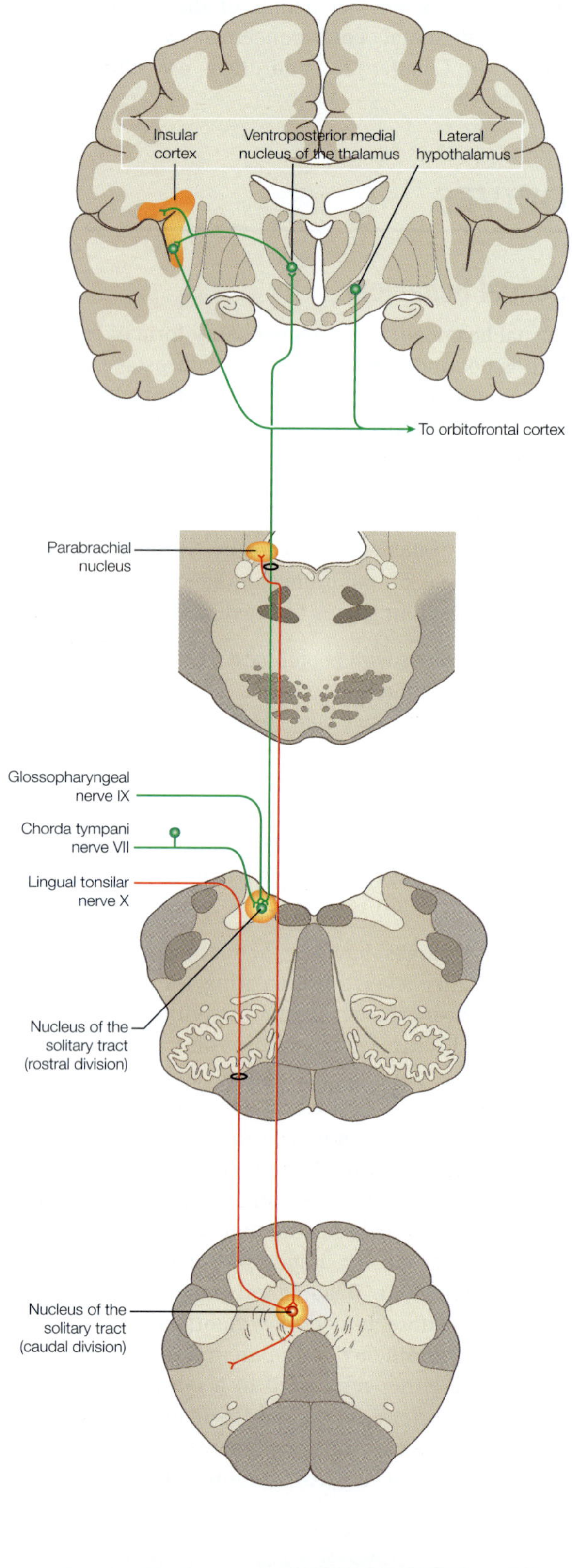

Figure 25.14 Anatomical overview of the central taste pathways. Electrical signals from cranial nerves VII, IX and X that contain information on the chemical properties of tastants are conveyed to the rostral division of the nucleus tractus solitarius (rNTS) of the medulla, the principal visceral-sensory nucleus of the brainstem. In the rat, second-order fibres (i.e. rNTS efferents) project ipsilaterally to gustatory centres in parabrachial nuclei (PBN) of the pons, from where a first (dorsal) pathway projects to the parvicellular part of the ventroposterior medial nucleus of the thalamus (VPMpc), the taste thalamic nucleus. The second (ventral) pathway includes direct projections from the PBN to the central nucleus of the amygdala and lateral hypothalamus. In primates, however, the NTS projection fibres bypass the PBN, only to join the central tegmental tract and synapse directly into the VPMpc, whereas the PBN seems to be dedicated to convey general visceral information (mainly through vagal afferents) to specialized thalamic nuclei. In either case, thalamic afferents then project to the primary gustatory cortex, which is defined as the VPMpc cortical target. The VPMpc also sends projections to regions neighbouring the primary somatosensory cortex, adjacent to the precentral gyrus, and that overlap with cortical somatotopic sites for the face and oral cavity. The primary taste cortex projects to the central nucleus of the amygdala, from where gustatory information reaches the lateral hypothalamus and midbrain dopaminergic regions. The primary taste cortex also projects anteriorly to the caudolateral orbitofrontal region, called the secondary taste cortex. Taste neurons in the caudolateral orbitofrontal cortex converge with cells receiving projections from the primary olfactory cortex, which might have implications for flavour perception. The orbitofrontal cortex is also targeted by projections from the lateral hypothalamus, allowing taste responses to be modulated by satiety states. Finally, cortical taste areas send afferents to the rNTS/PBN, allowing for top-down modulation of gustatory processing at the level of the brainstem

Blue, projections to rNTS; green, primary taste areas; red, projections to caudal NTS.

Modified, with permission, from ref. 11.

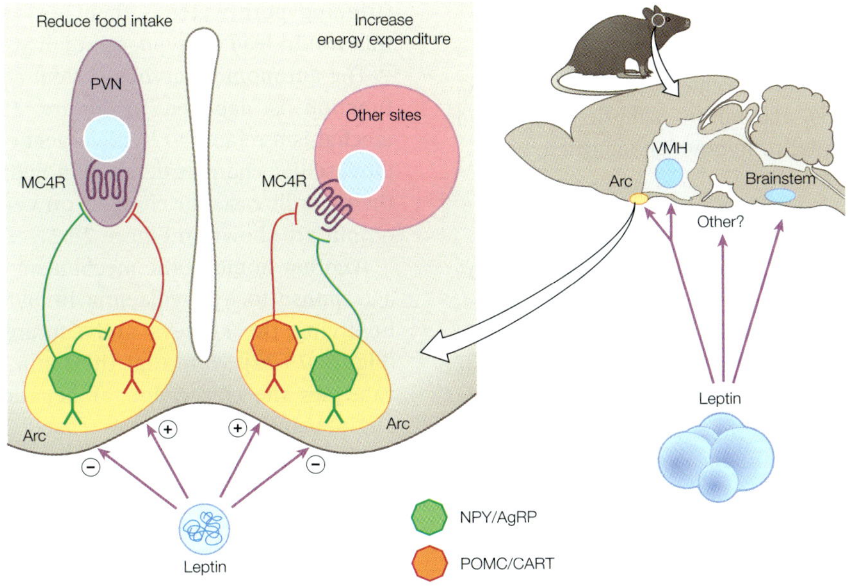

Figure 25.15 Control of food intake by the hypothalamus. Leptin acts as a peripheral signal of long-term energy stores to bring about changes in food intake and energy expenditure. The hypothalamus receives and integrates neural, metabolic and hormonal signals to regulate energy homeostasis. In particular, the adipocyte-derived hormone leptin and its downstream anorexigenic pathways have a critical role in the control of food intake

Arc, arcuate nucleus; AgRP, agouti-related protein; CART, cocaine- and amphetamine-related transcript; MC4R, melanocortin 4 receptor; NPY, neuropeptide Y; POMC, proopiomelanocortin; PVN, paraventricular nucleus; VMN, ventromedial nucleus.

Redrawn with permission from ref. 11.

Figure 25.16 details how hormonal signals derived from the gut and classical endocrine organs act in synergy to affect changes in feeding behaviour. During hunger, the smell (and then possibly also the taste) of food leads to aroma and taste signals, which impact, via olfactory and gustatory cortex, on the hypothalamus, sending signals to the dorsal motor nucleus of the vagus and, via vagal cholinergic fibres, causing secretion of insulin from B-cells of the pancreas. This cephalic phase of insulin secretion should be distinguished from the gastrointestinal phase of insulin secretion, in which further insulin secretion takes place as a result of food entering the stomach and duodenum. In due course, circulating breakdown products of food directly stimulate insulin secretion from the pancreas; this is the substrate phase of insulin secretion.

Ghrelin, a ligand for the growth hormone secretagogue receptor (GHSR), is an orexigenic octanoylated 28-amino-acid peptide produced and secreted by cells within the oxyntic glands of the stomach. Circulating ghrelin levels fluctuate over the course of the day in relation to food intake; ghrelin messenger RNA (mRNA) expression and peptide secretion are increased by weight loss, fasting and insulin-induced hypoglycaemia, while peripheral administration of ghrelin stimulates food intake and decreases fat utilization.[12,13] Hence, ghrelin has been proposed to be an enteric signal involved in energy homeostasis, being unique in that it stimulates appetite rather than acting as a satiety signal.[12,13]

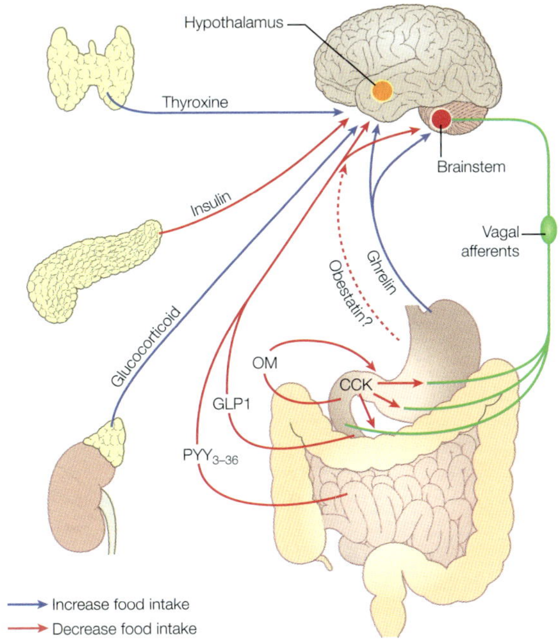

Figure 25.16 Hormonal signals derived from the gut and classical endocrine organs such as the pancreas, thyroid and adrenal glands act in synergy to effect changes in feeding behaviour

CCK, cholecystokinin; GLP-1, glucagon-like peptide 1; OXM, oxyntomodulin; PYY_{3-36}, peptide YY_{3-36}.

Redrawn with permission from ref. 11.

THIRST

The following two homeostatic mechanisms relate to drinking: osmotic homeostasis, related to osmotic thirst, and volume homeostasis, related to hypovolaemic thirst.

Osmotic thirst

This occurs when body fluid (e.g. plasma) solute concentrations rise too far, which may result from several causes, such as dietary sodium loading leading to increased plasma sodium ion concentration; dehydration; and high levels of sweating. The raised extracellular fluid osmolality (systemic hypertonicity) stimulates the lamina terminalis. Details of components of the lamina terminalis acted upon by this circulating factor and by other circulating factors are shown in Figure 25.17. Figure 25.18 details the subsequent neural and hormonal inputs into the brain and the central neural pathways that mediate sensory integration of signals for the generation of drinking (thirst).

A positron-emission tomography (PET) study of ten volunteers has demonstrated that the cingulate cortex is particularly activated in osmotic thirst induced by intravenous infusion of hypertonic saline.[14] The authors of this PET study concluded that the anterior and posterior cingulate, and the anterior wall of the third ventricle, are major elements of a pattern including thalamic, hippocampal, orbitofrontal, insula, and midbrain sites that subserve the genesis of consciousness of thirst when plasma [Na^+] increases.[14]

Hypovolaemic thirst

The volume of extracellular fluid may become lower because of haemorrhage or sodium depletion, for example. Drinking pure water is then not an adequate solution, as this would lead to hypo-osmolality.

The autonomic nervous system control of cardiovascular function is depicted in Figure 25.19. One homeostatic mechanism related to hypovolaemic thirst involves the cardiovascular changes detailed in Figure 25.20. The effects of these cardiovascular changes on venous return and cardiac output are shown in Figure 25.21.

Another homeostatic mechanism that comes into play as a response to hypovolaemia involves endocrine responses involving the kidneys and suprarenal or adrenal glands (Figure 25.22). Note that the renin secreted by the kidney catalyses the conversion of hepatic angiotensinogen into angiotensin I, which is itself then converted into angiotensin II (catalysed by pulmonary angiotensin-converting enzyme). In addition to causing vasoconstriction and stimulating suprarenal (adrenal) aldosterone secretion, angiotensin II also acts as a neurotransmitter in the brain (see Figure 25.18). Binding to type 2 (AT_2) receptors in the subfornical organ (SFO) leads, via the supraoptic and paraventricular nuclei, to secretion of arginine vasopressin (AVP; antidiuretic hormone, ADH) from the posterior pituitary gland, which in turn leads to stimulation of AVP V_2 renal receptors, causing increased water permeability in distal convoluted tubules and collecting ducts of nephrons and therefore increased water retention, increased urinary osmolality and reduced urinary volume. These last three changes act to reverse hypovolaemia. As shown in Figure 25.18, the central action of angiotensin II also stimulates thirst.

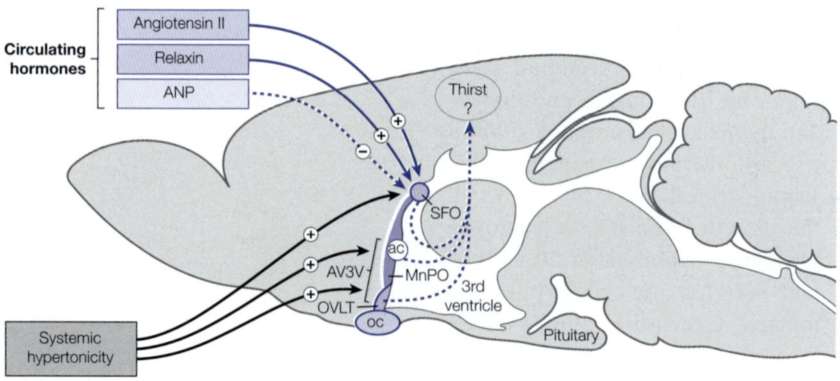

Figure 25.17 Diagram of the sagittal midline of the rat brain, showing circulating factors that act on the various components of the lamina terminalis to influence thirst. The two parts of the lamina terminalis that lack a normal blood–brain barrier, the subfornical organ (SFO) and organum vasculosum of the lamina terminalis (OVLT), are shaded with vertical lines, whereas the other component of the lamina terminalis, the median preoptic nucleus (MnPO), is indicated by the spotted area. The part of the lamina terminalis that is included in the anteroventral third ventricle region (AV3V) is indicated by the white bracket. The interrupted white line indicates an inhibitory influence of atrial natriuretic peptide (ANP), whereas angiotensin II, relaxin and hypertonicity have excitatory actions on the lamina terminalis. The question mark indicates that the efferent pathways from the lamina terminalis that mediate thirst are not yet known

ac, anterior commissure; oc, optic chiasm.

Reproduced with permission from McKinley and Johnson (2004). The physiological regulation of thirst and fluid intake. *News in Physiological Sciences* 19(1): 1–6

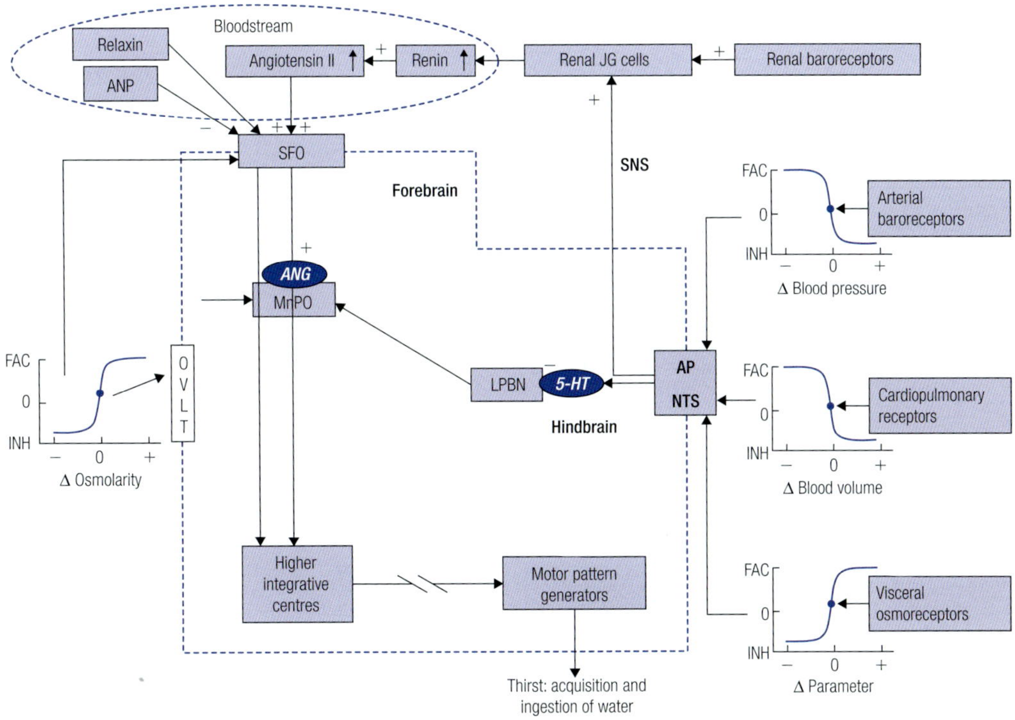

Figure 25.18 Diagram depicting neural and hormonal inputs into the brain and the central neural pathways that mediate sensory integration of signals for the generation of drinking (thirst). Both inhibitory and excitatory inputs from the periphery are derived from arterial and cardiopulmonary baroreceptors and other visceral receptors (e.g. gastric, hepatic/portal, renal). Information carried in afferent nerves projects mainly to the nucleus of the solitary tract (NTS). Angiotensin (ANG) acts in the form of ANG II on ANG type 1 (AT_1) receptors in the subfornical organ (SFO). Osmoreception takes place in structures along the organum vasculosum of the lamina terminalis (OVLT) (MnPO). Hormonal information to the SFO is subsequently carried in descending pathways, some of which are likely to use ANG in the mode of a neurotransmitter, to forebrain structures such as those in the anteroventral third ventricle region (AV3V). Ascending information to the forebrain is carried in projections from noradrenergic cell groups in the hindbrain, which are activated by arterial and cardiopulmonary receptor input under conditions of hypotension and/or hypovolaemia. ANG and noradrenergic inputs act synergistically in forebrain nuclei. A hindbrain inhibitory pathway originating in the area postrema (AP) and medial NTS ascends to the lateral parabrachial nucleus (LPBN). This projection uses serotonin (5-HT) as a neurotransmitter and prevents against excessive sodium and water intake to limit excess expansion of blood volume. Inhibitory input is likely to ascend the neuraxis either directly or indirectly to interact with forebrain structures

FAC, facilitation; INH, inhibition; SNS, sympathetic nervous system.

Reproduced with permission from McKinley and Johnson (2004). The physiological regulation of thirst and fluid intake. *News in Physiological Sciences* 19(1): 1–6

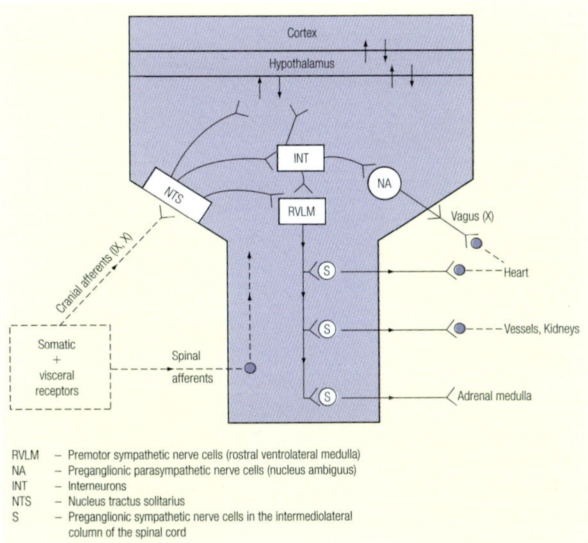

Figure 25.19 Sympathetic and parasympathetic nerves in the brain and spinal cord involved in cardiovascular control

Reproduced with permission from Power and Kam, *Principles of Physiology for the Anaesthetist*. Hodder, London. (2007).

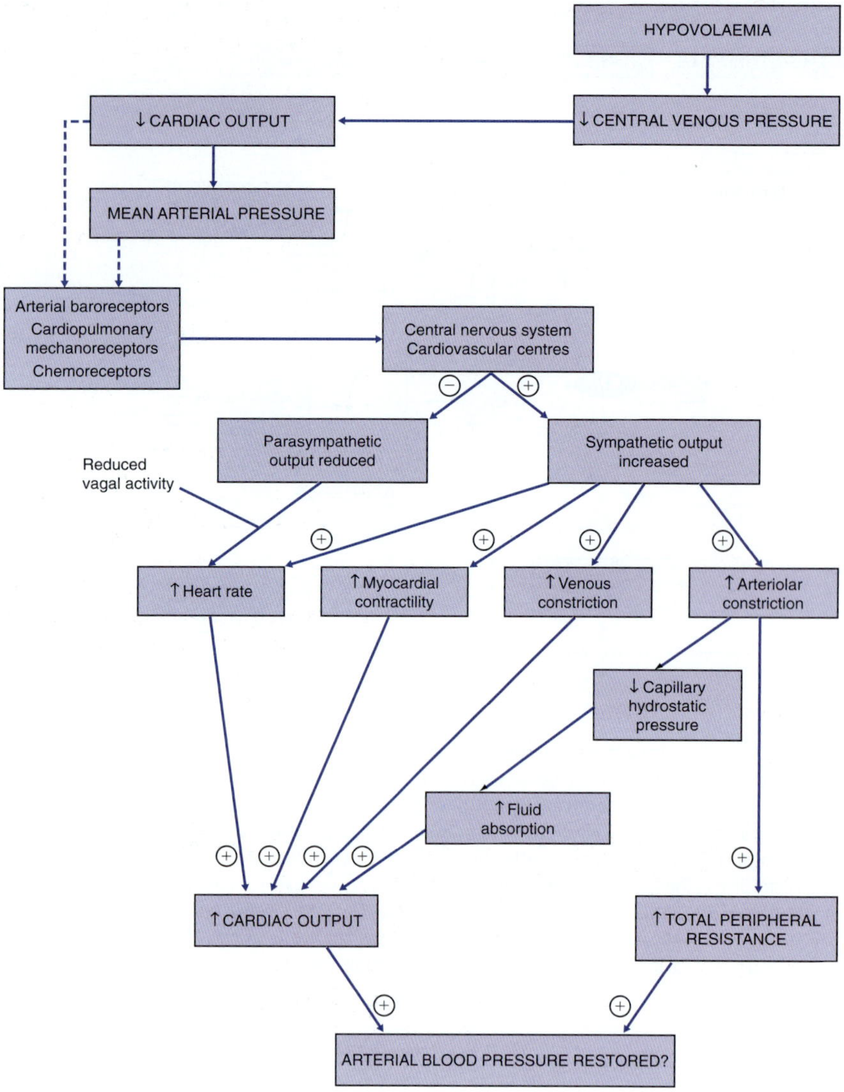

Figure 25.20 Cardiovascular changes following hypovolaemia

Reproduced with permission from Power and Kam, *Principles of Physiology for the Anaesthetist*. Hodder, London. (2007).

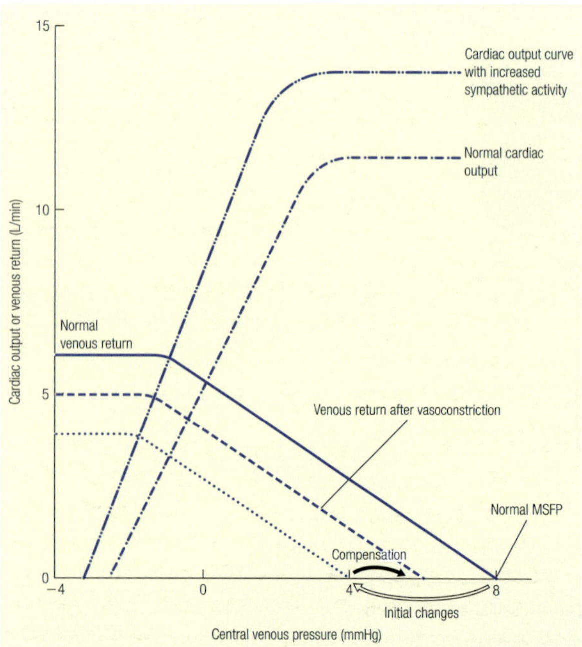

Figure 25.21 Effects on venous return and cardiac output curves of the cardiovascular changes that occur in response to hypovolaemia (e.g. haemorrhage)

MSFP, mean systolic filling pressure

Reproduced with permission from Power and Kam, *Principles of Physiology for the Anaesthetist*. Hodder, London. (2007).

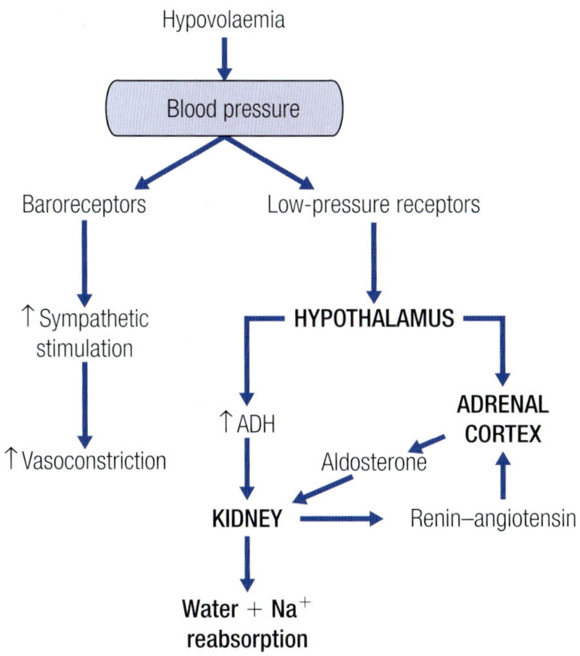

Figure 25.22 Endocrine responses to hypovolaemia

Reproduced with permission from Power and Kam, *Principles of Physiology for the Anaesthetist*. Hodder, London. (2007).

KEY POINTS

- Neural and endocrine systems are involved, sometimes together, in integrated behaviour.
- Such behaviours include perception, pain, memory, motor function and the drives of sexual behaviour, hunger and thirst.

REFERENCES

1. Solomon SG, Lennie P (2007) The machinery of colour vision. *Nature Reviews Neuroscience* **8**: 276–86.
2. Kanwisher N, Wojciulik E (2000) Visual attention: insights from brain imaging. *Nature Reviews Neuroscience* **1**: 91–100.
3. Griffiths TD, Warren JD (2004) What is an auditory object? *Nature Reviews Neuroscience* **5**: 887–92.
4. Power I, Kam P (2008) *Principles of Physiology for the Anaesthetist*, 2nd edn. London: Hodder Arnold.
5. Eichenbaum H, Lipton PA (2008) Towards a functional organization of the medial temporal lobe memory system: role of the parahippocampal and medial entorhinal cortical areas. *Hippocampus* **18**: 1314–24.
6. Hines M (2006) Prenatal testosterone and gender-related behaviour. *European Journal of Endocrinology* **155** (suppl. 1): S115–21.
7. Sherwin BB (1994) Sex hormones and psychological functioning in postmenopausal women. *Experimental Gerontology* **29**: 423–30.
8. Van Goozen SH, Wiegant VM, Endert E, *et al.* (1997) Psychoendocrinological assessment of the menstrual cycle: the relationship between hormones, sexuality, and mood. *Archives of Sexual Behavior* **26**: 359–82.
9. Beauregard M, Levesque J, Bourgouin P (2001) Neural correlates of conscious self-regulation of emotion. *Journal of Neuroscience* **21**: RC165.
10. Karama S, Lecours AR, Leroux JM, *et al.* (2002) Areas of brain activation in males and females during viewing of erotic film excerpts. *Human Brain Mapping* **16**: 1–13.
11. Simon SA, de Araujo IE, Gutierrez R, Nicolelis MA (2006) The neural mechanisms of gustation: a distributed processing code. *Nature Reviews Neuroscience* **7**: 890–901.
12. Coll AP, Farooqi IS, O'Rahilly S (2007) The hormonal control of food intake. *Cell* **129**: 251–62.
13. Williams DL, Cummings DE (2005) Regulation of ghrelin in physiologic and pathophysiologic states. *Journal of Nutrition* **135**: 1320–25.
14. Denton D, Shade R, Zamarippa F, *et al.* (1999) Neuroimaging of genesis and satiation of thirst and an interoceptor-driven theory of origins of primary consciousness. *Proceedings of the National Academy of Sciences USA* **96**: 5304–9.

FURTHER READING

Power I, Kam P (2008) *Principles of Physiology for the Anaesthetist*, 2nd edn. London: Hodder Arnold.

Chapter 26

Neurogenesis and cerebral plasticity

Basant K Puri

INTRODUCTION

This chapter begins with a consideration of corticoneurogenesis. This is followed by evidence that neurogenesis occurs in the adult human brain. Some aspects of synaptogenesis and synaptic elimination in the human brain are then described. Finally, the evidence for cerebral plasticity in adults in infrahuman mammalian species and humans is detailed.

CORTICONEUROGENESIS

Definition

Pasko Rakic has defined corticoneurogenesis as being the process of production, allocation, migration and settling of neurons into proper areal and laminar positions within the cortical sheet.[1]

Historical aspects

Historically, the important finding that cortical neurons migrate from their place of origin near the cerebral ventricles (in the ventricular zone) to their final destinations in the overlying cortex was discovered towards the turn of the nineteenth century by Wilhelm His, Ramón y Cajal and others. Cajal's original drawing of Golgi-stained neonatal human visual cortex showed transient neurons; these have been named Cajal–Retzius neurons in honour of their co-discoverers.[2]

This pattern of corticogenesis was confirmed in the 1960s by Angevine, Sidman, Rakic and others using the technique of tagging replicating DNA in dividing cells of developing mammalian cerebral cortex with radiolabelled tritiated thymidine (3H-TdR); only those mature neurons that derived from cells dividing at the time of the radiolabelling will contain this radioactive marker.

Main stages and zones of the cortical wall

The main stages in the formation of the layered structure of the human cerebral cortex are illustrated in Figure 26.1,

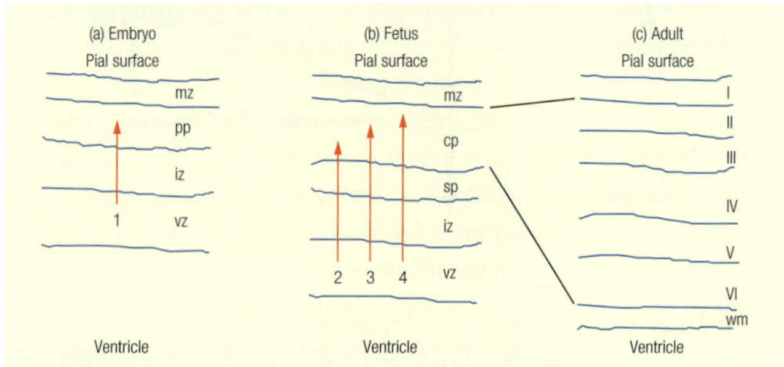

Figure 26.1 Main stages in the formation of the layered structure of the cerebral cortex. (a) The earliest migrating postmitotic neuroblasts (1) leave the ventricular zone (vz), crossing the intermediate zone (iz) to form the preplate (pp). (b) The preplate is subsequently split by the settling of later migrating neuroblasts. Successive waves of centrifugally migrating neuroblasts (2–4) establish the inside-out structure of the cortical plate (cp), situated between the subplate (sp), the remnant of the inner aspect of the preplate and the marginal zone (mz). (c) Mature layered structure of the cerebral cortex, demonstrating the origin of layers II–VI from the cortical plate, whereas layer I (mz) Cajal–Retzius neurons derive largely from the outer portion of the preplate white matter (wm)

Reproduced with permission from Love, Louis and Ellison, *Greenfield's Neuropathology* 8th edn. Hodder, London. (2008).

which also depicts the successive zones from the ventricular zone, adjacent to the cerebral ventricle, outwards to the marginal zone, adjacent to the pia mater (see also Chapter 23). The migrating neurons stop migrating in the cortical plate, which is just deep to and adjacent to the marginal zone. Neurons migrating later end up travelling past earlier neurons (which are no longer migrating) and end up nearer the pia mater. Hence, the cortical plate has an inside-out structure.

Using the fluorescent axon tracer dioctadecyl-tetramethylindocarbacyanine perchlorate (DiI) and the fluorescent DNA-binding molecular marker 4′,6-diamidino-2-phenylindole (DAPI), further details of the corticogenesis at mid-gestation in the human striate cortex (Brodmann area 17, primary visual cortex, V1) have been studied, including the occurrence of a waiting period, as shown in Figure 26.2.[3]

The different zones of the cortical wall described above were formalized by the Boulder Committee in 1970 and based in large measure on the work of Rakic. More recently,

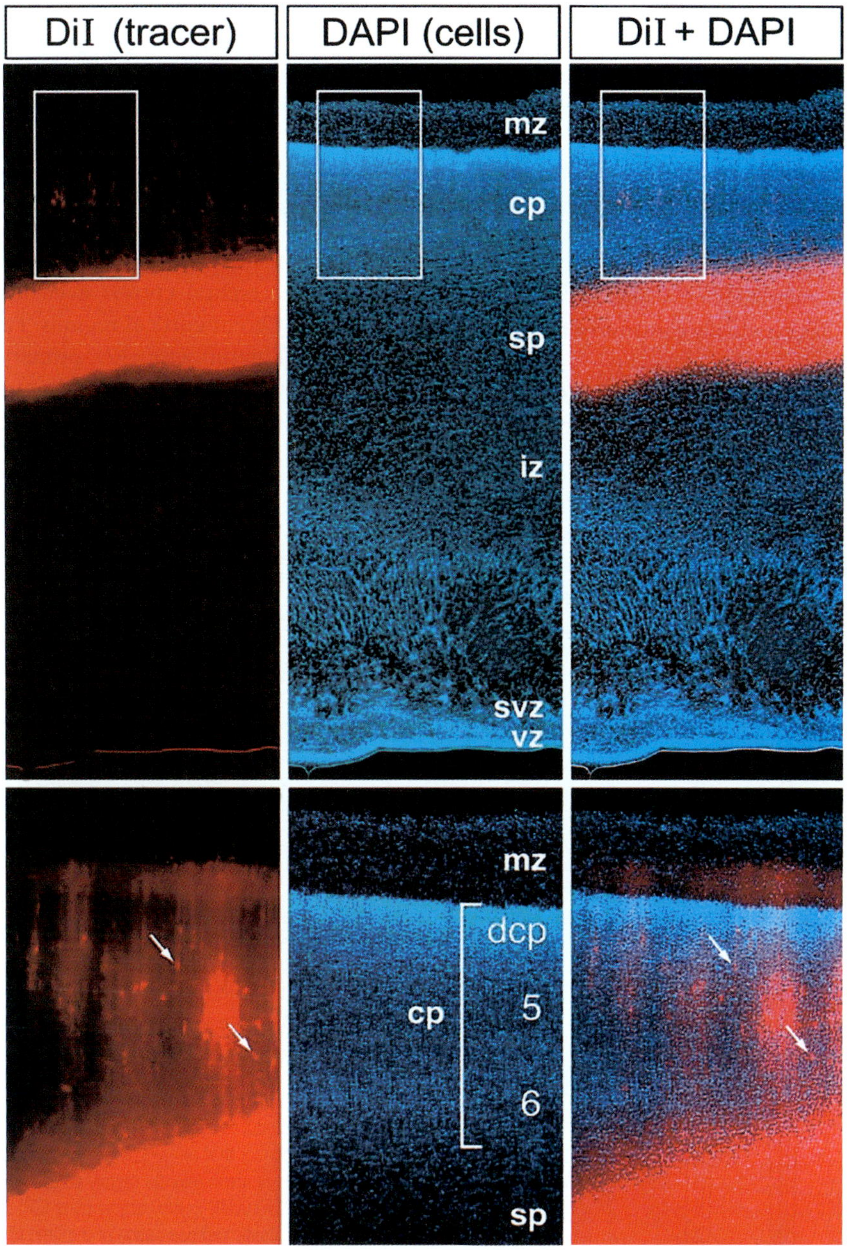

Figure 26.2 Human visual cortex (area 17): development of cortical connections at mid-gestation. Dioctadecyl-tetramethylindocarbacyanine perchlorate (DiI) was injected into the optic radiations between the lateral geniculate nucleus and visual cortex in a fixed brain. Labelled thalamocortical axons project heavily into the subplate (sp), a transient cellular compartment where thalamocortical axons wait for the arrival of layer IV neurons. At this age, the cortical plate (cp) contains only neurons belonging to layers V and VI, and a dense cortical plate (dcp) containing newly migrated neurons. Superficial cortical layers are 'born' later than deep layers, and thus corticogenesis proceeds in an inside-out gradient. The cerebral wall also consists of a ventricular zone (vz) and a subventricular zone (svz), where neurons and glia proliferate; an intermediate zone (iz), where neurons migrate and axonal pathways develop; and a marginal zone (mz), precursor of cortical layer I. At higher magnifications (bottom panels), the cortical plate is seen to contain some retrogradely labelled neurons (arrows), corresponding to corticobulbar and corticospinal projections from layer V and corticothalamic projections from layer VI. After layer IV neurons arrive and differentiate, the thalamocortical axons will invade the cortical plate and synapse in layer IV. This experiment exemplifies the dynamic processes of cortical cell proliferation, migration, and axon growth and pathfinding. Fluorescent axons tracer DiI, counterstained with 4′,6-diamidino-2-phenylindole (DAPI)

Reproduced with permission from Love, Louis and Ellison, *Greenfield's Neuropathology* 8th edn. Hodder, London. (2008).

in light of advances in our knowledge of corticoneurogenesis, the following revisions of the Boulder model have been proposed by Bystron and colleagues:[2]

- A transient layer with a diverse population of neurons forms between the neuroepithelium and the pial surface of the dorsal telencephalon before the appearance of the cortical plate (CP). We suggest that the term preplate, which is already widely used, should be adopted for this layer.
- The subventricular zone appears as a distinctive proliferative layer before the emergence of the CP, earlier than previously recognized.

- There is no distinct cell-sparse layer under the pial surface before the CP forms. Thus, the term marginal zone should be used only after the appearance of the CP, to refer to the residual superficial part of the preplate, which becomes the layer 1 of the mature cortex.
- The term intermediate zone (IZ) has been used in various ways. We propose that it should be reserved for the heterogeneous compartment that lies between the proliferative layers and the postmigratory cells above. The IZ contains radially and tangentially migrating cells and a thickening layer of extrinsic axons that eventually constitutes the white matter.
- The subplate (SP) is a distinct and functionally important transient layer, located directly below the cortical plate, which was not recognized by the Boulder Committee. In rodents and carnivores most SP neurons are born before the first CP cells. In humans, preplate cells also contribute to the SP, but its substantial thickening at later stages probably involves the addition of later-born neurons.

Time course

The above inside-out pattern of development holds for all areas of the cerebral cortex, even though the time course varies for different cortical regions. For example, the striate cortex (Brodmann area 17, primary visual cortex, V1) develops over a longer period of time than Brodmann area 24, say. Figure 26.3 shows the probable range of the time of

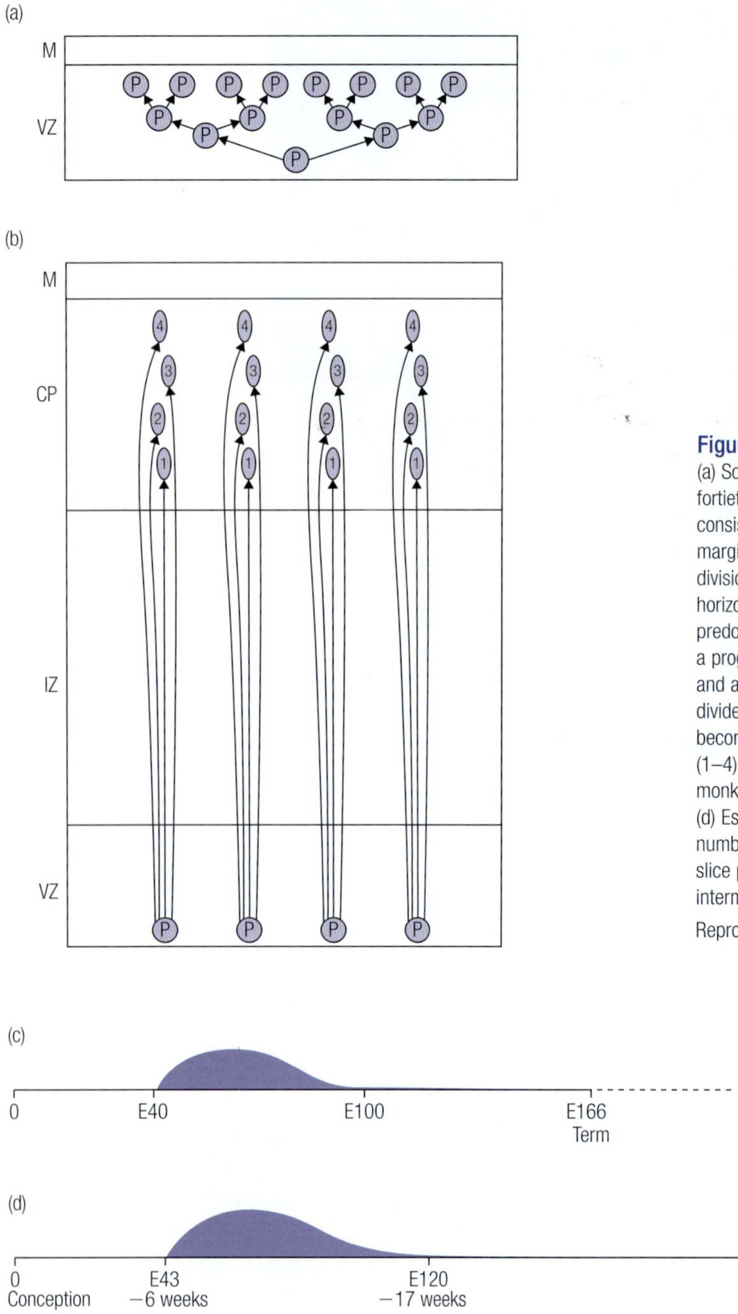

Figure 26.3 Relationships of modes of cell division to duration of corticogenesis. (a) Schematic model of symmetrical cell divisions that predominate before the fortieth embryonic day (E40). At this early embryonic age, the cerebral wall consists of only the ventricular zone (VZ), where all cells proliferate, and the marginal zone (M), where some of them extend their radial processes. Symmetrical division produces two progenitors (P) during each cycle and causes rapid horizontal lateral spread. (b) Model of asymmetrical or stem division that becomes predominant in the monkey embryo after E40. During each asymmetrical division, a progenitor (P) produces one postmitotic neuron that leaves the ventricular zone and another progenitor that remains within the proliferative zone and continues to divide. Postmitotic neurons migrate rapidly across the intermediate zone (IZ) and become arranged vertically in the cortical plate (CP) in reverse order of their arrival (1–4). (c) Diagrammatic representation of the time of neuron origin in macaque monkey. Data are obtained from [^{3}H]thymidine autoradiographic analyses. (d) Estimate of the time of neuron origin in the human neocortex based on the number of mitotic figures within the ventricular zone, supravital DNA synthesis in slice preparations of fetal tissue, and the presence of migrating neurons in the intermediate zone of the human fetal cerebrum

Reproduced with permission from ref. 6.

neuron origin in the human neocortex (Figure 26.3d), the corresponding time of origin in the macaque monkey (Figure 26.3c) and the relationships of modes of cell division to duration of corticogenesis.

Neuronal migration

Figure 26.4 is a schematic diagram of the composition of, and neuronal migration in, the developing cerebral wall. Note in particular that the radial glia appear to offer a form of scaffolding from the ventricular zone to the marginal zone of the developing cerebral cortex, along which postmitotic neuronal cells travel. A model of the cascade of molecular events that are thought to take place during this process of neuronal migration, as these cells extend leading processes that follow the contours of the radial glia, has been proposed by Rakic and colleagues and is shown in Figure 26.5.[1]

Subplate neurons are the first cortical neurons to mature. They direct migrating cortical plate neurons and targeting of their axonal projections, and are selectively vulnerable to early hypoxic-ischaemic brain injury in animal models. Timing of subplate neuron death determines the resulting defect in thalamocortical development: very early excitotoxic subplate neuron death results in failure of thalamocortical innervation, while later subplate neuron death interferes with the refinement of thalamocortical connections into mature circuits.[4,5]

Radial-unit hypothesis

According to Rakic:

> The manner by which postmitotic cells migrate and become distributed is crucial for understanding how the neocortex forms as a sheet rather than as a lump. The waves of postmitotic neurons that are generated within the same site in the ventricular zone arrive successively at the cortical plate where they pass by each other, and become arranged radially in the form of cell stacks – named ontogenetic columns. Therefore, a radial unit consists of cells that originate from several clones but share the same birthplace, migrate along the common pathway, and settle within the same ontogenetic column.[6]

Figure 26.6 illustrates how the developing cortical plate consists of these ontogenetic columns. The corresponding radial-unit hypothesis postulates that the size of the cerebral cortex depends on the number of contributing radial units, which in turn depends on the number of founder cells.[6]

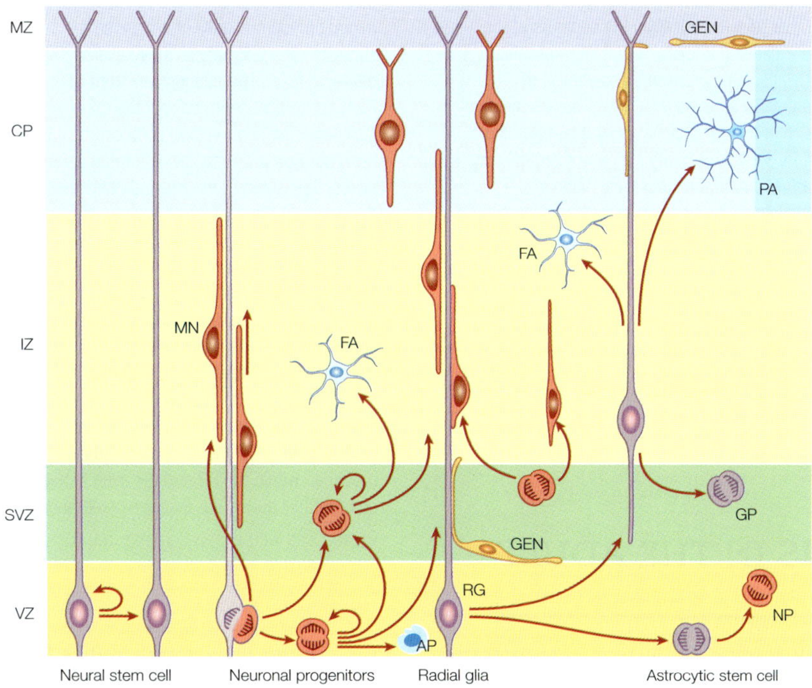

Figure 26.4 Schematic diagram of the composition, cellular events and the relationship in the developing cerebral wall, based on data obtained from species ranging from the mouse to human and non-primates. Initially, a homogeneous population of neural stem cells (green), which divide symmetrically, transform into radial glial cells (RG), which divide asymmetrically and over time produce migrating neurons (MN, red) and dedicated neuronal progenitors with short processes (red mitotic divisions) that populate the ventricular (VZ) and subventricular (SVZ) zones and produce all projection neurons and the majority of interneurons in humans and a small fraction in rodents. In addition, a population of tangentially migrating neurons from the ganglionic eminence (GEN, blue) arrives at the dorsal telencephalon from the ganglionic eminence, mostly via the SVZ and marginal zone (MZ), to supply the majority of interneurons in rodents and about one-third in humans. Eventually RGs undergo apoptosis (AP) or directly or indirectly generate ependymal cells, fibrillary astrocytes (FA), protoplasmic astrocytes (PA), glial progenitors (GP) or astrocytic stem cells that retain a neurogenic potential (NP)

Reproduced with permission from ref. 1.

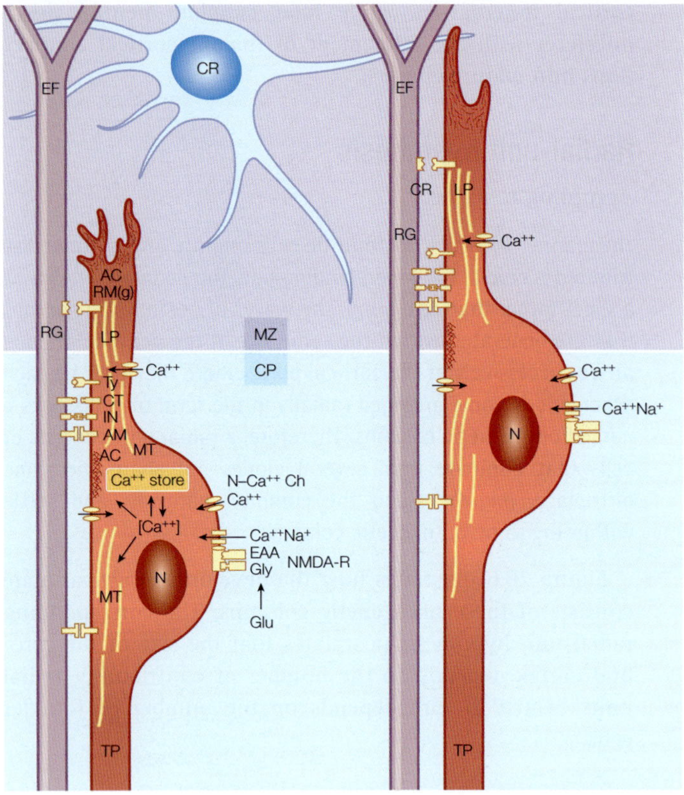

Figure 26.5 Model of a proposed cascade of molecular events that takes place during migration of postmitotic cells across the developing cerebral wall. Migrating cells extend a leading process (LP) that selectively follows the contours of the radial glial fibre (RF) as it spans the expanding cerebral wall. The cytoskeleton within the LP and trailing process (TP) contains prominent assemblies of microtubules (MT) and actin-like contractile proteins (AC), which are involved in elongation of the LP and translocation of the nucleus (N) and the surrounding cytoplasm. The leading process enters the cortical plate (CP) and marginal zone (MZ), but the nucleus stops at the CP/MZ interface (grey area). Various intracellular, membrane-bound and extracellular matrix molecules provide signals or are directly engaged in selection of the migratory pathway, rate of cell movement and the cessation of migration at the CP/MZ borderline

AC, actin-like filaments; AM, homotypic adhesion molecule; CR, Cajal–Retzius cell; CT, catenin; EAA, excitatory amino acids; EF, end-foot of radial glial fibre; Glu, glutamate; Gly, glycine; I, integrine; RM(g), gliophilic recognition molecule; RM(n), neurophilic recognition molecule.

Reproduced with permission from ref. 1.

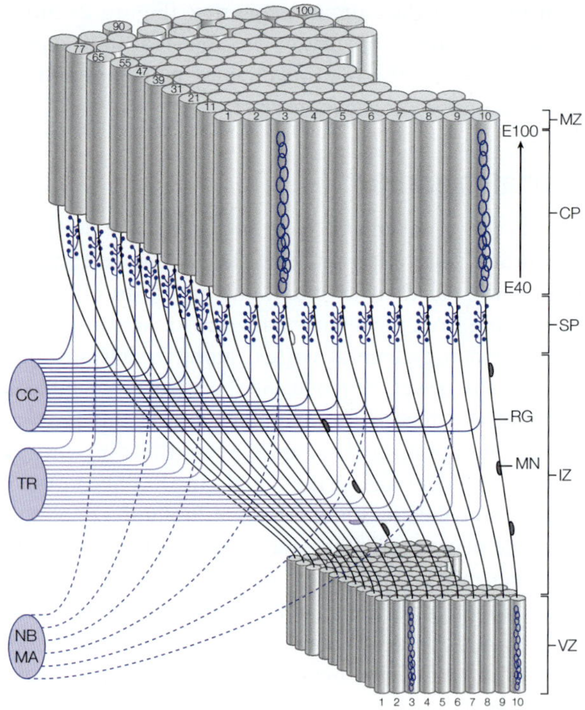

Figure 26.6 Basic developmental events and types of cell–cell interactions that occur during the early stages of corticogenesis, before formation of the final pattern of cortical connections. This diagram emphasizes radial migration, a predominant mode of neuronal movement that, in primates, underlies the elaborate columnar organization of the neocortex. After their last division, cohorts of migrating neurons (MN) first traverse the intermediate zone (IZ) and then the subplate zone (SP), where they have an opportunity to interact with waiting afferents that arrive sequentially from the nucleus basalis (NB) and monoamine (MA) subcortical centres, from the thalamic radiation (TR), and from several ipsilateral and contralateral corticocortical bundles (CC). After newly generated neurons bypass the earlier generated ones that are situated in the deep cortical layers, they settle at the interface between the developing cortical plate (CP) and the marginal zone (MZ) and, eventually, form a radial stock of cells that share a common site of origin but are generated at different times. For example, neurons that are produced between embryonic days E40 and E100 in radial unit 3 follow the same radial glial fascicle and form ontogenetic column 3. Although some cells, presumably neurophilic in nature of their surface affinities, might detach from the cohort and move laterally, guided by an axonal bundle (e.g. horizontally oriented, red cell leaving radial unit 3), most postmitotic cells are gliophilic (e.g. have affinity for the glial surface) and obey constraints strictly that are imposed by transient radial glial scaffolding (RG). This cellular arrangement preserves relationships between the proliferative mosaic of the ventricular zone (VZ) and the corresponding protomap within the SP and CP, even though the cortical surface in primates shifts considerably during the massive cerebral growth encountered in mid-gestation

Reproduced with permission from ref. 6.

NEUROGENESIS IN THE ADULT HUMAN BRAIN

Neurogenesis in the adult human brain was demonstrated by Eriksson and colleagues.[7] They studied the dentate gyrus and the subventricular zone in humans, since these regions had been shown to generate new neurons in the postnatal and adult period in infrahuman mammalian species. Patients with squamous cell carcinomas at the base of the tongue, in the larynx or in the pharynx received bromodeoxyuridine (BrdU) dissolved in saline and given as an intravenous infusion to assess the proliferative activity of the tumour cells, expressed as BrdU-labelling index. BrdU is a synthetic form of thymidine, which has been used as a marker of neurogenesis in infrahuman species. The brains of the patients were studied postmortem. No signs of macroscopic or microscopic metastases were found in autopsy material from the cerebrum in any of the patients.[7] Quantitation of newly generated cells in the hippocampus in each of five patients is shown in Figure 26.7. Labelling with NeuN, a neuronal marker, and comparison with the

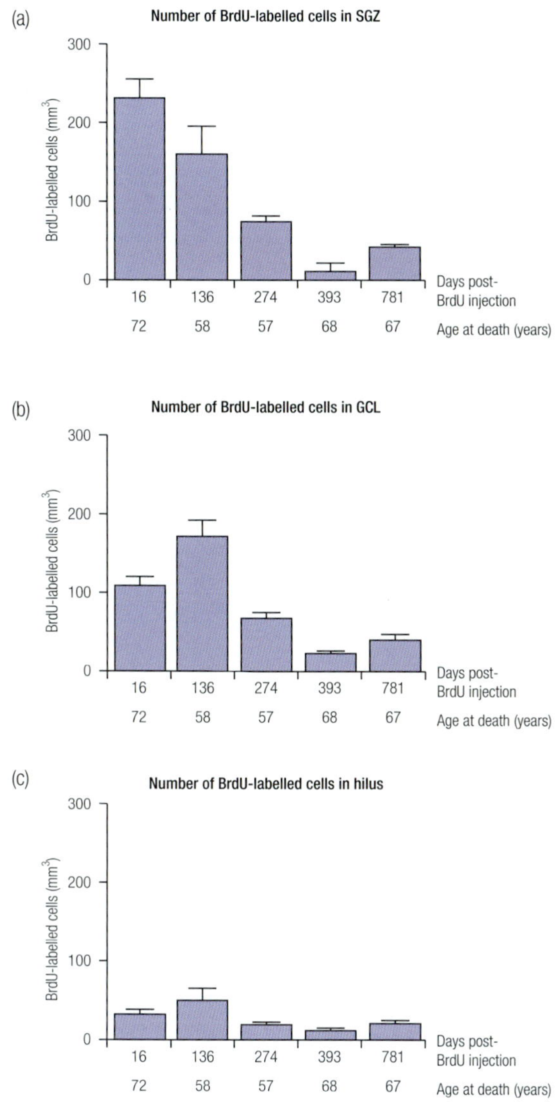

Figure 26.7 Quantitation of newly generated cells in the adult human hippocampus. The density of bromodeoxyuridine (BrdU) immunoperoxidase-stained cells in the subgranular zone (SGZ) (a), the granule cell layer (GCL) (b) and the hilus (c) was determined in five to seven sections per patient (mean number of BrdU-positive cells/mm^3 sample volume ± standard error of the mean (SEM)). The corresponding patient's age at the time of death and interval as BrdU infusion are given for each BrdU-treated patient ($n = 5$)

Reproduced with permission from ref. 7.

adult rat brain demonstrated that these newly generated cells were indeed neurons.

SYNAPTOGENESIS AND SYNAPTIC ELIMINATION IN THE HUMAN BRAIN

Huttenlocher and de Courten published the results of a postmortem study in 1987 in which synaptic density in human striate cortex was determined at various ages, together with measurement of total volume of striate cortex, making it possible to estimate the total number of synapses.[8] Their key findings included the following:

- Synaptogenesis in human striate cortex was found to be most rapid between the ages of 2 months and 4 months, a time that also is critical for the development of function in visual cortex of the infant.
- Synapse elimination occurred subsequently, with loss of about 40 per cent of synapses between the ages of 8 months and 11 years.
- Synapse numbers were stable in adults, except for a slightly lower value in a single brain at age 71 years.
- Analysis by individual cortical layers showed similar age-related changes in all strata of striate cortex, except for somewhat later synaptogenesis in cortical layers V and VI.
- Total volume of striate cortex reached adult size remarkably early, at about age 4 months.

These findings supported the hypothesis that exuberant synaptic connections are an anatomical substrate for plasticity in developing cerebral cortex.[8]

Subsequently, Huttenlocher and Dabholkar carried out a study in which they compared the formation of synaptic contacts in human cerebral cortex in two regions: the auditory cortex (Heschl's gyrus) and the prefrontal cortex (middle frontal gyrus).[9] Figure 26.8 shows the combined results of this study and the previous 1987 study of the striate cortex. It can be seen that the time course of synaptogenesis in the visual cortex resembles that in the auditory cortex, except that synapse elimination appears to begin earlier in the visual cortex.[9]

A plot of the difference between the synaptic density in auditory cortex and that in the middle frontal gyrus against conceptual age gave the distribution shown in Figure 26.9, suggesting earlier synaptogenesis and earlier synaptic elimination in auditory cortex compared with prefrontal cortex.[9] As the authors concluded:

> The present data show regional differences in synaptogenesis in human neocortex both in fetal brains and postnatally up to at least age 15 months (CA [conceptual age] 700 days) in cortical layers 2 to 3, and up to at least age 3 months (CA 363 days) in the lower cortical layers. A rapid burst in synaptogenesis occurs postnatally in visual and auditory cortex. Prefrontal cortex appears to acquire synaptic junctions more slowly. By age 3.5 years, prefrontal cortex has caught up to auditory cortex. In primary visual cortex net synapse elimination appears to have started already at that age.[9]

CEREBRAL PLASTICITY

Non-human mammalian adult brain

Reorganization of cortical representation in the adult has been demonstrated in different mammalian species. For

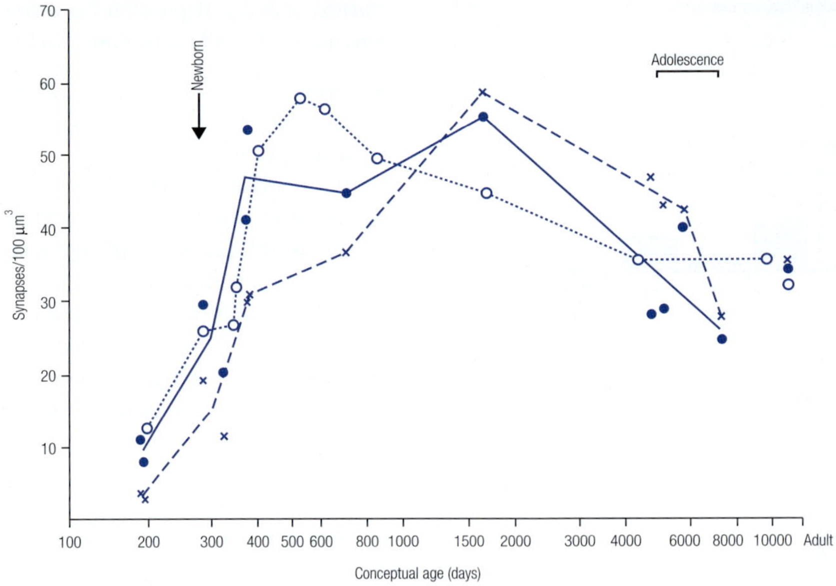

Figure 26.8 Mean synaptic density in synapses/100 μm³ in auditory, calcarine and prefrontal cortex at various ages
Open circles, visual cortex (area 17); filled circles, auditory cortex; x, prefrontal cortex (middle frontal gyrus).
Reproduced with permission from ref. 9.

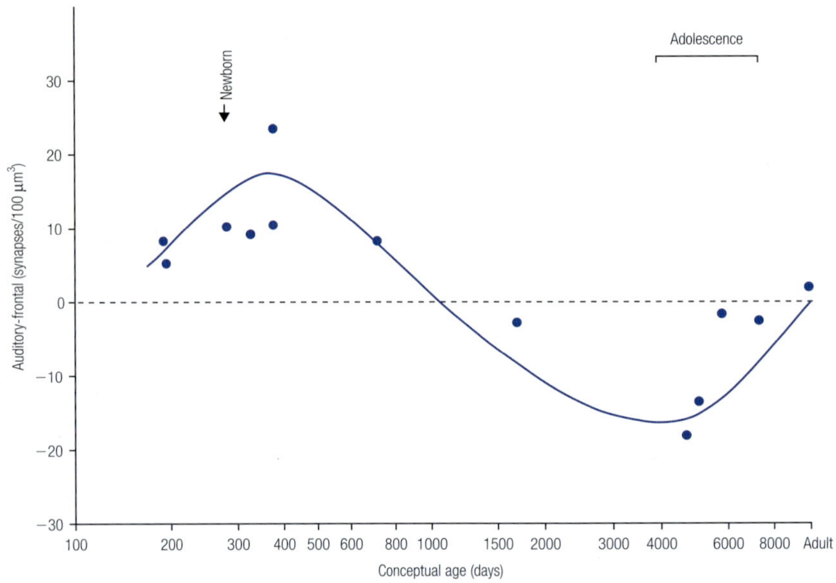

Figure 26.9 Difference scores (synaptic density in auditory cortex – synaptic density in middle frontal gyrus) plotted against conceptual age. The dotted line represents the line of zero difference in time course of synapse formation and elimination between the two cortical regions. The solid line represents a curve of best fit for the data
Reproduced with permission from ref. 9.

example, in the late 1980s, Robertson and Irvine examined the effect of restricted unilateral cochlear lesions on the orderly topographic mapping of sound frequency in the auditory cortex of adult guinea pigs.[10] These lesions, although restricted in spatial extent, resulted in a variety of patterns of histological damage to receptor cells and nerve fibres within the cochlea. Nevertheless, all lesions resulted in permanent losses of sensitivity of the cochlear neural output across a limited frequency range; 35–81 days after such damage to the organ of Corti, the area of contralateral auditory cortex in which the lesioned frequency range would normally have been represented was partly occupied by an expanded representation of sound frequencies adjacent to the frequency range damaged by the lesion.[10]

In the early 1990s, a demonstration of plasticity in the frequency representation of primary auditory cortex in the adult brain of owl monkeys was published by Recanzone and colleagues, who reported increased cortical area of representation of a restricted frequency range in primary auditory cortex that was correlated with performance at a frequency-discrimination task.[11] Monkeys trained for several weeks to discriminate small differences in the frequency of sequentially presented tonal stimuli revealed a progressive improvement in performance with training; at the end of the training period, the tonotopic organization of AI was defined by recording multiple-unit responses at 70–258 cortical locations, and these responses were compared with those derived from three normal monkeys and from two monkeys that received the same auditory stimuli but that were engaged in a tactile discrimination task. The cortical representation, sharpness of tuning and latency of the response were greater for the behaviourally relevant frequencies of trained monkeys when compared with the same frequencies of the control monkeys; the cortical area of representation was the only studied parameter that was correlated with behavioural performance.[11] This experiment showed that natural stimulation can modify the tonotopic organization of AI in the adult primate and that this alteration is correlated with changes in perceptual acuity.

To determine the relative contributions of intrinsic and extrinsic factors to the functional specification of different cortical regions, von Melchner and colleagues studied ferrets, for which it was known that, when retinal projections are redirected neonatally to the auditory thalamus, they have visually responsive cells in auditory thalamus and cortex, form a retinotopic map in auditory cortex and have visual receptive field properties in auditory cortex that are typical of cells in visual cortex. They found that this cross-modal projection and its representation in auditory cortex can mediate visual behaviour; when light stimuli were presented in the portion of the visual field that was seen only by this projection, 'rewired' ferrets (Figure 26.10) responded as if they perceived the stimuli to be visual rather than auditory (Figure 26.11).[12] The authors of this study deduced that the perceptual modality of a neocortical region is instructed to a significant extent by its extrinsic inputs. In addition gratings of different spatial frequencies could be discriminated by the rewired pathway, although the grating acuity was lower than that of the normal visual pathway.

Adult human brain

Plasticity has now been demonstrated in the living human cerebral cortex, using techniques such as functional magnetic resonance imaging (fRMI), positron-emission tomography (PET) and magnetic source imaging (MSI), the last of which involves combining structural magnetic resonance imaging (MRI) with magnetoencephalography (MEG). Some examples are now given.

Flor and colleagues showed that, following upper limb amputation, phantom-limb pain is a perceptual correlate of cortical reorganization.[13] They used MSI, as detailed in Figure 26.12, to study 12 men and 1 woman who had had an arm amputated (either post-traumatically or because of osteosarcoma). As shown in Figure 26.13, there was a large significant positive correlation between the amount of cortical reorganization and the degree of phantom-limb pain (but not non-painful phenomena). Phantom-limb pain was found to explain 83 per cent of the variance in cortical reorganization. These results indicated that phantom-limb pain is related to, and may be a consequence of, plastic changes in primary somatosensory cortex.[13] From Figure

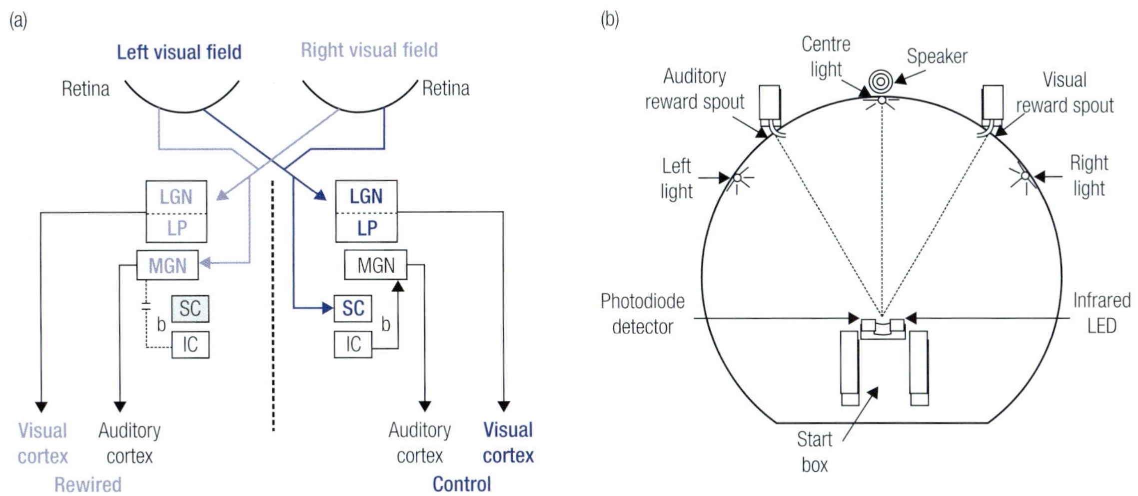

Figure 26.10 Behavioural role of retinal projections routed to the auditory pathway. (a) Pathway from the retina to the visual thalamus, including the lateral geniculate nucleus (LGN) and the lateral posterior nucleus (LP), and to the superior colliculus (SC) in the control hemisphere (right); and to the LGN/LP and medial geniculate nucleus (MGN) in the rewired hemisphere (left). The SC and adjacent brachium (b) of the inferior colliculus (IC) were ablated neonatally in the left hemisphere. Visual projections in each hemisphere represent the contralateral visual field. (b) Apparatus for experiment. Dashed lines denote the borders of the left and right monocular fields and the direction of central gaze. Animals were rewarded at the right spout after a light in the left monocular field, and at the left spout after a sound from a central speaker. Subsequently, their responses to light in the centre or the right monocular field were tested. Animals initiated trials by standing in the start box with their muzzle between an infrared light-emitting diode (LED) and a photodiode detector

Reproduced with permission from ref. 12.

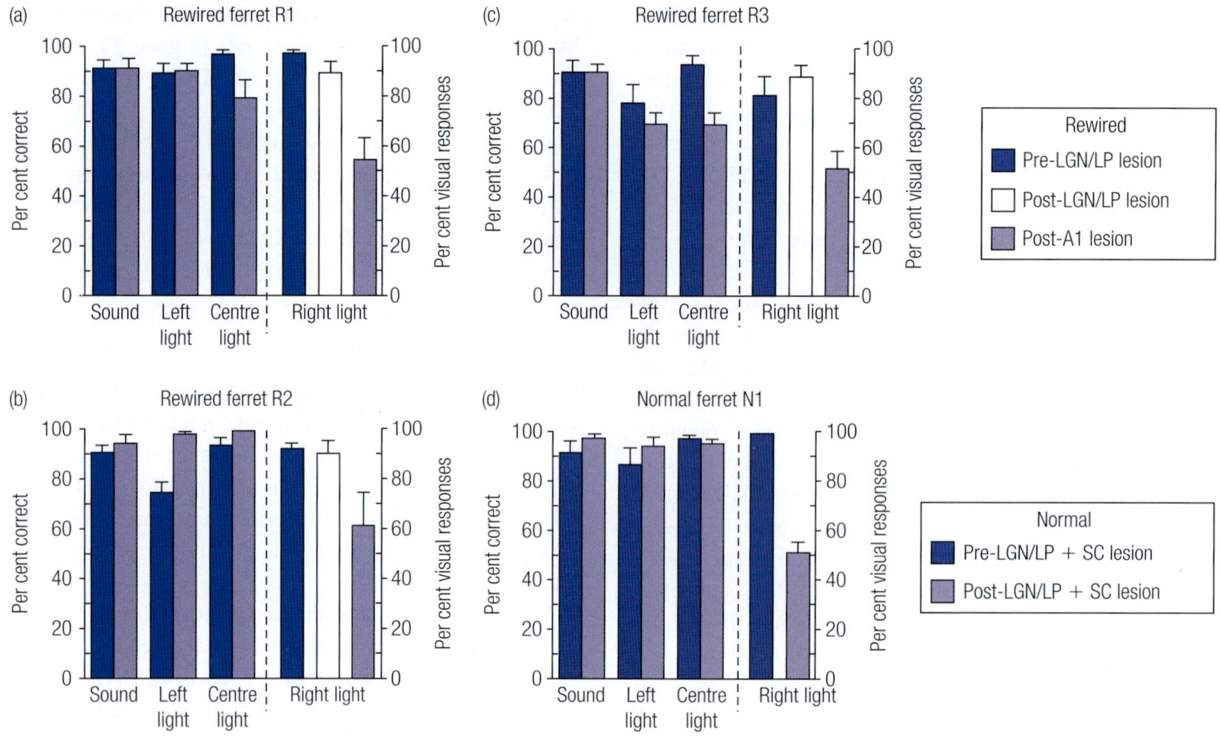

Figure 26.11 Responses of rewired and normal ferrets to sound and light stimuli. (a–c) Responses of rewired ferrets to the various stimuli under three separate conditions: after training with sound and left light stimuli, before the left lateral geniculate nucleus (LGN)/lateral posterior nucleus (LP) lesion (dark blue bars); after the left LGN/LP lesion (white bar; only the response to the right light is shown); and after the left A1 lesion (violet bars). Response bars (mean ± standard deviation) depict performance in the final 10–19 days in the pre-LGN/LP lesion condition, and in the first 10–18 days in the post-LGN/LP lesion and post-A1 lesion conditions. (d) Responses of normal ferret N1 to the stimuli before a lesion of the left LGN/LP and superior colliculus (SC) (blue bars) and after (red bars). Response bars depict performance in the final 9 days in the pre-LGN/LP + SC lesion condition, and in the first 12 days in the post-LGN/LP + SC lesion condition

Reproduced with permission from ref. 12.

26.13 it can be seen that five of the subjects were relatively free of phantom-limb pain. The mean shift in the focus of cortical responsivity to facial stimulation was 0.43 cm for these five pain-free subjects but almost five times higher, at 2.05 cm, for the eight remaining subjects who suffered phantom-limb pain.

When learning to play a stringed musical instrument, it is the digits of the left hand, apart from the thumb, that are used to find notes on the strings. (The right hand is used for bowing or plucking the strings.) The same group showed that the somatosensory cortical representation of the left hand of string-players is expanded compared with controls; the effect was smallest for the left thumb, and no such differences were seen for the representations of the right-hand digits.[14] The amount of cortical reorganization in the representation of the fingering digits was correlated with the age at which the person had begun to play. These results suggest that the representation of different parts of the body in the primary somatosensory cortex of humans depends on

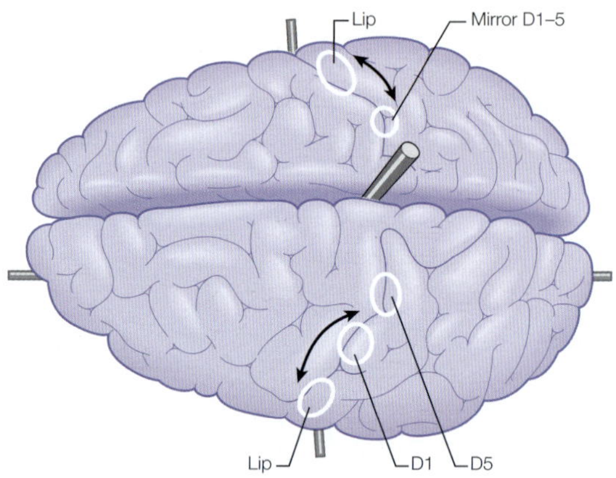

Figure 26.12 Illustration of the method used to determine the degree of cortical reorganization. The centres of the magnetic responses to stimulation on the face and digits are superimposed on to a magnetic resonance imaging (MRI) scan of an individual subject. Using a neuromagnetometer, magnetic fields were recorded from 37 locations over a circular concave area (14.4 cm diameter) above the parietotemporal cortex contralateral to the site of stimulation (first or fifth digit of the intact hand, chin, or lower lip). Magnetoencephalography (MEG) was sampled at 520.5 Hz. For each magnetic field distribution, a single equivalent current dipole (ECD) model was fitted. The ECD locations were mapped on to the cortical surface of Brodmann area 3b, which was reconstructed from an MRI scan. Distances between locations along the curved surface of the somatosensory map can be represented by the distance in the three cortical dimensions (black rods). The arrows connecting the cortical representation of the lip and (i) the midpoint between digits 1 (D1) and 5 (D5) on the intact side (lower arrow) and (ii) the midpoint between the mirror images of the first and fifth digit and the lip on the amputated side (upper arrow) represent the cortical-distance measure used

Reproduced with permission from ref. 13.

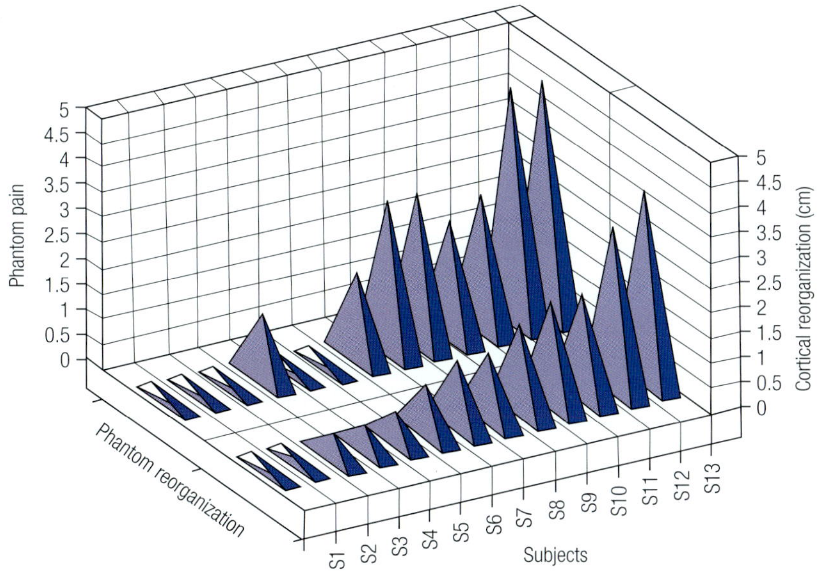

Figure 26.13 Amount of cortical reorganization (in cm) for each of the 13 subjects (S1–S13) plotted against the intensity of phantom-limb pain, as measured using the West Haven-Yale Multidimensional Pain Inventory

Reproduced with permission from ref. 13.

use and changes to conform to the current needs and experiences of the individual.[14]

Liepert and colleagues spatially mapped the motor cortex using focal transcranial magnetic stimulation (TMS) before and after 2 weeks of treatment with constraint-induced movement therapy following stroke.[15] Motor-output areas of the abductor pollicis brevis muscle, motor-evoked potential (MEP) amplitudes and the location of the centre of gravity of motor cortex output were studied. Changes observed after constraint-induced movement therapy included an improvement in motor performance substantially in all patients; an increase of motor output area size and MEP amplitudes, indicating enhanced neuronal excitability in the damaged hemisphere for the target muscles; and a considerable shift in the mean centre of gravity of the motor output maps, indicating the recruitment of motor areas adjacent to the original location. The authors concluded that, even in chronic stroke patients, reduced motor cortex representations of an affected body part can be enlarged and increased in level of excitability by an effective rehabilitation procedure. Furthermore, the cortical regions that produce abnormal slow waves, indicating dysfunctional cortex, become reduced after such rehabilitative therapy.[16]

From these and other studies demonstrating cerebral plasticity in adult humans, Elbert and Rockstroh have advanced the following general principles of cortical reorganization:[16]

- The abolition of sensory input or deafferentation, as produced by amputation or segregation of a sensory nerve, results in the invasion of adjacent cortical representations of intact parts of the sensorium into the cortical representation zone of the affected sensory part.
- Increased use of a receptor pool leads to an expansion of the respective cortical representation zone.
- Training of extremity use after central nervous system injury that affected the cortical tissue representing that body part results in improved extremity function and reorganization in brain activity.
- Cortical reorganization emerges in response to massed practice of behavioural relevant tasks. This generally implies an intense training schedule of several hours a day for several successive days. The absolute amount of training seems less important than the priority of training in daily activity.
- Reorganization through synchronicity of input leads to disarrangement of representational zones.

KEY POINTS

- Corticoneurogenesis is the process of production, allocation, migration and settling of neurons into proper areal and laminar positions within the cortical sheet. During this process, the cortical plate has an inside-out structure and radial glia offer a form of scaffolding from the ventricular zone to the marginal zone, along which postmitotic neuronal cells travel.
- The inside-out pattern of development holds for all areas of the cerebral cortex, even though the time course varies for different cortical regions.
- According to the radial-unit hypothesis, the size of the cerebral cortex depends on the number of contributing radial units, which in turn depends on the number of founder cells.
- Neurogenesis has been demonstrated in the adult human brain.
- Exuberant synaptic connections are an anatomical substrate for plasticity in the developing cerebral cortex.

- The time course of synaptogenesis in human visual cortex resembles that in auditory cortex, except that synapse elimination appears to begin earlier in the visual cortex.
- Reorganization of cortical representation in the adult has been demonstrated in different mammalian species.
- Plasticity has been demonstrated in the living human cerebral cortex using techniques such as fRMI, PET and MSI.
- In humans, cortical reorganization emerges in response to massed practice of behavioural relevant tasks.

REFERENCES

1. Rakic P (2006) A century of progress in corticoneurogenesis: from silver impregnation to genetic engineering. *Cerebral Cortex* **16** (suppl. 1): i3–17.
2. Bystron I, Blakemore C, Rakic P (2008) Development of the human cerebral cortex: Boulder Committee revisited. *Nature Reviews Neuroscience* **9**: 110–22.
3. Hevner RF, Daza RA, Rubenstein JL, *et al.* (2003) Beyond laminar fate: toward a molecular classification of cortical projection/pyramidal neurons. *Developmental Neuroscence* **25**: 139–51.
4. McQuillen PS, Ferriero DM (2005) Perinatal subplate neuron injury: implications for cortical development and plasticity. *Brain Pathology* **15**: 250–60.
5. Folkerth RD, Kinney HC (2008) Disorders of the perinatal period. In S Love, DN Louis, DW Ellison (eds) *Greenfield's Neuropathology*, 8th edn. London: Hodder Arnold.
6. Rakic P (1995) A small step for the cell, a giant leap for mankind: a hypothesis of neocortical expansion during evolution. *Trends in Neuroscience* **18**: 383–8.
7. Eriksson PS, Perfilieva E, Bjork-Eriksson T, *et al.* (1998) Neurogenesis in the adult human hippocampus. *Nature Medicine* **4**: 1313–17.
8. Huttenlocher PR, de Courten C (1987) The development of synapses in striate cortex of man. *Human Neurobiology* **6**: 1–9.
9. Huttenlocher PR, Dabholkar AS (1997) Regional differences in synaptogenesis in human cerebral cortex. *Journal of Comparative Neurology* **387**: 167–78.
10. Robertson D, Irvine DR (1989) Plasticity of frequency organization in auditory cortex of guinea pigs with partial unilateral deafness. *Journal of Comparative Neurology* **282**: 456–71.
11. Recanzone GH, Schreiner CE, Merzenich MM (1993) Plasticity in the frequency representation of primary auditory cortex following discrimination training in adult owl monkeys. *Journal of Neuroscience* **13**: 87–103.
12. Von Melchner L, Pallas SL, Sur M (2000) Visual behaviour mediated by retinal projections directed to the auditory pathway. *Nature* **404**: 871–6.
13. Flor H, Elbert T, Knecht S, *et al.* (1995) Phantom-limb pain as a perceptual correlate of cortical reorganization following arm amputation. *Nature* **375**: 482–4.
14. Elbert T, Pantev C, Wienbruch C, *et al.* (1995) Increased cortical representation of the fingers of the left hand in string players. *Science* **270**: 305–7.
15. Liepert J, Miltner WH, Bauder H, *et al.* (1998) Motor cortex plasticity during constraint-induced movement therapy in stroke patients. *Neuroscience Letters* **250**: 5–8.
16. Elbert T, Rockstroh B (2004) Reorganization of human cerebral cortex: the range of changes following use and injury. *Neuroscientist* **10**: 129–41.

Chapter 27

The neuroendocrine system

Peter Fitzgerald and Timothy G Dinan

INTRODUCTION

Neuroendocrinology is the study of the endocrine role of neuronal cells and the neural regulation of the endocrine system. Many psychiatric disorders are associated with disturbances in neuroendocrine axis function, which thus implicates abnormalities of this axis as being of possible aetiological significance to the development of the psychiatric disorder. Furthermore, understanding fully the biological sequelae of stress is important in determining why some individuals seem resilient to developing psychiatric illness in the face of significant stress while others seem especially vulnerable.

In general terms, the discipline of neuroendocrinology involves the study of the neural regulation of the hypothalamic, pituitary and peripheral end-organ hormone secretions and the study of the effects of each of the endocrine axes on the central nervous system (CNS). It is now recognized that the brain is the principal endocrine gland of the body, not only due to its seminal role in orchestrating the various axes but also because of the multiple target sites within it for hormonal action.

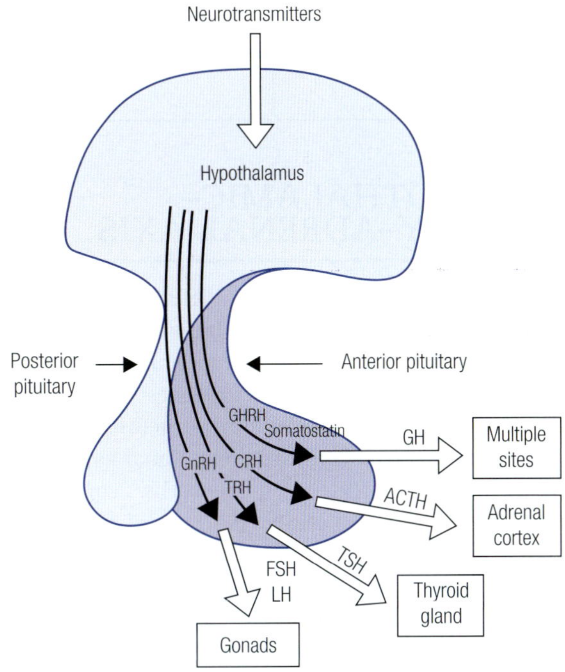

Figure 27.1 Outline of the neuroendocrine axis

ACTH, adrenocorticotropic hormone; CRH, corticotropin-releasing hormone; FSH, follicle-stimulating hormone; GH, growth hormone; GHRH, growth hormone-releasing hormone; GnRH, gonadotropin-releasing hormone; LH, luteinizing hormone; TRH, thyrotropin-releasing hormone; TSH, thyroid-stimulating hormone.

THE HYPOTHALAMIC–PITUITARY HORMONAL AXIS

The primary endocrine regulatory regions are the hypothalamus and pituitary (Figure 27.1).

The hypothalamus is a poorly defined anatomical area situated at the floor of the third ventricle. It consists of several discrete nuclei, which are grouped according to their anatomical location as follows:

- *Anterior:* supraoptic and preoptic nuclei
- *Central:* paraventricular, dorsomedial, ventromedial and arcuate nuclei
- *Posterior:* posterior and mamillary.

The hypothalamus functions as a command centre. It integrates information about the state of the brain and body by way of extensive neuronal projections throughout the CNS and intrinsic chemosensitive neurons that respond to circulating levels of various hormones. The hypothalamus thus plays a seminal role in the maintenance of homeostasis by coordinating the actions of the pituitary gland to respond appropriately to any changes that it detects in the body and environment.

The hypothalamus is the site of synthesis and secretion of a variety of releasing factors, which are released into the portal vasculature at the median eminence, where they pass down the portal veins to the sinusoids surrounding cells of the anterior pituitary and regulate the synthesis and release of various hormones (Table 27.1). In addition to their principal actions as release or release-inhibiting factors for pituitary hormones, the hypothalamic peptides also function in extra-hypothalamic brain regions as neurotransmitter substances, yielding direct brain effects independent of their pituitary actions.

Table 27.1 Hypothalamic and pituitary hormones

Hypothalamic stimulatory hormones	Inhibitory hypothalamic hormones	Anterior pituitary hormones	Posterior pituitary hormones
Corticotropin-releasing hormone (CRH)	Dopamine	Adrenocorticotropic hormone (ACTH)	Antidiuretic hormone (vasopressin)
Arginine vasopressin (AVP)	Somatostatin	Thyroid-stimulating hormone (TSH)	Oxytocin
Thyrotropin-releasing hormone (TRH)		Prolactin	
Growth hormone-releasing hormone (GHRH)		Growth hormone	
Gonadotropin-releasing hormone (GnRH)		Follicle-stimulating hormone (FSH)	
		Luteinizing hormone (LH)	

THE HYPOTHALAMIC–PITUITARY–ADRENAL AXIS

The hypothalamic–pituitary–adrenal (HPA) axis is the core endocrine stress system in humans. It plays a pivotal role in regulating metabolic and immune function and exerts profound effects on the brain (e.g. neurogenesis, neuronal survival, influencing the size of limbic structures, functional effects on memory and contextual emotional appraisal).[1]

Following any threat to homeostasis, corticotropin-releasing hormone (CRH) release is triggered from the parvocellular neurons of the paraventricular nucleus (PVN) in the hypothalamus. Under basal conditions, CRH is the dominant regulator of the axis; in situations of chronic stress, many parvocellular neurons co-express arginine vasopressin (AVP), which plays an important role in sustaining HPA activation (see below).[2,3] CRH and AVP act synergistically on the anterior pituitary corticotrophs to bring about the release of adrenocorticotropic hormone (ACTH), which in turn stimulates increased glucocorticoid (cortisol in humans) secretion from the adrenal glands.[3] The glucocorticoids control homeostasis and play a central role in the ability to cope with the threat or challenge. Glucocorticoids play an important role in both the onset and the termination of the stress response; their secretion is tightly controlled and limited by their own negative feedback effects at both pituitary and brain sites (Figure 27.2).[4] This negative feedback on CRH and ACTH secretion can occur within minutes after the onset of the stress response and thus prevents oversecretion of glucocorticoids and contributes to the reining in of the acute activation of the axis when the threat or stress has passed.[5]

In humans, the circadian rhythm in ACTH and cortisol secretion is entrained to the wake–sleep cycle and is pulsatile in nature, with a frequency of approximately one pulse per hour. The greatest amplitudes occur in the early morning, thus resulting in peak cortisol levels at this time,

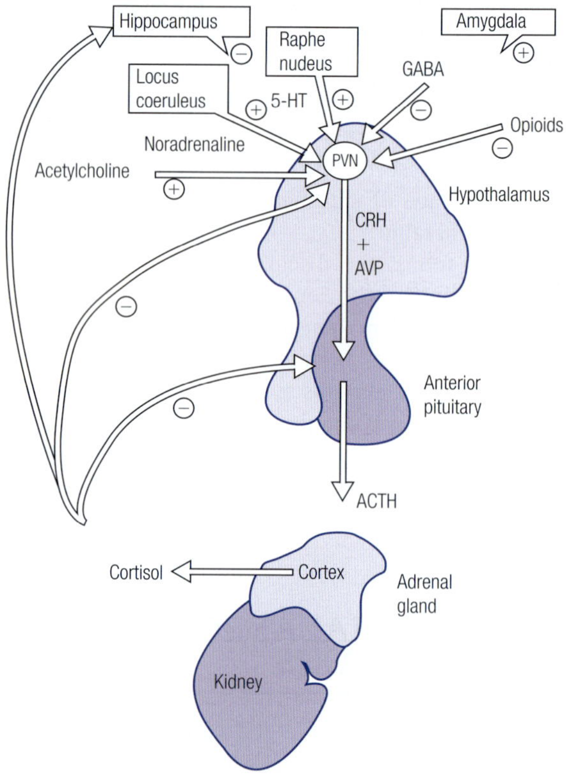

Figure 27.2 Hypothalamic–pituitary–adrenal axis

ACTH, adrenocorticotropic hormone; AVP, arginine vasopressin; CRH, corticotropin-releasing hormone; GABA, γ-aminobutyric acid; 5-HT, 5-hydroxytryptamine; PVN, paraventricular nucleus.

with a trough in secretion occurring in the evening and early night.

The principal mechanism of action of cortisol throughout the body is through activation of intracellular receptors, which subsequently translocate to the nucleus and bind to specific DNA sequences, thus modulating gene transcription.[6] There are two major receptors for cortisol: type 1 (or mineralocorticoid receptor, MR) and type 2 (or glucocorticoid receptor, GR). Centrally the MR is mainly expressed either alone or together with the GR in hippocampal neurons, while the GR receptor has a more ubiquitous distribution within brain neurons. The MR has a ten-fold higher affinity for cortisol than the GR does, and thus the MR monitors basal diurnal fluctuation in cortisol while the GR becomes progressively occupied only at peaks of cortisol secretion and after a stressful stimulus.[7,8] The GR is therefore believed to be more important in the regulation of the stress response when endogenous cortisol levels are high, such as in major depression (see below).

In addition to receiving negative feedback from cortisol, the hypothalamus is influenced by neuronal input from cortical pathways, including those derived from the hippocampus and the amygdala. Whether feedback on to the PVN is excitatory or inhibitory depends on the location and type of the activated receptor. For example, activation of the MR at the hippocampus and amygdala exerts negative feedback inhibition on CRH, while GR stimulation in the amygdala results in an increase in CRH in response to stress.[9,10] A wide variety of neurotransmitters also influence the hypothalamic PVN regulation of the HPA. These transmitters include serotonin, noradrenaline, acetylcholine and the opioids. Furthermore, the pro-inflammatory cytokines tumour necrosis factor alpha (TNF-α), interleukin 1 (IL-1) and interleukin 6 (IL-6) are primary HPA-stimulating cytokines that act directly on the hypothalamic paraventricular neurons to stimulate CRH production.[11]

It has become increasingly recognized that prolonged activation of the HPA axis exposes the brain and body to the deleterious effects of excessive glucocorticoid secretion, with pathological consequences, including hypertension, diabetes, formation of atherosclerotic plaques and impaired immune function. Centrally, the hippocampus suffers from atrophy of its neuronal dendrites and impaired neurogenesis, which is thought to mediate the disruption to long-term potentiation and impaired memory performance observed in states of chronic glucocorticoid excess.[12] Furthermore, chronic stress has been shown to increase dendritic arborization in the amygdala, which may in part be why individuals can have difficulty forgetting traumatic events.

HPA axis functioning in major depression

Multiple disturbances at different levels of the HPA axis have been described in patients with major depression, with hyperactivity of the axis in a significant subgroup of people with depression (50–70%) being one of the most consistent and important findings in biological psychiatry. This increase in cortisol levels has been explained by both increased forward drive in the axis and decreased negative feedback.

The following disturbances in HPA axis functioning (indicating an overactive axis) are documented in major depression.

- Elevated cortisol levels
- Dexamethasone non-suppression of cortisol
- Enhanced adrenal gland volume as measured by computed tomography (CT) or magnetic resonance imaging (MRI)
- Blunted ACTH release in response to CRH (CRH stimulation test)
- Enhanced ACTH release in response to CRH when pretreated with dexamethasone (DEX-CRH test)
- Elevated CRH in the cerebrospinal fluid
- Enhanced cortisol response to synacthen (ACTH stimulation test).

The dexamethasone suppression test (DST) was popularized in psychiatry by Bernard Carroll as a means of investigating the functional integrity of negative feedback control of the HPA axis.[13,14] Dexamethasone is a potent synthetic glucocorticoid that binds primarily to GRs in the anterior pituitary and thus suppresses ACTH and cortisol secretion via a negative feedback mechanism. The most common form of the test involves the administration of 1 mg dexamethasone at 11 p.m., with subsequent cortisol measurements at intervals over the following 24 h, thus testing the functional integrity of the GRs (i.e. GR responsiveness) in mediating inhibition on the axis. Low-dose DSTs (0.5 mg and 0.25 mg) have also been used, in particular to investigate disorders characterized by enhanced suppression (e.g. post-traumatic stress disorder, PTSD; see below). There are several hundred published studies reporting on DST in depression, all reporting that approximately 50 per cent of people with major depression fail to adequately suppress cortisol levels after administration of 1 mg dexamethasone.[15] The test lacks adequate specificity, however, and positive results are also seen in other disorders, including dementia, eating disorders and schizophrenia. The DST has also been used to follow the course of treatment in patients who had a positive DST while depressed. Those patients whose HPA axis recovers to normality after successful treatment for depression tend to remain in remission for longer than those who still have an abnormal DST.[16]

In addition to impaired negative feedback control of HPA in major depression, there is an increased forward drive promoting the hypercortisolism.[17] ACTH responses to exogenous CRH are often blunted in patients with depression, as demonstrated by the CRH stimulation test, in which 100 μg CRH is given intravenously with subsequent measurement of ACTH and cortisol response. This blunting is thought to reflect a down-regulation of CRH receptors on the corticotrophs of the anterior pituitary and a restricted secretory response of ACTH to CRH caused by elevated basal cortisol levels. Despite a blunted ACTH response to CRH, a normal cortisol response is maintained due to an overactive HPA axis inducing a hyperplastic adrenal cortex that is thus hypersensitive to ACTH stimulation. Furthermore, CRH neuronal hyperactivity is generally reduced by antidepressant therapy, and persistent alteration in HPA axis function despite compliance with antidepressant medication is a marker for a poor response to such treatment.

The CRH test has also been combined with pretreatment with dexamethasone (DEX-CRH test), which results in enhanced rather than blunted ACTH and cortisol responses in patients with depression compared with healthy controls.[18] A multicentre study by Kunugi and colleagues demonstrated significantly enhanced pituitary–adrenocortical responses to the DEX-CRH test in in-patients with depression. Furthermore, restoration of normal HPA axis response occurred with clinical responses to treatment of depression, particularly in patients who underwent electroconvulsive therapy (ECT).[19] Interestingly, a further DEX-CRH study by a different Japanese group demonstrated that the normalization of HPA axis dysfunction subsequent to successful treatment of depression correlated with a restoration of normal cerebral glucose metabolism in prefrontal cortical and limbic brain areas.[20]

We have previously focused on the role of vasopressin in the increased HPA forward drive seen in depression. We examined a cohort of subjects with depression on two separate occasions, with CRH alone, and with the combination of CRH and desmopressin (ddAVP), an analogue of AVP.[21] Consistent with previous findings, a significant blunting of ACTH output to CRH alone was noted. However, when ddAVP was combined with CRH in our study, the release of ACTH in patients with depression and in healthy volunteers became indistinguishable, thus indicating that, although CRH1 receptors are down-regulated in depression, a concomitant up-regulation of the V3 (also known as V1b) receptor takes place. In a further study assessing ACTH and cortisol responses to ddAVP in major depression, we observed increased responses in the patients with depression compared with the healthy controls, providing further support for up-regulation of the anterior pituitary V3 receptor in this disorder.[22] Interestingly, plasma AVP levels have been found to be correlated positively with cortisol in patients with depression,[23,24] and a single-nucleotide polymorphism (SNP) for the V3 receptor has been found to be protective against depression.[25]

A fact that distinguishes the hypercortisolaemia seen in major depression from that of Cushing's disease/syndrome (characterized by excessive glucocorticoid secretion secondary to a pituitary or adrenal tumour) is that in major depression the amplitude and timing of the circadian rhythm appear to remain intact, although the peak and nadir in circulating cortisol concentrations are elevated. In patients with Cushing's disease/syndrome, however, the ACTH and cortisol circadian rhythms are generally lost due to the constant production of either one or both of these hormones by the pituitary adenoma or adrenal tumour. This may be why hypercortisolaemic patients with depression do not develop the physical changes that are characteristic in Cushing's disease/syndrome. In addition, there is evidence that, in at least some tissues of the body, the GR is desensitized in patients with depression. In relation to this, we demonstrated a marked impairment in the normal cutaneous blanching response to topical corticosteroid administration in patients with major depression compared with healthy controls, thus implicating impaired GR function in mediating cutaneous vasoconstriction in this group.[26]

CRH derived from parvocellular neurons of the hypothalamus is the primary stimulus to ACTH secretion. CRH receptors are not limited to the pituitary corticotrophs, however, but are distributed widely throughout the cerebral cortex and limbic system.[27] CRH has thus been shown to modulate diverse neurotransmitter systems, including glutamate, dopamine, serotonin and noradrenaline. Reciprocal excitatory interactions exist between the CRHergic pathways and the brainstem sympathetic locus coeruleus–noradrenergic system. CRH activates the locus coeruleus and thus increases noradrenaline release from it; in turn, noradrenaline activates both hypothalamic CRH and the amygdala.[28] It is thought that such reciprocal stimulation may contribute to the sleep disturbance and anxiety symptoms seen in major depression.

HPA axis functioning in other psychiatric disorders

The HPA axis has been studied in a number of anxiety disorders, most notably PTSD. The findings in other anxiety disorders have been modest – cortisol secretion has not been associated with panic attacks per se, and dexamethasone non-suppression occurs in only approximately 17 per cent of patients with panic disorder.[29–31] CRH challenge studies have been inconsistent, with some demonstrating a decreased ACTH response when compared with healthy controls[32] but others finding a normal response.[33] Overall, studies of anxiety disorders other than PTSD would suggest either a normal or a modestly increased HPA axis function in these disorders.

With regard to PTSD, the majority of studies demonstrate reduced baseline cortisol levels in PTSD in addition to enhanced cortisol suppression to low-dose dexamethasone administration.[34] Furthermore, somewhat counterintuitively given the hypocortisolism above, there is considerable evidence that CRH levels are increased in PTSD.[35] There has been growing evidence that cortisol-related alterations in PTSD may reflect an underlying vulnerability to the development of the disorder following trauma exposure. In longitudinal studies, lower cortisol levels observed soon after the experience of trauma have been found to be associated with the future development of PTSD, and relative hypocortisolism has also been associated with prior trauma exposure (a risk factor for PTSD).[36,37] Genetic susceptibility may also be an important factor, and low cortisol levels have been shown to be related inversely to PTSD symptom severity in a subgroup of combat veterans displaying a particular glucocorticoid receptor polymorphism (the Bcl1 GC genotype) that results in increased glucocorticoid sensitivity.[38]

Dysfunction of the HPA axis characterized by hypocortisolism has also been consistently observed in chronic fatigue syndrome (CFS).[39,40] A case-control study, which recruited from a general population sample, compared childhood trauma rates and awakening salivary cortisol responses in patients with CFS and healthy controls. The study demonstrated that a decreased cortisol response was associated with childhood trauma in CFS.[41] Indeed, decreased cortisol responses to awakening were observed only in those subjects with CFS who reported exposure to childhood trauma and not in individuals with CFS but without such exposure. The authors suggested that hypocortisolism may reflect a marker for developmental risk for CFS rather than a correlate of the CFS itself. The role of childhood trauma in rendering an individual susceptible to future psychiatric disorder is discussed further below.

It has been suggested that the HPA axis may have some involvement in the development of psychotic disorders by increasing brain dopaminergic activity.[42–44] Generally, in relation to schizophrenia, similar abnormalities to those seen in depression are described in the literature, although with less consistency and to a lesser degree. Although there have been inconsistent reports of elevated cortisol levels in subjects with psychotic disorders,[45,46] the DST has been more consistent, with most studies demonstrating impaired negative feedback of the axis (i.e. higher levels of non-suppression) in subjects with schizophrenia compared with healthy controls.[47,48] Some studies have observed a greater degree of suppression in patients with a higher symptom load.[49,50] While antipsychotic medications can affect HPA activation in a general dampening manner, studies on drug-naive patients with schizophrenia have consistently observed HPA dysfunction characterized by overactivation of the axis.[51,52] The hippocampus has important inhibitory regulatory actions on the HPA axis as described above and, in relation to psychotic disorders, studies have demonstrated reduced hippocampal glucocorticoid receptor numbers in addition to a smaller hippocampal volume.[53,54] Furthermore, the pituitary gland has been found consistently to be larger in at least the early stages of psychotic disorders, a finding that is independent of treatment with antipsychotic medications, thus ruling out enlargement secondary to effects on prolactin (see below), but it is thought to be mediated by an increase in the size and number of the pituitary's ACTH-producing cells.[55] Research has observed that individuals at ultra-high risk of developing psychosis who go on to develop a psychotic disorder already have an enlarged pituitary gland in the months before psychosis onset compared with high-risk individuals who do not go on to develop psychosis.[56] Taking all of the above together, these lines of research suggest that HPA axis dysfunction may have an important role in the development of psychosis and is an interesting area of future research.

THE HYPOTHALAMIC–PITUITARY–THYROID AXIS

Thyroid hormones are fundamental to normal brain development and regulate neuronal growth and synaptogenesis. They are involved in maintaining optimal metabolism in multiple organ systems and play a vital role in temperature regulation.

The functioning of the hypothalamic–pituitary–thyroid (HPT) axis has been studied extensively in psychiatric illnesses, particularly in depressive disorders, due to the long-standing observation that patients with hypothyroidism and euthyroid patients with depression share many clinical features, including cognitive impairment, lethargy and low mood.[57] Indeed, it is recognized that 30 per cent of patients with mood disorders have some form of thyroid dysfunction.[58]

The HPT axis is driven centrally by secretion of thyrotropin-releasing hormone (TRH) from the parvocellular region of the PVN of the hypothalamus (Figure 27.3). TRH is released into the portal circulation and thereafter binds to receptors on thyrotroph cells of the anterior pituitary, where it stimulates the synthesis and release of thyroid-stimulating hormone (TSH). In addition to TRH, the hypothalamus also releases an inhibitory hormone of TSH called somatostatin. TSH stimulates the synthesis and secretion of two thyroid hormones from the thyroid gland – tri-iodothyronine (T3) and tetra-iodothyronine (T4). T3 is the more biologically active form. T4 is the predominant form released from the thyroid, and subsequent de-iodination to form T3 is performed by the target organs, including the brain. TRH synthesis and release are regulated primarily by T3 through a negative feedback mechanism. TRH release is inhibited by serotonergic input to the hypothalamic nucleus, while dopamine has a net stimulatory effect.

Centrally thyroid nuclear receptors are particularly abundant in the hippocampus, but they are expressed throughout the brain. There is extensive intraneuronal

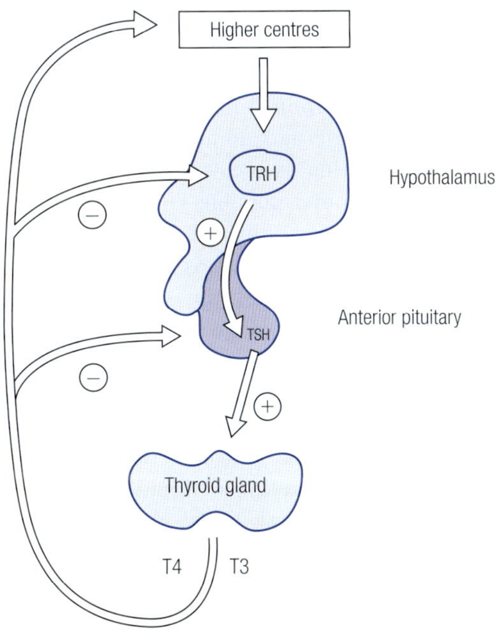

Figure 27.3 Hypothalamic–pituitary–thyroid axis
T3, tri-iodothyronine; T4, tetra-iodothyronine; TRH, thyrotropin-releasing hormone.

co-localization of TRH with other neuroactive substances, including 5-hydroxytryptamine (5-HT), substance P and dopamine.[59]

There has been extensive investigation of the HPT axis in major depressive disorder. About 15 per cent of patients with depression have evidence of autoimmune thyroiditis.[60] It has long been established that approximately a quarter of patients with major depression have an impaired TSH response to TRH administration, which has been suggested to indicate hypersecretion of TRH in this disorder (with subsequent down-regulation of anterior pituitary TRH receptors).[61] Furthermore, the normal nocturnal rise of TSH that occurs in the hours after midnight can be lost in patients with depression,[62] but sleep deprivation restores it.[63] Subclinical (or grade II) hypothyroidism, characterized by normal thyroid hormone concentrations but elevated basal TSH levels and an exaggerated TSH response to TRH, is also overrepresented in major depression and is a known risk factor for treatment resistance.[64]

Clinical studies have shown that exogenous thyroid hormone can augment treatment-resistant depression.[65,66] The evidence base has been improved by publication of the Sequenced Treatment Alternatives to Relieve Depression (STAR*D) programme, which was a pragmatic effectiveness study that used remission of symptoms as its main outcome measure. At stage 3 of this trial, 24.7 per cent of patients with treatment-resistant depression remitted with T3 augmentation (*v.* 15.9% of patients who received lithium augmentation), and T3 was found to be significantly better tolerated than lithium.[67] Sokolov and colleagues found that responders to T3 augmentation had lower circulating TSH and higher circulating T4 before antidepressant treatment compared with non-responders.[68] There have been inconsistent reports from small studies of concomitant T3 administration accelerating the response to antidepressant therapy when initiating treatment for depression.[69,70]

The mechanism of action of thyroid hormone augmentation has yet to be determined fully, but it may act through increasing serotonergic and noradrenergic neurotransmission (possibly by acting as a co-transmitter in the case of noradrenaline).[71] Another possible mechanism of action is via restoration of central thyroid hormone homeostasis, which may be disturbed in severe depression due to cortisol-induced inhibition of the enzyme 5-deiodinase. This enzyme converts T4 to T3 within the CNS, and therefore elevated cortisol levels seen in depression may impair optimum thyroid hormone functioning within the brain.[72] Finally, T3 augmentation may modulate cerebral blood flow. Functional imaging research has indicated that hypothyroid subjects display a significant reduction in brain activity and cerebral blood flow compared with euthyroid controls. In relation to mood disorders, Marangell and colleagues demonstrated an inverse relationship between TSH and cerebral blood flow in unmedicated patients with mood disorders who were free from overt thyroid disease, and found the greatest reduction in blood flow to be in those areas of the brain that have been implicated in depression: the left dorsolateral prefrontal cortex (PFC) and the medial PFC.[73]

The HPT dysregulation seen in mood disorders may be related to underlying HPA axis abnormalities. The blunted response of TSH to TRH administration in depression has been shown to be strongly correlated with the ACTH response to CRH challenge. Glucocorticoids have been shown to inhibit TSH secretion, and in vitro studies of cultured hypothalamic neurons have demonstrated glucocorticoid-induced stimulation of TRH gene expression, an action that is inhibited by tricyclic antidepressants and selective serotonin reuptake inhibitors (SSRI).[74–77]

THE PROLACTIN AXIS

Prolactin (PRL) is a polypeptide hormone that is predominantly synthesized and secreted from lactotroph cells of the anterior pituitary gland. It was discovered by Riddle and colleagues in 1933, who demonstrated its ability to elicit lactation in mammals, and has since been found to be involved in a vast array of functions, extending from reproduction and lactation to roles in metabolism, behaviour, immunoregulation and osmoregulation.[78]

Hyperprolactinaemia is a potentially serious adverse outcome associated with significant morbidity such as hypogonadism, leading to osteoporosis and increased risk of hip fracture.[79] A growing body of evidence has linked elevations in prolactin to a possible increased risk of certain cancers (most notably breast, but also prostate) and pituitary tumours.[80–83]

Secretion of PRL by pituitary lactotroph cells is predominantly under the control of dopamine, which exerts a tonic inhibitory influence on the hormone's synthesis and release. The dopamine is derived from a neuronal population in the arcuate nucleus of the hypothalamus and reaches the anterior pituitary via transport through the long portal veins. Dopamine exerts a direct effect on the lactotrophs by binding to the dopamine type 2 receptor expressed on their cell membranes, ultimately inhibiting both synthesis and secretion of PRL.[79] This tonic upstream inhibition conveys a unique characteristic to PRL secretion compared with other pituitary hormones, whose secretory tone is determined largely by stimulatory agents. This discrepancy stems from PRL's lack of a single target organ to provide a classical negative feedback loop (e.g. in contrast to ACTH). Also, lactotrophs have much higher basal secretory activity compared with other endocrine cells and are thus more responsive to inhibition than stimulation.

With respect to psychiatry, this is of clinical relevance due to the action of antipsychotic medications on the D2 receptor. All antipsychotic medications can affect prolactin levels via binding to dopamine receptors on the lactotroph cell membrane, with those that have potent D2 receptor antagonism and poorest blood–brain barrier permeability having the greatest and most sustained effect. Thus, the typical antipsychotic agents have all been associated with sustained hyperprolactinaemia; of the atypical medications, those that cross the blood–brain barrier easily and exhibit fast dissociation from the dopamine receptor have the least impact on serum prolactin concentrations (e.g. clozapine, quetiapine). All atypical antipsychotic agents result in at least a transient rise in PRL, however, and some can display persistent hyperprolactinaemia akin to the typical agents by virtue of their potent D2 antagonism (e.g. risperidone, paliperidone, amisulpride). Prevalence rates of hyperprolactinaemia in patients prescribed typical antipsychotics are high, with estimations ranging from 33 per cent to over 80 per cent.[84,85] In relation to depot formulations, studies have reported hyperprolactinaemia in approximately 35 per cent of patients.[84] Prevalence rates of hyperprolactinaemia in patients prescribed atypical antipsychotic agents vary significantly according to the individual drug, with those classified as 'prolactin-sparing' having rates from less than 5 per cent to 30 per cent.[86]

Abnormally high PRL levels may be clinically silent for many years, or the most common symptoms of hyperprolactinaemia such as sexual dysfunction may be undisclosed by the patient or erroneously ascribed to the underlying disease process rather than as an adverse effect of medication. Concerns regarding the possible impact of persistent hyperprolactinaemia have only recently come into focus as the widespread use of atypical antipsychotics as first-line agents has shifted attention away from the main problems of their forerunners (extrapyramidal side effects, tardive dyskinesia) to newer concerns regarding metabolic and endocrine abnormalities, including hyperprolactinaemia. There has been a growing awareness of the higher risk of a range of physical illnesses in patients with long-term mental illness, and consideration of the risk of physical disease complications must now be a prominent factor when selecting treatments for mental illness,[87] not least of these considerations being the potential for sustained hyperprolactinaemia.

THE HYPOTHALAMIC–PITUITARY–GROWTH HORMONE AXIS

The release of GH from the anterior pituitary is under the combined regulation of the hypothalamic pituitary peptides growth hormone-releasing hormone (GHRH) and somatostatin. The former has a stimulatory action and the latter an inhibitory action. These peptides in turn are regulated by classic neurotransmitters such as acetylcholine, noradrenaline, dopamine and γ-aminobutyric acid (GABA).

It was first demonstrated in 1982 that stimulation of noradrenergic alpha-2 receptors brought about the release of GH and that such a response is blunted in major depression.[88] This was interpreted as indicative of a subsensitivity of the alpha-2 receptor in depression. Ansseau and colleagues found blunted GH release following clonidine (an alpha-2 agonist) challenge in patients with mania.[89] Similar responses were reported by Dinan and colleagues in patients challenged with the noradrenergic reuptake inhibitor desipramine.[90] It is interesting to note that cholinergic inputs also regulate GH release, and that both depressed and manic patients challenged with the acetylcholinesterase inhibitor pyridostigmine show exaggerated release of GH. Through the use of such neuroendocrine challenge tests, the data indicate an imbalance between noradrenergic and cholinergic regulation in mood disorders.

RESILIENCE AND VULNERABILITY TO STRESS

Why some individuals seem impervious or resilient to the potential negative consequences of stressful life events while in others the same stress precipitates psychiatric illness is an area of increasing attention and research. A proposed model for understanding resilience and vulnerability for the development of stress-related disorders is the 'three-hit model' posited by de Kloet and colleagues.[91] This proposes that genetic variability in conjunction with early life experiences primes the brain's response to major stressful events in later life.

Genetic variants of the MR and GR that may potentially predispose an individual to an abnormal stress response have therefore been the subject of much investigation. One such type of genetic variant is the SNP, which gives rise to differential expression of the same gene (alleles). Several SNPs within the GR and MR genes have been tested for functionality and have been found to change the regulation of the HPA axis at different levels.[92] For example, Wust and colleagues demonstrated significantly different HPA axis responsivity dependent on genetic GR variant status in a male twin cohort study.[93] Carriers of the GR polymorphism N363S showed higher saliva and plasma cortisol responses compared with controls to both a psychological stressor (Trier social stress test) and following ACTH challenge, while homozygotes for another GR polymorphism (Bcl1) demonstrated lower cortisol responses as compared with controls. Marked sex differences also appear to exist with respect to GR polymorphisms on stress variability, as observed by Kumsta and colleagues, who found in their study that women with the Bcl1 G/G genotype had the highest cortisol levels, while men with the same genotype had the lowest cortisol levels.[94] Characterization of patients with stress-related psychiatric disorders according to different GR genotypes has been carried out, with as yet inconsistent findings. A German study of patients with depression found significantly elevated frequencies of the Bcl1 and ER22/23EK GR SNPs in their sample (n = 342) but failed to demonstrate a significant genotype effect when the reactivity of the HPA axis was tested in subjects by administration of a DEX-CRH challenge.[95] However, response to antidepressant treatment was improved in carriers of ER22/23EK. Brouwer and colleagues observed different treatment responses in their study that demonstrated substantially lower response rates in patients with depression who were carriers of the Bcl1 polymorphism.[96]

In relation to literature on the long-lasting physiological effects of early childhood trauma, a growing body of evidence is emerging to indicate that early life events can programme abnormal activation of CRHergic pathways, including HPA axis functioning into adulthood, which may thus confer a vulnerability for the development of psychiatric illness. Animal research employing maternal deprivation paradigms in neonatal rodents and non-human primates has demonstrated that maternally deprived animals exhibit HPA axis changes that persist into adulthood and that resemble depressed adult individuals (such as hyperactivity of the HPA axis and central CRH-containing pathways).[97,98] Human research has demonstrated that subjects who are abused during childhood exhibit a markedly enhanced stress response and that this remains into adulthood.[99–101] It seems that if significant stress is experienced early in life within a genetic window of vulnerability, then this permanently programmes the individual's subsequent responsiveness to future stressful events. It is also important to highlight that any such programming that may occur could apply to other closely related systems in addition to the HPA axis in a mutually permissive manner. Evidence that links childhood trauma with increased inflammatory markers in adulthood[102–104] may be part of the same pathophysiological process as that of sustained HPA axis abnormalities, given that both systems are intimately connected and bidirectionally influenced. Such a model provides a plausible and dynamic biological framework for understanding the link between early stressful life events and a sustained vulnerability for a range of stress-related illnesses throughout the lifespan.

KEY POINTS

- Neuroendocrinology is the study of the endocrine role of neuronal cells and the neural regulation of the endocrine system.
- The core components of the neuroendocrine axis are the hypothalamus, the pituitary gland and the various end-organ sites (e.g. adrenal gland, thyroid gland).
- Regulation of the axis is largely through a combination of forward drive by hypothalamic releasing factors and negative feedback control by the various end-organ hormones. Higher brain centres, neurotransmitters and the immune system also influence the axis.
- Many psychiatric disorders are associated with disturbances in neuroendocrine axis function, which thus implicates abnormalities of this axis as being of possible aetiological significance to the development of the psychiatric disorder.
- Early childhood traumatic events may result in permanent alterations to the neuroendocrine axis.

REFERENCES

1. Herbert J, Goodyer IM, Grossman AB, *et al.* (2006) Do corticosteroids damage the brain? *Journal of Neuroendocrinology* **18**: 393–411.
2. Vale W, Spiess J, Rivier C, Rivier J (1981) Characterisation of a 41 residue ovine hypothalamic peptide that stimulates secretion of the corticotropin and beta-endorphin. *Science* **213**: 1394–9.
3. Dinan TG, Scott LV (2005) Anatomy of melancholia: focus on the hypothalamic-pituitary-adrenal axis overactivation and the role of vasopressin. *Journal of Anatomy* **207**: 259–64.
4. De Kloet ER, Joels M, Holsboer F (2005) Stress and the brain: from adaptation to disease. *Nature Reviews. Neuroscience* **6**: 463–75.
5. Keller-Wood ME, Dallman MF (1985) Corticosteroid inhibition of ACTH secretion. *Endocrine Reviews* **5**: 1–24.
6. Schaaf M, Cidlowski JA (2002) Molecular mechanisms of glucocorticoid action and resistance. *Journal of Steroid Biochemistry and Molecular Biology* **83**: 37–48.
7. Ruel JM, de Kloet ER (1985) Two receptor systems for corticosterone in the rat brain: microdistribution and differential occupation. *Endocrinology* **117**: 2505–11.
8. De Kloet ER, DeRijk RH, Meijer OC (2007) Therapy insight: is there an imbalanced response of mineralocorticoid and glucocorticoid receptors in depression? *Nature Clinical Practice. Endocrinology and Metabolism* **3**: 168–79.
9. Muller MB, Wurst W (2004) Getting closer to affective disorders: the role of CRH receptor systems. *Trends in Molecular Medicine* **10**: 409–15.
10. Reul JM, Holsboer F (2002) Corticotropin-releasing factor receptors 1 and 2 in anxiety and depression. *Current Opinions in Pharmacology* **2**: 23–33.
11. Dentino AN, Pieper CF, Rao KMK, *et al.* (1999) Association of interleukin-6 and other biological variables with depression in older people living in the community. *Journal of the American Geriatric Society* **47**: 6–11.
12. Sheline YI, Wang PW, Gado MH, *et al.* (1996) Hippocampal atrophy in recurrent major depression. *Proceedings of the National Academy of Sciences of the USA* **93**: 3908–13.
13. Carroll BJ (1985) Dexamethasone-suppression test: a review of contemporary confusion. *Journal of Clinical Psychiatry* **46**: 13–24.
14. Carroll BJ, Feinberg M, Greden JF, *et al.* (1981) A specific laboratory test for the diagnosis of melancholia: Standardization, validation, and clinical utility. *Archives of General Psychiatry* **38**: 15–22.
15. Holsboer F (2003) Corticotropin-releasing hormone modulators and depression. *Current Opinion in Investigational Drugs* **4**: 46–50.
16. Kin NM, Nair NPV, Amin M, *et al.* (1997) The dexamethasone suppression test and treatment outcome in

elderly depressed patients participating in a placebo-controlled multicenter trial involving moclobemide and nortriptyline. *Biological Psychiatry* **42**: 925–31.
17. Heit S, Owens MJ, Plotsky P, Nemeroff CB (1997) Corticotropin-releasing factor, stress and depression. *Neuroscientist* **3**: 186–94.
18. Sher L (2006) Combined dexamethasone suppression-corticotropin-releasing hormone stimulation test in studies of depression, alcoholism, and suicidal behaviour. *Scientific World Journal* **31**: 1398–404.
19. Kunugi H, Ida I, Owashi T, *et al.* (2006) Assessment of the dexamethasone/CRH test as a state-dependent marker for hypothalamic-pituitary-adrenal (HPA) axis abnormalities in major depressive episode: a multicenter study. *Neuropsychopharmacology* **31**: 212–20
20. Aihara M, Ida I, Yuuki N, *et al.* (2007) HPA axis dysfunction in unmedicated major depressive disorder and its normalization by pharmacotherapy correlates with alteration of neural activity in prefrontal cortex and limbic/paralimbic regions. *Psychiatry Research* **15**: 245–56.
21. Dinan TG, Lavelle E, Scott LV, *et al.* (1999) Desmopressin normalizes the blunted adrenocorticotropin response to corticotrophin-releasing hormone in melancholic depression: evidence of enhanced vasopressinergic responsivity. *Journal of Clinical Endocrinology and Metabolism* **84**: 2238–40.
22. Dinan TG, Lavelle E, Scott LV (2004) Further neuroendocrine evidence of enhanced V3 receptor responses in melancholic depression. *Psychological Medicine* **34**: 169–72
23. Brunner J, Keck ME, Landgraf R, *et al.* (2002) Vasopressin in CSF and plasma in depressed suicide attempters: preliminary results. *European Neuropsychopharmacology* **12**: 489–94
24. De Winter RF, van Hemert AM, DeRijk RH, *et al.* (2003) Anxious-retarded depression: relation with plasma vasopressin and cortisol. *Neuropsychopharmacology* **28**: 140–47.
25. Van West D, Del-Favero J, Aulchenko Y, *et al.* (2004) A major SNP haplotype of the arginine vasopressin 1b receptor protects against recurrent major depression. *Molecular Psychiatry* **9**: 287–92.
26. Fitzgerald P, O'Brien S, Scott LV, *et al.* (2006) Cutaneous glucocorticoid receptor sensitivity and pro-inflammatory cytokine levels in antidepressant resistant depression. *Psychological Medicine* **36**: 37–44.
27. Aguilera G, Flores M, Carvallo P, *et al.* (1990) Receptors for corticotrophin-releasing factor. In EB De Souza, CB Nemeroff (eds) *Corticotropin-Releasing Factor: Basic and Clinical Studies of a Neuropeptide.* Boca Raton, FL: CRC Press.
28. Tsigos C, Chrousos GP (2002) Hypothalamic-pituitary-adrenal axis, neuroendocrine factors and stress. *Journal of Psychosomatic Research* **53**: 865–71.
29. Abelson JL, Cameron OG (1994) Adrenergic dysfunction in anxiety disorders. In OG Cameron (ed.) *Adrenergic Dysfunction and Psychobiology.* Washington, DC: AP Press.
30. Graeff FG, Garcia-Leal C, Del-Ben CM, *et al.* (2005) Does the panic attack activate the hypothalamic-pituitary-adrenal axis? *Anais da Academia Brasileira de Ciências* **77**: 477–91.
31. Heninger GR (1990) A biological perspective on comorbidity of major depressive disorder and panic disorder. In JD Maser, CR Cloninger (eds) *Comorbidity of Mood and Anxiety Disorders.* Washington, DC: AP Press.
32. Holsboer F, von Bardelehen U, Buller R, *et al.* (1987) Stimulation response to corticotrophin-releasing hormone (CRH) in patients with depression, alcoholism and panic disorder. *Hormone and Metabolic Research* **16** (suppl.): 80–88.
33. Abelson JL, Nesse RM, Vinik A (1994) Pentagastrin infusions in panic disorder II. *Biological Psychiatry* **36**: 73–8.
34. Yehuda R (2006) Advances in understanding neuroendocrine alterations in PTSD and their therapeutic implications. *Annals of the New York Academy of Science* **1071**: 137–66.
35. Kasckow JW, Baker D, Geracioti TD, Jr (2001) Corticotropin-releasing hormone in depression and posttraumatic stress disorder. *Peptides* **22**: 845–51.
36. Delahanty DL, Raimonde AJ, Spoonster E, *et al.* (2003) Injury severity, prior trauma history, urinary cortisol levels, and acute PTSD in motor vehicle accident victims. *Journal of Anxiety Disorders* **17**: 149–64.
37. Yehuda R, McFarlane AC, Shalev AY (1998) Predicting the development of posttraumatic stress disorder from the acute response to a traumatic event. *Biological Psychiatry* **44**: 1305–13.
38. Bachmann AW, Sedgley TL, Jackson RV, *et al.* (2005) Glucocorticoid receptor polymorphisms and posttraumatic stress disorder. *Psychoneuroendocrinology* **30**: 297–306.
39. Heim C, Ehlert U, Hellhammer DH (2000) The potential role of hypocortisolism in the pathophysiology of stress-related bodily disorders. *Psychoneuroendocrinology* **251**: 1–35
40. Cleare AJ (2003) The neuroendocrinology of chronic fatigue system. *Endocrine Reviews* **24**: 236–52.
41. Heim C, Nater UM, Maloney E, *et al.* (2009) Childhood trauma and risk for chronic fatigue syndrome: association with neuroendocrine dysfunction. *Archives of General Psychiatry* **66**: 72–80.
42. Walker EF, Diforio D (1997) Schizophrenia: a neural diathesis-stress model. *Psychological Review* **104**: 667–85.
43. Corcoran C, Walker E, Huot R, *et al.* (2003) The stress cascade and schizophrenia: etiology and onset. *Schizophrenia Bull* **29**: 671–92.

44. Walker E, Mittal V, Tessner K (2008) Stress and the hypothalamic-pituitary-adrenal axis in the developmental course of schizophrenia. *Annual Review of Clinical Psychology* **4**: 189–216.
45. Whalley LJ, Christie JE, Blackwood DH, *et al.* (1989) Disturbed endocrine function in the psychoses: I. Disordered homeostasis or disease process? *British Journal of Psychiatry* **155**: 455–61.
46. Meltzer HY, Lee MA, Jayathilake K (2001) The blunted plasma cortisol response to apomorphine and its relationship to treatment response in patients with schizophrenia. *Neuropsychopharmacology* **24**: 278–90.
47. Altamura C, Guercetti G, Percudani M (1989) Dexamethasone suppression test in positive and negative schizophrenia. *Psychiatry Research* **30**: 69–75.
48. Muck-Seler D, Pivac N, Jakovljevic M, *et al.* (1999) Platelet serotonin, plasma cortisol and dexamethasone suppression test in schizophrenic patients. *Biological Psychiatry* **45**: 1433–9
49. Newcomer JW, Faustman WO, Whiteford HA, *et al.* (1991) Symptomatology and cognitive impairment associate independently with post-dexamethasone cortisol concentrations in unmedicated schizophrenic patients. *Biological Psychiatry* **29**: 855–64.
50. Tandon R, Mazzara C, DeQuardo J, *et al.* (1991) Dexamethasone suppression test in schizophrenia: relationship to symptomatology, ventricular enlargement and outcome. *Biological Psychiatry* **29**: 953–64.
51. Walsh P, Spelman L, Sharifi N, *et al.* (2005) Male patients with paranoid schizophrenia have greater ACTH and cortisol secretion in response to metoclopramide-induced AVP release. *Psychoneuroendocrinology* **30**: 431–7.
52. Ryan MC,Sharifi N, Condren R, Thakore JH (2004) Evidence of basal pituitary-adrenal overactivity in first episode, drug naive patients with schizophrenia. *Psychoneuroendocrinology* **29**: 1065–70.
53. Webster MJ, Knable MB, O'Grady J, *et al.* (2002) Regional specificity of brain glucocorticoid receptor mRNA alterations in subjects with schizophrenia and mood disorders. *Molecular Psychiatry* **7**: 985–94.
54. Shenton ME, Dickey CC, Frumin M, *et al.* (2001) A review of MRI findings in schizophrenia. *Schizophrenia Research* **49**: 1–52.
55. Pariante CM (2008) Pituitary volume in psychosis: the first review of the evidence. *Journal of Psychopharmacology* **22**: 76–81
56. Garner B, Pariante CM, Wood SJ, *et al.* (2005) Pituitary volume predicts future transition to psychosis in individuals at ultra-high risk of developing psychosis. *Biological Psychiatry* **58**: 417–23.
57. Nemeroff CB (1989) Clinical significance of psychoneuroendocrinology in psychiatry: focus on the thyroid and the adrenal. *Journal of Clinical Psychiatry* **50**: 13–20.
58. Baumgartner A, Graf AA, Kurten I, Meinhold H (1988) The hypothalamic-pituitary-thyroid axis in psychiatric patients and healthy subjects: parts 1–4. *Psychiatry Research* **24**: 271–332.
59. Hokfelt T, Tsuruo Y, Ulfhake B, *et al.* (1989) Distribution of TRH-like immunoreactivity with special reference to co-existence with other neuroactive compounds. *Annals of the New York Academy of Science* **553**: 76–105.
60. Nemeroff CB, Simon JS, Haggerty JJ, *et al.* (1983) Antithyroid antibodies in depressed patients. *American Journal of Psychiatry* **142**: 840–43.
61. Prange AJ, Wilson LC, Lara PP, *et al.* (1972) Effects of thyrotropin releasing hormone in depression. *Lancet* **2**: 999–1002
62. Pinchera A (1990) Nocturnal serum thyrotropin (TSH) surge and the TSH releasing hormone: dissociated behaviour in untreated depressives. *Journal of Clinical Endocrinology and Metabolism* **71**: 650–55.
63. Baumgartner A, Graf AA, Kurten I, *et al.* (1990) Thyrotropin (TSH) and thyroid hormone concentration during partial sleep deprivation in patients with major depressive disorder. *Journal of Psychiatric Research* **24**: 281–92.
64. Hickie I, Bennett B, Mitchell P, *et al.* (1996) Clinical and subclinical hypothyroidism in patients with chronic and treatment-resistant depression. *Australian and New Zealand Journal of Psychiatry* **30**: 246–52.
65. Abraham G, Miliev R, Stuart Lawson J (2006) T3 augmentation of SSRI resistant depression. *Journal of Affective Disorders* **91**: 211–15.
66. Lojko D, Rybakowski JK (2007) L-Thyroxine augmentation of serotonergic antidepressants in female patients with refractory depression. *Journal of Affective Disorders* **103**: 253–6
67. Nierenberg AA, Fava M, Trivedi MH: *et al.* (2006) A comparison of lithium and T3 augmentation following two failed medication treatments for depression: a STAR*D report. *American Journal of Psychiatry* **163**: 1519–30
68. Sokolov ST, Levitt AJ, Joffe RT (1997) Thyroid hormone levels before unsuccessful antidepressant therapy are associated with later response to T3 augmentation. *Psychiatric Research* **69**: 203–6.
69. Prange AJ, Wilson LC, Rabon AM, *et al.* (1969) Enhancement of imipramine antidepressant activity by thyroid hormone. *American Journal of Psychiatry* **126**: 457–69.
70. Feighner JP, Robins E, Guze SB, *et al.* (1972) Diagnostic criteria for use in psychiatric research. *Archives of General Psychiatry* **26**: 57–63.
71. Gordon JT, Kaminski DM, Rozanov CB, *et al.* (1999) Evidence that 3,3′,5-triiodothyronine is concentrated in and delivered from the locus coeruleus to its noradrenergic targets via anterograde axonal transport. *Neuroscience* **93**: 943–54.
72. Hindal JT, Kaplan MM (1988) Inhibition of thyroxine 5-deiodination type II in cultured human placental

cells by cortisol, insulin, 3,5-cyclic adenosine monophosphate and butyrate. *Metabolism: Clinical and Experimental* **37**: 664–8.
73. Marangell LB, Ketter TA, George MS, *et al.* (1997) Inverse relationship of peripheral thyrotropin-stimulating hormone levels to brain activity in mood disorders. *American Journal of Psychiatry* **154**: 224–30.
74. Iovino M, Steardo L, Monteleone P (1991) Impaired sensitivity of the hypothalamic-pituitary-thyroid axis to the suppressant effects of dexamethasone in elderly subjects. *Psychopharmacology* **105**: 481–5.
75. Samuels MH, McDaniel PA (1997) Thyrotropin levels during hydrocortisone infusions that mimic fasting-induced cortisol elevations: a clinical research center study. *Journal of Clinical Endocrinology and Metabolism* **82**: 3700–704.
76. Luo LG, Bruhn TO, Jackson IMD (1995) Glucocorticoids stimulate thyrotropin-releasing hormone gene expression in cultured hypothalamic neurons. *Endocrinology* **136**: 4945–50.
77. Jackson IMD, Luo LG (1998) Antidepressants inhibit the glucocorticoid stimulation of TRH expression in cultured hypothalamic neurons. *Journal of Investigative Medicine* **46**: 470–74.
78. Freeman ME, Kanyicska B, Lerant A, *et al.* (2000) Prolactin: structure, function, and regulation of secretion. *Physiological Reviews* **80**: 1523–631.
79. Howard L, Kirkwood G, Lesse M (2007) Risk of hip fracture in patients with a history of schizophrenia. *British Journal of Psychiatry* **190**: 129–34.
80. Harvey PW, Everett DJ, Springall CJ (2008) Adverse effects of prolactin in rodents and humans: breast and prostate cancer. *Journal of Psychopharmacology* **22**: 20–27.
81. Tworoger SS, Eliassen AH, Rosner B, *et al.* (2004) Plasma prolactin concentrations and risk of postmenopausal breast cancer. *Cancer Research* **64**: 6814–19.
82. Tworoger SS, Eliassen H, Sluss P, *et al.* (2007) A prospective study of plasma prolactin concentrations and risk of premenopausal and postmenopausal breast cancer. *Journal of Clinical Oncology* **25**: 1482–8.
83. Szarfman A, Tonning JM, Levine JG, *et al.* (2006) Atypical antipsychotics and pituitary tumours: a pharmacovigilance study. *Pharmacotherapy* **26**: 748–58.
84. Bushe C, Shaw M (2008) Prevalence of hyperprolactinaemia in a naturalistic cohort of schizophrenia and bipolar outpatients during treatment with typical and atypical antipsychotics. *Journal of Psychopharmacology* **21**: 768–73.
85. Jakovljevic M, Pivac N, Mihaljevic-Peles A, *et al.* (2007) The effects of olanzapine and fluphenazine on plasma cortisol, prolactin and muscle rigidity in schizophrenic patients: a double blind study. *Progress in Neuropsychopharmacology and Biological Psychiatry* **31**: 399–402.
86. Bushe C, Shaw M, Peveler RC (2008) A review of the association between antipsychotic use and hyperprolactinaemia. *Journal of Psychopharmacology* **22**: 46–55.
87. Dinan TG, Thakore J, Citrome L, *et al.* (2005) Metabolic and lifestyle issues and severe mental illness: new connections to well-being? *Journal of Psychopharmacology* **19**: 118–22.
88. Charney DS, Heninger GR, Sternberg DE, *et al.* (1982) Adrenergic receptor sensitivity in depression: effects of clonidine in depressed patients and healthy subjects. *Archives of General Psychiatry* **39**: 290.
89. Ansseau M, von Frenckell R, Cerfontaine JL, *et al.* (1987) Neuroendocrine evaluation of catecholaminergic neurotransmission in mania. *Psychiatry Research* **22**: 193–206.
90. Dinan TG, Yatham LN, O'Keane V, *et al.* (1991) Blunting of noradrenergic stimulated growth hormone release in mania. *American Journal of Psychiatry* **148**: 936–8.
91. De Kloet ER, DeRijk RH, Meijer OC (2007) Therapy insight: is there an imbalanced response to mineralocorticoid and glucocorticoid receptors in depression? *Nature Clinical Practice. Endocrinology and Metabolism* **3**: 168–79.
92. DeRijk RH, de Kloet ER (2008) Corticosteroid receptor polymorphisms: determinants of vulnerability and resilience. *European Journal of Pharmacology* **583**: 303–11.
93. Wust S, van Rossum EFC, Federenko L, *et al.* (2004) Common polymorphisms in the glucocorticoid receptor gene are associated with adrenocortical responses to psychosocial stress. *Journal of Clinical Endocrinology and Metabolism* **89**: 563–74.
94. Kumsta R, Entringer S, Koper JW, *et al.* (2007) Sex specific associations between common glucocorticoid receptor gene variants and hypothalamus-pituitary-adrenal axis responses to psychological stress. *Biological Psychiatry* **62**: 863–9.
95. Van Rossum EFC, Binder EB, Majer M, *et al.* (2006) Polymorphisms of the glucocorticoid receptor gene and major depression. *Biological Psychiatry* **59**: 681–8.
96. Brouwer JP, Appelhof BC, van Rossum EF, *et al.* (2006) Prediction of treatment response by HPA-axis and glucocorticoid receptor polymorphism in major depression. *Psychoneuroendocrinology* **31**: 1154–63.
97. Sánchez MM, Ladd CO, Plotsky PM (2001) Early adverse experience as a developmental risk factor for later psychopathology: evidence from rodent and primate models. *Development and Psychopathology* **13**: 419–49.
98. Coplan JD, Andrews MW, Rosenblum LA, *et al.* (1996) Persistent elevations of cerebrospinal fluid concentrations of corticotrophin-releasing factor in adult nonhuman primates exposed to early life stressors: implications for the pathophysiology of mood and

anxiety disorders. *Proceedings of the National Academy of Science of the USA* **93**: 1619–23.

99. DeBellis MD, Chrousos GP, Dorn LD, *et al.* (1994) Hypothalamic-pituitary-adrenal axis dysregulation in sexually abused girls. *Journal of Clinical Endocrinology and Metabolism* **78**: 249–55.
100. Heim C, Newport DJ, Heit S, *et al.* (2000) Pituitary-adrenal and autonomic responses to stress in women after sexual and physical abuse in childhood. *Journal of the American-Medical Association* **284**: 592–7.
101. Heim C, Nemeroff CB (2002) Neurobiology of early life stress: clinical studies. *Seminars in Clinical Neuropsychiatry* **7**: 147–59.
102. Danese A, Pariante CM, Caspi A, *et al.* (2007) Childhood maltreatment predicts adult inflammation in a life course study. *Proceedings of the National Academy of Sciences of the USA* **104**: 1319–24.
103. Pace TW, Mletzko TC, Alagbe O, *et al.* (2006) Increased stress-induced inflammatory responses in male patients with major depression and increased early life stress. *American Journal of Psychiatry* **163**: 1630–33.
104. Taylor SE, Lehman BJ, Kiefe CI, *et al.* (2006) Relationship of early life stress and psychological functioning to adult c-reactive protein in the coronary artery risk development in young adults study. *Biological Psychiatry* **60**: 819–24.

Chapter 28

The neurophysiology and neurochemistry of arousal and sleep

John Shneerson

NATURE OF SLEEP

Sleep is a state of reduced awareness and responsiveness to internal and external stimuli. The reduced awareness is selective and it is stimuli of significance to the individual that are most likely to cause arousal from sleep.[1] Sleep is also a transient phase that alternates with wakefulness and from which, unlike coma, the subject can be aroused quickly. The transition between wakefulness and sleep, however, may last for several minutes, and it may be impossible to determine the exact moment of falling asleep. In these transitional states, some aspects of both sleep and wakefulness coexist. Similarly, physical incoordination, sometimes with confusion, is common after waking from sleep (sleep inertia), probably due to delayed activation of the prefrontal cortex at the transition from sleep to wakefulness. The hallucinations associated with delirium such as delirium tremens probably represent partial rapid eye movement (REM) sleep intrusion into wakefulness. Sleep paralysis is also intrusion of the skeletal muscle relaxation of REM sleep into wakefulness.

DURATION OF SLEEP

The mean duration of sleep in the UK is now around 7 h per night,[2] but there is probably a normal distribution, with around 8 per cent of people sleeping for less than 5 h and 2 per cent for more than 10 h. The duration of sleep that is obtained is often different from what is needed, and it should be sufficient to lead to a feeling of being refreshed on waking and remaining alert and able to function normally throughout the day.[3] Life expectancy is shorter in people who obtain little sleep at night and also in people with prolonged overnight sleep.[4] Both short- and long-sleepers have approximately the same duration of the deeper stages (3 and 4) of non-REM (NREM) sleep. After sleep deprivation, the duration of these sleep stages increases on the first night of more prolonged sleep, and an increase in REM sleep is seen subsequently.

Daytime naps are normal in young children and common in elderly people, particularly between 2 p.m. and 4 p.m., when the circadian rhythms favour sleep. Stages 3 and 4 NREM sleep usually occur only if there has been significant sleep deprivation or if a nap lasts longer than around 30 min. These long naps are more likely to be followed by sleep inertia; brief 'power naps' of around 20 min are usually more refreshing.

PHYSIOLOGY OF SLEEP AND WAKEFULNESS

Structure of sleep

Until the discovery of REM sleep in 1953, it was generally felt that sleep was a passive homogeneous state. Since then, it has been recognized that there are four to five cycles each night of NREM and REM sleep, alternating at around 60- to 90-min intervals. NREM sleep dominates early in the night, particularly its deeper stages (3 and 4), but REM sleep becomes more prolonged later in the night.

Physiology of NREM sleep

During NREM sleep, the cerebral cortical activity is synchronized. The synchronization of cortical activity is secondary to bursts of activity in thalamocortical neurons. These effectively disconnect the cortex from the brainstem, so that motor activity is largely reflex. Functional neuroimaging has shown that the prefrontal cortex and limbic system are inactivated. There is a relative increase in parasympathetic compared with sympathetic activity, and the metabolic rate is reduced by 5–10 per cent. The core body temperature falls as NREM sleep is entered, and the reduction in alveolar ventilation leads to a slight increase in arterial $P\text{CO}_2$. The heart rate and blood pressure fall. Protein synthesis and other anabolic processes are increased. Cell division is most rapid during NREM sleep. It has been considered to be a restorative or a recovery phase, particularly for the brain but probably in part for the rest of the body as well.

Physiology of REM sleep

REM sleep, in contrast, may have a primarily neurodevelopmental role. It is most prolonged pre- and postnatally. Both NREM and REM sleep also play a part in memory, particularly for motor tasks.

The cerebral cortex is active during REM sleep, but in a different pattern from that seen in wakefulness. The prefrontal cortex is inactivated, but several areas of the limbic system are active. This cortical activity is manifested as dreams. The cortex still reacts to sensory information from the brainstem, but there is intense skeletal muscle inhibition, which prevents the physical enactment of dream mentation. Autonomic function is very variable, with rapid fluctuations in heart rate, blood pressure and respiratory pattern.

Control of sleep and wakefulness

Whether the subject is awake or asleep depends on the balance of influences promoting and inhibiting each of these states.[5] The three known processes are:

- *Sleep homeostatic drive (process S):* the drive to enter sleep increases, probably exponentially with the duration since the end of the previous NREM sleep episode.[6] It therefore increases during prolonged wakefulness and decreases once NREM sleep has been entered at night. There is probably a similar homeostatic drive to enter REM sleep, which increases during NREM sleep but not during wakefulness.
- *Circadian rhythms:* the intrinsic circadian rhythm is usually around 24.2 h and is entrained by external timegivers to gear it to the environment. The suprachiasmatic nuclei (SCN) in the supraoptic anterior hypothalamus are the most important centres controlling the circadian rhythms. Each cell in the SCN is capable of spontaneous depolarization, and their coordination is the source of circadian rhythmicity. At least 12 genes have been identified that control the periodicity of the SCN cells. Impulses reach the SCN from the retinal ganglion cell receptors, which are distinct from the rods and cones that lead to the sensation of vision. The retinal ganglion cells are also particularly sensitive to wavelengths of around 460 nm (blue light). The output from the SCN reaches the centres controlling sleep and wakefulness, particularly the ventrolateral preoptic area (VLPO) of the anterior hypothalamus, and the centres controlling feeding, temperature, endocrine function and motor activity. Light exposure also inhibits secretion of melatonin from the pineal gland. This is usually secreted at night, with a peak level in adults at 3–5 a.m. Melatonin entrains the SCN and helps to synchronize circadian rhythms, for instance of temperature and cortisol secretion, with those of sleep.
- *Adaptive drive:* there are a variety of mechanisms that enable the sleep–wake cycle to adapt to environmental conditions.[7,8] These include behavioural factors, such as motivation and attention; psychological factors, such as mental activity and relaxation; and reflex factors, such as light exposure,[9,10] noise, pain, environmental temperature, physical exercise and food intake.

NEUROANATOMY OF SLEEP AND WAKEFULNESS

Cerebral cortical activity is critical in determining whether sleep or wakefulness occurs, but it does not generate the drive to enter sleep or wakefulness.[11,12] The most important anatomical structures (Figure 28.1) that regulate this are as follows:

- *Aminergic brainstem nuclei:* these include the locus coeruleus, raphe nuclei and tuberomamillary nuclei (TMN). These are most active during wakefulness, partially suppressed in NREM sleep and totally suppressed in REM sleep. They all favour wakefulness and inhibit REM sleep. They project to the hypothalamus, thalamus and basal forebrain, and together they form the ascending reticular activating system.
- *Laterodorsal tegmental (LDT) and pedunculopontine tegmental (PPT) nuclei:* these promote REM sleep when they are most active. They are inactive in NREM sleep, but activity returns during wakefulness. They also influence the sleep-related eye movements and the loss of muscle tone that are characteristic of REM sleep.
- *Higher centres promoting wakefulness:* these include the perifornical hypothalamus whose neurons release orexin (hypocretin) and have an excitatory effect on the brainstem aminergic nuclei. The mesolimbic dopaminergic system projects to the prefrontal cortex and limbic system, cholinergic neurons in the basal forebrain and the SCN.

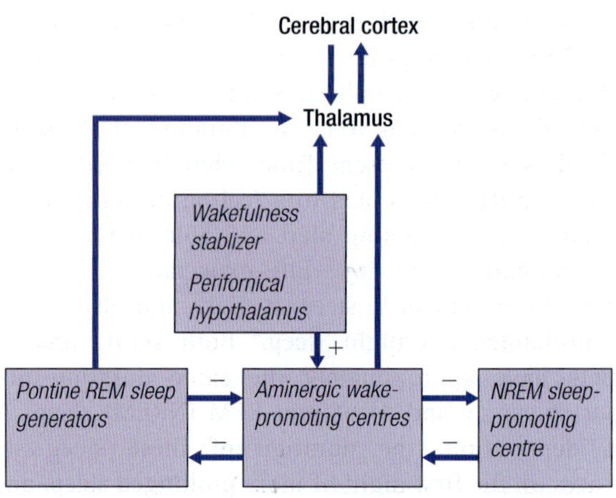

Figure 28.1 Structures involved in control of sleep and wakefulness

- *Sleep-promoting higher centres:* these include the VLPO and the anterior hypothalamus, which inhibits the aminergic nuclei and promotes NREM sleep. Accumulation of adenosine in the extracellular spaces in the basal forebrain also inhibits the wakefulness-promoting cholinergic neurons in this region and thereby promotes sleep.
- *Pathways to the cerebral cortex to enable sleep to occur:* these are mainly via the thalamus, especially during NREM sleep, and the basal forebrain and hypothalamus. These closely linked areas integrate the sleep and wakefulness drives with circadian influences.

NEUROCHEMISTRY OF SLEEP

The neurotransmitters and neuromodulators released at synapses strongly influence sleep, but other important chemicals are more diffusely present in the brain and cerebrospinal fluid and promote sleep or wakefulness. They act as local neurohormones influencing the threshold for depolarization of the postsynaptic membranes. Some of the systemically released classical hormones act in this way. The actions of the most important neurotransmitter amines are shown in Table 28.1, but there are also a wide variety of peptides and prostaglandins, as well as cannabinoids and adenosine,[13] which influence sleep and wakefulness.

CONCLUSION

The modern view of sleep as a complex fluctuating state of reduced awareness contrasts with the older view of it being a passive inactive phase purely for restoration of cerebral function. The differences between NREM and REM sleep and wakefulness underlie many of the manifestations of sleep disorders, as well as physiological process such as consolidation of memory.

Table 28.1 Effects of neurotransmitter amines on sleep and wakefulness

Effect	Noradrenaline	Acetylcholine	5-HT	Dopamine	Histamine
Promotes	Wakefulness	Wakefulness, REM	Wakefulness	–	Wakefulness
Inhibits	REM	–	REM	–	REM
Other actions	Influences mood and behaviour	Motor inhibition in REM	Influences mood, behaviour and motor control	Influences thoughts, emotions, behaviour and motor control	–

5-HT, 5-hydroxytryptamine; NREM, non-rapid eye movement; REM, rapid eye movement.

KEY POINTS

- The repetitive cycles of NREM and REM sleep during each night underlie the presentation of many sleep disorders.
- NREM sleep is primarily restorative and REM sleep helps to establish new neural networks.
- The anatomical and chemical substrate of sleep and wakefulness is complex and involves areas throughout the brain.

REFERENCES

1. Velluti RA (1997) Interactions between sleep and sensory physiology. *Journal of Sleep Research* 6: 61–77.
2. Ferrara M, de Gennaro L (2001) How much sleep do we need? *Sleep Medicine Reviews* 5: 155–79.
3. Horne J (2004) Is there a sleep debt? *Sleep* 27: 1047–9.
4. Bliwise DL, Young TB (2007) The parable of parabola: what the U-shaped curve can and cannot tell us about sleep. *Sleep* 30: 1614–15.
5. Johns M (1998) Rethinking the assessment of sleepiness. *Sleep Medicine Reviews* 2: 3–15.
6. Franken P (2002) Long-term vs short-term processes regulating REM sleep. *Journal of Sleep Research* 11: 17–28.
7. Roenneberg T, Kuehnle T, Juda M, *et al.* (2007) Epidemiology of the human circadian clock. *Sleep Medicine Reviews* 11: 429–38.
8. Van Someren EJW, Riemersma-Van Der Lek RF (2007) Live to the rhythm, slave to the rhythm. *Sleep Medicine Reviews* 11: 465–84.
9. Cajochen C, Krauchi K, Danilenko KV, Wirz-Justice A (1998) Evening administration of melatonin and bright light: interactions on the EEG during sleep and wakefulness. *Journal of Sleep Research* 7: 145–57.
10. Cajochen C (2007) Alerting effects of light. *Sleep Medicine Reviews* 11: 453–64.
11. Espana RA, Scammell TE (2004) Sleep neurobiology for the clinician. *Sleep* 27: 811–20.
12. Pace-Schott EF, Hobson JA (2002) The neurobiology of sleep: genetics, cellular physiology and subcortical networks. *Nature Reviews. Neuroscience* 3: 591–605.
13. Porkka-Heiskanen T, Alanko L, Kalinchuk A, Stenberg D (2002) Adenosine and Sleep. *Sleep Medicine Reviews* 6: 321–32.

Chapter 29

The electroencephalogram and evoked potential studies

Caroline Brown and Jonathan Bird

INTRODUCTION

The aim of this chapter is to introduce the basics of electroencephalographic (EEG) recording generally and outline both clinical and clinical-research practices. The use, analysis and interpretation of EEG and other neurophysiological measures require some commitment of time and resource,[1] and it is not the aim of this chapter to train the reader to expert level. Readers in pursuit of greater in-depth knowledge are referred to Binnie and Stefan[2] for an overall review of EEG in psychiatric settings and to specialist books such as Engel[3] on epilepsy and Luck[4] for further information on the event-related potential (ERP).

In essence, EEG measures the combined electrical output generated by cortical neurons and, as a consequence, clinicians should consider utilizing EEG recording if it is believed that there is an *organic* cause within the central nervous system (CNS) underlying the given symptoms.

This chapter gives an overall introduction to, and brief overview of, basic techniques in recording EEG. Some specific clinical uses are outlined, ranging from sensory deficit through to specific syndromes, including epilepsy and related symptomatology, which are based on visual interpretation of the electroencephalograph itself. Following this, some of the analytical methods available and how they may inform us of underlying changes in CNS function are given.

In the presentation of each section, current views and interpretations are referred to, where they are thought to offer some guidance in clinical decisions. Clinicians with expertise use such visual interpretation in diagnosis and treatment decisions. The use of mathematical analytical tools and statistical tests of difference between EEG components allows direct comparison between different research hypotheses, generated from clinical evidence.

RECORDING EEG

The basics: what does EEG measure?

Specifically, EEG measures electrical activity that is discharged by many thousands of cortical neurons as their activity synchronizes. The electrical potential of single neural cells changes, depending upon excitatory and inhibitory input from the dendrites of neighbouring presynaptic neurons; a measure of such activity using an intracellular single electrode is called the action potential. EEG can only measure activity from cells that are aligned similarly to one another and radial to the scalp. As voltage drops at distance from the source, currents from deep sources are less easy to detect than those from nearer the skull. Measures of cortical electrical activity taken at the scalp may well suffer from refractive errors due to changes at the margins between the cortical surface, cerebrospinal fluid, meningeal membranes, skull bone and scalp. These recording issues are shown diagrammatically in Figure 29.1.

EEG is more reliable when detecting neural communication differences at surface or cortical levels and less reliable for detection of deep or subcortical events.

EEG and its sister technology magneto-encephalography (MEG) have a tremendous advantage over other neurophysiological measures in terms of *temporal resolution*, as they can be recorded in the millisecond range. Indeed, the limiting factor underlying recording accuracy tends to be data storage capacity, as each channel (electrode) contributes a data point at each recording time over the entire period being measured, hence a sampling rate of 1000 Hz using 32 electrodes will generate 32 000 data points per second and 1.92 million data points after 1 min.

EEG is excellent at identifying *when* events occur. Although it can be (and is) used in assessment of location of epileptogenic focus, EEG alone is not considered sufficient

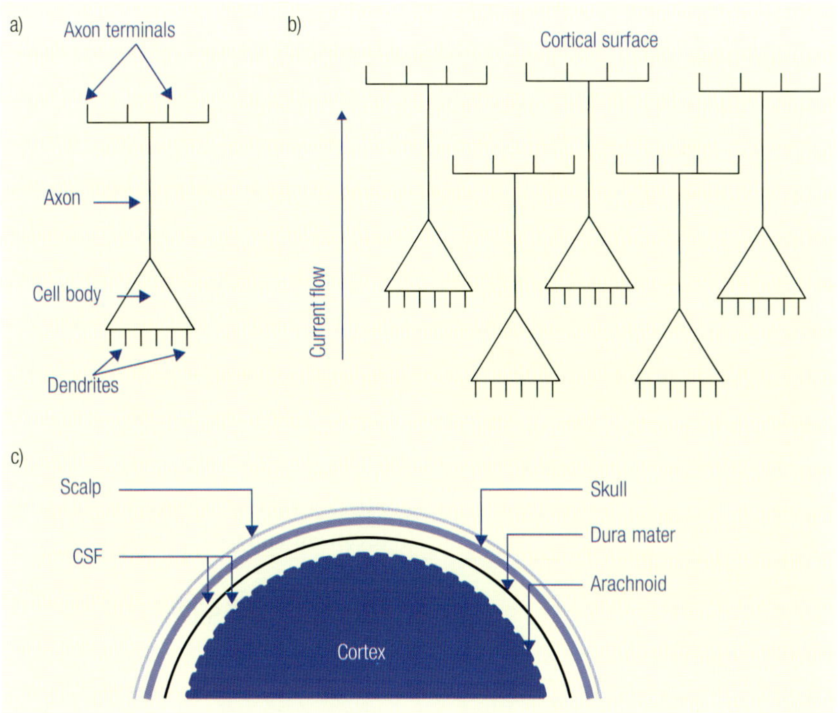

Figure 29.1 (a) Diagrammatic representation of neuron; (b) parallel and radial arrangement of pyramidal cells within cortex; (c) potential refraction errors as electrical signals pass from cortex via cerebrospinal fluid (CSF), meninges, bone and scalp

where precise spatial resolution is required but should be used when clinically necessary in cases of classification and diagnosis of suspected organically based disorder. Essential uses of EEG are highlighted in this chapter.

The temporal-sensitivity advantage makes EEG a particularly suitable tool for enabling support in the diagnosis and treatment in epileptic symptomatology, as changes in electrical activity before a seizure happen in the order of tens of seconds before its onset. As outlined below, the temporal sensitivity of EEG enables several methods of analysis that allow interpretation of underlying causality by direct interpretation of graphical output, or through indirect analysis of coherent activity and/or frequency spectra power and components, (see Spectral analysis, below; and Coherence: a mathematical measure of similarity of frequency between two cortical locations, below).

Absolute localization of current source is not possible because the electrodes at the scalp are detecting the summation of electrical voltage that may be generated in, mathematically speaking, many potential sites. The development of more sophisticated analytic tools,[5,6] and the use of high-density recording electrode montages, is improving spatial resolution, but it is generally considered that, for accurate spatial resolution, other, more expensive measures should be used, in particular magnetic resonance imaging (MRI) or positron-emission tomography (PET). Exciting developments utilizing the diamagnetic properties of electrical currents are now enabling the localization of electrical source within MEG, which retains the temporal resolution of EEG not available in other scanning technologies.

Recording EEG: a first tutorial

Cortical electrical activity is measured using highly electrosensitive electrodes, often, but not exclusively, utilizing a silver–silver chloride construction with electrolyte gels of varying composition. Regardless of whether these electrodes are held to the scalp by adhesive (glue) or by elastic caps, it is essential that impedance levels are reduced as much as possible in order to increase the *signal-to-noise* ratio. This entails the scalp being abraded to remove loose epidermal cells; patients and participants are asked to arrive without having used hair products previously or are asked to wash them out before recording. The advent of the elastic-based cap has enabled the process of readying the recording montage to become shorter, which in research settings has led to the development of high-density recording systems where montages of 64, 132 and even 256 electrode sites are not uncommon. In order to promote clarity and comparison between reports, there is an internationally accepted montage of electrodes, the 10–20 system (Figure 29.2).[7] The development of dense array systems leads to reports that refer findings back to the 10–20 system for clarity in understanding. Current use of dense and very dense arrays in epilepsy is focussed on EEG *source localization* of epileptogenic focus (see Plummer *et al.*[6] for a comprehensive review).

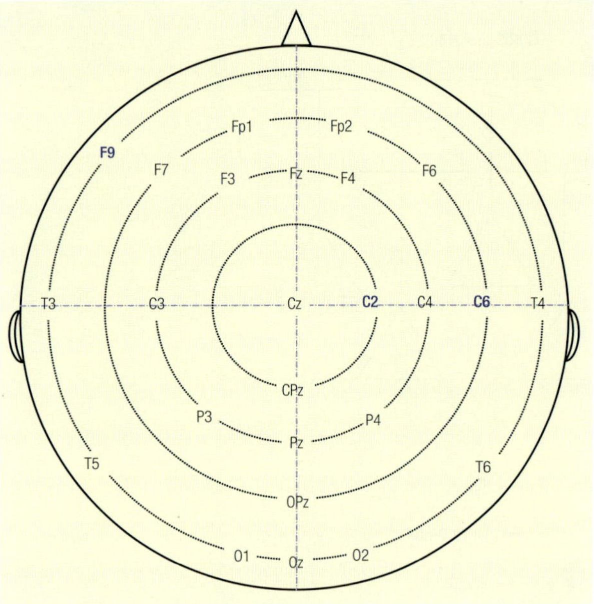

Figure 29.2 The scalp is measured from front to back (nasion to inion) and from side to side (pre-auricular points). Electrodes are placed at sites that are 10 per cent and 20 per cent respectively of these distances. Regions of the scalp are identified by lobe names and central locations: F, frontal; C, central; O, occipital; P, parietal; T, temporal. Left hemisphere sites are given odd numbers and right hemisphere sites even numbers. Electrodes placed on midline sites are given the suffix 'z'. As density of electrode montages increases, nomenclature has expanded by conjoining site letters; so, for instance, electrodes between central and parietal locations are given the prefix 'CP'

American Clinical Neurophysiology Society (1994) Modified combinatorial nomenclature: guideline 13 – guidelines for standard electrode position nomenclature. *Journal of Clinical Neurophysiology* **11**: 111–13.

CLINICAL USE OF EEG IN PSYCHIATRY

The most basic analysis of EEG is to look at the graphed output of all the recording channels. The spike-and-wave patterns of activity associated with epileptic syndrome are usually visual and time-measured. Although described as 'basic', the interpretation of these patterns and of differences between channels requires care and training. More complex forms of analysis involve mathematical algorithms to transform the digital data in some way.

The printout of an EEG presents, to the uninitiated, a frighteningly complex range of waveforms. It is important, therefore, to realize that a great deal of what is seen on the EEG is, to the experienced eye, of little clinical relevance. This is the very converse of what is seen on the electrocardiogram (ECG), which is the most similar tracing likely to have been seen by most doctors. While in the ECG almost everything on the page is of considerable importance, the reading of an EEG is much more a question of pattern recognition and observing the gestalt of the whole picture. Essentially, the EEG boils down to assessing for the following abnormalities:

- Slow waves
- Paroxysmal activity
- Maturational abnormalities
- Acute organic states
- Asymmetries of normal rhythms.

Both slow waves and paroxysmal activities can be divided into those that are generalized and those that are focal (localized).

Before reading an EEG, it is important to be aware that there is a wide range of biological and technical artefacts that may be seen and can be discounted. However, a number of artefacts can be very misleading; for instance, the rolling slow-wave pattern of a sweat artefact seen only over one side of the head might be mistaken for a cortical tumour, whereas a regular sharp-wave discharge of an ECG artefact seen only on some leads might be thought to be a localized epileptic discharge.

Generalized slow waves

These may be subdivided further into *synchronous* and *asynchronous.*

Synchronous generalized slow waves appear predominantly over both left and right frontal regions. Intermittent synchronous bilateral slow waves are seen as a result of brainstem damage, representing a decrease in activity in subcortical nuclei and subsequent corticothalamic activity. Such brainstem-damage related abnormalities are referred to as frontal intermittent rhythmical delta activity (FIRDA) (Figure 29.3).

Asynchronous but generalized slow waves – that is, slow waves that occur at a different rate and at different times in the two hemispheres – are typically seen with widespread cortical dysfunction, such as an organic confusional state. Such abnormalities would typically arise with toxic or metabolic encephalopathies. Such disorders may, in the first instance, present either as confusion or occasionally as a rather atypical psychosis. It is very important that the EEG be carried out in these circumstances.

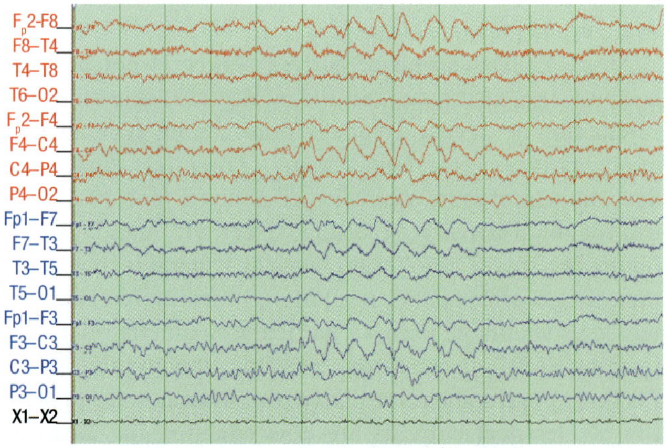

Figure 29.3 Frontal intermittent rhythmical delta activity (FIRDA)

Focal (localized) slow waves, particularly those in the delta range, are typically seen over a brain tumour but also as what is termed 'a breach rhythm' over a neurosurgical site, where the functioning cortex has been damaged or removed (Figure 29.4). They represent, essentially, an area of brain where the normal faster cortical activity is not occurring and, therefore, the slower rhythms from the subcortical regions can be seen.

Generalized paroxysmal activity may usefully be divided into those that show a regular three per second (3 Hz) of spike-and-wave pattern, those that show some atypical spike-and-wave pattern (Figure 29.5) and those that are generalized but not of either of the previous two types.

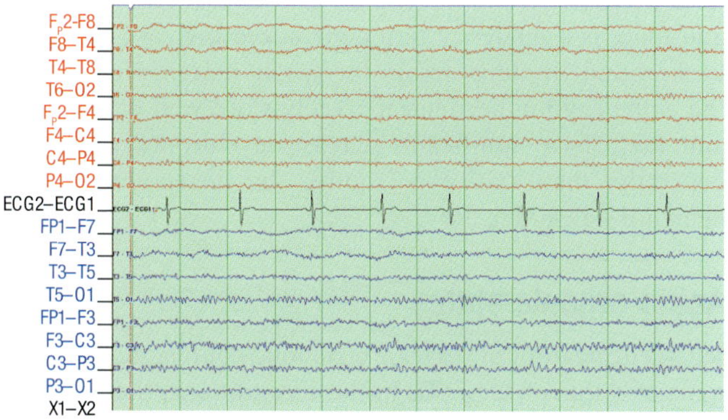

Figure 29.4 Breach rhythm over left central regions, following surgery

Paroxysmal activities

Likewise, these may be generalized or localized. Generalized paroxysmal activities in the form of three per second (3 Hz) spike-and-wave discharges are seen in typical and true 'absence epilepsies', also called true 'petit mal epilepsy'. This condition typically arises in childhood and is associated with brief absences of consciousness, often with slightly flickering eyelids and occasionally with brief jerking movements around the eyes and sometimes of the hands. During the absence, the 3-Hz spike-and-wave discharges are seen; when the discharge ceases, the individual returns to full consciousness and may not be aware of the episode at all. After a time, an individual with this sort of epilepsy will recognize that they are missing parts of the conversation. As in all generalized epilepsies, the patient has no aura or warning that the seizure is about to occur.

Generalized atypical spike-and-wave discharges tend to be slower, at 2 Hz or 2.5 Hz. They are often less regular and they often contain multiple spikes. Such discharges are seen in a range of generalized epilepsies, but particularly in the Lennox–Gastaut syndrome. This syndrome is associated with learning disabilities, multiple generalized seizure types (tonic, atonic, absence, tonic–clonic) and a poor prognosis for recovery. Lennox–Gastaut syndrome may emerge out of the early onset, in infancy, of West syndrome, with severe paroxysmal activities seen in a 'hypsarrhythmic' pattern and myoclonic or 'Salaam' attacks.

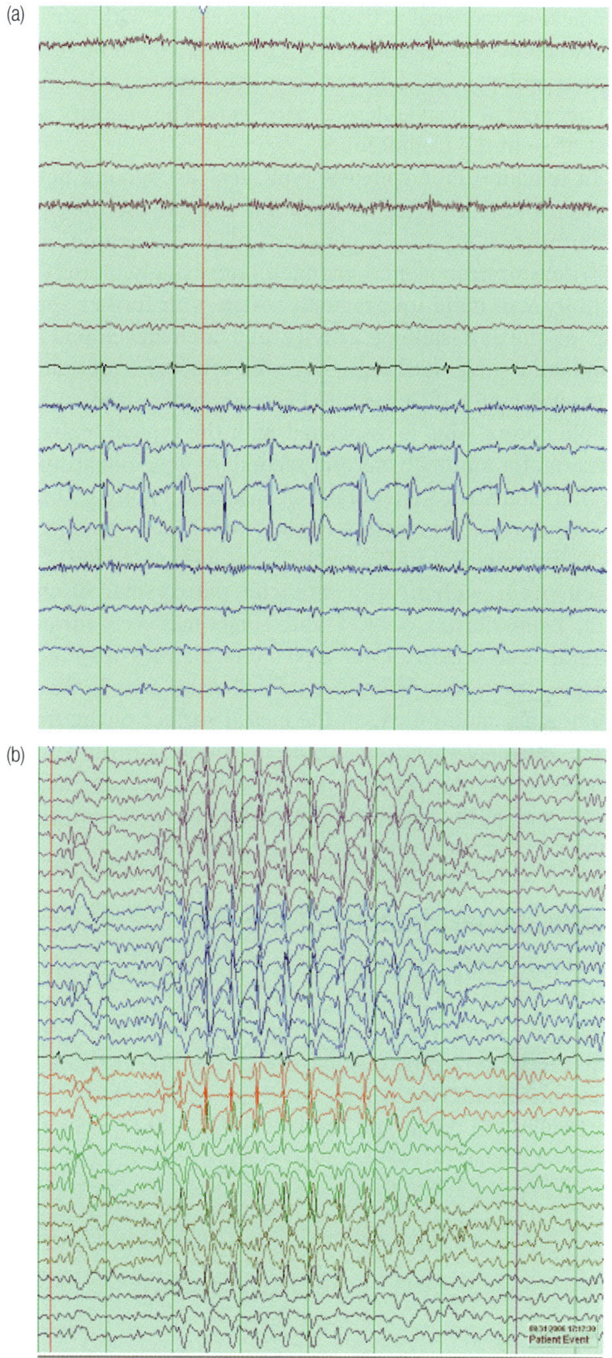

Figure 29.5 (a) Series of spike and slow-wave complexes; (b) atypical spike and slow-wave complexes

There is a range of generalized epilepsies that do not fall into either of the above groups and that may be associated with paroxysmal activity only during sleep.

It is essential to recognize whether an epilepsy is of a generalized nature from the outset of treatment, as certain anti-epileptic medications may make generalized epilepsies worse (phenytoin and carbamazepine on occasion), and patients with these sorts of epilepsy are unlikely to be suitable for any form of resective surgery. It is very important that the EEG be carried out in these circumstances.

Focal paroxysmal activities are associated with partial or localization-related epilepsies. The most common form of partial epilepsy arises in one or other temporal lobe. About 80 per cent of focal epilepsies arise here. The majority of the rest arise in the frontal lobes.

In temporal lobe epilepsy, typically, fast spiking activity is seen over the affected temporal lobe at the onset of a seizure, possibly after a period of relative quietude on the EEG (electrodecremental change). Increasingly, paroxysmal activity will build up gradually, often with further spreading of the fast-spiking activity and then development of spike-and-wave discharges over the affected temporal lobe and, eventually, if the seizure becomes generalized, over the whole cortex. This is associated with the typical 'march' of aura, motor automatisms and secondary generalization that is characteristic of temporal lobe seizures (Figure 29.6).

Partial epilepsies arising in the frontal lobes, as observed by carers, medical staff directly or through video EEG,[8] may often occur without any interictal paroxysmal discharge and, even during a brief and sometimes very dramatic frontal lobe seizure, clear EEG abnormalities may not be seen on the cortex. Many frontal epilepsies arise in the supplementary motor area, on the mesial surface of the frontal lobe, and may therefore not be detectable on the surface. Scalp recordings may also be obscured by movement artefacts, and so invasive recording with electrodes, at neurosurgery, over the cortex itself may be needed.

Maturational changes of the EEG

The 'maturational' changes of the EEG during an individual's lifetime are of importance. The EEG of a newborn infant is completely different from that of an adult. A picture characterized by a burst of activity and then by suppression of activity will be seen in normal newborn and particularly in premature babies. As the infant grows, faster activity is seen and eventually, during late childhood and early adolescence, an alpha rhythm will begin to emerge, initially seen over central regions and gradually localizing over the occipital regions. Before the age of 5 years, it is very common to have a number of asymmetries of the EEG, with one hemisphere perhaps developing before the other. It would be expected that the normal posterior alpha rhythm, at 8–14 Hz, would be established by about the age of 15 years. It is often felt that, if this has not happened, then the EEG may be regarded as relatively 'immature'. For further information, the reader is referred to Yordanova and Kolev.[9]

As an individual enters old age, there tends to be a slight slowing of the alpha rhythm, although it should still remain above 8 Hz. There may be more central fast (beta) activity, and there is a tendency to a generalized increase of slower background rhythms across the whole cortex. However, if the alpha rhythm becomes markedly slow, well below 8 Hz, and there is a significant increase in slow-wave activity generally, then this may signify the development of a dementing disorder.

Acute organic states

The identification of toxic or metabolic confusional states is a major value of the EEG. In these conditions, there is usually random synchronous and asynchronous slow-wave activity of a kind not seen in an individual with a functional psychiatric condition. On occasion, specific abnormalities are seen. Lateralized triphasic complexes are associated with herpes encephalitis; bifrontal triphasic waves are typically seen at some stage in hepatic encephalopathy, although this may occur later on. Periodic high-voltage complexes are seen in subacute sclerosing panencephalitis.

In dementing conditions, there is typically a slowing of

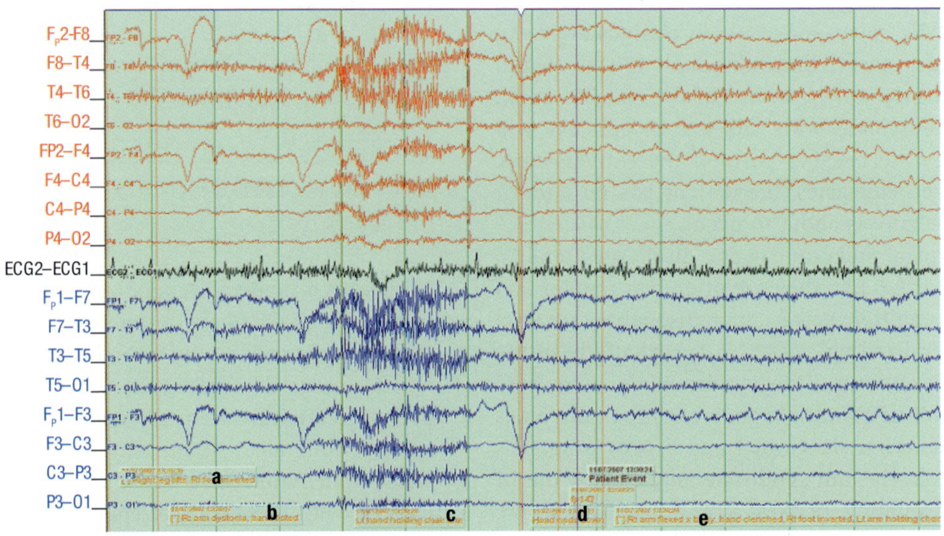

Figure 29.6 Left frontal seizure. **a** Right leg lifts. Right foot inverted. **b** Right arm dystonia, hand fisted. **c** Left hand holding chair arm. **d** Head nods down. **e** Right arm flexed x [across] body, hand clenched, Right foot inverted, Left arm holding chair.

the alpha rhythm and a polymorphic picture of slower waves (theta and delta). The slower the development of the dementia, the less likelihood there is of marked change in the EEG. However, slow-wave activity and a slowing of the alpha rhythm is a helpful discriminator from depression.

In Alzheimer's disease, there tends to be diffuse slowing, but there may be runs of frontal delta resulting from subcortical damage, and there is a later appearance of sharper waves and sometimes of paroxysmal activity focally. Multi-infarct dementia tends to show more localized and unilateral slow-wave activity.

The EEGs recorded in focal or lobar dementias are very frequently normal for the majority of the history.

Huntington's dementia is associated with a particularly low-amplitude EEG, a relative flattening of the EEG.

Creutzfeldt–Jakob disease is associated with an early loss of the alpha rhythm and the appearance of theta waves, but these are non-specific and may be missed. Later on in the disease, sometimes just briefly before death, the typical picture of periodic triphasic complexes is always seen. The appearance of these triphasic complexes appears to be associated with the rate of progression of the disorder, there being more abnormalities if the disease is progressing rapidly.

Asymmetries of normal rhythms

Asymmetries in EEG activity may be normal or pathological. A mu rhythm may show one-sided bias, which is of no diagnostic significance. A breach rhythm, on the other hand, of similar frequency and at times even similar outline to the mu, though not necessarily of the same location, indicates brain trauma and is often seen at the sites of previous surgery.

Neonates may show 50 per cent asymmetry in their various EEG activities; this is normal, but a 50 per cent disparity in amplitude between hemispheres of the adult alpha rhythm could indicate a unilateral thalamic or occipital problem.

The most significant pathological asymmetries involve slow activity within the delta and theta wavebands, except for posterior slow waves of youth, which generally present more abundantly in the right posterior quadrant than the left. As outlined above, asymmetrical slow activity, especially delta activity at the lower frequency end, is a strong indicator of pathology. Very slow undulating localized delta may indicate a focal lesion such as an acute collection or abscess. If surrounding brain tissue is distorted, it reacts functionally by slowing, so that a whole hemisphere may be affected. Conversely, generalized slow waves, if 'flattened' on one side, should raise the suspicion of an extradural collection.

Transient sharpened theta presenting temporally and asymmetrically may indicate temporal dysfunction or an epileptogenic site in young patients. This significance decreases with age and after the age of 50 years these transients rarely indicate new epileptogenicity.

Beta activity is present but scant in normal recordings but can increase during alcohol use or administration of benzodiazepines or barbiturates. The latter two drugs are often used in the intensive care unit (ICU) for patient sedation. Asymmetries of this induced beta activity may indicate that a brain area or side is not capable of generating faster frequencies due to underlying pathology or damage.

Thus, asymmetries have to be assessed in the context of the patient's age and history. There is a great deal of individual variability, and hence asymmetries are really significant only if they are very obvious and generally comprise an excess of slow activity.

ANALYTICAL TECHNIQUES IN EEG

Research activity in both typical and atypical (medical) arenas necessitates the use of analytical techniques that enable direct and precise comparison of EEG between groups of people. In this section, an overview is given of the main types of analysis available. The time-locking of EEG waveforms to a given event allows averaging over many trials and gives a waveform known as the ERP. Other forms of analysis can enable the constituent waveforms within EEG to be measured. In this section, the ERP, spectral analysis and coherence analysis are outlined briefly.

The event-related potential

Recording cortically generated electrical changes to a given stimulus tells us nothing from one trial. However, if patients (or volunteers in cognitive neuroscience experiments) are given many repetitions of each stimulus trial, and the resulting EEG is averaged over all trial epochs, then the resultant mean electrical signal shows characteristic patterns or changes in positive and negative activity. Such analysis is called an *evoked potential* (Figure 29.7). Sensory processing in the auditory, visual and somatosensory domains is called auditory evoked potential (AEP), visual evoked potential (VEP) and somatosensory evoked potential (SEP), respectively. Some experimental paradigms requiring correct responses are known as ERPs. The positive and negative deflections at given times are known as *components* and are nominated N for negative deflections and P for positive deflections. These are then either counted in order of appearance (e.g. N1, P1, N2) or, where particular components are reliably found at a given time, the component is named by that time (e.g. N170, which is found over ventral posterior regions during face-processing tasks).

Where practitioners need to identify sensory processing deficits, it is possible to use evoked potentials in visual, auditory and somatosensory modalities. Very early differences in the first 100 ms represent activity related to early neural pathways between receptor and sensory cortex and are linked to attentional processes. Hemispheric differences can indicate unilateral lesions (visual modality,[10] auditory modality,[11–15] somatosensory modality[16]).

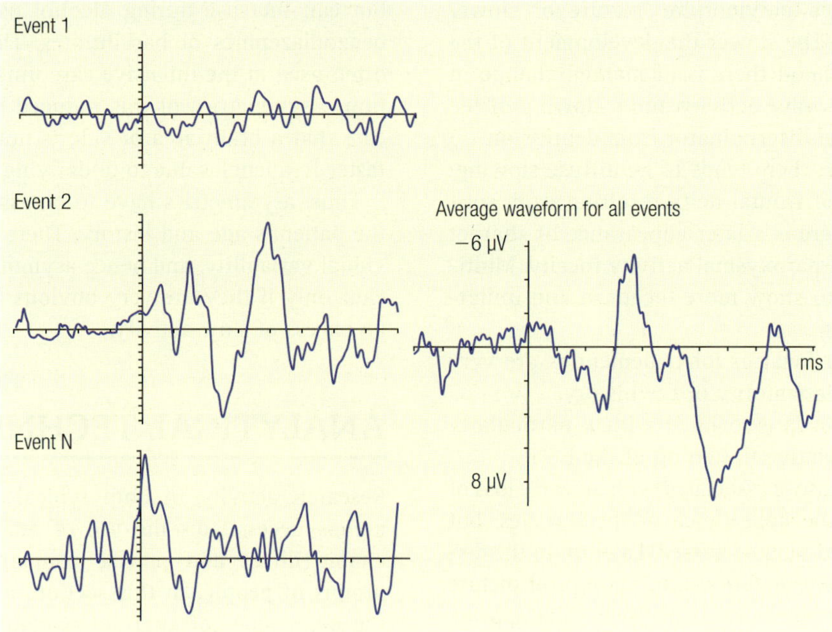

Figure 29.7 The evoked potential. Each event is recorded and the average waveform or evoked response potential calculated

Additionally, behavioural and cognitive links to these early and later components (100 ms onwards) may be of use in identifying underlying disorders. One such comparison is that of mismatch negativity (MMN), the result of an increase in negativity following a deviant stimulus (compared with a regular stimulus). This is thought to represent pre-attentional processes and as a consequence has been used to investigate psychiatric disorders where attentional deficits are contributory, such as Alzheimer's disease, schizophrenia, alcohol dependency and attention deficit hyperactivity disorder (ADHD). Readers are referred to Näätänen *et al.*[17] and Giard *et al.*[18] for further information on auditory MMN, and Tales *et al.*[19] for more on visual MMN.

Spectral analysis

In the previous section on the visual analysis of EEG, the frequency of spike-and-wave activity and of slow-wave rhythms as visualized on the output was outlined. In research settings where specific hypotheses are tested by measuring activity in many people, it is necessary to measure periodicity precisely. EEG can be mathematically decomposed into its component frequency bands (Table 29.1), using filtering online or mathematical forms of Fourier transform, fast Fourier transform or wavelet algorithms, the latter being most useful in ongoing or dynamic identification of spectral components. There are suggestions that independent component analysis might be a useful algorithm in frequency decomposition.[20,21] In general, the slower the frequency of the EEG wave, the higher the amplitude, which enables the detection of disease or atypicality when this pattern is not found.

Table 29.1 Frequency bands

Name	Frequency (Hz)
DC (direct current)	< 0.5
Delta	0–3
Theta	4–7
Alpha	8–12
Mu	7–11
Beta	12–25 (30)
Gamma	30–100 Hz
Lambda	Single, sharp waves

Direct current (DC) changes in negative or positive shift can determine the state of the nervous system metabolism;[22] these change with cognitive function and load[23] and correlate with blood oxygenation level-dependent (BOLD) responses measured in functional magnetic resonance imaging (fMRI).[24,25]

Delta-frequency waves are those measured between 0 Hz and 3 Hz and are therefore usually termed 'slow waves'; they tend towards greatest amplitude.

Theta-frequency waves are those measured between 4 Hz and 7 Hz. Theta is seen normally in young children, and in older children and adults when drowsy. Atypical increases and patterns of theta activation have been linked to the onset of Alzheimer's disease[26,27] and depression.[28]

Alpha-frequency waves are those measured between 8 Hz and 12 Hz. Predominantly measured over posterior regions in both hemispheres, alpha waves are elicited by asking participants to shut their eyes and can be seen when patients (and bored volunteers) become drowsy and over-relaxed. Likewise, the alpha rhythm usually attenuates with eye-opening or mental exertion.

Waves of similar frequency (7–11 Hz) measured over the precentral areas encompassing the sensorimotor cortex are known as mu rhythms. Characteristically, mu rhythms attenuate with contralateral limb movement;[29] likewise, during the imagined movement of a limb, the contralateral mu rhythm reduces.[30]

Beta-frequency waves are those measured from 12 Hz to 25–30 Hz. They are usually distributed symmetrically and frontally located, and are maximally measured in alert, eyes-open or anxious people. Some variances in beta waves are associated with effects of drugs, in particular benzodiazepines. Beta's association with anxious thinking is reflected in reports of increased and disordered patterns of beta activity in obsessive–compulsive disorders,[31] sleep disorders[32] and the control of ADHD via biofeedback.[33]

Gamma-frequency waves are those measured in the frequency range of approximately 26–100 Hz. Gamma rhythms are thought to represent the binding mechanism within and between different populations or networks of neurons, enabling cognitive or motor functions.[34,35] In autism, increased-amplitude gamma activity has been identified and is interpreted as an attenuation of inhibitory mechanisms;[36–38] in schizophrenia, disordered processing is linked to differences in gamma amplitude and coherence.[39–41]

Lambda waves are single sharp waves over the occipital pole, associated with scanning visual scenes or pictures. It has been suggested that they represent the start of passage of information from occipital to prefrontal areas,[42] while other negative waveforms over visual areas in response to patterns may represent local processing.[43]

Coherence: a mathematical measure of similarity of frequency between two cortical locations

Another potential source of information that can be identified through the use of spectral decomposition of the EEG signal is that of coherence, a form of analysis that compares the periodicity of a given frequency between two locations. This is thought to give information on the localization of network activity by enabling the identification of lead and lag assemblies of neurons. Current research utilizing coherence analysis is enabling the identification of malfunctioning circuits in Alzheimer's disease[44] and Parkinson's disease[45] and, by use of electrocorticograph (EcoG), potentially mapping epileptogenic circuits within temporal lobe epilepsy.[46]

CONCLUSION

The EEG is used in psychiatric conditions in order to assist in diagnosing and excluding certain organic brain diseases. It may be helpful in distinguishing between an acute toxic confusional psychosis and an acute functional psychosis. It is of major importance in distinguishing between epilepsy and various non-epileptic seizures (psychogenic seizures). It may be of assistance in the differential diagnosis of panic disorder or focal temporal seizures. Occasionally an EEG may be a pointer to a frontal lesion rather than a depressive disorder. It is helpful in the diagnosis of a dementing disorder in a patient who appears to be depressed, or vice versa.

The technological advances over the past three decades have improved data-handling capabilities exponentially, thus enabling far greater sophistication in analytical techniques. As a consequence, many relatively new research paradigms are being utilized in endeavouring to understand, classify and define brain activity, whether normal or atypical. The vast array of different measures and analyses, combined with the many syndromes and the underlying causes of such syndromes, may appear baffling at first glance. It is the aim of this chapter to introduce some of the main issues and some of the current interpretative views as reported in the literature.

KEY POINTS

- EEG is useful in psychiatric conditions where organic brain disease is suspected.
- EEG is of major importance in distinguishing between epileptic and non-epileptic (psychogenic) seizures.
- EEG is essential in identifying whether an epilepsy is of a generalized nature before giving medication.
- EEG is of major importance in differential diagnosis of focal temporal seizures.
- EEG may be of assistance in making the distinction between psychosis and acute functional psychosis.
- EEG may enable differential identification between frontal lesion depressive disorder and dementia.
- In research settings, there are a number of analytical techniques available enabling the direct comparison of specific phenomena between diagnostic groups across studies.

REFERENCES

1. Pillai J, Sperling MR (2006) Interictal EEG and the diagnosis of epilepsy. *Epilepsia* **47** (suppl. 1): 14–22.
2. Binnie CD, Stefan H (1999) Modern electroencephalography: its role in epilepsy management. *Clinical Neurophysiology* **110**: 1671–97.
3. Engel J, Jr (2005) *Epilepsy: Global Issues for the Practicing Neurologist.* New York: Demos Medical Publishing.

4. Luck SJ (2005) *An Introduction to the Event-Related Potential Technique*. Cambridge, MA: MIT Press.
5. Scherg M, Bast T, Berg P (1999) Multiple source analysis of interictal spikes: goals, requirements, clinical value. *Journal of Clinical Neurophysiology* **16**; 214–24.
6. Plummer C, Harvey AS, Cook M (2008) EEG source localization in focal epilepsy: where are we now? *Epilepsia* **49**: 201–18.
7. Homan RW, Herman J, Purdy P (1987) Cerebral location of international 10-20 system electrode placement. *EEG and Clinical Neurophysiology* **66**: 376–82.
8. Salinsky M, Kanter R, Dasheiff RM (1987) Effectiveness of multiple EEGs in supporting the diagnosis of epilepsy: an operational curve. *Epilepsia* **28**: 331–4.
9. Yordanova J, Kolev V (2007) Event-related brain oscillations in normal development. In LA Schmidt, SJ Segalowitz (eds) *Developmental Psychophysiology: Theory, Systems, and Methods*. New York: Cambridge University Press.
10. Mauguière F, Butler SR, Ceranic B, *et al.* (2004) Normal findings by modality. In CD Binnie, R Cooper, F Mauguière, *et al.* (eds) *Clinical Neurophysiology*, Vol. 1. Amsterdam: Elsevier.
11. Kraus N, Smith DI, Reed NL, Stein L, Cartee C (1985) Auditory middle latency responses in children: effect of age and diagnostic category. *Electroencephalography and Clinical Neurophysiology* **62**: 342–51.
12. Wolpaw JR, Wood CC (1982) Scalp distribution of human auditory evoked potentials: II. Evidence for overlapping sources and involvement of auditory cortex. *Electroencephalography and Clinical Neurophysiology* **54**: 25–38.
13. Deiber MP, Ibañez V, Fischer C, Perrin F, Mauguière F (1988) Sequential mapping favours the hypothesis of distinct generators for na and pa middle latency auditory evoked potentials. *Electroencephalography and Clinical Neurophysiology* **71**: 187–97.
14. Kileny P, Paccioreti D, Wilson AF (1987) Effects of cortical lesions on middle latency auditory evoked responses. *Electroencephalography and Clinical Neurophysiology* **66**: 108–20.
15. Ibañez V, Deiber MP, Fischer C (1989) Middle latency auditory evoked potentials in cortical lesions: criteria of interhemispheric asymmetry. *Archives in Neurology* **46**: 1325–32.
16. McComas AJ (1999) The world of touch: from evoked potentials to conscious perception. *Canadian Journal of Neurological Sciences* **26**: 7–17.
17. Näätänen R, Lehtokoski A, Lennes M, *et al.* (1997) Language-specific phoneme representations revealed by electric and magnetic brain responses. *Nature* **385**: 432–34.
18. Giard MH, Perrin F, Pernier J, Bouchet P (1990). Brain generators implicated in processing of auditory stimulus deviance: a topographic event-related potential study. *Psychophysiology* **27**: 627–40.
19. Tales A, Butler SR, Fossey J, *et al.* (2002) Visual search in Alzheimer's disease: a deficiency in processing conjunctions of features. *Neuropsychologia* **40**: 1849–57.
20. Onton J, Westerfield M, Townsend J, Makeig S (2006) Imaging human EEG dynamics using independent component analysis. *Neuroscience and Biobehavioral Reviews* **30**: 808–22.
21. Makeig S, Debener S, Onton J, Delorme A (2004) Mining event-related brain dynamics. *Trends in Cognitive Sciences* **8**: 204–10.
22. Murik SE, Shapkin AG (2004) Simultaneous recording of EEG and direct current (DC) potential makes it possible to assess functional and metabolic state of nervous tissue. *International Journal of Neuroscience* **114**: 977–97.
23. Pleydell-Pearce CW (1994) DC potential correlates of attention and cognitive load. *Cognitive Neuropsychology* **11**: 149–66.
24. Khader P, Schicke T, Roder B, Rosler F (2008). On the relationship between slow cortical potentials and BOLD signal changes in humans. *International Journal of Psychophysiology* **67**: 252–61.
25. Vanhatalo S, Tallgren P, Becker C, *et al.* (2003) Scalp-recorded slow EEG responses generated in response to hemodynamic changes in the human brain. *Clinical Neurophysiology* **114**: 1744–54.
26. Rodriguez G, Copello F, Vitali P, Perego G, Nobili F (1999) EEG spectral profile to stage Alzheimer's disease. *Clinical Neurophysiology* **110**: 1831–7.
27. Polikar R, Topalis A, Green D, Kounios J, Clark CM (2007) Comparative multiresolution wavelet analysis of ERP spectral bands using an ensemble of classifiers approach for early diagnosis of Alzheimer's disease. *Computers in Biology and Medicine* **37**: 542–58.
28. Wienbruch C, Moratti S, Elbert T, *et al.* (2003) Source distribution of neuromagnetic slow wave activity in schizophrenic and depressive patients. *Clinical Neurophysiology* **114**: 2052–60.
29. Pfurtscheller G, Neuper C, Krausz G (2000) Functional dissociation of lower and upper frequency mu rhythms in relation to voluntary limb movement. *Clinical Neurophysiology* **111**: 1873–9.
30. McFarland DJ, Miner LA, Vaughan TM, Wolpaw JR (2000) Mu and beta rhythm topographies during motor imagery and actual movements. *Brain Topography* **12**: 177–86.
31. Yasan A, Gurgen F (2004) Obsesif Kompulsif Bozuklukta Elektroensefalografı Bulgulari. [Electroencephalography findings in patients with obsessive compulsive disorder.] *Klinik Psikofarmakoloji Bulteni* **14**: 61–7.
32. Perlis ML, Kehr EL, Smith MT, *et al.* (2001) Temporal and stagewise distribution of high frequency EEG activity in patients with primary and secondary insomnia and in good sleeper controls. *Journal of Sleep Research* **10**: 93–104.
33. Strehl U, Leins U, Danzer N, *et al.* (2004) EEG feedback for children with attention-deficit/hyperactivity disorder

(ADHD): preliminary results from a randomized, controlled study. *Kindheit und Entwicklung* 13: 180–89.
34. Tallon-Baudry C, Bertrand O (1999) Oscillatory gamma activity in humans and its role in object representation. *Trends in Cognitive Sciences* 3: 151–62.
35. Müller MM, Bosch J, Elbert T, *et al.* (1996) Visually induced gamma-based responses in human electroencephalographic activity: a link to animal studies. *Experimental Brain Research* 112: 96–102.
36. Brock J, Brown CC, Boucher J, Rippon G (2002) The temporal binding deficit hypothesis of autism. *Development and Psychopathology* 14: 209–24.
37. Brown C, Gruber T, Boucher J, Rippon G, Brock J (2005) Gamma abnormalities during perception of illusory figures in autism. *Cortex* 41: 364–76.
38. Grice SJ, Spratling MW, Karmiloff-Smith A, *et al.* (2001) Disordered visual processing and oscillatory brain activity in autism and Williams syndrome. *Neuroreport* 12: 2697–700.
39. Gordon E, Williams L, Haig AR, Wright J, Meares RA (2001) Symptom profile and 'gamma' processing in schizophrenia. *Cognitive Neuropsychiatry* 6: 7–19.
40. Haig AR, Gordon E, De Pascalis V, *et al.* (2000) Gamma activity in schizophrenia: evidence of impaired network binding? *Clinical Neurophysiology* 111: 1461–8.
41. Light GA, Hsu JL, Hsieh MH, *et al.* (2006) Gamma band oscillations reveal neural network cortical coherence dysfunction in schizophrenia patients. *Biological Psychiatry* 60: 1231–40.
42. Thorpe SG, Nunez PL, Srinivasan R (2007) Identification of wave-like spatial structure in the SSVEP: comparison of simultaneous EEG and MEG. *Statistics in Medicine* 26: 3911–26.
43. Radhakrishnan K, Sunku AJ, Donat JF, Klass DW (2007) Pattern-induced negative occipital potentials (PINOP). *Journal of Clinical Neurophysiology* 24: 277–80.
44. Hidasi Z, Czigler B, Salacz P, Csibri E, Molnar M (2007) Changes of EEG spectra and coherence following performance in a cognitive task in Alzheimer's disease. *International Journal of Psychophysiology* 65: 252–60.
45. Timmermann L, Florin E, Reck C (2007) Pathological cerebral oscillatory activity in Parkinson's disease: a critical review on methods, data and hypotheses. *Expert Review of Medical Devices* 4: 651–61.
46. Ortega GJ, de la Prida LM, Sola RG, Pastor J (2008) Synchronization clusters of interictal activity in the lateral temporal cortex of epileptic patients: intraoperative electrocorticographic analysis. *Epilepsia* 49: 269–80.

Chapter 30

Neurochemistry

Gavin P Reynolds, Michael K Harte and Trisha A Jenkins

INTRODUCTION

The brain is a highly complex and specialized organ, and this complexity can be seen in its cellular composition. The cellular specialization of the brain, and of the other components of the central nervous system (CNS) and peripheral nervous system (PNS), inevitably reflects, and is ideally suited to, its function. This cellular specificity is built on a foundation of biochemical factors, processes and mechanisms; thus, there is also a neurochemical specificity in brain function. This is primarily but not solely associated with neurons, which are differentiated by the neurotransmitters they secrete and the receptors they express. It is this neurochemistry with which this chapter is mainly concerned.

The central component of this cellular structure is the neuron. The neuron is a highly specialized cell with unique features that enable it to generate and propagate electrical impulses and to translate those impulses into a chemical signal to pass information to an adjacent cell. This process is synaptic neurotransmission, and inevitably much of this chapter will be concerned with the specialized molecules and mechanisms of neurotransmission. Synaptic control of neuronal activity provides the complex, elaborate, subtle and flexible mechanisms by which the brain is able to process information. Thus, synaptic neurotransmission is the point at which we can modify neuronal function – distorting it or normalizing it when it goes awry. The great majority of psychiatric drugs act directly or indirectly to influence neurotransmitter function at the synapse.

Glial cells

The neuron is outnumbered in the CNS by the various glial cells, supporting neuronal function structurally or biochemically, although it has been shown that some glial cells can have direct effects on neurotransmission. The glia include oligodendrocytes, or Schwann cells in the PNS, forming the myelin sheath that provides electrical insulation for neuronal axons. The membranes of these cells are specialized for this function in having relatively high lipid content and less protein (20% protein rather than the more typical 50% in other cells).

Astroglia (or astrocytes) are the most common cells of the CNS, where they provide many of the necessary processes absent in the highly specialized neurons. They provide the neuron with glucose and regulate the extraneuronal environment by removing the products of neuronal activity. This includes uptake of potassium ions for which they express a high density of potassium channels. They also express transporters for fast-acting neurotransmitters such as glutamate and γ-aminobutyric acid (GABA), facilitating their rapid removal from the synapse after release. They are involved in subsequent decarboxylation of glutamate to glutamine and the return of glutamine to neurons as the precursor of glutamate. Astrocytes have also been shown to express certain glutamate receptors.

The intimate relationship of astrocytes with both the blood supply (see below) and neurons demonstrates their role in mediating neuronal control of blood flow, which is usefully employed as a surrogate indicator of neuronal activity in neuroimaging studies of brain function. Proliferation of astrocytes occurs in situations following neural damage; this gliosis, or gliotic reaction, results in the CNS equivalent of scar tissue.

Microglia are the CNS equivalent of monocytes: they are relatively mobile and continually monitor the brain environment to identify damage by detecting changes in K^+ ions, and act as phagocytic scavengers when activated, as can astrocytes.

The blood–brain barrier

The blood–brain barrier protects the brain from unwanted incursion by a variety of substances from bacteria and other cells to single proteins and small molecules, while permitting passage into the brain of many compounds necessary for its normal function, such as oxygen, glucose and amino acids. These protective and facilitatory processes use both passive and active mechanisms.

The blood–brain barrier is thus both a physical barrier and a series of biochemical processes associated with a dense layer of luminal epithelial cells having supportive 'astrocytic feet' behind them. The tight junctions between cells provide an effective physical barrier against cellular and subcellular species and plasma solutes. However, there are also efflux transporter mechanisms that actively exclude potentially toxic small molecules, such as the p-glycoprotein transporter (MDR1 or ABCB1). Although of benefit in protecting the brain from xenobiotics, this system can compromise drug delivery by diminishing drug availability to the brain; several psychiatric drugs (e.g. risperidone, paroxetine, citalopram) are p-glycoprotein substrates.

The blood–brain barrier contains active transport mechanisms that transfer small molecules from the blood into the brain. These include a large number of transporters for glucose, amino acids and other essential nutrients, some of which may also recognize certain drugs as substrates. Important in understanding neurotransmitter biochemistry is the large neutral amino-acid transporter system (system L), of which two components are LAT-1 and LAT-2. This is responsible for the transport of several amino acids essential to brain function, including tyrosine and tryptophan, precursors of the catecholamine neurotransmitters and serotonin, respectively.

Ion channels and ion pumps

The neuron is an excitable cell with unique physiological properties that are essential for its function in transmission of nerve impulses, the action potential, from cell body to axon terminal. There are also essential features at the axon, or neuronal, terminal that bring about release of stored neurotransmitter into the synapse in response to the arrival of the action potential. The immediate driving force behind these processes is the membrane potential across the neuronal membrane. It is maintained by an uneven distribution of ionic charge across the plasma membrane, with K^+ more concentrated on the inside of the cell, and Na^+ and Ca^{2+} more concentrated on the outside of the cell. These concentration gradients arise largely through the action of the energy-dependent sodium/potassium ATPase, an enzymic pump that breaks down adenosine triphosphate (ATP) in the presence of intracellular Na^+, driving the pump that exchanges this Na^+ for extracellular K^+ in order to maintain ionic concentration gradients and membrane potential. It is the ion channels in the cell membrane that determine how this membrane potential is used to propagate action potentials and stimulate neurotransmitter release.

Ion channels are formed of four to six channel proteins that assemble to form a pore. Each subunit has a hydrophobic surface that readily associates with the phospholipid layer of the membrane. The composition of proteins varies between channels, and this is what provides their different properties and selectivity. Ion channels are selectively permeable for particular ions (e.g. sodium, potassium, calcium, chloride); this selectivity, specified by the pore diameter and the nature of the amino acid residues lining it, is their most important property.

Ion channels can be rested (closed, but able to be opened upon a stimulus), activated (open) or inactivated (closed and not able to be opened by a stimulus). Most ion channels remain inactivated until specific signals dictate their opening. This property of gating is governed by changes in the local environment of the membrane, such as the membrane potential, leading the channel to be termed 'voltage-gated', or when they respond to changes in neurotransmitter concentrations, when they are known as 'ligand-gated'.

The voltage-gated Na^+ and K^+ channels control the production and propagation of the action potential. But when the action potential arrives at the neuronal terminal, voltage-gated Ca^{2+} channels are particularly important in the first stage of translating this electrical signal into chemical neurotransmission. These Ca^{2+} channels are concentrated at the synaptic cleft and open in response to the change in membrane potential associated with the arrival of an action potential. Ca^{2+} enters the cell down an electrical and chemical gradient – intracellular Ca^{2+} is held at about 10^{-7} M while outside the cell it is approximately 10^{-4} M.

The subsequent local increase in Ca^{2+} within the presynaptic cell membrane promotes fusion of vesicles containing neurotransmitter stores with the membrane, leading to exocytotic release of transmitter. This is brought about by effects on lipid metabolism and on the function of several structural and soluble proteins within the presynaptic terminal. Thus, vesicles that are attached to the cytoskeleton by synapsin I are released following a Ca-dependent phosphorylation of synapsin I, allowing them to move to the presynaptic active zone. Vesicles in the active zone are attached to, and fuse with, the plasma membrane by the action of several Ca^{2+}-sensitive structural and soluble proteins.

Ca^{2+} has multiple actions on the cell and these can have toxic effects if they are not controlled carefully. Thus, there are effective mechanisms for the removal of Ca^{2+} from the cytosol following transmitter release. There are buffering systems such as Ca^{2+} binding proteins, vesicular sequestration and mitochondrial storage, and there are also two pumping mechanisms to remove Ca^{2+} from the cell, including a Ca^{2+}-ATPase and a Ca^{2+}/Na^+ antiporter pump.

CHEMICAL NEUROTRANSMISSION

Neurotransmitters are generally small molecules that are released from a neuron into a synapse in response to an action potential to have an effect on a postsynaptic cell. This implies that there is substantial cellular specialization; neurons need to have mechanisms for synthesis and storage of neurotransmitter, and postsynaptic cells will have specific receptors. Thus, there is both pre- and postsynaptic specialization. In addition, there need to be mechanisms for transmitter release (as described above) and cellular processes for removal.

Classically, there are specific criteria suggested for the identification of a specific substance as a transmitter, including its presence in the neuron, its release following neuronal stimulation and specific removal mechanisms. In addition, the effect of the putative transmitter needs to be identical with its endogenous functional activity. However, as our understanding of the complexity of the brain has developed, increasingly more substances have been identified that meet some, but not necessarily all, of these criteria. Thus, compounds with synaptic actions may be secreted by glial cells, or stimulated release of a neuropeptide may not be associated with a rapid synaptic removal mechanism but may rely primarily on diffusion away to terminate its action.

The main classical transmitters to be discussed here are dopamine and noradrenaline, serotonin, acetylcholine, glutamate and γ-aminobutyric acid (GABA); some important neuropeptides are included in a further section. There are other compounds that also have 'classical' neurotransmitter activity, including histamine and glycine, and further molecules that have less conventional modes of action, such as nitric oxide (NO), adenosine and the endogenous cannabinoid anandamide. Neurotransmitters comprise a disparate group of compounds with different chemical structures and functional activities. The classical transmitters are often subdivided in a variety of ways, depending on various criteria, including chemical class (e.g. catecholamine, neuropeptide), duration of response (fast, slow) or postsynaptic effect (excitatory, inhibitory). However, it is the postsynaptic receptors that determine whether neurotransmitters are excitatory or inhibitory and that contribute to the rapidity of their response.

The classical neurotransmitters are synthesized from readily available precursors by specific and selective enzymatic processes. The ubiquity of neurotransmitter precursors is an important feature that enables the CNS to function even under conditions of extreme physiological stress. In, for example, situations of starvation, when the body may exhaust fat supplies and turn to protein breakdown for energy, the amino acids from which the monoamine neurotransmitters are produced remain available in the blood. Active transport processes across the blood–brain barrier ensure a ready availability of precursor for neurotransmitter synthesis.

The synthesis and storage processes determine the specificity of neurons for particular neurotransmitters (Table 30.1). Most of the enzymes responsible for the synthesis of transmitter molecules are found only in specific neurons. Similarly, the transporters responsible for uptake or reuptake of transmitter into the neuronal terminal and those mediating storage in vesicles are exclusive to neuronal subtypes.

Functional anatomy of neurotransmitter systems

The specificity that neurotransmitters impart to neurons contributes to the anatomical specificity of brain function. Some neurotransmitters appear ubiquitous throughout the

Box 30.1 The cannabinoid system

The effects on the brain of preparations from *Cannabis sativa*, the hemp plant, have been known for thousands of years. Low doses of cannabis can have effects that are both euphoric and calming, as well as being analgesic and impairing cognitive and psychomotor function. It can stimulate appetite and in high doses may be psychotogenic. These actions are primarily brought about by an active component of cannabis, Δ^9-tetrahydrocannabinol (THC), which has been shown to act as an agonist at specific cannabinoid receptors, of which CB1 is the major brain site. The naturally occurring agonists at the CB receptors, the endocannabinoids, include the derivatives of arachidonic acid, anandamide and 2-arachidonylglycerol. CB1 receptors are found primarily on presynaptic neuronal terminals, where they are thought to mediate retrograde signalling. This is a process of feedback inhibition across the synapse, whereby the endocannabinoid is synthesized in and released from postsynaptic cells in response to synaptic activity to have an inhibitory effect on further presynaptic release of transmitter.

The cannabinoid system interacts with glutamate, opioid, dopamine and other neurotransmitter systems, and these interactions are likely to be important in a variety of functions, including reward and drug dependence. Synthetic cannabinoid ligands have potential in the treatment of pain, nausea, obesity and drug dependence.

The high occurrence of cannabis abuse in people with schizophrenia is surprising considering the psychotogenic propensity of THC, although some of its other effects may be enjoyable and provide relief from symptoms. However, cannabis has other components beside THC; one of these, cannabidiol, has both CB1 antagonist effects and antipsychotic properties, indicating the potential of synthetic CB1 antagonists as antipsychotic drugs.

FURTHER READING

Laviolette SR, Grace AA (2006) The roles of cannabinoid and dopamine receptor systems in neural emotional learning circuits: implications for schizophrenia and addiction. *Cellular and Molecular Life Sciences* **63**: 1597–613.

Maldonado R, Valverde O, Berrendero F (2006) Involvement of the endocannabinoid system in drug addiction. *Trends in Neuroscience* **29**: 225–32.

Table 30.1 Major enzymes involved in the synthesis and degradation of transmitter molecules

Neurotransmitter	Major synthesis enzyme	Major degradation enzymes
Dopamine	Tyrosine hydroxylase	Catechol-O-methyl transferase, monoamine oxidase A and B
Noradrenaline	Dopamine b-hydroxylase	Catechol-O-methyl transferase, monoamine oxidase A
Serotonin	Tryptophan hydroxylase	Monoamine oxidase A
Acetylcholine	Choline acetyltransferase	Acetylcholinesterase
GABA	Glutamic acid decarboxylase	GABA transaminase
Glutamate	Glutaminase	Aspartate aminotransferase

GABA, γ-aminobutyric acid.

brain; this is true for glutamate and GABA, respectively the major excitatory and inhibitory neurotransmitters. Thus, glutamate is associated with most neuronal interconnections from, to and between cortical areas, while GABA is the primary transmitter within the interneurons that provide inhibitory control over the activity of these and other neuronal systems. Other neurotransmitters are highly specific in both anatomical distribution and function. This is illustrated by the various pathways of dopamine: the highest concentrations of brain dopamine are found in the caudate nucleus and putamen, the terminal regions of the nigrostriatal pathway, where it is essential to the control of motor function.

The catecholamine neurotransmitters

Dopamine and the biochemically related noradrenaline (norepinephrine) are the main catecholamine neurotransmitters, so-called because of their 3,4-dihydroxyphenyl (catechol) structure. Adrenaline (epinephrine) is a further member of this group but is only a relatively scarce transmitter in the human brain, despite its major role in adrenal gland function. With serotonin (and, strictly, histamine), they comprise the monoamine neurotransmitters. They may also be referred to as 'biogenic amines'.

Most dopamine and noradrenaline in the brain is found within neurons with their cell bodies in the brainstem: in the substantia nigra and adjacent ventral tegmental area (VTA) for dopamine, and primarily in the locus coeruleus for noradrenaline. The substantia nigra and locus coeruleus are the two melanin-pigmented nuclei of the human brain and a consequence of the high turnover of neurotransmitter in these structures; neuromelanin is a product of catecholamine oxidation.

The main dopaminergic pathways of the human brain are illustrated in Figure 30.1. The great majority of dopaminergic neurons project to the striatum, the caudate nucleus and putamen, from the substantia nigra. It is this pathway that degenerates profoundly in Parkinson's disease. The innervation of the limbic structures (e.g. nucleus accumbens, amygdala) and neocortical regions is from the VTA. A small hypothalamic tuberoinfundibular pathway secretes dopamine into the hypophyseal portal blood to have effects on dopamine receptors of the anterior pituitary gland, where it acts as the prolactin inhibitory factor.

Noradrenergic neurons have a more diffuse innervation, projecting to many brain regions, including the limbic structures of the hippocampus, amygdala and nucleus accumbens, and the thalamus, hypothalamus, neocortex and cerebellum.

Dopamine is synthesized from tyrosine and transported from the blood across the blood–brain barrier by the active large neutral amino-acid transporter system. Within the dopaminergic neuron, tyrosine is converted to L-dihydroxyphenylalanine (L-dopa) by the rate-limiting enzyme tyrosine hydroxylase (TH) (Figure 30.2). L-Dopa is rapidly

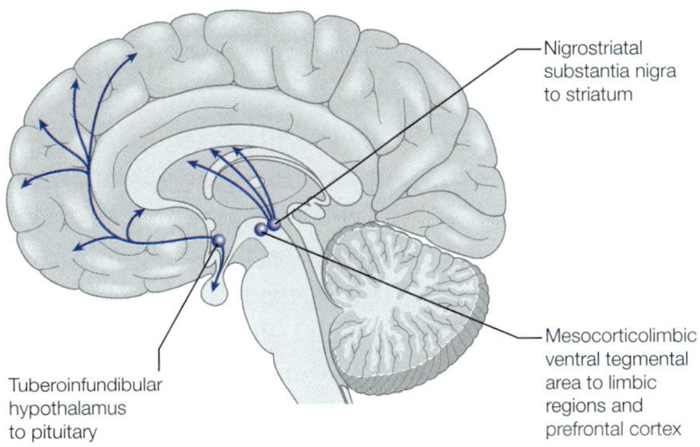

Figure 30.1 Dopaminergic tracts. There are four main dopaminergic tracts in the brain: (i) the nigrostriatal pathway from the substantia nigra to the striatum; (ii) the tuberoinfundibular providing dopamine via the blood of the hypothalamus neurons to the pituitary, which has a controlling effect on the release of the hormone prolactin; (iii) the mesolimbic tract from the ventral tegmental area to many parts of the limbic system; and (iv) the mesocortical tract from the ventral tegmental area to the neocortex, particularly to prefrontal regions

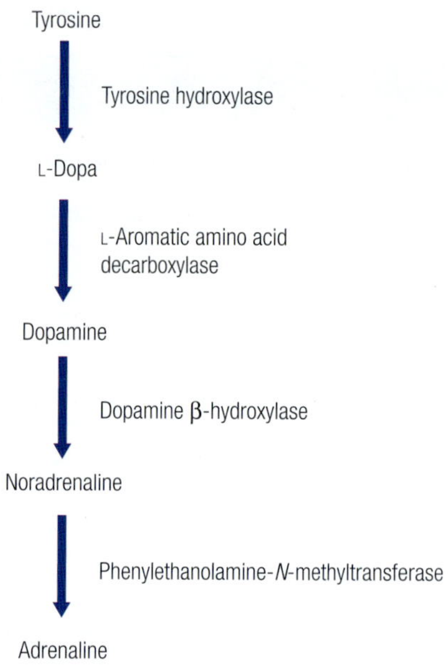

Figure 30.2 Pathway for synthesis of the monoamines

decarboxylated to dopamine by L-aromatic amino acid decarboxylase (AAAD); dopamine is then taken up and stored in vesicles by the vesicle monoamine transporter (VMAT). A further transporter for dopamine is found in the neuronal membrane, which modulates the temporal and spatial influence of dopamine, although the major removal process for released transmitter is diffusion away from the synapse.

Although neurotransmitter release from vesicles into the synapse is controlled in part by neuronal activity, the synthesis of new catecholamine transmitters is also carefully regulated by feedback mechanisms. The rate-determining TH enzyme provides the point for this control; it is subject to end-product inhibition by intracellular dopamine and noradrenaline. TH can also be regulated by receptors sensitive to extracellular transmitter (autoreceptors); there are synthesis-modulating autoreceptors sensitive to dopamine that influence the phosphorylation status of the enzyme. As the synthesis of its immediate precursor, L-dopa, is the rate-determining step in dopamine synthesis, bypassing this step by administration of L-dopa will increase the availability of dopamine, independent of the regulatory control provided by tyrosine hydroxylase. This is made use of in the treatment of Parkinson's disease with L-dopa.

There are also release-modulating autoreceptors that provide a usually inhibitory control over neurotransmitter release; for dopamine and noradrenaline, these are D2-like and α2 receptors, respectively.

Noradrenaline neurons are biochemically differentiated from those of dopamine by the additional presence of dopamine-β-hydroxylase in the synaptic vesicles (see Figure 30.2). These neurons also employ the VMAT, but the neuronal membrane has a specific noradrenaline transporter.

Adrenaline-containing neurons such as the chromaffin cells of the adrenal medulla and some isolated brainstem nuclei contain the enzyme phenylethanolamine-*N*-methyltransferase, responsible for adrenaline synthesis by methylation of noradrenaline (see Figure 30.2).

5-Hydroxytryptamine

5-Hydroxytryptamine (5-HT, serotonin) also has a widespread innervation in the human brain, with most projections arising from neuronal cell bodies in the dorsal and median raphe and neighbouring nuclei of the lower brainstem. There are projections to the hippocampus, amygdala, hypothalamus, thalamus, neocortex and striatum and other basal ganglia regions, including the substantia nigra, although most structures receive some serotonergic innervation.

5-HT is synthesized from tryptophan, also a substrate for the large neutral amino-acid transporter system across the blood–brain barrier. As with the catecholamine neurotransmitters, the enzyme responsible for initial hydroxylation of precursor amino acid represents the rate-determining step in transmitter synthesis (Figure 30.3). This enzyme, tryptophan hydroxylase (TPH), has been shown to occur in two forms with separate genes; the *TPH2* gene codes for the enzyme form that is found primarily in human brain. The resultant 5-hydroxytryptophan is decarboxylated by AAAD to 5-HT, which is taken up into vesicles by VMAT. Again, a specific 5-HT transporter is found in the neuronal membrane.

Although the initial tryptophan hydroxylation step is rate-determining, the TPH enzyme is not saturated and availability of tryptophan can determine the rate of 5-HT synthesis. Tryptophan is unusual among amino acids in that up to 90 per cent is bound to plasma albumin and hence unavailable for transport into the brain; this limits the tryptophan available for 5-HT synthesis. Also, in contrast to catecholamine synthesis, there is no end-product inhibition of TPH, although TPH activity may be influenced by neuronal firing, which can be modulated by autoreceptors of the 5-HT1A subtype.

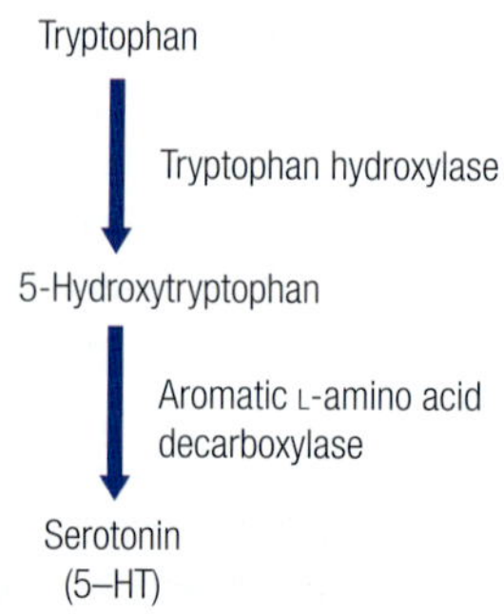

Figure 30.3 Pathway for synthesis of serotonin
5-HT, 5-hydroxytryptamine.

Melatonin

In a specific set of cells in the pineal gland, 5-HT is converted by two enzymes to form melatonin. This hormone is released from the pineal gland under the control of, and to have feedback effects on, the suprachiasmatic nucleus of the hypothalamus, the circadian clock of the brain. Melatonin release is enhanced at night to have, among other actions, inhibitory effects on 5-HT neuronal activity.

Synaptic removal of the monoamine neurotransmitters

Once released into the synapse to have effects on postsynaptic cells by binding to receptors, 5-HT and the catecholamine neurotransmitters are removed via neuronal transporters specific to each transmitter. These important sites for pharmacotherapeutic intervention are found on the presynaptic cell membrane and permit transmitter, at least in part, to be recycled by uptake into the neuronal terminal and re-stored in vesicles.

Excess transmitter can be metabolized, and all three transmitters are substrates for monoamine oxidase (MAO), which occurs in two main forms with different genes. MAO-A is responsible for 5-HT and noradrenaline, while dopamine can also be oxidized by MAO-B. The enzymes are present throughout the body, including the gut, kidneys and liver, and found in neurons and glial cells in the CNS, although there is some selectivity of MAO subtype within brain regions. In addition to its role in metabolizing transmitter, MAO has a function in metabolizing dietary xenobiotics and thereby protecting the brain from unwanted and potentially neuroactive compounds. This is demonstrated by the 'cheese effect', the hypertensive crisis occurring when both MAO subtypes are inhibited by an MAO inhibitor and a source of tyramine (e.g. mature cheese, pickled herrings, some red wines) is ingested. Tyramine, normally rapidly removed by MAO before it can reach neuronal terminals, acts as a 'false transmitter' and directly or indirectly (by transmitter release) can bring about a substantial and occasionally life-threatening increase in blood pressure.

Although MAO-A is the only metabolic removal mechanism for 5-HT, the catecholamines are substrates for another enzyme, catechol-O-methyltransferase (COMT). This enzyme also acts on the products of MAO (and vice versa) (Figure 30.4). It exists in soluble and membrane-bound forms; its cellular and subcellular localization is not fully understood, although the soluble enzyme may be localized primarily to glia while membrane-bound COMT appears to be present on intracellular membranes of postsynaptic cells. In regions where the innervation is relatively dense (such as the striatum for dopamine), COMT has little effect on transmitter availability, since reuptake via neuronal transporters and subsequent storage or oxidative metabolism is relatively more important in regulating synaptic transmitter. However, in regions such as the cortex where neuronal terminals are relatively sparse, COMT activity appears to have a relatively greater importance and can influence concentrations of dopamine. This has attracted interest since there are common genetic variants in COMT that influence its activity and are associated with (presumably dopamine-mediated) individual differences in frontal cortical cognitive function, particularly in the context of cognitive deficits in schizophrenia.

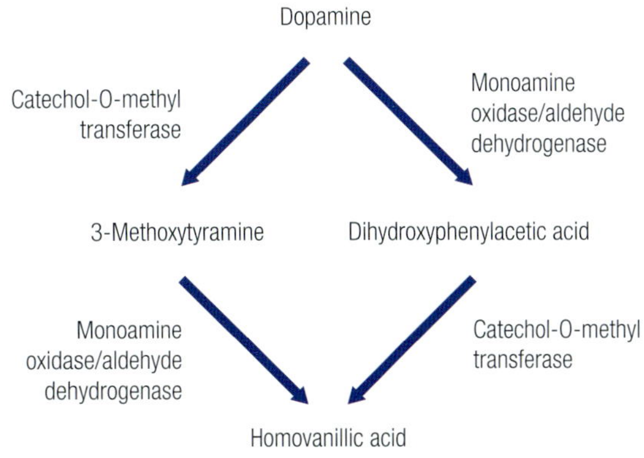

Figure 30.4 Pathway for degradation of dopamine

Acetylcholine

The first identified neurotransmitter was acetylcholine, detected as the substance released from the vagus nerve to diminish heart rate. In addition to its role in the PNS as a transmitter in parasympathetic nerves and at the neuromuscular junction, it also has a role in brain function, controlling motor and cognitive functions. It has a major cell group in the basal forebrain, where, from the basal nucleus of Meynert, there are projections to the cerebral cortex and parts of the amygdala, thalamus and basal ganglia. Adjacent nuclei (of the septum and the diagonal band of Broca) project to the hippocampus. This system is implicated in Alzheimer's disease, in which the degeneration of basal forebrain cholinergic neurons is thought to contribute to cognitive deficits.

Cholinergic neurons in the brainstem projecting rostrally are part of the reticular activating system. There are also cholinergic interneurons, notably in the striatum, where they play a major role in the control of motor function.

Acetylcholine is synthesized in neurons from readily available precursors: acetyl-coenzyme A (acetyl-CoA), deriving from glucose in intermediary metabolism, and choline, a component of membrane lipids. This enzymatic process requires choline acetyltransferase (ChAT), an enzyme specific to cholinergic neurons and present in excess in the neuronal terminal (Figure 30.5). Hence, it is the availability of precursors that normally determine rate of acetylcholine synthesis, although there appears to be some product inhibition of ChAT activity. Acetylcholine is stored in vesicles by a specific vesicular acetylcholine transporter.

Released acetylcholine is removed from the synapse by the hydrolytic enzyme acetylcholinesterase (AChE) to pro-

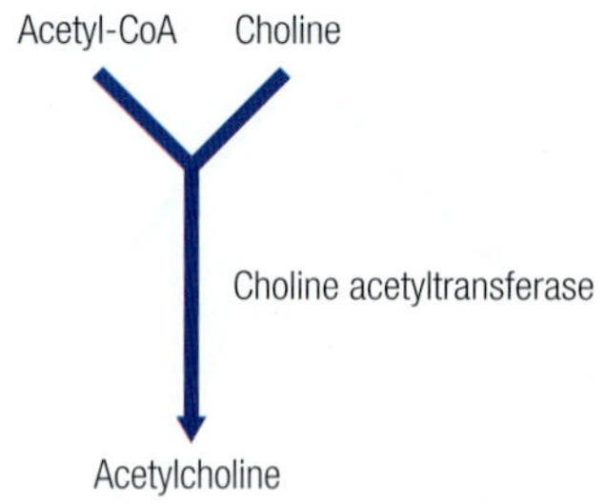

Figure 30.5 Pathway for synthesis of acetylcholine

duce acetic acid and choline. AChE is a glycoprotein that in one form is attached to the extracellular matrix of the cell membrane at the synapse and rapidly breaks down released acetylcholine. AChE inhibition can increase brain acetylcholine and is a target for the treatment of Alzheimer's disease. Much of the choline produced in this process is taken up into the presynaptic neuron by a high-affinity transporter specific to cholinergic cells, where it can be recycled into more acetylcholine. Release-modulating autoreceptors are present on cholinergic terminals; these are primarily of the muscarinic M2 subtype.

Glutamate

Glutamate (glutamic acid) is the major excitatory neurotransmitter in the brain and is involved in all aspects of brain function. It is found throughout the CNS, notably as the transmitter in the large pyramidal neurons (e.g. motor neurons) of the cortex that project to other regions of the brain or spinal cord. Aspartate (aspartic acid) is another excitatory neurotransmitter that is similarly distributed, albeit in somewhat lower concentrations; it may be a specific transmitter in certain cortical, hippocampal and cerebellar neurons. However, it is not easy to clearly differentiate aspartate and glutamate neurotransmission, since the two transmitters have common effects at several receptors and share many presynaptic mechanisms. It is thus common to refer to the effects of the two as excitatory amino acid (EAA) neurotransmission; often, discussion of glutamatergic action cannot distinguish effects of aspartate and is used to imply EAA, rather than solely glutamate, neurotransmission. This convention with be used in much of the following discussion, which will not specifically address aspartate as a transmitter.

The neuronal specificity of glutamatergic cells is provided by specific synthetic and transporter mechanisms. Glutamate is an important component of cellular metabolism, being an amino acid required for protein synthesis, and hence is found in all cells, where it is synthesized from glucose via the Krebs cycle. Neurotransmitter glutamate is formed primarily from glutamine by the enzyme glutaminase. Glutamate is then taken up into vesicles by specific transporters (vesicular glutamate transporters 1 and 2 primarily in brain) for storage before release on stimulation.

Released glutamate is removed very rapidly from the synapse by specific cell membrane transporters, the excitatory amino acid transporters (EAATs). These sodium-dependent transporters are found not only in presynaptic neurons (primarily EAAT3 in cerebral neurons) but also in postsynaptic cells (also EAAT3) and surrounding glial cells (EAAT1, EAAT2). Glial EAAT2 in particular is responsible for over 90 per cent of total glutamate uptake. These highly effective removal processes are essential not only in limiting the action of glutamate to transient effects on synaptic transmission after release but also in limiting the toxicity that comes from excessive extracellular glutamate (Box 30.2). Glutamate

Box 30.2 Excitotoxicity

It has long been known that the excitatory amino acid neurotransmitter glutamate can cause damage to neural tissue. Introduced systemically, it can cause damage to retinal cells and to regions of the hypothalamus in young animals; these effects can be blocked by antagonists of glutamate receptors. Glutamate receptor agonists such as kainic, ibotenic and quinolinic acids can also cause neuronal damage on injection into neural tissue, specifically to neuronal cell bodies and dendrites, while preserving axons passing through the area of lesion. This process demonstrates a close correlation between the excitatory receptor effects and neurotoxic potencies of these glutamate agonists, indicating a mechanism of excitatory neurotoxicity, or excitotoxicity.

Excitotoxicity is due to enhanced and excessive receptor-mediated Ca^{2+} entry into neurons via the glutamate/*N*-methyl-D-aspartate (NMDA) receptor. Neurons have mechanisms to minimize the cytosolic concentrations of Ca^{2+}, but when these buffering and transporter capacities are overcome by an excess of Ca^{2+} influx following excitatory stimulation of glutamate receptors, several toxic processes may be initiated:

- Activation of proteases and phospholipases
- Loss of mitochondrial function
- Loss of nuclear function
- Further glutamate release.

The concept and process of excitotoxicity have been valuable in developing models for the understanding of neurodegenerative disease. In addition, it may well contribute to neuronal damage following ischaemic stroke and epileptic seizures, and to the neurotoxic effects of inflammatory responses within the brain. Excitotoxic damage is also postulated to contribute to the structural changes and neuronal deficits in the brain reported in schizophrenia and affective disorders.

FURTHER READING

Nicholls D (2008) Oxidative stress and energy crises in neuronal dysfunction. *Annals of the New York Academy of Sciences* **1147**: 53–60.

Olney JW (1990) Excitotoxic amino acids and neuropsychiatric disorders. *Annual Review of Pharmacology and Toxicology* **30**: 47–71.

release is under inhibitory control by metabotropic autoreceptors, primarily of the mGluR2 subtype.

The glutamate removed from the synapse by uptake into glia is mainly metabolized to glutamine by the enzyme glutamine synthetase, which is absent in the neuron. This glial glutamine then serves as the precursor for further neuronal glutamate after active transport from the glial cell into the neuron. Thus, there is a 'glutamine cycle' providing for the synthesis and recycling of neurotransmitter glutamate, differentiating this pool of amino acid from the glutamate associated with cellular metabolism (Figure 30.6).

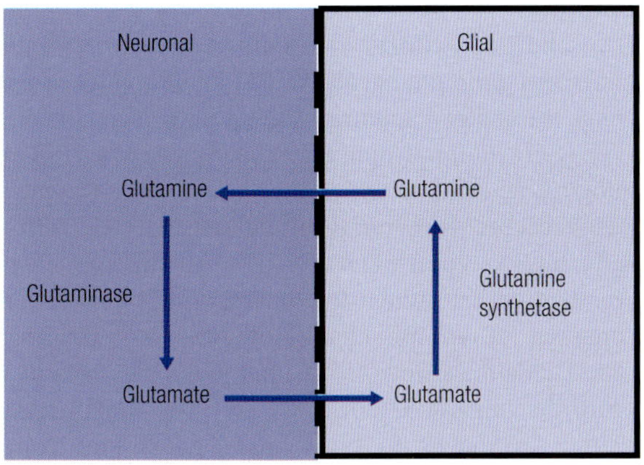

Figure 30.6 Pathway for glutamate synthesis and recycling

γ-Aminobutyric acid

GABA is the main inhibitory neurotransmitter in the brain. Like glutamate, GABA is ubiquitous in the CNS, where it is found in the majority of interneurons and also in some inhibitory projection neurons. For example, neurons projecting from the striatum to the pallidum and subsequently the thalamus are GABAergic; these are important in the control of motor function and selectively degenerate in Huntington's disease. Neurons containing GABA can be subdivided in many ways: on the basis of their electrical activity (fast-/slow-firing), the neuropeptides they contain (e.g. cholecystokinin (CCK), somatostatin), their morphology (e.g. chandelier cells) or their calcium-binding proteins (e.g. parvalbumin). Parvalbumin-containing GABAergic interneurons have been found to be diminished in the cortex and hippocampus in schizophrenia.

GABA is synthesized from glutamate in neuronal terminals by the enzyme glutamic acid decarboxylase (GAD). It is stored in vesicles by the specific vesicular GABA transporter. Synaptic released GABA is removed rapidly by sodium-dependent transporters, which, as for glutamate, are found not only in presynaptic neuronal membranes but also on adjacent astrocytes. GABA release, as with other neurotransmitters, is under inhibitory feedback control through autoreceptors, primarily of the $GABA_B$ subtype.

Metabolic breakdown of GABA occurs in both neurons and glia by the enzyme GABA-transaminase which, by transferring an amino group to α-ketoglutarate, results in the (re)formation of glutamate, the immediate synthetic precursor of GABA.

NEUROTRANSMITTER RECEPTORS

The various neurotransmitters and other signalling molecules in the brain bring about their effects by action at specific receptors. These receptors are proteins that respond to agonists – that is, molecules such as neurotransmitters and drugs that mimic neurotransmitter action at the receptor. Agonist action is due to binding of the molecule to a specific recognition site on the protein; this binding to the receptor initiates a process of biochemical or ionic effects that influence cellular function. Molecules including agonists that bind to receptors are called ligands; drugs and other ligands that block the binding of agonist to the receptor, or block the effects of agonist binding, are referred to as antagonists.

Receptors are generally membrane-bound, although certain hormonal receptors may be found in the cytoplasm. Although they can occur on intracellular membranes, this chapter focuses on receptors in the cell membrane and responding to extracellular neurotransmitters or hormones. There are two main groups of cell-surface receptors – the metabotropic receptors and the ionotropic receptors.

The archetypal neurotransmitter receptor is found within the synapse on the postsynaptic membrane, where it responds rapidly to released neurotransmitter to influence postsynaptic neuronal activity, typically increasing or decreasing likelihood of an action potential. However, there may be receptors on the presynaptic axon terminal that control neurotransmitter release; these respond to neurotransmitter released from that neuron (an autoreceptor) or are postsynaptic to another neurotransmitter terminal (a heteroreceptor). There may also be autoreceptors elsewhere on the neuron, such as the cell body or its surrounding dendrites, which control transmitter synthesis or neuronal activity.

Ionotropic receptors

Ionotropic receptors, also referred to as ligand-gated ion channels, are large proteins generally composed of five subunits that assemble in the membrane. They tend to exhibit considerable heterogeneity in their subunit composition, leading to a variation in function. These oligomeric proteins contain about 20 transmembrane segments arranged around a central aqueous channel. Ionotropic receptors open in response to the binding of a ligand (e.g. neurotransmitter) to the receptor protein. This causes a conformational change in the receptor, which generally results in the opening of an ion channel. When open, the ion channel is usually selective to one or more ions, primarily Na^+, K^+, Ca^{2+} or Cl^-. Because of the close linkage between ligand binding and ion channel opening, ionotropic receptors operate with a very short latency (a few milliseconds). Consequently, receptors of this type control fast synaptic transmission in the nervous system. However, when continuously exposed to ligand or transmitter, many ionotropic receptors exhibit rapid desensitization. This may be an adaptive response to limit postsynaptic response under conditions of high presynaptic activity.

The direct link to an ion channel, characteristic of the ionotropic receptors, is in contrast with the indirect action of metabotropic receptors, which commonly use second-messenger systems (see below). Members of the ionotropic family, including nicotinic receptors, $GABA_A$ receptors, NMDA and non-NMDA receptors and the 5-HT3 receptor, are discussed in more detail below.

$GABA_A$ receptors

GABA receptors are the major inhibitory receptor in the brain. The ionotropic $GABA_A$ receptor is the most prevalent of the known GABA receptor subtypes and demonstrates a ubiquitous distribution throughout the brain.

The $GABA_A$ receptor is composed of five subunits comprising an integral transmembrane ion channel. The channel is gated by the binding of two agonist (GABA) molecules. When open, the channel predominately conducts chloride ions, resulting in hyperpolarization in the postsynaptic cell.

Several classes of subunits have been cloned. These receptor subunits have been labelled with the Greek letters α, β, γ, δ, ε, θ and ρ. GABA requires both α and β components in order to bind. $GABA_A$ receptors are typically made up of two α and two β subunits among the five subunits, although the particular subunit composition often varies widely among brain regions and species. Furthermore, the existence of a large family of genes coding for diverse subunits (α_{1-6}, β_{1-4}, γ_{1-3}, δ_{1-6}, ε_{1-6}, θ_{1-6}, ρ_{1-2}) adds to the structural diversity of the receptor. The existence of multiple $GABA_A$ receptor subtypes differing in subunit composition, localization and functional properties underlies their role for fine-tuning of neuronal circuits.

Apart from the binding site for GABA, the receptor complex possesses sites of action for a number of clinically important drugs. These include the benzodiazepines, general anaesthetics and barbiturates. All of these drugs enhance the Cl^- current activated by GABA, thus increasing the inhibitory action of the receptor.

Subtle differences in subunit composition result in a number of subpopulations of $GABA_A$ receptors with different regional and cellular locations. The functional relevance of these subpopulations is the subject of continued research. For example, benzodiazepine ligands with high activity at α_1 subunits are associated with sedation, ataxia and amnesia, while those with greater activity at α_2 or α_3 subunits show greater anxiolytic activity. The development of subtype selective ligands may have pharmacological advantages in that they may allow dissociation of desired therapeutic effects from undesirable side effects. Although anticonvulsant effects can be produced by agonists acting at any of the $GABA_A$ subtypes, α_2-selective agonists would lack the side effects (e.g. sedation, amnesia) associated with the older drugs.

The heterogeneity of the $GABA_A$ receptor provides many avenues for the design and development of new chemical entities acting on subtypes of $GABA_A$ receptors to aid in the treatment of diseases, including epilepsy, alcohol dependence and certain psychiatric disorders.

NMDA and non-NMDA excitatory amino acid receptors

NMDA and non-NMDA (α-amino-3-hydroxy-5-methyliosoxazole-4-propionic acid (AMPA) and kainate) receptors make up the major excitatory amino acid receptors in the CNS. They are all ionotropic receptors named after the pharmacological agonists to which they selectively respond.

NMDA receptors are found throughout the CNS, with particularly high receptor densities found in the hippocampus and cerebral cortex. Activation of NMDA receptors results in the opening of an ion channel that is non-selective to cations. This allows flow of Na^+ and small amounts of Ca^{2+} ions into the cell and K^+ out of the cell. The NMDA receptor is distinct in that it is both ligand-gated and voltage-dependent. At resting membrane potentials, NMDA receptors are inactive. This is due to a voltage-dependent block of the channel pore by magnesium ions (Mg^{2+}), preventing ion flow through it.

NMDA receptor subunits are encoded by seven different genes – *NR1*, *NR2A–NR2D* and *NR3A–NR3B*. The NR1 subunit undergoes extensive splicing, which results in eight variants – NR1-1a,1b to NR1-4a,4b. It is the co-assembly of the obligatory NR1 subunit (glycine binding) with NR2 (glutamate binding) subunits and/or NR3 subunits that yields a functional receptor. Receptor pharmacology and channel properties vary depending on which NR2 isoform (i.e. A–D) is present. It has been suggested that the subunits probably assemble as tetramers with stoichiometry $(NR1)_2(NR2)_2$. The role of the NR3 subunit(s) that were discovered more recently remains unclear.

In addition to glutamate, the NMDA receptor requires a co-agonist, glycine, to bind to allow the receptor to function. The glycine binding site is found on the NR1 subunit. The NMDA receptor also contains a number of other recognition sites for endogenous and exogenous ligands. These include a unique recognition site for the dissociative anaesthetics phencyclidine and ketamine and for other non-competitive antagonists (e.g. MK801). Two other modulatory sites associated with the NMDA receptor are a site that binds zinc ions (Zn^{2+}), producing a voltage-independent block of NMDA responses, and a polyamine recognition site, whose activation by the endogenous polyamines spermine and spermidine facilitates NMDA receptor-mediated transmission, an effect brought about by increasing the affinity of the receptor for glycine.

NMDA receptors play an important role in long-term potentiation (LTP), long-term depression and synaptic plasticity, all cellular mechanisms involved in learning and memory. Overactivation of the receptor can result in damage and eventually cell death through the process of excitotoxicity (see Box 30.2).

Like NMDA receptors, AMPA and kainate receptors also mediate fast excitatory transmission and are associated with channels that, when open, primarily conduct Na^+ ions. Unlike NMDA receptors, however, these channels are not voltage-dependent, do not require the binding of a co-agonist and have a low permeability for Ca^{2+} ions.

As with NMDA receptors, the AMPA receptor assembly is also thought to be formed by a combination of four subunits termed $GluR_{1-4}$, each transcribed by a different gene. Splicing in the extracellular N-terminal regions of the transmembrane domain of the transcript results in each of the four subunits having a 'flip/flop' variant. AMPA receptors are found throughout the CNS with a similar distribution to NMDA receptors. Receptor diversity is brought about in a region-dependent manner through tissue-specific subunit compositions. This receptor type undergoes dynamic insertion and removal from the neuronal membrane, an effect that is dependent on neuronal activity in the synapse. Activation of AMPA receptors is critical for depolarization and regulation of NMDA receptor signalling. The ion channel of the NMDA receptor is blocked by Mg^{2+} under resting conditions; activation of AMPA receptors results in partial depolarization of the cell membrane leading to extrusion of the Mg^{2+} ions.

In common with NMDA and AMPA receptors, kainate receptors are composed of four subunits. These receptors are comprised of combinations of $GluR_{5-7}$ and KA_{1-2} subunits. Although classically described as having a distribution that was limited to specific regions, it is now evident that kainate receptors have a widespread distribution throughout the CNS, being located at both pre- and postsynaptic sites. Pharmacologically they are still difficult to distinguish from AMPA receptors, and very few kainate receptor-selective compounds have been identified. Key evidence is emerging to support a metabotropic-like action of some postsynaptic kainate receptors, suggesting a dual signalling mechanism for these receptors. This bimodal action is common with AMPA receptors but is completely distinct from the purely ionotropic NMDA receptors.

Nicotinic receptors

Nicotinic and muscarinic receptors, named after the selective exogenous agonists nicotine and muscarine respectively, are two types of receptor activated by the neurotransmitter acetylcholine. The muscarinic receptors are G-protein-coupled receptors and discussed below, while the nicotinic type are ionotropic receptors that mediate a fast synaptic transmission following agonist activation.

Nicotinic receptors are composed of five types of subunits (α, β, γ, δ, ε). These subunits are found in different combinations in the different types of nicotinic receptor. Muscle-type nicotinic receptors always contain two α subunits, which are critical in acetylcholine binding, and one of each of the other subunits. In contrast, neuronal nicotinic receptors contain only two types of subunit (α and β). However, the structural diversity of these receptors comes from the existence of diverse subunits – α_{2-7}, α_{9-10} and β_{2-4}. The neuronal nicotinic receptors have been further divided into two main groups based on their sensitivity to the snake venom toxin α-bungarotoxin. The α-bungarotoxin-sensitive receptors are homomeric, containing the α_7 or α_9 subunit, and are found primarily in pre- and postsynaptic neurons and in developing muscle. The α-bungarotoxin-insensitive receptors are heteromeric, containing combinations of α_{2-6} and β_{2-4}, and often modulate the release of other transmitters. The most common of the neuronal receptors is the $\alpha_4\beta_2$ subtype, which is ubiquitously expressed and is able to bind most nicotinic agonists with high affinity. The stoichiometry of the individual receptor subtype determines its biophysical and functional properties as well as its pharmacological profile.

Nicotinic receptors are involved in a wide range of physiological processes. Muscle-type nicotinic receptors are localized at neuromuscular junctions, where an electrical impulse from a neuron to a muscle cell signals contraction and is responsible for muscle tone; as such, these receptors are targets for muscle relaxants. The many types of neuronal nicotinic receptors are located on both pre- and postsynaptic neurons in the CNS, where they are involved in complex brain function such as cognitive function, learning and memory, arousal, reward, motor control and analgesia.

5-HT$_3$ receptors

The 5-HT$_3$ receptor is unique among the currently known serotonergic receptor subtypes in that it belongs to the ionotropic family. 5-HT$_3$ receptors are similar in structure to other ionotropic receptors, and agonist activation opens a cation channel that results in depolarization.

They have a widespread distribution in the PNS, where the highest concentrations in the brain are found in the area postrema, entorhinal cortex, amygdala and certain brainstem nuclei.

5-HT$_3$ postsynaptic receptors mediate fast excitatory transmission. They are also found on presynaptic terminals, where they modulate neurotransmitter release. 5-HT$_3$ receptor antagonists, through blockade of receptors in the CNS and gastrointestinal tract, are currently used in the treatment of postoperative and cytotoxic drug nausea and emesis.

Metabotropic receptors

These are the most common class of receptors. Of the neurotransmitters discussed previously, all act at specific metabotropic receptors. The major subgroup of metabotropic receptors that is employed for all these neurotransmitters is referred to as the G-protein-coupled receptors (GPCRs), short for guanine nucleotide diphosphate (GDP)-binding protein coupled receptors.

All have a characteristic structural design: seven hydrophobic (lipophilic) transmembrane regions within a single polypeptide chain, such that GPCRs wrap back and forth through the lipid cell membrane and are exposed to both the intracellular and extracellular surface of the cell. This gives rise to an alternative name for this group of receptors – the seven-transmembrane domain (7TM) receptors. The specific structure is determined by these hydrophobic polypeptide sequences alternating with hydrophilic regions that remain outside the membrane; these include a C-terminal region that resides within the intracellular cytoplasm and an N-terminal region that extends into the extracellular space. The extracellular domain of the GPCRs usually contains the neurotransmitter binding site, although some GPCRs bind ligands within the transmembrane of the receptor (Figure 30.7).

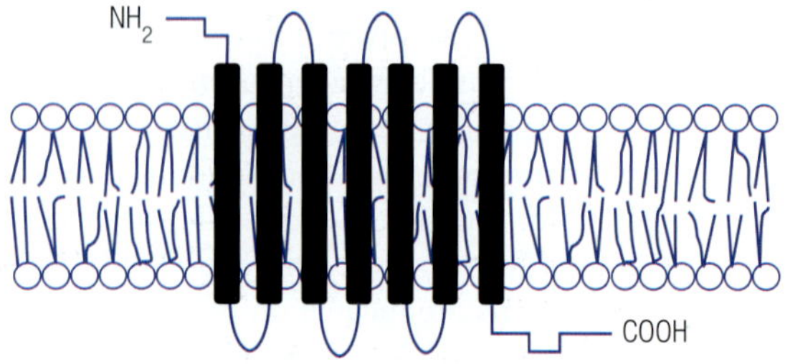

Figure 30.7 Schematic representation of a G-protein-coupled receptor. There are seven transmembrane helices. COOH is the C-terminal (intracellular), and NH_2 the X-terminal (extracellular)

G-proteins are the transduction components that are linked to GPCRs. G-proteins exist as a cluster of subunits (α and βγ). At rest, the α subunit is tightly bound to GDP. When a GPCR is activated (occupied by an agonist), it associates with its G-protein, initiating the exchange of GDP to guanine nucleotide triphosphate (GTP) by the α subunit, which in turn disassociates from the βγ subunit (Figure 30.8). The GTP-α and βγ subunits can then act with effector proteins, also known as secondary transduction components, inside the cell. These effectors include intracellular enzymes such as adenylate cyclase and phopholipase C, ion channels and other classes of proteins. Termination of the signal mediated by the G-protein is usually brought about by the hydrolysis of GTP to GDP by GTPase, which the α subunit possesses intrinsically. This leads to a re-association of the α subunit with the βγ subunit and the cycle can begin again. As the action of metabotropic receptors is mediated by biochemical processes, the effect of receptor stimulation is relatively long-lasting, with a typical timescale of seconds to minutes. This is in contrast to the fast-acting ionotropic receptors discussed above.

The modulation of intracellular enzymes by G-protein activation results in the production of second messengers, signalling molecules that communicate the agonist-mediated stimulation to effector proteins within the intracellular domain of the cell. The specific Gα protein subunit that is activated often determines which effector the G-protein will influence. There are a large number of identified Gα proteins. Two of the most common are $G\alpha_s$ and $G\alpha_q$, which stimulate adenylate cyclase and phopholipase C respectively, while $G\alpha_i$ results in adenylate cyclase inhibition. However, these G protein subtypes can also directly influence neighbouring ion channels; thus, $G\alpha_s$ can open Ca^{2+} channels and $G\alpha_i$ inhibits these but opens K^+ channels, with hyperpolarizing effects.

Adenylate cyclase, when stimulated by the $G\alpha_s$ subunit, converts ATP to cyclic adenosine monophosphate (cAMP). cAMP activates protein kinase A (PKA), which phosphorylates intracellular proteins, many of which are enzymes of the cAMP protein kinase class.

Phospholipase C (PLC), when activated, cleaves the phospholipid phosphatidyl 4,5-bisphosphate (PIP2) into inositol-1,4,5-triphosphate (IP3) and diacylglycerol (DAG). IP3 triggers the release of Ca^{2+} from intracellular stores, resulting in a rise in $[Ca^{2+}]$ within the cell and activation of

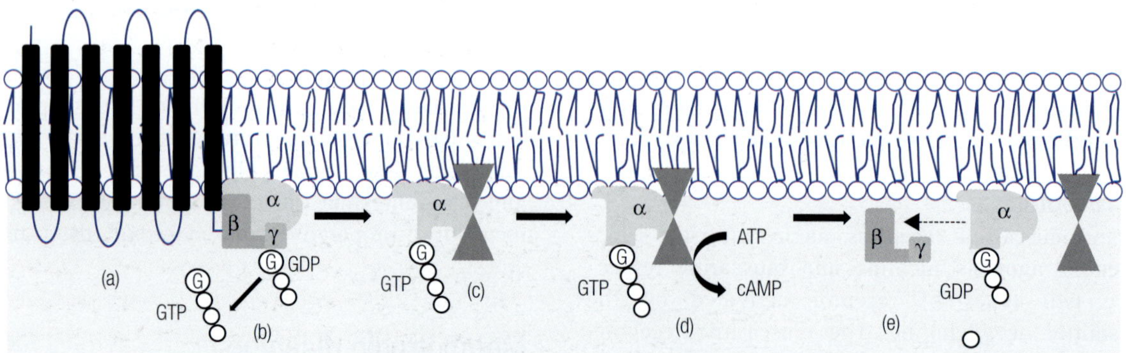

Figure 30.8 Schematic representation of the signalling mechanism of a G-protein-coupled receptor (GPCR). (a) In the cell membrane the G-protein exists as a complex of subunits (α, β and γ). Unactivated, guanine nucleotide diphosphate (GDP) is bound tightly to the α subunit of the G-protein. (b) Upon binding of an agonist to the receptor, there is a conformational change in the G-protein coupling domain, causing the bound GDP to exchange with intracellular guanine nucleotide triphosphate (GTP). (c) The α-GTP unit dissociates from the G-protein to interact with a target protein (e.g. an enzyme such as adenylate cyclase), (d) converting adenosine triphosphate (ATP) to cyclic adenosine monophosphate (cAMP) and increasing GTPase activity, leading to hydrolysis of GTP to GDP, and thus (e) the α subunit can recombine with the β subunit

downstream events. DAG activates protein kinase C, which then phosphorylates specific cellular proteins.

Several metabotropic receptor subtypes appear to have a constitutive activity – that is, they demonstrate effects on second-messenger systems while unoccupied by agonist. While agonists will enhance this effect by increasing the association of receptor with G-protein, some antagonists may not merely block the action of agonists but also diminish the constitutive activity of the receptor. Such an effect is called inverse agonism and is common for drugs that are antagonists at receptors including dopamine D2, 5-HT2A and 5-HT2C receptors.

Dopamine receptors

Dopamine D2-like receptors

The dopamine D2 receptor is found in the highest concentrations in the striatum, where it mediates dopamine's effects on motor and psychomotor function. It is also found in other regions of the brain, including the pituitary gland, where it is involved in the tonic inhibition of prolactin secretion. In the early 1990s, it was found to be one of a series of three structurally related gene products: D2, D3 and D4 receptors. The D3 receptors are also found in the striatum and notably the limbic structures. They may have a particular involvement as an autoreceptor in presynaptic control of dopamine release. D4 receptors, once thought to be overexpressed in schizophrenia and important in clozapine's action, are no longer major targets for antipsychotic drug development. They are found in the cerebral cortex but in substantial concentrations only in the retina.

Dopamine D2-like receptors are found on postsynaptic membranes and at presynaptic sites. Agonist action at presynaptic autoreceptors provides the means to regulate further transmitter synthesis and release; diffusion of dopamine to extrasynaptic D2-like receptors allows it to influence more neuronal systems than solely the postsynaptic cell.

Functional polymorphisms of the D2 and D3 receptor genes have been reported to be associated with aspects of antipsychotic drug effects, including response of positive symptoms and, for D3, tardive dyskinesia. Polymorphisms of the D4 receptor gene have been associated with various personality traits, including novelty-seeking behaviour and obsessive–compulsive disorder.

These D2-like receptors have generally inhibitory effects on neuronal function, primarily through inhibition of adenylate cyclase activity by the $G\alpha_i$ subunit, although the $G\beta\gamma$ subunit can influence a variety of further effector systems, including ion channels, phospholipases and protein kinases.

Dopamine D1-like receptors

The dopamine D1 receptor is distributed more widely, being present in the basal ganglia and other subcortical structures and in the cerebral cortex, where it has a greater role than D2-like receptors in mediating dopaminergic neurotransmission. Thus, it is important in the action of dopamine on cognitive function in the frontal cortex. D1 receptors have a lower affinity for dopamine than D2 receptors and may be involved primarily in more classical synaptic neurotransmission; they do not contribute to presynaptic control mechanisms via autoreceptor function.

As with D2-like receptors, molecular biological studies identified heterogeneity of D1-like receptors; a second gene encoding a receptor structurally related to the D1 receptor was identified. This D5 receptor is the least understood of the five dopamine receptors; it is found to be important in the central control of blood pressure, but it is intriguing in being reported to be genetically associated with the risk of schizophrenia and attention deficit hyperactivity disorder (ADHD).

The D1 receptor has long been considered as having opposing effects to the D2 receptor, with an excitatory action primarily through stimulatory effects (via $G\alpha_s$) on adenylate cyclase.

Adrenoceptors

Receptors to the neurotransmitter noradrenaline (and that also respond to adrenaline) were originally divided into α- and β-adrenergic receptor (adrenoceptor) subtypes, each of which have undergone further subdivision on the basis initially of pharmacological differences and, more recently, separate genes.

α_1 Adrenoceptors

α_1 Adrenoceptors within the CNS are found in high concentrations within the locus coeruleus, which contains the cell bodies for the ascending and descending noradrenergic neurons. Receptors are also found in the thalamic nuclei, amygdala and hippocampus, and cerebral cortex, corresponding to the regulation of mood and attention. The activation of α_1 adrenoceptors generally results in an excitatory effect via G_q-mediated pathways, but it is thought to reduce neuronal activity in the hippocampus. α_1 Adrenoceptors may also influence brain functions via non-neuronal mechanisms, as glial cells can express α_1 adrenoceptors. α_1 Adrenoceptors can be subdivided into A/C, B and D subtypes, based upon their differential affinities to adrenergic compounds.

α_2 Adrenoceptors

α_2 Adrenoceptors are found as autoreceptors, present in noradrenergic regions of the hindbrain, and postsynaptic α_2 receptors, as target receptors for noradrenergic projections, in the forebrain (cortex, limbic regions, hypothalamus) and in the spinal cord. Reflected by their widespread distribution, they are involved in many functions, including blood pressure regulation, analgesia and sedation, and temperature regulation. Furthermore, they appear to be involved in the regulation of behaviour, cognitive function and mood; the hyperactivity of brain monoaminergic neurons that occurs during stress can lead to psychopathologies such as anxiety disorders and depression. Three subtypes of the α_2

adrenoceptor have been characterized: A, B and C. Their cellular activity, typical of many auto- and heteroreceptors, is to decrease adenylate cyclase activity through coupling to G_i.

β Adrenoceptors

There are three classes of β adrenoceptor – 1, 2 and 3 – which have differing affinities for noradrenaline and adrenaline. The distribution of β adrenoceptor sites in the human brain has shown that β_1 receptors are found mostly in the striatum and globus pallidus, while β_2 sites are located predominating in the cerebellum and β_3 in the hippocampus, cerebral cortex and striatum. Within the CNS, noradrenergic transmission has long been implicated in stress-related changes in behaviour, and β adrenoceptor antagonists are used widely in anxiety disorders such as social phobia, post-traumatic stress disorder and panic disorder. All β adrenoceptors activate G_s to stimulate adenylate cyclase, although there is evidence of the involvement of other signalling pathways such as mitogen-activated protein kinases.

5-Hydroxytryptamine receptors

All but one subtype of the many 5-HT receptors are metabotropic GPCRs. Most important in the context of psychiatric disorders are the 5-HT1 and 5-HT2 receptor classes, although both 5-HT4 and 5-HT6 receptors are involved in CNS function and are potential targets for drug action.

5-HT1 receptors

5-HT1A receptors are found at postsynaptic sites in the hippocampus and cortex, where they mediate inhibitory effects of transmitter on adenylate cyclase. They are also present as autoreceptors on the cell bodies and dendrites of 5-HT neurons in the raphe nuclei, where they are important in regulating neuronal activity, notably in the context of antidepressant drug mechanisms. A polymorphism in the promoter region of the 5-HT1A receptor gene has been shown to influence control of gene expression by affecting the binding of a transcription factor; this functional polymorphism has been reported to be a risk factor for depression and suicide and to influence symptom response to antidepressant drugs.

5-HT1B and 1D receptors are primarily presynaptic autoreceptors providing an inhibitory control of 5-HT release, but they have been little studied in the context of psychopharmacology and mental illness.

5-HT2A receptors

5-HT2 receptors are excitatory postsynaptic receptors, working via stimulation of PLC. Of the two major subtypes, the 5-HT2A receptor is found in many regions of the brain, including the cortex and the basal ganglia, where, among other actions, they influence dopaminergic neurotransmission. They are thought to be involved in some of the beneficial effects of atypical antipsychotic drugs on cognitive and negative features of psychotic illness and in minimizing extrapyramidal side effects. Polymorphisms of the 5-HT2A receptor gene have been associated, albeit weakly, with a variety of psychiatric diagnoses and response to treatment, particularly relating to antidepressants and antipsychotics.

5-HT2C receptors

5-HT2C receptors, found in basal ganglia and limbic regions of the brain, may also contribute to effects of some of antipsychotic and antidepressant drugs. These receptors appear to inhibit dopaminergic activity, influencing motor function. They also have effects on food intake and other hormonally controlled behaviours, due to their presence in the hypothalamus. Functional polymorphisms of the 5-HT2C receptor gene are associated with several effects of psychiatric drug treatments, including the frequency of tardive dyskinesia and the severity of drug-induced weight gain.

5-HT4 and 6 receptors

5-HT4 and 5-HT6 receptors are excitatory receptors with effects mediated by stimulation of adenylate cyclase. 5-HT4 receptors are found in several subcortical regions, including basal ganglia and limbic systems, although pharmacological interest is mainly in their presence outside the CNS, in the gastrointestinal system in particular. Nevertheless, the receptors do appear to have effects on learning and memory and are a drug target for the treatment of cognitive and dementing disorders. 5-HT6 receptors, found in many cortical and subcortical brain regions, are closely involved in cognitive function through their ability to regulate cholinergic neurotransmission. They are also involved in anxiety, affect and control of body weight and are thus a drug target for the treatment of obesity and several neuropsychiatric indications.

Muscarinic acetylcholine receptors

The muscarinic acetylcholine-sensitive receptors have five subtypes, M1–M5. In terms of their activity, they can be divided into two groups: the M1, M3 and M5 subtypes with an excitatory action via stimulation of PLC, and the inhibitory M2 and M4 receptors, which act through adenylate cyclase. M1 receptors are found widely in brain tissue, where they are postsynaptic to cholinergic terminals in cortex and striatum and hence can influence cognitive and motor functions. M5 receptors are little studied, but one site at which they are found is on dopaminergic neurons and thus they can contribute to dopaminergic regulation.

The M2 and M4 subtypes function as inhibitory autoreceptors in the hippocampus and cortex (M2) and striatum (M4), where they may also have heteroreceptor effects. These muscarinic receptors are also involved in spinal cord function, notably nociception, and are also important outside the CNS. The M3 receptors are involved in stimulating secretion from various organs, including the salivary gland and the pancreatic beta cell, although they are also present in the CNS, where they can act as excitatory heteroreceptors. Several muscarinic receptor subtypes are found in smooth muscle, where they control gut motility and can influence various aspects of genitourinary function, among other effects.

Histamine receptors

Of the four subtypes of the GPCR histamine receptors, H1–3 are most studied in terms of brain function. H1 and H2 are excitatory receptors found postsynaptic to histamine projections in many parts of the brain: H1 in the hypothalamus and limbic structures, and H2 in the basal ganglia and cortex. H1 receptors in particular are thought to mediate drug effects on sedation and food intake. H3 receptors are primarily presynaptic, acting as inhibitory autoreceptors and as heteroreceptors controlling the release of other transmitters, including acetylcholine.

Metabotropic glutamate receptors

The metabotropic glutamate receptors (mGluRs) are dimeric GPCRs comprised of eight subtypes ($mGluR_{1-8}$) that fall into three main groups, based on sequence homology, signal transduction mechanism and receptor pharmacology. Group I receptors are $mGluR_1$ and $mGluR_5$, group II are $mGluR_2$ and $mGluR_3$, and group III contains $mGluR_4$ and $mGluR_{6-8}$. MGluRs are unusual in that they show no sequence homology with other GPCRs. They contain a large extracellular N-terminal tail that contains the glutamate binding site. Group I receptors stimulate Ca^{2+} release via IP3 formation, while group II and III receptors are negatively coupled to adenylate cyclase.

With the exception of $mGluR_6$, which is confined to the retina, all other mGluRs are expressed in the mammalian CNS, where they are found in both neuronal and glial cells. Individual family members exhibit distinct spatial and temporal expression profiles. Neuronally expressed group I mGluRs are typically localized postsynaptically, whereas group II and III receptors are predominantly presynaptic, localized in axon terminals where they can regulate neurotransmitter release. The role played by mGluRs in glial cells is unclear.

Development of drugs with greater subtype specificity and enhanced bioavailability has identified important roles played by mGluRs in the CNS. For example, preclinical studies have provided evidence for the potential use of group II mGluR agonists in the treatment of schizophrenia. Furthermore, selective agents acting as allosteric antagonists at the $mGluR_5$ subtype have demonstrated therapeutic potential for addiction.

$GABA_B$ receptors

$GABA_B$ receptors are metabotropic receptors that belong to the GPCR family. Although $GABA_B$ receptors are found throughout the CNS, they are present at lower levels than the ionotropic $GABA_A$ receptor. $GABA_B$ receptors are located both pre- and postsynaptically. Presynaptically they inhibit the release of excitatory and inhibitory transmitters. The functional importance of postsynaptic $GABA_B$ receptors is highlighted by segregation of $GABA_A$ and $GABA_B$ synapses in the mammalian brain. Two major $GABA_B$ subunits have been identified, $GABA_{B1}$ and $GABA_{B2}$; these two subunits form heterodimers together, where $GABA_{B1}$ contains the ligand binding site and $GABA_{B2}$ mediates G-protein signalling through $G\alpha_i$, opening K^+ channels postsynaptically and inhibiting Ca^+ channels at presynaptic sites.

Pharmacologically, $GABA_B$ receptors can be distinguished from $GABA_A$ receptors by their selective affinity for baclofen and the lack of affinity for muscimol and bicuculline. Baclofen is currently used as a muscle relaxant to decrease spasticity in a number of neurological disorders. Studies utilizing novel brain-penetrative $GABA_B$ receptor antagonists also suggest a role for this receptor in the improvement of cognitive function.

INTRODUCTORY PHARMACOLOGY OF THE MAJOR NEUROTRANSMITTER SYSTEMS

Synaptic chemical neurotransmission is the essential process in communication between neurons and hence is a core mechanism in brain function. It is also the major point at which we can influence neuronal activity with drug treatment. Each of the presynaptic processes of transmitter synthesis, storage, release and reuptake, the metabolic removal of transmitter, and the various presynaptic and postsynaptic receptor sites is a potential, if not actual, target for neuro- and psychoactive drugs (Figure 30.9). In addition, there are other ways in which drugs may influence neuronal activity, including direct effects on ion channels, on second-messenger systems, on neuronal metabolism and on membrane structure.

One such mechanism, which is independent of a direct effect on neurotransmitter function but which has effects

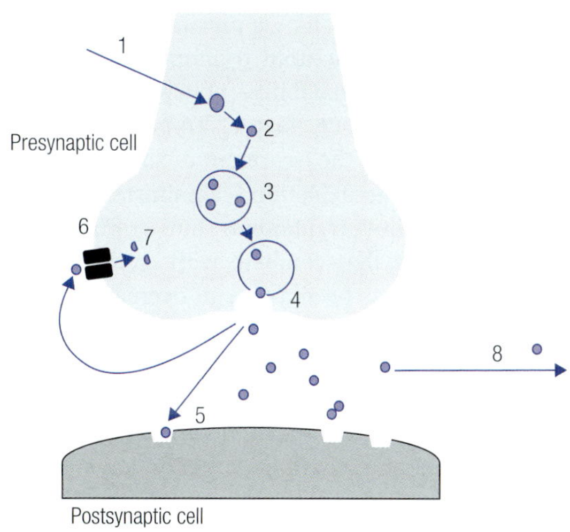

Figure 30.9 Potential targets for neuro- and psychoactive drugs: (1) transport of precursor, (2) enzymatic synthesis of transmitter, (3) vesicular transport and storage of transmitter, (4) release of transmitter, (5) postsynaptic binding, (6) reuptake of transmitter, (7) metabolic breakdown, (8) diffusion from synapse

on neuronal activity, is that of the local anaesthetics. These drugs cross the neuronal cell membrane to block the voltage-gated Na^+ channels that are so important for propagation of the nerve impulse. This mechanism is employed in some antiepileptic drugs, several of which are also effective in relieving symptoms of bipolar disorder. These anticonvulsants and mood stabilizers, including valproate, lamotrigine and carbamazepine, demonstrate a use-dependent blockade of Na^+ channels relatively selective for rapidly firing neurons. Some anticonvulsants are also inhibitors of Ca^{2+} channels, resulting in effects associated with diminished neurotransmitter release.

Neurotransmitter synthesis

Neurotransmitter synthesis is the initial process open to pharmacological intervention. Although inhibition of rate-determining enzymes is an effective mechanism of diminishing transmitter in experimental pharmacology, enhancement of transmitter synthesis by supplementation with precursor compounds has been an effective and clinically valuable approach. The key example here is L-dopa. Shortly after the identification of dopamine as a neurotransmitter in the basal ganglia, a region important in the control of motor function, a profound deficit of dopamine was found in the striatum of patients dying from Parkinson's disease. Providing L-dopa, which bypassed the rate-determining step of tyrosine hydroxylation, increased the availability of dopamine and relieved the motor symptoms. Co-administration of a peripherally acting dopa decarboxylase inhibitor was found to minimize the peripheral side effects of L-dopa at the same time as increasing its availability to the brain. This drug combination has been the mainstay of Parkinson's disease treatment for several decades.

Supplementation of serotonin synthesis by treatment with tryptophan is another example of effective enhancement of transmitter function by a precursor compound. This takes advantage of the fact that tryptophan hydroxylase is not saturated, so the availability of tryptophan from the blood is the rate-limiting factor. Tryptophan has been found to be effective in the treatment of some patients with depression. Tryptophan depletion – administering an amino acid mixture without tryptophan but containing large neutral amino acids that compete with tryptophan at the blood–brain barrier has been a way of decreasing serotonin synthesis in humans in the study of the role of serotonin function in mood and cognition.

Pharmacological manipulation of the availability or synthesis of excitatory amino acid neurotransmitters is not easily undertaken and could potentially have effects on other aspects of cell function, given the essential role of glutamate in non-transmitter aspects of cell function. However, synthesis of acetylcholine can be influenced by pharmacological effects on its precursor; acetylcholine concentrations can increase in response to administration of quantities of choline or choline-containing lipids, an approach that has been explored in the past for the treatment of dementia.

Neurotransmitter storage

Depletion of vesicular stores of neurotransmitter can have a profound effect on neuronal, and hence brain, function. This is seen with reserpine, a drug used for centuries as an antihypertensive and antipsychotic by blocking the vesicular monoamine transporter. This results in depletion of vesicular stores of catecholamines and serotonin and consequently substantial reduction in the synaptic activity of these neurotransmitters. Side effects of reserpine include, not surprisingly, parkinsonism, relating to its effect on dopamine, and depression, relating primarily to its effects on serotonin. Tetrabenazine, used in the treatment of dyskinetic motor disorders such as Huntington's disease, has similar action in inhibiting the vesicular monoamine transporter.

One of the actions of the dietary monoamine tyramine is to displace catecholamines from vesicular stores, resulting in the 'cheese effect' associated with MAO inhibition (see above). Amphetamines (see below) also displace endogenous transmitter from catecholamine-containing (and sometimes serotonin-containing) vesicles, with methylphenidate showing some greater selectivity for central dopaminergic terminals.

Neurotransmitter release and reuptake

Stimulant drugs such as cocaine and amphetamine, and amphetamine-related drugs such as methylphenidate and methylenedioxymethamphetamine (MDMA, ecstasy), also have effects on monoamine neurotransmitter release and reuptake. The effects of these and many other drugs in inducing dependence is associated with an increase in the activity of dopamine in the nucleus accumbens, a region involved in reward mechanisms. The increase in dopamine release in this and other areas by the stimulant drugs is brought about by an enhancement of dopamine release or a blockade of its reuptake.

The differences in action between these stimulant drugs reflect their differences in mechanism and neurotransmitter selectivity. Cocaine is an effective inhibitor of the neuronal dopamine transporter and, to a lesser extent, serotonin and noradrenaline transporters. Amphetamine can also interact with the dopamine and noradrenaline transporters but brings about a reversal of their transport processes, enabling cytosolic catecholamine to be transported out of the cell, in essence enhancing transmitter release.

The drug of abuse MDMA appears primarily to involve 5-HT systems in its action. Although it does appear to have amphetamine-like effects on dopamine release, MDMA enhances serotonin release, inhibition of reuptake through the serotonin transporter and depletion of stores, partly through effects on 5-HT synthesis by inhibition of tryptophan hydroxylase.

The major drugs influencing monoamine neurotransmitter reuptake are the antidepressants. The tricyclic antidepressants (TCAs) vary in selectivity between having primarily noradrenergic effects (e.g. desipramine) and those with relatively greater effects on serotonin reuptake (e.g. amitriptyline). However, the TCAs have wide and variable effects on other systems, including serotonin, muscarinic, alpha-adrenergic and histamine receptors, many of which may contribute to unwanted side effects. The selective serotonin reuptake inhibitor (SSRI) antidepressants primarily inhibit the serotonin transporter, with generally fewer effects on other systems, resulting in an improved side-effect profile. Effects on noradrenaline reuptake have been reintroduced more recently with the selective noradrenaline reuptake inhibitor (NRI) reboxetine, and selective serotonin and noradrenaline reuptake inhibitors (SNRIs) such as venlafaxine.

Tiagabine, an antiepileptic drug that has been proposed, like several other antiepileptic drugs, to have efficacy in bipolar disorder, inhibits GABA reuptake through a neuronal transporter, resulting in increased extraneuronal concentrations of transmitter.

Neurotransmitter metabolism

The removal of neurotransmitters by metabolizing enzymes is a process that provides further pharmacological opportunities to influence synaptic activity – inhibition of neurotransmitter breakdown is likely to result in its increased availability for release into the synapse. MAO, being the only enzyme for metabolic removal of serotonin and important for catecholamine metabolism, is a valuable target to enhance neurotransmitter activity. Inhibition of this enzyme (or enzymes – there are two forms of the enzyme, A and B, with different substrate selectivity) is the mechanism of action of several antidepressant drugs. These MAO inhibitors include the older and non-specific 'suicide' (i.e. irreversible) inhibitors phenelzine and tranylcypromine, which are susceptible to the 'cheese effect' (see above), as well as the newer, reversible and hence safer MAO type A inhibitor moclobemide. MAO-A is thus the target for antidepressant action, since it metabolizes 5-HT and noradrenaline. MAO-B inhibition with selegiline is an adjunctive treatment for Parkinson's disease; it enhances the efficacy of L-dopa by inhibiting dopamine breakdown.

COMT inhibition is not used routinely in psychiatry, although it has been proposed as a potential approach to alleviate cognitive deficits in, for example, schizophrenia. However, COMT inhibitors are used in the adjunctive treatment of Parkinson's disease, where they inhibit peripheral breakdown of L-dopa.

Acetylcholine neurotransmission can be enhanced by inhibition of the enzyme responsible for its synaptic removal, AChE. This can be beneficial in the treatment of Alzheimer's disease with drugs such as donepezil or galantamine, which are reversible inhibitors of AChE. However, the organophosphates that comprise many insecticides and the mustard nerve gases are inhibitors of AChE that can cause profound toxicity and fatality by reaction with the enzyme and subsequent uncontrolled accumulation of synaptic acetylcholine.

Many anti-epileptic drugs focus on increasing GABA function. One approach has been to inhibit GABA metabolism; vigabatrin blocks the breakdown of GABA by GABA transaminase to increase synaptic availability.

RECEPTOR PHARMACOLOGY

A comprehensive review of the role of neurotransmitter receptors in neuropharmacology is beyond the scope of this chapter. However, we have indicated below some relevant receptor-mediated effects of common drugs and have included some future prospects for improved treatments through novel receptor ligands.

Dopamine receptors

The D1-like (D1 and D5) receptors are very similar in structure and pharmacology, and few compounds can distinguish between them as yet. Ligands selective for D1-like receptors are primarily used scientifically, agonists producing an increasing behavioural responsiveness as shown by stimulatory effects on activity and finer motor movements. Conversely, D1-like receptor antagonists are potent inhibitors of these dopamine-mediated behaviours. Neither agonist nor antagonist classes of D1 receptor ligands are used clinically. The D5 receptor, in contrast to the D1 receptor, can occur directly coupled to the $GABA_A$ receptor, enabling functional interactions; however, there are as yet no selective D5 ligands.

Antagonism of dopamine D2-like receptors is the major mode of action of the antipsychotic drugs, resulting in a reduction in the positive psychotic symptoms in many patients, although this mechanism appears to have no great effect on the negative and cognitive features of schizophrenia. This action at striatal D2 receptors is also responsible for the acute extrapyramidal side effects, although various other pharmacological effects of the drugs, including partial agonism in the case of aripiprazole, are used to minimize the incidence of these side effects. The second-generation atypical antipsychotics such as risperidone, olanzapine and quetiapine have effects at many other receptors but are all antagonists of D2-like receptors, albeit with different relative affinities at the D2, D3 and D4 subtypes. Thus, amisulpride and clozapine have higher affinities for D3 and D4, respectively, than for the D2 receptor subtype. Several phenothiazine antagonists for the dopamine D2 receptor, and other antipsychotics, are also used for the prevention and treatment of iatrogenic nausea and vomiting and cytotoxic and radiation sickness.

Apomorphine is a strong dopamine receptor agonist that, as with non-selective ergot-derived D2 agonists such as bromocriptine and cabergoline, can be used for the treatment of Parkinson's disease, often as an adjunct to L-dopa. D2-agonists such as bromocriptine are also effective in treating the consequences of hyperprolactinaemia, such as hypogonadism and galactorrhoea.

Adrenoceptors

Many of the drugs interacting with the β adrenoceptor are widely used pharmaceutically for peripheral conditions: β adrenoceptor agonists including the non-selective isoprenaline and the β_1-selective dobutamine treat a variety of cardiac disorders, while β_2-selective agonists such as salbutamol are spasmolytics and widely used in asthma. β Adrenoceptor antagonists, β-blockers, such as propranolol (non-selective) and atenolol (β_1-selective antagonist), are used for the treatment of hypertension and angina, but they have central effects on anxiety by reducing the physiological symptoms (tremor, sweating, clammy palms) of the fight/flight response. More recently, β_3-specific agonists have become of interest in the potential treatment of anxiety and depression, after disappointing initial studies as potential anti-obesity drugs, which reflects their action in enhancing lipolysis.

α Adrenoceptor pharmaceuticals also have peripheral effects, focusing primarily on smooth muscle control; α_1 agonists are vasoconstrictor sympathomimetics. Centrally acting α_1 antagonists include phentolamine, which can affect the pain response, and prazosin, which as well as being antihypertensive and useful in urinary disturbances has been reported to reduce sleep disturbances in post-traumatic stress disorder. It is the α_1 antagonism of some antidepressant and antipsychotic drugs that underlies their side effect of postural hypotension.

Clonidine is a α_2-adrenergic agonist used in the treatment of hypertension and migraine; it may also be useful in controlling neuropathic pain. In addition, it has wide-ranging effects on sleep: increasing sedation, reducing insomnia and minimizing night sweats. Moreover, it is also used as adjunct therapy in Tourette's syndrome and attention deficit disorder to control hyperactivity, impulsivity and tics. Antagonism of α_2 receptors is an effect of the antidepressants mianserin and mirtazapine; by blocking these presynaptic auto- and heteroreceptors, these drugs stimulate release of noradrenaline and 5-HT. The α_2 antagonist idazoxan has been investigated scientifically as adjunct therapy with antipsychotics in schizophrenia, where it improves symptom response in previously poorly responding patients. This indicates that the α_2 antagonism of clozapine might contribute to its particular efficacy in this patient group. The naturally occurring α_2-adrenergic antagonist yohimbine has been reported to be useful in the treatment of erectile dysfunction.

5-HT receptors

The pharmacology of 5-HT receptors is relevant to treatment of the majority of psychiatric disorders. Depression, anxiety, bipolar disorder and schizophrenia all have 5-HT implicated in mechanisms of therapeutic drug action, if not in their pathology. Many psychiatric drugs have effects at 5-HT receptors, and those that do not, such as the antidepressants that act on transport processes, may still bring about therapeutic effects via 5-HT receptor-mediated effects.

5-HT1A receptors

One therapeutic mechanism with such indirect receptor regulation involves the 5HT1A autoreceptor. The action of SSRIs in blocking 5-HT reuptake into neurons results in increased extraneuronal 5-HT around the somatodendritic sites of the regulatory 5-HT1A receptors. The agonist effect on these inhibitory autoreceptors results initially in a compensatory decrease in neuronal firing, followed by an eventual down-regulation of receptor density and a return to normal, or elevated, receptor-stimulated neuronal activity. This is thought to account for the delay in clinical response to antidepressant treatment. A polymorphism (−1019G/C) within the 5-HT1A gene influences this receptor regulation, resulting in a diminished neurochemical and hence clinical response in some individuals.

The 5-HT1A receptor is a target for some anxiolytic drugs, such as buspirone, a partial 5-HT1A receptor agonist. 5-HT1A partial agonist activity is also a component of the pharmacological profile of some antipsychotic drugs, including aripiprazole, quetiapine and clozapine, although whether this contributes to their clinical effects on, for example, depressive symptoms remains unclear.

5-HT2 receptors

The 5-HT2A receptor is implicated in both antidepressant effects and antipsychotic action. A consequence of most antidepressant treatments is a decrease in the numbers of postsynaptic 5-HT2A receptors, despite an increase in neuronal sensitivity to 5-HT. More direct effects on 5-HT2A receptors occur with many antipsychotics, particularly the atypical drugs. It is thought that their antagonism of 5-HT2A receptors may contribute to diminished extrapyramidal side effects, as striatal 5-HT2A antagonism results in increased dopamine release. It is also suggested that the same mechanism in the frontal cortex might underlie an improved response of negative schizophrenia symptoms to treatment with some atypical drugs, although support for this relationship between pharmacology and clinical response is unimpressive.

Several antidepressants and antipsychotics have an antagonist action at the related 5-HT2C receptor, including mirtazapine, clozapine and olanzapine. Whether this action might contribute to some beneficial effects on symptoms is unclear, although there is a theoretical basis for it providing some protective effect against antipsychotic-induced extrapyramidal side effects. However, the role of the 5-HT2C receptor in controlling food intake is likely to be important in the substantial effects of 5-HT2C antagonists on weight gain.

5-HT6 receptors

Drugs acting on 5-HT6 receptors can have positive effects on learning and memory, an effect mediated through their regulation of glutamatergic and cholinergic activity. The high affinity of a wide range of psychiatric drugs, including several antipsychotics and antidepressants, for the 5-HT6 receptor, together with its almost exclusive expression in the CNS, being abundant in limbic and cortical regions, raises the possibility that such compounds could be developed as adjunct therapeutics with existing treatments to improve learning and memory deficits in Alzheimer's disease, schizophrenia and depression. A preliminary report that the cognitive enhancing properties of a 5-HT6 receptor antagonist extends to patients with Alzheimer's disease further highlights the therapeutic promise of this receptor subtype.

Acetylcholine receptors

Both muscarinic and nicotinic acetylcholine receptor families are involved in a number of physiological functions, including cognition, reward, motor activity and analgesia, and have been implicated in pathological conditions such as Alzheimer's disease, Parkinson's disease, some forms of epilepsy, depression, autism and schizophrenia.

Muscarinic receptors in the basal ganglia mediate action of anticholinergic drugs, including procyclidine and benzatropine, used in the treatment of iatrogenic parkinsonism and other acute extrapyramidal side effects. The side effects of these drugs limit their use, however. Muscarinic antagonists can suppress M3 receptor-mediated salivation, causing dry mouth, can decrease gut motility, causing constipation, and can inhibit cholinergic neurotransmission in the cortex and hippocampus, resulting in cognitive disturbances. Several antipsychotics, notably clozapine, have antimuscarinic effects, as do some of the older tricyclic antidepressants.

Agonist action at postsynaptic muscarinic receptors and selective antagonism at the M2 autoreceptor provide potential targets for treatment of cognitive dysfunction in Alzheimer's disease and other disorders, including schizophrenia. Nicotinic receptors too represent a target for cognition: nicotine in cigarettes or patches reportedly improves cognition in Alzheimer's disease. The $\alpha_4\beta_2$ subtype has a selective partial agonist, varenicline, used to support smoking cessation, while drugs acting at the α_7 receptor are under investigation for treating cognitive disturbances in schizophrenia.

GABA receptors

$GABA_A$ receptors contain a number of recognition sites for molecules other than GABA. A substantial number of centrally acting and clinically active drugs, including the benzodiazepines, barbiturates, steroids and anaesthetics, can modulate the activity of $GABA_A$ receptors and thereby affect the inhibitory neurotransmission mediated by GABA.

Reflecting the ubiquitous distribution of $GABA_A$ receptors, benzodiazepines can be muscle-relaxant, anticonvulsant, sedative and anxiolytic drugs. These drugs, and some non-benzodiazepine drugs such as zolpidem, appear to exert their effects by selectively potentiating the effects of GABA on the $GABA_A$ receptor. However, not all $GABA_A$ receptors are affected by benzodiazepines, because of the requirement of a particular α subunit.

The barbiturates exert their modulatory role on the $GABA_A$ receptor through increasing the duration of channel opening, but they have no effect on opening frequency or channel conductance.

Neuroactive steroids are potent positive allosteric modulators of $GABA_A$ receptors with sedative, anxiolytic and anticonvulsant properties. There is evidence that the δ subunit is involved in modulating the effect of neurosteroids, since their action is reduced in mice lacking the δ subunit.

$GABA_A$ receptors in particular have long been implicated in mediating at least some of the pharmacological actions of alcohol. More recently, a specific and pharmacologically relevant alcohol binding site on a subtype of $GABA_A$ receptor ($\alpha_4/_6\beta_3\delta$) has been identified. A putative behavioural alcohol antagonist, Ro15-4513, at this binding site has been identified that diminishes the actions of low to moderate concentrations of alcohol in potentiating GABA-induced Cl^- currents.

Picrotoxin is a pro-convulsant alkaloid that noncompetitively blocks the GABA-gated chloride flux by binding to a site located within the ion channel. The major agonists, antagonists and modulators are summarized in Table 30.2.

It is clear from the above that we are only starting to understand the complexity of the $GABA_A$ receptor and considerable work is needed to further understand the role played by the different subtypes in brain function. However, the development of drugs that are more selective for various subtypes may offer much in improved clinical specificity with reduced adverse effects.

Baclofen is a GABA analogue that was originally tested as a GABA-like substance that might prove useful in controlling epilepsy and other convulsive states. It was subsequently found that baclofen showed very little postsynaptic effect in the brain and the actions of the drug were not blocked by bicuculline. This led to the discovery, in the early 1990s, of the $GABA_B$ receptor. Activation of presynaptic $GABA_B$ receptors with baclofen decreases Ca^{2+} conductance and reduces neurotransmitter release. Baclofen has clinical efficacy as an antispasticity agent and may have analgesic properties in certain types of pain, such as trigeminal neuralgia.

The drug of abuse and anti-narcolepsy agent sodium oxybate (γ-hydroxybutyrate, GHB) is also thought to act via $GABA_B$ receptors. Brain-penetrative competitive antago-

Table 30.2 Major agonists, antagonists and modulators of $GABA_A$ receptors

Pharmacology	Receptor site	Benzodiazepine site	Other modulatory sites
Endogenous agonists	GABA	Diazepam binding inhibitor	Neurosteroids, e.g. progesterone
Agonists	Muscimol, gaboxadol	Anxiolytic benzodiazepines	Barbiturates, steroid anaesthetics
Antagonists	Bicuculline, gabazine	Flumazenil	–
Channel blocker	Picrotoxin		

GABA, γ-aminobutyric acid.

nists at $GABA_B$ receptors have been developed in the hope of better elucidating the role played by this receptor in the brain. Studies suggest that $GABA_B$ antagonists may suppress absence epilepsy seizures, improve cognitive impairment and even act as neuroprotective agents.

Glutamate receptors

Due to the multiple combinations of individual subunits, a feature characteristic of many ionotropic receptors, NMDA receptors exist in many different subtypes. However, compounds that can usefully discriminate between these multiple subtypes have still to evolve. The agonist homoquinolinic acid, a conformationally constrained analogue of glutamate, shows higher affinity for NMDA receptors that contain the NR_{2B} subunit, thus displaying some subtype selectivity.

Similar to $GABA_A$ receptors, various modulatory sites on the NMDA receptor offer several opportunities for pharmacological interaction. One example is the glycine co-agonist site, which increases the affinity of the NMDA receptor for glutamate. This potentiation of NMDA receptor function by glycine or glycine agonists (e.g. D-serine, cycloserine) has been shown in clinical trials to be a useful approach to enhancing symptom response in the treatment of schizophrenia, in which an NMDA receptor hypofunction is implicated.

Activation of the receptor can also be modulated by the binding of different polyamines. Antagonists of the polyamine modulatory site, specific for the NR_{2B} subunit, exhibit neuroprotective action in a number of biochemical models of ischaemia and trauma. The dissociative anaesthetics ketamine and phencyclidine belong to a group of NMDA receptor antagonists that act by binding to the pore of the open (activated) NMDA receptor channel and are thus non-competitive antagonists. However, none of these compounds shows subunit selectivity.

A number of AMPA receptor positive allosteric modulators, drugs that do not lead to receptor desensitization and do not activate the receptor when applied alone, have been identified. These AMPA receptor potentiators have demonstrated efficacy when explored in rodent models of cognition and are now entering clinical trials.

Initially the utility of drugs acting at the mGluRs as in vivo tools has been restricted by their limited CNS bioavailability following systemic administration. More recently, mGluRs have emerged as potential new drug targets for treatment of a range of CNS disorders. mGlu2/3 receptor agonists are reported to reduce panic anxiety in panic disorder, and animal and clinical studies also provide strong evidence that agonists at the same receptors have robust efficacy in treating positive and negative symptoms in patients with schizophrenia.

NEUROPEPTIDES

A neuropeptide is a short neuroactive protein of generally fewer than 100 amino acids. Neuropeptide transmitters are synthesized differently from classical neurotransmitters: instead of being produced enzymatically in the neuronal terminal from common precursor compounds, peptide neurotransmitters are synthesized from precursor proteins produced from specific genes. In most cases, these gene products give rise to a propeptide, which is then cleaved by peptidase enzymes to form the peptide neurotransmitter. This means that increases in production of neuropeptide require an increase in gene expression, a slow process that can take hours or even days. This limiting step means that an increase in neuronal demand for peptide synthesis cannot induce a rapid response.

Peptides are stored in large dense-core vesicles within neurons. These neurons very often contain both a conventional neurotransmitter and one or more neuropeptides; that is, they coexist within a neuron. Release of the large vesicles, containing the neuropeptide, and the small vesicles, containing the neurotransmitter, is regulated differentially in that peptides are typically released at a high neuronal firing frequency, while neurotransmitters are released at a low frequency.

These differences between the classical and neuropeptide transmitters have led some to argue that the neuropeptides do not always fulfil the criteria defining a neurotransmitter, and they should be better described as neuromodulators.

Thus, they may not always have effects alone on postsynaptic cells but require the action of a classical transmitter, which is enhanced or, in some cases, suppressed by neuropeptide action. This modulatory action thus differs from the direct effect often shown by classical transmitters, although in complex and dynamic neuronal circuitry these transmitters are often modulating other neurotransmitter effects. The semantic differences between neuromodulator and neurotransmitter are arbitrary; where neuropeptides act within synapses, we shall refer to them as neurotransmitters. However, it should be said that several neuropeptides have local or systemic hormonal activity, often in addition to neurotransmitter action. This too can be seen for classical transmitters such as noradrenaline, 5-HT and histamine, however.

Peptides bind with high specificity and high affinity to their receptors, which are generally G-protein-coupled or metabotropic receptors. Activation of the peptide receptors modulates the responsiveness of the postsynaptic membrane to the action of classical neurotransmitters, and hence many classical neurotransmitters localize with neuropeptides in the brain, for example dopamine with neurotensin (NT) or CCK. Moreover, many neuropeptides may act independently as neurotransmitters.

Unlike classical neurotransmitters, synaptic inactivation of neuropeptides is generally performed by enzymes, and there is no active reuptake process. Released neuropeptide transmitter molecules diffuse away from the synapse and are cleaved by peptidases, which may be cytosolic or membrane-bound. These enzymes are not specific to a single peptide neurotransmitter but instead show specificity for certain types of amino acids pairing, the building blocks of peptide transmitters. However, this 'inactivation' is not always all as it seems. Certain peptide fragments derived from enzymatic activation can also be biologically active.

Cholecystokinin

CCK is a peptide neurotransmitter that was originally isolated from the gut but that is distributed extensively and abundantly within the central nervous system. CCK is co-localized with dopamine in a significant subset of mesencephalic neurons originating within the ventral tegmental area and terminating in the nucleus accumbens. Neurochemical and behavioural studies demonstrate that CCK has significant modulatory effects on dopamine transmission within the mesolimbic system. In addition, CCK is thought to regulate the functional activity of postsynaptic GABAergic medium-sized spiny neurons in the nucleus accumbens.

CCK binds to two different subtypes of receptors, which are both GPCRs and display approximately 50 per cent homology. The CCK_1 receptor is found mainly in the gut but also in several brain nuclei, such as the interpeduncular nucleus, area postrema and nucleus of the solitary tract. Conversely, the CCK_2 receptor is distributed widely throughout the CNS and is found in the olfactory bulbs and tubercle, medial frontal and cingulate cortices, frontal and frontoparietal cortices, retrosplenial cortex, nucleus accumbens, striatum and hippocampus. The CCK_2 receptor binds CCK-8 and the peptide gastrin at equal potency.

CCK's actions include the induction of anxiety-related behaviour in humans and experimental animals, an action via stimulation of CCK_2 receptors. Antagonists of this receptor display intrinsic anxiolytic properties. Conversely, CCK produces a reduction in food intake, via the hindbrain CCK_1 receptors, while also inhibiting expression of orexigenic peptides in the hypothalamus.

CCK is found in various forms, dependent on the numbers of amino acids (e.g. CCK-58, sulphated CCK-8 (CCK-8S) and CCK-4, where CCK-8S is the major transmitter form), and their synthesis is reliant on post-translational modification of the CCK gene product preprocholecystokinin. The CCK-8 inactivating enzyme is a serine peptidase, tripeptidyl peptidase II.

Neurotensin

NT is a 13-amino-acid peptide. NT immunoreactive neurons and terminal systems and receptors are found in many parts of the brain, including the basal and anterior hypothalamus, nucleus accumbens, septum and several brainstem nuclei. Its actions include analgesia, hypothermia and release of growth hormone and prolactin. NT is present in midbrain dopaminergic neurons of the mesolimbic, mesocortical and nigrostriatal dopaminergic pathways.

There are currently three characterized receptors for NT in the CNS. NTS1 and NTS2 receptors are both GPCRs and found on neurons and glia within the CNS. NTS1 receptors have high affinity for NT, but NTS2 receptors have lower affinity and the role of NT at this receptor is unclear. The NTS3 receptor is a type I amino acid receptor single-transmembrane-spanning receptor and is found in adipocytes as well as neurons and glia.

Most studies on the role played by NT in the CNS indicate clearly that NTS1 regulates dopaminergic function in both the nucleus accumbens and dorsal striatum by reducing function of the D2 autoreceptor and the activity of postsynaptic D2 receptors located on glutamate terminals. The influence of NT on dopaminergic transmission in nigrostriatal and mesocortical pathways suggests that NT plays a role in the pathophysiology of several CNS disorders, including Parkinson's disease, schizophrenia and addiction.

NT is synthesized as part of a 170-amino-acid precursor protein that also contains the related hexapeptide neuromedin N. It is degraded by a number of peptidases, leading to the formation of biologically inactive fragments.

Substance P

The 11-amino-acid polypeptide substance P (SP) coexists with the neurotransmitter serotonin in bulbospinal and dorsal raphe neurons, and with GABA and dynorphin in the striatal medium spiny neurons. In the CNS, SP has been associated with the regulation of anxiety and stress, respiratory rhythm, nausea and vomiting, and particularly pain and nociception. Reducing levels of SP with compounds such as capsaicin produces an analgesic and anti-inflammatory effect.

SP and its GPCR, the NK_1 receptor, are believed to play an important role in the modulation of stress-related, affective and anxious behaviour. Both peptide and receptor are found in brain limbic regions such as the amygdala and hippocampus, areas associated with stress and affective response, and show significant spatial overlap with neurotransmitters such as serotonin and noradrenaline. Aversive and stressful stimuli have been shown to change SP brain tissue content and NK_1 receptor binding, while an increase in intracerebral SP concentration produces anxiogenic-like responses in various behavioural tasks. For this reason, NK_1 receptor antagonists are currently being developed for the treatment of anxiety and depressive disorders.

SP is one of the tachykinin peptides, which include neurokinin A (NKA) and neurokinin B (NKB), all synthesized from the same preprotachykinin gene. SP can be degraded by a number of peptidases, including neutral endopeptidase and angiotensin-converting enzyme (ACE).

Opioid neuropeptides

The opioid neuropeptides include the dynorphins, encephalins, endomorphins and nociceptin/orphanin FQ. They bind to a series of GPCRs termed the opioid receptors, which also bind opiate drugs such as morphine as ligands.

The dynorphins, dynorphin A, dynorphin B and α/β-neoendorphin, arise from the precursor protein prodynorphin. Within the CNS, they have the highest concentrations in the hypothalamus, medulla, pons, midbrain and spinal cord. Moreover, dynorphin and their G-protein-coupled κ-opioid receptor are highly expressed in dopaminergic-rich regions: the prefrontal corticostriatal loop, within the prefrontal cortex, nucleus accumbens and dorsal striatum, and the ventral tegmental area and substantia nigra pars reticulata. This localization is consistent with neurochemical data indicating that dynorphin and κ-opioid receptors regulate the activity of mesoaccumbal, mesocortical and nigrostriatal dopamine and GABAergic neurons, and regulate extracellular dopamine levels. In addition, dynorphins are important in the pain response and the maintenance of homeostatic control. The dynorphins arise from the precursor protein prodynorphin.

The encephalins, Met^5-encephalin and Leu^5-encephalin, are two pentapeptides whose sequences differ only in their C-terminal amino acid. Within the basal ganglia, encephalins play an important co-transmitter role in the GABAergic striatal output pathway projecting to the external segment of the globus pallidus. These striatopallidal medium spiny neurons also co-express dopamine D2 receptors. The encephalins bind to the μ and δ classes of opioid receptors. μ-Receptors are found in the thalamus, cortex and periaqueductal grey matter, where they modulate analgesia, respiratory depression and euphoria. δ-Receptors are found in the amygdala, pontine nuclei and cortical regions, where they modulate analgesia and antidepressant effects. Both receptors are also involved in drug dependence.

Exogenous opioids include the natural opiates such as morphine and codeine, and synthetic opiates such as oxycodone, diacetylmorphine (heroin), methadone and pethidine. Repeated exposure to increasing dosages of opioids can lead to opioid tolerance (the need to take higher dosages of drugs in order to achieve the same opioid effect due to receptor sensitization) and drug dependence (susceptibility to withdrawal symptoms). These effects involve the mesolimbic reward system – opioid tolerance reduces the ventral tegmental area's release of dopamine from an important brain system underlying craving and compulsive drug use. The locus coeruleus is involved in the expression of opiate physical dependence and withdrawal involving the neurotransmitter noradrenaline.

Corticotropin-releasing hormone

Corticotropin-releasing hormone (CRH) is an important neuropeptide that is highly involved in the stress response. The regions of the hypothalamic paraventricular nucleus (PVN) with CRH neurons, the medial and periventricular nuclei, receive heavy projections of catecholaminergic fibres from the brainstem nuclei. In addition to containing noradrenaline, these catecholamine cell groups projecting to the PVN also express glutamate and neuropeptide Y (NPY). These catecholamines are suggested to have stimulatory effects on both the release and the production of hypophysiotrophic CRH, while co-transmitters of the catecholaminergic afferents that innervate CRH neurons, including NPY and glutamate, may also have profound regulatory roles over hypophysiotrophic neurons.

In response to stress, CRH is produced by neuroendocrine cells in the PVN of the hypothalamus and is released from these neurons into the primary capillary plexus of the hypothalamo-hypophyseal portal system, a system of blood vessels that links the hypothalamus and the anterior pituitary. At the pituitary, CRH stimulates the release of the stress hormone adrenocorticotropic hormone (ACTH). ACTH then acts on the adrenal glands to produce glucocorticoid hormones, mainly cortisol. In a negative-feedback cycle, glucocorticoids act on the hypothalamus and pituitary to suppress CRH and ACTH production. This pathway, shown in Figure 30.10, is termed the hypothalamic–pituitary–adrenal (HPA) axis and is a major neuroendocrine system that controls reactions to stress. The HPA axis regulates many body processes, including mood, digestion, the immune system, sexuality and homeostatic control such as energy storage and use.

The HPA axis seems to have many cross-links with the

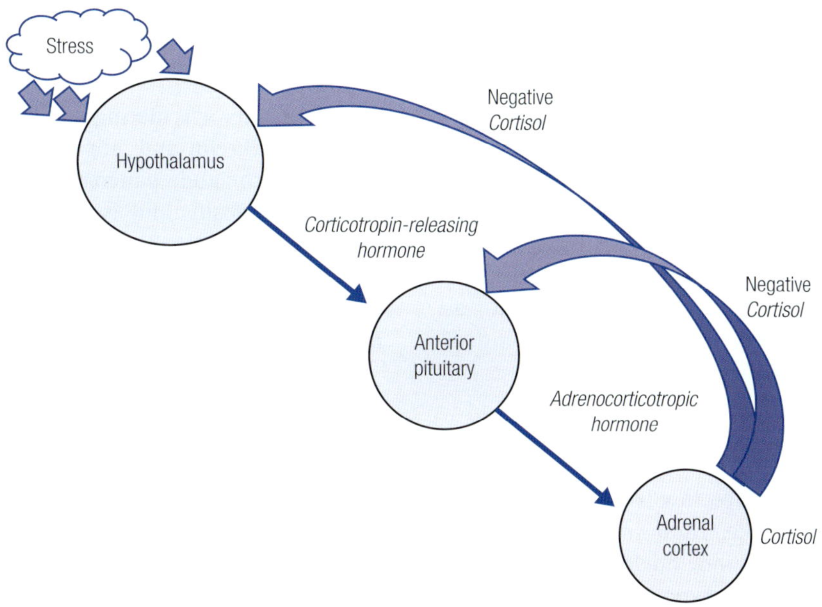

Figure 30.10 Schematic representation of the hypothalamic–pituitary–adrenal (HPA) axis. In response to stress, corticotropin-releasing hormone (CRH) is produced by neuroendocrine cells in the paraventricular nucleus of the hypothalamus and is released from these neurons into a system of blood vessels that links the hypothalamus and the anterior pituitary. Here, CRH stimulates the release of adrenocorticotropic hormone (ACTH). ACTH then acts on the adrenal glands to produce glucocorticoid hormones, mainly cortisol. In a negative-feedback cycle, glucocorticoids act back on the hypothalamus and pituitary to suppress CRH and ACTH production

neuroendocrine pathways that homeostatically regulate food intake: CRH-containing neurons are located in the PVN of the hypothalamus, the major centre in the control of feeding behaviour; CRH inhibits feeding in rats; CRH is suggested to be an important intermediate in the anorectic effects of leptin; and the hypophagic effect of central CRH may result in part from inhibitory control of the orexigenic neural pathways involving NPY. CRH exerts an opposite effect on appetite when compared with glucocorticoids, with the orexigenic effect of glucocorticoids, following the anorectic effect of CRH at the beginning of the stress response, playing a role in the recovery stage for the replacement of the replenishment of energy required during the fight or flight response.

CRH is a 41-amino-acid peptide synthesized from procorticotropin-releasing hormone. CRH binds to the corticotropin-releasing hormone receptor (CRHR), a GPCR.

Hypothalamic neuropeptides

Angiotensin II (Ang II) binds to two types of GPCR, namely AT1 and AT2. Brain AT1 receptors are found largely within the circumventricular structures and in hypothalamic and brainstem nuclei. There is a strong association between brain angiotensin and catecholaminergic systems, in particular in brain regions involved in autonomic and cardiovascular control and fluid balance with noradrenergic and adrenergic neurons and the nigrostriatal system with dopamine. Ang II is involved in the regulation of blood pressure and fluid and electrolyte balance, which it regulates peripherally and within the CNS. Ang II is synthesized from the precursor angiotensinogen via the enzyme ACE. Upon degradation by various propeptidases, a number of peptide fragments of Ang II are formed, which are also thought to be biologically active – Ang II (1–7), Ang III and Ang IV – with the latter suggested to produce positive effects on memory.

Vasopressin (AVP), also known as arginine vasopressin and antidiuretic hormone, is a 9-amino-acid peptide that binds to two types of receptor (1A and 1B) within the CNS. Acting largely within the pituitary and hypothalamus, AVP homeostatically controls plasma osmolality and regulation of blood pressure and temperature. AVP has also been suggested to have higher-order functions such as regulation of male-typical social behaviours, including scent-marking, aggression and paternal care. Additionally, AVP is suggested to be fundamental for the formation or expression of social learning and memory and in emotionality.

Oxytocin (OT) is a 9-amino-acid peptide with a similar structure to AVP whose sequence differs from OT by two amino acids. OT is synthesized in the nuclei of the hypothalamus and stored mainly in the posterior pituitary. Its major role is in female reproduction – uterine contractions, breastfeeding and maternal behaviour. It also plays an important role in the regulation of male and female sexual behaviour. Brain OT has generally been described as an important regulator of the stress response, with central administration of synthetic OT found to exert an anxiolytic effect in rodents. OT also plays a major role in the regulation of complex physiological stress responses, including stress-induced neuronal activation and activity of the HPA axis by inhibiting HPA axis responses to a wide variety of physical, emotional and pharmacological stressors, and may thus make an important contribution to the attenuated stress responsiveness found in pregnancy and during lactation.

Two related neuropeptides, orexin A and B, are produced in the lateral and posterior hypothalamus and send projections throughout the brain. A major role of the orexin system is the integration of circadian rhythm, tiredness and metabolic influences to promote wakefulness, thought to be through interaction with neurotransmitters such as dopamine, histamine and acetylcholine. Dysregulation of the orexin system causes narcolepsy.

Feeding neuropeptides

There are multiple neuropeptides involved in controlling satiety, appetite and food intake. These include neuropeptides found within the hypothalamic nuclei involved in the control of feeding (e.g. NPY, agouti-related peptide (AgRP)) and circulating peptides secreted peripherally into the blood to have effects on these areas of the hypothalamus (e.g. ghrelin, leptin, adiponectin). Some of these are described briefly here.

NPY is a 36-amino-acid peptide found in the hypothalamus and the autonomic nervous system. NPY binds to five GPCRs (Y1–Y5). Its main effect is increasing food intake; in rodents, stimulation of NPY activity increases eating, while blockade of hypothalamic NPY activity via the Y1 and Y5 receptor subtypes decreases food intake. NPY has been implicated in eating disorders: in obesity, an increase in NPY activity is thought to be brought about by high levels of glucocorticoids abolishing the negative feedback of CRH on NPY synthesis and release.

AgRP is produced in the arcuate nucleus in the hypothalamus and is co-localized with NPY in neurons. AgRP increases appetite and decreases metabolism and energy expenditure. α-Melanocyte-stimulating hormone (MSH) is an anorectic peptide also found in neurons of the arcuate nucleus in the hypothalamus and playing an inhibitory role in feeding and energy storage. Melanin-concentrating hormone is another peptide found primarily in the hypothalamus, where it is involved in the control of food intake and energy balance. Melanin-concentrating hormone knockout mice are lean and hypophagic and have increased metabolic rates.

Leptin is a protein hormone that plays a key role in regulating energy intake and energy expenditure, including appetite and metabolism. It is produced by adipose tissue; leptin secretion increases as fat is deposited and diminishes as the adipocyte stores of fat decrease. It interacts with the LepRb class of receptor, which are present in a number of hypothalamic nuclei. Leptin signals to the brain that the body has had enough to eat, by inhibiting the activity of neurons that contain NPY and AgRP and stimulating receptors containing MSH. First discovered in mutant obese mice, mutations in the leptin gene have been shown to have a role in obesity and in antipsychotic-induced weight gain. It has been shown that leptin may also be produced within the brain.

Two further circulating peptides with effects on food intake are ghrelin and adiponectin. Ghrelin is produced in the stomach and pancreas to stimulate appetite and increase adiposity and is thought to act in concert with leptin. Adiponectin has an import role in glucose regulation, fatty-acid breakdown and insulin sensitivity. Produced by adipose tissue, adiponectin has been shown to be decreased in obesity.

Neurotrophins

Neurotrophins or neurotrophic factors are a class of growth factors that stimulate the survival, growth and differentiation of cells in the CNS. Neurotrophins activate two distinct classes of transmembrane receptors, the tropomyosin-related kinase (Trk) family of receptors and the p75 receptor. The Trk family of receptor tyrosine kinases includes the TrkA, TrkB and TrkC receptors, which are activated preferentially by the neurotrophins nerve growth factor (NGF), brain-derived neurotrophic factor (BDNF), NT-4/5 and NT-3. Conversely, the p75 receptor binds both the mature form of the neurotrophins and their precursor peptides.

NGF mediates neuronal survival and differentiation. First characterized as a survival factor for developing sympathetic and sensory neurons, it is now clear that it plays an important role in the maintenance and regeneration of mature peripheral neurons. However, the highly restricted specificity of NGF for sympathetic and sensory neurons and striatal and basal forebrain cholinergic neurons suggests that NGF has an important selective role in the CNS. Cholinergic neurons of the nucleus basalis, medial septum and striatum are unique in that they express both NGF receptors TrkA and p75; it is thought that NGF maintains the function of cholinergic neurons in these regions. Accordingly, due to the loss of cholinergic neurons in Alzheimer's disease, investigations have also revealed alterations in various markers for NGF and its receptors in patients with Alzheimer's disease.

BDNF regulates synaptic plasticity, helping to support the survival of existing neurons and to encourage the growth and differentiation of new neurons and synapses, including hippocampal and cortical neurons and cholinergic, nigrostriatal dopaminergic and 5-HT neuron classes. BDNF and its receptor TrkB are also expressed widely in association with glutamatergic synapses. BDNF is synthesized, stored and released from glutamatergic neurons. It facilitates glutamate release and increases phosphorylation of the NR1 and NR2B subunits of the NMDA–receptor complex.

BDNF is involved in LTP. cAMP response element binding protein (CREB), a transcription factor consistently implicated in memory processing, is a major mediator of neuronal BDNF responses. This provides strong evidence for a role for BDNF in memory formation and storage, particularly in hippocampus-dependent learning.

The many actions of BDNF on different types of neuron have led to the view that malfunctioning of neurotrophins may be a contributing factor in the development of psychiatric disorders. This hypothesis is supported by studies showing that neurotrophins are abnormally regulated in animal models of psychiatric illness and changed after antipsychotic or antidepressant administration. In addition, human studies have demonstrated altered BDNF levels in both blood and the CNS in schizophrenia, while in depression plasticity-related changes such as hippocampal atrophy are thought to be related to a decreased expression or function of BDNF or the TrkB receptor (Box 30.3). In addition, a functional coding region polymorphism (Val66Met) of the BDNF gene, associated with smaller hippocampal volumes and poor performance on hippocampus-dependent memory tasks, has been proposed as a risk factor (albeit a weak one) for the development of bipolar disorder and schizophrenia.

KEY POINTS

- Synaptic control of neuronal activity provides the complex, elaborate, subtle and flexible mechanisms by which the brain is able to process information.
- Neurons are highly specialized cells with mechanisms for synthesis and storage of neurotransmitter, mechanisms for transmitter release and processes for removal of transmitter from the synapse.
- There are many substances that may be released from neurons to have a variety of effects on neuronal activity and cellular function: the fast amino acid neurotransmitters, the slower monoamine transmitters, the modulatory neuropeptides, and less conventional compounds such as cannabinoids (Box 30.1) and NO.
- The specificity that neurotransmitters impart to neurons contributes to the anatomic specificity of brain function. Some neurotransmitters are ubiquitous throughout the brain, while others are highly specific in both anatomical distribution and function.
- Neurotransmitters and other signalling molecules bring about their effects by action at specific cell membrane receptors, of which there are two main groups: the ionotropic receptors, which are ligand-gated ion channels influencing cell membrane polarization, and the metabotropic receptors, which, via G-protein-mediated production of second messengers, can have a wide variety of biochemical effects on cell function.
- Synaptic neurotransmission is the major point at which we can influence neuronal activity in the brain. Each of the processes of neurotransmitter synthesis, storage, release, reuptake and metabolism, and the receptors at which neurotransmitters act, are targets for neuropsychiatric drugs.

Box 30.3 Adult neurogenesis

Many organs of the body show a capacity to regenerate. For many years, it was understood that the neurons of the adult central nervous system (CNS) were unable to do this: neurons are postmitotic cells and, when lost from the developed brain, are not replaced. More recently, research has questioned this assumption. Neurogenesis, the process by which new neurons are formed, does occur in certain discrete areas of the adult mammalian brain, including the dentate gyrus of the hippocampus.

It has been shown that there are neural progenitor cells in the subgranular zone of the rat hippocampus that divide to produce young cells that mature into fully differentiated hippocampal neurons. Animal studies have shown that this process can be down-regulated by stress and glucocorticoids, while antidepressants, increased activity and an enriched environment can enhance neurogenesis. These environmental and pharmacological effects on neurogenesis appear to have effects on, and perhaps via, brain-derived neurotrophic factor (BDNF) expression, reflecting the importance of this neurotropic factor both in neurogenesis and in maintaining neuronal survival.

It has not been demonstrated unequivocally that neurogenesis occurs in the human adult. However, disturbances of neurogenesis may occur in major psychiatric disorders. Thus, depression has been hypothesized to reflect deficits in neurogenesis, resulting in neuronal deficits and hence volume loss in the hippocampus, an effect reversed by antidepressant drug treatment.

FURTHER READING

Eisch AJ, Cameron HA, Encinas JM, *et al.* (2008) Adult neurogenesis, mental health, and mental illness: hope or hype? *Journal of Neuroscience* **28**: 11785–91.

Zhao C, Deng W, Gage FH (2008) Mechanisms and functional implications of adult neurogenesis. *Cell* **132**: 645–60.

FURTHER READING

Neurotransmitter systems and neurochemical mechanisms

Webster RA ed (2001) *Neurotransmitters, Drugs and Brain Function.* Wiley Blackwell.

Pocock JM, Kettenmann H (2007) Neurotransmitter receptors on microglia. *Trends in Neuroscience* **30(10)**: 527–35.

Poo Mu-ming (2001) Neurotrophins as synaptic modulators. *Nature Reviews Neuroscience* **2**: 24–32.

Benes FM (2001) Carlsson and the discovery of dopamine. *Trends in Pharmacological Sciences* **22(1)**: 46–7.

Reynolds GP (2008) The neurochemistry of schizophrenia. *Psychiatry* **7(10)**: 425–29.

Berton O, Nestler EJ (2006) New approaches to antidepressant drug discovery: beyond monoamines. *Nature Reviews Neuroscience* **7**: 137–51.

Strand FL (1999) *Neuropeptides: Regulators of Physiological Processes.* Cambridge, Mass.: MIT Press.

Ionotropic & metabotropic receptors (general)

Barrera NP, Edwardson JM (2008) The subunit arrangement and assembly of ionotropic receptors. *Trends in Neurosciences* **31(11)**: 569–76.

Kew JNC, Kemp JA (2005) Ionotropic and metabotropic receptor structure and pharmacology. *Psychopharmacology* **179**: 4–29.

Sanders RD, Brian D, Maze M (2008) G-protein-coupled receptors. *Handbook of Experimental Pharmacology* **(182)**: 93–117.

Receptors and their pharmacology

Snyder SH (2004) Opiate receptors and beyond: 30 years of neural signaling research. *Neuropharmacology* **47** Suppl 1: 274–85.

Sieghart W (2006) Structure, pharmacology, and function of $GABA_A$ receptor subtypes. *Advances in Pharmacology* **54**: 231–63.

Paoletti P, Neyton J (2007) NMDA receptor subunits: function and pharmacology. *Current Opinion in Pharmacology* **7(1)**: 39–47.

Kalia LV, Kalia SK, Salter MW (2008) NMDA receptors in clinical neurology: excitatory times ahead. *Lancet Neurology* **7(8)**: 742–55.

Bowery NG (2006) $GABA_B$ receptor: a site of therapeutic benefit. *Current Opinion in Pharmacology* **6(1)**: 37–43.

Sacco KA, Bannon KL, George TP (2004) Nicotinic receptor mechanisms and cognition in normal states and neuropsychiatric disorders. *Journal of Psychopharmacology* **18(4)**: 457–74.

Van Hooft JA, Vijverberg HPM (2000) 5-HT_3 receptors and neurotransmitter release in the CNS: a nerve ending story? *Trends in Neurosciences* **23(12)**: 605–10.

Raiteri M (2008) Presynaptic metabotropic glutamate and $GABA_B$ receptors. *Handbook of Experimental Pharmacology* **(184)**: 373–407.

Sealfon SC, Olanow CW (2000) Dopamine receptors: from structure to behavior. *Trends in Neurosciences* **23(10)**: S34–40.

Millan MJ, Marin P, Bockaert J, la Cour CM (2008) Signaling at G-protein-coupled serotonin receptors: recent advances and future research directions. *Trends in Pharmacological Sciences* **29(9)**: 454–64.

Meltzer HY, Li Z, Kaneda Y, Ichikawa J (2003) Serotonin receptors: their key role in drugs to treat schizophrenia. *Progress in Neuropsychopharmacology and Biological Psychiatry* **27(7)**: 1159–72

King MV, Marsden CA, Fone KC (2008) A role for the 5-HT1A, 5-HT4 and 5-HT6 receptors in learning and memory. *Trends in Pharmacological Sciences* **29**: 482–92.

Reynolds GP (2004) Receptor mechanisms in the treatment of schizophrenia. *Journal of Psychopharmacology* **18(3)**: 340–5.

Iversen LL, Iversen SE, Bloom FE, Roth RH (2009) *Introduction to Neuropsychopharmacology.* New York: Oxford University Press.

Chapter 31

Neuropathology

Steve M Gentleman

INTRODUCTION

The aim of this chapter is to give a brief overview of the pathological changes that underlie key central nervous system (CNS) disorders that may be encountered in a clinical psychiatry setting.

PATHOLOGICAL CHANGE IN THE CENTRAL NERVOUS SYSTEM

Neurons

All of the cell types seen in the brain can be involved in the reaction to damage, but it is often the neurons that are the primary target for pathology in CNS disorders. Neurons are highly metabolically active cells, a fact that is clearly reflected in their morphology. They have a large nucleus with a prominent nucleolus, numerous mitochondria, a highly developed Golgi apparatus, and abundant rough endoplasmic reticulum (ER). It is these stacks of rough ER that form the characteristic Nissl substance, which can be stained with basophilic dyes such as cresyl violet and help to distinguish neurons from other cell types (Figure 31.1a).

Neurons can undergo a number of different morphological changes, depending on the nature of the insult. For example, in response to acute hypoxic or ischaemic changes, neurons become eosinophilic, with a shrunken cytoplasm and a hyperchromatic nucleus (Figure 31.1b). In more chronic conditions, neurons become atrophic, with pyknotic nuclei and diffusely basophilic cytoplasm.

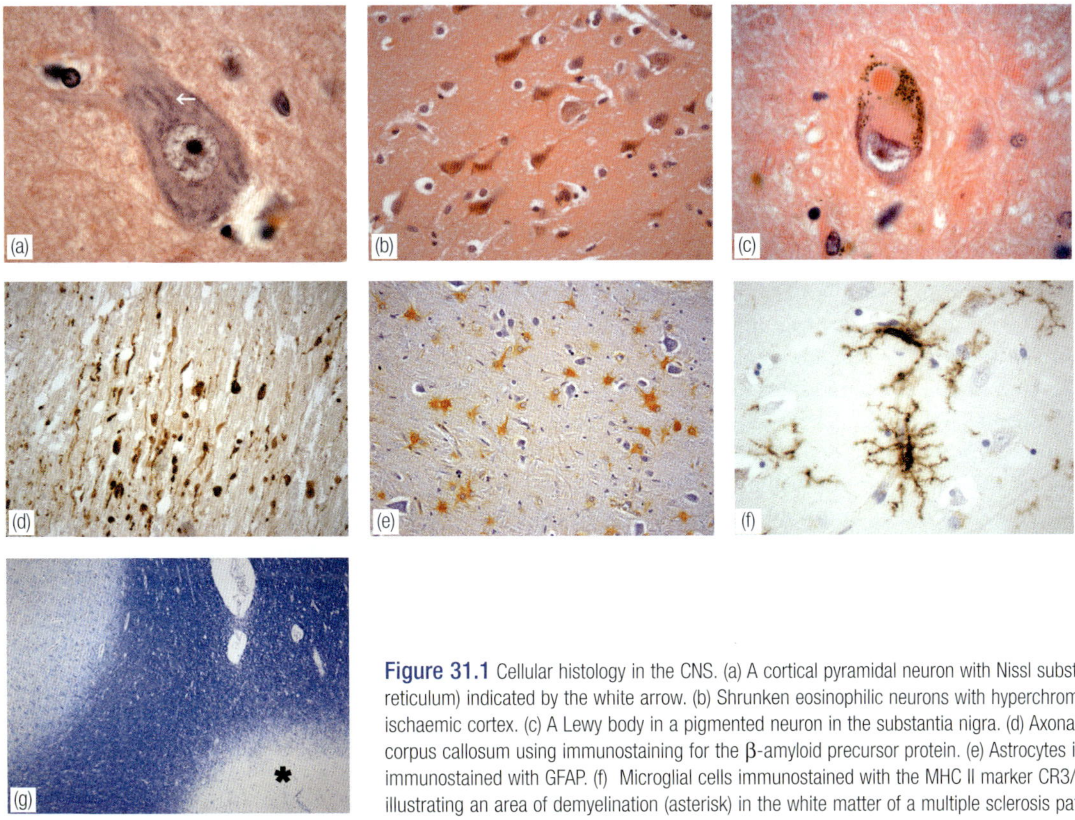

Figure 31.1 Cellular histology in the CNS. (a) A cortical pyramidal neuron with Nissl substance (rough endoplasmic reticulum) indicated by the white arrow. (b) Shrunken eosinophilic neurons with hyperchromatic nuclei in an area of ischaemic cortex. (c) A Lewy body in a pigmented neuron in the substantia nigra. (d) Axonal injury demonstrated in the corpus callosum using immunostaining for the β-amyloid precursor protein. (e) Astrocytes in the hilus of the hippocampus immunostained with GFAP. (f) Microglial cells immunostained with the MHC II marker CR3/43. (g) Luxol Fast Blue staining illustrating an area of demyelination (asterisk) in the white matter of a multiple sclerosis patient.

Whereas these morphological changes are generally associated with cell death, central chromatolysis, in which the cell body swells, the Nissl substance disperses and the nucleus moves to the edge of the cell, is associated with reparative processes, particularly in large motor neurons such as those seen in the ventral horn of the spinal cord. Another key manifestation of pathology, particularly in degenerative disorders, is the presence of intraneuronal inclusions, such as Lewy bodies in Parkinson's disease (PD) (Figure 31.1c), some of which will be discussed in more detail later in this chapter.

In addition to changes seen in the neuronal cell body, axons can also display pathological changes. Eosinophilic swellings or spheroids, composed of neurofilaments and cellular organelles, are found in axons where normal axonal transport has been interrupted as a result of trauma or hypoxia. Although these can be seen in routine haematoxylin and eosin (H&E)-stained sections, they are more easily detected using immunostaining for the β-amyloid precursor protein (Figure 31.d).

Astrocytes

Astrocytosis, observed as a proliferation and hypertrophy of astrocytes, is a reactive process initiated by damage to the CNS, irrespective of cause. These changes are accompanied by the production of large amounts of the intermediate filament protein glial acidic fibrillary protein (GFAP), immunostaining for which is used routinely to detect astrocytosis (Figure 31.1e). When astrocytes become activated, the cell processes become much more prominent and the enlarged cytoplasm becomes uniformly eosinophilic (gemistocytic). In some degenerative conditions, proteins can accumulate in astrocytes, for example tau in progressive supranuclear palsy (PSP) or corticobasal degeneration.

Microglia

Microglia are considered to be the immune sensor cells of the CNS, able to present antigen and to release a variety of cytokines and chemokines. They also have a key role in the phagocytosis of tissue debris after injury. It remains unclear whether activation of CNS microglia is a beneficial or deleterious process, although it seems likely that at least in the first instance it is a protective response; if it persists, however, it may drive the progression of longer-term degenerative processes. Microglia adopt different morphologies, depending on their activation state. Resting microglia have a highly ramified structure, whereas activated microglia have shorter thickened processes and a more obvious cell body. Activated cells can be immunostained using the MHC II marker CR3/43 (Figure 31.1f). Macrophage/microglial cells can be seen around old infarcts, where they often contain haemosiderin, and also around areas of active demyelination, where they can be seen to contain myelin debris.

Oligodendrocytes

Oligodendrocytes are the myelinating cells of the CNS. Damage to these cells is evident in demyelinating diseases such as multiple sclerosis (MS) (Figure 31.1g). However, as with astrocytes and neurons, they can also be affected by inclusions, such as the α-synuclein immunoreactive Papp-Lantos inclusions that are now considered diagnostic for multiple system atrophy (MSA) (see Movement disorders, below). Tau-positive coiled bodies are also characteristic of PSP and other tauopathies (see Movement disorders, below).

DEMENTIAS

Alzheimer's disease

There are estimated to be 700 000 people in the UK with dementia,[1] the most common form of which is Alzheimer's disease (AD). The distinctive pathology of the disease that was to take his name was originally described by Alois Alzheimer in 1907 and initially was restricted to cases of presenile dementia, where the age of onset was below the age of 65 years. However, the term AD is now used to cover dementia patients of all ages who reach a threshold level of neuropathological change.

Macroscopic pathology

Cerebral atrophy and low brain weight are commonly observed in AD, but these features are also seen in other degenerative disorders and so are not reliable diagnostic indicators. The atrophy tends to be more marked in the frontal, parietal and medial temporal lobes. The hippocampus in particular may be atrophic, with relative enlargement of the inferior horn of the lateral ventricle, a finding often picked up by in vivo imaging.

Microscopic pathology

The microscopic lesions that define the disease are extracellular senile plaques, intracellular neurofibrillary tangles and gliosis, all of which are associated to some extent with normal ageing and therefore none of which is pathognomonic. Diagnosis is therefore made on the basis of the number and distribution of plaques and tangles with respect to age.[2–6] Plaques consist of deposits of the 39- to 43-amino-acid amyloid-β (Aβ) peptide, which is derived from the processing of a longer membrane-bound protein called amyloid precursor protein (APP). The plaques have a varying morphology, ranging from diffuse, amorphous deposits to the more classical form with a condensed core surrounded by a neuritic halo (Figure 31.2a). In some cases, there may also be significant deposition of the Aβ peptide in the walls of the intraparenchymal and leptomeningeal blood vessels in the form of cerebral amyloid angiopathy (CAA) (Figure 31.2b).

Neurofibrillary tangles are composed primarily of a hyperphosphorylated form of the microtubule-associated

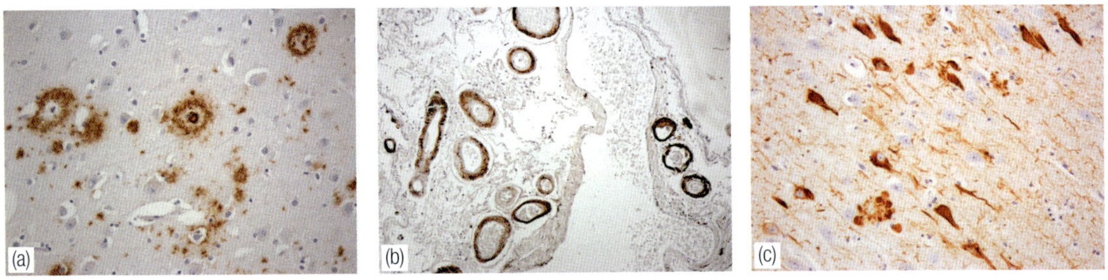

Figure 31.2 Alzheimer-type pathology. (a) Extracellular Aβ peptide plaques in the cerebral cortex. (b) Cerebral amyloid angiopathy in the form of Aβ peptide deposits in vessel walls. (c) Tau immunostaining of neurofibrillary tangles, neuritic plaques and neuropil threads in the entorhinal cortex of an Alzheimer's patient

protein tau. Aggregation of this protein causes disruption of the neuronal cytoskeleton and consequently impairs normal transport processes within the neurons. Tau pathology can also be seen in the neuritic clusters around classic plaques and the neuropil threads in the brain parenchyma (Figure 31.2c). Traditionally, both plaques and tangles were stained using silver impregnation techniques, but nowadays, with antibodies available against the key pathological proteins, immunostaining is the method of choice.

Although cortical pathology predominates in AD, both tangles and plaques can also be found in subcortical areas. Most notably, neuritic pathology and severe cell loss are seen in the nucleus basalis of Meynert. The cells in this basal forebrain nucleus provide the cholinergic innervation to the entire cerebral cortex, and it is the loss of this system that is thought to underlie some of the core cognitive and memory deficits observed in AD. Consequently, it is replacement of this cholinergic deficit that forms the basis for most currently available therapies for AD.

Dementia with Lewy bodies

Dementia with Lewy bodies (DLB) is the second most common form of dementia and is one of a group of disorders (including PD) that involves alterations to the protein α-synuclein. Clinically it can be distinguished from AD on the basis of a fluctuating course and the presence of symptoms such as hallucinations.[7] It can occur as a result of the presence of cortical Lewy bodies alone or, more commonly, in the presence of some degree of AD pathology. In fact, there is much current debate as to what is the precise pathological substrate for dementia in patients with DLB, DLB and AD, and Parkinson's disease dementia (PDD).[8]

Macroscopic pathology

Cerebral atrophy tends to be less severe than that seen in AD. Section of the midbrain reveals a pale substantia nigra, similar to that seen in PD, due to the loss of neuromelanin-containing dopaminergic neurons.

Microscopic pathology

Cortical Lewy bodies are smaller than those typically found in brainstem nuclei and are more irregular in shape. They are found most abundantly in the deeper layers of the cingulate, entorhinal and temporal cortices (Figure 31.3), whereas the occipital and primary sensory and motor cortices are generally spared. The substantia nigra shows variable degrees of neuronal loss and Lewy body pathology. Lewy neurites are also seen throughout the brain and within the hippocampus show a particular localization in the CA2 subfield. Both Lewy bodies and neurites can be detected using ubiquitin immunostaining, but the method of choice is now to use α-synuclein antibodies.[9]

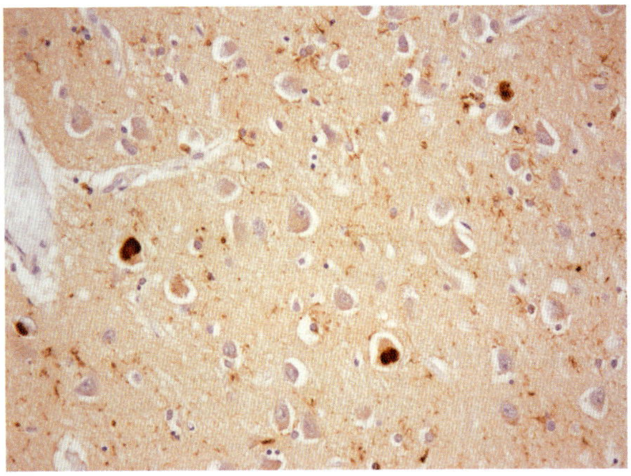

Figure 31.3 α-Synuclein immunostaining of cortical Lewy bodies in the cingulate cortex of a patient with dementia with Lewy bodies

Frontotemporal lobar dementias

As the name suggests, the frontotemporal lobar dementias (FTLDs) are a group of non-Alzheimer neurodegenerative disorders, including Pick's disease, in which the frontal and temporal cortex are the areas preferentially affected by pathology. They present clinically in many ways, but there are three main syndromes. The first involves behavioural changes, including social disinhibition, and subsequently language disturbances. In the other two syndromes, progressive non-fluent aphasia and semantic dementia, the language deficits are primary. In other FTLDs, parkinsonism or amyotrophic lateral sclerosis may also feature in the clinical presentation. Historically, a variety of terminologies has been used to describe these conditions, but in light of more recent genetic and biochemical findings and a greater understanding of their molecular biology there is now an emerging consensus in terms of nomenclature.[10]

Macroscopic pathology

Selective atrophy of the frontal or temporal lobes is typically observed in FTLD brains. This may or may not be associated with gross atrophy of the basal ganglia and loss of pigmentation of the substantia nigra, depending on the type of FTLD.

Microscopic pathology

By using immunocytochemistry for key proteins, it is possible to identify the various subtypes of FTLD based on the pathology seen. Tau immunostaining is observed in tangle-only dementia, Pick's disease and rare cases where there is a mutation in the gene for tau, *MAPT*. In tangle-only dementia, there is cortical neuronal loss, gliosis and numerous neurofibrillary tangles in the absence of any Aβ pathology (in contrast to AD). In Pick's disease, there are tau-immunoreactive inclusions called Pick bodies in cortical neurons and in neurons of the dentate gyrus of the hippocampus.

The other major subset of FTLD is those that are tau-negative but that exhibit ubiquitin-positive inclusions (FTLD-U). It has been discovered that the ubiquitinated protein present in these inclusions is TAR DNA-binding protein 43 (TDP-43).[11] Immunostaining with antibodies against TDP-43 highlights neuronal cytoplasmic inclusions, intranuclear 'cat's-eye' type inclusions (Figure 31.4), dystrophic neurites and glial cell inclusions and can be used to diagnose these conditions, some of which are associated with specific gene mutations.[12,13]

Vascular dementia

Despite numerous clinical and pathological studies, the precise relationship between vascular pathology and cognitive decline remains far from clear. One key problem is that pure vascular pathologies are relatively rare, and often there are signs of coexistent degenerative pathology, most frequently AD, giving rise to the concept of 'mixed dementia'. However, it is generally accepted that large-vessel disease, small-vessel disease and hypoperfusion may all contribute to cognitive impairment. Based on an assessment of the extent and location of these pathological changes, criteria for the neuropathological diagnosis of six subtypes of vascular dementia have been proposed.[14]

Macroscopic pathology

Dementia is common in individuals who have had a stroke, whether as a result of a single large infarct or multiple smaller infarcts. This led Hachinski and colleagues in 1974 to coin the term 'multi-infarct dementia',[15] a term that has now largely been superseded by the broader term of 'vascular dementia'. Pathological and imaging studies suggest that vascular dementia is related to the volume and location of cerebral lesions.[16,17] In some patients with 'strategic infarcts' in areas important for normal cognitive function, such as the hippocampus, this relationship breaks down and the effects can be disproportionate to the size of the lesion.

Microscopic pathology

Small-vessel disease, particularly arteriosclerosis (Figure 31.5), is a common feature of dementia in elderly people. This may be seen in the form of lacunes, small holes in the tissue, which arise as a result of ischaemic damage around occluded vessels and are most frequently associated with hypertension. Lacunar infarcts are most commonly seen in the basal ganglia, thalamus and cortical white matter. Depending on their precise location, they may be clinically silent and may be found incidentally only at postmortem. On magnetic resonance (MR) and computed tomography (CT) imaging, small-vessel disease in the white matter, along with its attendant myelin disruption and glial reaction, is known as leucoaraiosis. The severity of leucoaraiosis has been correlated with the extent of cognitive impairment, making imaging an important component of the clinical assessment of vascular dementia.

In addition to the common vascular conditions outlined above, a number of rarer familial vasculopathies have been

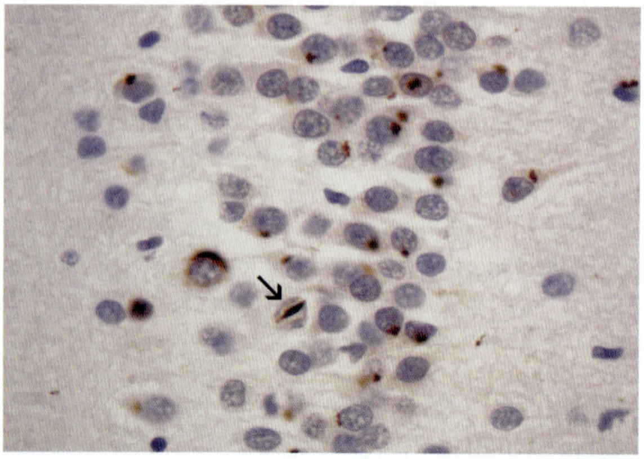

Figure 31.4 Intranuclear "cats-eye" inclusion in the dentate gyrus of a patient with an FTLD

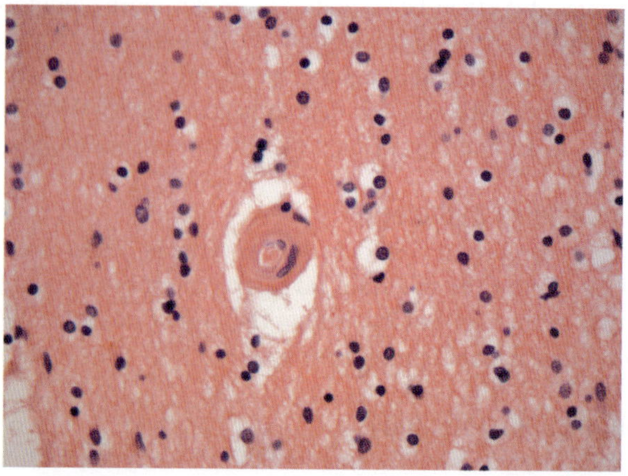

Figure 31.5 Small vessel disease. A small white matter artery showing thickened walls in a patient with hypertension

identified. Cerebral autosomal dominant arteriopathy with subcortical infarcts and leucoencephalopathy (CADASIL) is a disorder associated with mutations in the *NOTCH3* gene, resulting in multiple infarcts in the frontal white matter and basal ganglia.[18] There are then a string of rare conditions named according to the nationality of the families in which they were first described: hereditary cerebral haemorrhage with amyloidosis, Dutch type (HCHWA-D), which is due to a mutation in the same APP gene that is central to the pathology of AD;[19] hereditary cerebral haemorrhage with amyloidosis, Icelandic type (HCHWA-I), which is due to a mutation in the *CST3* gene that encodes for the cystatin C protein;[20] and familial amyloidosis, Finnish type, which is due to a mutation in the *GSN* gene that codes for gelsolin.[21]

Creutzfeldt–Jakob disease

Creutzfeldt–Jakob disease (CJD) is the most common form of human prion disease. The disease usually presents as a rapidly progressing dementia, often associated with ataxia, visual abnormalities and pyramidal and extrapyramidal features. Prion diseases, also known as transmissible spongiform encephalopathies, are unique in that they may be sporadic, inherited or acquired. The transmissible agent is defined as a prion (proteinaceous infectious particle), contains no nucleic acid and is composed entirely of a modified form of a normal cellular prion protein.[22] The mechanisms underlying the conversion of prion protein from its normal cellular form to the disease associated form in sporadic CJD are not well understood. However, inherited forms of prion disease such as Gerstmann–Straussler–Scheinker syndrome and fatal familial insomnia are associated with mutations in the prion protein gene, *PRNP*. Furthermore, varying susceptibility to prion diseases is associated with polymorphisms in the *PRNP* gene, most notably at codon 129. Acquired forms of prion disease, which require transfer of the pathological form of the prion protein but may have very long incubation times, include kuru, a disease associated with endocannibalism in the Fore tribe of Papua New Guinea; iatrogenic CJD, which has been associated with contaminated neurosurgical instruments, cadaveric dural grafts and pituitary hormones; and variant CJD,[23] which is thought to have arisen from infected beef entering the human food chain.

Microscopic pathology

Prion diseases are characterized by the presence of spongiform change in the cortex, thought to be the distension and swelling of neuronal cell processes (Figure 31.6a). There is also neuronal cell loss, prominent reactive astrogliosis and deposition of the pathological form of the prion protein (Figure 31.6b).

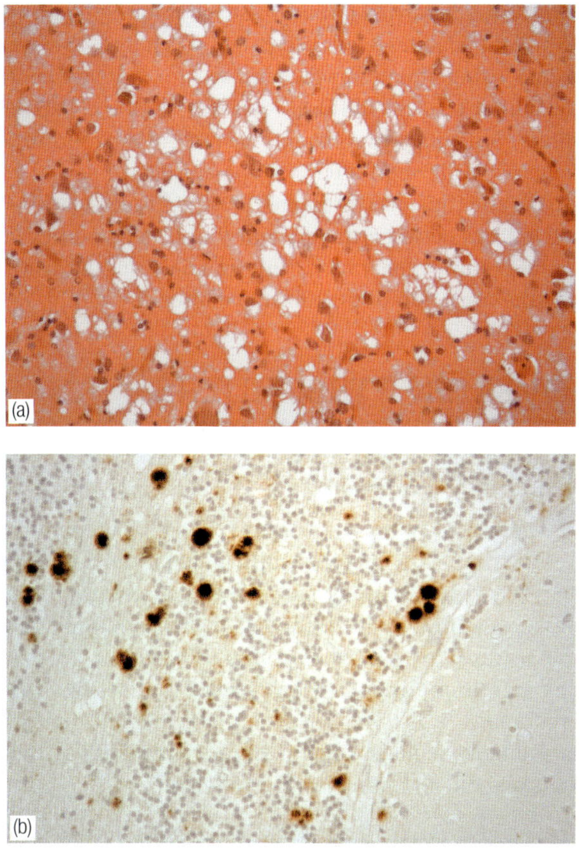

Figure 31.6 CJD. (a) Spongiform change in the cortex of a CJD patient. (b) Accumulation of the abnormal prion protein in the granule cell layer of the cerebellum

Dementia pugilistica

Boxers who are subjected to repeated blows to the head during the course of their career may develop neurological signs and a progressive dementia known as 'punch-drunk syndrome' or dementia pugilistica in later life.[24] Although this phenomenon was initially reported in boxers, there are now plenty of studies suggesting that longer-term cognitive impairment may also be a risk in other contact sports, such as rugby union and Australian rules football.[25]

Macroscopic pathology

Rotational acceleration as a consequence of repeated glancing blows to the head can lead to focal damage of midline structures. A fenestrated cavum septum pellucidum is often seen in boxers, whereas it is rarely seen in non-boxers unless there is a history of head injury. The ataxia and parkinsonism often seen in dementia pugilistica are caused by scarring to the inferior surface of the cerebellum and the loss of pigmented cells from the substantia nigra, respectively.

Microscopic pathology

The main microscopic changes associated with dementia pugilistica are neurofibrillary tangles throughout the cerebral cortex, particularly the medial temporal lobe, and the brainstem. These have been found to be biochemically very similar to those seen in Alzheimer brains. In the original boxer studies,[24] carried out using silver staining techniques, no amyloid plaques were seen; but when the cases were revisited using immunocytochemistry for the Aβ peptide, large numbers of diffuse deposits were observed.[26] Similarly, diffuse Aβ has been observed in a proportion of patients who die soon after a single episode of severe head injury,[27] and this has prompted further investigations of possible links between trauma and the subsequent development of neurodegeneration. One possible mechanism for this is the initiation of neuroinflammation.[28]

MOVEMENT DISORDERS

Parkinson's disease

PD is the most common of the movement disorders, affecting approximately 1 per cent of the population over the age of 65 years. The disease is characterized by tremor, rigidity, bradykinesia and abnormalities of posture and gait. These motor features are caused by a loss of normal nigrostriatal dopaminergic projections. However, as is described below, the pathology of PD is now known to be much wider spread than thought previously, and many patients will also manifest autonomic and psychiatric symptoms.

Macroscopic pathology

At gross examination, the brain of the patient with PD is likely to appear normal and be of normal weight. Distinctive pathology will be seen when the brainstem is examined. Cross-section of the midbrain reveals pallor of the substantia nigra, and a similar loss of pigmented cells from the locus coeruleus can be seen in pontine sections.

Microscopic pathology

PD, like DLB (see above), is an α-synucleinopathy, and immunostaining with antibodies against α-synuclein is now the method of choice for identifying the Lewy bodies that characterize the disease at the microscopic level (Figure 31.7). In the substantia nigra there is loss of pigmented dopaminergic cells, usually more marked in the lateral parts. There is also free pigment either lying in the neuropil or in macrophages. Other areas of the brain often showing pathological α-synuclein include the locus coeruleus, nucleus basalis of Meynert, dorsal nucleus of the vagus (associated with dysphagia) and the intermediolateral columns of the spinal cord (associated with autonomic deficits). Lewy bodies are not unique to PD and DLB but can also be seen in AD and sometimes in individuals with no clinical symptoms (incidental Lewy bodies), where they are assumed to represent preclinical PD.

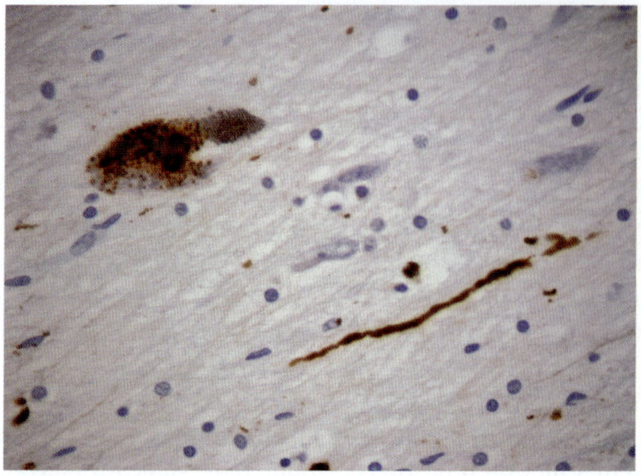

Figure 31.7 α-Synuclein immunostaining highlighting a Lewy body and a large Lewy neurite in the substantia nigra of a patient with Parkinson's disease

Progressive supranuclear palsy

PSP is an example of a so called 'parkinsonism-plus' syndrome and is much rarer than PD. The disease is associated with parkinsonism (usually without tremor), falls and vertical gaze problems. Unlike PD, PSP is a tauopathy, with the cellular changes due to pathological accumulation of tau protein.

Macroscopic pathology

As with PD, there is depigmentation of the substantia nigra, but in PSP there is generally sparing of the locus coeruleus. Other subtle changes that can help distinguish the two conditions are the presence of a mild atrophy of the midbrain, superior cerebellar peduncles and discolouration of the dentate nucleus of the cerebellum in PSP.

Microscopic pathology

Along with subcortical neuronal loss and gliosis, the main pathology in PSP is the accumulation of tau in both neurons and glial cells, particularly in the substantia nigra, subthalamic nucleus and globus pallidus. In the neurons the tau deposits form tangles and pretangles. Astrocytes in the striatum containing tau inclusions take on a tufted appearance, while oligodendrocytes in the white matter accumulate the tau in the form of coiled bodies (Figure 31.8).

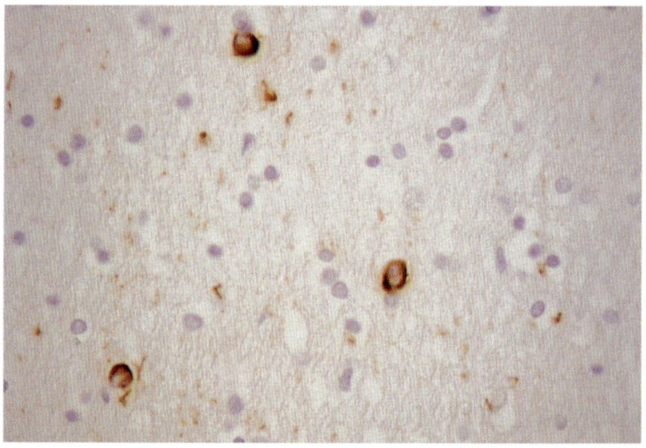

Figure 31.8 Tau immunostaining of coiled bodies in striatal oligodendrocytes in a case of PSP

Multiple system atrophy

MSA is another example of a 'parkinsonism-plus' syndrome, but in this case, as in PD, it is an α-synucleinopathy. The term MSA covers three previously distinct disorders: olivopontocerebellar atrophy (OPCA), which is characterized by prominent cerebellar ataxia; Shy–Drager syndrome, a primary autonomic failure; and striatonigral degeneration that presents with a prominent parkinsonism. More recently, the terms MSA-C (cerebellar) and MSA-P (parkinsonism) have come into general use and Shy–Drager syndrome has been dropped because autonomic failure is a feature in all MSA cases.

Macroscopic pathology

In cases where parkinsonism is prominent, there is atrophy of the brainstem and pons and a loss of pigmentation of the substantia nigra. There is often also a characteristic greenish discolouration and shrinkage of the putamen. Cerebellar atrophy is evident in cases with a prominent ataxia.

Microscopic pathology

The grouping of these previously separate conditions is based on the common presence of glial cytoplasmic inclusions. Specifically they are comma-shaped α-synuclein inclusions in oligodendrocytes, sometimes called Papp–Lantos bodies (Figure 31.9), and they are prevalent in the basal ganglia, substantia nigra and cerebellum.

Huntington's disease

Huntington's disease (HD) is a hyperkinetic disorder that is inherited in an autosomal dominant fashion and affects approximately 5 in 100 000 of the population. It is caused by an unstable CAG (glutamine) expansion in the *IT-15* gene on chromosome 4, which codes for the huntingtin protein. The disease occurs in people who have more than 37 repeats of the glutamine sequence. The age of onset shows an inverse correlation with the number of repeats, and there is anticipation – that is, there is expansion of the number of repeats on parental transmission.

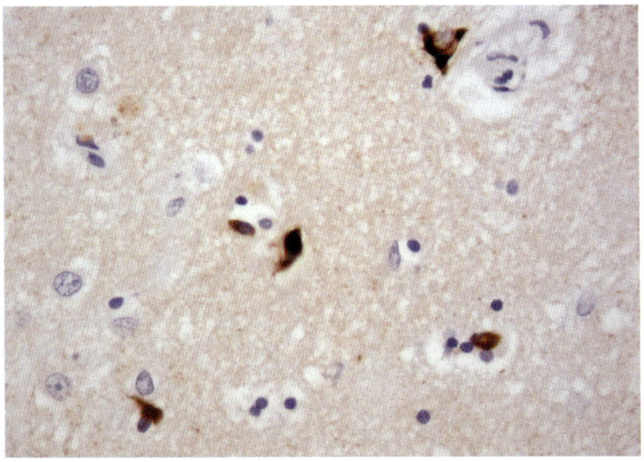

Figure 31.9 Papp-Lantos bodies (α-synuclein stained oligodendrocyte inclusions) in a patient with MSA

Macroscopic pathology

The frontal cortex is often mildly atrophic, but the cardinal pathology is seen on coronal slicing of the brain, when it becomes clear that there is marked atrophy of the caudate and putamen, with a corresponding increase in the size of the ventricles.

Microscopic pathology

In the striatum there is loss of the medium spiny neurons and a marked astrocytic reaction. There is also neuronal loss and gliosis in the cortex. Ubiquitin or huntingtin immunostaining reveals intranuclear inclusions and also accumulations of the protein in neurites in both the striatum and the cortex. The precise mechanisms of neurotoxicity associated with these inclusions remain unknown.

Motor neuron disease

Motor neuron disease (MND) is a chronic progressive disorder of motor neurons presenting as muscle wasting, weakness and eventually paralysis. The most common form of the disease is amyotrophic lateral sclerosis (ALS), in which both the upper and lower motor neurons are affected, leading to degeneration of the corticospinal tracts and a spastic paraparesis. Sometimes there is selective damage of the brainstem motor nuclei, leading to progressive bulbar palsy. Approximately 10 per cent of all MND cases are familial, and the best characterized genetic cause is a mutation in the copper-zinc-superoxide dismutase gene (*SOD1*).[29]

Macroscopic pathology

The brain appears normal in the majority of cases, unless there is particularly prominent upper motor neuron disturbance, in which case the precentral gyrus may be atrophic. Additionally, if there is associated dementia, there may be frontotemporal atrophy (see Frontotemporal lobar dementias, above). The main gross pathology is seen in the spinal cord, which is thinner than normal and where the anterior nerve roots appear atrophic and discoloured.

Microscopic pathology

Depending on the clinical subtype of the MND, the main microscopic pathology is the loss of motor neurons from the ventral horn of the spinal cord, lower brainstem motor nuclei and the Betz cells of the primary motor cortex. Luxol-fast blue staining of the spinal cord will show pallor of the corticospinal tracts. Some surviving motor neurons in the spinal cord contain inclusion bodies that can be detected with ubiquitin stains.

CEREBRAL TUMOURS

A detailed description of CNS tumours is way beyond the scope of this chapter, and so this section will be restricted to a very brief outline. For a more comprehensive account, the reader is directed to the World Health Organization (WHO) classification of tumours of the CNS.[30]

Tumours are classified histologically on the basis of their presumed cell of origin (see Figure 31.10), although biochemical and molecular studies are bringing some of these assumptions into question and the classification of tumour types is reviewed regularly in the light of new research information. The tumours can be either primary or secondary. Primary tumours arise from cells of the CNS (neuroepithelial) and meninges (non-neuroepithelial), whereas secondary tumours arise elsewhere in the body and metastasize to the CNS. In adults 70 per cent of tumours occur supratentorially, while in children this is reversed, with approximately 70 per cent of tumours affecting the brainstem and cerebellum. In adults the most common tumours are (in descending order) metastases, gliomas, meningiomas and Schwannomas. By contrast, in children tumours tend to be neuroectodermal in origin, for example medulloblastomas. Different tumour types are commonly found in certain anatomical locations, as shown in Table 31.1.

Intracranial tumours become clinically manifest for a number of reasons. Depending on their precise localization, they can produce focal dysfunction (e.g. hemiparesis if they impinge on the primary motor cortex), they can initiate epileptic activity in neighbouring tissue, and they can act as mass-occupying lesions, causing raised intracranial pressure. If they are located in the posterior cranial fossa, they can also interrupt normal flow of cerebrospinal fluid (CSF), causing hydrocephalus.

Tumours are graded histologically to give some prognostic indication to clinicians and to help them decide the most appropriate treatment regime. Grade I tumours have a low proliferative potential and, depending on their location, can be treated by neurosurgical resection alone. Grade II lesions tend to be infiltrative in nature, often recur and in some cases are able to transform into grade III lesions over time. Grade III lesions show clear evidence of malignancy in the form of nuclear changes and mitotic activity and in most cases will require adjuvant radiation or chemotherapy. Grade IV lesions are extremely malignant and generally carry a very poor prognosis.

Table 31.1 Common locations for neuroepithelial tumours

Tumour type	Location
Astrocytoma, glioblastoma	Cerebral hemispheres
Oilgodendroglioma	Cerebral hemispheres
Ependymoma	Ventricular walls
Central neurocytoma	Lateral ventricles
Pilocytic astrocytoma	Hypothalamus, cerebellum
Myxopapillary ependymoma	Conus medullaris, cauda equina
Paraganglioma	Cauda equina
Medulloblastoma	Cerebellum

SCHIZOPHRENIA

Schizophrenia has long been referred to as the 'graveyard of neuropathology'[31] because of the difficulty in identifying any precise neuroanatomical changes that might explain the neuropsychological symptoms of the disorder. Numerous detailed structural studies of the brains of patients with schizophrenia have been carried out, but the results have often been conflicting. This lack of a clear structural basis for schizophrenia has led to it being described as a functional ps§ychosis, with the problem being attributed to faulty neural circuitry. However, there are now some relatively robust findings to suggest that there may be subtle structural changes occurring in certain areas of the brain, and this is a research field that is likely to expand over the coming years.

Macroscopic pathology

The most consistent observation in patients with schizophrenia, based largely on imaging studies, is the presence of ventricular enlargement and reduction in brain volume.[32] At the neuropathological level, this is clearly not useful diagnostically because such changes are seen in a whole range of other disorders. However, the fact that there is some loss of brain substance is supported by the observa-

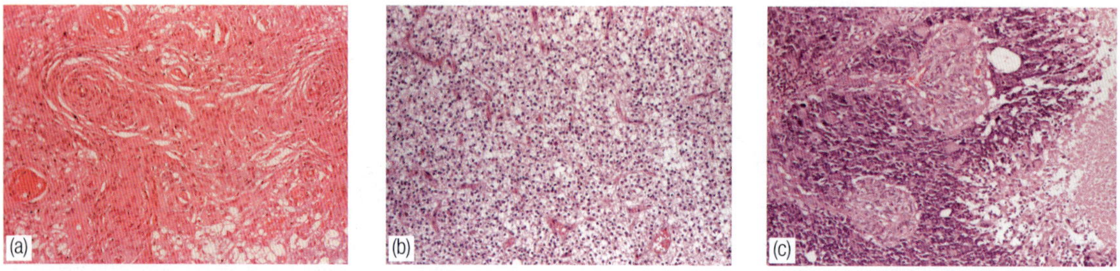

Figure 31.10 Tumours. (a) WHO grade I meningothelial meningioma. (b) WHO grade II oligodenodroglioma. (c) WHO grade IV glioblastoma
Photos courtesy of Dr F Roncardi.

tion that there is a reduction in brain weight of up to 5 per cent.[33] What remains unclear is what component of the tissue is actually being lost (neurons, glia, neuropil, etc.). Other macroscopic changes that have been proposed but that are not widely replicated are a loss of normal brain asymmetry, reduced size of the corpus callosum and disruption of normal gyrification.

Microscopic pathology

At the microscopic level, one of the key debates has been over the role of gliosis. Early studies suggested that periventricular gliosis may be found in 70 per cent of schizophrenia cases,[34] perhaps pointing to an ongoing degenerative process. However, the majority of studies carried out to look at the extent of gliosis do not replicate these findings, and the current consensus is that gliosis is not a feature of the disorder in most cases.[35] In the absence of a clear degenerative process, attention has shifted more towards a developmental aetiology for the disorder and, in particular, the presence of cytoarchitectural abnormalities in certain areas of the brain such as the thalamus, hippocampus and prefrontal cortex. For example, based on reproducible stereological studies, the mediodorsal nucleus of the thalamus appears to be smaller than normal and to contain fewer neurons in schizophrenic patients.[36] In the hippocampus and prefrontal cortex, there appear to be decreases in neuronal size and changes in synaptic proteins. Exactly how these subtle cytoarchitectural changes might give rise to the symptoms of schizophrenia remains unclear and the debate goes on, but the current state of the field, and the key controversies to be resolved, have been expertly reviewed by Harrison.[35]

For more in-depth discussion of the neuropathology underlying all of the disorders mentioned in this chapter, and a lot more that are not, the reader is referred to *Greenfield's Neuropathology*.[37]

KEY POINTS

- All cell types of the CNS may be involved in disease pathology.
- Alzheimer's disease (AD) is characterized by the presence of extracellular Aβ peptide plaques and intracellular neurofibrillary tangles.
- Dementia with Lewy Bodies (DLB) is an α-synucleinopathy.
- The pathology of AD and DLB can coexist in the same patient.
- Fronto-temporal lobar dementias are categorized according to the protein found in the pathological inclusions.
- Creutzfeldt–Jakob disease is a prion disease that may be inherited or acquired.
- Parkinsonism may be caused by different underlying pathologies.
- Parkinson's disease and multiple system atrophy are α-synucleinopathies.
- Progressive supranuclear palsy is a tauopathy.
- Schizophrenia does not have a definitive neuropathology.

REFERENCES

1. Knapp M, Prince M (2007) *Dementia UK: The Full Report*. London: Dementia UK.
2. Mirra SS, Heyman A, McKeel D, *et al.* (1991) The Consortium to Establish a Registry for Alzheimer's Disease (CERAD): part II. Standardization of the neuropathologic assessment of Alzheimer's disease. *Neurology* **41**: 479–86.
3. National Institute on Aging, Reagan Institute Working Group on Diagnostic Criteria for the Neuropathological Assessment of Alzheimer's Disease (1997) Consensus recommendations for the postmortem diagnosis of Alzheimer's disease: National Institute on Aging, and Reagan Institute Working Group on Diagnostic Criteria for the Neuropathological Assessment of Alzheimer's Disease. *Neurobiology of Aging* **18** (suppl.): S1–2.
4. Braak H, Braak E (1991) Neuropathological staging of Alzheimer-related changes. *Acta Neuropathologica* **82**: 239–59.
5. Alafuzoff I, Arzberger T, Al-Sarraj S, *et al.* (2008) Staging of neurofibrillary pathology in Alzheimer's disease: a study of the BrainNet Europe Consortium. *Brain Pathology* **18**: 484–96.
6. Alafuzoff I, Pikkarainen M, Arzberger T, *et al.* (2008) Inter-laboratory comparison of neuropathological assessments of beta-amyloid protein: a study of the BrainNet Europe consortium. *Acta Neuropathologica* **115**: 533–46.
7. McKeith IG, Dickson DW, Lowe J, *et al.* (2005) Diagnosis and management of dementia with Lewy bodies: third report of the DLB Consortium. *Neurology* **65**: 1863–72.
8. Jellinger KA (2009) Significance of brain lesions in Parkinson disease dementia and Lewy body dementia. *Frontiers of Neurology and Neuroscience* **24**: 114–25.
9. Alafuzoff I, Ince PG, Arzberger T, *et al.* (2009) Staging/typing of Lewy body related alpha-synuclein pathology: a study of the BrainNet Europe Consortium. *Acta Neuropathologica* **117**(6): 635–52.
10. Cairns NJ, Bigio EH, Mackenzie IR, *et al.* (2007) Neuropathologic diagnostic and nosologic criteria for frontotemporal lobar degeneration: consensus of the Consortium for Frontotemporal Lobar Degeneration. *Acta Neuropathologica* **114**: 5–22.
11. Neumann M, Sampathu DM, Kwong LK, *et al.* (2006) Ubiquitinated TDP-43 in frontotemporal lobar degeneration and amyotrophic lateral sclerosis. *Science* **314**: 130–33.
12. Baker M, Mackenzie IR, Pickering-Brown SM, *et al.* (2006) Mutations in progranulin cause tau-negative frontotemporal dementia linked to chromosome 17. *Nature* **442**: 916–19.
13. Cruts M, Gijselinck I, van der Zee J, *et al.* (2006) Null mutations in progranulin cause ubiquitin-positive frontotemporal dementia linked to chromosome 17q21. *Nature* **442**: 920–24.

14. Kalaria RN, Kenny RA, Ballard CG, *et al.* (2004) Towards defining the neuropathological substrates of vascular dementia. *Journal of the Neurological Sciences* **226**: 75–80.
15. Hachinski VC, Lassen NA, Marshall J (1974) Multi-infarct dementia: a cause of mental deterioration in the elderly. *Lancet* **2**: 207–10.
16. Tomlinson BE, Blessed G, Roth M (1970) Observations on the brains of demented old people. *Journal of the Neurological Sciences* **11**: 205–42.
17. Mielke R, Herholz K, Grond M, Kessler J, Heiss WE (1992) Severity of vascular dementia is related to volume of metabolically impaired tissue. *Archives of Neurology* **49**: 909–13.
18. Thomas NJ, Morris CM, Scaravilli F, *et al.* (2000) Hereditary vascular dementia linked to notch 3 mutations: CADASIL in British families. *Annals of the New York Academy of Sciences* **903**: 293–8.
19. Levy E, Carman MD, Fernandez-Madrid IJ, *et al.* (1990) Mutation of the Alzheimer's disease amyloid gene in hereditary cerebral hemorrhage, Dutch type. *Science* **248**: 1124–6.
20. Levy E, Lopez-Otin C, Ghiso J, Geltner D, Frangione B (1989) Stroke in Icelandic patients with hereditary amyloid angiopathy is related to a mutation in the cystatin C gene, an inhibitor of cysteine proteases. *Journal of Experimental Medicine* **169**: 1771–8.
21. Haltia M, Ghiso J, Prelli F, *et al.* (1990) Amyloid in familial amyloidosis, Finnish type, is antigenically and structurally related to gelsolin. *American Journal of Pathology* **136**: 1223–8.
22. Prusiner SB (1998) Prions. *Proceedings of the National Academy of Sciences, USA* **95**: 13363–83.
23. Will RG, Zeidler M, Stewart GE, *et al.* (2000) Diagnosis of new variant Creutzfeldt-Jakob disease. *Annals of Neurology* **47**: 575–82.
24. Corsellis JA, Bruton CJ, Freeman-Browne D (1973) The aftermath of boxing. *Psychological Medicine* **3**: 270–303.
25. McIntosh AS, McCrory P, Comerford J (2000) The dynamics of concussive head impacts in rugby and Australian rules football. *Medicine and Science in Sports and Exercise* **32**: 1980–84.
26. Roberts GW, Allsop D, Bruton C (1990) The occult aftermath of boxing. *Journal of Neurology, Neurosurgery, and Psychiatry* **53**: 373–8.
27. Roberts GW, Gentleman SM, Lynch A, *et al.* (1994) Beta amyloid protein deposition in the brain after severe head injury: implications for the pathogenesis of Alzheimer's disease. *Journal of Neurology, Neurosurgery, and Psychiatry* **57**: 419–25.
28. Griffin WS, Sheng JG, Royston MC, *et al.* (1998) Glial-neuronal interactions in Alzheimer's disease: the potential role of a 'cytokine cycle' in disease progression. *Brain Pathology* **8**: 65–72.
29. Rosen DR, Siddique T, Patterson D, *et al.* (1993) Mutations in Cu/Zn superoxide dismutase gene are associated with familial amyotrophic lateral sclerosis. *Nature* **362**: 59–62.
30. Louis DN, World Health Organization, International Agency for Research on Cancer (2007) *WHO Classification of Tumours of the Central Nervous System*. Lyon: IARC.
31. Plum F (1972) Prospects for research on schizophrenia: 3. Neurophysiology: neuropathological findings. *Neuroscience Research Program Bulletin* **10**: 384–8.
32. Lawrie SM, Abukmeil SS (1998) Brain abnormality in schizophrenia: a systematic and quantitative review of volumetric magnetic resonance imaging studies. *British Journal of Psychiatry* **172**: 110–20.
33. Bruton CJ, Crow TJ, Frith CD, *et al.* (1990) Schizophrenia and the brain: a prospective clinico-neuropathological study. *Psychological Medicine* **20**: 285–304.
34. Stevens JR (1982) Neuropathology of schizophrenia. *Archives of General Psychiatry* **39**: 1131–9.
35. Harrison PJ (2004) Schizophrenia and dementia. In MM Esiri, V M-Y Lee, JQ Trojanowski (eds) *The Neuropathology of Dementia*, 2nd edn. Cambridge: Cambridge University Press.
36. Pakkenberg B (1990) Pronounced reduction of total neuron number in mediodorsal thalamic nucleus and nucleus accumbens in schizophrenics. *Archives of General Psychiatry* **47**: 1023–8.
37. Love S, Louis DN, Ellison DW (2008) *Greenfield's Neuropathology*, 8th edn. London: Hodder Arnold.

Chapter 32

Neuroimaging

Basant K Puri

INTRODUCTION

In this chapter, an introductory account is given of some of the main features of computed tomography (CT), magnetic resonance imaging (MRI), blood oxygen level-dependent functional magnetic resonance imaging (BOLD fMRI), magnetic resonance spectroscopy (MRS), fluid-attenuated inversion recovery (FLAIR), diffusion tensor imaging (DTI) tractography, arterial spin labelling (ASL), single-photon-emission computed tomography (SPECT) and positron-emission tomography (PET), with an emphasis on their applications in modern psychiatry. The temptation to include mathematical equations has largely been resisted. Detailed aspects of the physics involved have been omitted, as have details of different magnetic resonance (MR) sequences, echo-planar imaging and the workings of the PET cyclotron. For readers interested in these details, a selection of suitable further reading is given at the end of the chapter.

COMPUTED TOMOGRAPHY

X-ray CT, previously known as computed axial tomography (CAT), is a digital form of structural neuroimaging that utilizes X-ray attenuation married to a tomographic technique that separates out axial or transverse images. It was developed in the UK by Sir Godfrey Hounsfield.[1,2] The basic design of a CT scanner is shown in Figure 32.1.

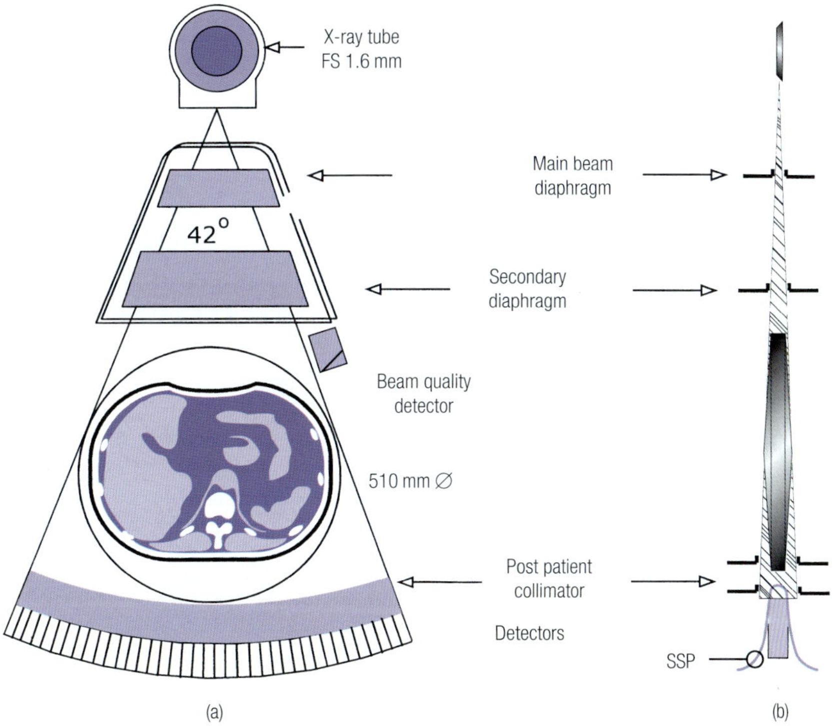

Figure 32.1 (a) Basic computed tomography (CT) design, showing an X-ray source collimated to a fan beam rotating around the patient's abdomen. The X-ray tube and detectors are fixed together as a single rotating unit. (b) The fan beam assembly, showing collimator and detector geometry. The slice has a greater thickness in the middle, and post-patient collimation defines the slice sensitivity profile

Reproduced from Dowsett *et al. The Physics of Diagnostic Imaging*, 2nd edn. Hodder, London. (2006).

After being scanned, the part of the body of interest is stored in a format digitally divided into voxels, which are cuboids. On any two-dimensional planar display, two-dimensional pixels are shown, as illustrated in Figure 32.2.

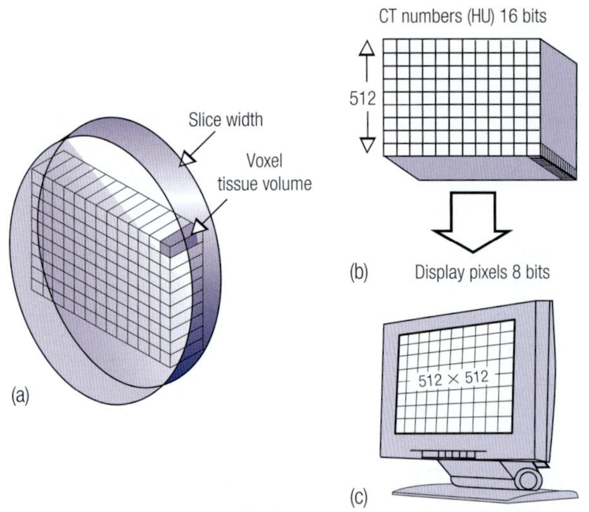

Figure 32.2 (a) The body slice represented as a digital matrix stored as computed tomography (CT) numbers. Each small tissue volume resolved by the matrix is a voxel, or volume element. (b) The voxel information is stored in memory by typically a 512 × 512 matrix. (c) The windowed display pixel is stored as a 512 × 512 matrix, which can be 4–8 bits deep

Reproduced from Dowsett *et al. The Physics of Diagnostic Imaging*, 2nd edn. Hodder, London. (2006).

From the viewpoint of psychiatric research and clinical practice, CT had the considerable advantage over plain X-ray radiography of allowing ready visualization of the ventricular system of the brain; the brain, including its ventricles, is almost radiotranslucent. Before the advent of CT, the ventricular system was visualized using pneumoencephalography, a procedure involving the replacement of some cerebrospinal fluid (CSF) with air; this is a cumbersome invasive procedure associated with several side effects, not least of which is the occurrence of headaches when the subject sits up (to allow the air to rise to the head). Soon after the introduction of CT, this non-invasive neuroimaging technique was used to study the relative size of the ventricular system in patients with schizophrenia. The first group to publish a major CT study in this area was that of Eve Johnstone, Timothy Crow, Christopher Frith and colleagues. They reported that, compared with age-matched controls, 17 patients with chronic schizophrenia had enlarged lateral ventricles, ascertained using CT; furthermore, increased ventricular size was highly related to indices of cognitive impairment.[3]

In general, given that MRI does not involve any ionizing radiation and permits high-resolution structural imaging, which is usually non-invasive (as contrast agents are not usually required), where available, MRI is taking over from CT in clinical psychiatric practice unless there is a contraindication for the use of MRI in a particular patient (see below). MRI is also now usually the structural neuroimaging modality of choice for research in psychiatry.

There is still controversy in the area of acute stroke imaging (in which the use of an intravenous contrast agent is usually needed for the MRI scanning) as to which of CT and MRI is better. The two are compared in Table 32.1.[4]

MAGNETIC RESONANCE IMAGING

Basic physics

Within a strong external magnetic field, B_0, there is a tendency for hydrogen protons, which possess the quantum property of spin and behave like magnetic dipoles, to line up with the external magnetic field, as depicted in Figure 32.3; a majority of these protons point in the same direction

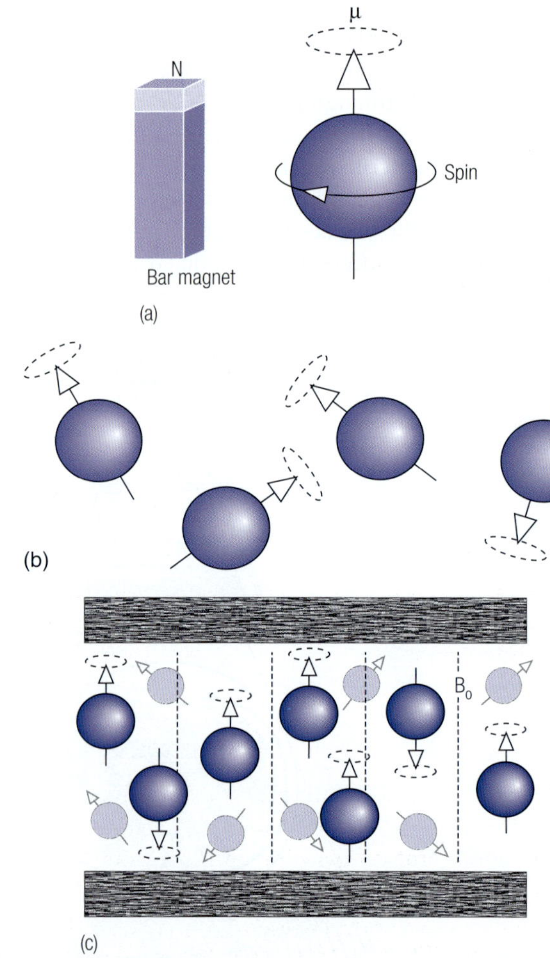

Figure 32.3 (a) The hydrogen proton compared with a bar magnetic, showing the proton spin creating a magnetic dipole μ, analogous to the magnetic pole of a bar magnet. (b) A group of three protons, showing various orientations of their axes in free space. (c) The proton axes are aligned in a strong external magnetic field, B_0. A smaller proportion take up the opposing direction

Reproduced from Dowsett *et al. The Physics of Diagnostic Imaging*, 2nd edn. Hodder, London. (2006).

Table 32.1 Comparison of computed tomography (CT) and magnetic resonance imaging (MRI) in acute stroke imaging

	CT	MRI
Availability	Widely available	Limited availability in most centres (especially for emergency use)
Scan duration	Short	Potentially longer
Cost	Low (standard non-contrast); high (CTA/CTP)	Very high
Radiation	Yes	No
Contrast type	Requires iodinated contrast for CT angiogram and perfusion	Gadolinium is water-soluble (risk of nephrogenic systemic fibrosis with renal insufficiency)
Sensitivity to early ischaemia	Poor	High
Posterior fossa visualization	Poor (bony artefact)	Good
Brain coverage (CT perfusion)	Limited	Whole brain
Contraindications	Renal insufficiency (iodinated contrast)	Severe renal insufficiency (gadolinium-based contrast); ferromagnetic material, e.g. pacemaker, aneurysm clips; claustrophobia; medical instability

CTA, computed tomography angiography; CTP, computed tomography perfusion.
After Hsia.[4]

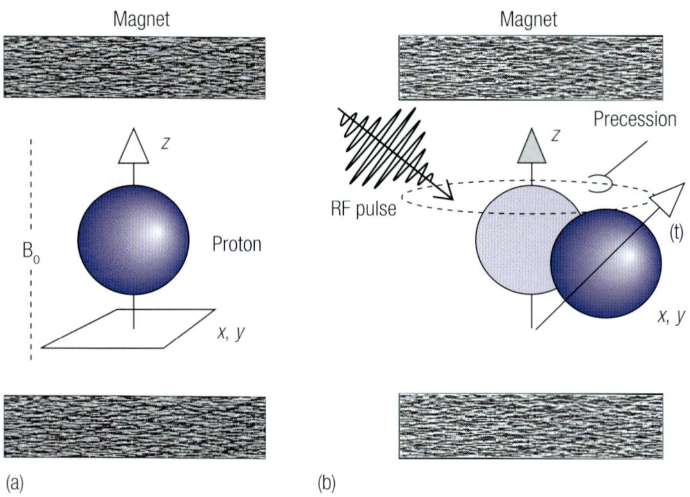

Figure 32.4 (a) The proton in a magnetic field aligned with the longitudinal *z*-axis; the transverse plane is the *x,y* plane. There are zero components in *x* and *y*. (b) A radiofrequency (RF) pulse displaces the proton axis, so that the *x* and *y* components are now both positive

Reproduced from Dowsett *et al. The Physics of Diagnostic Imaging*, 2nd edn. Hodder, London. (2006).

as the field, but a minority of the protons that line up are in the diametrically opposite direction. For simplicity, considering only those protons that line up in the same direction as the external magnetic field (i.e. those that are 'parallel' to the magnetic flux), when such protons are subjected to a radiofrequency (RF) pulse they are displaced (Figure 32.4). This can be thought of as being rather like the precession that a top or gyroscope undergoes when subjected to a small tangential force while spinning and being under the influence of an external gravitational field (Figure 32.5). Recovery from the recession gives rise to the nuclear magnetic resonance (NMR) signal, as shown in Figures 32.6 and

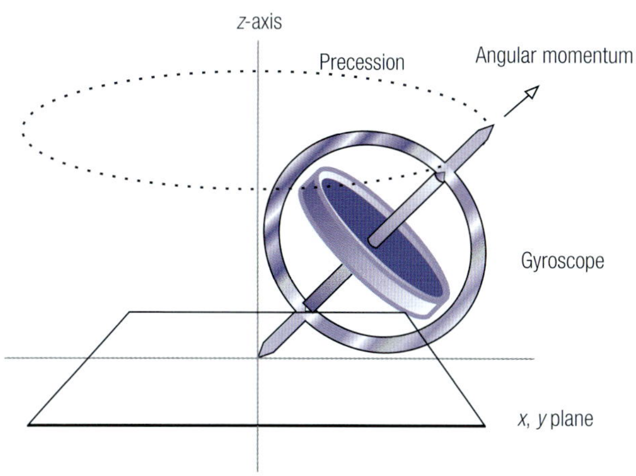

Figure 32.5 A disturbed spinning gyroscope, showing an off-centre wobble or precession and representing a very simple model of precession of a proton subjected to a radiofrequency (RF) pulse

Reproduced from Dowsett *et al. The Physics of Diagnostic Imaging*, 2nd edn. Hodder, London. (2006).

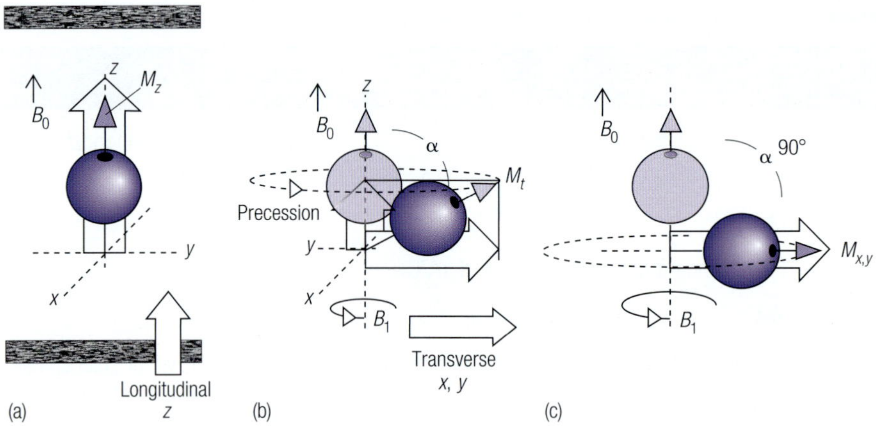

Figure 32.6 (a) The proton in an external magnetic field, B_0. The total proton contribution is represented by the vector M_z at equilibrium in the z-plane. Here, the z-component takes its maximum value and both the x and y components are zero. (b) A radiofrequency (RF) pulse creates the opposing field B_1, which displaces M by an angle α. The x and y components have now grown. (c) A sufficiently large RF pulse displaces M into the x,y plane (z-component is 0; the x and y components are maximum). Longitudinal recovery now takes place

Reproduced from Dowsett *et al. The Physics of Diagnostic Imaging*, 2nd edn. Hodder, London. (2006).

32.7; definitions of parameters used in these figures are given in Table 32.2.

For a given nucleus type (e.g. hydrogen proton), the angular frequency of precession of the nucleus is directly proportional to the external magnetic field strength (flux density), B_0, which is therefore the value of the main magnetic field strength of the MR scanner. The constant of proportionality is known as the gyromagnetic ratio and is denoted by γ. (The gyromagnetic ratio is calculated by dividing the value of the magnetic moment (μ in Figure 32.3) by the product of 2π and the modulus of the spin angular momentum of the nucleus.) Thus, the angular frequency of precession is given by γB_0; this frequency is the Larmor frequency, ω_L, and the equation $\omega_L = \gamma B_0$ is the Larmor equation. The unit of the magnetic field strength is the tesla, abbreviated to T in Système International d'Unités (SI units). (Note that, in MR papers and commercial MRI scanner literature, 'tesla' is often incorrectly rendered 'Tesla'.) Typical values of B_0 for MRI scanners in clinical use at the time of writing vary in value between 0.5 T and 3 T, while some scanners used for human or rodent in vivo research may have field strengths as high as 7 T or 9 T. MRI scanners used for studying tissue samples and inanimate objects tend currently to have a field strength of over 11 T; patients are not directly scanned using such scanners, and the instruments tend to be called NMR scanners. Note that MRI used to be referred to as NMR; one reason for the change in terminology was the concern that patients might be perturbed by the word 'nuclear' – in fact, MRI or NMR scanning does not use any ionizing radiation.

Further details of the physics of MRI are beyond the scope of this book; good accounts are given in some of the books mentioned under further reading at the end of this chapter.

Table 32.2 Definition of parameters relating to the origin of the nuclear magnetic resonance (NMR) signal

Symbol	Definition
B_0	Static magnetic field
z	Longitudinal plane
x,y	Transverse plane
M	Sum magnetization vector
M_z	Proportion of M in z (longitudinal magnetization)
M_{xy}	Proportion of M in x,y (transverse magnetization)
$M(t)$	M at time t after the RF pulse; magnitude $\propto$ spin density

RF, radiofrequency.

Reproduced from Dowsett DJ, Kenny PA, Johnston RE (2006) *The Physics of Diagnostic Imaging*, 2nd edn. London: Hodder Arnold.

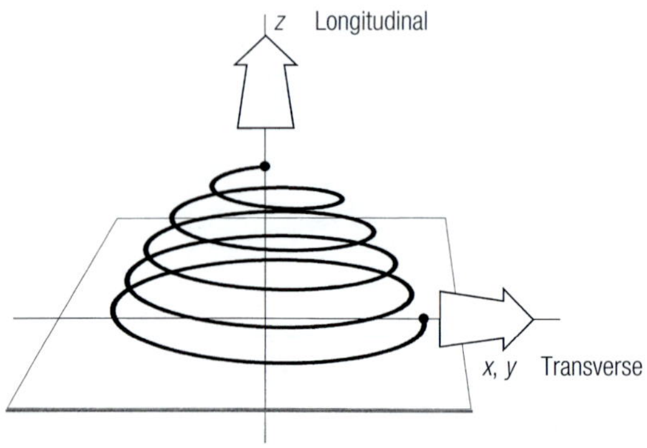

Figure 32.7 The magnetic vector tracing out a spiral path as it regains equilibrium with the z-plane

Reproduced from Dowsett *et al. The Physics of Diagnostic Imaging*, 2nd edn. Hodder, London. (2006).

T1- and T2-weighted imaging

T1 is the longitudinal time constant and indexes the rate at which the longitudinal magnetization, M_z, returns to its maximum value following an RF pulse, as shown in Figure 32.8. (It is measured when M_z reaches approximately 63 per cent of its maximum value after a 90° RF pulse brings it to zero. This is because $M_z = 1 - e^{-t/\mathrm{T1}}$, and setting $t = \mathrm{T1}$ gives $M_z = 1 - e^{-1}$, which is 0.632 to three decimal places.) The value of T1 varies with the magnetic field strength, as shown in Figure 32.9. At a given field strength, the T1 is longer for CSF than for grey matter, and in turn longer for grey matter than for white matter. It is particularly short for fat. (With its higher concentration of myelinated sheaths, white matter clearly has a higher density of fat than does grey matter.)

T2 is the transverse time constant and indexes the rate at which the transverse magnetization, M_{xy}, decays to its minimum value of zero following an RF pulse. (It is measured when M_{xy} decays to approximately 37 per cent of its maximum value because we can take $M_{xy} = e^{-t/\mathrm{T2}}$, and setting $t = \mathrm{T2}$ gives $M_z = e^{-1}$, which is 0.368 to three decimal places.)

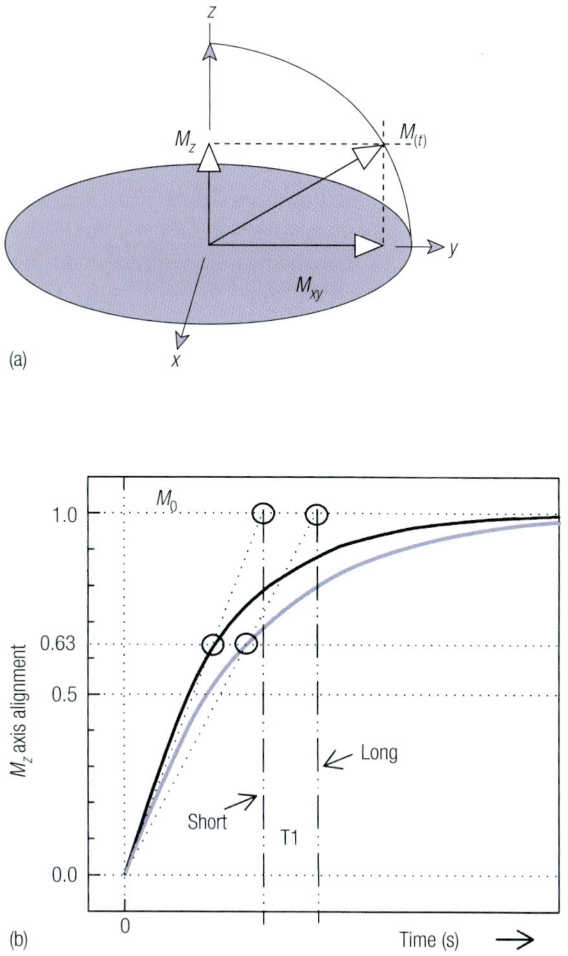

Figure 32.8 (a) Vector diagram identifying the proportion of M_z and M_{xy} in the proton magnetic vector M at time t. (b) M traces out an exponential decay curve as it regains equilibrium (achieved when $M_z = 1$). The value of T1 is measured at approximately 63 per cent recovery (see text). Both short and long T1 examples are shown

Reproduced from Dowsett *et al. The Physics of Diagnostic Imaging*, 2nd edn. Hodder, London. (2006).

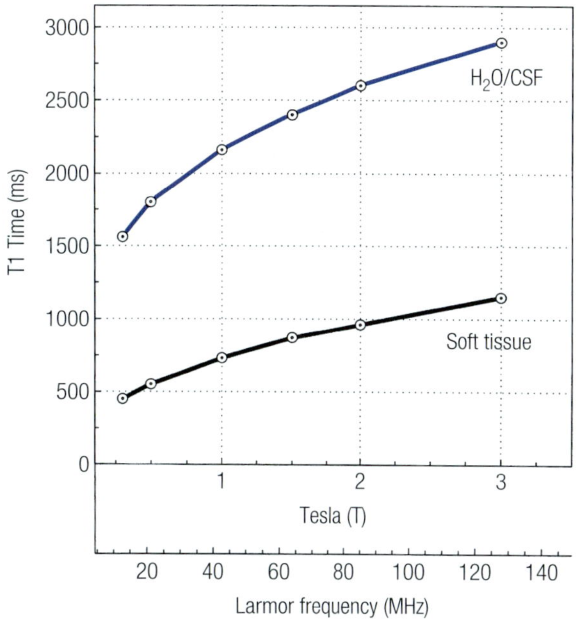

Figure 32.9 Variation of T1 (in milliseconds, ms) with magnetic field strength (in teslas, T) for liquid (water, cerebrospinal fluid) and soft tissue; grey matter and white matter in the brain have intermediate values

Reproduced from Dowsett *et al. The Physics of Diagnostic Imaging*, 2nd edn. Hodder, London. (2006).

In MRI scans of the brain, if scanning sequence parameters are chosen selectively to emphasize T1 characteristics (T1-weighted scans), white matter has a higher signal intensity (i.e. it appears 'whiter') than grey matter, which in turn has a higher signal intensity than CSF. In a T2-weighted MRI scan, CSF has a higher signal intensity than grey matter or white matter; such scans are also good for imaging cerebral oedema (which also has a high signal intensity). These differences are shown in Figure 32.10, which also shows how an intravenous contrast agent (in this case, based on gadolinium) may helpfully enhance the imaging of some cerebral tumours.

Receiver coils

The NMR signal is detected using a receiver or detector coil, usually specifically designed for the part of the body being investigated. Special coils are becoming available that allow parallel imaging to be carried out. These involve multiple imaging coils that record imaging data simultaneously using techniques such as sensitivity encoding for MRI (SENSE) and simultaneous acquisition of spatial harmonics (SMASH) so that the image acquisition time is shortened. There are also advantages from parallel imaging in terms of reducing certain types of MRI artefacts.

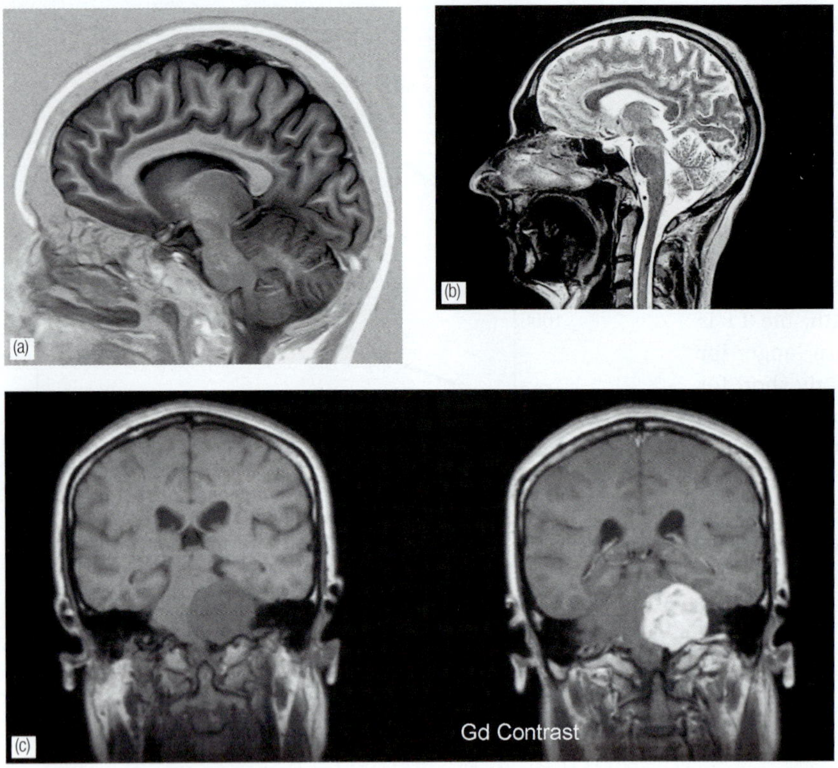

Figure 32.10 (a) Sagittal T1-weighted magnetic resonance imaging (MRI) scan of the brain. (b) Sagittal T2-weighted MRI scan of the brain. (c) A positive contrast agent (gadolinium–diethylenetriamine penta-acetic acid, Gd-DTPA) emphasizes the cerebral neoplasm by increasing the T1 effect

Reproduced from Dowsett *et al. The Physics of Diagnostic Imaging*, 2nd edn. Hodder, London. (2006).

Safety

The magnetic field strengths typically used during in vivo human scanning are very high compared with the strength of the earth's magnetic field. For example, while the strength of the latter, at the surface of the earth, is around 30–60 μT, a field strength of 3 T inside the bore of a modern 3-T MRI scanner is 50 000–100 000 times stronger. The strength of the magnetic field falls off with increasing distance from the main MRI magnet. Special magnetic shielding is also placed around the scanner. A warning contour, usually in yellow and black, is fixed to the floor around the scanner at the distance corresponding to a field strength of 500 μT. This corresponds to a field strength of 5 G using the previous unit of magnetic field strength (flux density) of the gauss (1 gauss (or 1 G) is one ten-thousandth of a tesla; i.e. 1 T = 10 000 G). Therefore, this contour is often still referred to as being the '5-gauss line'. It can be very dangerous to bring freely mobile ferromagnetic materials within the 5-gauss line. Even a small piece of metal such as a paperclip or a pen containing ferromagnetic components can turn into an extremely dangerous, and potentially even lethal, object if it is brought within this contour: there is a strong attraction to the bore of the magnet and such an object can fly into this part of the scanner, all the time accelerating while approaching the scanner, so that its momentum increases correspondingly. If a person happens to be lying in the scanner at the time, this can clearly be very dangerous. For similar reasons, in the event of a suspected cardiac arrest or other such emergency, it is important not to allow the ordinary hospital crash team into the scanning area within the 5-gauss area (their stethoscopes, pins for neurological examinations, etc. can turn into potentially lethal missiles) but instead to ensure that medical staff present during the MR scanning are properly trained to carry out emergency resuscitation in the MRI environment. The magnetic field from the scanner may also interfere with certain types of equipment that are nearby. For instance, older cathode ray tube monitors may show images that are permanently displaced, hospital equipment may not function properly, and mobile telephones (if their use is permitted in the area) may fail to receive a normal signal. Weaker contours (e.g. the 2.5-gauss line) also extend right around the scanner, at a greater distance from the main scanner magnet than the 5-gauss line, and so may extend beyond a wall at the back of the scanner; this may have implications for any equipment being operated on the other side of that wall.

In terms of the safety of individuals being considered for scanning, there are several aspects to bear in mind. The imaging safety checklist that I routinely use before scanning anyone checks for the presence of the following:

- Cardiac pacemaker
- Mechanical heart valve
- History of foreign body in the eye
- Occupation as a metal worker, grinder or welder
- Metallic implant, metal prosthesis, orthopaedic plates or screws
- Shrapnel
- Aneurysm clip/haemostatic clip
- Ear implant
- Artificial eye

- Coloured contact lens
- Interventional radiological device
- Pregnancy
- Intrauterine contraceptive device (IUCD)
- Implantable pump or neurostimulator
- Allergies (if the subject is to receive a contrast agent)
- A watch
- Any jewellery
- Anything in the patient's pockets (e.g. keys).

The presence of an artificial cardiac pacemaker is an absolute contraindication; failure of the pacemaker inside the scanner could clearly be fatal. Any person who has had a history of one or more small pieces of metal entering the eye (e.g. while carrying out metal grinding) should not be allowed near a scanner unless they have had orbital X-rays taken and cleared by a radiologist; just one small sliver of metal could tear through the cornea and the rest of the eye while the subject is inside the scanner. The presence of a metallic implant might not necessarily be an absolute contraindication, depending on factors such as the location of the implant and the field strength of the scanner; there is a danger not only of displacement but also of the metal heating during the scanning session. Indeed, MRI scanning does impart energy to the patient being scanned, and so during scanning it is important to monitor and regularly record the value of the specific absorption rate (SAR); one should also monitor the scanner room temperature and how uncomfortable the subject may be feeling. The presence of an aneurysm clip or haemostatic clip is an absolute contraindication; displacement of such a clip could be very dangerous and potentially fatal. A coloured contact lens might be dangerous, as some make use of metallic pigments. At the time of writing, MRI is not routinely permitted during pregnancy in many countries without strict permission of the local research ethics committee (indeed, there are some MRI studies specifically of pregnant women). If a female subject is using an IUCD (a 'coil'), the make of the IUCD should be checked carefully in advance; if the IUCD is not MRI-compatible, then the scanning session might cause the IUCD to be dislodged, potentially leading to failure of contraceptive cover. It is good practice to ask the patient to change into hospital pyjamas before being allowed into the scanner. Any underwear that contains metal should be removed first. For instance, ordinary bras that have metal fasteners should not be worn, while sports bras without such metal fasteners are usually safe. If the patient insists on wearing their own clothes, these should be checked carefully for the presence of any metal components, such as fasteners, zips, metal buttons, metal fasteners and sequins. The pockets of the clothing, even hospital pyjamas, should be checked for a final time before the patient enters the scanner area; under no circumstances should keys and other such objects be allowed into the scanner room.

Claustrophobic feelings inside the scanner are a relative contraindication. Some patients are able to go ahead after verbal reassurance. Others can do so if a second person (who should also be carefully metal-checked first) is present; this second person might sit by the subject (on a non-metallic chair) and perhaps hold gently on to a covered part of one of the subject's lower limbs during the scan.

It is important to ensure that leads (e.g. from headphones, a patient alarm and the scanner coil) do not make loops on the subject's body while they are lying in the scanner, as these could cause burns. For a similar reason (related to the need to prevent local electrical circuits from forming within the strong magnetic field), the patient should be asked not to allow bare parts of their body (e.g. the hands and lower arms) to touch each other and not to cross their arms or legs while being scanned. Particularly at field strengths of 3 T and above, care should be exercised with subjects who have tattoos present, and metal-based make-up should be removed completely before entering the scanner room. It is always worth carrying out one final check before the patient enters the scanner room: they may have picked up a pen and put it in a pocket, or they may have forgotten to remove a hairclip.

Advanced structural imaging

Structural MR neuroimaging can be used to carry out ventricular segmentation and thereby measure the volume of the ventricles of the brain. The cerebral tissue itself can be segmented into grey matter and white matter. The cortex can be analysed for features such as its degree of folding.

Voxel-based morphometry (VBM) is based on the distribution of grey matter in the brain and, in a group, may reveal areas of grey matter loss.[5]

It has been found that image registration is of particular use, both in terms of research and from a clinical perspective. This technique allows subtle changes in brain structure to be picked up and quantified between consecutive scans from the same patient; these scans may be several months or even years apart. This is helpful, for instance, in following the response of cerebral tumours to chemotherapy or radiotherapy. Image registration can also be used to compare groups, as shown in Figure 32.11. Here, analysis of the

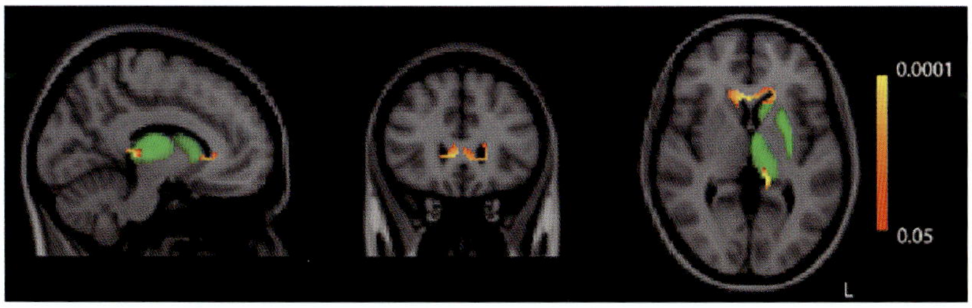

Figure 32.11 Image-registration techniques were applied to structural magnetic resonance imaging (MRI) scans in a Huntington's disease clinical trial. Voxel-wise local analyses of ethyl-eicosapentaenoic acid treatment versus placebo over 12 months showed significant changes at the head of the caudate nucleus and the posterior thalamus (shown in green along with the putamen; red–yellow colour bar shows the *P*-value under the null hypothesis of no change)

Reproduced from ref. 12.

MRI scans from patients with Huntington's disease taking part in a randomized, double-blind, placebo-controlled trial of a new intervention showed that, compared with the placebo, the active treatment was associated with significant group-level reductions in brain atrophy in the head of the caudate nucleus and the posterior thalamus.[6] These findings showed that the active treatment was associated with significant reduction in brain atrophy, particularly in the caudate and thalamus.

BLOOD OXYGEN LEVEL-DEPENDENT FUNCTIONAL MAGNETIC RESONANCE IMAGING

In 1991, Bruce Rosen's group at Harvard Medical School published the first quantitative determination of human brain activation using MRI. This fMRI study used the measurement of cerebral haemodynamics, following the injection of the MRI contrast agent gadolinium–diethylenetriamine penta-acetic acid (Gd-DTPA). During photic stimulation, localized increases in blood volume were detected in V1 in a study involving seven subjects.[7]

The following year, the same group published a non-invasive fMRI study that did not involve injections of a contrast agent.[8] Instead, the study relied on the BOLD effect. BOLD depends on the fact, that in contrast to oxyhaemoglobin (which is diamagnetic), deoxyhaemoglobin (which is paramagnetic, having unpaired electrons) may be used as an endogenous contrast agent. In theory, the greater the activation of a part of the brain, the greater is its use of oxygen. This in turn leads to a greater concentration of deoxyhaemoglobin. Hence, greater activation is associated with greater signal intensity in BOLD fMRI. In this first human study, V1 was again shown to be activated during photic stimulation in seven volunteers, while M1 was found to be activated during repetitive contralateral hand-squeezing; these results are shown in Figures 32.12–14 from the original paper by Kwong and colleagues.[8]

BOLD fMRI rapidly established itself as a standard non-invasive functional neuroimaging technique, which is now in widespread use. The detailed physics and methodology are beyond the scope of this book, but for those who are interested further good accounts are to be found in some of the texts recommended for further reading.

MAGNETIC RESONANCE SPECTROSCOPY

The above description of the physics of MRI confined itself to a consideration of hydrogen protons. There are other nuclei that also interact with the strong magnetic field of an MRI scanner. Some of these are shown in Table 32.3; it can be seen that they include the 13-carbon and 31-phosphorus isotopes. It can also be seen from Table 32.3 that the value of the gyromagnetic ratio, γ (vide supra), differs between the different nuclei.

The basic principles of MRS have been summarized by the author:[9]

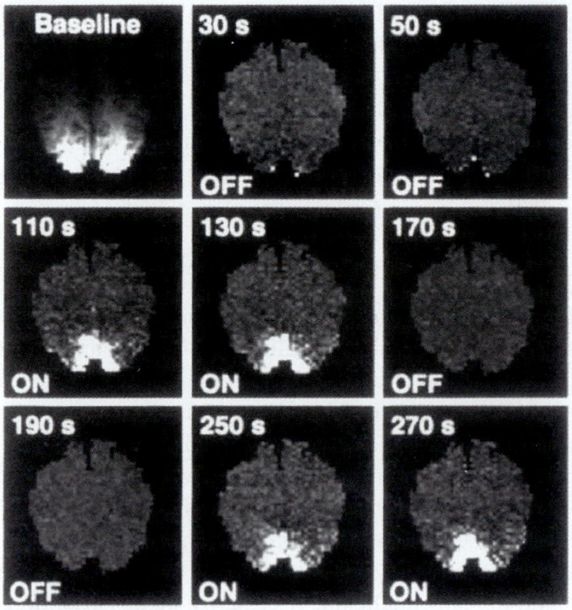

Figure 32.12 The first published human study of V1 activation during photic stimulation using blood oxygen level-dependent functional magnetic resonance imaging (BOLD fMRI). Images are obliquely aligned along the calcarine fissures, with the occipital pole at the bottom. Images were acquired at 3.5-s intervals. The upper left image was acquired during darkness (baseline). This baseline image was subtracted from subsequent images. Eight of these subtraction images are displayed, chosen when the image intensities (see Figure 32.15) reached a steady-state signal level, during darkness (OFF) and during photic stimulation at 8 Hz (ON). During stimulation, local increases in signal intensity were detected in V1.

Reproduced from ref. 8.

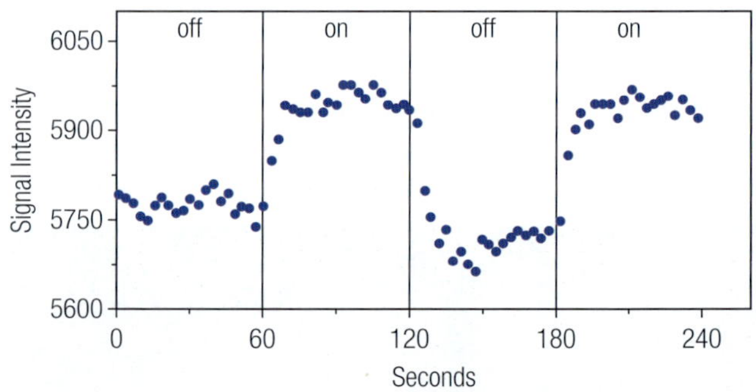

Figure 32.13 Signal intensity changes for a region of interest within the visual cortex during the experiment shown in Figure 32.14

Reproduced from ref. 8.

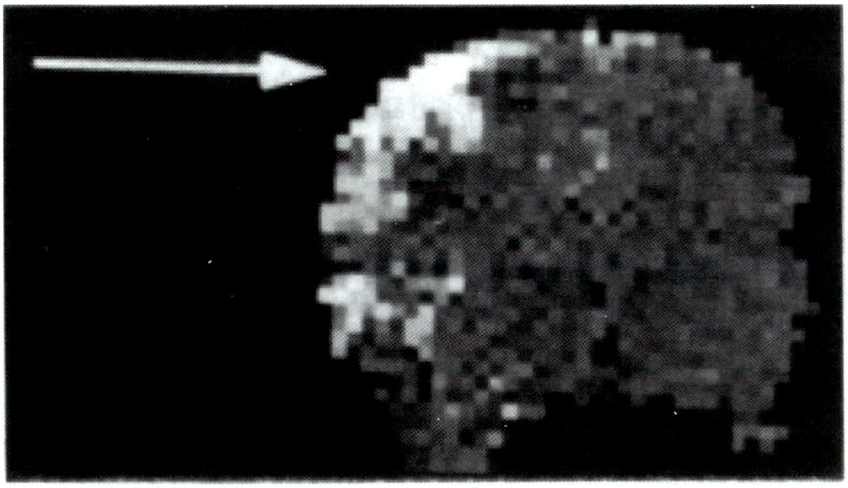

Figure 32.14 The first published human study of M1 activation (during repetitive contralateral hand squeezing) using blood oxygen level-dependent functional magnetic resonance imaging (BOLD fMRI). (a) Coronal subtraction image (stimulated minus unstimulated), showing M1 activation (arrow). (b) Temporal response

Reproduced from ref. 8.

Spectroscopy revolutionized the study of organic chemistry and biochemistry during the last century. While X-ray crystallography, mass spectrometry and infrared spectroscopy cannot be used non-invasively in the study of fatty acid metabolism in adult human brains, fortunately nuclear magnetic resonance spectroscopy can be so used. In the context of human in vivo studies, nuclear magnetic resonance spectroscopy is more commonly referred to as magnetic resonance spectroscopy, partly to avoid the potentially pejorative and upsetting word 'nuclear' when talking to human volunteers and patients, and partly because the technique involves the use of the same magnetic resonance imaging scanners as are employed to carry out structural magnetic resonance imaging.

The technique requires a strong magnetic field, preferably at least 1.5 T when applied to the adult human brain. Certain atomic nuclei in the brain interact with this strong static magnetic field. These include protons and the 13-carbon and 31-phosphorus isotopes. In lay terms, each of these nuclei can be considered to possess more than one possible energy level in the magnetic field. Upon exposure of the brain to a short pulse of radiofrequency energy in a magnetic resonance scanner, some of these nuclei absorb the radiofrequency energy and enter a higher quantum energy state. Recovery of the previous, lower, quantum energy state is associated with the reverse process of the release of energy. The latter is measured as an amplified signal by the head coil receiver.

With all such measurements, there is the phenomenon of 'noise'. For example, when a normal radio receiver is not tuned correctly to a radio station, then one hears a lot of static – noise. (Actually, some of this noise may derive from electromagnetic radiation which had its origin in the big bang.) Then, as one tunes in to a correct station frequency (a resonance frequency), the signal-to-noise ratio becomes high enough to allow the station to be heard clearly. The individual nuclei also

Table 32.3 Useful nuclei in nuclear magnetic resonance (NMR)

Isotope	Natural abundance (%)	γ (MHz)	Signal intensity
^{1}H (proton)	99.98	42.58	1.0000
^{19}F	100	40.05	0.8300
^{23}Na	100	11.26	0.0930
^{31}P	100	17.24	0.0660
^{17}O	0.037	5.77	0.0290
^{13}C	1.11	10.71	0.0160
^{35}Cl	75.5	4.17	0.0084
^{15}N	0.37	4.30	0.0010
^{39}K	93.1	1.99	0.0005

Reproduced from Dowsett DJ, Kenny PA, Johnston RE (2006) *The Physics of Diagnostic Imaging*, 2nd edn. London: Hodder Arnold.

have particular resonance frequencies. In order to improve the signal-to-noise ratio, multiple readings are taken. Since the noise is assumed to be random, successive additions of the readings lead to relative enhancement of the true signals against a diminishing background of noise signals which tend to cancel each other out. Furthermore, in a given molecule, all the protons do not usually resonate at the same frequency, and all the 31-phosphorus nuclei do not usually resonate at another single frequency (different from that for the protons). This is because the resonance frequencies for given nuclei are partly determined by the electron structure of the molecule. (In classical electromagnetic physics, one can consider that the motion of these charged electrons in a magnetic field gives rise to an electric current which in turn gives rise to an associated and opposing magnetic field, in accordance with Maxwell's equations; this causes varying levels of shielding of the nuclei from the applied external magnetic field.) The difference between the resonance frequencies of a given nucleus and of a reference nucleus is calculated and the chemical shift of the given nucleus is then defined in terms of the ratio of this difference to the resonance frequency of the reference nucleus. The chemical shift is usually expressed in parts per million (ppm). The signals from the brain are plotted as peaks against the chemical shift, the latter constituting the abscissa of the graph. The area under each peak is directly proportional to the concentration of the corresponding nucleus in the sample (for instance, a brain voxel) under study. Moreover, the shape of the peak(s) yields information about the electrochemical environment of the nucleus in the molecule. Further details of this technique are beyond the scope of this chapter but may be found in the paper by Cox and Puri.[10]

The chemical shift (conventionally denoted as δ) between water and lipid is illustrated in Figure 32.15.

Figure 32.16a shows a normal brain proton MR spectrum. Since water is by far the most abundantly occurring substance containing free hydrogen protons in the brain, the peak corresponding to water is much larger than that from other substances. Therefore, while acquiring proton MRS (^{1}H MRS) data, it is usually necessary to suppress this water peak, using a suitable spectroscopy sequence. Of the remaining peaks, that corresponding to *N*-acetyl-aspartate (NAA) is particularly prominent and may be thought of as being a neuronal marker. In Figure 32.16c, it can be seen that the NAA peak is reduced in area in a glioblastoma, as a result of there being fewer normally functioning neurons in the tumour. Choline (Cho), among other functions, acts as a polar head group in phospholipid molecules. Lactate is not normally seen in the human brain (apart from in some prematurely born infants), but it may become present during anaerobic respiration (Figure 32.16c). Proton MRS carried out at a stronger magnetic field (≥ 3 T) allows other peaks to be identified and is therefore more informative.

Figure 32.17a shows a spectrum from a 31-phosphorus MRS (^{31}P MRS) study of the brain in schizophrenia.[11] The peak labelled PME (phosphomonoesters) corresponds to the phosphoethanolamine and phosphocholine peaks and indexes membrane phospholipid anabolism, while the peak labelled PDE (phosphodiesters) corresponds to the glycerol 3-phosphoethanolamine and glycerol 3-phosphocholine peaks and indexes phospholipid catabolism. Other peaks shown in Figure 32.17a are inorganic phosphate (Pi), phosphocreatine (PCr) and γ, α and β nucleotide triphosphate (NTP). βNTP indexes adenosine triphosphate (ATP). (The majority of adenosine diphosphate (ADP) is 31-phosphorus NMR-invisible, although the γNTP signal overlaps with signals from βADP.) The broad component from the 31-phosphorus neurospectroscopy study shown in Figure 32.17b indexes brain cell motion-restricted membrane phospholipids; this has been reported as being unchanged in schizophrenia.[12]

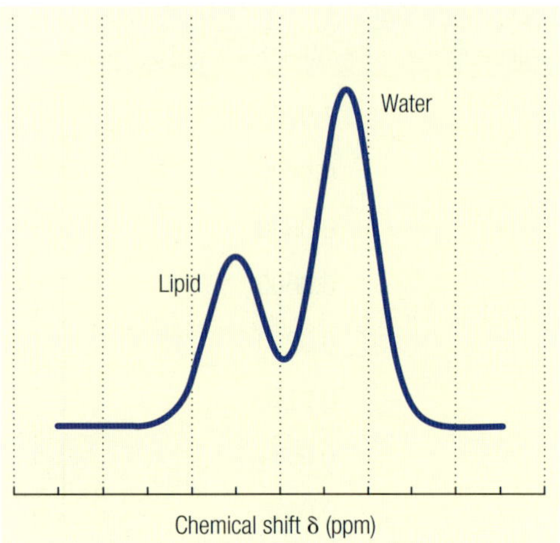

Figure 32.15 Chemical shift between water and lipid

Reproduced from Dowsett *et al. The Physics of Diagnostic Imaging*, 2nd edn. Hodder, London. (2006).

FLUID-ATTENUATED INVERSION RECOVERY

FLAIR refers to a particular type of MRI sequence that produces a strong T2-weighting, suppresses the signal from CSF, and minimizes the contrast between grey matter and white matter, thereby producing images with significantly increased lesion-to-background CSF contrast and enhancing the visibility and detectability of lesions, particularly in the peripheral subcortical and periventricular regions.[13,14] Figure 32.18 is a FLAIR MRI scan showing a hyperintense middle cerebral artery infarct.

DIFFUSION TENSOR IMAGING TRACTOGRAPHY

DTI can be used to infer the location of white matter tracts in the brain. Parker and colleagues have summarized the methodology:[15]

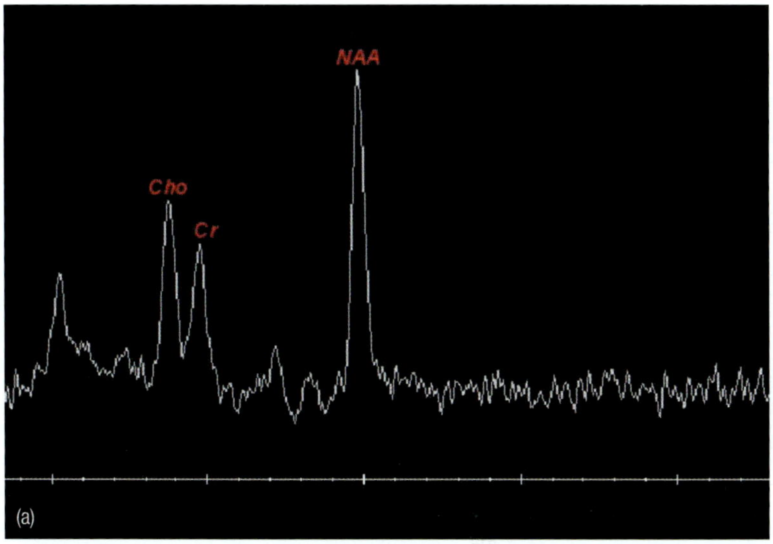

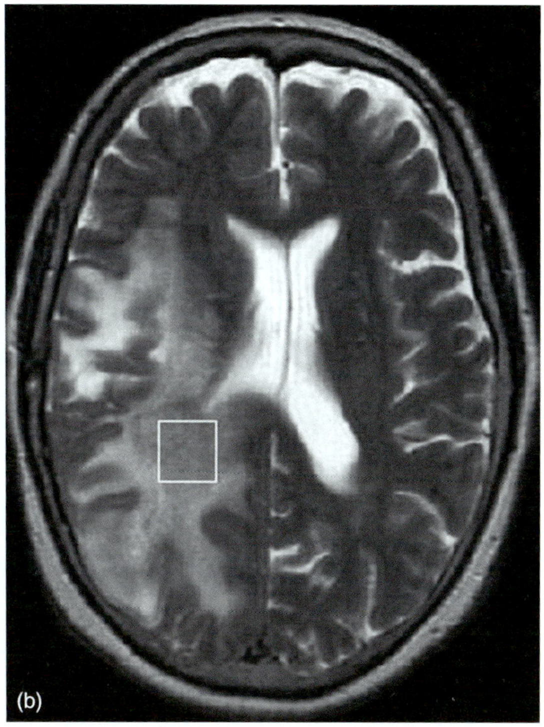

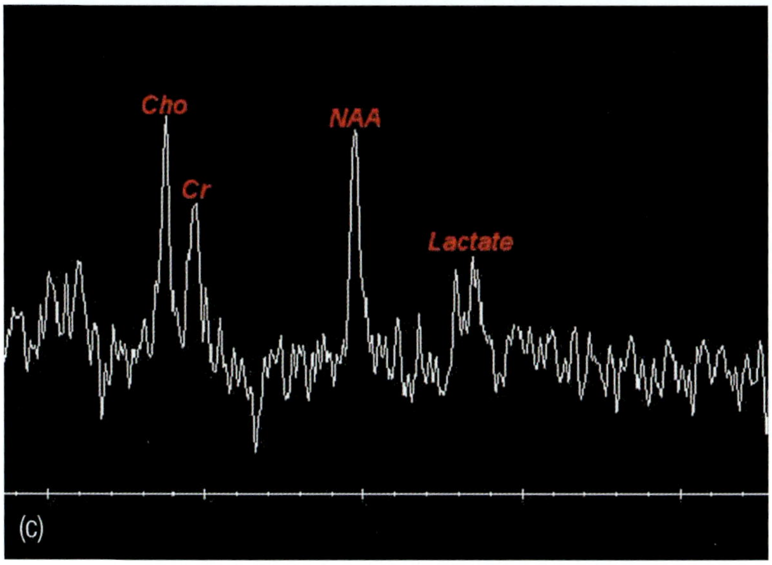

Figure 32.16 Proton magnetic resonance spectroscopy (MRS). (a) Normal proton spectrum of the brain showing the key metabolites *N*-acetyl-aspartate (NAA), creatine (Cr) and choline (Cho). (b) Mass lesion surrounded by vasogenic oedema on a T2-weighted transverse section, showing the voxel sampled in (c). (c) Typical spectrum from a glioblastoma showing reduced NAA, confirming a reduction in normally functioning neurons, a raised choline indicating an increased membrane turnover, and little change in creatine. The lactate peak indicates anaerobic respiration

Reproduced with permission from Graham *et al.*, *Adams & Graham's Introduction to Neuropathology*, 3rd edn. Hodder, London. (2006).

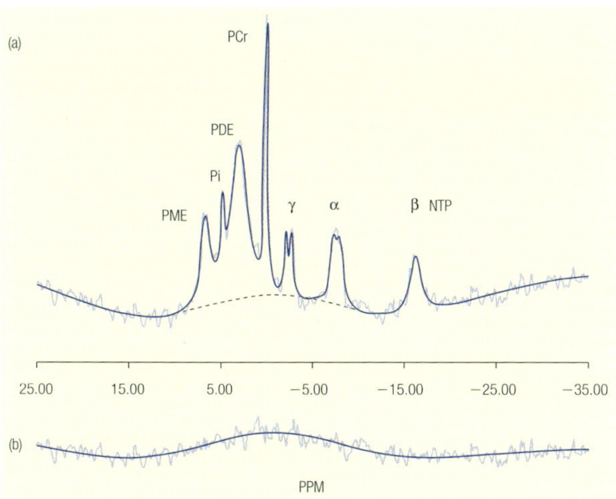

Figure 32.17 31-phosphorus magnetic resonance spectroscopy (MRS). (a) Fitting seven peaks (darker line) to the 31-phosphorus spectrum (lighter line). The dotted line shows the baseline from the broad component, which is also shown in (b)

Reproduced from ref. 11.

Diffusion tensor imaging probes the random thermal motion of water molecules in tissue. Obstructions to this motion, including cell cytostructure and membranes, cause restricted diffusion. When these microscopic obstacles are arranged coherently over the scale of an imaging voxel, the bulk diffusion properties within that voxel become directional or anisotropic; water molecules may be less restricted in their motion in certain orientations than others. DTI is sensitive to this anisotropy. The information gained from a DTI study may therefore be interpreted to provide information concerning the orientation of tissue microstructure. This microstructure has a high degree of regional directional coherence in white matter and low coherence in gray matter. Thus DTI is able not only to distinguish these tissue types, but also to elucidate the bulk orientation of microstructure therein. This information provides the basis of DTI *tractography* – methods developed to determine the pathways of anatomical CNS connections *in vivo*.

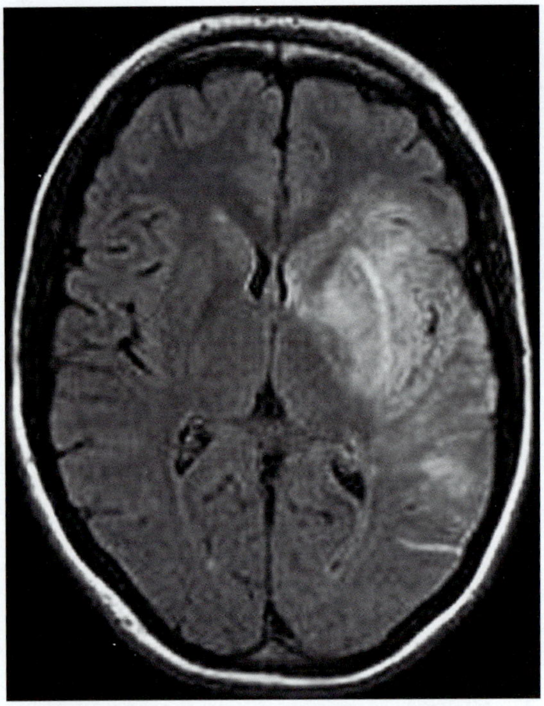

Figure 32.18 Middle cerebral artery infarct. Non-dominant hemisphere fluid-attenuated inversion recovery (FLAIR) magnetic resonance imaging (MRI) scan, showing a hyperintense infarct

Reproduced with permission from Graham *et al.*, *Adams & Graham's Introduction to Neuropathology*, 3rd edn. Hodder, London. (2006).

Tractography involves calculating the fractional anisotropy (FA), which is a measure of the anisotropy of the tensor that indicates the degree of directional preference of the fibre bundles in any given voxel.[15]

ARTERIAL SPIN LABELLING

ASL is a form of fMRI in which endogenous water molecules in arterial blood are given a special magnetization tag ('inversion') in the neck before entering the brain. The tagged images of the brain are then collected and allow cerebral blood flow to be determined. Owing to the lack of ionizing radiation, ASL is replacing PET in some studies.

SINGLE-PHOTON-EMISSION COMPUTED TOMOGRAPHY

SPECT, also known as single-photon-emission tomography (SPET), is a form of functional imaging that involves the use of a radioactive ligand. For assessing cerebral blood flow, the radioisotope or radiolabelled ligand needs to be introduced into the cerebral circulation, which can be carried out by, for example, injecting a solution of the radioactive ligand into the bloodstream or by asking the patient to inhale a gaseous form of the radioactive ligand. An example of the former is the radioligand 99m-technetium hexamethylpropylene amine oxime (^{99m}Tc-HMPAO), while an example of the latter is the gas 133-xenon (^{133}Xe).

The radioactive ligand emits single γ photons. These are detected using gamma cameras. In the case of SPECT neuroimaging, the reconstruction of the γ photon data may reflect cerebral blood flow or cerebral tissue binding, depending on the nature of the ligand used.

One particular advantage of SPECT is that some ^{99m}Tc-based ligands can be used to determine the cerebral blood flow at a time when the patient is not even in the same room as the gamma camera. For example, ^{99m}Tc-HMPAO may be injected into the bloodstream in its lipophilic form. In this form, it can readily cross the blood–brain barrier. However, having done so, it may then be converted into a hydrophilic form in a reaction that is almost irreversible (Figure 32.19).[16] As the hydrophilic form does not freely cross the blood–brain barrier, one has, as it were, obtained a binding of the radioligand in the brain that corresponds to the cerebral blood flow shortly after the time of injection into the bloodstream. There is then a window of opportunity of at least half an hour before the level of radioactivity has decayed too much, during which time the patient may undergo SPECT scanning. Clearly this is useful if one is trying to study unpredictable symptomatology, such as auditory hallucinations or epilepsy, which occurs when the patient is at a location different from that of the gamma camera (e.g. a patient with schizophrenia may be on a hospital ward at the time when he or she experiences auditory hallucinations). Although the spatial resolution of SPECT (of the order of 10 mm) is generally poorer than that of PET (around 5–7 mm) and fMRI, the advantage just mentioned of SPECT with radiotracers such as ^{99m}Tc-HMPAO has made it a useful neuroimaging modality in some neuropsychiatric research studies. For example, McGuire and colleagues used SPECT to demonstrate increased blood flow in Broca's area during auditory hallucinations in schizophrenia,[17] while our

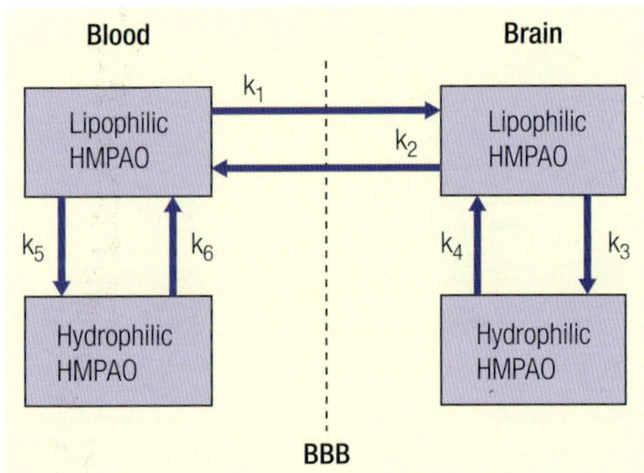

Figure 32.19 Four-compartment model describing the kinetics of 99m-technetium hexamethylpropylene amine oxime (^{99m}Tc-HMPAO) in the brain: k_1 to k_6 denote constants of first-order kinetics. Lipophilic HMPAO is freely diffusible from blood to brain; hydrophilic HMPAO is non-diffusible. Since the conversion from the lipophilic to the hydrophilic form is almost irreversible, $k_4 = k_6 = 0$

BBB, blood–brain barrier.

Reproduced with permission from ref. 16.

group have used it to study abnormal saccadic distractibility[18] and religious delusions[19] in schizophrenia.

Although largely taken over by PET and combined PET/CT (higher quality, higher spatial resolution, higher quantitative accuracy), and fMRI and ASL (no ionizing radiation), SPECT may have a role clinically in demonstrating early changes in cerebral blood flow in disorders such as Alzheimer's disease[20] and early dementia in Down syndrome.[21]

POSITRON-EMISSION TOMOGRAPHY

PET is a form of functional imaging that is currently being replaced in many centres by scanners that combine PET and multi-slice helical CT. These combined PET/CT scanners allow structural CT data to be collected rapidly and then allow the PET functional data to be registered accurately to the structural data. The patient being scanned does not need to change his or her position in respect of the table on which they are lying; the CT and PET components are adjacent to each other in the single scanner gantry, as shown in Figure 32.20.

Basic physics

In 1928 Paul Dirac derived an equation in quantum mechanics, which has become known as the Dirac equation, from which he deduced the existence of an anti-particle to the electron. This was purported to have similar properties to the electron (e^-), but with the opposite electrical charge (hence, e^+). Dirac was proved to be right, with the positron, as this anti-particle is called, being observed in 1932. When a particle and its anti-particle interact, they undergo an annihilation reaction and their joint mass is converted into energy, in accordance with Einstein's 1905 special theory of relativity. In the case of the interaction between a positron and an electron (each with mass 511 keV/c^2, where c is the velocity of electromagnetic radiation in vacuo and keV stands for kiloelectron volts), this energy, of 1022 keV, or approximately $2 \times 8.19 \times 10^{-14}$ joules, manifests itself as a dual γ photon emission, with each γ photon travelling in a direction that is diametrically opposite to that of the other, and each photon having an energy of 511 keV, or approximately 8.19×10^{-14} joules.

In PET neuroimaging, a positron-emitting radionuclide is introduced into the cerebral circulation; as with SPECT, common methods are via intravenous administration of a radiotracer in solution or by inhalation of a gaseous radiotracer. A difference from SPECT is that in the brain the radionuclide emits a positron and a neutrino. After the positron interacts with an electron, the PET scanner detects the resulting dual γ photon emission; with SPECT, only one γ photon is emitted. The PET scanner detects these two photons (which, since they travel in opposite directions, are termed 'anti-parallel') in coincidence; two suitable photons

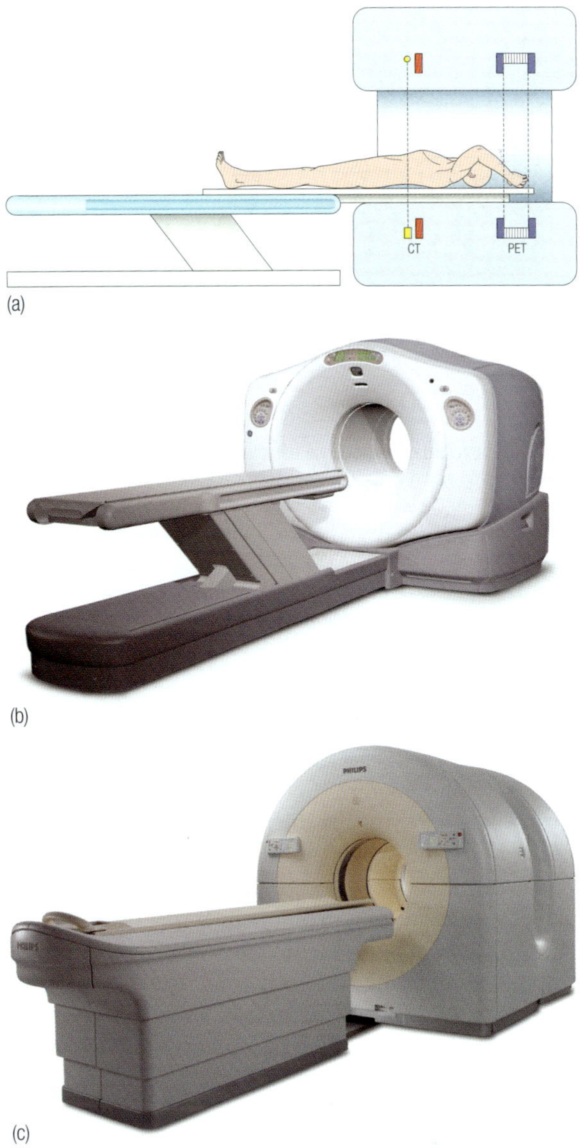

(a)

(b)

(c)

Figure 32.20 (a) Schematic diagram of a positron-emission tomography (PET)/computed tomography (CT) scanner, showing the CT and PET fields of view. (b) GE Discovery ST PET/CT scanner. (c) Philips Gemini PET/CT scanner Photographs courtesy of GE Healthcare and Philips Medical Systems

detected within a certain period of each other, the coincidence window, are assumed to originate from the same positron–electron interaction. This process is summarized in Figure 32.21.

Not all coincidence pairs of γ photons are true coincidences that pertain to the image. Some are caused by photon scattering or by random single-photon emissions, as shown in Figure 32.22. These scatter and random coincidences cause background noise in the imaging.

Radionuclides

Properties and production routes for radionuclides commonly used in PET are shown in Table 32.4. The table gives

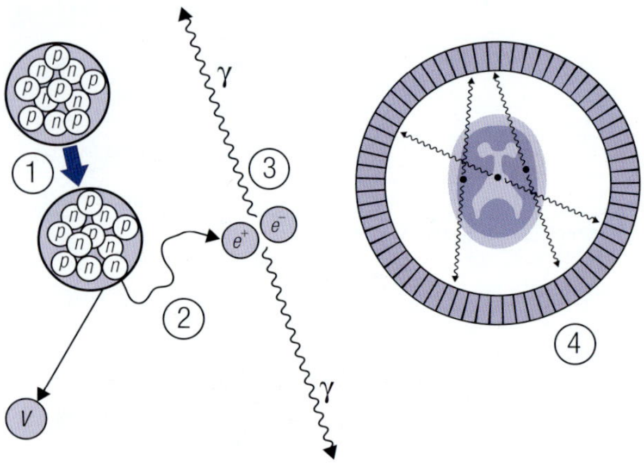

Figure 32.21 Annihilation coincidence detection. A positron and a neutrino are emitted by a proton-rich nucleus (1). The positron follows a convoluted path (2) of a millimetre or so. At the end of its path, the positron interacts with an electron to produce two anti-parallel 511-keV photons (3), which are detected in coincidence (4) by the positron-emission tomography (PET) scanner

Reproduced with permission from Barrington, *Atlas of Clinical Positron Emission Tomography*, 2nd edn. Hodder, London. (2005).

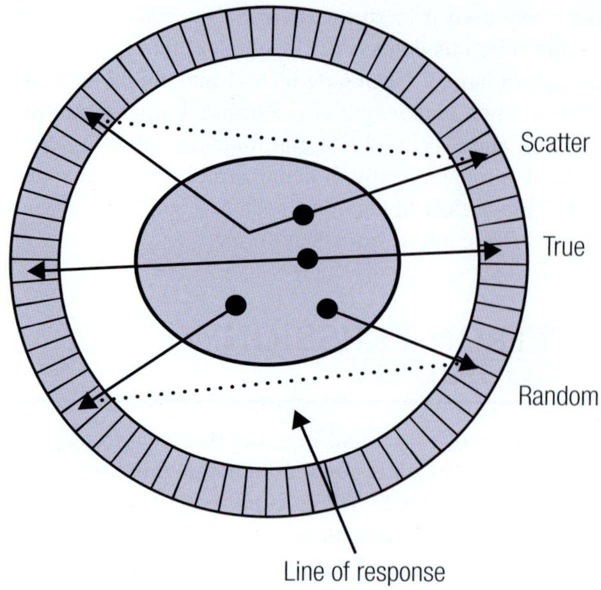

Figure 32.22 True, scatter and random coincidences

Reproduced with permission from Barrington, *Atlas of Clinical Positron Emission Tomography*, 2nd edn. Hodder, London. (2005).

the maximum energy, E_{max}, of positrons emitted from the radionuclides, in megaelectron volts (MeV). Note that 1 MeV is approximately 1.602×10^{-13} J. The higher the positron energy, the further the positron can travel in tissue and the poorer the spatial resolution of the corresponding PET image.

The positron-emitting radionuclides in Table 32.4 that have low atomic numbers (conventionally denoted by *Z*) – that is, low numbers of protons in the nucleus – can be produced in small cyclotrons. These radionuclides are ^{11}C, ^{13}N, ^{15}O and ^{18}F. Figure 32.23 shows a commercial PET cyclotron and the inner workings of one schematically; the dee is an electrode. Further details of how a cyclotron works are beyond the scope of this book. Once the radionuclides have been produced, the radionuclides have to be separated from non-radioactive by-products; this is achieved by a technique such as high-performance liquid chromatography (HPLC).

2-[^{18}F]Fluoro-2-deoxy-D-glucose

The radiotracer 2-[^{18}F]fluoro-2-deoxy-D-glucose (^{18}F-FDG, or just FDG), based on the radionuclide ^{18}F, is a marker for glucose metabolism. It is a synthetic analogue of the glucose molecule, in which a hydroxyl group is replaced with a radioactive fluorine-18 atom. Like glucose, ^{18}F-FDG is readily transported into cells from the plasma, but, unlike

Table 32.4 Properties and production routes for positron-emission tomography (PET) radionuclides

Radionuclide	Half-life	E_{max} (MeV)	Production reaction	Target	Product
^{11}C	20.4 min	0.96	${}^{14}_{7}N(p,\alpha){}^{11}_{6}C$	$^{nat}N_2$ gas	$^{11}CO_2$ gas
^{13}N	9.96 min	1.19	${}^{16}_{8}O(p,\alpha){}^{13}_{7}N$	^{nat}O water	$^{13}NH_4^+$ ion
^{15}O	2.07 min	1.72	${}^{15}_{7}N(p,n){}^{15}_{8}O$	$^{15}N_2$ gas	$^{15}O_2$ gas
			${}^{14}_{7}N(d,n){}^{15}_{8}O$	$^{nat}N_2$ gas	$^{15}O_2$ gas
^{18}F	109.8 min	0.635	${}^{18}_{8}O(p,n){}^{18}_{9}F$	^{18}O water	$^{18}F^-$ ion
			${}^{20}_{10}Ne(d,\alpha){}^{18}_{9}F$	^{nat}Ne gas	^{18}F–F_2 gas
^{68}Ga	68 min	1.9	$^{68}Ge \rightarrow {}^{68}Ga$	(Generator)	Ga metal
^{82}Rb	75 s	3.36	$^{82}Sr \rightarrow {}^{82}Rb$	(Generator)	RbCl

Reproduced from Barrington SF, Maisey MN, Wahl RL (2006) *Atlas of Clinical Positron Emission Tomography*, 2nd edn. London: Hodder Arnold.

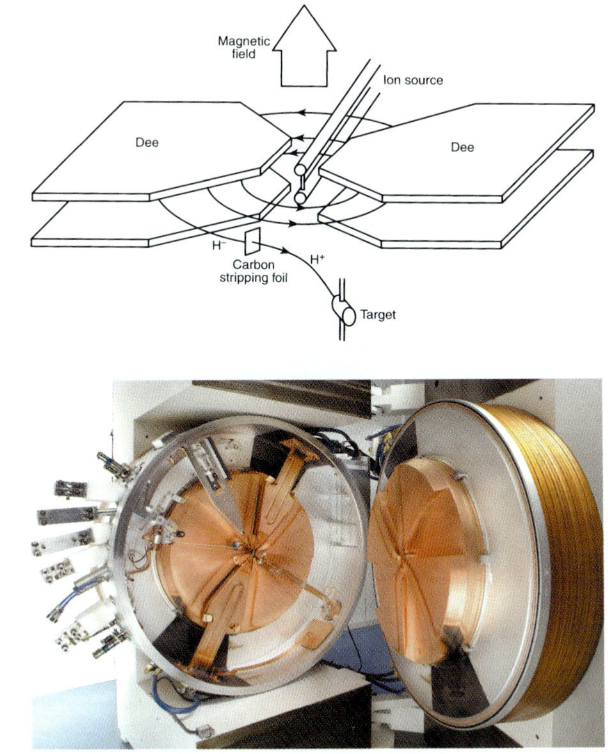

Figure 32.23 (a) Schematic diagram of the operation of a cyclotron. (b) A commercial positron-emission tomography (PET) cyclotron

Photograph courtesy of GE Healthcare.

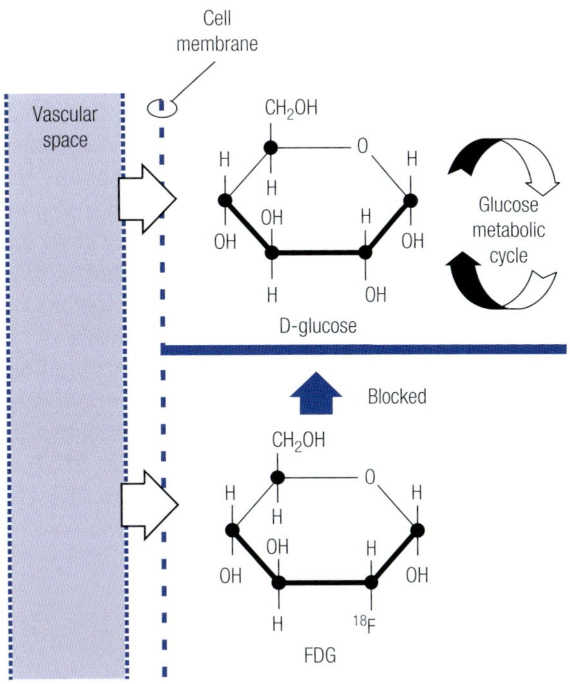

Figure 32.24 Blockage of 2-[^{18}F]fluoro-2-deoxy-D-glucose (^{18}F-FDG) from glucose metabolism after intracellular uptake

Reproduced with permission from Barrington, *Atlas of Clinical Positron Emission Tomography*, 2nd edn. Hodder, London. (2005).

glucose-6-phosphate, after intracellular phosphorylation by hexokinase ^{18}F-FDG-6-phosphate is not acted upon by glucose-6-phosphatase and so remains trapped intracellularly, as shown in Figure 32.24. With a relatively long half-life of approximately 110 min and a cellular uptake similar to that of glucose, ^{18}F-FDG is a particularly good radiotracer for use in PET neuroimaging. There is a relatively high uptake, of approximately 6 per cent, of administered ^{18}F-FDG by the brain. Another advantage of this radiotracer is that units are now available that allow automated synthesis from reagents of quantities of ^{18}F-FDG suitable for PET imaging in only around 40 min; Figure 32.25 shows one such unit.

The following techniques have been suggested to reduce physiological uptake of ^{18}F-FDG in PET neuroimaging:[22]

- Inject the patient in silence in a quiet darkened room
- Avoid stimulation during the uptake period
- Avoid any sedation for the uptake period
- The subject should avoid any glucose-containing sedation before visiting the PET centre.

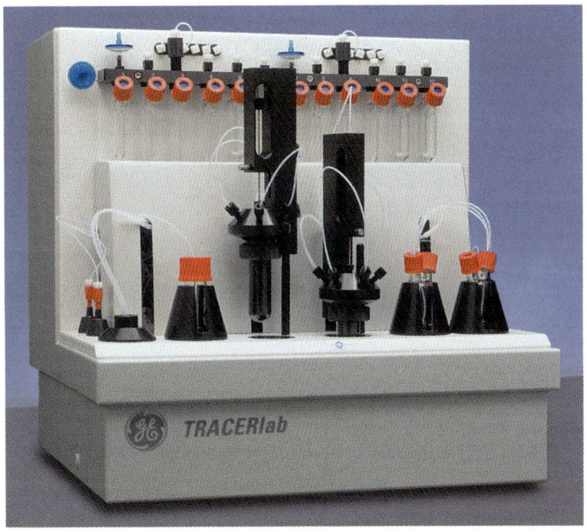

Figure 32.25 Automated 2-[^{18}F]fluoro-2-deoxy-D-glucose (^{18}F-FDG) synthesis unit

Courtesy of GE Healthcare.

Research with radioligands

PET neuroimaging has been used widely for psychiatric research. Specific radioligands are required when researching neurotransmission. For example, the study of dopamine (D2/D3) receptors in the brain using PET can be carried out with the dopamine receptor radioligand [^{11}C]raclopride; 5-hydroxytryptamine (5-HT)$_{1A}$ receptors can be studied with [carbonyl-^{11}C]WAY-100635 and [carbonyl-^{11}C]desmethyl-WAY-100635; cannabinoid CB$_1$ receptors (in non-human primates) can be studied with [^{11}C]MePPEP and [^{18}F]AM5144; and nicotinic acetylcholine receptors (nAChR) can be studied with the fluoropyridine derivatives 2-[^{18}F]FA and 6-[^{18}F]FA.

An example of the use of [^{11}C]raclopride is a study by Reeves and colleagues of the relationship between striatal dopamine (D2/D3) receptor availability and delusions in Alzheimer's disease.[23] This study tested the hypothesis that the symptom domains delusions and apathy are associated with striatal dopamine (D2) receptor function in Alzheimer's disease. In vivo dopamine (D2/D3) receptor availability was determined with [^{11}C]raclopride PET in 23 patients with mild or moderate probable Alzheimer's disease. Figure 32.30 shows the right-sided striatal regions of interest, derived from structural MRI, superimposed on a [^{11}C]raclopride PET image. The mean [^{11}C]raclopride binding potential in the striatum was found to be higher in patients with delusions than in those without delusions, as shown in Figure 32.26, showing that striatal dopamine (D2/D3) receptor availability is increased in Alzheimer disease patients with delusions.[23]

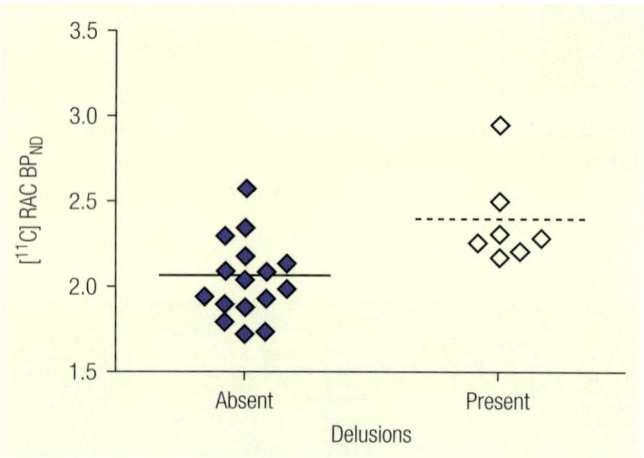

Figure 32.26 Mean [^{11}C]raclopride (RAC) binding potential (BP_{ND}) in the striatum, in the presence or absence of delusions

Reproduced with permission from ref. 23.

Clinical applications

PET can be useful in determining whether or not a lesion seen on structural MRI of the brain is a recurrence of a tumour in a patient with a history of malignancy. The use of PET to identify metabolic changes associated with a recurrent high-grade tumour is illustrated in Figure 32.27. These scans are from a patient with a history of treated glioblastoma multiforme, in whom a structural MRI scan (Figure 32.27a) showed a large mass with oedema, pointing to a possible diagnosis of recurrent tumour. The PET scan (Figure 32.27b) showed increased metabolic activity in the lesion, consistent with tumour recurrence.[22] The case illustrated in Figure 32.28 again shows how PET can be useful in differentiating between malignancy and, in this case, post-treatment changes. Here, although the MRI showed an enhancing region suggestive of recurrent tumour, this region did not take up ^{18}F-FDG, indicating that it was not in fact a recurrence but, probably, post-treatment fibrosis.[22]

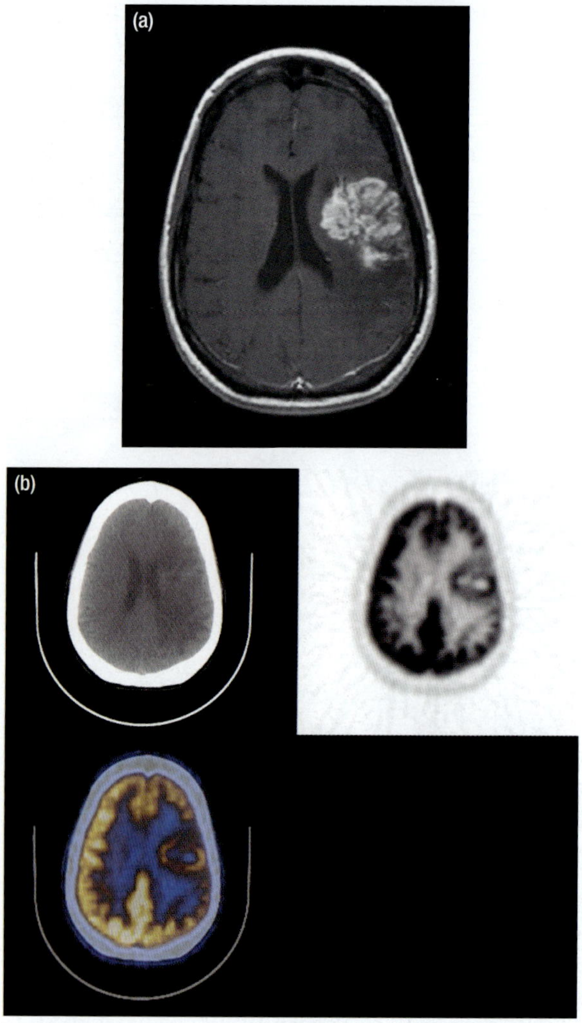

Figure 32.27 Magnetic resonance imaging (MRI) scan, showing a 50cm mass with oedema, suggestive of recurrent tumour, in a patient referred with a history of glioblastoma multiforme treated with surgery, chemotherapy and radiotherapy 4 years earlier. (b) Positron-emission tomography (PET) scans, showing increased metabolic activity associated with the mass in the inferoposterior aspect of the left frontal lobe compatible with recurrence. The diffuse decreased activity in the left frontal region is consistent with post-radiation changes

Reproduced with permission from Barrington, *Atlas of Clinical Positron Emission Tomography*, 2nd edn. Hodder, London. (2005).

PET is also useful in differentiating between intracerebral infection (commonly toxoplasmosis), which has no or low-grade ^{18}F-FDG uptake, and intracerebral malignancy (commonly lymphoma) in patients with human immunodeficiency virus (HIV) disease presenting with neurological illness.[22] This is illustrated in Figure 32.28, in which a focus of high ^{18}F-FDG uptake in a patient with HIV disease was consistent with the diagnosis of lymphoma, and Figure 32.30, in which the photopaenic defect corresponding to an MRI lesion in a patient newly diagnosed with HIV was consistent with toxoplasmosis and not lymphoma.[22]

PET is also useful in the diagnosis of dementia. Table 32.5 details the MRI and ^{18}F-FDG PET findings in various dementias (see also Chapters 37 and 72). In addition to

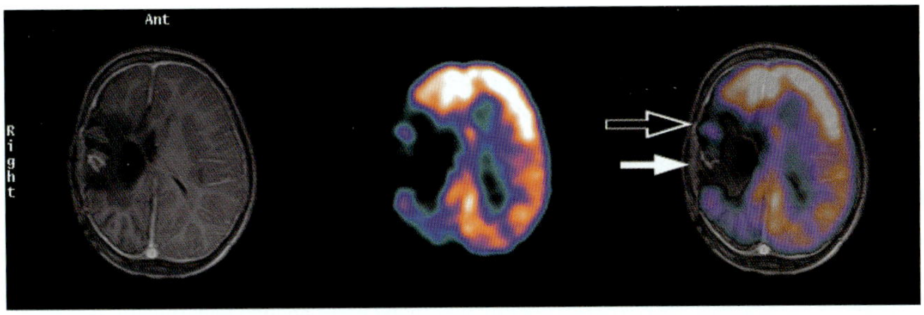

Figure 32.28 Magnetic resonance imaging (MRI) and positron-emission tomography (PET) scans of the brain of a child who had undergone multiple surgery, chemotherapy and radiotherapy for an anaplastic ependymoma. Although neurologically stable with a left hemiplegia, she complained of new headaches. The MRI scan (left) showed an enhancing region in the right parietal lobe suggestive of recurrent disease. 2-[^{18}F]Fluoro-2-deoxy-D-glucose (^{18}F-FDG) (middle) was registered to the MRI scan (right). The region of enhancing tissue on MRI did not take up ^{18}F-FDG (solid arrow), indicating that this was likely to be scar or inflammatory tissue. The small focus of ^{18}F-FDG uptake (broken arrow) in the right parietal region corresponded to an island of normal cortex on MRI

Reproduced with permission from Barrington, *Atlas of Clinical Positron Emission Tomography*, 2nd edn. Hodder, London. (2005).

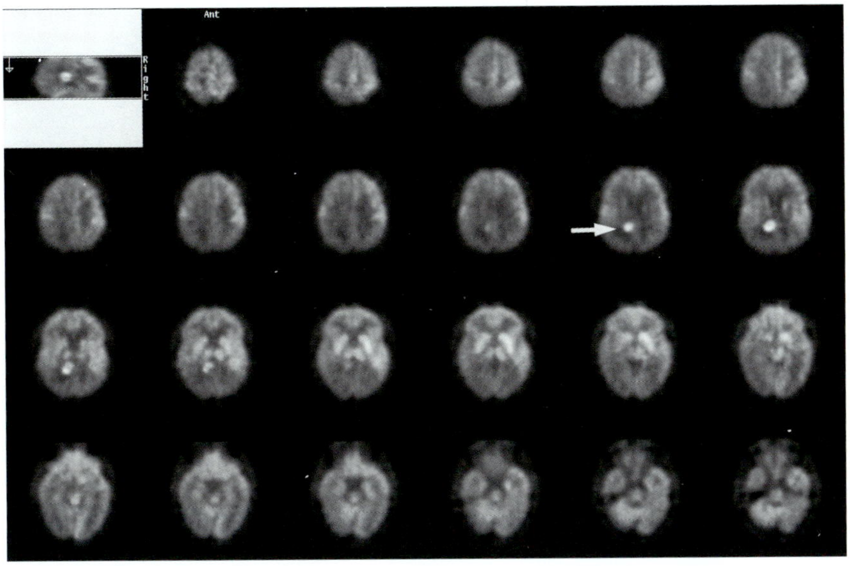

Figure 32.29 2-[^{18}F]Fluoro-2-deoxy-D-glucose (^{18}F-FDG) positron-emission tomography (PET) findings from a patient with human immunodeficiency virus (HIV) disease, who was referred with a magnetic resonance imaging (MRI) lesion of unknown nature in the right parietal lobe. There was a focus of intense uptake in the right parietal lobe posterior to the thalamus. Biopsy revealed lymphoma

Reproduced with permission from Barrington, *Atlas of Clinical Positron Emission Tomography*, 2nd edn. Hodder, London. (2005).

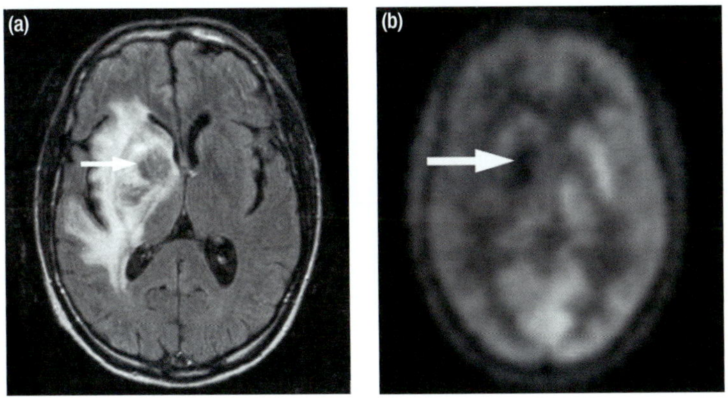

Figure 32.30 This patient with newly diagnosed human immunodeficiency virus (HIV) presented with a 6-week history of headache and increasing confusion associated with pyrexia. (a) Magnetic resonance imaging (MRI) showed a lesion centred on the right lentiform nucleus, with surrounding oedema and mass effect, consistent with toxoplasmosis or lymphoma. (b) There was a photopaenic effect on positron-emission tomography (PET) corresponding to the MRI lesion and consistent with toxoplasmosis and not lymphoma. The PET scan also shows diffuse reduction in the right frontoparietal region. The patient showed good clinical response to treatment with anti-toxoplasmosis therapy

Reproduced with permission from Barrington, *Atlas of Clinical Positron Emission Tomography*, 2nd edn. Hodder, London. (2005).

aiding in the differential diagnosis of dementia, ^{18}F-FDG PET is useful in differentiating between early Alzheimer's disease and benign memory loss, and also in differentiating dementia from pseudo-dementia or depression.[22] Three examples of the use of PET in different dementias follow.

Figure 32.31 shows ^{18}F-FDG PET images from a patient who presented with word-finding difficulties and memory impairment; cognitive testing revealed a global pattern of impairment, but with the left hemisphere more severely affected. The bitemporal, posterior parietal and temporal hypometabolism seen on PET were consistent with Alzheimer's disease; note that the preservation of cortical ^{18}F-FDG uptake in the posterior cingulate cortex weighs against a diagnosis of Lewy body dementia.[22]

Table 32.5 Magnetic resonance imaging (MRI) and 2-[^{18}F]fluoro-2-deoxy-D-glucose (^{18}F-FDG) positron-emission tomography (PET) findings in dementias

MRI	FDG-PET
Alzheimer's disease	
Early: normal or hippocampal atrophy	Temporoparietal and cingulate hypometabolism
Advanced: frontal, parietotemporal atrophy	Temporoparietal hypometabolism, with sparing of subcortical structures, primary visual and sensorimotor cortex; later also frontal hypometabolism, cortical atrophy and thalamic separation
Multiple infarct dementia	
White-matter signals and cortical and subcortical infarcts	Focal asymmetrical cortical and deep hypometabolic areas
Pseudo-dementia	
Normal	Normal or frontal hypometabolism
Frontal dementias	
Early: normal	Frontal: frontal lobe hypometabolism
Late: frontal atrophy	Pick: frontal + temporal hypometabolism
Trauma	
Mild: normal	Focal hypometabolism
Severe: atrophy	Focal hypometabolism
HIV	
Normal	Diffuse cortical hypometabolism with sparing of deep structures
Huntingdon's disease	
Early: normal	Hypometabolism of caudate nucleus
Late: caudate atrophy	
Lewy body disease	
Early: nil	Alzheimer disease-like picture, but with reduced visual cortex metabolism
Late: atrophy	

Reproduced from Barrington SF, Maisey MN, Wahl RL (2006) *Atlas of Clinical Positron Emission Tomography*, 2nd edn. London: Hodder Arnold.

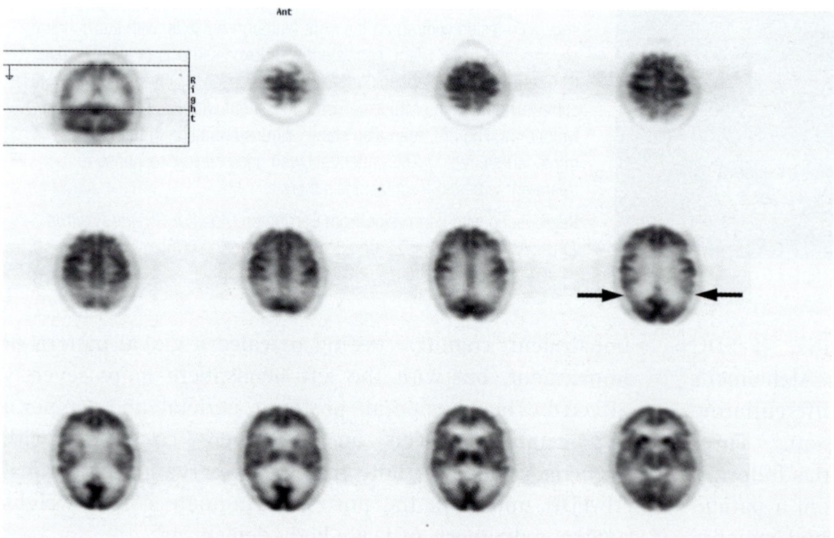

Figure 32.31 2-[^{18}F]Fluoro-2-deoxy-D-glucose (^{18}F-FDG) positron-emission tomography (PET) findings in a patient with word-finding difficulties and memory impairment. The bitemporal, posterior parietal and temporal hypometabolism seen on PET were consistent with Alzheimer's disease. The two black arrows on either side of the middle transverse image in the most right-hand column of images correspond to the level of the coronal scan shown at the top left

Reproduced with permission from Barrington, *Atlas of Clinical Positron Emission Tomography*, 2nd edn. Hodder, London. (2005).

Figure 32.32 shows ^{18}F-FDG PET images from a patient with Lewy body dementia; metabolism was reduced in the parietotemporal association cortices and frontal association cortex. The pattern of reduction in metabolism in the association cortices in Lewy body dementia is similar to that seen in Alzheimer's disease; although the cerebral hemispheres are involved bilaterally, the involvement may be asymmetrical in Lewy body dementia (in Figure 32.32 the metabolic reduction is more severe on the left); and metabolic reduction often occurs in the occipital cortex in Lewy body dementia.[22]

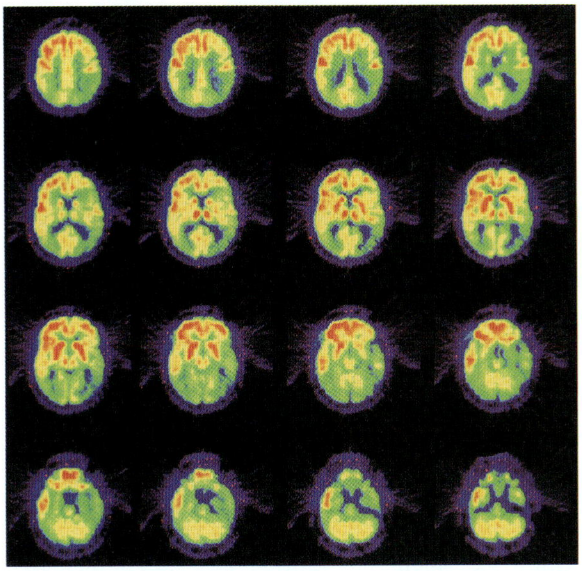

Figure 32.32 2-[^{18}F]Fluoro-2-deoxy-D-glucose (^{18}F-FDG) positron-emission tomography (PET) images from a patient with Lewy body dementia. Metabolism is reduced in the parietotemporal association cortices and frontal association cortex, and there is asymmetrical (more severe on the left) but bilateral involvement of the cerebral hemisphere

Reproduced with permission from Barrington, *Atlas of Clinical Positron Emission Tomography*, 2nd edn. Hodder, London. (2005).

Figure 32.33 shows PET images from a patient with Pick's disease (frontotemporal dementia), in which there is bilateral reduction in ^{18}F-FDG uptake in the frontal lobes. Reduced uptake in the temporal lobes is also sometimes seen.

KEY POINTS

- CT is a form of structural imaging that offers very high spatial resolution and uses X-rays.
- Structural MRI is a form of structural imaging that offers very high spatial resolution and does not involve the use of ionizing radiation. Image registration and voxel-based morphometry are just two of many advanced techniques that can be applied to MRI data.
- BOLD fMRI is a form of functional imaging that does not involve the use of ionizing radiation.
- MRS is a form of functional imaging that allows tissue chemistry to be studied in vivo.
- FLAIR is an MRI sequence that suppresses the signal from CSF and minimizes the contrast between grey matter and white matter.
- DTI tractography is an MR technique that allows the determination of the pathways of anatomical central nervous system connections in vivo.
- ASL is a form of functional imaging that allows cerebral blood flow to be determined without the use of ionizing radiation.
- SPECT is a form of functional imaging employing radiotracers to study regional cerebral blood flow and ligand binding.
- PET is a form of functional imaging employing radiotracers to study metabolic changes, regional cerebral blood flow and ligand binding.

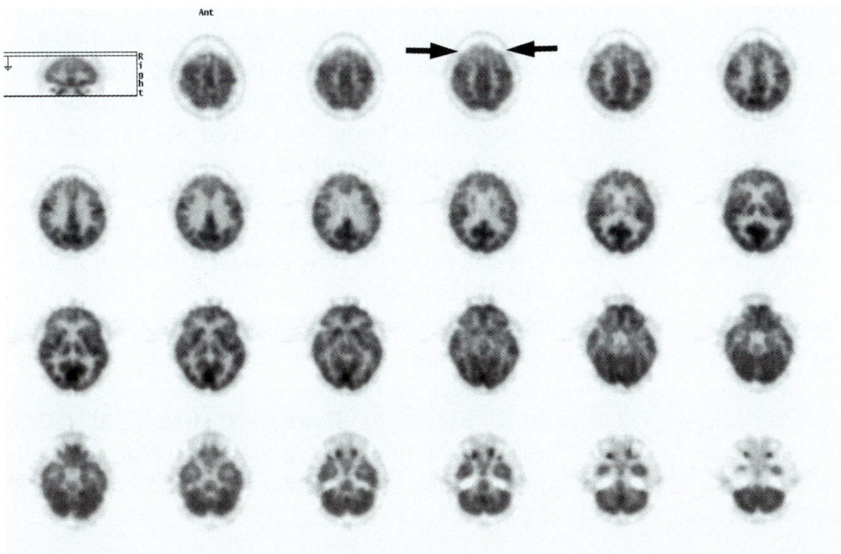

Figure 32.33 2-[^{18}F]Fluoro-2-deoxy-D-glucose (^{18}F-FDG) positron-emission tomography (PET) images from a patient with Pick's disease (frontotemporal dementia), in which there is bilateral reduction in uptake in the frontal lobes. The two black arrows on either side of a transverse image in the top row of images correspond to the level of the coronal scan shown at the top left

Reproduced with permission from Barrington, *Atlas of Clinical Positron Emission Tomography*, 2nd edn. Hodder, London. (2005).

FURTHER READING

Barrington SF, Maisey MN, Wahl RL (2006) *Atlas of Clinical Positron Emission Tomography*, 2nd edn. London: Hodder Arnold.

Buxton RB (2002) *Introduction to Functional Magnetic Resonance Imaging: Principles and Techniques.* Cambridge: Cambridge University Press.

Dowsett DJ, Kenny PA, Johnston RE (2006) *The Physics of Diagnostic Imaging*, 2nd edn. London: Hodder Arnold.

McRobbie DW, Moore EA, Graves MJ, Prince MR (2007) *MRI: From Picture to Proton*, 2nd edn. Cambridge: Cambridge University Press.

Port JD, Puri BK (2009) MR spectroscopy in psychiatry. In JH Gillard, AD Waldman, PB Barker (eds) *Clinical MR Neuroimaging: Diffusion, Perfusion and Spectroscopy*, 2nd edn. Cambridge: Cambridge University Press.

REFERENCES

1. Ambrose J, Hounsfield G (1973) Computerized transverse axial tomography. *British Journal of Radiology* **46**: 148–9.
2. Hounsfield GN (1973) Computerized transverse axial scanning (tomography): 1. Description of system. *British Journal of Radiology* **46**: 1016–22.
3. Johnstone EC, Crow TJ, Frith CD, *et al.* (1976) Cerebral ventricular size and cognitive impairment in chronic schizophrenia. *Lancet* **2**: 924–6.
4. Hsia AW (2009) 10 questions about acute stroke imaging: CT versus MRI – the controversy'. *Neurologist* **15**: 105–7.
5. Duncan J (2009) The current status of neuroimaging for epilepsy. *Current Opinion in Neurology* **22**: 179–84.
6. Puri BK, Bydder GM, Manku MS, *et al.* (2008) Reduction in cerebral atrophy associated with ethyl-eicosapentaenoic acid treatment in patients with Huntington's disease. *Journal of International Medical Research* **36**: 896–905.
7. Belliveau JW, Kennedy DN, Jr, McKinstry RC, *et al.* (1991) Functional mapping of the human visual cortex by magnetic resonance imaging. *Science* **254**: 716–19.
8. Kwong KK, Belliveau JW, Chesler DA, *et al.* (1992) Dynamic magnetic resonance imaging of human brain activity during primary sensory stimulation. *Proceedings of the National Academy of Science USA* **89**: 5675–9.
9. Puri BK, Tsaluchidu S, Treasaden IH (2009) Serial structural MRI analysis and proton and 31PMR spectroscopy in the investigation of cerebral fatty acids in major depressive disorder, Huntington's disease, myalgic encephalomyelitis and in forensic schizophrenic patients. *World Review of Nutrition and Dietetics* **99**: 31–45.
10. Cox IJ, Puri BK (2004) In vivo MR spectroscopy in diagnosis and research of neuropsychiatric disorders. *Prostaglandins, Leukotrienes and Essential Fatty Acids* **70**: 357–60.
11. Puri BK, Counsell SJ, Hamilton G, *et al.* (2004) Cerebral metabolism in male patients with schizophrenia who have seriously and dangerously violently offended: a 31P magnetic resonance spectroscopy study. *Prostaglandins, Leukotrienes and Essential Fatty Acids* **70**: 409–11.
12. Puri BK, Counsell SJ, Hamilton G (2008) Brain cell membrane motion-restricted phospholipids: a cerebral 31-phosphorus magnetic resonance spectroscopy study of patients with schizophrenia. *Prostaglandins, Leukotrienes and Essential Fatty Acids* **79**: 233–5.
13. Kates R, Atkinson D, Brant-Zawadzki M (1996) Fluid-attenuated inversion recovery (FLAIR): clinical prospectus of current and future applications. *Topics in Magnetic Resonance Imaging* **8**: 389–96.
14. De Coene B, Hajnal JV, Gatehouse P, *et al.* (1992) MR of the brain using fluid-attenuated inversion recovery (FLAIR) pulse sequences. *American Journal of Neuroradiology* **13**: 1555–64.
15. Parker GJ, Stephan KE, Barker GJ, *et al.* (2002) Initial demonstration of in vivo tracing of axonal projections in the macaque brain and comparison with the human brain using diffusion tensor imaging and fast marching tractography. *NeuroImage* **15**: 797–809.
16. Borch K, Greisen G (1997) 99mTc-HMPAO as a tracer of cerebral blood flow in newborn infants. *Journal of Cerebral Blood Flow and Metabolism* **17**: 448–54.
17. McGuire PK, Shah GM, Murray RM (1993) Increased blood flow in Broca's area during auditory hallucinations in schizophrenia. *Lancet* **342**: 703–6.
18. Crawford TJ, Puri BK, Nijran KS, *et al.* (1996) Abnormal saccadic distractibility in patients with schizophrenia: a 99mTc-HMPAO SPET study. *Psychological Medicine* **26**: 265–77.
19. Puri BK, Lekh SK, Nijran KS, *et al.* (2001) SPECT neuroimaging in schizophrenia with religious delusions. *International Journal of Psychophysiology* **40**: 143–8.
20. Nishimiya M, Matsuda H, Imabayashi E, *et al.* (2008) Comparison of SPM and NEUROSTAT in voxelwise statistical analysis of brain SPECT and MRI at the early stage of Alzheimer's disease. *Annals of Nuclear Medicine* **22**: 921–7.
21. Puri BK, Zhang Z, Singh I (1994) SPECT in adult mosaic Down's syndrome with early dementia. *Clinical Nuclear Medicine* **19**: 989–91.
22. Barrington SF, Wahl RL, Maisey M (2006) *Atlas of Clinical Positron Emission Tomography*, 2nd edn. London: Hodder Arnold.
23. Reeves S, Brown R, Howard R, Grasby P (2009) Increased striatal dopamine (D2/D3) receptor availability and delusions in Alzheimer disease. *Neurology* **72**: 528–34.

Chapter 33

Genetics

Michael Gill and Jane McGrath

BASIC CONCEPTS

Introduction

Genetics is the scientific study of the inheritance of traits both physical and behavioural. Genes provide the assembly code for the molecules that make up life and enable reproduction of living organisms. Genes are located on chromosomes, which are highly folded and compressed linear molecules of deoxyribonucleic acid (DNA) housed in the nuclei of cells. They pass from generation to generation, providing familial resemblance and individual variation, which, through evolution, is responsible for the diversity of life. This chapter describes the basic principles of genetics and their relevance to psychiatric disorders. The first use of the term 'genetics' was in 1906 by the biologist William Bateson, but the science of genetics began much earlier. Gregor Mendel, a monk working in the monastery in Brno in 1866, described laws of inheritance based on his observations of the inheritance of seven simple bimodal traits in pea plants. Mendel suggested that each parent plant had a pair of units of inheritance for each trait but contributed only one unit from each pair to its offspring.

Mendel's first law (the law of segregation) states that one of an individual's two units of inheritance (alleles) at any location is randomly distributed to each gamete. This is seen in the pattern of inheritance of autosomal dominant disorders such as Huntington's disease.

Mendel's second law (of independent assortment) states that the segregation of the alleles for any one trait to a gamete occurs independently of the segregation of the alleles for any other trait to that gamete. This law is true only for alleles not genetically linked (physically located close) to each other, and departure from it forms the basis of linkage analysis and has enabled genetic maps to be constructed and used to locate genes responsible for disorders.

Thomas Morgan demonstrated that genes were arranged linearly on chromosomes within cell nuclei and could be inherited together, depending on the physical distance between them and the frequency of recombination (see below) in the region. Morgan also demonstrated that linkage is rarely complete and that some traits are sex-linked.

In 1944, Oswald Avery, a Canadian bacteriologist, confirmed that genes were composed of DNA by transferring DNA from one strain of bacteria to another. He showed that the second strain acquired traits from the first and could pass these traits to future generations. In 1953, geneticists James Watson and Francis Crick discovered that the DNA molecule is composed of two long strands in the form of a double helix. Their deduction of the structure of DNA was made from X-ray photographs taken by a British scientist Rosalind Franklin and a New Zealander Maurice Wilkins. Crick and Watson deduced that DNA resembled a long spiral ladder with a sugar–phosphate backbone and rungs composed of pairs of complementary nucleotide bases. This structure immediately suggested that the molecule could unwind, separating at the nucleotide bases, and each half-strand could form a template for rebuilding the second strand and generating two identical copies. Thus, the genetic code could be replicated and transmitted to dividing cells and across generations.

By this time, it was known that genes produced proteins and scientists speculated that a genetic code, encrypted in the order of nucleotide bases, must determine the sequence of amino acids in proteins. Only four different nucleotides had been identified in DNA, but at least 20 different amino acids were known to occur in proteins. In 1962, Crick determined that the coding sequence is a series of three nucleotide bases and that each amino acid is specified by at least one of these sequences, called a codon.

More recent developments have made significant contributions to the new science of molecular genetics. Fredrick Sanger developed methods for analysing the molecular structure of proteins and for rapidly determining the nucleotide sequence of nucleic acids. Ed Southern provided a method for transferring DNA from a gel to a membrane, where it could be detected, and Kary Mullis developed the polymerase chain reaction (PCR), which allowed rapid enzymatic synthesis of multiple copies of a specific DNA sequence.

Chromosomes, cell division and genes

DNA is tightly packaged and protein-bound into 22 homologous pairs of chromosomes and two X chromosomes in females or an X and a Y in males (46 chromosomes in all). The total DNA complement in a cell is referred to as its genome. If placed end to end and unravelled, human DNA is over 2 m long and contains approximately 3.9×10^9 base pairs. Only 2–3 per cent of the genome consists of the coding sequences of approximately 30 000 genes. Much of the remaining DNA has no apparent function, but emerging possibilities include the regulation of DNA structure, repair and expression.

A gene is a length of DNA, some of which codes for a string of amino acids. Because chromosomes exist in homologous pairs, there are normally two copies of each gene in the human genome. The two copies are termed alleles. Due to mutations over time, the DNA base sequence throughout the genome, including within genes, varies between individuals and between the two copies possessed by an individual. This and the environment – the 'slings and arrows of outrageous fortune' – are what create differences between individuals. Thus, alleles may be the same (homozygous) or different (heterozygous). If different, the locus can be described as polymorphic. Mendel's first law states that only one allele for each gene may be inherited from each parent. At a given locus, the two alleles constitute the individual's genotype. If the locus is a gene, then the expression of the trait coded for by the genotype is called the phenotype. In this context, 'phenotype' is a broad term that would include the results of biochemical or protein analysis or might be outwardly observable in the form of a normally distributed trait (e.g. height) or the presence or absence of a disease state (e.g. Huntington's disease). If individuals with one copy of a given allele have the same phenotype as individuals with two copies, then the allele is said to be dominant. If two copies of an allele are required to produce the phenotype, then the allele is termed recessive. If the phenotype of individuals with one copy is intermediate between those with none and those with two, then the allele is co-dominant.

Somatic cells are the general cells throughout the body and are diploid, having 23 pairs of chromosomes, but sex cells (gametes) have only 23 chromosomes and are termed haploid. These differences in chromosome number, on which sexual reproduction depends, arise because somatic cells replicate by mitosis and gametes by a more complicated process called meiosis. In mitosis, chromosomes are duplicated in the prophase stage of the cell cycle. The duplicated chromosomes join at a constricted chromosomal region called the centromere to form sister chromatids. In metaphase, a spindle forms from a centriole at each cell pole to the centromere. During anaphase, the spindles retract, pulling a chromosome to each pole and distributing the chromosomes equally between two daughter cells identical to the parent cell (telophase).

Gametes are produced by meiosis, in which daughter cells receive only half the number of chromosomes. During the prophase stage of meiosis, each chromosome of each homologous pair duplicates itself, and the resulting sister chromatids are joined at the centromere. Each homologous pair of chromosomes produces a tetrad consisting of four chromatids. Non-sister (one from each parent) chromatids pair together and physically recombine (cross over), exchanging DNA. The cell now divides into four cells, each haploid and each containing a single chromatid from the tetrad. At fertilization, when gametes fuse, the normal diploid state of 46 chromosomes is restored. These two processes, recombination and random assortment of chromosomes at fertilization, contribute to individual differences and diversity within species.

Each chromosome is divided by the centromere into two arms, termed p and q, usually of different lengths. Staining procedures of chromosomes produce pale or dark bands of varying thickness specific to each chromosome, allowing individual chromosomes or chromosomal regions to be consistently identified. A standard nomenclature is used when studying chromosomal regions. For example, a locus in the second subdivision of the first band on the p arm of chromosome 8 would be termed 8p1.2.

Molecular genetics

Molecular genetics is the branch of genetics that investigates the chemical and physical nature of genes and the mechanisms by which genes control development, growth and physiology. Each chromosome contains a molecule of DNA composed of a backbone of sugar (deoxyribose) and phosphate, the purine bases adenine (A) and guanine (G), and the pyrimidine bases cytosine (C) and thymine (T). These repeating units of five-carbon sugar, phosphate and organic bases are called nucleotides. The DNA molecule is a double helix, resembling a spiral ladder, where each side is composed of alternating deoxyribose and phosphate molecules, with pairs of bases as rungs. Because bases can pair only by forming hydrogen bonds between T and A, or G and C, the sequence of one DNA strand is dependent on the sequence of the other, and so the strands are complementary. The DNA molecule unwinds during cell division, and each strand acts as a template for the production of a new strand with a complementary sequence of nucleotides. As this new sequence forms, DNA polymerase enzymes bind deoxyribonucleotides and fit them in place with the phosphate group of each incoming nucleotide being joined enzymatically to the 3′-deoxyribose group of the previous nucleotide. Because of the number of base pairs in a chromosome, replication is initiated at many different sites along each template and the segments of newly formed DNA are joined together with phosphodiester bonds by ligase enzymes. In mammalian chromosome replication, approximately 3000 nucleotides are added per minute, with an estimated accuracy of greater than 99.98 per cent. Errors in this process are called mutations; these can be occur naturally but are also induced by external agents (mutagens) such as radiation, ultraviolet light, and various chemicals.

The information for protein production contained in

DNA is decoded (transcripted) by a similar molecule (ribonucleic acid, RNA) and transported from the nucleus to ribosomes in the cytoplasm for translation into amino acids and protein construction.

Transcription begins when a section of the DNA molecule unzips and one of the DNA strands acts as a template for synthesis of an RNA transcript. The DNA gene sequence is preceded by an upstream signal region that initiates transcription and is succeeded by a downstream region containing a termination sequence. RNA differs from DNA by being single-stranded, having ribose instead of deoxyribose as its sugar, and having uracil (U) instead of the base thymine. Within a DNA gene sequence, there may be redundant, non-coding regions (introns) and coding regions (exons). After transcription, the introns are enzymatically removed and the exons spliced together in the correct order to form functional messenger RNA (mRNA). Exons can be spliced together in many different ways, so that different gene products can be generated in different tissues from the same structural gene. The Human Genome Project has shown that it is the complexity of gene regulation and alternative splicing rather than a large increase in the number of genes that largely explains the evolution of more complex organisms.

Translation involves transfer of genetic information from mRNA into a sequence of linked amino acids to form proteins. As described above, specific three-base sequences (codons) individually code for each amino acid, and this code is the same in all living organisms. The mRNA transcript initially attaches to a ribosome. Amino acids are brought to the ribosomes by transfer RNA (tRNA) molecules, which also have specific three-base sequences (called anticodons) complementary to the codons of mRNA. Thus, mRNA is translated into the amino acid sequence when tRNA anticodons line up along mRNA codons and construct the amino acid sequence specified by the mRNA. The ribosome moves along, 'reading' the mRNA until the protein specified by the original DNA sequence has been produced.

Cells require the ability to activate or repress transcription of genes during development or in response to the environment. Proteins called transcriptional factors can bind to DNA to activate or repress transcription, and extracellular factors such as hormonal activity can also influence transcription.

Mutations

A mutation that arises during mitotic division in non-gamete cells is called a somatic mutation and is not heritable. Mutations in cells that go on to produce gametes are called germ-line mutations and may be transmitted to the next generation. The simplest form of mutation involves a single base pair (a point mutation). The term 'mutation' refers to any change in sequence or structure, but it is sometimes taken to mean a change that causes or contributes to a disease or abnormal phenotype. If the DNA variant created by a mutation event becomes common in the population over time, then it is known as a polymorphism.

Point mutations are made up of base-pair changes or the loss (deletion) or gain (insertion) of a single base. If the change occurs in the coding region of a gene, then it may produce a codon that specifies a different amino acid (missense mutation) or that changes the sequence to a stop codon, causing production of an incomplete protein (a nonsense mutation).

Deletions, insertions and inversions involve larger sequences of DNA up to the point at which they become visible cytogenetically. It has become apparent that this type of mutation (and variation) is much more common in the human genome than previously considered. These types of submicroscopic chromosomal abnormality are called copy number variations (CNVs; see page 472).

Chromosomal mutations are often lethal, as they involve a change in the number of chromosomes or the translocation or rearrangement of large sections of chromosomes. The condition where the number of chromosomes is different from the normal diploid complement of 46 is called aneuploidy. Where embryonic development is possible, the phenotypic effects of aneuploidies are often clinically recognizable. Down syndrome (caused by an extra chromosome or rarely a translocation at chromosome 21), Edwards' syndrome (trisomy 18) and Patau syndrome (trisomy 13) are examples of autosomal aneuploidies. Aneuploidies that involve extra sex chromosomes often have less biological impact, although distinct phenotypes are recognized, such as Turner's syndrome (XO, females with one X chromosome) and Kleinfelter's syndrome (XXY).

Human Genome Project and DNA variation

Despite the description about DNA variation above, in any two randomly selected human genomes 99.9 per cent of DNA sequence is identical. The 0.01 per cent that is variable accounts for the genetic contribution to individuality, susceptibility to disease and population diversity. The Human Genome Project and the subsequent HapMap project have generated vast biological and database resources, including the sequence of the human genome and a catalogue of sequence, and more recently, structural variation. To date, many millions of DNA variants have been identified and are publicly available to researchers (see www.ncbi.nlm.nih.gov/SNP) seeking to map disease or trait genes.

Mendelian inheritance

Mendelian inheritance applies to the patterns of inheritance in human diseases caused by single mutations, where the mutation is both necessary and sufficient to cause the disease and is said to have a major gene effect.

Autosomal dominant disorders are the most common Mendelian disorders (7 per 1000 live births) and are apparent in individuals having one (heterozygous) or two (homozygous) mutant genes. Such conditions will, on average, affect half of all individuals in a sibship. If a proband has a dominant disorder, then one of their parents will also be affected, unless the disorder represents a new mutation. The extent to which a heterozygote shows features of the disorder is described as the penetrance of the condition; for example, the Huntington's mutation has an age-related penetration of almost 100 per cent.

Autosomal recessive disorders are less common (< 3 per 1000 live births), partly because the disorder is expressed only if the individual has two copies of the mutated gene. As with dominant disorders, the extent of expression depends on the penetrance of the mutations. If both parents are heterozygous for the mutant gene, then on average one in four children will be affected, as is the case in cystic fibrosis, for example.

X- (or sex-) linked disorders arise from mutations of the sex chromosomes and follow different inheritance patterns because males can only pass on their Y chromosomes to sons. Most X-linked conditions are recessive. A heterozygotic mother may pass on the mutant gene to her son, and he will be affected, while a heterozygote sister of the son will be a carrier. Affected males transmit the carrier state to half of their daughters but do not transmit the disease to their sons, as is the case with Duchenne muscular dystrophy.

Mitochondrial disorders are rare single-gene disorders caused by mutations in a mitochondrial gene. These follow a distinct maternal inheritance pattern because mitochondrial DNA in fertilized embryos is acquired exclusively from the ovum, as sperm do not contain mitochondria.

COMPLEX MODELS OF INHERITANCE

Common biological traits and behaviours are not categorical but are distributed quantitatively in the general population. These are likely to be determined by the interaction between many genes and the environment. Each gene (strictly speaking, each gene variant) contributes a small incremental effect, and these are known as genes of minor effect. Genes or locations on the genome that contribute to biological traits or behaviours that display these characteristics are called quantitative trait loci (QTLs).

Many common disorders with a demonstrated genetic component are thought to be due predominantly to genes of minor effect, which are neither necessary nor sufficient to cause the disorder but increase risk. Each minor or risk gene may have an effect independent of all other genes (an additive component), effects that are dependent on the other allele at that locus (a dominant interaction), or effects that are influenced by genotype at other loci (epistatic interactions). The proportion of the total variance of a trait in a population explained by additive genetic effects is called its heritability (h^2).

MOLECULAR GENETICS: TECHNIQUES AND TERMINOLOGY

Recombinant DNA technology

Recombinant DNA technology, or molecular cloning, is an umbrella term for the process of introducing a gene from an organism into a host cell, where it can be replicated and studied. When two different DNA samples are mixed together in the presence of a DNA ligase enzyme, the two ends anneal, forming a new DNA sequence that can be inserted into a cloning vector, often a plasmid, a small circular piece of DNA found naturally in bacteria and other organisms. This vector, when inserted into a host bacterial cell, replicates with the bacteria when cultured, allowing millions of copies of the original DNA sequence to be obtained (cloned).

Polymerase chain reaction: enzymatic DNA amplification

In the PCR, small pieces of DNA, called oligonucleotide primers, are chemically synthesized to be complementary to the DNA on either side of the sequence to be amplified. Mixing these primers with DNA containing the sequence to be amplified, a supply of individual nucleotides and a heat-stable DNA polymerase enzyme at a suitable temperature, these primers bind to their complementary sequences on each strand. Next, the individual DNA bases extend along the strand reforming the double helix. On heating to over 90 °C, the strands separate and the process begins again, with twice the number of molecules at the target. This procedure is automated by machines that cycle the reaction mixture through at the different temperatures to produce a large number of copies of the target DNA sequence.

Genotyping

Newer methods of detecting DNA variation have developed rapidly over the past 10 years, at least in part due to the Human Genome Project and HapMap. Using the DNA 'chip' technologies, the genotypes at thousands and even millions of locations across an individual's genome can now be produced rapidly. Recent developments include specialized chips designed to identify DNA CNVs across the genome. CNVs are now thought to contribute a substantial component of risk for many common disorders, including neuropsychiatric disorders.

Genomics and bioinformatics

Genetics is the study of individual genes and their effects. Genomics is the study of the functions and interactions of all the genes in the genome. Bioinformatics is a new science that has evolved to cope with the growing banks of molecular sequence and structural data. This involves computational methods for retrieval and analysis of data, including algorithms for sequence similarity searches, and prediction of the structure and function of genes. The available bioinformatics resources are now so extensive that, coupled with the increasing public availability of raw genomic data from government-funded research, much genetics research is being conducted in silico.

CONFIRMING A GENETIC CONTRIBUTION TO DISEASE: FAMILY, TWIN AND ADOPTION STUDIES SUPPORTING GENOMIC RESEARCH

Family studies can demonstrate that a disorder is familial, occurring more commonly in relatives of a proband than in the general population. This information can be collected either by taking a detailed family history from affected individuals or their relatives (the family history method), or more rigorously by using a family study approach, where all affected individuals are directly interviewed. Familiality may be due to shared genes or shared environment. For example, speaking the same language or going to medical school/being a doctor are familial but are due (mostly) to shared environment. Two natural forms of biological and social experiment, namely twin births and adoption, allow some separation of genetic and environmental effects.

Twin studies

Monozygotic (MZ) twins arise from a single fertilized ovum and so share identical genomes. Dizygotic (DZ) twins develop from different ova and, like any full siblings, share on average 50 per cent of their genes. Twin research assumes that twins share environmental effects equally. If both twins have a disease, then they are said to be concordant for that condition, but if only one twin is affected, then they are described as discordant. Higher concordance of disease in MZ twins than in DZ twins is strong evidence of a genetic contribution to disease, but there are several caveats. Ascertainment bias at recruitment is a potential flaw, but researchers try to overcome this problem by exploiting national or local twin registers to systematically screen all twin births. Twin studies assume that twins within a family share the same environment. This may not be completely true: environmental factors, including prenatal nutrition and birth trauma, may differ between twins. Being a twin in itself may contribute to illness.

Adoption studies

These studies examine the effect of being adopted into or out of a family with a specific disorder using a variety of designs. Adopted children who become ill may be identified and rates of illness compared in their adoptive and biological families (the adoptee family method). Adoption can also be studied prospectively, by using the parent as the proband. In this adoptee study method, the rates of illness in adopted offspring of affected individuals are compared with rates in adopted offspring of individuals without the disorder. As with twin studies, there are caveats. A child having affected biological parents may influence potential adoptive parents; adopted children may experience particular intrauterine effects; age at adoption is often overlooked; and adoption is a rare event.

If independent evidence from family, twin and adoption studies points to a significant genetic component for a disease or a trait, then it is reasonable to assume that one exists. An examination of the pattern of transmission in families coupled with twin results and general population frequency may suggest a particular Mendelian mode of inheritance or point to more complex patterns, including oligogenic models (5–20 genes) or polygenic models with hundreds of genes, each of very small effect. Genetic heterogeneity is also possible, with different genes causing the same or a similar disorder in different families, and mixed models are also likely. Few of these models can be determined conclusively in advance of molecular genetic studies.

QUANTITATIVE AND MATHEMATICAL ASPECTS OF GENETICS

Hardy–Weinberg law

This law states that the frequencies of alleles will, in the presence of random mating and in the absence of disturbances including mutation, natural selection, migration, inbreeding and random genetic drift, remain constant from generation to generation. Thus, let two polymorphic alleles A and a exist in a population. If their frequencies of occurrence (expressed in decimals) are p and q, respectively, then $p + q = 1$, and if mating between individuals is random, then after one generation the frequencies of the three genotypes will be p^2, $2pq$ and q^2. This generation will produce gametes A and a with frequencies p and q, similar to the previous generation. A sample of individuals is said to be in Hardy–Weinberg equilibrium if the frequencies of the observed genotypes AA, Aa and aa are statistically the same as the expected frequencies derived from allele frequencies using the above formula.

Recombination fraction

The process of recombination occurs during meiosis and, according to Mendel's second law, polymorphic DNA variants on separate chromosomes will segregate independently of each other. Even on the same chromosome, many variants will segregate independently if they are physically separated along the chromosome by some distance. The recombination fraction is defined as the number of recombinant gametes divided by the total number of gametes and, for independently segregating variants, takes the value 0.5. This measure is termed Morgans and 50 cM is the value relating to independent segregation between to variants (or between a variant and a disease mutation). This means that if the recombination fraction (θ) between two loci is less than 0.5, then they are not independently segregating and instead are linked, meaning in physical terms that they lie close together on the same chromosome. Genetic distance in cM is closely but not completely correlated with physical distance, because the probability of recombination varies across the genome. 1 cM is the genetic distance corresponding to a recombination fraction (θ) of 0.01, which is roughly equivalent to 1 million base pairs of DNA. The analysis of recombination in families is used in linkage analysis to identify polymorphic DNA variants that are linked to the disease mutation ($\theta < 0.5$), thus showing the approximate location of the mutation. Linkage analysis estimates θ and tests whether it is significantly less than 0.5. The conventional statistical method of doing this is to calculate a log of the odds (LOD) score. This is the common logarithm of the probability that the recombination fraction θ has some given value, divided by the probability that the value is 0.5. Where the mode of inheritance is known and the phenotype can be clearly defined, a LOD score of 3.0 (odds in favour of linkage 1000 : 1) is accepted as statistical proof of linkage and a score of −2.0 (odds against of 100 : 1) as proof of exclusion of linkage. However, the LOD score takes Bayesian theory into account, whereby the prior odds that two loci are linked is about 1 : 50. The observed odds ratio (OR) of a LOD score of 3 is 1000 : 1, leading to a posterior probability of about 20 : 1, roughly equivalent to a *P* value of 0.05. The LOD score method depends partly on the specified model of inheritance of the disease mutation and so may be less reliable when the model is unknown.

GENETIC ASSOCIATION METHODS AND LINKAGE DISEQUILIBRIUM

In their simplest form, association studies look for differences in allele frequencies between populations of patients and healthy controls. If the patient population has a specific allele more frequently than the control population, then that allele is said to be associated with the disorder. It is important to match populations carefully for studies of this type, because different allele frequencies among ethnic groups, called population stratification, can cause false positive results. To avoid this difficulty, many studies use ethnically homogeneous populations or a family-based approach including the non-transmitted parental allele as the control group. This design tests for departure from Mendel's first law. Until recently, association studies were hypothesis-driven and selected potential candidate genes or DNA variants based on genes associated with known biological systems. However, with technological advances, it has been possible to take a genome-wide hypothesis free approach. Apart from the technological advances required, this approach is also possible because of the presence of linkage disequilibrium (LD) within populations. LD is a form of linkage where the 'pedigree' selected is the entire population and the number of generations is unknown. If two genetic variants are in very close proximity, then they are said to be in LD when recombination between them is rare, even over many generations. Thus, a limited selection of DNA variants can statistically represent the majority of variation in the genome. Current DNA chips contain up to 1 million variants and the coverage of sequence variation is constantly improving.

CHROMOSOMAL ABNORMALITIES

Structural chromosomal abnormalities can result from deletions (part of the genetic material is lost), duplications (a portion of the chromosome is duplicated, leading to extra genetic material), inversions (a chromosomal rearrangement in which a segment of the chromosome is reversed), insertions (a portion of one chromosome is inserted into another chromosome) and translocations (reciprocal translocation occurs when there is exchange of material between two different chromosomes). Studying such chromosomal abnormalities in people with mental illness can lead to identification of candidate genes and help to refine areas of linkage.

Deletions and micro-deletion syndromes

Velocardiofacial syndrome (VCFS), Prader–Willi syndrome and Angelman syndrome are commonly caused by micro-deletions.

Velocardiofacial syndrome

In more than 90 per cent of cases, VCFS is caused by a hemizygous micro-deletion in chromosome 22q11.2. The phenotype of the syndrome is diverse but is of particular interest to psychiatry because of the behavioural and psychiatric aspects of the condition. Between 10 per cent and 30 per cent of individuals with VCFS are diagnosed with schizophrenia, bipolar affective disorder (BPAD), autism spectrum disorder or schizoaffective disorder. Attention deficit hyperactivity disorder (ADHD) and poor social skills are also observed at a higher than expected frequency in VCFS. Estimates of prevalence of VCFS vary, but it is thought to occur in 1 in 4000 live births.[1] The disorder can be inherited in an autosomal dominant fashion, but de novo mutations are more common. A large study investigating the cause of the deletion has reported that it appears to result from aberrant meiotic interchromosomal exchange.[2] The deleted region of 22q11.2 associated with VCFS contains approximately 35 genes. Within this deletion, the *TBX1* gene is thought to be largely responsible for the phenotype of VCFS. This gene plays a relatively clear role in cardiac development, but its influence on the behavioural and psychiatric phenotype is less well understood. Catechol-O-methyltransferase is another gene in the deleted region that been implicated in the psychiatric manifestation of the disorder.

Prader–Willi syndrome and Angelman syndrome

Prader–Willi syndrome and Angelman syndrome are rare neurogenetic disorders that result from loss of expression of paternal (Prader–Willi syndrome) or maternal (Angelman syndrome) genes on chromosome 15q11–13. Prevalence of Angelman syndrome is estimated to be between 1 in 20 000 and 1 in 10 000 live births, and prevalence of Prader–Willi syndrome is estimated to be between 1 in 15 000 and 1 in 12 000 live births.

Molecular mechanisms that can lead to the imbalance between maternal and paternal gene expression include micro-deletions, point mutations, uniparental disomy and imprinting. Micro-deletions are the most common cause of Prader–Willi syndrome and Angelman syndrome. Uniparental disomy occurs when a person receives two copies of a chromosome, or part of a chromosome, from one parent and no copies from the other parent. This is thought to account for about 20–30 per cent of cases. Imprinting refers to the phenomenon whereby genes are expressed only from the allele inherited from the mother or the father. Imprinting defects in Prader–Willi syndrome and Angelman syndrome are thought to result from abnormal methlyation status of important regions in the Prader–Willi syndrome/Angelman syndrome imprinting centre.

The most common genetic abnormality in Angelman syndrome is a maternal deletion of a region on chromosome 15q11–q13, which results in loss of functional expression of the gene *UBE3A*. This gene codes for an enzyme called ubiquitin protein ligase 3A, which attaches ubiquitin protein to proteins that should be degraded. However, the molecular mechanisms leading to the phenotype in Angelman syndrome are not yet understood.

In Prader–Willi syndrome, the majority (about 75%) of cases are due to de novo deletion of a region on the paternal chromosome 15q11–q13, with subsequent loss of functional expression of paternal copies of the small nuclear ribonucleoprotein polypeptide N (*SNRPN*) gene and *necdin* gene among others. The role of these genes is not well understood. The protein encoded by the *necdin* gene may suppress growth in postmitotic neurons, but to date little is known about how it influences the phenotype in Prader–Willi syndrome.

Translocation disrupting *DISC1* gene

Disrupted-in-schizophrenia 1 (*DISC1*) is a gene whose mutant truncation is associated with major psychiatric illness, in particular schizophrenia. Cytogenetic, linkage and association studies have identified the *DISC1* gene on chromosome 1 as a positional candidate conferring susceptibility to schizophrenia. *DISC1* may play a role in the regulation of cytoskeletal function. The variant of *DISC1* affects neuronal functions such as migration and intracellular transport, as these require intact cytoskeletal function.

Duplications and unstable repeat disorders

An interstitial duplication on chromosome 15 – dup(15)(q24q26) – has been associated with panic disorder, agoraphobia, social phobia, simple phobia and joint laxity.[3]

There are many nucleotide repeat sequences in the human genome. Pathogenic duplication, or expansion, of such repeat sequences results in a number of neuropsychiatric disorders including fragile X, myotonic dystrophy, Friedrich's ataxia, spinal and bulbar muscular atrophy, Huntington's disease, the spinocerebellar ataxias, dentatorubral-pallidoluysian atrophy and Machado–Joseph disease.

Unstable repeats can be coding (resulting in altered protein function) or non-coding (resulting in loss of protein function or altered RNA function). Unstable CAG repeats cause alteration of protein function in a number of disorders, including most of the spinocerebellar atrophies, Huntington's disease, dentatorubral-pallidoluysian atrophy and spinal and bulbar muscular atrophy. For example, Huntington's disease is caused by multiple copies (> 35 repeats) of a trinucleotide repeat sequence (CAG) within the coding region of the *huntingtin* gene on chromosome 4; the mutation leads to an abnormally expanded polyglutamine tract in huntingtin. Unstable trinucleotide repeats in fragile X syndrome (CGG repeat), fragile X syndrome E (CCG repeat) and Friedrich's ataxia (GAA repeat) result in loss of protein function (FMR1, FMR2 and FRDA proteins).

The myotonic dystrophies are caused by trinucleotide (CTG) and tetranucleotide (CCTG) expansions, which result in altered RNA function. Fragile X tremor/ataxia syndrome also results from an expanded repeat (CGG), which alters RNA function. In a number of other disorders, including some of the spinocerebellar atrophies, the pathogenesis of the nucleotide repeats remains unknown.

Genetic anticipation occurs in many of the nucleotide expansion disorders. This refers to the effect whereby a parent carrying a copy of the gene with a moderate number of repeats may not exhibit any (or only minor) symptoms of the disorder, and yet when the gene is inherited by their child the number of repeats expands dramatically, leading to disease manifestation at a young age.

Inversions

An inversion of chromosome 9 – inv(9)(p11q13) – has been associated with schizophrenia in a number of studies.[4]

Insertions

Insertion of 2q11.2–q21.1 into 8p21.3, leading to a partial trisomy of 2q, has been associated with schizoaffective disorder, psychotic illness and learning disability.[5]

Translocations

A reciprocal translocation – t(1;11)(q42;q14.3) – is associated with schizophrenia, BPAD and major depression.[6] Bipolar disorder and unipolar depression have also been associated with a reciprocal translocation between chromosomes 9 and 11 – t(9;11)(p24;q23.1).[7] Another reciprocal translocation – t(18;21)(p11.1;p11.1) – has been associated with schizophrenia, psychotic episodes and paranoid traits in one family.[8]

Copy number variants

A CNV is a structural chromosomal abnormality characterized by variation in the number of copies of a particular gene or sequences of DNA in a person's genome. Normally, humans have two copies of each region of the genome, one per chromosome. CNVs may be inherited, may result from aberrant replication, or may be caused by mutations including deletions, duplications, inversions, insertions and translocations. It is now thought that CNVs may have a significant influence on susceptibility to a number of common diseases, including neuropsychiatric conditions. CNVs have been reported in autism and schizophrenia (see below), and work is ongoing in the search for CNVs in other psychiatric conditions.

CLINICAL GENETIC SERVICES

In the UK and Ireland, there are centres providing clinical genetic services. In general, these services include genetic counselling, clinical cytogenetics and molecular genetics. Prenatal genetic testing may also be offered.

Genetic counselling

Genetic counselling has both a diagnostic and a supportive role and is offered to individuals with a genetic disorder or relatives at risk of developing a genetic disorder. People attending genetic counselling are provided with information about the causes and consequences of the disorder. The risk of developing and transmitting the condition is evaluated, and the options available in terms of tests, treatment or prevention are outlined and discussed in a supportive environment.

Clinical cytogenetics

In clinical cytogenetics, the chromosome complement of an individual is analysed to determine whether there is a change from the expected number of 46 chromosomes or whether there is a change in chromosome structure that could be of pathological significance.

Clinical molecular genetics

Molecular biological techniques are used to investigate individual genetic abnormalities associated with specific genetic disorders. Molecular genetic tests can be used to confirm or exclude diagnosis of a genetic disorder in a symptomatic individual, or to assess carrier status in asymptomatic relatives. However, molecular genetic testing is not used widely in psychiatric conditions because of the genetic complexity of the majority of these disorders.

Prenatal genetic testing

Prenatal genetic testing refers to screening for genetic conditions in a fetus before it is born. Chromosomal abnormalities (e.g. Down syndrome) and molecular genetic abnormalities (e.g. in cystic fibrosis) can be detected.

ETHICS IN GENETICS RESEARCH

There are a number of ethical issues in genetics research that differ from those that arise in other kinds of clinical research. These include privacy and confidentiality, informed consent and risks of harm.

Privacy and confidentiality are extremely important, due to the risk of bias, discrimination and stigma that could result if a person's genetic information were disclosed. It is essential that genetic researchers clearly inform study participants of all individuals or institutions who will have access to their data. DNA samples for research are commonly stored in repositories called DNA banks. Commonly, genetic researchers unlink personal identifiers from genetic data to reduce the threat to privacy and confidentiality.

In order to meet the criteria for informed consent, participants must be adequately informed, be free from coercion or undue influence, and be competent. In genetic research, it is often difficult to decide how much information is adequate; it is equally difficult to describe the risks of harm associated with the research. Risks in genetic research are generally not physical but instead are psychological, social or economic. For example, genetic testing can cause significant anxiety before and after testing, and disclosure of results could result in discrimination and stigmatization or increased cost of health/life insurance. In addition, family members of the participant may face similar problems even if they are not involved in the study. It has been suggested by many that genetic counselling should be mandatory in future genetic research in order to ensure fully informed consent. To give informed consent, the participant must understand the purpose of the research; how and where the specimens will be stored; who will have access to the information from the samples; whether the samples are anonymous or are linked to the participants with a code; whether the participants will be contacted about study findings; and whether the research will be used to develop any products for financial gain.

PRINCIPAL INHERITED CONDITIONS IN PSYCHIATRY

Alzheimer's disease

Epidemiology

Alzheimer's disease (AD) is the most common cause of dementia. Prevalence rises steeply from 5 per cent in the age group 65 years and older, to 22 per cent among those aged 95 years and older.[9] Women are at slightly higher risk of the disease, and it is more common in Europe and North America than in Asian countries.

Family, twin and adoption studies

Family studies and twin studies suggest a genetic aetiology. The risk of developing Alzheimer's disease is increased approximately 3.5-fold in first-degree relatives of probands with AD, and 25 per cent of people who develop late-onset AD have had a close relative with dementia.[10] Twin studies have reported an estimated heritability of AD of up to 80 per cent.[11] The disease appears to be a complex and genetically heterogeneous disorder.

Chromosomal abnormalities

Mutations in three genes – amyloid precursor protein (*APP*), presenilin 1 (*PSEN1*) and presenilin 2 (*PSEN2*) – are associated with rare forms of autosomal-dominant early-onset AD. APP is a cell-membrane protein cleaved by three proteolytic enzymes called secretases. Mutations in the *APP* gene on chromosome 21 cluster near sites where the beta-amyloid peptide is cleaved from APP (at beta and gamma secretase sites) and also where the beta-amyloid peptide itself is cleaved (alpha secretase site). Mutations in *PSEN1* (chromosome 14) and *PSEN2* (chromosome 1) affect the gamma-secretase cleavage of beta-amyloid from APP. The net result of mutations in these three genes is that proteolytic processing of the protein is disrupted and there is an increase in the deposition of abnormal beta-amyloid in the brain. The amyloid cascade hypothesis of AD holds that the formation of abnormal beta-amyloid is the primary deficit in the disorder, which leads to all other pathology (tau aggregation and phosphorylation, neuronal loss and cholinergic deficits).

Molecular genetics

Interestingly, mutations in *APP*, *PSN1* and *PSN2* have not been found in the more common late-onset AD, despite the fact that family history is the largest risk factor for AD. The only clearly identified genetic risk factor for late-onset AD involves the apolipoprotein E (*APOE*) gene. This gene has three common alleles (E2, E3, E4) and thus six possible genotypes. Presence of the *APOE4* allele is a susceptibility gene for AD, and it influences age of onset of the disorder. The most common genotype in the general population is E3/E3. In white people, E4/E4 genotype is associated with a significantly (15-fold) increased risk of AD compared with E3/E3 genotype. The E2/E4 and E3/E4 genotypes are also associated with an increased risk of AD (approximately three-fold). The E2 alleles are protective compared with E3/E3, with a reduction in risk of about 40 per cent. The pathogenic mechanism of the E4 allele is not fully understood. Higher serum cholesterol is reported in people with the E4 genotype, and altered lipid metabolism might affect AD pathogenesis. The APOE4 protein might also have differential binding to amyloid and tau proteins. However, many people without the *APOE4* allele develop AD, and many people with the *APOE4* risk allele do not develop AD.

Linkage studies

It is thought likely that there are at least four risk genes for AD that have not yet been localized,[12] and the search for these susceptibility genes is ongoing. For the more common, late-onset form of AD, a large number of chromosomal regions linked to or associated with the disease have been discovered, but their underlying genes have not been identified unequivocally. Large genetic linkage analysis studies have reported linkage at regions of chromosomes 6, 9, 10, 12 and 19.[13] However, investigation of these regions has not resulted in the identification of a definitive 'Alzheimer's gene'.

Association studies

A meta-analysis of all the genetic association studies in autism reported over a dozen potential Alzheimer susceptibility genes.[14] These authors have created a publicly available, continuously updated database that comprehensively catalogues all genetic association studies in the field of AD (www.alzgene.org).

Animal models

Animal models have been useful in unravelling the molecular pathogenesis of AD (see Gottz and Ittner[15] for a review). Much work has been carried out in transgenic mice, Drosphila (fruit flies) and nematodes. Work on animal models has yielded a number of important findings and identified therapeutic targets. For example, reduction of the intracellular protein tau was found to block beta-amyloid toxicity in mice models. Reduction of tau levels can be achieved by vaccination against tau in a mouse model, and it will be exciting to see whether this strategy will be safe and effective in humans. Abnormal beta-amyloid has also been targeted using vaccination strategies in animal models. An early trial in humans was discontinued prematurely after a number of participants developed meningoencephalitis. However, new vaccinations are under investigation and reports are eagerly awaited. The role of diet has also been investigated using mouse models, with reports that caloric restriction, the antioxidant ginkgo biloba and omega-3 polyunsaturated fatty acids are all associated with reduction of beta-amyloid.

Schizophrenia

Epidemiology

Schizophrenia affects between 0.5 per cent and 1 per cent of the population at some stage in their lives. It has a point prevalence of three to five cases per 1000. It is equally common in males and females, but with a peak onset of symptoms between age 15 and 25 years in males and between 20 and 30 years in females. It occurs in all parts of the world with approximately equal frequency. There is some evidence to suggest that the incidence of the disorder has decreased over recent decades.[16] There is a well-replicated seasonal variation in the birth rates of people who later develop the disease, with an excess in the late spring and early summer in the northern hemisphere.

Family, twin and adoption studies

Schizophrenia is a highly familial disorder. Lifetime risk for schizophrenia in first-degree relatives is 10–15 per cent; in monozygotic twins, it is about 50 per cent, as it is in the offspring of two parents with schizophrenia. Risk for monozygotic twins (40–60%) compared with risk for dizygotic twins (10–15%) suggests a heritability of approximately 80 per cent. Adoption studies have supported a genetic risk, with risk to biological offspring of schizophrenic parents greater than risk to adopted offspring, and risk in biological parents of adoptees who develop schizophrenia greater than risk in adoptive parents. Segregation analysis supports a polygenic, complex genetic aetiology in most affected families. The standard linkage approach to identify susceptibility loci of moderate effect may lack statistical power even for samples with thousands of families. Association studies of schizophrenia have a low prior probability because the neuropathology of schizophrenia is unknown (meaning that there are thousands of plausible candidates).

Chromosomal abnormalities

Cytogenetic studies have reported numerous associations between schizophrenia and chromosomal mutations such as translocations, inversions, deletions and trisomies. Because schizophrenia is relatively common, many may be coincidental. However, chromosome 22q deletions are more common in individuals with schizophrenia, and expression of the chromosome 22q deletion phenotype (VCFS) increases risk of psychosis. Strong evidence for linkage has also been reported for a balanced (1;11)(q42.1;q14.3) translocation that segregates with schizophrenia and related psychiatric disorders in a large Scottish pedigree.[17] This translocation disrupted a previously unknown gene on chromosome 1 (*DISC1*) expressed in the brain and involved in neurodevelopment. A translocation between chromosomes 1 and 16 in another family disrupts the phosphodiesterase-4 type B gene (*PDE4B*), the protein product of which is a binding partner to the DISC1 protein.

Molecular genetics: linkage studies

Many genome-wide linkage scans of schizophrenia have been performed. Individually, these have provided evidence suggestive of linkage to many different loci. A meta-analysis of these studies ($n \approx 2000$ affected individuals) provided statistical evidence that a number of these loci (including chromosome 6p, 8p and 22q) are true positive findings.[18] Linkage studies on a sample of Irish high-density schizophrenia families have identified linkage on chromosome 6p22.3, where later the Dysbindin gene was identified by genetic association,[19] and on chromosome 8p21–22 in Irish and Icelandic families, where later the Neuregulin 1 gene was identified.[20] Gene expression studies have also contributed to advances in the molecular genetics of schizophrenia. This approach looks for differences in expression of genes in postmortem brain tissue between affected individuals and controls. A review of 25 genome-wide linkage studies suggests eight chromosome regions with suggestive linkage evidence that contain promising candidate genes (in brackets) including 22q12–q13 (*COMT*, *PRODH2*, *ZDHHC8*), 8p22–p21 (*NRG1*, *PPP3CC*), 6p24–p22 (*DTNBP1*), 13q14–q32 (*G72*, *DAAO*), 6q21–q22 (*TRAR4*), 1q32–42 (*DISC1*) and 1q21–q22 (*RGS4*).

Molecular genetics: association studies

The literature on association studies in schizophrenia is very large. The Schizophrenia Forum hosts a database of potential candidate genes for schizophrenia emerging from association studies published in peer-reviewed journals.[21] There are 730 different gene/reference entries to date, showing the complexity of the task of making sense of the literature. Early candidate genes studies focused out of necessity on a limited number of genes and hypotheses, such as the dopamine hypothesis and the dopamine D2 and other receptor genes. These studies were limited, both by the lack of strength of the a priori hypothesis and by the sample sizes studied. Many studies reporting nominal evidence for association were followed by several negative reports. Stronger hypotheses have emerged, backed by linkage evidence (*NRG1*, *DTNBP1*, *G72*, *DAAO*) or cytogenetic evidence (*DISC1*). A meta-analysis of 12 'top' candidate genes selected from the Schizophrenia Forum database found genome-wide significant allelic association for seven, all with very small ORs for the associated risk allele. Statistical power and rigour, strong biological hypotheses and supportive genetic evidence may go some way to dissociate signal from noise in this literature.

Genome-wide association studies

These studies are under way and a small number have been reported to date. The first used a small sample but reported strong evidence for association with (colony-stimulating factor 2 receptor, type A (*CSF2RA*).[22] The second used a pooling strategy and identified a strong but not genome-wide significant signal in the coiled coil domain (*CCDC60*).[23] The Clinical Antipsychotic Trials of Intervention Effectiveness (CATIE) project reported a preliminary genome-wide association study of 738 cases and 733 controls, but with no signal reaching genome-wide significance.[24] O'Donovan and colleagues carried out a genome-wide association study of 479 cases and 2937 controls and followed up those signals with $P < 10^{-5}$ in more than 16000 additional cases and controls.[25] Of 12 loci followed up, three had strong independent support ($P < 5 \times 10^{-4}$), with the strongest reaching genome-wide significance at zinc finger protein 804A (*ZNF804A*).

Copy number variants

Smaller, submicroscopic CNVs have been shown to be more common in schizophrenia measured as total burden,[26] and at particular positions on the genome. More recently, two regions of the genome, one on chromosome 1q21.1 and another on chromosome 15q13.3, have been shown to occur in a small number of cases of schizophrenia at a frequency of similar order to the VCFS deletions.[27,28] Surprisingly, these deletions and their reciprocal duplications, are also found to cause a wide array of neurodevelopmental phenotypes, including mental retardation, minor physical abnormalities, cardiac abnormalities and autism.[29,30] The 1q21.1 and 15q13.3 CNVs are large at approximately 1.35 Mb and 1.5 Mb respectively, each containing many genes, including the A7 subunit of the nicotinic acetylcholine receptor (*CHRNA7*) gene on 15q, previously reported as showing evidence for linkage with schizophrenia. It is also becoming clear that small CNVs may disrupt individual genes, with a report from Rujescu and colleagues describing small (18–420 kb) deletions and duplications involving neurexin 1 (*NRXN1*) in approximately one in 200 cases of schizophrenia compared with 1 in 660 controls.[31]

Bipolar affective disorder

Epidemiology

BPAD is characterized by extreme mood dysregulation, with repeated episodes of elevated or depressed mood. BPAD occurs in 0.5–1 per cent of the population. The male/female ratio is equal.

Family, twin and adoption studies

Family, twin and adoption studies consistently indicate a strong genetic component to BPAD. Heritability of BPAD is high, in the region of 85 per cent.[32] Twin studies show a markedly elevated concordance rate of BPAD in monozygotic compared with dizygotic twins – 40 per cent versus 5 per cent.[32] BPAD is more common among biological parents than adoptive parents of adoptees with BPAD.[33] The mode of inheritance is unknown but is probably due to a number of genes, each of small effect.

Molecular genetics: linkage studies

A number of areas of the genome have repeatedly shown linkage with bipolar disorder. Some of these regions (4p16.1, 11p15.5, 12q24.31, 18p11.21, 21q22.2–3, 22q12.3) are particularly interesting because they contain genes that have been identified in association studies of BPAD. Linkage has also been replicated for regions of chromosome 5, 6, 8, 10, 13, 17, 18, 20 and the X chromosome, but these regions do not contain genes that have been implicated in association studies on BPAD (see Serretti and Madelli[34] for a review).

Molecular genetics: association studies

There have been an enormous number of studies over the past 20 years seeking to find the risk gene(s) for BPAD. There are now a number of genes that appear to be consistently associated with the disorder, including *SLC6A4*, *TPH2*, *DRD4*, *SLC6A3*, *DAOA*, *DTNBP1*, *NRG1*, *DISC1* and *BDNF*, which are discussed in more detail below. Other promising genes include *DRD1*, *HTR1A*, *HTR2A*, *HTR2C*, *COMT*, *MAOA*, *GABRA1* and *GABRA5* (see Serretti and Madelli[34] for a review).

One of the most widely studied genes in BPAD is the serotonin transporter gene (*SLC6A4*). This gene is located on chromosome 17 and is a strong functional candidate gene. The serotonin transporter coded for by the *SLC6A4* gene is a single protein responsible for serotonin uptake into presynaptic neurons. Tricyclic antidepressants and selective serotonin reuptake inhibitors (SSRIs) reduce serotonin reuptake by preventing serotonin binding to the protein. Variants of the promoter region of this gene affect transcriptional efficiency of the serotonin transporter protein. The neuronal tryptophan hydroxylase gene (*TPH2*) located on chromosome 12 codes for a rate-limiting enzyme in the synthesis of serotonin in the central nervous system. Genetic polymorphisms within this gene have been associated with BPAD in a number of studies.

Dopamine plays a key role in the regulation of emotion and motivation, and two genes involved in the dopamine system have shown consistent association with BPAD. *DRD4* located on chromosome 11 (11p15.5) codes for the D4 subtype of the dopamine receptor. Variants of the *DRD4* gene have shown association with BPAD in a number of studies. The dopamine transporter gene (*SLC6A3*/*DAT*), which has been mapped to 5p15.3, codes for a protein that mediates dopamine reuptake, and variants of this gene have shown association with BPAD.

The glutamate system has not been investigated widely in BPAD. However, two genes involved in the glutamatergic system have shown consistent association with BPAD. D-Amino acid oxidase activator (*DAOA*/*G72*) is a strong positional candidate gene in BPAD in that it is located in a region in positive linkage with BPAD (13q33.2).[35] A number of studies have shown association of this gene with BPAD. The biological mechanism is not understood, but *DAOA* is involved with the activation of *N*-methyl-D-aspartate (NMDA) receptors, a type of glutamate receptor.

Genetic association studies have provided strong evidence to support the theory that DNA variation at the *neuregulin*, *BDNF* and *DISC1* genes confers susceptibility to BPAD. These genes are all thought to play a role in cell growth or cell maintenance. A number of single nucleotide polymorphisms (SNPs) within the neuregulin 1 (*NRG1*) gene appear to be associated with BPAD. The mechanism by which neuregulin may influence disease susceptibility is unknown. It is hypothesized that abnormal neuregulin may lead to abnormal myelination, alter expression and activity of neurotransmitters, or cause synaptic destabilization. There is mounting evidence (11 studies to date) confirming an association between brain-derived neurotrophic factor (*BDNF*) and BPAD. This gene is located at 11p13, and the BDNF protein coded for is a neuronal growth factor that plays an important role in growth, development and survival of neuronal populations. A novel study demonstrated the potential functional importance of this gene. Poorer episodic memory and reduced hippocampal activation on functional magnetic resonance imaging (fMRI) were shown to be associated with a variant (val to met polymorphism) of this gene.[36] In addition, transcription of BDNF is modulated by antidepressants. BDNF has also been implicated in unipolar depression.

Linkage and association studies have identified the *DISC1* gene on chromosome 1 as a positional candidate conferring susceptibility to BPAD. This gene is located in 1q42.1. It is thought that *DISC1* may regulate cytoskeletal function. The variant of *DISC1* may therefore affect neuronal functions such as migration and intracellular transport, as these require intact cytoskeletal function.

Genome-wide association studies

Researchers at the National Institute of Mental Health (NIMH) have published a genome-wide association study in BPAD in which they report association with diacylglycerol kinase eta (*DGKH*) and several other genes in the aetiology of bipolar disorder.[37] The *DGKH* gene is particularly interesting, as it codes for a key enzyme in the lithium-sensitive phosphatidyl inositol pathway. In the landmark genome-wide association study carried out by the Wellcome Trust Case Control Consortium (WTCCC), there was only one association in BPAD (on 16p12) that met criteria for significance.[38] Results from a subsequent genome-wide association study have been compared with those of the WTCCC, and the report suggests that there are concordant signals for SNPs within the voltage-dependent calcium channel, L-type, alpha 1C subunit (*CACNA1C*) gene.[39] Since then, another genome-wide association study has identified association with *CACNA1C*.[40] Another gene, ankyrin G (*ANK3*), also showed significant association with BPAD. The authors theorize that dysfunction of ion channels may be involved in pathogenesis of bipolar disorder.[40]

Unipolar depression

Epidemiology

Unipolar depression or major depressive disorder is characterized by pervasive low mood, loss of interest and anhedonia. It is thought to be a multifactorial disorder involving predisposing personality traits, genetics and precipitating stressful life events. Point prevalence for unipolar depression is approximately 6 per cent.

Family, twin and adoption studies

Heritability is estimated to be 30–40 per cent when cases are ascertained from population surveys; however, heritability estimates are much higher (up to 70%) when probands with unipolar depression are ascertained from hospital or clinic settings (i.e. in more severe cases). Twin studies show that concordance rates for monozygotic twins are about 40 per cent and for dizygotic twins about 20 per cent.

An interesting consistent finding regarding the familiality of affective disorders is that first-degree relatives of probands with bipolar disorder have an increased risk of bipolar disorder and unipolar depression, whereas first-degree relatives of probands with unipolar depression have an increased risk of unipolar depression only.

Molecular genetics: linkage studies

Regions of interest have been identified in genome-wide linkage studies of unipolar depression. An area of chromosome 12 (12q22–23) shows linkage with unipolar depression; interestingly, this area overlaps with a region of interest in bipolar disorder.[41] A region of chromosome 2q also showed strong linkage with unipolar depression. This region is close to the gene coding for cyclic adenosine monophosphate (cAMP)-responsive element binding protein 1 (*CREB1*).[42]

Molecular genetics: association studies

Genes for major depression appear to overlap with those for anxiety and neuroticism.[43] In a study designed to investigate the relationship between personality and depression in women, it was reported that high trait neuroticism accounted for approximately 55 per cent of the genetic liability for major depression.[44]

As in BPAD, the serotonin transporter gene is a promising functional candidate gene in unipolar depression. One polymorphism of this gene (the short variant affecting the promoter region) causes reduced expression of the serotonin transporter protein and reduced presynaptic serotonin uptake. However, this polymorphism is not associated uniquely with major depression but also with anxiety-related personality traits.[45]

Gene–environment interactions

Gene–environment interactions are likely to be important in the aetiology of unipolar depression. Caspi and colleagues showed that the presence of one or two copies of the short allele of the serotonin transporter promoter polymorphism increases susceptibility to major depression occurring in relation to stressful life events,[46] and this finding has been replicated in two other samples. Hariri and colleagues reported that humans with one or two copies of the short allele have greater amygdalar activation when exposed to a fearful stimulus than individuals homozygous for the long allele.[47] Thus, human response to environmental stressors may, at least in part, be influenced by their genetic make-up.

Autism

Epidemiology

Autistic spectrum disorders (ASD) are devastating neurodevelopmental disorders of childhood characterized by deficits in social interaction and communication and restricted, repetitive patterns of behaviours, interest and activities. The term ASD is commonly used clinically to describe conditions on the autistic spectrum not meeting the strict criteria for autism as defined by *International Classification of Diseases*, 10th revision (ICD-10) or *Diagnostic and Statistical Manual*, 4th edition (DSM-IV). The reported prevalence of ASDs has increased over the past 20 years, with rates for childhood autism of 38.9 per 10 000, and 116.1 per 10 000 for all ASDs, from one study of 56 964 children in the south Thames region of the UK.[48] The male/female ratio in ASD is approximately 4 : 1, although when only severe cases of autistic disorder are considered the ratio approaches 1 : 1.

Family, twin and adoption studies

Autism has a strong genetic basis,[49] and the estimated heritability of autism is more than 90 per cent. The relative risk of a child being diagnosed with autism is increased at least 25-fold over the population prevalence in families in which a sibling is affected.[50] First-degree relatives of a child with ASD are more likely than controls to show subtle cognitive or behavioural features that are qualitatively similar to those observed in probands (the broader autism phenotype).[51,52] Twin studies report that concordance rates for monozygotic twins (70–90%) are very significantly higher than the corresponding values for dizygotic twins (0–10%).[53,54]

The aetiology of autism is poorly understood at both the cellular and the molecular level. However, there are theories about abnormal neuronal connectivity and defective synaptic function, which are gaining support from genetic findings and which may account for the core features of autism. Approximately 10–20 per cent of ASD cases are associated with defined mutations, genetic syndromes and de novo CNVs, none of which individually accounts for more than 1–2 per cent of cases.[55]

Chromosomal abnormalities

A number of chromosomal abnormalities have been identified in multiple patients with ASDs. However, such abnormalities are present in only 6–7 per cent of ASDs.[56] Important regions that have been identified include 15q11–13, 22q13 and 2q37. Within the 15q11–q13 locus, two genes (ubiquitin protein ligase, *UBE3A*; γ-aminobutyric acid A receptor beta 3, *GABRB3*) are thought to be central. Investigation of mutations in the 22q13 and 2q37 regions has led to the discovery of other genes, including *SHANK3*, which codes for a synaptic adaptor protein, and a gene coding for a GTPase-activating protein (*CENTG2*).

Molecular genetics: linkage studies

Linkage studies have not been particularly successful in the search for autism-susceptibility genes. Linkage of genome-wide significance has been replicated at only two regions – 17q11–q21 and 7q.[55] This reflects the genetic and phenotypic heterogeneity of autism. Current research is focusing on studying autism endophenotypes (measurable traits that are both heritable and related to a specific aspect of the condition under investigation).

Molecular genetics: association studies

Association studies have identified a number of potential susceptibility genes for autism. Strongest evidence exists for *CNTNAP2* (7q35, positional candidate), *EN2* (7q36, positional candidate linked to cerebellar abnormalities in animal studies), *GABRB3* (15q11–15q12, a positional candidate linked to neuroligin signalling), *ITGB3* (17q21, a positional candidate involved in regulation of serotonin), *OXTR* (3p25, an important gene in rodent social behaviour), *RELN* (7q22, a positional candidate), *SLC25A12* (2q24, a positional candidate related to neurite outgrowth and up-regulated in the prefrontal cortex of people with autism) and *SLC6A4* (17q11, a positional candidate involved in the regulation of serotonin).

DNA sequencing of candidate genes has allowed researchers to obtain evidence for the involvement of specific candidate genes in the ASDs. A number of genes involved in synaptic function (neuroligin 3, *NLGN3*; neuroligin 4-x linked, *NLGN4X*; *SHANK3*; neurexin 1, *NRXN1*) have been identified in this way, but the function of these genes is not fully understood. The interaction between neurexin and neuroligin proteins at the synapse is thought to play an important role in controlling the balance between excitatory glutamate and inhibitory γ-aminobutyric acid (IGABA) inputs.

Copy number variants

De novo and inherited CNVs are emerging as important causes of ASDs. Interesting CNVs that are under investigation are located at 16p11 (containing about 30 genes), 7q31 (containing 8 genes), and 20p13 (containing the oxytocin gene and arginine vasopressin gene, among 30 others).

Sebat and colleagues showed that de novo CNVs were significantly associated with autism.[57] They identified such CNVs in 10 per cent of patients with sporadic autism, in 3 per cent of patients with an affected first-degree relative, and in 1 per cent of the general population. Arising out of that work, a model for the genetic inheritance of autism has been proposed,[58] whereby sporadic autism might be caused by spontaneous mutations with high penetrance in males and multiply affected families occur when these mutations are transmitted to the next generation typically from females who are less likely to be affected.

Attention deficit hyperactivity disorder

Epidemiology

ADHD is a childhood-onset neurodevelopmental disorder characterized by inattention, hyperactivity and impulsiveness. ADHD affects 2–5 per cent of children and can persist into adolescence and adulthood. One study estimates the prevalence of current adult ADHD in the USA at 4.4 per cent.[59] Males are diagnosed with ADHD three to five times more frequently than females.

Family, twin and adoption studies

Family studies have found increased rates of ADHD in family members of affected probands.[60] Adoption studies support a genetic component to the familiality, with adopted children with ADHD more likely to have biological parents rather than adoptive parents with ADHD. Twin studies have consistently suggested a large (60–90%) genetic component when ADHD is considered a categorical diagnosis or a continuous trait.[61]

Chromosomal abnormalities

Bastain and colleagues assessed the prevalence of genetic abnormalities in an unselected population of 100 children with ADHD and intelligence quotient (IQ) over 80.[62] Only one subject had a clear cytogenetic abnormality (a girl with trisomy 47, XXX), but this was not different from the expected rate in the general population. No subjects were found with either the fragile X mutation or chromosome 22q11.2 VCFS deletion.

Molecular genetics: linkage studies

A small number of genome linkage scans in ADHD have been performed. Suggestive evidence (LOD scores of 3.73, 3.54 and 4.0) has been reported from American,[63] Dutch[64] and Colombian[65] family datasets. In only one region, 5p13, close to the dopamine transporter (*DAT1*), was there evidence for linkage (LOD score > 1) deriving from all three studies. This work was later extended by pooled analysis, indicating a common risk locus on chromosome 5p13. A further study found no evidence for linkage on the most established ADHD-linked genomic regions of 5p and 17, but it found suggestive linkage signals on chromosomes 9 and 16, respectively, with a LOD score of 2.13 at 9q22 and 3.1 at overlapping findings from previous studies.[66]

Molecular genetics: association studies

Most association studies followed a candidate gene approach targeting dopaminergic, serotonergic and noradrenergic system genes. In contrast to many other neuropsychiatric conditions, the a priori evidence for these hypotheses was reasonably substantial. Also in contrast to other disorders, many initial findings have stood the test of replication and meta-analysis. Beginning with Cook and colleagues, the dopamine transporter has been the target of many individual studies and meta-analyses.[67] This protein is the target of methylphenidate, the medication used to treat ADHD. Many individual studies and the majority of meta-analyses support a role for genetic variation at *DAT1* in the aetiology of ADHD.[68] Also supported by several individual studies and meta-analyses are *DRD4* and *DRD5* variants,[69] with overall ORs of approximately 1.3 for both risk variants. Serotonergic system gene variant with some consistent evidence for association with ADHD include 5-HT transporter (*5-HTT*), the 5-HT1B receptor and tryptophan hydroxylase 2 isoform. Noradrenergic candidate genes include dopamine beta hydroxylase (*DBH*) and the noradrenergic transporter (*NET*). One study reported from the large collaborative International Multi-center ADHD Genetics Project (IMAGE) group focused on 51 of the most likely candidate genes from a review of the literature.[70] The study reported nominal significance with one or more variants in 18 genes, including *DRD4*, *DAT1* and *TPH2*, mentioned above.

Genome-wide association studies

A large ADHD sample from the IMAGE study has been included in the Genetic Association Information Network (GAIN) study,[71] and the first publications are beginning to emerge. In the first of many expected reports, six quantitative phenotypes from 18 ADHD symptoms were used in genome-wide association analyses. Two variants, within genes *CDH13* and *GFOD1*, met the criteria for significance within a specified phenotype. The study also evaluated the association of variants from 37 candidate genes that were specified a priori, 17 of which had association *P* values lower than 0.01, including *DAT1*, *TPH2*, *DBH* and *5-HTR2A* mentioned above.

Anxiety disorders

Epidemiology

Anxiety disorders, including panic disorder, social phobia, specific phobias, generalized anxiety disorder, post-traumatic stress disorder (PTSD) and obsessive–compulsive disorder (OCD, discussed separately below), are the most prevalent class of DSM-IV disorders, with an overall lifetime prevalence of 28.8 per cent. Phobic disorders are the most common, having a lifetime prevalence of 12.5 per cent (specific phobia) and 12.1 per cent (social anxiety disorder). Lifetime prevalence of panic disorder is 4.7 per cent, agoraphobia without panic disorder 1.4 per cent, generalized anxiety disorder 5.7 per cent and PTSD 6.8 per cent.[72] There is a high degree of co-morbidity with each other and with other psychiatric disorders, especially affective disorders.

Family, twin and adoption studies

There is evidence from genetic epidemiological studies that anxiety disorders are familial and moderately heritable. Family studies show that there is an increased risk of anxiety disorders in first-degree relatives of probands; for example, phobic disorders are six to nine times more common in first-degree relatives with these disorders, and panic disorder is seven times more likely to occur in relatives of affected individuals.[73] Anxiety disorders appear to be moderately heritable, with estimates of heritability ranging from 30 per cent to 40 per cent,[74] implying that there are substantial environmental influences on the development of these disorders. As mentioned earlier, population twin studies have shown that genes for anxiety and neuroticism overlap with those for depression.[43]

Molecular genetics: linkage studies

Despite much research over the past years, susceptibility genes for anxiety disorders have remained elusive. Several whole-genome linkage studies investigating anxiety disorders have been published. However, there is limited overlap in the linkage sites between these studies. Linkage sites that do overlap include regions of chromosomes 7p, 16p and 8p. Loci on 7p and 16p may harbour susceptibility genes for panic disorder, and loci on 8p have been linked to anxiety-related personality traits.

Molecular genetics: association studies

Genetic association studies in large samples have looked promising, and replications in other samples are awaited.[75] Candidate gene studies in anxiety disorders are numerous. Most of the candidate genes studied are related to neurotransmitter systems known to be involved in anxiety and genes related to stress response.

SLC6A4 has been intensively investigated in anxiety disorders. This gene codes for the serotonin transporter, a protein of particular interest because it is the target for SSRI drugs in anxiety and because it is responsible for the uptake of serotonin from the synaptic cleft. There are two alleles of the gene; short and long. The short allele causes reduced expression and activity of the serotonin transporter. However, meta-analyses of the numerous association studies of *SLC6A4* have been inconclusive about the role of the gene in anxiety disorders or anxiety-related personality traits.[76,77] These inconclusive results may in part be due to differential exposure to environmental factors, which were not considered in the association studies. Association analysis by gene–environment interaction may be useful in future genetic studies of anxiety disorders.

Also of interest in panic disorders and anxiety-related personality traits are the genes for catechol-O-methyltransferase and cholecystokinin B receptor. The significance of these and other candidate genes in the aetiology of anxiety disorders is not yet known.

Genome-wide association studies

To date there has been only one genome-wide association study of neuroticism.[78] This study identified only a single locus, which explained less than 1 per cent of the variance. This would suggest that there are multiple genes contributing to the heritability of neuroticism.

Animal studies

A common polymorphism (val to met) in the *BDNF* gene has been implicated in the development of anxiety disorders. Modelling this polymorphism in mice gives rise to increased anxiety and changes in neuroanatomy (reduced hippocampal volume and deficient BDNF release from neurons) and reduced responsiveness to SSRI medication.[79] This variant of the *BDNF* gene may play a critical role in genetic predisposition to anxiety.

Obsessive–compulsive disorder

Epidemiology

Lifetime prevalence of OCD is estimated at 1.1–3.3 per cent.[80,81]

Family, twin and adoption studies

Twin and family studies provide convincing evidence for a genetic contribution to the disease. A review of all twin studies in OCD concludes that obsessive–compulsive symptoms are heritable, with genetic influences in children ranging from 45 per cent to 65 per cent and in adults from 27 per cent to 47 per cent.[82] That OCD is familial is evident from numerous family studies (see Pauls[83] for a review). Similar to the data from twin studies, evidence from family studies suggests that genetic influence is stronger for OCD that occurs in childhood. The rate of OCD in relatives of adult probands with OCD is increased approximately two-fold; however, in relatives of children and adolescents with OCD, the rate of OCD is increased ten-fold. In addition, OCD-spectrum disorders appear to be more common among relatives of probands with OCD. These include body dysmorphic disorder, somatoform disorders, grooming disorders and tic disorders.[84,85] The mode of inheritance is not fully understood, but it is likely that OCD is a complex genetic disorder with a number of genes important for the expression of the disease.

Molecular genetics: linkage studies

There have only been two genome-wide linkage studies in OCD, and both have had relatively small sample sizes.[86,87] Hanna and colleagues found linkage to regions on chromosomes 2, 9 and 16, with maximum linkage at a region on chromosome 9p24.[86] A subsequent study has also demonstrated linkage very close to this region of 9p24.[88] This area is particularly interesting because it includes the gene coding for the glutamate transporter that has been implicated in OCD in three independent association studies. However, the largest linkage study to date did not find evidence for linkage at 9p but reported that there was evidence for linkage on chromosomes 3q, 1q, 15q and 6q, with maximum linkage at 3q27–28. None of the linkage studies to date have achieved genome-wide significance.

Molecular genetics: association studies

Candidate gene studies have been focused on neurotransmitters thought to be involved in OCD. The serotonergic system has been of particular interest because of the well-documented efficacy of serotonin reuptake inhibitors in the treatment of OCD. Other neurotransmitter systems that have been investigated include the dopaminergic, glutamatergic and opioid systems. Two neuropeptides (arginine vasopressin and oxytocin) have also been implicated in the pathobiology of some forms of OCD. However, results from candidate gene studies of these systems have been disappointing. None has achieved genome-wide significance, and the majority have not been consistently replicated. Three independent studies have reported an association to the glutamate transporter (*SLCL1A1*).

The next step in molecular genetic studies of OCD will involve whole-genome association studies. Larger sample sizes are essential in future studies.

Anorexia nervosa

Epidemiology

Anorexia nervosa (AN) is a serious psychiatric condition characterized by an inability to maintain a normal body weight. Despite severe weight loss, individuals with AN perceive themselves to be heavier than they are in reality and engage in severe dieting, exercise and purging. The prevalence of narrowly defined AN is 0.3 per cent; including subthreshold cases, the prevalence ranges from 0.37 per cent to 1.3 per cent.

Family, twin and adoption studies

Along with female sex, a family history of AN is a strong risk factor, with first-degree relatives having a ten-fold increase in risk, not only for AN but also for a range of eating disorders, including bulimia nervosa.[89] Twin studies are not common in AN, but those conducted have been well designed, including studies that utilize twin registers. From these studies, the heritability of narrowly defined DSM-IV AN has been estimated at 56 per cent,[90] with shared environment and unique environment accounting for 5 per cent and 38 per cent, respectively.

Molecular genetics: linkage studies

A limited number of linkage studies with AN have been reported. The evidence that there is shows some support for a susceptibility locus on chromosome 1p36–1p34 when the phenotype is restricted to classical AN. This region contains two genes of interest in AN: the serotonin 1D receptor and the δ opioid receptor. An analysis of linkage taking into account AN traits such as obsessiveness, age at menarche and minimum body mass index (BMI) provides suggestive evidence for several other regions of the genome. Overall, the findings are not conclusive and further work is required.

Molecular genetics: association studies

Association studies have focused on candidate genes, including the serotonergic genes, thought to be involved in body weight regulation; and dopaminergic genes, thought to be involved in weight loss, hyperactivity, menstrual abnormalities, obsessive behaviours, and a range of additional genes including neuropeptide genes, growth genes and satiety-related genes. To date, variants at the serotonin 1D receptor gene, the dopamine D2 gene and the *BDNF* gene provide modest evidence for being associated with risk (see Bulik *et al.*[91] for a review).

Alcoholism

Epidemiology

Alcoholism is a worldwide public health problem that is costly both in human and in economic terms. In the USA, alcoholism costs the economy an estimated $185 billion per annum in healthcare, loss of productivity and legal/penal costs. The Epidemiological and Catchment area (ECA) study in the USA reported a 14 per cent lifetime prevalence of alcohol dependence, with a male/female ration of 2 : 1.[92] In the USA, prevalence of alcohol use disorder in the preceding 12 months is reported at 8.6 per cent.[93] There are major demographic and environmental influences, including age, type of drink, religion, culture, occupation, marital status and socioeconomic class.

Family, twin and adoption studies

There is an estimated four-fold increased risk of alcohol dependency in first-degree relatives of alcoholics. There is overlap of risk such that family members of alcoholics have increased risk of other substance use disorders, but there is also evidence of specificity of familial aggregation of the predominant drug of abuse, suggesting that there may be risk factors that are specific to the particular class of drug and risk factors that underlie substance abuse in general. Monozygotic twins have a higher risk of both being concordant for alcohol dependency than do dizygotic twins. Studies based on large population samples of twins confirm that there is a mixture of genetic and environmental factors. Adopted children of alcoholic parents have the same four-fold increased risk of alcohol dependency as do children raised by their alcohol-dependent parents.[94] Taken together, these studies confirm that alcohol dependence is substantially inherited, with estimated heritability of 50–60 per cent for both women and men.[95] Given the observed monozygotic/dizygotic twin ratio for alcohol dependency at approximately 2 : 1, likely modes of inheritance include an oligogenic model, or multiple alleles of strong individual effect, a genetic heterogeneity model. Genetic studies that cross compare risks for two phenotypes in twins or other relative pairs indicate that some risk factors are alcohol-specific whereas other are shared between different substances. For example, alcoholism and nicotine dependence are co-morbid, and it has been shown that about 50 per cent of the genetic liability to nicotine dependence is shared with alcoholism and about 15 per cent of the genetic liability to alcoholism is shared with nicotine dependence.

Molecular genetics: linkage studies

Several papers describe genome-wide linkage scans in alcohol abuse using phenotypes most supported by twin studies such as dependence diagnosis made according to DSM-IV criteria or estimates of quantity and frequency. Initially, few of the linkage 'peaks' from these scans appeared to overlap between studies. However, in the light of more recent genome-wide association studies, these linkage peaks are in the same regions as the variants identified by association.[96] In addition, the magnitude of the signal from each study at a given location was strongly correlated. Signals on chromosomes 1, 2, 4, 7, 10 and 11 appear to be the most consistent.[95]

Molecular genetics: association studies

The allelic variations most strongly associated with alcoholism are the functional variants at alcohol and acetaldehyde dehydrogenase genes, carriers of which flush in response to alcohol consumption. For the *ALDH*2* gene variant, carriers are incapable of metabolizing acetaldehyde at a rate sufficient to remove it from the blood, and in the case of the *ADH1B* and *ADH1C* variants, the variants produce an enzyme that metabolizes alcohol more rapidly, increasing the levels of acetaldehyde in the blood. Such individuals are highly unlikely to become alcoholic, the variants providing strong protection. However, because these variants are rare in white people, the impact at a population level is minimal. Candidate gene approaches have focused on GABA subunit genes that underlie some of the linkage peaks, the serotonin transporter and the *COMT* Val158Met variant.

Genes and behaviour

The monoamine oxidase A (MAOA) gene is a putative candidate gene for antisocial and other behavioural disorders in humans. MAOA is involved in serotonin degradation following its reuptake from the synaptic cleft. There is a variable-number tandem repeat polymorphism at the promoter of the *MAOA* gene, which is known to affect expression. Variants of *MAOA* can result in reduced enzymatic activity, and there is some evidence suggesting a link between low activity alleles of the *MAOA* gene and aggression and antisocial behaviour. Two separate studies have reported that in males exposed to maltreatment/childhood adversity, antisocial outcomes were more prevalent in those with the low activity *MAOA* allele; that, conversely, the high-activity allele conferred protection against antisocial behaviour.[97,98] Of note, in the absence of environmental adversity, there does not appear to be a simple association between low-activity MAOA and aggression or antisocial behaviour. Much work is still needed in this area.

PHENOTYPE–GENOTYPE CORRELATION

Phenotype definitions in psychiatry are descriptive and, even with more recently developed operational criteria, the focus is on reliability in the absence of biological validity. Given the level of symptom overlap between disorders, it is likely that there will be overlap of genetic susceptibility between disorders. This is particularly likely for the major psychoses, schizophrenia, bipolar disorder and the intermediate phenotype schizoaffective disorder. Here, genetic epidemiology and molecular genetic studies are challenging the Kraepelinian dichotomy. Twin studies have shown evidence of shared genetic susceptibility,[99] with cases of monozygotic twins where one individual is diagnosed with schizophrenia and one with bipolar disorder. Similarly, in the large Scottish family segregating the translocation disrupting the *DISC1* gene, some members with the translocation have schizophrenia, some bipolar disorder and some recurrent major depression.[6] Linkage and association studies have also produced evidence to suggest that there may be overlap in genetic susceptibility (see Owen *et al.*[100] for a review).

Extreme levels of phenotypic diversity have emerged from studies of structural variation in the genome. Mefford and colleagues tested for deletions and duplications at a locus on chromosome 1q21.1 previously reported to be deleted in individuals with mental and growth retardation and facial dysmorphism.[29] In a screen of more than 5000 patients, they found 25 with deletions and 9 with duplications of a region approximately 1.35 Mb in length. There was considerable variation in phenotype, including mild to moderate mental retardation, microcephaly and facial dysmorphism, cardiac abnormalities, cataracts and autism. Two large multicentre studies of copy number variation in schizophrenia, published about the same time, identified deletions of the same 1.35-Mb region in 10 from 3391 patients and in 11 from 4718 patients.[27,28] Similar findings were reported for a region on chromosome 15q13.3. These findings show that schizophrenia, a known neurodevelopmental disorder, might be one possible outcome of a chromosomal abnormality, the other outcomes including autism, mental retardation, cardiac abnormalities, cataracts, dysmorphism and other signs of aberrant development. It will be important to examine the phenotype carefully in the individuals identified as carrying these and other recently identified mutations to see whether and how they might differ with respect to other patients. Why the same genetic mutation might lead to so many different outcomes is unknown, but the answers will lead to significant insights into the genetic architecture of neurodevelopment.

There are likely to be implications for the future of psychiatric nosology, with disorder classification based increasingly on biological validity. With psychiatric disorders in individuals being characterized at a genetic and molecular level, it does not require much of a leap of the imagination to see the possibilities with respect to treatments and early interventions based on knowledge of underlying aetiology.

KEY POINTS

- Mendel's laws are important in understanding the principles of inheritance and the application of linkage and association methods.
- Complex patterns of inheritance generally apply to common traits and this is likely to be the case in neuropsychiatric disorders.
- Much of the genetic risk for psychiatric disorders will consist of multiple DNA variations each of small effect size. These are likely to be common throughout the population but in combination with other risk variants and environmental effects can produce the disorder phenotype.
- Identifying risk genes, even if their individual effect on risk is small, will provide important insights into disease pathophysiology.
- Major genes have been identified in Alzheimer' disease and in rare cases of schizophrenia and other major psychiatric disorders. In the case of the Disrupted in Schizophrenia 1 gene (*DISC1*) on chromosome 1, abnormal neuronal morphology and motility during neurodevelopment has been observed, underpinning the neurodevelopmental hypothesis of schizophrenia.
- Genome-wide association studies in sufficiently powered samples are beginning to emerge. Determining the function role of risk genes/DNA variations will be a major task for the neuroscience research community.
- Some DNA variation appears to be shared between disorders, in particular between schizophrenia and bipolar affective disorder.
- Sub-microscopic deletions and duplications, known as copy number variations (CNVs), play an important role in a significant proportion of cases of autism and schizophrenia. Apparently similar CNVs appear to underlie a diverse range of neurodevelopmental phenotypes, including autism and schizophrenia.
- Gene–environment studies will be increasingly important as risk genes are identified in the coming years.

REFERENCES

1. Wilson DI, Burn J, Scambler P, Goodship J (1993) DiGeorge syndrome: part of CATCH 22. *Journal of Medical Genetics* **30**: 852–6.
2. Saitta SC, Harris SE, Gaeth AP, *et al.* (2004) Aberrant interchromosomal exchanges are the predominant cause of the 22q11.2 deletion. *Human Molecular Genetics* **13**: 417–28.
3. Gratacos M, Nadal M, Martin-Santos R, *et al.* (2001) A polymorphic genomic duplication on human chromosome 15 is a susceptibility factor for panic and phobic disorders. *Cell* **106**: 367–79.
4. Kunugi H, Lee KB, Nanko S (1999) Cytogenetic findings in 250 schizophrenics: evidence confirming an excess of the X chromosome aneuploidies and pericentric inversion of chromosome 9. *Schizophrenia Research* **40**: 43–7.
5. Glass IA, Stormer P, Oei PT, Hacking E, Cotter PD (1998) Trisomy 2q11.2->q21.1 resulting from an unbalanced insertion in two generations. *Journal of Medical Genetics* **35**: 319–22.
6. Blackwood DH, Fordyce A, Walker MT, *et al.* (2001) Schizophrenia and affective disorders: cosegregation with a translocation at chromosome 1q42 that directly disrupts brain-expressed genes – clinical and P300 findings in a family. *American Journal of Human Genetics* **69**: 428–33.
7. Baysal BE, Potkin SG, Farr JE, *et al.* (1998) Bipolar affective disorder partially cosegregates with a balanced t(9;11)(p24;q23.1) chromosomal translocation in a small pedigree. *American Journal of Medical Genetics* **81**: 81–91.
8. Smith AB, Peterson P, Wieland J, Moriarty T, DeLisi LE (1996) Chromosome 18 translocation (18;21) (p11.1;p11.1) associated with psychosis in one family. *American Journal of Medical Genetics* **67**: 560–63.
9. Lobo A, Launer LJ, Fratiglioni L, *et al.* (2000) Prevalence of dementia and major subtypes in Europe: a collaborative study of population-based cohorts. Neurologic Diseases in the Elderly Research Group. *Neurology* **54** (suppl. 5): S4–9.
10. Bird TD (2005) Genetic factors in Alzheimer's disease. *New England Journal of Medicine* **352**: 862–4.
11. Gatz M, Reynolds CA, Fratiglioni L, *et al.* (2006) Role of genes and environments for explaining Alzheimer disease. *Archives of General Psychiatry* **63**: 168–74.
12. Daw EW, Payami H, Nemens EJ, *et al.* (2000) The number of trait loci in late-onset Alzheimer disease. *American Journal of Human Genetics* **66**: 196–204.
13. Kamboh MI (2004) Molecular genetics of late-onset Alzheimer's disease. *Annals of Human Genetics* **68**: 381–404.
14. Bertram L, McQueen MB, Mullin K, Blacker D, Tanzi RE (2007) Systematic meta-analyses of Alzheimer disease genetic association studies: the AlzGene database. *Nature Genetics* **39**: 17–23.
15. Gotz J, Ittner LM (2008) Animal models of Alzheimer's disease and frontotemporal dementia. *Nature Reviews Neuroscience* **9**: 532–44.
16. Der G, Gupta S, Murray RM (1990) Is schizophrenia disappearing? *Lancet* **335**: 513–16.
17. St Clair D, Blackwood D, Muir W, *et al.* (1990) Association within a family of a balanced autosomal translocation with major mental illness. *Lancet* **336**: 13–16.

18. Lewis CM, Levinson DF, Wise LH, *et al.* (2003) Genome scan meta-analysis of schizophrenia and bipolar disorder, part II: Schizophrenia. *American Journal of Human Genetics* **73**: 34–48.
19. Straub RE, Jiang Y, MacLean CJ, *et al.* (2002) Genetic variation in the 6p22.3 gene DTNBP1, the human ortholog of the mouse dysbindin gene, is associated with schizophrenia. *American Journal of Human Genetics* **71**: 337–48.
20. Stefansson H, Sigurdsson E, Steinthorsdottir V, Bjornsdottir S, *et al.* (2002) Neuregulin 1 and susceptibility to schizophrenia. *American Journal of Human Genetics* **71**: 877–92.
21. Allen NC, Bagade S, McQueen MB, *et al.* (2008) Systematic meta-analyses and field synopsis of genetic association studies in schizophrenia: the SzGene database. *Nature Genetics* **40**: 827–34.
22. Lencz T, Morgan TV, Athanasiou M, *et al.* (2007) Converging evidence for a pseudoautosomal cytokine receptor gene locus in schizophrenia. *Molecular Psychiatry* **12**: 572–80.
23. Kirov G, Zaharieva I, Georgieva L, *et al.* (2008) A genome-wide association study in 574 schizophrenia trios using DNA pooling. *Molecular Psychiatry* (forthcoming).
24. Sullivan PF, Lin D, Tzeng JY, *et al.* (2008) Genome-wide association for schizophrenia in the CATIE study: results of stage 1. *Molecular Psychiatry* **13**: 570–84.
25. O'Donovan MC, Craddock N, Norton N, *et al.* (2008) Identification of loci associated with schizophrenia by genome-wide association and follow-up. *Nature Genetics* **40**: 1053–5.
26. Walsh T, McClellan JM, McCarthy SE, *et al.* (2008) Rare structural variants disrupt multiple genes in neurodevelopmental pathways in schizophrenia. *Science* **320**: 539–43.
27. International Schizophrenia Consortium (2008) Rare chromosomal deletions and duplications increase risk of schizophrenia. *Nature* **455**: 237–41.
28. Stefansson H, Rujescu D, Cichon S, *et al.* (2008) Large recurrent microdeletions associated with schizophrenia. *Nature* **455**: 232–6.
29. Mefford HC, Sharp AJ, Baker C, *et al.* Recurrent rearrangements of chromosome 1q21.1 and variable pediatric phenotypes. *New England Journal of Medicine* (2008) **359**: 1685–99.
30. Miller DT, Shen Y, Weiss LA, *et al.* (2008) Microdeletion/duplication at 15q13.2q13.3 among individuals with features of autism and other neuropsychiatirc disorders. *Journal of Medical Genetics* (forthcoming).
31. Rujescu D, Ingason A, Cichon S, *et al.* (2009) Disruption of the neurexin 1 gene is associated with schizophrenia. *Human Molecular Genetics* **18**: 988–96.
32. McGuffin P, Rijsdijk F, Andrew M, *et al.* (2003) The heritability of bipolar affective disorder and the genetic relationship to unipolar depression. *Archives of General Psychiatry* **60**: 497–502.
33. Mendlewicz J, Rainer JD (1977) Adoption study supporting genetic transmission in manic-depressive illness. *Nature* **268**: 327–9.
34. Serretti A, Mandelli L (2008) The genetics of bipolar disorder: genome 'hot regions,' genes, new potential candidates and future directions. *Molecular Psychiatry* **13**: 742–71.
35. Craddock N, O'Donovan MC, Owen MJ (2005) The genetics of schizophrenia and bipolar disorder: dissecting psychosis. *Journal of Medical Genetics* **42**: 193–204.
36. Egan MF, Kojima M, Callicott JH, *et al.* (2003) The BDNF val66met polymorphism affects activity-dependent secretion of BDNF and human memory and hippocampal function. *Cell* **112**: 257–69.
37. Baum AE, Akula N, Cabanero M, *et al.* (2008) A genome-wide association study implicates diacylglycerol kinase eta (DGKH) and several other genes in the etiology of bipolar disorder. *Molecular Psychiatry* **13**: 197–207.
38. WTCCC (2007) Genome-wide association study of 14,000 cases of seven common diseases and 3,000 shared controls. *Nature* **447**: 661–78.
39. Sklar P, Smoller JW, Fan J, *et al.* (2008) Whole-genome association study of bipolar disorder. *Molecular Psychiatry* **13**: 558–69.
40. Ferreira MA, O'Donovan MC, Meng YA, *et al.* (2008) Collaborative genome-wide association analysis supports a role for ANK3 and CACNA1C in bipolar disorder. *Nature Genetics* **40**: 1042–4.
41. McGuffin P, Knight J, Breen G, *et al.* (2005) Whole genome linkage scan of recurrent depressive disorder from the depression network study. *Human Molecular Genetics* **14**: 3337–45.
42. Zubenko GS, Maher B, Hughes HB, *et al.* (2003) Genome-wide linkage survey for genetic loci that influence the development of depressive disorders in families with recurrent, early-onset, major depression. *American Journal of Medical Genetics. Part B: Neuropsychiatric Genetics* **123B**: 1–18.
43. Kendler KS, Neale MC, Kessler RC, Heath AC, Eaves LJ (1992) Major depression and generalized anxiety disorder: same genes, (partly) different environments? *Archives of General Psychiatry* **49**: 716–22.
44. Kendler KS, Neale MC, Kessler RC, Heath AC, Eaves LJ (1993) A longitudinal twin study of personality and major depression in women. *Archives of General Psychiatry* **50**: 853–62.
45. Lesch KP, Bengel D, Heils A, *et al.* (1996) Association of anxiety-related traits with a polymorphism in the serotonin transporter gene regulatory region. *Science* **274**: 1527–31.
46. Caspi A, Sugden K, Moffitt TE, *et al.* (2003) Influence of life stress on depression: moderation by a polymorphism in the 5-HTT gene. *Science* **301**: 386–9.

47. Hariri AR, Mattay VS, Tessitore A, *et al.* (2002) Serotonin transporter genetic variation and the response of the human amygdala. *Science* **297**: 400–403.
48. Baird G, Simonoff E, Pickles A, *et al.* (2006) Prevalence of disorders of the autism spectrum in a population cohort of children in South Thames: the Special Needs and Autism Project (SNAP). *Lancet* **368**: 210–15.
49. Bailey A, Phillips W, Rutter M (1996) Autism: towards an integration of clinical, genetic, neuropsychological and neurobiological perspectives. *Journal of Child Psychology and Psychiatry and Allied Disciplines* **37**: 89–126.
50. Jorde LB, Hasstedt SJ, Ritvo ER, *et al.* (1991) Complex segregation analysis of autism. *American Journal of Human Genetics* **49**: 932–8.
51. Bolton P, Macdonald H, Pickles A, *et al* (1994) A case-control family history study of autism. *Journal of Child Psychology and Psychiatry and Allied Disciplines* **35**: 877–900.
52. Bishop DV, Maybery M, Maley A, *et al.* (2004) Using self-report to identify the broad phenotype in parents of children with autistic spectrum disorders: a study using the Autism-Spectrum Quotient. *Journal of Child Psychology and Psychiatry and Allied Disciplines* **45**: 1431–6.
53. Bailey A, Le Couteur A, Gottesman I, *et al.* (1995) Autism as a strongly genetic disorder: evidence from a British twin study. *Psychological Medicine* **25**: 63–77.
54. Steffenburg S, Gillberg C, Hellgren L, *et al.* (1989) A twin study of autism in Denmark, Finland, Iceland, Norway and Sweden. *Journal of Child Psychology and Psychiatry and Allied Disciplines* **30**: 405–16.
55. Abrahams BS, Geschwind DH (2008) Advances in autism genetics: on the threshold of a new neurobiology. *Nature Reviews. Genetics* **9**: 341–55.
56. Marshall CR, Noor A, Vincent JB, *et al.* (2008) Structural variation of chromosomes in autism spectrum disorder. *American Journal of Human Genetics* **82**: 477–88.
57. Sebat J, Lakshmi B, Malhotra D, *et al.* (2007) Strong association of de novo copy number mutations with autism. *Science* **316**: 445–9.
58. Zhao X, Leotta A, Kustanovich V, *et al.* (2007) A unified genetic theory for sporadic and inherited autism. *Proceedings of the National Academy of Science of the USA* Jul 31;**104**: 12831–6.
59. Kessler RC, Adler L, Barkley R, *et al.* (2006) The prevalence and correlates of adult ADHD in the United States: results from the National Comorbidity Survey Replication. *American Journal of Psychiatry* **163**: 716–23.
60. Biederman J, Faraone SV, Keenan K, *et al.* (1992) Further evidence for family-genetic risk factors in attention deficit hyperactivity disorder: patterns of comorbidity in probands and relatives psychiatrically and pediatrically referred samples. *Archives of General Psychiatry* **49**: 728–38.
61. Faraone SV, Perlis RH, Doyle AE, *et al.* (2005) Molecular genetics of attention-deficit/hyperactivity disorder. *Biological Psychiatry* **57**: 1313–23.
62. Bastain TM, Lewczyk CM, Sharp WS, *et al.* (2002) Cytogenetic abnormalities in attention-deficit/hyperactivity disorder. *Journal of the American Academy of Child and Adolescent Psychiatry* **41**: 806–10.
63. Ogdie MN, Fisher SE, Yang M, *et al.* (2004) Attention deficit hyperactivity disorder: fine mapping supports linkage to 5p13, 6q12, 16p13, and 17p11. *American Journal of Human Genetics* **75**: 661–8.
64. Bakker SC, van der Meulen EM, Buitelaar JK, *et al.* (2003) A whole-genome scan in 164 Dutch sib pairs with attention-deficit/hyperactivity disorder: suggestive evidence for linkage on chromosomes 7p and 15q. *American Journal of Human Genetics* **72**: 1251–60.
65. Arcos-Burgos M, Castellanos FX, Pineda D, *et al.* (2004) Attention-deficit/hyperactivity disorder in a population isolate: linkage to loci at 4q13.2, 5q33.3, 11q22, and 17p11. *American Journal of Human Genetics* **75**: 998–1014.
66. Asherson P, Zhou K, Anney RJ, *et al.* (2008) A high-density SNP linkage scan with 142 combined subtype ADHD sib pairs identifies linkage regions on chromosomes 9 and 16. *Molecular Psychiatry* **13**: 514–21.
67. Cook EH, Jr, Stein MA, Krasowski MD, *et al.* (1995) Association of attention-deficit disorder and the dopamine transporter gene. *American Journal of Human Genetics* **56**: 993–8.
68. Yang MS, Gill M (2007) A review of gene linkage, association and expression studies in autism and an assessment of convergent evidence. *International Journal of Developmental Neuroscience* **25**: 69–85.
69. Li D, Sham PC, Owen MJ, He L (2006) Meta-analysis shows significant association between dopamine system genes and attention deficit hyperactivity disorder (ADHD). *Human Molecular Genetics* **15**: 2276–84.
70. Brookes K, Xu X, Chen W, *et al.* (2006) The analysis of 51 genes in DSM-IV combined type attention deficit hyperactivity disorder: association signals in DRD4, DAT1 and 16 other genes. *Molecular Psychiatry* **11**: 934–53.
71. Manolio TA, Rodriguez LL, Brooks L, *et al.* (2007) New models of collaboration in genome-wide association studies: the Genetic Association Information Network. *Nature Genetics* **39**: 1045–51.
72. Kessler RC, Chiu WT, Demler O, Merikangas KR, Walters EE (2005) Prevalence, severity, and comorbidity of 12-month DSM-IV disorders in the National Comorbidity Survey Replication. *Archives of General Psychiatry* **62**: 617–27.
73. Smoller JW, Gardner-Schuster E, Covino J (2008) The genetic basis of panic and phobic anxiety disorders.

American Journal of Medical Genetics. Part C: Seminars in Medical Genetics **148**: 118–26.

74. Hettema JM, Prescott CA, Myers JM, Neale MC, Kendler KS (2005) The structure of genetic and environmental risk factors for anxiety disorders in men and women. *Archives of General Psychiatry* **62**: 182–9.
75. Hovatta I, Barlow C (2008) Molecular genetics of anxiety in mice and men. *Annals of Medicine* **40**: 92–109.
76. Schinka JA, Busch RM, Robichaux-Keene N (2004) A meta-analysis of the association between the serotonin transporter gene polymorphism (5-HTTLPR) and trait anxiety. *Molecular Psychiatry* **9**: 197–202.
77. Sen S, Burmeister M, Ghosh D (2004) Meta-analysis of the association between a serotonin transporter promoter polymorphism (5-HTTLPR) and anxiety-related personality traits. *American Journal of Medical Genetics. Part B: Neuropsychiatric Genetics* **127B**: 85–9.
78. Shifman S, Bhomra A, Smiley S, *et al.* (2008) A whole genome association study of neuroticism using DNA pooling. *Molecular Psychiatry* **13**: 302–12.
79. Chen ZY, Jing D, Bath KG, *et al.* (2006) Genetic variant BDNF (Val66Met) polymorphism alters anxiety-related behavior. *Science* **314**: 140–43.
80. Karno M, Golding JM, Sorenson SB, Burnam MA (1988) The epidemiology of obsessive compulsive disorder in five United States Communities. *Archives of General Psychiatry* **45**: 1094–9.
81. Weissman MM, Bland RC, Canino GJ, *et al.* (1994) The cross national epidemiology of obsessive compulsive disorder. *Journal of Clinical Psychiatry* **55** (3 suppl.): 5–10.
82. Van Grootheest DS, Cath DC, Beekman AT, Boomsma DI (2005) Twin studies on obsessive-compulsive disorder: a review. *Twin Research and Human Genetics* **8**: 450–58.
83. Pauls DL (2008) The genetics of obsessive compulsive disorder: a review of the evidence. *American Journal of Medical Genetics. Part C: Seminars in Medical Genetics* **148**: 133–9.
84. Bienvenu OJ, Samuels JF, Riddle MA, *et al.* (2000) The relationship of obsessive-compulsive disorder to possible spectrum disorders: results from a family study. *Biological Psychiatry* **48**: 287–93.
85. Grados MA, Riddle MA, Samuels JF, *et al.* (2001) The familial phenotype of obsessive-compulsive disorder in relation to tic disorders: the Hopkins OCD family study. *Biological Psychiatry* **50**: 559–65.
86. Hanna GL, Veenstra-VanderWeele J, Cox NJ, *et al.* (2002) Genome-wide linkage analysis of families with obsessive-compulsive disorder ascertained through pediatric probands. *American Journal of Medical Genetics* **114**: 541–52.
87. Shugart YY, Samuels J, Willour VL, *et al.* (2006) Genome-wide linkage scan for obsessive-compulsive disorder: evidence for susceptibility loci on chromosomes 3q, 7p, 1q, 15q, and 6q. *Molecular Psychiatry* **11**: 763–70.
88. Willour VL, Yao Shugart Y, Samuels J, *et al.* (2004) Replication study supports evidence for linkage to 9p24 in obsessive-compulsive disorder. *American Journal of Human Genetics* **75**: 508–13.
89. Lilenfeld LR, Kaye WH, Greeno CG, *et al.* (1998) A controlled family study of anorexia nervosa and bulimia nervosa: psychiatric disorders in first-degree relatives and effects of proband comorbidity. *Archives of General Psychiatry* **55**: 603–10.
90. Bulik CM, Sullivan PF, Tozzi F, *et al.* (2006) Prevalence, heritability, and prospective risk factors for anorexia nervosa. *Archives of General Psychiatry* **63**: 305–12.
91. Bulik CM, Slof-Op't Landt MC, van Furth EF, Sullivan PF (2007) The genetics of anorexia nervosa. *Annual Review of Nutrition* **27**: 263–75.
92. Regier DA, Farmer ME, Rae DS, *et al.* (1990) Comorbidity of mental disorders with alcohol and other drug abuse: results from the Epidemiologic Catchment Area (ECA) study. *Journal of the American Medical Association* **264**: 2511–8.
93. Grant BF, Stinson FS, Dawson DA, *et al.* (2004) Prevalence and co-occurrence of substance use disorders and independent mood and anxiety disorders: results from the National Epidemiologic Survey on Alcohol and Related Conditions. *Archives of General Psychiatry* **61**: 807–16.
94. Prescott CA, Kendler KS (1999) Genetic and environmental contributions to alcohol abuse and dependence in a population-based sample of male twins. *American Journal of Psychiatry* **156**: 34–40.
95. Dick DM, Bierut LJ (2006) The genetics of alcohol dependence. *Current Psychiatry Reports* **8**: 151–7.
96. Uhl GR (2004) Molecular genetics of substance abuse vulnerability: remarkable recent convergence of genome scan results. *Annals of the New York Academy of Science* **1025**: 1–13.
97. Caspi A, McClay J, Moffitt TE, *et al.* (2002) Role of genotype in the cycle of violence in maltreated children. *Science* **297**: 851–4.
98. Foley DL, Eaves LJ, Wormley B, *et al.* (2004) Childhood adversity, monoamine oxidase a genotype, and risk for conduct disorder. *Archives of General Psychiatry* **61**: 738–44.
99. Cardno AG, Rijsdijk FV, Sham PC, Murray RM, McGuffin P (2002) A twin study of genetic relationships between psychotic symptoms. *American Journal of Psychiatry* **159**: 539–45.
100. Owen MJ, Craddock N, Jablensky A (2007) The genetic deconstruction of psychosis. *Schizophrenia Bulletin* **33**: 905–11.

PART 4

Mental health problems and mental illness

Chapter 34

Classification and diagnostic systems

Pesach Lichtenberg and RH Belmaker

INTRODUCTION

In this chapter we consider important issues in the psychiatric classification of disorders and then discuss how the World Health Organization's (WHO) *International Classification of Diseases* (ICD) and the American Psychiatric Association's (APA) *Diagnostic and Statistical Manual* (DSM) constructed their diagnostic systems.

What is 'mental disorder'? When are we justified in describing a behaviour or personality as 'abnormal'? These thorny questions have especially exercised psychiatrists since accusations by the anti-psychiatry movement in the 1960s that psychiatric diagnoses are actually stigmatic stamps of social deviations. Our determination of what is considered a mental disorder can have ramifications for diagnosis, treatment, forensics and healthcare coverage, and can not only reflect but also influence cultural mores. The history of psychiatry is littered with moral judgements disguised as medical diagnoses. Examples include drapetomania, described as a 'disease of the mind' causing black slaves in the nineteenth-century southern USA to betray their naturally submissive natures by absconding to freedom; and, more recently, homosexuality. Without a definition of mental abnormality, we will be hard-pressed to discern whether and when depression will be considered adaptive (as in grieving), sanctioned (as in religious penitents) or diseased; to distinguish between hearing voices as a mystical or a psychotic phenomenon; and to determine when the compulsive ingestion of an addictive substance will be normative (caffeine), disordered (alcohol) or verboten (heroin).

What, then, is a mental disorder? Here are some of the possible definitions, and their problems:

- Mere statistical deviation, as one might employ in determining a 'normal' level of serum liver enzyme or height, cannot suffice, lest anyone pursuing an unusual activity, or a usual activity with unusual persistence, be considered abnormal.
- Social deviation cannot serve as a criterion either, although some totalitarian regimes in the recent past have acted otherwise.
- Disruptive behaviour, were it to serve as a definition of abnormality, would logically lead to the massive transfer of the prison population to psychiatric wards.
- Personal distress seems necessary for determining abnormality, but it is hardly sufficient, for at least two reasons: How much distress is necessary? And, what about the individual, perhaps in the throes of a manic episode, or well settled in their home for the past couple of decades with agoraphobia and not suffering?
- Dysfunction is often invoked in the definition of disorder, but what, if anything, that term adds to our understanding is uncertain.
- Anchoring mental abnormality in an anatomical or physiological abnormality, as seems to be more easily done in other fields of medicine, will also not suffice. This is not just, because of the technical reason that we have yet to find any consistent biological substrate for mental disorder. It is also so because ultimately a mental disorder will be determined by behavioural or psychological function or dysfunction, in the absence of which no conceivable finding of brain imaging or receptor function can by itself justify a psychiatric diagnosis.
- Karl Jaspers, a German psychiatrist and phenomenologist, considered the sign of true mental disorder, as opposed to mere stressful reactions to trying circumstances, to be an inexplicable loss of understandable mental functioning and connections. When the form of the patient's cognitions and perceptions are no longer graspable by the attentive, empathic interview – for example, if the delusion cannot be found to carry any metaphoric meaning, or the depression is vastly disproportionate to any possible trigger – then we may speak of a primary mental disorder. This definition is perhaps narrow and depends upon very subjective judgements by the psychiatrist. Nevertheless, among many psychiatrists, especially in central Europe, Jaspers' influence remains strong today.
- A possible approach has been to define disorders and dysfunction in evolutionary terms. The argument goes that all functions, bodily as well as mental, have been honed by evolutionary forces, and when behaviour is maladaptive, we can diagnose a disorder. Although the wedding of evolutionary theory to psychiatry can enrich our understanding of health and pathology, this theory

also has its limitations. Some disorders may actually have been advantageous for the conditions under which they evolved. For example, hyperactive children are often considered disordered, but it is possible that roaming attention and constant movement, which are so disruptive in the modern classroom, may have been better adapted to the surroundings in the hostile environment of our origins in the African savannah.

The major diagnostic classification systems are well aware of the difficulties of defining disorder. The *International Classification of Diseases*, 10th revision (ICD-10) explains that '"Disorder" is not an exact term', while the *Diagnostic and Statistical Manual*, 4th edition (DSM-IV) admits:

> ... no definition adequately specifies precise boundaries for the concept of 'mental disorder'. The concept of mental disorder, like many other concepts in medicine and science, lacks a consistent operational definition that covers all situations.

The definitions of mental disorder nevertheless supplied by ICD-10 and DSM-IV are provided in Box 34.1. As the reader of the above will see, their definitions are subject to the problems we discussed. The seemingly straightforward stress upon subjective distress, an important part of both definitions, also raises an important question. Consider two individuals with a fear of heights, one living in a major metropolitan centre and rendered by her phobia unable to visit friends or seek work, and the other dwelling in a distant village of single-level huts. Their fear, and its psychological or biological substrate, may be identical, and yet only one would fulfil the proffered definitions of mental disorder.

Some will claim that the question is ultimately not important, that psychiatrists will simply treat whoever seeks treatment, and that ultimately our definitions will deductively adapt to that clinical reality. But that is a poor basis for providing therapy and hardly adequate for justifying what psychiatrists do when called upon to administer coercive treatment.

VALIDITY

In diagnosing mental illness, *essential validity* means that the names we give to psychiatric disorders are semantically capturing categories that are present in nature before we label them. This is a far-reaching claim, and many settle for *nominal* or *conceptual validity*, which demands of our category names only that they be internally coherent, consistent with empirical findings and of heuristic value. Either way, the disorders that we name provide a common language for communication among clinicians and researchers.

Other forms of validity assume one of the two types we have just mentioned. *Face validity* refers to the consensus of experts that the disorder named indeed exists. Experts can be wrong, and one should never be satisfied with face validity alone. *Descriptive validity* means that the different features of a syndrome indeed appear together. For example, individuals with dysphoric moods and reduced appetite will often also suffer from insomnia and have difficulty concentrating. A statistical method called *latent class analysis* examines whether certain clinical features tend to occur together. *Predictive validity* means that, based upon

Box 34.1 Definition of mental disorder

INTERNATIONAL CLASSIFICATION OF DISEASES, 10TH REVISION (ICD-10)

The term 'disorder' is used throughout the classification, so as to avoid even greater problems inherent in the use of terms such as 'disease' and 'illness'. 'Disorder' is not an exact term, but it is used here to imply the existence of a clinically recognizable set of symptoms or behaviour associated in most cases with distress and with interference with personal functions. Social deviance or conflict alone, without personal dysfunction, should not be included in mental disorder as defined here.

DIAGNOSTIC AND STATISTICAL MANUAL, 4TH EDITION (DSM-IV)

... each of the mental disorders is conceptualized as a clinically significant behavioral or psychological syndrome or pattern that occurs in an individual and that is associated with present distress (e.g. a painful symptom) or disability (i.e. impairment in one or more important areas of functioning) or with a significantly increased risk of suffering death, pain, disability, or an important loss of freedom. In addition, this syndrome or pattern must not be merely an expectable and culturally sanctioned response to a particular event, for example, the death of a loved one. Whatever its original cause, it must currently be considered a manifestation of a behavioral, psychological, or biological dysfunction in the individual. Neither deviant behavior (e.g. political, religious, or sexual) nor conflicts that are primarily between the individual and society are mental disorders unless the deviance of conflict is a symptom of a dysfunction in the individual, as described above.

our diagnosis, we can anticipate certain developments, such as clinical course or response to therapy. The surest form of validity, *construct validity*, implies that we know the aetiology of the disorder. This is the validity most sorely lacking in psychiatry, which is the major reason that psychiatry textbooks, as opposed to those in other fields of medicine, need to carry chapters exploring issues in classification.

One result of lacking a clear aetiological basis for mental disorders has been a proliferation of separate diagnoses according to varying clinical syndromes, which may actually share underlying mechanisms. For example, an individual may check the door 40 times at each exit to confirm that it is locked when leaving the flat; or she may check her reflection in the mirror from 40 different angles each morning to assess possible excess weight; or he may check his nose 40 times daily to evaluate whether it is crooked. These three cases will receive different diagnoses (obsessive–compulsive disorder, anorexia nervosa and dysmorphophobia, respectively), even though they share compulsive behaviours and respond to similar pharmacological treatments.

As a helpful contrast, one can consider the situation with, for example, myocardial infarction. The clinical symptoms and physical examination may vary from patient to patient, but the development of myocardial anoxia and death brought about by occlusion of the coronary arteries is a concept that unifies the differing presentations and outcomes of a single diagnostic entity. Of course, medicine is not free of its own diagnostic conundrums. One thinks of systemic lupus erythematosus (SLE) as a case where internal medicine, uncertain about pathophysiological mechanisms, seeks recourse in complex and changing criteria in an effort to provide nosological coherence.

These difficulties are an important reason that most psychiatrists are willing to consider their diagnostic labels as possessing conceptual rather than essential validity. Psychiatric diagnoses are best considered conceptual tools useful for organizing the current state of knowledge and for communicating in a common language.

RELIABILITY

Reliability refers to the extent to which different mental healthcare workers will arrive at the same diagnostic conclusion regarding a particular individual. A relatively simple mathematical formula for measuring inter-rater reliability, known as Cohen's kappa, is $\kappa = (P_o - P_c)/(1 - P_c)$, where κ is reliability, P_o is the observed agreement between raters, and P_c is the level of agreement expected between raters by chance.

High inter-rater reliability is a crucial part of any diagnostic system, because it permits clinicians and researchers to agree that a particular patient or subject is suffering from a particular diagnosis. Without such reliability, research into disorders cannot advance, since it will not be certain which disorder is actually being investigated.

It is well worth noting that reliability and validity can operate independently. Consider by illustration the following vignette:

A new syndrome is described as follows: a person, usually male, is bald, prefers open sandals, and resolutely and continuously listens to Radiohead music, to the detriment of his various occupational and familial obligations. Two of his friends are similarly afflicted. Have we discovered a new disorder?

The reliability of this purported syndrome would certainly be high; that is, we can easily elucidate the criteria so that different raters will agree whether the syndrome is present in any given individual. However, the validity would be doubtful, either in its essential sense – does such a concatenation of symptoms actually occur in nature? – or in its nominal sense – have we produced an idea that will withstand empirical testing or be of heuristic value? Any claims to predictive validity – for example, the prediction that a 'sufferer' will be found at the next Radiohead concert tour – derives from the individual symptom of Radioheadphilia and not from the syndrome.

This somewhat absurd example demonstrates the dilemma afflicting much of psychiatric nosology today, where considerations of reliability have taken precedence over those of validity. Depressive episodes, for example, can be reliably diagnosed, but its validity as a diagnosis, and not merely a collage of differing pathologies with overlapping clinical presentations, is being hotly disputed.

Nevertheless, if the inter-rater reliability is poor, then the validity of the diagnostic entity being examined is undermined, for the obvious reason that one cannot be certain to what exactly one is referring when using a diagnosis.

CATEGORICAL OR DIMENSIONAL DIAGNOSES?

The diagnoses used in psychiatry are usually categories: schizophrenia, anorexia nervosa, premature ejaculation, and so on. It is the use of categories, with assumptions that they describe psychopathological entities relatively well delineated from healthy personality traits, that raises the complex problems of validity. A different approach is to use dimensional diagnoses, either instead of or in addition to categorical diagnoses. Dimensional diagnoses describe the individual along a continuum. For example, reduced appetite may be rated on a scale; depressive syndrome might be assessed by scores on standardized rating scales such as the Beck Depression Inventory. In a purely dimensional diagnostic system, the patient will receive a number on a dimension rather than a diagnosis. No claim is made about the reification of the diagnostic category; on the contrary, an implication of a purely dimensional diagnostic system is that the disorder does not exist as a discrete entity but rather is an extreme case of normal variability, similar to hypertension in general medicine. The dimensional diagnosis can also supplement the categorical diagnosis, so that, for example, a patient may be said to suffer from a depressive episode with a severity of 30 on the Beck Depression Scale.

Studies utilizing various scales of symptom severity are in effect employing dimensional diagnoses. Dimensional diagnosis is also commonly used in scales of personality. A hint of dimensional diagnosis, tightly tethered to the categorical diagnosis, is found in the DSM and ICD codes for some disorders, which allow for the severity to be rated (e.g. mild, moderate, severe).

LUMPERS VERSUS SPLITTERS

A further issue in nosology is how broadly to define each diagnosis. Different diagnostic schemes include more or fewer patients, which can affect treatment decisions and epidemiological findings. 'Lumpers' tend to provide a broad definition of a disorder, allowing for manifestations varying in symptoms and severity, while 'splitters' distinguish between different narrowly and well-defined symptom clusters. An example of lumping coming under increasing scrutiny today is 'major depressive episode', which can include depressive syndromes of vastly varying symptomatology arising in a wide array of contexts, all receiving the same diagnosis. Proponents of purely dimensional diagnoses have less difficulty with this issue, since they can describe different clinical features without making claims for a specific diagnosis.

DIAGNOSTIC AND STATISTICAL MANUAL OF THE AMERICAN PSYCHIATRIC ASSOCIATION

First and second editions – DSM-I and DSM-II

The precursor to the first edition of the DSM was a classification for the treatment of soldiers developed in the middle of the twentieth century by the psychiatrist and psychoanalyst William Meninger. The APA was involved in the development of the DSM-I. DSM-I diagnoses frequently carried the phrase 'reaction', as in 'schizophrenic reaction', reflecting the ideas of Adolf Meyer (1866–1950), a prominent Swiss-born psychiatrist who stressed the social causation of much mental illness.

The second edition of DSM, prepared by the APA and published in 1968, was based upon the eighth edition of the ICD. The original 106 diagnoses in DSM-I grew to 182 in DSM-II. The term 'reaction' was no longer used. Nevertheless, like the first edition, the second also implied a largely psychoanalytical framework for understanding psychopathology, reflecting regnant professional opinion in the USA at the time.

Both DSM-I and DSM-II described in general terms, for each disorder, the way that a typical case of the disorder would appear. It was up to the clinician to decide how closely the description corresponded to a particular patient.

However, through the 1970s, dissatisfaction grew. One notable study in the early 1970s found that patients diagnosed by American psychiatrists as having schizophrenia were likely to be diagnosed as manic-depressive, neurotic or personality-disordered by their British counterparts. These and similar studies indicating abysmal reliability spurred efforts to improve reliability.

Third edition – DSM-III

In 1972, a group of researchers at Washington University established the Feighner criteria. This was a landmark in the way diagnosis was made. For 15 diagnoses, the researchers provided detailed inclusion and exclusion criteria. They also suggested criteria for validating a diagnosis, with five elements: a clearly defined clinical description (including demographic features, age of onset and precipitating events), delimitation from other disorders, biological and psychological tests, similar outcomes, and support from family studies.

The Research Diagnostic Criteria (RDC), published in 1978, modified the Feighner criteria, based on study findings. Robert Spitzer and colleagues, who developed the RDC, also established the Schedule for Affective Disorders and Schizophrenia (SADS), a structured interview intended for improving still further inter-rater reliability.

Robert Spitzer also headed the effort to produce the third edition of the DSM. When it appeared in 1980, it heralded a seismic shift in psychiatric nosology. Building upon the approach developed in the RDC, DSM-III provided criteria for 265 diagnoses, as well as information about clinical features, associated features, cultural considerations, course of illness and differential diagnosis.

Among the innovations instituted by DSM-III are the following:

- *Atheoretical formulations:* DSM-III attempted to detail the features and criteria for each diagnosis in a way that psychiatrists of varying and even contradictory theoretical schools could agree. For example, DSM-III deleted the term 'neurosis' from its diagnoses, in order to refrain from reliance upon a term associated with a particular school of thought and difficult to validate empirically.
- Diagnosing without dependence upon theories of aetiology required the use of *operationalized definitions*, wherein each disorder was diagnosed by empirically determined criteria indifferent to prior ideological assumptions. The idea of operationalized, atheoretical formulations had already been suggested in the late 1950s by the British psychiatrist Edward Stengel and reached full flower in the DSM-III.
- *Multi-axial diagnoses:* in keeping with the DSM's thoroughly empirical ambitions, they developed a scheme

(subsequently adopted by the ICD-10 as well) of diagnosing in various axes, or dimensions. The two ideas behind multi-axial diagnoses are (i) each individual is too complex to be grasped simply by a diagnosis of disorder; multi-axial diagnoses allow for greater complexity by including other aspects of the individual's condition and circumstances; and (ii) a biopsychosocial model of illness requires diagnosis on different levels, as can best be encompassed by multi-axial diagnoses. In principal, one can entertain an endless number of axes, each describing the patient from a different perspective. DSM-III settled for five axes, which have been altered slightly by DSM-IV and will be presented below.

- *Axis I:* clinical disorders or other disorders that may be a focus of clinical attention. These include the many disorders, usually not lasting a lifetime, that the psychiatrist can diagnose. If the patient fulfils criteria for various disorders, they should all be noted (Box 34.2).
- *Axis II:* personality disorders and developmental disorders (in DSM-IV, this became personality disorders and mental retardation). Personality disorders, like the axis I disorders, have operationalized criteria. However, because of the greater difficulty assessing personality characteristics than symptoms, the inter-rater reliability has generally been lower for axis II disorders (Box 34.3).
- *Axis III:* medical conditions, which can have any sort of bearing upon the patient's mental disorder. The non-psychiatric condition is listed using ICD codes. If, for example, a patient is depressed due to hypothyroidism, then they will receive a diagnosis of 'a mood disorder due to hypothyroidism' on axis I and hypothyroidism (E03) on axis III.
- *Axis IV:* severity of psychosocial stressors (in DSM-IV, this axis became 'psychosocial and environmental problems'). In DSM-III, the stress produced by these problems was quantified on a scale of 1–7, but in light of the great variety in responses to adversity, the illusion of quantifiable accuracy produced by numbers was replaced in DSM-IV by a verbal description of the stressful circumstances, listed in the relevant categories: primary support group, social environment, education, occupation, housing, economic, access to healthcare services, interaction with the legal system or being a victim of crime, and other psychosocial problem.
- *Axis V:* highest level of adaptive functioning past year (which in DSM-IV is called 'global assessment of function (GAF)'). This is a scale from 1 to 100 and intended to provide a generalized assessment of function (Box 34.4). In DSM-IV this may include level of functioning at the present time and be supplemented by assessments for past periods as well. The highest level of function attained during the past year can have prognostic significance.

DSM-III-R (revised), again led by Robert Sptizer, was published in 1987 and grew to 292 diagnoses. Criteria were amended based on new research findings.

Box 34.2 Axis I: clinical disorders

OTHER CONDITIONS THAT MAY BE A FOCUS OF CLINICAL ATTENTION

Disorders usually first diagnosed in infancy, childhood, or adolescence *(excluding mental retardation, which is diagnosed on Axis II)*
Delirium, dementia, and amnestic and other cognitive disorders
Mental disorders due to a general medical condition
Schizophrenia and other psychotic disorders
Mood disorders
Anxiety disorders
Somatoform disorders
Factitious disorders
Dissociative disorders
Sexual and gender identity disorders
Eating disorders
Sleep disorders
Impulse-control disorders not elsewhere classified
Adjustment disorders
Other conditions that may be a focus of clincal attention

Box 34.3 Axis II: personality disorders

MENTAL RETARDATION

- Paranoid personality disorder
- Schizoid personality disorder
- Schizotypal personality disorder
- Antisocial personality disorder
- Borderline personality disorder
- Histrionic personality disorder
- Narcissistic personality disorder
- Avoidant personality disorder
- Dependent personality disorder
- Obsessive–compulsive personality disorder
- Personality disorder not otherwise specified
- Mental retardation

Fourth edition – DSM-IV

Under the leadership of Allen Frances, DSM-IV arrived in 1994, with 297 diagnoses. It had several substantive changes from the DSM-III-R. 'Organic mental syndromes' no longer appeared, for such a term hinted at an untenable distinction between brain and mind. Instead, a new section appeared for 'mental orders due to a general medical condition'. A second important revision in DSM-IV was the addition for many disorders of the criteria that the symptoms cause 'clinically significant distress or impairment in social, occupational, or other important areas of functioning',

Box 34.4 Global assessment of function (GAF) scale

Consider psychological, social, and occupational functioning on a hypothetical continuum of mental health–illness. Do not include impairment in functioning due to physical (or environmental) limitations.

CODE	(NOTE: USE INTERMEDIATE CODES WHEN APPROPRIATE, E.G. 45, 68, 72.)
100–91	**Superior functioning in a wide range of activities, life's problems never seem to get out of hand, is sought out by others because of his or her many positive qualities. No symptoms.**
90–81	**Absent or minimal symptoms** (e.g., mild anxiety before an exam), **good functioning in all areas, interested and involved in a wide range of activities, socially effective, generally satisfied with life, no more than everyday problems or concerns** (e.g., an occasional argument with family members).
80–71	**If symptoms are present, they are transient and expectable reactions to psycho-social stressors** (e.g., difficulty concentrating after family argument); **no more than slight impairment in social, occupational or school functioning** (e.g., temporarily falling behind in schoolwork).
70–61	**Some mild symptoms** (e.g., depressed mood and mild insomnia) **OR some difficulty in social, occupational, or school functioning** (e.g., occasional truancy, or theft within the household), **but generally functioning pretty well, has some meaningful interpersonal relationships.**
60–51	**Moderate symptoms** (e.g., flat affect and circumstantial speech, occasional panic attacks) **OR moderate difficulty in social, occupational, or school functioning** (e.g., few friends, conflicts with peers or co-workers).
50–41	**Serious symptoms** (e.g., suicidal ideation, severe obsessional rituals, frequent shoplifting) **OR any serious impairment in social, occupational, or school functioning** (e.g., no friends, unable to keep a job).
40–31	**Some impairment in reality testing or communication** (e.g., speech is at times illogical, obscure, or irrelevant) **OR major impairment in several areas, such as work or school, family relations, judgment, thinking, or mood** (e.g., depressed man avoids friends, neglects family, and is unable to work; child frequently beats up younger children, is defiant at home, and is failing at school).
30–21	**Behavior is considerably influenced by delusions or hallucinations OR serious impairment in communication or judgment** (e.g., sometimes incoherent, acts grossly inappropriately, suicidal preoccupation) **OR inability to function in almost all areas** (e.g., stays in bed all day; no job, home, or friends).
20–11	**Some danger of hurting self or others** (e.g., suicide attempts without clear expectation of death; frequently violent; manic excitement) **OR occasionally fails to maintain minimal personal hygiene** (e.g., smears feces) **OR gross impairment in communication** (e.g., largely incoherent or mute).
10–1	**Persistent danger of severely hurting self or others** (e.g., recurrent violence) **OR persistent inability to maintain minimal personal hygiene OR serious suicidal act with clear expectation of death.**
0	Inadequate information.

thereby responding to criticism that too many people were diagnosable under DSM-III.

The evolution of a diagnosis across the subsequent editions of the DSM is offered in Box 34.5, with schizophrenia serving as the example.

Fourth edition (text revision) – DSM-IV-TR

DSM-IV-TR was published in 2000. It included revisions of the supporting information (e.g. clinical course) but not of the diagnostic criteria themselves.

DSM-V is scheduled to be published in 2012, and the results are eagerly awaited by many in the field. The proceedings of the many committees working on revising criteria are shrouded in secrecy, which is a source of controversy. The APA has made an effort to recruit researchers and clinicians relatively unmarked by pharmaceutical support in their work. It is possible that the categorical diagnoses will be complemented by dimensional subdiagnoses.

Box 34.5 Schizophrenia: an evolving definition

DIAGNOSTIC AND STATISTICAL MANUAL, FIRST EDITION (DSM-I)

This term is synonymous with the formerly used term dementia praecox. It represents a group of psychotic reactions characterized by fundamental disturbances in reality relationships and concept formations, with affective, behavioral, and intellectual disturbances in varying degrees and mixtures. The disorders are marked by strong tendency to retreat from reality, by emotional disharmony, unpredictable disturbances in stream of thought, regressive behavior, and in some, by a tendency to 'deterioration.' The predominant symptomatology will be the determining factor in classifying such patients into types.

DIAGNOSTIC AND STATISTICAL MANUAL, SECOND EDITION (DSM-II)

This large category includes a group of disorders manifested by characteristic disturbances of thinking, mood and behavior. Disturbances in thinking are marked by alterations of concept formation which may lead to misinterpretation of reality and sometimes to delusions and hallucinations, which frequently appear psychologically self-protective. Corollary mood changes include ambivalent, constricted and inappropriate emotional responsiveness and loss of empathy with others. Behavior may be withdrawn, regressive and bizarre. The schizophrenias, in which the mental status is attributable primarily to a *thought* disorder, are to be distinguished from the *major affective illnesses* ... which are dominated by a *mood* disorder. The *paranoid states* ... are distinguished from schizophrenia by the narrowness of their distortions of reality and by the absence of other psychotic symptoms.

DIAGNOSTIC AND STATISTICAL MANUAL, THIRD EDITION (DSM-III)

A. At least one of the following during a phase of the illness:

(1) bizarre delusions (content is patently absurd and has no possible basis in fact), such as delusions of being controlled, thought broadcasting, thought insertion, or thought withdrawal
(2) somatic, grandiose, religious, nihilistic, or other delusions without persecutory or jealous content
(3) delusions with persecutory or jealous content if accompanied by hallucinations of any type
(4) auditory hallucinations in which either a voice keeps up a running commentary on the individual's behavior or thoughts, or two or more voices converse with each other
(5) auditory hallucinations on several occasions with content of more than one or two words, having no apparent relation to depression or elation
(6) incoherence, marked loosening of associations, markedly illogical thinking, or marked poverty of content of speech if associated with at least one of the following:
- blunted, flat, or inappropriate affect
- delusions or hallucinations
- catatonic or other grossly disorganized behaviour

B. Deterioration from a previous level of functioning in such areas as work, social relations, and self-care

C. Duration

Continuous signs of the illness for at least six months at some time during the person's life, with some signs of the illness at present. The six-month period must include an active phase during which there were symptoms from A. with or without a prodromal or residual phase, as defined below.

Prodromal phase: A clear deterioration in functioning before the active phase of the illness not due to a disturbance in mood or to a Substance Use Disorder and involving at least *two* of the symptoms noted below, not due to a disturbance in mood or to a Substance Use Disorder.

Residual phase: Persistence, following the active phase of the illness, of at least *two* of the symptoms noted below, not due to a disturbance in mood or to a Substance Use Disorder.

Prodromal or Residual Symptoms

(1) social isolation or withdrawal
(2) marked impairment in role functioning as wage-earner, student, or homemaker
(3) markedly peculiar behavior (e.g., collecting garbage, talking to self in public, or hoarding food)
(4) marked impairment in personal hygiene and grooming
(5) blunted, flat, or inappropriate affect
(6) digressive, vague, overelaborate, circumstantial, or metaphorical speech

(7) odd or bizarre ideation, or magical thinking, e.g., superstitiousness, clairvoyance, telepathy, "sixth sense," "others can feel my feelings," over-valued ideas, ideas of reference

(8) unusual perceptual experiences, e.g., recurrent illusions, sensing the presence of a force or person not actually present

D. The full depressive or manic syndrome (criteria A and B of major depressive or manic episode), if present, developed after any psychotic symptoms, or was brief in duration relative to the duration of the psychotic symptoms in A.

E. Onset of prodromal or active phase of the illness before age 45.

F. Not due to any Organic Mental Disorder or Mental Retardation.

DIAGNOSTIC AND STATISTICAL MANUAL, FOURTH EDITION (DSM-IV)

A. Characteristic symptoms

(1) delusions
(2) hallucinations
(3) disorganized speech (e.g., frequent derailment or incoherence)
(4) grossly disorganized or catatonic behavior
(5) negative symptoms, e.g., affective flattening, alogia, or avolition

Note: Only one Criterion A symptom is required if delusions are bizarre or hallucinations are bizarre or hallucinations consist of a voice keeping up running commentary on the person's behavior or thoughts, or two or more voices conversing with each other.

B. Social/occupational dysfunction

For a significant portion of the time since the onset of the disturbance, one or more major areas of functioning such as work, interpersonal relations, or self-care are markedly below the level achieved prior to the onset (or when the onset is in childhood or adolescence, failure to achieve expected level of interpersonal, academic, or occupational achievement).

C. Duration

Continuous signs of the disturbance persist for at least 6 months. This 6-month period must include at least 1 month of symptoms (or less if successfully treated) that meet Criterion A (i.e., active-phase symptoms) and may include periods of prodromal or residual symptoms. During these prodromal or residual periods, the signs of the disturbance may be manifested by only negative symptoms or two or more symptoms listed in Criterion A present in an attenuated form (e.g., odd beliefs, unusual perceptual experiences).

D. Schizoaffective and Mood Disorder exclusion

Schizoaffective Disorder and Mood Disorder With Psychotic Features have been ruled out because either (1) no Major Depressive, Manic, or Mixed Episodes have occurred concurrently with the active-phase symptoms; or (2) if mood episodes have occurred during active-phase symptoms, their total duration has been brief relative to the duration of the active and residual periods.

E. Substance/general medical condition exclusion

The disturbance is not due to the direct physiological affects of a substance (e.g., a drug of abuse, a medication) or a general medical condition.

F. Relationship to a Pervasive Developmental Disorder

If there is a history of Autistic Disorder or another Pervasive Developmental Disorder, the additional diagnosis of Schizophrenia is made only if prominent delusions or hallucinations are also present for at least a month (or less if successfully treated).

INTERNATIONAL CLASSIFICATION OF DISEASES OF THE WORLD HEALTH ORGANIZATION

The ICD has far older roots than the DSM, starting out in the late nineteenth century as an internationally recognized list of causes of death. The sixth edition, appearing in 1948 under the auspices of the WHO, was expanded to include a classification of illness as well as causes of death. In this edition, psychiatric morbidity makes its first appearance, albeit with the single category 'mental illness and deficiency'. In the seventh edition, appearing in 1955, the chapter on mental disorders was unchanged.

The eighth (1966) and ninth (1978) editions of the ICD had an expanded chapter on mental disorders. ICD-8 also influenced the DSM-II, which appeared 2 years later.

The ICD-10, completed in 1992, had an enlarged Chapter V covering mental disorders. The ICD-10 has produced companion volumes (which may be downloaded free from the public domain at the WHO website, at www.who.int/classifications/icd/en). This includes the clinical descriptions and diagnostic guidelines, or the 'Blue Book', which contains diagnostic criteria intended for use mainly by clinicians, and the diagnostic criteria for research (DCR), or the 'Green Book', with more precise and restrictive criteria for use by researchers. The DCR has adopted several of the DSM-III innovations. A short glossary has also been published, for use alongside both works.

The ICD-10 adopted the DSM's multiaxial system. However, the axes are slightly different:

- Axis I included psychiatric disorders, personality disorders, mental retardation and medical illness – that is, the first three DSM-IV axes.
- Axis II assesses the disability resulting from the axis I diagnosis. Instead of the GAF of DSM's axis V, it uses a short disability assessment schedule (DAS-S).
- Axis III, corresponding to axis IV of the DSM-IV, refers to psychosocial problems confronting the patient.

The ICD-10 makes a greater effort to be adaptable to varying cultural environments, and seeks to be a basis for local schemes of classification.

The latest editions of the DSM and ICD show a great deal of cross-fertilization and a convergence of diagnostic approaches. DSM-IV-TR lists, in Appendix H, the ICD-10 codes for the DSM disorders. Nevertheless, differences between the two systems remain.

KEY POINTS

- No definition has been agreed upon for the term 'mental disorder'. Part of the difficulty lies in the lack of a clear aetiology.
- Similarly, the essential validity of the various diagnoses – that is, the claim that our diagnostic labels are semantically capturing categories that are present in nature – is uncertain.
- The value of a diagnosis is its conceptual validity, or internal coherence, providing a common language and a heuristic direction.
- Inter-rater reliability is the extent to which different clinicians will arrive at the same diagnostic conclusion.
- Diagnoses can be categorical, describing a well-delineated entity, or dimensional, along a continuum from health to disease with uncertain boundaries.
- DSM-IV features the use of operationalized diagnoses to improve reliability, and multiple axes to enhance biopsychosocial understanding.
- ICD-10 also uses multiple axes and attempts to provide an international basis for a common nosology.

INFORMATION SOURCES AND FURTHER READING

1. World Health Organization (1948) *Manual of the International Statistical Classification of Diseases, Injuries and Causes of Death*, 6th edn (ICD-6). Geneva: World Health Organization.
2. World Health Organization (1967) *Glossary of Mental Disorders and Guide to their Classification, for Use in Conjunction with the International Classification of Diseases*, 8th revision. Geneva: World Health Organization.
3. World Health Organization (1978) *Mental Disorders: Glossary and Guide to their Classification, for Use in Conjunction with the Ninth Revision of the International Classification of Diseases*. Geneva: World Health Organization.
4. American Psychiatric Association (1980) *Diagnostic and Statistical Manual of Mental Disorders*, 3rd edn. Washington, DC: American Psychiatric Association.
5. American Psychiatric Association (1987) *Diagnostic and Statistical Manual of Mental Disorders*, 3rd edn, revised. Washington, DC: American Psychiatric Association.
6. World Health Organization (1992) *International Statistical Classification of Diseases and Related Health Problems*, 10th revision. Geneva: World Health Organization.
7. World Health Organization (1993) *The ICD-10 Classification of Mental and Behavioural Disorders: Diagnostic Criteria for Research*. Geneva: World Health Organization.
8. American Psychiatric Association (1994) *Diagnostic and Statistical Manual of Mental Disorders*, 4th edn. Washington, DC: American Psychiatric Association.
9. American Psychiatric Association (2000) *Diagnostic and Statistical Manual of Mental Disorders*, 4th edn, text revision. Washington, DC: American Psychiatric Association.
10. American Psychiatric Association (2002) *A Research Agenda for DSM-V*. Washington, DC: American Psychiatric Association.
11. Bentall RP (1992) A proposal to classify happiness as a psychiatric disorder. *Journal of Medical Ethics* **18**: 94–8.
12. Bentall RP (2003) *Madness Explained: Psychosis and Human Nature*. London: Penguin.
13. Bolton D (2008) *What is Mental Disorder? An Essay in Philosophy, Science, and Values*. Oxford: Oxford University Press.
14. Cartwright SA (1851) Report on the diseases and physical peculiarities of the Negro race. *New Orleans Medical and Surgical Journal* **7**: 691–715.
15. Cosmides L, Tooby J (1999) Toward an evolutionary taxonomy of treatable conditions. *Journal of Abnormal Psychology* **108**: 453–64.

16. Feighner JP, Robins E, Guze SB, *et al.* (1972) Diagnostic criteria for use in psychiatric research. *Archives of General Psychiatry* **26**: 57–63.
17. Helzer JE, Kraemer HC, Krueger RF (2006) The feasibility and need for dimensional psychiatric diagnoses. *Psychological Medicine* **36**: 1671–80.
18. Horwitz AV, Wakefield JC (2007) *The Loss of Sadness.* New York: Oxford University Press.
19. Janca A, Kartrup M, Katsching N, *et al.* (1996) The World Health Organization Short Disability Assessment Schedule (WHO DAS-S): a tool for the assessment of difficulties in selected areas of functioning of patients with mental disorders. *Social Psychiatry* **31**: 349–54.
20. Jaspers K, Hoenig J, Hamilton M (1963) *General Psychopathology.* Manchester: Manchester University Press.
21. Kendell RE (1975) The concept of disease and its implications for psychiatry. *British Journal of Psychiatry* **127**: 305–15.
22. Kendell RE, Cooper JE, Gourlay AJ, *et al.* (1971) Diagnostic criteria of American and British psychiatrists. *Archives of General Psychiatry* **25**: 123–30.
23. Moller HJ (2008) Systematic of psychiatric disorders between categorical and dimensional approaches: Kraepelin's dichotomy and beyond. *European Archives of Psychiatry and Clinical Neuroscience* **258** (suppl. 2): 48–73.
24. Regier DA, Kaelber CT, Roper MT, Rae DS, Sartorius N (1994) The ICD-10 clinical field trial for mental and behavioral disorders: results in Canada and the United States. *American Journal of Psychiatry* **151**: 1340–50.
25. Reznick L (1987) *The Nature of Disease.* London: Routledge & Kegan Paul.
26. Robins E, Guze SB (1970) Establishment of diagnostic validity in psychiatric illness: its application to schizophrenia. *American Journal of Psychiatry* **126**: 983–7.
27. Sartorius N (1995) *Understanding the ICD-10 Classification of Mental Disorders.* London: Science Press.
28. Sartorius N, Kaelber CT, Cooper JE, *et al.* (1993) Progress toward achieving a common language in psychiatry: results from the field trial of the clinical guidelines accompanying the WHO classification of mental and behavioral disorders in ICD-10. *Archives of General Psychiatry* **50**: 115–24.
29. Spitzer RL, Endicott J, Robins E (1978) Research diagnostic criteria: rationale and reliability. *Archives of General Psychiatry* **35**: 773–82.
30. Spitzer RL, Endicott J, Robins E (1978) *Research Diagnostic Criteria (RDC) for a Selected Group of Functional Disorders*, 3rd edn. New York: New York State Psychiatric Institute.
31. Spitzer RL, Fleiss JL (1974) A re-analysis of the reliability of psychiatric diagnosis. *British Journal of Psychiatry* **125**: 341–7.
32. Stengel E (1959) Classification of mental disorders. *Bulletin of the World Health Organization* **21**: 601–63.
33. Wakefield JC, First MB (2002) Clarifying the distinction between disorder and nondisorder: confronting the overdiagnosis problem (false-positives) in DSM-IV. In KA Phillips, MB First, HA Pincus (eds) *Advancing DSM: Dilemmas in Psychiatric Diagnosis.* Washington, DC: American Psychiatric Publishing.
34. Zachar P, Kendler KS (2007) Psychiatric disorders: a conceptual taxonomy. *American Journal of Psychiatry* **164**: 557–65.

Chapter 35

Cognitive assessment

Adam Zeman and Lorna Torrens

WHAT IS COGNITION?

Cognition, briefly, is the capacity to acquire, store and use knowledge. Indeed, it shares its etymological origin with 'knowledge' in the Indo-European root *gno*. It has also been defined as 'the totality of capacities underlying complex adaptive behaviour'[1] and, more lengthily, as 'the capacity of the brain to process information accurately and to program adaptive behaviour, involving the abilities to solve problems, communicate, memorize information or focus attention'.[2]

Listing the elements of cognition is more revealing than providing abstract definitions: the major cognitive functions comprise consciousness, attention, perception, memory, language, numeracy, executive function and praxis.[3–5] In this chapter we explain what each of these functions involves, sketch their neural bases, describe how best to assess them, and mention their common pathologies, including the clinical features of the major varieties of delirium and dementia. We outline a practical approach to a brief but sensitive and wide-ranging cognitive assessment and explain what a neuropsychologist can add to the assessment of cognition, including the measurement of intelligence quotient (IQ).

Three common misconceptions about cognition are worth correcting at the outset:

- Cognition is not an entirely independent function. Although cognitive testing is a distinctive aspect of assessment, cognitive processes are tied closely to general medical, neurological and behavioural functioning. The clue to the cause of a cognitive disorder may come from general medical examination (e.g. the slow pulse and coarse skin of hypothyroidism), neurological examination (e.g. the choreiform movements of Huntington's disease), cognitive assessment itself (e.g. the pure anterograde memory deficit of early Alzheimer's disease) or neuropsychiatric observations of behaviour (e.g. the disinhibition of frontal lobe dementia).
- Cognitive processes are not restricted to certain higher brain regions. The belief that cognitive functions are localized in the association cortex has given way to the view that they depend on interconnected networks of regions distributed around the brain, both cortical and subcortical. Damage to the thalamus, for example, can profoundly disable cognition.[6] There is also a growing recognition of the cognitive, affective and behavioural importance of subcortical regions such as the cerebellum and basal ganglia, which have classically been associated with motor functions.[7,8] This richer understanding of the way in which cognition is represented in the brain should help to explain how cognitive processes arise from more basic sensorimotor functions.
- Cognitive functions are not entirely separate from one another, or from related neuropsychological functions such as personality, mood and motivation. Difficulty sustaining attention, for example, inevitably impacts on memory, and impairments of language have widespread effects on cognition. Low mood, apathy or a deliberate decision to withhold effort will also influence the results of cognitive testing. This is not to say that cognitive deficits cannot occur in relative isolation. Damage to the hippocampi, for example, causes predominant problems with memory. But the interdependence of neuropsychological functions does mean that individual test results must be interpreted in a broader cognitive and clinical context.

THE ELEMENTS OF COGNITION

Consciousness

Definition

Consciousness normally implies both a particular global behavioural state – wakefulness – and the occurrence of experience – awareness.[9]

Neural basis

The cycle of sleep and waking is controlled by a network of structures in the upper brainstem, thalamus, hypothalamus and basal forebrain.[10] These structures are the components of the ascending reticular activating system, which, it is now recognized, incorporates several neurochemically distinct subsystems, strategically placed to modulate the level

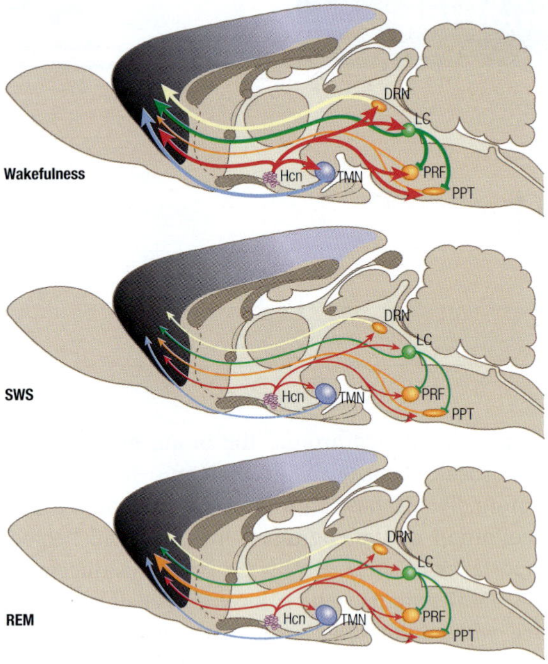

Figure 35.1 Schematic model of neurotransmitter circuits involved in the three states of vigilance. During wakefulness, hypocretin (Hcrt) activity excites noradrenergic (green), histaminergic (deep blue) and serotonergic (yellow) neurons, which give rise to enhanced cortical activity and arousal. Slow-wave sleep (SWS) is characterized by synchronous intrinsic cortical activity, and most subcortical afferents show reduced activity. During rapid-eye-movement (REM) sleep, low hypocretin activity results in disinhibition of REM-on cholinergic neurons (orange) DRN, dorsal raphe nucleus; LC, locus coeruleus; PPT, pedunculopontine tegmental nucleus; PRF, pontine reticular formation; TMN, tuberomamillary nucleus.

Box 35.1 Epworth Sleepiness Scale

Daytime sleepiness:

- Sitting and reading
- Watching television
- Sitting inactive in a public place, e.g. theatre, meeting
- Passenger in a car for an hour
- Lying down to rest in the afternoon
- Sitting and talking to someone
- Sitting quietly after lunch
- In a car while stopped in traffic.

– 0 = would never doze
– 1 = slight chance of dozing
– 2 = moderate chance
– 3 = high chance

and mode of function in the cerebral hemispheres (Figure 35.1). The key neurotransmitters involved in the control of conscious state are serotonin (raphe nuclei), noradrenaline (locus coeruleus), acetylcholine (nuclei at the pons–midbrain junction and in the basal forebrain), dopamine (ventral tegmentum), histamine (hypothalamus), hypocretin (hypothalamus) and glutamate (reticular nuclei).

It is possible to be awake but unaware, as in the vegetative state, in which brainstem function is relatively intact while the functioning of the cerebral hemispheres is severely impaired.[6] Awareness – the occurrence of experience – is thought to require adequate amounts of appropriately synchronized and widely distributed activity in the cerebral hemispheres.[9,11]

Assessment

The state and level of consciousness are usually assessed using the Glasgow Coma Scale (GCS),[12] which requires examination of the eyes and of verbal and motor responses (Figure 35.2). Although this is an extremely useful tool, it is important to remember, especially in the intensive care unit (ICU), that a paralysed patient may be fully conscious and yet score 3/15 on the GCS. Clues to the preservation of awareness in patients with apparently impaired consciousness include any evidence of perceptual distinctions (e.g. between relatives and strangers), of purposeful actions (e.g. sustained visual tracking or reaching for an object) and of communication (either expressive or receptive). Conscious state is not usually a major consideration during cognitive assessment in the clinic, but relative impairments of

COMA SCALE				
Eyes open	Spontaneously	4		Eyes closed by swelling = C
	To speech	3		
	To pain	2		
	None	1		
Best verbal response	Oriented	5		Endotracheal tube or tracheostomy = T
	Confused	4		
	Inappropriate words	3		
	Incomprehensible sounds	2		
	None	1		
Best motor response	Obey commands	6		Usually records the best arm response
	Localize pain	5		
	Normal flexion	4		
	Abnormal flexion	3		
	Extension to pain	2		
	None	1		
COMA SCALE TOTAL 3–15				

Figure 35.2 Glasgow Coma Scale

Table 35.1 Classification of states of impaired awareness

Condition	Vegetative state	Minimally conscious state	Locked-in syndrome	Coma	Death confirmed by brainstem tests
Awareness	Absent	Present	Present	Absent	Absent
Sleep–wake cycle	Present	Present	Present	Absent	Absent
Response to pain	±	Present	Present (in eyes only)	±	Absent
GCS score	E4, M1–4, V1–2	E4, M1–5, V1–4	E4, M1, V1	E1, M1–4, V1–2	E1, M1–3, V1
Motor function	No purposeful movement	Some consistent or inconsistent verbal or purposeful motor behaviour	Volitional vertical eye movements or eye-blink preserved	No purposeful movement	None or only reflex spinal movement
Respiratory function	Typically Preserved	Typically Preserved	Typically Preserved	Variable	Absent
EEG Activity	Typically slow wave activity	Insufficient data	Typically normal	Typically slow wave activity	Typically absent
Cerebral metabolism	Severely reduced	Insufficient data	Mildly reduced	Moderately to severely reduced	Severely reduced or absent
Prognosis	Variable: if permanent continued vegetative state or death	Variable	Depends on cause but full recovery unlikely	Recovery, vegetative state or death within weeks	Already dead

EEG, electroencephalogram; GCS, Glasgow Coma Scale.

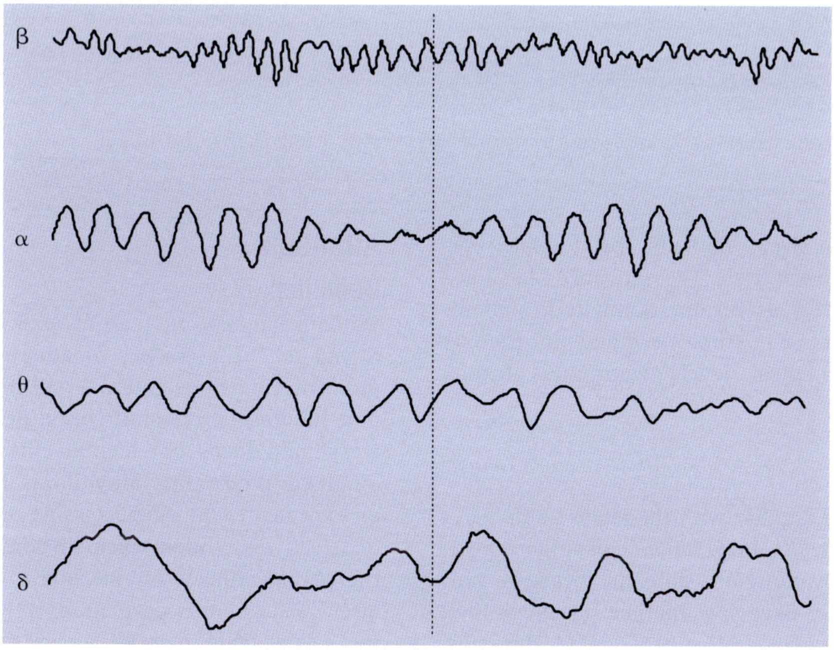

Figure 35.3 Basic rhythms of the electroencephalogram (EEG). Records from diagnostic EEGs performed in four different patients, exemplifying β rhythm (> 14 Hz), α rhythm (8–13 Hz), θ rhythm (4–7 Hz) and δ rhythm (4 Hz). In each case the dotted line bisects a 2-s sample

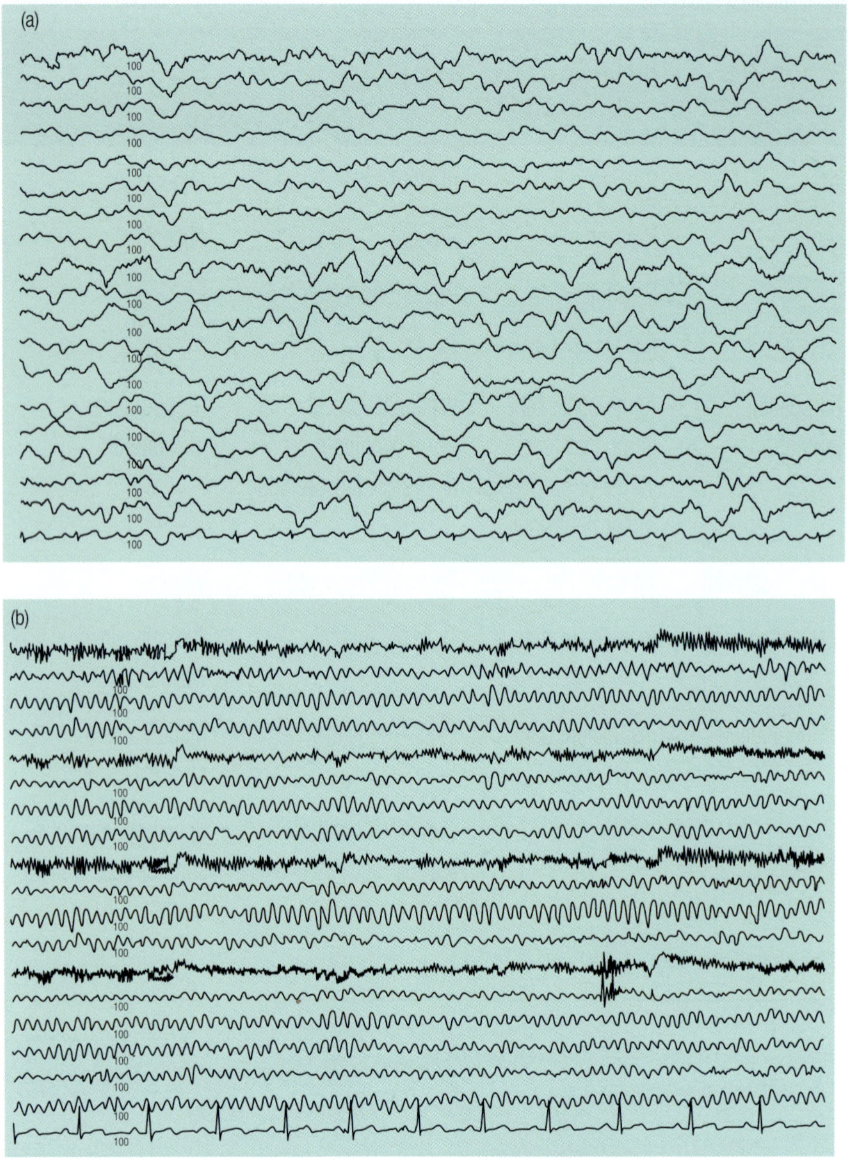

Figure 35.4 Electroencephalograms (EEGs) from the same patient during (a) and after recovery from (b) an episode of delirium

vigilance are common: sleepy patients, for example, perform poorly on cognitive tests. The Epworth Sleepiness Scale (Box 35.1) is a very useful questionnaire in patients who complain of excessive daytime sleepiness: scores over 10–11 indicate pathological levels warranting further assessment.

Pathologies

Psychiatrists should be familiar with the major pathologies of consciousness outlined in Table 35.1 – coma, the vegetative state, the minimally conscious state, the locked-in syndrome and brain death.[13] Excessive daytime sleepiness is an underrecognized cause of cognitive impairment, due most commonly to insufficient sleep, obstructive sleep apnoea or narcolepsy.[14]

Attention

Definition

William James wrote that 'my experience is what I agree to attend to'.[15] The essence of attention is selection. At any moment, numerous external and internal targets are available to consciousness: attention decides on which of these we should focus our mental energies. The term is often qualified: preparatory attention is deployed when we await an expected event, such as a ring on the doorbell; we speak of selective attention when we concentrate on the voice on the phone rather than the music on the radio; sustained attention, which is particularly relevant to cognitive testing, allows us to maintain mental focus on a task; and spatial attention refers to our ability to allocate attention in space or to the neural processes that allow this.

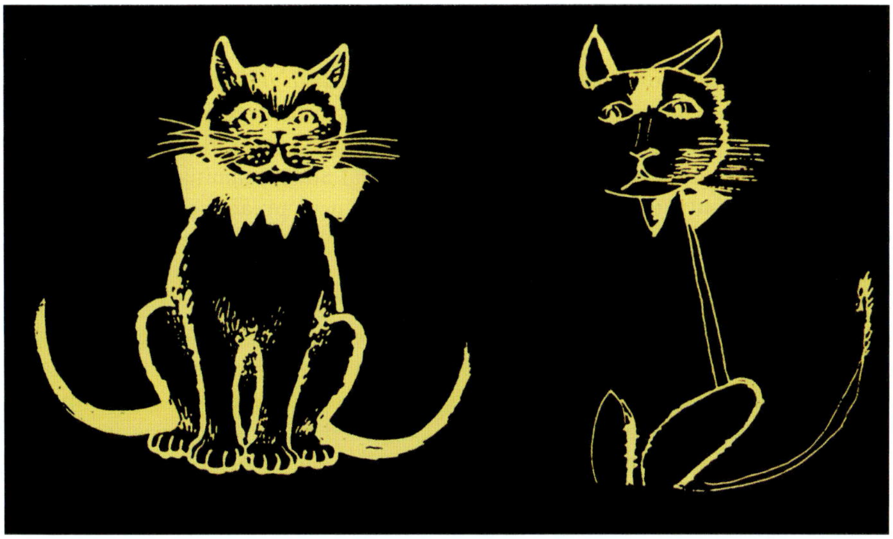

Figure 35.5 Copy of a two-tailed cat made by a patient with neglect of the left side of space

Neural basis

The neural basis of attention is both distributed and localized. It is distributed in the sense that it involves the concerted activity of widespread brain regions. Factors that disrupt the coherence of distributed brain activity – such as drugs, drug withdrawal, metabolic upset and confusion – are the most common causes of impaired attention.[3] The resulting global brain dysfunction is manifest clinically as a confusional state and, often, in the electroencephalogram (EEG) as a slowing of cerebral rhythms (Figures 35.3 and 35.4).

However, aspects of the neural basis of attention are localized.[16] The expression of attention in the brain is a heightening of activity in brain regions subserving the attended material, for example in visual areas if attention is directed toward vision. In the case of visual attention, the neural mechanisms by which attention is engaged and switched include the posterior parietal cortex, the pulvinar nucleus of the thalamus and the superior colliculus in the midbrain. Finally, the control of attention is tied to the frontal lobe systems involved in cognitive control – executive function – more generally (see below).

Assessment

Sustained attention is assessed clinically by asking the patient to perform a moderately demanding repetitive task, for example subtracting 7 from 100 five times, spelling the word 'world' backwards, or reciting the months of the year backwards. Clearly, specific difficulties with arithmetic or spelling can impair performance on the first and second of these tests: the results, as always, need to be interpreted in the context of the patient's cognitive performance as a whole.

Spatial attention is tested by giving the patient a task that requires an even allocation of attention across space, such as bisection of a straight line or the drawing of a clock face including its numbers and hands (Figure 35.5).

Pathologies

As indicated above, sustained attention is most commonly disrupted by factors that globally impair brain function, such as drugs, drug withdrawal, metabolic upset and confusion, giving rise to confusional states (also known as 'delirium'). Focal pathology in the structures that engage and switch specific forms of attention, for example visual attention, can, not surprisingly, impair that form of attention. Finally, impairment of attention is a common accompaniment of a dysexecutive syndrome in which the executive network that directs attention is impaired.

Spatial attention is most commonly impaired by right inferior parietal damage, causing neglect, the failure to attend to the contralateral (in this case, left) side of space.[17] The severity of neglect can vary from a minor failure to identify stimuli in a task requiring visual search to a disabling failure to act towards the left side of space or to use the left side of the body. Extinction is a related deficit, involving the failure to detect one of two stimuli presented simultaneously in matching positions in the two visual fields, although each is detected when present separately. Dressing dyspraxia is also associated with right parietal lesions and results from difficulty in orienting garments correctly with respect to body parts because of spatial disorientation.

Perception

Definition

Perception is the ability to gain knowledge of the world through the senses.

Neural basis

Much of the brain, especially the posterior parts of the cerebral cortex, is involved in the processing of sensory information.[18,19] There are now known to be around 30 maps of the visual world in the occipital, parietal and temporal lobes, dedicated to analysis of the principle features of visual stimuli – form, depth, colour and motion. Two major streams of visual perceptual processing have been distinguished: a ventral steam, running from the occipital into the temporal lobe, concerned particularly with object and person identification, and a dorsal stream, running from the occipital into the parietal lobe, concerned particularly with the visual guidance of action (Figure 35.6).[20] As information passes through the visual areas in these streams, it is gradually transformed in ways that correspond to the uses to which it is put; for example, cells in later areas in the ventral stream, which enable object recognition, respond to higher-order properties of objects such as their identity or colour, whereas cells in earlier visual areas respond to simpler properties such as the presence of edges. Similar general principles apply to the other senses. Although perception is less strongly lateralized than language (see below), the right hemisphere takes the leading role in some aspects of perception: disorders of face recognition, for example, and the syndrome of neglect are associated more strongly with right than with left hemisphere pathology.

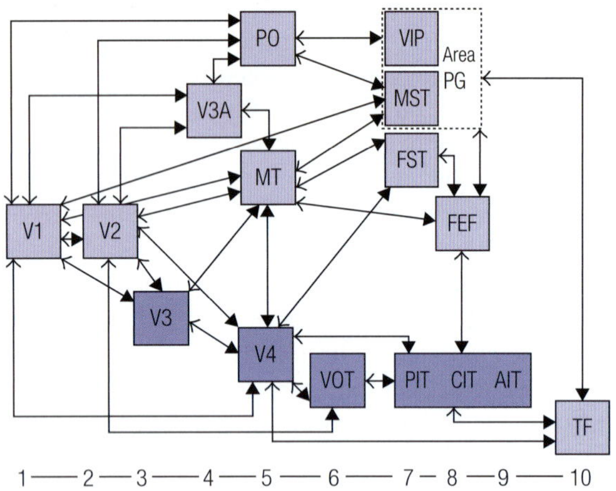

Figure 35.6 Two cortical visual systems. A dorsal pathway runs through area MT to the parietal cortex, and a ventral pathway (shaded) runs through V4 to the inferotemporal cortex. The dorsal pathway is thought to be concerned with where an object is, and the central pathway with what the object is. Numbers 1–10 indicate the hierarchical levels of the various areas in the alternative schema of Felleman and Vam Essen

AIT, anterior inferotemporal; CIT, central inferotemporal; FEF, frontal eye fields; FST, floor of superior temporal; LIP, lateral interparietal; MST, medial superior temporal; MT, middle temporal; PIT, posterior inferotemporal; PO, parieto-occipital; VIP, ventral intraparietal; VOT, ventral occipitotemporal; VP, ventral posterior.

TF and PG are the area nomenclature of Von Bonin and Bailey. TF lies in the parahippocampal gyrus. Area PG includes area 7a, a subdivision of Brodmann's area 7.

Only dominant connections are shown. Solid arrowheads indicate feed-forward projections; open arrowheads indicate feedback projections.

Assessment

Auditory perception is assessed incidentally by conversation and visual perception by naming tasks. The standard specific bedside test of visual perception involves copying a drawing, such as the overlapping pentagons of the Mini-Mental State Examination (MMSE).[21] This test can certainly reveal perceptual impairment, but it will also be affected by difficulty in producing or organizing the drawing.

Pathologies

Agnosias, literally 'failures of knowledge', are disorders in which the early stages of sensation are intact but the perception or knowledge to which they normally gives rise is impaired.[22] Visual agnosias are classically divided into apperceptive and associative types: apperceptive visual agnosias include specific impairments of colour, movement and form perception; associative visual agnosias include inabilities to recognize objects or faces, although these can, in many cases, be copied or matched. These disorders usually result from damage to the ventral stream of visual processing.

Balint's syndrome follows bilateral damage to the dorsal stream. It involves simultanagnosia (the inability to make out more than one item in the visual scene at a time), optic ataxia (difficulty reaching for a seen object) and oculomotor dyspraxia (difficulty in directing eye movements accurately).

Memory

Definition

Memory is the capacity that allows our behaviour and experience to change in response to what has happened to us in the past. Some familiarity with the terminology of memory is useful. Memories of every kind must be acquired (or encoded), stored and later retrieved if they are to be useful. Many memories undergo a complex process of consolidation by which they become less vulnerable to loss over time. Anterograde memory refers to the ability to acquire memories from a given point in time; retrograde memory refers to the ability to retrieve memories that were formed previously. Figure 35.7 shows a widely accepted contemporary classification of the types of memory: this classification maps on to the neural systems subserving the different kinds of memory (see below).[23,24] The key distinctions in this classification are between declarative memories (those we can articulate) and procedural memories (which underlie our know-how); short-term declarative memory, also known as working memory (memory for information with which we are actively working) and long-term declarative memory (memory for information that is in store and can be recollected but that may not be in consciousness currently); and episodic memory (memory for single events) and semantic memory (our database of knowledge about the world and language). Autobiographical memory, of particular importance in psychiatry, involves both personal semantic and personal episodic

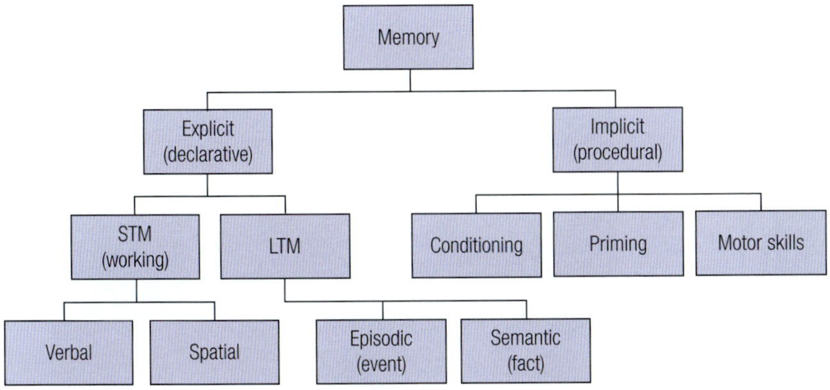

Figure 35.7 Taxonomy of memory

LTM, long-term memory; STM, short-term memory.

memory (you can probably remember where you lived when you were 8 years old – a semantic fact – and some of the first-hand details of an important event from your primary school – an episodic memory).[25]

Neural basis

Memory formation depends ultimately on modifications of the strengths of synaptic connections between neurons.[26] As modifiable synapses are present everywhere in the brain, memory, in a sense, is everywhere too. However, different kinds of memory involve different brain regions. Short-term, or working, memory depends on neural systems that represent the material with which we are working, for example language systems if we are repeating a name and address, and frontal executive systems that select what we work with at a given moment. Entering material from working memory into long-term declarative memory requires that the circuit of Papez is intact (Figure 35.8): this limbic circuit includes structures in the medial temporal lobe (MTL), especially the hippocampus, the fornix, the large fibre bundle that interconnects the MTL and the thalamus, and structures in the thalamus, particularly the anterior thalamic nuclei and mamillary bodies. Damage anywhere along the course of the circuit of Papez can give rise to an amnesic syndrome (see below). The long-term storage of semantic memories depends on the lateral temporal neocortex.[27] The frontal lobes play a strategic role in memory formation and retrieval. Rich recollection of past personal experiences activates a widespread network of brain regions in all four lobes of the brain.[28] There is lively current debate over whether or not intact MTLs are permanently required for such rich recollection.[29] Procedural memories are much less dependent on the MTLs. The cerebellum, basal ganglia and sensory cortices are required for conditioning, learning of motor skills and sensory priming, respectively.

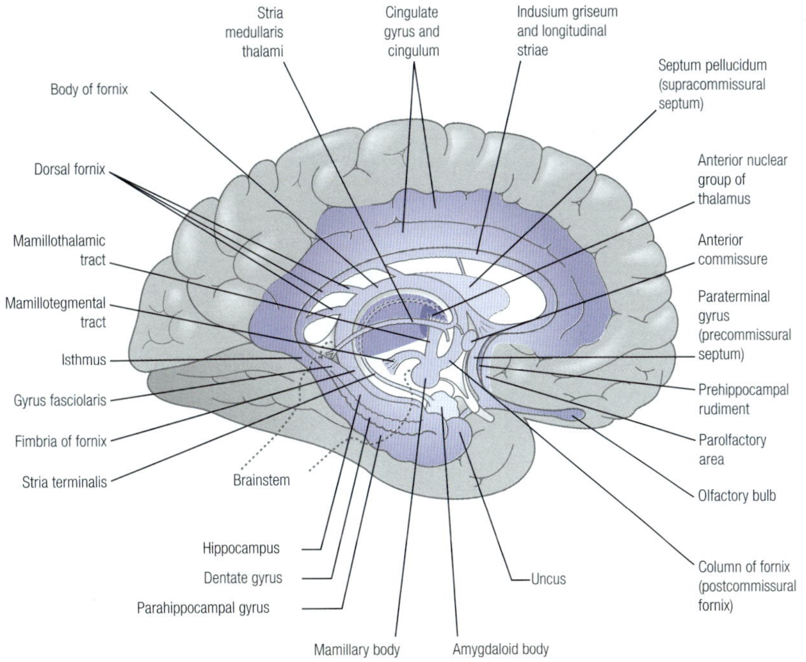

Figure 35.8 Partial dissection of the medial aspect of the right hemisphere, revealing key regions of the limbic system

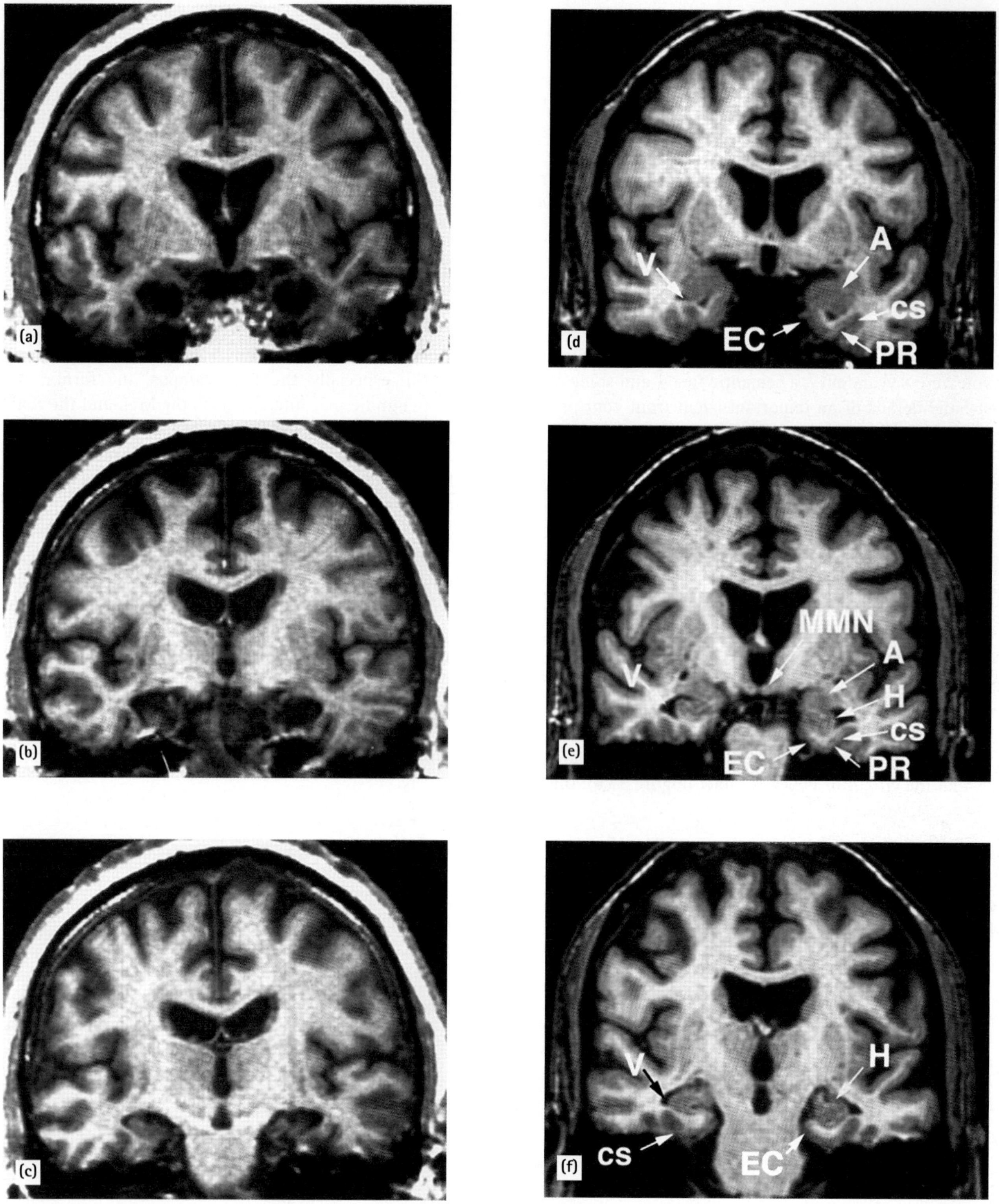

Figure 35.9 Coronal magnetic resonance imaging (MRI) scans from the patient 'HM' (a–c) and a control subject (d–f)
CS, collateral sulcus; EC, entorhinal cortex; H, hippocampus; LGN, lateral geniculate nucleus; MMN, medial mamillary nucleus; V, ventricle.

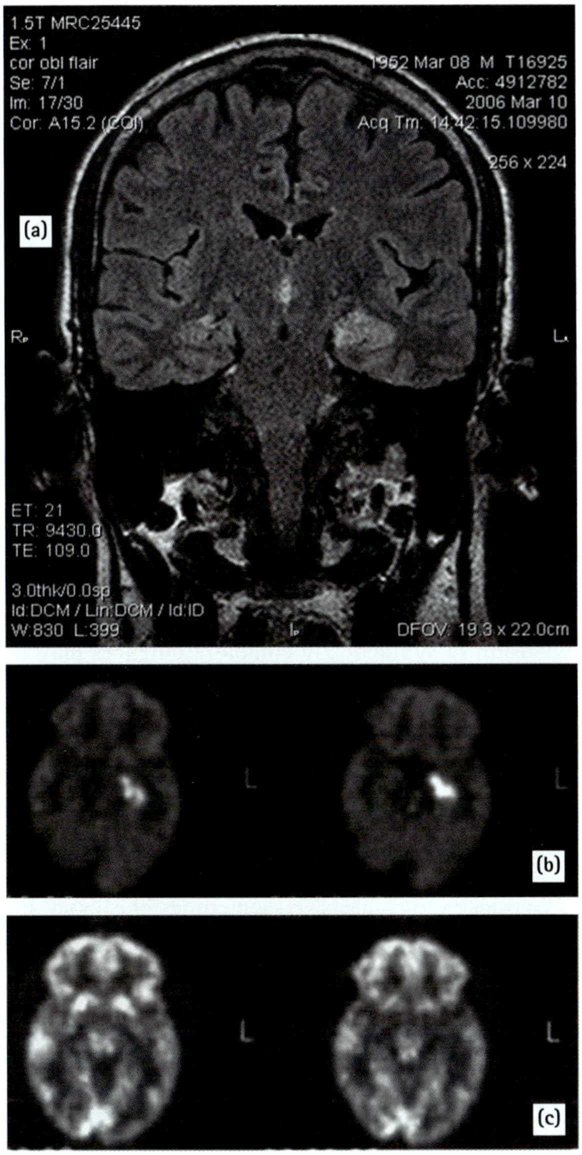

Figure 35.10 Magnetic resonance imaging (MRI) and positron-emission tomography (PET) scans from a patient with transient epileptic amnesia, showing (a) left hippocampal (on right on scan) oedema at the time of a flurry of attacks, with (b) left hippocampal hypermetabolism (demonstrated by PET) that (c) resolved with treatment of the epilepsy

Assessment

Short-term or working memory is assessed by asking the patient to repeat three words or a name and address. Long-term declarative memory is assessed by asking the patient to retrieve the three words or name and address after a period of distraction sufficient to 'wipe' the working memory. Semantic memory is assessed by asking the patient to name objects or to answer general knowledge questions. These simple tests are useful but fail to tap important aspects of memory, including longer-term retention, autobiographical memory and procedural memory.

Pathologies

Severe damage anywhere along the course of the circuit of Papez causes an amnesic syndrome – an inability to acquire new long-term declarative memories, associated with some degree of retrograde amnesia. Examples include the bilateral excision of the MTLs in the famous patient HM (Figure 35.9),[30] whose anterior MTLs were surgically removed as a treatment for epilepsy; the early pathology of Alzheimer's disease, which begins in the MTLs; and Korsakoff's syndrome, due to established thiamine deficiency, in which the causative lesion lies in the anterior thalamus. A transient amnesic syndrome occurs in disorders that transiently disable these structures, including concussion, transient global amnesia, transient epileptic amnesia (Figure 35.10) and drug-induced amnesia.[31,32] Damage to the temporal neocortex, most often seen in the temporal lobe variant of frontotemporal dementia, causes semantic memory impairment (Figure 35.11).[27] This affects knowledge of objects and language if the left temporal lobe is principally affected, and knowledge of people if the right temporal lobe is worse affected. The existence of focal retrograde amnesia (loss of past memories in the absence of any impairment of the ability to form new ones) as a result of brain damage is controversial,[33] and such cases often turn out to have a psychiatric or forensic explanation. However, there are now a few well-documented cases of this kind, suggesting that brain damage can occasionally give rise to this pattern of deficit.[34]

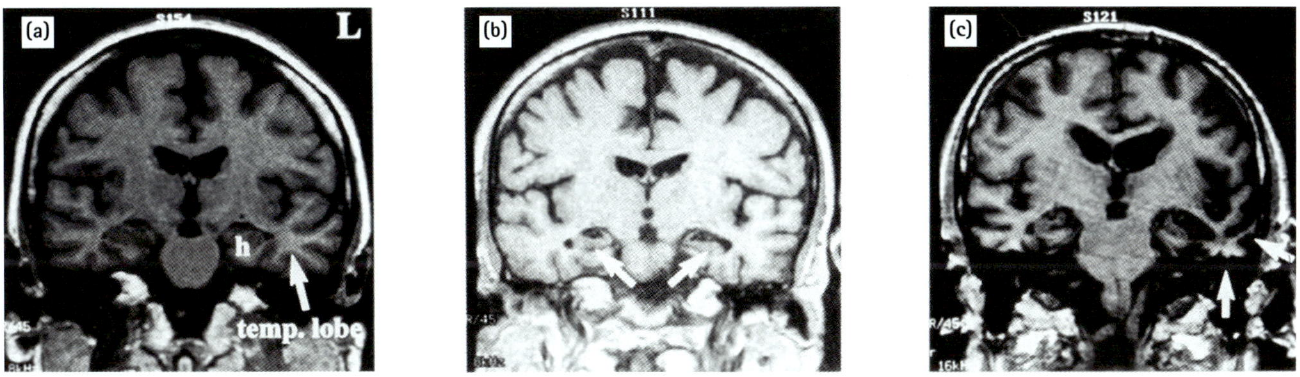

Figure 35.11 Coronal magnetic resonance imaging (MRI) scans from (a) a normal subject, (b) a patient with early Alzheimer's disease with bilateral hippocampal atrophy and (c) a patient with semantic dementia with atrophy of the inferior left temporal neocortex

Language

Definition

Language is the capacity to communicate using words. Language functions include the abilities to speak, understand, repeat, name, read, write and spell.

Neural basis

Language is the most clearly asymmetrical function of the human brain. It is predominantly represented in the left hemisphere in almost all right-handed people and in the majority of left-handed people. Broca's area, in the left inferior frontal lobe, processes fluent speech; Wernicke's area in the left superior temporal lobe is required for comprehension of one's own and others' speech (Figure 35.12). These areas are connected by a fibre bundle, the arcuate fasciculus. Cortical regions surrounding Broca's and Wernicke's areas contribute to their function. Although language is predominantly a dominant hemisphere function, the right hemisphere contributes to prosody, the musical and emotional aspects of speech and speech perception.

Assessment

The critical elements of assessment are to listen to the patient's spontaneous speech to establish whether it is fluent or dysfluent, and to determine whether the patient's comprehension is intact. Comprehension can be tested by using instructions of increasing complexity (one to several stages), or by using language of increasing sophistication to frame the request ('Please point to the drawing of the marsupial'). A more comprehensive assessment tests naming, repetition, reading, writing and spelling.

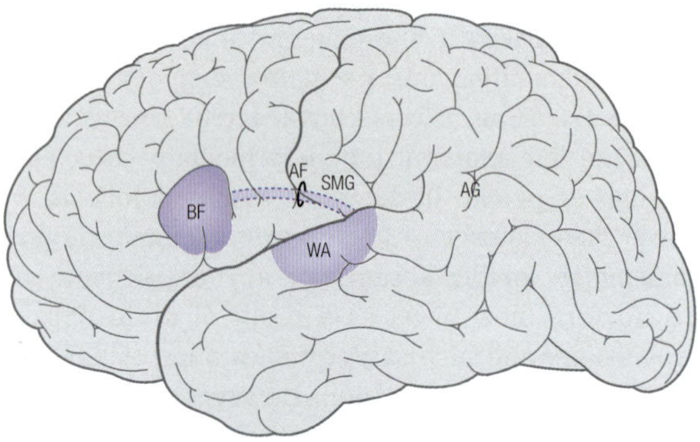

Figure 35.12 Key brain regions involved in language-processing
AF, arcuate fasciculus; AG, angular gyrus; BF, Broca's area; SMG, supramarginal gyrus; WA, Wernicke's area.

Pathologies

Dysphasia, or aphasia, is a disorder of language function that must be distinguished from dysarthria, a disorder of articulation (Table 35.2, Box 35.2). The term 'dyslexia' is specifically applied to disorders of reading, and the term 'dysgraphia' to disorders of writing. Damage to Broca's area particularly disrupts fluency and syntax, the grammatical ordering of language. Patients with Broca's dysphasia produce meaningful but dysfluent and effortful speech, from which function words (e.g. 'the', 'to') are often omitted. Patients may produce phonetic word approximations known as phonemic paraphasias (e.g. 'mister' for 'matter'). Comprehension of syntactically complex sentences may be impaired. Patients are usually aware of their deficit and frustrated by it. Damage to Wernicke's area disrupts the semantic aspect of language, impairing comprehension both of one's own and others' speech: this gives rise to fluent but empty or nonsensical output, containing paraphasic errors (semantic, e.g. 'hand' for 'foot', and phonemic, e.g. 'pot' for 'put'). Patients are usually unaware of their deficit. Wernicke's dysphasia is sometimes mistaken for thought disorder. Patients with thought disorder should, however, be able to follow instructions, indicating that their comprehension is relatively intact (although it is noteworthy that the region of the brain associated with thought disorder in schizophrenia overlaps Wernicke's area). Writing in Broca's aphasia and comprehension of the written word in Wernicke's aphasia are usually affected in similar ways to speech production and comprehension, respectively. Damage to the arcuate fasciculus causes conduction aphasia, impairing repetition out of proportion to other functions. Damage to surrounding cortical regions but sparing Broca's or Wernicke's area gives rise to aphasia with similar

Table 35.2 Main varieties of dysphasia

Type	Fluency	Comprehension	Repetition	Naming
Global dysphasia	+	+	+	+
Broca's dysphasia	+	–	+	+
Wernicke's dysphasia	–	+	+	+
Conduction dysphasia	–	–	+	+
Transcortical motor dysphasia	+	–	–	+
Transcortical sensory dysphasia	–	+	–	+

+ indicates affected; – indicates unaffected functions.

Box 35.2 Examples of dysphasic speech

BROCA'S DYSPHASIA

'Cinderella ... poor ... um ... 'dopted her ... scrubbed floor ... um ... tidy ... poor ... um ... 'dopted ... si-sisters and mother ... ball ... Ball ... prince ... um ... shoe ...'

WERNICKE'S DYSPHASIA

'I can't tell you what that is, but I know what it is, but I don't know where it is. But I don't know what it's under. I know it's ... you couldn't say it's ... I couldn't say what it is. I couldn't say what that is. This shu – that should be right in here. That's very bad in there. Anyway, this one here, and that, and that's it. This is the getting in here and that's the getting around here, and that, and that's it. This is getting in here and that's the getting around here, this one and one with this one. And this one, and that's it, isn't it? I don't know what else you'd want.'

characteristics to Broca's or Wernicke's aphasia, but with relative sparing of repetition (transcortical motor and transcortical sensory aphasias, respectively).

Dyslexia can occur as a result of damage to the left visual cortex and adjacent corpus callosum, disconnecting the left hemisphere from information about the written word (alexia without agraphia); as a result of visual neglect (neglect dysgraphia); or in central forms in association with left hemisphere damage, for example due to stroke or dementia, causing surface dyslexia (in which patients become dependent on letter-by-letter reading with resulting difficulty in reading irregular words such as 'pint', which are read to rhyme with 'mint'), or deep dyslexia, in which the ability to read letter by letter is lost (with resulting inability to read nonsense words such as 'proke', and semantic reading errors, e.g. 'brother' for 'sister').

Dysgraphia can occur in association with other types of dyspraxia (dyspraxic dysgraphia, see below), in association with neglect ('neglect dysgraphia') and in central forms due to left hemisphere damage analogous to surface and deep dyslexia (see above). Dysgraphia is particularly associated with damage to the angular gyrus, the focus of damage in Gerstmann's syndrome of central dysgraphia, acalculia (see below), right–left disorientation and finger agnosia (inability to name or point to indicated fingers).

Numeracy

Definition

Numeracy is the ability to recognize and manipulate numbers to solve arithmetical problems.[5]

Neural basis

Numeracy is principally dependent on the dominant hemisphere, is often but not always associated with dysphasia, and has a particularly strong association with the posterior left hemisphere, especially the parietal lobe, including the angular gyrus.

Assessment

Assessment is by oral addition, subtraction, multiplication and division.

Pathologies

Dyscalculia is an acquired disturbance of the ability to calculate.[5] It can result from an inability to comprehend, read or write numbers, generally associated with aphasia. Spatial dyscalculia involves difficulty with written calculations occurring in association with neglect. Anarithmetria, or primary dyscalculia, is the specific inability to perform calculations such as addition and subtraction. Spatial dyscalculia is associated with right hemisphere pathology, whereas impaired use of numerical symbols and anarithmetria occur in association with damage to the posterior left hemisphere, including the angular gyrus.

Executive function and social cognition

Definition

Executive function is the capacity to organize thought and behaviour. This includes the abilities to plan, initiate, monitor and adjust a course of action; to 'shift set', changing tack from one activity or approach to another; to reason; and to problem-solve. These abilities are linked closely to the capacities for appropriate social interaction and empathy,[35] capacities that are, in turn, important determinants of personality. As self-monitoring is a cardinal executive function, patients with dysexecutive disorders commonly lack insight into their predicament.

Neural basis

Executive functions are particularly associated with the frontal lobes (Figure 35.13).[19] Whereas the primary motor cortex and premotor areas are involved in the moment-to-moment control of action, the prefrontal cortex – lateral prefrontal, ventromedial prefrontal and anterior cingulate – plays a more strategic role. The lateral prefrontal cortex has been linked particularly with working memory functions, of the kind required, for example, to solve the Wisconsin Card Sort Test in which one must keep track of the correct criterion – symbol shape, colour or number – by which to sort a pack of cards and then make appropriate adjustments when the criterion changes. The ventromedial (or orbitofrontal) cortex is associated with the control of behaviour, especially social behaviour, under guidance by emotion, empa-

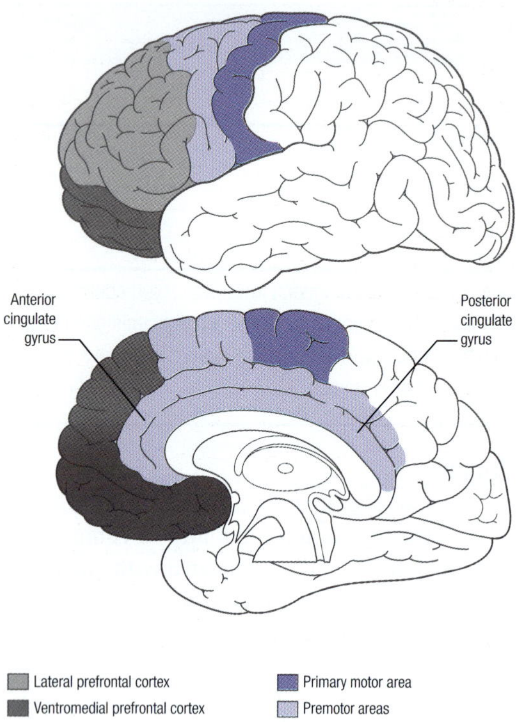

Figure 35.13 Major subdivisions of the frontal lobes

thy and theory of mind (our ability to impute mental states such as desires and beliefs to others). The anterior cingulate cortex is thought to play a key role in the allocation of attention. It mediates between arousal systems, the lateral prefrontal cortex and motor output, thus integrating arousal, cognition and action.

The control of executive function is not limited to the prefrontal cortex. The frontal lobes have crucial subcortical connections with the basal ganglia, thalamus and cerebellum (Figure 35.14). Disruption to these structures, or to the links between them, can also give rise to a dysexecutive syndrome.

Assessment

Executive function is notoriously difficult to test in the clinic: patients with dysexecutive syndromes severe enough to cause major disruption to long-term decision-making can score full marks on standard cognitive tests such as the MMSE. The single most useful simple clinical measure of executive function is verbal fluency: this task requires generation of as many examples as possible in a minute from a particular category, for example 'animals' or 'words beginning with the letter p'. This task requires an ability to search semantic memory flexibly, remembering for example that the category 'animals' includes fish as well as household pets. The lower limit of normal is ten exemplars. The ability to copy motor sequences is also dependent on frontal lobe function: Luria's fist–side–palm sequence and alternating bimanual sequences (Figure 35.15) can be used to assess this. Dysexecutive disorders commonly give rise to disinhibition: in the go–no go task, the patient is asked to tap the table when the examiner taps once, but not to tap when the examiner taps twice. A dysexecutive patient may find it difficult to withhold a response in the second situation. Confabulation, indifference to failure and perseveration of responses are common qualitative features of dysexecutive syndromes.

Pathologies

Focal damage to the frontal lobes occurs most commonly as a result of trauma, stroke or neurosurgical excision. The celebrated case of Phineas Gage involved a railwayman whose ventromedial frontal lobes were destroyed by a metal rod. Gage survived for some years, but with a much altered personality, such that his 'friends and acquaintances said he was "no longer Gage"'. The frontal variant of frontotemporal dementia presents with changes in personality and behaviour, often involving apathy, disinhibition, and loss of empathy and interest in others. Similar features can occur as a result of subcortical pathologies, because of disruption of the looping pathways mentioned above. These include

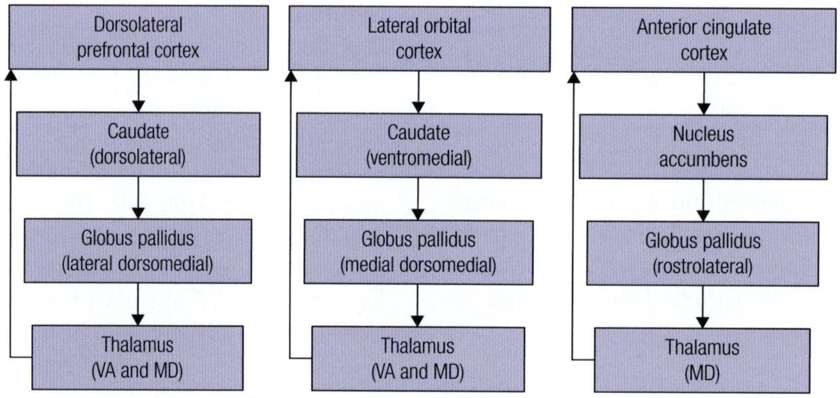

Figure 35.14 Subcortical connections of the frontal lobes
MD, mediodorsal; VA, ventral-anterior

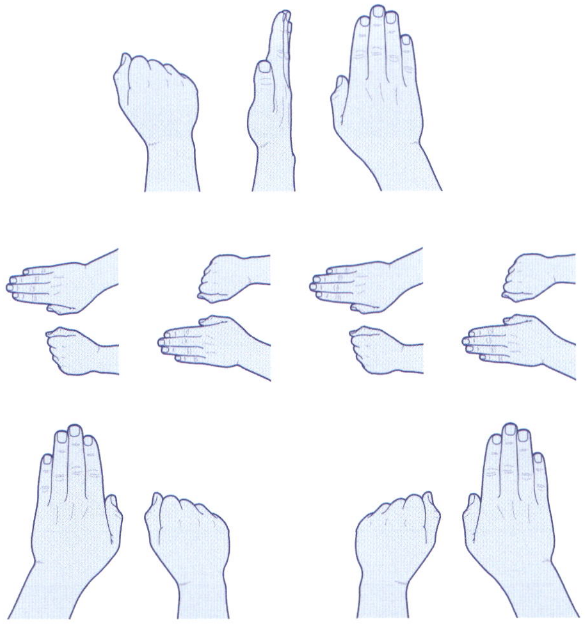

Figure 35.15 Luria three hand-position test (on top) and an alternating bimanual sequence (below)

From Luria AR (1996) *Higher Cortical Functions in Man.*

focal pathologies affecting the basal ganglia or cerebellum and diffuse pathologies affecting the white matter, for example disease of the small blood vessels of the brain and multiple sclerosis. The notion that cerebellar pathology can give rise to features similar to disorders of the frontal lobe has been enshrined in the concept of the 'cerebellar cognitive affective syndrome'. Bilateral damage restricted to the region of the anterior cingulate cortex can give rise to a state of profound 'will-less-ness' or abulia, akinetic mutism.

Praxis

Definition

Praxis is the ability to learn and perform skilled actions such as writing, gesturing, using a toothbrush or playing a musical instrument. Skilled actions may be transitive, involving another object such as a piano, or intransitive, such as waving. Although praxis may not be an obvious element of cognition, it clearly involves a form of knowledge, and it is crucial to our wellbeing, as it provides the output channel for all the other cognitive processes. 'Dyspraxia' involves a deficit in the higher-order control of motor function, not accounted for by sensory loss, by more basic motor deficits such as weakness, tremor, dystonia or ataxia, or by dementia.

Neural basis

Praxis is associated with the dominant hemisphere, which controls the more skilled hand and language. Regions of the left frontal and parietal lobes contain the motor engrams for skilled actions and are required to select and implement these. Performance of skilled oral movements depends particularly on the inferior frontal lobe and insula.

Assessment

Praxis is assessed by asking patients to copy arbitrary hand positions (e.g. tip of thumb touching tip of little finger), to perform mimes of transitive and intransitive actions (e.g. brushing hair, stopping traffic), and to perform learned skilled movements of the mouth (e.g. blowing out a match).

Pathologies

The terminology of dyspraxias has been used inconsistently.[36] The term 'limb kinetic dyspraxia' refers to a type of dyspraxia in which movements are performed adequately but dysfluently. The term 'ideomotor dyspraxia' has been used to refer to failure to produce intransitive gestures, impairment in the use of single objects or, more broadly, a disorder of the production system for skilled actions. 'Ideational dyspraxia' has been used to refer to failure to produce transitive actions, impairment in the use of a series of objects, as in striking a match or, more broadly, a disorder of the conceptual system that contains knowledge of tool functions and actions.

Dyspraxia can occur as part of the behavioural syndrome resulting from focal left hemisphere damage of whatever cause and early in the course of neurodegenerative diseases, including Alzheimer's disease and corticobasal degeneration. Oral (or buccofacial) apraxia may accompany Broca's aphasia.

These disorders of skilled movement imitation and selection are sometimes associated with symptoms of motor disinhibition: imitation behaviour (involuntary imitation of the examiner's movement), utilization behaviour (involuntary utilization of objects that come into view, e.g. the donning of several pairs of spectacles), and alien limb behaviour, involving apparently purposeful limb movements disavowed by the patient. Grasp, pout and palmomental reflexes can occur in association with dyspraxia and with dysexecutive syndromes, as they reflect a loss of the motor inhibition normally exercised by the frontal lobes (grasp: the patient's hand grasps the examiner's despite a request not to do so; pout: a puckering of the lips when a spatula is placed against them; palmomental: a puckering of the chin on stroking the ipsilateral thenar eminence).

DELIRIUM AND DEMENTIA

The two most commonly encountered forms of cognitive impairment are dementia and delirium (Table 35.3).[3,4] The distinction is important, as the two forms of disorder have very different causes and management. The hallmark of delirium is impairment of sustained attention, with resulting impairment of memory and reasoning. Delirium generally has a subacute onset over hours to days and is associated with alterations of arousal (high or low), disturbances of the sleep–wake cycle, fleeting delusions, hallucinations and disturbed behaviour. Dementia by contrast is usually of insidious onset, and the capacity for sustained attention is

Table 35.3 Features of delirium versus dementia

Feature	Delirium	Dementia
Onset	Abrupt/subacute	Insidious
Course	Fluctuating	Slow progression
Duration	Hours–weeks	Months–years
Alertness	Abnormally high or low	Typically normal
Sleep–wake cycle	Disrupted	Typically normal
Attention	Impaired	Relatively normal
Orientation	Impaired	Intact in early dementia
Working memory	Impaired	Intact in early dementia
Episodic memory	Impaired	Impaired
Thought	Disorganized, delusional	Impoverished
Speech	Slow/rapid, incoherent	Word-finding difficulty
Perception	Illusions/hallucinations common	Usually intact in early dementia
Behaviour	Withdrawn/agitated	Varies: often intact early on

relatively preserved.[37,38] The diagnosis of dementia requires the presence of progressive decline in two or more domains of cognition, giving rise to significant impairment of activities of daily living.

A broad-brush distinction between cortical dementia and subcortical dementia (Table 35.4) is useful in the diagnostic process. Cortical dementias such as Alzheimer's disease give rise to the classic neuropsychological deficit syndromes of amnesia, aphasia, agnosia and apraxia. Subcortical dementias,[39] such as the dementia of multiple sclerosis and subcortical cerebrovascular disease, are characterized by slowing of cognition, often associated with altered behaviour and personality and a dysexecutive syndrome.

Box 35.3 lists the common predisposing, facilitating and precipitating causes of delirium.

The most commonly encountered forms of dementia are Alzheimer's disease, vascular dementia, Lewy body dementia (DLB) and frontotemporal dementia. Boxes 35.4 and 35.5 list diagnostic criteria for Alzheimer's disease[40] and DLB.[41] Vascular dementia is heterogeneous as it can result (i) from multiple infarcts giving rise to cognitive impairments that depend on the brain regions affected; (ii) from disease of small blood vessels, causing diffuse white matter damage and a subcortical dementia; and (iii) from strategic infarction in a region crucial to cognition such as the thalamus. The Hachinski Ischaemic Scale (Table 35.5) has some value in identifying vascular dementia.[42] Frontotemporal dementia is a collective term used to describe a group of disorders in which the major pathological finding is atrophy of the frontal or temporal lobes, or usually both, causing three major dementia syndromes: a behavioural variant, presenting with alterations of personality and behaviour; a semantic dementia variant, presenting with gradual loss of vocabulary and associated knowledge of the world; and a progressive non-fluent aphasia variant.[27] Table 35.6 provides a more wide-ranging, but not comprehensive, list of the causes of dementia.

Table 35.4 Features of cortical versus subcortical dementia

Function	Cortical (e.g. Alzheimer's disease)	Subcortical (e.g. Huntington's disease)
Alertness	Normal	'Slowed up'
Attention	Normal early	Impaired
Executive function	Normal early	Impaired
Episodic memory	Amnesia	Forgetfulness
Language	Aphasic	Reduced output
Praxis	Apraxia	Relatively normal
Perception	Impaired	Impaired
Personality	Preserved (unless frontal type)	Apathetic, inert

Box 35.3 Causes of delirium

PREDISPOSING FACTORS

- Age
- Pre-existing brain damage/cognitive impairment
- Sensory impairment
- Multiple/severe associated physical/?psychiatric illness
- Alcoholism.

FACILITATING FACTORS

- Psychosocial stress
- Sleep deprivation
- Sensory deprivation/overload
- Immobility.

PRECIPITATING FACTORS

- Prescribed/recreational drugs, drug withdrawal
- Infection
- Organ failure
- Metabolic disturbance
- Surgery
- Pain, urinary retention, faecal impaction.

Box 35.4 Diagnostic criteria for the clinical diagnosis of probable Alzheimer's disease

The National Institute of Neurological and Communicative Disorders and Stroke (NINCDS)–Alzheimer's Disease and Related Disorders Association (ADRDA) criteria are intended to serve as a guide for the diagnosis of probable, possible and definite Alzheimer's disease.

CRITERIA FOR THE CLINICAL DIAGNOSIS OF PROBABLE ALZHEIMER'S DISEASE

- Dementia established by clinical examination and documented by the Mini-Mental Test, Blessed Dementia Scale or similar examination, and confirmed by neuropsychological tests
- Deficits in two or more areas of cognition
- Progressive worsening of memory and other cognitive functions
- No disturbance of consciousness
- Onset between ages 40 years and 90 years, most often after age 65 years
- Absence of systemic disorders or other brain diseases that in and of themselves could account for the progressive deficits in memory and cognition.

SUPPORTING SYMPTOMS FOR DIAGNOSIS OF PROBABLE ALZHEIMER'S DISEASE

- Progressive deterioration of specific cognitive functions such as language (aphasia), motor skills (apraxia) and perceptions (agnosia)
- Impaired activities of daily living and altered patterns of behaviour
- Family history of similar disorders, particularly if confirmed neuropathologically
- Laboratory results of:
  - normal lumbar puncture as evaluated by standard techniques;
  - normal pattern or non-specific changes in electroencephalogram (EEG), such as increased slow-wave activity
  - evidence of cerebral atrophy on computed tomography (CT), with progression documented by serial observation.

OTHER CLINICAL FEATURES CONSISTENT WITH THE DIAGNOSIS OF PROBABLE ALZHEIMER'S DISEASE, AFTER EXCLUSION OF CAUSES OF DEMENTIA OTHER THAN ALZHEIMER'S DISEASE

- Plateaus in the course of progression of the illness
- Associated symptoms of depression, insomnia, incontinence, delusions, illusions, hallucinations, catastrophic verbal, emotional or physical outbursts, sexual disorders and weight loss
- Other neurological abnormalities in some patients, especially with more advanced disease and including motor signs such as increased muscle tone, myoclonus or gait disorder
- Seizures in advanced disease
- CT normal for age.

FEATURES MAKING THE DIAGNOSIS OF PROBABLE ALZHEIMER'S DISEASE UNCERTAIN OR UNLIKELY

- Sudden apoplectic onset
- Focal neurological findings such as hemiparesis, sensory loss, visual field deficits, and incoordination early in the course of the illness
- Seizures or gait disturbances at the onset or very early in the course of the illness.

A PRACTICAL APPROACH: HISTORY-TAKING, THE MMSE AND BEYOND

History-taking

Cognitive assessment begins at the start of the clinical encounter.[3] Difficulties encountered in giving a history due to problems with attention, memory, language or executive function may reveal the presence of cognitive disorder. Cognitive symptoms should be clarified in the usual way, with enquiries about the precise nature of the problem (e.g. 'poor memory' may mean, among other things, absent-mindedness, word-finding difficulty, problems with spatial orientation or face recognition, or a true anterograde memory deficit), its duration and tempo, any precipitants, variability, and relieving or exacerbating factors. It can be helpful to enquire specifically about the following areas:

- Concentration: absent-minded errors
- Memory: for recent events, faces, routes
- Language: word-finding, comprehension, reading, writing, spelling

Box 35.5 Consensus criteria for the clinical diagnoses of probable and possible dementia with Lewy bodies

These operational diagnostic criteria for dementia of the Lewy body type (DLB) were developed at a consensus meeting bringing together proponents of the previous diagnostic criteria from healthcare professionals in Nottingham and Newcastle.

- The central feature required for a diagnosis of DLB is progressive cognitive decline of sufficient magnitude to interfere with normal social or occupational function. Prominent or persistent memory impairment may not necessarily occur in the early stages but is usually evident with progression. Deficits on tests of attention and of frontal subcortical skills and visuospatial ability may be especially prominent.
- Two of the following core features are essential for a diagnosis of probable DLB, and one is essential for possible DLB:
  - Fluctuating cognition with pronounced variations in attention and alertness
  - Recurrent visual hallucinations that are typically well formed and detailed
  - Spontaneous motor features of parkinsonism.
- Features supportive of the diagnosis are:
  - repeated falls;
  - syncope;
  - transient loss of consciousness;
  - neuroleptic sensitivity;
  - systematized delusions;
  - hallucinations in other modalities.
- A diagnosis of DLB is less likely in the presence of:
  - stroke disease, evident as focal neurological signs or on brain imaging;
  - evidence on physical examination and investigation of any physical illness or other brain disorder sufficient to account for the clinical picture.

Table 35.5 Hachinski Ischaemic Scale*

Abrupt onset	2
Stepwise progression	1
Fluctuating course	2
Nocturnal confusion	1
Relative preservation of personality	1
Depression	1
Somatic complaints	1
Emotional incontinence	1
History of hypertension	1
History of strokes	2
Evidence of associated atherosclerosis	1
Focal neurological symptoms	2
Focal neurological signs	2

*These criteria for vascular dementia are based upon the Hachinski Ischaemic Score, originally derived on the basis of cerebral blood-flow patterns in people with dementia. On the weighted scale, a score of 7 or more is taken to indicate vascular dementia, while a score of 4 or less suggests that this is an unlikely diagnosis.

Table 35.6 Causes of dementia

Inherited	HD, Wilson's, leucodystrophies
Primary degeneration	AD, DLB, FTD, PSP, CBD
Vascular	Multi-infarct, subcortical, strategic infarction
Infective	HIV, TSE, HSE, Whipple's, SSPE, syphilis
Inflammatory	MS, vasculitis, Hashimoto's, limbic encephalitis
Neoplastic	Primary/secondary CNS tumours, limbic encephalitis
Traumatic	After head injury
Structural	Hydrocephalus, chronic subdurals
Metabolism/endocrine	Hypothyroidism
Deficiency	Vitamin B12/folate
Sleep-related	OSA
Substances/drugs	Alcohol, anticholinergics, hypnotics
Psychiatric	Depression (pseudo-dementia)

AD, Alzheimer's disease; CBD, corticobasal degeneration; CNS, central nervous system; DLB, Lewy body dementia; FTD, frontotemporal dementia; HD, Huntington's disease; HIV, human immunodeficiency syndrome; HSE, herpes simplex encephalitis; MS, multiple sclerosis; OSA, obstructive sleep apnoea; PSP, progressive supranuclear palsy; SSPE, subacute sclerosing panencephalitis; TSE, transmissible spongiform encephalopathy.

- Calculation: finances
- Praxis: motor skills
- Activities of daily living: washing, dressing, shopping, cooking, housework, professional work, driving, social activities, hobbies.

Cognitive symptoms are often accompanied by other neuropsychiatric symptoms, which should be identified, in particular personality change, mood disturbance, psychotic phenomena, and altered eating habits, sexual behaviour or sleep.

Questions about the patient's life history, including their career, main relationships, children and grandchildren, can provide revealing information about their linguistic ability, memory and ability to organize their thoughts.

It is vital to interview an informant, and generally advisable to do so in the patient's absence. It is helpful, therefore, to explain at the start of the consultation that you generally speak to the patient and informant both together and separately. After initial history-taking in the presence of the informant, I usually speak to the informant on his or her own, before examining the patient on his or her own. It can be helpful to give the informant a questionnaire that systematically probes for relevant symptoms, such as the Cambridge Behavioural Inventory.[43,44]

Examination

The cognitive assessment should normally be part of a broadly based medical assessment including general history-taking, mental state, general medical examination and neurological examination.

Cognitive assessment is facilitated by using a pro forma that systematically samples the domains of cognition discussed above.[45] The MMSE is the most widely used brief tool for cognitive assessment and is invaluable.[21] It is insensitive, however, to mild or early deficits and to executive impairment. The Addenbrooke's Cognitive Examination (ACE) incorporates and builds on the MMSE, providing a score out of 100, with subscores for attention, orientation, memory, fluency, language and visuospatial ability.[46] It can usually be administered within about 15 min, and it provides a very useful profile of cognitive ability. Sensitivity, specificity and positive predictive values for dementia are available (Table 35.7).

Neither the MMSE nor the ACE tests praxis adequately. It can therefore be helpful to supplement the ACE with the clinical tests of praxis mentioned above.

WHAT CAN FORMAL NEUROPSYCHOLOGY ADD TO CLINICAL ASSESSMENT?

A clinical neuropsychologist is primarily a clinical psychologist who will usually, in the UK, have a post-qualification diploma conferring full practitioner membership of the British Psychological Society's Division of Neuropsychology. In addition to their more specialized skills in cognitive assessment, neuropsychologists possess the fundamental tools of the clinical psychologist, for example awareness of psychiatric diagnoses, that might provide additional or alternative explanations to neurological ones. Their remit has increasingly been extended to include evidence-based and functionally relevant rehabilitation.[47]

Cognitive assessment is part of a broader enquiry. The selection of tests administered will depend, for example, on the referral question being posed (which should be explicit), the approach to the question (e.g. battery *v.* hypothesis testing), the time available, the likely abilities and condition (both mental and physical) of the individual being tested, the relative importance of reliability and validity, and the question of whether and when repeat testing might be required.

At the outset it is crucial to establish a baseline – an estimate of an individual's likely premorbid ability. The measures used, which must be interpreted in the light of factors such as educational and occupational achievement, are typically reading-based tasks such as the National Adult Reading Test (NART)[48] and, more recently, the Wechsler Test of Adult Reading (WTAR).[49] These tests rely on the observation that reading skills are relatively robust in the face of most causes of cognitive decline. The usefulness of both measures is limited by ceiling effects, educational and cultural effects, and disorders such as dyslexia. Alternatives include the 'spot the word' component of the Speed and Capacity of Language Processing (SCOLP) test[50] or the 'best subtest score', where the Wechsler Adult Intelligence Scale (WAIS) has been administered.

The WAIS (in the UK, WAIS-III UK)[51] is the most widely used measure of adult intelligence.[52] Interestingly, test development was based not on theory but on practical and clinical perspectives[53] by David Wechsler, who defined an individual's intelligence as 'the capacity to act purposefully, to think rationally, and to deal effectively with his (or her) environment'. Fourteen subtests contribute to four indices,

Table 35.7 Sensitivity, specificity and positive predictive value of the Addenbrooke's Cognitive Examination (ACE): dementia positive predictive value (PPV) at different prevalence rates

ACE-R cut-off	Sensitivity	Specificity	5%	10%	20%	40%
88	0.94	0.89	0.31	0.48	0.68	0.85
82	0.84	1.00	1.0	1.0	1.0	1.0

two verbal (verbal comprehension and working memory) and two non-verbal (processing speed and perceptual organization). These results yield an overall full-scale IQ (FSIQ) and separate measures of verbal and performance IQ. It is important to recognize significant discrepancies between various abilities that might invalidate such overall averages. The Wechsler Abbreviated Scale of Intelligence (WASI) is a shorter, but reliable, four-subtest screening measure.[54]

The Wechsler Memory Scale (WMS-III) is conveniently co-normed with the WAIS-III.[55] It assesses diverse aspects of memory function across an age range of 16–89 years and yields index scores and a number of other functionally relevant measures in immediate, general (delayed) and working memory in both auditory (verbal) and visual domains. The Rivermead Behavioural Memory Test, now in its third revision, is a more straightforward tool.[56] The WAIS-III and WMS-III provide comprehensive overviews of current cognitive function and memory. Their results can indicate areas requiring more focused neuropsychological testing.

Thus, although one can assess attention informally during testing and with the help of working memory tasks on the WAIS-III and WMS-III, the Test of Everyday Attention (TEA) would allow a more detailed evaluation.[57] This test provides a broad-based measure of various aspects of attention, including sustained attention, visual and auditory selective attention, attentional switching and auditory-verbal working memory. The Trail Making Test,[58] now also available as Colour Trails,[59] is an alternative short, but highly sensitive, measure of attention, sequencing, mental flexibility, visual search and motor function. It is more appropriate for individuals with impaired literacy. Inattention, or neglect, can be assessed in detail with the help of the Behavioural Inattention Test (BIT).[60]

The presence of perceptual difficulties might be indicated by impaired performance on WAIS-III subtests from the Perceptual Organization Index (Picture Completion, Block Design and Matrix Reasoning). They could then be further elucidated using the Visual Object and Space Perception Battery (VOSP),[61] which makes separate assessments of object and spatial perception.

Detailed assessment of language abilities often involves collaboration between a neuropsychologist and a speech and language therapist. However, some appreciation of an individual's receptive and expressive language skills is required to interpret other cognitive strengths and weaknesses. The initial process of history-taking and interview will often highlight difficulties, for example with comprehension or word-finding. Thereafter, useful additional information may emerge from administration of the WAIS-III Vocabulary and Comprehension subtests or from a measure of word fluency such as the Controlled Oral Word Association Test (COWAT or FAS test).[62] Thought disorder may become apparent during the administration of the Silly Sentences component of the SCOLP test.[50] A wide range of language-assessment batteries is available.

The tests available to assess the concept of executive function are as heterogeneous as the concept itself. This is, without doubt, the most challenging area of neuropsychological assessment. Although the concept of a dysexecutive syndrome is currently popular, an individual impaired on some measures of executive function may be unimpaired on others: it is good practice to report which specific tasks or clusters of tasks are affected. The Behavioural Assessment of Dysexecutive Syndrome (BADS) is a functional, six-subtest battery that taps most of the important facets of executive function, including cognitive flexibility, action-planning, self-monitoring, temporal judgement and organization.[63] In addition, the battery contains a 20-item questionnaire assessing areas including emotional, personality, motivational behavioural and cognitive changes. As both the patient and someone who knows them well complete the measure, it is possible to assess insight. The Delis-Kaplan Executive Function System (D-KEFS) battery is a more comprehensive battery.[64] It now includes UK norms and incorporates many of the individual tests often used in isolation (the Colour–Word Interference Test, based on the Stroop Test, the Verbal Fluency Test and the Trail Making Test). The Hayling and Brixton Tests again address many of the relevant facets of executive function, including initiation, response suppression and rule detection/adherence.[65] Tests of social cognition, such as the faux pas test, are a recent addition to the neuropsychologists' armamentarium.[66]

No neuropsychological assessment is complete without an assessment of mood state, either informally or with the help of instruments such as the Hospital Anxiety and Depression (HAD) questionnaire.

Competent neuropsychological assessment is time-consuming, multifaceted and challenging. Neuropsychological assessment instruments, and their interpretation, are becoming increasingly sophisticated. With experience, medically trained clinicians can often make confident diag-

KEY POINTS

- Cognition involves the capacities to acquire, store and use knowledge.
- Its key elements are consciousness (wakefulness), attention, perception, memory, language, executive function and praxis.
- Its key disorders are delirium and dementia, which have distinctive features, causes and treatments.
- A broad-brush distinction between cortical and subcortical types of dementia is clinically useful.
- A systematic approach to history-taking and bedside cognitive assessment with standard tests such as the MMSE and the ACE often allow a confident clinical diagnosis.
- Formal neuropsychological assessment is indicated where a high or low baseline complicates interpretation of standard clinical tests, in detailed definition of unusual symptoms, and in planning and monitoring treatment programmes.

noses of cognitive disorders on the basis of clinical assessment and the use of a screening tool such as the ACE. Expert neuropsychological help is especially valuable in the assessment of high-performing individuals with cognitive complaints who score at ceiling on screening tests; in individuals with pre-existing learning difficulties in whom the interpretation of poor performance on screening tests is unclear; in individuals with highly specific or unusual neuropsychological symptoms requiring more detailed exploration; and in the development and monitoring of treatment programmes.

REFERENCES

1. Elger CE, Helmstaedter C, Kurthen M (2004) Chronic epilepsy and cognition. *Lancet Neurology* 3: 663–72.
2. Aldenkamp AP, Baker GA, Meador KJ (2004) The neuropsychology of epilepsy: what are the factors involved? *Epilepsy and Behavior* 5 (suppl. 1): S1–2.
3. Hodges JR (2007) *Cognitive Assessment for Clinicians*. Oxford: Oxford University Press.
4. Larner AJ (2008) *Neuropsychological Neurology*. Cambridge: Cambridge University Press.
5. Heilman KM, Valenstein E (2003) *Clinical Neuropsychology*, 4th edn. Oxford: Oxford University Press.
6. Zeman A (1997) Persistent vegetative state. *Lancet* **350**: 795–9.
7. Cummings JL (1993) Frontal-subcortical circuits and human behavior. *Archives of Neurology* **50**: 873–80.
8. Schmahmann JD, Sherman JC (1998) The cerebellar cognitive affective syndrome. *Brain* **121**: 561–79.
9. Zeman A (2001) Consciousness. *Brain* **124**: 1263–89.
10. Pace-Schott EF, Hobson JA (2002) The neurobiology of sleep: genetics, cellular physiology and subcortical networks. *Nature Reviews. Neuroscience* **3**: 591–605.
11. Baars BJ (2002) The conscious access hypothesis: origins and recent evidence. *Trends in Cognitive Sciences* **6**:47–52.
12. Teasdale G, Jennett B (1974) Assessment of coma and impaired consciousness: a practical scale. *Lancet* **2**: 81–4.
13. Working Party of the Royal College of Physicians of London (2003) *The Vegetative State: Guidance on Diagnosis and Management*. London: Royal College of Physicians of London.
14. Schneerson JM (2005) *Sleep Medicine: A Guide to Sleep and Its Disorders*. Oxford: Blackwell.
15. James W (1890) *The Principles of Psychology*. New York: Henry Holt.
16. LaBerge D (1995) *Attentional Processing*. Cambridge, MA: Harvard University Press.
17. Robertson IH, Marshall J (1993) *Unilateral Neglect: Clinical and Experimental Studies*. Hove: Lawrence Erlbaum Associates.
18. Zeki S (1993) *A Vision of the Brain*. Blackwell.
19. Gazzaniga M, Ivry RB, Mangun GR (2002) *Cognitive Neuroscience: The Biology of the Mind*, 2nd edn. New York: Norton.
20. Milner AD, Goodale MA (1995) *The Visual Brain in Action*. Oxford: Oxford University Press.
21. Folstein MF, Folstein SE, McHugh PR (1975) 'Mini-mental state': a practical method for grading the mental state of patients for the clinician. *Journal of Psychiatric Research* **12**: 189–98.
22. Farah MJ (2004) *The Cognitive Neuroscience of Vision*. Oxford: Blackwell.
23. Squire LR, Zola-Morgan S, Cave CB, *et al.* (1990) Memory: organization of brain systems and cognition. *Cold Spring Harbor Symposia on Quantitative Biology* **55**: 1007–23.
24. Squire LR (2004) Memory systems of the brain: a brief history and current perspective. *Neurobiology of Learning and Memory* **82**: 171–7.
25. Conway MA (2005) Memory and the self. *Journal of Memory and Language* **53**: 594–628.
26. Kandel ER, Schwartz JH, Jessell TM (1991) *Principles of Neural Science*, 3rd edn. East Norwalk, CT: Prentice Hall.
27. Hodges JR (2007) *Frontotemporal Dementia Syndromes*. Cambridge: Cambridge University Press.
28. Svoboda E, McKinnon MC, Levine B (2006) The functional neuroanatomy of autobiographical memory: a meta-analysis. *Neuropsychologia* **44**: 2189–208.
29. Moscovitch M, Rosenbaum RS, Gilboa A, *et al.* (2005) Functional neuroanatomy of remote episodic, semantic and spatial memory: a unified account based on multiple trace theory. *Journal of Anatomy* **207**: 35–66.
30. Corkin S, Amaral DG, Gonzalez RG, Johnson KA, Hyman BT (1997) HM's medial temporal lobe lesion: findings from magnetic resonance imaging. *Journal of Neuroscience* **17**: 3964–79.
31. Butler CR, Graham KS, Hodges JR, *et al.* (2007) The syndrome of transient epileptic amnesia. *Annals of Neurology* **61**: 587–98.
32. Hodges JR (1991) *Transient Amnesia*. London: WB Saunders.
33. Kopelman MD (2004) Focal retrograde amnesia and the attribution of causality: an exceptionally critical review. *Cognitive Neuropsychology* **17**: 585–621.
34. Evans JJ, Graham KS, Pratt KH, Hodges JR (2003) The impact of disrupted cortico-cortico connectivity: a long-term follow up of a case of focal retrograde amnesia. *Cortex* **39**: 767–90.
35. Rankin KP, Gorno-Tempini ML, Allison SC, *et al.* (2006) Structural anatomy of empathy in neurodegenerative disease. *Brain* **129**: 2945–56.
36. Graham NL, Zeman A, Young AW, Patterson K, Hodges JR (1999) Dyspraxia in a patient with corticobasal degeneration: the role of visual and tactile inputs to action. *Journal of Neurology, Neurosurgery, and Psychiatry* **67**: 334–44.

37. Scottish Intercollegiate Guidelines Network (SIGN) (2006) *Management of Patients with Dementia: A National Clinical Guideline*. Report no. 86. Edinburgh: Scottish Intercollegiate Guidelines Network.
38. National Institute for Health and Clinical Excellence (NICE) (2006) *Dementia: Supporting People with Dementia and their Carers in Health and Social Care*. Report no. 42. London: National Institute for Health and Clinical Excellence.
39. Albert ML, Feldman RG, Willis AL (1974) The 'subcortical dementia' of progressive supranuclear palsy. *Journal of Neurology, Neurosurgery, and Psychiatry* **37**: 121–30.
40. McKhann G, Drachman D, Folstein M, *et al.* (1984) Clinical diagnosis of Alzheimer's disease: report of the NINCDS-ADRDA Work Group under the auspices of Department of Health and Human Services Task Force on Alzheimer's Disease. *Neurology* **34**: 939–44.
41. McKeith IG, Galasko D, Kosaka K, *et al.* Consensus guidelines for the clinical and pathologic diagnosis of dementia with Lewy bodies (DLB): report of the consortium on DLB international workshop. *Neurology* (1996) **47**: 1113–24.
42. Hachinski V, Iliff L, Zilkha E, *et al.* (1975) Cerebral blood flow in dementia. *Archives of Neurology* **32**: 632–7.
43. Bozeat S, Gregory CA, Ralph MA, Hodges JR (2000) Which neuropsychiatric and behavioural features distinguish frontal and temporal variants of frontotemporal dementia from Alzheimer's disease? *Journal of Neurology, Neurosurgery, and Psychiatry* **69**: 178–86.
44. Wear HJ, Wedderburn CJ, Mioshi E, *et al.* (2008) The Cambridge Behavioural Inventory revised. *Dementia and Neuropsychologia* **2**(2): 102–107.
45. Cullen B, O'Neill B, Evans JJ, Coen RF, Lawlor BA (2007) A review of screening tests for cognitive impairment. *Journal of Neurology, Neurosurgery, and Psychiatry* **78**: 790–99.
46. Mioshi E, Dawson K, Mitchell J, Arnold R, Hodges JR (2006) The Addenbrooke's Cognitive Examination Revised (ACE-R): a brief cognitive test battery for dementia screening. *International Journal of Geriatric Psychiatry* **21**: 1078–85.
47. Goldstein LH, McNeil JE (2004) What is the relevance of neuropsychology for clinical psychology practice? In LH Goldstein, JE McNeil (eds) *Clinical Neuropsychology: A Practical Guide to Assessment and Management for Clinicians*. Chichester: John Wiley & Sons.
48. Nelson E (1982) *National Adult Reading Test (NART)*, 2nd edn. Windsor: NFER-Nelson.
49. The Psychological Corporation (2001) *The Wechsler Test of Adult Reading*. San Antonio, TX: The Psychological Corporation.
50. Baddeley A, Emslie H, Nimmo Smith I (1992) *The Speed and Capacity of Language-Processing Test*. Bury St Edmunds: Thames Valley Test Company.
51. Wechsler D (1997) *WAIS-III (UK) Administration and Scoring Manual*. London: The Psychological Corporation.
52. Kaufman AS (1990) *Assessing Adolescent and Adult Intelligence*. Boston, MA: Allyn & Bacon.
53. Kaufman AS, Lichtenberger EO (1999) *Essentials of WAIS-III Assessment*. New York: John Wiley & Sons.
54. The Psychological Corporation (1999) *The Wechsler Abbreviated Scale of Intelligence Manual*. San Antonio, TX: The Psychological Corporation.
55. Wechsler D (1997) *WMS-III (UK) Administration and Scoring Manual*. London: The Psychological Corporation.
56. Wilson B, Greenfield E, Clare L, *et al.* (2007) *Rivermead Behavioural Memory Test*, 3rd edn. Oxford: Harcourt Assessment.
57. Robertson IH, Ward T, Ridgeway V, Nimmo-Smith I (1997) *The Test of Everyday Attention Manual*. Bury St Edmunds: Thames Valley Test Company.
58. Partington JE, Leiter RG (1949) Partington's Pathway Test. *Psychological Service Centre Bulletin* **1**: 9–20.
59. D'Elia LF, Satz P, Uchiyama CL, White T (1996) *Colour Trails Test*. Odessa, FL: PAR.
60. Wilson B, Cockburn J, Halligan P (1987) *Behavioural Inattention Test Manual*. Bury St Edmunds: Thames Valley Test Company.
61. Warrington E, James M (1991) *The Visual Object and Space Perception Battery Manual*. Bury St Edmunds: Thames Valley Test Company.
62. Benton AL, Hamsher KdeS (1989) *Multilingual Aphasia Examination*. Iowa City, IA: AJA Associates.
63. Wilson B, Alderman N, Burgess P, Emslie H, Evans J (1996) *Behavioural Assessment of the Dysexecutive Syndrome*. Bury St Edmunds: Thames Valley Test company.
64. Wechsler D (1944) *The Measurement of Adult Intelligence*, 3rd edn. Baltimore, MD: Williams & Wilkins.
65. Burgess PW, Shallice T (1997) *The Hayling and Brixton Tests*. Bury St Edmunds: Thames Valley Test Company.
66. Gregory C, Lough S, Stone V, *et al.* (2002) Theory of mind in patients with frontal variant frontotemporal dementia and Alzheimer's disease: theoretical and practical implications. *Brain* **125**: 752–64.

Chapter 36

Neurology for psychiatrists

Peter Garrard

INTRODUCTION

The work of a neurologist consists of the diagnosis and treatment of a daunting array of disorders in a system of inconceivable complexity. Nevertheless, a systematic clinical approach, a working knowledge of common neurological conditions, and an informed, hypothesis-driven deployment of a few powerful investigations make the work not only possible but also enjoyable. This chapter begins by outlining a system for gathering relevant information from a patient so that a diagnostic problem can be formulated simply. It then discusses the disease processes that commonly give rise to these problems and how test results can help to distinguish between them. The chapter concludes with an outline of the principles of treatment of the common neurological conditions.

THE NEUROLOGICAL PATIENT

Neurological evaluation

A clear account of the symptoms and time course of a neurological complaint is without doubt the most valuable information that can be obtained during a clinical encounter. Many of the most common presenting symptoms – pain, sensory disturbance and dizziness – are subjective experiences, whose descriptions will differ in important ways, depending on the underlying cause, and therefore reward careful exploration. Episodes of blackout and collapse are usually described to, rather than seen by, the clinician, and different underlying mechanisms may be recognizable from the presence or absence of specific features. Although weakness can be quantified, and tremors or other movement disorders observed, knowledge of the circumstances of onset and the time course of any subsequent change is critical. Cognitive dysfunction can be tested informally with some specificity, but the patient's account of their problems will often reveal the domain or domains in which abnormalities are most likely to be found.

Pain

Three types of pain fall within the remit of neurology: headache, facial pain and neuropathic pain.

Headache

Headache is the most common neurological symptom and is typically associated with a degree of anxiety disproportionate to the gravity of the underlying cause. This is because the vast majority of headaches belong to one of the primary headache syndromes, which are benign and usually treatable. Headache syndromes are stereotyped and follow a pattern of attacks and remissions. A large number of stereotypic headache syndromes are now recognized, but the clinical distinctions most important for practical purposes are between migraine, cluster headache and cervicogenic tension headache. The features by which each of these syndromes can be differentiated are listed in Table 36.1.

In contrast to the primary headache syndromes, cases in which headache is secondary to an underlying lesion or process will usually be found to harbour serious cranial pathology. The history in these cases is usually shorter and the evolution of the discomfort progressive. At any age, the possibility of a space-occupying lesion causing an increase in intracranial pressure needs to be considered in a patient who describes waking daily with a global headache that is partially relieved by assuming an upright posture. If position-dependent visual obscurations are also described (due to pressure changes sufficient to disrupt the function of the optic nerves), raised intracranial pressure becomes a racing certainty.

Severe headaches with a sudden onset typically present to the emergency department, where occasionally, although by no means always, an immediate computed tomography (CT) scan reveals the presence of blood in the subarachnoid space. Subarachnoid bleeding should always enter into the clinical differential of sudden severe headache. Onset is explosively abrupt – often likened to a sudden blow to the head; the greater the precision with which the patient describes the headache onset (e.g. 'just as I was reaching for a tin of baked beans on the shelf'), the more likely it is to represent a haemorrhagic event. Obtaining a history of a primary syndromic headache in addition to the presenting event should not be considered reassuring in cases with a

Table 36.1 Headache syndromes

	Migraine	Cluster headache	Cervicogenic tension headache
Presentation	Teenage–early adulthood; more common in women	Middle age; more common in men	Any; both sexes equally
Mode of onset	Preceding aura in about 10%; slow build-up (30 min–several hours)	No warning; rapid build-up (minutes)	No warning; rapid build-up (minutes)
Distribution	Often unilateral	Orbital or temporal	Bifrontal or occipital
Quality	'Throbbing', 'pulsating'	'Intense', 'excruciating', 'drilling'	'Tight', 'squeezing', 'like a tight band around head'
Accompanying features	Intense nausea	Ptosis, conjunctival injection, lachrymation, rhinorrhoea	Mild nausea in some cases
Aggravating factors	Light *and* sound; sometimes smells	Light in some cases	Stress; light *or* sound
Duration	Rarely >24 h	Minutes to hours	30 min–7 days
Periodicity	Variable, but rarely more than monthly; can be catamenial	High degree of regularity of recurrence, by both time of day and season	Variable frequency; usually towards end of day
Sensitivity to treatment	Frequently and exquisitely to 5-HT agonists	May be aborted by inhaled oxygen	Usually sensitive to NSAIDs

5-HT, 5-hydroxytryptamine; NSAIDs, non-steroidal anti-inflammatory drugs.

high clinical suspicion: people with migraine have subarachnoid haemorrhages at the same rate as the rest of the population (about 10 cases per 100 000 person-years).

In patients over age 60 years, a unilateral persistent 'boring' discomfort associated with more widespread tenderness over the scalp, pain in the masseter muscles when chewing (jaw claudication) and a significantly raised erythrocyte sedimentation rate (ESR) may be secondary to giant cell arteritis. This frequently overlooked cause of headache is of great importance, as it often responds well to steroids and, untreated, may cause permanent loss of vision.

Facial pain

Trigeminal neuralgia is the archetypal facial pain syndrome. It is diagnosed on the strength of a classic history of paroxysmal, shooting discomfort in the distribution of one or more divisions of the fifth cranial nerve, typically in response to local stimulation (touching, shaving, eating or teeth-cleaning). Attacks occur in clusters punctuated by periods of spontaneous remission. Trigeminal neuralgia is commonly idiopathic, but it may be secondary to vascular or infiltrative lesions anywhere along the path of the nerve, or rarely to an inflammatory process in the brainstem. Secondary cases may be associated with a trigeminal sensory deficit.

Facial pain due to herpes zoster (post-herpetic neuralgia) can affect the branches of the trigeminal nerve, producing a vesicular eruption in the distribution of the affected branch (almost always the ophthalmic) in the active stages and residual scarring in the post-infectious period.

Patterns of facial pain that do not have any of the characteristics of primary or secondary trigeminal neuralgia are termed 'atypical', are seldom associated with identifiable pathology, and show a variable response to neuropathic pain medication.

Neuropathic pain

Pain is a common and potent cause of disability in neurological disorders and may be a feature of either central or peripheral nervous system disease. Pain of neuropathic origin is usually described as having a 'burning', 'electric' or 'tingling' quality and can be aggravated by superficial stimulation (e.g. contact with bedclothes). The latter phenomenon supports the idea that nociceptive hyperexcitability is the responsible mechanism, at least in peripheral nerve disease.

Visual symptoms

Although most patients with gradual visual failure are seen by an optician or ophthalmologist, those with a more rapid history, a fluctuating course, or symptoms of diplopia (double vision) or oscillopsia (visual instability) are usually considered to require neurological evaluation.

Visual failure

In the absence of any visible abnormalities in the external components of the eye, monocular visual impairment may be caused by damage (commonly inflammatory or infiltrative) to the optic nerves. Optic nerve fibres carrying information from the nasal half of the retina (which responds to changes in the outer, or temporal portions of the field of vision) cross the midline at the optic chiasm, joining fibres from the temporal half of the opposite eye, to form the optic tract. Damage to the visual system posterior to the chiasm therefore results in visual loss in one or other visual field (homonymous hemianopia). A lesion at the chiasm itself causes loss vision in both temporal fields (bitemporal hemianopia). These patterns of loss may be hinted at by a patient who 'can only see things on the left (or right)' or complains of 'blurring around the edges'. Visual deficits above or below a horizontal midline suggest damage to the retinal vessels. In common with many, if not all, neurological complaints, the pattern (complete, partial, variable, progressive or stuttering) and speed (sudden, over seconds to minutes, or over hours to days) is of crucial importance to a judgement of the likely pathology.

Diplopia

Diplopia arises from a change in the alignment of the eyes in relation to the visual world, due to limitation of movement of the orbit in one or more directions. Diplopia may be due to oculomotor nerve dysfunction, failure of transmission at the neuromuscular junction, distortion of the orbit by a solid mass, or infiltration of the 'strap muscles' of the eye. The relative positions of the two images may provide clues as to the aetiology: diplopia that is fatiguable or variable suggests a problem at the neuromuscular junction; progressive or painful diplopia suggests an infiltrative cause; horizontally spaced images are produced by limitation of abduction or adduction; vertical diplopia maximal on down-gaze is typical of an isolated fourth nerve palsy.

Oscillopsia

An inability to maintain stable fixation on the visual environment is a common symptom of loss of oculomotor control at the level of the cerebellum or its connections with the oculomotor centres in the brainstem. The symptom is usually accompanied by the other cardinal complaints of cerebellar dysfunction (walking and balance difficulties, clumsiness and slurring of speech), and nystagmus (see below) is an expected finding on examination. Nystagmus without an accompanying history of oscillopsia is long-standing and often congenital.

Weakness

Muscle weakness implies damage involving (i) the precentral gyrus of the cerebral cortex or the white-matter tracts that transmit impulses through the hemispheric subcortical white matter, midbrain, brainstem and spinal cord; (ii) any part of the network of lower motor neurons that convey impulses to effector muscles; or (iii) the muscles themselves.

Hemispheric lesions

A lesion affecting motor regions of the cerebral hemispheres will give rise to weakness of the face or limbs on the side opposite to the lesion. The arm, leg and face may be differentially impaired because of the somatotopic organization of the motor strip: weakness confined to a single leg can be due to pathology confined to the medial portion of the precentral gyrus. Lesions of the dominant hemisphere are usually accompanied by language disturbance (see below), and relatively mild language involvement in comparison to the degree of weakness suggests a predominantly subcortical localization of the lesion. The speed of onset of the problem is critically important to the likely process, which is most commonly vascular or neoplastic.

Brainstem lesions

Vascular, inflammatory or infiltrative lesions in the brainstem may also give rise to contralateral hemiplegia. In these instances, the weakness will be accompanied by additional difficulties, including incoordination, impaired motor control of the eyes, face, speech and swallow, disequilibrium, nausea and hemi-body sensory disturbance. More extensive brainstem lesions cause weakness affecting all four limbs (tetraparesis), together with one or more of these additional deficits.

Spinal-cord lesions

A lesion within the spinal cord produces weakness, and usually some form of sensory alteration, in structures whose innervation depends on the cord at or below the level of the lesion. Lesions involving only one half of the cord will produce weakness of one or both limbs on the same side (although sensory impairment may be bilateral – see below), but weakness or stiffness of both legs (spastic paraparesis) or all four limbs (tetraparesis), usually with accompanying bladder dysfunction, and without the additional features of a brainstem lesion (see above), infallibly implicates the spinal cord as the site of damage. The presence of paraparesis (i.e. sparing of the arms) implies that the lesion is below the T1 segment of the cord – the lowest level at which nerve fibres travelling to or from the arms form part of the motor or sensory tracts. A description of numbness or sensory alteration with an upper limit (sensory level) may indicate whether such a lesion lies within the thoracic or lumbar segments.

Lower motor neuron lesions

The lower motor neuron originates in the anterior horn of the spinal cord grey matter, emerging from the cord at segmental intervals, along with the posterior (sensory) roots, to form the spinal nerves. Those formed in cervical and lumbar regions are incorporated into plexuses, from which nerve trunks, carrying both efferent (motor) and afferent (sensory) information to and from the peripheries, emerge. It is rare for the motor components of any of these structures to be selectively disrupted. Unless the anterior horn itself or the ventral roots alone are the pathological focus, a lower motor neuron lesion is therefore accompanied by sensory change, whose distribution may suggest the location of damage. These patterns of sensory and motor loss are described below, in the section dealing with sensory symptoms.

Muscle pathology

In contrast to a lower motor neuron lesion, muscle pathology is never accompanied by sensory symptoms. Myopathy is suggested by a proximal distribution of weakness, resulting in symptoms such as difficulty rising from a chair or raising the arms above the head. Weakness may be accompanied by an aching discomfort in these regions.

Sensory symptoms

Subjective alteration of sensation can be either positive (usually described as 'tingling') or negative ('numbness') and can point the way to a range of important diagnoses if attention is paid to the anatomically relevant details.

Contiguous areas of numbness or tingling at the distal extremities (usually beginning with the soles of the foot, and often slowly progressive) raises the possibility of a peripheral neuropathy. More extensive involvement, including proximal regions of the upper and lower limbs at onset, suggests the presence of a more widespread process involving the plexus or the cell bodies of sensory neurons (dorsal root ganglionopathy).

When symptoms are more focal, radiculopathy (segmental damage to the nerve root in the intervertebral foramen) or mononeuropathy should be considered. The most common mononeuropathies are carpal tunnel syndrome (which commonly presents with tingling in the first three fingers) and ulnar neuropathy (tingling in the fourth and fifth fingers). Both presentations may overlap with those of compression of the lower cervical nerve roots, although the latter are normally accompanied by discomfort in the neck. The distinction is often clinically evident after exploration of the accompanying motor involvement and the distribution of insensitivity to cotton-wool or a metal point (see below). Analogous symptoms occur in the lower limbs, due to compression of the common peroneal nerve, tibial nerve (tarsal tunnel syndrome) and the lumbosacral nerve roots, which produce distinct patterns of altered sensation over the lower leg and foot. A list of landmark symptom sites that may be helpful in unravelling these distinctions is provided in Table 36.2.

Compression of the median or ulnar nerves may be bilateral, but other combinations of two or more discrete areas of sensory alteration in the limbs suggest a pattern of mononeuritis multiplex, which is frequently associated with more widespread systemic pathology.

Abnormal movement

The most common movement disorder is tremor, whose diagnosis requires distinction from the more unusual hyperkinetic patterns of involuntary (chorea, myoclonus and hemiballismus) and quasi-voluntary (tic disorders) phenomena.

Table 36.2 Mononeuropathies

	Median	Ulnar nerve	Common peroneal	Femoral
Common site and mechanism of compression	Carpal tunnel syndrome; wrist trauma	Acute or chronic low-grade elbow trauma	Single or repetitive trauma to lateral aspect of knee	Diabetes; posterior abdominal wall pathology
Symptoms	Forearm or hand pain; tingling in tips of first three digits; often nocturnal	Pain in fifth finger and adjacent palm; elbow pain	Often painless; usually presents with foot-drop	Severe anterior thigh pain; rapid-onset quadriceps wasting and weakness
Muscle-wasting	Thenar eminence: severe cases	Hypothenar eminence: severe cases	Rare	Anterior thigh: always
Weakness	Thumb abduction (movement away from hand in line with forearm)	Abduction and adduction of all digits	Foot dorsiflexion, inversion and eversion	Hip flexion and knee extension; loss of knee jerk
Objective sensory impairment	Distal portions of first three digits	Ulnar border of hand; tips of digits 4 and 5	Lateral border of leg and dorsum of foot	Entire anteromedial border of leg
Root origins of fibres	C5–T1	C8–T1	L4–S2	L2–L4
Overlapping spinal nerve root(s) syndrome: differences	C7: additional triceps and long finger flexor weakness; numbness involves forearm; triceps jerk reduced or absent	C8: additional triceps weakness; numbness extends up medial border of forearm; triceps jerk reduced or absent	L5/S1: inversion of foot and sensation over medial border (L4) both spared; ankle jerk reduced or absent	Lumbar plexus (L1–L4): more extensive sensory loss; adductor weakness

Tremor

Any rhythmic, repetitive, involuntary movement of the extremities or head may be classified as a tremor, the hand being the most common site. Many cases, particularly in patients under the age of 40 years, represent a benign physiological phenomenon ('essential tremor'): in these cases, the problem tends to be exaggerated by states such as stress, fatigue and anxiety and disappears after the intake of small quantities of alcohol. A clear history of isolated tremor in the previous generation is often obtained. Some forms of physiological tremor may be task- or activity-specific, such as writing, or orthostatic tremor.

A drug history is important: statins, inhaled β agonists, sodium valproate, lithium, tricyclic antidepressants and neuroleptic agents may be implicated and not infrequently prescribed in combination. Caffeine intake is another common modifiable factor.

In people in older age groups, tremor is more likely to be a manifestation of parkinsonism. A parkinsonian tremor is present at rest, typically worse during attention-demanding mental tasks, and not present during reflexive movements. Tremor may remain the dominant or even sole clinical feature of Parkinson's disease over many years.

Tremor can be purely factitious but, even in cases of unusually coarse or bizarre patterns, midbrain (rubral) or cerebellar pathology and Wilson's disease are important diagnostic considerations, especially in younger patients.

Chorea

A choreiform movement disorder is more complex and widespread than a tremor, in keeping with its derivation from the Greek word meaning 'dance'. In general terms, it is less predictable, in both spatial and temporal terms, than the simple oscillatory movements that characterize a tremor. Unilateral chorea may appear as a feature of a focal ischaemic or inflammatory lesion. Chorea is a recognized feature of autoimmune disease, including systemic lupus erythematosus (SLE) and the antiphospholipid syndrome. Sydenham's chorea refers to an immunologically mediated complication of streptococcal infection. Florid chorea is a feature of the autosomal dominant neurodegenerative condition Huntington's disease (HD) and is a presenting feature of inherited metabolic conditions such as Wilson's disease and storage disorders.

Myoclonus

Brief isolated involuntary small-volume movements are referred to as 'myoclonus' or 'myoclonic jerks'. The movements may be observed and in some instances elicited by startle, cutaneous stimulation or posture (asterixis). Commonly, however, the presence of myoclonic jerks is inferred from a history of intermittent acts of sudden clumsiness or from a description. The most dramatic and noticeable examples appear as movements of the shoulder girdle, limbs or face, but small-volume jerks may be observed in the outstretched fingers, axial musculature or the palate.

A history of myoclonus is associated with a number of primary epilepsy syndromes, including juvenile myoclonic epilepsy. Myoclonic jerks are seen following recovery from anoxic brain injury (post-anoxic myoclonus) and in metabolic encephalopathies: the prominence of the movement may correlate with the severity of the condition. Stimulus-sensitive small-volume jerks of the outstretched fingers are associated with the early stages of neurodegenerative disorders, including Alzheimer's disease (AD). Startle myoclonus is typical, but not diagnostic, of Creutzfeldt–Jakob disease.

Hemiballismus

Hemiballistic movements involve complexes of muscles acting in a coordinated but involuntary fashion to bring about dramatic 'flinging' movements of one arm or leg. Movements are of sudden onset and brief duration. They occur following injury to the contralateral subthalamic nucleus, typically ischaemic or haemorrhagic, and are usually self-limiting within a period of weeks. Hemiballismus is to be distinguished from the equally unusual 'alien limb phenomenon', in which a patient engages in complex goal-directed activities such as picking up objects or removing items of clothing without any sense of agency; the arm is described as having a life or will of its own. The alien limb syndrome may follow injury or degenerative change in the frontal or parietal cortical regions.

Tic disorders (stereotypies)

The movement disorders described above are involuntary phenomena, but a tic is a willed movement, executed in response to an irresistible impulse. Tic disorders are therefore a form of compulsive behaviour manifesting in brief motor acts involving the limbs, face or muscles of phonation (vocal tics). Although these acts may in some instances resemble myoclonic jerks, they are typically more complex, requiring the mutual coordination of more than one muscle group, and they may involve a pattern that develops in a predictable fashion over time. At the extreme end of a spectrum of severity lies Tourette's syndrome, characterized by multiple motor and vocal tics.

Disturbances of consciousness

The patient who has suffered their first ever blackout is usually eager to know whether they have epilepsy and the likelihood of recurrent events. The answers to these two important questions are clearly linked, and so the first clinical decision to be made is whether the event was due to cerebral or circulatory disturbance ('fit or faint').

This distinction may be difficult to make, but the greater the amount of first-hand information available from a witness to the attack, the easier it becomes. A witness's description of a convulsive epileptic seizure can be decisive: a period of unconsciousness with recovery over minutes, including a period of confusion, a prolonged postictal period of myalgia, headache and fatigue, all suggest epilepsy. In contrast, premonitory light-headedness, a rapid recovery, retained memory of events right up to the onset of the blackout, and awareness during emergence from unconsciousness are all suggestive of a faint. Shaking movements, even a brief convulsion, may be described during a faint, but a prolonged phase of tonic muscular contraction and clonic (convulsive) movements of the limbs, preceded or accompanied by vocalization, are all definite hallmarks of epilepsy. Urinary incontinence more commonly accompanies an epileptic event, but its description does not exclude a haemodynamic cause. Soreness of the sides of the tongue or mouth due to tonic contraction of the jaw muscles is a fit marker but by no means a feature of all cases.

A well-described complex partial seizure, characterized by sequences of purposeless movements of the face, hands or feet, often accompanied by a vacant, staring expression and an unresponsive state, and continuing for seconds to minutes (cf. stereotypies) should be easily recognizable. Complex partial seizures are often marked by the preceding occurrence of a sensory aura (e.g. a hallucination of smell, taste or familiarity – déjà vu). Epileptic auras may also occur in isolation (simple partial seizures).

In an absence attack, the phenomenon of vacancy and unrousability is not accompanied by abnormal movements and indeed may occur during the continued performance of other activities, such as walking or driving.

Bizarre motor phenomena, psychiatric morbidity – latent or declared – and evidence of awareness during the episode are suggestive of a factitious event, or 'pseudo-seizure'. It is important to remember that pseudo-seizures and genuine epileptic attacks may occur in the same individual, and that seizures of frontal origin are often associated with seemingly bizarre motor phenomena.

Cognitive decline

In unskilled hands clinical cognitive evaluation can be a frustratingly time-consuming exercise, but for the experienced observer it can be extremely diagnostically rewarding. An important principle is that clinical data should be gathered not only from the patient but also from a close associate, preferably not in the presence of each other, as this may inhibit the disclosure of diagnostically important information.

The differential diagnosis of cognitive decline varies with both the patient's age and the pattern and rate of progression of their symptoms. The incidence of AD increases exponentially with age, such that around one in five people over the age of 80 years is clinically affected, and an even higher number harbour presymptomatic plaque and tangle pathology. In common with all biological processes, higher brain function declines with normal ageing, leaving the principal diagnostic dilemma in an elderly patient with cognitive dysfunction one of distinguishing incipient AD from age-related decline. In such borderline cases, the diagnostic category of mild cognitive impairment (MCI) proves to be a useful compromise: patients with cognitive complaints but defective performance on only a single domain of performance are put into this category, in the knowledge that after a year as many as 50 per cent will have deteriorated to a condition consistent with early AD. Although a history of insidious cognitive decline in a patient over 65 years of age is more likely to represent the onset of AD than any other pathological process, below this cut-off AD and frontotemporal lobar degeneration (FTLD) are approximately equally common. The onset of vascular dementia is also more common in late middle age than old age and is particularly likely in people with one or more vascular risk factors.

Clinical examination

A great deal of critical diagnostic information will have been gathered during the interview stage of the clinical encounter, including the characteristics of the patient's gait and speech, the presence and characteristics of any abnormal movements, and a crude assessment of cognition. Formalizing, elaborating and, where possible, quantifying these observed abnormalities is one purpose of the clinical examination; the other is to look for clues to underlying pathology that cannot be seen without specific testing.

Higher cognitive function

Adequate bedside or clinic-based cognitive evaluation can be achieved using a minimum of equipment. The most effective and time-efficient tools are those that rely on more than one cognitive domain but that produce differential patterns of performance, depending on the nature of the deficit. Spontaneous speech, for instance, which contains myriad clues to the integrity of the language system (rate of production, phonological and syntactic integrity, vocabulary), can be examined while the patient is prompted to recall recent notable news items.

Similarly, both working and verbal episodic memory can be evaluated by asking the patient to repeat and, after a delay, recall a word list or name and address. Immediate recall is impaired by working memory dysfunction, while problems with delayed recall would implicate learning and storage. An analogous test of non-verbal memory (particularly useful when evaluating a patient with an aphasic disorder) consists of asking the patient to copy, and later reproduce from memory, three simple geometric designs (e.g. a wire cube, a five-pointed star and intersecting pentagons), a task that makes concurrent demands on visuospatial and constructional skills. Non-verbal memory may, in any case, be impaired independently of memory for verbal material.

Verbal fluency, using both initial letter and semantic category as a cue, is another clinical technique with compound utility: patients with executive deficits characteristically experience greater difficulty searching for words beginning with a particular letter than they do for words belonging to the same semantic category (essentially, an exaggeration of normal performance, presumably due to the fact that neural states corresponding to semantically related items are mutually activating). In contrast (and for similar reasons), patients with semantic dementia often produce more words per minute in the letter than the category condition. Patients with frontal variant FTLD may involuntarily perseverate on a single word and are often unable to inhibit a tendency to produce obscenities or words with sexual connotations. Patients with AD often repeat the same word several times during the course of the test, due to their defective memories.

Naming errors are a further source of diagnostically important information: a series of relatively low-frequency but visually distinct pictures can elicit several kinds of highly informative error pattern: phonological errors (i.e. distortions of the correct phonological form of the word) suggest that the patient has a problem in the verbal output system; circumlocutions ('a beautiful creature that jumps'), semantic errors, and overuse of category, generic or highly prototypical terms (e.g. 'animal', 'dog', 'item' or 'thing') implies a breakdown at the level of meaning, or semantic memory; and the patient who scrutinizes a line drawing or traces the outline with their finger before producing the name of something conceptually distinct but vaguely visually similar (e.g. 'ball' in response to a picture of an apple) is likely to have profound visuospatial impairment. These distinct patterns point clearly to dysfunction in the left inferior frontal, bilateral anterior temporal, and posterior occipitoparietal regions, respectively.

Cranial nerves

With the exception of cranial nerves I and II, which transmit special sensory modalities, the cranial nerves emerge from nuclei that are located in the upper (III–VIII) and lower (IX–XII) parts of the brainstem. They are best examined from the eyes downwards, beginning with visualization of the optic fundus.

The optic fundus

A normal optic disc (Figure 36.1a) appears pale pink in colour, with a smooth, well-defined border, flush with the surrounding retinal surface. The retinal vessels can be clearly seen radiating from its centre, with pulsation often visible. The disc may become swollen, as a result either of

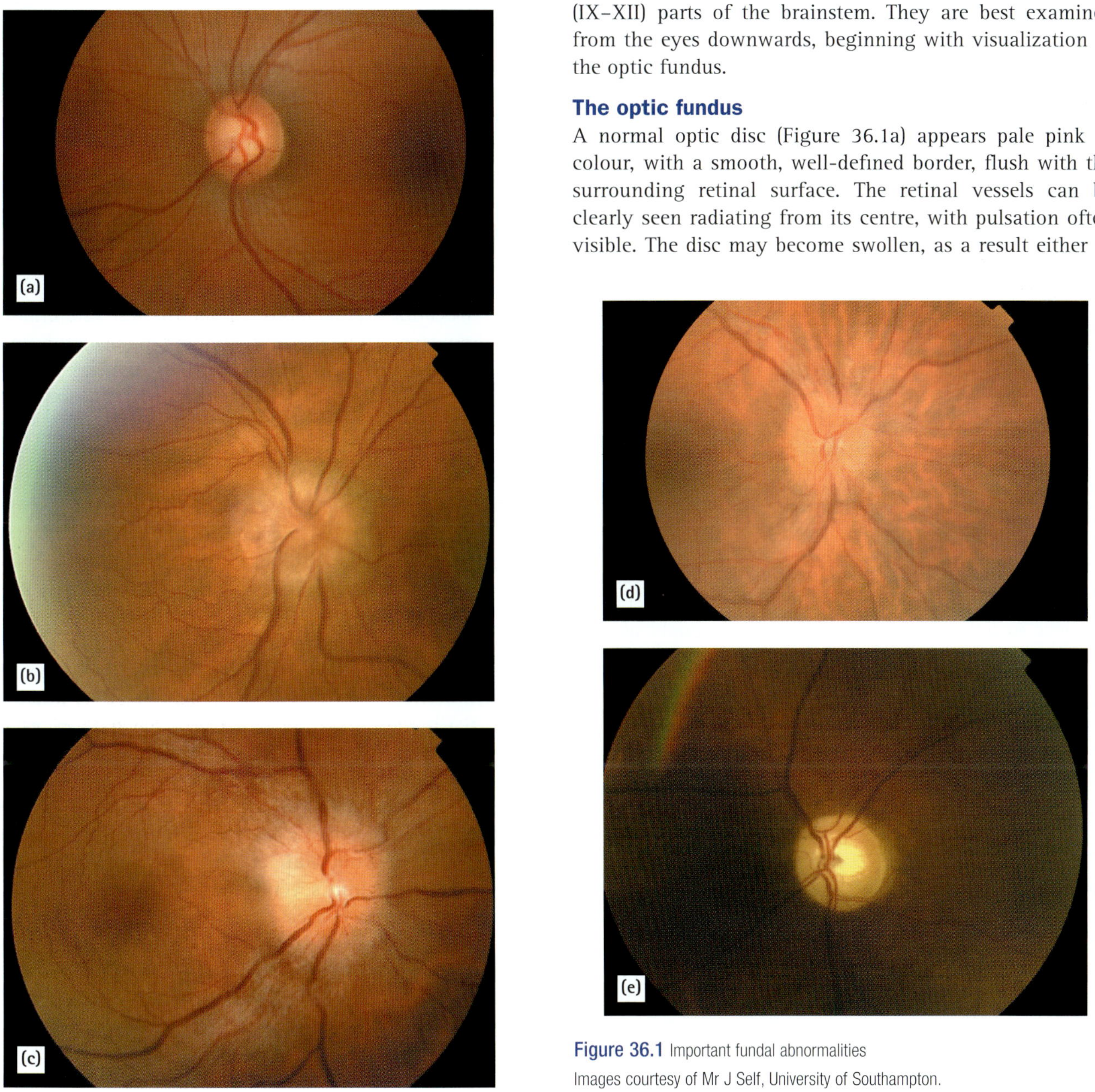

Figure 36.1 Important fundal abnormalities
Images courtesy of Mr J Self, University of Southampton.

inlammation in the nerve (optic neuritis) or of interstitial fluid accumulation caused by impaired venous drainage secondary to raised intracranial pressure. The edges of a subtly swollen disc (Figure 36.1b) lose their clarity, while more established swelling causes the surface to protrude away from the retina (Figure 36.1c). Haemorrhages may also be visible in severe cases (Figure 36.1d).

Optic disc swelling is a sign of an acute and active process and should never be ignored. Chronic damage to the optic nerve (usually following resolution of one or more inflammatory events) results in an atrophic appearance, recognizable by its sickly pale colour and shrunken area (Figure 36.1e).

Although identification or exclusion of optic nerve swelling is an essential goal of fundoscopy, the peripheries of the retinal surface may also reveal the presence of retinitis pigmentosa, whose spiculated appearance (Figure 36.2) is associated with a variety of metabolic disorders.

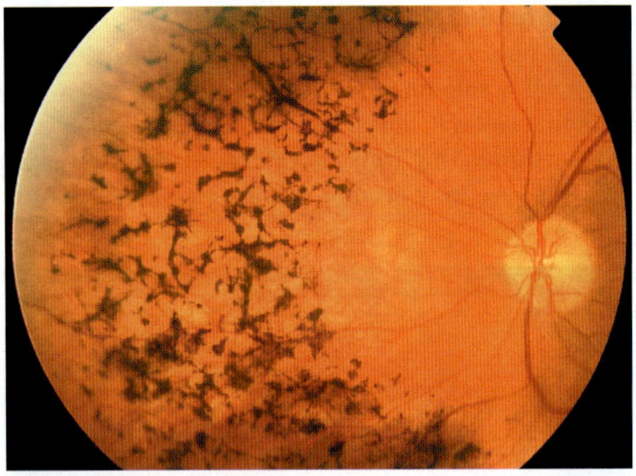

Figure 36.2 Retinitis pigmentosa
Image courtesy of Mr J Self, University of Southampton.

Before or after fundal examination, the pupils may be examined for shape, regularity, equality, and contraction in response to light. The level of the eyelids should also be noted: complete closure (ptosis) on one side will be obvious, but partial ptosis may require specific inspection. Partial ptosis, together with reduction in pupillary diameter (miosis) in the same eye, form the defining features of Horner's syndrome. This results from interruption of the long sympathetic pathway that runs from the hypothalamus to the smooth muscle of the eye, via the upper thoracic segments of the spinal cord.

Eye movements

Deviation of the orbit may be evident on immediate inspection and is not always pathological: sequentially occluding the two eyes and looking for a compensatory movement of the deviated eye towards the midline can confirm a lifelong squint. Uncompensated deviation indicates paralysis of the oculomotor muscle or muscles acting in the opposite direction. This may be due to infiltration of the muscle, but more commonly it indicates loss of innervation. Loss of function of the sixth nerve results in deviation of the globe towards the midline due to weakness of the lateral rectus muscle. An eye that is deviated laterally and inferiorly indicates weakness of the medial, superior and inferior recti, all of which are supplied by the third nerve, and is frequently accompanied by enlargement of the pupil, as it also transmits the fibres that mediate reflex constriction.

Pursuit movements in response to movement of a target in the vertical and horizontal planes confirm complete or partial failure in one or more of these directions and may bring out a previously unseen palsy of the fourth nerve by demonstrating loss of radial intortion of the globe (evident in the normal condition from subtle rotatory movement of the scleral vessels on down-gaze). Double vision will be reported with a paralytic, but not a compensated, squint: images are reported as separated horizontally in a sixth nerve palsy, diagonally in a third nerve palsy and obliquely in a fourth nerve palsy. In the latter, two images of a pen held horizontally in front of the eyes will form an arrowhead shape whose tip points to the side of the lesion.

Nystagmus (rhythmic oscillations of the eye) may be visible with the patient looking straight ahead (primary position of gaze) but is more commonly evoked by voluntary eye movement. The direction of oscillation is diagnostically important: horizontal nystagmus is caused by a lesion to the cerebellar circuitry on the side to which it is maximal. Down-beating nystagmus suggests a lesion at the base of the brainstem. Unilateral nystagmus combined with limitation of horizontal movement indicates interruption of the upper brainstem tracts between the third and sixth nerve nuclei (internuclear ophthalmoplegia).

Facial weakness

For most of its length, the seventh (facial) nerve consists only of motor fibres innervating the muscles of facial expression. For clinical purposes, a lesion of the facial nerve therefore results in an inability voluntarily to elevate the forehead (frontalis), forcibly close the eyelids (orbicularis oculi), widen the mouth, and purse or tighten the lips (orbicularis oris). A seventh nerve lesion may occur anywhere between the base of the pons (where its nucleus is situated in close proximity to that of the sixth nerve) and the main nerve trunk as it passes through the parotid gland. Facial weakness caused by a more central lesion (i.e. in the contralateral motor cortex or underlying white matter) is recognizable by sparing of the frontalis muscle, which receives input from both cerebral hemispheres. Thus, an upper motor neuron seventh nerve palsy affects only the muscles of the lower face.

The most common cause of an isolated global or lower motor neuron facial weakness is Bell's palsy, in which the nerve swells and becomes trapped by the bony stylomastoid foramen. Bilateral Bell's palsy rarely, if ever, occurs; bilateral facial weakness implies an alternative pathology such as sarcoidosis or Guillain–Barré syndrome.

Facial sensation

Sensation over the skin of the face, the buccal and nasal mucosa, the teeth and the nasal sinuses is mediated by the ophthalmic, maxillary and mandibular nerves, which are subdivisions of the trigeminal or fifth cranial nerve. The mandibular nerve also carries motor fibres to the muscles involved in opening and closing the jaw. Damage may occur to one or more of the three divisions; the trunk of the parent nerve; the sensory fibre tract, which extends caudally from the main nucleus in the pons to below the cervicomedullary junction; and to white matter of the contralateral hemisphere.

Patterns associated with all these lesion sites are clinically recognizable, and they are distinguishable from cases without an organic cause: the ophthalmic division has a distribution that includes the scalp as far back as the vertex (i.e. it does not terminate at the hairline), the nose, and the area between and around the eyes (including the corneas – tested by lightly stroking the cornea with a small twist of cotton-wool to elicit reflex closure of the eyelid); the maxillary division includes the upper lip and cheeks, and the mandibular the lower lip, chin and temples. Damage to the trigeminal tracts produces symptoms and signs that cross these boundaries, often forming a muzzle- or mask-like distribution. The skin over the angle of the jaw, the ear cartilage and the occiput fall outside the distribution of trigeminal divisions.

The lower cranial nerves

Brainstem lesions produce dysfunction in the nuclei of cranial nerves VIII–XII and accompanying deficits in the long motor and sensory tracts. Skull-base pathology can impinge directly on the extracranial portions of the nerves, causing isolated dysfunction in one or more of these structures: a lesion of the glossopharyngeal nerve causes loss of sensation over the posterior tongue and palatal regions, depriving the sensitive gag reflex of its afferent arm; a patient with tenth nerve dysfunction complains of hoarseness, swallowing difficulty and a tendency to aspirate, due to muscular weakness in the palate and vocal folds, and loss of the efferent arm of the gag reflex; damage to the accessory nerve (XI) produces weakness of shoulder-shrugging and head-turning (away from the side of the lesion); and damage to the glossopharyngeal nerve gives rise to weakness and wasting of the tongue.

More diffuse damage to the motor systems subserved by the lower cranial nerves produces a picture of generalized loss of function in the muscles of articulation and swallowing. Where the lesion involves central structures (e.g. bilateral internal capsular infarcts) or a combination of upper and lower motor neuron pathology (the progressive bulbar palsy of motor neuron disease), speech takes on a strangulated quality, the jaw jerk is exaggerated, and emotional lability is exhibited. These features are absent when the lower motor neuron or neuromuscular junction alone is involved (e.g. due to carcinomatous meningitis, Guillain–Barré syndrome or myasthenia gravis).

Evaluation of the limbs

Examination of the limbs includes observation of posture and muscle bulk, assessment of resting muscle tone, classification and distribution of any loss of power, and elicitation of the tendon reflexes. This information allows the critical distinction between upper and lower motor neuron weakness to be made. Gait, coordination and sensation are tested at the end of the examination.

Muscle posture and bulk

Involuntary posturing of the arms or legs suggests an upper motor neuron lesion as the cause of motor disturbance, while wasting of muscle implies damage to a peripheral component or lower motor neuron. By definition, the former is situated proximal to the anterior horn cell (i.e. in or above the descending motor tracts in the spinal cord) and the latter distal to it (i.e. in or below the exiting motor nerve root). Certain patterns of muscle wasting are strongly suggestive of an underlying lesion: distal symmetrical wasting implies degeneration of the peripheral nerves (peripheral neuropathy); unilateral thenar or hypothenar wasting suggests median and ulnar nerve lesions, respectively; and global atrophy of the small hand muscles implies a lesion to the T1 nerve root.

Muscle wasting occurs when individual motor neurons die back, depriving single muscle fibres of trophic support. When this process is widespread (as occurs in amyotrophic lateral sclerosis, ALS), focal contractions of small areas of denervated muscle (fasciculations) may be seen. The deltoids and triceps in the arms and the quadriceps in the legs are the best places to examine for this ominous sign.

Muscle tone

For normal posture to be maintained, skeletal muscle needs to maintain a baseline level of activity at rest, and it is the balance of activity in the extensors and flexors of the legs and arms that is evaluated when muscle tone is tested.

Testing is performed in the upper limbs by passively flexing and extending the arm at the elbow and then pronating and supinating the hand at the wrist. In the normal subject, a scarcely perceptible degree of resistance is detected, as compared with the heavy passivity associated with a chronic lower motor neuron lesion, and the increased resistance (often described as a 'catch') evident following upper motor neuron lesions. In the lower limb, the leg is picked up briskly at the knee joint; increased tone will cause the heel to be lifted off the examination couch, while normal tone allows the heel to be dragged along the surface.

Power

The ability to resist an appropriate force applied by the examiner against the direction of action of a muscle or muscle group is an indication of normal power. The important word here is 'appropriate', as applied both to the patient and to the muscle being tested: a healthy 30-year-old can usually generate more power than an octogenarian patient with arthritis, while biceps flexion generates more force than finger abduction.

The five-point grading system provides a convenient metric for quantifying muscle strength (Table 36.3). The distribution and the grade of weakness provide useful information as to the likely origin of the problem: symmetrical weakness affecting the proximal groups (including flexion and extension of the neck) suggests a disease of muscle, while distal weakness implies a neuropathic origin. Weakness disproportionately affecting the anti-gravity muscles (those that bend the arms and straighten the legs) is likely to arise from a central (upper motor neuron) lesion, while a global pattern is more typical of peripheral (lower motor neuron) dysfunction. Spastic weakness of both legs indicates a lesion in the cord; if there is no additional weakness in the arms or hands, then the lesion lies below the level of T1. A spastic quadriparesis suggests a lesion at or above C4. Hemiplegic weakness is usually due to a lesion in the contralateral hemisphere, but it may also be caused by a process compromising one half of the cord. Compression neuropathies also produce highly recognizable combinations of (usually unilateral) weakness, although they are easily confused with lesions at the level of the cervical and lumbar nerve roots. Disentangling these possibilities often relies on evidence gained from the tendon reflexes and the sensory examination.

Table 36.3 Medical Research Council (MRC) power grading

MRC grade	Definition
5	Normal power against resistance
4	Active movement against gravity and some against resistance
3	Active movement of the limb against gravity but not against resistance
2	Active movement of limb when gravity eliminated
1	Flicker or trace of muscle contraction
0	No contraction

Reflexes

The monosynaptic muscle stretch reflex is elicited by striking an anatomically accessible tendon and watching for reflex contraction in the muscle to which it attaches. The contraction may be normal, exaggerated or absent. Exaggerated (brisk) reflexes indicate loss of central modulation and thus indicate a central lesion at a level higher than the reflex being tested. Since the afferent and efferent arms of a monosynaptic stretch reflex are carried through one or two adjacent nerve roots, an isolated absent reflex suggests damage at root level, often due to impingement by a protruding intervertebral disc. Knowledge of the root levels through which commonly elicited reflex arcs are transmitted is therefore essential to interpretation (Table 36.4). A generalized absence of reflexes suggests a more widespread process, involving either multiple nerve roots or individual nerve fibres, or both. Absent or diminished reflexes may be brought out by asking the patient to perform a muscle-tensing manoeuvre. Contrary to popular belief, the effects of reinforcement are not evanescent but last for 5–10 s.

Table 36.4 Levels of reflex arcs

Reflex	Spinal root transmitting
Biceps	C5
Triceps	C6
Supinator	C7
Finger	C8
Knee	L4
Ankle	S1

Sensation

One rule transforms sensory testing from a painful exercise in time-wasting into a useful data-gathering process: know what you are trying to find. This is, after all, why it is performed at the end of the examination. A patient with symptoms and signs of a peripheral neuropathy often shows a 'glove and stocking' pattern of sensory loss – so look for one, using either a pin or a tuning fork. A patient with a spastic paraparesis probably has a lesion in the cord between T1 and L1, and the line on the torso below which sensation is reduced or absent provides more precise localizing information – so examine for a 'sensory level'; a spastic hemiparesis due to a cord rather than a hemispheric lesion will often be accompanied by a 'dissociated' sensory impairment (impairment of joint position sense on the side of the weakness, and reduction in light touch appreciation on the other) – a diagnosis clinched. Nerve and root entrapments can also be disentangled by exploring the skin over the distribution of, say, the ulnar nerve (fourth and fifth fingers) and the C8 nerve root (ulnar border of the hand and forearm) with the tip of a pin.

Some patients are, admittedly, poor sensory witnesses, and it is often better to hand them a pin and ask them to demonstrate the distribution of the sensory deficit themselves. Patients with a consistent and anatomically meaningful loss will quickly distinguish themselves from those with patchy and inconsistent impairments that are rarely if ever associated with organic disease.

NEUROLOGICAL ILLNESSES

Many of the diagnostic categories used in modern neurology have their origins in the remarkably astute observations of nineteenth- and early-twentieth-century clinicians. Since then, the understanding of neurological disease has benefited, perhaps more than any other branch of clinical medicine, from advances in the basic biological sciences. The categorization of neurological disease as it is currently understood is briefly outlined below, in order to orient the reader to the diversity of pathophysiological processes that underpin many of the common acute and chronic neurological conditions. In view of the size and diversity of the subject, what follows is intended as an index rather than a work of reference.

Chronic conditions

It is useful to consider the pathophysiological processes causing chronic neurological disease under a series of broad causative headings. A small but important subgroup of conditions affecting the nervous system consists of inherited disorders, which include diseases of both central and peripheral regions of the nervous system. Within acquired neurological disease, a large percentage of patients will turn out to have a primary degenerative pathology, and similarly large numbers of patients will be affected by vascular and inflammatory processes. Autoimmune processes are increasingly recognized as a mechanism underlying neurological dysfunction of various kinds. Several infectious agents continue to cause morbidity; and metabolic and nutritional deficiencies, although unusual, are potentially amenable to straightforward treatment, and should never, therefore, be overlooked.

Inherited disorders

The important groups of dominantly inherited neurological disease include the young-onset movement and cognitive disorders (HD, familial AD), and the inherited spinocerebellar ataxias (SCA), of which 29 genetically distinct varieties have so far been described and the most common of which are now susceptible to genetic testing. Cerebral autosomal dominant arteriopathy with subcortical infarcts and leucoencephalopathy (CADASIL) is an unusual cause of premature cerebrovascular disease but recognizable in patients with young-onset stroke, a background that includes classical migraine or depression, and imaging appearances of confluent white-matter lesions in the brainstem and hemispheres (particularly the temporal lobes). Diseases of peripheral nerve (the hereditary motor and sensory neuropathies) and muscle (the muscular dystrophies) have also been extensively subcategorized using molecular or genetic criteria, allowing many cases to be given highly specific diagnostic labels.

Few recessive conditions primarily affecting the central nervous system are known; though some of the familial neuropathy subtypes show this pattern of inheritance. Those with a neurological component are generally of metabolic origin and will be mentioned under that heading.

An important subgroup of inherited neurological disease is caused by mutations carried not in the cell's nucleus but in the mitochondria, producing abnormalities of cellular energy production. The effects of these disorders depend on the distribution of defective mitochondria within the organs, but almost all have some form of neurological involvement, which includes excessive muscle fatigue, optic nerve degeneration, and a severe and rapidly progressive encephalopathy.

Neurodegenerative disorders

Details of causation in many of the neurodegenerative conditions have not been defined completely, and in consequence few of these progressive illnesses are currently amenable to treatment. Improved understanding of the molecular basis of this group of conditions may well render the term obsolete, replacing it with a variety of mechanistic categories derived from molecular-level description. This process is already emerging: a number of clinical conditions that previously were considered to be of disparate origin (AD, frontotemporal dementia, corticobasal degeneration, progressive supranuclear palsy) are now considered under the umbrella term 'tauopathies', indicating the formation of abnormal aggregates of tau protein within the brain. Common neurodegenerative appearances that do not fall into the tauopathy category include prion disease, disorders of alpha synuclein, and appearances associated with ubiquitin-containing inclusions. Prion diseases (e.g. Creutzfeldt–Jakob disease in humans and scrapie in sheep) cause dysfunction and destruction of brain tissue by the relentless, self-catalysing propagation of prion protein aggregates. Pathological markers of other conditions are composed of aggregates of different material: alpha synuclein is seen in the brain of patients with Parkinson's disease and dementia with Lewy bodies. Ubiquitin inclusions are a more recently defined pathological entity and are found in the brain of a subset of patients with frontotemporal dementia and of patients with motor neuron disease.

Vascular disease

Sporadic cerebrovascular disease should always be considered as a potential cause of central nervous system symptomatology in patients over the age of 50 years and is particularly likely in heavy smokers, patients with a history of diabetes, lipid disorders or hypertension, and patients with a family history of vasculopathy. Both acute and chronic ischaemic injury can produce signs of dysfunction clinically localizable to the cerebral hemispheres and brainstem. Acute vascular injuries are dealt with below. Chronic damage, usually to the hemispheric white matter, is a potent and common cause of cognitive decline, often characterized by slowed but accurate mental processing ('subcortical dementia'). Vascular cognitive impairment does not, contrary to popular dogma, invariably proceed in a stepwise rather than a insidiously progressive fashion, and it frequently coexists with a degenerative pathology such as AD. Unlike pure neurodegenerative conditions, however, progression in vascular cognitive impairment is susceptible to modification by good risk-factor management. Vascular insufficiency causing injury to the spinal cord also occurs but is considerably less common than compressive or inflammatory processes.

Inflammatory conditions

Demyelination, or the loss of the myelin layer from nerve cells, is the final common pathway of neuronal damage from a number of processes, including inherited and acquired metabolic disorders, autoimmune conditions and infection. Sporadic cases of demyelinating illness are, however, most commonly associated with an immune-mediated inflammatory aetiology.

Myelin is a layer of phospholipid that ensheathes the axons of many neurons, both central and peripheral, providing electrical insulation and vastly increasing the speed of impulse transmission. The myelin sheath surrounding peripheral nerves is formed by Schwann cells, while axons in the central nervous system are myelinated by oligodendrocytes. This difference between central and peripheral myelin is critical, as demyelination due to an inflammatory process occurs either centrally (e.g. in multiple sclerosis, MS) or peripherally (the demyelinating polyneuropathies), but rarely in both together.

MS is the most common inflammatory disorder of the central nervous system and should be considered as significantly more likely than vascular disease in young adults with acute central deficits. MS is a complex diagnosis that requires clinical and magnetic resonance (MR) evidence of the dissemination of inflammatory lesions over time and space, and laboratory evidence of central nervous system inflammation. These data may be considered in relation to accepted diagnostic criteria, of which the revised McDonald criteria are currently the most commonly applied. The disease can affect any of the white-matter tracts of the central nervous system and can therefore produce most types of central deficit: common patterns include monocular visual loss (optic neuritis), cerebella ataxia, disorders of eye-movement control, and spastic paraparesis. Deficits due to inflammatory damage tend to evolve over a period of hours rather than the seconds to minutes characteristic of a vascular insult. In the majority of cases, the disease is manifested by a series of acute attacks, the effects of which may partially or fully resolve (relapsing and remitting MS) or result in further decline (secondary progressive MS). Primary progressive MS, in which the patient's functional status gradually declines without the occurrence of an acute episode, is also a recognized disease pattern. The cause or causes of MS are still poorly understood, but it probably involves a combination of inherited susceptibility and one or more environmental factors.

Inflammatory demyelination in peripheral nerves occurs acutely – in Guillain–Barré syndrome (see below) – and in the context of chronic inflammatory demyelinating polyneuropathy (CIDP). Patients with the latter condition give an insidious history of numbness and tingling of the peripheries, weakness and clumsiness of the limbs, and walking difficulty. Clinical examination reveals an absence of upper motor neuron or other central features, and diagnosis is based on exclusion of alternative causes of peripheral neuropathy (importantly, diabetes, vitamin B12 deficiency, monoclonal gammopathy and connective tissue diseases), elevated cerebrospinal fluid protein content, and characteristic appearances on peripheral nerve biopsy. Like MS, CIDP can follow a relapsing–remitting or chronically progressive course.

Infectious causes of chronic neurological disease

The transmissible causes of chronic neurological illness most important to consider are the human immunodeficiency virus (HIV) and *Treponema pallidum* (the infectious agent responsible for syphilis).

HIV infection can produce neurological manifestations at most levels in the nervous system. Moving from centre to periphery, it can be responsible for an acute encephalopathy or more prolonged dementia; central demyelinating lesions; a parkinsonian state and other movement disorders; chronic meningitis; a myelopathy with vacuolar imaging changes in the spinal cord; a mononeuritis multiplex; and an inflammatory myopathy. HIV infection also increases the likelihood of cerebral lymphoma and of acute viral and bacterial infections affecting the nervous system (see below).

Neurological manifestations of syphilis (neurosyphilis) occur as a late complication in under 10 per cent of the (currently few) patients in whom a primary treponemal infection was left untreated. The spectrum of neurosyphilis is broad, but patterns fall into one or more of three broad categories: chronic meningitis associated with obliterative vascular disease (meningovascular syphilis); tabes dorsalis (demyelination and degeneration within the posterior columns of the spinal cord); and general paresis (a neurodegenerative dementia associated with florid psychotic symptoms). Neurological infection with the infectious agent may also remain asymptomatic. Neurosyphilis still, therefore, enters into the differential diagnosis of stroke, myelopathy, myopathy and dementia, particularly in younger patients.

A diagnosis of syphilis infection can be made using a number of serological tests such as the sensitive Venereal Diseases Research Laboratory (VDRL) test or the more specific *T. pallidum* haemagglutination assay (TPHA). Suspected neurosyphilis can be confirmed by demonstrating additional changes (pleocytosis or high protein levels) and positive serological tests in the spinal fluid.

A less well-known spirochaetal cause of neurological illness is *Borrelia burgdorferi*, the agent responsible for Lyme disease. The organism is transmitted by tick bites, and its manifestations are initially systemic (diffuse muscular pain) and dermatological (a spreading erythematous discolouration of the skin). If infection is left untreated, bilateral facial weakness, mononeuritis multiplex, lymphocytic meningitis and encephalopathy may emerge. The early stages are responsive to treatment with doxycycline, but neurological involvement requires intravenous administration of an antibiotic that crosses the blood–brain barrier (usually ceftriaxone).

Nutritional deficiencies and metabolic disorders

The complex molecular-level structure of the nervous system means that it may, in principle, be vulnerable to chronically low levels of a number of nutrient types, including glucose, fatty acids and amino acids. In practice, however, it is the vitamins – specifically, those in the B, A and E groups – that are classically associated with chronic neurological disorders, as they are essential to widespread metabolic processes and are not manufactured by the body. Dietary deficiency or failure of absorption may therefore be associated with a group of disorders whose importance is emphasized by their complete reversibility.

Thiamine (vitamin B1) deficiency produces an acute syndrome of midbrain and brainstem dysfunction known as Wernicke's encephalopathy. In its classic form, the syndrome comprises acute confusion, eye-movement abnormalities and ataxia. It is a common complication of alcoholism, but it is also seen in association with anorexia nervosa and with hyperemesis of pregnancy, and following gastric surgery. The treatment of any acute encephalopathic illness, ophthalmoplegia and ataxia should include the intravenous administration of thiamine. If left untreated, this reversible deficiency state may give rise to an amnestic and psychotic state (Korsakoff's syndrome) or to coma and death.

Although one of the central functions of vitamin B12 is the maturation of red blood cells, neurological manifestations in the form of memory dysfunction may occur well before the development of a megaloblastic anaemia. More chronic deficiency can give rise to a peripheral neuropathy and a spinal-cord syndrome caused by degeneration ('subacute combined degeneration') of the posterior and lateral columns.

Among the metabolic causes of neurological (and often psychiatric) illness, Wilson's disease and porphyria are rare but effectively treatable and therefore important to consider in appropriate clinical settings.

Wilson's disease is a recessively inherited disorder of copper metabolism. Unbound circulating copper is deposited in the liver, cornea and brain (particularly the basal ganglia), giving rise to the major clinical features: liver dysfunction; corneal discolouration (Kayser–Fleischer rings); movement disorders, including tremor, rigidity, bradykinesia and bizarre dystonic posturing (often misdiagnosed as a functional phenomenon); and psychiatric symptoms, ranging from anxiety and depression to psychosis. Wilson's disease should be considered in all young patients with a movement disorder and in patients with psychiatric symptoms together with liver dysfunction.

Porphyria is a genetically determined disorder of haem biosynthesis. Its clinical manifestations are dominated by episodes of abdominal pain, but the frequently accompanying neurological and psychiatric symptoms include polyneuropathy, transient sensory or motor symptoms in the limbs, seizures, reversible cognitive decline and behavioural abnormalities. Porphyria is a rare condition but should be suspected in any patient with unexplained or atypical recurrent neurological episodes, psychotic behaviour in the context of acute abdominal pain, and a positive family history.

Acute neurological events

Stroke

Any acute and persistent neurological deficit of vascular origin, whether caused by cerebral ischaemia or intracerebral haemorrhage, is referred to as a stroke. Fully reversible deficits of vascular origin are always ischaemic and occur when perfusion to affected tissue is re-established before permanent neuronal damage has taken place. The majority of completed strokes also have an ischaemic basis, typically as a result of an atheromatous or cardioembolic thrombus occluding a cerebral end-artery (i.e. any portion of the anterior, middle or posterior cerebral arteries distal to the circle of Willis, or any of their branches). A stroke may also follow dissection of one of the vertebral or carotid arteries in the neck – a common aetiology in patients under the age of 40 years, usually presenting with a prior history of neck pain and trauma. Carotid dissection may be accompanied by Horner's syndrome on the side opposite the hemiparesis, due to disruption of the carotid sympathetic plexus. Around 15–20 per cent of strokes are caused by a haemorrhage into the substance of the brain, an event that is often difficult to distinguish clinically from an ischaemic event.

The neurological deficit that follows an ischaemic stroke depends on the distribution and extent of the lesion: the middle cerebral artery is implicated in a majority of cases, producing a contralateral hemiparesis (worse in the arm), homonymous quadrantanopia and dysphasia (when the dominant hemisphere is involved); isolated anterior cerebral artery territory infarction is rare but is associated predominantly with contralateral leg weakness and personality change (disinhibition); posterior cerebral artery stroke typically gives rise to brainstem-related and cerebellar signs, or a homonymous hemianopia; a small infarct of the internal capsule caused by obstruction of a penetrating branch of the middle cerebral artery typically causes complete contralateral hemiparesis.

It is now recognized that survival and recovery after stroke are optimized by management on an acute stroke unit under the care of a specialist team, with seamless transition through all stages of management, including initiation of secondary preventive strategies and rehabilitation pre- and post-discharge. Above all, it should be recognized that stroke is a medical emergency, for which strategies relying on the 'healing power of nature' alone are no longer acceptable. Acute management is aimed at identifying factors critical to recovery (particularly swallowing and communication ability), stabilizing or correcting critical physiological parameters such as blood pressure and cardiac rhythm, and establishing whether the mechanism of the stroke was ischaemic or haemorrhagic (on CT). If the mechanism is ischaemic, and symptom onset was less than 3 h previously, then thrombolytic therapy with intravenous Alteplase can be considered. Modern MR imaging modalities are used to define the location, vascular territory, extent of the hypoperfused area and of the wider region, or 'ischaemic penumbra' in which the reversible physiological changes of ischaemia are beginning to occur.

Epilepsy

The term 'epilepsy' is applied to any self-limiting disturbance of consciousness, cognition, motor function or sensation caused by a transient disturbance of normal electrochemical stability in the brain. For the sake of simplicity, epileptic attacks are further subclassified into generalized and partial seizures: in a generalized attack the electrical disturbance affects the entire brain and, as a result, consciousness is lost; when the disturbance is restricted to a localized area, the attack is referred to as partial. Most (though not all) generalized seizures are associated with stiffness and rhythmic jerking movements of the trunk and limbs (convulsions). Partial seizures include subjective sensory or psychological experiences (auras), uncontrollable muscular contractions affecting a single limb (focal motor or Jacksonian seizures); and automatic motor behaviours with reduced environmental awareness (complex partial or temporal lobe seizures).

Generalized attacks often develop from partial seizures as the focal electrical disturbance spreads (secondary generalized seizures), but they may also occur as a primary phenomenon. Primary generalized epilepsy is an idiopathic entity, probably with a genetic component, while partial and secondary generalized seizures usually indicate the presence of a structural lesion in the brain acting as an epileptogenic focus. The latter include congenital areas of neuronal dysplasia, sclerosis of the hippocampal formation, and later acquired changes such as vascular, traumatic and neoplastic disease.

The brain's electrochemical stability usually returns to normal, either spontaneously or in response to administration of a rapidly acting anticonvulsant drug (such as diazepam), within minutes of the onset of the attack and corresponds to the gradual recovery of normal function over minutes. When recovering from a generalized seizure, patients usually pass through a period of disorientation and confusion, and there may be postictal neurological deficits, including focal weakness (Todd's paralysis) or, in rare cases, psychotic behaviour, which may last for hours. Symptoms of exhaustion, headache, nausea, malaise and depression follow recovery (the postictal phase) and may take several days to clear.

Most seizures can be kept under satisfactory control with one or two anticonvulsant drugs. Carbamazepine is usually the drug of first choice for partial seizures, and sodium valproate for primary generalized attacks. Lamotrigine is often effective as second-line therapy in either situation. Special consideration is given to starting anticonvulsant treatment in women who use hormonal contraceptive methods, as carbamazepine, phenytoin and topiramate induce the metabolism of the hormones, whether delivered orally or by injection, resulting in reduced effectiveness. Sodium valproate and levetiracetam do not have this effect and so are drugs of choice in this patient group. Refractory seizures arising from a small underlying epileptogenic focus may, in selected cases, be brought under control by surgically resecting the lesion.

When a single seizure or consecutive series of seizures lasts for 30 min or longer, the situation – referred to as status epilepticus – is life-threatening and requires urgent medical intervention. Management of status epilepticus begins with the resuscitative stage of securing the airway, assessing for and treating cardiopulmonary problems, and treating hypo- or hyperglycaemia and other reversible metabolic derangements. A protocol of escalating intervention is then followed until the seizure terminates. A typical emergency schedule begins with an intravenous bolus of a rapidly acting agent such as lorazepam followed by an intravenous infusion of phenytoin. In refractory cases, the patient should be transferred to an intensive treatment unit (ITU) for general anaesthesia and the ventilatory support and continuous close monitoring that this necessitates.

Meningitis and encephalitis

The infectious meningitides are rapidly developing and potentially fatal infections involving the membranous material between the surface of the brain and the skull vault (the meninges). Bacterial meningitis is most often due to *Streptococcus pneumoniae* (pneumococcal meningitis), with *Neisseria meningitidis* (meningococcus), *Haemophilus influenzae* and *Listeria monocytogenes* accounting for most of the remainder. In certain groups, such as immune-compromised, homeless or alcoholic people and those from the developing world, mycobacterial infection (TB meningitis) is another common mechanism. Meningeal involvement with viral infection (viral meningitis) is not a grave condition, but diagnosis depends specifically on exclusion of the bacterial variety. In contrast, suspected viral encephalitis calls for the urgent initiation of antiviral therapy.

A patient with meningitis will be severely unwell, irritable, and sometimes drowsy, delirious or fitting. There may be signs of cardiovascular instability due to haematogenous infection. Symptoms (if they can be reported) will be dominated by intense photophobic headache, nausea, vomiting and neck stiffness. Meningeal pain results in severe restriction of movement in adjacent structures, resulting in stiffness of neck flexion or back pain on straight-leg-raising (Kernig's sign), or both.

A rapidly spreading purple and red rash over the trunk, limbs and mucous membranes accompanies (and may precede) meningococcal infection. Encephalitis may present in a similar fashion but usually manifests as mild to moderate confusion, fever and headache.

Management of suspected meningitis or encephalitis begins with prompt administration of broad spectrum intravenous antibiotics or aciclovir, or both: delaying to wait for the results of diagnostic tests may prove fatal. Confirmation and refinement of the diagnosis requires examination of the cerebrospinal fluid, obtained at lumbar puncture. If consciousness is impaired or there are focal neurological deficits, brain imaging is required to exclude obstructive hydrocephalus or an intracranial space-occupying lesion, which would make lumbar puncture hazardous. Definitive diagnosis depends on the results of culture, antigen detection or DNA analysis, which take days to obtain. Values obtained from emergency microbiological and biochemical assays within hours allow, however, for exclusion or further refinement of the suspected diagnosis (Table 36.5).

Acute neuromuscular syndromes

It is helpful to think of peripheral weakness as originating from dysfunction in some part of the motor pathway between the motor root and the effector muscle. Acute illnesses characterized by progressive neuromuscular weakness may be caused by pathology affecting the nerve, neuromuscular junction and muscle. Prompt recognition is vital in view of the potential involvement of bulbar and respiratory muscles, failure of which may have catastrophic consequences if not recognized at an early stage.

Acute inflammatory demyelinating polyneuropathy (AIDP, or Guillain–Barré syndrome) is a condition involving the peripheral nerves and nerve fibres. The syndrome usually follows a respiratory or gastrointestinal infection and is typically characterized by sensory change ('pins and needles' or numbness) and weakness in the feet, which spreads proximally, usually over a period of hours to days. Preceding low back pain is often described. A small proportion of patients begin to recover before profound motor weakness ensues, but the majority will develop weakness of all four limbs and the respiratory, facial and bulbar muscles and, in severe cases, autonomic involvement, causing haemodynamic instability. Each of these outcomes requires careful monitoring in the context of a specialist neurosciences unit, and in many cases ventilatory support will be required. The diagnosis is based on a typical clinical picture of ascending weakness and areflexia; a raised cerebrospinal fluid protein; and slowing of conduction times on nerve conduction studies, suggesting a peripheral demyelinating process. A variant of the condition in which the inflammatory target is the axon rather than the myelin sheath is also recognized. Other than supportive measures, the mainstay of treatment consists of intravenous immune globulin, which has been shown in clinical trials to shorten the duration of disability and dependence if started within 2 weeks of symptom onset. Long-term follow-up has shown that around 80 per cent of patients make a full functional recovery within 12 months, although the axonal variant carries a poorer prognosis for full recovery. Around 5 per cent of cases go on to suffer further episodes, following which their illness is classified as CIDP.

The neuromuscular junction is the point at which a motor axon synapses on to a muscle endplate (an excitable region of muscle fibre membrane from where action potentials are initiated, resulting in muscle contraction). Propagation of an action potential down the axon will cause release of a neurotransmitter (which in skeletal muscle takes the form of acetylcholine) that binds to receptors on the endplate. Myasthenia gravis is an autoimmune-mediated condition caused by antibodies directed against the acetylcholine receptor, blocking neurotransmission and causing variable weakness. At a clinical level, this mechanism is distinguishable from diseases of peripheral nerve or muscle by its characteristic fatiguability (i.e. the harder the muscle has to work, the weaker it becomes). Weakness may begin in the muscles of eye movement and opening, in the facial and bulbar muscles, or in the limbs. Diagnosis is based on the

Table 36.5 Cerebrospinal fluid contents

	Bacterial	Tuberculous	Viral
Appearance	Turbid, syrup-like	Fibrin web	Clear
Cell count and type	>1000 polymorphs	10–1000 lymphocytes	50–1500 lymphocytes
Glucose	<60% of value in plasma	Markedly lower than value in plasma	60–80% of plasma level
Protein	Mild to moderate elevation	Moderate to marked elevation	Normal range to mild elevation
Organisms	Visible on microscopy using Gram staining or grown on culture	Acid-fast bacilli sometimes seen on microscopy using Ziehl–Nielsen stain	None seen or grown

demonstration of antibodies directed against the cholinergic receptor, which are found in around 65 per cent of cases. Electrodiagnostic studies, including repetitive nerve stimulation to demonstrate the decremental muscle response analogous to fatiguability, and recording spontaneous activity in individual nerve fibres (single-fibre electromyography, EMG) are often helpful. In equivocal cases, intravenous infusion of a short-acting drug (edrophonium) that inhibits the metabolism of acetylcholine results in temporary restoration of movement or power in patients with the disease. Treatment consists of regular doses of longer-acting cholinesterase inhibitors to relieve the symptoms of weakness, together with immunosuppressive drugs to reduce the circulating receptor antibody load.

Diseases affecting muscle fibres themselves may be dystrophic or associated with other inherited conditions (see above), but it is the inflammatory myopathies that may present as an acute weakness. This group of conditions usually gives rise to proximal and symmetrical weakness, and muscle pathology typically causes an increase in the circulating levels of creatine kinase (CK), which is released from damaged muscle. Diagnosis usually depends on histological findings of a muscle biopsy specimen, at which two patterns of inflammatory process are described: polymyositis (a pure inflammatory muscle disorder), and dermatomyositis (in which associated skin abnormalities are additionally seen). In older patients, some cases of dermatomyositis turn out to be of paraneoplastic origin.

NEUROLOGICAL INVESTIGATIONS

Imaging

Neurological diagnosis has been revolutionized by the advent of modern brain imaging techniques. The localization of a brain or spinal-cord lesion, which formerly depended on demonstrating a clear-cut neurological deficit, is achievable earlier and with greater certainty, improving the likelihood of successful treatment – albeit at the cost of performing vast numbers of normal scans and of revealing symptomless and incidental anomalies. So, although neurologists have not been rendered redundant by imaging, our remit has changed: in the pre-imaging era, the neurologist was lead counsel for the prosecution; today, he or she is more like a judge, carefully sifting through evidence, evaluating it against clinical facts and deciding on its importance.

Neurological practice is aided by evidence from both structural and functional imaging techniques. Although MR imaging has become the modality of choice for most central nervous system disease, CT still has a place by virtue of its rapidity, making it suitable for emergency diagnosis. CT angiography is the favoured modality for non-invasive investigation of intracranial vascular disease. The large associated X-ray dose, however, limits its repeated use in a single individual. Using MR, high-resolution anatomical images of the brain or spinal cord are acquired by placing the site of interest within a powerful magnetic field and detecting the radiofrequency emissions of hydrogen ions within an array of small subdivisions (voxels). This information is used to create a three-dimensional image, which can be reconstructed in the three canonical planes (axial, coronal and sagittal). Pathological changes give rise to alterations in the signal obtained using different acquisition parameters (sequences), whose specificity to the underlying process (e.g. inflammation and infarction) can be diagnostically important.

Functional magnetic resonance imaging (fMRI) identifies regional changes in cerebral blood flow time-locked to periods of cognitive activity. The resulting signal change – known as the blood oxygen level-dependent (BOLD) effect – has been firmly established as spatially and temporally linked to regional changes in neural activity. fMRI is primarily a research tool used to investigate the cerebral basis of cognition, but it is beginning to find a clinical role, particularly in the fields of degenerative and vascular disease and rehabilitation.

Both structural and functional MR have the advantage of non-invasiveness, but other functional techniques, particularly positron-emission tomography (PET) and single-photon-emission computed tomography (SPECT), rely on measurements of energy emissions from intravenously injected metabolically active compounds that have been altered to incorporate a radioactive isotope into their molecular structure. The distribution and magnitude of radioactivity thus reflects the location and concentration of the compound. Interpretation also depends on the biological properties of the compound: regional radioactivity after inhalation of ^{15}O reflects changes in local blood flow (like fMRI). ^{18}F-Fluorodeoxyglucose (a glucose analogue incorporating a radioisotope of fluoride) will be taken up in proportion to a region's metabolic activity, which is a precursor of neurodegeneration and therefore an early diagnostic marker in dementia. Pittsburgh compound B (PiB) binds with high affinity to amyloid plaques and is consequently of interest as a disease-specific marker for Alzheimer's disease.

Information about regional cerebral blood flow can be obtained by mapping the emissions of gamma radiation following injection of technetium-99m-labelled hexamethylpropyleneamine oxime (^{99m}Tc-HMPAO) using a SPECT scanner. On the same principle, the marked reduction of striatal dopaminergic neurons that underlies Parkinson's disease can be demonstrated by mapping the uptake of a radiolabelled agent, ^{123}I-ioflupane, that binds to dopamine transporters. Although the resolution of SPECT is coarser than that of fMRI or PET, ^{99m}Tc has a half-life of approximately 6 h (compared with 2 min for ^{15}O and 1.5 h for ^{18}F), and emissions can be measured after, rather than during, the injection period, enhancing its suitability to the clinical context, particularly in the field of dementia.

Psychometry

Cognitive problems are an integral component of the neurodegenerative dementias and contribute to disability in other central nervous system pathologies, such as stroke, closed head injury and MS. Although useful clinical information can be acquired at the bedside, formal psychometric testing allows deficits of specific cognitive abilities (cognitive speed, attention, executive function, language, praxis, visuospatial processing) to be dissected and quantified with more accuracy and with reference to age- and premorbid intelligence quotient (IQ)-adjusted norms. The need to differentiate between incipient dementia and a potentially reversible depressive state, or an organic from a factitious memory problem, are other important clinical scenarios in which obtaining a psychometric profile can be helpful.

A neuropsychological report will contain summary information about a patient's intellectual performance (full-scale IQ), broken down into verbal and non-verbal components (verbal and performance IQ), together with an estimate, typically based on the National Adult Reading Test (NART), of their optimal level of intellectual functioning (premorbid IQ). Differences of 20 or more IQ points between verbal and performance subscores, or between full-scale score and premorbid estimates, give rise to concern.

Although differences across the six verbal and five performance subtests of the Wechsler Adult Intelligence Scale (WAIS; Table 36.6) may provide an indication of specific areas of cognitive weakness, including short-term working memory, the thoughtful and attentive reader will notice that these do not include any measures of long-term memory. Recognition memory is therefore tested using both verbal and non-verbal material. A series of items (pictures or words) are shown one by one to the subject during an initial exposure, and later re-presented, interspersed with previously unseen items (foils) during a test phase. The patient simply has to identify those items they have seen before. The more demanding task of freely recalling previously seen material can be assessed using a word-list learning paradigm, or by reproduction of a geometrical design from memory. A patient with a true isolated episodic memory deficit should still be capable of skill acquisition and other forms of automatic implicit learning, so failure on tasks that demonstrate implicit learning in a patient with an amnestic profile are highly suggestive of a factitious aetiology.

There is no single test for the integrity of semantic memory (the long-term store of information relating to word-meaning and general knowledge). However, patients who overgeneralize when given pictures to name (e.g.

Table 36.6 Wechsler Adult Intelligence Scale (WAIS) subtests

WAIS scale	Subtest	Notes and examples
Verbal	Information	Graded test of culturally specific general knowledge: e.g. 'How many months are there in a year?' (easy), 'How many MPs are there in the British parliament?' (difficult)
	Digit span	Ability to repeat a lengthening sequence of digits, first forwards and then backwards; both conditions place demands on attention and concentration, while the backward digit span additionally tests verbal short-term (working) memory
	Vocabulary	Graded test of word definition: e.g. 'bed' (easy), 'tirade' (difficult)
	Arithmetic	Graded test of mental arithmetic: e.g. 'What is £4 and £5?' (easy), 'How many hours would it take to walk 24 miles at a speed of 3 miles per hour?' (difficult)
	Comprehension	A test of practical reasoning: e.g. 'Why do people have to register their marriage?'
	Similarities	A graded test of concept formation requiring the subject to explain what two items have in common: e.g. orange and banana (easy), praise and punishment (difficult)
Performance	Picture completion	20 pictures of common objects with a missing detail, which the subject has to indicate: e.g. a pair of spectacles without a bridge
	Picture arrangement	Sequences of pictures, which the subject arranges to form a story
	Block design	A test of visuospatial and constructional abilities involving the assembly of patterns using coloured blocks
	Object assembly	Reconstruction of a picture (e.g. of an elephant) that has been cut into pieces like a jigsaw
	Digit symbol	A test of visuomotor coordination, and of motor and mental processing speed: the subject uses a key code that pairs digits 1–9 with a unique shape to transcode a random sequence of digits on a page into the correct sequence of shapes

responding 'animal' to all pictures of living things), and those who provide inaccurate or impoverished definitions of specific nouns (e.g. 'It's an animal; got four legs and a tail; I think they live abroad' when asked 'What is an ostrich?'), are likely to have a deficit in this domain.

Executive function describes the individual's ability to self-monitor, plan and implement strategies for completing tasks, follow a set of rules, and select or inhibit information depending on its current relevance. Clearly this is a complex construct but nonetheless one that appears to depend on the integrity of cortical regions in the dorsal and lateral regions of the frontal lobes. Tests such as the Wisconsin Card Sorting Test, in which the subject is asked to group a sequence of geometrical designs that vary in three dimensions (shape, colour and number), and then told to change strategies at various points in the test, are sensitive to executive dysfunction. An inability to switch from one rule to another is particularly suggestive of this functional deficit.

Electrophysiology

Clinical electrophysiology can provide information relevant to cerebral, peripheral nerve and muscle dysfunction and their aetiologies.

Electroencephalography (EEG) provides a record of the background activity and rhythmicity, and of transient additions to these patterns, within the cerebral cortex. The wave patterns in a normal record can be decomposed into four basic frequencies: the slowest activity (≤3 Hz), referred to as the delta rhythm, is prominent during deep (non-rapid eye movement, REM) sleep; waveforms with a frequency of 4–7 Hz (theta rhythm) may emerge during drowsiness; alpha activity (8–12 Hz) dominates the record in the posterior regions and is accentuated with eye closure; the beta rhythms (>12 Hz) are seen in frontal brain regions and dominate the record when the patient is alert. Disturbances of the normal distribution of these underlying rhythms, particularly in the form of excessive presence of the slower rhythms, are non-specifically indicative of a functional disturbance (encephalopathy). This information needs to be interpreted with reference to the clinical scenario, as it is rarely specific to a particular mechanism and may be related, for instance, to the cerebral effects of drugs, metabolic disturbances or neurodegenerative change. Periodic bi- or triphasic discharges are, however, typical of the later stages of sporadic Creutzfeldt–Jakob disease (sCJD) but are not seen in the variant form (vCJD), so this finding can have important diagnostic implications.

The emergence of other patterns of transients (termed spikes or sharp waves, depending on their amplitude and duration) represents intermittent, synchronous activity within a neuronal population and may suggest a predisposition to epilepsy; their distribution (i.e. widespread or localized to one hemisphere or lobar region) can provide evidence for an epileptic tendency of generalized or focal origin. One of the most important tasks for the clinical neurophysiologist is therefore to distinguish such epileptiform activity from other transient elements such as sleep spindles, which are normal physiological phenomena, and from the contaminating artefacts caused by body or eye movements.

Occasionally, cerebral activity may be recorded while a clinical seizure is occurring, either serendipitously or as part of a prolonged recording that aims to capture the cerebral basis of the event (video telemetry). The simultaneous occurrence of electrophysiological and clinical evidence of epilepsy enables a firm diagnosis of an epileptic seizure (rather than a predisposition to seizures) to be made, while clinical activity in the absence of a neurophysiological correlate is strongly suggestive of a factitious explanation.

The principle of recording cerebral activity from voltage changes detected by scalp electrodes is also employed in evoked potential studies. In this paradigm, EEG changes are time-locked to a sensory stimulus, such as a simply alternating visual pattern (e.g. an alternating chequerboard display), an auditory click or electrical stimulation of the peripheries. The time taken for the expected electrophysiological signal to emerge is indicative of the integrity of the white-matter pathways within the visual system, brainstem and spinal cord, respectively.

Peripheral neurophysiological testing relates to abnormalities of motor and sensory nerves and skeletal muscle. Following the application of an electrical stimulus to the skin directly overlying the course of a peripheral nerve, a response can be measured from an electrode overlying either a muscle or a portion of skin that is supplied by fibres carried in the stimulated nerve. These recordings provide information about the function of motor and sensory components, respectively, within the nerve being tested. The results are normally considered in terms of the amplitude of the response or its velocity (calculated by dividing the distance between stimulating and recording points by the millisecond delay between the two events). A reduction in amplitude is interpreted as indicating loss of or damage to individual axons, while slowed conduction times are caused by damage to the myelin sheath. Depending on the site or sites of any abnormal findings, nerve conduction studies can distinguish between diffuse processes (peripheral neuropathy), focal damage due to entrapment or trauma, and multifocal disruption of nerve integrity (mononeuritis multiplex).

Electromyography provides a recording of electrical activity within a muscle, either from a surface electrode or via a needle inserted into the body of the muscle itself (needle EMG). Observed activity relates to activity within a group of motor units (defined as a single motor neuron and the collection of individual muscle fibres on which it synapses), at rest and during contraction. In a normal motor unit, no activity is seen at rest, while damage to the axonal component of a motor unit results in spontaneous discharges (fasciculation and fibrillation). During slow incremental contraction, action potentials from increasing numbers of motor units are observed (recruitment), and any abnormal features during this process – such as increased or decreased amplitude and duration of the action potentials, the number of units recruited, and the rate of recruitment – are used to determine whether the pathology is in the muscle or in the axon (myopathic *v.* neuropathic EMG). The presence of spontaneous activity and neuropathic features in the absence of any evidence of peripheral nerve dysfunction on the nerve conduction study suggests pathology originating from a more proximal component of the motor neuron, up to and including the anterior horn cell.

The cerebrospinal fluid

Cerebrospinal fluid examination is routinely performed in acute neurological illness, particularly central nervous system infection, and in patients with more indolent neurological conditions affecting either central or peripheral structures. Cerebrospinal fluid is obtained from a patient by inserting a 20 or 22 gauge spinal needle through the lumbar theca, under local anaesthetic, between the spinous processes of the L4 and L5 vertebrae, which are palpable in the midline at the level of the top of the iliac crest. Cerebrospinal fluid pressure can be measured by collecting the initial specimen in a vertical glass tube and measuring the height of the column. A low-pressure headache (relieved by lying down) occurs in up to a third of patients due to continued cerebrospinal fluid leakage after withdrawal of the needle. It normally settles spontaneously within days but sometimes necessitates infusion of a sample of venous blood obtained from the patient to seal the defect (blood patch).

A number of important laboratory measurements can be made on the cerebrospinal fluid: suspected bacterial, mycobacterial or fungal infection may be confirmed by immediate microscopy; evidence of viral or partially treated bacterial infection may be inferred from the type and density of white cells present; malignant cells may be identified in cases of central nervous system lymphoma or malignant meningitis; a translucent yellow tinge due to the breakdown products of haemoglobin (xanthochromia) forms 12 h after leakage of blood into the subarachnoid space and persists for at least 2 weeks, allowing a diagnosis of subarachnoid haemorrhage to be made even if blood was not, or is no longer, visible on CT; elevated protein content suggests acute or chronic inflammation, and the appearance on a cerebrospinal fluid electrophoresis of immunoglobulin bands that are not matched by similar patterns in a serum analysis suggests an inflammatory process originating on the central nervous system side of the blood–brain barrier.

The presence of 14-3-3 protein is suggestive of, although not specific to, sCJD or vCJD. Cerebrospinal fluid tau and amyloid levels, and other biomarkers, can be useful adjuncts to the diagnosis of AD and other specific neurodegenerative diseases, although cerebrospinal fluid sampling is not a routine part of the standard diagnostic work-up for early dementia.

Tissue biopsy

Muscle and nerve

Nerve and muscle biopsy are minor procedures carried out under local anaesthetic in order to obtain diagnostic information that cannot be acquired by less invasive means. Almost all patients with clinical and electrophysiological evidence of myopathy will be submitted to muscle biopsy, allowing degenerative, metabolic, dystrophic and inflammatory conditions to be identified from typical histological features. The large bulk and easy identification make deltoid or quadriceps the usual muscles of choice, though there may be clinical reasons for targeting other specific muscles.

Nerve biopsies are typically taken from the ankle (sural) or wrist (radial), since at these sites the nerve bundles consist of sensory fibres, restricting the inevitable postoperative deficit to a small and non-disabling area of anaesthesia. Nerve histology enables a firm diagnosis of vasculitic neuropathy to be established or excluded, the former justifying prolonged use of powerful immunosuppressive drugs. Rarer infiltrative causes, such as amyloid or lymphomatous neuropathy, will also become evident on biopsy.

Brain

The hazardous nature of brain biopsy, and its obvious potential for causing permanent functional disability, means that a decision to perform it is restricted to those cases in which there is high clinical suspicion of either (i) a potentially treatable but otherwise unprovable pathological process or (ii) a condition that, for prognostic purposes, is important to demonstrate.

TREATMENT OF NEUROLOGICAL DISEASE

Many chronic neurological conditions are amenable to specific therapies, although most of these act by relieving symptoms. Those that ameliorate the clinical course of the disease (disease-modifying agents) are unfortunately few and far between. The main groups of symptomatic treatments are anticonvulsant drugs (which raise the epileptic seizure threshold, reducing the likelihood of an episode); anti-migraine drugs (particularly of the triptan group, which stimulate serotonin receptors in the brain and cranial blood vessels); dopamine analogues and agonists (which partially compensate for the dopaminergic neuron deficit that underpins the movement disorder in Parkinson's disease); and (underpinned by a similar principle) cholinergic agents in AD. Specific treatments for neuropathic pain include those with anticonvulsant and antidepressant properties, which may act by inhibiting overactivity in nociceptive fibres. Corticosteroids, usually in the form of intravenous methylprednisolone, are used to encourage resolution in acute exacerbations of relapsing conditions with an inflammatory basis, including MS. Immune-suppressant drugs, such as methotrexate and cyclophosphamide, have a role in reducing the frequency of relapses and hence the need for repeated steroid doses. A selection of the important symptomatic agents, together with their indications, modes of action and important adverse effects, is provided in Table 36.7.

Table 36.7 Neurological drugs

(a) Multiple sclerosis (MS)

Drug name/group	Methylprednisolone	Interferon beta	Baclofen	Oxybutynin
Mode of action	Suppression of cell-mediated and humoral immunity	Modification of immune response	Modulation of GABA receptor	Muscarinic acetylcholine receptor antagonist
Indication(s)	Acute onset or exacerbation of non-infectious inflammatory disorders	Relapsing–remitting MS	Symptomatic relief of muscle spasm and spasticity-related pain	Symptomatic treatment of urinary frequency and nocturia
Principal side effects and disadvantages	Immune suppression, weight gain, glucose intolerance, osteoporosis, myopathy	Flu-like symptoms, irritation due to need for subcutaneous injection	Drowsiness, delirium, seizures, gastrointestinal disturbances	Mucosal dryness, blurred vision, urinary retention

GABA, γ-aminobutyric acid.

(b) Other neuroinflammatory and autoimmune disorders

Drug name/group	Edrophonium	Pyridostigmine	Cyclophosphamide	Methotrexate
Mode of action	Short-acting inhibition of acetylcholinesterase	Long-acting inhibition of acetylcholinesterase	Suppression of cell metabolism and division	Inhibition of DNA and RNA synthesis
Indication(s)	Myasthenia gravis (diagnosis)	Myasthenia gravis (treatment)	Suppression of activity in autoimmune diseases	Suppression of activity in autoimmune diseases
Principal side effects and disadvantages	Parasympathomimetic effects (cardiac arrhythmias, nausea, abdominal cramps, diarrhoea, hypersalivation)	Parasympathomimetic effects (cardiac arrhythmias, nausea, abdominal cramps, diarrhoea, hypersalivation)	Immune suppression, infertility, susceptibility to malignancy	Pancytopenia, pulmonary fibrosis

(c) Epilepsy

Drug name/group	Phenytoin	Carbamazepine	Sodium valproate	Lamotrigine	Topiramate	Levetiracetam
Mode of action	Sodium channel blockade	Sodium channel blockade	Multiple	Multiple	Unknown	Unknown
Principal indication(s)	Treatment of status epilepticus (intravenous administration)	First-line treatment for all seizure types	First-line treatment for primary generalized epilepsy	First- or second-line treatment for partial seizures	Stand-alone or adjunctive treatment for all types of epilepsy	Stand-alone or adjunctive treatment for partial epilepsy
Principal side effects and disadvantages	Coarsening of facial features, hirsutism, gum hypertrophy, cerebellar ataxia	Confusion and mental blunting, leucopenia, hyponatraemia	Metabolic encephalopathy, cognitive decline, weight gain	Stevens–Johnson syndrome	Speech and language difficulties, weight loss	Headache, dizziness, mood swings
Potential for hepatotoxicity	Low	High	High	Low	Low	Low
Effect on oral contraceptive	Enzyme-inducing: reduced effectiveness	Enzyme-inducing: reduced effectiveness	No effect	No effect	Enzyme-inducing: reduced effectiveness	No effect

(d) Headache

Drug name/group	Triptan group	Beta-blockers	Amitriptyline	Topiramate	Acetazolamide	Indometacin
Indication(s)	Acute treatment of migraine	Migraine prophylaxis	Migraine and tension headache prophylaxis	Migraine and tension headache prophylaxis	Idiopathic intracranial hypertension	Acute treatment of paroxysmal hemicrania
Mode of action	Serotonin receptor agonist	Non-selective beta adrenergic receptor antagonist	Inhibition of serotonin and noradrenaline reuptake	Unknown, but includes inhibition of carbonic anhydrase	Inhibition of carbonic anhydrase leading to diuresis	Prostaglandin inhibition
Principal side effects and disadvantages	Hypotension, nausea	Depression, fatigue, bradycardia, exacerbation of asthma, arterial insufficiency	Mucosal dryness, fatigue, confusion, visual blurring	Speech and language difficulties, weight loss	Tingling in peripheries, altered taste sensation, visual blurring	Gastric irritation, fluid retention, renal impairment

(e) Neuropathic pain

Drug name/group	Amitriptyline	Gabapentin	Pregabalin	Carbamazepine
Indication(s)	Peripheral neuropathic pain	Central or peripheral neuropathic pain	Central or peripheral neuropathic pain	Central or peripheral neuropathic pain
Principal side effects and disadvantages	Mucosal dryness, fatigue, confusion, visual blurring	Fatigue, dizziness, mood swings	Fatigue, dizziness	Confusion and mental blunting, leucopenia, hyponatraemia

(f) Movement disorders

Drug name/group	Levodopa	Ropinirole	Entacapone	Trihexyphenidyl	Selegiline	Beta-blockers	Primidone
Indication(s)	Idiopathic Parkinson's disease	Idiopathic Parkinson's disease	Idiopathic Parkinson's disease, in conjunction with levodopa	Idiopathic Parkinson's disease	Idiopathic Parkinson's disease	Essential tremor	Essential tremor
Mode of action	Precursor of dopamine	Selective dopamine receptor agonist	Inhibits metabolism of levodopa by COMT	Muscarinic receptor antagonist	Inhibition of monoamine oxidase B mediated dopamine metabolism	Non-selective beta adrenergic receptor antagonist	Unknown
Principal side effects and disadvantages	Nausea, hypotension, sleep cycle disturbance, hallucinations, involuntary movements	Nausea, dizziness, gastrointestinal disturbances, confusion and hallucinations	Nausea, dizziness, gastrointestinal disturbances	Mucosal dryness, blurred vision, urinary retention, drowsiness	Nausea, dizziness, abdominal pain	Depression, fatigue, bradycardia, exacerbation of asthma, arterial insufficiency	Drowsiness, dizziness, ataxia

COMT, catechol-O-methyl transferase.

(g) Neurodegenerative diseases

Drug name/group	Cholinesterase inhibitors	Memantine
Indication(s)	Mild to moderate Alzheimer's disease	Moderate to severe Alzheimer's disease
Mode of action	Enhancement of central nervous system acetylcholine activity	NMDA glutamate receptor blockade
Principal side effects and disadvantages	Headache, fatigue, gastrointestinal disturbance	Drowsiness, confusion, agitation

NMDA, *N*-methyl-D-aspartate.

(h) Cerebrovascular disease

Drug name/group	Aspirin	Clopidogrel	Dipyridamole	Warfarin
Mechanism of action	Cyclooxygenase inhibition reducing platelet aggregation	Inhibition of platelet aggregation	Inhibition of platelet aggregation	Decreases blood coagulability by inhibition of vitamin K
Indication(s)	Primary and secondary cerebrovascular prophylaxis	Primary and secondary cerebrovascular prophylaxis	Primary and secondary cerebrovascular prophylaxis	Prevention of embolic stroke or TIA in atrial fibrillation
Principal side-effects and disadvantages	Gastric mucosal irritation	Gastric mucosal irritation, bleeding	Gastric mucosal irritation	Bleeding

TIA, transient ischaemic attack.

Drugs that act on the underlying mechanisms of disease, and either reverse or modify the process, would be of enormous public health benefit and greatly welcomed by patients. Unfortunately, such agents remain largely an aspiration rather than a reality. One exception is interferon beta, which has been shown to reduce the relapse rate and long-term disability in some patients with relapsing–remitting MS, although its precise mechanism of action remains poorly understood.

KEY POINTS

- A clear history of the onset (sudden or gradual), pattern (variable, stuttering, progressive) and time course (static, improving, worsening) of a patient's symptoms is the single most important neurological investigation: diagnosis can often be confidently based on this information alone; without it, the result of the most sophisticated laboratory tests are often uninterpretable.
- Neurological symptoms can be thought of as disturbances of (i) sensation (including pain), (ii) balance, (iii) consciousness, (iv) muscular control and (v) cognitive function.
- Headache is the most common neurological symptom and rarely has a sinister underlying cause. Subarachnoid haemorrhage, giant cell arteritis (in patients aged over 60 years) and raised intracranial pressure should, however, not be missed, as the consequences of delaying treatment may be devastating.
- Muscular weakness due to a lesion in the cerebral hemisphere, brainstem, spinal cord, lower motor neuron, neuromuscular junction or muscle are each associated with distinctive combinations of clinical features.
- Movement disorders can be classified into diagnostically helpful categories (tremor, chorea, myoclonus, hemiballismus, tic) on the basis of history or observation.
- A witness's description is essential to the evaluation of a first suspected 'fit'. Home video recordings are becoming more common as clinical evidence and are to be encouraged.
- An informative analysis of the nature of cognitive decline is possible using careful history-taking and a battery of simple neuropsychological instruments adapted for use in the clinic or at the bedside.
- Contrary to popular belief, many neurological illnesses, both acute and chronic, are amenable to effective symptomatic treatment. Drugs for modifying the course of chronic disease, however, remain a largely unachieved aspiration.

Chapter 37

Organic disorders

David P Moore and Basant K Puri

INTRODUCTION

This chapter describes the following groups of organic disorders, all of which are of importance in clinical neuropsychiatry: neurodegenerative and movement disorders; vascular disorders; trauma; hypoxic disorders; nutritional, toxic and metabolic disorders; infectious and related disorders; prion diseases; endocrinological disorders; immune-related disorders; and brain tumours and hydrocephalus. Psychiatric assessment is covered in Chapter 48.

NEURODEGENERATIVE AND MOVEMENT DISORDERS

Alzheimer's disease, Lewy body disease and frontotemporal dementia are detailed in Chapter 72.

Parkinson's disease

Parkinson's disease, also known as idiopathic parkinsonism and paralysis agitans, is common, with a prevalence of roughly 0.2 per cent. The male/female ratio is about 1.5 : 1.

Clinical features

The onset is gradual and insidious, with symptoms generally first appearing in the mid-50s. The range is from 20 years to 80 years.

It initially manifests with parkinsonism:[1,2] patients typically present with asymmetrical tremor or rigidity affecting an upper or, less commonly, lower extremity. Over time, the opposite side becomes involved, and eventually all four limbs are affected.

Once fully established, Parkinson's disease leaves a stamp on patients that is, once recognized, almost unforgettable. Patients stand in a stooped 'flexion' posture, with their arms and knees in flexion. A rhythmic (3–7 cycles/s – cps, hertz, Hz) rest tremor is present, most noticeably in the hands but also evident, when seated, in the feet; the jaw is also often tremulous. Of note, although the tremor typically resolves with sleep, in a minority of patients it may persist.[3,4] The face is often 'masked' and expressionless, and there is a reduced frequency of blinking; there may also be copious drooling. Speech is hypophonic, soft, monotonous and lacking in emotional inflection. Handwriting undergoes a micrographic change, producing scratchy, small letters. Passive extension of the limbs reveals the rigidity, which, although often 'cogwheel', may at times be 'lead pipe' in character.

While walking there is reduced arm swing, and patients often display *marche à petit pas*, wherein they take small, shuffling steps; furthermore, they often display festination, in which, as they walk, their steps become ever more rapid and closely spaced, to the point at which a catastrophic fall forward seems almost inevitable. Upon evaluating the station of these patients, one typically finds retropulsion, wherein a gentle push on the patient's chest will induce a gradual toppling backward that the patient cannot keep up with by backward steps. Bradykinesia manifests as slowness in virtually any activity. For example, even in the absence of tremor or significant rigidity, it may take many minutes to fasten a button. A related phenomenon is bradyphrenia, in which thoughts, although coherent and logical, move very slowly.

Another curious phenomenon is freezing: in this, patients on the brink of an intentional act suddenly become frozen and unable to move at all.[5] A patient standing in a doorway and desirous of walking down the hall may be unable to lift a foot, take a step or move at all. Amazingly, such freezing may be prevented by providing appropriate visual cues. For example, if the hallway is marked off with pieces of tape set about one footstep apart, the patient may well be able to begin and finish the walk down the hall without difficulty; furthermore, in some cases, patients may be able to lyse their own frozen state by simply imagining such cues.[6]

Akathisia may occur and may appear early in the course of the disease, before any pharmacological treatment.[7]

Autonomic symptoms such as dysphagia, constipation, urinary frequency or incontinence, and nocturia are common, occurring in over one-half of patients after 10 years or more of disease.[8]

Parkinson's disease is associated with dementia,[9] with overall reported prevalence figures ranging from 11 per cent[10] to 41 per cent.[11] Its prevalence rises with age: Mayeux and colleagues noted a prevalence of 0 for people under 50 years and 69 per cent for those over 80 years.[11] Similarly, over an 8-year follow-up, Aarsland and colleagues noted that 78 per cent became demented.[12] It also appears that dementia is more likely in patients with more severe motor symptoms. Importantly, the dementia does not appear until after the motor symptoms have been well established: one study found that the onset of dementia occurred at a mean of 13 years after the appearance of motor symptoms, with a range of 6–21 years.[13] The dementia is fairly non-specific: patients may experience difficulty with memory and concentration; less commonly, focal deficits such as aphasia or apraxia may appear.

Major depression has been reported in 3 per cent,[14] 5 per cent[15] and, in two separate studies, 21 per cent of patients.[16,17] Minor depressive symptomatology may be found in other patients[15] – indeed, up to 20 per cent.[17,18] The presence of depression worsens the cognitive deficits in patients who are also demented.[19] In patients with primarily unilateral motor symptomatology, depressive symptoms are more likely when the right side of the body is affected compared with the left, indicating an involvement of the left hemisphere in the genesis of depression.[17]

Rapid-eye-movement (REM) sleep behaviour disorder is fairly common.

Course

Untreated, most patients become incapacitated within 8–10 years, with death often from pneumonia. With treatment, survival of 15 years or more may be expected.

Pathology

Macroscopically, there is depigmentation of the substantia nigra and the locus coeruleus. Microscopically, neuronal loss is present not only in these structures but also in the dorsal raphe nucleus, the pedunculopontine nucleus, the dorsal motor nucleus of the vagus, the thalamus, hypothalamus, nucleus basalis of Meynert, the amygdala, and in various areas of the cortex, including the temporal, insular, and cingulate cortices. Remaining neurons typically display the hallmark of Parkinson's disease, namely the Lewy body, which is an intracytoplasmic inclusion, composed of alpha-synuclein, neurofilaments and ubiquitin.

Motor symptoms correlate with cell loss in the substantia nigra and generally do not appear until 60 per cent or more of these cells have been lost. Dementia correlates with cell loss and Lewy bodies in the cortex,[13] and depression with similar changes in the locus coeruleus[20] and the dorsal raphe nucleus.[21] Of note, the dorsal raphe nucleus serves as one of the main sources of serotonergic innervation to the cortex and a correlation has been found between cerebrospinal fluid (CSF) levels of 5-hydroxyindoleacetic acid, a metabolite of serotonin, and the presence of depression in patients with Parkinson's disease.[16,18]

Aetiology

Although the mechanism or mechanisms underlying cell loss and Lewy body formation are not known, it is theorized that, perhaps related to mitochondrial respiratory chain dysfunction, there is an increased formation of free radicals, with subsequent cell damage.

Genetic factors and environmental factors may both be involved. Although idiopathic Parkinson's disease has long been thought to be sporadic, epidemiological work strongly suggests the involvement of familial factors.[22] Furthermore, fluorodopa positron-emission tomography (PET) has demonstrated not only reduced dopamine uptake in the striatum of patients but also a reduced uptake in their clinically unaffected co-twins, suggesting that the co-twins had asymptomatic disease.[23] Environmental toxins have long been suspected, and suspicion has focused on exposure to pesticides.[24] Cigarette-smoking appears to reduce the risk of developing Parkinson's disease.[25]

Interest in genetic factors has been stimulated by the investigation of cases having a clear-cut, unequivocal familial basis. These constitute only a small percentage of cases, no more than 10 per cent, and the pattern of inheritance may be either autosomal dominant or autosomal recessive. Table 37.1 lists the various forms that have been discovered.

Psychiatric side effects of medication

Most patients treated with levodopa or dopamine agonists eventually develop significant neuropsychiatric side effects. The most common of these are visual hallucinations; others include psychosis, anxiety (during wearing-off of levodopa) and certain other, much less common phenomena, including impulsive behaviours, stereotypies, euphoria (with, rarely, mania) and delirium.

Visual hallucinations are very common with prolonged treatment with either levodopa or dopamine agonists: in one 6-year study, the percentage of patients with hallucinations increased gradually until, at the end of the study, 62 per cent of patients were experiencing them.[26] The hallucinations are typically complex, involving scenes, animals or people, and may last from minutes to hours or even days; importantly, early on, patients retain insight into the hallucinatory nature of these experiences and recognize that they are not real. Auditory hallucinations, or even olfactory or gustatory hallucinations, may also occur, but these are much less common.[26,27] Of note, in a very small minority of patients, visual hallucinations may occur before any treatment is administered. Furthermore, it appears that patients with greater cell loss and Lewy body pathology in the amygdala are more likely to develop hallucinations when treated with levodopa.[28] It may well be that amygdalar pathology not only renders patients more sensitive to the hallucinogenic effects of levodopa and dopamine agonists but may also, if severe enough, independently cause hallucinations.

Psychosis is said to be present when patients either experience hallucinations without insight or develop delusions. As noted above, visual hallucinations with preserved insight are very common; however, over a matter of several

Table 37.1 Classification of familial Parkinson's disease

Locus (omim)	Chromosome	Gene/protein	Inheritance
PARK1	4q21	*SNCA*/α-synuclein	Autosomal dominant
PARK2	6q25–27	*PRKN*/parkin	Autosomal recessive
PARK3	2p13	Not known	Autosomal dominant
PARK4	Original linkage was incorrect (see triplication of *SNCA*)		
PARK5	4p14	Ubiquitin C-terminal hydrolase L1	Autosomal dominant
PARK6	1p35–36	*PINK1*/PTEN-induced kinase 1	Autosomal recessive
PARK7	1p36	*DJ1*/DJ-1	Autosomal recessive
PARK8	12p11.2–13.1	*LRRK2*/Lrrk2 (Dardarin)	Autosomal dominant
PARK10	1p32	Not known	Genetic susceptibility
PARK11	2q36–37	Not known	Genetic susceptibility
GBA	1q21	*GBA*/glucocerebrosidase	Genetic susceptibility
SCA2	12q24	*ATXN2*/ataxin-2	Autosomal dominant
SCA3	14q24.3–q31	*ATXN3*/ataxin-3	Autosomal dominant
MAPT (FTDP-17)	17q21.1	*MAPT*/tau	Autosomal dominant
NR4A2/NURR1	2q22–23	*NR4A2 (NURR1)*/NURR1	Unknown
SNCAIP	5q23.1–23.3	*SNCAIP*/synphilin 1	Unknown

Reproduced with permission from Love S, Louis DN, Ellison D (eds) (1998) *Greenfield's Neuropathology*, 8th edn. London: Hodder Arnold.

years, the majority of patients who do have hallucinations will lose insight and begin to react to the visual hallucinations as if they were real.[29] Delusions, often of persecution, may also occur but are much less common.[27]

Treatment of hallucinations or psychosis should generally involve an attempt at reducing the dose of levodopa and/or dopamine agonists. These side effects are generally dose-responsive and in some cases it may be possible to reduce the dose sufficiently to allow for a substantial resolution of them without sacrificing control of the parkinsonism. When dose reduction is either ineffective or impractical, consideration may be given to treatment with an antipsychotic. Of the various second-generation antipsychotics that have been used, clozapine is the most successful; however, its side effects may make one hesitant to use it and, in such cases, consideration may be given to low-dose risperidone.

Anxiety may be seen during motor fluctuations of the 'wearing-off' type, and full anxiety attacks may occur; other symptoms seen during the 'off' period include depressed mood, irritability and sweating.

Impulsive behaviours, including pathological gambling, compulsive shopping and hypersexuality, may occur as side effects of treatment in a small proportion of patients and appear more likely in those treated with dopamine agonists; with discontinuation of treatment with the offending medication, symptoms resolve within days to months.

Stereotypies seen with treatment may be complex and socially disabling. Known as 'punding', these may include repeatedly taking apart and putting together machinery or engaging in other purposeless behaviours.

Euphoria may occur, and some patients may escalate the dose in order to achieve this side effect. In some cases, albeit rarely, a manic episode may occur.

Delirium has been noted as a side effect but is rare.

Amyotrophic lateral sclerosis

Amyotrophic lateral sclerosis (ALS), first clearly delineated by the French neurologist Jean-Martin Charcot in 1874, is classically characterized by a combination of upper and lower motor neuron signs; there is additional involvement of the frontal and temporal cortices in this disease, with, in a substantial minority of patients, the development of a dementia. Also known as Charcot's disease, motor neuron disease and Lou Gehrig's disease (after the famous

American baseball player who suffered from it), ALS has a lifetime prevalence of roughly 4–6 per 100 000 and is more common in men than women by a ratio of approximately 1.5 : 1.

Clinical features

Onset is gradual, most patients falling ill between the ages of 40 years and 70 years. Classically, patients present with weakness in one of the upper extremities, often in the hand, and there may be difficulty buttoning clothes or using small tools; over time, other limbs become involved. Eventually, with involvement of both upper and lower neurons, brisk deep tendon reflexes are found, with atrophic muscular weakness and fasciculations. With involvement of the upper motor neurons destined for the cranial nerve nuclei, a pseudo-bulbar palsy may appear, with dysarthria, dysphagia, and 'emotional incontinence', with forced laughter and crying; the jaw-jerk reflex tends also to be brisk. With involvement of the lower motor neurons in the cranial nerve nuclei, the tongue may become atrophic and demonstrate fasciculation. Sensory changes are generally absent.

Subsequent to the onset of the upper and lower motor neuron symptoms, dementia may gradually appear in up to one-quarter of all patients; in a significant minority of others, there will be a cognitive decrement of less severe degree, characterized by poor short-term memory and judgement.[30]

Although most patients present with a combination of upper and lower motor neuron signs and symptoms, in a small minority the presentation is weighted heavily towards either the upper motor neuron (producing primary lateral sclerosis) or the lower motor neuron (producing progressive muscular atrophy). Primary lateral sclerosis is characterized clinically by a progressive spastic paresis, accompanied in roughly one-half of patients by a pseudo-bulbar palsy. Progressive muscular atrophy, in contrast, presents with progressive weakness, atrophy and fasciculations. In most cases, patients with progressive lateral sclerosis or progressive muscular atrophy go on to develop clear clinical evidence of involvement of both upper and motor neurons, thus leaving no doubt as to the correct diagnosis.

Electromyography (EMG) typically reveals evidence of denervation, and nerve condition velocity studies are typically normal.

T2-weighted or fluid-attenuated inversion recovery (FLAIR) magnetic resonance imaging (MRI) may reveal increased signal intensity bilaterally in the centrum semiovale, corresponding to the corticospinal tracts. Rarely, atrophy may be noted in the prefrontal gyrus.

Course

ALS is almost invariably progressive, with death, often from respiratory failure or intercurrent pneumonia, generally occurring within about 3 years; survival past 5 years is uncommon.[31]

Aetiology

Ninety per cent of cases are sporadic; roughly 10 per cent are inherited in an autosomal dominant fashion, secondary to mutations in the gene for superoxide dismutase on chromosome 21,[32] and there are very rare cases of inheritance on a recessive basis. Although the mechanism underlying cell loss in ALS is not known, excitotoxicity is strongly suspected.

Progressive supranuclear palsy

Progressive supranuclear palsy, or the Steele–Richardson–Olszewski syndrome, is characterized by an atypical parkinsonism, usually accompanied by supranuclear ophthalmoplegia and, in about half of cases, dementia. It is uncommon and occurs somewhat more frequently in men than women.

Clinical features

The onset is insidious and generally occurs in the sixth decade. The disease typically presents with frequent unexplained falls owing to postural instability. An atypical parkinsonism then gradually appears, characterized by a more or less symmetrical onset of rigidity, generally without tremor, and an abnormal gait typified by a wide-based stance with short, shuffling steps. Importantly, rather than the typical flexion posture seen in most cases of parkinsonism, patients with progressive supranuclear palsy typically display a dystonic axial rigidity, which may also affect the neck. Dystonic rigidity also affects the facial musculature, at times creating an 'astonished' appearance.

Classically, 1–3 years after the parkinsonism is established, one also sees a supranuclear ophthalmoplegia for vertical gaze, wherein patients have difficulty voluntarily looking down, a difficulty that may make walking down stairs particularly treacherous. This feature, however, may be delayed for many years and in some cases may never appear.

Dementia occurs in about one-half of all patients, generally well after the parkinsonism has become established: patients have difficulty with concentration and memory, and there may be elements of a frontal lobe syndrome[33] with prominent apathy.[34] Rarely, dementia may constitute the presenting symptom of progressive supranuclear palsy.[35] Over time, pseudo-bulbar palsy with emotional incontinence may occur, and seizures may occur in a small minority. Aphasia, agnosia and apraxia are rare.

MRI may reveal atrophy of the midbrain and, in some cases, of the frontal and temporal cortices.

Course

The disease is progressive, with death within 5–7 years.

Pathology

Macroscopically there is atrophy of the midbrain, globus pallidus and, in some cases, the frontotemporal cortex.

Microscopically, cell loss is noted in the mesencephalic tectum, periaqueductal grey matter, locus coeruleus, substantia nigra, dentate nucleus, red nucleus, thalamus (especially in the caudal intralaminar nuclei), globus pallidus, subthalamic nucleus, and the temporal and inferior frontal cortices. This is accompanied by gliosis and, in surviving neurons, one finds neurofibrillary tangles dissimilar to those of Alzheimer's disease.[36]

Aetiology

Although definite autosomal dominantly inherited cases have been identified, the vast majority of cases appear to be sporadic. There does, however, appear to be a 'susceptibility genotype', composed of normal variants in the gene for tau, which predisposes to classic progressive supranuclear palsy.[37,38]

Corticobasal ganglionic degeneration

This rare disorder, apparently equally common in men and women, is characterized by atypical parkinsonism or dementia, or both.

Clinical features

The onset is gradual, usually in the sixth or seventh decade. Most patients present with a strikingly asymmetrical rigid akinetic parkinsonism affecting an upper limb; dystonic rigidity may also be present. Cortical sensory loss, apraxia and myoclonus are common. Dementia occurs in about one-half of patients and, although this usually follows the motor disturbance by years, it may at times be the presenting feature;[39,40] indeed, in two series, the majority of patients presented with dementia.[41,42] In patients who do develop dementia, depression is common; apathy and irritability may also occur.[43]

Corticobasal ganglionic degeneration may rarely present with primary progressive aphasia[44,45] or with a personality change with frontal lobe features.[44] Although the alien hand sign is said to occur, this sign is not in fact well described in this disorder: rather, patients display such purposeless movements as grasping, 'wandering' or levitation.

MRI may reveal asymmetrical cortical atrophy affecting primarily the parietal and frontal cortices.

Course

Over a long period of time, the parkinsonism gradually becomes bilateral; in some cases, cerebellar signs may appear and, rarely, supranuclear ophthalmoplegia has been noted. Death typically occurs within 6–10 years, generally secondary to aspiration pneumonia.

Pathology

Macroscopically there is asymmetrical cortical atrophy, affecting primarily the parietal lobe and the posterior portion of the frontal lobe; over time, the atrophy may spread to the contralateral side, and the temporal lobes and anterior portions of the frontal lobes may become involved. Microscopically, changes are seen in these areas and in the basal ganglia and substantia nigra, consisting of neuronal loss and astrocytosis; surviving neurons are large, ballooned and achromatic and contain tau-positive filaments.

Aetiology

The vast majority of cases are sporadic.

Multiple system atrophy

Three variants are generally recognized: the striatonigral, olivopontocerebellar and Shy–Drager variants. It is uncommon and somewhat more frequent in men than women.

Clinical features

The onset is gradual and typically occurs in the sixth decade.

The striatonigral variant, seen when the striatum and substantia nigra are most involved, is characterized by the gradual onset of parkinsonism, which is similar to that seen in Parkinson's disease, with the exceptions that the flexion posture is often extreme and tremor is seen in only a minority of patients and is typically not of the classic pill-rolling type. Furthermore, patients may have other signs not typical of Parkinson's disease, such as hyperreflexia and extensor plantar responses, myoclonus and, rarely, supranuclear ophthalmoplegia for downward gaze.

The olivopontocerebellar variant, seen with involvement of the inferior olives, basis pontis and cerebellar cortex, is characterized by the gradual onset of ataxia, intention tremor, dysarthria and scanning speech; reflex myoclonus is also commonly seen and emotional incontinence occurs in roughly one-third of cases.[46]

The Shy–Drager variant, seen when the intermediolateral grey matter of the spinal cord is heavily involved, is characterized by evidence of autonomic failure, such as urinary retention or incontinence, postural dizziness or syncope, erectile dysfunction and, rarely, faecal incontinence.

Dementia may occur in a minority of patients with multiple system atrophy and may be distinguished by elements of a frontal lobe syndrome.[47] Rarely, multiple system atrophy may present with a personality change and dementia, as has been noted in a case of the olivopontocerebellar variant.[48]

Regardless of which variant the disease presents with, over a matter of years most patients will eventually display features of all three variants. Many patients also eventually develop laryngeal stridor.

There is a strong association with REM sleep behaviour disorder:[49] one report noted that the vast majority of patients with multiple system atrophy had this disorder, which could precede the development of typical symptomatology by years.[50]

MRI may reveal atrophy of the striatum, pons, inferior olives and cerebellum. In some cases, especially in patients with the striatonigral variant, the putamen displays decreased signal intensity on T2-weighted scanning but laterally has a surrounding rim of increased signal intensity. In other cases, especially those with the olivopontocerebellar variant, the basis pontis will display the 'hot-cross bun sign' on axial T2-weighted images, wherein the base of the pons is marked by lines that give it the appearance of a hot-cross bun seen from above.

Course

It is gradually progressive, with death, often from aspiration pneumonia, generally within 6–9 years.

Pathology

Macroscopically, there is variable atrophy of the cerebral cortex (particularly the frontal area), striatum (more so the putamen than the caudate), pons, inferior olives and cerebellum. Microscopically, cell loss and astrocytosis are seen not only in these areas but also in the substantia nigra, locus coeruleus, ventrolateral medulla and intermediolateral grey matter of the spinal cord. Cytoplasmic inclusions containing alpha-synuclein are seen in oligodendroglia and in surviving neurons.

Aetiology

This is a sporadic disorder of unknown cause.

Huntington's disease (chorea)

The lifetime prevalence is 0.004–0.008 among white populations, one-third of that in black populations and one-tenth among Japanese populations.

Clinical features

The onset is generally highly insidious and may occur anywhere from childhood to the eighth decade, with most patients falling ill in their thirties. The presentation may be with either chorea or a personality change; over time, in the vast majority of patients, both these syndromes will become present and be joined by the gradual development of dementia.[51] Exceptions to this rule do occur, especially in people with late onset in the sixth decade or beyond, when one may see primarily chorea, with little or no cognitive deficit.[52]

Chorea may initially present as fidgetiness, clumsiness or a tendency to drop things; obvious choreiform movements are generally first visible on the face (including the forehead), from where they spread to involve the trunk and extremities. There may be facial grimacing, brow-wrinkling and blinking; upper extremity involvement may lead to shoulder-shrugging, abrupt flinging of the arms, or purposeless 'piano-playing' movements of the hands. In shaking the patient's hand, one may note the classic 'milkmaid grip', wherein the patient's grasping of the examiner's hand feels as if the patient is attempting to milk a cow. Lower extremity involvement may lead to a lurching, staggering or 'dancing and prancing' gait, which in some cases may so resemble the gait seen in alcohol intoxication that patients have been arrested for public intoxication. Importantly, these choreiform movements are quite brief, appearing and disappearing on a random basis from one location to another with lightning-like rapidity. Interestingly, although some patients seem fully aware of their chorea, it is not at all uncommon to find patients with obvious chorea denying that anything is amiss.

Early on, patients may attempt, with varying degrees of success, to disguise the choreic movements by merging them with purposeful movements: for example, a choreic fling of the arm up to the head may be purposefully extended to draw the fingers through the hair, as if the purpose had all along been to straighten the hair. Dysarthria often occurs, as does dysphagia, which may lead to aspiration. The chorea eventually makes almost all purposeful activity, whether eating, dressing or walking, almost impossible, and patients eventually become chair-bound or bedridden. At the end, the chorea may gradually disappear, to be replaced by a rigid, akinetic state. In advanced cases, seizures may also occur.

The personality change presents with poor judgement, impulsivity, irritability and an overall coarsening of behaviour. Over time, dementia develops, characterized by deficits in memory, concentration, calculation and abstraction; focal signs, such as aphasia and apraxia, are generally not seen. Associated symptoms are found in the vast majority of patients,[53–55] including depression of variable severity in roughly half, agitation, irritability, apathy and anxiety and, in a minority, euphoria or, rarely, mania. Delusions, generally of persecution, and, less commonly, hallucinations may be seen in a small minority; rarely, Huntington's disease may present with a psychosis.[53] Suicidal ideation is common,[56] and suicide itself occurs in a significant minority.[57]

When Huntington's disease presents in childhood or adolescence, one often sees the Westphal variant, in which, rather than chorea, there is a rigid, akinetic state generally accompanied by severe dementia, often with seizures, myoclonus and ataxia; in other cases, rather than parkinsonism, the presentation may be with chorea, myoclonus or dementia.

Structural neuroimaging may be normal early in the course; over time, however, because of atrophy of the caudate nuclei, there is a characteristic dilation of the frontal horns of the lateral ventricles, yielding a characteristic 'butterfly' configuration. Cortical atrophy, especially of the frontal lobes, may also be seen.

A positive family history is found almost universally. Exceptions may occur secondary to rarely occurring spontaneous mutations or, more commonly, to uncertain parentage.

Course

Huntington's disease is relentlessly progressive: most patients die within 10–30 years of onset, with an average life expectancy of about 15 years. Those with an earlier age of onset experience a more rapid course, with death within about 10 years; conversely, those with a late onset, in the fifth decade or beyond, typically experience a longer course.

Pathology

Macroscopically, atrophy is noted in the caudate, less so in the putamen, and to a degree in the frontal and parietal cortices. Neuronal loss and reactive astrocytosis are noted in these areas; in the caudate nucleus in particular, spiny neurons are lost first. Surviving neurons may display intranuclear inclusions, which contain huntingtin.

Aetiology

Huntington's disease is a fully penetrant autosomal dominant disorder. The affected gene, at 4p16, codes for huntingtin; in Huntington's disease there are increased CAG repeats (36 or more) at this locus.

Choreoacanthocytosis

This rare disorder is a member of the neuroacanthocytoses.

Clinical features

The onset is generally in the late twenties or early thirties but may occur anywhere from late childhood to the seventh decade. Clinically, most patients present with gradually progressive chorea, which, over time, is often joined by other abnormal movements, such as tics, dystonia or mild parkinsonism. A classic symptom, seen in only a minority, is self-mutilating lip- or tongue-biting, which is outside the patient's control: one patient despite attempting to 'restrain herself ... by placing her fingers or a folded towel in her mouth ... nevertheless had bleeding and scarred lesions of her oral mucosa and lips'.[58] Most patients will also develop a sensorimotor peripheral polyneuropathy and, in a minority, seizures may occur. Roughly half of all patients will also develop personality change or dementia, or both.

Acanthocytic erythrocytes, to a degree of 10 per cent or more, are seen on peripheral smears; importantly, the smears must be fresh wet preparations and, given the chance of false negatives, at least three smears should be examined. Genetic testing is available.

Creatine kinase is elevated in most cases and MRI may reveal caudate nucleus atrophy.

Course

The disease is gradually progressive, with death, on average, after 14 years.

Pathology

Macroscopically, there is atrophy of the caudate, putamen and, to a lesser degree, the globus pallidus. Microscopically, neuronal loss and gliosis are seen in these structures and in the substantia nigra. Axonal loss occurs in the peripheral nerves.

Aetiology

Choreoacanthocytosis is an autosomal recessive condition occurring secondary to mutations in the *VPS13A* gene at 9q21 (formerly known as *CHAC*), which codes for chorein. There may be considerable phenotypic heterogeneity in the same family.

Fragile X-associated tremor/ataxia syndrome

Fragile X-associated tremor/ataxia syndrome (FXTAS) is far more common in men than women.

Clinical features

Although the age of onset ranges from the fourth to the ninth decade, most patients fall ill in the seventh decade, with the gradual onset of ataxia and tremor. The tremor, although typically of the intention type, may also have a rest or postural component. Over time, mild parkinsonism may also accrue, with rest tremor, rigidity and bradykinesia. Peripheral neuropathy is common, and some patients may experience autonomic symptoms, such as erectile dysfunction.

Cognitive deficits eventually appear, and anywhere from one-quarter to one-half of patients may eventually become demented: short-term memory loss, poor concentration, concreteness and poor judgement are common. Frontal lobe symptomatology may also be seen, with disinhibition, perseveration and inappropriate jocularity, and mood changes are common, with agitation, irritability, apathy or depression.[59,60]

MRI may reveal both cerebral and cerebellar cortical atrophy. The most characteristic finding, however, is the 'middle cerebellar peduncle' sign: on T1-weighted scans these peduncles show decreased signal intensity, and on T2-weighted scans there is increased signal intensity.[61] This sign, although not universally present, becomes more likely later in the course of the disease. Genetic testing is available.

Course

Symptoms progress very slowly.

Pathology

Macroscopically, there is cerebral and cerebellar cortical atrophy. Microscopically, there is neuronal loss in these regions, and status spongiosus in the cerebellar white matter and the middle cerebellar peduncles. Intranuclear inclusions are found in both astrocytes and surviving neurons.

Aetiology

Like fragile X syndrome, FXTAS occurs as the result of a mutation in the fragile X mental retardation 1 (*FMR1*) gene, located on the long arm of the X chromosome, with an increase in the number of CGG repeats up into the premutation range of from 55 to 200.

Dentatorubropallidoluysian atrophy (DRPLA)

Clinical features

The onset of dentatorubropallidoluysian atrophy (DRPLA) is gradual and the clinical features are strongly influenced by the age of onset. Early-onset cases are characterized by ataxia, myoclonus, seizures and dementia.[62] Late-onset cases are typified by chorea or ataxia, or a combination of these; in a minority of cases, one may also see a mild degree of dystonia or parkinsonism.[62] In adults one also sees the eventual development of dementia, which may be accompanied by prominent hallucinations and delusions; rarely, DRPLA may present with a psychosis in adult years.[63] A small minority of adults may also have seizures. MRI may reveal superior cerebellar peduncular atrophy and, on T2-weighted scans, increased signal intensity in the globus pallidus.

Course

DRPLA is a gradually progressive disorder.

Pathology

Neuronal loss is found in the dentate nucleus, red nucleus, globus pallidus, subthalamic nucleus, striatum, substantia nigra, inferior olive, thalamus and cerebral cortex. In surviving neurons, intranuclear inclusions, formed of abnormal atrophin-1, may be found.

Aetiology

DRPLA is an autosomal dominantly inherited disorder: mutations exist in the gene for atrophin-1, on chromosome 12, which consist of an expansion of a normally occurring CAG repeat. There is considerable phenotypic heterogeneity within and between families.

Wilson's disease

Wilson's disease (hepatolenticular degeneration) occurs in around 1–2 per 100 000 of the general population.

Clinical features

The onset is typically between late childhood and early adulthood, although the range is wide, from early childhood to the sixth decade. The presentation may be with movement disorder, psychosis, personality change or dementia; over time, most patients eventually develop a combination of these. Other features include seizures, a Kayser–Fleischer ring, hepatitis and anaemia.

The movement disorder may consist of dystonia, chorea, tremor or parkinsonism; dysarthria may also appear. Dystonia may present with torticollis, dystonia of the upper or lower extremity, oculogyric crisis[64] or facial dystonia; classically, there is a fixed, vacuous, wide-mouthed dystonic smile. Chorea may involve either the upper or the lower extremities. The tremor may be rhythmic or irregular; at times, one may see the classic 'wing-beating' tremor in which a rhythmic elevation and lowering of the upper extremities, combined with flexion at the elbows, gives an overall appearance of a frightened bird flapping its wings.

Personality change is generally characterized by lability, disinhibition and, at times, bizarre behaviour.[65–67]

Psychosis is characterized by hallucinations and delusions[66,68] and may be bizarre, with Schneiderian first-rank symptoms. Indeed, one of Wilson's patients heard 'God and the devil talking to him simultaneously' and said that he was 'influenced, willed or hypnotized to do certain things'.[69] In one case, stuporous catatonia dominated the presentation.[70]

Seizures may occur but are rare, occurring in about 5 per cent of patients.

The Kayser–Fleischer ring is a golden-brown discolouration of the corneal limbus, visible either on slit-lamp examination or to the naked eye. Although present in the overwhelming majority of patients, cases of unequivocal Wilson's disease (with a movement disorder) without a Kayser–Fleischer ring do occur.

Hepatic damage may lead to clinical hepatitis, with fever, malaise, abdominal pain and elevated transaminase levels. With significant hepatic dysfunction, hepatic encephalopathy may occur.

A Coombs-negative haemolytic anaemia may occur.

The caeruloplasmin and total serum copper levels are both low, but the serum free copper is elevated, as is the 24-h urinary copper; in a small minority of patients, the caeruloplasmin level may be normal. Liver biopsy reveals an elevated copper level.

MRI may reveal characteristic findings.[71] On T2-weighted scans, increased signal intensity may be seen in the head of the caudate and lateral aspect of the putamen, with decreased signal intensity in the globus pallidus; in the midbrain, the 'face of the giant panda' sign may be seen, with increased signal intensity in the tegmentum and decreased signal intensity in the red nuclei. On T1-weighted scans, increased signal intensity may be seen in the caudate and putamen.

Given the large number of possible mutations, genetic testing is not practical.

Pathology

Biliary excretion is deficient and copper accumulates, first in the liver, where it causes hepatitis, and then, once it spills over into the systemic circulation, in the brain, where copper deposition occurs primarily in a pericapillary distribution. Macroscopically, there is atrophy and a brownish discolouration of the striatum, with, in advanced cases, cavitation and a mild degree of cortical atrophy. Microscopically, there is neuronal loss and astrocytosis in the striatum (more so in the putamen than in the caudate) and to a lesser degree in the globus pallidus; other affected structures include the cerebral cortex (especially the frontal lobes), thalamus, red nucleus, substantia nigra, dentate nucleus and cerebellar cortex. Copper deposition in Descemet's membrane produces the Kayser–Fleischer ring.

Aetiology

Wilson's disease is an autosomal recessive disorder resulting from mutations in the *ATP7B* gene on chromosome 13 that codes for the copper-binding ATPase; multiple different mutations have been identified.

Spinocerebellar ataxia

Spinocerebellar ataxia (SCA) is also known as autosomal dominant cerebellar ataxia.

Clinical features

The clinical hallmark is the appearance of gradually progressive cerebellar ataxia generally accompanied by dysarthria and nystagmus. The onset, although generally in the early to mid-adult years, may occur anywhere from childhood to senescence. With disease progression, almost all patients also develop one or more of the following associated features: hyperreflexia and extensor plantar responses; decreased vibratory sense, atrophy and fasciculations; supranuclear ophthalmoplegia; tremor (including titubation), dystonia, chorea, myoclonus or parkinsonism; or pigmentary retinopathy. Seizures are uncommon and may be grand mal, simple or complex partial in type.

Dementia may occur in a minority of patients, as may personality change (often frontal lobe type). Some patients may develop delusions and hallucinations. Rarely, SCA may present with dementia, personality change or psychosis.

Genetic testing is available.

MRI may reveal atrophy of the cerebellum, pons and inferior olives.[72,73]

Pathology

There is atrophy of the cerebellum, pons and inferior olives. Associated atrophy may also be found in one or more of the spinocerebellar tracts, Clarke's column, globus pallidus, subthalamic nucleus, substantia nigra and cerebral cortex.

Aetiology

SCA is an autosomal dominantly inherited syndrome, and approximately 26 different loci have been identified. For example, SCA19 (genetic locus 1p21–q21) is associated with cognitive impairment, while SCA13 (19q13.3–q13.4) is associated with early onset and developmental delay.

Pantothenate kinase-associated neurodegeneration

This disease was formerly known as Hallervorden–Spatz disease, but the use of this name is now discouraged, given the participation of Hallervorden and Spatz in the obscene Nazi 'euthanasia programmes' of the Third Reich.[74]

Clinical features

The onset is typically gradual and, although most patients fall ill in childhood or adolescence, adult-onset cases may occur. The clinical symptomatology is heavily influenced by the age of onset.

Childhood-onset cases are generally characterized by slowly progressive dystonic rigidity, prominent in both the extremities and the face; although this dystonia may be unilateral initially, bilateral involvement eventually occurs. Over time, other abnormal movements may appear, including tremor or choreoathetosis; tics have also been noted in a small minority of patients, as have obsessions and compulsions. Dementia occurs gradually.

Adult-onset cases may present with parkinsonism, dystonia or athetosis. Over time, and with progression of the abnormal movements, dementia may occur. Rarely, the presentation may be with dementia, followed years later by a movement disorder. In some cases depressive symptomatology may occur or, rarely, delusions and hallucinations.

In addition to the abnormal movements, many patients may also develop signs of spasticity, with hyperreflexia and the Babinski sign; in a minority, pigmentary retinopathy may occur.

MRI generally reveals the distinctive 'eye of the tiger' sign.[75] On T2-weighted scans, increased signal intensity is seen in the lateral aspect of the globus pallidus, whereas on the inner aspect there is a gross loss of signal intensity: the overall effect, seen on axial imaging, is of looking a tiger in the eye.

Course

Childhood-onset cases show gradual progression, with death occurring within 10–15 years; adult-onset cases tend to pursue a longer course, and some patients may remain ambulatory for decades.

Pathology

Macroscopically, the globus pallidus is atrophic and exhibits a yellow-brown discolouration. Microscopically, iron deposition and axonal spheroids are seen in the globus pallidus, cerebral cortex and pars reticulata of the substantia nigra.

Aetiology

This is a recessively inherited disorder, and mutations are found in the gene for pantothenate kinase, *PANK2*, on chromosome 20.

Dopa-responsive dystonia

It is important not to miss this diagnosis in clinical practice because, although dopa-responsive dystonia is uncommon, the dystonia tends to respond to levodopa.

Clinical features

The classic onset is in childhood, but later onsets in adolescence and adulthood have also been reported. Regardless of the age of onset, symptoms generally both appear and accrue gradually.

Childhood-onset cases generally present with an intermittent dystonia of one foot; over time, the dystonia spreads, eventually involving the other lower extremity and then the upper extremities; truncal and cervical dystonia may also eventually appear. A characteristic feature of the dystonia has been termed 'sleep benefit': after a good night's sleep, the dystonia may be very mild, or even absent, only to reappear gradually and worsen as the day wears on. In some cases, mild parkinsonism may appear; myoclonus has also been noted. The movement disorder may be accompanied by depression or obsessions and compulsions.

Later-onset cases may also be marked by more prominent parkinsonism. In some cases, the syndrome may present with depression or obsessions and compulsions without any abnormal movements.[76,77]

Course

In childhood-onset cases the dystonia eventually generalizes over about 3–4 years, after which it remains static.

Pathology

Reduced neuromelanin has been reported in the substantia nigra, without cell loss, in both DYT5a and DYT14 (see below).

Aetiology

Dopa-responsive dystonia is a genetically heterogeneous syndrome. The following diseases have so far been described: DYT5a, DYT5b and DYT14.

DYT5a (Segawa syndrome) is autosomal dominant and constitutes the most common cause of dopa-responsive dystonia. There is a mutation in the guanosine triphosphate cyclo-hydrolase 1 (*GCH1*) gene on chromosome 14. GCH1 is the rate-limiting enzyme for the synthesis of tetrahydrobiopterin, which is an essential co-factor for tyrosine hydroxylase. Hence, there is a reduction in dopamine production.

DYT5b is an autosomal recessive disorder caused by a mutation in the gene for tyrosine hydroxylase on chromosome 11.

DYT14 is an autosomal dominant disorder linked to a site on chromosome 14.

Tourette's syndrome

Described by Georges Gilles de la Tourette in 1885, this classic cause of chronic tics is also known as Gilles de la Tourette syndrome, *maladie des tics* and *tic convulsiv*. It has a lifetime prevalence of about 0.05 per cent and is about three times more common in males than females.

Clinical features

The onset is typically with a simple tic, more often motor than verbal, and more often on the head or face than elsewhere. Although the age of onset may be anywhere from infancy to the early adult years, most patients fall ill in childhood, around the age of 7 years.

In its fully developed form, both motor and verbal tics are present; these may be either simple or complex. Sensory tics are also usually present.

Motor tics are usually the first to appear. Simple motor tics include blinking, brow-wrinkling, grimacing and shoulder-shrugging; complex motor tics may include touching, smelling, hopping, throwing, clapping, bending over, squatting, or even such very complex acts as echopraxia or copropraxia (making obscene gestures). Motor tics usually appear first in the face or head and then spread in a caudal direction. In most cases, before having a tic, patients first experience an urge to tic,[78] an urge that may at times be resisted, albeit with difficulty. Some patients are able to abort a motor tic with a *geste antagoniste*, such as placing a hand under the chin to prevent the emergence of a tic of the head.[79]

Simple vocal tics include snorting, hissing, coughing, throat-clearing, grunting and, classically, barking. Complex vocal tics include uttering words, simple phrases or entire sentences. Echolalia or palilalia may occur; in a minority of patients, classic coprolalia, or involuntary swearing, may occur.

Sensory tics appear to exist in two forms. In one form, there is simply the experience of an itch or a tingle;[80] this is seen in perhaps one-quarter of patients. In the other form, the sensory tic appears more as a premonitory urge to a motor tic;[81,82] this has been reported in over 90 per cent of cases.[82] Remarkably, in one case a premonitory urge to itch was experienced by a patient as residing in another person, whom the patient then proceeded to scratch.[83]

Rarely, dystonic movements, especially cervical or facial dystonias, may appear, but not until 10–38 years have passed.[84]

Obsessions and compulsions are common, eventually appearing in nearly one-half of all patients.[85,86] They typically begin to appear about 5 years into the course. The compulsions often centre on getting things 'just right'.[87]

Attention-deficit hyperactivity disorder (ADHD) very commonly accompanies Tourette's syndrome. When this occurs, the hyperactivity usually precedes the tics by a little over a year.[88]

Course

In most cases, symptoms gradually worsen over a matter of a few years, peaking in severity around the age of 10 years; subsequently there is a gradual and progressive remission of symptoms, such that by the age of 18 years roughly one-half of patients are left with either no or only trivial tics.[89,90] In those cases where full remissions do occur, relapses may appear, sometimes decades later.

Pathology and aetiology

Tourette's syndrome is familial, with concordance rates rising from about 5 per cent in siblings to approximately 10 per cent in dizygotic twins and 50 per cent in monozygotic twins; indeed, if one accepts the presence of simple tics as evidence of the disorder, then the monozygotic concordance rises to over 75 per cent. It is a complex genetic disorder.

MRI studies strongly suggest a reduced size of the basal ganglia. Although neuropathological studies have not revealed distinctive microscopic findings, immunological studies have shown a decreased number of dopamine reuptake sites in the striatum and a decrease in dynorphin staining in fibres coursing from the striatum to the globus pallidus.

Some research suggests that, at least in a certain minority of cases, Tourette's syndrome may be an autoimmune disease, triggered, in turn, by a preceding beta-haemolytic streptococcal infection. Swedo and colleagues considered Tourette's syndrome to be part of a syndrome that they named paediatric autoimmune neuropsychiatric disorders associated with streptococcal infections (PANDAS).[91] In this condition, similar to Sydenham's chorea, a preceding group A beta-haemolytic streptococcal pharyngitis triggers an immune response that cross-reacts with the basal ganglia, leading to, among other symptomatologies, tics; increased levels of anti-streptococcal antibodies in patients support this notion. Furthermore, most studies have also found an increased incidence of serum anti-basal ganglia antibodies.

Myotonic dystrophy type 1

The lifetime prevalence of myotonic dystrophy type 1 (DM1) is around 5 per 100 000. It is equally common in males and females.

Clinical features

The onset is gradual and insidious. Most patients fall ill in their late teens or early twenties, but the age of onset ranges from childhood to the sixth decade.

The cardinal symptoms are myotonia and weakness. Myotonia may go unnoticed or manifest in difficulty in, for example, letting go of a doorknob or disengaging from a handshake. Myotonia may be elicited by tapping the thenar eminence with a percussion hammer and observing for the characteristic muscle dimpling. Weakness is eventually accompanied by atrophy, which is more prominent distally, being seen first in the upper extremities. Other signs may also accrue. Many patients have a distinctive 'myopathic facies', with frontal balding, ptosis, and wasting of the face and neck musculature; the voice often becomes nasal and monotone. Cataracts occur in over 90 per cent of patients, and there may be deafness and gonadal failure, with erectile dysfunction or menstrual irregularity. Cardiac conduction abnormalities and arrhythmias may occur, including atrioventricular block, fascicular block, intraventricular conduction block, atrial fibrillation and ventricular premature contractions; less commonly, cardiomyopathy with congestive heart failure may occur. Alveolar hypoventilation may occur.

Cognitive impairment is eventually seen in the majority of patients;[92,93] although generally mild, this may progress to dementia.[94] Personality change may also occur and, although tending to be mixed in type, avoidant traits may predominate.[95,96] Apathy is more common than among comparable controls.[97] Depression appears to be no more common than in comparable controls; in considering the diagnosis of depression, one must guard against misinterpreting the expressionless 'myopathic facies' as a depressed affect.[98–100]

Hypersomnia is not uncommon[101] and indeed may be the presenting complaint:[102] some patients may literally sleep for days.[103] Although some of these hypersomnic patients demonstrate sleep apnoea (of either the central or obstructive type), the number of apnoeic episodes is not high enough to account for the degree of hypersomnolence.[104]

As noted below, 'anticipation' may occur in this disease, and some children may be born with 'congenital' myotonic muscular dystrophy, characterized, among other symptoms, by mental retardation.[105]

Computed tomography (CT) and MRI may reveal a mild degree of cortical atrophy. On magnetic resonance (MR) scanning, patchy areas of increased signal intensity on T2-weighed scans may be seen in the white matter.[106] Genetic testing is available.

Course

Myotonic muscular dystrophy is gradually progressive and, although patients with later onsets and milder symptoms may experience a normal lifespan, cases of early onset and severe symptoms are often associated with premature death in early or middle adult years, often from cardiac or respiratory causes.

Aetiology and pathology

DM1 is inherited in an autosomal dominant fashion with almost 100 per cent penetrance but a quite variable expressivity, even within the same family. Mutations consist of an expansion of a normally occurring CTG triplet in the myotonic dystrophy protein kinase (*DMPK*) gene on 19q13.3. 'Anticipation' may occur, in which in succeeding generations, and with expansion of the triplet repeat, the disease becomes more severe and has an earlier onset. Anticipation is more likely with maternal transmission than paternal cases.

Dystrophic muscle shows characteristic changes, including internal nuclei in muscle fibres. Neuronal heterotopias have been noted in the cerebral cortex and neurofibrillary tangles in the hippocampus. In cases characterized by hypersomnolence, cell loss was noted in the midbrain superior central nucleus; in cases marked by alveolar hyperventilation, cell loss was seen in the medullary reticular formation.

Other rare disorders

Cerebrotendinous xanthomatosis

This recessively inherited lipid storage disease (mutations in *CYP27*, a gene on chromosome 2 coding for sterol 27-

hydroxylase) may cause dementia. The onset is very gradual and, although most patients begin to have symptoms in late childhood or early adolescence, the range in age of onset is wide. The fully developed disease is characterized by dementia, seizures, long-tract signs, ataxia, peripheral sensorimotor polyneuropathy, gross tendon enlargement, especially evident in the Achilles tendon, cataracts and chronic diarrhoea. Although the disease may present with any one of these various features, in most cases the presentation will be with juvenile cataracts or with chronic, intractable diarrhoea.

Thalamic degeneration

This is characterized clinically by dementia and pathologically by relatively selective degeneration of the thalamus, in the absence of known causes such as Creutzfeldt–Jakob disease. This syndrome probably subsumes several or more different disease processes. The age of onset may range from adolescence to the seventh decade, and the mode of onset from subacute to insidious. Dementia may be accompanied by apathy and somnolence, emaciation or myoclonus.

Metachromatic leucodystrophy

This is a recessively inherited disorder, secondary to any of a large number of mutations in the chromosome 22 gene for arylsulfatase A (which normally converts sulfatides into cerebroside, a normal constituent of myelin). Demyelination and accumulation of sulfatides in the brain, peripheral nerves, kidneys and gallbladder result. When appearing in adolescents or adults, it may present with a psychosis, personality change or dementia.

Adrenoleucodystrophy

This X-linked disorder (mutations in the *ALD* gene) is characterized pathologically by the accumulation of very-long-chain fatty acids in the brain, spinal cord, peripheral nerves and adrenal glands, and clinically by a variable combination of dementia, spasticity and adrenal failure.

Kufs' disease

This typically presents in early adult years in one of two fashions. Type A patients present with grand mal and myoclonic seizures and dementia, often accompanied by ataxia or abnormal movements, such as athetosis or parkinsonism. Type B patients typically present with personality change or dementia, which may also be accompanied by ataxia and other abnormal movements. The disease is relentlessly progressive, with death occurring on average after 12 years.

VASCULAR DISORDERS

Vascular dementia is described in Chapter 72.

Vascular (arteriosclerotic) parkinsonism

This disorder, which is probably uncommon, is characterized by atypical parkinsonism occurring on the basis of lacunar infarctions in either the mesencephalon or the basal ganglia.

Clinical features

The onset is generally in the seventh or eighth decade. Clinically, the parkinsonism is characterized by bradykinesia, lead-pipe rigidity, instability and a tendency to fall. The posture may or may not be in flexion; the gait is either shuffling or 'magnetic', in that the feet seem 'stuck' to the floor. Overall, these parkinsonian features may be symmetrical or asymmetrical. Notably, both tremor and cogwheeling are generally absent, and the response to levodopa is generally poor. Vascular (lacunar) dementia may occur, and typically there is damage to corticospinal tracts (e.g. spasticity) and corticobulbar tracts, with pseudo-bulbar palsy.

MRI reveals multiple lacunes, with at least some of them involving either the basal ganglia or the mesencephalon.[107]

Course

The overall course is generally one of progression and may be either stepwise or more or less gradual.

Aetiology and pathology

In most patients, vascular parkinsonism occurs in the setting of multiple lacunes affecting not only the basal ganglia or substantia nigra but also the corticospinal and corticobulbar tracts as they course through the internal capsule.

Binswanger's disease

First described by Otto Binswanger in 1894,[108] this is characterized by a slowly progressive dementia occurring in elderly people on the basis of a diffuse microangiopathic ischaemic leucoencephalopathy or leucoaraiosis. It is considered to be one of the vascular dementias.

Clinical features

The onset is generally gradual, occurring in the sixth or later decades. Clinically, as described by Binswanger, there is a 'slow development of the deterioration of the intellectual capacities',[109] and patients present with a non-specific dementia, with slowness of thought, decreased short-term memory, disorientation and concreteness. In advanced cases, a pseudo-bulbar palsy may occur. Minor focal signs, such as asymmetrical deep tendon reflexes or a Babinski sign, may be seen, but in uncomplicated Binswanger's disease major clear-cut syndromes such as aphasia or apraxia do not occur.

CT reveals widespread areas of radiolucency in the periventricular white matter and centrum semiovale. MRI is more sensitive and on FLAIR or T2-weighted images one finds multiple patchy and confluent areas of increased signal intensity in the periventricular region and the centrum semiovale, extending close to the cortex but sparing the U-fibres. In advanced cases, these patchy areas may coalesce to the point of creating a virtual 'white-out'.

Aetiology and pathology

At autopsy, the small penetrating medullary vessels display lipohyalinosis and, in some cases, the lumens are obliterated. There is widespread demyelination, with some associated axonal loss; in severe cases, cystic changes may occur. Although it is suspected that these microangiopathic changes occur on the basis of long-standing hypertension, other factors are probably also at work, as Binswanger's disease may occur in normotensive individuals.

Cranial arteritis

Cranial arteritis is also known as giant-cell arteritis and temporal arteritis. In people over 50 years of age, it is a not uncommon disorder; it is seen primarily in white people, especially those of Nordic descent.

Clinical features

The symptomatology varies according to which arteries are inflamed.[110] Branches of the external carotid artery are commonly involved, and inflammation of the temporal artery is classic, causing a severe headache in the temporal region, which, although generally unilateral, can be bilateral. If the occipital artery is involved, the headache may be localized to the neck. Involvement of the facial artery may lead to jaw claudication, with facial pain upon chewing; involvement of the lingual artery may cause tongue necrosis. Of the branches of the internal carotid artery, the ophthalmic artery is classically involved; in such cases, unilateral blindness may occur, which may or may not be preceded by episodes of amaurosis fugax.

In about 10 per cent of cases, strokes or transient ischaemic attacks (TIAs) may occur;[111] this may be seen with involvement of either the vertebral artery or the internal carotid artery. With vertebral artery involvement, clots may form, which may then embolize further downstream, for example to the posterior cerebral artery. Small branches of the vertebral arteries may also be occluded, leading to medullary infarction. With involvement of the internal carotid artery, clots may also form, with embolization downstream, causing occlusion of the middle or anterior cerebral arteries or their branches. Small penetrating arteries may be involved, causing multiple lacunes. In some cases, if the number and location of infarctions are appropriate, vascular dementia may ensue.

Most cases are further characterized by constitutional symptoms such as malaise, fatigue, anorexia and a low-grade fever. Most patients also have an associated polymyalgia rheumatica, with muscle aching and stiffness, which, although diffuse, is most prominent in the neck and shoulders.

With rare exceptions the erythrocyte sedimentation rate (ESR) is elevated, generally above 50 mm/min and often above 100 mm/min. Mild anaemia is common, and the alkaline phosphatase may also be elevated. The diagnosis is confirmed by biopsy of an involved artery, such as the temporal artery; given the segmental nature of the inflammation, however, false negatives are possible and multiple biopsies may be required.

Aetiology and pathology

Involved arteries show a graulomatous inflammation characterized by the presence of giant cells. The inflammation is segmental, and between the involved segments the artery may be normal. Thrombi may form over the inflamed areas and emboli may be generated; in some cases the artery may become occluded. Although the mechanism underlying the inflammation is not known, an autoimmune process is suspected.

Cerebral amyloid angiopathy

Also known as congophilic amyloid angiopathy, this a not uncommon disorder characterized by amyloid angiopathy.

Clinical features

Onset is typically in the seventh or later decades. The disorder may present with either spontaneous lobar intracerebral haemorrhages or gradually progressive dementia.

The lobar intracerebral haemorrhages present with a gradual evolution, over perhaps half an hour, of headache, nausea and vomiting, and a focal deficit appropriate to the location of the haemorrhage. Classically, the haemorrhage occurs spontaneously and recurrences are the rule. With multiple recurrences, a stepwise accrual of cognitive deficits may occur, eventually leading to a picture of multi-infarct dementia.

Dementia may also be of gradual onset and progression, and in this instance it is non-specific in character, with decreased short-term memory, variable disorientation, and deficits in abstracting and calculating ability.

Cerebral micro-haemorrhages may occur; these may be silent or present with relatively minor focal findings that, in most cases, resolve over time. Residual deposits of haemosiderin may serve as seizure foci, and partial seizures may also occur.

MRI will reveal evidence of any old intracerebral haemorrhages; in cases with a leucoencephalopathy, T2-weighted or FLAIR images reveal bilateral, more or less symmetrical, patchy or confluent areas of increased signal intensity that spare the U-fibres. Gradient echo images may reveal punctate areas of decreased signal intensity, corresponding to old micro-haemorrhages.[112] In some cases, one finds large asymmetrical areas of increased signal intensity on T2-weighted or FLAIR imaging in the subcortical white matter, which fail to enhance and which may represent vasogenic oedema.

Course

This depends on the preponderance of the underlying pathology. With repeated intracerebral haemorrhages, a stepwise course may occur, whereas cases with leucoencephalopathy are characterized by a gradual progression of cognitive deficits. The combination of these two courses may also occur and is distinctive for this disease.[113]

Aetiology and pathology

Amyloid deposition occurs in the walls of small and medium-sized cortical arterioles, resulting in fibrinoid degeneration and the formation of microaneurysms.[114] Affected vessels are congophilic, staining well with Congo red dye, thus accounting for the alternative name for this disorder, 'congophilic amyloid angiopathy'. The aneurysmal dilations of these vessels are fragile and account for both spontaneous lobar intracerebral haemorrhages and micro-haemorrhages. Within the areas of distribution of the affected arteries, rarefaction of the white matter occurs, probably on an ischaemic basis.

Although the vast majority of cases are sporadic, cerebral amyloid angiopathy may also occur on an autosomal dominant basis as hereditary cerebral haemorrhage with amyloidosis, of either the Dutch or Icelandic type.

CADASIL

Cerebral autosomal dominant arteriopathy with subcortical infarcts and leucoencephalopathy (CADASIL) is a rare autosomal dominantly inherited arteriopathy.

Clinical features

CADASIL is characterized by the onset of recurrent migraine headaches, typically with aura, in the third or fourth decade, followed by recurrent strokes or TIAs in the fourth or fifth decade, and a dementia in the sixth or seventh decade. A pseudo-bulbar palsy may occur and, in a small minority of patients, seizures may appear. The strokes are typically of the lacunar type, reflecting infarcts that occur primarily in the basal ganglia. The dementia, although generally reflecting the effects of multiple lacunar infarctions, at times may also be caused by progressive leucoencephalopathy, and in rare instances CADASIL may present with dementia secondary to the leucoencephalopathy in the absence of stroke.[115,116]

Two unusual manifestations of CADASIL must also be kept in mind, namely intracerebral haemorrhage and reversible delirium. Intracerebral haemorrhage, primarily of the thalamus or basal ganglia, may occur but is uncommon. Delirium is rare. Patients present with a subacute delirium, often accompanied by seizures and fever, which may progress to coma; recovery is spontaneous and occurs after 1–2 weeks.[117]

MRI reveals prior lacunar infarctions. Most patients also have diffuse leucoencephalopathy and, indeed, this may be present early on, even before the first stroke. The leucoencephalopathy is evident on either T2-weighted or FLAIR imaging: patchy, confluent areas of increased signal intensity are seen in the centrum semiovale and the periventricular white matter and also, classically, in the external capsule and, most notably, in the white matter of the anterior temporal lobe. Gradient echo imaging has also identified evidence for old micro-haemorrhages in the thalamus and basal ganglia.

Diagnosis may be made by genetic testing. Skin biopsy may also be performed, but false negatives are common.

Course

The course is described above. Death occurs in the seventh to ninth decade, often from pneumonia.

Aetiology and pathology

In this autosomal dominant disorder mutations are found in the *Notch3* gene on chromosome 19. Pathologically, there is concentric fibrous thickening of small penetrating arteries, leading to both subcortical infarcts and widespread leucoencephalopathy.

Granulomatous angiitis of the central nervous system

This rare disorder is also known as primary angiitis of the central nervous system (PACNS).

Clinical features

Although the disease may present at any age, most patients are in their thirties or forties. The onset is generally subacute, spanning a few weeks. Clinically, patients typically have severe, generalized headache, and in this setting they develop delirium, which may be accompanied by focal deficits or, uncommonly, seizures. Although focal deficits such as hemiparesis may have a stroke-like onset, in most cases they appear gradually. Sometimes the spinal cord may be involved.

The ESR is generally either normal or only mildly elevated. MRI may initially be normal; however, over time areas of increased signal intensity on FLAIR or T2-weighted imaging appear in the cerebrum or cerebellum. Angiography may be normal or may disclose typical beading. Lumbar puncture should be performed in all suspected cases: there is typically a lymphocytic pleocytosis, an elevated protein and a normal glucose.[118] Brain biopsy, sampling both the leptomeninges and the cerebrum from the tip of the non-dominant temporal lobe, is the gold standard; however, even this may be falsely negative, missing affected tissue.

Course

Untreated, progressive deterioration occurs in almost all cases and perhaps half of all patients will die within months, with the remainder surviving for up to 2 years or more.

Aetiology and pathology

The cause is unknown. A granulomatous angiitis affects both small leptomeningeal vessels and small or medium-sized parenchymal vessels. The cerebrum is most commonly affected, although the cerebellum, brainstem and even the cord may be involved.

Polyarteritis nodosa

Also known as periarteritis nodosa, this is a rare systemic vasculitis.

Clinical features

The onset is generally subacute or gradual in middle years with constitutional symptoms and evidence of involvement of the kidneys, gastrointestinal tract or muscles; renal disease may lead to hypertension or renal failure. The respiratory tract is not involved.

Nervous system involvement generally occurs only after other evidence of the disease is well established. Peripheral nervous system involvement, which is most common, typically involves a mononeuritis multiplex. In a minority of patients, central nervous system (CNS) involvement may occur, most commonly presenting with lacunar strokes; larger territorial infarctions and intracerebral haemorrhages are rare. In a very small minority of patients, delirium[119] or dementia[120] may occur; seizures have also been noted.

Both the white cell count (WCC) and the ESR are elevated. Anti-neutrophil cytoplasmic antibodies (ANCA), especially perinuclear ANCA (pANCA), are found in the majority of cases. The Venereal Disease Research Laboratory (VDRL) test may be falsely positive. MRI will reveal infarctions. Definitive diagnosis is made by biopsy of an affected muscle or peripheral nerve.

Course

Although spontaneous remissions do occur, they are rare, and most cases are characterized by relentless progression, with only about 10 per cent of patients surviving past 5 years.

Aetiology and pathology

There is a systemic, segmental panarteritis affecting medium and small arteries, with, at times, extension into arterioles. With intimal proliferation, thrombosis and occlusion of arteries may occur; with involvement of the muscular layer, microaneurysms may form. These microaneurysms may rupture occasionally; however, they typically undergo fibrosis, thus creating nodules along the course of the artery, thereby providing the characteristic that gives the disease its name.

Involvement of the peripheral vasa nervorum leads to the mononeuritis multiplex. Within the CNS, involvement of small perforating arteries leads to lacunar infarctions; in uncommon cases involving larger arteries, territorial infarctions may occur and, with rupture of an aneurysm, intracerebral haemorrhage may be seen.

Although the mechanism underlying the arteritis is not known with certainty, deposition of immune complexes probably plays a role, and in this regard there is an association with hepatitis B antigenaemia.

Behçet's disease

This was first described in 1937 by the Turkish dermatologist Hulusi Behçet. There is evidence of CNS involvement in one-tenth to one-third of patients. Although not uncommon in Japan and the eastern Mediterranean region, Behçet's disease is rare in Europe and the USA.

Clinical features

Behçet's disease typically presents in the twenties or thirties, and almost all patients have oral aphthous ulcers and some form of uveitis. Genital ulcers are somewhat less common. Another distinctive sign, not seen in all patients, is pathergy: here, within 1–2 days of minor skin trauma, for example phlebotomy, a large pustule forms at the site of the trauma. Other symptoms include furuncles, erythema nodosum, migratory thrombophlebitis and a non-deforming polyarthritis. Within the context of these symptoms, evidence of CNS involvement may appear.

When the CNS is involved, a wide variety of symptoms may appear, including delirium, dementia, pseudo-bulbar palsy with emotional incontinence, hemiplegia, ataxia, cranial nerve palsies, abnormal movements (e.g. chorea), personality change of the frontal lobe type and, rarely, seizures. In addition to vasculitis, both meningitis and dural sinus thrombosis may occur, and in such cases one may see headache; in cases of dural sinus thrombosis, one may also see signs of increased intracranial pressure, with nausea, vomiting and papilloedema.

T2-weighted or FLAIR MRI may reveal areas of increased signal intensity in the brainstem, cerebellum or, less commonly, cerebrum; these areas may demonstrate enhancement with gadolinium. MR venography may be required to demonstrate dural sinus thrombosis. The CSF may be abnormal, with an elevated total protein and/or a pleocytosis, which is generally lymphocytic. The ESR and WCC may be elevated.

Course

Most cases demonstrate an episodic course. The first attack tends to occur in the twenties or thirties, and most attacks last in the order of weeks or a month or more, after which there is a spontaneous remission. These remissions, however, are generally not complete, and most patients are left with residual symptoms. Recurrent attacks are the rule, and after each attack the overall burden of residual symptoms increases. In some cases, this typical episodic course may evolve into one of steady, waxing and waning progression; rarely, Behçet's disease may pursue a chronic, non-episodic course from the outset, as was seen in a case of progressive dementia with aphthous and genital ulcers.[121]

Aetiology and pathology

The aetiology is unknown, but an autoimmune process is suspected.

CNS perivenular vasculitis occurs. Meningeal inflammation may also occur, possibly accompanied by dural sinus thrombosis.

Hypertensive encephalopathy

This relatively common disorder is sometimes subsumed under the syndrome reversible posterior leucoencephalopathy.

Clinical features

In the setting of sustained diastolic pressure elevations, often 130 mm Hg or higher, delirium and headache evolve over a matter of 1–3 days. Most patients also experience nausea and vomiting, and a majority experience bilateral visual blurring, which may progress to cortical blindness. Seizures may also occur and, in a minority of patients, focal signs such as aphasia or hemiplegia may occur. Untreated, patients may become comatose. Fundoscopy may reveal papilloedema or retinal haemorrhages. Acute cardiac and renal failure may accompany the cerebral symptomatology.

CT may reveal bilaterally symmetrical areas of hypodensity in the occipitoparietal white matter. MRI is more sensitive and, on T2-weighted or FLAIR imaging, increased signal intensity will be seen in the same areas; gradient echo imaging may reveal evidence of petechial haemorrhages. Rarely, these MRI findings may be found in the brainstem and cerebellum.

Course

Untreated hypertensive encephalopathy may be fatal. In cases in which the blood pressure is corrected, symptoms gradually resolve over a matter of days, and white-matter abnormalities seen on CT/MRI typically clear within a week or so. In those cases in which focal findings were noted, these may persist, and MRI will show persistent abnormalities consistent with infarction. With a sufficient number of strategically placed infarctions, patients may be left with vascular dementia.

Aetiology and pathology

As blood pressure rises above a critical level, autoregulation of small and medium-sized cerebral arteries fails and there is extravasation of proteinaceous fluid into the surrounding white matter; some vessels may also rupture, causing petechial haemorrhages, and others may undergo fibrinoid necrosis and occlusion, causing infarction.

Reversible posterior leucoencephalopathy syndrome

Clinical features

The syndrome presents acutely, over hours, and manifests with delirium or lethargy, accompanied typically by headache, nausea or vomiting, and grand mal seizures, which may have a focal onset.[122] Cortical blindness is common. Other symptoms may also occur, such as hemianopia, hemiparesis, abulia or asterixis.

T2-weighted or FLAIR MRI reveals areas of increased signal intensity bilaterally in the white matter of the occipital and parietal lobes, with similar findings, in many cases, noted in the posterior aspects of the temporal lobes.

Course

With prompt and adequate treatment, clinical findings resolve within days to weeks.

Aetiology and pathology

This syndrome has been noted secondary to treatment with a variety of chemotherapeutic and immunomodulatory agents, including tacrolimus, ciclosporin, vincristine, methotrexate, bevacizumab, cyclophosphamide, asparaginase, cisplatin, cytarabine, interferon-alpha, and immunoglobulins. Although the mechanism of toxicity is not clear, it probably involves damage to the vascular endothelium.

Vasogenic oedema is seen within the white matter. In cases with an unfavourable outcome, white-matter infarction occurs.

Other uncommon vascular disorders

Thrombotic thrombocytopenic purpura

This typically occurs in young or middle-aged adults. It is marked by the subacute onset of delirium and thrombocytopenia. The delirium is marked by a pronounced fluctuation in the severity of symptoms throughout the day. Other symptomatology includes focal signs, such as hemiparesis or aphasia, which are typically transient, and seizures, with, in a small minority, complex partial status epilepticus.

The platelet count is generally reduced below 30 000/mm^3, and there is an accompanying microangiopathic haemolytic anaemia with schistocytes or Burr cells. Renal failure with proteinuria and azotaemia is common, as are fever and purpura.

Fat embolism syndrome

This syndrome represents an uncommon complication of fractures or surgery to the long bones, or trauma to fatty tissues, in which showers of fat globules pass to and through the lungs, leaving the patient in respiratory distress and with delirium.

Anywhere from 1 to 3 days after relevant trauma or surgery, patients develop dyspnoea and confusion; there may also be seizures and strokes and, in severe cases, coma. In some cases, a petechial rash may appear on the trunk.

Diffusion-weighted MRI reveals multiple punctate areas of increased signal intensity, primarily scattered throughout the white matter, with variable involvement of the cortex or subcortical structures. Chest radiography reveals bilateral 'fluffy' infiltrates; in a minority of cases, fat globules may be observed on urinalysis.

Transient global amnesia

The first episode of transient global amnesia generally occurs in the sixth or seventh decade. Episodes are generally of abrupt onset and may be associated with various precipitating events, such as strong emotion, sexual intercourse, pain, physical exertion, the Valsalva manoeuvres or even immersion in cold water. Whether or not a precipitating event is present, the patient suddenly experiences amnesia that has retrograde and anterograde components. The retrograde component covers at least the previous few hours and in many cases may stretch much further into the past: typically, this retrograde amnesia displays a temporal gradient, such that, whereas the amnesia may be quite dense for events of the very recent past, it becomes patchy for events further back.[123] The anterograde component is fairly dense, and patients are unable to keep track of any ongoing events during the episode. Most patients, although not confused, are more or less alarmed at their state, and many will anxiously and repeatedly ask where they are and how they got to be where they are. Formal mental status testing reveals that patients are coherent, alert and not confused. Although digit span is intact, patients are unable to recall any of three words after 5 min; furthermore, they will be unable to recall events of the recent past leading up to the onset of the episode. In essence, cognitive ability, other than memory, remains normal, and indeed some patients may engage in quite complex activity, such as playing an organ piece, during the episode itself.[124] Neurological examination is generally normal. The episode generally lasts 4–18 h, averaging about 6 h, and terminates gradually.

After the episode has cleared, patients are once again able to keep track of ongoing events, and their ability to recall words after 5 min is fully restored. When they try to recall what happened, however, they often find an 'island' of amnesia that covers not only the duration of the event itself but also any events that occurred anywhere from a few minutes to an hour or so just before the onset of the episode. Although clinically patients are thus fully restored, detailed testing may reveal some subtle decrements in memory.[125,126]

Although the aetiology of this disorder is unknown, it is included here because of the strong suspicion that it may result from either transient ischaemia or venous congestion of medial temporal structures.

TRAUMA

Subdural haematoma

Clinical features

Acute subdural haematoma typically occurs following traumatic brain injury and is often accompanied by other intracranial injuries, such as diffuse axonal injury, contusions, intracerebral haemorrhages and subarachnoid haemorrhage. Patients may develop delirium or may present in stupor or coma.

Subacute subdural haematoma tends to present with drowsiness and delirium,[127] and symptoms may fluctuate for days; when the haematoma occurs secondary to trauma, the latent interval between trauma and onset of symptoms may last from days to around a week. Focal signs such as hemiparesis may or may not be present. With progression, uncal herniation may occur, with the development of an ipsilateral third nerve palsy and hemiparesis.

Chronic subdural haematoma may be caused by trivial head injury and, indeed, anywhere from one-quarter to one-half of patients may not recall any head trauma. After a latent interval of months to years, patients gradually develop dementia, often accompanied by headache; personality change may occur;[128] rarely, chronic subdural haematoma may present with depression.[127] Focal signs such as hemiparesis may or may not be present; when present, they may be mild. Rarely, seizures may occur.

CT/MRI is diagnostic. In the case of acute and subacute haematomas, blood may be demonstrated for a week or two, after which, with haemolysis, a proteinaceous fluid remains. In chronic cases, the fluid has the same imaging characteristics as CSF. Most cases of subdural haematoma occur over the frontal or parietal convexities, and the haematoma itself has a convex shape; in a minority of patients, haematomas may also be found in the interhemispheric fissure or layering on top of the tentorium cerebelli.

Course

Acute subdural haematomas tend to enlarge rapidly and may become immediately life-threatening. Subacute subdural haematomas tend to evolve over a matter of weeks and may either progress to stupor or coma or may stabilize, after which there may be a greater or lesser degree of gradual improvement. Chronic subdural haematomas tend to undergo very gradual progression.

Aetiology and pathology

Most cases occur secondary to trauma, either a blow to the head or an acceleration–deceleration injury. This may be obvious and severe, for example in a motor vehicle accident; however, in elderly patients, the trauma need not be severe and indeed may appear trivial. Acute subdural haematomas generally occur secondary to arterial bleeding, which explains their rapid evolution and grave prognosis. Subacute and chronic subdural haematomas, however, typically appear secondary to venous bleeding owing to rupture of the delicate bridging veins that span from the surface of the cortex to the overlying dural sinuses. Regardless of the source of the bleeding, blood accumulates in the virtual space between the dura and the arachnoid. Haemolysis occurs and, within a week or two of the initial bleed, a relatively clear fluid remains. The further evolution may then take one of two paths. In cases in which the haematoma is relatively small, the fluid may simply be resorbed, with little in the way of anatomical sequelae. However, in cases of larger fluid collection, fibroblastic activity may either create a fibrotic scar that replaces the fluid, or one may see the creation of a pseudo-membrane that encapsulates the remaining fluid. The appearance of a pseudo-membrane sets the stage for the clinical occurrence of a chronic subdural haematoma. These encapsulated fluid collections tend to enlarge very gradually, probably as a result of bleeding from fragile capillaries found in the pseudo-membrane itself, which accounts for the gradual progression of symptoms.

Chronic subdural haematomas are more likely in patients who are prone to falls, such as those with alcoholism or epilepsy, and in those on anticoagulants or with blood dyscrasias. Old age also increases the risk of a chronic subdural haematoma, perhaps because normal atrophy with ageing leads to stretching of the bridging veins, making them more vulnerable to rupture.

Diffuse axonal injury

With a sudden and severe acceleration–deceleration injury, axons and arterioles are subjected to substantial shearing and rotational stresses, leading to widespread damage typically accompanied by other traumatic lesions such as contusions and intracerebral haemorrhages.

Clinical features

Typically, patients are rendered immediately unconscious at the moment of injury. Some may never regain consciousness; those that do may develop a persistent vegetative state or may emerge into delirium, which, upon clearing, typically leaves the patient with significant cognitive deficits, in some cases amounting to dementia.[129,130] Other sequelae may include agitation and personality change.

CT may demonstrate multiple petechial haemorrhages, typically in the centrum semiovale or corpus callosum; however, in many cases the scan may look unremarkable. MRI is more sensitive and typically displays multiple abnormalities in the centrum semiovale, corpus callosum, internal capsules, dorsolateral quadrants of the brainstem, and the superior cerebellar peduncles; gradient echo imaging enables identification of micro-haemorrhages.

Course

Most improvement is seen over the first 6 months post-injury, with some further, but less substantial, progress over the following 6 months. After a year, however, little further spontaneous improvement may be expected.

Aetiology and pathology

With either sudden impact or severe whiplash injury, the head undergoes an acceleration–deceleration injury and tremendous shearing and rotational forces are exerted intracranially, resulting in immediate damage to long axons and penetrating arterioles. Axons acutely display retraction balls and microglial clusters and, over time, microglial scars appear. Damage to arterioles leads to petechial haemorrhages of various sizes. Certain areas of the brain are more susceptible to such injuries, including the corpus callosum, the white matter of the centrum semiovale near the grey–white junction, the internal capsules, the dorsolateral quadrants of the brainstem, and the superior cerebellar peduncles.

Dementia pugilistica

This disorder is also known as punch-drunk syndrome, punch-drunkenness and chronic traumatic encephalopathy.

Clinical features

Onset of symptoms is gradual and occurs 5–40 years after there has been an accumulation of a sufficient number of blows to the head, which, in the case of professional boxers, equates to perhaps a dozen or so knockouts. Thus, in most cases, symptoms are delayed until long after the boxer has left the ring.

When the syndrome is fully developed, patients present with dementia, ataxia, some dysarthria and parkinsonism. The presence of ataxia and dysarthria often gives the impression of alcohol intoxication ('punch drunk'). The dementia is non-specific, except perhaps for an undue amount of irritability.

CT/MRI typically displays an enlarged cavum septi pellucidi, cerebral cortical atrophy and ventricular dilation.

Aetiology and pathology

The cause is repeated blows to the head. Although the disorder is found most commonly in boxers, other individuals may also be at risk, for example professional jockeys. The cavum septi pellucidi and ventricles are enlarged, and the cerebral cortex and cerebellum are atrophied. Microscopically, there are widespread neurofibrillary tangles, identical to those found in Alzheimer's disease. Neuritic (senile) plaques are also present; however, in contrast to Alzheimer's disease, they are diffuse. Cell loss occurs in the substantia nigra and locus coeruleus, but Lewy bodies are absent.

Post-concussion syndrome (post-concussional disorder)

Clinical features

Concussion may be associated with loss of consciousness that generally lasts only a minute or so; in other cases, patients may remain conscious but appear dazed and mildly confused, with these symptoms resolving quickly. The amnesia following concussion extends in a retrograde fashion for up to hours and in an anterograde fashion from minutes to, in rare cases, hours. In a very small minority of cases, concussion may be associated with a grand mal seizure occurring within seconds of the impact; also known as 'concussive convulsions', these events do not recur and do not portend the development of epilepsy. Although the grosser aspects of concussion clear immediately, there may be some subtle and mild difficulty with memory and concentration, which typically resolves gradually within a week;[131] in patients with a history of prior concussion, however, these symptoms may take longer to resolve.[132]

In a minority of patients, concussion may be followed by the post-concussion syndrome, in which, in addition to the above cognitive difficulties, other symptoms become evident within the first day and then persist. Headache tends to be severe and may be continuous or episodic; it may be dull and continuous, or throbbing, and may be exacerbated by loud noises, coughing or sneezing. Fatigue may be constant or may become evident only on exertion. Dizziness may consist of mere light-headedness, or there may be a true vertigo; when vertigo is present, patients may complain that it is exacerbated or precipitated by changes in position or by any sudden movements. Depression may occur and be marked by severe insomnia. Irritability may be prominent, and patients may complain of great difficulty controlling their temper. Less commonly, anxiety may also be seen. Other symptoms may occur, including photophobia, hyperacusis, and hyperhidrosis. Many patients report that alcohol exacerbates their symptoms.

Course

In most cases, a gradual remission of symptoms occurs from a few weeks up to 3 years after the concussion, with the majority of patients recovering in a matter of months. When symptoms persist for more than 3 years, a chronic, indefinite course may be anticipated.

Aetiology

Although concussion probably occurs secondary to a fully reversible disruption of axonal function, post-concussion syndrome probably occurs secondary to a mild degree of diffuse axonal injury, as indicated by MRI[133] and in one autopsy case of a patient with the syndrome who died 7 months after the concussion of an unrelated cause.[134]

HYPOXIC DISORDERS

Post-anoxic (post-hypoxic, post-ischaemic or ischaemic–hypoxic) encephalopathy

Clinical features

Among those patients who survive an ischaemic–hypoxic event and emerge from coma, some may be left in a persistent vegetative state; others emerge into a delirium of variable duration. After the delirium clears, some patients may recover entirely; however, most will be left with either dementia or amnesia. The dementia may or may not be accompanied by delusions and hallucinations; many patients will be restless, and in some cases there may be a significant degree of agitation. In some cases, rather than dementia, patients will be left with an isolated amnestic syndrome, with both anterograde and retrograde components.

Action (or intention) myoclonus may occur and may appear independently or in concert with dementia or amnesia. Parkinsonism, dystonia or athestosis (or a combination of these) may also appear.

MRI may reveal a variety of findings, including laminar cortical necrosis, watershed infarctions and abnormalities in the basal ganglia.

Course

Dementia and amnesia may show some improvement over the first 6 months or so, after which these features tend to remain stably chronic. Parkinsonism and dystonia may show gradual progression over many years.

Aetiology and pathology

Common causes include cardiac arrest, haemorrhagic or septic shock, carbon monoxide (CO) poisoning, strangulation and drowning. After 5 min or more of global ischaemia or anoxia, permanent damage occurs. In patients who develop post-anoxic encephalopathy, one finds cortical atrophy, ventricular dilation and, within the cerebral cortex, either a laminar or a multifocal pattern of cortical necrosis. In cases characterized by isolated amnesia, the temporal lobes, in particular the hippocampi, are heavily involved; in cases of parkinsonism or dystonia, the basal ganglia show similar changes. In some cases of global ischaemia, watershed infarctions may also occur.

Delayed post-anoxic leucoencephalopathy

This may occur in a small minority of those patients who make a more or less complete recovery after emergence from coma following a global hypoxic or ischaemic insult.

Clinical features

The lucid interval averages about 2–3 weeks, ranging from 2 days to 2 months. The onset of the encephalopathy is fairly sudden, occurring over a matter of a day or two, and patients generally present with a combination of delirium and a movement disorder. Confusion, amnesia, apathy, irritability and incontinence are prominent, and some patients may become mute. Parkinsonism is the most common movement disorder, but some patients may develop dystonia and some may experience a combination of both syndromes. Spasticity is common, with hyperreflexia and extensor plantar responses. Delirium may occasionally be absent and patients may present only with a movement disorder, such as parkinsonism, dystonia or chorea.

T2-weighted MRI reveals increased signal intensity in the white matter in patients with delirium; acutely, diffusion-weighted imaging (DWI) shows increased signal intensity in the same area. In patients with a movement disorder, T1-weighted scanning may reveal decreased signal intensity in the striatum.

Course

In a small minority of patients the course is fulminant, with coma and death. In most, however, the course is favourable, with patients experiencing a more or less complete recovery of cognitive abilities over 6–12 months, with only a minority being left with residual dementia. The movement disorder, however, may persist and in some cases may progressively worsen.

Pathology

At autopsy there is a massive, symmetrical, diffuse demyelination of the white matter, with variable involvement of the basal ganglia.

Carbon monoxide poisoning

Clinical features

The onset of intoxication may be gradual or sudden. Given that CO is colourless and odourless, victims may be unaware of their plight. In general, although the correlation between carboxyhaemoglobin level and clinical symptomatology is only a rough one, headache and delirium appear at a carboxyhaemoglobin level of 10–30 per cent, worsening and being joined by nausea and vomiting as the level rises to 40 per cent.[135] At levels of 40–50 per cent, stupor and ataxia appear, and cyanosis may be seen. When the level rises above 50 per cent, coma and convulsions occur. Levels over 60 per cent are often fatal. Although it is traditional to associate CO poisoning with a cherry-red discolouration of the lips, nails and skin, this is in fact rare; if anything, most patients display a degree of cyanosis.

In survivors, characteristic CT/MRI changes may be seen in the globus pallidus.

Course

In general, if intoxication ceases before the onset of stupor, recovery is typically complete within anywhere from hours to weeks.[136] If coma occurs, and even in some cases in which only delirium has occurred, a minority of patients may experience significant sequelae, such as post-anoxic encephalopathy or delayed post-anoxic encephalopathy.

Aetiology and pathology

CO poisoning may be accidental, as may occur with poorly ventilated gas, wood or charcoal stoves, or by suicidal intent, such as when patients hook a hose to the car exhaust and then funnel it into the tightly windowed car or simply leave the car running in an enclosed garage. The affinity of CO for haemoglobin is over 200 times greater than that of oxygen and, when a high fraction of haemoglobin exists as carboxyhaemoglobin, tissue anoxia supervenes. CO also binds to mitochondrial cytochrome oxidase, thereby impairing cellular respiration; furthermore, CO also binds to iron-rich CNS areas such as the globus pallidus and substantia nigra. In fatal cases, widespread petechial haemorrhages are found throughout the cerebrum.

NUTRITIONAL, TOXIC AND METABOLIC DISORDERS

Wernicke's encephalopathy and Korsakoff's psychosis are considered in Chapter 69.

Vitamin B12 deficiency

Clinical features

Symptoms referable to the cerebrum or spinal cord tend to appear subacutely over weeks or months.

Cerebral involvement manifests most commonly with dementia, which may be marked by hallucinations and delusions.[137] Personality change may also occur, and, rarely, depression[138] or mania.[139] Another rare manifestation is psychosis ('megaloblastic madness'): in one case, a 46-year-old woman developed delusions of persecution and jealousy and was correctly diagnosed only when symptoms of subacute combined degeneration became evident;[140] in another case, a 47-year-old woman became withdrawn, guarded and suspicious, heard the voice of God commanding her to board a spaceship, and prayed fervently, with all symptoms resolving upon vitamin B12 (cobalamin) administration.[141]

Subacute combined degeneration reflects demyelination of the peripheral nerves, posterior columns and lateral corticospinal tracts. Patients present with acral paraesthesiae, followed by ataxia, a positive Romberg test and eventually spasticity. The plantar responses are generally extensor, but the deep tendon reflexes may be either increased or depressed, depending on the peripheral neuropathy severity.

Macrocytosis, with or without anaemia, is common; however, both of these findings may be absent. Indeed, in one large study, both the red blood cell count and the mean corpuscular volume were normal in approximately one-fifth of patients.[142]

MRI reveals patchy, confluent areas of increased signal intensity in the centrum semiovale in patients with cerebral symptomatology, while electroencephalography (EEG) may show generalized slowing.

It is customary to obtain a serum B12 level; it is also appropriate to obtain levels of methylmalonic acid and homocysteine. In B12 deficiency, both methylmalonic acid and homocysteine levels are elevated, and this combination of findings is extremely sensitive and specific for B12 deficiency;[142] when the serum B12 level is borderline, these two findings should be relied on when deciding whether intracellular B12 deficiency is present.

Course

Most cases are gradually progressive.

Aetiology and pathology

The most common cause of vitamin B12 deficiency is pernicious anaemia; anti-parietal cell antibodies lead to destruction of gastric parietal cells, with a consequent lack of intrinsic factor and deficient uptake of ingested B12 by ileal cells. Most patients also have anti-intrinsic factor antibodies. Other antibodies may also be present, including antibodies against the thyroid and adrenal/suprarenal gland, and patients may develop Hashimoto's thyroiditis with hypothyroidism, or adrenocortical insufficiency.

Other causes of B12 deficiency include strict vegetarianism, severe malnutrition (e.g. in patients with chronic alcoholism), total or partial gastrectomy, inherited abnormalities of the R binder or intrinsic factor, achlorhydria, pancreatic insufficiency, steatorrhoea or malabsorption of any cause, tapeworm infestation, bacterial overgrowth (e.g. after a Billroth II operation), ileal diseases (e.g. Crohn's disease), ileal resection, and chronic treatment with omeprazole or metformin. All of these causes lead to intracellular B12 deficiency because of a failure of B12 absorption and are associated with decreased serum B12 levels. There are also some very rare diseases characterized by intracellular B12 deficiency or malutilization; in these disorders, the serum B12 level will be normal, but with elevated serum methylmalonic acid and homocysteine levels. Examples include inherited abnormalities in transcobalamin II and abnormalities in the intracellular metabolism of cobalamin. There may also be an association between acquired immunodeficiency syndrome (AIDS) and B12 deficiency.

Clinical B12 deficiency can be precipitated by inhalation of nitrous oxide, for example during dental procedures or in drug abusers. In cases in which there is already a subclinical B12 deficiency, nitrous oxide inhalation can acutely precipitate symptoms; in other cases, for example in young, well-nourished drug abusers, symptoms may not occur until nitrous oxide has been abused for a long time.

When B12 deficiency has been confirmed by elevated methylmalonic acid and homocysteine levels, efforts should be made to determine the cause of this deficiency. Given that pernicious anaemia is the most common cause, all patients should be tested for anti-parietal cell and anti-intrinsic factor antibodies. If these are absent, then the other causes noted above should be considered.

Neuropathologically, demyelination is seen within the centrum semiovale and in the posterior columns and lateral corticospinal tracts.

Folate deficiency

Clinical features

Reynolds and colleagues demonstrated an association of folate deficiency with dementia,[143] and Strachan and Henderson described two convincing cases of dementia secondary to folate deficiency, one occurring in combination with a peripheral neuropathy and the other without any other symptoms.[144] Folate deficiency is also a cause of megaloblastic anaemia. The serum homocysteine level is elevated.

Course

It appears that, in the absence of treatment, the course is progressive.

Aetiology

Folate is needed in DNA biosynthesis and is found in fresh green vegetables, some fruits, yeast, kidney and liver. Dietary deficiency, as in chronic alcoholism, is the most common cause of deficiency; intestinal malabsorption (e.g. in sprue) may also be a factor. Given the limited hepatic storage of folic acid, symptoms of deficiency may appear within a few months of poor oral intake or malabsorption. Medicines that reduce folate levels include oral contraceptives, phenytoin, primidone, phenobarbital, carbamazepine, pyrimethamine, trimethoprim, pentamidine, sulfasalazine and methotrexate. Marginal folic acid reserves may be depleted rapidly in conditions of increased metabolic demand, for example during pregnancy and lactation, and during the reticulocytosis seen with treatment of vitamin B12-induced anaemia.

Pellagra

This may occur clinically, as either acute (encephalopathic) or chronic pellagra.

Clinical features

Encephalopathic pellagra presents fairly acutely, over days to a week. When fully developed, it is characterized by delirium, dysarthria, cogwheel rigidity, gegenhalten and myoclonus.[145–147]

Pellagra of gradual onset appears insidiously over many months. When fully developed, it is characterized by dementia, dermatitis and diarrhoea ('3 Ds').[148] The dementia may present with apathy, depression or anxiety; however, over time, typical cognitive deficits, such as decreased memory and poor concentration, eventually appear. The dementia at times may also be marked by delusions or hallucinations.[149] The dermatitis is characterized initially by erythematous lesions in sun-exposed areas. Eventually, the skin becomes hyperpigmented and roughened, and it is from the Italian for 'rough' (*pelle*) 'skin' (*agra*) that the disease gains its name. Diarrhoea may be severe and the fluid blood-tinged. Most cases of pellagra do not, however, present with the full '3 Ds': some patients with pellagrous dementia may have only one of the other 'Ds', and in some cases there may only be dementia, without any rash or diarrhoea.

EEG shows generalized slowing.

Although the serum niacin level is low, a more reliable test is a 24-h urine test for niacin metabolites.

Course

The encephalopathic form may be rapidly progressive, and coma and death may occur in a matter of weeks. The chronic form pursues a slower course, with death in a matter of years.

Aetiology and pathology

Niacin deficiency occurs most commonly as a result of dietary deficiency. In developed countries, this is seen primarily in malnourished patients with alcoholism as the encephalopathic form. The chronic form was endemic in the American south among people subsisting primarily on corn. As corn contains niacin in a bound, biologically less active form, and also lacks tryptophan, these individuals very gradually became niacin-deficient. Since the introduction of corn flour enriched with niacin, the chronic form of pellagra has almost disappeared in the USA. Other causes of niacin deficiency include bowel resection, Crohn's disease and anorexia nervosa.

Pellagra has also been noted in conditions in which the normal endogenous conversion of tryptophan to niacin is impaired, for example following isoniazid treatment. The normal enzymatic conversion of tryptophan to niacin is dependent on the activated form of pyridoxine (vitamin B6); isoniazid impairs the conversion of the inactive form of B6 to the active form and by this indirect mechanism reduces the endogenous production of niacin. Another example is in cases of carcinoid tumour, in which the gross overutilization of tryptophan by the tumour leaves less available for conversion to niacin.

Within the CNS, neurons are swollen and display chromatolysis, with eccentric nuclei and a loss of Nissl substance, seen particularly in neurons of the pontine nuclei, cerebellar dentate nuclei, cerebral cortex, basal ganglia and anterior horn of the spinal cord.

Manganism

Clinical features

The onset of symptoms is typically gradual, occurring after months or years of exposure to manganese. Patients may present with personality change or parkinsonism, or both.[150]

The personality change[150,151] typically consists of asthenia, fatigue, irritability, emotional lability, and a peculiar kind of 'incongruous' laughter, reminiscent of the emotional incontinence seen in pseudo-bulbar palsy: patients may smile without cause, or burst out in laughter, again for no apparent reason.[152] Insomnia or hypersomnia may accompany these changes.

The parkinsonism is characterized by rigidity, bradykinesia, postural instability, and a tendency to 'freeze' and fall upon turning. Cogwheeling is often seen and, although tremor may also be present, it is generally not of the 'pill-rolling' type. The parkinsonism may also be accompanied by dystonia, often affecting the cervical musculature or face. The most characteristic feature is a distinctive dystonic gait abnormality known as 'cock-walk': patients walk on their metatarsophalangeal joints as if they were wearing high heels; at times, the elbows may be flexed, creating the overall appearance of the walk of a rooster.

Dementia may occur concurrent with the parkinsonism and may be characterized by a marked degree of memory loss.[151]

Psychosis ('manganese madness') may occur and is characterized by excitation, hallucinations and delusions.[150]

T1-weighted MRI may reveal increased signal intensity within the globus pallidus bilaterally. Manganese levels are increased in the serum, hair or 24-h urine sample.

Course

With ongoing exposure, symptoms gradually worsen. With cessation of exposure, however, rather than a gradual reduction of parkinsonian signs and symptoms, these actually continue gradually to worsen over the next 10 years or so,[153,154] after which they persist in a stable chronicity.[155] A similar progression has been noted for the 'cock-walk'.[156]

Aetiology and pathology

Most cases of chronic manganese exposure result from inhalation among manganese miners and people who work in steel or battery factories. Cases have also been reported secondary to drinking contaminated well water or, very rarely, to prolonged intravenous total parenteral nutrition with manganese-containing solutions.

Neuronal loss and gliosis, although most prominent in the globus pallidus, are also found in the putamen, pars reticulata of the substantia nigra, thalamus, hypothalamus and cerebral cortex.

Intoxication with other metals

Thallium intoxication

Although thallium can be absorbed through either the lungs or the skin, industrial exposure is rare and most cases of thallium intoxication are by ingestion. Since thallium was banned as a rodenticide, current cases generally represent a deliberate, often homicidal, poisoning.

Acute intoxication generally presents with abdominal pain, vomiting and diarrhoea. Within days or a week or so, patients develop delirium and painful peripheral sensorimotor polyneuropathy, which may progress to quadriplegia. Cranial neuropathies, with facial palsy or ophthalmoplegia, may also develop; rarely, grand mal seizures may occur. Within 1–3 weeks, patients develop severe, generalized alopecia.

Gradual intoxication presents with dementia, sensorimotor polyneuropathy and alopecia.

Thallium may be found in the urine and serum and, in long-standing cases, the hair.

Acute intoxication may be fatal in up to one-tenth of cases. In survivors, there is a gradual, more or less complete recovery; in some cases there may be persistent cognitive deficits (which may be severe enough to produce dementia) or personality change.

Arsenic intoxication

Although elemental arsenic causes relatively little CNS toxicity, arsenic salts are toxic. Arsenic salts are found in certain herbicides and rodenticides, and ingestion may occur accidentally or with suicidal or homicidal intent.

Acute ingestion is followed rapidly by delirium, nausea, vomiting and diarrhoea, which may be bloody; convulsions may also occur. Classically there is an odour of garlic on the breath. Arrhythmias, renal failure and hypotension may occur. Within 1–3 weeks, painful peripheral sensorimotor polyneuropathy appears.

Chronic exposure to small amounts of arsenic salts may cause both dementia and polyneuropathy. Hyperkeratosis of the palms and soles may occur, and Mees' lines – transverse white discolouration of the nails – may appear. Occasionally there is mild alopecia.

Arsenic may be found in a 24-h urine sample and, within weeks of exposure, is also found in the hair and nails.

Bismuth intoxication

Bismuth is found in a number of preparations and is used for the control of diarrhoea and in the treatment of *Helicobacter pylori* infection.

The onset may be gradual or acute, depending on the dosage. Gradual onset is marked by insomnia and mood changes, with depression, irritability or, uncommonly, euphoria; rarely, delusions or hallucinations may occur. With high dosage, there may be an acute onset of delirium, accompanied by myoclonus, ataxia and, in a minority of patients, seizures.

CT may reveal patchy areas of cortical radiolucency in the cortex.

Tin intoxication

Exposure to tin compounds may occur in certain industries or by ingestion.

Delirium and seizures have been reported after intoxication with trimethyltin and triethyltin. With phenyltin ingestion, delirium and ataxia occur.

Although most patients survive trimethyltin intoxication, the mortality rate after triethyltin intoxication is approximately 50 per cent. Among patients who survive tin intoxication, residual symptoms are common and may be severe.

Lead encephalopathy

Toxic accumulations of lead may occur in a number of ways. Children may eat lead-based paint chips. Among adults, exposure may occur in certain occupations, for example in welders and in people who work in battery factories or lead smelters; 'moonshine' whiskey, made with the help of old car radiators, may also be a source. Other less common sources include lead-glazed pottery, certain alternative medications and retained bullets. Leaded petrol (gasoline) used to be a major source, but since lead additives were banned this has essentially ceased to be a problem.

In children, acute lead encephalopathy may be preceded by a prodrome of irritability, abdominal pain and lethargy that lasts for weeks. In both children and adults, the full syndrome is marked by delirium, which may be accompanied by excitation, hallucinations, delusions, ataxia and seizures; classically, patients complain of a metallic taste in the mouth. Haemolysis and renal failure may occur.

Chronic lead encephalopathy in children may present with very gradual cognitive decline, which may range in severity from a drop of a few intelligence quotient (IQ) points to dementia. There is also an association between lead exposure and the development of a syndrome virtually identical to attention-deficit hyperactivity disorder (ADHD). Occasionally seizures may occur.

Chronic lead encephalopathy in adults may present with either personality change or dementia of variable severity; patients also may complain of colicky abdominal pain and a metallic taste in the mouth. In some cases, depressive symptoms may be seen. Motor peripheral neuropathy may occur, with, classically, wrist- and foot-drop.

Whole blood lead levels of over 80 µg/dL are associated with an acute presentation, whereas levels of 10–20 µg/dL, if chronically maintained, produce chronic encephalopathy. The zinc protoporphyrin level is also increased. In both children and adults, 'lead lines' may be seen at the border of the gingiva and teeth; in childhood cases, lead lines may also be seen in radiographs of the tibia or other long bones.

Acute lead encephalopathy runs a rapid course, with mortality rates approaching 25 per cent. Survivors may be left with dementia, seizures or spasticity. Chronic lead encephalopathy shows little improvement over time.

Mercury intoxication

Three forms of mercury are potentially toxic to humans, namely elemental mercury (e.g. in gold miners), salts of mercury (in people employed in the manufacture of plastics, fungicides and electronics), and organic mercury as methylmercury (e.g. from contaminated fish and contaminated seed grain), ethylmercury and phenylmercury.

With acute exposure to elemental mercury via inhalation, a pneumonitis may occur. Acute exposure to either mercury salts or to organic mercury may cause vomiting, which may be quite severe in the case of mercury salts and may also be accompanied by renal failure.

Among patients who survive the acute exposure, and in cases of chronic, low-level exposure, various sequelae may gradually ensue, including personality change, dementia and abnormal movements. The personality change, erethism, is classically characterized by emotional lability, shyness and anxiety, all of which may be accompanied by insomnia. The dementia occurs generally only with greater exposure. Of the abnormal movements, tremor is perhaps the most classic and may affect the hands, lips, and tongue. Ataxia is common and may be accompanied by an intention tremor and dysarthria. Choreoathetosis may occur, as may parkinsonian features. A sensorimotor polyneuropathy may also appear, which may be quite painful. Visual scotoma or tunnel vision may also occur.

Whole blood levels of mercury are elevated, but the correlation between blood levels and clinical symptomatology is rough at best. In chronic cases, neuroimaging may reveal atrophy of the cerebral cortex (most prominently the calcarine cortex) and the cerebellar cortex.

Pathologically, there is widespread neuronal loss throughout the cerebral and cerebellar cortex, especially involving the calcarine cortex and, in the cerebellum, the granule cell layer.

Dialysis dementia (progressive dialysis encephalopathy)

This dementia is caused by aluminium intoxication and used to occur with chronic haemodialysis. With the routine purification of the dialysate, this disorder has almost disappeared; occasional cases, however, still occur, for example with the use of aluminium-containing medications in patients with chronic renal failure who are not on haemodialysis.

The onset of dementia is gradual, occurring on average after 37–40 months of dialysis. Patients present with a peculiar stuttering type of aphasia, followed by myoclonus, seizures and dementia. In a minority of patients, psychotic symptoms may occur, with delusions, hallucinations and bizarre behaviour.

Hypoglycaemia

Clinical features

As the blood glucose level falls below 2.5 mmol/L (45 mg/dL), autonomic symptoms appear fairly promptly, including anxiety, palpitations, tremulousness and diaphoresis; patients may also complain of hunger, nausea, headache and generalized weakness.

Neuroglycopaenic symptoms are associated with blood glucose levels of 1.67 mmol/L (30 mg/dL) or lower[157,158] but, unlike the autonomic symptoms, tend to appear only after this degree of hypoglycaemia has been sustained for approximately 30 min. Initially, patients may experience light-headedness or depersonalization. Delirium is common and may be associated with unusual behaviour: in one case, the patient 'was restless, opening and closing his eyes, and thrashing about with his arms and legs, occasionally hitting onlookers and spitting in their faces';[159] in another case, the patient, a soldier, 'walked into the mess hall ... [dressed] in his underwear'.[160] Partial or grand mal seizures may occur. A very small minority of patients also have focal findings such as hemiplegia or aphasia. With sustained hypoglycaemia, coma may ensue.

Although in most cases neuroglycopaenic symptoms are preceded by autonomic symptoms, exceptions occur, and some patients may present with neuroglycopaenic symptoms alone.[158,161,162] This may occur in patients with diabetes who have developed a diabetic autonomic neuropathy or in patients being treated with beta-blockers, which mask autonomic symptoms. Such a scenario may also occur in patients in which the blood glucose level drops very slowly, for example as may occur with fasting.

Course

Whereas autonomic symptoms respond promptly to glucose treatment, delirium may take up to an hour to subside. Patients who have developed coma may not recover consciousness and those who do may be left with dementia. In cases characterized by a residual dementia, a greater or lesser degree of recovery may occur over the following year or two.

Aetiology

Symptomatic hypoglycaemia may occur in the fasting state, for example early in the morning before breakfast or in people who skip meals, or postprandially, several hours after a meal. Fasting hypoglycaemia is seen most commonly in people with diabetes on insulin or oral antidiabetic agents; it may also occur in patients with insulinomas or in those who undertake a prolonged fast, for example during a hunger strike or in patients with anorexia nervosa.[163] Liver disease, by impairing gluconeogenesis, may also set the stage for fasting hypoglycaemia. Gluconeogenesis is also inhibited by alcohol and, after a bout of binge drinking when little food is consumed, hypoglycaemia is common. Postprandial hypoglycaemia may be seen in early type II diabetes; after vagotomy, gastrectomy, pyloroplasty or gastrojejunostomy; and rarely in functional or essential postprandial hypoglycaemia.

Hypoglycaemia may also be intentionally produced by malingerers who inject themselves with insulin or take high doses of oral antidiabetic agents. Whenever this is suspected, as well as checking the glucose level, one should also determine the insulin and C-peptide levels and obtain a toxicology screen for oral agents.

Central pontine myelinolysis

Originally described by Adams and Foley in 1953, this disorder is classically characterized clinically by the development of a combination of flaccid quadriplegia and delirium, and pathologically by demyelination in the central portion of the pons, all occurring within 2–3 days of overly rapid correction of chronic hyponatraemia.[164] Exceptions to this classic picture do occur, with prominent demyelination in extrapontine sites associated with movement disorders or delirium in the absence of quadriplegia. The existence of these exceptions has led some authors to propose the alternative names 'central pontine and extrapontine myelinolysis' or, more generally, 'osmotic demyelination syndrome'.

Uraemia

Clinical features

When caused by severe renal failure, the onset reflects the rapidity with which the kidneys fail, and hence the onset of uraemic encephalopathy may range from acute to gradual. Patients may initially experience some lassitude or a mild degree of somnolence; however, eventually delirium appears that is often marked by visual hallucinations. Asterixis and multifocal myoclonus are common, and in some cases one may see diffuse multifocal muscle twitching; dysarthria may also occur. In a minority of patients, seizures, typically grand mal, may appear. In one rare case, uraemia presented with only mania.[165]

A sensorimotor polyneuropathy may occur and may be acute or gradual in onset; the motor component may be severe and patients may become quadriparetic. In a little under 50 per cent of patients with a polyneuropathy, there may be prominent dysaesthesiae and restlessness, similar to that seen in the restless legs syndrome.

The severity of the encephalopathy correlates with the level of blood urea nitrogen (BUN) and also with the rapidity with which the BUN rises. For example, although in cases of acute renal failure levels of 35.7 mmol/L (100 mg/dL) are typically associated with delirium, in renal failure of very gradual onset levels of 71.4 mmol/L (200 mg/dL) may be tolerated with few if any symptoms.

The EEG typically shows generalized slowing; triphasic waves may also be seen.

Course

Typically the symptoms of delirium show marked fluctuations throughout the day. The overall course parallels that of the renal failure, and in some progressive cases coma may ensue.

Aetiology and pathology

Urea itself is not the cause of the CNS dysfunction, and the delirium probably results from an 'auto-intoxication' by as yet unidentified substances. In chronic cases that come to autopsy, an excess of protoplasmic astrocytes has been found.

Hepatic encephalopathy

Clinical features

Acute-onset cases typically present with delirium. In gradual-onset cases, although delirium eventually occurs, it is often preceded by a prodrome characterized by impaired judgement, difficulty with abstracting, and mood changes, often tending toward euphoria. The delirium is characterized by confusion, drowsiness, sleep reversal, asterixis and myoclonus.[164,166–168] A small minority of patients may have seizures, which may be partial or grand mal, and a minority may also have focal signs such as hemiparesis. Rarely, catatonic symptoms such as waxy flexibility may occur.[169] Fetor hepaticus occurs in about half of cases. With progression of hepatic failure, stupor and coma may occur, accompanied by rigidity and bilateral Babinski signs.

The EEG shows generalized slowing, often accompanied by triphasic waves; interictal epileptiform discharges may occasionally be seen.[170]

Although the blood ammonia level is elevated in most cases, there is only a rough correlation between the degree of elevation and the severity of the encephalopathy.

Course

Without treatment, the course mirrors the severity of the underlying hepatic failure. With treatment, provided that coma has not supervened, recovery is generally good; in cases that have progressed to coma, the mortality rate is high.

With repeated episodes, patients may develop acquired hepatocerebral degeneration (see below).

Aetiology and pathology

With significant disease or dysfunction of hepatocytes, or with significant shunting of blood past the liver and directly into the systemic circulation, toxins normally removed by the liver reach the brain. In chronic cases, there may be an increased number of Alzheimer type II astrocytes. In acute cases characterized by coma, cerebral oedema occurs, sometimes with transtentorial herniation.

The most common causes of hepatic failure are viral hepatitis and alcoholic cirrhosis. Often the onset of delirium may be traced to an event that increased the nitrogenous load in the gut beyond the diminished detoxifying capacity of the liver. Examples include high-protein meals, blood (as may occur with bleeding oesophageal varices or peptic ulcer disease), constipation, infection, anaesthesia, hypokalaemia, uraemia, and exposure to alcohol or sedative-hypnotics, especially benzodiazepines.

Acquired hepatocerebral degeneration

Clinical features

The onset is typically gradual and often punctuated by repeated episodes of hepatic encephalopathy. Cognitive deficits may occur and range from mild to dementia. The movement disorder is often complex, with variable admixtures of chorea, facial grimacing, postural tremor, parkinsonism and ataxia. Chorea, when present, often affects the head and neck, and the resulting movements may be tic-like in character.

T1-weighted MRI typically reveals increased signal intensity in the globus pallidus; similar changes may be seen in the striatum and in the substantia nigra.

Course

In general, the overall course is marked by slow progression.

Aetiology and pathology

This rare disorder occurs secondary to repeated or prolonged bouts of hepatic encephalopathy.

At autopsy, spongiform change or laminar cortical necrosis may be found in the cerebral and cerebellar cortices; spongiform change is also noted in the basal ganglia, and this may be accompanied by microcavitation. Alzheimer type II astrocytes are present in the cortex and basal ganglia.

Hepatic porphyria

Of the hepatic porphyrias, four can cause delirium. Acute intermittent porphyria is found worldwide and may have a prevalence as high as 5–10 cases per 100 000. Variegate porphyria may be found in Sweden and among white people in South Africa. Hereditary coproporphyria is rare and delta-aminolaevulinic acid (ALA) dehydratase deficiency extremely rare.

From a clinical viewpoint, the first three hepatic porphyrias are essentially the same, with the exception that both variegate porphyria and hereditary coproporphyria may cause a photosensitive rash, a symptom not seen in acute intermittent porphyria.

Of interest, it appears that the periodic 'madness' of King George III represented attacks of hepatic porphyria.

Clinical features of the first three porphyrias

These are episodic disorders; the first episode usually appears in late adolescence or early adulthood. The attacks tend to present fairly acutely and are often precipitated by one of the factors mentioned below.

Classically, episodes are characterized by abdominal pain with vomiting, constipation or diarrhoea, accompanied, in about half of cases, by delirium, which is often marked by affective lability, delusions of persecution and visual hallucinations, which may be quite compelling;[171,172] in some cases, stupor or coma may supervene. Uncommonly, rather than delirium there may be psychosis with auditory hallucinations, delusions of persecution and bizarre behaviour, all occurring in a clear sensorium without confusion or cognitive deficits.[173,174] Other symptoms, seen in a minority of patients, include a primarily motor polyneuropathy (which may progress to quadriparesis), cranial neuropathy (most commonly with ophthalmoplegia or facial palsy), partial or grand mal seizures, hypertension, tachycardia and fever. A small minority of patients may also have significant hyponatraemia, which in turn may form a syndrome of inappropriate antidiuretic hormone (ADH) secretion or intestinal or renal sodium loss.

T2-weighted MRI may reveal scattered areas of increased signal intensity within the subcortical white matter.

During episodes, a 24-h urine test shows elevated levels of porphobilinogen and ALA in all three of these porphyrias. In addition, patients with variegate porphyria and hereditary coproporphyria also display elevated urinary coproporphyrin; distinguishing between these two requires a 24-h stool collection for protoporphyrin and coproporphyrin. In variegate porphyria, protoporphyrin levels are higher than those of coproporphyrin; in hereditary coproporphyria, the converse holds true. Importantly, in between episodes all these measurements may be normal.

Course

The duration of episodes usually ranges from days to weeks. Although most patients recover completely, death may occur as a result of respiratory failure owing to motor neuropathy or an arrhythmia. Repeat episodes are common and typically occur in response to a specific precipitating factor.

Aetiology

The first three porphyrias are inherited in an autosomal dominant pattern; acute intermittent porphyria occurs secondary to mutations in the gene for porphobilinogen deaminase (chromosome 11); variegate porphyria to mutations in the gene for protoporphyrinogen oxidase (chromosome 1); and hereditary coproporphyria to mutations in the gene for coproporphyrinogen oxidase (chromosome 3). When the haem biosynthetic pathway becomes stressed in the presence of these mutated proteins, upstream proteins accumulate and an episode occurs. The fourth porphyria, ALA dehydratase deficiency, is an autosomal recessive disorder.

Precipitating factors include infection, menstruation, pregnancy, fasting (or a low-carbohydrate diet), surgery, and many drugs, including barbiturates, phenytoin, valproic acid, carbamazepine, nortriptyline, sulphonamides, griseofulvin, meprobamate, ergot derivatives, synthetic oestrogens and progestins, danazol, alpha-methyldopa, chlorpropamide and alcohol. Importantly, the following drugs appear to be safe: phenothiazines, opioid analgesics, chloral hydrate, gabapentin, levetiracetam, diazepam, diphenhydramine, aspirin and paracetamol (acetaminophen).

Fahr's syndrome (idiopathic striopallidodentate calcinosis, idiopathic calcification of the basal ganglia)

Clinical features

The presentation is generally gradual and may be characterized by either a movement disorder or a neuropsychiatric syndrome. Over long-term follow-up, most patients display a combination of these symptoms.

Of the movement disorders seen, the most common is parkinsonism; choreoathetosis or dystonia may also occur, and in a small minority of patients there may be ataxia or dysarthria.

Neuropsychiatric syndromes most commonly include

dementia.[175–177] Personality change, which may be of the frontal lobe type,[178,179] may also occur. Psychosis, similar to that of schizophrenia,[180,181] has been reported, especially in elderly patients.[182] Other presentations include depression or mania[183] and obsessions and compulsions.[184] Seizures have also been noted.

CT displays bilateral basal ganglia calcification. One also sees bilateral calcification in other structures, such as the dentate nuclei, the thalamus and the grey–white junction of the cerebral and cerebellar cortices.

Aetiology

The calcification may either be secondary to some other disorder, such as hypoparathyroidism, or occur on a primary basis as an idiopathic or inherited disorder, in which case one speaks of 'Fahr's disease'.

INFECTIOUS AND RELATED DISORDERS

The neurological and psychiatric sequelae of AIDS are considered in Chapters 36 and 49.

Cytomegalovirus encephalitis

The great majority of adults show evidence of prior infection with cytomegalovirus (CMV). In immunocompromised patients, for example those with AIDS or those undergoing transplantation, the virus may reactivate and, among other syndromes, produce delirium. Autopsy studies have demonstrated evidence of CMV infection of the CNS in approximately one-third of patients with AIDS, making it one of the most common opportunistic infections seen in this condition. The delirium typically presents subacutely and is of variable severity; in some cases, however, the onset may be fulminant and the delirium quite severe, and in such cases there are often signs of brainstem involvement, such as nystagmus, ophthalmoplegia and ataxia. Some patients may also have cord involvement or a peripheral neuropathy.

Progressive multifocal leucoencephalopathy

In almost all cases patients have depressed cell-mediated immunity, most commonly owing to AIDS, in which 2–5 per cent of patients are afflicted.

Clinical features

The onset is typically subacute, generally over approximately 2 weeks. In most cases, patients present with a slowly progressive focal sign, such as hemianopia, aphasia, apraxia, hemisensory loss or hemiplegia; rarer focal findings such as Balint's syndrome have also been reported. Over time, these initially unilateral deficits become bilateral, and many patients then go on to develop personality change, dementia or, rarely, delirium. Seizures may occur in up to 20 per cent of patients and may be simple partial, complex partial or grand mal. Rarely, the disorder may present with dementia,[185,186] delirium[187] or personality change.[188] Cerebellar signs are uncommon. Other rare signs include quadriparesis secondary to brainstem involvement, dystonia, chorea and parkinsonism.

The EEG may show diffuse or focal slowing.

MRI reveals one or more focal lesions, generally in the subcortical white matter (signal intensity decreased on T1 and increased on FLAIR).

The CSF, although characteristically normal, may occasionally reveal a mild lymphocytic pleocytosis. The polymerase chain reaction (PCR) assay for JC virus is generally, but not always, positive. Serum testing for antibodies to JC virus is not helpful, given that most adults will be positive. In doubtful cases, brain biopsy may be required.

Course

The disorder is generally relentlessly progressive, with death occurring after about 4 months on average. Rarely, the course may stretch out for years; even more rarely, there may be spontaneous remissions

Aetiology

The disorder occurs secondary to a CNS opportunistic infection by the JC virus. Approximately 80 per cent of the adult US population have latent JC virus infection. In a very small minority of patients with depressed cell-mediated immunity, this virus reactivates and spreads to the brain. Although the most common cause of immunoincompetence in these patients is AIDS, progressive multifocal leucoencephalopathy has also been noted in Hodgkin's disease, other lymphomas, leukaemia, other cancers, tuberculosis, sarcoidosis, systemic lupus erythematosus (SLE), post-transplantation therapeutic immunosuppression and natalizumab pharmacotherapy. Very rarely, it may occur in otherwise healthy individuals.

Pathology

Within the CNS, oligodendrocytes and, to a lesser degree, astrocytes are infected by the JC virus. With destruction of oligodendrocytes, demyelination with only relative axonal sparing occurs and foci of demyelination begin to appear. Within and surrounding these foci there is a variable, and typically slight, degree of inflammation. At least initially, these foci are generally few in number and confined to one hemisphere; most commonly, they are seen in the subcortical white matter and the centrum semiovale; however, rarely, they may be prominent in the cerebellar white matter or the brainstem. Over time, the foci increase in size and number, and bilateral involvement occurs.

Herpes simplex encephalitis

Clinical features

Herpes simplex encephalitis can occur at any age, but most patients are middle-aged or older. The onset generally spans several days; however, the range is wide, from explosive onsets over several hours to gradual onsets lasting weeks or more. In some cases the onset may be preceded be a prodrome, lasting several days, of malaise, headache, irritability and mild fever.

Typically, patients present with fever, headache and delirium. Most also develop focal signs, such as hemiparesis or aphasia, and approximately two-thirds have complex partial or grand mal seizures. Although meningeal signs, such as a stiff neck or photophobia, are common, they are generally not severe. Notably, bizarre behaviour is common and, although this usually occurs in the context of the delirium, there are rare reports of the encephalitis presenting with either mania[189] or psychosis.[190] Untreated, coma develops in about one-third of patients.

CT scanning may show radiolucent areas in the medial aspects of one or both temporal lobes, but it may be normal for up to a week. MRI is much more sensitive, showing increased medial temporal lobe signal intensity on FLAIR or T2-weighted scanning, although this too may be normal for the first few days. DWI may show increased signal intensity in the same regions, which may be evident earlier than that seen on T2-weighted or FLAIR imaging. Gadolinium enhancement may also occur.

The EEG is usually normal for the first few days but will eventually show delta slowing in one temporal area, which may be accompanied by periodic complexes;[191] with progression of the disease, bilateral involvement may be seen.

PCR assay of the CSF is almost 100 per cent sensitive for herpes simplex DNA and is the diagnostic procedure of choice. The CSF itself may be normal during the first few days but will in most cases show an elevated total protein with a lymphocytic and polymorphonuclear pleocytosis; red cells may also be present, reflecting the haemorrhagic nature of the inflammatory process. Although the glucose level is typically normal, it may rarely be reduced.

If lumbar puncture is not possible, brain biopsy may be necessary in order to make a definitive diagnosis; however, treatment should rarely await such a procedure.

Course

Untreated, over 50 per cent of patients die within days or a few weeks. In survivors, the clinical picture usually stabilizes in a matter of weeks; exceptionally, the acute illness may be prolonged for months or even longer.

Although most patients have only one episode, recurrences may occur occasionally.

Among survivors, the vast majority are left with significant sequelae, most commonly a chronic amnestic syndrome, dementia or personality change. Other sequelae include focal signs (e.g. aphasia, hemiplegia) or epilepsy; rarely, there may be a Kluver–Bucy syndrome. There is also a case report in which complex motor and vocal tics occurred.[192]

Aetiology

Although most cases are caused by type 1 herpes simplex virus (which usually causes orolabial infections), type 2 virus may be causative in a small minority. Most adults have at some time been infected with herpes simplex type 1, and the virus may remain in a latent state in various sites, including the trigeminal ganglion.

Pathology

There is intense inflammation (which may progress to haemorrhagic necrosis) affecting initially the medial portions of the temporal lobe, with, in most cases, eventual spread to other regions, including the lateral aspects of the temporal lobe, insula, inferior portions of the frontal lobes, and cingulate cortex. Although involvement is typically unilateral early on, with time both temporal lobes become involved. There may be substantial oedema, and both uncal and subfalcine herniation may occur. In survivors, scarring, cavitation and cystic change are seen in affected regions.

Encephalitis lethargica

Also known as von Economo's disease and European sleeping sickness, this was first described by Baron Constantin von Economo at a meeting of the Vienna Psychiatric Society in 1917. It swept the world in an epidemic during 1917–28, and sporadic cases still occur.

Clinical features

Acute encephalitis lethargica is characterized by headache, fever, sleep reversal (nocturnal wakefulness and diurnal somnolence), delirium, various oculomotor pareses and, classically, oculogyric crises; some patients also display euphoria, psychosis or stuporous catatonia.

The CSF may be normal or may reveal a lymphocytic pleocytosis and an elevated total protein; oligoclonal bands may also be present.

Course

The mortality rate for acute encephalitis was about 25 per cent; among survivors, the encephalitis gradually cleared over about a month.

Post-encephalitic parkinsonism occurred in over 50 per cent of survivors after a latent interval of 1–20 years. Patients gradually developed a syndrome similar to that seen in idiopathic Parkinson's disease. In addition, other motor abnormalities, including dystonia, blepharospasm and oculogyric crises, were often present. Interestingly, these transient oculogyric crises could also be accompanied by classic obsessions or compulsions; in some cases, palilalia or agitation and excitation were noted to accompany the oculogyric crises. Oculogyric crises, although most commonly seen in conjunction with post-encephalitic parkinsonism, at times occurred independently.

Other sequelae, seen in a minority of patients, included dementia, narcoleptic and cataplectic attacks and, in children, restlessness and inattentiveness.

Pathology and aetiology

Autopsies of patients dying in the acute stage revealed inflammation with a perivascular accumulation of lymphocytes and plasma cells in the midbrain, basal ganglia, and cortex. In patients with sequelae, autopsy studies have revealed neuronal loss, gliosis and, in the remaining neurons, neurofibrillary tangles similar to those of Alzheimer's disease, in the substantia nigra, locus coeruleus, hippocampus, basal ganglia, thalamus and cerebral cortex. Macroscopically, there was cortical atrophy and depigmentation of the substantia nigra and locus coeruleus.

Given that the pandemic of encephalitis lethargica coincided with the Spanish influenza epidemic, it was long suspected that encephalitis lethargica was secondary to influenza. Work on archived specimens, however, has failed to find any evidence of influenza RNA.[193]

Infectious mononucleosis

In about 5 per cent of cases of infectious mononucleosis, the central or peripheral nervous system may be involved, producing, variously, delirium, seizures, meningismus, ataxia, a cord syndrome, or a cranial or peripheral neuropathy. The disorder is caused by the Epstein–Barr virus and is transmitted primarily via oral secretions passed during intimate contact such as kissing. The virus gains access to the bloodstream and infects lymphocytes, spreading later to various other organs, including the brain. Although mononucleosis may occur in adults, it is most commonly seen in children and adolescents. Typically there is a prodrome, lasting for 1–2 weeks, of fatigue, malaise and headache, after which one sees the classic development of sore throat, fever and cervical adenopathy; splenomegaly and hepatomegaly may also occur.

Rabies

Rabies typically occurs after a patient is bitten by a rabid animal, for example a dog, cat, wolf, fox, skunk, raccoon or vampire bat; cases have also been reported secondary to respiratory transmission in spelunkers within bat-infested caves and in a veterinarian who was working with the homogenized brain of a rabid animal; more recently, rabies has been reported secondary to solid-organ transplantation from a donor with an unsuspected case.[194] Although rabies is very rare in developed countries, it remains a significant problem in India and parts of Asia.

After the patient is bitten by an infected animal, there is a latent, asymptomatic period, generally of 1–3 months, with a range of weeks to a year or more; the duration of the latency appears related not only to the severity of the bite but also to the distance from the bitten area to the brain, with bites on the feet having the longest latency and facial bites the shortest.

With resolution of the latent interval, there is usually a prodrome, lasting days, characterized by headache and malaise; pain or paraesthesiae may also develop at the site of the original bite. Subsequently, the illness may evolve in one of two forms, namely furious rabies or dumb (or paralytic) rabies.

Furious rabies is seen in perhaps 80 per cent of cases and is characterized by restlessness, agitation, excitability, excessive startability and convulsions; delirium is typical, and patients may engage in bizarre behaviour, including biting. The combination of excessive salivation and dysphagia caused by pharyngeal spasm may literally cause the patient to foam at the mouth. Pharyngeal spasm may also be provoked by swallowing water or even by the sight of water, giving rise to the classic symptom of hydrophobia. Dumb rabies is characterized by a flaccid paralysis that typically begins in one limb and rapidly becomes generalized and symmetrical.

Subacute sclerosing panencephalitis

Subacute sclerosing panencephalitis (SSPE) occurs in 5–10 out of 1 000 000 people with a history of measles and in approximately 1 out of 1 000 000 people who receive the measles immunization. It is three to four times more common in males than females.

Clinical features

The vast majority of cases occur in children. In these cases, the average latency from the preceding infection or immunization is about 8 years and the average age of onset about 13 years. In adults, the latency ranges from 8 years to 33 years, and the average age of onset is in the early twenties.

The onset is generally gradual, even insidious, and typically the disease evolves through three stages. In the first stage, the patient may become restless, distractable and forgetful; irritability and moodiness may be noted. In some cases, particularly in those with adult-onset disease, this first stage may be characterized by a psychosis that may mimic schizophrenia, with delusions (including Schneiderian first-rank symptoms) and stuporous catatonia. In the second stage, dementia evolves, accompanied by myoclonus, ataxia and partial or grand mal seizures; abnormal involuntary movements such as chorea, athetosis or dystonia are occasionally seen at this point. In the third and final stage, there is stupor and generalized rigidity, and eventually coma. There are many exceptions to this typical picture. In some cases, the onset may be relatively fulminant, with severe symptomatology seen in a matter of months. Furthermore, there may be considerable overlap among the various stages.

MRI may reveal cortical atrophy and, on T2-weighted

imaging, multiple areas of increased signal intensity in the cerebral grey and white matter, with a predilection for the periventricular area.

The EEG in the second and third stages will display a classic burst-suppression pattern in the majority of cases.[195]

The CSF is generally acellular, with a mildly elevated total protein. The immunoglobulin G (IgG) level is increased, sometimes greatly so, oligoclonal bands may be found, and, most importantly, anti-measles antibodies are present.

Course

Although the course is variable, most patients pass through the three stages and die within 1–3 years. In fulminant cases, however, a fatal outcome may occur within several months. Occasionally the course is prolonged, up to a decade or more, and there may at times be periods of relative stability, lasting many years; however, these inevitably give way to further progression.

Aetiology

SSPE occurs secondary to a reactivation of a dormant measles virus that lacks a normal M-protein; rather than undergoing 'budding', these defective viruses spread by means of cell fusion within the CNS.

Pathology

There is widespread perivascular inflammation accompanied by patchy demyelination and neuronal loss. Within surviving neurons, inclusions are found within nuclei, which, by electron microscopy, appear similar to measles nucleocapsids.

General paresis of the insane

Details of neurosyphilis, including neurological symptomatology, are given in Chapter 36. General paresis of the insane (GPI; also known as dementia paralytica and paretic neurosyphilis) is not necessarily associated with meningovascular syphilis and, indeed, it may be the only manifestation of tertiary neurosyphilis. GPI typically manifests with dementia of gradual onset and slow progression. Although the dementia may be non-specific, certain cases may be marked by frontal-lobe-type personality change; mood changes, tending towards either mania or depression; or delusions and hallucinations. Rarely, GPI may present with psychosis. Regardless of the typology of the dementia, other signs and symptoms gradually accrue. Seizures, either partial or grand mal, are common. Dysarthria and anomia may occur, and handwriting becomes very poor. Coarse tremor is common and may be present not only in the hands but also in the lips and tongue. Very typically the facial musculature loses its tone, giving the patient a vacant, dull facial expression. The Argyll Robertson pupil is present in most cases. With further progression, the gait becomes unsteady and a true 'general paresis' occurs, with profound widespread weakness of almost all of the voluntary musculature. The plantar responses become extensor and, unless tabes dorsalis is present, there is a generalized hyperreflexia.

Whipple's disease

This is found mostly in white males.

Clinical features

The disorder typically presents in middle years. Migratory large-joint polyarthralgia is common; patients also typically have abdominal pain, diarrhoea, weight loss and mild fever. In a minority of patients, the CNS is involved and, although such involvement generally occurs within the context of long-standing arthralgia or abdominal symptomatology, there are cases in which Whipple's disease has presented with CNS involvement alone.

When the CNS is involved, patients typically present with gradually progressive dementia, delirium or personality change. In most cases, other symptoms are also present, including upper motor neuron signs, ataxia, nystagmus, myoclonus, seizures, supranuclear ophthalmoplegia, and various manifestations of hypothalamic dysfunction, including sleep disturbance (with either hypersomnolence or, less commonly, insomnia), hyperphagia, decreased libido or diabetes insipidus. A small minority of patients may also display oculomasticatory myorhythmia, in which pendular eye movements occur in concert with rhythmic jaw movements.

T2-weighted MRI may reveal multifocal areas of increased signal intensity within the cerebral cortex, basal ganglia, thalamus, midbrain and cerebellar cortex; in some cases, these lesions may show enhancement with gadolinium.

The CSF may show a lymphocytic pleocytosis or an elevated total protein, or both, with a normal glucose. In rare instances, some of the white cells may be periodic acid–Schiff (PAS)-positive. PCR assay is typically, but not always, positive for *Tropheryma whippelii* DNA.

The diagnosis may also be established by small-bowel biopsy, which may reveal not only PAS-positive macrophages but also a positive PCR assay; however, it must be kept in mind that, albeit rarely, CNS Whipple's disease can occur with a negative small-bowel biopsy.

Course

CNS involvement is a grave sign in Whipple's disease; in most cases, there is steady progression, with death occurring within 6–12 months.

Aetiology and pathology

The disorder occurs secondary to infection with the bacillus *T. whippelii*. Within the CNS, focal areas of inflammation and necrosis, with glial scars, are found in the cerebral cortex, basal ganglia, hypothalamus, brainstem (especially the periaqueductal grey matter) and cerebellar cortex.

PAS-positive macrophages are found in these regions, and electron microscopy may reveal the bacillus within the macrophage.

Malaria

Malaria occurs secondary to infection with any one of four species of the protozoon *Plasmodium*, including *P. malariae*, *P. vivax*, *P. ovale* and *P. falciparum*. Of these four, only *P. falciparum* invades the CNS, causing cerebral malaria. Malaria is endemic in Haiti, much of Asia and Oceania, and tropical and subtropical areas of Africa and South America; although it has been eradicated from most of North America and Europe, cases may still be seen in people returning from travel in endemic areas who did not take adequate prophylactic medication.

About 1–4 weeks after infection via the bite of an *Anopheles* mosquito, patients fall ill with fever, headache, malaise and myalgia. A small minority of those whose malaria has occurred secondary to *P. falciparum* may then develop cerebral malaria, with delirium, stupor or coma, and seizures. Focal signs such as hemiparesis may uncommonly occur. Diagnosis is by examination of peripheral blood smears.

Toxoplasmosis

Infection by *Toxoplasma gondii* is common in birds and mammals; cats serve as the definitive hosts and oocysts found in cat faeces may remain viable for up to a year. Primary infection in humans occurs secondary to eating contaminated food or undercooked lamb, pork or beef from infected animals and is very common: serological studies indicate that about one-third of adults in North America and Europe have been infected. In the vast majority, host defences are capable of rapidly controlling the infection and, during primary infection, patients are either asymptomatic or suffer a self-limited mononucleosis-like syndrome. Toxoplasma, however, may not be eradicated but remain latent in cysts, often in muscle.

CNS infection is very rare in immunocompetent adults. In immunocompromised patients, however, CNS toxoplasmosis does occur, either during a primary infection or, more commonly, with reactivation of a latent infection. In the pre-AIDS era this was noted in patients with cancer and in patients undergoing therapeutic immunosuppression, but it was rare; with the advent of AIDS, however, CNS toxoplasmosis has become common and indeed is the most common opportunistic infection in patients with AIDS, where it typically appears only when the CD4 count falls below 200/mm^3.

In most cases, CNS toxoplasmosis presents subacutely, over a matter of weeks. The presentation is variable, depending on the number and location of toxoplasma abscesses, and may include headache, fever, delirium, dementia, seizures and various focal signs, including hemianopia, hemiparesis, aphasia or, uncommonly, abnormal movements such as dystonia or chorea.

PRION DISEASES

Creutzfeldt–Jakob disease

Creutzfeldt–Jakob disease (CJD) occurs at an annual rate of 1–2 cases per 1 000 000 and is equally common in males and females. About 85 per cent of cases occur on a sporadic basis (sporadic CJD, sCJD), 10 per cent are inherited on an autosomal dominant basis, and the remainder represent iatrogenic infections (iatrogenic CJD, iCJD).

Clinical features

On average, sporadic cases appear in the early sixties, but the range is wide, from late teenage years to the tenth decade. Inherited cases tend to appear a bit earlier, mostly in the early fifties. Iatrogenic cases appear anywhere from 1 years to 30 years after the infectious event. Although most cases appear subacutely, over weeks to months, fulminant onsets spanning only a few days have been reported.

The presentation may be with dementia, personality change, psychosis,[196,197] cerebellar ataxia, or visual symptomatology such as hemianopia or cortical blindness; rare presentations include aphasia,[198] the 'alien hand sign'[199] or mania.[200] With progression, almost all patients become profoundly demented, and the dementia is accompanied by myoclonus (which may be stimulus-responsive) in almost 90 per cent of cases. Parkinsonism of the rigid, akinetic variety may occur, as may upper motor neuron signs; in a small minority of patients, evidence of lower motor neuron dysfunction, such as fasciculations, may be seen. Seizures occur in a small minority of patients.

MRI generally discloses cortical atrophy, the progression of which may be monitored with registration of serial scans. T2-weighted, FLAIR imaging and DWI may display increased signal intensity in the striatum and cerebral and cerebellar cortices; within the cortex, the increased signal intensity follows the cortical ribbon, displaying a gyriform pattern.

The EEG may show generalized slowing, and in some cases frontal intermittent rhythmic delta activity (FIRDA) has been noted.[201] The most characteristic EEG findings, however, are periodic triphasic spike-and-slow-wave complexes at around 1 Hz,[202] which are eventually seen in the majority of cases of sCJD and in some cases of genetic CJD and iCJD. The EEG may become abnormal only as the disease progresses; consequently, when the initial EEG fails to reveal this finding, it may be appropriate to perform serial EEGs.

The CSF is acellular with a normal glucose; in a very small minority of patients, the total protein level may show a mild elevation. Most importantly, the 14-3-3 protein is found in 50–95 per cent of cases.

Course

CJD progresses rapidly, and often one may see a decline from week to week, with death occurring within about 6 months on average. The overall range is relatively wide, with some patients dying in as little as a month and others surviving for up to 3 years.

Pathology and aetiology

Microscopically there is widespread spongiform change within the grey matter of the cerebral cortex, basal ganglia, thalamus and cerebellar cortex, which in turn is accounted for by grossly swollen dendrites and axons. In perhaps 5–10 per cent of cases, plaques may be found, which are, at least in part, composed of prions. There is also neuronal loss and astrogliosis but very little, if any, inflammation. Prions are also found in peripheral nerves, olfactory neuroepithelium, spleen and muscle.

The prion protein is a normally occurring cellular protein coded for by the *PRNP* gene on chromosome 20. The agent responsible for CJD is a pathological form of the prion protein.

The aetiology of sCJD is not clear. Some authors think there may be spontaneous, age-related transformations of normal cellular prion proteins into pathogenic prion proteins, whereas others suspect that sCJD may represent infections with a long incubation period.

Inherited cases occur secondary to any one of a large number of mutations in *PRNP*. Mutations may occur spontaneously, in which case the family history will be negative.

iCJD has occurred upon inadvertent exposure to tissue from patients with CJD via the following procedures: corneal transplants, dura mater grafts, the use of contaminated electrodes during neurosurgical procedures, injections of human growth hormone, and the injection of human pituitary gonadotropins. Interestingly, a case also occurred secondary to the use of lyophilized dura mater in the treatment of a nasopharyngeal angiofibroma, a procedure in which the dura mater remained extracranial.[203] The persistence of prions cannot be overemphasized: in one case, electrodes that had been used during neurosurgery on a patient with CJD 2 years earlier were cleaned three times and repeatedly sterilized in ethanol and formaldehyde vapour and yet were still able to transmit the disease to a chimpanzee.[204]

New-variant Creutzfeldt–Jakob disease

New-variant CJD (nvCJD; also known simply as variant CJD) is a very rare infectious prion disease acquired by eating meat derived from cows that had bovine spongiform encephalopathy (BSE), or 'mad cow disease'. Currently, most cases have occurred in the UK (Table 37.2).

Clinical features

The incubation period between ingestion of contaminated meat and disease development is probably less than 20 years. Disease onset is subacute and, although most patients have been in their late twenties, the range of age of onset is wide, from early adolescence to the eighth decade.

Most patients present with behavioural changes such as depression or, less commonly, personality change, withdrawal, agitation, insomnia, apathy, emotional lability

Table 37.2 Variant Creutzfeldt–Jakob disease (vCJD) cases worldwide (August 2007)

Country	Total number of primary cases (number alive)	Total number of secondary cases: blood transfusion (number alive)	Cumulative residence in UK >6 months during period 1980–1996
UK	163 (6)	3 (0)	166
France	22 (2)	–	1
Republic of Ireland	4 (1)	–	2
Italy	1 (0)	–	0
USA	3 (0)	–	2
Canada	1 (0)	–	1
Saudi Arabia	1 (1)	–	0
Japan	1 (0)	–	0
Netherlands	2 (0)	–	0
Portugal	2 (1)	–	0
Spain	1 (0)	–	0

Reproduced with permission from Love S, Louis DN, Ellison D (eds) (1998) *Greenfield's Neuropathology*, 8th edn. London: Hodder Arnold.

or psychosis, which in turn may comprise visual and auditory hallucinations and Schneiderian first-rank symptoms.[205–207] The remainder of patients present with ataxia, dysaesthesiae or memory loss, or a combination of these and behavioural changes. With progression, dementia eventually appears, which is often accompanied by myoclonus.[206–209]

FLAIR MR scanning displays a distinctive pulvinar sign in approximately three-quarters of all patients, characterized by increased signal intensity in the pulvinar of the thalamus. In addition, increased signal intensity may occur in the basal ganglia and cerebral and cerebellar cortices.

The EEG may demonstrate generalized slowing.[206] With rare exceptions, periodic spike-and-slow-wave complexes are absent.

The CSF is acellular, with a normal total protein. The 14-3-3 protein is found in about 50 per cent of cases.

Tonsil biopsy appears to be sensitive and specific.[210]

Course

nvCJD is relentlessly progressive, with most patients dying within a little over a year, with a range of 18 months to 3 years.

Aetiology and pathology

nvCJD occurs secondary to eating beef from cows that had BSE; in turn, cows contract the disease by eating meal made from the offal of sheep that had the transmissible spongiform encephalopathy scrapie. Almost all patients have been homozygous for methionine at codon 129 of *PRNP*.

Within the thalamus, basal ganglia, and cerebral and cerebellar cortices, there are widespread prion plaques surrounded by spongiform change. Prions are also found in tonsils, lymph nodes and the spleen. It also appears that prions are present in the blood, and there have been cases of nvCJD occurring secondary to blood transfusion.[211]

Other prion diseases

Gerstmann–Sträussler–Scheinker disease

Gerstmann–Sträussler–Scheinker disease (GSS) is a very rare, autosomal dominantly inherited prion disease occurring occur secondary to any one of several mutations in the *PRNP* gene. The onset is subacute or gradual, and usually in the sixth decade, with a wide range from the third to the eighth decades. Classically, patients present with progressive ataxia, with the eventual development of dementia; in some cases, parkinsonism or long-tract signs may also occur. Death occurs, on average, after 5–6 years.

The EEG may show generalized slowing, but there are no periodic complexes. The CSF is normal and the 14-3-3 protein is absent.

Fatal familial insomnia

Onset is typically subacute or gradual and occurs in middle years, with a wide range from late adolescence to the seventh decade. In general, patients develop intractable insomnia, followed in many cases by oneiroid states in which they appear confused, experience visual hallucinations, and behave as if they were acting out dreams. In one case, 'the patient performed movements of sawing with a virtual saw and stopped bewildered when told there was no saw'.[212] Rarely, the presentation may be with a psychosis coupled with insomnia.[213] Paroxysms of autonomic disturbance often occur, with hyperhidrosis, tachycardia, hypertension and irregular respiration. Over time, dementia appears, accompanied, variously, by ataxia, myoclonus and spasticity. Although insomnia is the initial hallmark of this disease, in some cases it may appear late in the course and, rarely, it may be absent.

The EEG shows slowing, but there are no periodic complexes. The CSF is generally normal, although in a small minority of patients the 14-3-3 protein may be found.

Most cases occur on an autosomal dominant basis, with mutations found at codon 178 of *PRNP*.

Kuru

Kuru is a unique human prion disease, spread by ritual cannibalism that included ingestion of brain, and present only in the Fore people of New Guinea. With the elimination of cannibalism in the 1950s, new infections stopped, but, given the long incubation period, the disease itself is still present. After a long incubation period, spanning 4–50 years or more, patients gradually develop ataxia and tremor, followed, in a minority, by dementia.

Pathologically there is atrophy of the cerebellar vermis and flocculonodular lobe. Microscopically there is widespread spongiform change, neuronal loss and astrocytosis, together with kuru plaques, which are distinguished from the amyloid plaques of Alzheimer's disease, for example, by the presence of spikes radiating out around the plaque circumference.

ENDOCRINOLOGICAL DISORDERS

Cushing's syndrome

Clinical features

The mode of onset is dependent on the underlying cause. Cases caused by exogenous steroid use are of the most rapid onset and may appear within days. Cushing's disease secondary to a pituitary adenoma may present very gradually, over years, and cases of Cushing's syndrome secondary to ectopic adrenocorticotropic hormone (ACTH) production may present over months.

Neuropsychiatric features include depression, mania or hypomania, anxiety, psychosis, dementia and/or delirium.

Depression is the most prominent neuropsychiatric feature;[214] it occurs in one-half to three-quarters of patients with Cushing's syndrome and may be the presenting feature.[215] Anxiety commonly accompanies the depression, as agitated depression. The depression at times may be severe, with psychotic features,[216] which may be either mood-congruent[217] or mood-incongruent,[218] with Schneiderian first-rank symptoms of thought broadcasting and thought insertion. Both suicide attempts and completed suicides may occur.[219]

Mania is less common than depression in Cushing's syndrome of endogenous origin,[215,219,220] but the converse holds true in exogenous cases, in which mania is common.[221]

Anxiety of pathological degree has been noted in about one-tenth of patients[215] but is most often seen in the context of depression.

Psychosis, although rare, can occur secondary to Cushing's syndrome. One patient presented with delusions of persecution, auditory and visual hallucinations, and bizarre behaviour, which all cleared with adrenalectomy;[222] another patient experienced agitation, auditory hallucinations, and religious and grandiose delusions, which again cleared with adrenalectomy.[223]

Delirium may occur but is rare, being noted in only about 1 per cent of cases.[215] Dementia is rare and is often characterized by prominent memory loss.

These neuropsychiatric features classically occur in the setting of a Cushingoid habitus, with moon facies, truncal obesity and violaceous abdominal striae. Other features include acne, hirsutism, proximal myopathy, easy bruisability, hypertension, diabetes mellitus, amenorrhoea and, rarely, pseudo-tumour cerebri. All these features, however, take time to develop and thus may not be present in cases of Cushing's syndrome secondary to exogenous steroid use, which may develop over days. Furthermore, in cases of Cushing's syndrome secondary to ectopic ACTH secretion by an oat-cell carcinoma, one may see emaciation rather than obesity.

When Cushing's syndrome occurs secondary to exogenous steroid administration, the diagnosis is fairly obvious, as symptoms appear within days of using high-dosage steroids, for example more than 60 mg/day of prednisone. However, when endogenous steroid overproduction is suspected, laboratory testing is essential to confirm the diagnosis. Confirmation of suspected endogenous hypercortisolaemia is sought via a 24-h urine test for free cortisol. Serum cortisol levels show pulsatile fluctuations during the day and hence should not be relied on. If the 24-h urine free cortisol level is normal, the diagnosis is effectively ruled out.

In cases in which the 24-h urinary free cortisol level is elevated, further testing is required to determine the cause. The first step is to obtain an ACTH level. In hypercortisolaemia secondary to an adrenal tumour the ACTH is low, whereas in all other cases it is elevated. If the ACTH is elevated, the next step is to determine whether the ACTH is derived from an ectopic source, for example lung carcinoma, or from a pituitary tumour, and this is accomplished with the high-dose dexamethasone suppression test. In this test, patients are given 2 mg of dexamethasone orally every 6 h over 2 days; during the second day, a 24-h urine sample is collected for measurement of free cortisol. In cases of ectopic ACTH production, the tumour secreting the ACTH is not sensitive to the feedback of dexamethasone and hence continues to secrete ACTH, resulting in an increased free cortisol level in the 24-h urine sample; in such cases, one speaks of 'non-suppression of cortisol by dexamethasone'. By contrast, pituitary adenomas do remain sensitive to dexamethasone and, in these cases, ACTH output falls with a resulting fall in the 24-h urine free cortisol level; in such cases, one speaks of 'suppression of cortisol by dexamethasone'. An alternative, or supplementary, test is the corticotropin-releasing hormone (CRH) stimulation test: ectopic ACTH-secreting tumours are not sensitive to CRH, and cortisol and ACTH levels do not rise significantly; pituitary adenomas, however, are sensitive, and here cortisol and ACTH levels do rise.

In some cases, the dexamethasone test may be equivocal, and differentiating between an ectopic ACTH-secreting tumour and a pituitary tumour may depend on sampling venous blood flow from the pituitary using sampling from the superior petrosal sinus or internal jugular vein.

If a pituitary tumour is suspected, MRI with gadolinium enhancement is in order, and, if positive, may obviate the need for superior petrosal or internal jugular sampling. Unfortunately, however, most ACTH-secreting pituitary tumours are microadenomas and about 50 per cent will escape detection by MRI.

Course

This depends on the underlying cause. Once cortisol levels are returned to normal, either by stopping exogenous steroids or by virtue of treatment of endogenous causes, neuropsychiatric features gradually resolve; although such resolution may occur within weeks to days in cases secondary to relatively short-term treatment with high-dose exogenous steroids, months may be required in endogenous cases.

Aetiology

There are various causes for endogenous hypercortisolaemia. Adrenal tumours, which may be either adenomas or carcinomas, account for about 15 per cent of cases. Ectopic ACTH-secreting tumours likewise account for about 15 per cent; although small-cell lung cancer is the most common of these, other tumours may also be at fault, including cancer of the thymus, pancreas or thyroid, and phaeochromocytoma. Pituitary adenomas are by far the most common cause, accounting for about 70 per cent. There are also very rare reports of CRH-secreting tumours, which may be located in the hypothalamus or ectopically, as for example in thyroid cancer.

Adrenocortical insufficiency

Clinical features

Acute adrenocortical insufficiency presents with nausea, vomiting and abdominal pain, with rapidly falling blood pressure, postural dizziness and eventually hypovolaemic shock. Delirium develops, followed by stupor and coma.

Chronic adrenocortical insufficiency presents gradually with fatigue, listlessness, poor concentration, anorexia, nausea, diarrhoea or constipation, and abdominal pain. Depression may occur;[224] rarely, there may be delirium[224] or psychosis.[225,226] Blood pressure is low and postural dizziness common. In primary cases, with a lack of cortisol feedback on the pituitary, excessive stimulation of melanocytes by ACTH may lead to hyperpigmentation, especially prominent in sun-exposed areas and on the buccal and gingival mucosa. Chronic adrenocortical insufficiency may also be complicated by an acute episode, as may occur when chronic patients are subjected to a significant physiological stress such as surgery.

Serum cortisol is reduced. In primary cases ACTH levels are increased because of a lack of feedback inhibition on the pituitary, whereas in secondary cases the ACTH level is low. In cases in which ACTH levels are equivocal, further testing may be conducted with a synthetic ACTH analogue in order to determine whether such cases are primary or secondary; in primary cases there is little or no rise in ACTH, whereas in secondary cases, presuming that the adrenal/suprarenal glands have not atrophied owing to chronic non-stimulation, there should be a robust rise in ACTH.

Further laboratory abnormalities may be seen in primary cases in which destruction of the adrenal/suprarenal glands causes decreased mineralocorticoid levels, with resulting hyponatraemia and hyperkalaemia.

Course

Acute adrenocortical insufficiency is a life-threatening emergency. The course of chronic adrenocortical insufficiency is determined by the underlying cause: in the case of primary chronic adrenocortical insufficiency resulting from autoimmune destruction of the adrenals, there is a gradual progression of symptoms, with death occurring in perhaps 2 years.

Aetiology

Primary adrenocortical insufficiency is most commonly caused by autoimmune destruction of the adrenal/suprarenal glands. In this disorder, other endocrine glands may also be targeted by the autoimmune process, and patients may develop Hashimoto's thyroiditis (with either hyperthyroidism or hypothyroidism), pernicious anaemia with vitamin B12 deficiency, hypoparathyroidism with hypocalcaemia, or diabetes mellitus. Other causes of primary adrenocortical insufficiency include adrenoleucodystrophy, tuberculosis, CMV infection (e.g. in AIDS), sarcoidosis, amyloidosis, metastatic disease and haemorrhagic infarction (e.g. during septicaemia or with overvigorous anticoagulation). With the exception of haemorrhagic infarction, all of these forms of primary adrenocortical insufficiency cause a chronic presentation.

Secondary adrenocortical insufficiency most commonly occurs secondary to abrupt discontinuation of long-term corticosteroid treatment. Any patient taking supraphysiological corticosteroid doses for more than a month will have some suppression of ACTH output from the pituitary coupled with some atrophy of the adrenal cortex. Other causes of secondary adrenocortical insufficiency include infarction, and tumours or granulomas of the pituitary or, rarely, the hypothalamus. These secondary cases may present either acutely (e.g. with abrupt discontinuation of steroid treatment) or chronically (e.g. with slowly growing pituitary tumours).

Hyperthyroidism

Clinical features

The age of onset varies according to the underlying aetiology: Graves' disease typically appears in the twenties or thirties, while toxic multinodular goitre generally has an onset in old age. Although symptoms usually appear gradually, over weeks or months, subacute onsets may be seen, especially in relation to various physiological stressors.

Typically, patients are apprehensive and anxious and, although fatigued and tired, often experience restlessness and an inability to sit still. Anxiety often stands out and may represent the presenting complaint. Patients typically complain of diaphoresis, heat intolerance and an increased frequency of bowel movements; despite an often increased appetite with increased caloric intake, there may be substantial weight loss. On examination, one finds tachycardia, widened palpebral fissures and proptosis, a fine postural tremor, and generalized hyperreflexia; there may also be a proximal myopathy. Women may complain of menstrual irregularity and men may experience erectile dysfunction. Rarely, there may be chorea, grand mal seizures or a motor peripheral neuropathy.

Apathetic hyperthyroidism represents a variant of hyperthyroidism that is generally only seen in elderly people and that is characterized by apathy and, in some patients, lethargy.[227] Remarkably, of the autonomic signs and symptoms seen in typical cases, only tachycardia is common in this apathetic variant: diaphoresis, tremor and hyperreflexia are generally absent. Many patients also develop atrial fibrillation and congestive failure.

Of the neuropsychiatric features seen in hyperthyroidism, depression is the most common and is seen in a substantial minority,[228] especially in patients with apathetic hyperthyroidism,[229] in whom the only clue to the correct diagnosis may be tachycardia or congestive heart failure. Depression may be accompanied by mood-congruent delusions[230] or considerable agitation.[231]

Mania is less common than depression[232] and, in some cases, may be of the mixed variety.[233]

Psychosis, although only rarely caused by hyperthyroidism, may occur: one patient developed a delusion of jealousy and, convinced that his wife was having an affair, had her followed; when his hyperthyroidism was treated, his psychosis resolved.[234]

Dementia may occur in typical hyperthyroidism[235] but is rare. By contrast, a significant minority of patients with the apathetic variant will develop cognitive deficits that may be severe enough to constitute dementia.[236] Rarely, delirium may also occur.

Thyroid storm is a complication that typically appears in a patient with untreated hyperthyroidism who is subjected to some significant physiological stress (e.g. surgery, infection). There is a rapid escalation of all of the typical signs and symptoms, followed by hyperthermia, delirium, stupor and coma. In some cases, seizures may occur. Rarely, thyroid storm has presented with psychosis.[237,238] Thyroid storm may also occur in the setting of apathetic hyperthyroidism and in such cases may present with coma in the absence of any autonomic features.[239]

In almost all cases of hyperthyroidism the free thyroxine (T4) level will be elevated and the thyroid-stimulating hormone (TSH) level reduced. Exceptions occur in cases of triiodothyronine (T3) thyrotoxicosis, in which the free T4 level is normal; in cases in which the clinical suspicion of hyperthyroidism is high and the free T4 is normal, the free T3 level should be determined. Other exceptions include the very rare cases of a hypothalamic tumour secreting thyrotropin-releasing hormone (TRH) or a pituitary adenoma secreting TSH: in both cases, both the free T4 and the TSH levels are elevated.

Course

This is dictated by the underlying cause. Thyroid storm, regardless of the underlying cause, may pursue a fulminant course, with death in hours or days.

Aetiology

Most cases result from Graves' disease. Other causes include toxic multinodular goitre, toxic solitary adenoma and the thyroiditides, including lymphocytic thyroiditis, subacute (De Quervain's) thyroiditis and Hashimoto's thyroiditis. The thyroiditides are characterized by 'leakage' of T4 from the inflamed thyroid and, typically, cause hyperthyroidism that is time-limited and that may, depending on the amount of inflammatory damage and scarring, be followed by hypothyroidism. Rare causes include hypothalamic tumours, pituitary adenomas, inherited pituitary resistance to T4, production of ectopic TSH by various tumours (hydatidiform mole, uterine choriocarcinoma, testicular choriocarcinoma), and production of T4 by various tumours (struma ovarii or metastatic follicular carcinoma of the thyroid). Finally, hyperthyroidism may occur as a side effect of amiodarone and may also be intentional, as in thyrotoxicosis factitia.

Hypothyroidism

Clinical features and course

The age of onset is determined by the underlying cause. Cases secondary to Hashimoto's thyroiditis typically appear in the late thirties or early forties, and cases occurring after thyroidectomy may first appear within weeks postoperatively. The onset and evolution of symptoms are typically gradual.

Typically, patients develop psychomotor retardation, with slowed speech and movements; in some cases, lethargy and somnolence may occur. When asked a question, up to a minute may pass before the patient responds; the response itself, when it does come, is slow. Simple activities such as unfastening a button may take an inordinate amount of time to complete. Patients may appear apathetic and lacking in initiative, and often there may be difficulty with concentration and 'fogginess' of thought and memory.[240] The overall appearance is often distinctive: skin becomes thickened, puffy and even boggy, and this is particularly obvious on the face, in the supraclavicular fossae, and on the dorsal surfaces of the hands and feet. The hair becomes thin and brittle, and there may be considerable hair loss, including the lateral thirds of the eyebrows. Other symptoms include a voice change towards hoarseness, cold intolerance, constipation, weight gain, decreased libido, erectile dysfunction and menorrhagia. Vibratory sense may be lost and the deep tendon reflexes are often reduced; the ankle jerk is often 'hung up', with a delayed relaxation phase. Cranial nerves may be involved, with partial deafness and, rarely, a peripheral facial palsy; cerebellar ataxia ('myxoedema staggers')[241] occurs in up to 20 per cent. Very rarely, seizures may occur. Myxoedematous infiltration may cause carpal or tarsal tunnel syndrome; macroglossia may also occur and, if severe, may be followed by obstructive sleep apnoea. Bradycardia and hypotension are common, and there may be a degree of hypothermia; pericardial and pleural effusions may also occur. In a small minority of cases, a syndrome of inappropriate ADH secretion may occur, with hyponatraemia.

In severe cases, 'myxoedema coma' may develop. Typically this occurs in patients with long-standing hypothyroidism who are subjected to a physiological stress (e.g. surgery, infection) or who are given phenothiazines[242] or any medications with prominent sedative effects. Stupor or coma develops, accompanied by hypothermia (which may be severe), significant bradycardia, respiratory depression and, in a significant minority, grand mal seizures.

Of the neuropsychiatric features seen in hypothyroidism, depression is most common; this may be severe and may be accompanied by hallucinations and delusions.[243]

Psychosis occurring secondary to hypothyroidism has traditionally been referred to as 'myxoedema madness'[244] and is often characterized by delusions of persecution and reference and auditory hallucinations.[245,246]

Dementia may present with failing memory,[247,248] followed by deficits in calculation and orientation; in some cases, the dementia may be accompanied by delusions of persecution and auditory hallucinations.

The EEG typically shows generalized slowing.

Free T4 is reduced in all cases. In primary hypothyroidism, the TSH is increased; in both secondary and tertiary cases, however, TSH is reduced. Distinguishing secondary from tertiary cases generally requires a TRH-stimulation test. In cases of secondary hypothyroidism, given a lack of pituitary cells capable of producing TSH, the TSH response to exogenous TRH is blunted. By contrast, in tertiary hypothyroidism, in which a chronic lack of endogenous TRH allows for an up-regulation of TRH receptors on pituitary cells, there is an enhanced response of TSH to TRH.

In subclinical primary hypothyroidism, although the free T4 level is within normal limits, the TSH level is mildly elevated. These indicate that, although the free T4 may be within broadly defined limits of normal, it is nevertheless below the individual patient's 'normal' as indicated by the rise in TSH. Although patients may not have symptoms directly related to these findings, the findings are significant for two reasons. First, they may indicate that the patient is in the very early stages of what will become clinically evident hypothyroidism, and therefore close monitoring is required. Second, such subclinically reduced free T4 levels, although not causing symptoms per se, will nevertheless blunt the response to antidepressants or mood-stabilizing agents in patients with major depression or bipolar disorder.

Aetiology

Primary hypothyroidism accounts for over 90 per cent of cases. The most common cause is Hashimoto's thyroiditis, indicated by the presence of anti-thyroid antibodies. Other causes include thyroidectomy, radioactive iodine treatment, neck irradiation, iodine deficiency and various medications, including amiodarone and lithium, in which case the occurrence of hypothyroidism is most likely in patients with anti-thyroid antibodies.[249]

Secondary hypothyroidism may occur with tumours or infarction of the pituitary gland.

Tertiary hypothyroidism may occur with tumours or infarction of the hypothalamus; other causes include granulomatous disease and carbamazepine.

IMMUNE-RELATED DISORDERS

Multiple sclerosis

In this chapter neuropsychiatric manifestations of multiple sclerosis (MS) will mainly be considered; other aspects are detailed in Chapter 36.

Fatigue may occur and may be severe. Sexual dysfunction is very common, with decreased libido, erectile dysfunction or decreased vaginal lubrication. Uncommon symptoms and signs include aphasia and seizures, which may be either partial or grand mal in type, and various paroxysmal phenomena, such as hemifacial spasm, Lhermitte's sign, trigeminal neuralgia, and lancinating pains in the extremities.

Dementia of variable severity, ranging from mild, almost subclinical impairment to debilitating, is eventually seen in the majority of patients. In rare cases, dementia may constitute the sole or predominant presenting feature of MS.[250] In one case, for example, the only symptom in addition to the dementia was optic neuritis,[251] and in two other cases it was unsteady gait.[252] In one very rare case, a gradually progressive dementia constituted the only clinical evidence of MS.[253] Although the correlation of dementia and plaque location and number has not been worked out definitively, it appears that cognitive deficits correlate both with the total burden of plaques within the cerebral white matter and with atrophy of the corpus callosum, which in turn may merely reflect overall disease activity in the hemispheric white matter.

Depression is eventually seen in perhaps one-quarter of patients.[254] Depression may occur on a reactive basis in any debilitating disease, and MS is no exception. Certain facts, however, suggest strongly that depression in MS may also be a direct result of plaque formation. Patients with MS are more likely to experience depression than are normal control subjects[255] or patients with comparably disabling neurological diseases that generally spare the cerebrum, such as amyotrophic lateral sclerosis.[256,257] Furthermore, in contrast to what one might expect if the depression were reactive, there is little or no correlation between the occurrence of depression and the extent of the patient's disability,[258] and, regardless of the degree of overall disability, patients are more likely to experience depression when the plaques are in the cerebrum than when they are in the cerebellum or spinal cord.[259,260] Furthermore, there is a correlation between depression and the presence of plaques in the inferior left frontal white matter,[261] left arcuate fasciculus[262] and right temporal white matter.[263]

Euphoria may occur and is typically of the 'bland' or non-infectious type; it has been noted in anywhere from one-quarter[254] to the vast majority of patients[264] and is correlated with cerebral rather than spinal plaque formation.[259] The contrast between this euphoria and the patient's actual condition can be quite dramatic: one of Wilson's patients, 'bedridden and unable to stand, remarked, "you will not believe me when I say I feel thundering well"'.[265] This bland euphoria is typically not accompanied by hyperactivity or pressure of speech and is often seen in concert with some degree of intellectual impairment.[254] Although they are unusual, definite manic episodes may also occur in addition to this bland euphoria;[266,267] indeed, out of all of the reasons for admission to psychiatric hospital for patients with MS, mania is the most common.[268]

Emotional incontinence, with uncontrollable laughter or crying in the absence of a corresponding affect, is seen in about one-tenth of patients,[254,269] generally only in far-advanced cases.

Psychosis may, rarely, dominate the clinical picture;[270,271] in one very rare case, MS presented with a psychosis characterized by social withdrawal, 'mystic' visual hallucinations and various delusions.[253]

Almost all plaques demonstrate increased signal intensity on T2-weighted or FLAIR MRI, and active plaques show enhancement with gadolinium. In some cases, severe plaques may undergo cystic change, and on T1-weighted MRI such plaques will appear as 'black holes' with greatly reduced signal intensity. Plaques are typically found in the centrum semiovale and in a periventricular distribution, where they tend to favour the occipital horns.

The CSF is abnormal in almost all cases. A mild lymphocytic pleocytosis, in the range of 6–30 cells/mm^3, is seen in about one-third of cases, and the total protein is mildly elevated (rarely over 100 mg/dL) in about one-half. The IgG index is elevated in over two-thirds, and oligoclonal bands are present in over 90 per cent. The myelin basic protein is elevated in over three-quarters of cases. The 14-3-3 protein may be found in a little over one-tenth of all cases.[272]

Systemic lupus erythematosus

SLE occurs in 0.015–0.05 per cent of the general population. It is far more common among females than males, and among black populations than white populations; in black females, the prevalence rises to 0.4 per cent.

Clinical features

Although lupus may appear at almost any age, the majority of patients fall ill between puberty and 40 years of age.

SLE is a systemic disease and in most cases cerebral lupus occurs in the setting of other symptoms, including constitutional symptoms (fatigue, fever, weight loss) and those referable to other organ systems, such as the musculoskeletal system, skin, heart, lungs or kidneys. Musculoskeletal symptomatology is very common and includes myalgia, arthralgia and a non-deforming polyarthritis. Cutaneous manifestations include photosensitivity, rashes (especially a malar rash) and alopecia. Cardiac symptomatology incorporates pericarditis and Libman–Sacks endocarditis. Pulmonary involvement may manifest with pleurisy, which may or may not be accompanied by pleural effusion. Renal involvement may manifest initially with proteinuria and cellular casts; over time, renal failure may occur. Various cytopenias, including anaemia, leucopenia and thrombocytopenia, may also occur.

Cerebral lupus may manifest with depression, mania, psychosis, delirium or dementia, seizures, chorea, or focal signs such as hemiparesis. Although these findings may occur independently, patients often have a mixture.

Depression, in some cases accompanied by hallucinations or delusions, has been found commonly by some authors[273,274] but not others.[275,276] Mania, although reported,[277] appears rarely. Psychosis is relatively uncommon;[274,275,278] although typically characterized by delusions and hallucinations, it may rarely present with stuporous catatonia. Rarely, psychosis may constitute the presenting feature.[279]

Delirium may occur[274,276,280] and is often accompanied by hallucinations, either visual or auditory. Dementia may also be seen but is relatively uncommon.[280]

Seizures are relatively common[280] and may be partial (complex partial or simple partial) or grand mal in type. Chorea may occur and indeed may constitute the presentation of SLE. Focal deficits are common[280] and may include hemiparesis, aphasia or hemianopia. Thrombotic thrombocytopenic purpura has been noted, but this is usually a terminal event.[280]

In addition to cerebral involvement, the peripheral nervous system may also be involved, with either peripheral polyneuropathy or mononeuritis multiplex.

The anti-nuclear antibody (ANA) test is positive in approximately 95 per cent of patients, and the serum VDRL test may be falsely positive. As the ANA lacks specificity, however, a positive result here must be followed up by a more specific test, such as anti-native DNA (also known as anti-double-stranded DNA) or anti-Sm. During active disease, the ESR is often elevated and one or more complement levels (C3, C4, CH50) are generally decreased. Consideration may also be given to testing for the presence of serum anti-ribosomal P antibodies and for the anti-phospholipid syndrome, including lupus anticoagulant and anti-cardiolipin antibodies of both the IgG and immunoglobulin M (IgM) types. Anti-ribosomal P antibodies may be associated with the occurrence of psychosis, and anti-phospholipid antibodies may be associated with infarction.

MRI may be normal or may show evidence of infarction. When infarctions are present, they tend to occur in one of two patterns. Either there are multiple small infarcts in either the cerebral cortex or the subcortical white matter, or one finds relatively large territorial infarctions in the areas of distribution of large pial vessels.

The EEG may be normal or show slowing, which may be generalized or focal. In patients with seizures, interictal epileptiform discharges may or may not be present.

Course

Overall, the course is characterized by a gradual waxing and waning of symptoms; full remissions are unusual and generally not permanent. Although SLE is in general compatible with long-term survival, the appearance of cerebral or renal disease is an ominous sign.

Aetiology

Lupus is characterized by the presence of a large number of autoantibodies directed at various tissues in multiple organ systems. Although the cause is not known, it is strongly suspected that the autoimmune response occurs secondary to some environmental trigger in genetically susceptible individuals.

Pathology of neuropsychiatric features

It appears that most cases of depression, mania, psychosis and delirium occur on the basis of cerebritis; however, these syndromes may also occur with appropriately placed infarctions (e.g. depression with frontal lobe; mania with frontal or temporal lobe, thalamus or caudate; psychosis with temporal lobe or thalamus; delirium with temporal lobe or thalamus). Dementia may occur on the basis of cerebritis but appears more commonly due to multiple infarctions. Seizures may likewise occur with cerebritis or with infarction.

Susac's syndrome

Susac's syndrome (retinocochleocerebral vasculopathy), first described by Susac in 1979,[281] is a rare disorder, typically seen in young adult females.

Clinical features

Classically one sees the subacute onset of delirium, often accompanied by headache, in the setting of sensorineuronal hearing loss and visual disturbances.

MRI typically reveals multiple areas of increased signal intensity on FLAIR and T2-weighted images, scattered throughout the white and grey matter with a predilection for the corpus callosum. In some cases these lesions may demonstrate contrast enhancement.

Course

There is usually a more or less complete remission of symptoms after 2–4 years. Recurrences, although not common, may occur.

Pathology and aetiology

In the setting of a widespread cerebral microangiopathy, there are multiple micro-infarcts affecting the white matter (especially the corpus callosum) and the grey matter. Retinal and cochlear infarctions also occur.

Although the aetiology of the angiopathy is not known, an autoimmune mechanism is suspected.

Limbic encephalitis

In the vast majority of cases, limbic encephalitis occurs on a paraneoplastic basis, most often in patients with small-cell lung cancer. It is rare, occurring in less than 0.1 per cent of all patients with cancer.

Clinical features

The onset of symptoms is typically subacute, spanning days or weeks. It is often the presenting symptom of cancer, and in some cases the tumour itself may remain undetected for years after the onset of the encephalitis.

The most common presentation is with delirium marked by prominent anterograde and retrograde amnesia, often accompanied by seizures and personality change or hallucinations. Other, less common presentations include depression, isolated amnesia, seizures, somnolence and catatonia (with 'confusion, stereotypy, echolalia, stiffness, verbigeration, formal thought disorder, and negativism'[282]). Rare symptoms include abnormal movements such as chorea, narcoleptic attacks with cataplexy, rapid eye movement (REM) sleep behaviour disorder, and, especially in association with ovarian cancer, hypoventilation with respiratory failure.

In cases occurring on a paraneoplastic basis, one may also see other paraneoplastic syndromes, including cerebellar degeneration with ataxia; brainstem encephalitis with nystagmus, ataxia, oculomotor palsies and vertigo; opsoclonus–myoclonus; sensory neuropathy; Lambert–Eaton myasthenic syndrome; and the stiff-person syndrome.

Early in the course, MRI is often normal; over time, however, most cases will have increased signal intensity in the medial aspects of the temporal lobes on T2-weighted or FLAIR imaging; these abnormalities, although initially unilateral, typically become bilateral.

The EEG is abnormal in almost all cases and typically shows temporal slowing, which may initially be unilateral, only to become bilateral later.

The CSF may be normal or may display any one of a number of findings, including a mild lymphocytic pleocytosis, a mildly elevated total protein, or oligoclonal bands.

Although in the vast majority of cases of limbic encephalitis abnormalities will be found on MRI, EEG or CSF assay, exceptions do occur, especially early on. In cases in which the clinical findings are strongly suggestive of the diagnosis but these tests are negative, PET scanning should be considered; even in cases in which all other tests are negative, PET may reveal focal hypermetabolism in one or both temporal lobes.

A wide variety of anti-neuronal antibodies have been identified, including anti-Hu (or ANNA-1), anti-Ri (or ANNA-2), ANNA-3, anti-Ma1, anti-Ma2 (or anti-Ta), anti-amphiphysin, anti-CRMP-5 and anti-voltage-gated potassium channel (or anti-VGKC). In paraneoplastic cases, various tumours have been found, including cancer of the lung (most commonly of the small-cell type), breast, testicle, colon, pancreas, ovary, thymus, prostate and bladder; cases have also been associated with lymphoma.

Course

Although the overall course is one of progression, at times there may be plateaux; however, these almost always give way to further decline. True spontaneous remissions, although reported, are rare, and most patients die within months to a year or more, either of complications of the limbic encephalitis or from the underlying cancer.

Pathology and aetiology

There is a lymphocytic perivascular inflammation, with neuronal loss and gliosis within the limbic system, primarily involving medial temporal structures. In the vast majority of cases, this inflammation occurs on a paraneoplastic basis, with antibodies raised against the cancer cross-reacting with normal neuronal tissue. However, there are cases of limbic encephalitis occurring in the context of anti-VGKC antibodies in which no cancer is found, and the mechanism underlying the genesis of this autoimmune response remains unknown.

Sarcoidosis

Sarcoidosis is somewhat more common in females than males. In the USA it is far more common in black people than white people, and in Europe people from northern countries are more commonly affected than people from southern countries.

Clinical features

Although onset in adolescence or the middle or later years may occur, most patients fall ill in their twenties or thirties. The onset is often gradual, and many cases are discovered serendipitously on chest radiography.

Sarcoidosis may be protean in its manifestations, but certain presentations deserve note. Perhaps 90 per cent of patients have pulmonary involvement, which may manifest with symptoms such as cough or dyspnoea or may be asymptomatic and discovered only incidentally by chest radiograph, which may reveal bilateral hilar lymphadenopathy or a diffuse reticulonodular appearance. Other symptoms include erythema nodosum, lupus pernio, lymphadenopathy, arthropathy and parotid gland enlargement. Hepatic involvement occurs in almost three-quarters of patients, although hepatic failure is rare. Hypercalcaemia occurs in a majority of patients, and some may develop nephrocalcinosis and eventual renal failure.

Involvement of the nervous system occurs in 5–25 per cent of patients, and in a very small minority of cases it may represent the only manifestation of sarcoidosis. With a basilar meningitis, cranial neuropathies may occur; with obstruction of the outflow foramina of the fourth ventricle, hydrocephalus may occur; involvement of arteries may be followed by stroke. Cerebral involvement may be characterized by multiple granulomas or by relatively few large lesions, or even by a solitary lesion; in these cases there may be dementia, delirium, seizures or focal signs. Hypothalamic or pituitary granulomas may present with endocrinological syndromes. The cord may also be compressed and the peripheral nervous system is often involved.

Cranial neuropathies occur in approximately one-half of cases and, although various cranial nerves may be involved, one most commonly sees a peripheral facial palsy, which may be unilateral or bilateral. The eighth cranial nerve may also be involved, with deafness, as may the optic nerve or chiasm with blindness or hemianopia.

Hydrocephalus occurs in about 5 per cent of patients and may present with dementia and gait disturbance.

Stroke is rare and appears generally to present with a lacunar syndrome, reflecting granulomatous involvement of the penetrating arteries.

Dementia may occur and may be accompanied by a frontal lobe syndrome[283] or by delusions and hallucinations.[284] Cognitive deficits of variable degree may occur in close to 50 per cent of patients with neurosarcoidosis.[285] Delirium has also been noted but appears to be rare.

Seizures occur in about 15 per cent of patients and may be grand mal or partial. Focal signs may occur and reflect the location of any cerebral granulomas.

Endocrinological changes have been noted in up to one-third of patients and may consist of diabetes insipidus, hyperprolactinaemia, hypothyroidism, hypogonadism and adrenocortical insufficiency. Hypothalamic involvement may also manifest with disturbances of appetite or with somnolence; rarely, symptomatic narcolepsy may occur.[286]

MRI typically reveals any basilar meningitis or macroscopic parenchymal granulomas.

The CSF is abnormal in only about 50 per cent of cases; abnormalities include a mild lymphocytic pleocytosis, a mildly elevated total protein and, in a minority of patients, oligoclonal bands or an elevated IgG index. In a very small minority of patients, the glucose level is mildly reduced. The level of CSF angiotensin-converting enzyme is elevated in a little over 50 per cent of patients. The serum angiotensin-converting enzyme level is likewise elevated in over 50 per cent of patients.

Definitive diagnosis requires biopsy evidence of typical sarcoid granulomas, and in most cases lung biopsy is performed.

Course

This is variable. Spontaneous remission of neurosarcoidosis occurs after many months in about one-half of cases, although relapses may occur; in the remaining cases the disease pursues a chronic, often fluctuating course.

Pathology

The cardinal lesion is a non-caseating granuloma. The pathology of neurosarcoidosis is described above.

Other disorders

Hashimoto's encephalopathy

Although most patients with Hashimoto's encephalopathy (steroid-responsive encephalopathy associated with autoimmune thyroiditis, SREAT) are in their forties, the age of onset varies widely, from childhood to the eighth decade. The onset is typically subacute, over days or perhaps weeks. The overwhelming majority of patients have delirium, which in most cases is accompanied by any or all of tremor, myoclonus, ataxia and seizures. Stroke-like episodes are common and are typically characterized by aphasia; hemiplegia or hemisensory loss may also occur. These stroke-like episodes are of brief duration, lasting in the order of hours or a day or more, and typically undergo a full remission. Very rarely Hashimoto's encephalopathy may present with psychosis[287] or dementia.[288]

Sydenham's chorea

Sydenham's chorea, also known as St Vitus' dance, rheumatic chorea and chorea minor, is one of the major manifestations of rheumatic fever, occurring in about one-quarter of patients. Because of the widespread treatment of streptococcal pharyngitis with penicillin, Sydenham's chorea is currently uncommon; it occurs more frequently in females than males, with a ratio of approximately 7 : 3.

Neuropsychiatric features are very common. Obsessions and compulsions occur most notably:[289] one prospective study reported them in 70 per cent of patients,[290] and another study in 82 per cent.[291] The course of these obsessions and compulsions is of interest. Although they tend to peak in severity along with the worsening of the chorea and to remit before the chorea does, in fact they generally make their appearance before the chorea sets in.[291] Importantly, it appears that in cases of rheumatic fever it is only those patients who develop Sydenham's chorea who develop obsessions and compulsions; patients without chorea remain free of them.[290]

Tics, similar to those seen in Tourette's syndrome, may also occur during Sydenham's chorea.[292]

Delirium is seen in less than 10 per cent of patients,[293] but it may be profound.[294]

Mania is a rare manifestation[295,296] and may present as either pure mania or mixed mania or, rarely, be coupled with a depression.[295,297] Depression is even rarer than mania in Sydenham's chorea.[295]

Psychosis, with hallucinations and delusions, may occur in a small minority of patients[298] and may symptomatically resemble the psychosis seen in schizophrenia.[299,300]

BRAIN TUMOURS AND HYDROCEPHALUS

Brain tumours

Clinical features

Although brain tumours may occur at any age, most patients are middle-aged or older. The onset ranges from acute to insidious, depending in large part on the aggressiveness of the tumour involved. Certain gliomas, such as glioblastoma multiforme, may evolve rapidly over several weeks or months, whereas some meningiomas may attain a large size without ever causing symptoms and may indeed be found incidentally on imaging for other reasons or at autopsy. The overall symptomatology may be divided into the following domains: headache; non-focal symptoms; focal signs and specific syndromes, such as dementia or personality change; and seizures. In this chapter we consider primarily the neuropsychiatric manifestations.

Dementia is classically seen with tumours of the frontal lobe or corpus callosum, when it is often accompanied by apathy, dullness and somnolence, or by frontal lobe syndrome. Tumours of the thalamus and hypothalamus may also cause dementia, and with hypothalamic tumours one often sees additional symptoms such as hypersomnolence, weight gain or diabetes insipidus.

Personality change may be seen with tumours of the frontal lobe or temporal lobe and, rarely, with tumours of the thalamus or hypothalamus. Although this personality change may be non-specific, in cases of frontal lobe tumours one classically sees an accompanying frontal lobe syndrome.[301]

Delirium may occur with tumours of the temporal lobe[302] or the hypothalamus.[303]

Amnesia, with isolated short-term memory loss, may be seen with tumours that impinge on any part of the circuit of Papez, for example the fornix (e.g. by a subsplenial tumour), the mamillary bodies (e.g. by a craniopharyngioma) and the thalamus.

Mania may uncommonly occur with tumours of the mesencephalon, hypothalamus, thalamus, cingulate gyrus or frontal lobe.

Depression may rarely constitute the presentation of a tumour, as has been noted with a tumour of the anterior portion of the corpus callosum.[304]

Psychosis may occur with tumours, most commonly of the temporal lobe; other locations include the frontal lobe and the corpus callosum.

Tumours located in the hypothalamus may present with dementia, personality change, delirium, amnesia or mania. Other symptoms may also be seen, including diabetes insipidus, anorexia with profound weight loss, and hyperphagia with extreme weight gain, which may, in rare instances, be accompanied by episodic rage.[305]

With growth of the tumour and enlargement of the area of peri-tumoural oedema, the clinical picture evolves, with worsening of initial symptoms and addition of new ones. In some cases, hydrocephalus may occur, with symptoms as discussed below. In other cases, there may be acute clinical exacerbations resulting from either intra-tumoural haemorrhage or infarction secondary to arterial compression.

MRI should be obtained in all cases, generally with gadolinium enhancement.

Course

The natural course varies widely, depending on the malignancy of the tumour itself, ranging from as little as months in the case of glioblastoma multiforme up to a decade or more with low-grade gliomas.

Aetiology

Brain tumours may be either primary to the CNS or, more commonly, metastatic.

Of the primary brain tumours, gliomas and meningiomas constitute the vast majority of cases. Primary CNS lymphoma, once rare, has become increasingly common, both in immunocompromised and in immunocompetent patients. Other primary brain tumours, seen in a small minority, include neuromas, medulloblastoma, gangliocytoma, pituitary adenoma, craniopharyngioma, pineal tumours, hemangioblastoma, and colloid cyst of the third ventricle.

Metastases may arise from various different primary tumours and almost always reach the brain via haematogenous spread. By far the most common source is lung cancer, primarily the non-small-cell type, followed by breast cancer and melanoma, and then by various other tumours, including those of the colon and rectum, kidney, gallbladder, liver, thyroid, testicle, prostate, uterus or ovary and pancreas; both systemic lymphoma (primarily of the non-Hodgkin's type) and leukaemia may also metastasize to the brain. Of all these primaries, melanoma and testicular cancer, although not common, exhibit the greatest propensity for metastasis to the brain.

Two-thirds of metastases eventually settle in the brain parenchyma, whereas the remainder lodge either in the leptomeninges (where they create leptomeningeal carcinomatosis) or in the dura. Parenchymal metastases may be found throughout the cerebrum; they are found in the hemispheres in about three-quarters of cases, in the cerebellum in about one-eighth, and in the brainstem or thalamus in the remainder; of the metastases lodging in the hemispheres, all lobes may be involved, including, in descending order, the frontal, parietal, occipital and temporal lobes.

Adult hydrocephalus

Clinical features

Acute hydrocephalus is a form of non-communicating hydrocephalus in which there is a complete, or near-complete, obstruction of CSF flow. It is characterized clinically by a rapid onset of symptoms, over days, hours or even quicker. Patients present with headache, stupor and vomiting; without treatment, coma and death may ensue rapidly.

Chronic hydrocephalus may represent either a communicating or a non-communicating condition; when it occurs as a result of non-communicating hydrocephalus, one finds only a partial obstruction. Clinically, chronic hydrocephalus typically presents gradually, or even insidiously, and is characterized by dementia marked by forgetfulness, apathy and a generalized slowing of thought and behaviour; rarely, akinetic mutism may occur.[306] Gait disturbance also occurs and may either precede or follow the onset of dementia. The gait may be shuffling, apraxic or 'magnetic' in type. Urinary urgency, frequency or incontinence may also occur. There may be generalized hyperreflexia and bilaterally positive Babinski signs.

Although ventriculomegaly is evident on CT or MRI, MR scanning is preferred as it is more likely to reveal the underlying cause of any obstructive hydrocephalus. In addition, on T2-weighted or FLAIR images, one typically sees evidence of transependymal flow of CSF from the ventricles into the immediately subjacent white matter, producing a hazy rim of increased signal intensity in a periventricular distribution.

Lumbar puncture may or may not be necessary. In cases of non-communicating hydrocephalus, the opening pressure is normal; in cases of communicating hydrocephalus, except normal-pressure hydrocephalus (see below), it is generally increased.

Course

Acute hydrocephalus is a catastrophic event, with rapid evolution of symptoms. Chronic hydrocephalus, by contrast, is marked by a very slow progression of symptoms as CSF pressure very slowly increases. In most cases, however, a new 'equilibrium' is eventually reached between CSF production and outflow; in this situation, although the ventricles remain under increased pressure, they do not undergo any further expansion. When this development occurs, the previously 'active' hydrocephalus is said to have undergone 'arrest'; such 'arrested' cases of hydrocephalus clinically manifest a plateau of symptoms, with a subsequently stable clinical course.

Aetiology

In non-communicating hydrocephalus the obstruction may occur at various sites and may be caused by various different lesions. Thus, the foramen of Monro may be obstructed by a tumour such as an astrocytoma, or by a colloid cyst of the third ventricle, and the third ventricle may be occluded by a tumour. The aqueduct of Sylvius may be stenotic or may suffer post-infectious scarring; it may also be compressed by adjacent tumours such as pineal tumours. The fourth ventricle may be compressed by cerebellar lesions such as tumours, haemorrhages or infarctions. The exit foramina of Magendie and Luschka may be occluded by scarring, as may occur after an episode of viral or bacterial meningitis, or in the course of an indolent basilar meningitis, as may be seen in meningovascular syphilis, tuberculosis and fungal infections; scarring and obstruction may also occur after a subarachnoid haemorrhage, either spontaneous or as may be seen with traumatic brain injury.

Communicating hydrocephalus is most commonly seen with obstruction of outflow at the arachnoid granulations. Although such obstruction most commonly occurs after subarachnoid haemorrhage, it may also occur in leptomeningeal carcinomatosis; rarely, egress of CSF through the arachnoid villi may be slowed in cases of extremely elevated total protein values, as in some cases of spinal tumour or polyneuritis. Another rare mechanism underlying communicating hydrocephalus is CSF overproduction, as with papilloma of the choroid plexus. Normal-pressure hydrocephalus (see below) is an important cause of communicating hydrocephalus.

Normal-pressure hydrocephalus

Normal-pressure hydrocephalus is a form of chronic communicating hydrocephalus that occurs on an idiopathic basis.

Clinical features

Classically, the disorder presents with the triad of gait disturbance, dementia and urinary incontinence or urgency.[307,308] The onset of symptoms is typically gradual and generally occurs in late middle age or later.

Of the classic triad of symptoms, gait disturbance typically constitutes the first evidence of this disorder. Patients may walk with short steps on a somewhat widened base, and sometimes there is a degree of shuffling, but the distinctive feature is a 'magnetic' gait; some may complain that it feels as if their feet are 'glued to the floor'.

The dementia is characterized by forgetfulness, slowness of thought and action, apathy, and indifference. Rarely, the clinical picture may be dominated by personality change or depression; even more rarely, the picture is dominated by aggressiveness or mania.

Urinary incontinence may be only intermittent and patients may not complain of it. At times, rather than incontinence there may only be urinary urgency.

On examination, there may be generalized hyperreflexia, and the Babinski sign may be positive bilaterally; snout and grasp reflexes may also be present.

CT or MRI reveals lateral ventricular enlargement out of proportion to any sulcal enlargement that may be present. If lumbar puncture is performed, then the opening pressure is typically normal.

Course

In most cases there is a gradual progression of symptoms, and some patients may eventually develop akinetic mutism and an inability to stand. Often, however, the hydrocephalus may become arrested, and symptoms may 'plateau out'.

Aetiology

Although the opening pressure on lumbar puncture is generally normal, it appears that in these patients there are indeed elevations in CSF pressure but that these elevations occur only intermittently, typically at night. In this condition, the hydrocephalus is of the communicating type and it appears that the intermittently increased pressure occurs secondary to an impaired outflow of CSF through the arachnoid villi.[309] The mechanism underlying this impaired outflow, however, is not known.

The mechanism whereby symptoms appear probably relates to stretching of the long periventricular axonal fibres.

KEY POINTS

Organic disorders that may manifest neuropsychiatric symptomatology include the following:

- Neurodegenerative and movement disorders
- Levodopa or dopamine agonist medication used in the treatment of parkinsonism
- Vascular disorders
- Trauma
- Hypoxic disorders
- Nutritional, toxic and metabolic disorders
- Infectious and related disorders
- Prion diseases
- Endocrine disorders
- Immune-related disorders
- Brain tumours
- Hydrocephalus.

FURTHER READING

Love S, Louis DN, Ellison DW (2008) *Greenfield's Neuropathology*, 8th edn. London: Hodder Arnold.

Moore DP (2008) *Textbook of Clinical Neuropsychiatry*, 2nd edn. London: Hodder Arnold.

REFERENCES

1. Hoehn MM, Yahr MD (1967) Parkinsonism: onset, progression and mortality. *Neurology* **17**: 427–42.
2. Hughes AJ, Daniel SE, Blankson S, *et al.* (1993) A clinicopathologic study of 100 cases of Parkinson's disease. *Archives of Neurology* **50**: 140–48.
3. April RS (1966) Observations on parkinsonian tremor in all-night sleep. *Neurology* **16**: 720–24.
4. Stern M, Roffwarg H, Duvoisin R (1968) The parkinsonian tremor in sleep. *Journal of Nervous and Mental Disease* **147**: 202–10.
5. Giladi N, McMahon D, Przedborski S, *et al.* (1992) Motor blocks in Parkinson's disease. *Neurology* **42**: 333–9.
6. Morris ME, Iansek R, Matyas TA, *et al.* (1996) Stride length regulation in Parkinson's disease: normalization strategies and underlying mechanisms. *Brain* **119**: 551–68.
7. Lang AE, Johnson K (1987) Akathisia in idiopathic Parkinson's disease. *Neurology* **37**: 477–81.
8. Verbaan D, Marinus J, Visser M, *et al.* (2007) Patient-reported autonomic symptoms in Parkinson disease. *Neurology* **69**: 333–41.
9. Biggins CA, Boyd JL, Harrop FM, *et al.* (1992) A controlled, longitudinal study of dementia in Parkinson's disease. *Journal of Neurology, Neurosurgery, and Psychiatry* **55**: 566–71.

10. Mayeux R, Stern Y, Rosenstein R, *et al.* (1988) An estimate of the prevalence of dementia in idiopathic Parkinson's disease. *Archives of Neurology* **45**: 260–62.
11. Mayeux R, Denaro J, Hemenegildo N, *et al.* (1992) A population-based investigation of Parkinson's disease with and without dementia: relationship to age and gender. *Archives of Neurology* **49**: 492–7.
12. Aarsland D, Andersen K, Larson JP, *et al.* (2003) Prevalence and characteristics of dementia in Parkinson disease: an 8-year prospective study. *Archives of Neurology* **60**: 387–92.
13. Aarsland D, Perry R, Brown A, *et al.* (2005) Neuropathology of dementia in Parkinson's disease: a prospective, community-based study. *Annals of Neurology* **58**: 773–6.
14. Hantz P, Caradoc-Davies G, Caradoc-Davies T, *et al.* (1994) Depression in Parkinson's disease. *American Journal of Psychiatry* **151**: 1010–14.
15. Tandberg E, Larsen JP, Aarsland D, *et al.* (1996) The occurrence of depression in Parkinson's disease: a community-based study. *Archives of Neurology* **53**: 175–9.
16. Mayeux R, Stern Y, Cote L, *et al.* (1984) Altered serotonin metabolism in depressed patients with Parkinson's disease. *Neurology* **34**: 642–6.
17. Starkstein SE, Preziosi TJ, Bolduc PL, *et al.* (1990) Depression in Parkinson's disease. *Journal of Nervous and Mental Disease* **178**: 27–31.
18. Mayeux R, Stern Y, Williams JBW, *et al.* (1986) Clinical and biochemical features of depression in Parkinson's disease. *American Journal of Psychiatry* **143**: 756–9.
19. Kuzis G, Sabe L, Tiberti C, *et al.* (1997) Cognitive functions in major depression and Parkinson disease. *Archives of Neurology* **54**: 982–6.
20. Chan-Palay V, Asan E (1989) Alterations in catecholamine neurons of the locus coeruleus in senile dementia of the Alzheimer type and in Parkinson's disease with and without dementia and depression. *Journal of Comparitive Neurology* **287**: 373–92.
21. Becker T, Becker G, Seufert J, *et al.* (1997) Parkinson's disease and depression: evidence for an alteration of the basal limbic system detected by transcranial sonography. *Journal of Neurology, Neurosurgery, and Psychiatry* **63**: 590–96.
22. Sveinbjornsdottir S, Hicks AA, Jonsson T, *et al.* (2000) Familial aggregation of Parkinson's disease in Iceland. *New England Journal of Medicine* **343**: 1765–70.
23. Piccini P, Burn DJ, Ceravolo R, *et al.* (1999) The role of inheritance in sporadic Parkinson's disease: evidence from a longitudinal study of dopaminergic function in twins. *Annals of Neurology* **45**: 577–82.
24. Ascherio A, Chen C, Weisskopf MG, *et al.* (2006) Pesticide exposure and risk for Parkinson's disease. *Annals of Neurology* **60**: 197–203.
25. Thacker EL, O'Reilly EJ, Weisskopf MG, *et al.* (2007) Temporal relationship between cigarette smoking and risk of Parkinson disease. *Neurology* **68**: 764–8.
26. Goetz CG, Wuu J, Curgian LM, *et al.* (2005) Hallucinations and sleep disorders in PD: six-year prospective longitudinal study. *Neurology* **64**: 81–6.
27. Holroyd S, Currie L, Wooten GF (2001) Prospective study of hallucinations and delusions in Parkinson's disease. *Journal of Neurology, Neurosurgery, and Psychiatry* **70**: 734–8.
28. Harding AJ, Stimson E, Hernderson JM, *et al.* (2002) Clinical correlates of selective pathology in the amygdala of patients with Parkinson's disease. *Brain* **125**: 2431–45.
29. Goetz CG, Fan W, Leurgans S, *et al.* (2006) The malignant course of 'benign hallucinations' in Parkinson disease. *Archives of Neurology* **63**: 713–16.
30. Rippon GA, Scarmeas N, Gordon PH, *et al.* (2006) An observational study of cognitive impairment in amyotrophic lateral sclerosis. *Archives of Neurology* **63**: 345–52.
31. Del Aguila MA, Longstreth WT, McGuire V, *et al.* (2003) Prognosis in amyotrophic lateral sclerosis: a population-based study. *Neurology* **60**: 813–19.
32. Rosen DR, Siddique T, Patterson D, *et al.* (1993) Mutations in Cu/Zn superoxide dismutase gene are associated with familial amyotrophic lateral sclerosis. *Nature* **362**: 59–62.
33. Verny M, Jellinger KA, Hauw J-J, *et al.* (1996) Progressive supranuclear palsy: a clinicopathological study of 21 cases. *Acta Neuropathologicaologica* **91**: 427–31.
34. Litvan I, Mega MS, Cummings JL, *et al.* (1996) Neuropsychiatric aspects of progressive supranuclear palsy. *Neurology* **47**: 1184–9.
35. Davis PH, Bergeron C, McLachlan DR (1985) Atypical presentation of progressive supranuclear palsy. *Annals of Neurology* **17**: 337–43.
36. Takahashi H, Oyanagi K, Takeda S, *et al.* (1989) Occurrence of 15-nm wide straight tubules in neocortical neurons in progressive supranuclear palsy. *Acta Neuropathologicaologica* **79**: 233–9.
37. Higgins JJ, Adler RI, Loveless JM (1999) Mutational analysis of the tau gene in progressive supranuclear palsy. *Neurology* **53**: 1421–4.
38. Morris HR, Gibb G, Katzenschlager R, *et al.* (2002) Pathological, clinical and genetic heterogeneity in progressive supranuclear palsy. *Brain* **125**: 969–75.
39. Bergeron C, Pollanen MS, Weyer L, *et al.* (1996) Unusual clinical presentation of cortical-basal ganglionic degeneration. *Annals of Neurology* **40**: 893–900.
40. Schneider JA, Watts RL, Gearing M, *et al.* (1997) Corticobasal degeneration: neuropathologic and clinical heterogeneity. *Neurology* **48**: 959–69.
41. Grimes DA, Lang AE, Bergeron CB (1999) Dementia as the most common presentation of cortical-basal ganglionic degeneration. *Neurology* **53**: 1969–74.
42. Murray R, Neumann M, Forman MS, *et al.* (2007) Cognitive and motor assessment in autopsy-proven corticobasal degeneration. *Neurology* **68**: 1274–83.

43. Litvan I, Cummings JL, Mega M (1998) Neuropsychiatric features of corticobasal degeneration. *Journal of Neurology, Neurosurgery, and Psychiatry* **65**: 717–21.
44. Geda YE, Boeve BF, Negash S, *et al.* (2007) Neuropsychiatric features in 36 pathologically confirmed cases of corticobasal degeneration. *Journal of Neuropsychiatry and Clinical Neurosciences* **19**: 77–80.
45. Ikeda K, Akiyama H, Iritani S, *et al.* (1996) Corticobasal degeneration with primary progressive aphasia and accentuated cortical lesion in superior temporal gyrus: case report and review. *Acta Neuropathologica* **92**: 534–9.
46. Parvizi J, Joseph J, Press DZ, *et al.* (2007) Pathological laughter and crying in patients with multiple system atrophy – cerebellar type. *Movement Disorders* **22**: 798–803.
47. Robbins TW, James M, Lange KW, *et al.* (1992) Cognitive performance in multiple system atrophy. *Brain* **115**: 271–91.
48. Critchley M, Greenfield JG (1948) Olivo-ponto-cerebellar atrophy. *Brain* **71**: 343–64.
49. Iranzo A, Santamaria J, Rye DB, *et al.* (2005) Characteristics of idiopathic REM sleep behavior disorder and that associated with MSA and PD. *Neurology* **65**: 247–52.
50. Plazzi G, Corsini R, Provini F, *et al.* (1997) REM sleep behavior disorder in multiple system atrophy. *Neurology* **48**: 1094–7.
51. Pflanz S, Besson JAO, Ebmeier KP, *et al.* (1991) The clinical manifestation of mental disorder in Huntington's disease: a retrospective case record study of disease progression. *Acta Psychiatrica Scandinavica* **83**: 53–60.
52. Britton JW, Uitti RJ, Ahlskog JE, *et al.* (1995) Hereditary late-onset chorea without significant dementia: genetic evidence for substantial phenotypic variation in Huntington's disease. *Neurology* **45**: 443–7.
53. Caine ED, Shoulson I (1983) Psychiatric symptoms in Huntington's disease. *American Journal of Psychiatry* **140**: 728–33.
54. Folstein SE, Abbott MH, Chase GA, *et al.* (1983) The association of affective disorder with Huntington's disease in a case series and in families. *Psychological Medicine* **13**: 537–42.
55. Paulsen JS, Ready RE, Hamilton JN, *et al.* (2001) Neuropsychiatric aspects of Huntington's disease. *Journal of Neurology, Neurosurgery, and Psychiatry* **71**: 31–4.
56. Paulsen JS, Hoth KF, Nehl C, *et al.* (2005) Critical periods of suicide risk in Huntington's disease. *American Journal of Psychiatry* **162**: 725–31.
57. Schoenfeld M, Myers RH, Cupples LA, *et al.* (1984) Increased rate of suicide among patients with Huntington's disease. *Journal of Neurology, Neurosurgery, and Psychiatry* **47**: 1283–7.
58. Medalia A, Merriam A, Sandberg M, *et al.* (1989) Neuropsychological deficits in choreoacanthocytosis. *Archives of Neurology* **46**: 573–83.
59. Bacalman S, Farzin F, Bourgeois JA, *et al.* (2006) Psychiatric phenotype of the Fragile X-associated tremor/ataxia syndrome (FXTAS) in males: newly described fronto-subcortical dementia. *Journal of Clinical Psychiatry* **67**: 87–94.
60. Bourgeois JA, Cogswell JB, Hessl D, *et al.* (2007) Cognitive, anxiety and mood disorders in the fragile X-associated tremor/ataxia syndrome. *General Hospital Psychiatry* **29**: 349–56.
61. Brunberg JA, Jacquemont S, Hagerman RJ, *et al.* (2002) Fragile X premutation carriers: characteristic MR imaging findings of adult male patients with progressive cerebellar and cognitive dysfunction. *American Journal of Neuroradiology* **23**: 1757–66.
62. Becher MW, Rubinsztein DC, Leggo J, *et al.* (1997) Dentatorubral and pallidoluysian atrophy (DRPLA): clinical and neuropathological findings in genetically conformed North American and European pedigrees. *Movement Disorders* **12**: 519–30.
63. Adachi N, Arima K, Asada T, *et al.* (2001) Dentatorubral-pallidoluysia atrophy (DRPLA) presenting with psychosis. *Journal of Neuropsychiatry and Clinical Neurosciences* **13**: 258–60.
64. Lee MS, Kim YD, Lyoo CH (1999) Oculogyric crisis as an initial manifestation of Wilson's disease. *Neurology* **52**: 1714–15.
65. Bridgman O, Smyth FS (1944) Progressive lenticular degeneration. *Journal of Nervous and Mental Disease* **99**: 534–43.
66. Dening TR, Berrios GE (1989) Wilson's disease: psychiatric symptoms in 195 cases. *Archives of General Psychiatry* **46**: 1126–34.
67. Walshe JM, Yealland M (1992) Wilson's disease: the problem of delayed diagnosis. *Journal of Neurology, Neurosurgery, and Psychiatry* **55**: 692–6.
68. Gysin WM, Cooke ET (1950) Unusual mental symptoms in a case of hepatolenticular degeneration. *Diseases of the Nervous System* **11**: 305–9.
69. Wilson SAK (1912) Progressive lenticular degeneration: a familial nervous disease associated with cirrhosis of the liver. *Brain* **34**: 295–509.
70. Davis EJB, Borde M (1993) Wilson's disease and catatonia. *British Journal of Psychiatry* **162**: 256–9.
71. Sinha S, Taly AB, Ravishankar S, *et al.* (2006) Wilson's disease: cranial MRI observations and clinical correlation. *Neuroradiology* **48**: 613–21.
72. Arpa J, Cuesta A, Cruz-Martinez A, *et al.* (1999) Clinical features and genetic analysis of a Spanish family with spinocerebellar ataxia 6. *Acta Neurologica Scandinavica* **99**: 44–7.
73. Ueyama H, Kumanoto T, Nagao S, *et al.* (1998) Clinical and genetic studies of spinocerebellar ataxia type 2 in Japanese kindreds. *Acta Neurologica Scandinavica* **98**: 427–32.

74. Shevell M (2003) Hallervorden and history. *New England Journal of Medicine* **348**: 3–4.
75. Angelini L, Nardocci N, Rumi V, *et al.* (1992) Hallervorden–Spatz disease: clinical and MRI study of 11 cases diagnosed in life. *Journal of Neurology* **239**: 417–25.
76. Hahn H, Trant MR, Brownstein MJ, *et al.* (2001) Neurologic and psychiatric manifestations in a family with a mutation in exon 2 of the guanosine triphosphate-cyclohydrolase gene. *Archives of Neurology* **58**: 749–55.
77. Van Hove JLK, Steyaert J, Matthijs G, *et al.* (2006) Expanded motor and psychiatric phenotype in autosomal dominant Segawa syndrome due to GTP cyclohydrolase deficiency. *Journal of Neurology, Neurosurgery, and Psychiatry* **77**: 18–23.
78. Lang AE (1991) Patient perception of tics and other movement disorders. *Neurology* **41**: 223–8.
79. Wojcieszek JM, Lang AE (1995) Gestes antagonistes in the suppression of tics: 'tricks for tics'. *Movement Disorders* **10**: 226–8.
80. Chee KY, Sachdev P (1997) A controlled study of sensory tics in Gilles de la Tourette syndrome and obsessive-compulsive disorder using a structured interview. *Journal of Neurology, Neurosurgery, and Psychiatry* **62**: 188–92.
81. Cohen AJ, Leckman JF (1992) Sensory phenomena associated with Gilles de la Tourette's syndrome. *Journal of Clinical Psychiatry* **23**: 319–23.
82. Leckman JF, Walker DE, Cohen DJ (1993) Premonitory urges in Tourette's syndrome. *American Journal of Psychiatry* **150**: 98–102.
83. Karp BI, Hallett M (1996) Extracorporeal 'phantom' tics in Tourette's syndrome. *Neurology* **46**: 38–40.
84. Stone LA, Jankovic J (1991) The coexistence of tics and dystonia. *Archives of Neurology* **48**: 862–5.
85. Frankel M, Cummings JL, Robertson MM, *et al.* (1986) Obsessions and compulsions in Gilles de la Tourette's syndrome. *Neurology* **36**: 378–82.
86. Robertson MM, Trimble MR, Lees AJ (1988) The psychopathology of Gilles de la Tourette's syndrome: a phenomenological analysis. *British Journal of Psychiatry* **152**: 388–90.
87. Leckman JF, Walker DE, Goodman WK, *et al.* (1994) 'Just right' perceptions associated with compulsive behavior in Tourette's syndrome. *American Journal of Psychiatry* **151**: 675–80.
88. Cardoso F, Veado CCM, de Oliveira JT (1996) A Brazilian cohort of patients with Tourette's syndrome. *Journal of Neurology, Neurosurgery, and Psychiatry* **60**: 209–12.
89. Leckman JF, Zhang H, Vitale A, *et al.* (1998) Course of tic severity in Tourette syndrome: the first two decades. *Pediatrics* **102**: 14–19.
90. Pappert EJ, Goetz CG, Louis ED, *et al.* (2003) Objective assessment of longitudinal outcome in Gilles de la Tourette's syndrome. *Neurology* **61**: 936–40.
91. Swedo SE, Leonhard HL, Garvey M, *et al.* (1998) Pediatric autoimmune neuropsychiatric disorders associated with streptococcal infections: clinical description of the first 50 cases. *American Journal of Psychiatry* **154**: 264–71.
92. Modoni A, Silvestri G, Pomponi MG, *et al.* (2004) Characterization of the pattern of cognitive impairment in myotonic dystrophy type 1. *Archives of Neurology* **61**: 1943–7.
93. Perini GI, Colombo G, Armani M, *et al.* (1989) Intellectual impairment and cognitive evoked potentials in myotonic dystrophy. *Journal of Nervous and Mental Disease* **177**: 750–54.
94. Huber SJ, Kissel JT, Shuttleworth EC, *et al.* (1989) Magnetic resonance imaging and clinical correlates of intellectual impairment in myotonic dystrophy. *Archives of Neurology* **46**: 536–40.
95. Delaporte C (1998) Personality patterns in patients with myotonic dystrophy. *Archives of Neurology* **55**: 635–40.
96. Winblad S, Lindberg C, Hansen S (2005) Temperament and character in patients with classical myotonic dystrophy type 1 (DM-1). *Neuromuscular Disorders* **15**: 287–92.
97. Rubinsztein JS, Rubinsztein DC, Goodburn S, *et al.* (1998) Apathy and hypersomnia are common features of myotonic dystrophy. *Journal of Neurology, Neurosurgery, and Psychiatry* **64**: 510–15.
98. Adie WJ, Greenfield JG (1924) Dystrophia myotonica (myotonia atrophica). *Brain* **47**: 73–127.
99. Billings EG, Ravin A (1941) A psychiatric study of patients manifesting dystrophica myotonica. *American Journal of Psychiatry* **97**: 1116–34.
100. Bungener C, Jouvent R, Delaporte C (1998) Psychopathological and emotional deficits in myotonic dystrophy. *Journal of Neurology, Neurosurgery, and Psychiatry* **65**: 353–6.
101. Manni R, Zucca C, Martinetti M, *et al.* (1991) Hypersomnia in dystrophica myotonica: a neurophysiological and immunogenetic study. *Acta Neurologica Scandinavica* **84**: 498–502.
102. Hansotia P, Frens D (1981) Hypersomnia associated with alveolar hypo-ventilation in myotonic dystrophy. *Neurology* **31**: 1336–7.
103. Phemister JC, Small JM (1961) Hypersomnia in dystrophia myotonica. *Journal of Neurology, Neurosurgery, and Psychiatry* **24**: 173–5.
104. Van der Meche FGA, Bogaard JM, van der Sluys JCM, *et al.* (1994) Daytime sleep in myotonic dystrophy is not caused by sleep apnoea. *Journal of Neurology, Neurosurgery, and Psychiatry* **57**: 626–8.
105. Koch MC, Grimm T, Harley HG, *et al.* (1991) Genetic risks for children of women with myotonic dystrophy. *American Journal of Human Genetics* **48**: 1084–91.
106. Di Costanzo A, De Salle F, Santoro L, *et al.* (2002) Pattern and significance of white matter abnormalities

in myotonic dystrophy type 1: an MRI study. *Journal of Neurology* **249**: 1175–82.

107. Zijlmans JCM, Thijssen HOM, Vogels OJM, *et al.* (1995) MRI in patients with suspected vascular parkinsonism. *Neurology* **45**: 2183–8.
108. Binswanger O (1894) Die abgrenzung des allgemeinen progressiven. *Paralysie Klin Wochenschr* **31**: 1103–5, 1137–9, 1180–86.
109. Blass JP, Hoyer S, Nitsch R (1991) A translation of Otto Binswanger's article 'The delineation of the generalized progressive paralyses'. *Archives of Neurology* **48**: 961–72.
110. Wilkinson IMS, Russell RWR (1972) Arteries of the head and neck in giant cell arteritis: a pathological study to show the pattern of arterial involvement. *Archives of Neurology* **27**: 378–91.
111. Caselli RJ, Hunder GG, Whisnant JP (1988) Neurologic disease in biopsy-proven giant cell (temporal) arteritis. *Neurology* **38**: 352–9.
112. Greenberg SM, O'Donnell HC, Schaefer PW, *et al.* (1999) MRI detection of new hemorrhages: potential marker of progression in cerebral amyloid angiopathy. *Neurology* **53**: 1135–8.
113. Nobuyoshi I, Nishihara Y, Horie A (1984) Amyloid angiopathy and lobar cerebral haemorrhage. *Journal of Neurology, Neurosurgery, and Psychiatry* **47**: 1203–10.
114. Okazaki H, Reagan TJ, Campbell RJ (1979) Clinicopathologic studies of primary cerebral amyloid: angiopathy. *Mayo Clinic Proceedings* **54**: 22–31.
115. Filley CM, Thompson LL, Sze CI, *et al.* (1999) White matter dementia in CADASIL. *Journal of the Neurological Sciences* **163**: 163–7.
116. Mellies JK, Baumer T, Muller JA, *et al.* (1998) SPECT study of a German CADASIL family: a phenotype with migraine and progressive dementia only. *Neurology* **50**: 1715–21.
117. Schon F, Martin RJ, Prevett M, *et al.* (2003) 'CADASIL coma': an underdiagnosed acute encephalopathy. *Journal of Neurology, Neurosurgery, and Psychiatry* **74**: 249–52.
118. Vollmer TL, Guarnaccia J, Harrington W, *et al.* (1993) Idiopathic granulomatous angiitis of the central nervous system: diagnostic challenges. *Archives of Neurology* **50**: 925–30.
119. Ford RG, Siekert RG (1965) Central nervous system manifestations of periarteritis nodosa. *Neurology* **15**: 114–22.
120. MacKay ME, McLardy T, Harris C (1950) A case of periarteritis nodosa of the central nervous system. *Journal of Mental Science* **96**: 470–75.
121. Borson S (1982) Behçet's disease as a psychiatric disorder: a case report. *American Journal of Psychiatry* **139**: 1348–9.
122. Hinchey J, Chaves C, Appignani B, *et al.* (1996) A reversible posterior leukoencephalopathy syndrome. *New England Journal of Medicine* **334**: 494–500.
123. Kritchevsky M, Squire LR (1989) Transient global amnesia: evidence for extensive, temporally graded retrograde amnesia. *Neurology* **39**: 213–18.
124. Byer JA, Crowley WJ (1980) Musical performance during transient global amnesia. *Neurology* **30**: 80–82.
125. Guillery-Girard B, Quinette P, Desgranges B, *et al.* (2006) Long-term memory following transient global amnesia: an investigation of episodic and semantic memory. *Acta Neurologica Scandinavica* **114**: 329–33.
126. Steinmetz EF, Vroom FQ (1972) Transient global amnesia. *Neurology* **22**: 1193–200.
127. Black DW (1984) Mental changes resulting from subdural hematoma. *British Journal of Psychiatry* **145**: 200–203.
128. Cameron MM (1978) Chronic subdural hematoma: a review of 114 cases. *Journal of Neurology, Neurosurgery, and Psychiatry* **41**: 834–9.
129. Scheid R, Walther K, Guthke T, *et al.* (2006) Cognitive sequelae of diffuse axonal injury. *Archives of Neurology* **63**: 418–24.
130. Strich SJ (1956) Diffuse degeneration of the cerebral white matter in severe dementia following head injury. *Journal of Neurology, Neurosurgery, and Psychiatry* **19**: 163–85.
131. McCrea M, Guskiewicz KM, Marshall SW, *et al.* (2003) Acute effects and recovery time following concussion in collegiate football players: the NCAA Concussion Study. *Journal of the American Medical Association* **290**: 2556–63.
132. Guskiewicz KM, McCrea M, Marshall SW, *et al.* (2003) Cumulative effects associated with recurrent concussion in collegiate football players: the NCAA Concussion Study. *Journal of the American Medical Association* **290**: 2459–55.
133. Hofman PA, Stapert SZ, von Kroonenburgh MJ, *et al.* (2001) MR imaging, single-photon emission CT, and neurocognitive performance after mild traumatic brain injury. *American Journal of Neuroradiology* **22**: 441–9.
134. Bigler ED (2004) Neuropsychological results and neuropathological findings at autopsy in a case of mild traumatic brain injury. *Journal of the International Neuropsychological Society* **10**: 794–806.
135. Sayers PR, Davenport SJ (1930) *Review of Carbon Monoxide Poisoning.* Public Health Bulletin no. 195. Washington, DC: US Government Printing Office.
136. Smith JS, Brandon S (1970) Acute carbon monoxide poisoning: 3 years experience in a defined population. *Postgraduate Medical Journal* **46**: 65–70.
137. Lurie LA (1919) Pernicious anemia with mental symptoms: observations on the variable extent and probable duration of central nervous system lesions in four autopsied cases. *Archives of Neurology Psychiatry* **2**: 67–109.
138. Fraser TN (1960) Cerebral manifestations of addisonian pernicious anemia. *Lancet* **2**: 458–9.

139. Goggans FC (1984) A case of mania secondary to vitamin B12 deficiency. *American Journal of Psychiatry* **141**: 300–301.
140. Smith LH (1929) Mental and neurologic changes in pernicious anemia. *Archives of Neurology and Psychiatry* **22**: 551–7.
141. Evans DL, Edelsohn GA, Golden RN (1983) Organic psychosis without anemia or spinal cord symptoms in patients with B12 deficiency. *American Journal of Psychiatry* **140**: 218–21.
142. Lindenbaum J, Healton EB, Savage DG, *et al.* (1988) Neuropsychiatric disorders caused by cobalamin deficiency in the absence of anemia or macrocytosis. *New England Journal of Medicine* **318**: 1720–28.
143. Reynolds EH, Rothfeld P, Pincus JH (1973) Neurological disease associated with folate deficiency. *British Medical Journal* **2**: 398–400.
144. Strachan RW, Henderson JG (1967) Dementia and folate deficiency. *Quarterly Journal of Medicine* **36**: 189–204.
145. Ishii N, Nishihara Y (1981) Pellagra among chronic alcoholics: clinical and pathological study of 20 necropsy cases. *Journal of Neurology, Neurosurgery, and Psychiatry* **44**: 209–15.
146. Jolliffe N, Bowman K, Rosenblum L, *et al.* (1940) Nicotinic acid deficiency encephalopathy. *Journal of the American Medical Association* **114**: 307–9.
147. Serdaru M, Hausser-Hauw C, Laplane D, *et al.* (1988) The clinical spectrum of alcoholic pellagra encephalopathy: a retrospective analysis of 22 cases studied pathologically. *Brain* **111**: 829–42.
148. Spivak JL, Jackson DL (1977) Pellagra: an analysis of 18 patients and a review of the literature. *Johns Hopkins Medical Journal* **140**: 295–309.
149. Pierce LB (1924) Pellagra: report of a case. *American Journal of Psychiatry* **81**: 237–43.
150. Abd El Naby S, Hassanein M (1965) Neuropsychiatric manifestations of chronic manganese poisoning. *Journal of Neurology, Neurosurgery, and Psychiatry* **28**: 282–8.
151. Cook DG, Fahn S, Brairt KA (1974) Chronic manganese intoxication. *Archives of Neurology* **30**: 59–64.
152. Charles JR (1927) Manganese toxaemia, with special reference to the effects of liver feeding. *Brain* **50**: 30–43.
153. Huang C-C, Lu C-S, Chu N-S, *et al.* (1993) Progression after chronic manganese exposure. *Neurology* **43**: 1479–83.
154. Huang C-C, Chu N-S, Lu C-S, *et al.* (1998) Long-term progression in chronic manganism: ten years of follow-up. *Neurology* **50**: 698–700.
155. Huang C-C, Chu N-S, Lu C-S, *et al.* (2007) The natural history of neurological manganism over 18 years. *Parkinsonism and Related Disorders* **13**: 143–5.
156. Huang C-C, Chus N-S, Lu C-S, *et al.* (1997) Cock gait in manganese intoxication. *Movement Disorders* **12**: 807–8.
157. Hart SP, Frier BM (1998) Causes, management and morbidity of acute hypoglycaemia in adults requiring hospital admission. *Quarterly Journal of Medicine* **91**: 505–10.
158. Malouf R, Brust JCM (1985) Hypoglycemia: causes, neurological manifestations, and outcome. *Annals of Neurology* **17**: 421–30.
159. Bosboom WMJ, Frijns CJM, Gijn J (1996) Yelling attacks and wasted hands. *Lancet* **348**: 238.
160. Zivin I (1970) The neurological and psychiatric aspects of hypoglycemia. *Diseases of the Nervous System* **31**: 604–7.
161. Case Records of the Massachusetts General Hospital (1988) *New England Journal of Medicine* **318**: 1523–8.
162. Moersch FP, Kernohan JW (1938) Hypoglycemia: neurologic and neuropathologic studies. *Archives of Neurology and Psychiatry* **39**: 242–57.
163. Rich LM, Caine MR, Findling JW, *et al.* (1990) Hypoglycemic coma in anorexia nervosa: case report and review of the literature. *Archives of Internal Medicine* **150**: 894–5.
164. Adams RD, Foley JM (1953) The neurological disorder associated with liver disease. *Research Publications – Association for Research in Nervous and Mental Disease* **32**: 198–237.
165. El-Mallakh RS, Shrader SA, Widger E (1987) Single case study: mania as a manifestation of end-stage renal disease. *Journal of Nervous and Mental Disease* **175**: 243–5.
166. Fraser CL, Arieff AI (1985) Hepatic encephalopathy. *New England Journal of Medicine* **313**: 865–73.
167. Read AE, Laidlaw J, Sherlock S (1961) Neuropsychiatric complications of portocaval anastamosis. *Lancet* **1**: 961–4.
168. Summerskill WHJ, Davidson EA, Sherlock S, *et al.* (1956) The neuropsychiatric syndrome associated with hepatic cirrhosis and extensive portal collateral circulation. *Quarterly Journal of Medicine* **25**: 245–66.
169. Jaffe N (1967) Catatonia and hepatic dysfunction. *Diseases of the Nervous System* **28**: 606–8.
170. Ficker DM, Westmoreland BF, Sharbrough FW (1997) Epileptiform abnormalities in hepatic encephalopathy. *Journal of Clinical Neurophysiology* **14**: 230–34.
171. Cross TN (1956) Porphyria: a deceptive syndrome. *American Journal of Psychiatry* **112**: 1010–14.
172. Paredes A, Jones H (1959) Psychopathology of acute intermittent porphyria: case report. *Journal of Nervous and Mental Disease* **129**: 291–301.
173. Hirsch S, Dunsworth FA (1955) An interesting case of porphyria. *American Journal of Psychiatry* **111**: 703.
174. Mandoki MW, Sumner GS (1994) Psychiatric manifestations of hereditary coproporphyria in a child. *Journal of Nervous and Mental Disease* **182**: 117–18.
175. Kobari M, Nogawa S, Sugimoto Y, *et al.* (1997) Familial idiopathic brain calcification with autosomal dominant inheritance. *Neurology* **48**: 645–9.

176. Slyter H (1979) Idiopathic hypoparathyroidism presenting as dementia. *Neurology* **29**: 393–4.
177. Wszolek ZK, Baba Y, Mackenzie IR, *et al.* (2006) Autosomal dominant dystonia-plus with cerebral calcifications. *Neurology* **67**: 620–25.
178. Lam JS, Fong SY, Yiu GC, *et al.* (2007) Fahr's disease: a differential diagnosis of frontal lobe syndrome. *Hong Kong Medical Journal* **13**: 75–7.
179. Weisman DC, Yaari R, Hansn LA, *et al.* (2007) Density of the brain, decline of the mind: an atypical case of Fahr disease. *Archives of Neurology* **64**: 756–7.
180. Chabot B, Roulland C, Dollfus S (2001) Schizophrenia and familial idiopathic basal ganglia calcification: a case report. *Psychological Medicine* **31**: 741–7.
181. Francis A, Freeman H (1984) Psychiatric abnormality and brain calcification over four generations. *Journal of Nervous and Mental Disease* **172**: 166–70.
182. Ostling S, Andreasson LA, Skoog I (2003) Basal ganglia calcification and psychotic symptoms in the very old. *International Journal of Geriatric Psychiatry* **18**: 983–7.
183. Trautner RJ, Cummings JL, Read SL, *et al.* (1988) Idiopathic basal ganglia calcification and organic mood disorders. *American Journal of Psychiatry* **145**: 350–53.
184. Lopez-Villegas D, Kulisevsky J, Deus J, *et al.* (1996) Neuropsychological alterations in patients with computed tomography-detected basal ganglia calcification. *Archives of Neurology* **53**: 251–6.
185. Sellal F, Mohr M, Collard M (1996) Dementia in a 58-year-old woman. *Lancet* **347**: 236.
186. Zunt JR, Tu RK, Anderson DM, *et al.* (1997) Progressive multifocal leukoencephalopathy presenting as human immunodeficiency virus type 1 (HIV)-associated dementia. *Neurology* **49**: 263–5.
187. Davies JA, Hughes JT, Oppenheimer DR (1973) Richardson's disease (progressive multifocal leukoencephalopathy). *Quarterly Journal of Medicine* **42**: 481–93.
188. Astrom KE, Mancall EL, Richardson EP (1958) Progressive multifocal leuko-encephalopathy: a hitherto unrecognized complication of chronic lymphatic leukaemia and Hodgkin's disease. *Brain* **81**: 93–111.
189. Fisher CM (1996) Hypomanic symptoms caused by herpes simplex encephalitis. *Neurology* **47**: 1374–8.
190. Wilson LG (1976) Viral encephalopathy mimicking functional psychosis. *American Journal of Psychiatry* **133**: 165–70.
191. Upton A, Gumpert J (1970) Electroencephalography in diagnosis of herpes-simplex encephalitis. *Lancet* **1**: 650–52.
192. Northam RS, Singer HS (1991) Postencephalitic acquired Tourette-like syndrome in a child. *Neurology* **41**: 592–3.
193. McCall S, Henry JM, Reid AH, *et al.* (2001) Influenza RNA not detected in archival brain tissues from acute encephalitis lethargica cases or in postencephalitic Parkinson cases. *Journal of Neuropathology and Experimental Neurology* **60**: 696–704.
194. Srinivasan A, Burton EC, Kuehnert MJ, *et al.* (2005) Transmission of rabies virus from an organ donor to four transplant recipients. *New England Journal of Medicine* **352**: 1103–11.
195. Wulf CH (1982) Subacute sclerosing panencephalitis: serial electroencephalographic studies. *Journal of Neurology, Neurosurgery, and Psychiatry* **45**: 418–21.
196. Dervaux A, Laine H, Czermak M, *et al.* (2004) Creutzfeldt–Jakob disease presenting as psychosis. *American Journal of Psychiatry* **161**: 1307–8.
197. Zeng S, Kim CH, Rahman H (2001) Psychotic symptoms presented in familial Creutzfeldt–Jakob disease, subtype E220K. *Journal of Clinical Psychiatry* **62**: 734–5.
198. Mandell AM, Alexander MP, Carpenter S (1989) Creutzfeldt–Jakob disease presenting as isolated aphasia. *Neurology* **39**: 55–8.
199. MacGowan DJL, Delanty N, Petito F, *et al.* (1997) Isolated myoclonic alien hand as the sole presentation of pathologically established Creutzfeldt–Jakob disease: a report of two patients. *Journal of Neurology, Neurosurgery, and Psychiatry* **63**: 404–7.
200. Lendvai I, Saravay SM, Steinberg MD (1999) Creutzfeldt–Jakob disease presenting as secondary mania. *Psychosomatics* **40**: 524–5.
201. Wieser HG, Schwarz U, Blatter T, *et al.* (2004) Serial EEG findings in sporadic and iatrogenic Creutzfeldt–Jakob disease. *Clinical Neurophysiology* **115**: 2467–78.
202. Steinhoff BJ, Zerr I, Glatting M, *et al.* (2004) Diagnostic value of periodic complexes in Creutzfeldt–Jakob disease. *Annals of Neurology* **56**: 702–8.
203. Antoine JC, Michel D, Bertholon P, *et al.* (1997) Creutzfeldt–Jakob disease after extracranial dura mater embolization for a nasopharyngeal angiofibroma. *Neurology* **48**: 1451–3.
204. Gibbs CJ, Asher DM, Kobrine A, *et al.* (1994) Transmission of Creutzfeldt–Jakob disease to a chimpanzee by electrodes contaminated during neurosurgery. *Journal of Neurology, Neurosurgery, and Psychiatry* **57**: 757–8.
205. Will RG, Zeidler M, Stewart GE, *et al.* (2000) Diagnosis of new variant Creutzfeldt–Jakob disease. *Annals of Neurology* **47**: 575–82.
206. Zeidler M, Stewart GE, Barraclough CR, *et al.* (1997) New-variant Creutzfeldt–Jakob disease: neurological features and diagnostic tests. *Lancet* **350**: 903–7.
207. Zeidler M, Johnstone EC, Bamber RWK, *et al.* (1997) New-variant Creutzfeldt–Jakob disease: psychiatric features. *Lancet* **350**: 908–10.
208. Collinge J, Rossor M (1996) A new-variant of prion disease. *Lancet* **347**: 916–17.
209. Will RG, Ironside JW, Zeidler M, *et al.* (1996) A new-

variant of Creutzfeldt–Jakob disease in the UK. *Lancet* **347**: 921–5.

210. Hill AF, Butterworth RJ, Joiner S, *et al.* (1999) Investigation of variant Creutzfeldt–Jakob disease and other human prion diseases with tonsil biopsy specimens. *Lancet* **353**: 183–9.
211. Wroe SJ, Pal S, Siddique D, *et al.* (2006) Clinical presentation and pre-mortem diagnosis of variant Creutzfeldt–Jakob disease associated with blood transfusion; a case report. *Lancet* **368**: 2061–7.
212. Almer G, Hainfellner JA, Brucke T, *et al.* (1999) Fatal familial insomnia: a new Austrian family. *Brain* **122**: 5–16.
213. Dimitri D, Jehel L, Durr A, *et al.* (2006) Fatal familial insomnia presenting as psychosis in an 18-year-old man. *Neurology* **67**: 363–4.
214. Spillane JD (1951) Nervous and mental disorders in Cushing's syndrome. *Brain* **74**: 72–94.
215. Kelly WF (1996) Psychiatric aspects of Cushing's syndrome. *Quarterly Journal of Medicine* **89**: 543–51.
216. Cohen SI (1980) Cushing's syndrome: a psychiatric study of 29 patients. *British Journal of Psychiatry* **136**: 120–24.
217. Maclay WS, Stokes AB (1939) Mental disorder in Cushing's syndrome. *Journal of Neurology, Neurosurgery, and Psychiatry* **1**: 110–18.
218. Trethowan WH, Cobb S (1952) Neuropsychiatric aspects of Cushing's syndrome. *Archives of Neurology Psychiatry* **67**: 283–309.
219. Jeffcoate WJ, Silverstone JT, Edwards CRW, *et al.* (1979) Psychiatric manifestations of Cushing's syndrome: response to lowering of plasma cortisol. *Quarterly Journal of Medicine* **191**: 465–72.
220. Haskett RF (1985) Diagnostic categorization of psychiatric disturbance in Cushing's syndrome. *American Journal of Psychiatry* **142**: 911–16.
221. Wolkowitz OM, Rubinow D, Doran AR, *et al.* (1990) Prednisone effects on neurochemistry and behavior. *Archives of General Psychiatry* **47**: 963–8.
222. Hickman JW, Atkinson RP, Flint LD, *et al.* (1961) Transient schizophrenic reaction as a major symptom of Cushing's syndrome. *New England Journal of Medicine* **264**: 797–800.
223. Hertz PE, Nadas E, Wojtkowiki H (1955) Case report: Cushing's syndrome and its management. *American Journal of Psychiatry* **112**: 144–5.
224. Engel GL, Margolin SG (1941) Neuropsychiatric disturbances in Addison's disease and the role of impaired carbohydrate metabolism in the production of abnormal cerebral function. *Archives of Neurology and Psychiatry* **45**: 881–4.
225. Cleghorn RA (1951) Adrenal cortical insufficiency: psychological and neurological observations. *Canadian Medical Association Journal* **65**: 449–54.
226. McFarland HR (1963) Addison's disease and related psychoses. *Comprehensive Psychiatry* **4**: 90–95.
227. Lahey FH (1931) Non-activated (apathetic) type of hyperthyroidism. *New England Journal of Medicine* **204**: 747–8.
228. Kathol RG, Delahunt JW (1986) The relationship of anxiety and depression to symptoms of hyperthyroidism using operational criteria. *General Hospital Psychiatry* **8**: 23–8.
229. Thomas FB, Mazzaferri EL, Skillman TG (1970) Apathetic thyrotoxicosis: a distinctive clinical and laboratory entity. *Annals of Internal Medicine* **72**: 679–85.
230. Taylor JW (1975) Depression in thyrotoxicosis. *American Journal of Psychiatry* **132**: 552–3.
231. Van Uitert RL, Russakoff LM (1979) Hyperthyroid chorea mimicking psychiatric disease. *American Journal of Psychiatry* **136**: 1208–10.
232. Trzepacz P, McCue M, Klein I, *et al.* (1988) A psychiatric and neuropsychological study of patients with untreated Graves' disease. *General Hospital Psychiatry* **10**: 49–55.
233. Ingham SD, Nielsen JM (1931) Thyroid psychosis: difficulties in diagnosis. *Journal of Nervous and Mental Disease* **74**: 271–7.
234. Hodgson RE, Murray D, Woods MR (1992) Othello's syndrome and hyperthyroidism. *Journal of Nervous and Mental Disease* **180**: 663–4.
235. Bulens C (1981) Neurologic complications of hyperthyroidism: remission of spastic paralysis, dementia, and optic neuropathy. *Archives of Neurology* **38**: 669–70.
236. Martin FI, Deam DR (1996) Hyperthyroidism in elderly hospitalized patients: clinical features and treatment outcomes. *Medical Journal of Australia* **164**: 200–203.
237. Bursten B (1961) Psychosis associated with thyrotoxicosis. *Archives of General Psychiatry* **4**: 267–73.
238. Greer S, Parsons V (1968) Schizophrenia-like psychosis in thyroid crisis. *British Journal of Psychiatry* **114**: 1357–62.
239. Ghobrial MW, Ruby EB (2002) Coma and thyroid storm in apathetic thyrotoxicosis. *Southern Medical Journal* **95**: 552–4.
240. Nickel SN, Frame B (1958) Neurologic manifestations of myxedema. *Neurology* **8**: 511–17.
241. Jellinek EH, Kelly RE (1960) Cerebellar syndrome in myxoedema. *Lancet* **2**: 225–7.
242. Mitchell JRA, Surridge DHC, Willison RG (1959) Hypothermia after chlorpromazine in myxoedematous psychosis. *British Medical Journal* **2**: 932–3.
243. Whybrow PC, Prange AJ, Treadway CR (1969) Mental changes affecting thyroid gland dysfunction: a reappraisal using objective psychological measurement. *Archives of General Psychiatry* **20**: 48–63.
244. Asher R (1949) Myxoedematous madness. *British Medical Journal* **2**: 555–62.
245. Crowley RM (1940) Psychoses with myxedema. *American Journal of Psychiatry* **96**: 1105–16.
246. Karnosh LJ, Stout RE (1935) Psychoses of myxedema. *American Journal of Psychiatry* **91**: 1263–74.

247. Akelaitis AJE (1936) Psychiatric aspects of myxedema. *Journal of Nervous and Mental Disease* **83**: 22–36.
248. Uyematsu S (1920) A case of myxedematous psychosis. *Archives of Neurology Psychiatry* **3**: 252–76.
249. Calabrese JR, Gulledge AD, Hahn K, *et al.* (1985) Autoimmune thyroiditis in manic-depressive patients treated with lithium. *American Journal of Psychiatry* **142**: 1318–21.
250. Bergin JD (1957) Rapidly progressive dementia in disseminated sclerosis. *Journal of Neurology, Neurosurgery, and Psychiatry* **20**: 285–92.
251. Jennekens-Schinkel A, Sanders EACM (1986) Decline of cognition in multiple sclerosis: dissociable artifacts. *Journal of Neurology, Neurosurgery, and Psychiatry* **49**: 1354–60.
252. Mendez MF, Frey WH (1992) Multiple sclerosis dementia. *Neurology* **42**: 696.
253. Fontaine B, Seilhean D, Tourbah A, *et al.* (1994) Dementia in two histologically confirmed cases of multiple sclerosis: one case with isolated dementia and one case associated with psychiatric symptoms. *Journal of Neurology, Neurosurgery, and Psychiatry* **57**: 353–9.
254. Surridge D (1969) An investigation into some psychiatric aspects of multiple sclerosis. *British Journal of Psychiatry* **115**: 749–64.
255. Fassbender K, Schmidt R, Mofsner R, *et al.* (1998) Mood disorders and dysfunction of the hypothalamic-pituitary-adrenal axis in multiple sclerosis. *Archives of Neurology* **55**: 66–72.
256. Schiffer RB, Babigian H (1984) Behavioral disorders in multiple sclerosis, temporal lobe epilepsy and amyotrophic lateral sclerosis: an epidemiologic study. *Archives of Neurology* **41**: 1067–9.
257. Whitlock FA, Siskind MM (1980) Depression as a major symptom of multiple sclerosis. *Journal of Neurology, Neurosurgery, and Psychiatry* **43**: 861–5.
258. Moller A, Wiedemann G, Rohde U, *et al.* (1994) Correlates of cognitive impairment and depressive mood disorder in multiple sclerosis. *Acta Psychiatrica Scandinavica* **89**: 117–21.
259. Rabins PV, Brooks BR, O'Donnell P, *et al.* (1986) Structural brain correlates of emotional disorder in multiple sclerosis. *Brain* **109**: 585–97.
260. Schiffer RB, Caine ED, Bamford KA, *et al.* (1983) Depressive episodes in patients with multiple sclerosis. *American Journal of Psychiatry* **140**: 1498–500.
261. Feinstein A, Roy P, Lobaugh N, *et al.* (2004) Structural brain abnormalities in multiple sclerosis patients with major depression. *Neurology* **62**: 586–90.
262. Pujol J, Bello J, Deus J, *et al.* (1997) Lesions in the left arcuate fasciculus region and depressive symptomatology in multiple sclerosis. *Neurology* **49**: 1105–10.
263. Berg D, Supprian T, Thomas J, *et al.* (2000) Lesion patterns with multiple sclerosis and depression. *Multiple Sclerosis* **6**: 156–62.
264. Cottrell SS, Wilson SAK (1926) The affective symptomatology of disseminated sclerosis: a study of 100 cases. *Journal of Neurology Psychopathology* **7**: 1–30.
265. Wilson SAK (1954) *Neurology*, 2nd edn. London: Butterworths.
266. Joffe RT, Lippert GP, Gray TA, *et al.* (1987) Mood disorder and multiple sclerosis. *Archives of Neurology* **44**: 376–8.
267. Schiffer RB, Wineman M, Weitkamp LR (1986) Association between bipolar affective disorder and multiple sclerosis. *American Journal of Psychiatry* **143**: 94–5.
268. Pine DS, Douglas CJ, Charles E, *et al.* (1995) Patients with multiple sclerosis presenting to psychiatric hospitals. *Journal of Clinical Psychiatry* **56**: 297–306.
269. Feinstein A, Feinstein K, Gray T, *et al.* (1997) Prevalence and neurobehavioral correlates of pathological laughing and crying in multiple sclerosis. *Archives of Neurology* **54**: 1116–21.
270. Mathews WB (1979) Multiple sclerosis presenting with acute remitting psychiatric symptoms. *Journal of Neurology, Neurosurgery, and Psychiatry* **42**: 859–63.
271. Parker N (1956) Disseminated sclerosis presenting as schizophrenia. *Medical Journal of Australia* **1**: 405–7.
272. Martinez-Yelamos A, Saiz A, Sanchez-Valle R, *et al.* (2001) 14-3-3 protein in the CSF as prognostic marker in early multiple sclerosis. *Neurology* **57**: 722–4.
273. Ganz VH, Gurland BJ, Deming WE, *et al.* (1972) The study of the psychiatric symptoms of systemic lupus erythematosus: a biometric study. *Psychosomatic Medicine* **34**: 207–20.
274. Miguel EC, Rodriguez Pereira RM, de Braganca Pereira CA, *et al.* (1994) Psychiatric manifestations of systemic lupus erythematosus: clinical features, symptoms, and signs of central nervous system activity in 43 patients. *Medicine* **73**: 224–32.
275. Guze SB (1967) The occurrence of psychiatric illness in systemic lupus erythematosus. *American Journal of Psychiatry* **123**: 1562–70.
276. Hugo FJ, Halland AM, Spangenberg JJ, *et al.* (1996) DSM-III-R classification of psychiatric symptoms in systemic lupus erythematosus. *Psychosomatics* **37**: 262–9.
277. Johnson RT, Richardson EP (1968) The neurological manifestations of systemic lupus erythematosus: a clinical–pathological study of 24 cases and review of the literature. *Medicine* **47**: 337–69.
278. Lim L, Ron MA, Ormerod IEC, *et al.* (1988) Psychiatric and neurological manifestations in systemic lupus erythematosus. *Quarterly Journal of Medicine* **66**: 27–38.
279. Agius MA, Chan JW, Chung S, *et al.* (1997) Role of antiribosomal P protein antibodies in the diagnosis of lupus isolated to the central nervous system. *Archives of Neurology* **54**: 862–4.
280. Devinsky O, Petito CK, Alonso DR (1988) Clinical and

neuropathological findings in systemic lupus erythematosus: the role of vasculitis, heart emboli, and thrombotic thrombocytopenic purpura. *Annals of Neurology* **23**: 380–84.

281. Susac JO, Hardman JM, Selhorst JB (1979) Microangiopathy of the brain and retina. *Neurology* **29**: 313–16.
282. Tandon R, Walden M, Falcon S (1988) Catatonia as a manifestation of paraneoplastic encephalopathy. *Journal of Clinical Psychiatry* **49**: 121–2.
283. Hook O (1954) Sarcoidosis with involvement of the nervous system. *Archives of Neurology Psychiatry* **71**: 554–75.
284. Thompson C, Checkley S (1981) Short term memory deficit in a patient with cerebral sarcoidosis. *British Journal of Psychiatry* **139**: 160–61.
285. Scott TF, Yandora K, Valeri A, *et al.* (2007) Aggressive therapy for neurosarcoidosis. *Archives of Neurology* **64**: 691–6.
286. Rubinstein I, Gray TA, Moldofsky H, *et al.* (1988) Neurosarcoidosis associated with hypersomnolence treated with corticosteroids and brain irradiation. *Chest* **94**: 205–6.
287. Bostantjopoulou S, Zafiriou D, Katsarou Z, *et al.* (1996) Hashimoto's encephalopathy: clinical and laboratory findings. *Functional Neurology* **11**: 247–51.
288. Galluzzi S, Geroldi C, Zanetti O, *et al.* (2002) Hashimoto's encephalopathy in the elderly: relationship to cognitive impairment. *Journal of Geriatric Psychiatry and Neurology* **15**: 175–9.
289. Swedo SE, Rapoport JL, Cheslow DL, *et al.* (1989) High prevalence of obsessive-compulsive symptoms in patients with Sydenham's chorea. *American Journal of Psychiatry* **146**: 246–9.
290. Asbahr FR, Negrao AB, Gentil V, *et al.* (1998) Obsessive-compulsive and related symptoms in children and adolescents with and without chorea: a prospective 6-month study. *American Journal of Psychiatry* **155**: 1122–4.
291. Swedo SE, Leonard HL, Schapiro MB, *et al.* (1993) Sydenham's chorea: physical and psychological symptoms of St Vitus dance. *Pediatrics* **91**: 706–13.
292. Creak M, Guttmann E (1935) Chorea, tics, compulsive utterances. *Journal of Mental Science* **81**: 834–9.
293. Nausieda PA, Grossman BJ, Koller WC, *et al.* (1980) Sydenham chorea: an update. *Neurology* **30**: 331–4.
294. Diefendorf AR (1912) Mental symptoms of acute chorea. *Journal of Nervous and Mental Disease* **39**: 161–72.
295. Abt IA, Levinson A (1916) A study of two-hundred twenty-six cases of chorea. *Journal of the American Medical Association* **67**: 1342–7.
296. MacKenzie S (1887) Report on inquiry: II. Chorea. *British Medical Journal* **1**: 425–36.
297. Haskell RH (1914) Mental disturbance associated with acute articular rheumatism. *American Journal of Insanity* **71**: 361–81.
298. Hammes EM (1922) Psychoses associated with Sydenham's chorea. *Journal of the American Medical Association* **79**: 804–7.
299. Leys D (1946) Rheumatic encephalopathy. *Edinburgh Medical Journal* **53**: 444–9.
300. Putzel L (1879) Cerebral complications of chorea. *Medical Record* 220–22.
301. Avery TL (1971) Seven cases of frontal tumor with psychiatric presentation. *British Journal of Psychiatry* **119**: 19–23.
302. Keschner M, Bender MB, Strauss I (1936) Mental symptoms in cases of tumor of the temporal lobe. *Archives of Neurology and Psychiatry* **35**: 572–96.
303. Alpers BJ (1940) Personality and emotional disorders associated with hypothalamic lesions. In JF Fulton, SW Ranson, AM Frantz (eds) *Research Publications: Association for Research in Nervous and Mental Disease. The Hypothalamus and Central Levels of Autonomic Function.* Baltimore, MD: William & Wilkins.
304. Ironside R, Guttmacher M (1929) The corpus callosum and its tumors. *Brain* **52**: 442–83.
305. Reeves AG, Plum F (1969) Hyperphagia, rage and dementia accompanying a ventromedial hypothalamic neoplasm. *Archives of Neurology* **20**: 616–24.
306. Messert B, Henke TK, Langheim W (1966) Syndrome of akinetic mutism associated with obstructive hydrocephalus. *Neurology* **16**: 635–49.
307. Adams RD, Fisher CM, Hakim S, *et al.* (1965) Symptomatic occult hydrocephalus with 'normal' cerebrospinal fluid pressure. *New England Journal of Medicine* **273**: 117–26.
308. Hill ME, Lougheed WM, Barnett HJM (1967) A treatable form of dementia due to normal-pressure, communicating hydrocephalus. *Canadian Medical Association Journal* **97**: 1309–11.
309. Borgesen SE, Gjerris F (1987) Relationships between intracranial pressure, ventricular size, and resistance to CSF outflow. *Journal of Neurosurgery* **67**: 535–9.

Chapter 38

Schizophrenia and paranoid psychoses

Peter F Buckley and Peter Jones

INTRODUCTION

Schizophrenia is the most severe of all of the mental illness, although thankfully it is not as common as other conditions such as depression and anxiety disorders. Although schizophrenia clearly runs in families, the genetic basis for this condition is poorly understood. Many patients have no family history of psychosis. Other factors such as brain trauma and obstetric complications are also considered important. The prevailing view of schizophrenia is that this is a disorder (or perhaps even a collection of disorders of similar presentation) that has its origins in faulty brain development in utero. Treatment for schizophrenia needs to be comprehensive and sustained. Medications are the bedrock of treatment, but medications alone are not sufficient and patients need many supports towards their recovery. This chapter provides a current overview of our understanding of the aetiology, course and treatment of schizophrenia.

HISTORICAL AND CONCEPTUAL CONTEXT

Although it is clear that mental illness existed in ancient times, the first clinical characterization of schizophrenia is credited to the German psychiatrist Kraepelin (1855–1926).[1] He differentiated 'dementia praecox' [the dementia of youth], which later evolved into the schizophrenia concept, from bipolar disorder or 'manic depressive insanity'. Schizophrenia was characterized by Kraepelin as having a protracted, downward-spiralling clinical course. The prominence of psychotic symptoms (delusions and hallucinations) was also acknowledged. However, schizophrenia actually got its name from Eugen Bleuler (1857–1959). This Swiss psychiatrist coined the term 'schizophrenia' to describe the fragmentation of mental processes that occurs with the illness. The term has been misused widely, and ascribed to ideas of schizophrenia as a 'split personality' and a 'Jekyll and Hyde' person. Since the name is now stigmatizing and conjures such negative ideas, there have been attempts to rename the condition.

Bleuler was less focused on positive symptoms as the hallmark of schizophrenia. He considered other aspects of greater importance. His fundamental symptoms became known as the 'four As': ambivalence, loosening of associations, affective incongruity and blunting, and autism, by which he meant emotional withdrawal. Bleuler had meant to narrow the diagnostic criteria but, inadvertently, his ideas led to a nondescript, diffuse concept of schizophrenia. Another influential clinician turned philosopher, Karl Jaspers, took this notion to another extreme and proposed that schizophrenia was characterized and recognizable by the clinician's inability to understand the patient's world and mental processes – the so-called 'Praecox feeling'.

In contrast, Kurt Schneider took a much more strict phenomenological approach and determined that, in the absence of an organic cause, the presence of the following symptoms (so called 'first-rank symptoms') were diagnostic of schizophrenia. These first-rank symptoms were:

- hearing third-person voice hallucinations;
- hearing running-commentary hallucinations;
- hearing one's own thoughts spoken aloud;
- feeling that one's body is under the control or influence of somebody or something else;
- actions or feelings that are experienced or behaved as coming from the influence of somebody or something else;
- feeling that one's thoughts are being broadcast to others (thought-broadcasting);
- feeling that one's thoughts are being taken away or external thoughts are being put into one's mind (thought withdrawal or insertion);
- delusional perception (the belief that something 'ominous' has changed but one cannot figure out what it is; this is the period of perplexity, just before the patient becomes frankly delusional).

These descriptions by Schneider have been highly influential, although on their own they are not really diagnostic or pathognomonic of schizophrenia. Schneider was, in fact, quite humble about their significance, merely considering them to be particularly useful to the clinician making a judgement about the presence or absence of schizophrenia.

More recent contributions have focused on aetiology and potential types of schizophrenia. Timothy Crow, in England, ascribed aetiological relevance to the pattern of symptoms in schizophrenia, describing how positive symptoms were associated with more neurochemical changes while negative symptoms were evidence of structural brain changes.[2] Crow and his colleague Eve Johnstone were the first to show brain changes on the computed tomography (CT) scans of patients with schizophrenia, findings that they called the 'dementia of dementia praecox'. Crow described a type 1/type II classification of schizophrenia:

- *Type I:* more florid presentation; more positive symptoms; probably due to dopamine dysregulation; shows a good response to antipsychotic therapy.
- *Type II:* more chronic; predominantly negative symptoms; associated with enlarged brain ventricles and cortical tissue loss; shows a poor response to antipsychotic therapy.

William Carpenter in the USA has asserted that people who have an illness with predominantly negative symptoms (the so-called 'deficit syndrome') have a distinct subtype of schizophrenia that differs on brain chemistry, structural brain changes, treatment responsivity and course.[3] Peter Liddle in England described three syndromes of schizophrenia: (i) a positive syndrome – 'reality distortion – characterized by delusions and hallucinations; (ii) a negative syndrome (broadly similar to the concept of deficit syndrome; see above); and (iii) a 'disorganization' syndrome characterized by positive formal thought disorder, inappropriate affect and poverty of speech content. Robin Murray in England and Daniel Weinberger in the USA have emphasized the notion that schizophrenia is a disorder of faulty brain development.[4] Evidence from many studies over the past 30 years supports their neurodevelopmental hypothesis of schizophrenia. This evidence includes:

- postmortem brain changes of under- or maldeveloped cells and brain structures;
- brain imaging findings at the time of diagnosis;
- gene abnormalities, especially among those that code for brain development;
- obstetric complications;
- season of birth phenomenon – a curious, well-replicated, excess of births of people with schizophrenia in the first 3 months of the year;
- heightened associations of schizophrenia with prenatal (first trimester) infections, malnutrition and other prenatal insults;
- presence of minor physical anomalies that signify brain maldevelopment.

Today, this is the prevailing theory of schizophrenia, having been supported by direct evidence of abnormalities of motor and language milestones, cognition and social performance that occur in early childhood, antedating florid psychosis; it is the focus of much of the current research. Weinberger has even developed 'prenatal-lesioned' (rat) animal models of schizophrenia that simulate some of the neurochemical abnormalities in schizophrenia. Crow has also suggested that this faulty brain development is genetically based and that it is related to speech development and to sexual dimorphism. Nancy Andreasen in the USA has proposed that schizophrenia is a disorder of brain dysconnectivity. She has described a series of imaging studies of pattern of brain abnormalities that are associated with schizophrenia.[5]

This brief historical overview provides a useful context for considering what we currently know about schizophrenia and how we treat the condition. The reader is also directed to several excellent reviews on schizophrenia and some authoritative books.[6–13] Sadly, the reality is that schizophrenia remains an enigmatic condition. Because of this and because of its association (albeit overstated and misunderstood by the lay public) with violence, schizophrenia remains a highly stigmatizing condition. One study evaluated 'potential discriminatory experiences' among 732 people with schizophrenia in 27 countries:[14] positive discrimination was rarely noted, and the majority of patients had experienced some form of negative discrimination. Over 70 per cent of patients did not wish to reveal their mental illness in public. Patients felt they were discriminated against in getting (29% of patients) and keeping (29%) a job, and most patients (64%) said they would decline to even apply for a job because of the certainty of discrimination. Stigma is a pervasive problem.

DIAGNOSIS

Schizophrenia is a complicated diagnosis. Current operational criteria for the disorder, such as those of the fourth edition of the *Diagnostic and Statistical Manual of Mental Disorders* (DSM-IV) in the USA and the tenth revision of the *International Statistical Classification of Diseases and Related Health Problems* (ICD-10) in Europe emphasize a Schneiderian view of the condition being characterized by delusions (fixed, false beliefs), hallucinations (typically 'hearing voices' in the absence of any sensory input), disturbances of speech (illogicality, non-linearity of thought and conversation), restricted affect and emotionality, and impairments of thinking (memory, attention, reasoning, awareness). It is important to distinguish this psychosis from other psychotic conditions, which it can resemble in presentation (Table 38.1). It is also important to note that many patients may not present with florid symptoms. Additionally, patients may present with depressive symptoms first as part of a prodromal state, and then there is the later emergence of delusions and hallucinations.[15]

Table 38.1 Conditions that can resemble schizophrenia

Major depression with psychotic features
Bipolar disorder
Drug-induced psychoses
Organic-related psychoses:
– infections
– toxins
– cerebrovascular
– metabolic
– endocrine
Delusional disorder

Given the impact of symptoms, the condition is typically associated with a decline in social or occupational performance. Indeed, this may be what parents, friends or colleagues notice first – a withdrawal, dropping out of college, or inability to cope with the stress of work. For many patients, the onset of such 'disintegration' is insidious. Other people experience a more a florid presentation, manifest by prominent delusions, hallucinations and bizarre behaviours, leading to disruptive public behaviour and emergency contact with the police. There are also cognitive impairments (in executive functioning, attention, reasoning, comprehension, and both short- and long-term memory) that, although in many cases are more subtle and 'overshadowed' by the delusions and hallucinations, are still quite disabling aspects of the illness.

Patients can be ill for many months or even years before they come into treatment, and there is increasing evidence linking the duration of untreated psychosis (DUP) with poorer outcome,[16] now confirmed in systematic reviews (Figure 38.1). There are a variety of reasons as to why this may be, including neurobiological concepts of kindling and the strengthening of neural circuits involved in psychopathology with time, psychological notions linking continued trauma from frightening psychotic experiencing leading to further morbidity, and social explanations of increasing loss of social capital (education, family ties, occupational and vocational opportunity) the longer a young adult remains ill. It is likely that each plays a part.

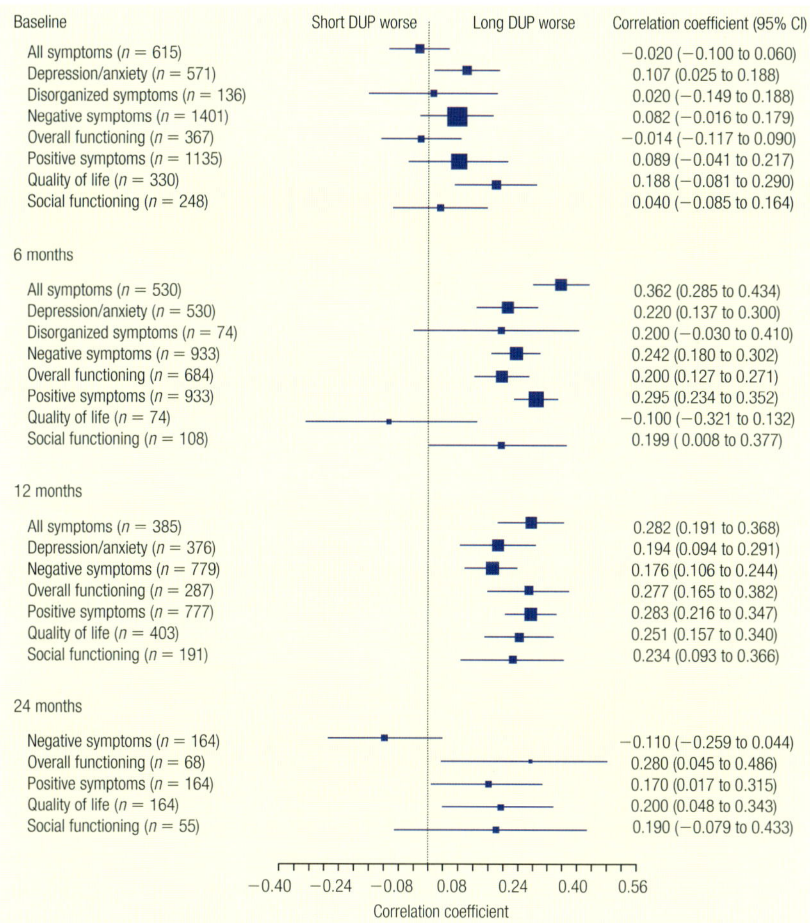

Figure 38.1 Summary correlations between duration of untreated psychosis (DUP) and outcomes by follow-up point in months. The size of the squares is roughly proportional to the amount of data available in the systematic review. Note the consistency of findings with longer DUP associated with poorer outcomes in a variety of domains

CI, confidence interval.

Reproduced with permission from ref. 16.

Thus, while there is a lack of strong evidence that reducing DUP will improve outcome (although evidence is accumulating, e.g. Power *et al.*[17]), this notion of intervening early engenders great zeal and determination among many disciplines who find reasons to support it. This observation has led to considerable developments in service delivery. Early intervention services for young adults with a first episode of psychosis are now becoming common around the world. The interventions that these and other services should deliver are reviewed later in this chapter.

Taken to another stage, early intervention through an effort to identify people with prodromal symptoms (e.g. oddities of behaviour and speech, strange non-delusional ideas) or early fragments of the schizophrenia syndrome, so-called 'at-risk mental states' (ARMS), have begun. Some studies have suggested that giving antipsychotics (or perhaps even antidepressants, alone) to these patients might forestall a psychotic break. However, there are serious ethical considerations with this approach.[18] The earlier the intervention is delivered, the lower the proportion of a group of people with ARMS will actually develop a psychotic syndrome; the positive predictive value for such a syndrome may be relatively low, although in a treatment-seeking group that, by definition, has disability of some sort, there are other morbidities that merit intervention. This complex context is compounded by costs to all those treated with antipsychotics in terms of side effects, which may be serious and even life-threatening; even follow-up and 'watchful waiting' may have down-sides in terms of anxiety and stigma.

Although a dramatic presentation may lead some to wonder 'how hard can it be to diagnose this person as psychotic?', the presentation could (and in fact is likely to) be complicated by abuse of drugs. This complicates things considerably. Also, as stated above, many people who develop schizophrenia become depressed as the illness evolves. It can be difficult to determine whether the person has major depression or is in the early stages of a psychotic illness. It is therefore best to wait to see how things play out definitively over months before making such a serious diagnosis as schizophrenia. Practically, the ICD mandates that clinicians consider this illness as 'schizophreniform disorder' if the duration is less than 6 months.[19] This is because some patients may have only a single psychotic episode, which looks indistinguishable from schizophrenia, but they will regain normal functioning without any recurrence. Similarly, patients who abuse drugs such as cannabis can have a psychotic break that appears like schizophrenia, but they too may regain normal functioning without further episodes once they stop taking the drugs; this is known as 'drug-induced psychosis'.[6] Thus, these recent classifications build in to the diagnosis the notion of poor prognosis first emphasized by Kraepelin (who would have seen mainly people with poor prognosis in his asylum setting). This excludes schizophrenia syndromes that either are brief with a good prognosis or have a putative aetiological association with drugs. Others suggest that the schizophrenia syndrome should merely reflect the psychological phenomena rather than comment on cause or course.

Schizophrenia typically begins in adolescence or in early adulthood. This is one of the most robust findings about the disorder that shapes its huge personal and societal impact and probably betrays a great deal about its biology and the vulnerability of the postpubertal brain to generate the syndrome. This is an important developmental period involving the maturation of myelinated connections bringing cognitively important cortical areas such as the dorsolateral prefrontal cortex 'online', and the sculpturing of those connections at the ultra-structural, synaptic level.

Schizophrenia is often said to occur equally in men and women, although the more one defines the disorder to exclude affective disturbance, the more there is a preponderance of men. Most affected young men and women develop schizophrenia at a similar age in their later teens and twenties, but the risk period for women goes on for longer, such that their average age at onset is around 4 years later. In addition, the illness tends to be milder in women, with, on average, a better outcome. The reasons for these gender differences are not known. However, it has been suggested that overall the illness is milder in females and that this might be because of some moderating effect of sex hormones upon the dopamine system.

CAUSES

Ultimately, we do not know what causes schizophrenia.[6–10] However, we consider that schizophrenia runs in families and is associated with birth complications, head injury, epilepsy and drug abuse. Cannabis abuse raises one's risk for schizophrenia by 2- to 4.5-fold. The initial evidence by Andreasson and colleagues in a longitudinal study of Swedish conscripts caused controversy, as it was one of the first pieces of evidence to support an environmental 'cause' of schizophrenia.[20] The debate has continued with valuable findings from other cohort studies but remains controversial because of the difficulties in the distinction between the effects of acute intoxication, after which a psychotic syndrome may wear off, as in the drug-induced psychoses mentioned above, and the question as to whether cannabis use can precipitate an ongoing schizophrenia syndrome that persists even once cannabis is cleared from the body. Given that cannabis use is common in people with the disorder and that some people are reluctant to stop using cannabis, probably because of an underlying and under-recognized dependence syndrome, these two issues are difficult to tease apart. A meta-analysis of all relevant studies confirmed an association, although more modest than some authorities had been arguing (Figure 38.2).[21] However, it is possible that, overall, average results such as these mask individuals at particularly strong risk who are mixed in with others at low or even no risk. Some studies suggest

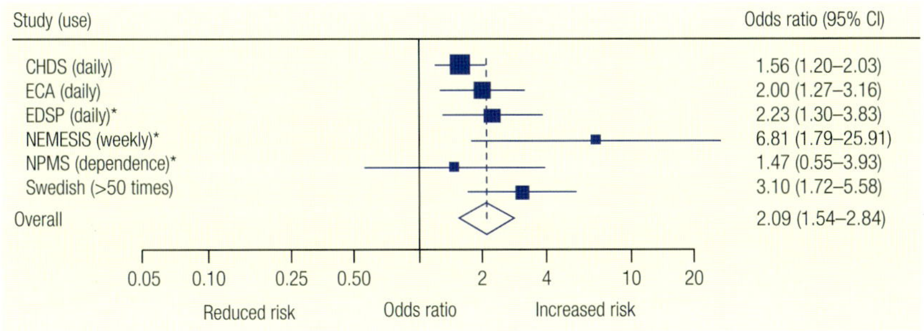

Figure 38.2 Forest plot showing adjusted odds ratios and 95 per cent confidence interval (CI) for any psychosis outcome according to most frequent use of cannabis in individual studies

Results not adjusted for other drug use.

that people who also have a genetic vulnerability are 16 times more likely to become psychotic when they abuse cannabis. The relationship of cannabis to the risk of schizophrenia has become an important research and even political issue for healthcare policy.

Schizophrenia is not due to a single cause. However, it is not known whether schizophrenia is a disease with many causes or whether schizophrenia is a collection of similar diseases, each with a different single (or simple) cause.[22] An ongoing debate about the causes of schizophrenia is whether any particular event (e.g. genetic defects, birth complications) leads to this condition (like the model of multiple causes of epilepsy) or alternatively, whether each of these can cause a psychotic condition that has a different cause but is similar in presentation and fits under the general profile of schizophrenia (as in pneumonia, whether caused by a virus or by bacteria).

Genetic component

Whether schizophrenia is a single illness or multiple illnesses has not been teased out, but we do know that it has a strong genetic basis that puts relatives at risk.[22,23] We know that the condition is overrepresented, in a complex manner, in families. Also, bipolar disorder appears to be overrepresented – albeit not to the same extent – in the families of people who have schizophrenia. In a study by Lichtenstein and colleagues, the heritability of schizophrenia and bipolar disorder was estimated at 64 per cent and 59 cent, respectively, and first-degree relatives of people with either condition had an increased risk for these disorders.[24] Environmental influences were estimated at 4.5 per cent for schizophrenia and 3.4 per cent for bipolar disorder. There appears to be substantial overlap between these disorders, attributable to shared genetic effects rather than environmental influences. However, the genetics of schizophrenia are highly complex. Genetic studies have shown abnormalities on several chromosomes (e.g. chromosome 5, 8, 11, 13, 22).[24] As with many aspects of schizophrenia, the findings are inconclusive and do not point to a precise gene involved. More recent genetic studies have focused on the search for abnormalities in genes or their related proteins that are involved in development (e.g. dysbindin, neuregulin, synaptosome-associated protein of 25 000 Da (SNAP-25), brain-derived neurotrophic factor (BDNF)).[22] These approaches seek candidate regions based upon prior studies and for known pathophysiological links, with many now focusing on gene regions that are involved in neurodevelopment. Additionally, new approaches also apply genome-wide single-nucleotide polymorphism arrays, exploring for rare copy number variants (CNVs). A study group found evidence for rare genetic variants in an extremely large patient sample (3391 patients with schizophrenia) compared with matched control subjects ($n = 3181$).[25] In addition to the anticipated deletions in the region on chromosome 13 that have already been implicated in velocardiofacial syndrome (a genetic condition in which 30% of patients develop a psychosis that is indistinguishable from schizophrenia), the study found small deletions on chromosomes 1 and 15 that had not been reported previously. A separate consortium also found small deletions in the same areas on chromosome 15.[26] Although these variants are rare and represent deletion of sections of DNA, they substantially increase the risk of schizophrenia. Nevertheless, they still account for only a small amount of the total number of cases of schizophrenia.

Birth and other environmental factors

One of the most reproducible findings in schizophrenia is that affected patients are far more likely to have been born in the first 3 months of the year – the so-called 'season of birth effect'.[27] This curious, yet robust, association points to birth or to the time in utero as relevant to the development of schizophrenia. It has been reliably estimated that about 20 per cent of people who develop schizophrenia have had some sort of birth complication. These include events such as prenatal exposure to influenza, haemolytic anaemia, severe malnutrition, pre-eclampsia, asphyxia or fetal distress. A study examined BDNF from umbilical cord and maternal blood samples collected in a large cohort of people who later developed schizophrenia. It was observed that BDNF was significantly reduced in those patients who experienced fetal hypoxia, further emphasizing the importance of obstetrical complications as an aetiological event in schizophrenia.[28] The birth complication may occur because of some problem in pregnancy or labour or the fetus may be neurodevelopmentally challenged in some way. Brain development in utero might have gone wrong in some way due to genetic misprogramming or due to some external injury (e.g.

a mother with an infection during the critical first 3 months of pregnancy). Another study found that mothers who were exposed to the death of a relative during the first trimester of their pregnancy were 1.67 times more likely to have offspring who later developed schizophrenia or related psychoses.[29] Interestingly, the study did not find any higher risk of schizophrenia if the death of the relative occurred in the 6 months before conception or even after the first trimester. There are several lines of evidence that point to the vulnerability of the fetal brain to the physiological impact of stress, especially the effects of glucocorticoids early in brain development. There is a confluence of evidence that these risk factors (in utero stress, infection, malnutrition, vitamin D) may play a role in the aetiology of schizophrenia.[27]

People with schizophrenia frequently abuse alcohol or illicit drugs. This occurs throughout the illness. This relationship is also often seen at the time of the person's first presentation of psychosis, raising the vexing 'chicken and egg' question. Indeed, it is a key question as to whether substance abuse can 'cause' schizophrenia, whether it is some epiphenomenon or the result of people self-medicating to cope with the symptoms of schizophrenia. The preponderance of evidence points to some likely causative role for some drugs, particularly cannabis;[30] as argued above, part of this association may be explained by genotype–environment interaction.

Other aspects of the environment undoubtedly influence the genesis of schizophrenia. We have been through a period where received wisdom was that the incidence or first occurrence of schizophrenia was the same everywhere. The evidence for this notion came mainly from the highly influential study in ten countries by the World Health Organization that indicated similar incidence of the disorder in the different sites.[31] However, the point of the study was, in fact, to indicate that the disorder occurred at all in different settings and cultures, not that the incidence was the same. When the syndrome was defined fairly broadly (so numbers of cases and statistical power were higher), there were significant differences, also hinted at with more narrow definitions but with far lower precision or ability to differentiate. This should have come as no surprise given that Farris and Dunham, two Chicago social scientists, had identified in the 1920s marked gradients in the first occurrence of paranoid schizophrenia, but not bipolar disorder, according to the socioeconomic characteristics of small areas of that city.[32] The incidence over 10 years was obviously higher in the central, poorer districts than in the more affluent, peripheral districts. Although it is accepted that people with chronic illness tend to drift into less affluent areas (so-called 'social drift'), the contribution of the social environment to the first occurrence of the illness is more challenging.

A series of studies from the UK have reinvigorated interest in the influence of the social environment, building on the evidence of the associations that Faris and Dunham identified, including their apparent distinction between non-affective psychosis (schizophrenia) and affective illness. There is considerable evidence linking social adversity at the neighbourhood level and evidence linking lower social bonds (social cohesion) in communities with an increased risk of first-episode schizophrenia.[33–36] It is the areas in which people live and interact with others that are important, rather than the country level.

Another dimension of the environmental aspect of risk comes from studies of migrant populations, a paradigm combining aspects of person and place. Just like the link with cannabis, the finding that migrant groups are at increased risk has been contentious, particularly because, in the UK and in the rest of Europe, the phenomenon linked perhaps the most stigmatizing disorder, schizophrenia, with one of the most socially disadvantaged groups, the black Caribbean migrant community. Several decades of research have been necessary to ensure that the association is not due to diagnostic bias, under-enumeration of the migrant population and other biases, but it is now clear that the link does exist and that it survives adjustment for obvious alternative explanations such as poverty and cannot be explained by reasons such as different patterns of drug use in these groups. Not only has a systematic review shown uncanny consistency in the findings of studies throughout the world and including many migrant groups in many countries,[37] but also studies in the UK now demonstrate that this is not a phenomenon confined to Afro-Caribbean people.[38,39] Rather, it seems as if being a migrant, and perhaps particularly a 'visible' minority in a host community, leads to an increased risk of schizophrenia and other psychotic disorders; the effects are huge, with relative risks of five-fold or so. The fact that the incidence of schizophrenia appears unremarkable in the country of origin, the lack of obvious familiality or selective migration to suggest purely genetic explanations, and the apparent normal development of children from migrant groups destined to develop schizophrenia all point towards the explanation of this phenomenon being in the realm of a psychosocial trigger related to the experience of being a minority in a host community.

Thus, studies of the social environment not only show large effects but also offer insights into new mechanisms, such as 'social defeat',[40,41] in which psychological experience can itself become toxic, particularly perhaps in an individual (brain) that is vulnerable for other reasons, whether genetic or related to the very early environment. One can see the necessity to develop realistically complex models that are not confined to either genetic or environmental models.

BRAIN ABNORMALITIES AND THE NEURODEVELOPMENTAL HYPOTHESIS

There is evidence that brain development is disturbed in schizophrenia. The evidence comes from postmortem brain studies of people with schizophrenia who died from natural causes (e.g. heart attack, although this could also influence or bias postmortem brain findings) or from suicide (which could also affect the brain).[42] Although this type of research has its own methodological problems, these studies have shown convincing evidence of abnormal (underdeveloped) cells and of cells that are misplaced or misaligned in the brains of people with schizophrenia. More recent studies have shown deficits in the expression of neurodevelopmental genes and BDNF in several postmortem brain collections.[22]

Imaging studies of patients show a range of brain abnormalities: smaller cortex overall, preferentially less grey matter than white matter, enlarged ventricles (especially the lateral ventricles), enlarged caudate nucleus and putamen (these latter findings are likely due to the effect of antipsychotic medications), smaller thalamus and reduced temporal lobes (especially reductions in the hippocampal regions).[43,44] These subtle findings occur more often in the temporal lobes than in any other brain regions, with perhaps more left hemisphere involvement. Magnetic resonance imaging (MRI) studies have also included relatives of patients with schizophrenia as a comparison group. These reveal much milder, but similar, findings in healthy relatives (who do not have the illness but may have genes susceptible to schizophrenia).[45] This raises the question of whether such brain abnormalities are present from birth or even before the onset of schizophrenia. Studies of patients in their first episode of psychosis show the same patterns of abnormalities on brain imaging, but in a more attenuated form.[46] Studies of prodromal populations show even milder, barely detectable brain abnormalities. In one such study, the prodromal patients who went on to have a psychotic break had more temporal lobe abnormalities on MRI than patients who did not progress to psychosis.[47] There are also many functional imaging studies that include the use of positron-emission tomography (PET), single-photon-emission computed tomography (SPECT), functional magnetic resonance imaging (fMRI) and magnetic resonance spectroscopy (MRS).[43] These confirm a pattern of underactivity of the frontal lobes. Studies have also shown that hearing voices is associated with overactivity in the (left) temporal lobe regions. Also, both MRS studies of first-episode patients and longitudinal MRS studies reveal a decrement in *N*-acetyl-aspartate (NAA), a putative marker of neuronal integrity.

Collectively, these findings have led many people to consider schizophrenia as a neurodevelopmental disorder.[48] Cortical vulnerabilities may become exposed at adolescence when the brain shows heightened plasticity. Drugs or stress during adolescence may be other critical events.

Seemingly in direct opposition to the brain-imaging evidence that supports the neurodevelopmental hypothesis in schizophrenia, other, long-term imaging studies report a progressive loss of brain tissue.[43,48] For example, MRI studies in patients with first-episode schizophrenia who are then rescanned years later demonstrated that progressive brain changes occur in patients who relapse and are more symptomatic. A more recent study tested the relationship between vulnerability in the expression of BDNF polymorphism and progressive brain tissue loss on MRI. Their results showed that patients who possess the met-met allele had the most reduction in frontal lobe tissue. Interestingly, patients who received most medications had the most frontal tissue loss, an effect that proved independent of BDNF polymorphism status.[49]

OTHER THEORIES ABOUT THE CAUSES OF SCHIZOPHRENIA

Oxidative stress has been proposed as another mechanism to understand how schizophrenia occurs and how the disease has such a broad constellation of effects.[7–10] It is proposed that, through vulnerability to oxidative damage, there are free radical effects that impact on cellular processes, especially mitochondrial, prostaglandin and cell-membrane functioning. This hypothesis has been studied in a variety of ways, including plasma and cerebrospinal fluid assays for breakdown products of oxidative stress, brain imaging of neurochemistry using MRS, and treatment studies using vitamin E or fish-oil products. There continue to be other, more speculative ideas about schizophrenia. Some authors have suggested that infections might cause schizophrenia, either through prenatal efforts (see earlier) or through retroviral or genetic encoding effects;[27] *Toxoplasmosa gondii* has been studied as an example.[6] It is also suggested that urban factors might be causative for schizophrenia;[6,22] exactly what these factors are is unclear at present. One study suggested that schizophrenia might be caused by irritation of the brain that could occur from middle-ear disease.[50] The study determined that people who had middle-ear disease were over 3.6 times more likely to have a later diagnosis of schizophrenia (or over 4 times more likely if the middle-ear disease was on the left side). It is no longer believed that parents can cause schizophrenia through their communication styles; these old hypotheses (the 'double-blind' hypothesis, the 'schizophrenogenic matter' hypothesis) were highly damaging.

BRAIN CHEMISTRY AND SCHIZOPHRENIA

Overactivity of the dopamine neurotransmitter system is the most compelling neurochemical abnormality in schizophrenia.[51,52] This is also the most easily explained theory:

people become psychotic because their dopamine is overactive. There is certainly evidence for this, including functional brain-imaging studies that show excess of dopamine in the brain of patients when they are acutely psychotic. But, like all the other explanations of schizophrenia, it is not quite as simple as 'too much dopamine'. Some researchers have suggested that there is overactivity of dopamine in one brain region (e.g. temporal lobes), concomitant with underactivity in another area (e.g. frontal lobes). Also, the fault may not be across all dopamine receptors but perhaps may be selective in some of the subclasses of dopamine receptors or even beyond the actual receptors, as a downstream deficit in cell signalling. It is clear that other neurotransmitter systems are affected in schizophrenia; the neurotransmitter systems implicated in this disease include cholinergic, glutamatergic, noradrenergic and serotonin. Deficits in these other neurotransmitter systems (e.g. glutamate receptors) may be primary or may underlie schizophrenia directly or indirectly through their interrelated effects on the dopamine system.[53] Thus far, the dopamine system has been the most pronounced neurochemical abnormality. Additionally, dopamine dysregulation plays a role in how antipsychotic drugs work.[51] The neuropharmacology of antipsychotics is described later.

TREATMENT: GENERAL CONSIDERATIONS

Schizophrenia is a difficult illness to treat.[54] Antipsychotic drugs work best on positive symptoms but have generally limited impact on negative or cognitive symptoms. This is a real drawback since, in the long run, negative and cognitive symptoms tend to be more disabling. These are the features that most limit functional outcome and the patient's capacity to work. Additionally, antipsychotic medications have a substantial side-effect burden. This includes both distressing side effects (e.g. sedation, restlessness) and life-shortening effects (e.g. myocarditis, pulmonary embolism, obesity, metabolic syndrome). It is perhaps not surprising, given the inadequate efficacy combined with adverse effects of these medications, and the inherent impairment of insight among patients, that many patients become non-adherent with their treatment. This adds further complexity to the care of people with schizophrenia. It is also important to appreciate that the medications alone are ineffective and that patients need counselling, support, family involvement, care advice and job skills training. Most services struggle to provide the breadth of personnel, skills and resources that are needed for comprehensive care.[54,55] Additionally, there is considerable variability in the access to care and in the medication practices (e.g. variability between practitioners with underdosing of medications, patients staying too long on a medication, with patients receiving two or more antipsychotics simultaneously). A well-constructed comprehensive plan, delivered over time in a consistent and collaborative manner, compiled with the support of family members and a strong sense of hope and personal resilience, collectively offers the best chance for a successful long-term outcome for patients with this chronic, relapsing condition.

Treatment expectations: from relapse to recovery

Although many patients will relapse over time, especially if they stop their medication (there is a one in five risk of relapse over 1 year when patients stop their medications), it is nevertheless equally important to emphasize that patients can recover and lead a satisfying life, albeit often with diminished lifetime goals.[56] A clinical US study by Harding and colleagues found that 68 per cent of patients met defined recovery criteria when they were contacted again some 32 years after their (lengthy) hospitalization.[57] More recently, Harrow and colleagues, in an ongoing Chicago study, found that 41 per cent of patients had recovered when contacted after 15 years.[58] In an effort to raise the bar in treatment in order to enhance remission and recovery, Andreasen and colleagues proposed criteria for remission.[59] There are also operational criteria for recovery.[60] There is also a growing consumer perspective that views 'recovery' less as an outcome and more as a recovery process.[61] In this recovery model, patients are less focused on the symptoms and disability of schizophrenia and instead are focused on living a meaningful life in the community. This is a more personal and optimistic model that places greater emphasis on individual choice and collaboration in treatment, on personal resilience and self-determination, on hope and on spirituality. It is akin to how somebody copes with having multiple sclerosis, diabetes mellitus or coronary artery disease: the medicines are key, but what really matters is the patient's own resilience, hope and personal outlook. We have a poor understanding of how all of these potentially powerful individual strengths and effects ultimately impact the course of schizophrenia. Much of our focus is on the prevailing medical model, whereby we seek to diligently quantify and compare the effects of medicines.

Treatment settings

Most people with schizophrenia receive their care as outpatients in community facilities or programmes that they attend regularly, sometimes daily or weekly. Many patients live at home and their care is in effect overseen by their families, a visiting nurse or a multidisciplinary (assertive community treatment, ACT) team.[62] Many patients live in supported housing, group homes or personal care homes overseen by counsellors or care managers. Patients do best when they have regular contact with their treatment team, especially when they can also access their treatment team in times of stress or relapse.

Unfortunately, many people with schizophrenia need to be hospitalized when they get sick. This is best achieved on a voluntary basis. Hospital stays are generally short (on average, a week or less), and the patients are then returned to their community setting with a (revised) treatment plan and the support to avert another hospitalization. The construction and range of community services are covered in chapter 73. Hospital admission is indicated when the patient poses a risk to him- or herself or to others. Patients who have bizarre and highly disturbing behaviour often need to be hospitalized. Patients may also have to be hospitalized for worsening of their illness due to side effects of medications or due to medical co-morbidities. For some patients, simply staying out of the hospital is a laudable outcome; these patients require the most intensive community support. For a minority of patients, long-term hospital care is a sad and hard-to-come-by necessity.

When a patient refuses to come into the hospital and they truly pose a risk to self or others, then the clinician may commit the patient involuntarily to in-patient care. The circumstances and procedures for involuntary committal are covered in chapter 79.

Treatment team and resources

'It takes a village!' Although the patient and psychiatrist might together decide on medications and other aspects of treatment, successful care requires much more than that. It requires a team of mental health professionals working collaboratively with the patient and their family. Increasingly, patients also help themselves by organizing into self-help groups (e.g. Schizophrenia Anonymous, analogous to Alcoholics Anonymous) or by helping each other as trained peer counsellors (peer-support specialists). Patients also turn to the Internet for education, support and resources. A European study showed how patients could use a Web-based self-monitoring system to detect when they were relapsing and to communicate this more effectively to their psychiatrists.

MEDICATION CHOICES

Antipsychotic medications, in spite of their limitations, are truly the bedrock of treatment. Unfortunately, clinicians and patients struggle greatly together to find the best fit among the choices of available medications. Medication choice remains highly variable and individualized. It is not driven by neurobiological considerations. Indeed, medication choice remains a trial-and-error process, with the patient's risk for particular side effects associated with any given medication generally being taken into consideration.[7,8] We know generally what dose of medication to prescribe, but we have little scientific understanding to guide actual dosing decisions for a particular patient. By perhaps too simply an analogy, it is important to learn in general how to drive a car, but it is crucial to know how best to drive your own car. This wide variability in medication choices and treatment decisions, underlying an inability to predict response or tolerability for the particular patient, is a major obstacle in treating schizophrenia. There is some hope that pharmacogenetics will offer greater predictability of treatment response and side-effect liability. Initial pharmacogenetic studies of clozapine have shown the promise of this strategy.[63]

Mechanism of action of antipsychotics

Exactly how antipsychotics work remains a mystery. Most evidence points to effects on blocking dopamine receptors in the mesolimbic system. For first-generation antipsychotics (FGAs; see below), it has been proposed from neuroimaging (PET, SPECT) studies that the drugs need to achieve at least a 60 per cent occupancy rate of dopamine receptors in order to be clinically effective.[51] The dilemma is that at 70 per cent occupancy rate of dopamine receptors, these drugs cause muscle side effects.[64] Some drugs, such as haloperidol, are more potent in their binding and can saturate the dopamine receptors at relatively low doses. Other antipsychotics are low-potency agents and are generally given at higher doses. Among second-generation antipsychotics (SGAs; see below), the situation is even more complex. These drugs are highly variable in the extent and manner that they bind to dopamine receptors. Risperidone, olanzapine and ziprasidone bind to dopamine (D_2) receptors at proportionately lower rates than FGAs and at relatively lower rates compared with each other (risperidone is the most potent in D_2 binding among these three drugs). Clozapine generally reaches only a 40–50 per cent D_2 occupancy rate, and giving more medication will not exceed this rate ('glass-ceiling effect'). Quetiapine has an even lower rate (28% average) of D_2 binding, although Kapur and colleagues have proposed the elegant 'kiss-and-run' theory to explain that quetiapine appears to saturate D_2 receptors.[65] In contrast, aripiprazole virtually saturates D_2 receptors with a 90–95 per cent D_2 occupancy rate, even at low doses;[66] this agent, however, has a partial agonist effect – that is, it functions more as a dopamine agonist when the synapse has insufficient dopamine, and it becomes more of a dopamine antagonist when there is an excess of dopamine. The dopamine hypothesis of antipsychotic action is complicated further by the existence of multiple subtypes of dopamine receptors, and these medications have variable affinities for these receptors. Efforts to design highly selective dopamine antagonists with sensitivity to a particular subtype alone have not produced clinically robust antipsychotic agents.[67]

Kapur has also emphasized that dopamine antagonism alone is 'necessary but not sufficient' for antipsychotic effects. In truth, these drugs have wide-ranging effects on other neurotransmitter systems – cholinergic, noradrenergic, serotonergic and histaminergic. This may explain some variability in their effects on symptoms, although it is generally considered that these binding profiles are more discriminatory of the side-effect burden of each drug. More recently, research efforts have focused selectively on these neurotransmitters as a target to add specific drugs to treat specific symptoms. As an example, anticholinesterase agents have been tried as augmenting agents alongside antipsychotic medications in an effort to enhance cognition.[68] An exciting new development is the advent of a completely new class of antipsychotic drugs,[69] acting via glutamate and related receptors, which have shown promising results in early (phase II) clinical trials. Not only is their action through a non-dopaminergic (in the first instance) mechanism, suggesting new understanding of the disease and also freedom from the side-effect profiles of current drugs, but also they may have efficacy against the particularly disabling cognitive deficits that define poor outcome for many people. Further evidence is eagerly awaited.

Nevertheless, all of the currently available antipsychotics bind to D_2 receptors at least to some extent, providing at least some unifying hypothesis as to their mechanism of action. On the other hand, clozapine, the most effective antipsychotic, binds the least of all antipsychotics to D_2 receptors. Clozapine has a highly complex binding profile to multiple neurotransmitters. Meltzer has suggested that its relative antagonism at dopamine and serotonin receptors is key to clozapine's mode of action. To that end, risperidone, ziprasidone and sertindole were developed with a predominance of dopamine/serotonin antagonism. Conversely, olanzapine most closely resembles clozapine in its complex pharmacology at multiple receptors. There is intense interest in new drugs that are in development.[67] There are several selective antagonists that act at glutamate receptors, and one has already shown a favourable clinical profile.[69] The neuropharmacology of many FGAs and SGAs is summarized in Table 38.1.

First- and second-generation antipsychotics

The classification of antipsychotics is awkward and confusing. Older ('typical', 'conventional') antipsychotics are now being increasingly referred to as 'FGAs'. Clozapine and the newer drugs ('atypicals') that have come after it are referred to as 'SGAs'. This classification suggests a class effect, although none really exists. It is now generally appreciated that, leaving aside clozapine, which usually is considered unique, there is no major difference in efficacy between FGAs and SGAs. Moreover, there is no overwhelming evidence of superiority of one drug over another within either the earlier FGA class of drugs or the current SGAs. These points are hotly debated. An appraisal of the current literature is helpful here. Geddes and colleagues in Oxford conducted a highly influential meta-analysis of studies comparing FGAs and SGAs.[70] They suggested that the clinical benefits of SGAs were 'overemphasized' and that too high doses of FGAs were used in these studies, thereby 'stacking the deck' in favour of SGAs. Conversely, Davies and colleagues reported similarity between FGAs and SGAs in another meta-analysis.[71] Leucht and colleagues examined 1-year relapse rates in studies comparing FGAs and SGAs.[56] In their meta-analysis, SGAs were superior to FGAs. More recently, Leucht and colleagues reported another meta-analysis, showing no difference between antipsychotics.[72] Another study suggested that source of funding was the major determinant of whether one drug fared better than another in comparative clinical trials among SGAs.[73]

Several large, often independently funded studies have produced comparative data to inform this key consideration of relative merits among available antipsychotics. In the USA, Lieberman and colleagues reported the results of the 1457-patient pragmatic study Clinical Antipsychotic Trials of Intervention Effectiveness (CATIE).[74] Although open to multiple interpretations, the 18-month study found that on the primary study measure ('all cause discontinuation'), the SGAs (risperidone, quetiapine, ziprasidone) were similar to perphenazine. In contrast, olanzapine proved to be the most robust and yet also the least well-tolerated antipsychotic. In England, Jones and colleagues reported the results of the 314-patient pragmatic study Cost Utility of the Latest Antipsychotic drugs in Schizophrenia Study 1 (CUtLASS 1). This group hypothesized that randomization to prescription of an SGA compared with an FGA would result in a benefit in terms of quality of life (and a variety of secondary outcomes) at 1 year. Such a benefit was definitely excluded (Figure 38.3), leading to a clear cost-effectiveness for the FGA and possibly at least clinical equipoise between the two groups; patients showed no preference for SGA drugs.[75]

In a parallel study of treatment-resistant schizophrenia (CUtLASS 2), clozapine stood out as the most effective drug.[76] Phase II of the CATIE study also reported clozapine's superiority.[77] The Treatment of Early Onset Schizophrenia Study (TEOSS) provides comparative date on FGAs versus SGAs for the treatment of schizophrenia.[78] In this study of childhood schizophrenia, 116 children and adolescents aged 8–19 years were randomized to 8 weeks of treatment with olanzapine, risperidone or molindone. Efficacy was generally similar across all three groups, with response

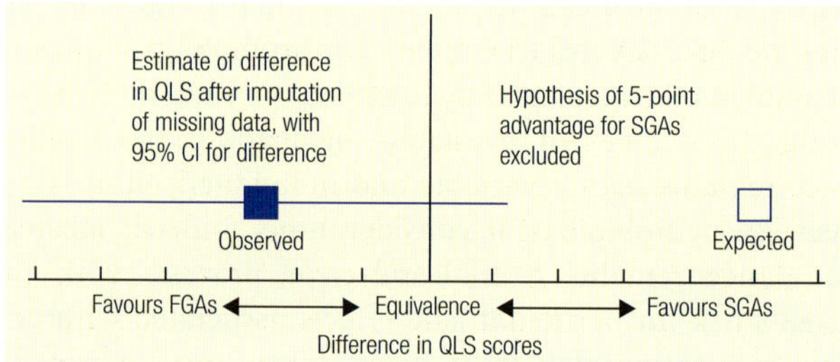

Figure 38.3 Differences in Quality of Life Scale (QSC) scores at 1 year between patients taking first-generation antipsychotics (FGAs) and second-generation antipsychotics (SGAs)

CI, confidence interval.

rates of 50 per cent, 46 per cent and 34 per cent for patients receiving molindone, risperidone and olanzapine, respectively. Olanzapine was associated with most weight gain and risperidone with some gain; molindone, chosen originally because of historical information suggesting that it had a low liability for weight gain, was not associated with weight gain in the study. Another European study, the European First Episode Schizophrenia Trial (EUFEST), showed some advantage in 1-year efficacy for SGAs over the FGA haloperidol.[79] Another US study showed equal efficacy between quetiapine and risperidone and olanzapine in patients with first-episode schizophrenia.[80]

It should be appreciated that inadequate understanding of the optimum and individualized dosing for all of these drugs greatly hampers both their utility and comparisons between the agents. It is also plausible, although not supported by any research data, that these drugs perform differently in different groups of patients, despite appearing broadly similar in overall outcomes. Getting the 'right fit' of drug, and its best dose, for any patient still remains more art than science. It is also important to appreciate that very often patients do not take their medication, and this is a major barrier in the treatment of schizophrenia.[81]

Clozapine

Clozapine is indicated for patients who are treatment-refractory – that is, they have not responded well enough to prior medications.[82] It is also indicated for patients with schizophrenia who are suicidal.[83] Psychiatrists vary widely in which medicines they choose, in what doses they use them and in how long they treat the patient with any given drug; hence, there is uncertainty as to when it is time to use clozapine. Many experts feel that clozapine is underutilized.[84] These variable medication practices, real concern about the adverse-effect profile of clozapine, and the cumbersome procedures for administering and monitoring of clozapine therapy collectively contribute to this powerful drug being either unused or relegated to the treatment of last resort. This contrasts with the evidence for clozapine's efficacy, first confirmed in the seminal clozapine/chlorpromazine study[82] and now well replicated.[85]

Antipsychotic formulations

Many of the FGAs and SGAs are available in formulations other than tablets. Liquid and dissolvable-wafer formulations are useful in acutely psychotic patients who (often as in-patients) refuse to take their medicines. Likewise, acute intramuscular preparations can be given to patients who are agitated and dangerous when they are refusing to take any medications orally. These options are typically short-term, with the intent of transition to oral tablet formulations as the situation stabilizes.

Some antipsychotics are available in long-acting injectable formulations. These are typically given every 2 weeks or once a month. They offer the patient and clinician the assurance that the medication is 'on board', although if the patient does not turn up for their regular injection, then non-compliance is declared. Studies generally suggest lower relapse rates with long-acting injectable antipsychotics, especially if patients are followed for beyond 1 year.[86] However, some patients dislike injections and find this approach stigmatizing, coercive and potentially painful. Other research confirms high tolerability and satisfaction among those patients who commit to this treatment approach. It is likely that other formulations and delivery systems (intranasal, transdermal, surgical) will be developed in the future. Because medication non-adherence is such an obstacle to effective treatment, further breakthroughs in formulations as well as newer drugs that are more efficacious or better tolerated are sorely needed.

Combining medications

It is common for psychiatrists to give patients two antipsychotic medications simultaneously. The rationale for this is invariably either to boost the effectiveness of the first antipsychotic or to reduce its side-effect burden by adding a different drug and thus lowering the required dose of the first drug. Many clinicians like this approach.[87] Many patients also prefer this approach and achieve clinical stability with this trial-and-error cocktail. However, scientific evidence to support the validity of this approach is remarkably lacking.[6,13]

Another commonly used strategy is to combine some other psychotropic drug with the antipsychotic. This is done to augment or boost the antipsychotic effect.[88] Augmenting agents include antidepressant medications, anticonvulsants, lithium and benzodiazepines. Antidepressants are given to augment the antipsychotic effect, but they are most commonly prescribed for co-morbid depression or anxiety. Benzodiazepines are typically used for co-morbid anxiety. Although these approaches appear reasonable and are commonplace in practice, the scientific evidence to support any of these augmentation strategies is, at best, inconclusive. Cholinergic agents and glutamatergic agents are being studied as adjunctive treatments to target cognitive features.[68] Several large-scale studies of these agents are in progress. Most recently, the approach of giving *N*-acetylcysteine in a precursor of glutathione (a key element in the phospholipid pathway) showed some benefit in a 24-week placebo-controlled, double-blinded study in patients with schizophrenia.[89]

Switching medications

It is generally considered that 4–6 weeks of treatment with an antipsychotic given at adequate dose is required before determining that the drug is ineffective and moving on to another choice. The drug to choose next is a matter of considerable debate, in the relative absence of guidance from available research.[90] It is recommended that patients are switched gradually, ideally over weeks, from one drug to another, in some form of cross-tapering strategy. Abrupt changes in medication risk withdrawal effects combined with acute tolerance effects of the new drug. Also, if the transition is unsuccessful, the patient can relapse. Drug-free holidays and intermittent antipsychotic therapy are not recommended because of the acknowledged heightened risk of relapse with these strategies.[91]

Managing medication side effects

Patients are highly variable in their tolerance and propensity to experience the wide range of side effects with antipsychotic medications. In general, side effects are often dose-related, and so judicious prescribing is warranted to minimize exposure to these side effects. On the other hand, some side effects (e.g., agranulocytosis with clozapine therapy) are not related to dose and appear to be largely idiosyncratic in occurrence.

A point of distinction between FGAs and SGAs is the higher rate of muscular side effects observed during treatment with FGAs. Acute effects such as dystonia and akathisia are highly distressing for patients and greatly increase the risk that the patient will stop taking that medication. In long-term care, tardive dyskinesia (TD) is a major worry and was seen at an incident rate of 5 per cent per year during the first 5 years of treatment with a FGA. TD is disfiguring, is often distressing to patients and has been associated with a shortened lifespan. TD can still occur during treatment with an SGA, although available evidence suggests that the risk of TD is ten times lower with SGAs than with FGAs.[92]

On the other hand, SGAs are generally much worse than FGAs in causing obesity and a host of metabolic disturbances. These are now major considerations in the treatment of schizophrenia.[93,94] Clozapine is the worst drug for these side effects;[95] olanzapine appears to be second. The more recent drugs (ziprasidone, aripiprazole) may be less likely to induce obesity or metabolic disturbances; however, patients are certainly not immune to these effects on either drug. The occurrence of obesity and metabolic disturbances (elevated glucose, insulin intolerance, diabetes mellitus, hyperlipidaemia, hypercholesterolaemia) has greatly complicated the management of schizophrenia.[96] Choice of medications is also influenced powerfully by these considerations. Patients may be switched from one drug to another in order to reduce weight gained or to reduce metabolic disturbances that have emerged in therapy.[97] These individual decisions seem clinically intuitive; however, scientific evidence has not caught up with clinical practice around these matters. Similarly, patients are increasingly being prescribed statins along with their antipsychotic medications. This approach has yet to be validated scientifically.[98] There are also non-pharmacological approaches to reduce the burden of these side effects;[99] these approaches appear to be beneficial. However, implementing lifestyle changes is difficult.

PSYCHOLOGICAL TREATMENTS

Patients require tremendous support to cope with this disabling condition. Family members also require education about the illness and support.

Individual therapies

Patients benefit from supportive counselling and practical psychotherapy. A focus on coping strategies, education about schizophrenia, and developing awareness of risk factors and the patient's individual pattern of relapse are helpful aspects of therapy. Cognitive-behavioural therapy (CBT) has been modified with some success in treating patients with schizophrenia.[100] A large multicentre British study found only a minimal impact of CBT in maintenance treatment.[101] A variant of CBT, compliance therapy (CT), has also been studied. Kemp and colleagues found a 20 per cent reduction in relapse compared with non-specific supportive therapy in an 18-month clinical trial.[102] The results of subsequent studies have been less conclusive. The impact of peer support has not been scientifically validated. Psychoeducation remains a major therapy.[103]

Group therapies

Psychoanalytically oriented group therapy or individual psychoanalysis is not an appropriate approach for patients with schizophrenia. Group therapy aimed at socialization, illness psychoeducation, and developing support is appropriate and helpful. Social skills training is also effective in boosting the patient's community engagement, developing social skills and reducing relapse.[104]

Family therapies

There is ample and compelling evidence that giving support, psychoeducation and specific instructions to family members can reduce relapse in the patient. This is one of the most evidence-based interventions in schizophrenia. A Cochrane systematic review synthesized data from randomized controlled trials involving 4124 people with schizophrenia and their families.[105] They found evidence for benefit such that about eight families had to be involved in the intervention in order to prevent one relapse (number needed to treat (NNT) 8; 95% confidence interval (CI) 6 to 11), with a similar effect for reduction in hospital admission, possibly through, in part, increased adherence to medication. Family members also benefit from, and do good work in, advocacy and self-help organizations.[106]

Cognitive remediation

Initially based upon the literature on cognitive retraining for patients who have suffered head trauma, there is now a growing literature on the impact of cognitive remediation in healing patients with schizophrenia. The results of several studies are generally positive and hold out the promise that cognition can be enhanced through computerized training modules. However, a recurrent problem seen in these studies is that learning does not appear to sustain and generalize from the computer to everyday life.[107]

VOCATIONAL AND SUPPORT SERVICES

Although most patients with schizophrenia are not in active employment, there is evidence from several health services research studies and demonstration projects that patients can work if supported adequately. Even patients who are hallucinating can sometimes hold down a job that is low in stress. On the other hand, patients with cognitive problems or negative symptoms do not do well in the work environment. Also, although patients may attain a job, staying employed and staying stable while employed is a major challenge for many people with schizophrenia. A study by McGurk and colleagues showed a better employment rate when cognitive remediation was also used for people who were returning to work.[108]

Some patients need highly intensive monitoring in the community. This community outreach, called assertive community therapy (ACT), is delivered in the patient's home on a daily basis by a highly specialized multidisciplinary team. It is an effective treatment for patients with severe schizophrenia.[109]

OTHER TREATMENT CONSIDERATIONS

Electroconvulsive therapy (ECT) is an uncommon treatment for people with schizophrenia, given adjunctively with antipsychotic medications. Patients with catatonia and patients who are recurrently suicidal are the best candidates for ECT.[110] Transcranial magnetic stimulation (TMS) has been shown in research to reduce auditory hallucinations in patients with schizophrenia.[111] Psychosurgery and deep brain stimulation are not acceptable treatments for schizophrenia.

KEY POINTS

- Schizophrenia is extraordinarily complex.
- Genetic causative influences predominate but by no means tell the complete story.
- Current thinking on schizophrenia sees it as a neurodevelopmental disorder.
- Dopamine dysregulation is important but by no means the complete picture neurochemically.
- Treatment is challenging, with medications as a bedrock of (but not the only) treatment.
- Maximizing recovery potential for people with schizophrenia requires clinically assertive and optimistic care.
- Clinicians must be continuously appraised of therapeutic advances.

FURTHER READING

van Os J, Kapur S (2009) Schizophrenia. *Lancet* **374**: 635–45.

REFERENCES

1. Castle DJ, Buckley PF (2008) *Schizophrenia*. Oxford: Oxford University Press.
2. Crow TJ (1980) Molecular pathology of schizophrenia: more than one disease process? *British Medical Journal* **280**: 66–8.
3. Carpenter WT, Heinnichs DW, Wagman AM (1988) Deficit and non deficit forms of schizophrenia: the concept. *American Journal of Psychiatry* **145**: 578–583.
4. Murray RM, O'Callaghan E, Castle DJ, Lewis SW (1992) A neurodevelopmental approach to the classification of schizophrenia. *Schizophrenia Bulletin* **18**: 319–32.
5. Andreasen NC (1999) A unitary model of schizophrenia: Bleuler's 'fragmented phrene' as schizencephaly. *Archives of General Psychiatry* **56**: 781–7.
6. McDonald AW, Schulz SC (2009) What we know: findings that every theory of schizophrenia should explain. *Schizophrenia Bulletin* **35**: 493–508.
7. Tandon R, Nasrallah HA, Keshavan MS (2009) Schizophrenia, 'just the facts' 4: clinical features and conceptualization. *Schizophrenia Research* **110**: 1–23.
8. Keshavan MS, Tandon R, Boutros NN, Nasrallah HA (2008) Schizophrenia, 'just the facts': what we know in 2008 – part 3. Neurobiology. *Schizophrenia Research* **106**: 89–107.
9. Tandon R, Keshavan MS, Nasrallah HA (2008) Schizophrenia, 'just the facts': what we know in 2008 – part 2. Epidemiology and etiology. *Schizophrenia Research* **102**: 1–18.
10. Tandon R, Keshavan MS, Nasrallah HA (2008) Schizophrenia, 'just the facts': what we know in 2008 – part 1. Overview. *Schizophrenia Research* **100**: 4–19.
11. Lieberman J, Stroup S, Perkins DO (2006) *Textbook of Schizophrenia*. Washington, DC: American Psychiatric Press.
12. Jones PB, Buckley PF (2006) *Schizophrenia*. London: Elsevier.
13. Castle DJ, Copolov D, Wykes T, Mueser K (eds) (2008) *Pharmacological and Psychosocial Treatments for Schizophrenia*, 2nd edn. London: Informa.

14. Thornicroft G, Brohan E, Rose D, *et al.* (2009) Global pattern of experienced and anticipated discrimination against people with schizophrenia: a cross-sectional survey. *Lancet* **373**: 408–15.
15. Ihara K, Morgan C, Fearon P, *et al.* (2009) The prevalence, diagnostic significance and demographic characteristics of Schneiderian first-rank symptoms in an epidemiological sample of first-episode psychoses. *Psychopathology* **42**: 81–91.
16. Marshall M, Lewis S, Lockwood A, *et al.* (2005) Association between duration of untreated psychosis and outcome in cohorts of first-episode patients: a systematic review. *Archives of General Psychiatry* **62**: 975–83.
17. Power P, Liacoponi E, Reynolds N, *et al.* (2007) Assessment Team Study: general practitioner education and access to an early detection team in first-episode psychosis. *British Journal of Psychiatry* **51**: S133–9.
18. McGorry PD, Killackey E, Yung A (2008) Early intervention in psychosis: concepts, evidence and future directions. *World Psychiatry* **7**: 148–56.
19. World Health Organization (1992) *International Classification of Diseases*. Geneva: World Health Organization.
20. Andreasson S, Allebeck P, Engstrom A, Rydberg U (1987) Cannabis and schizophrenia: a longitudinal study of Swedish conscripts. *Lancet* **2**: 1483–6.
21. Moore TH, Zammit S, Lingford-Hughes A, *et al.* (2007) Cannabis use and risk for psychotic or affective mental health outcomes: a systematic review. *Lancet* **370**: 319–28.
22. Harrison PJ, Weinberger DR (2005) Schizophrenia genes, gene expression, and neuropathology; on the matter of their convergence. *Molecular Psychiatry* **10**: 40–68.
23. McClellan JM, Susser E, King MC (2007) Schizophrenia: a common disease caused by multiple rare alleles. *British Journal of Psychiatry* **190**: 194–9.
24. Lichtenstein P, Yip BH, Bjork C, *et al.* (2009) Common genetic determinants of schizophrenia and bipolar disorder in Swedish families: a population-based study. *Lancet* **373**: 234–9.
25. The International Schizophrenia Consortium, Stone JL, O'Donovan MC, *et al.* (2008) Rare chromosomal deletions and duplications increase risk of schizophrenia. *Nature* **455**: 237–41.
26. Stefansson H, Rujescu D, Cichon S, *et al.* (2008) Large recurrent microdeletions associated with schizophrenia. *Nature* **455**: 232–6.
27. McGrath JJ, Murray RM (2003) Risk factors for schizophrenia: from conception to birth. In SR Hirsch, DR Weinberger (eds) *Schizophrenia*. Oxford: Blackwell.
28. Cannon TD, Yolken R, Buka S, Torrey EF, Collaborative Study Group on the Perinatal Origins of Severe Psychiatric disorders (2008) Decreased neuro response to birth hypoxia in the etiology of schizophrenia. *Biological Psychiatry* **64**: 797–802.
29. Khashan AS, Abel KM, McNamee R, *et al.* (2008) Higher risk of offspring schizophrenia following antenatal maternal exposure to severe adverse life events. *Archives of General Psychiatry* **65**: 146–52.
30. Moore TH, Zammit S, Lingford-Hughes A, *et al.* (2007) Cannabis use and risk of psychotic or affective mental health outcomes: a systematic review. *Lancet* **370**: 319–28.
31. Jablensky A, Sartorius N, Ernberg G, *et al.* (1992) Schizophrenia: manifestations, incidence and course in different cultures – a World Health Organization ten-country study. *Psychological Medicine. Monograph Supplement* **20**: 1–97.
32. Farris REL, Dunham HW. (1960) *Mental Disorders in Urban Areas: An Ecological Study of Schizophrenia and Other Psychoses*, 2nd edn. New York: Hafner.
33. Kirkbride JB, Boydell J, Ploubidis GB, *et al.* (2008) Testing the association between the incidence of schizophrenia and social capital in an urban area. *Psychological Medicine* **38**: 10083–94.
34. Kirkbride JB, Fearon P, Morgan C, *et al.* (2007) Neighbourhood variation in the incidence of psychotic disorders in Southeast London. *Social Psychiatry and Psychiatric Epidemiology* **42**: 438–45.
35. Kirkbride JB, Morgan C, Fearson P, *et al.* Neighbourhood-level effects on psychoses: re-examining the role of context. *Psychological Medicine* **37**: 1413–25.
36. Morgan C, Fisher H, Hutchinson G, *et al.* (2009) Ethnicity, social disadvantage and psychotic-like experiences in a healthy population based sample. *Acta Psychiatrica Scandinavica* **119**: 226–35.
37. Cantor-Graae E, Selten JP (2005) Schizophrenia and migration: a meta-analysis and review. *American Journal of Psychiatry* **162**: 12–24.
38. Fearon P, Kirkbride JB, Morgan C, *et al.* (2006) Incidence of schizophrenia and other psychoses in ethnic minority groups: results from the MRC AESOP Study. *Psychological Medicine* **36**: 1541–50
39. Cold JW, Kirkbride JB, Barker D, *et al.* (2008) Raised incidence rates of all psychoses among migrant groups: findings from the East London first episode psychosis study. *Archives of General Psychiatry* **65**: 1250–58. [Erratum in **66**: 161.]
40. Selten JP, Cantor-Graae E, Kahn RS (2007) Migration and schizophrenia. *Current Opinion in Psychiatry* **20**: 111–15.
41. Selten JP, Cantor-Graae E (2007) Hypothesis: social defeat is a risk factor for schizophrenia? *British Journal of Psychiatry Supplement* **51**: S9–12. [Erratum in *British Journal of Psychiatry* **192**: 234.]
42. Iritani S (2007) Neuropathology of schizophrenia: a mini review. *Neuropathology* **27**: 604–8.

43. Pearlson GD, Calhoun V (2007) Structural and functional magnetic resonance imaging in psychiatric disorders. *Canadian Journal of Psychiatry* **52**: 158–66.
44. Wright IC, Rabe-Hesketh S, Woodruff PW, *et al.* (2000) Meta-analysis of regional brain volumes in schizophrenia. *American Journal of Psychiatry* **57**: 16–25.
45. Lawrie SM, McIntosh AM, Hall J, Owens DG, Johnstone EC (2008) Brain structure and function changes during the development of schizophrenia: the evidence from studies of subjects at increased genetic risk. *Schizophrenia Bulletin* **34**: 330–40.
46. Tanskanen P, Ridler K, Murray GK, *et al.* (2008) Morphometric brain abnormalities in schizophrenia in a population-based sample: relationship to duration of illness. *Schizophrenia Bulletin*, in press.
47. Pantelis C, Velakoulis D, McGorry PD (2003) Neuroanatomical abnormalities before and after onset of psychosis: a cross-sectional and longitudinal MRI comparison. *Lancet* **361**: 281–8.
48. Lieberman JA, Perkins D, Belger A, *et al.* (2001) The early stages of schizophrenia: speculation on the pathogenesis, pathophysiology, and therapeutic approaches. *Biological Psychiatry* **50**: 884–97.
49. Ho BC, Andreasen NC, Dawson JD, Wassink TH (2007) Association between brain-derived neurotrophic factor Val66Met gene polymorphism and progressive brain volume changes in schizophrenia. *American Journal of Psychiatry* **164**: 1890–99.
50. Mason P, Rimemr M, Richman A, *et al.* (2008) Middle-ear disease and schizophrenia: case–control study. *British Journal of Psychiatry* **193**: 192–6.
51. Kapur S, Remmington G (2001) Dopamine (D2) receptors and their role in atypical antipsychotic action: still necessary and may even be sufficient. *Biological Psychiatry* **50**: 873–83.
52. Di Forti M, Lappin JM, Murray RM (2007) Risk factors for schizophrenia: all roads lead to dopamine. *European Neuropsychopharmacology* **17** (suppl. 2): S101–7.
53. Meador-Woodruff J, Kelinmen J (2002) Neurochemistry of schizophrenia: glutamate abnormalities. In K Davis, D Cheney, J Coyle, CD Nemeroff (eds) *Neuropsychopharmacology as fifth generation of progress*. Philadelphia: Lippincott Williams & Wilkins.
54. Lehman AF, Lieberman JA, Dixon LB, *et al.* (2004) Practice guidelines for the management of patients with schizophrenia, second edition. *American Journal of Psychiatry* **161** (2 suppl.): 1–56.
55. Buckley PF (2007) Factors that influence treatment success in schizophrenia. *Journal of Clinical Psychiatry* **115**: 93–100.
56. Leucht S, Barnes TR, Kissling W, *et al.* (2003) Relapse prevention in schizophrenia with new-generation antipsychotics: a systematic review and exploratory meta-analysis of randomized, controlled trials. *American Journal of Psychiatry* **160**: 1209–22.
57. Harding CM, Brooks GW, Ashikaga T, Strauss JS, Breier A (1987) The Vermont longitudinal study of persons with severe mental illness I: methodology, study sample, and overall status 32 years later. *American Journal of Psychiatry* **144**: 718–26.
58. Strauss GP, Harrow M, Grossman LS, Rosen C (2008) Periods of recovery in deficit syndrome schizophrenia: a 20-year multi-follow-up longitudinal study. *Schizophrenia Bulletin*, in press.
59. Andreasen NC, Carpenter WT, Jr, Kane JM, *et al.* (2005) Remission in schizophrenia: proposed criteria and rationale for consensus. *American Journal of Psychiatry* **12**: 441–9.
60. Substance Abuse and Mental Health Services Administration (2006) *National Consensus Statement on Mental Health Recovery*. Rockville, MD: US Department of Health and Human Services.
61. Davidson L, Chinman M, Sells D, *et al.* (2006) Peer support among adults with mental illness: a report from the field. *Schizophrenia Bulletin* **32**: 443–50.
62. Fiander M, Burns T, McHugo GJ, Drake RE (2003) Assertive community treatment across the Atlantic: comparison of model fidelity in the UK and USA. *British Journal of Psychiatry* **182**: 248–54.
63. Foster A, Miller D, Buckley PF (2007) Pharmacogenetics and schizophrenia. *Psychiatric Clinics of North America* **30**: 417–35.
64. Howes OD, McGuire PK, Kapur S (2008) Understanding pathophysiology is crucial in linking clinical staging to targeted therapeutics. *World Psychiatry* **7**: 162–3.
65. Kapur S, Zipursky R, Jones C, *et al.* (2003) A positron emission tomography study of quetiapine in schizophrenia: a preliminary finding of an antipsychotic effect with only transiently high dopamine D2 receptor occupancy. *Archives of General Psychiatry* **57**: 553–9.
66. Carlsson Ml, Carlsson A, Nilsson M (2004) Schizophrenia: from dopamine to glutamate and back. *Current Medicinal Chemistry* **11**: 267–77.
67. Biedermann F, Fleischhacker WW (2009) Antipsychotics in the early stage of development. *Current Opinion in Psychiatry* **22**: 326–30.
68. Harvey PD, Cornblatt B (2008) Pharmacological treatment of cognition in schizophrenia: an idea whose time has come. *American Journal of Psychiatry* **165**: 163–5.
69. Patil St, Zhang L, Martenyl F, *et al.* (2007) Activation of mGlu2/3 receptors as a new approach to treat schizophrenia: a randomized phase 2 clinical trial. *Nature Medicine* **13**: 1102–7.
70. Geddes J, Freemantle N, Harrison P, *et al.* (2000) Atypical antipsychotics in the treatment of schizophrenia: systematic overview and regression analysis. *British Medical Journal* **321**: 1371–6.
71. Davis J, Chen N, Glick ID (2003) A meta-analysis of the efficacy of second-generation antipsychotics. *Archives of General Psychiatry* **60**: 553–64.

72. Leucht S, Corves C, Arbter D, *et al.* (2009) Second-generation versus first-generation antipsychotic drugs for schizophrenia: a meta-analysis. *Lancet* **373**: 31–41.
73. Heres S, Davis J, Maino K, *et al.* (2006) Why olanzapine beats risperidone, risperidone beats quetiapine, and quetiapine beats olanzapine: an exploratory analysis of head-to-head comparison studies of second-generation antipsychotics. *American Journal of Psychiatry* **163**: 185–94.
74. Lieberman JA, Stroup TS, McEvoy JP, *et al.* (2005) Effectiveness of antipsychotic drugs in patients with chronic schizophrenia. *New England Journal of Medicine* **353**: 1209–23.
75. Jones PB, Barnes TR, Davies L, *et al.* (2006) Randomized controlled trial of the effect on quality of life of second- vs. first-generation antipsychotic drugs in schizophrenia. *Archives of General Psychiatry* **63**: 1079–87.
76. Lewis SW, Barnes TR, Davies L, *et al.* (2006) Randomized controlled trial of effect of prescription of clozapine versus other second-generation antipsychotic drugs in resistant schizophrenia. *Schizophrenia Bulletin* **32**: 715–23.
77. McEvoy JP, Lieberman JA, Stroup TS, *et al.* (2006) Effectiveness of clozapine versus olanzapine, quetiapine, and risperidone in patients with chronic schizophrenia who did not respond to prior atypical antipsychotic treatment. *American Journal of Psychiatry* **163**: 600–610.
78. Sikich L, Frazier JA, McClellan J, *et al.* (2008) Double-blind comparison of first- and second-generation antipsychotics in early-onset schizophrenia and schizo-affective disorder: findings from the treatment of early-onset schizophrenia spectrum disorder (TEOSS) study. *American Journal of Psychiatry* **165**: 1420–31.
79. Kahn RS, Fleischhacker WW, Boter M, *et al.* (2008) Effectiveness of antipsychotic drugs in first-episode schizophrenia and schizophreniform disorder: an open randomized clinical trial (EUFEST). *Lancet* **371**: 1085–97.
80. McEvoy JP, Lieberman JA, Perkins DO, *et al.* (2007) Efficacy and tolerability of olanzapine, quetiapine, and risperidone in the treatment of early psychosis: a randomized, double-blind 52-week comparison. *American Journal of Psychiatry* **164**: 1050–60.
81. Buckley PF, Foster A, Patel N, Ernnert A (2009) *Nonadherence with Mental Health Treatments*. New York: Oxford University Press.
82. Kane J, Honigfeld G, Singer J, *et al.* (1988) Clozapine for the treatment-resistant schizophrenic: a randomized comparison with chlorpromazine. *Archives of General Psychiatry* **45**: 789–96.
83. Meltzer HY, Alphs L, Green, *et al.* (2003) Clozapine treatment for suicidality in schizophrenia. International Suicide Prevention Trial (InterSePT). *Archives of General Psychiatry* **60**: 82–91.
84. Troy M, Buchanan B, Buckley PF, *et al.* (2007) The Texas Medication Algorithm Project antipsychotic algorithm for schizophrenia: 2006 update. *Journal of Clinical Psychiatry* **68**: 1751–62.
85. Kumra S, Kranzler H, Gerbino-Rosen G, *et al.* (2008) Clozapine and 'high-dose' olanzapine in refractory early-onset schizophrenia: a 12-week randomized and double-blind comparison. *Biological Psychiatry* **63**: 524–9.
86. Adam, CE, Fenton M, David AS (2001) Systematic meta-review of depot antipsychotic drugs for people with schizophrenia. *British Journal of Psychiatry* **179**: 290–99.
87. Goff DC, Freudenreich O (2004) Focus on polypharmacy in schizophrenia: does anyone truly benefit. *International Journal of Neuropsychopharmacology* **7**: 109–11.
88. Schulz S, Buckley PF, Barnes TRE (2003) Treatment refractory schizophrenia. In SR Hirsch, ER Weinberger (eds) *Schizophrenia*, 2nd edn. Oxford: Blackwell Science.
89. Berk M, Copolov D, Dean O, *et al.* (2008) *N*-acetyl cysteine as a glutathione precursor for schizophrenia: a double-blind, randomized, placebo-controlled trial. *Biological Psychiatry* **64**: 361–8.
90. Weidan PJ, Buckley PF (2007) Switching antipsychotic medications. *Journal of Clinical Psychiatry* **68**: 14–23.
91. Robinson DG, Woener MG, Napolitano B, *et al.* (2008) Randomized comparison of olanzapine versus risperidone for the treatment of first-episode schizophrenia: 4-month outcomes. *American Journal of Psychiatry* **163**: 2096–102.
92. Correll CU, Leucht S, Kane JM (2004) Lower risk for tardive dyskinesia with second-generation antipsychotics: a systematic review of 1-year studies. *American Journal of Psychiatry* **161**: 414–25.
93. Buckley PF, Miller BJ, Foster A (2008) Schizophrenia and metabolic disturbances: host vulnerability and the risk of antipsychotic therapy. *Focus* **6**: 172–9.
94. Newcomer J (2007) Antipsychotic medications: metabolic and cardiovascular risk. *Journal of Clinical Psychiatry* **68**: 813.
95. Henderson DC, Cagliero E, Gray C, *et al.* (2000) Clozapine, diabetes mellitus, weight gain and lipid abnormalities: a five year naturalistic study. *American Journal of Psychiatry* **157**: 975–81.
96. Marder SR, Essock SM, Miller AL, *et al.* (2006) Physical health monitoring of patients with schizophrenia. *American Journal of Psychiatry* **161**: 1334–49.
97. Stroup TS, McEvoy JP, Swartz MS, *et al.* (2007) Comparison of antipsychotics for metabolic problems (CAMP): a NIMH schizophrenia trials network study. *Clinical Schizophrenia and Related Psychosis* **1**: 69–72.

98. Wu RR, Zhao JP, Guo XF, *et al.* (2008) Metformin addition attenuates olanzapine-induced weight gain in drug-naive first-episode schizophrenia patients: a double-blind, placebo-controlled study. *American Journal of Psychiatry* **165**: 352–8.
99. Faulkner G, Cohn T, Remington G (2007) Interventions to reduce weight gain in schizophrenia. *Schizophrenia Bulletin* **33**: 654–6.
100. Wykes T, Steel C, Everitt B, Tarrier N (2008) Cognitive behavior therapy for schizophrenia: effect sizes, clinical models, and methodological rigor. *Schizophrenia Bulletin* **34**: 523–37.
101. Sellwood W, Wittkowski A, Tarrier N, Barrowcough C (2007) Needs-based cognitive-behavioural family intervention for careers of patients suffering from schizophrenia: 5-year follow-up of randomized controlled effectiveness trial. *Acta Psychiatrica Scandinavica* **116**: 447–52.
102. Kemp R, Kirov G, Everitt B, Hayward P, David A (1998) Randomised controlled trial of compliance therapy: 18-month follow-up. *British Journal of Psychiatry* **172**: 413–19.
103. Pitshel-Walz G, Baumi J, Bender W, *et al.* (2006) Psychoeducation and compliance in the treatment of schizophrenia: results of the Munich psychosis information project study. *Journal of Clinical Psychiatry* **57**: 443–52.
104. Bellack AS, Meuser KT, Ginerich S, Agresta J (2004) *Social Skills Training for Schizophrenia*. New York: Guilford Press.
105. Pharoah F, Mari J, Rathbone J, Wong W (2006) Family intervention for schizophrenia. *Cochrane Database of Systematic Reviews* (4): CD000088.
106. Huey LY, Lefley HP, Shern DL, Wainscott CA (2007) Families and schizophrenia: the view from advocacy. *Psychiatric Clinics of North America* **30**: 549–66.
107. Bell M, Bryson G, Greig T, *et al.* (2001) Neurocognitive enhancement therapy with work therapy. *Archives of General Psychiatry* **58**: 763–8.
108. McGurk SR, Meuser KT, Feldman K, Wolfe R, Pascaris A (2007) Cognitive training for supported employment: 2–3 year outcomes of a randomized controlled trial. *American Journal of Psychiatry* **164**: 437–41.
109. Nelson G, Aubry T, LaFrance A (2007) A review of the literature on the effectiveness of housing and support, assertive community, treatment, and intensive case management interventions for persons with mental illness who have been homeless. *American Journal of Orthopsychiatry* **77**: 350–61.
110. Elkis H (2007) Treatment resistant schizophrenia. *Psychiatric Clinics of North America* **30**: 511–33.
111. Thirthalli J, Bharadwaj B, Kulkarni S, *et al.* (2008) Successful use of maintenance rTMS for 8 months in a patient with antipsychotic-refractory auditory hallucinations. *Schizophrenia Research* **100**: 351–2.

Chapter 39

Mood disorders/affective psychoses

Ewa Wisniewska Young, Nicol Ferrier, Brian Lunn and Andrew Brittlebank

INTRODUCTION

Mood disorders are characterized by a significant and pervasive change in mood to either depression or elation that goes beyond the normal experience of happiness during auspicious times and unhappiness during inauspicious times. Typically, mood disorders are recurrent and onset of episodes is often associated with stressful events or situations. Symptoms of depression and less frequently elation are commonly associated with physical illnesses and other psychiatric disorders.

CLASSIFICATION SYSTEMS

The two main classification systems for mental disorders are the World Health Organization (WHO) *International Classification of Diseases*, version 10 (ICD-10)[1] and the American Psychiatric Association's *Diagnostic and Statistical Manual*, version 4, text revision (DSM-IV-TR).[2] In their classification of affective disorders, these systems are broadly similar but have some significant differences.

They both have separate categories for single and recurrent episodes of mood disorders. The persistent but mild mood disturbances of cyclothymia (repeated depressed and elated mood) and dysthymia (sustained depressed mood) are also recognized in both.

The most notable difference between DSM-IV and ICD-10 is that that ICD-10 recognizes only one type of bipolar affective disorder (BAD) whereas DSM-IV separates this condition into bipolar I disorder, bipolar II disorder and cyclothymia. Another difference is DSM-IV's inclusion of mood disorders secondary to medical conditions in a subcategory of mood disorders, whereas ICD-10 separates 'organic mental disorders' into a separate category. The DSM-IV classification refers to 'major depressive episodes', whereas ICD-10 names them 'depressive episodes'. Additionally, DSM-IV has subcategories for 'partial remission' and 'full remission of a major depressive episode', whereas ICD-10 specifies only 'full remission'.

Both classification systems distinguish mania and hypomania according to severity of symptoms. DSM-IV allows a diagnosis of BAD with the presence of just a single episode of mania or hypomania, whereas ICD-10 requires at least two episodes of mood disturbance, one of which must be hypomanic, manic or mixed. In DSM-IV, bipolar I is diagnosed following the occurrence of at least one manic episode or mixed episode, with or without depressive episodes. Bipolar II requires depressive episodes and at least one hypomanic episode but the absence of any manic episodes. DSM-IV categorizes cyclothymia as a type of BAD, whereas both dysthymia and cyclothymia are included under persistent mood disorders in ICD-10. DSM-IV includes rapid cycling as a specifier for bipolar disorders, but it is not mentioned in ICD-10.

AETIOLOGY OF AFFECTIVE DISORDERS

The aetiology of affective disorders is multifactorial, even in individual patients, and there are many ways to group the different factors. For example, the biopsychosocial model takes account of biological, psychological and social factors that influence a person over their lifespan. These factors can also be grouped into predisposing factors, precipitating factors and perpetuating factors. Another way to view the aetiology of affective disorders is to separate the components into genetic and environmental factors. In this chapter we have used the biopsychosocial model.

Biological factors

The biological factors contributing to affective disorders have been investigated from a number of different perspectives: genetic factors, neurochemical changes, neuroendocrine abnormalities, cellular factors and cerebral pathophysiology.

Genetics

Family studies show the risk of mood disorders to be increased in first-degree relatives of patients with depression, and that the earlier the age of onset, the higher the risk. Relatives of patients with bipolar disorder have a higher risk of both bipolar disorder and unipolar depression, whereas relatives of patients with unipolar depression have a higher risk only of unipolar depression.

Although family studies show heritability, they do not show whether this is due to genetic factors or behavioural and environmental factors within certain families. It is from the work of twin studies that evidence has emerged of genetic factors contributing to the heritability of affective disorders. Twin studies have looked at the discrepancy in the concordance of the rate of affective disorders between monozygotic and dizygotic twins. These studies show concordance rates of 40–50 per cent in monozygotic twins and 20–25 per cent in dizygotic twins for depression.[3] In bipolar disorder, the results have been even more marked. The approximate lifetime risk of bipolar disorder in relatives of a bipolar proband has been shown to be: monozygotic co-twin, 40–70 per cent; first degree relative, 5–10 per cent; unrelated person, 0.5–1.5 per cent.[4]

One of the most influential twin studies looking at the heritability of depression and attempting to separate environmental and genetic factors in the causation of depression was published by Kendler and colleagues at the University College of Virginia.[5] They interviewed a large number of female twins and found considerable heritability of depression, with the extent of heritability proportional to the severity of depression. They also found that members of adult twin pairs do not share most environmental experiences of causative importance for depression. From this, they concluded that shared genetic factors are considerably more important than shared environmental factors in the tendency for depression to aggregate in families.

It is likely that genetic susceptibility to depression is polygenic. For example, twin studies have shown both a correlation between depression in women and neuroticism[6] and also a correlation between depression in women and heritability of neurotic traits.[7]

Adoption studies support a combined genetic and environmental aetiology of affective disorders.[8] The rate of bipolar disorder in biological parents of probands with bipolar disorder has been shown to be higher than for non-related adoptive parents in some studies.[9]

To date, molecular genetics has contributed only modestly to the understanding of the genetic component of affective disorders. It is assumed that the genetic component of affective disorders is related to alleles, variations of normal genes. The presence of different forms of the same gene, causing different phenotypes within a population, is known as genetic polymorphism. Linkage studies search for linkage of a disorder to a known gene. An early linkage study suggested linkage of bipolar disorder to markers on chromosome 11 in an Old Order Amish population;[10] however, this result has not been confirmed in subsequent studies on the same population. More recent, larger studies have consistently suggested a linkage of bipolar disorder to loci on chromosomes 4, 12 and 18 and 21[4].[11] These studies also support the theory that the inheritance of susceptibility to affective disorders is polygenic.

Allelic association studies compare the genotypes of patients and controls, with the aim of identifying an excess of certain alleles in patient populations. These studies have focused particularly on genes that code for monoamine transporters, but to date results have been inconclusive. Although some studies have shown an association between different alleles of the serotonin transporter gene (*SERT*) in both unipolar depression and bipolar disorder, the association is weak and not confirmed in some subsequent studies. Another finding has been that patients with rapid cycling bipolar disorder may be more likely to express a low activity allele of the catecholamine-O-methyl transferase gene. It has been suggested that this might contribute to rapid changes in mood.

Neurochemistry

The monoamine theory of affective disorders arose from observations that certain drugs, such as reserpine, that depleted monoamine neurotransmitters could induce depression, while chemicals, such as amphetamine and ecstasy, that cause release of monoamines induce euphoria. Antidepressants increase monoamine transmitter levels by increasing release, reducing reuptake or reducing breakdown. Monoamines include serotonin (5-hydroxytryptamine, 5-HT), noradrenaline, dopamine and acetylcholine.

Much research has focused on the role of serotonin in depression. Studies have shown that levels of tryptophan, a substrate of serotonin synthesis, are reduced in patients with untreated depression. It is not clear whether this is related to the cause of depression or is an effect of depression. Tryptophan depletion has been shown to induce depression in females[12] and also to cause a return of severe depressive symptoms in patients recovering from and in remission after a depressive episode.[13] Other studies have shown a serotonin metabolite to be reduced in the cerebrospinal fluid (CSF) of depressed patients.[14] Further studies showed that this is only the case for some depressed patients and that these patients have a higher risk of suicide attempts, suggesting that the association is more with impulsivity.[15] Perhaps the best evidence of the role of serotonin in depression is the efficacy of selective serotonin reuptake inhibitors (SSRIs) in treating depression.

Although there is no consistent evidence that levels of noradrenaline are altered in patients with depression, some antidepressants inhibit noradrenaline uptake while having little effect on 5-HT uptake, suggesting that noradrenaline does play an important aetiological role.

The dopamine system has also been associated with depression. The psychostimulants amphetamine and cocaine stimulate dopamine release and cause euphoria in normal volunteers. Parkinson's disease, which is due primarily to dopamine depletion, is associated with an increased risk of depression, and the dopamine agonist bromocriptine has been shown to have antidepressant properties. Furthermore, the antidepressant effects of bupropion are attributed primarily to its effects on the dopamine system, and electroconvulsive therapy (ECT) tends to increase dopaminergic function.

The dopamine system appears to be particularly important in bipolar disorder. Prodopaminergic stimulants can trigger mania and anti-manic medications tend to block the effects of dopamine. Patients with bipolar depression have been found to have reduced CSF levels of the dopamine metabolite homovanillic acid (HVA); conversely, some manic patients have been found to have increased levels of CSF HVA.[16]

The idea that affective disorders can be attributed to levels of neurotransmitters alone is clearly an oversimplification. Antidepressants cause rapid changes in neurotransmitter levels, but therapeutic effects take considerably longer to emerge. There are likely to be a number of interconnected neurotransmitter abnormalities present in affective disorders. Activity of one monoamine system influences the activity of the other monoamine systems via positive and negative feedback loops. These observations have led to the development of the neurotransmitter receptor hypothesis, which theorizes that depression is related to abnormalities in the receptors of monoamine neurotransmitters, with depletion of one or more neurotransmitters causing compensatory up-regulation of postsynaptic neurotransmitters.

Neuroendocrinology

The hypothalamic–pituitary–adrenal (HPA) axis is intrinsically involved in the physiological response to stress. Simplistically, the HPA axis involves corticotropin-releasing factor (CRF) from the hypothalamus, promoting the release of adrenocorticotropic hormone (ACTH) from the anterior pituitary. ACTH in turn stimulates glucocorticoid release from the adrenal cortex. Negative feedback loops provide regulatory control. One of these negative feedback loops involves cortisol, which binds to glucocorticoid receptors in various areas of the HPA axis and the hippocampus, reducing further HPA activity. The involvement of the hippocampus in regulation of the HPA axis has led some researchers to refer to it as the 'HHPA axis'.

A large amount of research has focused on the role of the HPA axis in depression. Some 50 per cent of patients with depression show hyperactivity of the HPA axis,[17] and studies have shown evidence of increased CRF, impaired pituitary response to CRH administration, increased levels of ACTH, adrenal gland enlargement, raised serum cortisol, and dexamethasone suppression test non-suppression in patients with depression. It is not understood whether the effect on the brain of raised cortisol levels is depressant or antidepressant. Excessive cortisol secretion in Cushing's syndrome is associated with an increased risk of depression. However, studies have shown that large doses of cortisol administered to patients with depression can be mood-enhancing. Additionally, hypercortisolaemia is also associated with psychotic illness and, in particular, mania.

The primary actions of glucocorticoids are intracellular. It has been suggested that transport across the cell membrane may be disturbed in depression, leading to low intracellular levels of intracellular cortisol. Furthermore, it has been proposed that antidepressants may influence this mechanism to increase intracellular levels of cortisol.[18]

Hyperactivity of the HPA axis in depression has a number of implications. It may have effects on cellular resilience, neuronal atrophy and, in turn, cognitive function. Elevated plasma cortisol may both suppress some aspects of cellular immunity and increase the levels of pro-inflammatory cytokines, which in turn are associated with raised levels of C-reactive protein (CRP). Raised CRP is an important risk factor for ischaemic heart disease, and perhaps this is part of the link between depression and heart disease. Antidepressant therapy has been shown to reduce the levels of these pro-inflammatory cytokines and CRP.

It has long been recognized that patients with hypothyroidism frequently exhibit cognitive impairment and depression, and patients with depression have higher than normal rates of hypothyroidism. A quarter of patients with major depression have a blunted thyroid stimulating hormone (TSH) response to thyrotropin-releasing hormone (TRH).[19] Studies have shown that patients with uncorrected hypothyroidism have a poor response to antidepressants, and there have been reports of tri-iodothyronine (T3) accelerating the rate of onset of antidepressant response. It is on the basis of this that thyroxine (T4) and T3 have been proposed as agents to augment antidepressant therapy, although this is specifically not recommended in the National Institute for Health and Clinical Excellence (NICE) 2004 guidance for depression[20] that applies to National Health Service (NHS) provision in England and Wales.

The hypothalamic–growth hormone axis is also likely to be involved. Patients with depression have been shown to have a reduced growth-hormone response to stimulation with α2-adrenergic agonists such as clonidine.[21] This may persist after recovery, suggesting that it may be a marker for depression vulnerability.

Cellular factors

Neurotransmitters in the brain such as the catecholamines are located in the extracellular space. The cellular response is determined by intracellular signalling pathways. When neurotransmitters bind to receptors on the outer membrane of cells, their message is carried either by ion channel effects or by influencing the levels of small molecules, originally called 'second messengers', such as cyclic adenosine monophosphate (cAMP) and protein kinase A (PKA). There is some evidence that antidepressants may modify intracellular signalling pathways by influencing intracellular messengers such as cAMP. There is also evidence of cell-signalling abnormalities in bipolar disorder. For example, concentrations of the PKA regulatory subunits in the cytoplasm are significantly lower in cells of various parts of the brain in bipolar disorder. Studies have also shown a higher concentration of cAMP-stimulated phosphorylation of

Rap1, a protein found in the platelets of patients with bipolar disorder.[22] Lithium treatment has been associated with changes to the phosphatidylinositol system and also to other components of the intracellular messaging system, although the exact relationship between lithium's intracellular effects and its therapeutic effect is not yet clear.

The molecular and cellular theory of depression suggests that a decrease in survival promoting neurotrophic factors may occur in depression. Changes to growth factors and neurotrophins such as brain-derived neurotrophic factor (BDNF) have been considered to influence cellular resilience and result in neuronal atrophy in patients with depression. Clinical imaging studies have supported this by demonstrating a decreased volume of certain brain structures in the brains of patients with depression. This in turn may affect cognitive function. The molecular and cellular theory also suggests that, via secondary messenger signalling systems, antidepressants increase the concentration of neurotrophic factors, which are essential for neuronal survival.[23,24]

It may be through mechanisms such as these that the observed phenomenon of 'kindling' occurs in depression. Kindling refers to a process in which repeated stimulation causes an escalating response. Although it is classically applied to epilepsy, it can also be applied to depression. After a single depressive episode, 85 per cent of patients will experience a recurrence; and although the first episode is often provoked by a negative life event, subsequent episodes are often unprecipitated. Recurrent depressive episodes also typically increase in frequency and duration.

Cerebral pathophysiology

Based on limited postmortem studies of patients with mood disorders, there is some evidence of changes in cortical and subcortical structures.

Structural brain imaging studies have shown that patients with unipolar depression have a tendency to smaller basal ganglia, hippocampi, cerebella and possibly frontal lobes. In bipolar disorder, imaging studies have shown a tendency to reduction in prefrontal cortex volume and enlargement of cerebral ventricles.

Functional neuroimaging studies of patients with depression have shown hypoperfusion in frontal, temporal and parietal areas. Other studies have shown reduced global cerebral activity in patients with depression. Patients with bipolar depression have been shown to have reduced amygdala activity. Few conclusions have been able to be made from this work regarding cause and effect at this stage.

Physical illness

Various medical illnesses increase the risk of depression. For some of these, it is likely to be due to the effect of having a significant life event (see Social factors, below), but some conditions have a particular association with affective disorders.

Depression is common following a stroke. Some 30–40 per cent of patients who survive intracerebral haemorrhage develop depression,[25] and depression probably impairs rehabilitation.[26]

Up to 33 per cent of patients develop depression after a myocardial infarction,[27] and prognosis in heart disease is worse for patients with depression.[28] The relationship between cause and effect is not clear and probably goes both ways.

Multiple sclerosis, temporal lobe epilepsy and early traumatic brain injury are associated with increased risk of bipolar disorder.

Although it is not a physical illness, there are a lot of physiological changes at the time of childbirth, and during the months following this there is a significantly raised risk of bipolar disorder.

Psychological factors

Psychological factors are clearly important in the aetiology of depression. Most of the literature comes from the ideas of psychoanalysis and cognitive-behavioural theory.

Psychoanalytical theory

Psychoanalytical theories of depression focus on loss, overdependence on external approval and internalization of anger.

Karl Abraham is credited with beginning psychoanalytical theory with the publication of a paper in 1911, but it was the work of Freud and in particular the publication of *Mourning and Melancholia* in 1917 that established the psychoanalytical theory of depression, which primarily interprets depression as a reaction to loss. Freud noted the similarities between grief and depression and suggested that, just as mourning results from loss by death, so melancholia (depression) results from loss of other kinds. Klein contributed to the theory in the 1930s by developing the idea of the 'depressive position' (developmental stage), whereby during the period around age 4–12 months the infant recognizes the mother as a 'whole object' and that she will return, even following episodes when the infant has been angry. Klein suggested that depression was more likely in people who failed to pass through the depressive position.

Bibring and Jacobson wrote about the importance of self-esteem in depression and how problems with self-esteem are related to both experiences at the oral stage and failures at later stages of development.

Further developments by Bibring in the 1950s and Blatt in the 1970s hold that the depressed person reacts intensely to a loss in later life due to it bringing back the fears of a loss during childhood of parental affection, either through actual loss of the parent or inappropriate parenting. The loss in later life causes the person to regress to the helpless and dependent state of childhood that they were at when the original loss occurred. The display of helplessness and appeal for affection and security is a cry for love.

Psychodynamic theory explains mania as a defence against depression.

Although psychoanalytical theories provide reasonable explanations for some of the behaviours exhibited by patients with mood disorders, there is little objective evidence to support or refute them.

Cognitive-behavioural theory

Cognitive-behavioural theories attribute depression to pessimistic views about oneself and the world.

The beginning of the cognitive model for depression originated from work by Seligman in the 1960s involving giving electric shocks to dogs following a warning, in a situation where they could not escape. The dogs learned to whimper and accept the shocks, and they continued with this behaviour later even when they had the opportunity to escape. This was described as 'learned helplessness'. According to the helplessness model of depression described by Peterson and Seligman, vulnerability to depression derives from a habitual pattern of explaining the causes of life events, which they called 'attributional style'.[29]

Beck grouped the negative thoughts of depressed patients into the three categories ('cognitive triad'): about the self, about present experiences, and about the future. Beck proposed that the negative self-beliefs including worthlessness are formed during childhood as a result of negative experiences, such as loss of a parent or rejection by peers, and these become 'core beliefs'. Beck also developed the idea that people with depression misperceive reality through the following cognitive distortions, and this contributes to their negative beliefs about themselves:

- Overgeneralization
- Magnification of bad events and minimizing good events
- Personalization to assume responsibility for bad events that were in reality outside the person's control
- Selective abstraction – focusing on the bad things and ignoring the good
- Arbitrary interference – drawing conclusions when there is little evidence to support them.

Abramson and others proposed that people have consistent 'attributional styles'. People with negative attributional styles have been shown to be more likely to have depressed reactions to difficult events.[30] Negative cognitive styles have also been shown to precede and predict depressive episodes.[31] More behaviourally oriented approaches theorize that a person becomes depressed when he or she ceases producing behaviour that elicits positive reinforcement.[32]

Social factors

Social factors in the aetiology of depression come into play at a very early stage. Longitudinal studies have shown an association between impaired fetal growth and low birth weight with depression.[33] Neurodevelopmental problems may be associated with an increased risk of depression, possibly exemplified in the 1946 British birth cohort study, which showed that children with low educational test scores were at increased risk for childhood and adult affective disorder.[34]

Childhood disadvantage has been linked with increased risk of depression, with some of the strongest evidence for this coming from Brown and Harris' surveys of inner-city populations.[35]

Mental illness is linked strongly to several aspects of social inequality. Unemployment is associated with increased risk of depression. Being married has been shown to be protective, particularly for men.

Life events, particularly losses, are often the precipitating factor for a depressive episode. Situations of 'entrapment' and 'humiliation' appear to be particularly important.[36] In the 6-month period following a life event, risk for depression and deliberate self-harm is increased six-fold. There are, however, methodological difficulties in assessing life events. Studies show that people suffering from a variety of physical illnesses report relatively high levels of adverse events in the years preceding onset of the illness. It may be that illness leads people to exaggerate their life difficulties, or that healthy people downplay their problems. Or it may be that life events are associated with the decision to seek help rather than the actual illness itself. Both Brown and Harris' studies of inner-city women in London and Kendler's twin studies showed that the association between stressful life events and depressive episodes declines as the number of previous depressive episodes increases.[37,38]

Stressful life events can also precipitate manic episodes in bipolar disorder,[39] with such events more common in the 6 months before first presentation. There is less association between milder episodes of hypomania and life events.

Social risk factors for bipolar disorder include single marital status, unemployment and possibly low income. Studies show social class to be stable over time for people with a diagnosis of bipolar disorder; however, unrecognized subsyndromal illness effects may confound assessment of presumed premorbid socioeconomic status.

Dysfunctional relationships within families have been associated with increasing the risk of bipolar disorder, but it is unclear whether this is cause or effect of illness in subjects and possibly also other family members.

DEPRESSION

Introduction

The concept of depression has evolved over time. Current classification systems owe a lot to the German psychiatrist Emil Kraepelin, known as the father of descriptive psychiatry, who coined the term 'depressive states' in the 1920s. The concept of cognitive and intrapsychic factors in depressive disorders was introduced by Freud in 1917 with the publication of *Mourning and Melancholia*, which shifted the focus from objective behavioural signs to subjective symptoms. The introduction of antidepressants in the 1950s reinforced biological models of depression. George Engel is credited with introducing the concept of illnesses having biological, psychological and social components, and the biopsychosocial model is generally accepted as the current model for depression.

Clinical features

The core symptoms of depression include sustained depressed mood, loss of interest and enjoyment, and reduced energy and activity. Symptoms are often divided into groups according to their nature.

Emotional symptoms include the following:

- Depressed mood, which should be present most days and throughout the day
- Anhedonia – loss of ability to experience pleasure
- Loss of interest in activities
- Irritability
- Diminished emotional reactivity
- Anxiety
- Tearfulness.

Biological symptoms of depression include the following:

- Diurnal variation in mood, with mood commonly improving as the day progresses
- Sleep disturbance, most commonly insomnia, classically involving early-morning wakening. Patients with atypical depression have hypersomnia
- Reduced energy, fatigue and decreased activity
- Change of appetite, which is usually decreased and may result in loss of weight. In atypical depression appetite is increased
- Reduced libido
- Constipation.

Cognitive symptoms include the following:

- Reduced concentration and attention, often with indecisiveness
- Impaired memory
- Slowness of thought processes.

Behavioural features include the following:

- Social withdrawal
- Reduced eye contact
- Psychomotor retardation or agitation
- Reduced facial expression
- Self-neglect.

Depressive cognitions include the following:

- Pessimism involving negative ideation about the future, with feelings of hopelessness and helplessness, and often thoughts of suicide and self-harm
- Feelings of guilt, with inappropriate self-blame
- Feelings of worthlessness and being a failure, resulting in loss of confidence and low self-esteem.

In severe depressive episodes, patients often experience psychotic symptoms, which are usually mood-congruent, including the following:

- Hallucinations, which are usually auditory and typically in the form of second-person auditory hallucination. Other modalities of hallucinations can also be present
- Delusions, which are usually mood-congruent, and the content typically including thoughts of guilt, poverty, persecution and illness. Cotard's syndrome describes patients who experience extreme nihilistic delusions of death and disintegration.

Epidemiology

The epidemiology of depressive disorders is complicated by difficulties in defining the boundaries of depression, dysthymia and euthymia due to diagnostic criteria imposing discrete diagnoses on a symptom continuum of varying severity and duration.

Studies show considerable variability in the lifetime rates of depression, ranging from under 5 per cent to 30 per cent, but it is generally accepted that the lifetime prevalence is between 10 per cent and 20 per cent. The 6-month prevalence rate is considered to be between 2 per cent and 5 per cent based on surveys in several countries. A cross-sectional WHO world health survey carried out in 60 countries covering all regions of the world showed a 1-year prevalence of depressive episode (ICD-10 criteria) of 3.2 per cent, with a 95 per cent confidence interval of 3.0 per cent to 3.5 per cent.[40] The prevalence of depression is higher in patients with medical conditions, with 10–14 per cent of patients under general hospital care affected.[41] Women are twice as likely as men to suffer from depression. There is increasing evidence that the prevalence of depression is increasing and that the age of onset is decreasing.[42]

Risk factors

Risk factors for depression include the following:

- Past history of a depressive episode – depression tends to be a recurrent illness
- Family history – studies show that genetics are a major factor in the aetiology of depression, with heritability of depression estimated to be between 40 per cent and 70 per cent
- Personality traits of neuroticism, obsessionality and impulsivity
- Being from a lower social class
- Living in an urban area
- Unemployment
- Being divorced, although the association is less clear for women than for men

- Lack of a confidant
- Adverse life events, in particular events of loss in vulnerable individuals
- Other psychiatric disorders – co-morbidity with depressive episodes is particularly common with anxiety disorders, substance misuse and personality disorders
- Physical illness – certain neurological illnesses, particularly cerebrovascular disease, Parkinson's disease, multiple sclerosis and epilepsy, may increase the rate of depression through shared neurotransmitter abnormalities. Endocrinological disorders, notably Cushing's syndrome, Addison's disease and disorders of thyroid function, have a particular association with increased rates of depression. Having any severe or prolonged medical condition can increase the risk of depression.

Brown and Harris' often quoted paper 'Social origins of depression: a study of psychiatric disorders in women' identified having three or more children under the age of 11 years, lack of paid employment and lack of a confiding relationship as risk factors for depression,[35] although subsequent studies have not consistently supported the first two of these factors.

Impact

Depression is one of the major causes of disability globally. The WHO has estimated that depression is currently the fourth leading cause of disease burden in the world, after perinatal conditions, lower-respiratory tract infections and human immunodeficiency virus (HIV)/acquired immunodeficiency syndrome (AIDs), and predicts that by 2020 it will be second, after ischaemic heart disease.[43,44]

Patients with depression have elevated standardized mortality ratios compared with the general population. Suicide is the main reason for this, but also contributing are increased rates of cardiovascular disorders, some other medical conditions, and substance misuse and dependence. The presence of depression in patients with coronary artery disease is associated with a doubling of the risk of cardiac death,[45] and in the 2 years following a myocardial infarction the presence of depression is associated with a more than two-fold increase in incidence of cardiac and all-cause mortality.[46] Although the relationship of cause and effect is not clear, suggested mechanisms include that heart disease may increase the likelihood of depression; depression may make heart disease more likely through unhealthy behaviours such as physical inactivity, smoking and poor adherence to medical advice. Other possibilities are that both disorders may share a biological basis, such as alterations in autonomic or hypothalamic–pituitary–adrenal axis function, abnormal platelet function or systemic inflammation.[47]

Course and outcome

Onset

Depression can start at any time in life. The age of onset is usually later than for bipolar disorder. Genetic factors play a more important role in early-onset depression. Late-onset depression is less likely to be associated with a family history and tends to be milder but more likely to become chronic than early-onset depression. A significant number of patients suffer prodromal depressive symptoms before diagnosis. The first manifestations of depressive symptoms are often mild and brief and are recognized only retrospectively.

Early detection of symptoms and appropriate treatment can prevent the development of more severe episodes.

Outcome

The average length of a single depressive episode is about 6 months. Longer episodes are less likely to end with full remission. Chronicity (defined as a non-remitting episode of major depression of at least 2 years' duration) occurs in 10–25 per cent of patients with depression. The rate of recovery from an index episode of depression declines over time. The course of depressive disorder for the majority of patients is recurrent. Approximately 25 per cent of patients have a recurrence of a depressive episode within 1 year of an index episode, and the proportion increases to around 75 per cent at 10 or more years. The first interval between episodes is longer than subsequent intervals, and a later age of onset of depression correlates with shorter first and subsequent intervals. The length and severity of episodes tend to increase with subsequent episodes.[48]

Studies in primary care show that a considerable proportion of patients diagnosed with depression have a poor prognosis, with only about 25 per cent fully recovered after 12 months. About 50 per cent have intermittent symptoms and another 25 per cent have persistent symptoms over the same period.[49] In the longer term, over 50 per cent of patients are still unwell 11 years later, with nearly 40 per cent having a relapsing or chronic course over this time.[50] Some 45 per cent of severely depressed patients recognized by their general practitioner (GP) remained depressed after 12 months, and of these nearly 30 per cent remained severely depressed.[51]

There are several factors increasing the risk of recurrence of depressive episodes, including early age of onset, substance misuse, personality disorder, diagnosis of dysthymia, history of previous depressive episodes, and lack of social support.

The incidence of recurrence is much less in patients on prophylactic treatment.

Patients admitted to hospital with depression with psychotic features have different short- and long-term outcomes than patients admitted with 'neurotic depression'. In the short term, patients with depression with psychotic features tend to improve more quickly, responding to biological and short-term pragmatic therapies. However, in the long term, patients admitted with depression with psychotic features have a considerably worse prognosis, with much higher rates of re-admission and long-term social dysfunction.[52]

About 10 per cent of patients with an initial diagnosis of unipolar depression will have a subsequent manic or hypomanic episode and be re-diagnosed with bipolar disorder.

Suicide

The rate of suicide is significantly increased in patients suffering from depression compared with the general population. It is also higher than in other mood disorders.

Risk of suicide is generally higher in patients who require hospitalization compared with those treated in the community. The risk of suicide in depressive disorder may be at its highest early in the course of the illness. The standardized mortality rate (SMR) for suicide in major depression has been estimated at 20 compared with suicide in the general population (SMR = 1.0).[53] It is generally accepted that 15 per cent of patients hospitalized with depression subsequently die from suicide.[54]

Diagnosis of depression

Classification systems

The two widely used classification systems for making the diagnosis of depression are ICD-10 and DSM-IV.

ICD-10

ICD-10 depression diagnoses are as follows:

Depressive episode (F32)
- Mild depressive episode (F32.0)
- Moderate depressive episode (F32.1)
- Severe depressive episode without psychotic symptoms (F32.2)
- Severe depressive episode with psychotic symptoms (F32.3)
- Other depressive episodes (including atypical depression) (F32.8)

Recurrent depressive disorder (F33)
- Recurrent depressive disorder, current episode mild (F33.0)
- Recurrent depressive disorder, current episode moderate (F33.1)
- Recurrent depressive disorder, current episode severe without psychotic symptoms (F33.2)
- Recurrent depressive disorder, current episode severe with psychotic symptoms (F33.3)
- Recurrent depressive disorder, currently in remission (F33.4).

The diagnosis of depression in ICD-10 is based on the presence of particular symptoms and the impact of those symptoms on the individual. ICD-10 lists ten symptoms that an individual with a depressive episode typically has. The ten symptoms are divided into a group of three symptoms that an individual with depression will usually have, and seven other symptoms:

Core symptoms:

- Depressed mood
- Loss of interest and enjoyment
- Reduced energy and decreased activity.

Other common symptoms:

- Reduced concentration and poor attention
- Reduced self-esteem and confidence
- Ideas of guilt and unworthiness
- Pessimistic thoughts
- Ideas or acts of self-harm or suicide
- Disturbed sleep
- Diminished appetite.

The severity of the episode is based primarily on the number of symptoms present, the level of distress caused by the symptoms and the impact of the symptoms on social function.

For the diagnosis of mild depressive episode, at least two core symptoms and at least two of the other symptoms should be present. The patient is usually distressed by the symptoms and has some difficulty in continuing with ordinary work and social activities.

Moderate depressive episode requires at least two core symptoms and at least three other symptoms. There will usually be considerable difficulty in continuing with social, work or domestic activities.

Severe depressive episode requires all three of the main symptoms and at least four of the other symptoms. The patient will usually show considerable distress or agitation, unless retardation is a marked feature.

Symptoms should be present for at least 2 weeks for a diagnosis of mild or moderate depressive episode. A diagnosis of severe depressive episode may be made following a shorter duration of symptoms if they are particularly severe or if psychotic symptoms are present.

For the diagnosis of recurrent depressive disorder, presence of at least two episodes lasting a minimum of 2 weeks is required. There should be several months without significant mood disturbance between them.

DSM-IV

DSM-IV sets out criteria for the diagnosis of major depressive episode or major depressive disorder, recurrent, and then uses *specifiers* to further categorize the severity:

Major depressive disorder, single episode
- Mild
- Moderate
- Severe (with or without psychotic symptoms)

Major depressive disorder, recurrent.

If a patient with recurrent major depressive disorder currently meets the full criteria for a major depressive episode, its current severity should be specified.

DSM-IV also includes specifiers that can be used to clarify the features of the episode, such as 'with catatonic features', 'with melancholic features' and 'with post partum onset'. Additionally, if the full criteria are not currently met for a major depressive episode, the following specifiers are available to describe the current clinical status: 'in partial remission', 'in full remission' and 'chronic'. The longitudinal course specifiers 'with/without full interepisode recovery' can be used, as can 'with seasonal pattern'.

DSM-IV sets out the following criteria for a major depressive episode:

- Five or more of the following nine (compared with ten in ICD-10) symptoms have been present during the same 2-week period and represent a change from previous functioning; at least one of the symptoms is either depressed mood or loss of interest or pleasure:
  - Depressed mood most of the day, nearly every day
  - Markedly diminished interest or pleasure, in all or almost all activities most of the day, nearly every day
  - Significant weight loss when not dieting, or weight gain, or decrease or increase in appetite nearly every day
  - Insomnia or hypersomnia nearly every day
  - Psychomotor agitation or retardation nearly every day
  - Fatigue or loss of energy nearly every day
  - Feelings of worthlessness or excessive or inappropriate guilt nearly every day
  - Diminished ability to think or concentrate, or indecisiveness, nearly every day
  - Recurrent thoughts of death or recurrent suicidal ideation.
- The symptoms do not meet criteria for a mixed (affective) episode.
- The symptoms cause clinically significant distress or impairment in social, occupational or other important functioning.
- The symptoms are not due to the direct physiological effects of a substance or medical condition.
- The symptoms are not better accounted for by bereavement.

The severity specifier to be used depends on the number of criteria symptoms present, the severity of the symptoms and the degree of functional disability or distress:

- Mild major depressive episode is characterized by the presence of five symptoms and minor social and either mild disability or capacity for normal function but with substantial and unusual effort.
- Moderate major depressive episode has a severity that is in between mild and severe.
- Severe major depressive episode without psychotic features is characterized by the presence of most of the criteria symptoms and clear-cut observable disability.

Age, culture and diagnosis

There are significant differences in the way people of different ages and cultural backgrounds tend to present when they have depression. Elderly people sometimes present with agitation, confusion and functional decline and may mistakenly be considered to have dementia. Children often present with irritability, social withdrawal and deterioration in performance at school.

Since the 1970s many ethnographic studies have shown that the presentation, attribution, classification, prevalence and prognosis of mental disorders vary greatly between cultures.[55] This can create significant difficulties if Western classifications are used without taking into consideration these cultural differences. Definitions of depression in classification systems such as ICD-10 and DSM-IV are descriptive syndromes that are highly heterogeneous and socially shaped. In view of this, some commentators disagree with the way organizations such as the WHO denote depression as a universally valid mental disorder that is amenable to a standard mental health toolkit.[56]

Symptoms of depression show some differences across cultures. People from the Indian subcontinent are more likely to report somatic symptoms while suffering from a depressive episode. Patients from China are more likely to report weakness or tiredness, while Middle Eastern cultures often associate depression with heart problems. A number of studies have shown ubiquity of somatic presentations worldwide, whereas 'psychologization' may be more culturally specific to Western cultures.[57]

Somatization is an important mechanism for many patients with depression and may involve both patient and doctor factors. Both anxiety and depression tend to amplify pain. There are a number of reasons why somatic symptoms may continue even in the absence of dysphoria. Somatic symptoms may secure advantages from partners, family and employers. Somatization may be inadvertently encouraged by doctors. Goldberg and Bridges have suggested three functions that somatization performs. First, it allows people who are unsympathetic to psychological illness or who live in cultures where mental illness is stigmatized to occupy the sick-role while psychologically unwell. Second, it enables the people to avoid blame by casting the individual as the suffering victim. Third, by reducing blame, it may save patients from being as depressed as they might otherwise have been.[58]

Thought content in depression is also influenced by cultural background. It is not unusual for patients from some African countries suffering from severe depression to have delusions about evil spirits and other themes that are not commonly seen in European cultures. Patients from cultures where mental illness is associated with considerable stigma will perceive their depressive symptoms in a very different way and may not spontaneously present them.

Differential diagnosis

Before making a diagnosis of depressive episode, it is important to consider:

- the onset of the disorder, concentrating on any potential precipitating factors such as recent life events (the highest risk being associated with loss or entrapment);
- the course and severity of the symptoms;

- previous episodes of mental illness (especially previous hypomanic or manic symptoms to identify patients who have bipolar disorder);
- any associated medical problems (low mood secondary to a general medical condition);
- substance misuse;
- recent bereavement (normal bereavement is not a mental disorder);
- use of pharmacological agents that can cause mood disturbance.

Differential diagnoses for a depressive episode include the following:

- *Other mental disorders:* depressive symptoms are common in almost all psychiatric disorders, but in particular it is important to consider the following:
  - Other mood disorders, including bipolar disorder, cyclothymia and dysthymia
  - Anxiety disorders, including generalized anxiety disorder, mixed anxiety and depressive disorder, obsessive–compulsive disorder, panic disorder and phobias
  - Schizophrenia and schizoaffective disorder (especially with negative symptoms and post-schizophrenic depression)
  - Eating disorders (anorexia nervosa, bulimia nervosa)
  - Stress-related disorders, including adjustment disorders, bereavement and post-traumatic stress disorder
  - Personality disorders, especially borderline personality disorder
  - Substance-induced depressive disorder.
- *Neurological disorders:*
  - Cerebrovascular disease
  - Parkinson's disease
  - Epilepsy
  - Multiple sclerosis
  - Huntington's disease
  - Tumours
  - Head injury.
- *Endocrine disorders:*
  - Thyroid disorders (hyper- and hypothyroidism)
  - Parathyroid disorders (hyperparathyroidism causes 'moans, bones and abdominal groans', referring to depression, bone pain and constipation)
  - Adrenal (Cushing's syndrome, Addison's disease, hyperaldosteronism)
  - Menstrual, menopausal and postpartum-related symptoms.
- *Infectious and inflammatory disorders:*
  - HIV/AIDS
  - Syphilis
  - Infectious mononucleosis
  - Tuberculosis
  - Systemic lupus erythematosus (SLE)
  - Rheumatoid arthritis.
- *Other physical conditions:*
  - Malignancy
  - Cardiopulmonary disease
  - Porphyria
  - Uraemia
  - Vitamin deficiency
  - Anaemia
  - Sleep apnoea.
- *Medication-related:*
  - Steroids
  - Antihypertensives (beta-blockers, methyldopa, reserpine, calcium channel blockers)
  - H_2 blockers (ranitidine, cimetidine)
  - Sedatives and hypnotics.
- *Substance misuse:*
  - Opiates, benzodiazepines, cannabis, alcohol
  - Stimulants, including amphetamine and methylenedioxymethamphetamine (MDMA, ecstasy).

Investigations

There are no specific tests that can be used to diagnose depression. Investigations are used mainly to exclude other independent problems or to identify treatable causes of depression. It is appropriate to check full blood count, urea, creatinine, electrolytes, serum calcium, liver function tests, thyroid function tests, glucose, erythrocyte sedimentation rate (ESR), plasma viscosity and, especially in older patients, vitamin B12/folate levels. More specific tests should be considered if indicated by history of symptoms or physical examination.

Management

General principles

The aim of managing depressive disorder is to treat the acute symptoms to ease distress, re-establish the patient's normal level of psychosocial functioning and reduce the likelihood of future relapse. The majority of patients with depression are treated in primary care. Patients referred to specialist psychiatric services usually have more severe depression, are treatment-resistant or have depression complicated by other factors such as co-morbidity. The most severely affected patients are usually managed in in-patient settings, sometimes on a compulsory basis. Reasons for hospital admission include significant suicide risk, risk to others, serious self-neglect, severe distress perhaps due to psychotic symptoms, lack of social support, and for initiation of ECT.

Patients with treatment-resistant depression can benefit from an in-patient assessment and close monitoring while new treatments are initiated. Depressive disorder complicated by a serious medical condition is often best treated in a hospital with close liaison with medical teams.

It is often possible to manage even severely depressed patients in the community with intensive support by specialist teams, often including home-based assessment and treatment. Patients with mild and moderate depression are usually managed in primary care settings, ideally by a multidisciplinary team.

The establishment of a collaborative relationship is an important foundation for effective care of patients with depression. Management needs to include regular monitoring of mental state and risk, review of concordance with treatment, and checking for side effects and efficacy of medication. Core to any management of mental disorders is psychoeducation, as this allows better understanding of the specific nature of their illness. There is evidence that active case management can improve outcomes in depression.[59] Active case management includes:

- proactively following up patients;
- assessing patient adherence to psychological and pharmacological treatments;
- monitoring the patient's progress;
- taking action when treatment is unsuccessful;
- delivering psychological support.

Assessment

Assessment of a patient with a depressive episode is performed according to the general principles of any psychiatric assessment; however, there are several specific areas that should be addressed. It is essential to enquire about possible psychosocial precipitants of the current episode as well as predisposing and potential perpetuating factors. Understanding these factors is crucial for the development of an appropriate management plan that targets the specific needs of the individual patient. Assessment should always include a full risk assessment, including history of previous deliberate self-harm and suicide attempts. Enquiry should be made regarding physical illness and medication. While assessing a patient with symptoms of depression, it is very important to ask specifically about past history of manic or hypomanic symptoms in order to exclude the possibility of bipolar disorder.

Treatment

It is useful to divide the treatment of depression into two phases. Acute treatment is aimed at symptom control and achieving remission. The long-term treatment focuses on maintenance and prevention of relapse. Treatment should include biological and psychosocial approaches.

Pharmacological treatment – acute phase

The risk/benefit ratio for use of antidepressant drugs in mild depression is poor. These drugs are therefore not currently recommended as a first-line treatment in mild depression. There is much stronger evidence for their efficacy in moderate and severe depressive episodes.

The efficacy of different antidepressants is similar; however, the side-effect profile varies. Current UK guidelines recommend SSRIs as first-line treatment of depression, although choice of medication should also take into account previous responses to medication. The UK Committee on Safety of Medicines advises using the lowest possible dose of an SSRI and monitoring closely for potential side effects in the early stages of treatment (especially restlessness, agitation and presence of suicidal thoughts).[60] If for any reason antidepressants need to be stopped, the doses should be reduced gradually in order to reduce the likelihood of discontinuation reaction symptoms.

The first-choice antidepressant should be continued at an initial dose for at least 4–6 weeks before any decision about its efficacy is made. If there is no improvement after that time, and there are no concerns about compliance or side effects, it may be appropriate to gradually increase the dose. If there is still no effect, then changing to another antidepressant should be considered. The drugs that should be prescribed as a second choice include another SSRI, a serotonin and noradrenaline reuptake inhibitor (SNRI), mirtazapine, moclobemide, reboxetine or a tricyclic antidepressant. Whenever possible, it is important to take into consideration the patient's choice following discussion about benefits and potential problems that may be encountered for the individual patient.

When changing from one antidepressant medication to another, it is important to take into account the possibility of discontinuation reactions and interactions between the two antidepressants. Most antidepressants have the potential for causing symptoms when they are discontinued if they have been taken regularly for more than a short period of time. Because of this, antidepressants should be phased out gradually unless a serious adverse event has occurred. Simultaneous administration of some antidepressants may lead to problems caused by pharmacodynamic interactions, such as serotonin syndrome, hypotension or drowsiness, or pharmacokinetic interactions, such as increased plasma levels due to enzyme inhibition.

There are three ways of changing from one antidepressant to another, with the rapidity of change depending on the risk of interactions between the medications. The first is a direct switch from one drug to another. Generally this is tolerated when changing from one SSRI to another because their effects are so similar that the administration of the new drug is likely to prevent significant discontinuation symptoms. The second way of changing antidepressants is by cross-tapering, whereby the dose of the antidepressant being discontinued is reduced slowly while the new antidepressant dose is introduced slowly. The third way is to phase out the first antidepressant completely before introducing the new drug, often having a washout period in between finishing one drug and starting the next to ensure complete elimination of the first medication. A washout period is particularly important when changing to a monoamine oxidase inhibitor (MAOI) from any other class of antidepressant, and vice versa.

Treatment of severe depression with psychotic symptoms requires antidepressant therapy to be augmented with an antipsychotic. Care needs to be taken because of the increased potential for side effects due to interactions between antidepressants and antipsychotics. The most common problems are anticholinergic effects and sedation. Atypical antipsychotics are less likely to cause these problems. Careful dose titration is important.

Routine use of benzodiazepines in the treatment of depression is not recommended. For patients presenting with severe anxiety symptoms, a short course at the lowest possible dose may be considered.

To reduce the risk of relapse, treatment with antidepressants should be continued for at least 6 months after achieving remission. It is important to maintain the dose of antidepressant that was originally effective. Six months following remission, the need for continuing medication should be reviewed carefully. Important factors to consider include the number of previous episodes, residual symptoms and ongoing psychosocial stressors. Patients who have a history of two or more depressive episodes should be treated for at least 2 years. Continuation of treatment for more then 2 years should be considered for patients with a more complicated history and higher chances of relapse.

Treatment-resistant depression

Treatment resistance is defined as a failure to respond to two different antidepressants given for a sufficient period of time and at an adequate dose. Patients meeting these criteria for treatment resistance should be reassessed carefully and the diagnosis reviewed. Attention should be paid to previous treatment history, perpetuating factors, adherence to current treatment, co-morbidities and suicide risk. Treatment should be continued within the multidisciplinary team if appropriate.

Very complex cases may require referral to specialist mental health services with expertise in the treatment of mood disorders.

Drug treatment options for treatment-resistant depression include the following:

- Augmentation with lithium should be considered.
- Venlafaxine may be more effective than some other antidepressants in treatment-resistant cases.
- Augmenting antidepressant treatment with another antidepressant is often effective, but the risk of side effects is increased. The most widely used combination is adding mirtazapine to an SSRI.
- Phenelzine may be used if patients are willing to comply with the dietary restrictions. Phenelzine may not be appropriate for individuals with a high risk of suicide due to its significant toxicity in overdose.

Electroconvulsive therapy

The efficacy of ECT in severe depression is well established from long-term trials. It is usually used only when there are psychotic or severe endogenous features present, and usually after a failed trial of pharmacological treatment. ECT is also indicated when depression has become life-threatening as a result of refusal of food and fluids.

A systematic review and meta-analysis in 2003 by the UK ECT Review Group concluded that ECT was significantly more effective than simulated ECT and pharmacotherapy. They also found that bilateral ECT was more effective than unipolar ECT, and that high-dose ECT was more effective than low-dose ECT.[61]

NICE published a technology appraisal *Guidance on the Use of ECT* in May 2003 for England and Wales.[62] It recommends that ECT is used to achieve rapid and short-term improvement of severe symptoms after an adequate trial of other treatment options has failed and when the condition is considered to be life-threatening. ECT is not recommended as a maintenance therapy in depressive illness because the long-term risks and benefits of ECT have not been established. There are several risks that should be considered before using ECT for treatment of depression, including those associated with anaesthesia and of cognitive impairment following ECT.

Neurosurgery

Surgical treatment of depression started in 1935, and some 12 000 procedures were carried out in the UK between 1936 and 1961.[63] Initially the procedure was fairly crude (prefrontal leucotomy), but over time more evidence-based procedures were performed, targeting very specific parts of the brain. Adverse effects from this surgery were considerable, including severe amotivation and personality change, and some 15 per cent of patients developed epilepsy.

Psychosurgery declined rapidly in the 1960s with the advent of antidepressants and a changing social climate. There are now very few psychosurgical operations carried out in the UK. It is illegal in some countries. It is used only in exceptional cases where all other treatments have repeatedly failed and the patient remains ill but retains capacity to consent to the procedure. Stereotactic subcaudate tractotomy (SST) is the treatment of choice for severe mood disorders. New techniques are associated with fewer adverse effects than the earlier procedures, and good outcomes with respect to the depressive illness being treated have been reported as ranging from 34 per cent to 68 per cent,[64] although of course there were no control subjects in these studies.

Treatment of post-stroke depression

Depression is commonly seen in patients following cerebrovascular accident. Treatment with antidepressants is effective and leads to faster rehabilitation. There is particularly good evidence for the efficacy of fluoxetine,[65] citalopram[66] and nortriptyline.[67] As with all patients, it is important to consider the possible interaction of antidepressants with other prescribed medication, such as warfarin.

Treatment of depression in diabetes mellitus

There is a 24 per cent lifetime prevalence of co-morbid depression in individuals with diabetes mellitus,[68] approximately three times higher than the prevalence of depression in the general population. The presence of depression is associated with poorer metabolic control, and there is evidence that treatment of depression may improve glycaemic control.[69] Therefore, early detection and appropriate treatment is important. The NICE guideline for depression recommends screening for depression in high-risk groups such as patients with diabetes mellitus in primary care.[20] This was taken further in 2006, with the introduction to the Quality and Outcomes Framework (QOF), a performance-related pay scheme for GPs in the UK. The QOF requires screening individuals on GPs' registers of patients with diabetes for depression.[70] SSRIs are recommended for first-line treatment. Due to their effects on glucose control and weight, tricyclic antidepressants and MAOIs should not be prescribed routinely. It is important to monitor blood glucose closely while starting, changing the dose or discontinuing antidepressant treatment.

Psychological treatment of depression

Patients with mild depression should be offered psychological therapy before considering antidepressant medication (see NICE guidance, below). It can be offered as the only treatment for patients with mild depressive disorder and in combination with medication for moderate and severe episodes. A number of different types of treatment are available, and the choice should be based on availability, patient preference and past experience. The appropriate treatment should be delivered by a trained healthcare professional.

Cognitive-behavioural therapy (CBT) should be considered for patients who prefer this type of intervention to medication and to those who, despite an adequate treatment with antidepressants, still experience some depressive symptoms. In more severe cases, it is appropriate to offer CBT in combination with medication, as this appears to be more effective than either treatment alone. A course of CBT is usually given over 10–12 weeks, although for patients with more severe depression the course is often longer. Sometimes follow-up sessions are considered, usually two to four sessions over a year after the initial course of treatment.

CBT for depression is typically directive and short-term. It focuses upon changing the depressed patient's negative thoughts regarding his or her self, world and future.[71] With depression tending to be a relapsing condition, relapse prevention is an important part of CBT treatment. Relapse prevention includes identifying high-risk situations, learning and practising coping skills and creating lifestyle balance.

CBT has been shown to be more effective than pill-placebo and equivalent to antidepressant medication. It is effective across a wide range of patient severity and can prevent relapse as effectively as continuous antidepressant medication.[71] CBT combined with antidepressant medication has been shown to be more effective at reducing depressive symptoms in chronically depressed patients than either treatment alone.[72]

Interpersonal therapy (IPT) aims to achieve symptomatic relief for patients with depression by addressing current interpersonal problems associated with the onset of the disorder. Treatment is usually of a similar duration to that for CBT. There is less evidence of efficacy for IPT than there is for CBT, but studies have shown IPT to be superior to placebo and equivalent to CBT and antidepressant therapy for mild depression and superior to placebo but less effective than antidepressants in severe depression.[73] IPT has also been shown to increase the length of time between episodes of depression in patients not receiving antidepressants.[74] As

Who is responsible for care?	What is the focus?	What do they do?
Step 5: In-patient care, crisis teams	Risk to life, severe self-neglect	Medication, combined treatments, ECT
Step 4: Mental health specialists, including crisis teams	Treatment-resistant, recurrent, atypical and psychotic depression, and patients at significant risk	Medication, complex psychological interventions, combined treatments
Step 3: Primary care team, primary care mental health worker	Moderate or severe depression	Medication, psychological interventions, social support
Step 2: Primary care team, primary care mental health worker	Mild depression	Watchful waiting, guided self-help, computerized CBT, exercise, brief psychological interventions
Step 1: GP, practice nurse	Recognition	Assessment

Figure 39.1 National Institute for Health and Clinical Excellence (NICE) stepped care model

CBT, cognitive-behavioural therapy; ECT, electroconvulsive therapy.

with CBT, there is evidence that combined IPT and antidepressant therapy is superior to either treatment alone.[75]

It may be appropriate to consider psychodynamic psychotherapy for patients with mild to moderate depressive illness in more complex cases where there is co-morbidity with personality disorders.[76] It should not be offered to patients suffering from severe depressive disorder, especially if psychotic symptoms are present. Treatment is lengthy but some benefits are seen while in therapy, including a reduction in treatment-seeking and need for medication. Due to the nature of psychodynamic psychotherapy, there is a paucity of trials with adequate methodology and statistical power to show efficacy or otherwise of this treatment in depression.

NICE guidance

NICE, an organization that produces guidance on public health, health technologies and clinical practice for England and Wales, released the guideline *Depression: Management of Depression in Primary and Secondary Care* in December 2004.[20] The guideline's recommendations are presented via a stepped care model (Figure 39.1).

Stepped care is a model of healthcare delivery that has been applied to a range of disorders, particularly those of a chronic nature. There are two main features of a stepped care system. First is that the recommended treatment offered for the condition should be the least intensive of those currently available but still likely to provide significant health gain. More intensive treatments are reserved for patients who do not benefit from simpler first-line treatments. Second, stepped care is self-correcting, in that the results of treatments and decisions about treatment provision are monitored systematically, and changes are made ('stepping up') if current treatments are not achieving significant clinical improvement.

In the NICE depression guideline, there are five steps with each step up, representing increased complexity of intervention. With higher steps, it is assumed that interventions in previous steps have been considered or implemented before the higher step is used.

The key priorities for implementation recommended in the NICE guideline are as follows:

- Screening for depression in primary care and general hospital settings in high risk groups: NICE recommends use of the following two questions for screening in these settings. The test is negative if both are negative, but if either is positive, further assessment is recommended:
  - During the past month, have you often been bothered by feeling down, depressed or hopeless?
  - During the past month, have you often been bothered by having little interest or pleasure in doing things?
- Watchful waiting as opposed to intervention is recommended as the initial step for patients with mild depression.
- Antidepressants are not recommended for the initial treatment of mild depression, because the risk/benefit ratio is poor.
- Guided self-help based on cognitive-behavioural therapy is recommended for patients with mild depression.
- Short-term psychological treatment is recommended for patients with mild and moderate depression.
- An SSRI is recommended as the first-line antidepressant if one is to be prescribed, because SSRIs are as effective as tricyclic antidepressants but less likely to be discontinued due to side effects.
- Patients should be informed about discontinuation symptoms if antidepressants are prescribed.
- A combination of antidepressants and individual CBT should be considered for patients at initial presentation with severe depression.
- Maintenance treatment with antidepressants for 2 years is advised for patients who have had two or more depressive episodes in the recent past and who have experienced significant functional impairment during the episodes.
- A combination of antidepressant medication and CBT should be considered for patients with treatment-resistant depression.
- CBT should be considered for patients with recurrent depression who have relapsed despite antidepressant treatment.

NICE makes a number of specific recommendations for treatment-resistant depression. Venlafaxine may be considered for patients who have failed two adequate trials of alternative antidepressants. When prescribing venlafaxine, be aware of the increased likelihood of patients stopping treatment because of side effects, its higher cost, its high propensity for discontinuation symptoms if stopped abruptly, and its toxicity in overdose. NICE recommends that an electrocardiogram (ECG) is carried out and blood pressure checked before starting venlafaxine. NICE recommends that a trial of lithium augmentation should be considered for patients who have failed to respond to several antidepressants. Augmentation of one antidepressant with another, such as addition of mirtazapine or mianserin to SSRIs, should be considered, but patients on these combinations should be monitored carefully, particularly for serotonin syndrome. NICE recommends phenelzine for patients who have failed to respond to alternative antidepressants and are prepared to tolerate the side effects and dietary restrictions, and the risk of toxicity in overdose has been considered.

NICE specifically recommends against augmentation of antidepressants with carbamazepine, lamotrigine, buspirone, pindolol, valproate or thyroid hormone due to insufficient evidence of efficacy and, particularly in relation to carbamazepine, significant risk of adverse effects due primarily to effects on the metabolism of other medications. Dosulepin is also not recommended due to increased cardiac risk and toxicity in overdose.

BIPOLAR AFFECTIVE DISORDER

Introduction

The Greek physician Aretaeus of Cappadocia (c.AD81–138)[77] is credited with the first description of what is now known as bipolar affective disorder.[78] The German psychiatrist Emil Kraepelin's distinction between manic–depressive psychosis and dementia praecox (schizophrenia) in the late 1800s was an enormous breakthrough in the understanding of bipolar disorder. Kraepelin did not distinguish between patients with psychotic unipolar depression and patients with both mania and depression. The understanding of unipolar depression and bipolar affective disorder as separate disease entities came in the 1960s from the work of Leonard and Angst.

Clinical features of mania

Typical features of mania include:

- elevated mood (excitement usually not in keeping with the current situation), but also commonly irritability and aggression, especially if confronted;
- increased self-esteem, which may manifest as grandiosity, inappropriate optimism, overfamiliarity and reduced social inhibition;
- increased energy manifesting as decreased need for sleep, overactivity, racing thoughts and pressured speech;
- distractibility and reduced attention span;
- inappropriate behaviour, particularly engagement in activities that are high risk for detrimental consequences, such as reckless spending, inappropriate sexual encounters and dangerous driving;
- significant disruption to occupational functioning and in family and social life.

Patients with mania may also experience dysphoria and some depressive symptoms. Sometimes they become suspicious. Psychotic symptoms can occur in more severe manic episodes. Patients can present with delusions, which are nearly always mood-congruent, and hallucinations. Some grandiose ideas can be delusional, such as of having a special role or power, and frequently have a religious content. Persecutory delusions can develop from extreme suspiciousness.

Due to the severity of disruption in functioning and the potential serious consequences, mania usually requires an admission to hospital, sometimes with compulsory detention.

Hypomania

Hypomania occurs when symptoms are less severe and do not meet criteria for mania, although mood during a hypomanic episode is still clearly different from the individual's usual mood. Patients with hypomania do not require hospitalization (DSM-IV criteria) and there are no psychotic symptoms present. The disturbance in a hypomanic episode is not severe enough to cause marked impairment in social and occupational functioning. There is often increased productivity or creativity, although distractibility and poor concentration may lead to impaired social or occupational functioning.

Course

Manic and hypomanic episodes typically begin suddenly, with symptoms developing rapidly over a few days. Episodes last from a few weeks to several months. They tend to be briefer and end more abruptly than depressive episodes. Some 50–60 per cent of manic episodes immediately follow or are followed by a depressive episode. A similar pattern applies to hypomanic episodes. About 5–15 per cent of individuals who have a hypomanic episode will develop a manic episode at some time in the future.

Clinical features of depression in bipolar disorder

In bipolar disorder, depressive episodes usually present with low mood, loss of interest and enjoyment, reduced energy, poor concentration, disturbed sleep and loss of appetite. Confidence and self-esteem are usually low, and hopelessness and ideas of guilt may be present. Psychotic symptoms may occur in severe episodes, and these are usually mood-congruent.

In comparison with unipolar depression, bipolar depression may be more likely to present with melancholic symptoms such as worthlessness, psychomotor retardation and mood-congruent psychotic symptoms. Atypical features such as hypersomnia are more often present.

Course

Depressive episodes in bipolar disorder are typically shorter than in unipolar depression, but they are usually less responsive to treatment.

Clinical features of a mixed affective episode

Manic or hypomanic symptoms occur along with depressive symptoms within the same episode of illness. Depressive symptoms and symptoms of mania or hypomania may alternate from day to day or even from hour to hour. A typical episode may consist of depressive mood being accompanied by increased activity and pressured speech. Manic symptoms can be accompanied by loss of energy and libido.

Course

Mixed affective episodes can develop in isolation or may evolve from a manic or depressive episode. Mixed affective episodes last from weeks to several months. They may resolve back to euthymia or may evolve into a depressive episode or, much less commonly, into a manic episode.

Clinical features of rapid-cycling bipolar disorder

The term 'rapid cycling' is applied to bipolar disorder when four or more separate mood episodes occur within a 12-month period. Apart from their frequency, the mood episodes are no different from mood episodes that occur in non-rapid-cycling bipolar disorder. Of patients with bipolar disorder seen in mood clinics, it is estimated that 10–20 per cent will have rapid cycling. A rapid-cycling pattern is seen predominantly in women. This pattern can occur at any time during the course of bipolar disorder and is associated with a poorer long-term prognosis. In some individuals it can be associated with antidepressant use.

Course of bipolar disorder

Bipolar disorder is a recurrent condition, with 90 per cent of individuals who have a manic episode having a future manic episode.[2] Manic episodes frequently precede or follow depressive episodes, and in many patients a clear pattern is evident. Studies suggest that, without long-term treatment, patients with bipolar I disorder would average four episodes over a 10-year period. The interval between episodes for both bipolar I and bipolar II disorder tends to decrease as the age of the individual increases, and in both conditions 5–15 per cent of individuals have four or more mood episodes within a given year (rapid cycling). Individuals who have psychotic symptoms during manic episodes are more likely to have psychotic symptoms in subsequent manic episodes.[2]

Although most individuals with bipolar disorder have resolution of symptoms between episodes, 20–30 per cent of patients with bipolar I disorder and 15 per cent of patient with bipolar II disorder continue to suffer mood symptoms. Up to 60 per cent of patients with bipolar I disorder have ongoing social impairment between episodes.[2]

Epidemiology

The epidemiology of bipolar disorder is complicated by issues related to defining cases. As with other mental disorders, defining cases depends on imposing discrete diagnoses on a symptom continuum of varying severity and duration. With case definition being fundamental to epidemiology, variation in defining cases has influence on prevalence rates and understanding of risk factors.

Diagnosis in individual patients may change over time due to changing presentation of symptoms. As bipolar disorder can be diagnosed only after a manic, hypomanic or mixed episode, a significant number of patients who present initially with depressive episodes are subsequently diagnosed with bipolar disorder following a manic pole episode. Additionally, although many patients have classic presentations, many do not. A patient may initially be considered to have bipolar disorder but over time the pattern of illness may become more clearly that of schizoaffective disorder and the diagnosis changed accordingly. In an adult cohort of patients experiencing a first psychotic episode, only 75 per cent kept their diagnosis of bipolar disorder after 6 months.[79] Therefore, the true incidence of bipolar disorder can only be estimated retrospectively.

Diagnosis also depends on interpretation of symptoms. The boundaries of bipolar disorder are not clear. Bipolar disorder with marked psychotic features overlaps with schizoaffective disorder. Patients with recurrent depressive episodes and mild or brief episodes of hypomania may or may not be diagnosed with bipolar disorder. Bipolar II disorder is receiving increasing recognition and as a result is being diagnosed more frequently. There are moves to lower the threshold for diagnosis of hypomania, which would result in increasing the prevalence of bipolar II disorder and reducing the prevalence of recurrent depressive disorder. There is an overlap of bipolar disorder with some personality disorders such as borderline personality disorder.

Prevalence rates for bipolar disorder across different studies are considerably more consistent than for depression. Large population studies such as the US National Institutes of Mental Health (NIMH) Epidemiologic Catchment (ECA) Study and the National Comorbidity Survey (NCS) (carried out in the USA) have shown a lifetime prevalence of bipolar disorder of 0.3–1.5 per cent.[80,81] The lifetime prevalence of bipolar I disorder (0.8%) is perhaps slightly higher than that of bipolar II disorder (0.5%), although increasing awareness of bipolar II disorder may increase the rate of this diagnosis. Poor recognition of and uncertainty about diagnosis of hypomania may currently result in underdiagnosis of this condition.[82]

Studies show the 6-month prevalence of bipolar disorder to be only slightly lower than the lifetime prevalence reflecting a high degree of chronicity and recurrence. The male to female ratio is approximately equal. The median age of onset is in late adolescence and early twenties, but a significant proportion of later-onset cases brings the mean age of onset up to late twenties. There is speculation that many patients actually exhibit symptoms in childhood but are not diagnosed. Ninety per cent of patients have their first episode before the age of 50 years. In patients who present later in life, organic factors are more likely to be involved.

A significant number of patients having their first manic, hypomanic or mixed affective episode have experienced a previous depressive episode. The risk of patients with depression having a subsequent manic pole episode and conversion to a diagnosis of bipolar disorder appears to increase in proportion to the severity of the depression. Of patients presenting with depression requiring hospitalization, the estimated risk of a subsequent manic episode is

5 per cent.[83] Factors in patients with depression that are associated with an increased likelihood of subsequent conversion to a diagnosis of bipolar disorder include early age of onset, postpartum onset and depression with psychomotor retardation.

There is some divergence between Europe and North America in the diagnosis of children and adolescents with bipolar disorder. Rates of diagnosis of bipolar disorder in children and adolescents in North America are considerably higher than in Europe.

Risk factors

Genetic factors are probably the predominant factor in relation to lifetime vulnerability to bipolar disorder, but other factors are more important as risk factors for determining when episodes of illness will occur. Genetic factors are discussed in the earlier section Aetiology of affective disorders.

There appears to be a seasonal pattern to bipolar disorder, with studies showing an increase in the number of manic episodes in the late spring and early summer. Disruption to biological rhythms such as from international travel or shift work is associated with increased risk of manic or depressive episodes. The postpartum period is a time of increased risk of illness for patients with bipolar disorder. Adverse life events are a risk factor for both depressive and manic episodes. Organic disease of the central nervous system may be a risk factor, particularly for-late onset bipolar disorder.

Family studies have suggested that many patients who go on to be diagnosed with bipolar disorder exhibit subsyndromal symptoms for some time before they develop diagnostic illness. Therefore, there are patients who exhibit mood swings and cyclothymia who are probably at higher risk of subsequent bipolar disorder.

Co-morbidity

Co-morbid psychiatric conditions are common in patients with bipolar disorder. Studies have shown considerably increased rates of alcohol and substance misuse and dependence. Panic disorder and, to a lesser extent, anxiety disorder are also more common in patients with bipolar disorder.

Impact

The economic cost to society of bipolar disorder is huge. The ECA study concluded that, over a 6-month period, about 10 per cent of patients with bipolar disorder received in-patient treatment. The NCS study showed that 45 per cent of patients with bipolar disorder had received psychiatric treatment within the past 12 months.[84]

Suicide

Individuals with bipolar disorder are at substantially increased risk of completed suicide than the general population. A meta-analysis of studies containing a total of 2257 cases of suicide by Harris and Barraclough gave an SMR for suicide in bipolar disorder of 15 compared with the general population (SMR = 1.0).[53] Nearly a third of patients with bipolar disorder admit to at least one previous suicide attempt. It is estimated that 10–15 per cent of patients with bipolar I disorder die from suicide.[85] Nearly 80 per cent of patients with bipolar disorder who commit suicide have experienced a depressive episode immediately before death. Mixed affective states are associated with a particularly high risk of suicide.[86]

Diagnosis

Classification systems

The two widely used classification systems for making the diagnosis of bipolar disorder are ICD-10 and DSM-IV.

ICD-10

The ICD-10 diagnoses for manic and mixed episodes and bipolar affective disorder are as follows:

- Manic episode (F30)
  - Hypomania (F30.0)
  - Mania without psychotic symptoms (F30.1)
  - Mania with psychotic symptoms (F30.2)
  - Other manic episodes (F30.9)
  - Manic episode, unspecified
- Other mood disorders (F38)
  - Mixed affective episode (F38.00)
- Bipolar affective disorder (F31)
  - Bipolar affective disorder, current episode hypomanic (F31.0)
  - Bipolar affective disorder, current episode manic with/without psychotic symptoms (F31.1/F31.2)
  - Bipolar affective disorder, current episode mild/mod depression (F31.3)
  - Bipolar affective disorder, current episode severe depression with or without psychotic symptoms (F31.4/F31.5)
  - Bipolar affective disorder, current episode mixed (F31.6)
  - Other bipolar affective disorders (F31.8)
  - Bipolar affective disorder, unspecified (F31.9).

ICD-10 requires a manic episode of any of the three severities as requiring elevated mood and an increase in the quantity and speed of physical and mental activity. The diagnosis of manic episode should be used only for a single episode. If there are previous or subsequent affective episodes, then the diagnosis should be bipolar affective disorder.

Hypomania is described as a lesser degree of mania but too persistent and marked for the diagnosis of cyclothymia. It requires persistent mild elevation of mood, increased levels of energy with increased activity, and usually strong feelings of wellbeing in physical and mental efficiency. Other features include talkativeness, overfamiliarity, increased sociability and sexual drive, and reduced need for sleep. Sometimes irritability and antisocial behaviour replace euphoric sociability. Concentration and attention are usually reduced. ICD-10 states that symptoms are severe enough to cause interference in social function but not to severely disrupt work or cause social rejection.

A diagnosis of mania requires elevated mood out of keeping with the individual's circumstances, with increased energy, overactivity, pressure of speech and reduced need for sleep. There is also social disinhibition, reduced attention span, distractibility, and grandiosity or overoptimism. There may be perceptual disorders such as subjective hyperacusis or increased appreciation of colour or texture. Symptoms must be present for at least 1 week and severe enough to cause almost complete disruption of ordinary work and social function.

Mania with psychotic symptoms is used when a patient fulfilling the criteria for a manic episode also has delusions or hallucinations. In these circumstances the manic symptoms tend to be severe. The delusions should be specified as congruent or incongruent with the mood.

A mixed affective episode requires at least 2 weeks of a mixture, sometimes with rapid alternation (usually within a few hours), of hypomanic, manic and depressive symptoms.

Bipolar affective disorder requires at least two episodes of affective disorder, one of which must be manic, hypomanic or mixed.

DSM-IV

DSM-IV sets out criteria for the diagnosis of mood episodes and bipolar disorders and uses specifiers to further categorize the severity of the current clinical state:

- Mood episodes
  - Major depressive episode
  - Manic episode
  - Mixed episode
  - Hypomanic episode
- Bipolar disorders
  - Bipolar I disorder
  - Bipolar II disorder
  - Cyclothymic disorder
  - Bipolar disorder not otherwise specified.

The following specifiers are used to describe the clinical status of the current or most recent mood episode:

- Mild, moderate, severe with/without psychotic features
- In partial remission
- In full remission.

The following specifiers are used to indicate the pattern of episodes in bipolar disorders:

- With/without full interepisode recovery
- With rapid cycling.

Manic episode criteria in DSM-IV are as follows:

- A distinct period of abnormally and persistently elevated, expansive, or irritable mood, lasting at least 1 week (or any duration if hospitalization is necessary).
- During the period of mood disturbance, at least three of the following symptoms have persisted (four if mood is only irritable) to a significant degree:
  - Inflated self-esteem and grandiosity
  - Decreased need for sleep
  - More talkative than usual or pressure to keep talking
  - Flight of ideas or subjective experience that thoughts are racing
  - Distractibility
  - Increase in goal-directed activity
  - Excessive involvement in pleasurable activities that have a high potential for painful consequences.
- The symptoms do not meet criteria for mixed episode.
- The mood disturbance is sufficiently severe to cause marked impairment in occupational functioning or in usual social activities or relationships with others, or to necessitate hospitalization to prevent harm to self or others, or there are psychotic features.
- The symptoms are not due to the direct physiological effects of a substance.

Mixed episode criteria in DSM-IV are as follows:

- The criteria are met for both a manic episode and for a major depressive episode nearly every day during at least a 1-week period.
- The mood disturbance is sufficiently severe to cause marked impairment in occupational function or in usual social activities or relationships with others, or to necessitate hospitalization to prevent harm to self or others, or there are psychotic features.
- The symptoms are not due to the direct physiological effects of a substance.

Hypomanic episode criteria in DSM-IV are as follows:

- A distinct period of abnormally and persistently elevated, expansive, or irritable mood, lasting at least 4 days, that is clearly different from the usual non-depressed mood.
- During the period of mood disturbance, at least three of the following symptoms have persisted (four if mood is only irritable) to a significant degree:
  - Inflated self-esteem and grandiosity
  - Decreased need for sleep
  - More talkative than usual or pressure to keep talking
  - Flight of ideas or subjective experience that thoughts are racing
  - Distractibility
  - Increase in goal-directed activity
  - Excessive involvement in pleasurable activities that have a high potential for painful consequences
- The episode is associated with an unequivocal change in function that is uncharacteristic of the person when not symptomatic.
- The disturbance in mood and the change in functioning are observable by others.
- The episode is not severe enough to cause marked impairment in social or occupational functioning, or to

Table 39.1 Diagnostic scales for bipolar disorder

Scale	Sensitivity	Specificity
Clinician-Administered Rating Scale for Mania (CARS-M)	0.85	0.87
Mini International Neuropsychiatric Inventory (MINI)	0.89	0.97
Psychosis Screening Questionnaire (PSQ)	0.96	0.95
Mood Disorder Questionnaire (MDQ)	0.72	0.90
Brief Psychiatric Rating Scale (BPRS)	0.67	0.72

necessitate hospitalization, and there are no psychotic features.

- The symptoms are not due to the direct physiological effects of a substance.

Bipolar I disorder requires the occurrence of one or more manic or mixed episode with or without a history of major depressive episodes.

Bipolar II disorder requires the occurrence of one or more major depressive episodes with at least one hypomanic episode.

The rapid-cycling specifier can be applied to bipolar I and bipolar II diagnoses. The criteria for this are that there have been at least four episodes of a mood disturbance in the previous 12 months that meet the criteria for a major depressive, manic, mixed or hypomanic episode. Episodes must be separated by partial or full remission for at least 2 months or a switch to an episode of opposite polarity.

Screening tools and rating scales

A number of instruments have been developed for use as diagnostic tools or severity rating scales. There is little evidence about use of screening tools for early detection of bipolar disorder. The gold standard against which to compare diagnostic tools is clinical assessment by experts, although even this is not perfectly consistent. Table 39.1 shows the diagnostic scales for bipolar disorder.[87]

Differential diagnoses for manic/hypomanic episode

- Depression with agitation
- Schizoaffective disorder
- Schizophrenia and other psychotic disorders
- Anxiety disorders
- Alcohol or drug misuse, especially stimulants and hallucinogens
- Attention deficit hyperactivity disorder and conduct disorder
- Physical illness, such as Cushing's syndrome, SLE, hyperthyroidism, epilepsy, multiple sclerosis, head injury, brain tumour, encephalitis, HIV
- Medication-induced.

Medication-induced mania/hypomania

A range of medications may induce symptoms of mania, including the following:

- Antidepressants: all antidepressants may trigger a manic episode, although the risk, many clinicians believe, is less with SSRIs and bupropion. Currently DSM-IV excludes mania induced by antidepressants as being diagnostic for bipolar disorder, but it is possible that patients who develop mania as the result of antidepressants do actually have bipolar disorder
- Other psychotropic medication: mania has been observed to result from treatment with some antipsychotics, mood stabilizers, anti-epileptic medications and stimulants (methylphenidate)
- Antiparkinsonian medications, including amantadine, bromocriptine, levodopa and Procyclidine
- Corticosteroids and anabolic steroids
- Respiratory medications, including salbutamol, aminophylline and ephedrine
- Analgesics, including opioids, nefopam and indometacin
- Antimicrobial agents, including some tuberculosis medications, zidovudine, dapsone, chloroquine and clarithromycin
- Others, including cimetidine, metoclopramide, baclofen, cyclizine and interferon.

Investigations

There are no specific tests that can be used to diagnose mania. Investigations are used mainly to exclude other independent problems or to identify causes of the manic symptoms.

Physical checks usually performed for a patient with mania include the following:

- A thorough physical examination
- Blood tests, including full blood count, urea, creatinine, electrolytes, serum calcium, liver function tests, thyroid function tests, glucose, ESR and plasma viscosity. More specific tests may be indicated by features of the history, findings on clinical examination or results of the initial tests
- Drug screen.

In specific circumstances, such as when there is a high index of suspicion of intracranial pathology, late onset or fluctuation course, it is appropriate to also arrange the following:

- Computed tomography (CT) or magnetic resonance imaging (MRI) scan of the brain
- Electroencephalogram (EEG).

Management

General principles

Treatment of bipolar affective disorder is aimed at treating acute episodes, reducing the severity and frequency of future episodes, and improving psychosocial functioning between episodes. A number of different treatment strategies can be used to substantially decrease morbidity and mortality. Management consists of pharmacological treatments, psychological therapies, and education for the individual, family and carers. It is important that the management plan not only covers treatment of the acute episode but also includes long-term strategies to maintain optimum mental health and social function between episodes.

The establishment and maintenance of collaborative relationships with patients with bipolar disorder and their families and carers is fundamental to achieving the above goals of treatment. When appropriate, patients should be encouraged to involve their families and carers in their treatment. They should be given full and clear information about the illness and treatment at each step, and this may include the use of self-help resources and support groups. Patients and carers should be advised about self-monitoring for early warning signs of relapse, given education about lifestyle that may help to reduce relapse such as sleep hygiene and work patterns, and given information about coping strategies. Patients and carers must be aware of a clear route of contact to services for times of relapse and crisis.

Patients and their carers often have useful knowledge gained from their experience of previous episodes that can be taken into account when planning future management. Patients should be given the opportunity to make informed decisions about their care and treatment. Respect for patients' preferences is likely to improve concordance. Patients should be encouraged to develop advance directives, particularly if they have had severe episodes or detention under mental health legislation. An advance directive should contain details of early warning signs from the patient's perspective that may indicate a possible relapse and the patient's preferred course of action in the event of a relapse, including who to contact and wishes around medication. To be useful, advance directives need to be reviewed regularly, recorded in the patient's care plan, and copied to the patient, care coordinator and GP.

It is particularly important to maintain a collaborative relationship with patients and carers and to provide education about the illness and support during the maintenance phase. Patients frequently discontinue treatment when they feel well, but relapses are common. Patients are also frequently unwilling to accept anti-manic medication at times when they have higher levels of activity, especially if their performance is not impaired by distractibility.

Clinicians caring for patients with bipolar disorder should take account of the needs of patients' family members and carers. Regular assessment should be made of the impact of the disorder on relationships, the welfare of dependent children, and the physical, social and mental health needs of carers. Families and carers may benefit from contact with support groups.

The place of treatment for a patient with bipolar disorder having an acute episode will depend on the nature of the episode, severity of symptoms, risk to the patient or others, and availability of support in the community. It is often possible to treat hypomanic and severe depressive episodes in the home environment, with the support of crisis intervention teams. Hospitalization may be required to protect the patient from physical harm to self or others, to protect against the consequences of injudicious behaviour, or to avoid overstimulation. It must be remembered that mania can be a life-threatening condition, not only from suicide but also from the complications of exhaustion, dehydration and hyperthermia. Hospitalization may have to be against the patient's wish, using mental health legislation.

Treatment of acute manic and hypomanic episodes

Manic patients frequently have marked behavioural disturbance, and initially treatment may need to focus on this. Very disturbed patients should be managed in a supportive environment with minimal stimulation balanced against provision of facilities for using up excess energy. Using distraction techniques and avoiding confrontation are important. The patient's physical health needs to be reviewed regularly, particularly checking for adequate hydration. Benzodiazepines such as lorazepam and antipsychotics, either alone or in combination, may be required to control severe behaviour disturbance. Restraint and rapid tranquilization using intramuscular medication may be required.

Treatment of mania and hypomania is predominantly based on pharmacotherapy. Both antipsychotics and mood stabilizers are effective. Patients with bipolar disorder may be quite sensitive to antipsychotics, so it is appropriate to start with a low dose. Benzodiazepines are useful in the short term for ameliorating behavioural disturbance and agitation, and their addition allows antipsychotic medications to be initiated at a low dose rather than at tranquillizing doses, which are associated with significant side effects and increased risk of sudden death due to their effects on myocardial transmission. Medications initiated in the acute phase are often continued as anti-manic prophylaxis, and this should be taken into account when treatment is initiated.

Carbamazepine has been used for long-term treatment of bipolar disorder, but recent trials have shown it to be substantially less beneficial than lithium at preventing relapse. Enzyme induction can be another complicating factor with carbamazepine. It is no longer generally recommended for routine use in acute mania.

If a patient is taking antidepressant medication at the onset of an acute manic episode, the antidepressant should be stopped. The rate of withdrawal of antidepressant medication depends on balancing the severity of manic episode with the likelihood of discontinuation symptoms.

If the patient is not already taking anti-manic prophylaxis, the following considerations should be taken into account when selecting anti-manic medication:

- Previous responses to anti-manic medication.
- Antipsychotic medications may be more effective when there are severe symptoms or behavioural disturbance. The side effects of weight gain and metabolic disturbance should be taken into account, especially in individuals at risk of diabetes.
- Valproate should generally be avoided in women of childbearing potential.
- Lithium has a slower onset of action, usually taking a week to achieve a response, so generally it should be avoided if symptoms are severe.
- Lithium has a narrow therapeutic window and requires monitoring of blood levels, and so it should be avoided in patients who are unlikely to be able to cooperate with this.

When patients develop a manic episode while being prescribed anti-manic medication, the following steps should be taken:

- Check concordance with medication.
- If on antipsychotic prophylaxis, consider increasing the dose. If there is no response to this, consider adding lithium or valproate.
- If on lithium, check serum levels and increase the dose if needed in order to achieve serum levels of 0.8–1.0 mmol/L. If there is inadequate response to optimum lithium levels, consider augmentation with an antipsychotic.
- If on valproate, increase the dose until there is clinical improvement or side effects limit further dose increase. Patients on doses higher than 45 mg/kg should be monitored carefully for liver toxicity. If there is inadequate response to maximum tolerated doses of valproate, consider augmentation with an antipsychotic.
- If the patient is prescribed carbamazepine for manic prophylaxis, the dose should not be increased routinely, but addition of an antipsychotic should be considered.

Treatment of acute depressive episodes in bipolar disorder

The drug treatment of depressive episodes in bipolar disorder is complicated by limited information from well-conducted randomized controlled trials. The main risk when treating depressed patients who have bipolar disorder is of causing a 'switch' to mania. Current guidance in the UK recommends prescribing anti-manic medication concurrently if antidepressants are to be prescribed.

In patients who are on anti-manic medication at the time of developing a depressive episode, concordance should be checked and the dose increased if necessary.

If the depressive episode is mild, it is often appropriate to delay medication changes, particularly if previous episodes of mild depression have not developed into more severe depression, because the episode may be self-limiting or may respond to supportive psychosocial measures. If symptoms persist, or if there is perceived to be significant risk of deterioration at the initial assessment, the patient should be treated in the same way as patients with moderate or severe depressive episodes.

Treatment for moderate or severe depressive episodes in patients with bipolar disorder generally involves initiation of an antidepressant. SSRI antidepressants are considered to be less likely than tricyclic antidepressants to cause switching to mania and so are generally recommended as first-line drugs. Antidepressant treatment should be initiated at a low dose and titrated up gradually. If an antidepressant is being initiated and the patient is not already taking anti-manic medication, this should also be initiated, with the choice of anti-manic medication being based on the same considerations as when starting it for a manic episode.

Because of the risk of causing a switch to mania in bipolar disorder, consideration should be given to discontinuing antidepressant therapy soon after the patient achieves remission from depressive symptoms and sometimes even symptoms have been less severe for a few weeks. The antidepressant should be withdrawn slowly over a number of weeks. Anti-manic therapy should be continued.

Antidepressant therapy should generally be avoided in patients with rapid-cycling bipolar disorder or a recent hypomanic episode because these patients are at particularly high risk of having a manic switch.

An alternative to starting an antidepressant may be the addition of quetiapine as monotherapy or in addition to existing antimanic medication if it is not an antipsychotic. Two randomized controlled trials showed quetiapine to be effective monotherapy for depression in both bipolar I disorder and bipolar II disorder. Quetiapine is not associated with switching to mania.[88]

Lamotrigine has been shown to be effective in treating bipolar depression and is commonly prescribed for this in North America. Studies have shown that lamotrigine may be effective prophylaxis against future episodes and does not cause switching or rapid cycling. Lamotrigine is increasingly prescribed for patients with a history of rapid-cycling bipolar disorder. Evidence supports its use in bipolar II disorder, but current UK guidelines recommend against its use in bipolar I disorder.

When depression is resistant to treatment, consider the following:

- Check concordance with medication.
- Check for evidence of substance misuse, ongoing psychosocial stressors, and co-morbid disorders such as anxiety or severe obsessional symptoms.
- Review physical health.
- Consider individual psychological therapy focused on depressive symptoms.
- Increase antidepressant therapy up to maximal recommended dose.
- Change antidepressant therapy. Mirtazapine and venlafaxine are recommended in UK guidance. There is some evidence that venlafaxine may be more likely than some other antidepressants to cause a switch to mania from studies comparing it with sertraline and bupropion.
- Consider addition of quetiapine or olanzapine if the patient is not already taking one of these.
- Consider addition of lithium.
- Consider using ECT.

Treatment of mixed episodes

Patients with a mixed affective episode should be treated in the same way that a manic episode is treated. Antidepressants should be avoided, as they may exacerbate symptoms.

Rapid-cycling bipolar disorder and acute treatment

Although the general principles of care are the same as with patients with non-rapid-cycling bipolar disorder, there are particular considerations that should be taken into account. The main risk is inducing a switch from one pole to the other. This is particularly likely when treating depressive episodes. Antidepressants should generally be avoided, as they are particularly likely to cause a switch to mania in these patients. It is recommended to focus on long-term treatment, putting less emphasis on the treatment of individual episodes. Trials of medication should be longer than usual – usually for a minimum of 6 months.

Electroconvulsive therapy in bipolar disorder

ECT can be useful in some patients in order to achieve rapid improvement in severe symptoms of depression or mania. It is generally indicated only when an adequate trial of other treatment options has been ineffective or when the episode is severe enough to be potentially life-threatening. When considering ECT, the risks of anaesthetic and coexisting medical conditions must be taken into account, along with the risk of cognitive impairment and causing a switch to the other affective pole. Lithium therapy in combination with ECT has been associated with increased risk of memory impairment and acute confusion, and so some authorities recommended a reduction in dose or withdrawal of lithium therapy before giving ECT, or starting ECT with a lower electrical stimulus.[88] Anticonvulsants and benzodiazepines raise the seizure threshold and therefore oppose the desired effect of the ECT, and so it is important to monitor the length of fits carefully if these medications are being prescribed.

Long-term management of bipolar disorder

Long-term management of bipolar disorder is aimed at preventing or reducing the frequency of acute episodes, minimizing symptoms between episodes and optimizing social functioning. It should include pharmacological and psychological treatment, education about the illness, and social interventions.

There is disagreement about the appropriate label for long-term medication in bipolar disorder. 'Anti-manic' treatment or prophylaxis and 'mood stabilizer' are terms that are also used to describe long-term treatment.

Long-term medication is recommended in the following situations:

- After a manic episode that was associated with significant risk and adverse consequences
- When a patient with bipolar I disorder has had two or more acute episodes
- When a patient with bipolar II disorder has significant functional impairment, is at significant risk of suicide, or has frequent episodes.

Long-term medication generally should be continued for a period of at least 2 years after an acute episode. Longer-term treatment may be appropriate if the patient has a history of frequent relapses or very severe episodes, or there are ongoing risk factors for relapse such as psychosocial stressors or substance misuse.

It is important that patients are involved in decisions about long-term medication, because there are considerable risks of adverse effects from most of the medications used. Patients should be educated about bipolar disorder and the risks of future episodes and be made aware of the possible harms from long-term medication. Patient participation in decision-making is likely to improve concordance.

A number of medications are now used for long-term treatment of bipolar disorder. Lithium was the first psychotropic agent shown to prevent recurrent episodes, but valproate, antipsychotics, carbamazepine and lamotrigine are also used. Current guidance for England and Wales recommends lithium, olanzapine or valproate for first-line therapy. If there are frequent relapses or there are ongoing symptoms causing functional impairment, alternative monotherapy or combination therapy from within this group should be considered.

The following factors must be taken into account when choosing medication for long-term bipolar treatment:

- Patient choice
- Previous response to treatment
- Clinical history, including affective pole and frequency of episodes
- Physical health, including renal function, obesity and risk of diabetes
- Whether the patient is of childbearing potential
- Likelihood of being able to cooperate with drug monitoring

- Cognitive state
- Risk of overdose
- Treatment advantages and side-effect profiles of the different medications.

Chronic and recurrent depressive symptoms may require long-term antidepressant therapy. This should generally be considered only for patients who have not had a recent manic or hypomanic episode, and it should usually be in combination with prophylactic medication. SSRI antidepressants at the minimum therapeutic dose are probably safest. Lamotrigine may be appropriate for patients with bipolar II disorder who have recurrent depression.

Lithium therapy

Lithium was discovered to be useful in treating mania by the Australian psychiatrist John Cade in 1949, and it has been used to treat bipolar disorder ever since. There has been considerably more research into the effects of lithium treatment than other medications used in bipolar disorder. Lithium is effective at preventing manic and depressive episodes, although it is more effective at preventing mania than depression. A review in 2001 showed that patients on lithium have a 1-year relapse rate of 40 per cent compared with 61 per cent for placebo.[89] A systematic review and meta-analysis in 2004 calculated that the number need to treat (NNT) with lithium in order to prevent relapse into mania or depression is 10 and 14, respectively.[90] Rebound mania following rapid discontinuation of lithium occurs in 50 per cent of patients, and intermittent lithium therapy may worsen the natural course in bipolar disorder, so it is generally appropriate to start lithium only if there is intention to continue with it long-term and concordance is likely. The current recommendation for duration of therapy is at least 3 years.[91] Lithium should be discontinued over at least a month to reduce the chances of rebound mania.

Long-term treatment with lithium has been shown to be associated with a reduced rate of suicide, although it is unclear whether this is due to the effects of lithium or the closer monitoring that patients taking lithium require.

Lithium has a narrow therapeutic index, requiring monitoring of serum levels on a regular basis. Common side effects include mild thirst, polyuria and a fine tremor. Longer-term adverse effects that occur not uncommonly are lithium-induced hypothyroidism and nephrotoxicity, both of which require regular blood test monitoring.

Lithium interacts with a number of other medications, co-administration of which can rapidly induce toxic levels of lithium or be associated with adverse reactions. Commonly encountered interacting medications include diuretics, angiotensin converting enzyme (ACE) inhibitors, non-steroidal anti-inflammatory drugs (NSAIDs), haloperidol, carbamazepine and SSRI antidepressants.

Valproate

Valproate has been shown to be effective in the treatment of acute mania, although there is less good-quality evidence of efficacy for long-term prevention of relapse in bipolar disorder. Side effects include significant weight gain and possibly a rare risk of hepatic failure and of causing polycystic ovaries. Valproate is teratogenic and should routinely be avoided in women of childbearing potential.

Antipsychotics

There is increasing evidence of the efficacy of antipsychotics in long-term treatment of bipolar disorder. Olanzapine, risperidone and quetiapine have the most evidence of efficacy and are the only antipsychotics currently licensed for use in bipolar disorder in the UK. Antipsychotics are associated with weight gain and metabolic effects, including dyslipidaemia, impaired glucose tolerance and hypertension. Patients taking these medications should have regular assessment for these effects.

Lamotrigine

There is evidence that long-term treatment with lamotrigine can reduce the risk of depressive episodes in bipolar disorder, but there is less effect against manic episodes. A particular indication for lamotrigine is patients with bipolar II disorders who predominantly have depressive episodes. The rare but serious side effects of bone marrow failure and Stevens–Johnson syndrome need to be considered. Stevens–Johnson syndrome is more likely with rapid dose escalation, high dose and concomitant use of valproate. Lamotrigine is not licensed for use in bipolar disorder in the UK.

Carbamazepine

Carbamazepine was the first medication after lithium to be used routinely for long-term treatment of bipolar disorder. Recent studies have shown it to be substantially less effective than lithium in preventing relapse. Because of this, it is now generally considered a third-line agent.

Psychological therapy in bipolar disorder

There is evidence of efficacy for psychological interventions in the treatment of depression in bipolar disorder, but there is little evidence for psychological treatment in mania, hypomania or mixed affective states.

Structured psychological interventions such as CBT should be considered for patients with bipolar disorder once they are past the acute phase of a relapse, with the aim of reducing the likelihood of future relapses. CBT focuses on conscious cognitive biases that may lead patients to make negative interpretations of events or situations and routines such as sleep–wake cycles, which may impact on mood fluctuations. The interventions aim to enhance patients' engagement with the environment via a combination of psychoeducation about the disorder and medication, mood monitoring for episode cues and triggers, strategies to help prevent progression when mild symptoms appear, and behavioural activation and cognitive restructuring to improve general coping ability.[92] Compared with mood stabilizer treatment alone, combination treatment of CBT and mood stabilizer has been shown to reduce the number of bipolar episodes, reduce the duration of episodes that do occur, and reduce the number of hospital admissions due to episodes. Patients treated with the combination also showed higher social functioning.[93]

Self-management

An important part of the management of bipolar disorder is empowering patients to contribute to the management of their condition. Through education and psychological therapy, patients can acquire skills to monitor their mood and behaviour and initiate an action plan when they recognize signs indicating relapse. For many patients, sleep disturbance is one of the first symptoms they become aware of. It is appropriate for some patients to have a small supply of hypnotics or neuroleptics that they can take at the first sign of relapse, or a plan to increase the dose of their long-term antipsychotic treatment.

Physical health

Patients with serious mental health problems, including bipolar disorder, are at considerably increased risk of physical ill-health compared with the general population. People with bipolar disorder are more likely to smoke, have smoking-related diseases and die prematurely than the general population.[94] There is increasing recognition of the importance of this problem, and strategies are now being put in place to address it. In the UK, the 2004 contract for GPs (revised 2006) included annual reviews of the physical health of patients with severe mental health problems, including bipolar disorder, in a performance-related pay scheme QOF.[70] Guidance from NICE for England and Wales also recommends an annual physical health review,[95] although this is not covered in the 2005 Scottish Intercollegiate Guidelines Network guideline for bipolar disorder.[87] Table 39.2 shows the recommended annual review checks for patients with bipolar disorder

Table 39.2 Recommended annual review checks for patients with bipolar disorder

	QOF[70]	NICE bipolar guideline
Blood pressure	Yes	Yes
Weight/body mass index	Yes	Yes
Smoking	Yes	Yes
Alcohol	Yes	Yes
Drug use	Yes	
Cholesterol	Yes[a]	Yes[b]
Glucose	Yes[c]	Yes
Cervical screening	Yes[a]	

[a]Where clinically indicated.

[b]All patients over age 40 years.

[c]Assessment of the risk of diabetes, especially if on olanzapine or risperidone.

NICE, National Institute for Health and Clinical Excellence; QOF, Quality and Outcomes Framework.

It is important that the results of the annual review are shared with appropriate healthcare professionals and that clear responsibility is established for treating any problems that are detected.

National guidance

In July 2006, NICE published the guideline *Bipolar Disorder: The Management of Bipolar Disorder in Adults, Children and Adolescents, in Primary and Secondary Care.*[95] This was the first time NICE had reviewed this topic, although it had previously released the technology appraisal *Olanzapine and Valproate Semisodium in the Treatment of Acute Mania Associated with Bipolar I Disorder.*[96] NICE's bipolar disorder guideline is based on the guideline development group's (GDG) analysis of the best available evidence and takes into account cost-effectiveness information where possible. The GDG acknowledged that there had been an increase in the research of bipolar disorder in the past decade, but it also emphasized the paucity of data in a number of areas and the lack of long-term studies in naturalistic settings.

The NICE guideline sets out a number of general principles relating to working with patients and their families, and considerations relating to specific groups of patients with bipolar disorder. Emphasis is put on the importance of establishing and maintaining collaborative relationships with patients, families and carers, and being accessible at times of crisis. Educating patients to help them manage and live with their condition is mentioned, as is the importance of having an advance directive. Patients with learning disabilities and personality disorders should have the same care as other patients. Psychosocial interventions targeted at drug and alcohol use should be considered for patients with these conditions. The guideline recommends having a robust protocol for transferring patients to services for people older than 65 years, but referral should be based primarily on patient need rather than just chronological age.

Key priorities for implementation set out in the guideline are as follows:

- Valproate should not be prescribed routinely for women of childbearing potential and, if it is chosen, precautions should be taken.
- Lithium, olanzapine and valproate should be considered for long-term treatment, with the choice depending on previous response, risk of relapse, physical health, patient preference, gender and cognitive state.
- If frequent relapses occur or there are ongoing symptoms impairing function, consider switching to alternative monotherapy or adding a second prophylactic agent.

- If combination prophylactic therapy is ineffective, consider referral to an expert in bipolar disorder, or a trial of lamotrigine (especially if bipolar II disorder) or carbamazepine.
- If a patient is taking an antidepressant at the onset of acute mania, the antidepressant should be stopped.
- Antidepressant therapy should not routinely be continued long term following a depressive episode because of the risk of switching to mania.
- People with bipolar disorder should have an annual physical health review, normally in primary care. This should include lipid levels in patients over age 40 years, glucose, weight, smoking, alcohol use and blood pressure.
- When diagnosing bipolar I disorder in adolescents, the adult criteria should be used, except that mania must be present, euphoria must be present most of the time on most of 7 days, and irritability may be helpful in making the diagnosis.

The Scottish Intercollegiate Guidelines Network released guidance for the management of bipolar disorder for Scotland in 2005.[87]

DYSTHYMIA

The core clinical feature of dysthymia is a chronically depressed mood that lasts for most of the day and is present most of the time for at least 2 years. Other clinical features that may be found include the same symptoms typically present in depression; however, symptoms are not severe enough to meet the criteria for a diagnosis of recurrent depressive disorder. Patients with dysthymia are usually able to maintain a basic level of social and occupational functioning.

Dysthymia usually begins in early adulthood and lasts for at least several years. It is more common in women.

The ICD-10 classification system places dysthymia within a category of mood disorders called 'persistent mood disorders', which also includes cyclothymia. DSM-IV-TR classifies dysthymia as a separate category within mood disorders.

Antidepressant drugs are effective in some patients, and CBT may be beneficial.

CYCLOTHYMIA

The essential feature of cyclothymia is a persistent instability of mood involving periods of hypomanic symptoms and periods of depressive symptoms. The severity and duration of the hypomanic and depressive symptoms are below the threshold for diagnosis of bipolar affective disorder. Mood swings are usually unrelated to life events.

Similar to dysthymia, cyclothymia is included in 'persistent mood disorders' in ICD-10 and as the separate category of 'cyclothymic disorder' in DSM-IV.

Cyclothymia usually develops early in adult life and has a chronic course. It is more common in individuals who have a family history of bipolar disorder. During the course of the illness there may be superimposed depressive, manic or hypomanic episodes, and in some cases the criteria for a diagnosis of bipolar disorder are met later in life.

Management of cyclothymia includes pharmacological treatment, usually with mood stabilizers. There is no evidence that any particular mood stabilizer is superior. Individuals with cyclothymia may benefit from psychoeducation and insight-oriented psychotherapy to help them understand and live with their condition.

ATYPICAL DEPRESSION

The term 'atypical depression' is generally applied to patients with a depressive episode who also have a predominance of the following symptoms:

- Preserved mood reactivity generally enabling the individual to still enjoy certain things but to a lesser extent
- Hyperphagia and weight gain
- Hypersomnia
- Extreme fatigue ('leaden paralysis'), described as a heavy feeling in the arms and legs
- Tendency to an exaggerated reaction to real or perceived rejection ('rejection sensitivity') that must be longstanding and not limited to episodes of mood disturbance and significant enough to cause functional impairment.

Atypical depression is included in ICD-10 in 'other depressive episodes', a subgroup of F32, depressive episode. DSM-IV delineates atypical features as an episode specifier, which can be applied to major depressive disorder, bipolar I or II disorder and dysthymic disorder.

There is evidence that the MAOI antidepressant phenelzine may be more effective than other antidepressants for women with atypical depression.[97]

SEASONAL AFFECTIVE DISORDER

Seasonal affective disorder (SAD) was initially proposed and described by Rosenthal in 1984.[98] He proposed that the essential clinical feature is a clear seasonal pattern to recurrent depressive episode with onset in winter in most cases and remission usually in spring. Rosenthal described a clinical picture where symptoms tended to be mild to moderate and included fatigue, hypersomnia, overeating with a craving for carbohydrates, and weight gain. Low self-esteem and decreased functioning are also typical. This clinical pattern was said to be five times more common in females than males.

Neither ICD-10 nor DSM-IV has a separate category for SAD. DSM-IV includes seasonal pattern as one of the specifiers that can be applied to the course of recurrent major depressive disorder and major depressive episodes in both bipolar I disorder and bipolar II disorder. There is a requirement that, in order for this specifier to be used, the seasonal pattern must have occurred during the previous 2 years without any non-seasonal episodes within the same time. It is also important to exclude episodes clearly precipitated by psychosocial stressors. A seasonal pattern appears to be more likely in bipolar II disorder.

ICD-10 includes seasonal depressive disorder within recurrent depressive disorder, which is the diagnosis that should be made if a seasonal pattern of depression is observed.

There is ongoing debate over whether SAD is a type of a depressive disorder or whether it should be considered as a description of a specific form of an atypical depressive episode.

Some authors have suggested that light therapy, also known as phototherapy, is beneficial in SAD. This involves exposure to bright artificial light and is thought to be most effective when given early in the morning. The claim is that improvement is usually seen within the first few days; however, in order to prevent relapse, it needs to be continued until the time of the year when natural remission would have occurred. It is inevitably difficult to design a randomized controlled trial that can test this using a double-blind methodology. There is limited evidence that antidepressants are effective in the treatment or prevention of SAD.

SCHIZOAFFECTIVE DISORDER

Schizoaffective disorder is characterized by equally prominent affective and schizophrenic symptoms that are simultaneously present during an episode of illness. The symptoms must meet the criteria for both schizophrenia and either a manic or a depressive episode. The diagnosis should not be used when patients have schizophrenic symptoms and affective symptoms in different episodes of illness. Schizoaffective disorder also needs to be distinguished from post-schizophrenic depression, whereby depressive symptoms occur following a psychotic episode. Episodes may be recurrent and can be manic, depressive or mixed. If patients have occasional schizoaffective episodes interspersed between recurrent typical episodes of mania or depression, then the diagnosis of bipolar affective disorder or recurrent depressive disorder rather than schizoaffective disorder should be used.

First-degree relatives of patients with schizoaffective disorder have an increased risk of schizophrenia. Some evidence suggests they also have an increased risk of mood disorders.

In schizoaffective disorder, psychotic symptoms are treated in the same way as are patients with schizophrenia. Manic or depressive symptoms are treated in the same way as they are in bipolar disorder.

The prognosis for schizoaffective disorder is generally worse than that for mood disorders but better than that for schizophrenia. Patients typically make a full recovery between episodes, with this being more likely with manic than with depressive schizoaffective episodes. Despite this, schizoaffective disorder is often associated with occupational and social dysfunction.

POSTNATAL DEPRESSION

The majority of women experience some degree of tearfulness and emotional lability in the week following childbirth, and this is commonly known as 'baby blues'. It is a self-limiting condition and usually lasts for a couple of days.

Postnatal depression is a depressive episode that occurs in women in the postnatal period. ICD-10 allows this diagnosis if symptoms begin within 6 weeks of delivery. Although the clinical features are similar to other depressive episodes, there is a particular preponderance for the mother to have worries about her ability to cope with her baby or concerns about her baby's health. It is now recognized that there is a significant anxiety component to postnatal depression.

Postnatal depression occurs in 10 per cent of women. Follow-through studies have shown a slight increase in point prevalence at 3–6 months postpartum compared with pregnancy, but overall there is little difference in the prevalence following childbirth and that in non-pregnant women.[99]

Precipitating factors for postnatal depression tend to include psychological adjustment to the changes following childbirth, sleep deprivation, and the hard work and stresses of parenthood.

Risk factors for postnatal depression are generally the same as those for depression at any other age and include having a family history of depression, previous depressive episodes, adverse social conditions including social isolation, and relationship problems. Other risk factors include older age, being a single mother, unwanted pregnancy, severe baby blues and previous postpartum psychosis.

Early detection is crucial in the management of postnatal depression. Education about postnatal depression is an important part of antenatal care. Women with risk factors should be monitored closely. The Edinburgh Postnatal Depression Scale has high sensitivity and is now used routinely in primary care in the UK.[100] Risk assessment is essential and must include risks to both the mother and the baby.

Treatment should generally start with organizing an appropriate support network. Psychological therapy, usually in the form of CBT, should be considered before starting pharmacological treatment. If antidepressant therapy is indicated, the same principles apply as when treating any other depressive episode. However, if the mother wishes to continue breastfeeding, an appropriate medication should be prescribed according to current evidence of safety for the baby. If there is significant risk of harm to either the mother or the baby, hospitalization may be required. ECT is used in severe cases.

Postnatal depression may have considerable negative effects on the relationship between mother and baby. Reduced quality and quantity of interaction between mother and baby can have a negative impact on the emotional development of the baby.

KEY POINTS

- Typically mood disorders are recurrent and onset of episodes is often associated with stressful events or situations.
- The aetiology of affective disorders is multifactorial.
- Various medical illnesses increase the risk of depression.
- The core symptoms of depression include sustained depressed mood, loss of interest and enjoyment, and reduced energy and activity.
- The lifetime prevalence of depression is between 10% and 20%.
- The World Health Organisation (WHO) has estimated that depression is currently the fourth leading cause of disease burden in the world.
- The rate of suicide is significantly increased in patients suffering from depression.
- Biological, psychological and social interventions should all be considered for inclusion in the treatment plan for patients with depression.
- Bipolar disorder usually causes severe disruption to patients' lives with manic episodes usually requiring inpatient treatment.
- Following a manic episode, long term antimanic therapy is required to reduce the likelihood of subsequent episodes.
- Patients with bipolar disorder are at considerably increased risk of morbidity and mortality due to physical health conditions.

REFERENCES

1. World Health Organization (1992) *The ICD-10 Classification of Mental and Behavioural Disorders.* Geneva: World Health Organization.
2. American Psychiatric Association (2000) *Diagnostic and Statistical Manual of Mental Disorders*, 4th edn, text revision. Washington, DC, American Psychiatric Association.
3. McGuffin P, Katz R, Watkins S, Rutherford J (1996) A hospital-based twin register of the heritability of the DSM-IV unipolar depression. *Archives of General Psychiatry* **53**: 129–36.
4. Craddock N, Jones I (1999) Genetics of bipolar disorder. *Journal of Medical Genetics* **36**: 585–94.
5. Kendler KS, Neale MC, Kessler RC (1992) A population-based twin study of major depression in women: the impact of varying definitions of illness. *Archives of General Psychiatry* **49**: 257–66.
6. Kendler KS, Gardner CO, Prescott CA (2002) Toward a comprehensive developmental model for major depression in women. *American Journal of Psychiatry* **159**: 1133–45.
7. Andrews G, Stewart G, Allen R, Henderson AS (1990) The genetics of six neurotic disorders: a twin study. *Journal of Affective Disorders* **19**: 23–9.
8. Cadoret RJ, Winokur G, Lengbehn D, *et al.* (1996) Depression spectrum disease: I. The role of gene-environment interaction. *American Journal of Psychiatry* **153**: 892–9.
9. Craddock N, Jones I (1999) Genetics of bipolar disorder. *Journal of Medical Genetics* **36**: 585–94.
10. Egeland JA, Gerhard DS, Pauls DL, *et al.* (1987) Bipolar affective disorders linked to DNA markers on chromosome 11. *Nature* **325**: 788–7.
11. Owen MJ, Cardno AG, O'Donovan MC (2000) Psychiatric genetics: back to the future. *Molecular Psychiatry* **5**:22–31.
12. Ellenbogen MA, Young SN, Dean P, *et al.* (1996) Mood response to acute tryptophan depletion in healthy volunteers, sex differences and temporal stability. *Neuropsychopharmacology* **15**: 465–74.
13. Delgado PL, Charney DS, Price LH, *et al.* (1990) Serotonin function and the mechanism of antidepressant action: reversal of antidepressant-induced remission by rapid depletion of plasma tryptophan. *Archives of General Psychiatry* **47**: 411–18.
14. Francis PT, Pangalos MN, Stephens PH, *et al.* (1993) Antemortem measurements of neurotransmission: possible implications for pharmacotherapy of Alzheimer's disease and depression. *Journal of Neurology, Neurosurgery, and Psychiatry* **56**: 80–84.
15. Brown GL, Linnoila MI (1990) CSF serotonin metabolite (5-HIAA) studies in depression, impulsivity and violence. *Journal of Clinical Psychiatry* **51**:31–41.
16. Goodwin FK, Jamison KR (2007) *Manic-Depressive Illness: Bipolar Disorders and Recurrent Depression*, 2nd edn. Oxford: Oxford University Press.
17. Goodwin G (2000) Neurobiological aetiology of mood disorders. In MG Gelder, JJL Ibor, NC Andreasen (eds) *New Oxford Textbook of Psychiatry.* Oxford: Oxford University Press.
18. Pariante CM, Miller AH (2001) Glucocorticoid receptors in major depression: relevance to pathophysiology and treatment. *Biological Psychiatry* **49**: 391–404.
19. Nemeroff CB (2000) Neuroendocrinology. In MG Gelder, JJL Ibor, NC Andreasen (eds) *New Oxford Textbook of Psychiatry.* Oxford: Oxford University Press.
20. National Institute for Health and Clinical Excellence (2004) *Depression: Management of Depression in Primary and Secondary Care.* Clinical guideline 23. London: National Institute for Health and Clinical Excellence.
21. Chekley SA, Slade AP, Shur P (1981) Growth hormone and other responses to clonidine in patients with

endogenous depression. *British Journal of Psychiatry* **138**: 51–5.
22. Manji HK, Lenox RH (2000) The nature of bipolar disorder. *Journal of Clinical Psychiatry* **61**: 42–57.
23. Duman RS, Heninger GR, Nestler EJ (1997) A molecular and cellular theory of depression. *Archives of General Psychiatry* **54**: 597–606.
24. Duman RS (2002) Synaptic plasticity and mood disorders. *Molecular Psychiatry* **7**: S29–34.
25. Gainotti G, Antonucci G, Marra C, Paolucci S (2001) Relation between depression after stroke, antidepressant therapy, and functional recovery. *Journal of Neurology, Neurosurgery, and Psychiatry* **71**: 258–61
26. Paolucci S, Antonucci G, Grazia Grasso M, *et al.* (2001) Post-stroke depression, antidepressant treatment and rehabilitation results: a case–control study. *Cerebrovascular Disease* **12**: 264–71.
27. Davies SJC, Jackson PR, Potokar J, Nutt DJ (2004) Treatment of anxiety and depressive disorders in patients with cardiovascular disease. *British Medical Journal* **328**: 939–43.
28. Barth J, Schumacher M, Herrmann-Lingen C (2004) Depression as a risk factor for mortality in patients with coronary heart disease: a meta-analysis. *Psychosomatic Medicine* **66**: 802–13.
29. Peterson C, Seligman MEP (1981) The reformulated model of helplessness and depression: parts I and II. *Tidsskrift for Norsk Psykoilogforening* **18**: 3–18, 53–9.
30. Seligman PEP, Abramson LY, Semmel A, von Baeyer C (1979) Depressive attributional style. *Journal of Abnormal Psychology* **88**: 242–7.
31. Abramson LY, Alloy LB, Hogan ME, *et al.* (1999) Cognitive vulnerability to depression: theory and evidence. *Journal of Cognitive Psychotherapy* **13**: 5–20.
32. Lewinsohn PM, Gotlib IH (1995) Behavioural theory and treatment of depression. In EE Beckham, WR Leber (eds) *Handbook of Depression*. New York: Guilford Press.
33. Gale CR, Martyn CN (2004) Birth weight and later risk of depression in a national birth cohort. *British Journal of Psychiatry* **184**: 28–33.
34. Van Os J, Jones P, Lewis G, Wadsworth M, Murray R (1997) Developmental precursors of affective illness in a general population birth cohort. *Archives of General Psychiatry* 54: 625–31.
35. Brown GW, Harris TO (1993) Aetiology of anxiety and depressive disorders in an inner-city population: 1. Early adversity. *Psychological Medicine* **23**: 143–54.
36. Brown GW, Harris TO, Hepworth C (1995) Loss, humiliation and entrapment among women developing depression: a patient and non-patient comparison. *Psychological Medicine* **25**: 7–21.
37. Brown GW, Harris TO, Hepworth C (1994) Life events and endogenous depression: a puzzle re-examined. *Archives of General Psychiatry* **51**: 525–34.
38. Kendler KS, Thornton LM, Gardner CO (2001) Genetic risk, number of previous depressive episodes, and stressful life events in predicting onset of major depression. *American Journal of Psychiatry* **158**: 582–6.
39. Hunt N, Bruce Jones W, Silverstone T (1992) Life events and relapse in bipolar affective disorder. *Journal of Affective Disorders* **25**: 13–20.
40. Moussavi S, Chatterji S, Verdes E (2007) Depression, chronic diseases and decrements in health: results from the world health surveys. *Lancet* **370**: 851–8.
41. Katon WJ (2003) Clinical and health services relationships between major depression, depressive symptoms, and general medical illness. *Biological Psychiatry* **54**: 216–26.
42. Cross National Collaborative Group (1992) The changing rate of major depression: cross national comparisons. *Journal of the American Medical Association* **268**: 3098–105.
43. Ustün TB, Ayuso-Mateos JL, Chatterji S, Mathers C, Murria CJ (2004) Global burden of depressive disorders in the year 2000. *British Journal of Psychiatry* **184**: 386–92.
44. Murray CJ, Lopez AD (1997) Alternative projections of mortality of disability by cause 1990–2020: Global Burdon of Disease Study. *Lancet* **349**: 1498–504.
45. Nicholson A, Kuper H, Hemingway H (2006) Depression as an aetiologic and prognostic factor in coronary heart disease: a meta-analysis of 6362 events among 146 538 participants in 54 observational studies. *European Heart Journal* **27**: 2763–74.
46. Van Melle JPD, de Jonge P, Spijkerman TA, *et al.* (2004) Prognostic association of depression following myocardial infarction with mortality and cardiovascular events: a meta-analysis. *Psychosomatic Medicine* **66**: 814–22.
47. Carney RM (2002) Depression as a risk factor for cardiac mortality and morbidity: a review of potential mechanisms. *Journal of Psychosomatic Research* **53**: 897–902.
48. Angst J (1997) A regular review of the long term follow up of depression. *British Medical Journal* **315**: 1143–6.
49. Mann AH, Jenkins R, Belsey E (1981) The twelve-month outcome of patients with neurotic illness in general practice. *Psychological Medicine* **11**: 535–50.
50. Lloyd KR, Jenkins R, Mann A (1996) Long-term outcome of patients with neurotic illness in general practice. *British Medical Journal* **313**: 26–8.
51. Goldberg D, Privett M, Ustun B, *et al.* (1998) The effects of detection and treatment on the outcome of major depression in primary care: a naturalistic study in 15 cities. *British Journal of General Practice* **48**: 1840–44.
52. Lee AS, Murray RM (1988) The long-term outcome of Maudsley depressives. *British Journal of Psychiatry* **153**: 741–51.

53. Harris EC, Barraclough B (1997) Suicide as an outcome for mental disorders: a meta-analysis. *British Journal of Psychiatry* **170**: 205–28.
54. Guze SB, Robins E (1970) Suicide and primary affective disorders. *British Journal of Psychiatry* **117**: 437–8.
55. Summerfield D (2008) How scientifically valid is the knowledge base of global mental health? *British Medical Journal* **336**: 992–4.
56. Summerfield D (2006) Depression: epidemic or pseudoepidemic? *Journal of the Royal Society of Medicine* **99**: 161–2.
57. Ryder AG, Yang J, Zhu X, *et al.* (2008) The cultural shaping of depression: somatic symptoms in China, psychological symptoms in North America? *Journal of Abnormal Psychology* **117**: 300–313.
58. Goldberg DP, Bridges K (1998) Somatic presentations of psychiatric illness in primary care setting. *Journal of Psychosomatic Research* **32**: 137–44.
59. Von Korff M, Goldberg D (2001) Improving outcomes in depression. *British Medical Journal* **323**: 948–9.
60. Committee on Safety of Medicines (2004) Report of the CSM Expert Working Group of the Safety of Selective Serotonin Reuptake Inhibitor Antidepressants. www.mhra.gov.uk.
61. UK ECT Review Group (2003) Efficacy and safety of electroconvulsive therapy in depressive disorders: a systematic review and meta-analysis. *Lancet* **361**: 799–808.
62. National Institute for Health and Clinical Excellence (2003) *Guidance on the Use of Electroconvulsive Therapy*. Technology appraisal 59. London: National Institute for Health and Clinical Excellence.
63. Semple D, Smyth R, Burns J, Darjee R, McIntosh A (2005) Psychosurgery/neurosurgery for mental disorder (NMD). In D Semple *et al.* (eds) *Oxford Handbook of Psychiatry*. Oxford: Oxford University Press.
64. Malizia AL (2000) Neurosurgery for psychiatric disorders. In MG Gelder, JJL Ibor, NC Andreasen (eds) *New Oxford Textbook of Psychiatry*. Oxford: Oxford University Press.
65. Wiart L, Petit H, Joseph PA, Mazaux JM, Barat M (2000) Fluoxetine in early poststroke depression: a double-blind placebo-controlled study. *Stroke* **31**: 1829.
66. Anderson G, Vestergaard K, L Lauritzen L (1994) Effective treatment of poststroke depression with the selective serotonin reuptake inhibitor citalopram. *Stroke* **25**: 1099–104.
67. Robinson RG, Schultz SK, Castillo C, *et al.* (2000) Nortriptyline versus fluoxetine in the treatment of depression and in short-term recovery after stroke: a placebo-controlled, double blind study. *American Journal of Psychiatry* **157**: 351–9.
68. Goldney RD, Phillips PJ, Fisher LJ, Wilson DH (2004) Diabetes, depression and quality of life: a population study. *Diabetes Care* **27**: 1066–70.
69. Lustman PJ, Anderson RJ, Freedland KE, *et al.* (2000) Depression and poor glycemic control: a meta-analytic review of the literature. *Diabetes Care* **23**: 934–42.
70. British Medical Association and NHS Employers (2006). *Revisions to the GMS Contract, 2006/07: Delivering Investment in General Practice*. London: British Medical Association and NHS Employers.
71. Grant P, Young PR, DeRubeis RJ (2005) Cognitive and behavioural therapies. In GO Gabbard, JS Beck, J Holmes (eds) *Oxford Textbook of Psychotherapy*. Oxford: Oxford University Press.
72. Keller MB, McCullough JP, Klein DN, *et al.* (2000) A comparison of nefazodone, the cognitive behavioural-analysis system of psychotherapy, and their combination for the treatment of chronic depression. *New England Journal of Medicine* **342**: 1462–70.
73. Klein DF, Ross DC (1993) Reanalysis of the National Institute of Mental Health Treatment of Depression Collaborative Research Program General Effectiveness Report. *Neuropsychopharmacology* **8**: 241–51.
74. Frank E, Kupfer DJ, Perel JM (1989) Early recurrence in unipolar depression. *Archives of General Psychiatry* **46**: 397–400.
75. Reynolds CF III, Frank E, Perel JM, *et al.* (1999) Nortriptyline and interpersonal psychotherapy as maintenance therapies for recurrent major depression: a randomized controlled trial in patients older than 59 years. *Journal of the American Medical Association* **281**: 39–45.
76. Bateman A, Fonagy P (1999) Effectiveness of partial hospitalization in the treatment of borderline personality disorder: a randomized controlled trial. *American Journal of Psychiatry* **156**: 1563–9.
77. Anderson DM, Dorland WAN (2000) *Dorland's Illustrated Medical Dictionary*. Philadelphia, PA: W.B. Saunders.
78. Porter R (2002) *Madness: A Brief History*. Oxford: Oxford University Press.
79. Fennig S, Kovasznay B, Rich C, *et al.* (1994) Six-month stability of psychiatric diagnoses in first-admission patients with psychosis. *American Journal of Psychiatry* **151**: 1200–208.
80. Kessler RC, Rubinow DR, Holmes C, Abelson JM, Zhao S (1997) The epidemiology of DSM-III-R bipolar I disorder in a general population survey. *Psychological Medicine* **27**: 1079–89.
81. Weissman MM, Bland RC, Canino GJ, *et al.* (1996) Cross national epidemiology of major depression and bipolar disorder. *Journal of the American Medical Association* **276**: 293–9.
82. Goodwin GM (2002) Hypomania: what's in a name? *British Journal of Psychiatry* **181**: 94–5.
83. Angst J, Sellaro R (2000) Historical perspectives and natural history of bipolar disorder. *Biological Psychiatry* **48**: 445–57.
84. Joyce PR (2000) Epidemiology of mood disorders. In

MG Gelder, JJL Ibor, NC Andreasen (eds) *New Oxford Textbook of Psychiatry.* Oxford: Oxford University Press.
85. Muller-Oerlinghausen B, Berghofer A, Aauer M (2002) Bipolar disorder. *Lancet* **359**: 241–7.
86. Stakowski SM, McElroy SL, Keck PE, West SA (1996) Suicidality among patients with mixed and manic bipolar disorder. *American Journal of Psychiatry* **153**: 674–6.
87. Scottish Intercollegiate Guidelines Network (2005) *Bipolar Affective Disorder: A National Clinical Guideline.* Edinburgh: Scottish Intercollegiate Guidelines Network.
88. Taylor D, Paton C, Kerwin R (2007) *The Maudsley Prescribing Guidelines*, 9th edn. London: Informa Healthcare.
89. Burgess S, Geddes J, Hawton K, *et al.* (2001) Lithium for maintenance treatment of mood disorders. *Cochrane Database Systematic Review* (3): CD003013.
90. Geddes JR, Burgess S, Hawton K, Jamison K, Goodwin GM (2004) Long-term lithium therapy for bipolar disorder: systematic review and meta-analysis of randomized controlled trials. *American Journal of Psychiatry* **161**: 217–22.
91. Goodwin GM (1994) Recurrence of mania after lithium withdrawal: implications for the use of lithium in the treatment of bipolar affective disorder. *British Journal of Psychiatry* **164**: 149–52.
92. Lam DH, Jones S, Bright J, Hayward P (1999). *Cognitive Therapy for Bipolar Disorder: A Therapist's Guide to Concepts, Methods and Practice.* Chichester, New York: John Wiley & Sons.
93. Lam DH, Watkins ER, Hayward P, *et al.* (2003) A randomized controlled study of cognitive therapy for relapse prevention for bipolar affective disorder: outcome of the first year. *Archives of General Psychiatry* **60**: 145–52.
94. Seymour L (2003) *Not All in the Mind: The Physical Health of Mental Health Service Users.* London: Mentality.
95. National Institute for Health and Clinical Excellence (2006) *Bipolar Disorder: The Management of Bipolar Disorder in Adults, Children and Adolescents, in Primary and Secondary Care.* Clinical guideline 38. London: National Institute for Health and Clinical Excellence.
96. National Institute for Health and Clinical Excellence (2003) *Olanzapine and Valproate Semisodium in the Treatment of Acute Mania Associated with Bipolar I Disorder.* Technology appraisal 66. London: National Institute for Health and Clinical Excellence.
97. Anderson IM, Nutt DJ, Deakin JFW (2000) Evidence-based guidelines for treating depressive disorders with antidepressants: a revision of the 1993 British Association for Psychopharmacology guidelines. *Journal of Psychopharmacology* **14**: 3–20.
98. Rosenthal NE, Sack DA, Gillin JC, *et al.* (1984) Seasonal affective disorder: a description of the syndrome and preliminary findings with light therapy. *Archives of General Psychiatry* **41**: 72–80.
99. Cox, JL, Murray D, Chapman D (1993) A controlled study of the onset, duration and prevalence of postnatal depression. *British Journal of Psychiatry* **163**: 145–50.
100. Cox JL, Holden JM, Sagovsky R (1987) Detection of postnatal depression: development of the 10-item Edinburgh Postnatal Depression Scale. *British Journal of Psychiatry* **150**: 782–6.

Chapter 40

Neurotic and stress-related disorders

Ian Treasaden

CONCEPT OF NEUROSIS

The term 'neurosis' was first used by William Cullen (1710–90) in 1784 for disorders of the nervous system for which there appeared no physical cause.[1] The term replaced Robert Whytt's 1768 'illness of the nerves', which itself superseded the term 'vapours'.[2]

Mental illness, which implies previous health, has been divided into psychoses and neuroses. In *psychoses*, there is loss of contact with reality, and the symptoms, such as delusions or hallucinations, are not understandable and cannot be empathized with. Psychoses are regarded as severe mental illnesses and in lay terms are referred to as 'madness'.

Neuroses or *psychoneuroses*, on the other hand, have symptoms that are both understandable (reality-based) and can be empathized with. Insight is usually maintained. They are regarded as milder and, in lay terms, are referred to as 'nerves'. They are quantitatively but not qualitatively different from 'normal', involving for instance, inappropriate or excessive anxiety. Neuroses are most usually (but not invariably) short-lived, but they can be chronic, impairing and accompanied by a change, characteristically in symptoms and often, secondarily, in behaviour.

Neuroses can be defined as abnormal psychogenic (psychologically caused) reactions. An anxiety neurosis would have predominantly anxiety symptoms; in phobic disorder or neurosis there would be predominantly phobic symptoms. Neuroses typically have two components:

- a vulnerable personality;
- stress factors triggering the reaction.

Neuroses can thus be seen as exaggerated forms of normal reactions to stressful events – that is, they are inappropriate to the situation or the stress, or the reaction occurs at a greater frequency or severity than normal. Classically, neurosis should have no demonstrable organic basis and there should be no loss of contact with external reality, such as occurs in psychosis. Neurotic symptoms are thus maladaptive reactions to stress and reflect excessive and inappropriate use of psychological defence mechanisms.

Neurotic symptoms are unpleasant and lead to the individual seeking relief. They are often accompanied by a decrease in social functioning. Individuals with a neurosis have an increased mortality rate, including suicide and fatal head injuries.

A distinction should be made between people with neuroses, which are a group of mental illnesses, and people who are sometimes referred to, particularly by the lay population, as 'neurotic' individuals, who most often have lifelong personality difficulties such as overanxiousness or overemotionality.

OVERVIEW OF NEUROTIC AND STRESS-RELATED DISORDERS

Epidemiology

Individual neurotic symptoms are common in the community, as well as in primary and secondary care, and thus can be regarded as normal. These symptoms include:

- inappropriate fears;
- anxiety and panic;
- brief bouts of depressive feelings;
- tension headaches;
- irritability;
- sleeplessness.

Neurotic symptoms are often seen in general practice, resulting in significant societal burden; they may be the predominant symptoms in one-sixth of individuals seen there and relevant in up to one-third. Patients with neurosis often present with physical symptoms. Individuals with neurosis are more frequently seen in a psychiatric outpatient clinic than as in-patients in a psychiatric hospital. Neurotic disorders are the most common psychiatric condition, at any one time affecting up to 10 per cent of all individuals and affecting over 15 per cent in a lifetime.

With the high incidence of neurotic symptoms in the general population, questions arise in individual cases as to whether such symptoms should be regarded as abnormal or such individuals as mentally ill. Should these symptoms be viewed merely as the individual's way of dealing with the problems of everyday life, or do they represent a formal mental illness? Mild neuroses, in fact, often remit spontaneously or with mild reassurance. However, individuals with neurosis are more likely to seek medical consultation, often owing to fear of physical illness, and accurate diagnosis avoids inappropriate medical investigations.

Co-morbidity, especially with depression, substance misuse or personality disorder, is common. Neurotic disorders often precede the development of depression.

In the differential diagnosis of neurosis, one should ask why this particular patient is presenting at this particular time with this particular symptom. If an individual presents with neurotic symptoms for the first time after the age of 35–40 years, it is probable that the symptoms may be due to a depressive disorder or, alternatively, to underlying organic disease.

Aetiology

Predisposing factors leading to the development of neurosis are often similar to those important in the development of personality disorder. In fact, neuroses often arise in people with abnormal personalities, leading such individuals into social and emotional difficulties to which they overreact emotionally.

Environmental factors such as family and early background are important, but there is increasing evidence for a genetic inherited predisposition to neurosis.[3]

The vulnerability of people in the general population to developing a neurosis under stress follows a normal distribution, as for height or weight (Figure 40.1). The incidence of neurosis rises with increasing environmental stress (Figure 40.2). Even people with normal stable personalities will develop neurosis under severe environmental stress, as can be seen in individuals involved in natural disasters and in wartime. The incidence of neurosis approached 100 per cent in individuals in the First World War trenches for prolonged periods, and in bomber crews in the Second World War after more than 30 missions. Although one person's stress may be another's pleasure, due to the individual's background and personality, certain situations such as combat are experienced as stressful by over 95 per cent of individuals. Lower percentages of people experience stress in examinations or public speaking, and up to 50 per cent of the population find job interviews stressful. Although not associated with external stresses, sensory deprivation (either experimentally or as experienced by hostages kept in solitary confinement) and, to a lesser extent, boredom can also result in extreme stress and anxiety.

A number of theories have been developed to explain neuroses. In Freudian psychoanalytical theory, neurotic symptoms are seen as the expression of intrapsychic anxiety due to unresolved emotional conflicts dating from childhood. Freud initially proposed that anxiety represented

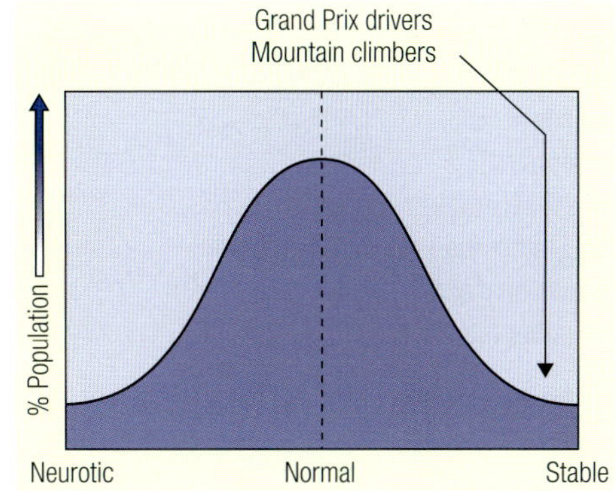

Figure 40.1 Vulnerability to developing neurosis

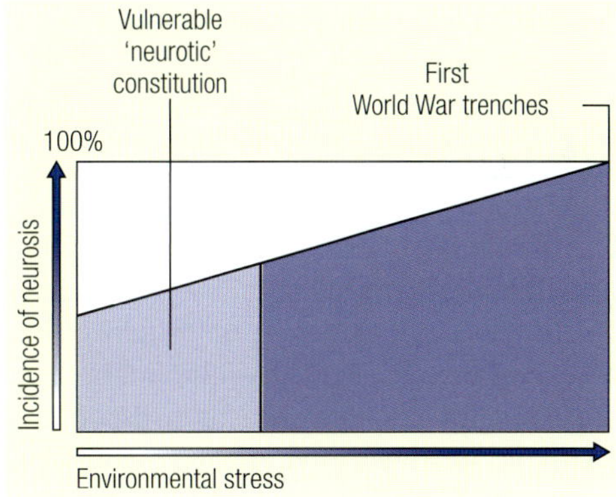

Figure 40.2 Incidence of neurosis with environmental stress

repressed libido (mental energy or drive). Later, he considered that anxiety reflected the birth experience, but he eventually replaced this theory with that of anxiety being a response of the ego to instinctual emotional tension. Freud differentiated the term 'anxiety neurosis', which he thought had a biological causation, from 'psychoneurosis', which included anxiety hysteria (phobic or situational anxiety), obsessive–compulsive neurosis and hysteria, all of which he saw as arising from unconscious conflicts. Learning theory has conceptualized the neuroses as learned maladaptive responses associated with a temporary reduction in anxiety. There is also evidence to suggest some genetic predisposition for the development of individual types of neuroses, although this may be predominantly through genetic influence on the development of personality.

As stated above, stress factors can be precipitating factors for neuroses in vulnerable individuals, and environmental factors, including family and marital factors, and social conditions, such as poor housing and unemployment, may be perpetuating factors for such disorders. Box 40.1 summarizes the factors associated with the development of neurotic and stress-related disorders.

Treatment

Evidence-based guidelines, such as from the National Institute for Health and Clinical Excellence (NICE) in the UK, are available. Cognitive-behavioural therapy (CBT) and

Box 40.1 Factors associated with development of neurotic and stress-related disorders

- Lower social class
- Unemployment
- Divorced, separated or widowed
- Renting rather than owning own home
- No educational qualifications
- Urban rather than rural.

Homeless people and prisoners have twice the risk of the general population.

selective serotonin reuptake inhibitor (SSRI) antidepressants are often effective treatments. SSRI antidepressants should be continued for 1 year after response. However, CBT may be more effective in preventing relapse.

Prognosis

The overall prognosis in these conditions is generally regarded as good, with up to 50 per cent of individuals recovering without treatment within 2 years and up to 70 per cent with treatment. However, up to half of individuals seen by a general practitioner (GP) will remain symptomatic 1 year later, and for patients seen by a psychiatrist about half will still be disabled after 4 years. Good prognostic indicators include a stable premorbid personality and the development of acute symptoms in response to transitory stresses. Poor prognostic factors include chronic or severe symptoms at presentation, persisting social problems and inadequate social support. There is an excess of mortality among people with neurotic disorders, largely due to increased rates of completed suicide.

CLASSIFICATION

The tenth revision of the *International Classification of Diseases* (ICD-10) has not retained the concept of a neurosis as a major organizing principle in classification, although it groups together three types of disorder because of their historical association with the concept of neurosis and also their association with psychological causation. These are the neurotic and stress-related disorders (which are considered in this chapter) and the somatoform and dissociative disorders, which are described in Chapter 41. Table 40.1 summarizes the neurotic and stress-related disorders on the basis of ICD-10. Mixed neurotic states are more common than the discrete syndromes. Panic disorder with or without agoraphobia and generalized anxiety disorder are the most disabling. Table 40.2 shows the frequency of neurotic conditions. The fourth edition of the *Diagnostic and Statistical Manual of Mental Disorders* (DSM-IV) uses the term 'anxiety disorders' rather than 'neurotic disorders' and, indeed, neurosis was absent from DSM-III. Table 40.3 compares DSM-IV with ICD-10 in relation to neurotic and stress-related disorders.

The basis for the current categorical classification for non-psychotic disorders has been criticized for lack of evidence, and a dimensional classification, for example with dimensions for anxiety and depression, has been proposed.[4]

ANXIETY DISORDERS

Normal anxiety

Anxiety is a mood, usually unpleasant in nature, accompanied by bodily (somatic) sensations and occurring with a subjective feeling of uncertainty and threat about the future. The term 'fear' is used to describe a normal and

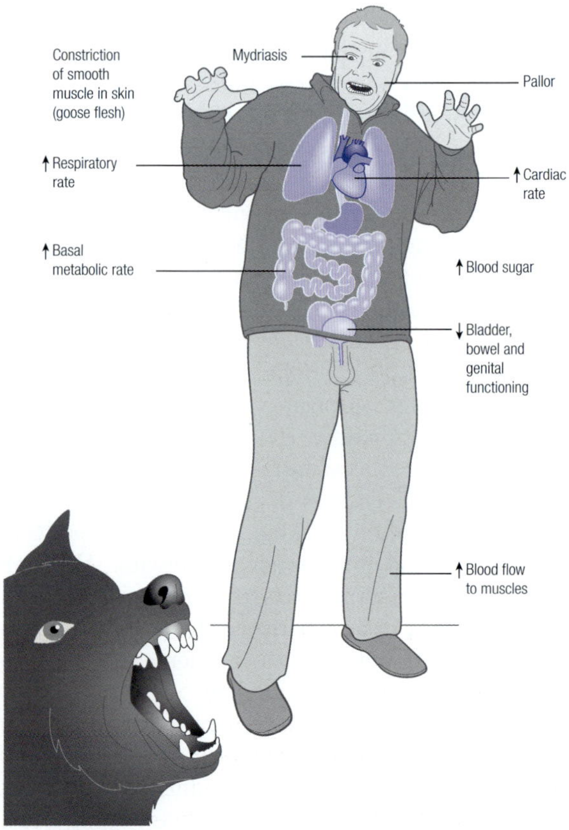

Figure 40.3 Physiological changes in Cannon's fight or flight reaction

Table 40.1 Neurotic and stress-related disorders based on *International Classification of Diseases*, 10th revision (ICD-10)

Disorders	Features
Generalized anxiety disorder	Generalized and persistent 'free-floating' anxiety symptoms involving elements of the following:
	Apprehension, e.g. worries about future misfortunes, 'feeling on edge', difficulty in concentrating
	Motor tension, e.g. restless fidgeting, tension headaches, trembling, inability to relax, etc.
	Autonomic overactivity, e.g. light-headedness, sweating, tachycardia or tachypnoea, epigastric discomfort, dizziness, dry mouth
Mixed anxiety and depressive disorder	Symptoms of anxiety and depression both present, but neither clearly predominates
Panic disorder	Recurrent attacks of severe anxiety (panic) not restricted to any particular situation or set of circumstances, and therefore unpredictable
	Secondary fears of dying, losing control or 'going mad'
	Attacks usually last for minutes only, and patients often experience a crescendo of fear and autonomic symptoms
	Comparative freedom from anxiety symptoms between attacks, although anticipatory anxiety is common
Phobic disorders	Anxiety is evoked only or predominantly by certain well-defined situations or objects external to the subject, which are not currently dangerous, and these are characteristically avoided or endured with dread
Specific (isolated) phobias	Restricted to highly specific situations, e.g. proximity to particular animals, heights, thunder, flying, blood
Agoraphobia	Fear not only of open spaces but also of related aspects, such as the presence of crowds and difficulty of immediate easy escape back to a safe place, usually home
	May occur with or without panic disorder
Social phobias	Fear of scrutiny by other people in comparatively small groups (as opposed to crowds), leading to avoidance of social situations
Obsessive–compulsive disorder	Recurrent obsessional thoughts or compulsive acts
	At least one thought or act still unsuccessfully resisted
	Thought of carrying out the act is not pleasurable
	Thoughts, images or impulses must be unpleasantly repetitive
Post-traumatic stress disorder	Delayed or prolonged response to stressful event or situation of threatening or catastrophic nature, likely to cause distress in anyone
	Episodes of repeated reliving of the trauma in intrusive memories (flashbacks), dreams or nightmares
	Sense of 'numbness' and detachment from other people
	Avoidance of activities and situations reminiscent of trauma
	Usually autonomic hyperarousal with hypervigilance, an enhanced startle reaction and insomnia

appropriate mood when the danger can be perceived and defined. Most of the bodily changes seen in anxiety are caused by increased sympathetic adrenergic nervous system discharges – Cannon's fight or flight reaction[5] (Figure 40.3) – which results in the release of adrenaline and other catecholamines. In our ancestral past such a reaction would prepare us to deal with a real physical threat, but today we may merely experience such reactions when under stress in everyday life, for instance in a traffic jam.

We all attempt to adjust our lives to maintain anxiety at an optimal level for us as individuals. However, like pain, anxiety is a useful warning and should not be suppressed

Table 40.2 Frequency of neurotic conditions

Condition	Frequency (%)
Mixed anxiety and depression	48
Generalized anxiety disorder	28
Depression	14
Phobia	12
Obsessive–compulsive disorder	10
Panic disorder	6

with drugs or alcohol. It is the central nervous system's alarm system to protect us from threat and is activated by environmental cues. There is an inverted U-shaped relationship between anxiety and performance developed by Hebb in 1955[6] known as the Yerkes–Dodson law[7] (Figure 40.4). This was based on an experiment on white mice being encouraged by low-, medium- and high-intensity electric shocks to learn to locate a compartment in a box. Medium-intensity shocks produced the fastest learning. Performance is reduced at low and very high levels of anxiety: thus, poor examination results are obtained by people with low anxiety levels who do not care whether they pass or fail and by people who become so highly anxious that they cannot concentrate. The Yerkes–Dodson law predicts that anxiolytic drugs reduce performance in a person with a low

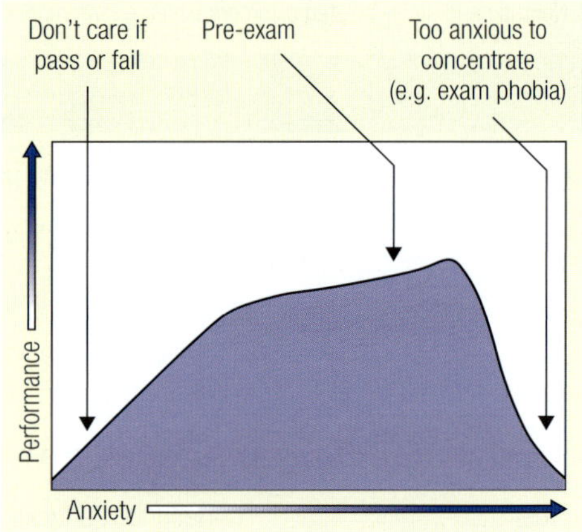

Figure 40.4 Neurotic and other stress-related anxiety disorders

anxiety level, but when a deterioration in performance is caused by high anxiety the reduction of symptoms by anxiolytic drugs should improve performance, for example in examination phobia. In assessing an individual's true level of anxiety, one should bear in mind that the complaint of symptoms of anxiety may lie anywhere along the Yerkes–Dodson curve. The individual may also be very anxious during a formal interview, but not so for long periods during the day, or vice versa. It is useful to distinguish between *trait anxiety*, which is a lifelong personality characteristic, and *state anxiety*, which is a temporal disorder with a discernible time of onset.

Table 40.3 Comparison of neurotic and stress-related disorders in the *International Classification of Diseases*, 10th revision (ICD-10) with anxiety disorders in the *Diagnostic and Statistical Manual of Mental Disorders*, 4th edition (DSM-IV)

ICD-10	DSM-IV
F40 Phobic anxiety disorders	
F40.00 Agoraphobic without panic disorder	300.22 Agoraphobia without history of panic disorder
F40.01 Agoraphobic with panic disorder	300.21 Panic disorder with agoraphobia
F40.1 Social phobias	300.23 Social phobia
F40.2 Specific (isolated) phobias	300.29 Specific phobia
F41 Other anxiety disorders	
F41.0 Panic disorder (episodic paroxysmal anxiety)	300.01 Panic disorder without agoraphobia
F41.1 Generalized anxiety disorder	300.02 Generalized anxiety disorder
F41.2 Mixed anxiety and depressive disorder	300.00 Anxiety disorder not otherwise specified (NOS)
F42 Obsessive–compulsive disorder	300.3 Obsessive–compulsive disorder
F43 Reaction to severe stress and adjustment disorders	
F43.0 Acute stress reaction	308.3 Acute stress disorder
F43.1 Post-traumatic stress disorder	309.81 Posttraumatic stress disorder
F43.2 Adjustment disorders	309.9 Adjustment disorders

GENERALIZED ANXIETY DISORDER

This is also known as anxiety neurosis, anxiety state or anxiety reaction, and is characterized by unrealistic or excessive anxiety and worry that is generalized and persistent and not restricted to particular environmental circumstances – that is, it is 'free-floating'.

Epidemiology

Community surveys suggest about 1.6 per cent of the adult population has generalized anxiety disorder at any one time, with a 1-year prevalence range of 3–8 per cent and a lifetime prevalence of 21 per cent. The female/male ratio is 2 : 1.[8] Around 15 per cent of patients attending GP surgeries and 25 per cent attending medical settings in general are 'anxious'. Generalized anxiety disorder often begins in early adult life, between the ages of 15 and 25 years, but rates continue to increase after the age of 35 years. Being older than 24 years, separated, widowed, divorced, unemployed or a home-maker correlates with general anxiety disorder. Pure generalized anxiety disorder is, however, rare compared with the much more common mixed picture of anxiety and depression. Co-morbidity is common, perhaps up to 90 per cent, for example with panic disorder and social phobia.

Clinical features

These are summarized in Figure 40.5 and Table 40.4. Individuals will not have all the psychic (affective) and

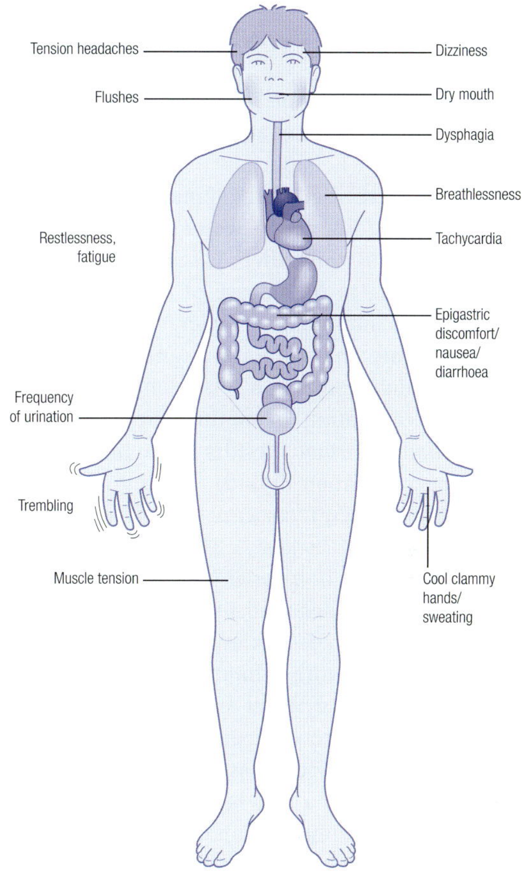

Figure 40.5 Somatic clinical features of generalized anxiety disorder

Table 40.4 Psychological features of generalized anxiety disorder

Symptoms	Characteristics
Psychic	Feelings of threat and foreboding
	Difficulty in concentrating or 'mind going blank'
	Distractable
	Feeling keyed up, on edge, tense or unable to relax
	Early insomnia and nightmares
	Irritability
	Noise intolerance, e.g. of children or music
Panic attacks	Unexpected severe acute exacerbations or psychic and somatic anxiety symptoms with intense fear or discomfort
	Not triggered by situations
	Individuals cannot 'sit out' the attack
Other features	Lability of mood
	Depersonalization (dream-like sensation of unreality of self or part of self)
	Derealization (dream-like sensation of unreality of world)
	Hypnogogic and hypnopompic hallucinations (when, respectively, going to sleep or waking)
	Perceptual distortion, e.g. distortion of walls or the sound of other people talking

somatic symptoms but will tend to have the same symptoms during each exacerbation, for example palpitations or trembling.

Males and individuals from lower social classes and some cultures are more likely to complain of somatic rather than psychic symptoms. It is important to understand that these are real and not merely 'all in the mind', and it is reassuring to the patient to be told this. In keeping with Cannon's fight or flight reaction, in which there is stimulation of adrenergic neurons leading to the release of adrenaline and other catecholamines, autonomic hyperactivity results in increased heart rate and palpitations and an increased rate of breathing, which results in a sensation of breathlessness. In turn, hyperventilation (sometimes referred to as the *'hyperventilation syndrome'*) results in the individual excessively blowing off carbon dioxide, leading to hypocapnia, which induces peripheral vasoconstriction and a 'pins and needles' sensation (paraesthesia). This can be countered by breathing into and out of a paper bag.

It is thus easy to understand how a patient, unaware of the normal physiology of anxiety, can get into a vicious cycle of anxiety and worry about somatic symptoms. The patient may forget the original stress that precipitated the episode and become preoccupied about dying from a heart attack (sometimes referred to as *'cardiac neurosis'* or the *'effort syndrome'*). Such a fear is increased if chest pain is also experienced owing to anxiety-induced increased muscle tension. Muscle tension is caused by increased blood flow to the muscles and increased tone, and contributes to the complaint of fatigue. The term *'neurasthenia'* (*fatigue syndrome*) has been used in the past to refer to a neurosis where fatigue is the predominant symptom.

Depersonalization and *derealization* are sometimes associated with anxiety neurosis and are disorders of self-awareness. In depersonalization, the individual has an altered or lost sense of personal reality or identity. In derealization, the individual's surroundings feel unreal. Individuals find these symptoms unpleasant and difficult to describe and are relieved when they are acknowledged by professionals. Such feelings can occur in normal individuals, especially those suffering loss of sleep, as well as in a *primary depersonalization–derealization syndrome*. They are also seen in individuals with depression, schizophrenia, alcohol and drug intoxication and withdrawal, and epilepsy. The feelings may also be induced by prescribed medication. Although unpleasant, they are bearable compared with panic attacks, which are associated with higher levels of anxiety (Figure 40.6).

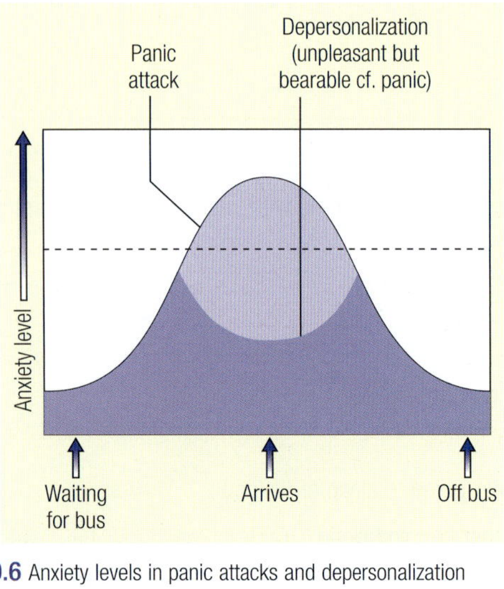

Figure 40.6 Anxiety levels in panic attacks and depersonalization

History-taking should explore the use of alcohol, caffeine and illicit drugs as possible explanations for anxiety symptoms, as well as any association of symptoms with precipitating events. The individual may have a tense and worried facial expression and posture, and may be tremulous, pale or sweaty. There may be overbreathing and evidence of agitation (purposeless activity due to anxiety), with pacing of the floor and fidgeting. Physical examination should exclude organic causes such as thyrotoxicosis. Although investigations for thyrotoxicosis might be justified, other physical causes of anxiety, such as phaeochromocytoma, are sufficiently rare for routine investigation not to be cost-effective unless clinically indicated.

Differential diagnosis

Many disorders and nearly all psychiatric conditions may present primarily with symptoms of anxiety (Box 40.2). Generalized anxiety disorder very rarely begins after age 35 years; individuals presenting for the first time after this age are more likely to have depressive or other psychiatric disorders, but the distinction between general anxiety disorder and depression can be difficult.[9] Rotational vertigo is not a symptom of anxiety.

Aetiology

Predisposing factors

There is some evidence of a genetic inherited influence on anxiety proneness associated with a vulnerability to depression, with environmental factors influencing presentation.[10] Environmental factors, such as through social learning, are also important in themselves (e.g. anxious insecure mothers raise anxious insecure children). Individuals with a premorbid anxious (avoidant) personality disorder are more prone to develop a chronic generalized anxiety disorder. There is also an association with early childhood separation experiences, especially separation from either parent. Bowlby's attachment theory suggests that such separations result in feelings of insecurity, which are reactivated in later life. Freudian psychoanalytical theory suggests that intrapsychic anxiety due to emotional conflict may be expressed directly as a generalized anxiety disorder.

Biological models of general anxiety disorder have been hypothesized, and involve the following:

Box 40.2 Disorders that can present primarily with symptoms of anxiety

- Generalized anxiety disorder
- Panic disorder
- Phobic disorders
- Obsessive–compulsive disorder
- Depressive disorder
- Schizophrenia and other paranoid psychoses
- Drug and alcohol withdrawal syndromes, e.g. delirium tremens
- Early dementia, e.g. catastrophic reactions upon psychometric testing
- Ictal anxiety due to epilepsy, especially temporal lobe epilepsy
- Thyrotoxicosis
- Phaeochromocytoma
- Unexpressed complaints of physical illness, e.g. lump in breast
- Drug and alcohol abuse, dependency and withdrawal symptoms, e.g. delirium tremens, caffeinism.

- Noradrenergic pathways (locus coeruleus–noradrenergic sympathetic autonomic nervous system), which are associated with fear and arousal
- Septo-hippocampal system and Papez circuit, which mediate anxiety and are where anxiolytic drugs act. Benzodiazepines act on γ-aminobutyric acid (GABA) type A receptor complexes.

The galvanic skin response of sweat glands to sympathetic stimulation is associated with a reduction in habituation in anxiety, but not thyrotoxicosis.

Precipitating and perpetuating factors

These include current stresses and life events, especially those associated with fear of loss. However, cognitive theories are now increasingly cited to explain the onset of generalized anxiety disorder.

Management

Most patients with generalized anxiety disorders are treated in the primary care setting. Counselling alone may be very effective, for example explanation of and reassurance about somatic symptoms of anxiety, such as palpitations, which the patient may believe are indicative of an imminent heart attack, or, more generally, reassurance that the individual is not going to lose control, 'go mad' or end up in a psychiatric hospital for life. Self-help materials, such as books and relaxation tapes and leaflets, reinforce counselling and can be a treatment in their own right.

Psychological treatments

There is good evidence that cognitive therapy and anxiety management techniques are effective, and these should be the first choices in treatment. Cognitive therapy is based on the idea that thoughts and feelings are related and that anxious thinking provokes or maintains the problem. The individual is taught to recognize and re-examine their anxious thoughts in order to find alternative and more helpful ways of thinking, which are then tested out in practice. Cognitive therapy also aims to identify and modify dysfunctional assumptions or beliefs that underlie anxious thinking. The aim is to replace automatic morbid anticipatory thoughts with realistic cognitions.

A cognitive-behavioural approach additionally includes exposure relaxation[11] and is superior to other forms of psychological treatment.[12]

Anxiety management training is based on the rationale that anxiety can be managed by breaking into the vicious cycles that keep the problem going. Education is via the explanation of anxiety and its causes and consequences. Relaxation exercises and, if indicated, breathing exercises are encouraged, and new ways of coping, such as distraction and cognitive techniques, are taught.

In both cognitive therapy and anxiety management, homework assignments for the patient may be required, and the patient should be warned that temporary setbacks may occur. Both cognitive therapy and anxiety management training may also be conducted effectively in a group setting.

Relaxation techniques are based on the assumption that mental relaxation follows physical relaxation. This may involve the use of progressive muscular relaxation, with or without the use of relaxation tapes. However, it is less effective than CBT.

The term 'autogenic training' (e.g. by biofeedback techniques) means learning to self-monitor anxiety levels and then apply relaxation techniques to daily activities. Yoga and transcendental meditation work as relaxation techniques and can be useful in generalized anxiety disorder.

In addition to non-directive and directive counselling and supportive psychotherapy, insight-oriented dynamic psychotherapy has been used for individuals with chronic generalized anxiety disorder who are unresponsive to other approaches. The technique aims to uncover and resolve unconscious emotional conflicts that result in intrapsychic anxiety, which is expressed as symptoms of generalized anxiety disorder. In particular, brief focal psychotherapy, which focuses on a specific problem and sets an agenda and time limits of therapy, has been found to be useful. In this technique, the individual is encouraged to talk freely, but the therapist interprets the content of the talk to reveal a deeper meaning, which can be understood and accepted by the patient.

Where interpersonal conflicts and stresses underlie the generalized anxiety disorder, marital or family therapy may be required. Similarly, environmental causes, such as poor housing, may have to be tackled.

Drug treatment

In the past, most patients presenting with generalized anxiety disorder were treated with tranquillizers, mainly benzodiazepines such as diazepam (Valium®). However, it is now recognized that such drugs can cause dependence, and their role is limited to brief periods of use to overcome symptoms so severe that they obstruct the initiation of more appropriate psychological treatments. Acutely disabled patients may require benzodiazepine drug therapy for up to 4 weeks, but even in these circumstances additional counselling, self-help and support are also required. Chronic use of minor tranquillizers should generally be avoided, although evidence is emerging that antidepressants, and possibly buspirone, may have a role in the longer-term management of severe persistent forms of anxiety.

Benzodiazepines are still the first choice when a rapid anxiolytic effect (as opposed to first-line treatment in general) is required. They should be used in the lowest dose possible and only as required, rather than routinely. In the absence of anxiety, they may merely result in sedation and increase the risk of dependency. Benzodiazepines should not be prescribed as hypnotics for more than 10 nights, or as anxiolytics for more than 2–4 weeks. Diazepam and chlordiazepoxide are used as anxiolytics, whereas temazepam and nitrazepam are used as hypnotics. Diazepam is the most prescribed drug ever in the history of prescribing. Flurazepam has been used by astronauts in space. Longer-acting compounds, such as diazepam, are preferred to those with a shorter half-life, such as lorazepam, which have a greater risk of withdrawal symptoms. Benzodiazepines may impair the effectiveness of psychological therapies and also the performance of skilled tasks and driving; patients should therefore be warned of these effects. Patients should also be warned about the potentially dangerous interactions of benzodiazepines with drugs and alcohol. Benzodiazepines have a definite abuse potential, with a risk of dependence and withdrawal symptoms on discontinuing long-term use. Prescribing benzodiazepines for a period of as little as 2 weeks can be associated, on cessation, not only with the re-emergence of the original symptoms, which the patient may then blame on the drug, but also with rebound anxiety and insomnia. Thus, patients on such a short course of a benzodiazepine night sedative should be warned that they will find it difficult to sleep for a few days after stopping their medication.

Only about one-third of long-term benzodiazepine users will experience a withdrawal syndrome upon stopping their medication. Numerous symptoms have been identified as characteristic of a benzodiazepine withdrawal syndrome. These include:

- neurotic symptoms, such as panic, agoraphobia, anxiety and insomnia;
- neurological symptoms, such as ataxia, paraesthesia, hyperacusis and micropsia;
- other major symptoms, such as hallucinations, psychosis and, in 1 per cent of patients, epilepsy.

The emergence of three new symptoms on discontinuation of benzodiazepine medication, or any symptom not part of the psychiatric disorder for which it was prescribed, such as epilepsy, is indicative of dependency. It should be noted, however, that before the benzodiazepines became available, barbiturates were widely used as anxiolytics and were associated with a much greater degree of dependency, as well as being more dangerous in overdose. Benzodiazepines are rarely fatal in overdose in normal individuals, unless combined with alcohol abuse or other drugs.

Ideally, the second choice of (but first-line drug) treatment of generalized anxiety disorder, if anxiety management training and cognitive treatment fail, is to use *SSRI antidepressants* or *selective noradrenergic reuptake inhibitor (SNRI) antidepressants*, which are often better tolerated than tricyclic or monoamine oxidase inhibitor (MAOI) antidepressants, which are also effective. It is unclear whether the combination of SSRI antidepressants and CBT is superior to either alone.

Buspirone is a serotonin 5-HT_{1A} receptor agonist and is suitable for the short-term management of severe anxiety when a rapid onset of effect is not essential, and for the treatment of anxious patients with a history of dependence on alcohol or sedatives/hypnotics. It has a progressive onset of action. It has diminished efficacy in previous benzodiazepine users and produces the side effects of dizziness, headache and nausea. It results in minimal sedation and psychological impairment and has no interactions with alcohol or other psychotropic drugs. It has a low or absent risk of dependence or abuse.

Beta-adrenergic antagonists (beta-blockers) are effective in patients with somatic anxiety symptoms caused by autonomic hyperactivity, such as palpitations, tremor and blushing. Patients may have found that blushing is also countered by cigarette-smoking. Beta-blockers do not affect symptoms caused by increased motor tension, such as headache; nor do they affect sweating, dry mouth, nausea, diarrhoea or frequency of micturition. They have side effects of tiredness, occasional nightmares and possibly depression, and they are contraindicated in cases of asthma and heart block. They are non-sedative and do not result in psychological impairment, abuse or dependence.

Low-dose antipsychotic medications, such as trifluoperazine and flupentixol, have also been used to some effect.

Antipsychotic medication can augment a limited response to SSRIs. Although there is probably no risk of true dependence, they can produce extrapyramidal side effects and have a slight risk of tardive dyskinesia.

Pregabilin, which has been used in neuropathic pain, has been found to be of use more recently.

Course and prognosis

The more chronic the generalized anxiety disorder, the worse the prognosis. A stable premorbid personality is a good prognostic sign. Generalized anxiety disorder can be complicated by the development of agoraphobia, secondary depression and abuse of alcohol and anxiolytics. Overall the course is variable and fluctuating, but chronic.

Anxiety is present usually where there is some possibility of choice of action. This may explain why some individuals facing execution, where there is no hope, do not appear anxious. Other factors such as depersonalization and denial may also be relevant, as may a paranoid attitude to circumstances in that the individual believes that others will 'get' them anyway, sooner or later.

PANIC DISORDER (EPISODIC PAROXYSMAL ANXIETY)

Panic disorder is characterized by acute and unprovoked (spontaneous) discrete periods of intense fear or discomfort (panic attacks) due to intense acute psychic and somatic anxiety symptoms, which are unexpected and not triggered by situations. During an attack, patients experience a sudden crescendo of fear and autonomic symptoms, resulting in a usually hurried exit from wherever they are: they are unable to sit out such attacks. They may also experience feelings of impending doom or death (*angor animus*) and somatic symptoms such as shortness of breath, palpitations, chest pain, tremor, faintness, dizziness, choking or smothering sensations. Fears of dying, 'going mad' or losing control are cardinal features. The attacks usually last for less than 30 min, with a peak of intensity around 10 min. Nocturnal panic attacks during sleep and non-fearful panic attacks with no psychological but only physiological symptoms can rarely occur.

If panic attacks occur in a specific situation (situational), such as on a bus or in a crowd, the patient may subsequently avoid and develop a phobia (inappropriate fear) of that situation, and even generalized agoraphobia. A panic attack is often followed by a persistent fear of having another attack and of being alone. Between attacks there is comparative freedom from anxiety symptoms, although anticipatory anxiety is common and may itself precipitate an attack. Table 40.1 (page 653) summarizes the ICD-10 diagnostic criteria for panic disorder. DSM-IV allows for both spontaneous and situational panic disorder – that is, with or without agoraphobia.

The frequency of panic attacks is not an accurate measure of the severity of panic disorder or the likely treatment response.

Panic disorder is maintained because the individual fears the somatic sensations associated with panic attacks. However, the only danger is subjective, due to the individual's interpretations of panic or its meaning or consequences (e.g. as threatening or dangerous). Catastrophic interpretations lead to anxious apprehension of future episodes and an increased vigilance regarding bodily sensations. Increasing autonomic nervous system arousal results and is then noted and responded to with fear, which in turn results in a further panic attack. Thus, a conditioned fear of fear pattern develops, with anxiety itself becoming a phobic (feared) stimulus. Individuals may stop undertaking physical exercise because this results in a raised heart rate, which sets the pattern into operation again and results in further panic attacks. The fear response may also increase muscle tension and lead to hyperventilation, exacerbating the overall experience and further aggravating the vicious cycle.

Panic disorder may also be the cause of unexplained medical symptoms.[13]

Panic originates from the Greek god Pan, who frightened humans and animals out of the blue.

Epidemiology

Although the lifetime prevalence for isolated panic attacks without agoraphobia has been found to be up to 27.7 per cent,[14] panic disorder occurs in only 1–2 per cent of the general population. It is more common (by two to three times) in females than males and may be worse premenstrually. The lifetime prevalence is around 4 per cent, compared with 8 per cent for panic attacks alone.[15,16] The age of onset is bimodal, an inverted U, with the highest peak around age 15–25 years and a second peak around age 45–54 years.

Co-morbidity

Agoraphobia occurs in 30–50 per cent of cases, with higher rates in patients seen in psychiatric settings. The risk of attempted suicide is raised where there is co-morbid depression (two-thirds of patients), alcohol misuse (up to one-third of patients) or substance misuse. Co-morbidity with medical conditions and bipolar disorder is also seen.

Differential diagnosis

Panic attacks can occur in established phobic disorders (situational anxiety with avoidance) in relation to the corresponding phobic situation, and also secondarily to depressive disorders, particularly in males. Some studies suggest a co-morbidity with depression or dysthymia of 45 per cent. Panic attacks may also result from intoxication with caffeine or amphetamines or withdrawal from substances such as barbiturates.

Physical disorders such as hypoglycaemia, phaeochromocytoma and hyperthyroidism must also be considered.

Aetiology

There is evidence of a genetic inherited predisposition, with increased concordance rates for monozygotic compared with dizygotic twins. Ninety-five per cent of patients with panic disorder have been found to have a genomic duplication (DUP25) on chromosome 15, compared with 7 per cent of the general population.[17] Such a predisposition may result from a biological vulnerability to this disorder related to ease of autonomic arousal, a lower threshold for initial panic attacks, and ease of anxious apprehension elicited by stress. There is an increased family history of agoraphobia, depression and suicide. An association has also been found between panic disorder and childhood parental death or separation from the mother. Premorbid overanxious personalities or otherwise high levels of anxiety predispose an individual to panic disorder. Panic disorder and agoraphobia also follow in about 16.7 per cent of cases after the implantation of a cardioverter/defibrillator, increasing in rate to one in five if it has been discharged.[18]

An association with benign joint laxity has been described, with an apparent 15 times increase in incidence. Panic attacks may also be provoked by excessive caffeine intake, injections of sodium lactate,[19] sympathomimetic drugs and carbon dioxide inhalation. The suffocation alarm theory of panic disorder postulates a central carbon dioxide hypersensitivity.[20]

Other theories include increased postsynaptic response to serotonin, increased adrenergic activity, and decreased inhibitory reactive sensitivity due to GABA. Pentagastrin and lactate[21] both induce panic. It is also postulated that the amygdala, hypothalamus and brainstem areas that mediate fear may also have a role.

Management

Advances in treatment have led to success rates of 80–100 per cent with CBT. A success rate of 50–60 per cent has been achieved with pharmacological treatments alone such as antidepressants and benzodiazepines.

Psychological treatments

There is good evidence for the efficacy of both behavioural methods (exposure to counter phobic avoidance, relaxation and control of hyperventilation) and cognitive methods (education about anxiety and panic and thinking errors).[22] The CBT approach is the first-line treatment and involves an initial education in the nature of panic attacks and the generation of fear of fear cycles. Cognitive restructuring is undertaken to enable the individual to identify particular catastrophic interpretations and to substitute more adaptive cognitions in their place. This is often achieved by a question-and-answer technique to detect flaws in logic, for example asking the individual to look at the actual frequency of fainting, which is usually zero, compared with the number of panic attacks experienced.

As thoughts are difficult to change without corrective experiences, interoceptive exposure techniques are used to achieve a controlled exposure of the individual to somatic sensations of anxiety and panic, with the goal of habituation to such symptoms, so they can be experienced without fear. Carbon dioxide inhalation and physical exercise have been used to this end. For instance, running on the spot produces a rapid heart rate and heavy legs. Dizziness and disorientation can be produced by the individual spinning or turning the head quickly, and hyperventilation will generate blurred vision, feelings of light-headedness, tingling, numbness and hot flushes. Depersonalization can be produced by staring at a fixed object or mirror for a prolonged period. Such exercises can be practised for 1–2 min, during which the patient's catastrophic thoughts are also elicited to demonstrate that catastrophic experiences do not follow. This process is called 'hypothesis testing'.

Cognitive restructuring and interoceptive exposure can be undertaken individually or in groups, and often involve homework practice with more diverse, prolonged and natural interoceptive exposure exercises.

Secondary agoraphobic avoidance due to panic disorder is treated by situational exposure, and anxiety management techniques and skills are taught where appropriate. For example, the patient can be instructed in muscle relaxation techniques and breathing retraining (i.e. to teach diaphragmatic and slow breathing skills to patients who hyperventilate).

This approach to panic disorder can be completed successfully within about 12–15 sessions, and its effect is maintained over time, as such skills can leave the individual with a sense of mastery of the condition, compared with the feelings of loss of self-control that often accompany the use of drugs. Individuals can also have occasional group CBT booster sessions from time to time.

Brief panic-focused psychodynamic psychotherapy to counter fears of being trapped and abandoned has also been used.

Drug treatments

Pharmacological treatments have proven efficacy but present discontinuation difficulties in up to 50 per cent of cases due to the re-emergence of symptoms upon stopping treatment. Antidepressants, especially the SSRIs (the first-line drug treatment in the NICE guidelines[23]), and also clomipramine, a tricyclic with a similar action on serotonin, are effective. Indeed, SSRI antidepressants should be regarded as the second-line treatment if CBT fails. Antidepressants may affect autonomic reactivity. They have a slower onset of action than the benzodiazepines, which tend to be effective only in the short term, although tolerance to anti-panic effects is said not to develop (as it does with sedation), and they can cause dependency with long-term use. NICE states that benzodiazepines should not be used in panic disorder. Pharmacological treatments are currently more commonly prescribed than cognitive-behavioural approaches, which require a skilled therapist. CBT, also recommended by NICE, may be used as an

Table 40.5 Differential diagnosis between generalized anxiety and depressive disorders

Generalized anxiety disorder	Depressive disorder
Common in early adult life	More common in later adult life
Onset age 20–40 years	Onset age 20–60+ years
More frequent in people with premorbid anxious personality	More frequent in people with previous stable personality
Previous episodes of anxiety	Previous episodes of depression or mania
Panic attacks frequent	Panic attacks rare
Lack of concentration	Loss of interest (anhedonia)
Minor loss of appetite	Major loss of appetite or increased appetite
Sexual performance reduced	Reduced libido
No diurnal variation of mood	Marked diurnal variation of mood
Initial insomnia	Early-morning wakening
Somatic symptoms common	Ideas of reference, guilt and hopelessness common
More related to external precipitants	Less frequently related to external precipitants
Chronic course	Episodic course

N.B. The diagnostic category often changes over time and in medical records; 90 per cent of individuals will at some point be labelled 'depressed'.

adjunct to or replacement for pharmacological treatment if this alone has been unsuccessful after 2–3 months. Drug treatment can improve the efficacy of CBT.[24]

Prognosis

With treatment, the prognosis is good (50–60% of patients remit with medication; 80–100% of patients remit with CBT). However, follow-up over 20 years shows less than 50 per cent of patients remain entirely panic-free. Untreated panic disorder frequently develops into other psychiatric conditions, such as depressive disorder.

MIXED ANXIETY AND DEPRESSIVE DISORDER (OR ANXIETY DEPRESSION)

In this disorder, symptoms of anxiety and depression are both present but neither is clearly predominant. Mixed pictures of neurotic disorders are much more common than discrete entities, such as generalized anxiety disorder. Mixed anxiety and depressive disorder is seen frequently, with up to half of patients with anxiety disorder meeting diagnostic criteria for depression. It is the most common psychiatric disorder in primary care. There are many more individuals in the population with this condition but who never come to medical or psychiatric attention. Anxiety is a mood about the future, while depression is a mood about the past. Table 40.5 demonstrates the theoretical differential diagnosis between pure anxiety and pure depressive disorders.

Management

Treatment of mild mixed anxiety and depressive disorder may be best undertaken by counselling, cognitive therapy or psychotherapy, especially interpersonal therapy, but it is also frequently treated in general practice by medication. Treating the depression usually relieves anxiety symptoms. Antidepressant medication is more effective than anxiolytic medication. The SSRI antidepressants are often tolerated better than standard tricyclics. It may, however, be necessary to treat both the depression and the anxiety.[25] In clinical practice, a common error is to misdiagnose depressive disorder or mixed anxiety and depressive disorder as merely a generalized anxiety disorder, and to prescribe minor tranquillizers such as benzodiazepines, often for long periods, with the associated increased risk of dependency. Such misdiagnosis often occurs because anxiety is present in nearly all cases of depression and may appear to be the predominant symptom.

PHOBIC DISORDERS

Fear is a normal prudent situational anxiety, for instance if one is under threat of attack. A phobia is an inappropriate situational anxiety with avoidance. The degree of avoidance is a useful measure of the severity of the disorder. The three main groups of phobic disorders and the lifetime prevalence rates are as follows[26]:

- Specific (isolated) phobias: 11.3%
- Agoraphobia: 6.7%
- Social phobias: 13.3%.

Table 40.1 outlines the ICD-10 diagnostic criteria for these three groups.

Specific (isolated) phobias or simple or monosymptomatic phobias

In specific phobias there is a persistent inappropriate fear of a circumscribed external object or situation, which leads to avoidance. Animal phobias occur equally in children of both sexes but are more common in women in adulthood. An individual with a phobia of cats will develop an immediate anxiety response in their presence and will avoid them, for instance by crossing to the other side of the road. Such specific phobias often start and are statistically normal in children. They often clear in early adulthood but are still common in a mild form in adults (e.g. fears of heights, the dark and spiders). For instance, half of adults are fearful of snakes. About 10 per cent of the general population have clinically significant specific phobias, most having developed in childhood, but only a small proportion seek professional help. The resultant incapacity depends on the frequency with which the phobic situation is encountered in daily life. For instance, an individual with a flying phobia may rarely have to confront this situation, unless air journeys are important to their work or social life, and treatment may not be necessary, at least for most of the year. However, avoidance of more common specific phobic objects, such as dogs and cats, may greatly interfere with an individual's daily activities, although specific phobias are less handicapping than other types of phobia. Also incapacitating is space phobia, which is a fear of falling when there is no nearby support.

Phobias of blood and bodily injury lead to bradycardia and hypotension upon exposure, in contrast to the tachycardia and increased blood pressure seen with other phobias. Such physiological changes on seeing blood could have conferred evolutionary advantage. This type of specific phobia is associated with a strong family history, often going back generations, and may be associated with a strong vasovagal reflex.

Agoraphobia

The term 'agoraphobia' originates from the Greek for 'fear of the marketplace', but it now has a wider meaning than fear only of open or public spaces: it also involves fear of being far from home, family and friends. The individual is fearful of being in places or situations where escape may be difficult or help unavailable if a panic attack were to occur. Individuals become anxious in anticipation of going out, particularly when unaccompanied, and this may restrict their activities. Avoidance, including an inability to enter shops, usually develops and in its extreme form results in individuals becoming housebound. Not all individuals who develop avoidance have a history of panic attacks, but around two-thirds do. Agoraphobia can either precede or follow panic attacks.[27] Shortness of breath is more common in panic attacks in agoraphobia. Breathlessness, dizziness, feelings of suffocation and fear of dying are common. Individuals with agoraphobia often feel worse the further they are from their home, and when out, they may be better in the company of someone else, unlike in social phobia. In its extreme form, individuals may even be unable to open the front door to retrieve items from the doorstep.

The clinical picture often includes claustrophobia (fear of closed spaces), as well as of crowded places, main roads and public transport. Individuals may abuse alcohol or drugs in an effort to overcome their phobia. Others become depressed as a result of the restrictions on their lifestyle, which in turn further exacerbates the agoraphobia.

Although specific (isolated) phobias are the most common in the general population, agoraphobia is the cause of 60 per cent of the phobic patients seen by psychiatrists. Such individuals often have a history of childhood fears and school phobia. Over two-thirds to three-quarters are female. They are often married and have a high incidence of sexual problems. However, pure agoraphobia is rare compared with co-morbid presentations with panic disorder or major depression.

Social phobia

Social phobia is characterized by the persistent fear of situations in which the person is subject to possible scrutiny by others, and also by fears that he or she may act in a humiliating or embarrassing way. Such situations include eating in a restaurant and public speaking. Social phobias may be specific, such as speaking or urinating in public, or generalized, with the individual experiencing distress in any social setting, even speaking on the telephone. Symptoms may include blushing and muscle twitching.

Social phobia can be precipitated by stressful or humiliating experiences, the death of a parent, separation or chronic exposure to stress, or it may have an insidious onset. Twin studies suggest a genetic vulnerability. There is little spontaneous remission, and chronicity is associated with co-morbidity with depression, other anxiety disorders and substance abuse in 75 per cent of cases. Blushing is particularly characteristic of panic attacks in social phobia. Palpitations, trembling and sweating are also common.

Social phobia is more common than previously considered and occurs in 3–4 per cent of the general population. First-degree relatives are three times more likely to be affected. It is associated with panic disorder and other

Table 40.6 Age of onset, sex ratio, characteristics and treatment response of phobias

	Specific phobias	Agoraphobia	Social phobia
Age of onset	3–8 years	15–30 years, most early to mid-20s	Peaks at 5 years and between 11 and 15 years. Presentation often delayed until late teenage/early 20s to 35 years
Sex ratio	Females > males	2.5 : 1 females : males	2.5 : 1 females : males (females = males in those seeking treatment[57])
Feared objects	Animals (zoophobia)	Open spaces	Formal social occasions
	Thunder (tonitrophobia)	Crowded places	Eating in public
	Heights (acrophobia)	Main roads	Talking socially
	Spiders (arachnophobia)	Public transport	
	Bees (apiphobia)	Housebound syndrome	
	Birds (ornithophobia)		
Cognitive-behavioural therapy	+++	+	++
SSRI or MAOI antidepressants	–	+	+

MAOI, monoamine oxidase inhibitor; SSRI, selective serotonin reuptake inhibitor.

Table 40.7 Differential diagnosis of social phobia and depression

	Social phobia	Depression
Loss of interest (anhedonia)	–	+
Energy	Normal	Reduced

anxiety disorders, which may have led to its delayed recognition as a syndrome apart from agoraphobia. Social phobics may abuse alcohol or drugs to counter social anxiety before social interaction. Social phobics who may have competent social skills should be differentiated from those with poor social skills that lead to social anxiety. They may as children have had temperaments of behavioural inhibition. Although individuals with social phobia may well have been shy adolescents, this should be distinguished from anxious (avoidant) personality disorder, although there is co-morbidity in 50 per cent of cases of each condition. People with avoidant personality disorder are shy and lack social confidence; people with social phobia show marked anxiety and avoidance. Social avoidance may also be caused by depression, panic disorder, schizophrenia and physical illness. People with schizoid personality disorder lack an interest in socializing. Table 40.6 shows the age of onset, sex ratio, characteristics and treatment of specific (isolated) phobias, agoraphobia and social phobias. Table 40.7 shows factors relevant to the differential diagnosis of social phobia and depression. Table 40.8 shows factors relevant to the differential diagnosis of general social phobia and panic disorder.

High rates of co-morbidity are, however, seen in social phobia, such as with other neurotic disorders, depression, post-traumatic stress disorder and substance abuse.[28]

On mental state examination in a clinic, an individual with a phobia may appear relaxed and otherwise normal, as the phobic object or situation is not present.

Aetiology

There is some limited evidence of a genetic inherited predisposition to develop agoraphobia (heritability 0.30), social phobia and phobia of small animals (heritability 0.47), but not of other phenomena.[29] In agoraphobia there is an increased concordance for monozygotic compared with dizygotic twins and an increased family history of panic

Table 40.8 Differential diagnosis of general social phobia and panic disorder

	General social phobia	Panic disorder
Panic attacks	In feared social situation	Unpredictable
Fear	Appearing foolish or awkward	Losing control or death
Social encounter if with friends	Little difference	Can enjoy

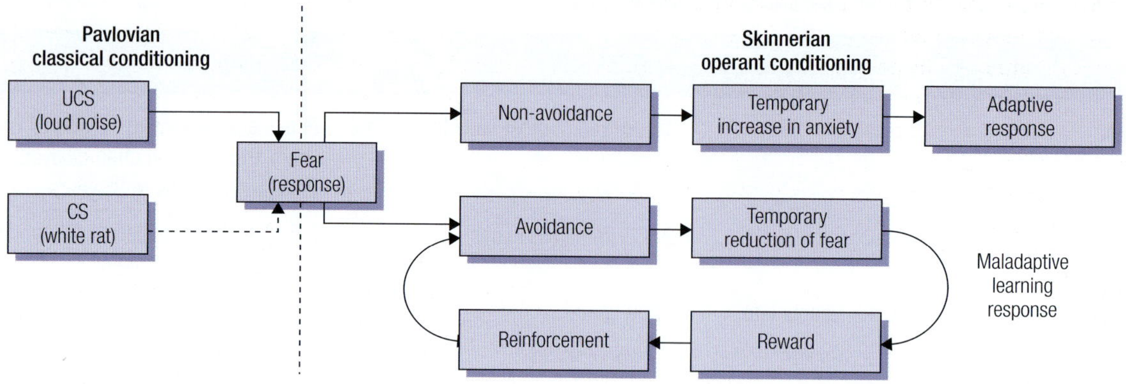

Figure 40.7 Behavioural learning theory and the development of phobias
CS, conditioned stimulus; UCS, unconditioned stimulus.

disorder and agoraphobia. In social phobia there is an increased concordance rate for monozygotic compared with dizygotic female twins (24.4% *v.* 15.3%). For simple or specific animal phobias there is evidence of increased concordance for monozygotic compared with dizygotic twins (25.9% *v.* 11%),[30] but not for situational phobias, which seem more environmentally determined. Specific phobias may originate in normal childhood fears. Even 1-year-old babies are fearful of writhing and darting animals and heights, but not, for instance, of manufactured dangerous objects such as guns. Such inborn fears may have been of evolutionary value.

Phobias can perhaps be best understood in terms of behavioural learning theory (Figure 40.7). The Pavlovian classical conditioning model is illustrated by the case of 'Little Albert'. In 1920 the American psychologist Watson caused Albert, then 11 months old, to develop a fear of his favourite furry toy rat by making a loud noise behind Albert when he attempted to touch the toy. This fear later generalized to a fear of all furry objects, and even to men with beards and his mother's fur neckpiece. Pavlovian classical conditioning with generalization might thus explain the development of a phobia that is, in effect, the pairing of a conditioned stimulus – the phobic situation – with an unconditioned stimulus (e.g. unexpected noise) to produce the response of fear. This seems to apply in social phobias where the conditioned fear response may be determined environmentally and triggered by the social situation in which anxiety first occurred.[31] However, only some individuals with specific animal phobias can recall their phobias being precipitated, for instance by being frightened or bitten by such animals in childhood.

Skinnerian or operant conditioning argues that the frequency of a behaviour can be altered by its consequences, such as reward or punishment. For example, avoidance of a phobic situation would be associated with a temporary reduction in anxiety, which is rewarding and thus reinforces the avoidance. This is a maladaptive learning response. The adaptive response would be to confront the phobic situation, even though this would produce a temporary increase in anxiety. The individual would then learn that such fear is excessive and inappropriate, the anxiety level would decrease and the phobia should thereafter be extinguished.

In Freudian psychoanalytical theory, phobic neuroses arise from intrapsychic anxiety caused by emotional conflict being concentrated into a specific situation by the defence mechanism of displacement. This leaves the individual free and able to cope with other situations in life. Other defence mechanisms such as projection and avoidance may also be pertinent. In 1909, Freud described the development of a phobia of horses in a 5-year-old child called 'Little Hans'. Freud postulated that Hans' fear of his father, and specifically of castration, was displaced on to horses in general after seeing a male horse urinate in the street. Freud's assessment, however, was based on information from Hans' father and not on the basis of an interview with Hans himself. Psychoanalytical explanations conceptualize phobias as symbolic representations of conflict, frequently of a sexual nature, that prevent the individual from going into a situation symbolic of that conflict. In agoraphobia, for example, a road with much traffic may represent sexual intercourse to an individual afraid of developing a sexual relationship. However, in spite of such theories, psychoanalysis is a very ineffective treatment of phobias in general.

The 'preparedness theory' suggests that fear of some objects may be evolutionarily adaptive to increase survival of the individual or species and may thus be difficult to extinguish.[32] An ethological theory of an evolutionarily determined genetic vulnerability to unfamiliar territory has also been proposed to account for agoraphobia.[33]

Predisposing, precipitating and perpetuating factors

The development of phobias may follow childhood parental death. Individuals with phobic disorder are also more likely to have a dependent, emotionally immature and possibly introverted premorbid personality, but this is not invariable. In the case of agoraphobia, although this can arise spontaneously, it is frequently precipitated by traumatic events such as bereavement, illness or divorce. Social phobias are said to develop from adolescence, and more commonly in shy, anxious and avoidant individuals with low self-esteem, and also in people who have experienced parental separation, overcontrolling maternal upbringing and childhood sexual abuse.[34]

Phobias might be prevented by generally encouraging children to face rather than avoid feared situations. Fears may be passed on from one generation to another within a family and, similarly, they vary according to cultural background.

Perpetuating factors may include alcohol and drug abuse, and also the collusion of family members. For instance, an agoraphobic female may obtain from her condition secondary gain from her spouse having to accompany her on outings or do the shopping instead of her, and he may collude in this because of his desire to have his wife be dependent on him. In addition, phobic disorders get worse with intercurrent depressive episodes, which may be in reaction to the phobias and the limitations they impose on the individual, or which may coexist with them or indeed predate them.

Management

Psychological treatment

Behaviour therapy is the treatment of choice for phobias, but it requires the patient's commitment. It is most effective, in 75 per cent of cases, for specific phobias. Exposure techniques are the most widely used, where the way in which avoidance maintains anxiety is explained and the individual is encouraged to face rather than avoid the phobic situation. This can be done in a graded way, tackling easier situations first and practising this repeatedly before confronting more difficult situations.

Exposure techniques developed from the behavioural technique of systematic desensitization (originally described by Wolpe[35]), in which relaxation training is combined with gradual exposure to the phobic stimulus over a number of sessions. The stimulus is presented in a progressively more anxiety-provoking form (graded hierarchy), either in fantasy but more effectively in vivo. It is based on the principle of reciprocal inhibition – that is, if a response incompatible with anxiety, such as relaxation, is produced while the subject is exposed to the source of this anxiety, then the fear and avoidance response will be extinguished. Thus, a systematic desensitization programme for an individual with a phobia of spiders (arachnophobia) might involve a graded hierarchy from thinking about spiders to being in the presence of a dead spider in a room, and then a live spider being brought progressively nearer to the individual until, with agreement, the individual might tolerate touching and holding the spider. Treatment goals should be agreed with the individual; for example, the goal for someone with a spider phobia might be merely to be in the same room as a spider, or it may be to hold the spider in the hand. 'Applied tension' may be additionally required in phobias of blood and bodily injury in order to counter the bradycardia and hypotension.

Flooding (implosion) is a behavioural technique in which the individual is maximally exposed to the feared stimulus, under supervision, until anxiety reduction or exhaustion occurs. This is based on the assumption that an individual cannot maintain a maximum level of anxiety indefinitely (in fact, beyond about 40 min). For instance, an individual with a phobia of heights may be taken, with consent, to the top of a tower block and asked to remain there with a therapist until the anxiety subsides. Such procedures can, of course, be distressing and the individual must be physically well enough (e.g. with no cardiac disease) to tolerate them. They are probably no more effective than other exposure techniques in the long term.

In modelling, the individual observes the therapist engaging in non-avoidant behaviour in relation to the phobic stimulus. The idea is that the individual should later copy such behaviour. Modelling may sometimes be usefully added to exposure and other behavioural treatments.

Behavioural techniques may be undertaken in groups. For instance, a group of agoraphobic patients may be taken together to the feared situation of a town centre. Such techniques also frequently involve elements of self-help, including homework in which the family members may also have to participate. It is also of note that many sexual dysfunctions have phobic elements and can be treated behaviourally.

Where agoraphobia is accompanied by panic disorder, CBT is the treatment of choice, using graded self-exposure, cognitive therapy or behavioural experiments to test catastrophic beliefs and cease safety behaviours.

For social phobia, CBT is the treatment of choice. This involves explanation, structured exercises for recognizing maladaptive thinking, exposure to simulated situations provoking anxiety, cognitive restructuring of the patient's maladaptive thoughts, homework assignments and self-administered cognitive restructuring routines. Undertaken in groups, CBT is moderately beneficial. There is no evidence of specific benefit from social skills or relaxation training.

It is important to be aware that the behaviour of family members may reinforce the phobia and obstruct treatment, and that family members may need to be counselled accordingly.

Drug treatments

Agoraphobia and depression sometimes coexist, and antidepressant drugs are often used. SSRI antidepressants and MAOIs such as phenelzine are superior to placebo in specifically relieving symptoms of agoraphobia and social phobia, perhaps reflecting underlying abnormalities in the serotonergic and dopaminergic systems. Tricyclic antidepressants may be effective in people with depressive features. CBT is the treatment of choice for people with agoraphobia with panic disorder, but high-dose SSRI antidepressants are the second-line treatment, although response may not appear for 6 weeks and reach a maximum level of benefit only after 12 weeks.

Benzodiazepines can be used to prevent the reinforcement of fear through avoidance; diazepam, for instance, can be given 1 h before an individual enters a phobic situation. However, anticipatory anxiety may sometimes be the main reinforcer of a phobia, so that benzodiazepines, for instance, taken 4 h before a phobic situation, may be more effective. Benzodiazepines are, in any case, most effective when used in combination with behavioural techniques, especially in the initial stages (e.g. to allow the individual to enter a phobic situation).

Beta-adrenergic antagonists (beta-blockers), such as propranolol, are effective if somatic symptoms predominate and reinforce a phobia, especially in specific social phobia. They do not work well in generalized social phobia.[36] As they are non-sedative, these drugs can be particularly useful for driving tests, examinations and for people in the acting or music professions, where sedation may impair performance. Beta-blockers have been used by snooker players to steady trembling arms and are certainly preferential to the use of alcohol for the same effect in professional darts players.

Although providing emotional support can be beneficial, psychoanalytical psychotherapy is considered to be very ineffective in the specific treatment of phobias.

Prognosis

Animal phobias have the best outcome. Social phobias tend to improve gradually and agoraphobias do worse, with a tendency towards chronicity.

OBSESSIVE–COMPULSIVE DISORDER

Obsesssive–compulsive disorder is a non-situational preoccupation in which there is subjective compulsion despite conscious resistance. Such preoccupations can be thoughts (ruminations or obsessions) or acts (rituals or compulsions).

Ruminations are like 'tunes' stuck in one's head. The content is often absurd or alien to the individual's normal personality, such as preoccupations with sex, violence, accidents or death, although such thoughts are recognized as the individual's own (*cf.* thought insertion in schizophrenia, where there is a delusional belief that thoughts are externally inserted into the individual's mind). Ruminations may be recurrent words, thoughts, ideas or mental images that are persistent, unwelcome, egodystonic and intrusive or that may be pointless or abstract. However, in general, patients do not act on their ruminations.

Rituals are akin to the childhood compulsion to walk between cracks in the pavement. They are repetitive and time-consuming and usually cause the patient distress. After an initial decrease in anxiety, rituals tend to increase anxiety further. Examples include obsessive washing or cleaning behaviour, and checking light switches or locks. Checking on three occasions is particularly common and has been related to the Holy Trinity. Individuals may also count to a certain number before undertaking an activity. Although rituals are sometimes referred to as 'compulsions', both ruminations and rituals are compulsive.

In obsessive–compulsive disorder, insight is maintained: individuals regard their ruminations or rituals as 'silly', but they are unable to stop. This is in contrast to delusional ideas, which may be recurrent and preoccupying, but where insight is lost and the ideas are regarded as true. Also in contrast to rituals, stereotypies are regular repetitive non-goal-directed movements, such as foot-tapping or utterances. These occur in conditions where insight is lost, such as chronic schizophrenia, infantile autism and mental handicap.

Particularly in chronic cases of obsessive–compulsive disorder, resistance to intrusive thoughts frequently abates and, indeed, may be absent and is therefore not an essential component of the disorder. In children, resistance is often absent. However, when conscious resistance is present, it is this that helps to generate the anxiety and tension, which are relieved only by ruminating again or performing the rituals.

Rituals may arise from obsessional doubts (*folie de doute*) and have been referred to as a small area of organization in the chaos of the individual's life. It is of note that when one normally checks switches or locks, one does not usually register (i.e. precisely remember) the activity, hence the capacity for obsessional doubting.

It is often helpful to individuals with obsessive–compulsive disorder to point out that anxiety comes first, before the ruminations or rituals, which are seen as a defence against anxiety. The patient may otherwise regard them as evidence of 'madness'. It should also be noted that depression and anxiety are common in obsessive–compulsive disorder.

So-called 'illness phobias' can better be understood as obsessive–compulsive disorders because such individuals ruminate on whether they have, for instance, cancer, acquired immunodeficiency syndrome (AIDS) or venereal disease. These are non-situational preoccupations, as compared with a true phobia, where there is an inappropriate external situational anxiety with avoidance.

The most common pattern involves obsessions about contamination followed by washing.

Individuals with washing rituals are often actually germ-phobic, but as it is not possible to see germs, the patient becomes dirt-phobic and generates washing rituals, to the extent that they might wash up to 40 times a day.

Screening questions include enquiring about:

- worry about contamination, dirt and germs;
- washing and checking excessively;
- unwanted thoughts of which one cannot be rid;
- doing things slowly in order to do them carefully;
- overconcern about routine, orderliness and symmetry.

Extreme slowness out of proportion to other symptoms (primary obsessional slowness) is rare.

Epidemiology

Past estimates of the prevalence of obsessive–compulsive disorder have included 0.5 per cent of the general population, 10 per cent of all patients with neurotic disorders and about 1 per cent of the psychiatric out-patient population. However, the disorder is now considered to be much more common than previously thought, and studies from the USA suggest that 2–3 per cent of the population may have obsessive–compulsive disorder at some time in their lives. Rates across the world are similar, although symptom themes vary. Minor obsessive–compulsive symptoms may be present in up to 17 per cent of the population; 1-month prevalence rates suggest it affects 1 per cent of males and 1.5 per cent of females. Males have an earlier onset. Two-thirds of individuals have an age of onset in the early twenties, before 25 years, with a mean age of about 22 years. It can even begin in childhood, with a peak age of onset of 12–14 years. Patients with checking rituals have an earlier mean age of onset of 18 years compared with other groups, with a mean age of onset of 27 years. The course tends to be chronic with exacerbations.

Differential diagnosis

Obsessional symptoms may be seen in up to 20–30 per cent of patients with depressive disorder and also in schizophrenia, where it has been suggested that premorbid obsessional symptoms, arising even in childhood, might represent defences against psychosis. Obsessional symptoms also occur in organic psychoses, including early dementia, and in anorexia nervosa and generalized anxiety disorder. Obsessional ruminations about harming one's baby occur as part of puerperal psychiatric disorders and, especially in cases of depression, should be taken very seriously in order to prevent them being acted on.

As discussed previously, delusional ideas may be recurrent and preoccupying, but insight is lost and they are regarded as true. Similarly, insight is lost in stereotypies, unlike obsessional rituals.

It is clinically useful to distinguish between the compulsions of obsessive–compulsive disorder and the impulsive behaviour of people with low impulse control and lack of resistance, such as individuals with psychopathic or eating disorders, disorders of sexual preference or gambling addiction.

Aetiology

The aetiology of obsessive–compulsive disorder is some way from being understood, and it is probable that its aetiology is different from other neurotic disorders. There is an increased genetic predisposition in first-degree relatives (3–7%) and a greater concordance between monozygotic (50–80%) compared with dizygotic (25%) twins.[37] However, types of rumination and ritual are not always the same in different affected family members. There is also a genetic association between Tourette's syndrome, chronic motor tic disorder and obsessive–compulsive disorder.[38] Indeed, up to 20 per cent of individuals with obsessive–compulsive disorder may have tics, which in turn are suggestive of basal ganglia disorder.

There is an increased incidence of obsessive–compulsive disorder in people with brain injury, for example due to head injuries, encephalitis, including encephalitis lethargica, or syphilis. Neuropsychological studies show abnormalities in executive function. Evidence for a neurobiological basis has been accrued from positron-emission tomography (PET) and magnetic resonance imaging (MRI) techniques, in which orbitofrontal and cingulate cortices and basal ganglia abnormalities have been found, as have reductions bilaterally in the size of the caudate nuclei and retrocallosal white matter. These findings all suggest structural abnormalities in the brain in at least some cases of obsessive–compulsive disorder. Increased glucose metabolism in the caudate nucleus and orbitofrontal cortex has also been found. There is also evidence for abnormalities in serotonin (5-HT) transmission or in its interaction with dopamine (DA) in the central nervous system. Some children and adolescents develop obsessive–compulsive disorder and motor tics after beta-haemolytic streptococcal infections, suggesting a cell-mediated autoimmune aetiology against basal ganglia peptides affecting the corticostriatal-thalamic-cortical circuits.[39]

A premorbid anankastic (obsessive–compulsive) personality disorder is said to predispose to the subsequent development of obsessive–compulsive disorder but is present in only 15–35 per cent of cases. Some studies suggest that a majority of patients have a premorbid anankastic personality, while others suggest that it is only a minority who do. People with an anankastic personality are characteristically obsessional, rigid, orderly, punctual and stubborn. However, they do not resist their obsessionality and their thoughts are not alien to them. Certain obsessional personality traits, such as conscientiousness, can be useful unless they result in insecure dithering and indecisiveness.

In Freudian psychoanalytical theory, anankastic personality disorder originates at the anal training stage of development (e.g. due to harsh toilet training). Obsessive-compulsive disorder is seen as a regression back from the

Oedipal to the anal-sadistic phase of development. Magical thinking (the belief that thinking about an event can cause that event) is also cited (omnipotence of thought). Obsessional symptoms are considered to arise from intrapsychic anxiety due to emotional conflicts being expressed via the defence mechanisms of displacement, reaction formation and undoing (e.g. checking to feel secure). Obsessive–compulsive disorder may represent a defence against anxiety associated with sexual and aggressive impulses, and also a defensive regression to the anal stage of development.

Learning theory cannot account fully for obsessive-compulsive disorder, but it does aid cognitive-behavioural treatment. Anxiety comes first; obsessions follow. The latter give rise to more anxiety, which leads to compulsions to reduce the feared consequences of the obsession and level of anxiety, but this is only short-lived and serves only to reinforce the compulsion.

Management

In the treatment of obsessive–compulsive disorder, any depressive component or other co-morbid intercurrent mental illness should also be treated effectively. The most common cause of ruminations is depression, not primary obsessive–compulsive disorder.

Psychological treatment

Supportive psychotherapy may be of value in pointing out to the individual that he or she is not 'going mad' and that anxiety comes before symptoms, which are seen as a defence against anxiety. However, psychoanalytical psychotherapy is ineffective, as the patient shows poor free association and may unprofitably ruminate during therapy, although people with an anankastic personality may benefit. This ineffectiveness may be further evidence in favour of a neurobiological basis for the condition.

CBT is, however, effective. This involves graded self-exposure and self-imposed response prevention of the 'undoing' of obsessions through compulsions, and/or cognitive therapy.

In general, rituals are easier to treat than ruminations. One behavioural approach for rituals is response prevention, whereby individuals learn to cope with the increasing tension associated with resistance when they are prevented from undertaking their rituals. Prevention is by distraction, discussion and, occasionally, mild physical restraint. In-patient treatment may be required for such treatment to be effective. Modelling can also be useful.

An alternative to response prevention is mass practice, in which the individual is told to keep repeating the rituals to a degree beyond what even he or she would wish to undertake voluntarily, until the anxiety reduces and the compulsion subsides.

Ruminations are less easy to treat. The technique of thought-stopping can, however, be helpful. In this, an individual is asked to relax and ruminate, whereupon the therapist will shout 'Stop!', at which point the patient must alter the content of those thoughts. Shouting of the word 'stop' is later replaced by the individual merely thinking of the word. The technique is repeated until the individual can learn thought control and to employ the technique as required. Smelling salts have also been used as an aversion technique to achieve thought-stopping. Individuals have also been taught to restrict their ruminating to a fixed period each day and thereafter to get on with their everyday lives.

Drug treatments

SSRI antidepressants at high doses are the drug treatment of choice. Their use developed from the observation that the tricyclic antidepressant clomipramine (the tricyclic with the most powerful 5-HT reuptake inhibition) was helpful over months (e.g. 8–16 weeks) in 40–60 per cent of cases.[40] Their beneficial effect is not dependent on their antidepressant properties. They are superior to other tricyclic antidepressants, although these too have produced improvement, perhaps because they treat the often-associated depression. Clomipramine causes significant anticholinergic side effects and sexual difficulties and can produce seizures at high doses. Clomipramine may be marginally superior, but SSRIs are better tolerated.[41] MAOI antidepressants have also been used successfully.

Low-dose atypical antipsychotic medication appears to be more effective than benzodiazepines, possibly because of its effect on conditioned responses. However, the use of atypical antipsychotics is as an adjunct in cases resistant to SSRI antidepressants, not as a monotherapy.[42] Benzodiazepines may be helpful in the short term.

Placebo response rates in studies are low (about 5%) compared with other psychiatric disorders.

Overall, for severe cases of obsessive–compulsive disorder, it is usual in the UK to combine CBT with SSRIs or to use an SSRI alone, but the combination may be superior.[43]

Psychosurgery

In severe, intractable, chronic and incapacitating cases, where all other treatments have failed, stereotactic site-specific brain surgery has been reported to be successful, although there is a lack of adequate trials and such procedures carry stigma. Radioactive yttrium implants and, more recently, non-invasive proton, electron and X-ray techniques have also been used.

Anterior cingulotomy, capsulotomy and limbic leucotomy have been found to be effective in 25–30 per cent of such cases. Cingulotomy carries a 1 per cent risk of epilepsy. All these procedures involve a separation of the frontal cortex from the deep limbic structures. A prerequisite for any such surgery is a stable premorbid personality, as patients with a history of antisocial behaviour and alcoholism may be further disinhibited in their behaviour as a result of the procedure. In England and Wales, under the Mental Health Act 1983, Section 57, neurosurgery for this

Table 40.9 Treatment of neurotic and stress-related disorders (treatment of choice given in italics)

Neurosis	Cognitive-behavioural therapy	Drugs
Generalized anxiety disorder	*Cognitive therapy*	SSRI or SNRI
	Anxiety management	Benzodiazepine, e.g. diazepam
	Applied relaxation techniques	β-Adrenoceptor antagonist
Panic disorder	*Cognitive-behavioural therapy*	SSRI
Specific phobia	*Behavioural therapy* with graded self-exposure and cessation of safety behaviours	–
Agoraphobia	*Cognitive-behavioural therapy*	SSRI
Specific social phobia	*Cognitive-behavioural therapy*	β-Adrenoceptor antagonist
General social phobia	*Cognitive-behavioural therapy*	SSRI
Obsessive–compulsive disorder	*Cognitive-behavioural therapy*	
	Thought-stopping	SSRI
	Ritual prevention	Clomipramine
	Mass practice	
Post-traumatic stress disorder	*Cognitive-behavioural therapy, EMDR*	SSRI or mirtazapine

EMDR, eye movement desensitization processing; SNRI, selective noradrenergic reuptake inhibitor; SSRI, selective serotonin reuptake inhibitor.

condition requires both the consent of the patient and the agreement of a second opinion in addition to that of the patient's responsible clinician (consultant). Neurosurgery is banned for this purpose in some other countries.

Prognosis

Obsessive–compulsive disorder can now be treated effectively in up to 70 per cent of cases. The more reasonable the preoccupation, the worse the prognosis tends to be – for example, checking that the house is locked before leaving home has a poorer prognosis than pointless rituals such as walking between the cracks in the pavement. Other poor prognostic factors include early age of onset, the coexistence of obsessions and rituals, low social function at baseline, magical obsessions and rituals.[44]

Table 40.9 summarizes the treatments for generalized anxiety disorder, panic disorder, phobic disorders and post-traumatic stress disorder.

NEUROTIC DISORDERS IN ELDERLY PEOPLE

In people aged over 65 years, the incidence and prevalence of neurotic disorders are reduced (generalized anxiety disorder 4%, simple phobia 4%, agoraphobia ≤8%, social phobia 1%, obsessive–compulsive disorder ≤0.8%). The onset of panic disorder in old age is unusual, and depression and underlying physical disorders should be excluded.[45] In elderly people, anxiety symptoms are often associated with depression and may be secondary to physical disorders or to prescribed drugs. Hypochondriacal symptoms are prominent.[46]

REACTIONS TO SEVERE STRESS AND ADJUSTMENT DISORDERS

ICD-10 provides a classification for a group of disorders that are a direct consequence of exceptionally stressful life events, producing acute stress reactions, or significant life changes leading to continued unpleasant circumstances, which result in adjustment disorders. Whereas psychosocial stresses can precipitate the onset or contribute to the presentation of many psychiatric conditions, the disorders in this group would not occur without the impact of such stresses. They can be regarded as maladaptive responses to severe or continued stress, in that they interfere with successful coping mechanisms and lead to impaired social functioning. Acts of self-harm, most commonly self-poisoning by a prescribed medication, may be associated closely in time with the onset of either an acute stress reaction or adjustment disorders.

Acute stress reaction/disorder

Acute stress reaction in ICD-10 or acute stress disorder[47] in DSM-IV is a transient disorder that develops in an individual with no other apparent mental disorder in response to exceptional physical or mental stress; it usually subsides within hours or days. The stress may be an overwhelming traumatic experience involving serious threat to the patient or a loved one, or an unusually sudden and threatening change in their social position or network, such as multiple bereavement or a domestic fire. The risk of developing this disorder is increased if physical exhaustion or other organic factors are present. Clearly, individual vulnerability and coping capacity are important, as not all people exposed to exceptional stress develop such a disorder. There is a mixed and usually changing picture of symptoms, typically including an initial state of 'daze', followed by depression, anxiety, anger, despair, overactivity (flight reaction or fugue) or withdrawal. No one symptom predominates for a long time, and the condition resolves rapidly within a few hours at most when the patient is removed from the stressful environment. When the stress continues or cannot be reversed, symptoms usually begin to diminish after 24–48 h and are usually minimal after 3 days.

This disorder was originally introduced into DSM-IV in 1994 to identify people who would develop post-traumatic stress disorder. However, only about half of cases do so, and the condition may be removed from DSM-V.

Post-traumatic stress disorder

This is a common reaction of normal individuals, usually within 6 months, to an extreme trauma ('an exceptionally threatening or catastrophic experience') that is likely to cause pervasive distress to almost anyone, such as experiencing a natural or manmade disaster, being involved in combat or a serious accident, witnessing the violent death of others, or being the victim of torture, terrorism, rape or other crime. Manmade disasters are more likely than natural disasters to cause post-traumatic stress disorder. Although predisposing factors such as personality traits and a previous history of neurotic or affective illness may lower the threshold for the development of the syndrome or aggravate its course, they are neither necessary nor sufficient to explain its occurrence. The syndrome is characterized by five elements:

- Experience of a major trauma
- Intrusive recollections in the form of thoughts, nightmares and flashbacks
- Sense of numbness and emotional blunting, which represent an attempt to avoid reminders of the trauma
- Increased arousal and hypervigilance, with an enhanced startle reaction and insomnia
- Onset follows trauma with a latency period of a few weeks to months, but not more than 6 months, and the condition lasts for at least 1 month.

Note that incomplete memory of the trauma can occur but is not characteristic.

The condition is seen as arising from the overwhelming and overloading of normal emotional processing. Emotional numbing/dissociation following traumatic events is predictive of post-traumatic stress disorder at 6 months.[48]

Epidemiology

The lifetime prevalence has been estimated as 7.8 per cent in the USA, with women twice as commonly affected as men. It occurs after a traumatic event in 8–13 per cent of men and 20–30 per cent of women. In men the traumatic event is more likely to be that of combat, while in women it is more likely to be rape. The exposure rates for significant traumatic events are much higher (60.7% of men, 51.2% of women).[49]

Neurobiology

Abnormalities in the hypothalamic-pituitary-adrenal axis, including hypocortisolaemia and supersuppression in the dexamethasone suppression test, the opposite to that seen in depression, together with abnormalities in regional blood flow in the basal ganglia and orbitofrontal cortex, as seen in obsessive–compulsive disorder, have been found, as have increased noradrenergic and serotonergic central activity.

Reduced hippocampal volume was reported in post-traumatic stress disorder in Vietnam veterans. The hippocampus mediates conscious memory, including of traumatic events, while the amygdala mediates unconscious memories, for example autonomic aspects of trauma. Decreased medial prefrontal and anterior cingulate areas have been found in neuroimaging studies, which correlate with increased activity in the amygdala, resulting in hypersensitivity to external threats, which is seen in post-traumatic stress disorder.[50]

Co-morbid psychiatric diagnoses are present in up to 80 per cent of patients. Anxiety and depression are commonly associated, and suicidal ideation may also occur. Both major depression and dysthymia may develop. The condition may be complicated by drug or alcohol abuse. Rarely, there may be dramatic acute episodes of fear, panic or aggression, triggered by stimuli that arouse a sudden recollection or a re-enactment of the trauma, or of the original reaction to it. Simple phobias, agoraphobia and social phobia may also develop.

Post-traumatic stress disorder, although not always referred to by that term, has been recognized throughout history. During the Second World War it was known as 'shell shock', but it was the Vietnam War that provided the major impetus for research into and description of the condition,[51] and since 1980 a number of natural disasters have led to its increasing recognition.

Prevention

Primary prevention has been attempted through stress inoculation in high-risk groups (e.g. exposure to dead bodies).

Secondary prevention strategies that have been found to be of value in aiding early emotional processing include early meetings of groups of survivors, within 1–2 days if possible, where group discussion can set the individual's emotional reactions within the normal range, and critical incident debriefing. The long-term efficacy of such measures is, however, unproven, and inappropriate and ill-timed interventions or interventions that lead to inappropriate rumination on the trauma can be harmful. NICE in the UK does not recommend brief single-session interventions.

Management

Many cases go undetected owing to the individual's reluctance to discuss symptoms and seek help. A high level of clinical suspicion is therefore required. Making the diagnosis can be reassuring to the individual, who often feels that no one can understand what he or she has been through. Specific treatment is indicated where symptoms have persisted for more than 6 months and social handicaps are significant. Self-help and mutual support groups, such as Rape Crisis Centres, can be of benefit. Central to most treatment approaches is the rehearsal of the 'trauma story', either in a cognitive-behavioural approach, which may include imaginal or in vivo exposure and may be combined with adjunctive anxiety management, or in a technique called 'testimony'. The aim is to rehearse the trauma and reawaken associated emotions, but in a way that can be tolerated and processed without leading to avoidance. Verbal recall represents behavioural exposure to a traumatic event, and the aim is to achieve habituation to it. Audiotape desensitization using the individual's own account of the trauma may also be of value. For survivors of torture, the pain is often compounded by guilt and fear, for instance over actions they may have been forced to carry out. They are encouraged to reframe their thinking and to see that such actions were due not to their betrayal of others but to the conditions to which they were subjected.

In the UK, NICE has made recommendations for sequential treatment in primary and secondary care settings and recommended either a CBT approach or eye movement desensitization processing (EMDR).[52] EMDR involves rapid and rhythmic eye movements induced by the patient visually tracking the therapist's finger moving back and forward for about 20 s, during which time the patient focuses on the traumatic image and associated negative emotions, sensations and thoughts, and discusses such associated emotions.[53] Once the distress begins to reduce, reference to positive thoughts for the event are encouraged. However, eye movement may not, in fact, be necessary,[54] with the procedure perhaps merely inducing desensitization.

Antidepressant medication, although not recommended as a routine first-line treatment, has also been found to be effective in the management of post-traumatic stress disorder, treating the commonly associated depression, facilitating sleep and reducing intrusive memories. SSRIs at high doses for 5–8 weeks have been cited as especially beneficial for core symptoms. Tricyclic antidepressants help the intrusive symptoms of anxiety and depression. However, the MAOI phenelzine may be better than the tricyclic imipramine. Response may be delayed for up to 8 weeks. NICE recommends the noradrenergic and specific serotonergic antidepressant (NaSSA) mirtazapine or the SSRI paroxetine. Benzodiazepines should be avoided because of their high dependency potential, especially in the first 2 weeks following the trauma, as their use may interfere with the memory processing necessary to reduce symptoms.

Hospital disaster plans should also take into account the psychological responses of victims.

Adjustment disorder

Adjustment disorders are states of emotional distress and disturbance, usually interfering with social functioning, arising in a period of adaptation to a significant life change or stressful life event such as bereavement or separation.[55] Onset is usually within 1 month of the event and the symptoms do not usually last more than 6 months. In contrast to an acute stress reaction, individual predisposition or vulnerability plays a greater role in the risk of developing such a disorder and in shaping its manifestations. However, it is assumed that the condition would not have arisen without the stress. There may be a brief or prolonged depressive reaction, a mixed anxiety and depressive reaction, or disturbance of conduct, for example in adolescence. Other predisposing factors include culture shock and hospitalization in children. As a condition, it has been little researched. Its management has been informed by the treatment of other conditions with similar symptomatology. It may respond better than major depression to antidepressant medication.[56]

KEY POINTS

- The term 'neurosis' encompasses a group of mental illnesses in which anxiety, phobic, panic and obsessional symptoms predominate. The dominant symptom determines the formal diagnosis, but several commonly coexist.
- Neurotic symptoms differ from normal symptoms such as anxiety only by their intensity, not qualitatively.
- Neuroses are abnormal psychogenic (psychologically caused) reactions.
- Most neuroses are precipitated by normal life stressors and are often associated with a vulnerable personality, especially dependent and anankastic (obsessional) personality disorders.
- Neurosis is twice as common in females as in males.
- Anxiety is a normal mood and, like pain, is a warning.
- Anxiety is accompanied by bodily (somatic) symptoms due to Cannon's (adrenergic) fight or flight reaction.
- Primary generalized anxiety disorder is rare compared with mixed anxiety and depressive disorder.

- Anxiety is more often associated with other psychiatric disorders, such as depression, than generalized anxiety disorder, especially when the onset is after the age of 35 years.
- Cognitive therapy and anxiety management techniques are effective treatments for generalized anxiety disorder.
- Benzodiazepines should not be prescribed as hypnotics for more than 10 nights, or as anxiolytics for more than 4 weeks, due to the risk of dependency.
- Panic attacks are discrete periods of intense fear or discomfort caused by acute psychic and somatic anxiety symptoms, which are unexpected and not triggered by situations.
- Panic disorder is effectively treated by cognitive-behavioural approaches.
- Antidepressants, especially the SSRIs and clomipramine, are also beneficial in panic disorder.
- A diagnosis of mixed anxiety and depressive disorder is made when symptoms of both anxiety and depression are present but neither symptom is severe enough to justify a separate diagnosis.
- Neurotic disorders do not include depression if this is the predominant symptom. It is instead classified under mood (affective) disorders as a depressive episode.
- Fear is a normal prudent situational anxiety.
- A phobia is an inappropriate situational anxiety with avoidance.
- Specific (isolated) phobias, such as of animals, are the most common phobias, but agoraphobia, a fear not only of open spaces but also of crowds and difficulty in making an easy escape, is the phobia most commonly seen by psychiatrists.
- Exposure techniques are the psychological treatment of choice for phobias and may involve homework assignments.
- SSRI and MAOI antidepressants such as phenelzine specifically relieve symptoms of agoraphobia and social phobia.
- Obsessive–compulsive disorder involves non-situational preoccupations with subjective compulsion despite conscious resistance. The preoccupations may be thoughts (ruminations/obsessions) or acts (rituals/compulsions).
- Insight is maintained in obsessive–compulsive disorder: 'It's silly, but I can't stop it.'
- Obsessional symptoms are common in depressive disorder, and any depressive component should always be treated adequately.
- Cognitive-behavioural therapy treatments for obsessive–compulsive disorder include thought-stopping for ruminations and response prevention for rituals.
- SSRIs and clomipramine specifically treat obsessional symptoms.
- Post-traumatic stress disorder is a reaction of normal individuals to a major trauma. Intrusive recollections, emotional numbing, increased autonomic arousal and hypervigilance occur.
- Meetings of groups of survivors and critical incident debriefing within 1–2 days may be preventive of post-traumatic stress disorder.
- Self-help and mutual support groups are helpful for people with post-traumatic stress disorder.
- Psychological treatments for post-traumatic stress disorder include rehearsal of the 'trauma story', such as 'testimony'.
- Antidepressant drugs are effective in the treatment of post-traumatic stress disorder, although their main effect may be on the associated depressed mood.

REFERENCES

1. Cullen W (1784) *First Line in the Practice of Physic.* Edinburgh: Elliott.
2. Whytt T (1768) Observations of the nature, causes and cure of those disorders which are commonly called nervous, hypochondriac, or hysteric: to which are prefixed some remarks on the sympathy of the nerves. In R Whytt (ed.) *The Works of Robert Whytt,* 3rd edn. Edinburgh: Balfour.
3. Hetterma JM, Neale MC, Kendler KS (2001) A review and meta-analysis of the genetic epidemiology of anxiety disorders. *American Journal of Psychiatry* **158**: 1568–78.
4. Goldberg DA (1996) A dimensional model for common mental disorders. *British Journal of Psychiatry Supplement* **30**: 40–49.
5. Cannon WE (1929) *Bodily Changes in Pain, Hunger, Fear and Rage: An Account of Recent Research into the Function of Emotional Excitement,* 2nd edn. New York: Appleton-Century-Crofts.
6. Hebb DO (1955) Drives and the C. N. S. (conceptual nervous system). *Psychological Review* **62**: 243–54.
7. Yerkes RM, Dodson JD (1908) The relation of strength of stimulus to rapidity of habit-formation. *Journal of Comparative Neurology and Psychology* **18**: 459–82.
8. Wittchen HU, Jacobi F (2005) Size and burden of mental disorder in Europe: a critical review and appraisal of 27 studies. *European Neuropsychopharmacology* **15**: 357–76.
9. Tyrer PJ, Baldwin DS (2006) Generalised anxiety disorder. *Lancet* **368**: 2156–66.
10. Kendler KS, Neale MC, Kessler RC, Heath AC, Eaves LJ (1992) Major depression and generalized anxiety disorder: same genes, (partly) different environments. *Archive of General Psychiatry* **49**: 716–22.
11. National Institute for Health and Clinical Excellence (2004) *The Management of Panic Disorder and Generalised Anxiety Disorder in Primary and Secondary Care.* London: National Collaborating Centre for Mental Health.
12. Durham RC, Chambers JA, MacDonald RR, Power KG, Major K (2003) Does cognitive-behavioural therapy influence the long-term outcome of generalized anxiety disorder? An 8–14 year follow-up of two clinical trials. *Psychological Medicine* **33**: 499–509.
13. Katon W (1984) Panic disorder and somatization: review of 55 cases. *American Journal of Psychiatry* **77**: 101–6.
14. Kessler RC, Chiu WT, Jin R, *et al.* (2006) The epidemiology of panic attacks, panic disorder, and agoraphobia in the National Comorbidity Survey Replication. *Archives of General Psychiatry* **63**: 415–24.
15. Simon GE, van Korff M (1991) Somatization and psychiatric disorder in the NIMH epidemiologic catchment area study. *American Journal of Psychiatry* **148**: 1494–1500.

16. Eaton WW, Kessler RC, Wittchen HU, Magee WJ (1994) Panic and panic disorder in the United States. *American Journal of Psychiatry* **151**: 413–20.
17. Gratacos M, Nadal M, Martin-Santos R, *et al.* (2001) A polymorphic genomic duplication on human chromosome 15 is a susceptibility factor for panic and phobic disorders. *Cell* **106**: 267–379.
18. Godemann F, Butter C, Lampe F, *et al.* (2004) Panic disorders and agoraphobia: side effects of treatment with an implantable cardioverter/defibrillator. *Clinical Cardiology* **27**: 321–6.
19. Pitts FN, McClure JN (1967) Lactate metabolism in anxiety neurosis. *New England Journal of Medicine* **13**: 29–36.
20. Klein DF (1993) False suffocation alarms, spontaneous panics, and related conditions: an integrative hypothesis. *Archives of General Psychiatry* **50**: 306–17.
21. Pitts FN, McClure JN (1967) Lactate metabolism in anxiety neurosis. *New England Journal of Medicine* **277**: 1329–36.
22. Barlow DH, Craske MG (1998) *Mastery of your Anxiety and Panic*. Albany, NY: Graywind Publications.
23. National Institute for Health and Clinical Excellence (2004) *Anxiety: Management of Anxiety (Panic Disorder, with or without Agoraphobia, and Generalised Anxiety Disorder) in Primary, Secondary and Community Care*. London: National Institute for Health and Clinical Excellence.
24. Mitte K (2005) A meta-analysis of the efficacy of psycho- and pharmacotherapy in panic disorder with and without agoraphobia. *Journal of Affective Disorder* **88**: 27–45.
25. Baldwin DS, Anderson IM, Nutt DJ, *et al.* (2005) Evidence-based guidelines for the pharmacological treatment of anxiety disorders: recommendations from the British Association for Psychopharmacology. *Journal of Psychopharmacology* **19**: 567–96.
26. Magee WJ, Eaton WW, Wittchen HU, McGonagle KA, Kessler RC (1996) Agoraphobia, simple phobia and social phobia in the National Comorbidity Survey. *Archives of General Psychiatry* **53**: 159–68.
27. Bienvenu OJ, Onyike CU, Stein MB, *et al.* (2006) Agoraphobia in adults: incidence and longitudinal relationship with panic. *British Journal of Psychiatry* **188**: 432–8.
28. Schneier ER, Johnson J, Hornig CD, *et al.* (1992) Social phobia. Comorbidity and morbidity in an epidemiological sample. *Archives of General Psychiatry* **49**: 282–8.
29. Skre I, Onstad S, Torgersen S, *et al.* (2000) The heritability of common phobic fear: a twin study of a clinical sample. *Journal of Anxiety Disorders* **14**: 549–62.
30. Kendler KS, Neale MC, Kessler RC, *et al.* (1992) The genetic epidemiology of phobias in women: the interrelationship of agoraphobia, social phobia, situational phobia and simple phobia. *Archives of General Psychiatry* **49**: 273–81.
31. Rapee RM, Heinberg RG (1997) The cognitive behavioural model of anxiety in social phobia. *Journal of Behaviour Research and Therapy* **35**: 741–56.
32. Marks IM (1969) *Fears and Phobias*. New York: Academic Press.
33. Lelliott P, Marks I, McNamee G, Tebena A (1989) Onset of panic disorder with agoraphobia: towards an integrated model. *Archives of General Psychiatry* **46**: 1000–1004.
34. Bandelow Bl, Charimo Torrente A, Wedekind D, *et al.* (2004) Early traumatic life events, parental rearing styles, family history of mental disorders, and birth risk factors in patients with social anxiety disorder. *European Archives of Psychiatry and Clinical Neuroscience* **254**: 397–405.
35. Wolpe J (1973) *The Practice of Behaviour Therapy*, 2nd edn. New York: Pergamon.
36. Blanco C, Raza MS, Schneier F, Leibowitz MR (2003) The evidence-based pharmacotherapy of social anxiety disorder. *International Journal of Neuropsychopharmacology* **6**: 427–42.
37. Hetterma JM, Neale MC, Kendler KS (2001) A review and meta-analysis of the genetic epidemiology of anxiety disorders. *American Journal of Psychiatry* **158**: 1568–78.
38. Pauls DL, Alsobrook JP, 2nd (1999) The inheritance of obsessive–compulsive disorder. *Child Adolescent Clinics in North America* **8**: 481–96.
39. Leonard HC, Swedo SE (2001) Paediatric autoimmune neuropsychiatric disorders associated with Streptococcal infection (PANDAS). *International Journal of Neuropsychopharmacology* **4**: 191–8.
40. Rappaport J (1990) *The Boy Who Couldn't Stop Washing: The Experience and Treatment of Obsessive–Compulsive Disorder*. London: HarperCollins.
41. Fineberg NA, Gale TM (2005) Evidence-based pharmacotherapy of obsessive-compulsive disorder. *International Journal of Neurosychopharmacology* **8**: 107–29.
42. Skapinakis P, Papatheodorou T, Mavreeas V (2007) Antipsychotic augmentation of serotonergic antidepressants in treatment-resistant obsessive–compulsive disorder: a meta-analysis of the randomised controlled trials. *European Neuropsychopharmacology* **17**: 79–93.
43. Foa EB, Liebowitz MR, Kozak MJ, *et al.* (2005) Randomized, placebo-controlled trial of exposure and ritual prevention, clomipramine and their combination in the treatment of obsessive–compulsive disorder. *American Journal of Psychiatry* **152**: 151–61.
44. Skoog G, Skoog I (1999) A 40 year follow-up of patients with obsessive compulsive disorder. *Archives of General Psychiatry* **56**: 121–7.
45. Flint AJ, Gagnon N (2003) Diagnosis and management of panic disorder in older patients. *Drugs in the Ageing* **20**: 881–91.
46. Lindesay J, Marudkar M (2001) Neurotic disorders. *Reviews in Clinical Gerontology* **11**: 51–70.

47. Bryant RA, Harvey AG (2000) *Acute Stress Disorder: A Handbook of Theory, Assessment and Treatment.* Washington, DC: American Psychiatric Association.
48. Murray J, Ehlers A, Mayou RA (2002) Dissociation and post-traumatic stress disorder: two prospective studies of road traffic accident survivors. *British Journal of Psychiatry* **180**: 363–8.
49. Kessler RC, Sonnega A, Bromet E, Hughes M, Nelson CB (1995) Post traumatic stress disorder in the National Comorbidity Survey. *Archives of General Psychiatry* **52**: 1048–60.
50. Hall AM (2002) Neuro-imaging finding in post traumatic stress disorder: systematic review. *British Journal of Psychiatry* **181**: 102–10.
51. Jones E (2006) Historical approaches to post-combat disorders. *Philosophical Transactions of the Royal Society of London. Series B, Biological Sciences* **361**: 533–42.
52. National Collaborating Centre for Mental Health (2005) *Post-Traumatic Stress Disorder: The Management of PTSD in Adults and Children in Primary and Secondary Care.* National clinical practice guideline. no. 26. London: Gaskell and the British Psychological Society.
53. Shapiro F (1995) *Eye Movement Desensitization and Reprocessing: Basic Principles, Protocols and Procedures.* New York: Guilford Press.
54. Davidson PR, Parker KCH (2001) Eye movement desensitization and reprocessing (EMDR): a meta-analysis. *Journal of Consulting and Clinical Psychology* **69**: 305–16.
55. Casey P (2001) Adult adjustment disorder: a review of the current diagnostic status. *Journal of Psychiatric Practice* **7**: 32–40.
56. Hameed U, Schwartz T, Malhotra K (2005) Antidepressant treatment in the primary care office: outcome for adjustment disorders vs. major depression. *Annals of Clinical Psychiatry* **17**: 77–81.
57. Robbins LN, Reiger DA (1991) *Psychiatric Disorders in America: The Epidemiologic Catchment Area Study.* New York: Free Press.

Chapter 41

Dissociative (conversion), hypochondriasis and other somatoform disorders

Ian Treasaden

INTRODUCTION

This chapter deals with the various types of neurotic and stress-related disorder previously included under the term 'hysteria'. This now redundant term referred to physical or mental symptoms not of organic origin and created and maintained for unconscious psychological motives.

The term 'hysteria' has now been replaced by the terms 'dissociative disorders' (mental and sometimes neurological symptoms for which no organic cause can be found) and 'somatoform disorders' (physical symptoms with no apparent organic basis). The term 'conversion' refers to medically unexplained symptoms affecting voluntary motor or sensory function, for example limb paralysis or psychogenic blindness or deafness, where mental stress has been converted into a physical symptom.

The term 'hysteria' has been in use for 2000 years and stems from the Greek word for womb, *husteria*. The ancient Greeks believed that the womb could wander through the body and cause malfunction in various organs by pressing on them. The term has been used in psychiatry with many and varied meanings, and it is still used today in some circumstances.[1]

The old hysterical neurosis is now described in the tenth revision of the *International Classification of Diseases* (ICD-10) under the term 'Dissociative (Conversion) Disorders' (Box 41.1) and includes the following concepts:

Box 41.1 Dissociative (conversion) disorders as described in ICD-10

COMMON THEMES

- Partial or complete loss of normal integration between memories of the past, awareness of identity and immediate sensations and control of bodily movements
- The term 'conversion' is applied to some of these disorders and implies that unresolved problems and conflicts are transformed into symptoms, e.g. paralysis and anaesthesias
- Denial of problems and difficulties that are obvious to others
- No evidence of physical disorder that might explain symptoms
- Evidence of psychological causation in form of association in time with stressful events and problems or disturbed relationships.

SPECIFIC DISORDERS

- *Dissociative amnesia:* loss of memory (partial or complete) for recent events of a traumatic or stressful nature
- *Dissociative fugue:*
  - Features of dissociative amnesia
  - Purposeful travel beyond everyday range
  - Maintenance of self-care and simple social interactions with strangers
- *Dissociative stupor:* profound diminution or absence of voluntary movement and normal responsiveness to external stimuli
- *Trance and possession states*
- *Dissociative disorders of movement and sensation:* e.g. loss of ability to move all or part of limb(s); sometimes accompanied by calm acceptance (*la belle indifférence*)
- *Dissociative convulsions* (pseudo-seizures)
- *Other dissociative and conversion disorders:* e.g. Ganser's syndrome, multiple personality.

- *Conversion hysteria*, in which there is a loss of or change in bodily function due to the conversion of unconscious intrapsychic anxiety, caused by emotional conflict, to physical bodily symptoms of symbolic significance (e.g. paralysis or anaesthesia of the limbs)
- *Dissociative states*, in which there is dissociation of the normally integrated functions of consciousness such that one mental activity may be dissociated from another, for example dissociative (hysterical) amnesia, in which stressful or traumatic events cannot be recalled while other memories, such as those required for everyday living, may be preserved.

Box 41.2 Varied meanings of the term 'hysteria'

HYSTERICAL NEUROSIS

This is now described in ICD-10 under the term 'Dissociative (Conversion) Disorders'.

HYSTERICAL SYMPTOMS

These may occur in other mental illnesses, such as depression and anxiety, and may also complicate organic disease.

EPIDEMIC (COMMUNICABLE) HYSTERIA OR MASS HYSTERIA

In this condition, there may be a widespread outbreak of particular hysterical or other symptoms, such as fainting, hyperventilation, emotional distress and abdominal pain. This often occurs among young females and in institutions such as schools. There is often a background of tension or apprehension, and the initial symptoms may appear in an influential or powerful figure and then spread, by suggestion, to younger or less influential individuals, while excluding outsiders or more intellectually able people. Food or chemical poisoning or infection may initially be suspected, which only increases the emotional tension. In the Middle Ages, dancing mania swept through Europe, although alternative explanations have been given for this in terms of an infective neurological disorder causing limb restlessness.

HYSTERICAL OR HISTRIONIC PERSONALITY DISORDER

Such individuals have overemotional and overdramatic personality traits. They may crave attention and be manipulative. Under stress they have an increased vulnerability to developing dissociative (conversion) disorders and are also prone to parasuicidal acts.

HYSTERICAL (HISTRIONIC) BEHAVIOUR

This term is used frequently, not only by the general public, to refer to behaviour where there is 'acting out' of problems and also loss of or poor control of impulses. Such behaviour occurs particularly in people with histrionic or psychopathic personalities. It is useful to distinguish the conscious motivation for such behaviour from the unconscious motivation underlying hysterical symptoms in dissociative (conversion) disorders.

HYSTERICAL PATIENT

This is a term of abuse often applied by doctors to patients, usually female, when the doctor is irritated because of a belief that the patient may be exaggerating her symptoms or the doctor has a feeling of being manipulated. Similar male patients tend to be labelled 'psychopaths'. The use of the term 'hysterical' in this way usually reflects an unsatisfactory doctor–patient relationship.

ST LOUIS HYSTERIA (BRIQUET'S SYNDROME)

Also known as 'somatization disorder', this refers to individuals with recurrent and multiple unexplained physical symptoms commencing before the age of 30 years and of chronic duration.

HYSTERICAL PSYCHOSIS OR HYSTERICAL PSEUDOPSYCHOSIS

This is a group of pseudopsychotic disorders, with pseudodelusions and pseudohallucinations, which occur suddenly after severe emotional stress and usually end abruptly within a few days. Such pseudohallucinations are experienced as arising within the mind, rather than being perceived by actual sense organs. They are a form of vivid imagery, located in subjective rather than objective space, but not subject to conscious control. Included in such disorders are a number of culture-bound disorders, such as 'running amok' in South-East Asia and, from history, the Vikings 'going berserk'. It has been suggested that Joan of Arc had an hysterical psychosis.

ANXIETY HYSTERIA

This is a psychoanalytical term for phobic anxiety.

Table 41.1 Comparison of ICD-10 and DSM-IV somatoform and dissociative disorders

ICD-10	DSM-IV
F44. Dissociative (conversion) disorders	300. Dissociative disorders
F45. Somatoform disorders	300. Somatoform disorders
F45.0 Somatization disorder	300.81 Somatization disorder
F45.2 Hypochondriacal disorder	300.7 Hypochondriasis
F45.4 Persistent somatoform pain disorder	307.80 Pain disorder

Box 41.2 shows the varied meanings of the term 'hysteria' used in the present and the past.

There are, however, significant interrelationships between the varied concepts of hysteria. For instance, people with a hysterical personality disorder are more likely than normal to develop conversion symptoms, conversion disorders and somatization disorder, and are more likely to be the influential figure instigating mass hysteria in others. Also, many females with St Louis hysteria, or Briquet's syndrome, have conversion symptoms. In addition, nearly all those in the above categories are prone to irritate their doctors and develop unsatisfactory doctor–patient relationships.

In ICD-10, the category of dissociative (conversion) disorders includes conversion disorder (previously hysterical neurosis, conversion type). In the fourth revised edition of the *Diagnostic and Statistical Manual of Mental Disorders* (DSM-IV-TR), the category of dissociative disorders does not include conversion disorder, which is subsumed under the category of somatoform disorders. Table 41.1 compares the nomenclature for these disorders in ICD-10 and DSM-IV.

For clarity, dissociative disorders will be described here separately from the conversion disorders. However, both dissociative and conversion disorders are usually temporarily related to a trigger and are of sudden onset; the link between psychological stress and resulting symptoms is not consciously known to the patient, and both disorders are increased in females, in people under age 40 years and in people with vulnerable personalities.

DISSOCIATIVE DISORDERS

These disorders are characterized by a psychogenic (psychologically caused) alteration in an individual's state of consciousness or personal identity. Box 41.1 summarizes the description of dissociative disorders given in ICD-10.

Dissociation is a state in which two or more mental processes coexist without becoming integrated. Emotional conflict and distress are thus segregated from normal consciousness, as in dissociative amnesia, or even to a separate distinct personality, which may take control of the person's behaviour, as in multiple personality disorder. Historically, Janet particularly emphasized the defence mechanism of dissociation following traumatic experiences in cases of hysteria.[2] Doubts, however, remain about the definition and measurement of dissociation.[3]

Dissociative amnesia

In this condition, the severity of loss of memory (whether partial or complete) for recent events of a traumatic or stressful nature contrasts with the otherwise very good preservation of other cognitive functions and the individual's ability to utilize memories that are not of a personal nature. Complete recovery may occur within a few days once the precipitating stress is removed. In contrast to amnesia of organic aetiology, dissociative amnesia may respond to anxiolytic medication. Included in the differential diagnosis would be transient global amnesia due to temporal lobe ischaemia caused by vertebrobasilar insufficiency.

Classically, in dissociative amnesia, episodic memory is present and does not involve problems in procedural memory or in memory storage, as in Wernicke–Korsakoff syndrome. The amnesia is reversible, including by hypnosis. The memory loss is for discrete periods of time, ranging from days to years, and usually for traumatic or stressful events, which it follows. Onset may be gradual or sudden, and people in the third or fourth decades of life are most often affected. Usually only one episode is involved, but multiple periods of lost memory are seen. Co-morbidity occurs with conversion disorders, depression, alcohol abuse and bulimia nervosa; personality disorders of histrionic, dependent or borderline type occur in a minority of patients with dissociative amnesia.

Dissociative fugue

In this condition, in addition to the features of dissociative amnesia, there is purposeful travel beyond the usual everyday range and maintenance of basic self-care. Simple social interactions with strangers are usually preserved. The unconscious motivation (primary gain) may be to avoid arrest for criminal activities or intolerable stresses at home or at work.

This is effectively amnesia with wandering and an inability to recall personal past history, sometimes combined with a partial or new identity. Memory of recent traumatic or stressful events may be lost. The differential diagnoses include organic fugue, where basic self-care and activities of daily living are not characteristically preserved, and postictal states, where there is an absence of current stressors and travel is without purpose.

Dissociative stupor

In this disorder, voluntary movement is severely reduced but the individual responds to external stimuli in a normal way. In spite of apparent reduction in consciousness, the individual is neither sleeping nor unconscious.

Other dissociative disorders

Included in this ICD-10 category is *Ganser's syndrome*, which is characterized by approximate or ridiculous answers to questions (e.g. Elizabeth III is the queen of England; a horse has five legs) and which occurs in the setting of diminished consciousness (a hysterical twilight state). There may also be somatic conversion signs and pseudo-hallucinations. The condition was described by Ganser in 1898 in three prisoners. It is considered to be very rare nowadays.

Also included in this category is *multiple personality*,[4] or, in DSM-IV, *dissociative identity disorder*, where there exist within the person two (the most common type) or more distinct personalities or personality states, at least two of which recurrently take full control of the person's behaviour. Switches between personalities are usually rapid. No personality has any awareness of any of the others. Sometimes a personality will be that of the individual at an earlier age. Multiple personality has been recognized since the early 1900s and was well described in the 1957 film *The Three Faces of Eve* (based on a book by Drs CH Thigpen and HM Cleckley). Patients may have a past history of childhood abuse. Some patients meet the criteria for dissocial personality disorder. Other patients have a history of substance abuse. It remains a controversial diagnosis[5] and is made more often in the USA than in the UK. It can be iatrogenic if reinforced during psychotherapy.

Reflecting the influence of culture, *dissociative trance* and *possession disorder* are more common in the East.

Predisposing and precipitating factors

Predisposing factors include severe childhood emotional trauma and abuse (often sexual), and a borderline personality disorder. The condition is usually triggered by severe psychological stress.

CONVERSION DISORDERS

Conversion disorders are characterized by loss of or alteration in bodily function arising from psychological conflict or need and are not explicable by a medical disorder.[6] Symptoms are typically neurological, affecting the voluntary nervous system. Typically, one or two neurological symptoms are seen. They are not, however, under voluntary control, as the individual is not conscious or aware of their psychological basis – that is, the individual is not intentionally producing symptoms or otherwise malingering. Such symptoms arise via the unconscious defence mechanism of displacement. This group of disorders was central in the history of the development of psychoanalytical theory.

Classically, symptoms in dissociative (conversion) disorders are of symbolic significance and have an unconscious motivation or primary gain, such as relief from intolerable intrapsychic conflict or the reduction or loss of anxiety, which may present as a calm acceptance (*la belle indifférence*) of what appears to be a serious disability. Internal conflicts are kept away from awareness. The gain is primary psychological, not financial, legal or social. Thus, an individual who is fearful both of battle and of being thought a coward may solve this conflict unconsciously by developing paralysis of the lower limbs, thus symbolizing the conflict. Similarly, individuals who unconsciously do not wish to see or hear what is going on may develop hysterical blindness or deafness. In the past, 'hysterical fits' (dissociative seizures) in females were related to sexual 'frigidity'. Individuals may also achieve secondary gain from their symptoms, such as attention, care and affection from others, including relatives, by the manipulation of relationships and by avoiding unwanted everyday tasks or situations – that is, adopting the advantages of the sick role.

Theoretically, in dissociative and conversion disorders the motivation is unconscious, whereas in malingering it is conscious. In clinical practice, however, such a differentiation may be less clear cut and it is often better to assess the degree of unconsciousness of motivation, which itself may vary over time.

Family and early background, and cultural factors, may determine the choice of hysterical symptoms, which may be modelled closely on symptoms experienced during a childhood illness, when the rewards of attention resulting from the sick role may have been learned. Similarly, an individual may develop a conversion symptom when a close relative develops similar symptoms, such as paralysis of one side as the result of a stroke.

In the past, hysterical fainting by females was common, but this is now a rare event. Similarly, in developed countries, gross paralysis of the limbs is now less common, while more subtle neurological conversion symptoms are more apparent. Gross conversion symptoms, however, still occur frequently in some developing countries.

Neurophysiological studies show that although an

individual with a conversion disorder may say that no feeling in an area is experienced, corresponding cortical evoked responses to tactile stimulation may be detected in the brain using an electroencephalogram. Individuals with conversion disorder (e.g. with limb paralysis) are suggestible and may 'take up their bed and walk' upon suggestion from a respected other. Alternatively, they may respond to physiotherapy, thereby unconsciously saving face.

Epidemiology

The age of onset is usually in adolescence or early adulthood, but the disorder may appear for the first time during middle age or even later. However, it should be emphasized that symptoms suggestive of a conversion disorder occurring in middle age or beyond are very likely to be due to organic illness. Although conversion disorder was considered common several decades ago, it is now encountered much more rarely. It is considered to be more common in women than in men. Most cases are seen in neurological or orthopaedic practice, and in military settings, especially at times of war. It may be more common in lower socioeconomic groups. The incidence is falling in developed countries, but it remains high in developing countries.

Clinical features

To summarize the above, symptoms have a primary gain that reduces anxiety and helps to resolve emotional conflict. They may be associated with secondary gain (e.g. attention of others), and symptoms may be symbolic and determined by, or modelled on, cultural, family or early background factors. Classically, symptoms may be calmly accepted (*la belle indifférence*), although in practice this is not seen frequently. However, the diagnosis is not dependent on the demonstration of gain or indifference. There is usually only one conversion symptom present in one episode of conversion disorder. Symptoms include the following:

- *Sensory symptoms:* these are incompatible with peripheral or central nervous system disorders and may include anaesthesias and paraesthesiae, especially of the extremities, e.g. 'stocking and glove' anaesthetic areas of the hands and feet (Figure 41.1).
- *Special sense organ symptoms:* these may include deafness and either unilateral or bilateral blindness or tunnel vision.
- *Motor signs:* see Figure 41.2.

Conversion symptoms may be distinguished from organic symptoms by their variability, their nature (which often reflects the individual's concept of anatomy and physiology) and their inconsistency with known anatomy and physiology (e.g. areas of stocking and glove anaesthesia). For example, individuals with hysterical aphonia are able to use the same muscles to cough that they would normally use to speak, while individuals with hysterical blindness may avoid colliding with objects. Areas of anaesthesia may be increased by suggestion from a doctor during an examination. Apparently paralysed extensor muscles of one leg may contract when the individual is asked to lie supine and raise the opposite leg.

History taking should concentrate on eliciting precipitating stress factors. A close relative or friend should also be interviewed, as this may help to elucidate, among other matters, the individual's use of the sick role. Physical examination and investigations should be completed quickly

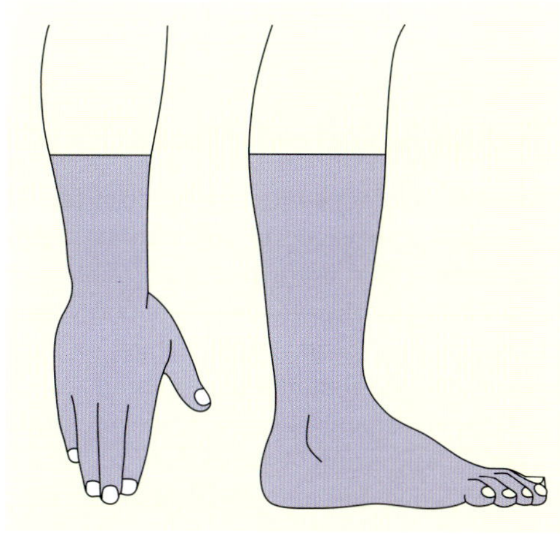

Figure 41.1 Typical areas of sensory loss in conversion disorders

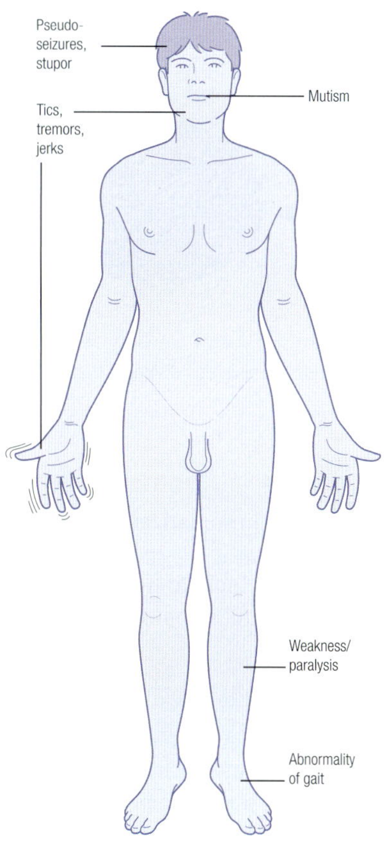

Figure 41.2 Common motor symptoms of conversion disorders

and, if normal, the physical symptoms themselves ignored thereafter.

Differential diagnosis

This includes any undiagnosed physical disorder, especially one that presents with vague multiple somatic symptoms, such as systemic lupus erythematosus (SLE) or multiple sclerosis. Undiagnosed physical disorders may be either difficult to diagnose (e.g. haemangioblastoma of the cerebellum or tumours of the foramen magnum) or not routinely considered (e.g. myasthenia gravis, acute intermittent porphyria). One classic study carried out at the National Hospital for Nervous Diseases in London on 85 patients diagnosed as having hysteria showed that after a follow-up period of 9 years, the diagnosis of hysteria had been replaced in one-third by that of an organic disorder.[7] For example, hysterical pain had been replaced by a diagnosis of trigeminal neuralgia or basilar artery migraine; hysterical paraesthesia and weakness by Takayasu's disease; and hysterical fits by epilepsy (Figure 41.3). However, subsequent studies have found lower rates (1–3%) of development of neurological disorders.[8,9] In another 24 individuals, the diagnosis of hysteria coexisted at the outset with that of an organic disorder. Overall, only 39 per cent had no significant organic disorder, and these included seven patients with recurrent depression, two with schizophrenia and four who had committed suicide.

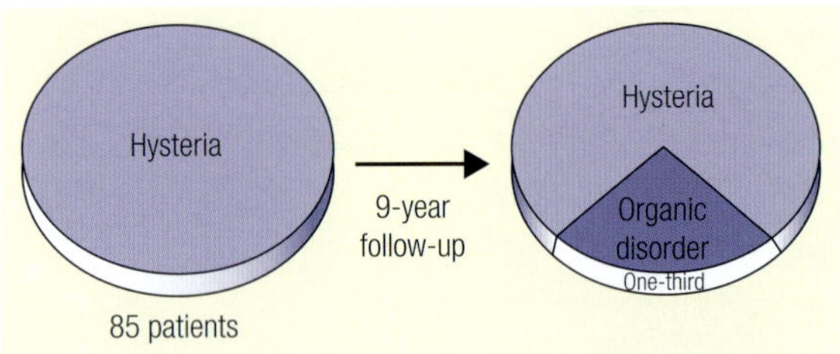

Figure 41.3 Results of Slater's 1965 study on conversion disorder ('hysteria') outcomes

Conversion symptoms can occur in somatization disorder and, more rarely, in schizophrenia.

Other diagnoses to be considered include hypochondriacal disorder and malingering, where symptoms are consciously produced.

Aetiology

Predisposing factors

There is little evidence in favour of a genetic predisposition to conversion disorders.

Freud initially used the term 'conversion'.[10] He had observed the French neurologist Charcot producing conversion hysteria in susceptible individuals by the use of hypnosis and even suggestion. The mechanisms underlying this condition have been sought, unsatisfactorily, ever since.[11] Freud saw these disorders as arising from mental or psychological energy and anxiety being repressed and converted into physical symptoms, which were often suggestive of a neurological disease and which resulted in avoidance of emotional conflict and thus a reduction in intrapsychic anxiety. The conflict is between instinctual impulses, for example aggressive or sexual, and inhibition against their expression.

A premorbid histrionic, dependent, passive–aggressive or antisocial personality disorder may be present in up to one-fifth of cases. Traits of suggestibility and increased capacity to dissociate may predispose towards the development of conversion symptoms.

Learning theory explains conversion disorders in terms of classical conditioning.

Previous physical disorders or exposure to such disorders in other people may be a predisposing factor by providing a model for the choice of conversion symptom. For instance, dissociative convulsions (pseudoseizures) are more likely to occur in people with epilepsy, as this provides a model for their symptoms; they have also learned the advantages of the sick role as a result of their condition.

The increased incidence of conversion disorder in young and immature people may reflect the fact that they have emerged only recently from the privileged dependent state of childhood. Similarly, it has been suggested that the greater proportion of women with the disorder apparent in the past perhaps reflected their overall greater dependence on men. In keeping with this theory, the ratio of females to males with the disorder has fallen considerably in recent decades.

Precipitating and perpetuating factors

Precipitating factors include severe stress, such as the recent death of a close relative, whose physical symptoms may be modelled by the patient, and at times of war. In fact, experience of warfare suggests that all individuals are capable of developing a conversion disorder. Head injury and temporal lobe epilepsy have also been suggested as precipitating factors. Impaired action generation with decreased activity in the left dorsolateral prefrontal cortex has also been found.[12]

The condition is perpetuated by secondary gain and the advantages of the sick role (see above).

The possibility of financial gain, such as in compensation neurosis, may also perpetuate the disorder. Table 41.2 summarizes the aetiology of conversion disorders.

Management

Most cases remit with non-specific supportive measures, particularly if suggestion is used. To prevent secondary

Table 41.2 Aetiology of conversion disorders

Predisposing factors	Childhood experience of illness
Precipitating factors	Physical illness, e.g. epilepsy
	Guillain–Barré syndrome
	Negative life events
	Relationship conflict
	Modelling of others' illness
Perpetuating factors	Behavioural responses, e.g. avoidance, disuse, reassurance-seeking
	Cognitive responses, e.g. fear of worsening, fear of serious disease

gain, chronicity or relapse, early resolution of symptoms is important. Physical investigations should be undertaken only if indicated, not merely as reassurance. In the absence of any abnormalities, the patient should be firmly reassured that there is no serious illness present and that the symptoms are familiar to the doctor and will remit. Any associated psychiatric disorder should be treated in its own right. Relaxation training, hypnosis and anxiolytics may also be of value.

If the symptoms do not remit, or precipitating or perpetuating factors continue, then it is necessary to help the patient to recognize these and to take action to counter them in order to prevent chronicity. Cognitive-behavioural therapy (CBT) has been found to be the most effective specific treatment. Cognitive-behavioural and physiological factors interrelate. Therefore, cognitive-behavioural treatments can result in physiological changes. Behaviour therapy alone has clinically been found to be effective. Psychotherapy may be indicated to gain insight into and explore the origins of the symptoms (e.g. by linking them to mood). However, the severe stresses may prevent the individual from discussing these problems.

Abreaction may also be indicated. This is the recall to consciousness of the underlying and causative repressed trauma, with the simultaneous re-experiencing of the emotion that originally accompanied it. Methods of achieving abreaction (catharsis) include psychotherapy alone, hypnosis[13] and the use of drugs, most safely with intravenous diazepam, although intravenous barbiturates and amphetamines have also been used.

Secondary gain may need to be countered by behavioural therapy and environmental manipulation. The advantages of the sick role should be minimized and those of health maximized. The involvement and help of family members and other individuals important to the patient may have to enlisted.

Prognosis

In general, the prognosis for most patients is good, with complete and rapid recovery either spontaneously or upon removal of the precipitating factors. Good prognosis is associated with acute onset and a clear and resolvable emotional conflict. If the condition persists after 1 year, the course is likely to be more intractable. Intractability is also associated with personality difficulties and poor motivation. About one-quarter of patients will have another conversion symptom within 6 years.

The prognosis is also better for a sustained disabling conversion disorder, such as paralysis, than for the intermittent use of symptoms such as dissociative convulsions (pseudoseizures), or where the symptom produces little disability in everyday life.

SOMATOFORM DISORDERS

ICD-10 divides the somatoform disorders into somatization disorder, hypochondriacal disorder and persistent pain disorder (Table 41.3). DSM-IV-TR also includes conversion disorder, which has already been described, and body dysmorphic disorder (dysmorphophobia) (Box 41.3).

Hypochondriacal disorder (hypochondriasis or hypochondriacal neurosis or severe health anxiety)

This is characterized by a persistent belief in the presence of one or more serious physical illnesses underlying the presenting symptom or symptoms, even though repeated examination and investigations have identified no adequate physical explanation. There is a persistent refusal to accept

Box 41.3 Somatoform disorders as described in DSM-IV-TR

- Somatization disorder
- Undifferentiated somatoform disorder
- Body dysmorphic disorder
- Conversion disorder
- Hypochondriasis.

Table 41.3 Somatoform disorders as described in ICD-10

Disorder	Characteristics
Somatoform disorder	At least 2 years of multiple and variable physical symptoms for which no adequate physical explanation has been found
	Persistent refusal to accept the advice or reassurance of several different doctors that there is no physical explanation for the symptoms
	Some degree of impairment of social and family functioning attributable to the nature of the symptoms and resulting behaviour
Hypochondriacal disorder	Persistent belief in the presence of one or more serious physical illnesses underlying the presenting symptom(s), despite strong evidence to the contrary, or a persistent preoccupation with a presumed disfigurement
	Persistent refusal to accept the advice or reassurance of several different doctors that there is no physical illness underlying the symptoms
Persistent pain disorder	Severe and distressing pain that cannot be explained fully by a physiological process or physical disorder
	Occurs in association with emotional conflict or psychosocial problems sufficient to allow the conclusion that they are the main causative influences
	Usually results in marked increase in support and attention

the advice and reassurance of doctors that no such physical illness exists.

Hypochondriacal disorder can thus be defined as an excessive concern about having a serious disease and morbid preoccupation with one's body or state of health, which is out of proportion to actual medical morbidity and is present for a major part of the time. Characteristic features include the following:

- Somatic (bodily) symptoms without medical explanation
- Disease conviction (belief in an occult medical illness, which is, in fact, not present)
- Disease fear
- Bodily preoccupation.

The term 'hypochondriasis' is also used to refer to a personality trait or a symptom in a number of psychiatric disorders (e.g. depression). Hypochondriacal symptoms are, in fact, most often seen as a feature of depressive disorder. The term 'hypochondriasis' originates from the ancient belief that it was associated with physical disorder of the organs below (*hypo-*) the costal margin (*chondrica*).

Epidemiology

This disorder can begin at any age but most commonly between the ages of 20 years and 30 years. It occurs slightly more commonly in males, or at least equally to females, in contrast to other somatoform disorders, which are more common in women. Its exact prevalence in the general population is unknown, and this is compounded by the fact that hypochondriacal complaints occur more commonly as part of another psychiatric syndrome, such as depressive disorder. Although hypochondriacal disorder is commonly seen in general medical practice (estimates of 4–15%), such individuals often refuse referral to mental health services and so are not frequently seen in psychiatric facilities.

Primary hypochondriacal disorder is said to occur more often in lower social classes, very young people, elderly people, Jewish people and people associated with disease, including medical students. It may be more common in non-European cultures, where depressive disorder presents more commonly with hypochondriacal/somatic features.

Clinical features

Individuals experience symptoms that strongly suggest disease to them but not to their examining doctors. Even if organic disease is present, symptoms will be disproportionate and typically refer to a number of anatomical locations and organs. Individuals are very concerned as to the exact significance of the symptoms and their aetiology, and also with their authenticity being accepted by others. They are convinced that they have a serious disease that is yet to be detected, and they cannot be persuaded otherwise, in spite of adequate reassurance, negative investigation results and a benign course of their condition over time.

Patients have a disease fear that is intense and persistent. They are vigilant to the slightest indication of illness, which alarms them greatly. Their bodily preoccupation is profound and extends to their general health status. They scrutinize themselves intensely. They habitually visit general practice and hospital clinics and accumulate a long history of medical contact. Ultimately, they always remain dissatisfied by their contact with the medical profession, whom they often criticize and blame for their continuing complaints, and a deteriorating doctor–patient relationship is common.

Differential diagnosis

This includes true organic disease, especially the early stages of neurological disorders such as multiple sclerosis, endocrine disorders such as thyroid or parathyroid disease, and also disorders that frequently affect multiple body systems (such as SLE). The presence of true organic disease does not, however, rule out coexisting hypochondriacal disorder.

Hypochondriacal symptoms are most often seen, in up to 80 per cent of cases, in depressive disorder. Somatic delusions of physical disease may be present in psychotic disorders, including depression and schizophrenia. In hypochondriacal disorder, beliefs are characteristically not of delusional intensity, in that the individual will accept the possibility that the disease may not be present, although such distinctions may be difficult to make, especially initially. Hypochondriacal concerns may also be present in generalized anxiety disorder, panic disorder and somatization disorder. In somatization disorder, the preoccupation is with the symptoms rather than the fear of having a specific disease or diseases.

Aetiology

Hypochondriasis is a polythetic disease – that is, it has numerous interacting causes. It has been argued that it is a variant form of other mental illnesses, such as depression or anxiety disorder, rather than a primary neurotic disorder.[14] However, the validity of primary hypochondriasis has been confirmed.[15]

Predisposing factors

Past experience of true organic disease, especially in childhood, in either oneself or a family member, predisposes to the development of this disorder (e.g. by modelling or reinforcement). Illness may have been a particular focus of attention and source of concern for family members of such patients.

Psychodynamic theory holds that hypochondriacal symptoms and associated suffering are assumed to have an unconscious meaning and gratification for an individual. Hypochondriacal disorder has been viewed as a somatic expression of oral dependency needs, including nurturing, attention, physical contact and sympathy. It has also been viewed as a transformation, through repression and displacement, of aggressive and hostile wishes arising from the past towards other people in the present, to whom such individuals make numerous and persistent physical complaints.

Hypochondriacal disorder has been seen as a hypochondriacal personality disorder.[16] It has also been viewed as a non-verbal communication from individuals with interpersonal problems. For an individual feeling overwhelmed by apparently insoluble problems, such complaints may represent a request to be placed in the sick role, in order to avoid normal obligations, postpone unwelcome events, and attract support and sympathy with no implications of blame.

Precipitating and perpetuating factors

Precipitating factors are usually significant psychosocial stresses. The condition is perpetuated by the persistence of such stresses, unresolved psychodynamic factors and the advantages of the sick role.

Management

This is usually undertaken by a general practitioner (GP), as such individuals often do not find psychiatric referral acceptable. Organic disease should be excluded, and any primary psychiatric disorder, such as depression, should be treated vigorously.

Specific psychiatric treatment may be of benefit if the individual can acknowledge emotional difficulties underlying the physical complaints. Psychiatric treatment is better undertaken in a non-psychiatric medical setting, with an emphasis on the reduction of psychosocial stresses and education about the role of psychological factors in the development of symptoms, and how to cope with such symptoms. The psychodynamic meaning of the symptoms should be sought, as should their relationship to the family and social situation. However, one should be cautious if it is clear that the symptoms are acting as a last-ditch powerful psychological defence.

CBT is the specific treatment of first choice. Misinterpretations should be identified and challenged and realistic interpretations substituted. Graded exposure to illness cues and illness related situations with response prevention should be undertaken, and core illness beliefs modified. Such an approach can result in up to 75 per cent symptom reduction.[17]

Antidepressant medication, particularly of the selective serotonin reuptake inhibitor (SSRI) type, is recommended by some for all such patients, particularly as most hypochondriacal symptoms in the general population are secondary to depression, which may explain the response. Antidepressant treatment is certainly the second-line treatment of choice if CBT fails or if there is significant comorbidity or severe symptoms.

Group psychotherapy is the psychotherapeutic approach of choice, although the primary aim is usually supportive rather than curative. The evidence for this and for individual insight-oriented psychotherapy is lacking.

Overall, it is worth remembering that the patient is symptomatic for psychological and social reasons, and no specific medical or surgical intervention will cure the need to be sick. The aim is to concentrate on the person as a whole. The patient should be seen regularly and attention given to any social and personal factors from which the complaints are considered to arise.

Specific medical interventions should be kept to a minimum, for example a simple physical examination. The main treatment is the physician's personal attention. Elaborate and invasive diagnostic and therapeutic procedures should be undertaken only when there is objective evidence for their use, and incidental abnormalities and equivocal findings should not be treated.

Prognosis

The prognosis is often poor, with individuals having chronic mild disability for most of their adult life. The more chronic the condition, the worse the prognosis. Where symptoms are associated with depressive or generalized anxiety disorder, the prognosis is better.

Somatization disorder (Briquet's syndrome, St Louis hysteria)

This is a chronic syndrome of multiple somatic (physical) symptoms, which have persisted for several years with no adequate medical explanation associated with psychosocial distress, impairment and medical help-seeking. There is no autonomic overstimulation. The alternative terms of 'Briquet's syndrome' and 'St Louis hysteria' arose from Briquet's 1859 concept of hysteria, which was revived by psychiatrists at Washington University, St Louis.[18]

The ICD-10 description of somatization disorder is given in Table 41.3. It will be seen that at least 2 years of multiple and variable physical symptoms are required for diagnosis. DSM-IV-TR criteria for somatization disorder indicate that the disorder should begin before the age of 30 years, must be of several years' duration, must not be caused or explained fully by organic disease, medication, illicit drugs or alcohol, and has caused the individual to seek treatment or resulted in significant impairment of social, occupational or other important areas or functions. For the diagnosis to be, made the individual must have had:

- two gastrointestinal symptoms, e.g. vomiting;
- four pain symptoms, e.g. pain in extremities;
- one sexual symptom other than pain;
- one pseudo-neurological symptom, e.g. amnesia or difficulty in swallowing.

These symptoms must not be intentionally produced or feigned (as in, respectively, factitious disorder or malingering).

Epidemiology

This disorder is diagnosed very rarely in males; for females, prevalence rates of up to 2 per cent have been found. Women have been found to outnumber men with this condition 5- to 20-fold. Symptoms begin in the teenage years or, rarely, in the twenties, usually before the age of 30 years.

Clinical features

Patients have long and complicated medical histories, with many diagnoses having usually been considered. Even if some benign organic disorders have been diagnosed, the complaints and disabilities are excessive and the individual is severely disabled. The majority are unable to work and may spend up to one-quarter of each month in bed. They may consult a number of doctors, at a number of institutions, even at the same time.

Associated features include the following:

- Anxiety, depression, threats of suicide and parasuicide attempts
- Increased incidence of antisocial personality disorder, and alcohol and drug abuse
- Interpersonal discord.

History-taking often reveals poor childhood adjustment, school difficulties, a disturbed adolescence, menstruation difficulties and dysmenorrhoea from menarche, sexual activity from an early age with sexual problems common, interpersonal discord, unstable relationships, a number of marriages, and inconsistent or neglectful parenting of any children.

Differential diagnosis

Physical disorders should be ruled out, particularly those with vague, multiple or confusing somatic symptoms, such as hyperparathyroidism, porphyria, multiple sclerosis and SLE. Multiple physical symptoms of late onset in life are almost always due to physical disease. In somatization disorder, there is an early onset of multiple symptoms involving a number of body systems and a long but benign course without the development of serious medical illnesses.

Unlike hypochondriasis, in somatization disorder there is less disease conviction, less disease fear and less bodily preoccupation. In addition, somatization disorder primarily affects females, whereas in hypochondriacal disorder males are affected at least equally.

The differential diagnosis also includes conversion disorder, depressive disorder, panic disorder and schizophrenia with multiple somatic delusions. Such disorders may coexist with somatoform disorder, particularly depression, and increase physical symptoms and negative appraisal of them.

Aetiology

Genetic and environmental factors probably both have a role. Monozygotic compared to dizygotic twin concordance in somatoform disorders was found to be 29 : 10 in one study.[19] Somatization disorder occurs in 10–20 per cent of first-degree female relatives. First-degree male relatives, however, have an increased incidence of alcoholism, drug abuse and antisocial personality disorder. Such genetic predisposition is in contrast to its absence in conversion disorder. Abnormal regulation of the cytokine system has also been hypothesized. Parental example may lead to behavioural learning of this condition, and physical illness in childhood may result in somatic rather than emotional responses for attention, care and countering hostility in adulthood.[20]

Management

Ideally, the diagnosis should be made early and unnecessary organic investigations and interventions avoided, as these are likely to result in further complaints arising from complications of the procedures, side effects of medication and iatrogenic disease. Medical practitioners are reluctant to diagnose somatoform disorder but are inclined to search for rare medical illnesses. The gallbladder, uterus, appendix and teeth may all be needlessly removed. The aim should be to direct attention to the associated psychosocial stresses in the patient's life and away from the symptoms. 'Doctor shopping' should be discouraged, and instead an attempt should be made to engage the patient in a long-term supportive therapeutic relationship with the GP, who can be advised, as required, by a psychiatrist as to the nature of the disorder and the feasible goals of treatment. Although the goal is to move the patient beyond somatization, a complete elimination of symptoms is unlikely, and general support and care of the patient is more important. Specific CBT may assist, by leading to the reattribution of physical symptoms,[21] for example through behavioural experiments with hyperventilation. Fixed beliefs by patients that their physical symptoms are due to environmental hypersensitivity and Candida are, however, difficult to alter. Psychodynamic psychotherapy has also been used. Psychotropic medication and analgesics tend not to be effective and such patients often concentrate on the resulting side effects.

Prognosis

This is generally poor, with a chronic course, repeated recurrences of symptoms, and disability persisting for most of the patient's life. Symptoms do tend to be more florid in early adult life, but the course is often fluctuating. Spontaneous remission is very rare. It is unlikely that such individuals will go more than 2 years without medical attention.

Dissociation, conversion and somatization have been integrated into a *unified model of medically unexplained symptoms*, including as regards its treatment.[22]

Persistent somatoform pain disorder (psychogenic pain)

The essential feature of this disorder is the preoccupation with persistent, severe and distressing pain in the absence of adequate physical findings to account for the pain or its intensity.[23] Pure psychogenic pain is, in fact, rare compared with psychological elaboration of pain associated with existing or previous injuries.

Pain always has a psychological component to it and has been defined as an unpleasant sensory and emotional experience associated with actual or potential tissue damage. Psychiatric consultation is often requested for people with chronic pain, which is not an uncommon complaint. Although many patients may have a past history of injuries, they often show no current evidence of tissue or nerve damage. In normal circumstances healing takes place within 3 months, or more rarely up to 6 months, and the correlation between pain and injury is poor after that period.

Epidemiology

The disorder is considered to be common in general medical practice. It is diagnosed almost twice as frequently in females as in males. Onset can occur at any age but is most frequent in the thirties and forties.

Clinical features

The normal course is for pain to appear suddenly and to increase in severity over a few weeks to months. Such pain is inconsistent with the anatomical distribution of the nervous system. Characteristically, the pain is continuous for much of the day, may cause difficulty in getting off to sleep but does not cause wakening, and has symbolic significance, for example chest pain in an individual who had a relative who died from a heart attack.

The common sites of pain are summarized in Figure 41.4. There is limited insight into associated psychological factors and patients characteristically respond less well to analgesics than to psychotropic medication. Persistent pain

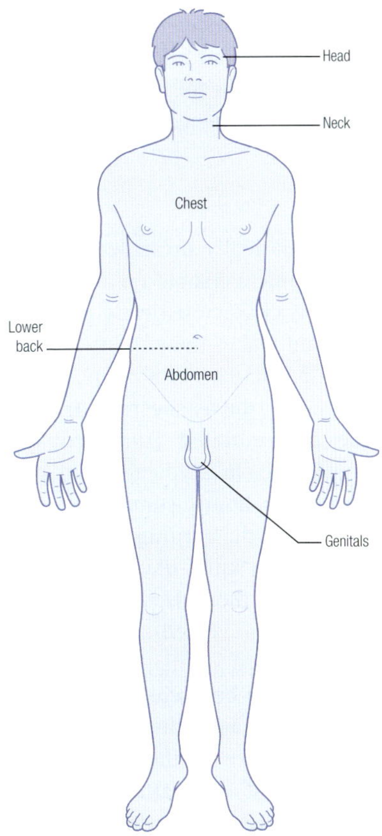

Figure 41.4 Common sites of psychogenic pain

disorder may be accompanied by local sensory and motor changes, such as paraesthesiae and muscle spasm. 'Doctor shopping' and excessive use of analgesics without relief are often seen. A past history of conversion symptoms is common, as is an associated depressive disorder.

The pain solves a psychological problem for the patient and may be ameliorated by psychological and environmental changes. It also corresponds to ideas held by the patient about the condition. The degree of resulting disability reflects these beliefs rather than the severity of any previous injury or organic disease. The more uncertain the patient is of the cause of this pain, or the greater the belief that the pain will endure, the worse the disability and the associated demoralization. The complaint often increases following extensive investigations with negative results, which merely frustrates the patient.

The history may reveal a vulnerable hypochondriacal personality with a low pain threshold. Getting a history from an informant is also useful and previous hospital records will need to be examined. The previous psychiatric history may reveal similar episodes, including similar causes and precipitants.

Physical examination is required, not only to exclude organic disease but also to gain credibility in the patient's eyes and to appreciate more fully the complaints. Persistent pain disorder is characterized on examination by overreaction to the examination itself, diffuse superficial tenderness, and weakness of all muscle groups in the region.

Investigations might also include requesting the patient to complete a diary of pain and associated behaviour and activities. This may reveal, for instance, that the pain is worse if the patient's partner is present and being sympathetic. Following assessment, it may be harmful to continue with a diary, as this may merely increase the patient's attention to the pain.

Differential diagnosis

True organic pain may be dramatically presented, particularly in patients with a histrionic personality. A physical cause is suggested if the pain is characteristically described as 'sore, boring or nagging' and wakes the patient at night, and also if it is localized to a particular dermatome.

Atypical facial pain, which may be as severe as trigeminal neuralgia, should be differentiated from temporomandibular joint (TMJ) syndrome. In atypical facial pain, the pain usually lasts minutes to hours, sometimes being continuous. The pain is aching, dull, burning or crushing, although occasionally it is sharp or knife-like. In TMJ syndrome there is focal tenderness of the TMJ, aggravated by talking, chewing or lateral jaw movement; this requires referral to an oral surgeon.

Other psychiatric illnesses should be excluded, in particular depressive disorder and somatization disorder, but pain rarely dominates the clinical picture of these conditions, although patients often complain of aches and pains. Some psychotic individuals, such as those with schizophrenia, may have a delusional pain syndrome. Generalized anxiety disorder may present with muscle pain and tension headaches. Malingering should also be excluded. Individuals dependent on narcotics may complain of pain in order to obtain opioids.

Aetiology

Predisposing factors

Patients with this disorder are more likely to have begun working at an unusually early age, held jobs that were physically strenuous or overly routinized, or been workaholics and rarely taken time off. In many cases, however, the pain is shaped by organic, psychological, personal and cultural factors.

A pain-prone personality profile has been proposed. Such personalities court injuries and unsuccessful surgery. However, such a profile, for example the inverted V profile on the Minnesota Multiphasic Personality Inventory (MMPI) (high scores for hypochondriasis and hysteria and a low score for depression), is often secondary to the impact of chronic pain.

A further theory suggests that such individuals come from an abusive parental family background, where the child is subject to physical abuse from parents who subsequently show remorse and comfort, so that the child grows up associating parental love with pain and suffering. However, such a background is infrequently seen in clinical practice, although an increased history of childhood physical and sexual abuse has been identified. Some ethnic and cultural groups, such as Asians, are said to somatize problems more frequently.

Precipitating and perpetuating factors

These include physical trauma, which occurs in about half of cases, and dissatisfaction with employment before injury.

A background of litigation with a view to compensation makes the resolution of the pain very unlikely while litigation is in progress. Even after a satisfactory legal settlement, a number of patients will continue to complain of chronic pain.

This disorder has also been considered as a variant of depressive disorder.[24]

Management

Organic disease should be excluded and, if it cannot, a full evaluation of the degree and extent of physical pathology and its contribution to the presentation of pain should be made.

Adequate medical treatment of any organic basis to pain is essential. Multidisciplinary pain clinics, with an anaesthetist, psychiatrist and physician present, may facilitate management. Current psychosocial stresses will need to be resolved. Antidepressants that affect both serotonin and noradrenaline reuptake, such as amitriptyline, are more effective than those that act mainly on noradrenaline uptake. Tricyclic antidepressants also have an analgesic action of faster onset than, and that is independent of, their antidepressant effects. Cognitive-behavioural methods of treatment have also been found to be of value.

Prognosis

In most cases the symptom has persisted for many years by the time the individual comes to the attention of psychiatrists. Patients who express emotional distress with physical symptoms tend to do poorly, whereas those who are able to accept the pain and appreciate that their own efforts to improve the quality of their life are of the utmost importance tend to do better.

Body dysmorphic disorder (dysmorphophobia)

This is a distressing preoccupation with some imagined or slight defect of appearance in a normal-appearing person. If a slight physical anomaly is present, the person's concern is grossly excessive. However, there is no correlation between body dysmorphic disorder and the degree of deformity. The belief in the defect is not of delusional intensity, although in clinical practice this distinction is often difficult to make and may not be valid, as the belief may vary from an overvalued idea to a delusion.[25] The term 'dysmorphic' originates from the Greek word for 'ugliness of face'. Although patients do often fear ridicule, and even fear upsetting others and thus show avoidance, the European term 'dysmorphophobia' is not used in the American DSM-IV-TR, as it is argued that there is no pure phobic avoidance.[26] In ICD-10, both dysmorphophobia and body dysmorphic disorder are included under the category of hypochondriacal disorder.

Epidemiology

The most common age of onset is from adolescence through to the third decade. Psychiatrists see only a small proportion of cases, and the disorder may actually be more common than thought previously. Women are affected slightly more often than men. Patients are more likely to go to a plastic surgeon or dermatologist than to a psychiatrist. Studies of US college students have suggested that a quarter may meet DSM-IV-TR criteria for body dysmorphic disorder.

Clinical features

The most common imagined defects are of the face, including wrinkles, the shape of the nose, excessive facial hair and facial asymmetries. More rarely, the complaint involves the feet, hands, back, breasts or genitals. Any preoccupation with the genitals and breasts must be more than is normal. Women are more preoccupied with breast and legs and are more likely to use make-up as camouflage and check their appearance in the mirror. Men are more preoccupied with their genitals, height and excess body hair.[27] There is never a disturbance of the whole body image, as is seen in anorexia nervosa, but more than one imagined defect in appearance may occur at one time, or a series may occur over time. The disorder can be markedly disabling, resulting in repeated visits to plastic surgeons or dermatologists in an effort at 'correction'. There is avoidance of social or occupational situations because of anxiety and fear of attention. Worry, dysphoria and depressive disorder frequently occur. Co-morbidity is frequent; in women this is often with generalized anxiety disorder, panic disorder and bulimia, while in men there is a lifetime co-morbidity increase in bipolar disorder. The individual's whole lifestyle may be affected: they become socially isolated, restrict their activities and are usually unmarried. They may frequently check their appearance in the mirror and may often change their hairstyle to alter their appearance.

Feeling grossly disfigured, such individuals often fear seeking help or present to a plastic surgeon or dermatologist before a psychiatrist. They may also fear being viewed as vain about their appearance. They are very sensitive to, and feel confused about, their internal, ideal and actual self-image. They may become socially isolated, unemployed and suicidal. One-quarter of the patients attempt suicide.

Differential diagnosis

Anorexia nervosa or transsexualism do not fulfil the diagnostic criteria for body dysmorphic disorder, as these two conditions are characterized by a disturbance of the whole body image and not some imagined defect in appearance. Concern about minor defects in appearance, such as acne, is common but not grossly excessive in normal adolescence. Individuals may exaggerate defects in appearance in major depression, as may individuals with an anxious (avoidant) personality disorder and social phobia, but such symptoms are not the predominant disturbance.

In delusional disorders, an individual's belief in a defect of appearance is of delusional intensity, which by definition is not the case in body dysmorphic disorder. Studies have suggested that up to 50 per cent of people complaining of a large nose and requesting plastic surgery are 'neurotic', but an increased incidence of schizophrenia and depression has also been found.

Aetiology

There is little definitive information on predisposing factors of body dysmorphic disorder. In psychodynamic theory, body dysmorphic disorder has been considered to represent an unconscious displacement on to body parts of sexual or emotional conflicts, or more general feelings of inferiority, poor self-image or guilt. Alternatively, the disorder may be used to explain the individual's failures with, and suffering in relation to, the opposite sex. In Freud's classic case history of 'the Wolf Man', the patient is described as neglecting his daily life and work because of his perception of a defect in appearance of his nose.

Some individuals have a sudden onset of body dysmorphic disorder precipitated after distressing experiences, including abandonment by their partner.

Increased family history of affective disorder and obsessive–compulsive disorder and high co-morbidity with depressive disorder are seen. The pathophysiology may involve serotonin, given the response of the condition to SSRI antidepressants.

Relationship with other psychiatric disorders

A relationship between body dysmorphic disorder and a number of other psychiatric disorders has been postulated, including mood disorder, obsessive–compulsive disorder and schizophrenia. It has been suggested that body dysmorphic disorder may, in fact, be only a non-specific symptom of such conditions. The links appear to be greatest with obsessive–compulsive disorder, but in that disorder preoccupying thoughts are more intrusive and unnatural than in body dysmorphic disorder.

The condition may also be related to delusional disorders, although by definition the defect is not of delusional intensity in body dysmorphic disorder. Where the belief is of delusional intensity, the terms 'monosymptomatic hypochondriasis' and 'monosymptomatic hypochondriacal psychosis' have been used. In fact, the delusional intensity of such beliefs can vary with time, and thus the clinical picture overlaps with body dysmorphic disorder.

Management

Although CBT and psychodynamic psychotherapy have been described as being of benefit, and CBT should be the first-line treatment of choice, with proven benefit over 2 years,[28] it appears that the best results may be obtained by using SSRI antidepressants.[29,30] Surgery is not generally effective, as patients often express dissatisfaction with the results, requesting and obtaining repeated operative procedures. However, where there is a slight physical anomaly and the defect in appearance is well circumscribed, some studies have shown good results from plastic surgery alone (e.g. rhinoplasty for a large nose).

Prognosis

The course is often chronic, persisting for several years, and often worsens over time in spite of treatment.

OTHER ASSOCIATED CONCEPTS

Undifferentiated somatoform disorder

This category, included within the somatoform disorders in DSM-IV-TR, is for individuals whose clinical picture does not meet the full criteria of somatization disorder. There may be either single circumscribed symptoms, such as difficulty in swallowing or, more commonly, multiple physical complaints, such as fatigue, loss of appetite or gastrointestinal problems. The duration of disturbance must be at least 6 months in order for this diagnosis to be made. The main categories of somatoform disorders are narrow, and most patients in clinical practice will be in this residual subcategory,[31] a reflection of the current unsatisfactory classification, or, alternatively, have another primary psychiatric disorder, such as depression or anxiety.

Medically unexplained physical symptoms

Most patients in clinical practice with such symptoms will, as described previously, have either undifferentiated somatoform disorder or another primary psychiatric disorder, such as anxiety, producing real somatic anxiety symptoms due to autonomic hyperactivity, or depression, producing for example, facial pain, (a depressive equivalent that is sometimes considered psychodynamically to equate to an emotional 'slap in the face'). The various terms used to refer to symptoms with no organic cause are listed in Box 41.4. Such terms are often used loosely and overlap.

About one in five new consultations in primary care will be with medically unexplained symptoms. This latter term avoids making assumptions about their cause. Many symptoms are transient, but one-third persist and cause distress and disability. They result from interactions between biological, psychological, social and cultural factors. All patients should be asked about low mood and biological symptoms of depression, their beliefs about their symptoms

Box 41.4 Terms applied to medically unexplained symptoms

- Hysterical
- Hypochondriacal
- Neurasthenia
- Chronic fatigue syndrome
- Myalgic encephalomyelitis (ME)
- Functional overlay
- Psychophysiological reaction
- Psychosomatic reaction
- Factitious
- Münchausen (hospital addiction) syndrome
- Malingering.

(e.g. fear of cancer), why they are seeking help now, and the relationship between symptoms, mood and social factors, with a view to the patient re-attributing the cause of their symptoms (e.g. relating overbreathing to anxiety or lower pain threshold to depression). The reality for patients of their symptoms should be accepted and an explanation of these should be provided if possible.

CBT can be of benefit, as can antidepressants for chronic pain and associated poor sleep, even in the absence of depression.

Somatization and medically unexplained symptoms

Somatization, from the Greek word *soma* ('body'), is a helpful concept in understanding patients with medically unexplained symptoms.[32] It is a tendency to experience physical distress and symptoms unaccounted for by pathological findings, to attribute them to physical illness, to communicate them and to seek medical help for them. It may be an earlier phenomenon than psychologization, which is especially prevalent in developed countries.[33]

Individuals in general may characteristically view symptoms as having physical, psychological or external causes. There may be a spectrum in the way individuals experience stress (Figure 41.5): at one extreme, this may be with pure psychic symptoms, such as worry about the stress; further along the spectrum, certain individuals may have free-floating anxiety, with both psychic and somatic symptoms; at the other extreme, individuals experience only somatic symptoms, which may be anxiety or depressive equivalents. The latter patients do not perceive such symptoms as having a psychological basis, which leads to their resisting psychological help and rather seeking a medical explanation. Somatization may be facultative and cease when help is received, or it may be a chronic true somatization of psychosocial distress.

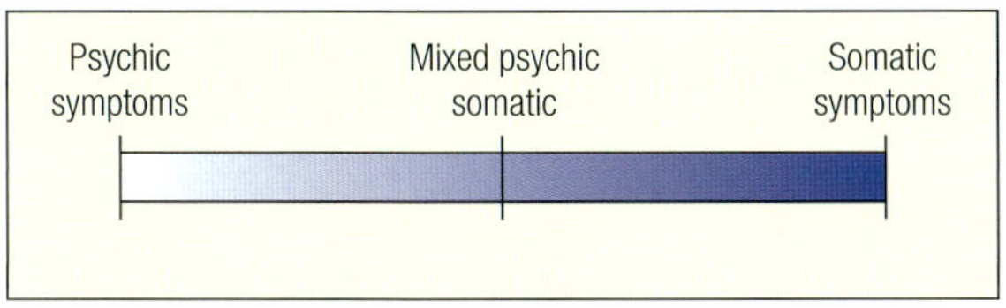

Figure 41.5 Spectrum of stress response

Autonomic hyperactivity accounts for the genuine somatic anxiety symptoms. In conversion disorders, physiological changes can be demonstrated in the voluntary nervous system. In hypochondriacal disorder, individuals are abnormally sensitive to normal sensations in the body.

Patients with medically unexplained physical symptoms exert disproportionately high financial and service burdens on health and social services. In any one week, 60–80 per cent of healthy people experience bodily symptoms, but only a small proportion of these will visit their GP; in 20 per cent, the physical symptoms will be due to minor emotional disorders. Patients who visit their GP may then be referred to hospital specialists, despite the absence of any abnormal physical findings on examination. Up to 40 per cent of patients seen by hospital medical specialists have medically unexplained physical symptoms and receive no organic diagnosis.

Such patients are resistant to any psychological interpretation, which they perceive as implying that their symptoms are not real but 'all in the mind'. However, it is important to remember that the causes of such symptoms do not have to be either physical or psychological – that is, if no organic disorder is found, it does not therefore have to be assumed to be a purely psychological problem. A medical model of disease does not, and should not, have to be restricted to organic or biological causes alone. Often psychiatric disorders are not looked for if any possible organic causative factor is found. In contrast, another investigation can always be proposed if no causative organic factor has been identified.

It is always important to consider not only the symptoms but also the patient's understanding of any illness and anxieties about it (i.e. thoughts) and the way the patient's daily life is affected by the symptoms (i.e. behaviour). A good doctor–patient interaction can be achieved only if the patient feels understood. With this in mind, it is possible to work with such patients' thoughts and behaviours via CBT.

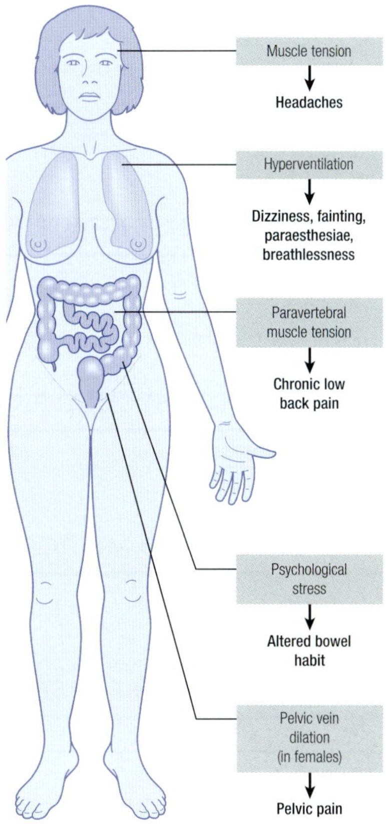

Figure 41.6 Pathophysiological mechanisms proposed for specific medically unexplained symptoms

Box 41.5 Interaction between psychiatric and physical disorders

ORGANIC MENTAL DISORDERS

Physical illness has direct effect on brain function:

- Delirium/acute confusional state/organic psychosis, e.g. liver failure
- Dementia/chronic organic psychosis
- Postoperative psychosis.

MALADAPTIVE PSYCHOLOGICAL REACTIONS TO ILLNESS

- Depression, e.g. amputation, mastectomy (due to loss)
- Guilt, e.g. fear of burden on relatives
- Anxiety, e.g. before operation, unpleasant procedure
- Paranoid reaction, e.g. if deaf or blind
- Anger
- Denial
- Preoccupation with illness
- Prolongation of sick role (fewer responsibilities, more attention).

PSYCHOSOMATIC DISEASE

Multiple (i.e. biopsychosocial) causes. For example life events/stress on physically and emotionally vulnerable, lead to changes in nervous, endocrine systems, etc. and disease. For example, bereavement may precipitate a heart attack, or stress may precipitate asthma, eczema or peptic ulcer.

PSYCHIATRIC CONDITIONS PRESENTING WITH PHYSICAL COMPLAINTS

- Somatic (physical) anxiety symptoms due to autonomic hyperactivity, e.g. palpitations
- Conversion disorders (via voluntary nervous system)
- Depression leading to facial pain, constipation, hypochondriacal complaints and delusions, e.g. of cancer, venereal disease
- Hypochondriacal disorder: excessive concern with health and normal sensations
- Somatization disorder
- Monosymptomatic hypochondriacal delusions, e.g. delusions of infestation or smell; other psychotic disorders, e.g. schizophrenia
- Münchausen (hospital addiction) syndrome
- Alcoholism, leading to liver disease
- Self-neglect.

PHYSICAL CONDITIONS PRESENTING WITH PSYCHIATRIC COMPLAINTS

- Depressive disorder precipitated by cancer, e.g. of pancreas
- Anxiety in hyperthyroidism
- Postviral depression, e.g. post-hepatitis, glandular fever, influenza.

MEDICAL DRUGS LEADING TO PSYCHIATRIC COMPLICATIONS

- Antihypertensive drugs leading to depression
- Corticosteroids leading to depression, euphoria.

PSYCHIATRIC DRUGS LEADING TO MEDICAL COMPLICATIONS

- Overdose
- Chlorpromazine leading to jaundice.

COINCIDENTAL PSYCHIATRIC AND PHYSICAL DISORDER

Box 41.6 Factors influencing response to physical illness

- *Patient:*
  - Personality, e.g. overanxious, obsessional
  - Illness behaviour, e.g. at what severity does the patient present?
- *Illness:*
  - Meaning and significance of illness, e.g. cancer.
- *Social environment:*
  - Threat to finances and employment
  - Welcomed if resolves conflict, e.g. marital.

Pathophysiological mechanisms proposed for specific medically unexplained symptoms

Figure 41.6 shows the proposed pathophysiological mechanisms for some specific medically unexplained symptoms.

Emotional arousal may lead to increased paravertebral muscle tension, which can be detected by an electromyogram, and results in chronic low back pain. Pelvic vein dilation may result in pelvic pain in females. Hyperventilation, with resetting of respiratory control mechanisms to a reduced $P\text{CO}_2$, may result in breathlessness or hyperventilation syndrome (HVS; also known as da Costa's Syndrome, cardiac neurosis, effort syndrome and circulatory neurasthenia). About one-quarter of patients with HVS have symptoms of panic disorder; 50–60 per cent of those with panic disorder or agoraphobia have symptoms of HVS. Inactivity, which reduces the capacity for further activity, and increased muscle tension may result in fatigue. Psychological stress produces irregular contractile activity of the smooth muscle in cases of altered bowel habit.

Box 41.5 outlines the interactions between psychiatric and physical disorders. Box 41.6 gives some examples of the factors influencing a patient's response to a physical illness.[34]

Psychological defensiveness, such as having a repressive coping style, may be associated with lower rates of psychopathology and psychiatric disorder, but this is counterbalanced by a restriction in self-awareness and interpersonal and social functioning, and a trade-off in physical ill-health, for example increased blood pressure and heart rate reactivity, reduced cell-mediated and humoral immunity responses, and possibly even progression of certain tumours, such as breast cancer.

Chronic fatigue syndrome

This is covered in detail in Chapter 51. In brief, chronic fatigue syndrome is characterized by the onset of unexplained physical and often mental fatigue, and heightened awareness of this, lasting for over 6 months and not related to ongoing exertion or alleviated by rest.[35] Prevalence is about seven in 100 000. It usually presents between 20 years and 50 years of age. Biopsychosocial factors contribute to the aetiology, and there is some evidence of genetic vulnerability.[36,37] Many patients relate the onset to an infection, which may indeed trigger the condition. In some cases, it may be a variant of the less chronic postviral infection fatigue. Some cases follow immunization. Evidence of Epstein–Barr virus infection is present in 10 per cent of cases. Most severe viral infections are associated with immunological abnormalities, especially in T-cell-mediated immunity.

Sixty per cent of patients have no previous psychiatric history, but one-half to two-thirds have a current co-morbid psychiatric disorder, especially minor depression in 40–50% of these cases, anxiety and somatization disorder. Diagnosis is based primarily on clinical history. The differential diagnosis includes depression. Co-morbidity with depression may be due to primary depression or depression secondary to chronic fatigue syndrome itself. Some authors argue that the condition is synonymous with the ICD-10 diagnosis of neurasthenia.[38] However, patients and their families frequently fear the stigma of a psychiatric diagnosis.

The condition is exacerbated, often a day or two later, by increased activity and by alcohol consumption. The essence of treatment is early paced activity management, avoiding over- and underactivity, and gradual rehabilitation with emotional support. CBT incorporating a rehabilitation approach and graded exercise can be offered as a more formalized approach and has been recommended by the National Institute for Health and Clinical Excellence (NICE).[39] Biofeedback approaches, self-help groups (attendees at these have a poorer prognosis), and psychodynamic therapy have also been used. Patients with chronic fatigue syndrome are sensitive to drug side effects, but low doses of tricyclic antidepressants can be helpful in improving sleep and alleviating pain. SSRI antidepressants in contrast may not be helpful unless depression is present. There is some evidence that treatment with essential fatty acids may be beneficial. Poor outcome is associated with personality disorder and prolonged convalescence.

Psychosomatic disorders

Rheumatoid arthritis, ulcerative colitis, bronchial asthma, essential hypertension, thyrotoxicosis and peptic ulcer have all been described as psychosomatic disorders, a category developed in the 1950s by analysts in the USA.[40] These are physical disorders aggravated or precipitated by psychological factors. Past theories that there are direct causal links between specific unconscious conflicts, psychological methods employed by individuals in coping with them and the development of specific organic diseases have now fallen into disrepute, for example for asthma,[41] and a more general theory has evolved, linking psychological stress in people with a vulnerable personality and an inherent vulnerability of certain of their bodily systems, leading to autonomic, endocrine or immunological changes, which in turn precipitate an organic disease to which they are predisposed. For instance, life events may precipitate a myocardial infarction, although the underlying coronary artery disease would already have been present. An increased vulnerability to cardiovascular conditions has been demonstrated in the first year after the death of a spouse. A link has also been suggested between coronary heart disease and type A personality (ambitious, aggressive and competitive, with a chronic sense of time urgency). Some authors also regard obesity and anorexia nervosa as psychosomatic disorders.

Other concepts and disorders related to physical complaints

These are described here for comparison, but are not by definition somatization disorders.

Monosymptomatic hypochondriacal psychosis

Those conditions where hypochondriacal delusions occur may take various forms.[42] There may be a delusion of insect infestation of the skin (Ekbom's syndrome),[43] delusions of lumps under the skin, delusions of internal parasitosis and a delusion that the individual is emitting a foul smell. Delusionally believing that there is a physical cause, the patient attempts to gather evidence for this and seeks multiple medical opinions, perhaps with themselves suggesting bizarre treatments. Although such patients may become paranoid and angry towards their doctors, there may be an otherwise encapsulated systematized hypochondriacal delusional system. Such individuals are difficult to manage and may be resistant to treatment, although the antipsychotic oral medication pimozide has been found to be especially effective. Some patients have also been reported to respond to antidepressant medication; in other cases, the disorder is part of a paranoid psychosis, depressive disorder or organic brain disorder.

The sick role

This was described by Parsons in 1951 and derived from learning and role theories.[44] If an individual adopts the sick role, there are two rights (exemption from normal social responsibilities and not being held responsible for one's condition) and two obligations (the obligation of wanting to recover and an obligation to seek appropriate help, usually from a doctor, and to cooperate with such help). An individual is liable to find the sick role attractive and adopt it when its advantages outweigh its disadvantages. For instance, an individual may be unable to respond adequately to the demands of daily life or may otherwise feel that adopting the sick role is the only way to receive sufficient sympathy, attention and love. Patients who as children had indulgent parents may find the sick role particularly attractive, due to their having learned that status and power can be achieved by manipulative behaviour strategies. Individuals may be especially prone to adopt the sick role at times of increased responsibility and stress (see also Chapter 11).

Illness behaviour

Illness behaviour is the way in which symptoms are perceived, evaluated and acted on.[45] Factors such as religion and social class affect how an individual responds to these symptoms, for example the tendency to seek, and the threshold for seeking, medical advice. Such behaviour may be judged inappropriate, given the individual's degree of disability and the situation. It may then be referred to as 'abnormal illness behaviour'.[46] Figure 41.7 illustrates the suggested relationship between organic disease and illness behaviour.

Accident neurosis

This condition overlaps with post-traumatic neurosis, which is often used to refer to neurotic symptoms following head injury (post-concussional syndrome). True malingering is uncommon following head injury. Gross 'neurotic' symptoms

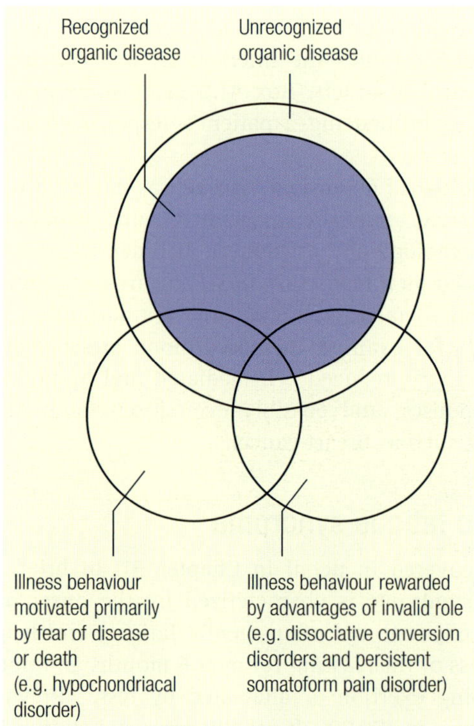

Figure 41.7 Relationship between organic disease and illness behaviour

are inversely related to the severity of the head injury and occur most often when the cause of the injury is perceived by the individual as someone else's fault or if financial compensation is possible. It is more likely to occur in males of lower social class following industrial injuries. Sexual dysfunction may be marked. It is now realized that even in cases of so-called 'compensation neurosis', symptoms may persist independent of seeking and achieving compensation, and the resulting disability is often underestimated. However, the longer compensation disputes continue, the worse the prognosis.

Factitious disorders

The term 'factitious' means not genuine, real or natural, and such disorders are characterized by physical or psychological symptoms that are intentionally produced or feigned, associated with a psychological need to assume the sick role, as evidenced by the absence of external incentives for such behaviour, such as economic gain, better care or physical wellbeing. This contrasts with malingering, where symptoms are also produced intentionally but for an external goal that is obviously recognizable when the environmental circumstances are known, for example financial compensation. Examples of physical symptoms in factitious disorders include self-inflicted injuries to the skin and symptoms arising from the acceptance of medication, despite the individual being aware of having an abnormal sensitivity to the drug. It usually begins before the age of 30 years. The main treatments used have been psychological, either confrontatory or non-confrontatory. Table 41.4 summarizes the differences between somatoform, conversion, dissociative and factitious disorders and malingering.

Münchausen syndrome (hospital addiction syndrome)

This is the best-studied form of factitious disorder with physical symptoms. It was described by Asher in 1951,[47] who coined the term after a fictional German cavalry officer, described by Raspe in 1785, Baron Karl von Munchausen, who harmlessly lied about his extraordinary military exploits. Patients feign illness to bring about repeated hospital admissions, investigations and operations for no obvious gain.[48] Although symptoms are consciously produced, motivation is largely unconscious but directed to achieving the sick role. It is an abnormal illness behaviour, a disorder of both illness behaviour and sick role. The patients simulate symptoms suggestive of serious physical illness and deceive medical staff. Men appear to be affected more than women. Patients' histories are often plausible but overdramatic. Patients may inflict injuries on themselves or simulate symptoms in a bizarre way, such as swallowing needles. Abdominal symptoms are the most common. Pathological lying (*pseudologia fantastica*[49]) is often present. Variants include presenting with psychiatric complaints, including a false history of bereavement. Patients may seek analgesic drugs and, more generally, attention. The condition is conceptualized as histrionic or hysterical behaviour in a severely disordered, sometimes masochistic, personality. Such individuals become impostors as a defence against feelings of inferiority and may masochistically play out a game with staff involving aggressive and sexual elements, perhaps to counter unconscious guilt and the psychological disintegration of the individual. Their behaviour may induce a sadistic response from staff. However, physical illness may predispose, coexist with or result from Münchausen syndrome.

When their feigning comes to light, such individuals may abscond from hospital but then travel to another hospital ('peregrination') and present with the same clinical scenario. Patients frequently change their names and the hospitals they approach, and they have a characteristic lack of visitors. Consistent management is thus made very difficult, with considerable associated costs,[50] morbidity and even mortality. Patients who wander usually have a longer history, are more often men, often are unemployed or frequently change jobs, and are more likely to present with abdominal or psychological symptoms, to have abused drugs and alcohol, and to have criminal convictions. Non-wanderers tend to be female, to be more stable socially, to be nurses, and to have less dramatic symptoms.

Aetiological factors may include parental abuse, neglect, early experience of chronic illness or hospitalization, paramedic employment, and experience of medical

Table 41.4 Difference between somatoform, conversion, dissociative and factitious disorders and malingering

	Physical symptoms	Psychological symptoms	Unconscious motivation	Conscious motivation	Voluntary production of symptoms	Involuntary production of symptoms
Somatoform disorders	+++	–	+	–	–	+
Conversion disorders	++	–	+	–	–	+
Dissociative disorders	–	++	+	–	–	+
Factitious disorders	++	+	+	–	+	–
Malingering	++	+	–	+	+	–

mismanagement with an associated grudge. Organic mental disorder should be excluded.

Treatment of coexisting depressive disorder may sometimes be of benefit. Psychological treatment is the ideal treatment of choice, either non-confrontatory or confrontatory.

A further variant is *Münchausen by proxy*, in which physical symptoms are intentionally produced in others, for instance by a mother in her child.[51–53] Such children do not show symptoms when in the care of others or when the mother is supervised. There may be a similar history of unexplained symptoms or even death in a sibling of the child. The mother may have medical experience, such as being a nurse, and have an emotionally distorted relationship with her partner. Through her behaviour, the mother becomes the centre of attention and herself receives care, which may underlie the motivation for such behaviour. Such women rarely ever admit to having produced physical symptoms in their children, often due to underlying feelings of deep humiliation.

Malingering

This is the conscious production of physical or psychiatric symptoms for external gain, for example to avoid prison, to obtain benefits or to avoid military service. It is not a mental disorder in ICD-10 or DSM-IV, although the latter describes it as an 'additional condition that may be the focus of clinical attention'.

KEY POINTS

- '*Hysterical*' symptoms occur not only in dissociative (conversion) disorders but also in other psychiatric disorders, such as depression and anxiety, and true organic disease.
- In epidemic (communicable) or mass hysteria, there is often a background of tension in an institution. Initial symptoms appear in an influential figure and spread to others by suggestion.
- Histrionic personality disorder is associated with an increased vulnerability to dissociative (conversion) disorders.
- Hysterical (histrionic) behaviour is consciously motivated, unlike the unconscious motivation underlying symptoms in dissociative (conversion) disorders.
- In dissociative states, such as amnesia or fugue (unexpected journeying with amnesia), there is partial or complete loss of normal integration between two or more mental processes.
- In conversion disorders, there is loss or change in bodily function, usually affecting the voluntary nervous system, such as paralysis or anaesthesia.
- Dissociative and conversion disorders have an unconscious motivation to resolve intrapsychic conflict and may show the following features:
  - Primary gain, e.g. to resolve conflict or reduce anxiety
  - Secondary gain, e.g. the attention of others
  - Symptom choice may be symbolic of the conflict and reflect modelling of symptoms that the individual or others have experienced
  - *La belle indifférence* (calm acceptance of symptoms).
- Hypochondriacal disorder is a disease conviction in spite of medical reassurance. There is intense persistent fear of disease and a profound preoccupation with body and health status.
- In hypochondriacal disorder, the patient is abnormally sensitive to normal physical signs and sensations and has a tendency to interpret them as abnormal.
- Hypochondriacal symptoms are most frequently secondary to depressive illness.
- Somatization disorder is a chronic syndrome of multiple physical symptoms not explainable medically.
- There is an increased incidence of somatization disorder in first-degree female relatives.
- In somatization disorder, first-degree male relatives have an excess of alcoholism, drug abuse and antisocial personality disorder.
- Unlike in hypochondriacal disorder, in somatization disorder there is less disease conviction, less fear of disease and less bodily preoccupation.
- Somatization disorder occurs primarily in females, compared with the at least equal incidence in males of hypochondriacal disorder.
- Somatization disorder has an onset before 30 years of age and has a long course without serious medical illness emerging.
- In body dysmorphic disorder (dysmorphophobia), there is a preoccupation with some imagined defect in appearance in a normal-appearing person that is not of delusional intensity.
- In clinical practice, most medically unexplained symptoms are due to undifferentiated somatoform disorder or to another primary psychiatric disorder, e.g. somatic anxiety symptoms, facial pain in depression.
- Somatization is the tendency to experience somatic (physical) symptoms unaccounted for by organic causes, to attribute such symptoms to physical illness and to seek medical help.
- Psychosomatic disorders are physical conditions aggravated or precipitated by psychological factors, e.g. bronchial asthma, peptic ulcer, ulcerative colitis.
- In monosymptomatic hypochondriacal psychosis, there are hypochondriacal delusions, such as skin infestation by insects or an emission of a foul smell.
- Adopting the sick role exempts an individual from normal responsibilities and from being held responsible for their condition.
- Illness behaviour refers to the way in which symptoms are perceived and acted upon by an individual.
- Accident neurosis overlaps with post-traumatic neurosis. Post-concussional syndrome refers to neurotic symptoms following a head injury.
- In cases of compensation neurosis, symptoms may persist after compensation.
- In malingering, symptoms are consciously produced for an obvious goal, which is lacking in factitious disorders.
- Münchausen (hospital addiction) syndrome is a factitious disorder in which patients repeatedly present at and get admitted to hospitals with feigned symptoms suggestive of serious physical illness.

REFERENCES

1. Lewis A (1975) The survival of hysteria. *Psychological Medicine* 5: 9–12.
2. Janet P (1907) *The Major Symptoms of Hysteria.* New York: Macmillan Press.
3. Holmes E, Brown RJ, Mansell W, *et al.* (2005) Are there two qualitatively distinct forms of dissociation? A review and some clinical implications. *Clinical Psychology Review* 25: 1–33.
4. Kluft RP (1991) Clinical manifestations of multiple personality disorder. *Psychiatric Clinics of North America* 14: 605–29.
5. Merskey H (1992) The manufacture of personalities: the production of multiple personality disorder. *British Journal of Psychiatry* 160: 327–40.
6. Toone BK (1990) Disorders of hysterical conversion. In C Bass (ed.) *Somatisation: Physical Symptoms and Psychological Illness.* Boston: Blackwell Scientific.
7. Slater E (1965) The diagnosis of hysteria. *British Medical Journal* 1: 1395–9.
8. Marsden CD (1986) Hysteria: a neurologist's view. *Psychological Medicine* 16: 277–88.
9. Stone J, Zeman A (2001) Hysterical conversion: a view from clinical neurology. In P Halligan, C Bass, J Marshall (eds) *Contemporary Approaches to the Science of Hysteria.* Oxford: Oxford University Press.
10. Breuer J, Freud S (2001) Studies on hysteria. In J Strachey, A Strachey (eds) *The Penguin Freud Library,* Vol. 3. London: Penguin.
11. Merskey H (1995) *The Analysis of Hysteria: Understanding Conversion and Dissociation.* London: Gaskell.
12. Spence SA, Crimlisk HC, Cope H, Ron MA, Grasby PM (2000) Discrete neurophysiological correlates in prefrontal cortex during hysterical and feigned disorder of movement. *Lancet* 355: 1243–4.
13. Oakly D (2001) Hypnosis and suggestion in the treatment of hysteria. In P Halligan, C Bass, J Marshall (eds) *Contemporary Approaches to the Science of Hysteria.* Oxford: Oxford University Press.
14. Kenyon F (1964) Hypochondriasis: a clinical study. *British Journal of Psychiatry* 100: 478–88.
15. Pilowsky I (1970) Primary and secondary hypochondriasis. *Acta Psychiatrica Scandinavica* 46: 273–88.
16. Tyrer P, Fowler-Dixon R, Ferguson B (1990) The justification for the diagnosis of hypochondriacal personality disorder. *Journal of Psychosomatic Research* 34: 637–42.
17. Warwick HM, Clark DM, Cobb AM, Salkovskis PM (1996) A controlled trial of cognitive-behavioural treatment of hypochondriasis. *British Journal of Psychiatry* 169: 189–95.
18. Guze S (1975) The validity and significance of hysteria (Briquet's syndrome). *American Journal of Psychiatry* 132: 138–41.
19. Torgerson S (1986) Genetics of somatiform disorders. *Archives of General Psychiatry* 43: 502–5.
20. Craig TKJ, Boardman AP, Mills K, *et al.* (1993) The South London somatisation study: I. Longitudinal course and the influence of early life experiences. *British Journal of Psychiatry* 163: 579–88.
21. Mayou R, Bass C, Sharpe M (eds) (1995) *Treatment of Functional Somatic Symptoms.* Oxford: Oxford University Press.
22. Brown RJ (2004) Psychological mechanisms of medically unexplained symptoms: an integrative conceptual model. *Psychological Bulletin* 130: 793–812.
23. Merskey H, Spear F (1961) *Pain: Psychological and Psychiatric Aspects.* London: Baillière, Tindall & Cassell.
24. Blumer D, Heilbron M (1982) Chronic pain as a variant of depressive disease: the pain-prone disorder. *Journal of Nervous and Mental Diseases* 170: 381–409.
25. McElroy SL, Phillips KA, Keck PE, *et al.* (1993) Body dysmorphic disorder: does it have a psychotic sub-type? *Journal of Clinical Psychiatry* 54: 389–95.
26. Munro A, Stewart M (1991) Body dysmorphic disorder and DSM-IV: the demise of dysmorphophobia. *Canadian Journal of Psychiatry* 36: 91–6.
27. Perugi G, Akiskal HS, Giannotti D, *et al.* (1997) Gender-related differences in body dysmorphic disorder (dysmorphophobia). *Journal of Nervous and Mental Diseases* 185: 578–82.
28. National Institute for Health and Clinical Excellence (2005) *Obsessive–Compulsive Disorder: Core Interventions in the Treatment of Obsessive–Compulsive Disorder and Body Dysmorphophobic Disorder.* London: National Collaborating Centre for Mental Health.
29. Perugi G, Giannotti D, di Vaio S, *et al.* (1996) Fluvoxamine in the treatment of body dysmorphic disorder (dysmorphophobia). *International Clinical Psychopharmacology* 11: 247–54.
30. Hollander E, Allen A, Kwon J, *et al.* (1999) Clomipramine vs. desipramine crossover trial in body dysmorphic disorder: selective efficacy of a serotonin re-uptake inhibitor in imagined ugliness. *Archives of General Psychiatry* 56: 1033–9.
31. Escobar JI, Golding JM, Hough RL, *et al.* (1987) Somatisation in the community: relationship to disability and use of services. *American Journal of Public Health* 77: 837–40.
32. Bass C (ed.) (1990) *Somatisation.* Oxford: Blackwell Scientific.
33. Goldberg D, Bridges K (1988) Somatic presentations of psychiatric illness in primary care setting. *Journal of Psychosomatic Research* 32: 137–44.
34. Sensky T (1990) Patients' reaction to illness: cognitive factors determine responses and are amenable to treatment. *British Medical Journal* 300: 622–3.
35. Wessely S, Hotopf MH, Sharpe M (1998) *Chronic Fatigue and Its Syndromes.* Oxford: Oxford University Press.

36. Prins JB, Van der Meer JW, Bleyesberg C (2006) Chronic fatigue syndrome. *Lancet* **367**: 346–55.
37. Afari N, Buchwald D (2003) Chronic fatigue syndrome: a review. *American Journal of Psychiatry* **160**: 221–36.
38. Wessley S (1990) Old wine in new bottles? Neurasthenia and ME. *Psychological Medicine* **20**: 35–53.
39. Baker R, Shore EJ (2007) Diagnosis and management of chronic fatigue syndrome or myalgic encephalomyelitis (or encephalopathy): summary of NICE guidance. *British Medical Journal* **335**: 446–8.
40. Alexander F (1950) *Psychosomatic Medicine*. New York: Norton.
41. Zeally AK, Aitken RC, Rosenthal JU (1970) Asthma: a psychophysiological investigation. *Proceedings of the Royal Society of Medicine* **644**: 825–9.
42. Munro A (1975) Monosymptomatic hypochondriacal psychosis. *British Journal of Hospital Medicine* **24**: 34–8.
43. Van Moffaert M (1992) Psychodermatology: an overview. *Psychotherapy and Psychosomatics* **58**: 125–36.
44. Parsons T (1951) *The Social System*. Glencoe, IL: Free Press.
45. Mechanic D (1962) The concept of illness behaviour. *Journal of Chronic Disease* **15**: 189–94.
46. Pilowsky I (1969) Abnormal illness behaviour. *British Journal of Medical Psychology* **42**: 347–51.
47. Asher R (1951) The Munchausen syndrome. *Lancet* **1**: 339–41.
48. O'Shea B, McGennis A, Cahill M, Falvey J (1984) Munchausen's syndrome. *British Journal of Hospital Medicine* **31**: 269–74.
49. King B, Ford C (1988) Pseudologica fantastica. *Acta Psychiatrica Scandinavica* **77**: 1–6.
50. Powell R, Boast N (1993) The million dollar man: resource implications for chronic Munchausen's syndrome. *British Journal of Psychiatry* **162**: 253–6.
51. Meadow R (1982) Munchausen syndrome by proxy. *Archives of Diseases of Childhood* **57**: 92–8.
52. Meadow R (1989) Munchausen syndrome by proxy. *British Medical Journal* **299**: 248–50.
53. Sheridan M (2003) The deceit continues: an updated literature review of Munchausen's syndrome by proxy. *Childhood Abuse and Neglect* **27**: 431–51.

Chapter 42

Eating disorders

Kate Webb, Ewa Zadeh, Victoria Mountford and J Hubert Lacey

INTRODUCTION

It is often easier to say what eating disorders are not rather than what they are. People with eating disorders do not have a problem with their eating. They can chew or eat their food as well as anyone else. People with anorexia nervosa do not have anorexia; indeed, they are usually ravenous. Despite the repeated claims in the media, anorexia nervosa is not a 'slimmer's disease'; nor does it develop because people want to look attractive.

The diagnosis of anorexia nervosa is at three levels. First, there needs to be a behaviour, such as dieting, overexercising or self-induced vomiting, that leads to weight loss. Second, the weight loss has to be sufficient that the person (if a woman) stops menstruating and, irrespective of gender, has a low sexual drive. Third, the thinking of people with anorexia nervosa changes: they are terrified of being at a normal weight.

It is a common clinical mistake to believe that the patient with anorexia nervosa is attempting to avoid 'being fat'; rather, she has a phobia of being at a normal weight, and this is the pathognomonic feature of anorexia nervosa. None of the other eating disorders have, strictly speaking, pathognomonic features; the behavioural features occur in other clinical conditions, particularly the mood states and disorders of personality.

Bulimia nervosa involves frequent binge eating coupled with compensatory behaviours designed to avoid gaining weight. People with bulimia nervosa do wish to weigh less, and this view is more entrenched than in the general population, but it does not have the intensity of anorexia nervosa.

Patients with bulimia nervosa feel out of control – a feeling that often extends beyond the eating behaviour itself. They feel unsure about social and interpersonal matters. They are sad and apprehensive, but the dominant emotion is anger – anger towards themselves or to a particular person, such as their mother or partner. Their feelings and the eating disorder fluctuate. A large minority are multi-impulsive; that is, their eating disorder has become mixed with addictive and self-damaging behaviour.

Anorexia nervosa invariably begins in adolescence, while bulimia nervosa is usually a condition of adulthood. People with bulimia nervosa are at normal weight, whereas people with anorexia nervosa are emaciated. Anorexia nervosa has a specific psychopathology, while people with bulimia nervosa, although wishing to be slim, rarely lose much body weight and certainly do not maintain a low weight.

There have been attempts to arrange people with eating disorders into one diagnostic group.[1] There is logic to this, as there is some overlap and sometimes patients can move from one diagnosis to another. Many clinicians have resisted this, however, because although eating-disordered individuals share a number of commonalities, such as overevaluation of control of eating, shape and weight, there are differences in the demographics, pathogenesis and treatment approaches of the main syndromes.

In addition to anorexia nervosa and bulimia nervosa, other diagnostic groups include binge-eating disorder (BED) and eating disorder not otherwise specified (EDNOS). BED involves frequent binge eating without any compensatory behaviours; it is usually associated with obesity. Apart from body weight, the disorder is similar to bulimia nervosa, but not all obese patients binge eat. EDNOS is a range of eating disorders including BED and other eating disturbances that show some, but not all, of the features of anorexia and bulimia nervosa.

The treatment of eating disorders has been the subject of much research. Somewhat flippantly, it has been suggested that there are only three significant findings: first, that bulimia nervosa responds to a cognitive-behavioural approach; second, that family-based treatments are to be recommended for adolescents with eating disorders; and third, that some patients with bulimia nervosa benefit from antidepressant medication. We do not know what will get any particular person with anorexia nervosa better, although there are complex multidisciplinary treatment approaches that benefit many. Unfortunately, severe and enduring anorexia is becoming an increasing problem, as is the multi-impulsive form of both anorexia and bulimia nervosa.

DIAGNOSIS

Anorexia nervosa

International Classification of Diseases, 10th revision (ICD-10) (F50.0)

The disorder is characterized by a deliberate weight loss associated with specific psychopathology, and resulting in malnourishment, with endocrine and medical disturbances. It occurs mostly in young women and girls, but men and adolescent boys may also be affected by anorexia nervosa.

- Weight loss leading to a body weight at least 15 per cent below the normal/expected for age and height body weight (or Quetelet's body mass index (BMI) at 17.5 kg/m^2 or less, used for age 16 years and over). Prepubertal patients may show failure to make the expected weight gain during the period of growth.
- Weight loss self-induced by avoidance of 'fattening foods' and other methods such as excessive exercising, use of appetite suppressants or diuretics, and purging behaviours such as self-induced vomiting or laxative misuse.
- Distorted body image: self-perception of being too fat and intrusive dread of fatness persisting as intrusive, overvalued ideas, which leads to self-imposed low weight threshold.
- Endocrine disturbances of hypothalamic–pituitary–gonadal axis (HPA), manifesting as amenorrhoea in women and loss of sexual interest and potency in men.
- In prepubertal onset, the sequence of pubertal events is delayed or arrested (e.g. growth, breast development and primary amenorrhoea in girls; juvenile genitals in boys). With recovery, puberty is often completed normally but menarche is late.[2]

Diagnostic and Statistical Manual of Mental Disorders, 4th edition, text revision (DSM-IV-TR)

- Refusal to maintain minimally normal body weight (<85%).
- Fear of gaining weight.
- Disturbance in perception of shape or size of body.
- Amenorrhoea (absence of three or more menstrual cycles).[3]

Subtypes

- *Restrictive:* predominant features – dieting, fasting or excessive exercising.
- *Binge eating/purging:* regular bingeing or purging; very likely to have other impulse-control problems.

NB: anorexia nervosa 'trumps' the diagnosis of bulimia nervosa.

Bulimia nervosa

ICD-10 (F 50.2)

- Recurrent episodes of overeating, when large amounts of food are consumed in short periods of time.
- Persistent preoccupation with eating, and strong desire/compulsion to eat (craving).
- Attempts to counteract the 'fattening' effects of food by one or more of the following:
  - Self-induced vomiting
  - Self-induced purging
  - Alternating periods of starvation
  - Use of medications (appetite suppressants, diuretics, etc.).
- Morbid dread of fatness, usually normal weight, may be a history of anorexia nervosa or obesity.[2]

DSM-IV-TR

- Recurrent episodes of binge eating, characterized by:
  - Eating in a discrete period of time an amount of food that is larger than for most people under the same circumstances
  - Feelings of lack of control over eating during the episode.
- Recurrent behaviours to prevent weight gain (e.g. self-induced vomiting, misuse of laxatives/diuretics/enemas/other medications, fasting or excessive exercise).
- All above occurs, on average, at least twice a week for 3 months.
- Self-evaluation unduly influenced by body shape and weight.
- Disturbance not occurring exclusively during episodes of anorexia nervosa.[3]

Subtypes

- *Purging:* regular self-induced vomiting or misuse of laxatives, diuretics or enemas during the current episode.
- *Non-purging:* compensatory behaviours such as fasting or excessive exercising used, but no regular self-induced vomiting or use of laxatives/diuretics/enemas.

Eating disorder not otherwise specified

This category in DSM-IV represents eating disorders of clinical severity, psychopathology and presence of social impairment that are similar to other eating disorder diagnoses but that do not meet all diagnostic criteria for either anorexia nervosa or bulimia nervosa.[3] For example, there could be a weight marginally above the diagnostic criteria for anorexia nervosa, or frequency of binge eating could be below that required by DSM-IV.[3] The main ICD-10 equivalents would be atypical anorexia nervosa (F50.1) and atypical bulimia nervosa (F 50.3): disorders that meet some but not all of the criteria for anorexia nervosa and bulimia nervosa, respectively, and where the overall clinical picture does not justify the diagnosis (e.g. lack of amenorrhoea or significant weight loss or does not meet the frequency criteria for bingeing and vomiting).[2] There should not be a weight loss secondary to a known physical illness.

EDNOS is the most common eating disorder in the outpatient setting and is widely used by clinicians, and yet it is not as well researched as other eating disorders. Perhaps the most well researched subcategory is BED – recurrent episodes of binge eating, in the absence of the regular use of compensatory behaviours aimed at weight control that are characteristic of bulimia nervosa and anorexia nervosa. People with BED usually have a BMI above the normal range of 20–25.

Some clinicians point out that there are certain problems of nosology that would need to be addressed when formulating diagnostic criteria for the fifth edition of the DSM.[4] EDNOS is the most widely seen eating disorder in clinical practice, and yet it has the 'residual' category in the major classification systems. Some proposals for DSM-V involve changing diagnostic criteria for anorexia nervosa (e.g. to drop amenorrhea as a criteria, or to upwardly adjust the weight threshold for anorexia nervosa); reclassifying EDNOS to several categories in their own right; and even creating one dimensional category of eating disorder, including all types and subtypes.

EPIDEMIOLOGY

The incidence of anorexia nervosa is approximately 8 cases per 100 000 population per year and is highest in women aged 15–19 years, who account for approximately 40 per cent of all diagnosed cases.[5] Incidence rates of anorexia nervosa in men have been reported less frequently, at below 0.1 cases per 100 000 population per year.[6] According to Hoeken, the average prevalence rate for anorexia nervosa is 0.3 per cent,[7] although it has varied in studies between 0 per cent and 0.9 per cent, with an average point prevalence of 0.29 per cent in young women.[5] There is less information about the incidence rates for men, but it has been reported at less than 1 per 100 000 population per year (around 10% of cases).[7]

The incidence of bulimia nervosa is 12 cases per 100 000 population per year, with a prevalence rate of 1 per cent. The average age of onset is 19 years – slightly older than in anorexia nervosa.

In a community setting, eating disorders tend to be divided into 60 per cent EDNOS, 14.5 per cent anorexia nervosa and 25.5 per cent bulimia nervosa.[7]

AETIOLOGY

There is no single cause for the development of an eating disorder. There seems to be a genetic predisposition/vulnerability, which, together with adverse life events and other environmental influences, could manifest as inappropriate dieting or emotional difficulties. This vulnerability may also predispose to particular personality traits or affective disorder (particularly associated with binge eating/purging). All the factors described below play an important role in the predisposing, precipitating and maintaining aetiological factors for eating disorders and will commonly interact as part of one complex aetiological model.

Genetic factors

Family studies have shown that there is an increased incidence of eating disorders in first-degree relatives by 7–12 times. Several studies have shown an increased concordance ratio for monozygotic and dizygotic twins,[8,9] with Holland and colleagues showing a concordance ratio of 56 : 5. The heritability of binge eating was estimated to be 50 per cent and broad bulimia nervosa 60 per cent, with the remaining variance attributable to individual specific environment.[10]

Sociocultural factors

Assimilation to a new culture with a higher prevalence of eating disorders may play a mediating role in the development of anorexia nervosa in a vulnerable person. This may occur as a result of the pursuit of thinness seen as ideal in Western cultures.[11] In vulnerable individuals, internalization of this ideal may result in feelings of discrepancy between self and ideal, which in turn can lead to body-image dissatisfaction and dietary restriction.[12] Experimental evidence suggests that media exposure or social pressures to the idealized thin can increase body-image concerns, at least in the short term. It could be considered a causal factor in models and media industries, but there is no evidence that it is so in a general population. Dieting, which may be culturally driven, is often a trigger for eating disordered behaviour in a vulnerable individual. Ethnic background does not appear to be a protective factor. Urbanization seems to be a risk factor for bulimia nervosa but not for anorexia nervosa.[13] There have been studies to suggest that anorexia nervosa is more common in people from higher socioeconomic groups, but no such association has been found in people with bulimia nervosa or in studies combining people with all eating disorders.[12]

Family factors

Family studies, such as those by Minuchin, were very influential in the 1970s and 1980s. Certain parenting styles ('anorexogenic mother') were thought to increase the risk for anorexia nervosa. These findings, however, are not supported in the newer studies, and current research suggests that patterns observed within the family, for example enmeshment, may be a result of the eating disorder rather than the cause of it. Blair and Freeman found that disordered eating may cause family disturbances.[14]

Sexual, physical and emotional abuse

Early studies focused predominantly on the role of sexual abuse in the development of eating disorders. Connors and Worse found a 30 per cent rate of sexual abuse in patients with eating disorders,[15] although many studies that have looked into associations between eating disorders and reported sexual abuse did not find a strong specific relationship. The generally held view is that sexual abuse is no higher in the eating disorders than in other neurotic conditions, save for the multi-impulsive form – that is, where the eating disorder occurs in conjunction with addictive or self-damaging behaviours. Later studies have highlighted the importance of examining sexual, physical and psychological abuse, particularly as it is often the case that more than one form of abuse will be present.[16] All forms of abuse may be seen as moderators of other factors, which may predispose an individual to develop an eating disorder, rather than as being a sufficient factor alone to cause the eating disturbance.[17] It has been suggested that the experience of emotional abuse may lead to a number of related manifestations, such as difficulties in tolerating distress, which are later implicated in the development of the eating disorder.[17]

Personality

Personality factors have been considered with regard to onset and manifestation of symptoms, maintenance of eating disorders and treatment response. Perfectionism is a risk factor for anorexia nervosa and bulimia nervosa, whereas obsessive–compulsive personality disorder has been found to be a risk factor only for anorexia nervosa.[18] Cluster C personality disorders (obsessive–compulsive, dependent, avoidant) are the most common among individuals with eating disorders, followed by cluster B (borderline, histrionic, narcissistic, antisocial).

Biological factors

Hypothalamic dysfunction and neuropsychological deficits (e.g. visuospatial processing) have been studied. Some of the deficits, for example cognitive functioning, improve with weight gain. However, there are some studies suggesting non-nutrition-related brain changes. For example, Gordon and colleagues found unilateral temporal lobe hypoperfusion demonstrated by a regional cerebral blood flow isotope scan.[19]

PATHOGENESIS

Few people would accept that the eating disorders have a single pathogenesis. The differences in demography, symptomatology and age of presentation for each disorder belie this.

There are, however, certain personal and social cultural factors that are common. Low self-esteem, perfectionism, rigidity and negative affect are frequent, but these are probably secondary rather than primary to the disorder. Some authors have noted a season of birth affect (April and June), and being slightly overweight before the illness. More relevant for anorexia nervosa is an early puberty, which leaves the girl without peers who are going through a similar experience. Family factors, particularly family dieting or disordered eating, or a family history of neurosis or addictive behaviour, are described by a few authors. Sexual abuse is not thought to be associated specifically with eating disorders, apart from the multi-impulsive form of bulimia nervosa.[20,21] A first-degree relative with an eating disorder has been implicated, as has chromosome 10 for bulimia nervosa and chromosome 1 for anorexia nervosa.[22] The overwhelming biological feature, however, is that primarily girls and women have these conditions. Further, the conditions occur in adolescence in anorexia and in early adulthood in bulimia.

Hilde Bruch was the first to attempt to explain the development of anorexia nervosa.[23] She emphasized the severe disturbance of body image rather than disordered eating. She related the development to the changing role of women after the Second World War. She saw anorexia nervosa occurring in those women who were casualties of the social, economic and political freedom that followed universal opportunities, expectations and the contraceptive pill. They were, she said, within 'a golden cage' where contradictions were played out. Their disorder seemed to control them, and yet they in turn had control over their families and starving bodies.

Crisp was influenced by Bruch, although he emphasized the powerful effect of the anorectic patient's own pubertal hormonal changes. In his model, the future person with anorexia nervosa found the passage to adult expectations and sexuality difficult.[24] Certain events – social, medical, familial – provided the seeds of the disorder around the age of 13 years, but the precipitating event would occur anytime in the following 5 years. Restriction would lead to weight loss and what Crisp referred to as 'pubertal regression', by which he meant that emotionally the patient returns to a prepubertal state. Further, she becomes trapped by her own biology, which is the hormonal status associated with low body weight. Crisp identified a threshold weight of approximately 40–42 kg above which plasma luteinizing hormone (LH) and follicle-stimulating hormone (FSH) can be stimulated. These hormones are associated with libido. The patient with anorexia nervosa, terrified of her low weight, attempts weight gain. On reaching this threshold, she becomes aware again of adult feelings and the unresolved conflicts that she experienced around puberty. Unsurprisingly, she seeks safety below the threshold. It is for this reason that most people with anorexia nervosa can be cajoled to gain some weight and reach approximately 40 kg. Beyond that, Crisp said it was only those patients who received a sophisticated psychotherapy, coupled with practical therapies, who could make the full journey to recovery and normal body weight.

The implications of this model are that the disorder is egosyntonic and that the patient rarely seeks change. Any weight gain is minor and the therapeutic task of the clinician is to achieve emotional maturity. Crisp said:

> Whatever the patient's chronological age, her psychological age has been arrested at or been regressed to, a pre-pubertal level since the onset of the illness. Her target-weight should represent this fact.

The implications of this are that the family needs empowerment and their involvement is essential. It was from Crisp that the core role of family therapy developed.

Cognitive-behavioural models of the eating disorders have developed over time and tend to focus on the maintenance of the disorders, while acknowledging the importance of aetiological factors. Fairburn and colleagues propose that once attempts to restrict eating begin, these are reinforced through three main feedback mechanisms that vary in influence over time.[25] First, dietary restriction enhances the sense of being in control. Second, aspects of starvation encourage further dietary restriction, through the physiological and psychological changes bought about by starvation (including impaired concentration, intense hunger and heightened sense of fullness), which all threaten the individual's sense of control. Third, control over shape, weight and eating become inextricably bound up in the individual's perception of their self-worth. The individual engages in behaviours such as hypervigilant body-checking or avoidance, further reinforcing distorted beliefs and assumptions regarding eating, shape and weight. Biases in information-processing contribute to these distorted beliefs. Thus, the overevaluation of control of eating, shape and weight is seen as the core maintaining mechanism of the eating disorder. Among individuals with bulimia nervosa, the vicious cycle of restriction, bingeing and purging serves further to undermine sense of control and contribute to sense of failure. Therefore, it is suggested that the onset of the disorder may be related to a need for self-control in general. In patients with a restrictive presentation this may be a result of an interaction between the individual's perfectionism and long-standing low self-esteem, while in more bulimic presentations the need may be for control over intolerable emotion.

As described below, cognitive-behavioural theory forms the basis of a successful range of treatments, particularly for bulimia nervosa. As researchers have become aware of the importance of deeper, core beliefs, the cognitive-behavioural therapy (CBT) model has been extended. Waller and colleagues have developed a schema theory model for eating disorders, based on good data.[26] Schemas are extremely stable, negative, rigid and global core beliefs that develop during childhood and that are expanded upon throughout an individual's lifetime. When a schema is triggered, the individual experiences intense affect such as a high level of anger, anxiety, shame or sadness. The model proposes two processes by which individuals attempt to avoid this intolerable affect. In people with a restrictive presentation, primary avoidance of affect, whereby the individual uses compensatory schema (e.g. perfectionism, emotional inhibition) to avoid triggering early maladaptive schema, is prominent. In people with a bulimic presentation, secondary avoidance of emotion occurs, in which the individual uses recognized behaviours (e.g. bingeing, vomiting) to escape or block the intolerable emotion.

TREATMENT OPTIONS FOR EATING DISORDERS

National Institute for Health and Clinical Excellence (NICE) guidelines recommend the following:[27]

Anorexia nervosa

- Most people with anorexia nervosa should be managed on an out-patient basis, with psychological treatment provided by a service that is competent in giving that treatment and assessing the physical risk of people with eating disorders.
- People with anorexia nervosa requiring in-patient treatment should be admitted to a setting that can provide the skilled implementation of refeeding with careful physical monitoring (particularly in the first few days of refeeding) in combination with psychosocial interventions.
- Family interventions that directly address the eating disorder should be offered to children and adolescents with anorexia nervosa.

Bulimia nervosa

- As a possible first step, patients with bulimia nervosa should be encouraged to follow an evidence-based self-help programme.
- As an alternative or additional first step to using an evidence-based self-help programme, adults with bulimia nervosa may be offered a trial of an antidepressant drug.
- Cognitive-behavioural therapy for bulimia nervosa (CBT-BN), a specifically adapted form of CBT, should be offered to adults with bulimia nervosa. The course of treatment should be for 16–20 sessions over 4–5 months.

- Adolescents with bulimia nervosa may be treated with CBT-BN, adapted as needed to suit their age, circumstances and level of development, and including the family as appropriate.

Atypical eating disorders

- In the absence of evidence to guide the management of atypical eating disorders (EDNOS) other than BED, it is recommended that the clinician considers following the guidance on the treatment of the eating problem that most closely resembles the individual patient's eating disorder.
- Cognitive-behavioural therapy for binge-eating disorder (CBT-BED), a specifically adapted form of CBT, should be offered to adults with BED.

All eating disorders

- Family members, including siblings, should normally be included in the treatment of children and adolescents with eating disorders. Interventions may include sharing of information, advice on behavioural management and facilitating communication.

PSYCHOLOGICAL INTERVENTIONS FOR ANOREXIA NERVOSA

Much research into eating disorders has been done since the 1970s. However, the research has concentrated largely on delineating the bulimia nervosa syndrome and determining and testing treatment approaches to it. Little has meaningfully changed in the treatment of anorexia nervosa, and yet this remains the mental illness with the highest mortality. Treatments for multi-impulsive eating disorders are reasonably promising on an in-patient basis, but out-patient treatments have yet to be developed. Overall, the treatment response of anorexia nervosa is erratic. The treatment for the acute phases of anorexia nervosa and for severe and enduring anorexia nervosa must be the highest priority.

The evidence base for the psychological treatment of anorexia nervosa is poor. The NICE guidelines for eating disorders found that the strength of evidence for psychological therapies was level C (expert committee reports or opinion or clinical experiences of respected authorities, or extrapolated from indirectly related randomized controlled trials (RCTs) or other well-designed studies) in the hierarchy of evidence, except for family therapy that directly addresses the eating disorder for children and adolescents with anorexia nervosa, which was graded as level B (well-conducted clinical studies but no RCTs).[27]

A systematic review of treatments for anorexia nervosa found serious weaknesses in the literature for psychological treatments.[28] The authors concluded that there was some evidence to suggest that CBT may be superior to nutritional counselling after restoration of weight,[29] but that it was unclear whether CBT was useful in the acute phase of illness in very underweight patients. The authors of the review found one unreplicated study that showed that manual-based non-specific clinical management (NSCM) was more effective than CBT or interpersonal psychotherapy (IPT) in improving global outcome in an out-patient setting.[30] They also reported that there was no significant evidence for family therapy in adults, although the evidence is supportive for family therapy in children and adolescents, as indicated in the NICE guidelines.[27] A study looking at psychoanalytical psychotherapy, cognitive analytical therapy (CAT) and family therapy with a control group of 'routine' management, in out-patient management of anorexia nervosa, found that psychoanalytical and family therapies were superior to routine management in terms of weight gain.[31]

Many studies have small sample sizes and high dropout rates, and it is difficult to come to firm conclusions about the efficacy of one psychological treatment over another. However, it is clear that treatment with a psychological therapy in a specialist eating disorder setting is superior to no treatment or a non-specialist treatment.[31,32] Establishing a positive therapeutic alliance is perhaps the most important factor in terms of engagement and outcome for psychological therapies for anorexia nervosa. More research is needed to look at the specific benefits of psychoanalytical psychotherapy, CBT, IPT, CAT, NSCM, motivational enhancement therapy and family therapy in the treatment of anorexia nervosa. Most patients should be treated in an out-patient setting,[27] although day-hospital and in-patient settings are suitable for patients who need more intensive or emergency treatment.

The aims of psychological treatment for anorexia nervosa vary, depending on the motivational stage of change: many patients are ambivalent about change and may not have sought help independently. It may be that motivational enhancement work and help to improve quality of life are all that the patient can manage at the moment, particularly in patients with severe and enduring anorexia nervosa, although it is important to persist with instilling the hope of recovery for all patients. For patients aiming at full recovery from anorexia nervosa, the aim will be to look at the underlying psychological predisposing, precipitating and maintaining aetiological factors for the eating disorder psychopathology and behaviours, as well as reintroducing regular eating and avoided foods and encouraging weight gain. Different psychological and behavioural issues may arise at each stage of recovery, and patients continue to need intensive out-patient psychological support for at least a year after weight restoration has been achieved,[27] whether as an in-patient, day patient or out-patient. Weight gain without psychological input is unlikely to achieve full and sustained recovery.

PSYCHOLOGICAL INTERVENTIONS FOR BULIMIA NERVOSA

In contrast to anorexia nervosa, treatment for bulimia nervosa has been well researched and a number of modalities have some empirical support. Indeed, the only level A recommendation for adults with eating disorders in the NICE guidelines is for CBT-BN.[27] For individuals with bulimia nervosa, a stepped-care approach, in which treatments are provided sequentially, according to need, is recommended.[27]

Self-help

The vast majority of patients with bulimia nervosa can be treated as out-patients. The first step of psychological treatment is self-help, which can be guided or unguided. Self-help has a number of advantages, including being more disseminable and less costly than individual treatments.[33] Guided self-help appears promising in the treatment of bulimia nervosa. In guided self-help, the patient is typically given a treatment manual and invited for a few brief out-patient appointments, where their progress is reviewed.

A systematic review identified four self-help trials for bulimia nervosa.[34] Outcomes are generally positive, with guided self-help demonstrating short- and long-term improvements. Although some studies appear to suggest that dropout may be higher in guided self-help than with face-to-face treatments,[35] others report no such difference.[36] An RCT of 121 patients entered into self-help with minimal guidance, self-help with face-to-face guidance, self-help with telephone guidance or waiting list demonstrated improvements in those who received additional guidance, particularly face to face.[37] Self-help with minimal guidance was not superior to the waiting-list condition. New technologies such as Internet-assisted self-help are also showing promise.[38]

In summary, it is likely that a subgroup of patients will respond well to guided self-help and may not need further intervention.[33] Guided self-help may therefore be most appropriate as part of a stepped-care approach within a primary care setting or as a cost-effective first response to patients presenting to a secondary care service, particularly if the alternative is a long wait for one-to-one therapy.[37]

Face-to-face therapy

There is general agreement within the field, supported by NICE,[27] that CBT is the treatment of choice for bulimia nervosa, delivered in group or individual format.[39–41] The aims of CBT are to modify behaviours and cognitions that maintain the eating disorder, focusing on the implementation of regular eating and reduction of the core pathology, the overevaluation of eating shape and weight. Food-monitoring diaries, cognitive restructuring and behavioural experiments are key strategies.

Despite this endorsement, the rates for complete remission are low,[39] leaving a substantial number of patients with continued difficulties. Thus, there is still need to improve current therapies and to develop sequential or alternative treatments. Fairburn and colleagues are developing a new enhanced form of CBT, building on existing theory by incorporating four additional maintaining mechanisms – clinical perfectionism, interpersonal differences, core low self-esteem and mood intolerance.[1] This treatment relates to a transdiagnostic model of eating disorders and highlights the use of individualized formulations. One trial compared 20 sessions of two types of enhanced CBT: *focused*, which focuses exclusively on modification of eating disorder symptomatology, and *broad*, which also addresses the four maintaining mechanisms, as relevant for the individual patient, with waiting-list controls for all eating-disorder patients with BMI above 17.5.[42] Both enhanced CBT treatments were found to be superior to waiting-list controls and earlier CBT treatments. Such changes were well maintained across the substantial 60-week follow-up period – important, as eating disorders are prone to relapse.

IPT is the only therapy that has been demonstrated to provide outcomes comparable to CBT, although the speed of response is slower.[39] Adapted for bulimia nervosa, IPT was originally developed as a short-term psychotherapy for depression. The focus is in assisting patients to identify and modify current interpersonal problems that may be maintaining the disorder. Thus, IPT may be appropriate for people with interpersonal difficulties or who are reluctant to engage in or are unsuccessful with CBT. A further treatment that shows promise is dialectical behaviour therapy (DBT),[43] an affect-regulation treatment originally developed for borderline personality disorder. An RCT comparing DBT with waiting-list controls demonstrated significant decreases in bingeing and purging.[44] A small case series provides preliminary support for a time-limited integrative psychodynamic behavioural approach, with significant reductions in bulimic symptoms.[45] Treatment studies have focused on women and therefore little is known about outcomes for men; clinicians are advised to adapt current models as appropriate.

In contrast to the adult literature, evidence-based treatment trials for adolescents with bulimia nervosa are largely absent.[46] The success of family-based therapy with adolescent patients with anorexia suggests that this may be applicable. An RCT comparing family-based therapy and supportive psychotherapy with 80 adolescents with bulimia nervosa found that family-based therapy showed a clinical and statistical advantage over supportive psychotherapy at post-treatment and 6 months follow-up.[46] Another trial compared family-based therapy with cognitive-behavioural guided self-care (GSC) and found GSC to be superior in terms of cessation of binge–purge episodes at 6 months, although patients in both treatment groups showed significant improvement over time and were indistinguishable at 1 year follow-up.[47] A small body of case series supports the use of CBT with adolescents with bulimia nervosa,[48] and NICE recommends CBT-BN, adapted to suit the circumstances.[27]

Research into bulimia nervosa is beginning to focus on the identification of predictors of treatment response, with Fairburn and colleagues demonstrating early change in frequency of purging as the best predictor of response at treatment end and 8 month follow-up.[49] More recently, there has been a focus on disseminating CBT for bulimia nervosa to routine clinical settings using individualized formulations, demonstrating outcomes comparable to those found in research trials.[50,51]

Psychological treatments for EDNOS

With the exception of BED, there is an absence of research for EDNOS. Treatments for BED are often similar to those for bulimia nervosa, and self-help is recommended as the first step.[27] Research suggests that, for some patients, self-help is effective in reducing binge-eating episodes and psychological features associated with BED and in promoting abstinence from binge eating.[52] With regard to face-to-face contact, a number of studies provide support for both group and individualized CBT, and this is recommended as the treatment of choice. DBT also shows promise, leading to greater reduction in binge days and in weight, shape and eating concerns.[52,53] IPT has also been demonstrated to significantly reduce binge days at end and 4 month follow-up.[54] Treatment of BED is often complicated by co-occurring obesity and associated medical concerns. It is of note that none of the studies has found significant reduction in BMI, and NICE advises that patients should be warned that all psychological treatments for BED have limited impact on weight.[27]

For the remaining EDNOS disorders, it is suggested that the clinician considers following the guidance for the disorder that the patient's presentation most closely resembles. This is supported by data on patients with BMI above 17.5.[42] A case series design study that included patients with atypical bulimia nervosa found that the majority of these patients responded to CBT as well as those with bulimia nervosa, with the exception of those with normal-weight purging disorder.[51]

Summary of psychological treatments for eating disorders

Since the original description of bulimia nervosa,[55] significant progress has been achieved in the development and evaluation of evidence-based psychological treatments for the eating disorders. Most notably, CBT is recognized as the treatment of choice for bulimia nervosa and BED, and there is evidence for family therapy with adolescents with anorexia nervosa. However, many challenges remain. Substantial numbers of patients fail to get better with these treatments, and the lack of research regarding anorexia nervosa and EDNOS is remarkable. Adolescent, EDNOS, male and chronic patients remain poorly researched. The enhancement of current therapies and development of newer therapies is highlighted above.

Models of service delivery are also important, with the UK favouring a stepped-care model. The research does not inform as to which patients will benefit from which, if any, of the treatments detailed above – for example, which patients are suitable for guided self-help compared with individual treatment. A potential limitation of this model is patients becoming demoralized as they step further up the care pathway. Reliable predictors of treatment outcomes also remain unclear.[56]

PHYSICAL PRESENTATION AND MANAGEMENT

Eating disorders, particularly anorexia nervosa, have one of the highest standardized mortality rates (SMRs) of any psychiatric disorder.

Patients with an eating disorder may present to healthcare professionals from many different medical specialties due to the fact that the physical consequences affect many different organ systems. Organic causes for unexplained weight loss should be excluded, but all clinicians should have knowledge of eating disorders sufficient to recognize likely cases and to refer on appropriately.

An initial physical examination and investigations should be carried out, but physical risk assessment in patients with eating disorders must be a longitudinal process. A general medical history and examination should be carried out, of which the specific elements will be described below.

Body mass index (normal 20–25 in adults)

BMI should not be used alone to assess physical risk, due to factors such as patients falsifying their weight through practices such as water-loading or carrying heavy objects in their clothes. A BMI below 17.5 meets the criteria for anorexia nervosa, and immediate risk to patients increases significantly as the BMI falls below 13.[57,58] However, speed of weight loss increases risk, particularly if it is more than 1 kg a week. Other behaviours such as purging and overexercise also exacerbate the risk of a low BMI. The BMI is less useful in children and adolescents (in whom standard growth charts may be used instead), in pregnancy and in people with a height at the limits of normal. Co-morbid physical illness may also increase physical risk, such as omission of insulin to cause weight loss in patients with diabetes mellitus.[59]

Proximal myopathy

Starvation will eventually cause breakdown of muscle for energy, and increasing proximal myopathy is a good indicator of weight loss and may be useful if a clinician suspects weight falsification. It can be assessed by using the squat test or sit-up test.[57,58]

Core temperature

Inadequate autonomic response to temperature variations in anorexia nervosa can cause low core temperature, which if below 34.5 °C is an indicator of significant physical risk.

Blood tests

Full blood count

Mild, usually normocytic (occasionally macrocytic) anaemia is common in patients with anorexia nervosa, although haemoconcentration due to dehydration may mask it. Anthrocytosis has been reported in anorexia nervosa and results in a low erythrocyte sedimentation rate (ESR). A low white cell count may occur, particularly neutropenia, which is concerning in anorexia nervosa. Severe infection may occur as a result of this and other immunological factors. Mild thrombocytopenia may also occur. Bone-marrow changes such as fat-cell depletion have a significant effect on haemopoiesis and are likely to be a major cause of haematological complications in patients with anorexia nervosa.[60]

Urea, creatinine and electrolytes

A raised urea and creatinine in patients with eating disorders may be due to dehydration, either through restriction of fluids or through purging behaviours. Regular vomiting usually causes a hypokalaemic, hypochloraemic metabolic alkalosis, with varying disturbances of sodium. Laxative and diuretic misuse can also cause hypokalaemia, with disturbances of pH, sodium and chloride. Hypokalaemia can cause cardiac arrhythmias, muscle weakness, cramps, renal and gastrointestinal disturbances, tetany and absent reflexes.[61] Oral supplements may be used but, if the serum potassium is less than 3, particularly alongside electrocardiogram (ECG) changes, hospital admission may be necessary. Purging commonly causes hypovolaemia, which activates the angiotensin–renin–aldosterone system. Sudden cessation of purging can cause rebound oedema and consequent rapid weight gain. The oedema usually settles with conservative management, although short-term potassium-sparing diuretics are occasionally used in persistent oedema.[62] Malnutrition, purging behaviours, alcohol misuse and refeeding syndrome may also cause hypophosphataemia, hypomagnesaemia and hypocalcaemia. Water-loading can cause hyponatraemia and, in the most serious cases, may result in clinical symptoms of water intoxication, which include confusion, ataxia, seizures, coma and occasionally death as a result of brainstem coning due to cerebral oedema.[63]

Liver function tests

Starvation can adversely affect liver function tests (LFTs), possibly associated with fatty infiltration of the liver.[64] Initial refeeding in patients with anorexia nervosa or co-morbid alcohol misuse may also affect LFTs.

Albumin

Together with severity of weight loss, low serum albumin (due to starvation or severe infection) is a predictor of death in anorexia nervosa.[27,65]

Glucose

Starvation-induced hypoglycaemia may be asymptomatic, but rarely, in the most serious cases, it can cause coma and death. Dumping syndrome – excessive insulin production in response to food – may cause hypoglycaemia during refeeding. Vomiting following bingeing may also result in hypoglycaemia, therefore maintaining the binge–purge cycle, as hypoglycaemia may precipitate bingeing.[61]

Endocrine

Thyroid functions tests are useful to rule out hyperthyroidism as a differential for weight loss, co-morbid thyroid dysfunction or thyroxine misuse. Eating disorders, particularly anorexia nervosa, affect the thyroid axis; the common pattern is low tri-iodothyronine (T3; thyroxine (T4) is sometimes low) and normal thyroid-stimulating hormone (TSH). Eating-disorder-related abnormalities should normalize with weight gain and will not need treating routinely. Raised growth hormone and cortisol with normal or low adrenocorticotropic hormone (ACTH) may also occur but do not need to be checked routinely unless there is concern about an endocrine disorder as a differential for anorexia nervosa.[61] Reproductive hormones may need to be measured alongside other investigations, following weight restoration, if the female patient does not begin menstruating.

Cardiac

Blood pressure

Starvation or hypovolaemia due to fluid restriction or purging commonly causes postural hypotension, and blood pressure should be monitored regularly. Concerning features are a blood pressure below 90/70 mmHg and a postural drop of more than 10 mmHg.[58]

Electrocardiogram: prolonged QTc interval

Prolongation of the QTc interval and QT variability are good predictors of life-threatening ventricular arrhythmias. Prolonged starvation with a low BMI, causing atrophy and histological changes in cardiac muscle and collagen fibres, and purging behaviours, resulting in hypokalaemia and hypomagnesaemia, may be directly arrhythmogenic or may prolong the QTc interval in patients with eating disorders.[66,67] A genetic or medication-related prolonged QTc interval may increase this risk, and medications (many psychotropic) should be used with caution in patients with eating disorders.

Bradycardia

Bradycardia is a common feature in patients with anorexia nervosa, possibly due to electrolyte disturbances, atrophy and reduced glycogen content of cardiac tissue cells, and thyroid dysfunction. It is particularly concerning if the pulse rate is less than 40 bpm, due to the consequent risk of arrhythmias. Resting tachycardia is an unusual and concerning feature in anorexia nervosa and should be investigated appropriately. Reduced variability of heart rate can also occur in anorexia nervosa and may be a predictor of sudden death, especially in patients with pre-existing cardiac disease.[66]

ECG: ST segment and T-wave abnormalities

ST segment and T-wave changes are usually related to the effects on cardiac muscle of starvation, hypothermia or electrolyte abnormalities and should be investigated and treated appropriately.[57,67]

Echocardiography

Patients with anorexia nervosa often have reduced left ventricular mass with reduced cardiac output. Mitral valve prolapse and pericardial effusion are other cardiac complications associated with eating disorders. Ipecac, an emetic sometimes used by patients with bulimia nervosa, causes potentially fatal toxic cardiomyopathy.[66,67]

Gynaecological

Eating disorders have significant behavioural, psychological and physiological effects on reproduction. In anorexia nervosa, amenorrhoea results from hypogonadotrophic hypogonadism. The ovaries regress to a prepubertal state, although this is usually reversed with weight restoration. Amenorrhoea or oligomenorrhoea also occurs in many patients with bulimia nervosa without weight loss. Bulimia nervosa has been found to be associated with polycystic ovarian syndrome, but with an unclear causal relationship. Pregnancy occurs rarely in patients with anorexia nervosa and is associated with higher miscarriage rates, suboptimal maternal weight gain and fetal growth retardation. Pregnancy in bulimia nervosa is associated with being unintentional, due to an assumption of infertility because of oligomenorrhoea or amenorrhoea, or due to associated risky sexual behaviour. It is also associated with higher rates of miscarriage, prematurity, hyperemesis gravidarum and some fetal abnormalities. Eating disorder symptoms may improve temporarily during pregnancy in patients with eating disorders but often relapse postnatally. Gynaecologists should be careful in offering fertility treatments to women with anorexia nervosa. Treatment for the eating disorder should be the prime concern; if pregnancy occurs, regular physical and nutritional monitoring and liaison with primary care and obstetric services are vital.[68]

Bone mineral density

Osteopenia and osteoporosis are serious complications of anorexia nervosa and are not fully reversible. Bone metabolism is a continuous dynamic process, and oestrogen normally inhibits certain cytokines that encourage excessive bone resorption. The teenage years are a peak time for bone mineral to be laid down, similar to the time of onset for anorexia nervosa. The consequent amenorrhoea is therefore involved in the aetiology of osteoporosis or osteopenia in anorexia nervosa as well as other factors, including reduced levels of insulin growth factor (which normally promotes bone formation), increased cortisol levels and other nutritional deficiencies. Dual-energy X-ray absorptiometry (DEXA) is used to measure bone density at the hip and spine. It is probably appropriate to carry out DEXA scans on patients who have been amenorrhoeic for 1 year or more due to weight loss, as significant deterioration of bone density will take this long to occur. Scanning may be motivational in some patients, and knowledge of the current fracture risk may be useful in terms of lifestyle planning. Significant changes to bone density are likely to take at least 2 years, and therefore more frequent scanning is thought to be unnecessary.

Weight restoration is the key intervention to preventing further deterioration and partly improving bone mineral density. Weight-bearing exercise may improve bone density in a person of normal weight but can be detrimental to bone health in an underweight patient due to the fracture risk, contributing to further weight loss and continued amenorrhoea. Bisphosphonates should not be used in young women due to the potential for serious side effects such as teratogenicity (based on animal studies). They also have a poor evidence base for the treatment of premenopausal osteoporosis associated with anorexia nervosa. Other medications sometimes used in osteoporosis associated with anorexia nervosa are hormone-replacement therapy (HRT), the oral contraceptive pill (OCP), and calcium and vitamin D supplements, but the evidence base for these treatments is weak. Children should not be given hormone replacement, as there is a risk of stunted growth due to premature closure of the epiphyses.[27,69]

Gastroenterological complications

Gastroenterological complications are very common in patients with eating disorders. Delayed gastric emptying in anorexia nervosa may cause bloating after meals, early satiety and reflux symptoms. Constipation is common in all eating disorders and may be related to poor food intake and colonic transit.[70] Hypokalaemia is also a cause of constipation and paralytic ileus.[61] Self-induced vomiting can cause complications such as Mallory–Weiss tears, reflux symptoms, oesophagitis and hiatus hernia. Gastric or oesophageal dilation/rupture due to bingeing and vomiting is rare.[62] Haematemesis is relatively common as a result of a mild tear, but serious causes must always be excluded. Rare but serious complications of refeeding include acute gastric dilation, rupture of the stomach and acute pancreatitis. Patients with eating disorders are also more prone to functional gastrointestinal disorders such as irritable bowel syndrome.[70] Chronic laxative misuse may also resemble a functional gastrointestinal problem.[62] Misuse of stimulant laxatives may cause atonic colon over time, due to disruption of the colonic nerve supply. Stimulant laxatives may cause serious abnormalities in electrolyte and fluid balance; in order to prevent rebound oedema, patients are advised to wean off laxatives slowly. Bulk laxatives may be required during the weaning-off process, but a regular dietary structure and appropriate exercise should help to restore normal bowel function.[27] Most complaints improve with recovery from the eating disorder.

Neurological complications

Neuroimaging in patients with anorexia nervosa has consistently shown widening of the sulci and ventricular enlargement. These generally appear to be reversible with recovery from the eating disorder, but certain functional abnormalities remain, which are possibly due to primary deficits. Electrolyte abnormalities can cause neurological complications and should be monitored and managed appropriately. Thiamine deficiency from malnutrition or alcohol misuse may cause Wernicke's encephalopathy, and vitamin B12 and folic acid deficiency can rarely result in subacute combined degeneration of the spinal cord.[71] During initial refeeding of patients with eating disorders, a general multivitamin supplement is usually sufficient.[27] Specific supplementation with thiamine or vitamin B compound should be given in Wernicke's encephalopathy (medical emergency), alcohol misuse, and cases of severe and enduring malnutrition.

Dermatological manifestations

Lanugo hair (hypertrichosis lanuginose) is common in anorexia nervosa – there is soft downy hair, usually on the lower back, abdomen and forearms (Figure 42.1).[72] Russell's sign (calluses/abrasions on the back of the hands) is an early sign in patients who induce the gag reflex with their fingers (Figure 42.2). Patients with anorexia nervosa may develop acne, particularly during weight restoration; acne may also be associated with polycystic ovarian syndrome in bulimia nervosa. Peripheral oedema during starvation or refeeding may cause skin changes. Changes to hair and nail structure, acrocyanosis, dermatitis, carotenoderma and dryness of the skin may also occur in patients with eating disorders.[73]

Oral manifestations

Enamel erosion is a very common oral problem in patients who chronically induce vomiting, although salivary pH and flow and acidity of diet may influence the development of erosion. Eating disorders may also cause problems with oral

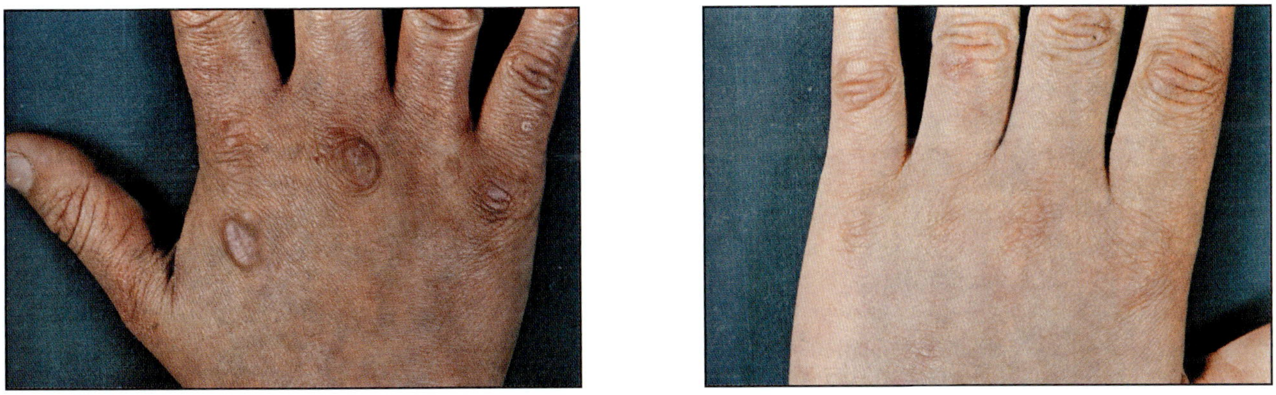

Figure 42.1 Presentations of Russell's sign. Reproduced with permission of Cambridge University Press from Gerald Russell's original paper. (ref.55)

mucosal and gingival tissues through poor oral hygiene, nutritional deficiencies, infection and self-induced vomiting. Self-induced vomiting can cause non-inflammatory hypertrophy of the salivary glands, most commonly the parotids, and also disturb the gag reflex.[74] Advice concerning oral health should be given to patients in order to limit oral damage. This includes using a non-acid mouth wash and fluoride toothpaste; rinsing the mouth with water and delaying brushing teeth after vomiting; reducing the amount of acidic foods and fluids in the diet; and regular check-ups with a dentist.[27]

Compulsory treatment

It is preferable that a patient with anorexia nervosa enters into treatment through their own free will. However, when a patient has become so seriously physically and mentally unwell that they lack the capacity to make an informed decision about life-saving treatment, it is the responsibility of the clinician to appropriately assess the need for refeeding under the Mental Health Act.

Treatment under the Mental Health Act should be considered before it is too late to start refeeding in a patient in a life-threatening condition. Intervention in children may be particularly urgent, as they will reach a dangerous physical state faster than adults, due to having fewer fat reserves.[27] A treatment section can be used in patients with anorexia nervosa in order to refeed, because the physical deterioration is related directly to the psychopathology that characterizes the disorder.[75] Compulsory refeeding is often initiated with nasogastric tube feeding, which can be emotionally and physically demanding for nursing staff. Patients need one-to-one nursing care on a specialist eating disorders unit or medical ward. If control and restraint are necessary, local or national guidelines should be followed. Mild sedation may be necessary, but BMI and cardiovascular and respiratory functioning must be taken into consideration when calculating the dose.

Refeeding and refeeding syndrome

Refeeding syndrome is most common in patients with a BMI below 12, recent rapid weight loss of more than 1 kg a week, alcohol misuse, bingeing and purging, and co-morbid physical illness.[27] Endogenous energy stores are catabolized during starvation as a means of providing energy, and insulin production is reduced. Despite sometimes normal serum levels, intracellular electrolyte levels, particularly phosphate, are often low. Insulin production increases on refeeding, in response to the move to exogenous carbohydrate metabolism. Insulin stimulates electrolyte uptake into cells, which may result in a sudden drop in serum electrolytes, most importantly phosphate. Peripheral oedema that usually settles with conservative management may occur during refeeding, but cardiac failure should be excluded.

Oral or intravenous phosphate supplementation may be used if necessary. Serum phosphate levels below 0.5 mmol/L may cause the most serious clinical features of refeeding syndrome. These comprise acute haemolysis, hypotension, cardiac failure, arrhythmias, rhabdomyolysis, respiratory failure, seizures, coma and sudden death.[76] Calorie intake during initial refeeding should be below the patient's basal metabolic requirements and should be increased gradually to reduce the risk of refeeding syndrome. Refeeding syndrome may also occur in patients at particular risk who are refeeding in an out-patient department. Careful monitoring of daily blood tests and diet are necessary for all high-risk patients in the initial stages of refeeding.

Further refeeding involves a gradual increase in dietary intake to encourage weight gain of approximately 1 kg a week on an in-patient unit and 0.5–1 kg a week in out-patients and day patients. To gain 1 kg a week, a patient will need approximately 1000 extra calories a day, on top of their normal requirements. This will mean a diet of approximately 2500–3000 calories/day, depending on the stage of weight gain, and should be achieved as far as is possible with a normal oral diet. Supplement high-calorie drinks are sometimes used for patients who are not aiming at full recovery from their eating disorder and are struggling with a full oral diet.

PHARMACOLOGY FOR EATING DISORDERS

One systematic review found that no medications trialled (antidepressants, hormonal and nutritional supplements) made a significant impact on weight gain in patients with anorexia nervosa.[28] Appropriate use of vitamin and electrolyte supplements and other medications to prevent or reduce physical risk is described above (see Physical presentation and management).

Olanzapine has been used for patients with anorexia nervosa in an attempt to reduce the intensity of the anorectic psychopathology, particularly fear of normal body weight and overvalued ideas about weight and shape. A literature review found that the limited evidence suggests that olanzapine at doses of 2.5–15 mg daily may be helpful in reducing anorectic psychopathology and helping weight gain.[77] However, more research is needed to clarify these findings, and refeeding alongside psychological therapies should be the mainstay of treatment for anorexia nervosa. Antidepressants may be used to improve mood in a patient with co-morbid depression, but low mood is common as a result of weight loss and malnutrition and may improve with refeeding.

Fluoxetine, a selective serotonin reuptake inhibitor (SSRI), has been licensed for the treatment of bulimia nervosa and is thought to help to reduce the urge to binge and vomit. A study found that fluoxetine 60 mg once a day is helpful in the treatment of bulimia nervosa, irrespective of the presence of co-morbid depression, and therefore suggested that its effect on the eating-disorder symptoms is not only secondary to the antidepressant effect.[78] SSRIs may also be useful in improving symptoms such as aggression, instability of mood, rejection sensitivity, anger, sexual disinhibition, illicit substance misuse and impulsive spending[79] and therefore may be helpful in treating symptoms in patients with multi-impulsive eating disorders.

Topiramate, an anticonvulsant, has been suggested as a treatment for BED in obese patients. A study found that CBT efficacy improved with added topiramate (at a maximum dose of 200 mg) compared with CBT and placebo, with significantly reduced bingeing and increased weight loss in the short term, and found that topiramate was well tolerated in terms of adverse effects.[80] More research is needed, particularly to look at whether the benefits are sustained in the longer term.

Medication is usually used in eating disorders alongside psychological therapies and aimed at specific symptoms rather than the core disorder.[81] When using medications in patients with eating disorders, particular care needs to be taken with regard to physical monitoring and dosage.

COURSE AND OUTCOME

Anorexia nervosa

A systematic review of the literature looked at outcomes of eating disorders.[82] It found that case series studies have shown that 24–82 per cent of patients have recovered at 5–15 years' follow-up. Two case series with comparison groups showed 27 per cent and 30 per cent recovery at 10 years and 12 years' follow-up, respectively, and a prospective cohort study with comparison group showed 59 per cent recovery at 5 years' follow-up. There were also concerns that, despite 'recovering' from their eating disorder, many patients continued to have significant concerns about weight and appearance, higher scores in the eating attitudes test, and dietary restriction. In all studies, up to 24 per cent of patients continued to have anorexia nervosa and many had traversed eating-disorder diagnoses or relapsed after a period of remission. Predictors of poor outcome in various studies included greater family hostility; extreme compulsion to exercise; poor social relationships before illness onset; psychiatric co-morbidity, particularly cluster C personality disorders, obsessive–compulsive disorder (OCD), autism-spectrum disorders, depression and substance misuse (associated with binge–purge subtype); more bingeing and purging behaviours; longer duration of disorder before presentation; older age at presentation; longer duration of amenorrhoea; and low albumin levels and lower BMI, haemoglobin and alkaline phosphatase at follow-up. The review also found higher rates of recovery for binge–purge subtype than for restrictive subtype at 4 years but no difference at 8 years; those patients who had the illness longer were more likely to have the binge–purge subtype. This fits with the finding that 52 per cent of patients with restrictive subtype were found to develop binge–purge subtype, usually within the first 5 years of follow up.

Berkman and colleagues also looked at mortality outcomes. The SMR for anorexia nervosa ranged from 1.36 to 30.5 and the SMR for suicide was 58.1 in one study.[83] Crude mortality rates vary from study to study but have been found to be as high as 20 per cent over 20 years. Predictors for death in anorexia nervosa in various studies included weight below 35 kg at presentation; more than one in-patient admission; a history of psychiatric hospitalization for anorexia nervosa; substance and alcohol misuse; longer duration of illness at start of treatment; poor social adjustment; hospitalization for an affective disorder; and suicidality associated with co-morbid mental illness.[82]

Bulimia nervosa and multi-impulsive eating disorders

A study showed that, at 12-year follow-up after in-patient treatment (common in Germany), 70.1 per cent of patients with an original diagnosis of bulimia nervosa had no eating disorder diagnosis (most of whom had a BMI below 30), 10.8 per cent had bulimia nervosa, 1.8 per cent had BED, 1.8 per cent had anorexia nervosa and 13.2 per had EDNOS.[84] In a systematic review of the literature,[82] predictors for poor outcome in bulimia nervosa were found to be substance misuse, poor impulse control, premorbid obesity, lifetime history of anorexia nervosa, older age at illness onset, co-morbid affective disorder and poor social adjustment. Many studies showed that BMI increased over time but remained largely within the normal range. The SMR for patients with bulimia nervosa was similar to that of the general population, throughout the studies.

Patients with multi-impulsive eating disorders have been found to have a poorer outcome, although there have been relatively few outcome studies. A study found that impulsive behaviours such as alcohol or substance misuse, recent suicide attempt, bingeing or stealing were the strongest predictor of a poor prognosis for patients with both anorexia and bulimia nervosa over a 4- to 6-year follow-up.[85]

Binge eating disorder and other EDNOS

There is a limited literature for outcome in BED. A study looked at 12-year outcome after in-patient admission for BED and found that 67.2 per cent of patients had no diagnosable eating disorder at 12 years (although 53.4 per cent of these had a BMI above 30), 7.8 per cent had BED, 9.4 per cent had a diagnosis of bulimia nervosa, none had anorexia nervosa and 12.5 per cent had other EDNOS.[84] Co-morbid psychiatric illness, high presenting BMI, a history of sexual abuse and impulsivity appear to be poor prognostic indicators. The SMR for BED is unclear.

There is a very limited literature on outcomes in other EDNOS. However, one study found that patients with atypical anorexia nervosa, who lacked the intense fear of normal body weight and body image disturbance, had a better outcome than those with typical anorexia nervosa.[86]

CONCLUSION

Eating disorders have high morbidity and mortality rates especially anorexia nervosa. They have a complex aetiology and pathogenesis. Although there are clearly distinct eating disorder syndromes, many patients traverse diagnoses over the course of their illness. Psychological treatment for bulimia nervosa is well researched, with cognitive-behavioural psychotherapy being the gold standard. The evidence base for psychological treatment for anorexia nervosa is less clear, perhaps due to factors such as difficulty engaging patients in treatment and high attrition rates. All patients with eating disorders need careful physical investigation and monitoring over time. Early detection and treatment are important, as this may lead to better prognosis.

KEY POINTS

- Eating disorders have a complex and multifactorial aetiology and pathogenesis.
- Most people with eating disorders should be treated in an out-patient setting.
- Day-patient or in-patient treatment may be required, particularly for patients with anorexia nervosa.
- CBT is the recommended treatment for bulimia nervosa.
- Psychological treatment in any modality should be offered to patients with anorexia nervosa and EDNOS.
- Anorexia nervosa has the highest standardized mortality rate of any psychiatric disorder.
- Patients with any eating disorder may present with high physical morbidity.
- All organ systems may be affected, and careful physical monitoring should be carried out in all patients with eating disorders.
- Treatment for an eating disorder should aim for the patient to gain or stabilize weight within the normal BMI range and deal with underlying psychological problems contemporaneously.

REFERENCES

1. Fairburn CG, Cooper Z, Shafran R (2003) Cognitive behaviour therapy for eating disorders: a 'transdiagnostic' theory and treatment. *Behaviour Research and Therapy* **41**: 509–28.
2. World Health Organization (1992) *The ICD-10 Classification of Mental and Behavioural Disorders: Clinical Description and Diagnostic Guidelines*. Geneva: World Health Organization.
3. American Psychiatric Association (1994) *Diagnostic and Statistical Manual of Mental Disorders*, 4th edn. Washington, DC: American Psychiatric Association.
4. Fairburn CG, Bohn K (2005) Eating disorder NOS (EDNOS): an example of the troublesome 'not otherwise specified' (NOS) category in DSM-IV. *Behaviour Research and Therapy* **43**: 691–701.
5. Hoeken D (2003) Review of the prevalence and incidence of eating disorders. *International Journal of Eating Disorders* **34**: 383–96.
6. Lucas AR, Crowson CS, O'Fallon WM, Melton LJ 3rd (1999) The ups and downs of anorexia nervosa. *International Journal of Eating Disorders* **26**: 397–405.
7. Hoek HW, Wijbrand H (2006) Incidence, prevalence and mortality of anorexia nervosa and other eating disorders. *Current Opinion in Psychiatry* **19**: 389–94.
8. Holland AJ, Sicotte N, Treasure JL (1988) Anorexia nervosa: evidence for a genetic basis. *Journal of Psychosomatic Research* **32**: 561–71.
9. Holland AJ, Hall A, Murray R, Russell GFM, Crisp AH (1984) Anorexia nervosa: a study of 34 twin pairs and one set of triplets. *British Journal of Psychiatry* **145**: 414–19.
10. Bulik CM, Sullivan PF, Kendler KS (1998) Heritability of binge-eating and broadly-defined bulimia nervosa. *Biological Psychiatry* **44**: 1210–18.
11. Becker AE, Burwell RA, Gilman SE, *et al.* (2002) Eating behaviours and attitudes following prolonged exposure to television among ethnic Fijian adolescent girls. *British Journal of Psychiatry* **180**: 509–14.
12. Striegel-Moore RH, Bulik CM (2007) Risks factors for eating disorders. *American Psychologist* **3**: 181–98.
13. Hoek HW, Bartelds AJ, Bosveld JJ, *et al.* (1995) Impact of urbanization on detection rates of eating disorders. *American Journal of Psychiatry* **152**: 1272–8.
14. Blair C, Freeman CPL, Cull A (1995) The families of anorexia nervosa and cystic fibrosis patients. *Psychological Medicine* **25**: 985–93.
15. Connors ME, Worse W (1993) Sexual abuse and eating disorders: a review. *International Journal of Eating Disorders* **13**: 1–11.
16. Rorty M, Yager J, Rossotto E (1994) Childhood sexual, physical and psychological abuse in bulimia nervosa. *American Journal of Psychiatry* **151**: 1122–6.
17. Waller G, Corstorphine E, Mountford V (2007) The role of emotional abuse in the eating disorders; implications for treatment. *Eating Disorders* **15**: 1–15.
18. Johnson C, Wonderlich SA (1992) Personality characteristics as a risk factor in the development of eating disorders. In JH Crowther, DL Tennenbaum (eds) *The Etiology of Bulimia Nervosa: The Individual and Familial Context*. Kent, OH: Kent State University Press.

19. Gordon I, Lask B, Bryant Waugh R, *et al.* (1997) Childhood-onset anorexia nervosa: towards identifying a biological substrate. *International Journal of Eating Disorders* **22**: 159–65.
20. Lacey JH, Evans CDH (1986) The impulsivist: a multi-impulsive personality disorder. *British Journal of Addiction* **81**: 641–9.
21. Lacey JH (1993) Self damaging and addictive behaviour in bulimia nervosa: a catchment area study. *British Journal of Psychiatry* **163**: 190–94.
22. Collier DA, Treasure JL (2004) The aetiology of eating disorders. *British Journal of Psychiatry* **185**: 363–5.
23. Bruch H (1978) *The Golden Cage: The Enigma of Anorexia Nervosa*. Cambridge, MA: Harvard University Press.
24. Crisp, AH (1980) *Anorexia Nervosa: Let Me Be*. London: Academic Press.
25. Fairburn CG, Shafran R, Cooper Z (1999) A cognitive behavioural theory of anorexia nervosa. *Behaviour Research and Therapy* **37**: 1–13.
26. Luck A, Waller G, Meyer C, Ussher M, Lacey H (2006) The role of schema processes in the eating disorders. *Cognitive Therapy and Research* **29**: 717–32.
27. National Institute of Health and Clinical Excellence (2004) *Eating Disorders: Core Interventions in the Treatment and Management of Anorexia Nervosa, Bulimia Nervosa and Other Related Eating Disorders*. National clinical practice guideline no. CG9. London: National Institute of Health and Clinical Excellence.
28. Bulik CM, Berkman ND, Brownley KA, *et al.* (2007) Anorexia nervosa treatment: a systematic review of randomized controlled trials. *International Journal of Eating Disorders* **40**: 310–20.
29. Pike KM, Walsh BT, Vitousek K, *et al.* (2003) Cognitive behaviour therapy in the post hospitalization treatment of anorexia nervosa. *American Journal of Psychiatry* **160**: 2046–9.
30. McIntosh VV, Jordan J, Carter FA, *et al.* (2005) Three psychotherapies for anorexia nervosa: a randomized controlled trial. *American Journal of Psychiatry* **162**: 741–7.
31. Dare C, Russell G, Treasure J, Dodge L (2001) Psychological therapies for adults with anorexia nervosa. *British Journal of Psychiatry* **178**: 216–21.
32. Nielsen S, Moller-Madsen S, Isager T, *et al.* (1998) Standardized mortality rates in eating disorders: a quantitative summary of previously published and new evidence. *Journal of Psychosomatic Research* **44**: 413–34.
33. Wilson GT, Vitousek KM, Loeb KL (2007) Stepped care treatment for eating disorders. *Journal of Consulting and Clinical Psychology* **68**: 564–72.
34. Shapiro JR, Berkman ND, Brownley KA, *et al.* (2007) Bulimia nervosa: a systematic review of randomised controlled trials. *International Journal of Eating Disorders* **40**: 321–36.
35. Thiels C, Schmidt U, Treasure J, Garthe R, Troop N (1998) Guided self change for bulimia nervosa incorporating the use of a self care manual. *American Journal of Psychiatry* **155**: 947–53.
36. Bailer U, de Zwann M, Leisch F, *et al.* (2004) Guided self help versus cognitive behavioural group therapy in the treatment of bulimia nervosa. *International Journal of Eating Disorders* **35**: 522–37.
37. Palmer RL, Birchall H, McGrain L, Sullivan V (2002) Self-help for bulimic disorders: a randomised controlled trial comparing minimal guidance with face to face or telephone guidance. *British Journal of Psychiatry* **181**: 230–35.
38. Ljotsson B, Lundin C, Mitsell K, *et al.* (2007) Remote treatment of bulimia nervosa and binge eating disorder: a randomized trial of internet-assisted cognitive behavioural therapy. *Behaviour Research and Therapy* **45**: 649–61.
39. Agras WS, Walsh BT, Fairburn CG, Wilson GT, Kraemer HC (2000) A multicenter comparison of cognitive behavioural therapy and interpersonal psychotherapy for bulimia nervosa. *Archives of General Psychiatry* **57**: 459–66.
40. Leung N, Waller G, Thomas G. (2000) Outcome of group cognitive-behaviour therapy for bulimia nervosa: the role of core beliefs. *Behaviour Research and Therapy* **38**: 145–56.
41. Mitchell JE, Agras S, Wonderlich S (2007) Treatment of bulimia nervosa: where are we and where are we going? *International Journal of Eating Disorders* **40**: 95–101.
42. Fairburn CG, Cooper Z, Doll HA, *et al.* (2009). Transdiagnostic cognitive-behavioural therapy for patients with eating disorders: a two-site trial with 60 week follow up. *American Journal of Psychiatry* **166**: 311–19.
43. Linehan MM (1993) *Cognitive Behavioral Treatment of Borderline Personality Disorder*. New York: Guilford Press.
44. Safer DL, Telch CF, Agras WS (2001) Dialectical behaviour therapy for bulimia nervosa. *American Journal of Psychiatry* **158**: 632–4.
45. Murphy S, Russell L, Waller G (2005) Integrated psychodynamic therapy for bulimia nervosa and binge eating disorder: theory, practice and preliminary findings. *European Eating Disorders Review* **13**: 383–91.
46. Le Grange D, Crosby RD, Rathauz P, Levethal BL (2007) A randomized controlled comparison of family-based treatment and supportive psychotherapy for adolescent bulimia nervosa. *Archives of General Psychiatry* **64**: 1049–56.
47. Schmidt U, Lee S, Beecham J, *et al.* (2007) A randomized controlled trial of family therapy and cognitive behavior therapy guided self-care for adolescents with bulimia nervosa and related disorders. *American Journal of Psychiatry* **164**: 591–8.
48. Schapman-Williams AM, Lock J (2007) Using cognitive behavioural therapy with adolescent onset bulimia nervosa. *Clinical Case Studies* **6**: 508–24.

49. Fairburn CG, Agras WS, Walsh BT, Wilson GT, Stice E (2004) Prediction of outcome in bulimia nervosa by early change in treatment. *American Journal of Psychiatry* **161**: 2322–4
50. Ghaderi A (2006) Does individualization matter? A randomized trial of standardized (focused) versus individualized (broad) cognitive behavior therapy for bulimia nervosa. *Behaviour Research and Therapy* **44**: 273–88.
51. Waller G, Patient E, Corstorphine E, *et al.* (2005) Cognitive behaviour therapy for bulimic disorders: effectiveness in non-research settings. Presented at the Eating Disorders Research Society Meeting, Toronto, Canada, September 2005.
52. Brownley KA, Berkman ND, Sedway JA, Lohr KN, Bulik CM (2007) Binge eating disorder treatment: a systematic review of randomised controlled trials. *International Journal of Eating Disorders* **40**: 337–48.
53. Telch CF, Agras WS, Linehan MM (2001) Dialectical behaviour therapy for binge eating disorder. *Journal of Consulting and Clinical Psychology* **69**: 1061–5.
54. Wilfley DE, Welch RR, Stein RI, *et al.* (2002) A randomised comparison of group cognitive behavioural therapy and group interpersonal therapy for the treatment of overweight individuals with binge eating disorder. *Archives of General Psychiatry* **59**: 713–21.
55. Russell G (1979) Bulimia nervosa: an ominous variant of anorexia nervosa. *Psychological Medicine* **9**: 429–48.
56. Fairburn CG, Wilson GT (eds) (1993) *Binge Eating: Nature, Assessment and Treatment.* New York: Guilford Press.
57. Robinson PH (2006) *Community Treatment of Eating Disorders.* Chichester: John Wiley & Sons.
58. Treasure J (2004) *A Guide to the Medical Risk Assessment for Eating Disorders.* London: Kings College London, University of London.
59. Crow SJ, Keel PK, Kendall D (1998) Eating disorders and insulin dependent diabetes mellitus. *Psychosomatic* **39**: 233–43.
60. Lambert M, Boland B (2000) Haematological complications. *European Eating Disorders Review* **8**: 158–61.
61. Connan F, Lightman S, Treasure J (2000) Biochemical and endocrine complications. *European Eating Disorders Review* **8**: 144–57.
62. Lasater LM, Mehler PS (2001) Medical complications of bulimia nervosa. *Eating Behaviours* **2**: 279–92.
63. Rome ES, Ammerman S (2003) Medical complications of eating disorders: an update. *Journal of Adolescent Health* **33**: 418–26.
64. Winston AP, Gowers S, Jackson AA, *et al.* (2005) *Guidelines for the Nutritional Management of Anorexia Nervosa.* Council report. London: Royal College of Psychiatrists.
65. Herzog W, Deter HC, Fiehn W, Petzold E (1997) Medical findings and predictors of long term physical outcome in anorexia nervosa: a prospective, 12-year follow-up study. *Psychological Medicine* **27**: 269–79.
66. Casiero D, Frishman W (2006) Cardiovascular complications of eating disorders. *Cardiology Review* **14**: 227–31.
67. McCallum K, Bermudez O, Ohlemeyer C, *et al.* (2006) How should the clinician evaluate and manage the cardiovascular complications of anorexia nervosa? *Eating Disorders* **14**: 73–80.
68. Webb K, Morgan J, Lacey JH (2009) Physical consequences of eating disorders. In N Agrawal, J Bolton (eds) *Current Themes in Psychiatry*, Vol. 5. London: Palgrave Macmillan. (In press)
69. Mehler PS (2003) Osteoporosis in anorexia nervosa: prevention and treatment. *International Journal of Eating Disorders* **33**: 113–26.
70. Chial HJ, McAlpine DE, Camilleri M (2002) Anorexia nervosa: manifestations and management for the gastroenterologist. *American Journal of Gastroenterology* **97**: 255–69.
71. Chowdhury U, Lask B (2000) Neurological correlates of eating disorders. *European Eating Disorders Review* **8**: 126–33.
72. Mitchell JE, Crow S (2006) Medical complications of anorexia nervosa and bulimia nervosa. *Current Opinion in Psychiatry* **19**: 438–43.
73. Strumia R (2002) Bulimia and anorexia nervosa: cutaneous manifestations. *Journal of Cosmetic Dermatology* **1**: 30–34.
74. Frydrych AM, Davies GR, McDermott BM (2005) Eating disorders and oral health: a review of the literature. *Australian Dental Journal* **50**: 6–15.
75. Mental Health Act Commission (2008) *The Treatment of Anorexia Nervosa Under the Mental Health Act 1983.* Guidance note 13. London: Mental Health Act Commission.
76. Hearing SD (2004) Refeeding syndrome. *British Medical Journal* **328**: 908–9.
77. Duncan KC (2007) The role of olanzapine in the treatment of anorexia nervosa. *Annals of Pharmacotherapy* **41**: 111–15.
78. Goldstein DJ, Wilson MG, Ascroft RC, Al-Banna M (1999) Effectiveness of fluoxetine therapy in bulimia nervosa regardless of comorbid depression. *International Journal of Eating Disorders* **25**: 19–27.
79. Fagin L (2004) Management of personality disorders in acute inpatient settings: part 1. Borderline personality disorders. *Advances in Psychiatric Treatment* **10**: 93–9.
80. Claudino AM (2007) Double-blind, randomized, placebo-controlled trial of topiramate plus cognitive-behaviour therapy in binge eating disorder. *Journal of Clinical Psychiatry* **68**: 1324–32.
81. Sansone RA, Sansone LA (2004) The use of psychotropic medications in eating disorder patients with personality disorders. *Eating Behaviours* **13**: 123–34.
82. Berkman ND, Lohr KN, Bulik CM (2007) Outcomes of eating disorders: a systematic review of the literature. *International Journal of Eating Disorders* **40**: 293–309.

83. Herzog DB, Greenwood DN, Dorer DJ, *et al.* (2000) Mortality in eating disorders: a descriptive study. *International Journal of Eating Disorders* **28**: 20–26.
84. Fichter MM, Quadflieg N, Hedlund S (2008) Long-term course of binge eating disorder and bulimia nervosa: relevance for nosology and diagnostic criteria. *International Journal of Eating Disorders* **41**: 577–86.
85. Sohlberg S, Norring C, Holmgren S, Rosmark, B (1989) Impulsivity and long-term prognosis of psychiatric patients with anorexia nervosa/bulimia nervosa. *Journal of Nervous and Mental Disease* **177**: 249–58.
86. Strober M, Freeman R, Morrell W (1999) Atypical anorexia nervosa: separation from typical cases in course and outcome in a long term prospective study. *International Journal of Eating Disorders* **25**: 135–42.

Chapter 43

Personality disorders

Peter Tyrer

INTRODUCTION

Personality disorders are odd. They are common (affecting around 7–10% of the population[1,2]), have a major influence on society[3] and yet are almost universally neglected in ordinary psychiatric practice. It is also odd that they are the least stable diagnoses in psychiatric practice[4] and yet regarded as conditions that are stable, arising in late adolescence and persisting to late middle or old age. This is also an essential element in their general description: people with personality disorder have an 'enduring pattern of inner experience and behaviour that deviates markedly from the expectations of the individual's culture'.[5] This dissonance between the notional lay impression of personality as the bedrock of psychic functioning that make the person's sense of 'self', and empirical data that suggest the diagnosis is unstable, is one of the major puzzles behind the diagnosis, and perhaps helps to explain why its measurement is such a perennial issue for psychiatrists and psychologists within and outside the research area. This is why researchers and clinicians are very much involved in questioning the reliability of personality disorder, and in this context the lay meaning of 'reliable' becomes the same as the statistical one of agreement. If people cannot agree on what constitutes personality disorder, then there is little confidence in those who are diagnosed as having the condition. For psychiatrists in training, it is important to start with the existing classification, to explain why it fails and what is likely to be offered as an alternative that is better suited to clinical practice. The course and treatment of these conditions is then discussed in the light of both new and old classifications, and readers can then come to their own conclusions as to which is superior.

CURRENT CLASSIFICATION

There are four elements that underpin the classification of personality disorders: (i) they are primarily disturbances of behaviour, not symptoms; (ii) they are persistent; (iii) they are associated with poor interpersonal relationships; and (iv) they create problems for both society and the individual. It will be apparent immediately that these features are not necessarily confined to personality disorders alone, and there has long been debate over the dividing line between mental state disorders (Axis I in the *Diagnostic and Statistical Manual of Mental Disorders* (DSM) classification) and personality disorders (Axis II). The current classification systems of personality disorder in the *International Classification of Diseases*, 10th revision (ICD-10)[6] and the fourth edition of DSM (DSM-IV)[5] both describe personality disorders as forming in childhood and adolescence and continuing through adulthood. A formal diagnosis of personality disorder cannot be made before the age of 18 years.

The clinician making an assessment of personality disorder is advised to make the diagnosis in two stages: (i) the identification of the condition as a personality disorder, and (ii) the categorization of the disorder into one of nine or ten categories – paranoid, schizoid, dissocial, emotionally unstable (borderline and impulsive), histrionic, anxious, dependent and anankastic in ICD-10, and paranoid, schizoid, schizotypal, antisocial, narcissistic, borderline, histrionic, avoidant, dependent and obsessive–compulsive in DSM-IV. In practice, most clinicians tend to plump for the categories first because they are so seductive and then try to justify the general criteria for general personality disorder second. Unfortunately, because the categories are not very good and there is a great deal of overlap between them, the diagnosis of personality disorder not otherwise specified (PD-NOS) is often chosen as the most appropriate diagnosis.[7,8] The four characteristics needed for the diagnosis of personality disorder in ICD-10 are evidence that:[6]

- the 'individual's characteristic and enduring patterns of inner experience and behaviour deviate markedly from the culturally expected and accepted range in one of more of the following areas – (a) cognition (ways of perceiving and interpreting things, people and events; forming attitudes and images of self and others), (b) affectivity (range, intensity and appropriateness of emotional arousal and responses), (c) control over impulses and gratification of needs, (d) manner of relating to others and of handling interpersonal situations';
- the deviation is pervasive as 'behaviour that is inflexible, maladaptive or otherwise dysfunctional across a broad range of personal and social situations';

- the disorder creates personal distress or an 'adverse effect on the social environment attributable to the deviant behaviour';
- the deviation is stable and long standing, with 'onset in late childhood or adolescence'.

In addition, there are two exclusion criteria: the condition cannot be explained as a manifestation or consequence of other mental disorders, and organic disorders should be excluded as these may give rise to personality change (e.g. in dementia) but are not personality disorders.

PROBLEMS WITH THE EXISTING CLASSIFICATION

The main problems with the existing classification are that (i) the specific diagnosis is temporally unreliable; (ii) there is too much overlap with other personality disorders; (iii) the characteristics defining the disorder (operational criteria) are not specific to each disorder (one of the reasons for the overlap); (iv) there appears to be reluctance, probably amounting to stigma, to use the diagnosis; and (v) the high use of PD-NOS as a diagnosis suggests that what clinicians identify as personality disorder cannot be fitted easily into the present classification.

The unreliability of the diagnosis is clearly shown in service statistics,[4] and this might be thought to be due to sloppy recording or inadequate assessment. However, even when assessors have been trained with interview schedules that are recommended for the assessment of personality disorder, diagnostic agreement is only at a level of around 0.45–0.50 (kappa).[9] The reason for this seems to be that formal personality assessment pretends that it can assess personality status over a period of years, but in practice only present personality status, or personality function,[10] is measured, and this changes from month to month.

The problem with overlap is that although each individual personality disorder appears to have face validity, the descriptions of each disorder are somewhat stereotyped and rarely exist alone. Factor analysis of the criteria for the different DSM personality disorders reveals a completely different structure from that postulated by the DSM system.[11] In an attempt to reduce this overlap, the personality disorders have been separated into three clusters in many research studies assessing personality disorder. These have now passed into common parlance, but it is worth stressing that the clusters are not actually described in the ICD-10 system of classification. The three clusters are the odd and eccentric group (cluster A), the flamboyant or dramatic group (cluster B) and the anxious and fearful group (cluster C) (Table 43.1). A fourth group, the obsessional or rigid cluster (cluster D), is also sometimes identified, but formally this is included within cluster C, in spite of good evidence that a four-group model is similar to the classification of normal personality variance in the community.[10]

However, even the cluster system does not remove overlap greatly, for when there is severe personality disorder it is possible to satisfy the criteria for almost all those present in the classification. What is somewhat surprising is that as personality disorder gets more severe in terms of its impact on the individual and on society, the numbers of personality disorders also seem to increase, and this is accommodated in a classification of severity (Table 43.2).

This classification of severity is not an accepted one, but as there is no alternative available it can be regarded as a working option[12] until another is found to be superior.

DIMENSIONAL VERSUS CATEGORICAL ASSESSMENT OF PERSONALITY DISORDER

Box 43.1 shows the DSM-IV criteria for antisocial personality disorder.

Table 43.1 Grouped classification of personality disorders by clusters

Cluster	Personality disorders included
A	ICD-10: schizoid, paranoid
	DSM-IV: schizoid, schizotypal, paranoid
B	ICD-10: dissocial, emotionally unstable (borderline and impulsive), histrionic
	DSM-IV: antisocial, borderline, histrionic, narcissistic
C	ICD-10: anxious, dependent
	DSM-IV: avoidant, dependent
D (but usually subsumed within cluster C)	ICD-10: anankastic
	DSM-IV: obsessive–compulsive

DSM-IV, *Diagnostic and Statistical Manual of Mental Disorders*, 4th edn; ICD-10, *International Classification of Diseases*, 10th revision.

Table 43.2 System to record severity of personality disorder

Level of severity	Description	Definition by categorical system
0	No personality disorder	Does not meet actual or subthreshold criteria for any personality disorder
1	Personality difficulty	Meets subthreshold criteria for any or several personality disorders
2	Simple personality disorder	Meets actual criteria for one or more personality disorders within the same cluster
3	Complex (diffuse) personality disorder	Meets actual criteria for one or more personality disorders within more than one cluster
4	Severe personality disorder	Meets criteria for creation of severe disruption to both individual and to many in society (antisocial personality disorder plus other criteria for level 3)

Serious consideration is being given to dimensional systems of classification in all parts of psychiatry, but it is particularly strong with personality disorder. There are many advantages of dimensional systems, not least of which is that when there is no clear distinction between the presence and absence of a disorder, then a dimensional system gives steadily better levels of agreement up to seven groups with no gain in reliability subsequently.[13] But better reliability does not necessarily mean better validity, and there is also some doubt as to whether clinicians would use a dimensional classification. It seems likely that if a dimensional system does enter either the ICD-11 or DSM-V classification in 2012–13, then it will show some similarity to the cluster system described above.

One main advantage of dimensional systems is that they remove the stigmatic label of personality disorder. The reluctance of clinicians to use the diagnosis is not only because it is unreliable; the reluctance to use the diagnosis in only about 10 per cent of the population who qualify for significant personality abnormality[14] suggests that the stigma attached to the diagnosis is the main reason, so that a clinician might baulk at crossing the dividing line between two of the criteria in Box 43.1 and three criteria, which qualifies the person for the diagnosis of antisocial personality disorder.

NATURAL HISTORY OF PERSONALITY DISORDER

Psychiatrists seldom have the opportunity to study the natural history of the disorders they treat, but this is not so true of personality disorders. Until recently no specific treatments were available, and so long-term follow-up studies of personality disorder were, in effect, a record of the natural course of these conditions. In almost every study in which long-term follow-up has taken place, there has been a steady fall in the number of people having the disorder, with a gradual reduction in the prevalence over time.[15] This can be a dramatic reduction, with more than half failing to reach the criteria for a personality disorder diagnosis after 5 years or more.[16–18] There is some variation in the course of different disorders. Disorders in the cluster B group tend to manifest earlier in life, with onset in late childhood, almost always diagnosed as conduct disorder, and have earlier resolution, whereas disorders in clusters A and C arise later but persist for longer (Figure 43.1). There are also suggestions that cluster A disorders may become more prominent later in life.[19]

No good explanation exists for this variation. The aetiology of cluster B disorders includes childhood abuse,

Box 43.1 Operational criteria for one personality disorder (the *Diagnostic and Statistical Manual of Mental Disorders*, 4th edn (DSM-IV) diagnosis of antisocial personality disorder)

A pervasive pattern of disregard for and violation of the rights of others occurring since the age of 15 years as indicated by at least three of the following:

- Failure to conform to social norms with respect to lawful behaviours, as indicated by repeatedly performing acts that are grounds for arrest
- Deceitfulness, as indicated by repeated lying, use of aliases or conning others for personal profit or pleasure
- Impulsivity or failure to plan ahead
- Irritability and aggressiveness, as indicated by repeated physical fights or assaults
- Reckless disregard for the safety of self or others
- Consistent irresponsibility, as indicated by repeated failure to sustain consistent work behaviour or honour financial obligations
- Lack of remorse, as indicated by being indifferent to or rationalizing having hurt, mistreated or stolen from another.

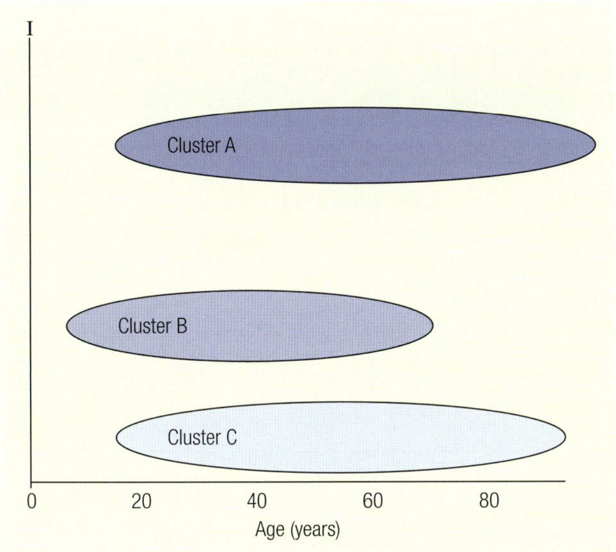

Figure 43.1 Differences in onset and course of clusters of personality disorders

physical, mental and sexual, and this is said to be particularly prominent in borderline personality disorder. Despite this claim, the prospective follow-up of populations necessary to test this hypothesis has not revealed a marked preponderance of borderline personality disorder as opposed to other personality disorders. Part of this problem is related to the severity of disorder. As noted above, when personality disorders become very severe, the people concerned satisfy the criteria for a large number of personality disorders, and so it is difficult to know which is primary. There has long been interest in the notion of psychopathy as a core element of antisocial personality. Oddly, it does not appear in the official psychiatric classifications, but it shows great overlap with antisocial personality disorder. Robert Hare invented the Psychopathy Checklist,[20] which itself was derived from the descriptions in a celebrated book by Hervey Cleckley, called *The Mask of Sanity* because Cleckley believed that behind the glib, charming, remorseless front of the true psychopath was a serious mental flaw, or disorder.[21] The revised form of the Psychopathy Checklist (PCL-R) is now in common use in the assessment of both risk and personality disorder.[20]

The most serious form of personality disorder in the UK is dangerous and severe personality disorder (DSPD). Although this originally masqueraded as a diagnosis, it now describes the DSPD programme in England. The programme allows for the detention of individuals in a secure setting if they satisfy all three of the following characteristics:

- They are more likely than not to commit an offence within 5 years that might be expected to lead to serious physical or psychological harm from which the victim would find it difficult or impossible to recover
- They have a significant disorder of personality
- The risk presented appears to be functionally linked to the significant personality disorder.[22]

Three hundred people are currently being treated in the programme in two high-security prisons (HMP Whitemoor and Frankland) and two special hospitals (Broadmoor and Rampton) in England. The assessment procedure has been defective in many respects[23] and expensive,[24] and the long-term feasibility of this initiative is far from certain.

TREATMENT

The successful treatment of personality disorder is probably the key to it being accepted as a proper diagnosis in psychiatry. As Kendell puts it:

> If, therefore, the psychiatrists and politicians who maintain that 'antisocial personality disorder' has as good a claim to being accepted as a mental disorder as schizophrenia can demonstrate that it responds to some form of treatment that is not simply a disciplined environment, it is likely that the opposition will melt away, and the same will be true for other types of personality disorder.[25]

It is fair to say that we do not yet have a satisfactory treatment for any form of personality disorder and so have not approached this point. Some of the reasons for this are apparent from our poor understanding of the genesis of normal personality and the reasons why its variation tends to be self-correcting.

Drug treatments

Every psychotropic drug has been used to treat personality disorder at some time in practice, and this only serves to reinforce the interpretation that nothing works. It is true that many drug trials have been carried out with some positive results,[26] the results of which are summarized below (Tables 43.3 and 43.4), but the total evidence base is very slim and as most of the studies have been industry funded the positive ones with only small numbers should be viewed with some scepticism, particularly when they have not been replicated. One of the main problems is that most of those with personality disorder are very poor at adhering to drug therapy so even when a treatment may be effecaceous it is only under conditions of supervised adherence that it is effective.[27,28] Because of the risks of drug treatment and only marginal advantage there is no strong reason for prescribing drugs except as a crisis measure. Unfortunately in practice a very large number of people with borderline personality disorder take these drugs[18] and it is likely that much of this polypharmacy is counter-productive.

Psychological treatments

In general, psychological treatments have been preferred to all others in the treatment of personality disorder. This

Table 43.3 Summary of randomized trials of antipsychotic drugs in the treatment of personality disorder

Antipsychotic drug tested	Personality diagnosis	Ref.	Type of study	Main results
Haloperidol	Borderline	28	Randomized controlled trial	Haloperidol (7 mg/day) superior to both amitriptyline and placebo
Trifluoperazine	Borderline	29	Crossover trial	No clear advantages of trifluoperazine over other (active) treatments
Thiothixene	Borderline and schizotypal	30	Randomized controlled trial	Thiothixene superior to placebo in both groups
Haloperidol		31	Randomized controlled trial	Haloperidol superior for irritability symptoms alone
Olanzapine	Borderline	32	Randomized controlled trial	Olanzapine somewhat superior to placebo in small trial (only 9 patients received placebo)
Olanzapine	Borderline	33	Randomized controlled trial (314 patients recruited – the only trial with an adequate sample size)	No advantages of olanzapine over placebo, apart from slight increase in speed of resolution of symptoms

Table 43.4 Summary of randomized trials of antidepressants in the treatment of personality disorder

Drug tested	Personality diagnosis	Ref.	Type of study	Main results
Amitriptyline	Borderline	28	Randomized controlled trial	Haloperidol (7 mg/day) superior to both amitriptyline and placebo
Tranylcypromine	Borderline	29	Crossover trial	No clear advantages over other (all active) treatments
Phenelzine	Borderline and schizotypal	34	Randomized controlled trial	Phenelzine significantly superior to haloperidol and placebo for symptoms of depression, borderline psychopathologic symptoms and anxiety
Fluoxetine	Inadequately specified, but most likely to be within antisocial group	35	Randomized controlled trial	Fluoxetine reduced impulsive and aggressive behaviour after 2–3 months of treatment compared with placebo
Lithium carbonate	Antisocial (presumed)	27	Randomized controlled trial	Some
Carbamazepine	Borderline	29	Crossover trial	No clear advantages of trifluoperazine over other (active) treatments
Sodium valproate (divalproex sodium)	Borderline	60, 61 62	Small randomized controlled trials	Marginal superiority of valproate only

preference is largely supported by the evidence from data and is perhaps a natural consequence of personality disorder being a complex disorder with an allegedly prolonged course with much variation. Psychodynamic, both individual and group, transference-focused psychotherapy, cognitive-behavioural therapy (CBT), schema-focused therapy, social problem-solving therapy and nidotherapy are the most commonly used treatments that have some degree of evidence base, but there are many variations of these treatments that are practised with conviction and enthusi-

Table 43.5 Summary of psychological treatments for personality disorder separated by types of disorder

Type of personality disorder	Personality category	Potential treatments
Type S (treatment-seeking)	Borderline	MBT, DBT, CAT, CBT, schema-focused therapy, transference focused psychotherapy, therapeutic community, social problem-solving
	Anxious (avoidant)	
Type R (treatment-resisting)	Antisocial	Positive reinforcement treatment programmes (of all sorts), nidotherapy
	Schizoid	
	Histrionic	No evidence
	Paranoid	Nidotherapy
	Dependent	No evidence
Intermediate	Impulsive	Social problem-solving
	Anankastic	

CAT, cognitive analytical therapy; CBT, cognitive-behavioural therapy; DBT, dialectical behaviour therapy; MBT, mentalization-based treatment.

asm. Although there are many treatments and, with a recent surge, many more randomized trials, the standard method of summarizing the results, combining data in the form of meta-analysis, is not very satisfactory. Although several meta-analyses have been published, the most influential being that of Leichsenring and Liebing,[36] in the National Institute for Health and Clinical Excellence (NICE) guideline for borderline personality disorder there was too much disparity and study methodology variation to justify using this approach.

In examining the value of each of these treatments, some simplification is needed, as there are many named personality disorders and differences in choice of treatment. Most of the psychological treatments are time-consuming and need a considerable degree of motivation, but unfortunately for the therapeutic enthusiast only a minority of patients, mainly with borderline pathology, are strong treatment-seeking people (type S personalities). Apart from the avoidant anxious group, which still contains many patients who avoid treatment, people with other personality problems (75% of the total) are treatment-rejecting (type R) patients.[37] It is therefore not surprising that most of the psychotherapies are competing with others for a small proportion of the total population with personality disorders (Table 43.5).

Borderline personality disorder

Dynamic psychotherapies

These therapies have been the mainstay of the management of borderline personality disorder ever since it was first identified as a clear disorder in the 1950s. Unfortunately, the evaluation of this has, until very recently, been confined to naturalistic studies; now that it has been shown that personality disorders have a tendency to improve irrespective of therapy (see above), such studies hardly constitute evidence of efficacy. Thus, the report by Michael Stone[16] of nearly 550 patients followed up for 20 years showed that most had improved significantly, but it was impossible to tell whether this was a consequence of the psychological treatment they had received.

The first influential randomized trial was carried out by Bateman and Fonagy[38,39] and was described as a combination of psychoanalytical psychotherapy combined with partial hospitalization (i.e. day hospital care). However, the authors have subsequently called this treatment 'mentalization-based treatment' (MBT).[40,41] Mentalization is described as:

> ... making sense of the actions of oneself and others on the basis of intentional mental states, such as desires, feelings, and beliefs. It involves the recognition that what is in the mind is in the mind and reflects knowledge of one's own and others' mental states as mental states.[42]

In short, mentalization involves awareness of complex mental functions in the self and others, and MBT aims to promote its development. The ability to mentalize is impaired in borderline personality disorder; the group and individual therapies focus on this facet but not exclusively, as a great deal of additional therapy goes into day hospital attendance and group therapy. In the original study of 38 patients, improvement in the MBT group was delayed until after 6 months, but its benefits have persisted up to 8 years.[38,41]

There were many outcomes in the study – hospital admissions and their duration, frequency of suicide attempts and acts of self-harm, drug treatment use, and changes in clinical symptoms – all of which showed greater improvement in the MBT group compared with treatment as usual. The treatment has now been developed fully in a manualized form[40] and has been adopted in many centres in the UK, particularly in day hospital settings. As yet, however, it has a very slim evidence base, with the results of a single small trial dominating many other, more substantial trials. What is needed is evidence that the effects of treatment can generalize to other centres.

Dialectical behaviour therapy (DBT) is an evidence-based multimodal treatment programme[43] developed specially for women who self-harm but since applied to other populations. Five stages of treatment are outlined: pre-treatment, achieving behavioural control, emotionally processing the past, resolving ordinary problems in living, and capacity to experience sustained joy; most of the research evidence is concerned with the first two of these stages. Much of the treatment is concerned with reducing impulsive acts such as substance misuse, binge eating and, particularly, suicidal behaviour. The treatment is a complex one and involves weekly individual therapy and group psychoeducational and skills training, usually for a contracted period of 1 year in the first instance. The central component of the dialectic is the combination of change and acceptance, the former involving behavioural change and the finding of solutions, and the latter encapsulated in the concepts of validation (acknowledgment of behaviour as logical and understandable) and mindfulness, a feature not completely separate from mentalization, in which thinking and feelings are allowed expression and put into a situational context without the need for immediate action.

Behavioural change also follows a complex pathway, with combinations of skills training, contingency management, exposure and cognitive modification. DBT also includes a structured team of therapists who have weekly supervision and consultation, and the option for patients to have telephone consultation, particularly in times of crisis.

Psychodynamic and psychoanalytical psychotherapies

These methods are generally less structured than MBT, CBT and cognitive analytical therapy (CAT) and have an emphasis on unconscious conflict that provokes disharmony in the relationships between people that create personality problems. Problems in relationships are classically seen to be repeated within the therapy relationship in the form of transference and counter-transference, which is interpreted by the therapist. In working with people with borderline personality disorder, this has changed in recent years, so that the therapist is now much more than a listener and interpreter. Transference-focused therapy[44] is probably the best form of a structured and manualized form of psychoanalytical therapy that links dysfunctional patterns of current interpersonal relationships to the transference relationships within therapy, with promotion of stronger identity relationships and reflection.

Therapeutic communities

A therapeutic community is difficult to define but is primarily a social and group-based intervention that leads to change through its own impetus rather than one imposed from outside. It is permissive in its approach but democratic in principle (although in the USA it has also been used to describe a compulsory programme of care for drug dependence). There are no adequate evaluations of therapeutic communities, but a randomized trial has been mounted.

The proponents of the approach are dedicated to its values, and there is no doubt that some users of the service do very well, but this does not provide a justification in itself for the approach.

Cognitive-behavioural therapy

Cognitive-behavioural therapy adapted for borderline personality disorder has been shown to have some value in reducing suicidal behaviour, both in individual therapy over 15–30 sessions[45] and also when combined with educational sessions in improving impulsive behaviour.[46,47] It is a treatment that requires additional training to that given for CBT in general, and the approach shows promise. It has also been extended to antisocial personality disorder, where it has been shown to be a feasible intervention worthy of development.[48]

Schema-focused therapy[49] is a variant of CBT that also involves an element of reparenting. It is somewhat more intensive than standard CBT for borderline personality disorder. Social problem-solving is a related intervention that has good evidence of efficacy from a randomized trial.[50]

Cognitive analytical therapy

This treatment, introduced by Anthony Ryle,[51,52] is a well-constructed and theoretically sound treatment for borderline personality disorder that overlaps with CBT and psychodynamic approaches but that has some clear distinguishing features that make it quite separate. CAT has been subjected to a randomized evaluation where it performed at least as well as the best available alternative,[53] but a low- or no-treatment comparison group was not tested – and needs to be.

Nidotherapy

This treatment (named after the Latin *nidus*, or 'nest'), based on the systematic adjustment of the environment to fit the person rather than vice versa,[54–56] is alleged to be particularly valuable in all forms of chronic mental illness that have failed to respond to treatment and for treatment-resisting (type R) personality disorders.[37] It is very different from psychotherapeutic approaches, in that the emphasis is on making environmental, rather than person, changes. A randomized controlled trial in assertive outreach services, where type R personalities predominate,[57] showed that it had a marked reduction in in-patient service provision.[58]

SUMMARY OF THE CLINICAL VALUE AND IMPORTANCE OF PERSONALITY DISORDER IN PRACTICE

Assessment

Personality disorder is currently very badly assessed in clinical practice, and it is not assessed much better in research assessments. The main problem is the gross unreliability of individual personality disorders; the assessment of personality as a general concept is better. The diagnosis should always be considered when a psychiatric problem appears to be much more complex than expected and its outcome unpredictable. However, these should not be regarded as diagnostic features. When making an assessment, it is important to regard the personality disorder, if considered present, as a provisional diagnosis or as a disorder of current personality function[10] that could be challenged if needed in the future.

Importance

Although assessment may be inaccurate, it is much better than not making an assessment at all. If there is any evidence of malfunction of personality, it should immediately give rise to the following questions:

- Is my mental state assessment of other problems presented an accurate one?
- Is the personality problem, even if not admitted or complained about, a major feature in the presentation?
- How should I accommodate the personality features in recommending treatment?

The answers to these questions lead to self-evident changes in the way that treatment is planned: an impulsive person with cluster B pathology should not be given an antidepressant that is dangerous in overdosage; an anxious person with clear dependent cluster C pathology should have clear instructions about the duration and ending of both psychological and drug treatment; and a meticulous person with obsessional personality features should have clear instructions about all treatments prescribed and, where possible, written material to help achieve the best results.

Treatment

Referral for formal treatment for personality disorder should be undertaken only when (i) it is part of a compulsory requirement (a court order) or (ii) it is specifically requested by the patient after a full discussion of the advantages and potential handicaps. In this context, it is worthwhile remembering the subtext of the formal recommendations from NICE for both borderline and antisocial personality disorders, which, although not referring to other groups, could almost certainly apply to them also:

When providing psychological treatment, especially for people with multiple comorbidities or severe impairment (or both), include:

- An explicit and integrated theoretical approach used by both the treatment team and the therapist, and shared with the service user
- Structured care in accordance with this guideline
- Provision for supervision by a therapist.

Although the frequency of psychotherapy sessions should be adapted to the person's needs and context of living, consider twice weekly sessions. Do not use brief psychological interventions (of less than three months' duration) specifically for borderline personality disorder or for its individual symptoms outside a service that has the characteristics outlined above.[59]

The message here is that a specific intervention to change personality structure and functioning should not be taken lightly. In most cases, accommodation needs to be made to the personality characteristics rather than an attempt to change it, and in the case of nidotherapy this 'accommodation' in a systematic form becomes a treatment in itself. If personality treatment is required, it must be a planned, determined and well-resourced intervention.

KEY POINTS

- Personality may be reasonably stable, but personality disorder is not, as the problems created by an abnormal personality are very dependent on situation and setting. Any cross-sectional assessment of personality should be regarded as one of current personality functioning only.
- The current classification of personality disorders is grossly defective but can be partly rescued by grouping into clusters and using these to measure severity.
- The different clusters of personality disorder are manifest at different ages, with cluster B (antisocial, borderline, histrionic, impulsive, narcissistic) becoming manifest in childhood earlier than other disorders and ending during middle age.
- There is no good evidence that drug treatment is of significant benefit in the management of personality disorder, except as short-term management in a crisis.
- Psychological treatments are preferable to drug treatments but need to be given in a well-supervised structured format to be effective. DBT, MBT, CBT and CAT all show promise for people with borderline personality disorder, but only DBT has a sufficient database to suggest real evidence of value.
- Nidotherapy – the systematic adjustment of the environment to fit the patient – has some evidence of cost-effectiveness and may be more suitable for treatment-resisting (type R) personality disorders.

FURTHER READING

Bateman A, Fonagy P (2006) *Mentalization-Based Treatment for Borderline Personality Disorder: A Practical Guide.* Oxford: Oxford University Press.

Binks CA, Fenton M, McCarthy L, *et al.* (2006) Psychological therapies for people with borderline personality disorder. *Cochrane Database of Systematic Reviews* (1): CD005652.

Holmes J (1999) Psychotherapeutic approaches to the management of severe personality disorder in general psychiatric settings. *CPD Bulletin Psychiatry* **2**: 35–41.

Moran P (1999) *Antisocial Personality Disorder: An Epidemiological Perspective.* London: Gaskell.

Paris J (1996) *Social Factors in the Personality Disorders: A Biopsychosocial Approach to Etiology and Treatment.* New York: Cambridge University Press.

Sampson M, McCubbin R, Tyrer P (2006) *Personality Disorder and Community Mental Health Teams: A Practitioner's Guide.* Chichester: John Wiley & Sons.

Tyrer P (2009) *Nidotherapy: Harmonising the Environment with the Patient.* London: Royal College of Psychiatrists Press.

REFERENCES

1. Torgersen S, Kringlen E, Cramer V (2001) The prevalence of personality disorders in a community sample. *Archives of General Psychiatry* **58**: 590–96.
2. Coid J, Yang M, Tyrer P, Roberts A, Ullrich S (2006) Prevalence and correlates of personality disorder in Great Britain. *British J ournal of Psychiatry* **188**: 423–31.
3. Coid J (2003) Epidemiology, public health and the problem of personality disorder. *British Journal of Psychiatry* **182** (suppl. 44): S3–5.
4. Baca-Garcia E, Perez-Rodriguez MM, Basurte-Villamor I, *et al.* (2007) Diagnostic stability of psychiatric disorders in clinical practice. *British Journal of Psychiatry* **190**: 210–26.
5. American Psychiatric Association (1994) *Diagnostic and Statistical Manual of Mental Disorders*, 4th edn. Washington, DC: American Psychiatric Association.
6. World Health Organization (1992) *International Classification of Diseases*, 10th revision. Geneva: World Health Organization.
7. Verheul R, Widiger TA (2004) A meta-analysis of the prevalence and usage of the personality disorder not otherwise specified (PDNOS) diagnosis. *Journal of Personality Disorders* **18**: 309–19.
8. Verheul R, Bartak A, Widiger T (2007) Prevalence and construct validity of personality disorder not otherwise specified. *Journal of Personality Disorders* **21**: 359–70.
9. Clark LA, Harrison JA (2001). Assessment instruments. In WJ Livesley (ed.) *Handbook of Personality Disorders: Theory, Research and Treatment.* New York: Guilford Press.
10. Tyrer P, Coombs N, Ibrahimi F, *et al.* (2007) Critical developments in the assessment of personality disorder. *British Journal of Psychiatry* **190** (suppl. 49): S51–9.
11. Livesley WJ, Jang KL, Vernon PA (1998) The phenotypic and genetic structure of traits delineating personality disorder. *Archives of General Psychiatry* **55**: 941–8.
12. Tyrer P, Johnson T (1996) Establishing the severity of personality disorder. *American Journal of Psychiatry* **153**: 1593–7.
13. Cicchetti DV, Showalter D, Tyrer P (1985) The effects of number of rating scale categories on levels of inter-rater reliability: a Monte Carlo investigation. *Applied Psychological Measurement* **9**: 31–6.
14. Newton-Howes G, Weaver T, Tyrer P (2008) Attitudes of staff towards patients with personality disorder in community health teams. *Australian and New Zealand Journal of Psychiatry* **42**: 572–7.
15. Shea MT, Stout R, Gunderson J, *et al.* (2002) Short-term diagnostic stability of schizotypal, borderline, avoidant, and obsessive-compulsive personality disorders. *American Journal of Psychiatry* **159**: 2036–41.
16. Stone MH (1993) Long-term outcome in personality disorders. *British Journal of Psychiatry* **162**: 299–313.
17. Zanarini MC, Frankenburg FR, Hennen J, Silk K (2003) The longitudinal course of borderline psychopathology: 6-year prospective follow-up of the phenomenology of borderline personality disorder. *American Journal of Psychiatry* **160**: 274–83.
18. Zanarini MC, Frankenburg FR, Hennen J, *et al.* (2006) Prediction of the 10-year course of borderline personality disorder. *American Journal of Psychiatry* **163**: 827–32.
19. Seivewright H, Tyrer P, Johnson T (2002) Change in personality status in neurotic disorders. *Lancet* **359**: 2253–4.
20. Hare RD (1991) *The Psychopathy Checklist Revised.* Toronto: Multi-Health Systems.
21. Cleckley H (1941) *The Mask of Sanity.* London: Kimpton.
22. Home Office and Department of Health (1999) *Managing Dangerous People with Severe Personality Disorder: Proposals for Policy Development.* London: Department of Health.
23. Tyrer P, Cooper S, Rutter D, *et al.* (2009) The assessment of dangerous and severe personality disorder: lessons from a randomised controlled trial linked to qualitative analysis. *Journal of Forensic Psychology and Psychiatry* **20**: 132–46.
24. Barrett B, Byford S, Seivewright H, *et al.* (2009) The assessment of dangerous and severe personality disorder: service use, cost and consequences. *Forensic Psychology and Psychiatry* **20**: 120–31.
25. Kendell R (2002) The distinction between personality disorder and mental illness. *British Journal of Psychiatry* **180**: 110–15.
26. Newton-Howes G, Tyrer P (2003) Pharmacotherapy for personality disorders. *Expert Opinion on Pharmacotherapy* **4**: 1643–9.

27. Sheard MH, Marini JL, Bridges CI, Wagner E (1976) The effect of lithium on impulsive aggressive behavior in man. *American Journal of Psychiatry* **133**: 1409–13.
28. Soloff PH, George A, Nathan RS, *et al.* (1986) Progress in pharmacotherapy of personality disorders: a double blind study of amitriptyline, haloperidol and placebo. *Archives of General Psychiatry* **43**: 691–7.
29. Cowdry RW, Gardner DL (1988) Pharmacotherapy of borderline personality disorder: alprazolam, carbamazepine, trifluoperazine and tranylcypromine. *Archives of General Psychiatry* **45**: 111–19.
30. Goldberg SC, Shulz SC, Shulz PM, *et al.* (1986) Borderline and schizotypal personality disorders treated with low dose thiothixene versus placebo. *Archives of General Psychiatry* **43**: 680–86.
31. Cornelius JR, Soloff PH, George A, Ulrich RF, Perel JM (1993) Haloperidol vs. phenelzine in continuation therapy of borderline disorder. *Psychopharmacology Bulletin* **29**: 333–7.
32. Zanarini MC, Frankenburg FR (2001) Olanzapine treatment of female borderline personality disorder patients: a double-blind, placebo-controlled pilot study. *Journal of Clinical Psychiatry* **62**: 849–54.
33. Schulz SC, Zanarini MC, Bateman A, *et al.* (2008) Olanzapine for the treatment of borderline personality disorder: variable dose 12-week randomised double-blind placebo-controlled study. *British Journal of Psychiatry* **193**: 485–92.
34. Soloff PH, Cornelius J, George A, *et al.* (1993) Efficacy of phenelzine and haloperidol in borderline personality disorder. *Archives of General Psychiatry* **50**: 377–85.
35. Coccaro EF, Kavoussi RJ (1997) Fluoxetine and impulsive aggressive behavior in personality-disordered subjects. *Archives of General Psychiatry* **54**: 1081–8.
36. Leichsenring F, Leibing E (2003) The effectiveness of psychodynamic therapy and cognitive behavior therapy in the treatment of personality disorders: a meta-analysis. *American Journal of Psychiatry* **160**: 1223–32.
37. Tyrer P, Mitchard S, Methuen C, Ranger M (2003) Treatment-rejecting and treatment-seeking personality disorders: Type R and Type S. *Journal of Personality Disorders* **17**: 265–70.
38. Bateman A, Fonagy P (1999) Effectiveness of partial hospitalization in the treatment of borderline personality disorder: a randomized controlled trial. *American Journal of Psychiatry* **156**: 1563–9.
39. Bateman AW, Fonagy P (2001) Treatment of borderline personality disorder with psychoanalytically oriented partial hospitalisation: an 18 month follow-up. *American Journal of Psychiatry* **158**: 36–42.
40. Bateman A, Fonagy P (2006) *Mentalization-Based Treatment for Borderline Personality Disorder: A Practical Guide.* Oxford: Oxford University Press.
41. Bateman A, Fonagy P (2008) 8-year follow-up of patients treated for borderline personality disorder: mentalization-based treatment versus treatment as usual. *American Journal of Psychiatry* **165**: 631–8.
42. Bateman A, Zanarini M (2008) Personality disorder. In: P Tyrer, KR Silk (eds) *Cambridge Textbook of Effective Treatments in Psychiatry.* Cambridge: Cambridge University Press.
43. Linehan MM (1993) *Cognitive-Behavioural Treatment for Borderline Personality Disorder.* New York: Guilford Press.
44. Clarkin JF, Levy KN, Lenzenweger MF, Kernberg OF (2007) Evaluating three treatments for borderline personality disorder: a multiwave study. *American Journal of Psychiatry* **164**: 922–8.
45. Davidson K, Norrie J, Tyrer P, *et al.* (2006) The effectiveness of cognitive behavior therapy for borderline personality disorder: results from the borderline personality disorder study of cognitive therapy (BOSCOT) trial. *Journal of Personality Disorders* **20**: 450–65.
46. Blum N, St John D, Pfohl B, *et al.* (2008) Systems Training for Emotional Predictability and Problem Solving (STEPPS) for outpatients with borderline personality disorder: a randomized controlled trial and 1-year follow-up. *American Journal of Psychiatry* **165**: 468–78.
47. Black DW, Allen J, St John D, *et al.* (2009) Predictors of response to Systems Training for Emotional Predictability and Problem Solving (STEPPS) for borderline personality disorder: an exploratory study. *Acta Psychiatrica Scandinavica*, in press.
48. Davidson KM, Tyrer P, Tata P, *et al.* (2009) Cognitive behaviour therapy for violent men with antisocial personality disorder in the community: an exploratory randomized controlled trial. *Psychological Medicine* **39**: 569–77.
49. Young JE (1990) *Cognitive Therapy for Personality Disorders: A Schemas-Focused Approach.* Sarasota, FL: Professional Resource Exchange.
50. Huband N, Duggan C, Evans C, Duggan C (2007) Social problem-solving plus psychoeducation for adults with personality disorder: pragmatic randomised controlled trial. *British Journal of Psychiatry* **190**: 307–13.
51. Ryle A (1997) The structure and development of borderline personality disorder: a proposed model. *British Journal of Psychiatry* **170**: 82–7.
52. Ryle A (1997) *Cognitive Analytic Therapy of Borderline Personality Disorder: The Model and the Method.* Chichester: John Wiley & Sons.
53. Chanen AM, Jackson HJ, McCutcheon LK, *et al.* (2008) Early intervention for adolescents with borderline personality disorder using cognitive analytic therapy: randomised controlled trial. *British Journal of Psychiatry* **193**: 477–84.
54. Tyrer P (2002) Nidotherapy: a new approach to the treatment of personality disorder. *Acta Psychiatrica Scandinavica* **105**: 469–71.
55. Tyrer P, Sensky T, Mitchard S (2003) The principles of

nidotherapy in the treatment of persistent mental and personality disorders. *Psychotherapy and Psychosomatics* **72**: 350–56.

56. Tyrer P (2009) *Nidotherapy: Harmonising the Environment with the Patient*. London: Royal College of Psychiatrists Press.
57. Ranger M, Methuen C, Rutter D, *et al.* (2004) Prevalence of personality disorder in the caseload of an inner city assertive outreach team. *Psychiatric Bulletin* (2004) **28**: 441–3.
58. Ranger M, Tyrer P, Milošeska K, *et al.* (2009) Cost-effectiveness of nidotherapy for comorbid personality disorder and severe mental illness: randomized controlled trial. *Epidemiologia e Psichiatria Sociale*, in press.
59. Kendall T, Pilling S, Tyrer P, *et al.* (2009) Borderline and antisocial personality disorders: summary of NICE guidance. *British Medical Journal* **338**: b93.
60. Frankenburg FR, Zanarini MC (2002) Divalproex sodium treatment of women with borderline personality disorder and bipolar II disorder: a double-blind placebo-controlled pilot study. *Journal of Clinical Psychiatry* **63**: 442–6.
61. Hollander E, Allen A, Lopez RP, *et al.* (2001) A preliminary double-blind placebo-controlled trial of divalproex sodium in borderline personality disorder. *Journal of Clinical Psychiatry* **62**: 199–203.
62. Hollander E, Tracey KA, Swann AC, *et al.* (2003) Divalproex in the treatment of impulsive aggression: efficacy in cluster B personality disorders. *Neuropsychopharmacology* **28**: 1186–97.

Chapter 44

Perinatal psychiatry

Ian Brockington

INTRODUCTION

The psychiatry of childbearing (synonyms: mother–infant psychiatry, perinatal psychiatry) has advanced greatly in the past 20 years. The world literature on the subject has more than doubled. The nosological framework provided by the *International Classification of Diseases*, version 10 (ICD-10) and the *Diagnostic and Statistical Manual*, 4th edition (DSM-IV) no longer covers the wide variety of disorders closely or specifically related to pregnancy, parturition and the puerperium. Most of the research has been conducted in Europe and North America, but the pattern of disease in these places, where maternal mortality has fallen to less than 20 in 10^5 births, with a corresponding fall in morbidity, may not match that seen in countries whose maternal mortality is 100 times that figure. It is in the latter countries that most of the infants are born, and their morbidity may be similar to that seen in Europe in the nineteenth century.

PSEUDOCYESIS

When a woman incorrectly believes herself to be pregnant and develops symptoms and signs of pregnancy, this is called pseudocyesis.[1] The differential diagnosis includes delusions of pregnancy occurring in women (also men) with a variety of psychoses, but without the somatic changes of pregnancy. There is also pregnancy simulated for social, mercenary or legal purposes. Occasionally organic disease (such as tumours) can mimic pregnancy.

The clinical features include:

- a firm belief in the pregnancy, which may last until the onset of a false labour at 9 months;
- amenorrhoea;
- morning sickness and/or pica;
- enlargement of the breasts and nipples, and even a discharge of colostrum;
- abdominal enlargement, caused by muscular contraction, tympanites, fat, retained faeces or pathological lesions;
- an illusion of fetal movements;
- enlargement of the uterus to the size of a 6-week pregnancy.

Modern diagnostic tests have greatly reduced the frequency of pseudocyesis. Where radiology or ultrasound is unavailable, an examination under anaesthetic is recommended, in the presence of a family member in order to avoid accusation of abortion.

The psychological basis is usually an intense desire for children. In some cases, however, a guilty fear of pregnancy has been the background; this has occasionally led to dangerous attempts at abortion by non-pregnant women. Pseudocyesis is a demonstration of the influence of psyche over soma, mediated by hormonal secretion. It occurs in at least a dozen other mammals. Persistence of the corpus luteum would explain breast changes, moderate uterine enlargement and secretory endometrium, but it is not the only basis: hormonal measurements have been made in at least 30 patients, some of whom had chronic anovulatory states, hyperprolactinaemia or androgen excess.

These women require psychotherapy. Simply revealing the diagnosis is unsatisfactory because the patient may misinterpret the advice, consult another doctor or develop a recurrence. The underlying conflicts must be explored, helping the patient to accept that she is not pregnant.

THE PSYCHIATRY OF PREGNANCY

Pregnancy adjustment

The psychopathology of pregnancy needs to be understood in terms of the adjustment all women must make when they conceive. Pregnancy is not only a biological event but also an adaptive process. A pregnant woman must carry the baby safely and prepare for the birth. She must ensure the acceptance of the child by the family, and develop a somewhat different relationship with the child's father and her inner circle of relatives and friends.

She must adjust to the sacrifices that motherhood demands; these include the loss of figure and facial bloom, weight gain and stretch marks. Some women take pride and pleasure in these changes, but others are embarrassed by them; dysmorphophobia, with ideas of reference and social avoidance, can ensue.[2]

Pregnancy may be accompanied by medical disorders, and there is often an interaction between physical and psychological factors. Pica is common, especially geophagia (eating earth or clay) and amylophagia (eating starch), which can lead to iron-deficiency anaemia, bowel obstruction and worm infections; other forms of pica can lead to lead poisoning and hypokalaemia. Although thiamine treatment has been readily available since 1936, hyperemesis gravidarum still causes Wernicke's encephalopathy. Delirium can complicate chorea gravidarum.[3] Obstructive sleep apnoea can occur in late pregnancy.[4]

About half of all conceptions are intended, but the planning of pregnancy and its acceptance are two different things: a small proportion of those who plan their pregnancies subsequently regret them. Most unplanned pregnancies are welcomed, sometimes after a delay and sometimes with ambivalence. Unwanted pregnancies are often terminated. A sizeable minority, however, are carried to term; although there are difficulties about definition, nomenclature and methodology, and differences in degree of negative feelings, the median figure is about 10 per cent.[5] This figure is higher in adolescents, and in countries where abortion is hazardous and hard to obtain. There is a hard core of rejected pregnancies that are at risk of various disorders.

Denial of pregnancy

In women who do not realize they are pregnant, one must distinguish between three different phenomena:

- Unnoticed pregnancy in women who are obese or near the menopause
- Deliberate concealment
- Dissociative denial.

A German survey of 29 000 births found an incidence of 1 in 475 women who failed to recognize pregnancy until the twentieth week; 12 of 62 cases were not diagnosed until labour began.[6] Welsh and American studies have obtained similar figures.[7,8]

The late discovery of an unwelcome pregnancy carries a small risk of suicide. The mother is also at risk of all those complications of delivery that, with modern antenatal care, have become rare. For the child, there are increased hazards, including prematurity and neonaticide.

Prenatal attachment

A pregnant woman 'bonds' or 'affiliates' to the unborn child in a way analogous to the formation of the mother–infant relationship after birth. The mother begins to have fantasies about the baby and talks affectionately to it. She may engage the husband and other children in 'playing' with the baby. At the same time, she prepares for the birth and motherhood ('nesting behaviour'). In some mothers, however, there is minimal attachment even at term, and some who deeply resent their pregnancy try to harm the fetus by pounding and bruising their abdomen (fetal abuse). A poor mother–fetus relationship is one of the predictors of impaired mother–infant bonding,[9,10] and, in clinical experience, fetal abuse predicts later child abuse.

Prepartum anxiety

For many mothers, pregnancy is a time of much anxiety. The first trimester may involve an anguished decision over whether to continue or terminate the pregnancy. Later, women who have experienced infertility, multiple miscarriages or fetal loss may be preoccupied by fears that they will lose this baby.[11] In the third trimester, anxiety is focused on fetal abnormality and coping with motherhood. In addition, fear of parturition (tocophobia) may be a reason for elective Caesarean section. Prepartum anxiety is an independent predictor of postpartum depression.[12]

These anxieties will usually be managed by ventilation and support, but anxiolytic medication can be used cautiously. Benzodiazepines carry the risk of fetal intoxication ('floppy infant syndrome').[13] Beta-adrenergic blocking agents risk neonatal hypoglycaemia.[14]

Depression

Prepartum depression is no less common than postpartum depression.[15] It can be recurrent, and case studies show an association with puerperal mania.[1] Some postpartum depression is a continuation of depression starting in pregnancy.

There are claims that prepartum anxiety and depression influence fetal outcome and child development, but there is a lack of consistency in the findings.[16,17]

The frequency of suicide is a vexed question. There are problems about the data since suicide and pregnancy are often concealed. Unwanted pregnancy is a factor in attempted and completed suicide. An increasing tolerance of single motherhood led to a decline of pregnancy-related suicide in Europe in the twentieth century, but this may not be true in countries that still stigmatize illegitimate pregnancy. Self-poisoning, usually in the first trimester, often results in fetal death[18] but not fetal abnormality.[19] Suicide is now (following the great reduction in fatalities from obstetric causes) the third most frequent cause of maternal death in the UK, after thromboembolism and heart disease,[20] but the prepartum suicide rate is below that in the general population.[21]

Prepartum depression is sometimes left untreated because of fears about the effect of drugs on the fetus. There is evidence of a slightly increased risk of congenital cardiac lesions in infants exposed to paroxetine in the first trimester. Tricyclic antidepressants increase the risk of preterm birth, respiratory distress, neonatal convulsions and other complications;[22,23] toxic and withdrawal effects are seen occasionally, especially after clomipramine treatment. Selective serotonin reuptake inhibitors (SSRIs) have toxic effects on the newborn, including agitation, altered muscle tone, problems with breathing and sucking, neonatal pulmonary hypertension[24] and other complications;[23] there are slight effects on birth weight and gestational age.[25] Withdrawal symptoms are often seen.[26] These risks must be balanced against those of depression, but particular caution should be exercised in prescribing these drugs during the last trimester. Electroconvulsive therapy (ECT) has been given safely to pregnant women many times. Complications are rare, but occasional patients have developed premature uterine contractions, which can be treated with a tocolytic drug such as ritodrine. The mother must be well oxygenated during anaesthesia and should be screened for rare syndromes of pseudocholinesterase deficiency.

Substance abuse

Ethanol

Heavy ethanol abuse has severe effects on the fetus. The main effect is retardation of intrauterine growth: although ethanol shortens gestation, the low birth weight is not explained by prematurity; rather, the infant is small for gestational age. The infant becomes addicted and may suffer neonatal withdrawal symptoms. Ethanol is also teratogenic, causing fetal alcohol syndrome (or 'spectrum disorder'), which includes growth retardation, microcephaly and facial anomalies due to maxillary hypoplasia (short palpebral fissures, thin vermilion border and short philtrum).[27] There is long-term cognitive and language impairment[28] and an association with behavioural disorders such as attention deficit hyperactivity disorder (ADHD).[29]

Narcotics

Narcotic addicts, like alcoholics, have multiple emotional and social problems. Many do not seek antenatal care. The infants may be affected by maternal malnutrition and infections such as venereal disease, hepatitis and acquired immunodeficiency syndrome (AIDS). Narcotics are not teratogenic, but a high proportion of the infants are of low birth weight, explained partly by prematurity and partly by intrauterine growth retardation. A withdrawal syndrome develops in most babies. Hair and meconium analysis improves the diagnosis of opiate (and also cocaine) abuse in mothers who present unexpectedly in labour. The perinatal mortality rate and frequency of sudden infant death are increased. There is an increased incidence of microcephaly, and there may be impaired mental development, although other factors in the maternal lifestyle may account for this. Methadone maintenance improves the birth weight, but it may depress respiration in the newborn and lead to a more severe and prolonged withdrawal syndrome, with a greater frequency of seizures. Buprenorphine may be a more suitable maintenance therapy, with milder withdrawal effects, but low birth weight and abstinence syndromes still occur.[30] If it is decided to withdraw heroin, this should be done in the second trimester, replacing it by methadone. Naloxone, which can be given by implant, has been used, although there are concerns about fetal abstinence syndromes. Newborn infants should be kept in hospital for at least 14 days. Respiratory depression can be treated by naloxone, and seizures and withdrawal symptoms by sedatives such as diazepam or by morphine itself. All these mothers should receive close psychiatric supervision and social casework.

Cocaine and amphetamines

Some of cocaine's effects are similar to those of narcotics – premature delivery, intrauterine growth reduction and an increased incidence of microcephaly. There is an association with rupture of membranes before 34 weeks. The withdrawal syndrome is less severe than with narcotics. The specific effects are cardiovascular: it causes uterine vasoconstriction, leading to placental abruption, and fetal cerebral infarcts. There is little evidence of toxic effects in the newborn,[31] but 1-month-old infants show subtle neurobehavioural anomalies such as reduced arousal and increased excitability.[32] Long-term effects on language development and behaviour are disputed and may be due to confounding factors such as low birth weight, maternal depression, poor parenting, abuse of other drugs, maternal education and poverty.[33] An increased risk of sudden infant death is also *sub judice*.

The effects of amphetamine abuse in pregnancy are similar to those of cocaine, including placental abruption and fetal brain infarcts. Papers have only recently begun to appear on pregnancy abuse of 3,4-methylenedioxymethamphetamine ('ecstasy').

Other abused substances

Cannabis is the illicit drug most frequently abused by pregnant women: it may affect fetal growth and have long-term neurobehavioural and cognitive deficits, but it is difficult to exclude the effect of confounding factors. Lysergic acid diethylamide (LSD) may have teratogenic or mutagenic effects, but this is based on case reports in offspring from deviant subcultures, whose parents also abuse 'street drugs'. Phencyclidine ('angel dust') addiction leads to neonatal withdrawal symptoms.

Eating disorders

Most anorexic women recover and start to menstruate again when their weight reaches about 80 per cent of the standard weight. Their desire for motherhood is shown by the frequency of infertility treatment and planned pregnancy. Ovulation can be induced by clomiphene or gonadotropins in women who fail to menstruate. There are numerous case reports and several long-term studies showing that many women with a history of anorexia nervosa give birth to children in the normal way.

Several studies have found that anorexia and bulimia are associated with low birth weight,[34–37] but this is disputed.[38,39] The only consistent finding is an increase in miscarriages, in common with women underweight for other reasons.[40]

A minority of anorexic women become pregnant while in the throes of the disease. The diagnosis may be delayed by their amenorrhoea. If the mother continues to restrict her diet, the fetus may suffer from malnutrition, and occasionally it has been necessary to rescue the infant by elective Caesarean section.

Eating disorders tend to improve during pregnancy, but they often relapse in the puerperium,[41] sometimes to a degree worse than before conception.[42] When the mother is actively anorexic, there is often conflict at mealtimes; occasionally, children suffer from their mother's asceticism, with stunted growth.[43] Bulimic mothers may also show deviant mothering – ignoring or excluding their children while overeating or vomiting, restricting food supplies, or exerting too much control during play and mealtimes;[42] video-feedback can be used to treat these disturbances.[44]

Obstetric factitious disorder

Self-induced illness behaviour can extend into the obstetric domain. Women may induce bleeding to simulate threatened miscarriage, placenta praevia or postpartum haemorrhage. They may stimulate rupture of the membranes or manipulate instruments such as an external tachodynamometer. In some cases this seems to be motivated by a desire for early delivery.

Psychosis

Pregnancy has no effect on chronic delusional states but may have a beneficial effect on menstrual, bipolar[45] and cycloid (acute polymorphic) psychoses. Nonetheless, acute manic and cycloid episodes occur during pregnancy, and some seem remarkably similar to puerperal psychosis. They would be regarded as sporadic or random, except that they have been observed in women with a history of puerperal psychosis (at least 13 in the literature). There is an association with multiparity, with the postpartum episode occurring first.

Many pregnant women with chronic psychoses require neuroleptic treatment. Butyrophenones are not teratogenic, but low-dose phenothiazines, used to treat hyperemesis in early pregnancy, are associated with a slightly increased risk of congenital abnormalities.[46] The main (but infrequent) hazard found with phenothiazines, butyrophenones and risperidone is sedation and extrapyramidal symptoms in the newborn. The newer neuroleptics have been in use for only 10–15 years. Clozapine seems safe, although there have been some cases of gestational diabetes, and there is a theoretical risk of fetal agranulocytosis. One study reported low birth rate and more neonatal admissions after olanzapine exposure.[47]

Lithium is relatively dangerous; at least 12 cases of the rare Ebstein's anomaly have been reported. After cardiac development has been completed, lithium is probably safe until delivery. Stopping lithium during pregnancy has a relapse rate similar to withdrawing treatment in non-pregnant women.[48] As delivery approaches, reduced renal clearance can result in toxicity with normal doses; eight cases of alarming blood levels (up to 5 mmol/L) have been reported, with coma and convulsions in the mother; even at normal blood levels, babies exposed to lithium have suffered lethargy, hypotonicity, nephrogenic diabetes insipidus and other effects. It is therefore advisable to withhold lithium for 1–2 days before delivery.[49]

Anti-epileptic drugs are often used in the prophylaxis of bipolar disorders. Carbamazepine has been associated with increased rates of congenital abnormality, including orofacial clefts. Sodium valproate is the most teratogenic of the anti-epileptic drugs after primidone. It was first noticed to cause spina bifida, with a frequency of 1–2 per cent; this is a dose-dependent effect, the threshold being more than 1100 mg/day. Folic acid is prophylactic, and the advice to women on this treatment (after excluding undiagnosed vitamin B12 deficiency) is to take 5 mg folic acid/day.[50] Valproate is now known to have wider effects. A fetal valproate syndrome has been described, with major malformations (especially congenital heart disease and limb defects), developmental delay and dysmorphic features, including a long upper lip with flat philtrum, and small nose, ears and jaw.[51] Some studies have found low intelligence quotient (IQ)[52] and early infantile autism,[53] but it is too early to be sure that environmental confounding factors are not at least partly responsible.[54] After the birth, infants may show withdrawal symptoms such as jitteriness and seizures. Lamotrigine clearance is 300 per cent greater in pregnancy, so blood levels are lower than expected; this is corrected rapidly after delivery. Given in normal doses in the first trimester, lamotrigine does not cause major congenital abnormalities.[55]

Obstetric liaison services

In view of the complexity of the psychological response to pregnancy, and the frequency of anxiety, depression and other psychiatric disorders, there should be a close liaison between obstetric and psychiatric services. In addition to the need to diagnose and treat prepartum psychiatric disorders, the high level of supervision in the antenatal clinics offers an opportunity for preventive psychiatry, by screening for vulnerabilities such as unwanted pregnancies, severe social problems and a history of psychosis, addictions and depression.

THE PSYCHOPATHOLOGY OF PARTURITION

Childbirth is among the severest of human ordeals, and, in spite of its brevity, carries a risk of various forms of psychopathology.[3] In countries with advanced obstetric care, these complications are rare, but may still be common where delivery is unsupervised or pregnancy is denied. Acts of desperation, such as auto-Caesarean section, suicide and rage attacks endangering the fetus, are fully described. Delirium is well documented; in most cases, it lasts a few hours, starting shortly before delivery and disappearing after the birth, with amnesia for the event; it can also continue into the puerperium or start immediately after the birth. Unexplained stupor and coma have also been described during and immediately after delivery.

Neonaticide

The term 'infanticide' covers the killing of infants and children by their parents in a wide variety of circumstances, broadly divided into neonaticide (killing the newborn) and filicide (the later murder of a child). Neonates (especially females) have been suppressed at various times in history, and in various societies, as an official policy or grass-roots custom to control population ('customary neonaticide'). This is quite different from criminal neonaticide, in which a mother, who has concealed her pregnancy and given birth in secret, murders the newborn. A major public health problem in Europe during the nineteenth century, its frequency has dwindled as a result of contraception, legal termination and changed attitudes to single motherhood, but it does still occur.[56] Neonaticide may be more common in countries that forbid abortion and stigmatize pregnancy, but data are lacking. The mental state of the mother can be deduced from the methods used: suffocation is the most common and testifies to the mother's panic when faced with a crying baby. In a minority of cases, brutal head injuries, stabbing and decapitation testify to rage and hatred. There has been much debate over whether the defence of insanity can be invoked. Most of these babies die when the mother is in the grip of an emotional crisis. This is not generally acceptable in law as insanity. Delirium, however, which is rare in hospital practice, may be more common in clandestine deliveries and is hard to exclude. If the defence is burdened with the proof of insanity, then there can be no valid evidence in unwitnessed deliveries; but there is the possibility of a miscarriage of justice – that a mother who killed her baby when her consciousness was clouded is wrongly condemned.

INFANT LOSS

The child may be lost for a variety of reasons:

- Termination of pregnancy at the behest of the mother
- Miscarriage, ectopic pregnancy or late termination of a wanted child for medical reasons
- Fetal death in utero, stillbirth, neonatal death or sudden infant death
- Relinquishment to adoption.

Termination of pregnancy

The indications for abortion include the following:

- *Medical:* to preserve the health and life of the mother.
- *Humanitarian:* when pregnancy has resulted from rape or incest.
- *Eugenic:* where there is a risk of congenital abnormality.
- *Psychiatric:* where there is a perceived risk of suicide or severe mental illness.
- *Social:* because pregnancy is untimely and disruptive.
- *On demand:* where there is belief that women should be free to decide when to have children.

There has been a debate on the validity of the psychiatric indications; this turns on the psychiatric consequences of a refusal to terminate. Suicide threats are common but are rarely carried out. A history of puerperal psychosis is not an indication because it is equally likely to follow abortion. There are other, arguably more serious puerperal complications, such as mother–infant relationship disorders, which are more common and severe after unwanted pregnancy. These can be avoided by adoption, but the psychological effects of relinquishment are not negligible.

In the run-up to termination, shame, anxiety and emotional turmoil are common,[57] but the abortion itself is often followed by relief. Most women who have made a personal choice suffer no adverse effects, either in the short or the long term. A minority experience regret and self-reproach over the 'murder' of the baby. Some feel like criminals and worry about punishment, a nemesis of sterility or congenital malformations. A few develop clinical depression, and a Finnish study showed that the suicide rate was raised.[21]

Many of these women have to make this decision in isolation. They do not inform their parents, or they face censure and unwelcome pressure. The attitude of the child's father is crucial but often unhelpful. It is essential that a woman makes her own decision – one of the most difficult she will ever take. It often has to be taken hastily, in an atmosphere of conflict and turmoil. The best outcomes are found when the woman makes a prudent decision in a context of respect and support from the child's father, parents, friends and counsellor.

Various organic psychoses occur after abortion, including infective delirium after criminal abortion and Wernicke–Korsakoff syndrome after hyperemesis. Shame-related psychogenic psychosis has been reported. In addition, manic and acute polymorphic episodes are seen, especially in women who have suffered similar episodes after childbirth; several have requested termination in order to prevent a recurrence of puerperal psychosis.

Miscarriage

Spontaneous abortion and ectopic pregnancy have the same psychological effects. Their emotional consequences are far from trivial and can be compared to perinatal death – less severe, but still the loss of a greatly desired child. The event itself may be disturbing, and some of the psychological symptoms resemble post-traumatic stress disorder. The incidence of depression in these women is four times the rate found in the general population, and it is even higher in childless women. There may be depressive episodes at the time of the expected delivery, anniversary reactions, and increased anxiety during and after the next pregnancy.[58] Another sequel is obsessional neurosis.[59] Helping the woman who has suffered a miscarriage is a variant of grief therapy, in which her distress is shared and her sadness, guilt and anger ventilated.

Late termination for medical reasons, although a deliberate intervention, is psychologically similar to miscarriage and to fetal death in utero. Some women wish to continue the pregnancy in the full knowledge that the baby will be abnormal. Depression is common and grief long-lasting. All these women require counselling before and after the termination.

Fetal death in utero, stillbirth, neonatal death and sudden infant death

Reactions to these events are generally more severe than to miscarriage, and each has its special characteristics. When the baby dies in late pregnancy, the mother carries a corpse within her and must undergo a futile labour. If the baby dies during labour, the loss is sudden and the shock pronounced, with a strong sense of unreality. When the child dies in the first week, the parents have to endure great anxiety, with dwindling hope; they may be involved in the decision to switch off the respirator and witness the child dying. The later death of an infant, when the maternal emotional response is fully developed, especially sudden infant death, is at the very top of the catalogue of calamities; there is no warning or preparation, the cause of death is perplexing, and there is a forensic investigation.

The grief of these parents is similar to other grieving but has its own special character: there may be grief hallucinations related to the infant – of fetal movements, the baby's face, or the infant crying or playing in the cot. There are the crises of disposing of the baby's belongings and of meeting friends and relatives, some of whom, floundering in embarrassment, are unable to comfort or sympathize ('wall of silence'). Especially after sudden infant death, there may be stigma, ostracism or malicious speculation. Envy of successful mothers is a problem; there may even be a temptation to steal another baby. Surviving children may be confused by their parents' grief and upset by family turmoil; they are also grieving and searching for the meaning of death.

When helping the parents, the principles are as follows:

- *Honesty and openness:* the admission of errors is delicate, but the parents' guilt should not be increased by the obstetric team's refusal to accept responsibility. Recrimination, litigation and complaining reactions are common. Staff should accept this as normal and try not to be defensive. One or more interviews with the consultant obstetrician are indicated.
- *Continued support:* after a stillbirth, most women prefer to be segregated from other patients and discharged from hospital as soon as possible. The woman must be visited by a member of the primary care team. A lactating woman may need bromocriptine or to donate milk to a milk bank. Hypnotics may help the woman troubled by insomnia. The woman's general practitioner (GP) should be alert for secondary psychiatric disorder.
- *Parents want to know why the baby died:* they should be warned that often no explanation is found. Necropsies in sudden infant death syndrome (SIDS) are specialized; the pathologist can play a vital psychological role and should be available for discussion.
- *Mementoes, including a photograph, should be kept:* the dignity of naming the baby and a burial ceremony is helpful. The value of seeing and holding the dead baby has been challenged: a controlled trial showed that these women had more anxiety, depression and post-traumatic stress disorder than women who had minimal contact with the stillborn infant.[60] However, what is wrong for some parents may be right for others.[61]
- *The bereaved mother needs to share her distress:* a sensitive and sympathetic listener can help the woman to grieve and accept her loss. This may be her husband or partner (who is also grieving), a family member or a friend. If not, professionals, especially chaplains and nurses, should step in. Self-help groups and voluntary agencies are invaluable for some bereaved mothers.
- *The next pregnancy:* no dogmatic advice can be given about the timing of the next pregnancy. Bereaved parents will be very anxious during pregnancy and in the puerperium and generally more anxious about their other children.
- *The grieving sibling:* the routine and rhythm of family life should be disturbed as little as possible. The parents should not be afraid to acknowledge their sadness. They should give a factual account of what happened, avoiding euphemisms. They should reassure their other children that they are not responsible and will not lose their parents' love; they should understand that neither they nor their parents are in imminent danger of death. The child can be helped to grieve by looking at pictures of the dead sibling, attending the funeral and visiting the graveyard.

Relinquishment

Adoption used to be the main way to handle accidental pregnancy and satisfy the longing to rear children. In the past 30 years, the number of children born to single mothers has climbed steeply, but European and North American society has developed a new tolerance, and the number of adoptions has fallen. International adoption has developed in response.

Although adoption is on the wane, attention has been focused on the psychological effects of relinquishment. For some adolescent mothers, giving up the child is a painful, loving and selfless action. In others, it is the enforced loss of a wanted child, with a charade of informed consent. As with termination, there is often loneliness and ostracism instead of understanding and support. Time is no healer; the child exists and can be seen again, and there is often a fantasy of restitution. After a decade, there is a new component: the adolescent child may seek its biological mother – an event the mother cannot influence. There are organizations to help relinquishing parents to find their offspring, and it has been necessary to legislate for reunions. In order to avoid adverse effects, a relinquishing mother needs counselling during the pregnancy and for at least 6 months after delivery. She may wish to see the newborn infant, and photographs should be filed. Information on the child's progress should be available, and some birth-mothers wish to reciprocate. 'Open adoption', where both sets of parents remain in contact, is under consideration. The aim is that a relinquishing mother emerges from the experience with self-respect and dignity.

The coercive removal of a child from abusive parents is a different situation. Where maternal mental illness is the reason, relinquishment is among the most unfortunate events that mothers can experience; it may also be traumatic for the child.

THE PSYCHIATRY OF THE POSTPARTUM PERIOD

The normal puerperium

For many mothers, giving birth is a supreme moment. Feelings of elation, peace and fulfilment help to sustain the mother during the weeks of strain that follow; but prolonged euphoric reactions, lasting a week or more, raise the possibility of puerperal hypomania and often switch to depression.[62]

Newly delivered mothers have to face a number of challenges, including the following:

- *Exhaustion and perineal trauma.*
- *Breastfeeding:* although this has many advantages, it is often difficult to establish. Breast abscesses (and uterine sepsis) can cause delirium.
- *Insomnia:* Sleep deprivation and disruption, especially during the first month, are common.
- *Recovery of normal figure and attractiveness:* bodily changes, especially weight gain, disturb some women, occasionally to the point of dysmorphophobia.[2]
- *Loss of libido:* episiotomy and vaginal trauma often cause dyspareunia, and fatigue may depress sexual activity. Sexual relations are usually resumed within 1–3 months, although reduced in frequency and with a delayed return of orgasm.
- *Loss of employment and leisure, and relative social privation.*

Against this background of rapid biological, social and emotional transition, a variety of psychiatric disorders occur. The psychiatric complications of childbirth are more numerous and complex than those of any other life event.

The maternity 'blues'

Often, between the third and fifth days postpartum, mothers experience a sudden, fleeting and unexpected period of sensitivity and uncharacteristic weeping. In the majority of women, this passes within a few hours or a day or two.

Reactions to severe labour

Post-traumatic stress

After an excessively painful labour, a labour with a disturbing loss of control,[63,64] fear of infant loss[65] or complications requiring emergency Caesarean section,[66] some mothers suffer nightmares and intrusive images and memories ('flashbacks'), similar to those occurring after other harrowing experiences. These flashbacks can last for months.[67] Some women avoid further pregnancy (secondary tocophobia), while those who become pregnant again may experience a return of symptoms, especially in the last trimester. Rates of up to 5.9 per cent of deliveries have been reported.[64] There is some evidence that early counselling reduces these symptoms.[68] Enduring symptoms require specific psychological treatment.

Querulant reactions

Another reaction to a severe labour experience is pathological complaining. These women complain bitterly about perceived mismanagement, and angry rumination and vengeful fantasies may continue for weeks or months, interfering with infant care. This disorder can be treated by a psychotherapeutic approach that distracts the mother from her grievances and reinforces productive child-centred activity.

Postpartum anxiety disorders

The frequency of postpartum anxiety disorders is comparable to that of postpartum depression.[69] A review of eight studies of panic disorder showed that 44 per cent of anxious women had an exacerbation and 10 per cent a new onset in the puerperium.[70]

Benzodiazepines should be used with caution in lactating mothers. The drugs are well absorbed from the gut and are metabolized more slowly in the neonatal liver; the neonatal blood–brain barrier is not fully developed. Sedation, poor suckling and weight loss have been described with diazepam; oxazepam is preferred.[71]

It is important to identify the focus as well as the form of anxiety, because there are several themes that require specific psychological therapies.

Infant-centred anxiety

Some mothers, especially *primiparae* in isolated nuclear families, are overwhelmed by the responsibility of caring for the newborn. In severe cases, this can result in panic, agitation and phobic avoidance of the infant; without intervention, these mothers risk losing their mothering role. This anxiety can often be handled by the wider family, without invoking professional help: contact with the baby should be encouraged, but always with the support of a competent adult. In severe cases, treatment is by systematic desensitization. While the infant is cared for by family or staff, the mother gradually takes over, at her own pace, undertaking the easiest tasks first, and involved in all decisions. With correct diagnosis and management, the prognosis is excellent.

Anxieties about infant health and survival

In women prone to anxiety and excessive worrying, and in those who have suffered years of infertility, recurrent miscarriage or infant loss, motherhood can lead to excessive solicitude about banal tasks such as bathing, and sensitivity to the slightest indication of childhood illness. In some women, the anxiety is focused on the possibility of sudden infant death.[72] These mothers lie awake listening to the baby's breathing, sleep with their hand on the infant's chest, check the infant many times each night, or even wake the baby to ensure that it is still alive. This results in excruciating tension, insomnia and exhaustion. Clinical experience suggests that day-hospital attendance, with anxiety management therapy and group support, is helpful, as are devices to monitor the infant's breathing. The vicious cycle of insomnia and hypervigilance can be interrupted by involving relatives and friends so that the mother can sleep under sedation. The support of other mothers who have recovered from similar problems is helpful.

Puerperal obsessional disorders

The puerperium is one of the main precipitants of obsessive–compulsive disorders.[73–75] In addition to rituals, there is a specific puerperal symptom – obsessions of infanticide. These mothers are gentle and devoted, but they experience extravagant thoughts, images or impulses of destroying their babies by fantastic methods, such as decapitation or throwing them in the fire. They are afraid to be left alone with their infants and may take extraordinary precautions.[76] It is important to distinguish these impulses from the pathological anger felt by irritable mothers with impaired bonding, which is a harbinger of child abuse. Ventilation, explanation and psychotropic medication are part of the treatment but are rarely sufficient. It is important to discourage avoidance of the child and to encourage cuddling and play, thus strengthening positive maternal feelings. Cognitive-behavioural treatment can help to achieve mastery over irrational impulses.

Depression

Over 1800 works have been published on postpartum depression, including more than 1600 in the past 12 years. But 'postpartum depression' is a term with two levels of meaning. For laypeople it covers all mental illness appearing after childbirth. As a household term, 'postnatal depression' has been valuable in drawing attention to the plight of mothers in poor mental health, providing a valid explanation for role failure, diminishing stigma, enabling mothers to accept that they are ill and to come forward for treatment, and persuading authorities to fund the necessary services. Some practitioners also use the term in this sense: much research is based on self-rating scores from which a diagnosis of 'postnatal depression' is made, without the confirmation of an interview.

In the strict sense, the postpartum illness must meet widely accepted criteria for depression. Focusing on confirmed diagnoses, the following facts have emerged:

- There is no clinical picture characteristic of postpartum depression.[77]
- Taking an overview of many studies, the incidence of depression is not raised in the puerperium.[78,79] Depression is common in women during the reproductive years, whether they are infertile, pregnant, puerperal, menopausal or involved in childrearing.
- The suicide rate is below the female rate in the general population.[80]
- Postpartum depression is not a homogeneous disorder. It includes the depressive pole of a bipolar illness as well as stress-induced depression and chronic dysthymia.
- Patients presenting with 'postpartum depression' often have co-morbid disorders, which also require diagnosis and their own specific treatment. Many mothers with anxiety, obsessional, post-traumatic or substance abuse disorders,[2,81] or with a disturbed infant relationship, are depressed.

Studies of the aetiology have found the same causal associations as for depression occurring in other circumstances: heredity, a history of previous attacks of depression, adverse events or social conditions, difficult relationships especially marital dysharmony, and social isolation. If depression were associated strongly with childbirth, then one would expect to find specific pregnancy-related factors, and there is some evidence for these:

- Depression during pregnancy is a predictor of postpartum depression.
- There is some evidence of genetic factors: an Australian twin study found genetic factors distinct from lifetime major depression.[82] Other studies have found a familial tendency,[83] but only if onset is within the first 6–8 weeks after delivery.[84]
- Two studies have implicated sex steroid hormones: in one, hypogonadism was induced in euthymic volunteers; oestrogen and progesterone were added back and then abruptly withdrawn: women with a history of postpartum depression became depressed.[85] An extension of this experiment, using corticotrophin releasing factor, showed that the pituitary–adrenal axis of women with a history of postpartum depression was more sensitive to gonadal steroids.[86]
- Unwanted pregnancy predicts both antepartum and postpartum depression.[87–89]
- In some cultures, having a female child[90] and in others polygamy increases the risk.

Whatever the epidemiological evidence, the effects of depression on family life and the emotional climate in which children are reared is of great concern. A growing child needs emotional support, attention, approbation and stimulation. The mother is the child's primary environment, and the mother's state of mind dominates the child's world. Even very young infants are disturbed by deviant maternal behaviour. Although deficits are not universal, the mother's depression can lead to anergia, brooding, reduced quantity, quality and variety of interaction, and loss of reinforcement of the mother's gaiety and tenderness.[91] The mother's anger may be misdirected at her children. Frequent irritability, impatience and criticism induce social withdrawal, anxiety and resentment. Moreover, depression may affect persistence in breastfeeding, the requirement for acute paediatric care[92] and, especially in developing countries, nutritional status.[93,94]

There have been attempts to study the long-term effects of maternal depression on the child's cognitive development. The results are inconsistent: at one extreme the timing and duration of depression had no effect,[95] and at the other extreme deficits in language or full-scale IQ were detectable at 5 and 11 years.[96,97] These investigations are bedevilled by many confounding factors, including social class, parental IQ, chronicity and severity of depression, life events, parental conflict and the quality of the mother–infant relationship. This latter factor has been examined by only one study,[98–100] and then only by a 5-min videotaped study of play at 2 months: the conclusion was that early postpartum depression, and associated disturbances in the mother–infant relationship, posed a risk to the development of the child; in one analysis, infant engagement with the mother at 2 months was the only variable predicting cognitive functioning at 5 years.[98]

In extreme cases, maternal depression can lead to the tragedy of combined suicide and filicide. Filicide has other rare causes, including delusions or command hallucinations involving the child, the late murder of an unwanted child, euthanasia, epileptic automatism and somnambulism, but only child abuse and depression are relatively common (in combination, $2–3/10^5$ children under 5 years of age per year). In child abuse, death results from ill-tempered assaults or overzealous punishment, without homicidal intent. In depression, filicide is committed in the belief that the child's best interests are being served (delusional mercy-killing). These mothers, if they survive, usually make no attempt to conceal the crime; they confess and seek punishment. Mothers may kill more than one child, but family murder seems more common in men.

Many more mothers are depressed than ever make their way to the surgery. The reasons for the failure to seek help are not fully understood: some recover early, some do not realize they are ill, and some are ashamed of confessing their symptoms, suffering in silence because of ignorance, stigma or fears of losing their baby. Screening procedures help the primary care services to identify cases. Patients identified by screening or self-referral require a detailed interview to identify vulnerability factors and all the components of the postpartum illness. The interview should explore the symptoms and course of the illness, and its context in the mother's life history, personality, circumstances and relationships with spouse, baby, other children and family of origin. It should systematically review this pregnancy, starting with conception and reactions to it, and exploring physical health and events trimester by trimester, paying particular attention to the experience of parturition. It is essential to probe the mother's developing relationship with the fetus and the infant. There are advantages in conducting this initial interview at home, because clinic attendance is an obstacle for mothers fettered with the care of young children, and because domiciliary assessment has a quality that cannot be achieved in the surgery.

Treatment is focused on depression and any underlying vulnerability. It will always involve psychotherapy, if only in the form of a single interview; it will usually include medication or other specific treatments; a few women require ECT. Working with the baby's father, potentially the main supporter, is important; fathers can come under strain, either because their partner's intimacy with the baby disturbs conjugal dynamics or because her depression has a domino effect on him. Home visits by community nurses are an ideal way of delivering continuing care and psychotherapy. An extensive literature has accumulated on the efficacy of psychological treatments. A wide variety of treatments have been tried, including psychodynamic and interpersonal psychotherapy, cognitive-behavioural therapy, peer and partner support, non-directive counselling, group therapy, midwife-led debriefing, psychoeducational groups, relaxation and massage therapy, exercise and light therapy.[101] As for drug treatment, there is no evidence that any drug is superior to others. There are at least 50 reviews of drug treatment in lactating mothers. The suckling infant has little body fat, less plasma protein-binding, an immature liver and kidney, and an undeveloped blood–brain barrier, but the risks are minor. Occasional babies have developed adverse effects such as sedation, respiratory depression and colic (with doxepin, nefazodone and fluoxetine). With most antidepressants, only a minute dose is delivered to the infant. Tricyclic antidepressants have the advantage of long usage, with no reports of adverse outcomes. Among the SSRIs, fluoxetine and citalopram deliver relatively high doses to the infant, and occasional infants develop significant serum levels and a decline in platelet 5-hydroxytryptamine (5-HT) concentrations.[102] Sertraline treatment, in contrast to treatment with paroxetine or fluvoxamine, leads to detectable levels in some breastfed infants[103] but does not affect infant serotonin levels.[104] The serotonin–noradrenaline reuptake inhibitor venlafaxine produces a higher drug level in breast milk than in maternal serum.[105] Bearing these reports in mind, it is not recommended that antidepressant agents be withheld, or that breastfeeding be stopped, but it is wise to use these drugs cautiously, and it may be helpful to administer the drug after breastfeeding. Among the hormonal treatments, progestogens given after delivery increase the risk of depression.[106] There is some evidence that oestrogens are antidepressive[107] and may be efficacious in postpartum depression, but only one or two trials have been published.

Postpartum depression has a recurrence rate of about 40 per cent.[108] Pregnant women often request advice or prophylaxis. If they are already symptomatic, or have risk factors such as marital friction or social isolation, they need support from community psychiatric nurses, voluntary agencies or other groups. If they are well, it is necessary only to establish contact, so that a recurrence is diagnosed and treated promptly. Prophylactic antidepressant medication can be considered: although a prophylactic trial of nortriptyline failed to affect the recurrence rate,[109] sertraline had a beneficial effect.[110]

MOTHER–INFANT RELATIONSHIP DISORDERS

The growth of the mother–infant relationship is the key psychological process in the puerperium. 'Bonding' is a popular term; professionals prefer the term 'attachment'. One must not confuse mother–infant with infant–mother attachment, which develops much more slowly. The mother–infant relationship consists essentially of ideas and emotions aroused by the infant, which find their expression in affectionate and protective behaviour. Its inner presence is betrayed by external signs, such as touching and fondling, kissing, cuddling and comforting, prolonged gazing and smiling, baby talk and cooing, recognizing signals, tolerating demands and resisting separation. No single activity defines it: particular behaviours wax and wane, but the relationship endures. Its power is revealed in self-sacrifice and the pains of separation. This emotional response enables the mother to withstand the never-ending vigilance and exhausting toil of the nurture of the newborn.

There is no critical period in the development of the maternal response. Close proximity from the start ('rooming-in') helps the mother to gain confidence, and breastfeeding may help. The infant plays an important part. The infant reacts preferentially to the human face and voice. Eye-to-eye contact mediates the interaction, and mutual gazing becomes an absorbing activity. The baby's smile and laughter are catalysts. Videotape studies have shown the infant contributing to a dialogue with its caregiver. Sometimes the maternal response is immediate, primed by affiliation to the fetus, but sometimes there is a worrying delay. For the first 3–4 weeks many mothers feel bruised, tired and insecure, and their babies seem strange and distanced. Some mothers are distressed by a temporary absence of affection for their babies. As the baby begins to respond socially, a normal relationship develops rapidly.

The term 'mother–infant relationship (or bonding, attachment) disorder' is appropriate for severe and persistent states in which the maternal emotional response is dominated by either or both of the following:

- *A negative emotional response:* the mother regrets the pregnancy and expresses dislike or hatred of her baby. She may try to persuade a relative to take over, and may demand that the infant be fostered or adopted. The most poignant manifestation is a secret wish that the baby 'disappear' – be stolen or die. Rejection of the infant is *threatened* when the mother seeks its temporary removal, and *established* when she persistently demands permanent placement.
- *Pathological anger:* the infant's demands anger the mother and provoke aggressive impulses, which may lead to shouting, cursing, screaming or assaults.

The frequency of these disorders in the general community can be estimated at about 1 per cent of children born. It is much higher in mothers who seek help for 'postnatal depression' – about 10 per cent at the level of established rejection and another 15 per cent for threatened rejection.[111]

There is a close relationship between these disorders and postpartum depression. Both are often present in mothers who present to services. Treatment of depression (e.g. by ECT) sometimes simultaneously cures an aversion to the infant. The onset of a late postpartum depression can be accompanied by the loss of a bond, even to the extent of rejection of the infant. But it is not appropriate, clinically or scientifically, to subsume this disorder under 'postnatal depression'. Some of these mothers are not depressed,[112,113] and in other mothers the severity, course and treatment response[114] differ. In the clinic, the relationship disorder must be diagnosed because it often requires specific psychological treatment. Without treatment, many cases become chronic. The children are insecurely attached[115] and develop behavioural problems.[116] Scientifically, the mother's relationship to her infant, and especially its severe malfunction, deserves close study. Unwanted pregnancy, impaired affiliation to the fetus and rejection of the infant are risk factors for child neglect and abuse and can contribute to their prevention.

The diagnosis can be facilitated by self-rating questionnaires.[117,118] The main resource is an interview probing the mother's emotional response and behaviour. In severe cases and in research, the gold standard is direct observation, preferably over a substantial length of time – a 5-min videotape may not be sufficient to distinguish between impaired interaction due to aversion and that due to anxiety, obsessional impulses or depression. In the day hospital or in-patient unit, 24 h/day, 7 days/week nursing observations are invaluable. In the future, functional magnetic resonance imaging (MRI) may provide objective correlates of the mother's emotional response.[119]

The treatment proceeds in stages:

- Where there is merely an absence of maternal emotional response, explanation and reassurance are appropriate.
- When hostility, rejection and anger are prominent, the primary decision is whether or not to attempt treatment. The infant's safety and wellbeing are the first consideration. The mother must not be trapped in unwelcome motherhood. The father also has his rights. The option of relinquishing the infant must be openly acknowledged and discussed fully with both parents.
- If it is decided to embark on treatment (as in most cases), depression should be treated with psychotherapy, drugs or ECT.
- The specific therapy is working on the dyadic relationship. This relationship, like others, grows through mutual pleasure, and the aim is to create circumstances in which mother and child can enjoy each other. They must therefore be treated together. Completely separating them (e.g. by hospitalizing the mother on her own) compounds the problem by adding an element of avoidance. But, if there is any hint of pathological anger, she must never be left alone with her infant and must be spared the irksome burdens of infant care. When mother and baby are calm, the mother is encouraged and helped to interact with the baby – to cuddle, talk, play and bring out the baby's smile and laughter. Participant play therapy and baby massage[120,121] may assist.

Treatment can take place at home, provided there is enough competent adult support to relieve the mother of night care and stressful duties. Day-hospital treatment is ideal for disorders of moderate severity. In severe and refractory cases, it may be necessary to admit the mother and infant to a psychiatric mother-and-baby unit, where an experienced team of psychiatric and nursery nurses can bring their skills to maximum effect. Even in the most severe cases, one can feel optimistic about a successful outcome.

Research on the prevention of these disorders is in its infancy. A controlled study showed that a videotape advising mothers how to interact affectionately with their infants had a significant positive effect on mother–infant interaction.[122]

POSTPARTUM PSYCHOSES

Postpartum psychoses fall into two main groups – organic psychoses and bipolar disorders; a third group – reactive or psychogenic psychosis – is most convincingly seen in adoptive mothers and fathers.

Among the organic psychoses,[3] two prepartum disorders – Wernicke–Korsakoff syndrome and chorea psychoses – can also present after childbirth. The most important causes of postpartum delirium are eclampsia and infection. The rarer causes are arterial occlusion, postpartum cerebral angiopathy, subdural and subarachnoid haemorrhage, cerebral venous thrombosis (common in India), epilepsy, ethanol withdrawal, Sheehan's syndrome, water intoxication and urea cycle disorders causing hyperammonaemia. Before 1925, a considerable proportion of postpartum psychoses were organic, but they are now hardly ever diagnosed in Europe or North America. They may still be important in Africa,[123] India, South-East Asia and Latin America, where most of the world's children are born.

The form of psychosis still seen in Europe and North America is related to the bipolar spectrum and to acute polymorphic (cycloid) psychosis.[124] These psychoses are acute, rapidly reaching a climax of severity. The onset is usually between 2 and 14 days after delivery. Mania is severe, often with schizoaffective symptoms or extreme excitement. Almost every psychotic symptom is seen – the whole gamut of delusions, verbal hallucinations, disorders of the will and self, and catatonic features. There is often an apparent confusion or perplexity. Since the advent of ECT and neuroleptic medication, the duration has fallen to a few weeks. A minority of patients show a tendency to relapse in rhythm with menstruation. Puerperal recurrences occur after 20–80 per cent of subsequent pregnancies,[125–128] or 100 per cent of subsequent pregnancies if depressive episodes are included.[129] Non-puerperal recurrences are also common.

These are biological brain disorders, with high heritability and an inborn tendency to develop episodes throughout life. The problem of causation can be broken down into three subsidiary questions: the nature of the diathesis, the determinants of clinical polarity (mania, depression or cycloid), and the trigger that provokes the episode. The first two questions belong to the wider study of bipolar and acute polymorphic disorders. The third is specific to puerperal psychosis. Clinical observations suggest not one, but several, triggers related to the female reproductive process – abortion, pregnancy itself (especially the last trimester), the early puerperium (especially the first 10 days), postpartum menstruation, menstruation in general, and possibly weaning. These triggers can be added to other biological events that trigger bipolar episodes, including surgery, steroid treatment and seasonal climatic changes. The incidence is less than one in 1000 pregnancies.[130,131] There is no association with twin pregnancies, breastfeeding, single parenthood or stillbirth, but higher rates are found in first-time mothers.[132] This psychosis has high heritability – not only for bipolar disorder but also for the puerperal trigger.[133] Molecular genetic studies are proceeding, and there is evidence of linkage with chromosomes 16p13 and 8q24.[134]

For treatment, the first resource is sedation by neuroleptic agents, but haloperidol should be used with caution because of the risk of severe extrapyramidal side effects, which include neuroleptic malignant syndrome. There have been few studies of breastfeeding mothers, but occasional infants have had haloperidol levels in the adult range.[135] Clozapine may accumulate in breast milk. Lithium has been used increasingly since the link with manic–depressive psychosis was recognized, and there is some evidence for its prophylactic value in women at high risk. Given to lactating mothers, it has rarely had adverse effects on the infant,[136] and is not absolutely contraindicated. Carbamazepine and valproate produce low serum levels in breastfed infants.[137] Electroconvulsive therapy is effective.[138] The location of treatment is an issue. Hospitalization is disruptive to the family, and it is possible to treat moderately severe cases at home, where the patient can maintain her role as partner, homemaker and mother, and her relationship with the newborn. If hospital admission is necessary, there are advantages in conjoint mother and baby admission.

SERVICES FOR MOTHERS WITH MENTAL ILLNESS

An outline of the services required for this area of psychiatry is slowly emerging. Its aims are prevention in those who are vulnerable, early and accurate diagnosis, and rapid effective intervention, with minimal disruption of family life. These aims require the following:

- *A multidisciplinary specialist team:* this team is of universal value – a key resource whatever the cultural background. It should include psychiatrists, nursing staff of various kinds, psychologists and social workers. It can serve a population of several million inhabitants, handling severe and intractable illness, training staff, developing services and conducting research.
- *A community service:* domiciliary assessment and home treatment are appropriate for mothers.
- *Day care:* a day hospital can provide a full range of interventions, including groups, play therapy, motherhood classes, anxiety management and occupational therapy, with minimal family disruption. The presence of mothers with similar disorders is an additional support. The children are cared for in a crèche.
- *In-patient facilities:* clinical experience suggests that conjoint admission of mother and infant is superior to the admission of the mother alone, and wards dedicated to conjoint admission also have advantages over admissions to general psychiatric wards. But there have been no objective comparisons of these state-of-the-art, expensive units with other forms of care.[139]
- *An obstetric liaison service:* apart from treating prepartum mental illness, this provides an opportunity for preventive psychiatry, by detecting vulnerability during pregnancy.
- *Links with other agencies providing services for mothers:* the social services have a key role. They can relieve the burden on the mother and safeguard the child by providing emergency foster care, and their family centres fulfil a similar function to mother-and-baby day hospitals. Other agencies that care for mothers and their infants include the National Society for the Prevention of Cruelty to Children (NSPCC), midwifery services, primary care teams and child psychiatry services.
- *A network of voluntary organizations:* these lay organizations can have close cordial ties with the professional service. Support from another mother who has suffered a similar problem and is now well is particularly appropriate – she knows the stratagems or words of comfort that were helpful, and she is proof of the possibility of recovery. For each disorder, a panel of recovered mothers is an important resource.
- *Medicolegal expertise:* expert advice is often required in cases of child abuse or infanticide, and where a mother with mental illness is seeking custody or access to her children.

KEY POINTS

- Knowledge of the psychiatry of pregnancy, parturition and the puerperium has advanced greatly during the past 20 years, with the publication of thousands of papers. Most have emerged from Europe and North America, where the birth rate and complications are low. The disease picture in the developing world may be very different.
- The most serious consequences of maternal mental illness are adverse effects on the child. Unwanted pregnancy and maladaptation to motherhood can have disastrous outcomes, including neglect (emotional and physical), abuse and infanticide.
- Depression, during pregnancy and after delivery, is not specific and is often accompanied by other disorders that require diagnosis and their own treatment.

- Anxiety disorders are common and often have themes specific to childbearing, such as tocophobia, infant-centred anxiety and the pathological fear of cot death.
- Obsessional disorders are common, and obsessions of infanticide are important, partly because of the differential diagnosis from anger-based abusive impulses.
- Pregnancy in women with eating disorders or substance abuse presents particular challenges.
- Traumatic delivery and infant loss have lasting consequences that require skilled psychological handling.
- There are many forms of prepartum and postpartum psychosis, most of which are rare complications of organic brain disease. The non-organic psychoses are linked to bipolar and acute polymorphic psychosis.
- Drug treatment has an extra dimension of unwanted effects on the developing fetus and the breastfed infant.
- The complexity of this field of psychiatry demands the deployment of specialist teams. Their resources (community services, day hospitals, conjoint admission) vary from one country to another, but their expertise is of universal value.

REFERENCES

There are approximately 10 000 published works on the psychiatry of childbearing. Works published up to 1995 were reviewed and referenced in my monograph *Motherhood and Mental Health.*[1] Limited to about 150 references, I have therefore cited only more recent publications.

1. Brockington IF (1996) *Motherhood and Mental Health.* Oxford: Oxford University Press.
2. Brockington IF, Macdonald E, Wainscott G (2006) Anxiety, obsessions and morbid preoccupations in pregnancy and the puerperium. *Archives of Women's Mental Health* **9**: 253–64.
3. Brockington IF (2006) *Eileithyia's Mischief: The Organic Psychoses of Pregnancy, Parturition and the Puerperium.* Bredenbury: Eyry Press.
4. Edwards N, Blyton DM, Hennessy A, Sullivan CE (2005) Severity of sleep-disordered breathing improves following parturition. *Sleep* **28**: 737–41.
5. Joyce TJ, Kaestner R, Korenman S. The effect of pregnancy intention on child development. *Demography* (2000) **37**: 83–94.
6. Wessel J, Buscher U (2002) Denial of pregnancy: a population based study. *British Medical Journal* 324: 458.
7. Nirmal D, Thijs I, Bethel J, Bhal PS (2006) The incidence and outcome of concealed pregnancies among hospital deliveries: an 11-year population-based study in South Glamorgan. *Journal of Obstetrics and Gynaecology* **26**: 118–21.
8. Friedman SH, Heneghan A, Rosenthal M (2007) Characteristics of women who deny or conceal pregnancy. *Psychosomatics* **48**: 117–22.
9. Siddiqui A, Hägglöf B (2000) Does maternal prenatal attachment predict postnatal mother–infant interaction? *Early Human Development* **59**: 13–25.
10. Damato EG (2004) Prenatal attachment and other correlates of postnatal maternal attachment to twins. *Advances in Neonatal Care* **4**: 274–91.
11. Armstrong DS (2002) Emotional distress and prenatal attachment in pregnancy after perinatal loss. *Journal of Nursing Scholarship* **34**: 339–45.
12. Sutter-Dallay AL, Giaconne-Marcesche V, Glatigny-Dallay E, Verdoux H (2004) Women with anxiety disorders during pregnancy are at increased risk of intense postnatal depressive symptoms: a prospective survey of the MATQUID cohort. *European Psychiatry* **19**: 459–63.
13. Swortfiguer D, Cissoko H, Giraudeau B, Jonville-Béra A (2005) Neonatal consequences of benzodiazepines used during the last month of pregnancy. *Archives de Pédiatrie* **12**: 1327–31.
14. Cissoko H, Jonville-Béra AP, Swortfiguer D, *et al.* (2005) Neonatal outcome after exposure to beta-adrenergic blockers late in pregnancy. *Archives de Pédiatrie* **12**: 543–7.
15. Kitamura T, Yoshida K, Okano T, *et al.* (2006) Multicentre prospective study of perinatal depression in Japan: incidence and correlates of antenatal and postnatal depression. *Archives of Women's Mental Health* **9**: 121–30.
16. Bánahidy F, Áces N, Puhó E, Czeizel AE (2006) Association between maternal panic disorders and pregnancy complications and delivery outcomes. *European Journal of Obstetrics and Gynecology and Reproductive Biology* **124**: 47–52.
17. Andersson L, Sundström-Poromaa I, Wulff M, *et al.* (2004) Implications of antenatal depression and anxiety for obstetric outcome. *Obstetrics and Gynecology* **104**: 467–76.
18. Czeizel AE, Timara L, Susanszky E (1999) Timing of suicide attempts by self-poisoning during pregnancy and pregnancy outcomes. *International Journal of Gynaecology and Obstetrics* **65**: 39–45.
19. Flint C, Larsen H, Nielsen GL, *et al.* (2002) Pregnancy outcome after suicide attempt by drug use: a Danish population-based study. *Acta Obstetrica Gynaecologica Scandinavica* **81**: 516–22.
20. Royal College of Obstetricians and Gynaecologists (2001) *Why Mothers Die 1997–1999: The Fifth Report of the Confidential Enquiries into Maternal Deaths in the United Kingdom.* London: Royal College of Obstetricians and Gynaecologists.
21. Gissler M, Berg C, Bouvier-Colle MH, Buerkens P (2005) Injury deaths, suicides and homicides associated with pregnancy, Finland 1987–2000. *European Journal of Public Health* **15**: 459–63.

22. Källen B (2004) Neonate characteristics after maternal use of antidepressants in late pregnancy. *Archives of Pediatric and Adolescent Medicine* **158**: 312–16.
23. Davis RL, Rubanowice D, McPhillips H, *et al.* (2007) Risks of congenital malformations and perinatal events among infants exposed to antidepressant medications during pregnancy. *Pharmacoepidemiology and Drug Safety* **16**: 1086–94.
24. Chambers CD, Hernandez-Dias S, van Marter LJ, *et al.* (2006) Selective serotonin-reuptake inhibitors and risk of persistent pulmonary hypertension in the newborn. *New England Journal of Medicine* **354**: 579–87.
25. Oberlander TF, Warburton W, Misri S, *et al.* (2006) Neonatal outcomes after prenatal exposure to selective serotonin reuptake inhibitor antidepressants and maternal depression using population-based linked health data. *Archives of General Psychiatry* **63**: 898–906.
26. Sanz EJ, De-las-Cuevas C, Kiuru A, *et al.* (2005) Selective serotonin reuptake inhibitors in pregnant women and neonatal withdrawal syndrome: a database analysis. *Lancet* **365**: 482–7.
27. Hoyme HE, May PA, Kalberg WO, *et al.* (2005) A practical clinical approach to diagnosis of fetal alcohol spectrum disorders: clarification of the 1996 Institute of Medicine Criteria. *Pediatrics* **115**: 39–47.
28. Cohn-Wesson B (2005) Prenatal alcohol and cocaine exposure: influences on cognition, speech, language and hearing. *Journal of Communication Disorders* **38**: 279–302.
29. Knopik VS, Heath AC, Jacob T, *et al.* (2006) Maternal alcohol use disorder and offspring ADHD: disentangling genetic and environmental effects using a children-of-twins design. *Psychological Medicine* **36**: 1461–71.
30. Kahila H, Saisto T, Kivitier-Kallio S, *et al.* (2007) A prospective study on buprenorphine use during pregnancy: effects on maternal and neonatal outcome. *Acta Obstetrica et Gynecologica* **86**: 185–90.
31. Eyler FD, Behnke M, Garvan CW, *et al.* (2001) Newborn evaluations of toxicity and withdrawal related to prenatal cocaine exposure. *Neurotoxicology and Teratology* **23**: 399–411.
32. Lester BM, Tronick EZ, LaGasse L, *et al.* (2002) The Maternal Lifestyle Study: effects of substance exposure during pregnancy on neurodevelopmental outcome in 1-month-old infants. *Pediatrics* **110**: 1182–91.
33. Messinger DS, Bauer CR, Das A, *et al.* (2004) The Maternal Lifestyle Study: cognitive, motor and behavioral outcomes of cocaine-exposed and opiate-exposed infants through three years of age. *Pediatrics* **113**: 1677–84.
34. Conti J, Abraham S, Taylor A (1998) Eating behavior and pregnancy outcome. *Journal of Psychosomatic Research* **44**: 465–77.
35. Bulik CM, Sullivan PF, Fear JL, *et al.* (1999) Fertility and reproduction in women with anorexia nervosa: a controlled study. *Journal of Clinical Psychiatry* **60**: 130–34.
36. Sollid CP, Wisborg K, Hjort J, Secher NJ (2004) Eating disorder that was diagnosed before pregnancy and pregnancy outcome. *American Journal of Obstetrics and Gynecology* **190**: 206–10.
37. Kouba S, Hällström T, Lindholm C, Hirschberg AL (2005) Pregnancy and neonatal outcomes in women with eating disorders. *Obstetrics and Gynecology* **105**: 255–60.
38. Ekéus C, Lindberg L, Lindblad F, Hjern A (2006) Birth outcomes and pregnancy complications in women with a history of anorexia nervosa. *British Journal of Obstetrics and Gynaecology* **113**: 925–9.
39. Franko DL, Blais MA, Becker AE, *et al.* (2001) Pregnancy complications and neonatal outcomes in women with eating disorders. *American Journal of Psychiatry* **158**: 1461–6.
40. Helgstrand S, Andersen AMN (2005) Maternal underweight and the risk of spontaneous abortion. *Acta Obstetrica and Gynecologica Scandinavica* **84**: 1197–201.
41. Blais MA, Becker AE, Burwell RA, *et al.* (2000) Pregnancy: outcome and impact on symptomatology in a cohort of eating-disordered women. *International Journal of Eating Disorders* **27**: 140–49.
42. Stein A, Fairburn CG (1996) Eating habits and attitudes in the postpartum period. *Psychosomatic Medicine* **58**: 321–5.
43. Russell GFM, Treasure J, Eisler I (1998) Mothers with anorexia nervosa who underfeed their children: their recognition and management. *Psychological Medicine* **28**: 93–108.
44. Stein A, Woolley H, Senior R, *et al.* (2006) Treating disturbances in the relationship between mothers with bulimic eating disorders and their infants: a randomized, controlled trial of video feedback. *American Journal of Psychiatry* **163**: 899–906.
45. Grof P, Robbins W, Alda M, *et al.* (2000) Protective effect of pregnancy in women with lithium-responsive bipolar disorder. *Journal of Affective Disorders* **61**: 31–9.
46. Altshuler LL, Cohen L, Szuba MP, *et al.* (1996) Pharmacologic management of psychiatric illness during pregnancy: dilemmas and guidelines. *American Journal of Psychiatry* **153**: 592–606.
47. Newport DJ, Calamaras MR, DeVane CL, *et al.* (2007) Atypical antipsychotic administration during late pregnancy: placental passage and obstetrical outcomes. *American Journal of Psychiatry* **164**: 1214–20.
48. Viguera AC, Nonacs R, Cohen LS, *et al.* (2000) Risk of recurrence of bipolar disorder in pregnant and nonpregnant women after discontinuing lithium maintenance. *American Journal of Psychiatry* **157**: 179–84.

49. Newport DJ, Viguera AC, Beach AJ, *et al.* (2005) Lithium placental passage and obstetrical outcome: implications for clinical management during late pregnancy. *American Journal of Psychiatry* **162**: 2162–70.
50. Wilson RD, Davies G, Désilets V, *et al.* (2003) The use of folic acid for the prevention of neural tube defects and other congenital abnormalities. *Journal of Obstetrics and Gynaecology of Canada* **25**: 959–73.
51. Kozma C (2001) Valproic acid embryopathy: report of two siblings with further expansion of the phenotypic abnormalities and a review of the literature. *American Journal of Medical Genetics* **98**: 168–75.
52. Vinten J, Kini U, Gorry J, *et al.* (2005) Neuropsychological effects of exposure to anticonvulsant medication in utero. *Neurology* **64**: 949–54.
53. Rasalam AD, Hailey H, Williams JHG, *et al.* (2005) Characteristics of fetal anticonvulsant syndrome associated autistic disorder. *Developmental Medicine and Child Neurology* **47**: 551–5.
54. Gaily E, Kantola-Sorsa E, Hiilesmaa V, *et al.* (2004) Normal intelligence in children with prenatal exposure to carbamazepine. *Neurology* **62**: 28–32.
55. Cunnington M, Tennis P, International Lamotrigine Pregnancy Registry Scientific Advisory Committee (2005) Lamotrigine and the risk of malformations in pregnancy. *Neurology* **64**: 955–60.
56. Putkonen H, Weizmann-Henelius C, Collander J, *et al.* (2007) Neonaticides may be more preventable and heterogeneous than previously thought: neonaticides in Finland 1980–2000. *Archives of Women's Mental Health* **10**: 15–23.
57. Bradshaw Z, Slade P (2003) The effects of induced abortion on emotional experiences and relationships: a critical review of the literature. *Clinical Psychology Reviews* **23**: 929–58.
58. Tsartsara E, Johnson MP (2006) The impact of miscarriage on women's pregnancy-specific anxiety and feelings of prenatal maternal-fetal attachment during the course of a subsequent pregnancy: an exploratory follow-up study. *Journal of Psychosomatic Obstetrics and Gynaecology* **27**: 173–82.
59. Geller PA, Klier CM, Neugebauer R (2001) Anxiety disorders following miscarriage. *Journal of Clinical Psychiatry* **62**: 432–8.
60. Hughes P, Turton P, Hopper E, Evans CD (2002) Assessment of guidelines for good practice in psychosocial care of mothers after stillbirth: a cohort study. *Lancet* **360**: 114–48.
61. Matthews M, Kohner N (2002) Psychosocial care of mothers after stillbirth. *Lancet* **360**: 1600.
62. Heron J, Craddock N, Jones I (2005) Postnatal euphoria: are 'the highs' an indicator of bipolarity? *Bipolar disorders* **7**: 103–10.
63. Soet JE, Brack GA, Dilorio C (2003) Prevalence and predictors of women's experience of psychological trauma during childbirth. *Birth* **30**: 36–46.
64. Adewuya AO, Ologun YA, Ibigbami OS (2006) Post-traumatic stress disorder after childbirth in Nigerian women: prevalence and risk factors. *British Journal of Obstetrics and Gynaecology* **113**: 284–8.
65. Slade P (2006) Towards a conceptual framework for understanding post-traumatic stress symptoms following childbirth and implications for future research. *Journal of Psychosomatic Obstetrics and Gynaecology* **27**: 99–105.
66. Ryding EL, Wijma B, Wijma K (1997) Posttraumatic stress reactions after emergency Caesarean section. *Acta Obstetrica Scandinavica* **76**: 856–61.
67. Söderquist J, Wijma B, Wijma K (2006) The longitudinal course of post-traumatic stress after childbirth. *Journal of Psychosomatic Obstetrics and Gynaecology* **27**: 113–19.
68. Gamble J, Creedy D, Moyle W, *et al.* (2005) Effectiveness of a counseling intervention after a traumatic childbirth: a randomized controlled trial. *Birth* **32**: 11–19.
69. Wenzel A, Haugen EN, Jackson LC, Brendl JR (2005) Anxiety symptoms and disorders at eight weeks postpartum. *Journal of Anxiety Disorders* **19**: 295–311.
70. Hertzberg T, Wahlbeck K (1999) The impact of pregnancy and puerperium on panic disorder: a review. *Journal of Psychosomatic Obstetrics and Gynaecology* **20**: 59–64.
71. Spigset O, Hägg S (1998) Excretion of psychotropic drugs into breast milk: pharmacokinetic overview and therapeutic implications. *CNS Drugs* **9**: 111–34.
72. Weightman J, Dalal BM, Brockington IF (1999) Pathological fear of cot death. *Psychopathology* **167**: 246–9.
73. Leckman JF, Mayes LC, Feldman R, *et al.* (1999) Early parental preoccupations and behaviors and their possible relationship to the symptoms of obsessive-compulsive disorder. *Acta Psychiatrica Scandinavica* **100**: 1–26.
74. Maina G, Vaschetto P, Ziero S, *et al.* (2001) Il postpartum come fattore di rischio specifico per l'esordio del disturbo ossessivo-compulsivo: studio clinico controllato. *Epidemiologia e Psichiatria Sociale* **10**: 90–95.
75. Labad J, Menchon JM, Alonso P, *et al.* (2005) Female reproductive cycle and obsessive-compulsive disorder. *Journal of Clinical Psychiatry* **66**: 428–35.
76. Jennings KD, Ross S, Popper S, Elmore M (1999) Thoughts of harming infants in depressed and non-depressed mothers. *Journal of Affective Disorders* **54**: 21–8.
77. Cooper C, Jones L, Dunn E, *et al.* (2007) Clinical presentation of postnatal and non-postnatal depressive episodes. *Psychological Medicine* **37**: 1273–80.
78. Najman JM, Andersen MJ, Bor W, *et al.* (2000) Postnatal depression: myth and reality – maternal depression before and after the birth of a child. *Social Psychiatry and Psychiatric Epidemiology* **35**: 19–27.

79. Evans J, Heron J, Francomb H, *et al.* (2001) Cohort study of depressed mood during pregnancy and after childbirth. *British Medical Journal* **323**: 257–60.
80. Gissler M, Hemminki E, Lönnqvist J (1996) Suicides after pregnancy in Finland, 1987–1994: register linkage study. *British Medical Journal* **313**: 1431–4.
81. Battle CL, Zlotnick C, Miller IW, *et al.* (2006) Clinical characteristics of perinatal psychiatric patients: a chart review study. *Journal of Nervous and Mental Disease* **194**: 369–77.
82. Treloar SA, Martin NG, Bucholz KK, *et al.* (1999) Genetic influences on post-natal depressive symptoms: findings from an Australian twin sample. *Psychological Medicine* **29**: 645–54.
83. Murphy-Eberenz K, Zandi PP, March D, *et al.* (2006) Is perinatal depression familial? *Journal of Affective Disorders* **90**: 49–55.
84. Forty L, Jones L, Macgregor S, *et al.* (2006) Familiarity of postpartum depression in unipolar disorder: results of a family study. *American Journal of Psychiatry* **163**: 1549–53.
85. Bloch M, Schmidt PJ, Danaceau M, *et al.* (2000) Effects of gonadal steroids in women with a history of postpartum depression. *American Journal of Psychiatry* **157**: 924–30.
86. Bloch M, Rubinow DR, Schmidt PJ, *et al.* (2004) Cortisol response to ovine corticotrophin-releasing hormone in a model of pregnancy and parturition in euthymic women with and without a history of postpartum depression. *Journal of Clinical Endocrinology and Metabolism* **90**: 695–9.
87. Beck CT (2001) Predictors of postpartum depression. *Nursing Research* **50**: 275–85.
88. McLennan JD, Kotelchuck M, Cho H (2001) Prevalence, persistence, and correlates of depressive symptoms in a national sample of mothers of toddlers. *Journal of the American Academy of Child and Adolescent Psychiatry* **40**: 1316–23.
89. Rich-Edwards JW, Kleinman K, Abrams A, *et al.* (2006) Sociodemographic predictors of antenatal and postpartum depressive symptoms among women in a medical group practice. *Journal of Epidemiology and Community Health* **60**: 221–7.
90. Patel V, Rodrigues M, DeSouza N (2002) Gender, poverty and postnatal depression: a study of mothers in Goa, India. *American Journal of Psychiatry* **159**: 43–7.
91. Paulson JF, Dauber S, Leiferman JA (2006) Individual and combined effects of postpartum depression in mothers and fathers on parenting behavior. *Pediatrics* **118**: 659–68.
92. Minkovitz CS, Strobino D, Scharfstein D, *et al.* (2005) Maternal depressive symptoms and children's receipt of health care in the first 3 years of life. *Pediatrics* **115**: 306–14.
93. Rahman A, Iqbal Z, Bunn J, *et al.* (2004) Impact of maternal depression on infant nutritional status and illness. *Archives of General Psychiatry* **61**: 946–52.
94. Stewart RC (2007) Maternal depression and infant growth: a review of recent evidence. *Maternal and Child Nutrition* **3**: 94–107.
95. Kurstjens S, Wolke D (2001) Effects of maternal depression on cognitive development of children over the first 7 years of life. *Journal of Child Psychology and Psychiatry* **42**: 623–36.
96. Brennan PA, Andersen MJ, Hammen C, *et al.* (2000) Chronicity, severity and timing of maternal depressive symptoms: relationships with child outcomes at age 5. *Developmental Psychology* **6**: 759–66.
97. Hay DF, Pawlby S, Sharp D, *et al.* (2001) Intellectual problems shown by 11-year old children whose mothers had postnatal depression. *Journal of Child Psychology and Psychiatry* **42**: 871–89.
98. Murray L, Fiori-Cowley A, Hooper R, Cooper P (1996) The impact of postnatal depression and associated adversity on early mother–infant interactions and later infant outcome. *Child Development* **67**: 2512–26.
99. Murray L, Hipwell A, Hooper R (1996) The cognitive development of 5-year-old children of postnatally depressed mothers. *Journal of Child Psychology and Psychiatry* **37**: 927–35.
100. Murray L, Sinclair D, Cooper P, *et al.* (1999) The socioemotional development of 5-year-old children of postnatally depressed mothers. *Journal of Child Psychology and Psychiatry* **40**: 1259–71.
101. Dennis CLE (2004) Treatment of postpartum depression, part 2: a critical review of nonbiological interventions. *Journal of Clinical Psychiatry* **65**: 1252–65.
102. Epperson CN, Jatlow PI, Czarkowski K, Anderson GM (2003) Maternal fluoxetine treatment in the postpartum period: effects on platelet serotonin and plasma drug levels in breastfeeding mother-infant pairs. *Pediatrics* **112**: e425–9.
103. Hendrick V, Fukuchi A, Altshuter L, *et al.* (2001) Use of sertraline, paroxetine and fluvoxamine by nursing women. *British Journal of Psychiatry* **179**: 163–6.
104. Epperson CN, Czarkowski KA, Ward-O'Brien D, *et al.* (2001) Maternal sertraline treatment and serotonin transport in breast-feeding mother-infant pairs. *American Journal of Psychiatry* **158**: 1631–7.
105. Wisner KL, Parry BL, Piontek CM (2002) Postpartum depression. *New England Journal of Medicine* **347**: 194–9.
106. Lawrie TA, Hofmeyr GJ, De Jager M, *et al.* (1998) A double-blind randomized placebo controlled trial of postnatal norethisterone enanthate: the effect on postnatal depression and serum hormones. *British Journal of Obstetrics and Gynaecology* **105**: 1082–90.
107. De Novaes Soares C, Almeida OP, Joffe H, Cohen LS (2001) Efficacy of estradiol for the treatment of depressive disorders in perimenopausal women. *Archives of General Psychiatry* **58**: 529–34.

108. Wisner KL, Perel JM, Peindl KS, Hanusa BH (2004) Timing of depression recurrence in the first year after birth. *Journal of Affective Disorders* **78**: 249–52.
109. Wisner KL, Perel JM, Peindl KS, *et al.* (2001) Prevention of recurrent postpartum depression: a randomized clinical trial. *Journal of Clinical Psychiatry* **62**: 82–6.
110. Wisner KL, Perel JM, Peindl KS, *et al.* (2004) Prevention of postpartum depression: a pilot randomized clinical trial. *American Journal of Psychiatry* **161**: 1290–92.
111. Brockington IF, Aucamp HM, Fraser C (2006) Severe disorders of the mother–infant relationship: definitions and frequency. *Archives of Women's Mental Health* **9**: 243–52.
112. Righetti-Veltema M, Conne-Perréard E, Bousquet A, Manzano J (2002) Postpartum depression and mother–infant relationship at 3 months. *Journal of Affective Disorders* **70**: 291–306.
113. Bernazzani O, Marks MN, Bifulco A, *et al.* (2005) Assessing psychosocial risk in pregnant/postpartum women using the Contextual Assessment of Maternity Experience (CAME). *Social Psychiatry and Psychiatric Epidemiology* **40**: 497–508.
114. Forman DR, O'Hara MW, Stuart S, *et al.* (2007) Effective treatment for postpartum depression is not sufficient to improve the developing mother–child relationship. *Development and Psychopathology* **19**: 585–602.
115. Tomlinson M, Cooper P, Murray L (2005) The mother–infant relationship and infant attachment in a South African peri-urban settlement. *Child Development* **76**: 1044–54.
116. Bor W, Brennan PA, Williams GM, *et al.* (2003) A mother's attitude towards her infant and child behaviour five years later. *Australian and New Zealand Journal of Psychiatry* **37**: 748–55.
117. Nagata M, Nagai Y, Sobajima H, *et al.* (2000) Maternity blues and attachment to children in mothers of full-term normal infants. *Acta Psychiatrica Scandinavica* **101**: 209–17.
118. Brockington IF, Fraser C, Wilson D (2006) The postpartum bonding questionnaire: a validation. *Archives of Women's Mental Health* **9**: 233–42.
119. Nitschke JB, Nelson EE, Rusch BD, *et al.* (2004) Orbitofrontal cortex tracks positive mood in mothers viewing pictures of their newborn infants. *Neuroimage* **21**: 583–92.
120. Field T, Grizzle N, Scafidi F, *et al.* (1996) Massage therapy for infants of depressed mothers. *Infant Behavior and Development* **19**: 107–12.
121. Onozawa K, Glover V, Adams D, *et al.* (2001) Infant massage improves mother–infant interaction for mothers with postnatal depression. *Journal of Affective Disorders* **63**: 201–7.
122. Wendland-Carro J, Piccinini CA, Millar WS (1999) The role of early intervention on enhancing the quality of mother-infant interaction. *Child Development* **70**: 713–21.
123. Ndosi NK, Mtawali ML (2002) The nature of puerperal psychosis at Muhimbili National Hospital: its co-morbidity, and associated main obstetric and social factors. *African Journal of Reproductive Health* **6**: 41–9.
124. Pfuhlmann B, Stöber G, Franzek E, Beckmann H (1998) Cycloid psychoses predominate in severe postpartum psychiatric disorders. *Journal of Affective Disorders* **50**: 125–34.
125. Pfuhlmann B, Franzek E., Beckmann H, Stöber G (1999) Long-term course and outcome of severe postpartum psychiatric disorders. *Psychopathology* **32**: 192–202.
126. Robling SA, Paykel ES, Dunn VJ, *et al.* (2000) Long-term outcome of severe puerperal psychiatric illness: a 23 year follow-up study. *Psychological Medicine* **30**: 1263–71.
127. Garfield P, Kent A, Paykel ES, *et al.* (2004) Outcome of postpartum disorders: a 10 year follow-up of hospital admissions. *Acta Psychiatrica Scandinavica* **109**: 434–9.
128. Robertson MMA, Jones I, Haque S, *et al.* (2005) Risk of puerperal and non-puerperal recurrence of illness following affective puerperal (post-partum) psychosis. *British Journal of Psychiatry* **186**: 258–9.
129. Freeman MP, Wosnitzer Smith K, Freeman SA, *et al.* (2002) The impact of reproductive events on the course of bipolar disorder in women. *Journal of Clinical Psychiatry* **63**: 284–7.
130. Terp IM, Mortensen PB (1998) Post-partum psychoses: clinical diagnoses and relative risk of admission after parturition. *British Journal of Psychiatry* **172**: 521–6.
131. Harlow BL, Vitonis AF, Sparen P, *et al.* (2007) Incidence of hospitalization for postpartum psychotic and bipolar episodes in women with and without prior prepregnancy or prenatal psychiatric hospitalizations. *Archives of General Psychiatry* **64**: 42–8.
132. Monk-Olsen T, Laursen TM, Pedersen CB, *et al.* (2006) New parents and mental disorders: a population-based register study. *Journal of the American Psychiatric Association* **296**: 2582–9.
133. Jones I, Craddock N (2001) Familiarity of the puerperal trigger in bipolar disorder: results of a family study. *American Journal of Psychiatry* **158**: 913–17.
134. Jones I, Hamshere M, Nangle JM, *et al.* (2007) Bipolar affective puerperal psychosis: genome-wide significant evidence for linkage to chromosome 16. *American Journal of Psychiatry* **164**: 1–6.
135. Yoshida K, Smith B, Craggs M, Kumar R (1998) Neuroleptic drugs in breast-milk: a study of pharmacokinetics and of possible adverse effects in breast-fed infants. *Psychological Medicine* **28**: 81–91.

136. Viguera AC, Newport DJ, Ritchie J, *et al.* (2007) Lithium in breast mild and nursing infants: clinical implications. *American Journal of Psychiatry* **164**: 342–5.
137. Piontek CM, Baab S, Peindl KS, Wisner KL (2000) Serum valproate levels in 6 breastfeeding mother-infant pairs. *Journal of Clinical Psychiatry* **61**: 170–72.
138. Reed P, Sermin N, Appleby L, Faragher B (1999) A comparison of clinical response to electroconvulsive therapy in puerperal and non-puerperal psychoses. *Journal of Affective Disorders* **54**: 255–60.
139. Joy JB, Saylan M (2007) Mother and baby units for schizophrenia. *Cochrane Database Systematic Review* (1): CD006333.

Chapter 45

Psychosexual medicine

Sandy Goldbeck-Wood

CONTEXT

Sex and the mind–body split

For better and for worse, we live in a post-Cartesian world. When René Descartes philosophically divided mind from body, or *res cogitans* from *res externa*, in 1641, he gave the Western world a powerful tool for thinking clearly about physical and mental health and illness as separate entities.[1] This divide has often served us well; but wherever mind and body illnesses are most deeply interconnected, this split in our thinking is apt to confuse rather than clarify. Sex, not uniquely, but par excellence, is almost impossible to think about usefully within separate categories of mind and body. Although a whole panoply of experts, including religious leaders, politicians, anthropologists, psychologists, psychotherapists, psychiatrists, gynaecologists, urologists, sexual health doctors and epidemiologists, each with differing languages and agendas, all consider sex their legitimate business, none has a real monopoly on relevant knowledge. There are, therefore, no true 'experts' on sex. Patients with sexual troubles are often at a loss as to where to turn, caught between sometimes contradictory-seeming agencies and approaches. And although for many patients the doctor will be a first port of call, it is unsurprising that doctors often feel out of their depth.

Sex and the medicine–psychotherapy split

Sometimes a simple, treatable, single cause can be found for a sexual difficulty, but more often the picture is complex, entangled and unamenable to a straightforward disease-based approach on the one hand, or a purely psychological approach on the other. While medicine adopts a disease-based view of illness, with specific aetiologies, epidemiologies and treatments attaching to the *disease*, in which the *doctor* is the expert and the relevant data are drawn from *outside* the consulting room, psychotherapy takes an *individually* centred view, in which symptoms are no more than pointers to an underlying illness, whose causes and solutions are *personal*, and in which the *patient*, with privileged access to the full data, is the expert and the doctor a facilitator of the self-investigatory process. Sexual distress, biopsychosocial in its very nature, calls for a crossing of this intellectual and clinical divide.

Bridge-building in doctor and patient

Hence, in encountering patients' psychosexual difficulties, we cannot stick either purely to the disease-based categorization of organic medicine and psychiatry, or purely to the narrative-based language of psychotherapy. We are forced out into an uncomfortable no-man's land between scientific discourses, because this is the place where our patients find themselves. Just as the psychosexual patient needs to open his or her mind to possible mind–body connections that could not hitherto be made, so the psychosomatic doctor needs to build intellectual and cultural bridges that join those objective and subjective, medical and psychotherapeutic, empirical and narrative-based, quantitative and qualitative approaches that have become disconnected and at times held artificially apart by factionalism and mutual suspicion. Psychosomatic work is therefore, to an extent, a process of post-Cartesian academic and clinical peace and reconciliation.

HISTORY

Sex research has traditionally been conducted in a political and moral battle zone. All early research into sex met with fierce political, moral or religious opposition, and, of the seven key contributors outlined in Box 45.1, all suffered strong political criticism, two had their works banned, one was imprisoned, and one felt obliged to change nationality. Whatever scientific criticisms we may legitimately make with the benefit of hindsight, modern psychosexual medicine owes each of these pioneers a debt.[2–14]

BIOLOGY

Anatomy

Normality in genital anatomy (Figures 45.1 and 45.2) is wide-ranging. Markedly differing lengths and diameters of

Box 45.1 Key figures from the history of sex research

VON KRAFFT EBING (1840–1902), SEXOLOGIST AND PSYCHIATRIST

- *Methodology:* Theoretician.
- *Key contributions:* Classified mental illness. Named and classified homosexuality. Promoted non-prosecution for 'innate' homosexuality. Coined the terms 'homosexuality', 'heterosexuality', 'sadism', 'masochism', 'necrophilia' and fetishism.
- *Key scientific criticisms:* Lacks an underlying theoretical framework to his classifications. Concept of 'degeneracy' – sexual activity not leading to procreation – later criticised by Havelock Ellis and Freud.
- *Principal works: Textbook of Insanity* (1879), *Psychopathia Sexualis* (1886, transl. 1902).

HENRY HAVELOCK ELLIS (1859–1939) SEXOLOGIST, PHYSICIAN AND SOCIAL REFORMER

- *Methodology:* Theoretician.
- *Key theoretical contributions:* Co-authored the first English-language textbook on homosexuality. Regarded homosexuality as neither a disease nor a crime. Championed women's rights and sexual education. Tolerant of childhood and adolescent sexuality. Sought the demystification of sex. Suggested psychological origin for most 'frigidity' and 'impotence'. Coined the terms 'narcissistic' and 'autoerotic'.
- *Key scientific criticisms:* Observations were purely theoretically based.
- *Principal works: Studies in the Psychology of Sex* (7 vols, 1897–1928), *Sexual Inversion* (1896).

SIGMUND FREUD (1856–1939), NEUROLOGIST, SEXOLOGIST AND FOUNDER OF PSYCHOANALYSIS

- *Methodology:* Theory based on clinical case studies.
- *Key theoretical contributions:* Postulated blocked libido as a cause of neurotic/hysterical/psychosomatic symptoms. Developed a theory of childhood sexuality, including a stage model of psychosexual development.
- *Key criticisms:* At times, makes sweeping theoretical and therapeutic claims on the basis of small numbers of cases.
- *Principal psychosexual text: Three Essays on the Theory of Sexuality* (1905).

WILHELM REICH (1897–1957)

- *Methodology:* Observation of clinical case material and that of colleagues.
- *Key theoretical contributions:* Elaboration of the psychosomatic mechanisms connecting blocked sexual energy and neurosis. Development of a theory of character based on these blocks. His work gave rise to the tradition of body psychotherapies.
- *Key criticisms:* Mental breakdown in later life and political discreditation cast a shadow retrospectively on his earlier, more cogent work.
- *Principal works: The Function of the Orgasm* (1927).

ALFRED KINSEY (1894–1956) PHYSICIAN AND SEXOLOGIST

- *Methodology:* Personal interview and filming of sexual acts.
- *Key theoretical contributions:* Two first large-scale surveys of sexual behavior: the **Kinsey Reports**. First statistical reports of childhood masturbation. Elucidated the high prevalence of extra- and premarital sex, the ubiquity and harmlessness of masturbation, and the high level of homosexual encounters.
- *Key scientific criticisms:* The use of personal interview rather than observation, and a focus on counting the frequency of sexual events rather than focusing on the whole experience. Ethically, the presentation of data that could probably not have been obtained without observation of **child sexual abuse** or through collaborations with child molesters.
- *Principal works: Sexual Behaviour in the Human Male* (1948), *Sexual Behaviour in the Human Female* (1953).

WILLIAM MASTERS (1915–2001), OBSTETRICIAN AND GYNAECOLOGIST, AND VIRGINIA JOHNSON (b. 1925), PSYCHOLOGIST

- *Methodology:* Direct observation of sexual acts in the laboratory, sometimes using 'assigned partners'.
- *Key theoretical contributions:* Originators of biological sex research. Observational data on the anatomy and physiology of the sexual response during intercourse and masturbation. Elucidation of the four-fold model of arousal, plateau, orgasm and resolution. Recognition of the refractory period in men and the capacity for multiple orgasm in women. Debunking of myths about vaginal lubrication, vaginal and clitoral orgasm, and loss of sexual responsiveness in older adults. Confirmation of masturbation as near-universal and impotence as largely psychological. 'Normalization' of discourse about sex. Development of first couples-based, focused sex therapy in 1970.

- *Key scientific criticisms:* Unrepresentative research participants. Uncritical acceptance of cultural assumptions such as that it is 'normal' for a woman to orgasm through penile thrusting.
- *Principal works: Human Sexual Response* (1966), *Human Sexual Inadequacy* (1970), *Homosexuality in Perspective* (1979).

SHERE HITE (b. 1942), SEX EDUCATOR AND FEMINIST

- *Methodology:* Individualistic, large-scale, questionnaire-based research. Development of a discourse on human responses to gender and sexuality.
- *Key theoretical contributions:* Focus on individual subjective sexual experience of sex. Incorporation of key feminist theoretical perspectives. Showed that 70% of women do not have **orgasms** through in–out thrusting **intercourse** but are able to achieve orgasm easily by **masturbation** or other direct clitoral stimulation.
- *Key criticisms:* Low response rates and possible response bias.
- *Principal works: The Hite Report on Female Sexuality* (1976, 2004), *The Hite Report on Men and Male Sexuality* (1981).

penis and sizes of labia majora and minora are all capable of being functionally normal in both sexual and reproductive terms, as well as attractive and pleasurable to the individual and their partner. Abnormalities certainly exist, such as marked Peyronie's disease, hypogonadism and vaginal stenosis, and are dealt with in detail in the gynaecological, urological and paediatric literature. On these, the doctor and patient usually agree, although even here the agreement on anatomical difference is not so much the end as the beginning of the exploration of what this means to the patient, how it affects him or her, and what treatment is appropriate. Far more common than frank anatomical abnormality is the *fear* of abnormality. As psychosexual doctors, we frequently encounter people who are worried that their genitalia might be abnormal when, on examination, we do not find them so. In the extreme case of body dysmorphia, the patient may be passionately convinced that his or her genitalia are abnormal or grotesque and strongly request treatment such as labial reduction surgery or penile enlargement, while the doctor, perplexed, can find no abnormality at all.[15] The pressure to endorse the patient's negative self-image and comply with requests for 'treatment' can be strong, and the fear of seeming unsympathetic or arrogant if we do not act looms large; but it is particularly important for psychological as well as physical reasons that the doctor is able to trust his or her clinical and medical judgement and remain truthful and congruent. Reporting our findings of normality in a way that does not dismiss the patient's concern, but instead invites curiosity and conversation about the discrepancy between the doctor's and the patient's judgement, can help the patient to reflect on the origins of his or her own dissatisfactions.

Physiology

Our understanding of the physiology of sexual response has travelled in just over a century from theory and speculation (see Box 45.1), via empirical and qualitative methods of data-gathering, to direct imaging via magnetic resonance imaging (MRI) scans made during sexual intercourse. Masters and Johnson were the first to characterize the human sexual response, in four stages of arousal, plateau, orgasm and resolution, which are summarized in Boxes 45.2 and 45.3.[9,16]

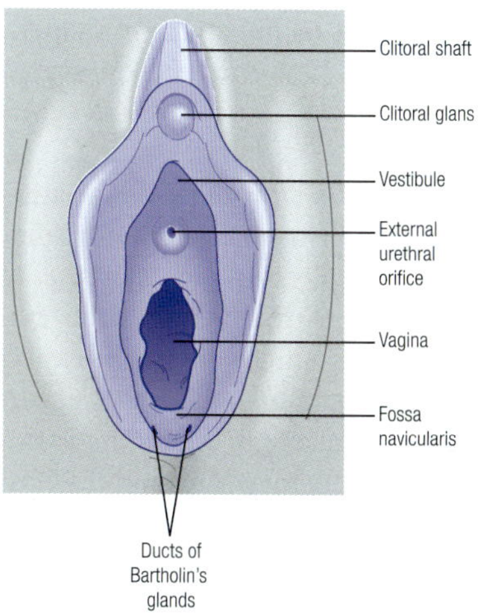

Figure 45.1 Normal female genital anatomy

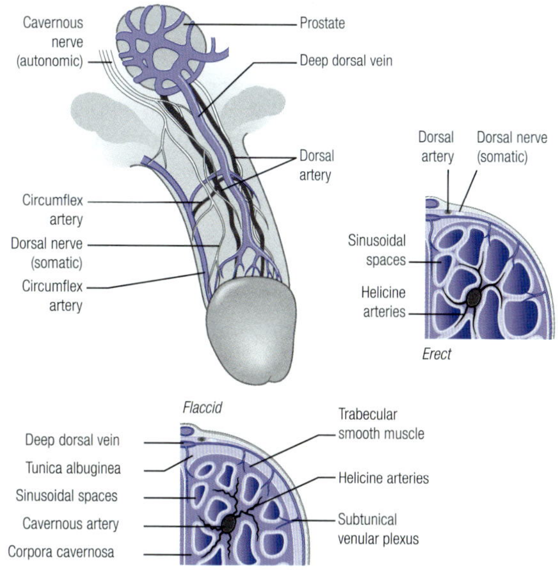

Figure 45.2 Normal male genital anatomy, showing mechanism of penile erection

Box 45.2 Masters and Johnson's four stages of sexual arousal

1. Excitement phase (in initial arousal)
2. Plateau phase (at full arousal, but not yet at orgasm)
3. Orgasm
4. Resolution phase (after orgasm).

Box 45.3 Physical aspects of the sexual response in women and men

IN WOMEN

The excitement phase draws on physical and psychological stimuli and involves vasocongestion of the external genitalia, clitoral erection, colour changes in the genital skin, and flattening and opening of the labia majora. Increased vaginal transudate reduces friction during intercourse. A turgid cuff of engorged tissue forms in the lower third of the vagina, the nipples and areoles become erect, and there is often a pink flush over the breasts, abdomen and limbs, known as the 'sex flush'.

The plateau phase draws more strongly on physical stimulus, which must continue if orgasm is to be achieved. The vagina lengthens and distends, with ballooning or tenting at the proximal end, the turgid cuff at its distal end increases, the uterus elevates, and the clitoris retracts.

Orgasm is characterized by brief myotonic contractions of the pelvic floor muscles of about 1 in every 0.8 s, and the release of genital vasocongestion. It varies markedly in intensity within and between women, has no definite endpoint, and is followed by the resolution phase, during which some women are able to return rapidly to orgasm ('multiple orgasm').

IN MEN

The excitement phase draws on physical or psychological stimuli, or both, and leads to vasocongestion of the penile corpora cavernosa, causing erection of the penis. Erection is dependent on the integrated action of psychological, endocrine, neural vascular and anatomical elements, and damage in any of these pathways can result in erectile dysfunction. In general terms, the ability to have spontaneous nocturnal or early morning erections, or erections during masturbation, precludes serious neurovascular causes of erectile dysfunction. At full penetration, the penis appears boomerang-shaped, with an average length of 22 cm from root to tip, reaching mid-sacrum or the sacral promontory, and filling the whole anterior or posterior fornix of the vagina. The plateau phase draws more strongly on physical stimulus and leads to orgasm, which is characterized by brief myotonic contractions of the pelvic floor muscles every 0.8 s, the release of genital vasocongestion, and ejaculation. Orgasm is followed by a refractory period, during which a return to orgasm is physiologically impossible. Orgasm and ejaculation are neurologically distinct, and it is possible for a man to ejaculate without experiencing satisfactory orgasm.

Non-biological influences on sexual response

A number of cultural and life-stage factors can affect sexual response and practice. The age of first sexual activity, the willingness to have sex during menstruation or before marriage, the use of contraception, attitudes to pregnancy, infidelity and divorce, and sexual activity in later life are all highly culture-bound. For example, the age of first adult sexual experience has moved steadily downwards across the Western world, with figures from the USA suggesting that one in five under-15s, and from the UK one in five under-16s, are sexually active,[17] with teenage pregnancy rates rising steadily in parallel.[18–20] Cultural attitudes within and between societies vary widely, from the extremely liberal, as exemplified by the 'free love' movement in the 1960s, which promoted unrestricted sex, to the extremely conservative, such as countries and subgroups that punish homosexuality with the death penalty or ostracize unmarried mothers. Sex is heavily mythologized in all ages and cultures, and some sexual myths can get in the way of sexual health and functioning (Box 45.4). Similarly, large-scale societal changes, such as the introduction of the contraceptive pill, the legalization of first homosexuality and then abortion, and the advent of human immunodeficiency virus (HIV) and acquired immunodeficiency syndrome (AIDS), have revolutionized sexual attitudes and practices (Box 45.5).

At a more personal level, there is considerable variation in sexual activity through the menstrual cycle, with some questionnaire-based evidence suggesting an increase in sexual activity pre- and post-menstrually and little evidence for an increase at ovulation, which one might expect based on the analogy with other mammals.[21] There appears to be widespread cultural avoidance of sex during menstruation, although this is less marked in white middle-class women. A minority of women use menstruation as a 'safe' period of presumed reduced fertility. Where menstruation is heavy, painful or irregular, this can affect sexual relating.

Box 45.4 Myths and taboos can interfere with sexual health and function:

- 'Sex during pregnancy might damage the baby'
- 'You can't get pregnant from first ever sexual intercourse'
- 'Orgasm is normally or should be mutual and simultaneous'
- 'Women should orgasm from penile thrusting only'
- 'Sex during menstruation or postpartum bleeding is impermissible/undesirable/dirty'
- 'Men should always feel like sex'
- '"Nice" women are not too interested in sex'
- 'Gay men are more promiscuous than straight men'
- 'Masturbation makes you blind'

Box 45.5 Key historical influences on sexual behaviour and attitudes

- *1844:* mass production of vulcanized rubber condom. Latex introduced in 1880s but widely available from 1930s.
- *1861:* legislation (Offences Against the Person Act) abolishes death penalty for buggery.
- *1885:* legislation (Criminal law Amendment Act) to completely criminalize male homosexuality.
- *Early 1900s:* vibrators available to public (previously restricted to doctor's consulting rooms) – fifth available household electrical appliance predating iron and vacuum cleaner.
- *1921:* publication of *Wise Parenthood* by Marie Stopes – a brief guide to contraception. First Marie Stopes clinic opened.
- *1960:* introduction of contraceptive pill (1961 in UK – married women only).
- *1960:* publication in UK of *Lady Chatterley's Lover* by DH Lawrence (written in 1928). Publisher prosecuted unsuccessfully under the 1959 Obscene Publications Act.
- *1963:* publication of *The Feminine Mystique* by Gloria Friedan (early feminist challenge to the idea that women could derive satisfaction only through devotion to home, husband and children).
- *1964:* first use of the term 'women's liberation' (Women's Liberation Movement coined 1968).
- *1967:* legislation (Abortion Act) to allow limited abortion in UK.
- *1973:* homosexuality removed from DSM-II by American Psychiatric Association.
- *1984:* approval of morning-after pill in UK (over-the-counter availability since 2001).
- *1981:* first cases of AIDS in the USA (term coined in 1982).
- *1987:* male homosexuality partly decriminalized in England and Wales (Sexual Offences Act). Separate legislation in Scotland (1980) and Northern Ireland (1982). Male homosexual age of consent 21 years (reduced to 18 years in 1993). No female homosexual age of consent before 2001.
- *2001:* equalization of homosexual and heterosexual age of consent (at 16 years, except in Northern Ireland, where it is currently 17 years but in the process of being equalized).

AIDS, acquired immunodeficiency syndrome; DSM-II, *Diagnostic and Statistical Manual of Mental Disorders*, 2nd edn.

The influence of contraception on sexual activity can range from positive effects of liberation from the fear of pregnancy, through hormonal side effects such as decreased libido or breast tenderness, to psychological unease about the loss of 'naturalness' associated with exogenous hormones or 'foreign bodies,' or even an unconscious desire for the very pregnancy that is consciously being prevented. Reliable data are difficult to gather in this area, since the attitudes, desires and cultural backgrounds of two partners both simultaneously influence the nature and timing of sexual activity.

Pregnancy can affect sexual desire and function in both partners, in both positive and negative ways. A couple's general feelings about the pregnancy, specific fears and fantasies about miscarriage or preterm labour, changes in the woman's body such as increased breast size and tenderness, increased genital congestion and lubrication, exhaustion, physical discomfort, uterine irritability, and milk spurting from the breasts during orgasm can all influence sex. On average, sexual activity appears to reduce in the first and third trimesters, when exhaustion, sickness and fear of miscarriage are greatest, but to increase, even in relation to the non-pregnant state, in the second trimester, but with wide variations between women.[21] Sex postpartum will depend on the pre-pregnancy state of the sexual relationship and on factors such as both partners' experience of the labour, the degree of exhaustion due to sleep deprivation or breastfeeding, physical discomfort relating to aspects of the delivery, and any postnatal depression or low mood. Breastfeeding, described by some women as sexually pleasurable, is experienced by others as neutral or even uncomfortable. Sexual desire often returns before the menstrual cycle, confirming that a cycle is essential for neither libido nor sex.

Menopause, with its associated symptoms of vaginal dryness, hot flushes and reduced libido, can represent a challenge or crisis in many women's sexual lives, although some suffer only minimally. In general, the motto 'use it or lose it' appears to apply to a degree, in that regular sexual activity appears to preserve the ability to lubricate and to tolerate and enjoy intercourse and orgasm. Uterovaginal prolapse and age-related urological symptoms can inhibit sexual activity, as can relationship factors such as sexual boredom, erectile dysfunction, illness in oneself or one's partner, and the inhibitory effects of perceived societal attitudes to sexual activity in older people. However, recent evidence confirms that sexual activity can continue in a satisfying, albeit modified, form beyond the menopause and into late life, and suggests that older people nowadays are enjoying more frequent and satisfying sex than that reported in previous generations.[22]

SEX AND EVIDENCE

Cultural challenges

Because sex is biopsychosocial, its study is spread across disciplines, no one of which can claim full expertise. This makes it challenging to research, at the level of both the individual study and the institution. Each discipline has evolved its own scientific culture, from the nuanced case-reporting and supervisory self-reflection of psychotherapy, through the qualitative research methodologies of the social sciences, to the numerical, population-level objectivity of randomized controlled trials and systematic reviews. Each approach contributes a different perspective on sexual dysfunction, and each has its own passionately defended ethic of rigour. It can be hard for differing disciplines to agree on the important research questions, never mind the correct methodologies for addressing them and the outcomes of interest. Both in the consulting room and in the university department, the resolution of sexual problems requires individuals who are willing to bridge the gap between biological and psychological approaches by learning each other's languages and research methodologies.[23,24]

Bias

Sex research is particularly bias-prone. Aside from *subcultural biases* based on the researcher's scientific background, researchers and clinicians are inevitably prone to *personal biases* based on their own sexual beliefs, feelings, experiences and preferences, however liberal or conservative, conscious or unconscious these may be.

Since direct observation of sexual activity is practically difficult, ethically questionable and almost by definition non-representative, research relies heavily on self-reporting, which is prone to the usual biases that this entails: the relationship between what people do and what they say they do is known to be unreliable, and the more socially unacceptable or controversial the behaviour, the more likely *underreporting bias* is to play a role. This complicates the investigation of anything from homosexual sex, anal sex or extramarital affairs to minority sexual practices such as paedophilia or fetishes. As well as underreporting bias, generally *poor response rates* common to all questionnaire surveys often limit the external validity, or generalizability, of research findings.

In addition, it is helpful to remember that most sex research is born of experience with individuals with sexual problems who present to doctors, which many, but not all, do, leading to possible *selection bias*. By definition, we know nothing about the number of people who do not present to doctors, and how and with what success they address their sexual problems. All of these biases place limits on the internal validity of sex research – that is, its accuracy in reflecting the research population – and its external validity – that is, its generalizability to a wider population. This means that caution in interpreting individual studies is particularly important, and the use of 'triangulation' whereby a picture is assembled using data from a variety of different sources and methodologies, much like the piecing together of a mosaic from fragments, is particularly helpful.

As sexual dysfunction has become more widely recognized, in part due to pharmaceutical company research interest, a number of validated and reliable measures of sexual function/dysfunction have been developed, usually brief, self-report questionnaires taking 10–20 min to complete.

In summary, just like work with an individual patient's psychosexual difficulty, scientific work around psychosexual distress is a multilayered reconstructive process, closer to the reassembling of fragments of data from different disciplines, using different methodologies and a variety of outcome measures, whether of biological function, self-reported physical experience, self-reported emotional experience, or broader factors such as quality of life.

What is known?

Although a wealth of rich, narrative-based and qualitative information exists on sexual function and dysfunction, there is a dearth of high-quality quantitative data, such as randomized controlled trials and systematic reviews with patient-centred outcomes. A critical review of the evidence relating to the efficacy of psychological interventions for sexual dysfunction carried out in 2004 by a body of international experts concluded that:[25]

- the best available evidence (levels 3, 4 and 5) supports the use of a multidisciplinary and/or biopsychosocial approach;
- more high-quality research into the efficacy of psychosexual treatments, and in particular combined biopsychosocial approaches, is needed;

- outcome studies are notoriously difficult to design and conduct in ways that meet high evidence standards while respecting the complexity of sexual life;
- many studies have a narrow view on genital function/dysfunction or performance, and an overemphasis on frequency counts of various sexual acts, as opposed to more subtle measures of satisfaction or health-related quality of life;
- even function-oriented studies disagree as to what constitutes a good treatment outcome (does the achievement of a single orgasm count as success in treating anorgasmia in women? Or should one count orgasm on some specified percentage of occasions – and from manual or oral stimulation or from coitus? Similarly, is frequency of heterosexual coitus a satisfactory measure of treatment for erectile dysfunction?);
- love, widely regarded as important especially in Western counties in fostering relational and sexual intimacy, is not typically discussed in scientific discourse or evidence-based research.

THE PSYCHOSOMATIC TRADITION AND PSYCHOSEXUAL MEDICINE

Psychosexual medicine: deep penetration on a narrow front

Psychosexual medicine arose in response to the needs of British doctors and patients struggling to understand and treat sexual difficulties. It is based on the work of two doctor-psychoanalysts, Michael Balint and Tom Main, who founded the Institute of Psychosexual Medicine in 1974, which offers training to somatic doctors and psychiatrists (Box 45.6).[26] Psychosexual medicine is an integrated approach that presupposes competence in taking a medical history and identifying underlying or coexisting organic disease, and treating or referring appropriately, but adds to these the skills and methods of psychodynamic psychotherapy. It is therefore intercultural, and firmly rooted in a wider academic tradition of psychosomatic medicine.[27]

Psychosomatic medicine in the UK and elsewhere

Although psychosomatic medicine exists as an independent clinical and academic specialty in many countries, such as the USA and parts of mainland Europe, the treatment of psychosomatic illness in the UK is spread across medical specialties. Individual pools of expertise have grown piecemeal in subspecialist areas such as liaison psychiatry, psychosexual medicine, pain management and general practice. The management of psychosomatic illness in the UK therefore depends on strong interdisciplinary liaison and is at particular risk from each specialty's pressures to deliver on 'core' targets and of being treated in inappropriate ways.

Psychosexual medicine differs both from other forms of sex therapy usually practised by non-doctors, where cognitive-behavioural methods, often involving the use of exercises, are used to modify unhelpful sexual attitudes and behaviours,[28] and from general psychotherapy, with its broader scope and often longer-term work. Each of these has a useful place, and in general the evidence is good that a skilled psychotherapist trained in a theoretically grounded model delivers effective results irrespective of primary orientation,[29] and that the differences between approaches are less sharply delineated in the clinical practice of experienced practitioners than in theory.[30] However, the Institute of Psychosexual Medicine's (IPM) brief, psychodynamic, sex-focused, medically grounded work is particularly suited for the time- and resource-constrained environment of the medical consultation and was described by IPM founder Dr Tom Main, with the wartime analogy: 'deep penetration on a narrow front'.

Box 45.6 Real-time questions in the psychosexual doctor's mind

- What, in detail, is the sexual problem? When does it occur and whom does it distress? For example, the answer 'I love my boyfriend and get aroused, but when I get close to orgasm I burst into tears, and he gets upset, and this puts me off having sex at all' is more informative than 'I don't feel like having sex'.
- When did it all start, and was anything else emotionally significant happening at the time, such as a death, an operation, an affair or a traumatic birth?
- Why is the patient presenting now (e.g. desire for a baby or fear for the relationship), especially when the problem has been long-term?
- How has the patient managed the problem so far, and what can you learn about the patient from this?
- How does the patient behave with you and make you feel (e.g. protective, warm, irritated, frustrated)? How might this relate to the patient's sexual life?
- How might the feelings or behaviours in the room reflect the patient's sexual life?
- What might the patient's body be 'saying' or 'thinking' that they have struggled to say or think?
- How is the patient responding to the examination or to your interpretive comments?

The psychosomatic tradition and medicine

When the psychic system fails, the organism begins to think – Sandor Ferenczi

Psychosomatic medicine is the study of genuine physical illness caused by mental or emotional rather than biological processes. Wherever the mind is not able to contain or metabolize distress, according to psychoanalytical theory the body takes over and, in Ferenczi's words, 'begins to think'.[31] The more 'unthinkable' the thought – be it too painful, shameful or frightening, or simply embarrassing – whether past abuse, ambivalence in relation to one's spouse or guilt about an affair, the more likely it is to be pushed beneath the surface of conscious awareness, only to burst out in unconscious, somatic ways that present to a doctor and not a psychotherapist. It is helpful if the doctor is alert to this possibility, so that he or she can offer an integrated medical and psychological approach to diagnosis and treatment.

The key idea behind analytical psychotherapy is that restoring hidden distress to awareness, however painful, delivers the patient from the need for his or her neurotic symptom and restores a kind of psychological homeostasis – the psychosomatic equivalent of lancing an abscess or debriding a wound of necrotic tissue, which superficially protects but actually impedes healing. In other words, much like some of the simpler surgical interventions, analysis is both the diagnostic imaging modality and the cure, at the same time.

So, although psychosomatic illness is also treated widely by psychotherapists, some of whom are specialized in a body-centred approach,[32] and to whose academic tradition we owe much of the useful literature on the mind–body connection, it remains a medical concern. This is recognized by the inclusion of these syndromes in the World Health Organization's International Statistical Classification of Diseases and Related Health Problems as 'neurotic, stress related and somatoform disorders'.[33]

How do psychosexual problems present to doctors?

Because sex is an intensely private activity, which many people find hard to speak about openly, sexual problems may present directly or indirectly, via an associated physical or psychological symptom, referred to by psychosexual doctors as a 'calling card',[21] such as pelvic pain, recurrent vaginal discharge, difficulty with having a smear test, depression or anxiety. The ritual of excluding organic pathology, while useful in itself, can also be an opportunity for the patient to test the doctor's perceived suitability to being entrusted with the full story.

Making an assessment can be complicated by the patient's or the doctor's feelings of embarrassment in discussing the problem, resistance to considering psychological causes because of the stigma surrounding mental illness, which includes the fear of being labelled 'mad,' of having their views dismissed, or of having a biological diagnosis missed. Add to this the shame some people feel, despite great efforts they have not been able to solve the problem themselves, and a perhaps understandable despair that an anonymous doctor could possible help where their own attempts have failed, and it is clear that establishing a therapeutic connection with the patient is a challenge.

The psychotherapeutic approach to consultation

Psychotherapy was described by Donald Winnicott, a paediatrician and psychoanalyst, as 'extended history taking'.[34] It differs from general medical history-taking in having a more open-ended approach and a greater interest in the kind of 'asides' that most doctors learn to screen out when taking a medical history, such as 'I know it was 14 December when the pain started because I'd just got back from my father's funeral.' Whether we find it interesting or merely banal, this kind of material is extraneous in the routine medical history because it is unlikely to be biologically relevant, but it can contain important psychological clues. The psychotherapist or psychosomatic doctor learns, without leaping to premature conclusions, to bear these in mind.

Indeed, the 'bearing in mind', during the period of the consultation, of a wide variety of information relating to the presenting difficulty and associated material, all presented piecemeal in an apparently random way, as dictated by the patient rather than the doctor's questions, without either losing sight of too much information or trying to structure things prematurely and losing of raw data, is a core psychotherapeutic skill. It requires some self-awareness and tolerance and a degree of practice, much like playing the party game of memorizing the objects on a tray, in order to be able to write them down afterwards.

In general, it is helpful to approach the patient in a spirit of interested ignorance, rather than with the preformed mental map of differential diagnoses that is often helpful in approaching organic illness. The map, in psychotherapeutic work, is drawn in collaboration with the patient as the consultation unfolds.

The skills of psychosexual medicine

Psychosexual medicine uses this extended history-taking to elicit both biological and psychological data.[21] In distinction from pure psychotherapy, it also includes physical examination, usually genital examination, or at least the possibility of this, and this too is used as an opportunity to reflect on the patient's body language and behaviour: is the patient happy to be examined, or is mere suggestion of examination resisted (e.g. 'I've got my period')? Does the patient settle comfortably on the couch and appear present and comfortable during the examination? Or does the patient flinch or shrink, become impassive or 'absent', or stretch out in an elaborate display of confidence? How does the patient describe his or her experience during and after the examination, and in response to the doctor's finding? Was the patient less fearful than expected? Is the patient relieved or anxious?

To the general consulting and counselling skills used in good medical and psychiatric history-taking, psychosexual medicine adds some specific skills, learned experientially over a 2- to 4-year period of reflective practice and derived from psychodynamic theory (see below).

The psychodynamic approach is most straightforwardly summarized in Malan's image of the 'triangle of person' (Figure 45.3) in which the patient's current relationship difficulties both mirror their past relationships (e.g. with parents in childhood) and are echoed in their relationship with the doctor in the consulting room.[35] For example, a patient who has been violently penetrated during sexual abuse by a parent may quite involuntarily resist all penetration, however much needed or desired, by both her partner who wants to make love with her and her doctor who wants to take a swab or a smear test or perform a vaginal examination. The patient may dearly want the intimacy of lovemaking or the reassurance of the examination, and fear the consequences of not being able to tolerate these, but she may find herself unable to allow a penis or a speculum anywhere near her vagina. The 'echo' might be detectable in the doctor–patient relationship both in physical ways, involving resistance of examination, and in more symbolic or psychological ways, such as a tendency to shut down or become distressed in response to probing questions. These responses can be noticed.

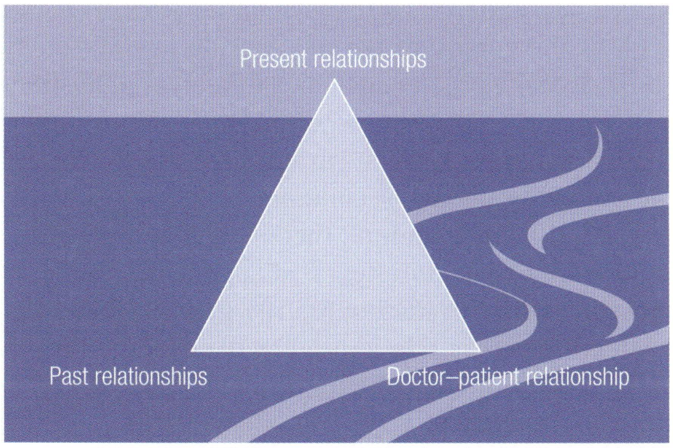

Figure 45.3 The psychodynamic triad

In short, the most important clinical tools of psychosexual medicine are those learned from reflected-on experience, rather than those acquired from reading books, even those based on high-quality evidence. Psychodynamic work requires a capacity for symbolization – the decoding of symbolic connections between emotional and physical worlds – and is not suitable for work with people suffering from psychotic illness, in which the capacity for symbolization – with the 'stepping back' that this implies – is impaired, and who are likely to experience attempts at analytical work as unhelpful at best and distressing at worst.

Psychosexual medicine uses general communication skills, such as:

- active listening;
- observation;
- letting the patient tell the story in their own way;
- the ability to tolerate silence;
- a non-judgemental attitude;
- an ability to discuss sexual events and body parts in a straightforward and relaxed way.

It also uses specialized psychodynamic skills, such as:

- observation and reflective use of the doctor–patient relationship: noticing how the patient behaves in relation to the doctor, and how the doctor finds him- or herself feeling or behaving in relation to the patient (known in wider analytical psychotherapy as analysis of the transference and countertransference);
- observation and reflective use of body language;
- psychodynamic, interpretive use of the physical, genital examination;
- retaining an awareness of the main thrust of the work: conversation about the sexual difficulty and physical examination and noticing where this is not adhered to, and attempting to understand why not (when is a digression helping to make important connections and when it is acting as a distraction?);
- awareness of the doctor's defences (e.g. recourse to overly medicalized language or unnecessary investigation or prescription) and interpretation of their relation to the sexual problem;
- awareness of the patient's defences (e.g. bringing a third party – a mother, baby or partner) to the consultation, or unwillingness to stay with the subject.

(See Table 45.1 overleaf and Box 45.6 on page 749 for a summary.)

NORMAL AND ABNORMAL

Normal variants

Variants of sexual expression now accepted as normal include homosexuality (sexual attraction to people of the same sex), bisexuality (sexual attraction to both the opposite and the same sex) and asexuality (no sexual desire at all). The word 'lesbian' is widely used to denote female homosexuality, 'gay' to denote male homosexuality or sometimes homosexuality in general, and 'straight' to denote heterosexuality. There is a worldwide prevalence of between 1.5 per cent and 10 per cent for homosexuality and around 0.1 per cent for bisexuality,[36] with studies con-

Table 45.1 Key elements of the psychosomatic approach

General counselling/communication skills	Specific psychodynamic skills
Observation	Observation and reflective use of body language
Active listening	Observation and reflective use of the doctor–patient relationship
Tolerating/using silence	Interpretive use of the physical examination
Adopting an attitude of attentive ignorance rather than of prior knowledge	Awareness of the doctor's defences to working (e.g. overmedicalization)
Maintaining a non-judgemental stance	Awareness of the patient's defences against working (e.g. distraction, avoidance of examination, use of a third party to the consultation as a barrier)
Discussing sexual events and body parts in a straightforward and relaxed way	Alertness to possible parallels between early experience and symptoms presented

ducted by gay rights groups showing higher figures and those conducted by anti-gay campaigners lower figures. In general, homosexuality and heterosexuality appear to exist on a spectrum, with only a large minority of people falling within a totally heterosexual category.[7,8]

Homosexuality has historically been the focus of widespread prejudice and persecution, ranging from criminalization and the death penalty at one extreme, through widespread legal and social discrimination, to pathologization with a variety of aetiological theories and largely ineffective and humiliating 'treatments' applied.

Homosexuality was finally decriminalized in the UK in 1967 and removed from the American Medical Association's list of mental disorders in the fourth edition of the *Diagnostic and Statistical Manual of Mental Disorders* (DSM-IV) in 1974, following decriminalization campaigning in the 1960s and the gay rights movement in the 1970s. There is no evidence that homosexuality either predisposes to or protects against psychosexual distress, although its presentation and assessment can be complicated by fear of prejudice. There is some evidence that homosexuality is associated with higher rates of mental illness, suicidality and psychosocial stressors, but as these data are cross-sectional no conclusions as to direction of causality can be drawn.[37]

Common psychosexual problems

A psychosexual problem by definition involves a level of distress to the individual or within his or her relationship, since there is and can be no legitimate scientific consensus about the 'normal' or 'correct' nature and frequency of sexual activity between consenting adults. Needs, desires and expectations vary widely. Even an objectively discernible biological problem such as erectile dysfunction or vaginismus becomes a psychosexual problem only when it is causing actual unhappiness. Hence the most useful focus in psychosexual work is a pragmatic one, based on what works and what does not, and what is satisfactory and what is distressing, for the individual or couple concerned.

The prevalence of sexual dysfunction is high – as high as 31 per cent according to population-based data from the USA.[38] Against a background of high prevalence and a lack of outcome data on the majority of sexual dysfunction, an evidence-based expert review of the psychological and interpersonal dimensions of sexual function came to the following general conclusions:[25]

- A variety of biopsychosocial factors may play a role in the development of sexual dysfunctions, including patient variables such as performance anxiety or depression; partner variables such as poor mental or physical health or disinterest; interpersonal non-sexual variables such as the quality of the relationship overall; interpersonal sexual variables such as the interval of abstinence, and specific sexual 'scripts' or presuppositions; and contextual variables such as current life stresses, for example involving money or children.
- Despite this recognition, there are few well-designed randomized trials on integrated approaches to the treatment of sexual dysfunctions. The greatest good-quality evidence exists in relation to erectile dysfunction. There is little good-quality research conducted on sexual dysfunction in women.

Because sexual pathology is seldom purely biological, a preformed disorder-based focus is seldom helpful in clinical practice, whatever the presenting complaint. One person's anorgasmia or erectile dysfunction will have a very different biopsychosocial signature from the next person's, and hence the most useful stance is one of 'interested ignorance'. In fact, a central element of psychosexual work is helping the patient to move beyond the collusive reductionism whereby sexual symptoms are assumed to arise from a physical disease that the doctor can 'fix', and towards a position where the patient can understand and begin to modify his or her own problem. However, symptom-based classifications are traditional, have wide currency especially in a research context, and are therefore useful to be aware of.

Sexual difficulties have traditionally been divided into disorders of sexual function, disorders of sexual preference and paraphilias, and disorders of gender identity, each appearing in a different section of the tenth revision of the World Health Organization's *International Classification of Diseases* (ICD-10).[33] Functional sexual disorders currently appear in ICD-10 category F5, 'behavioural difficulties and physical disorders and factors', while disorders of sexual identity and preference belong to Chapter 6, 'personality and behavioural disorders'. The following list of common sexual disorders is not exhaustive but reflects those seen most commonly in the psychosexual medical clinic: for men, erectile dysfunction, ejaculatory problems and loss of libido; and for women, loss of libido and sexual aversion, pain during sex, and anorgasmia. Painful sex occurs rarely in men, usually in the forms of ejaculatory pain or anal pain experienced during anal-receptive gay sex, known as anodyspareunia.

Common disorders of sexual function

Erectile dysfunction

Erectile dysfunction is the persistent inability to attain and maintain an erection sufficient to permit satisfactory sexual intercourse. Its aetiology can be biological or psychological but is usually mixed. Its worldwide prevalence is high, with the Massachusetts Male Aging Study quoting a combined prevalence of 52 per cent (17.2%, 25.2% and 9.6%, respectively, for mild, moderate and complete erectile dysfunction),[39] while a more recent Cologne-based study quotes an overall prevalence of 19.2 per cent, rising to 53.4 per cent in older men.[40] It can be acquired or lifelong.

Although benign in a narrow, biological sense, erectile dysfunction is often malign in its effects on quality of life, as well as increasingly recognized as a possible early warning sign of vascular disease, with which it shares common risk factors such as lack of exercise, smoking, obesity, hypercholesterolaemia and the metabolic syndrome.[41] Of all psychosexual disorders, erectile dysfunction is the most intensively researched, and it is the only psychosexual disorder for which effective pharmacological therapy is available.

Erection is a neurovascular function under hormonal control and is susceptible to neurological, vascular, endocrine and psychological interruption (Figure 45.4).[41] Part of the physiological process of erection involves the release of nitric oxide (NO) in vasculature of the corpus cavernosum as a result of sexual stimulation. NO activates the enzyme guanylate cyclase, which results in increased levels of cyclic guanosine monophosphate (cGMP), leading to smooth-muscle relaxation in blood vessels supplying the corpus cavernosum, and resulting in increased blood flow and an erection. Phosphodiesterase type 5 (PDE5) inhibitors inhibit the degradation of cGMP by PDE5, increasing blood flow to the penis during sexual stimulation. This mode of action means that PDE5 inhibitors are ineffective without sexual stimulation.

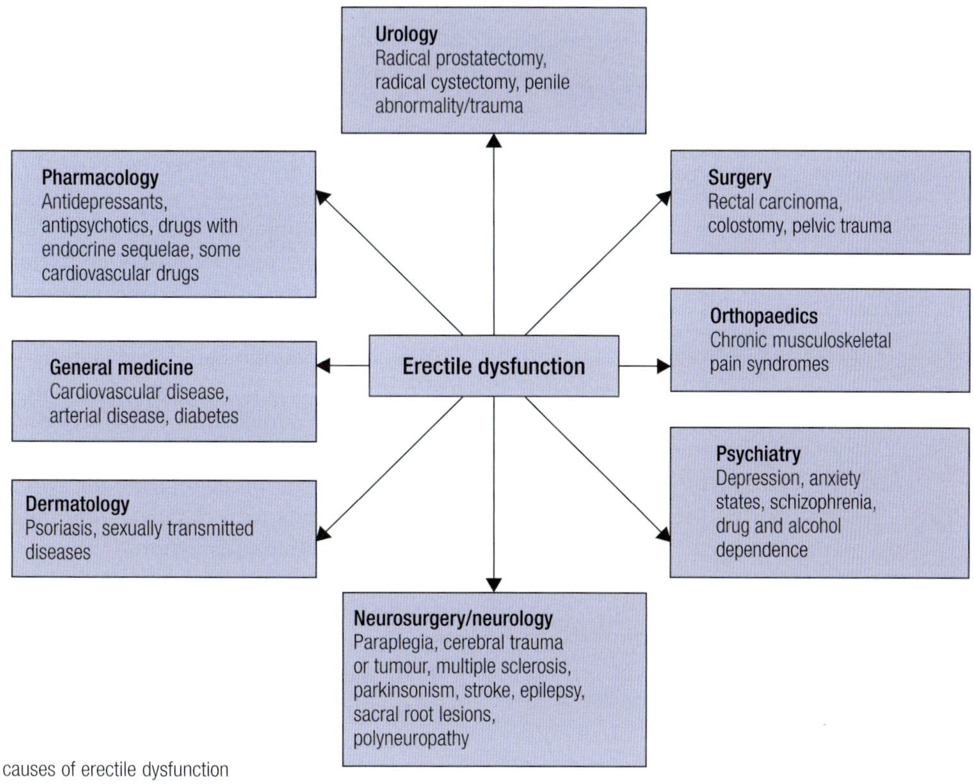

Figure 45.4 Organic causes of erectile dysfunction

Both the urological and the psychosexual communities agree on the biopsychosocial nature of most erectile dysfunction and the need for a joint psychological, biological and interpersonal approach to management.[41] This should include addressing modifiable lifestyle factors, optimizing the treatment of any underlying medical or psychological illnesses diseases such as diabetes, obesity or depression, and considering the use of PDE5 inhibitors for symptom relief and psychosexual therapy to address underlying psychological causes.[39]

Pharmacological treatment should not be used without proper investigation and, where possible, treatment of underlying psychological or neurovascular causes, but it can play a helpful role in both short- and longer-term treatment. The three available PDE5 inhibitors work by increasing blood flow to the penis and promoting smooth muscle relaxation (Figure 45.5). The biological efficacy of the PDE5 inhibitors is extremely good, with efficacies of 50–90 per cent measured on validated objective scales such as the International Index of Erectile Function (IIEF). Despite this, 50 per cent of men fail to continue treatment, in part due to failure to address relevant psychological and interpersonal issues.[40]

In general, men with both acquired and lifelong erectile dysfunction benefit from psychosexual interventions, but with greater benefit on average for those who have

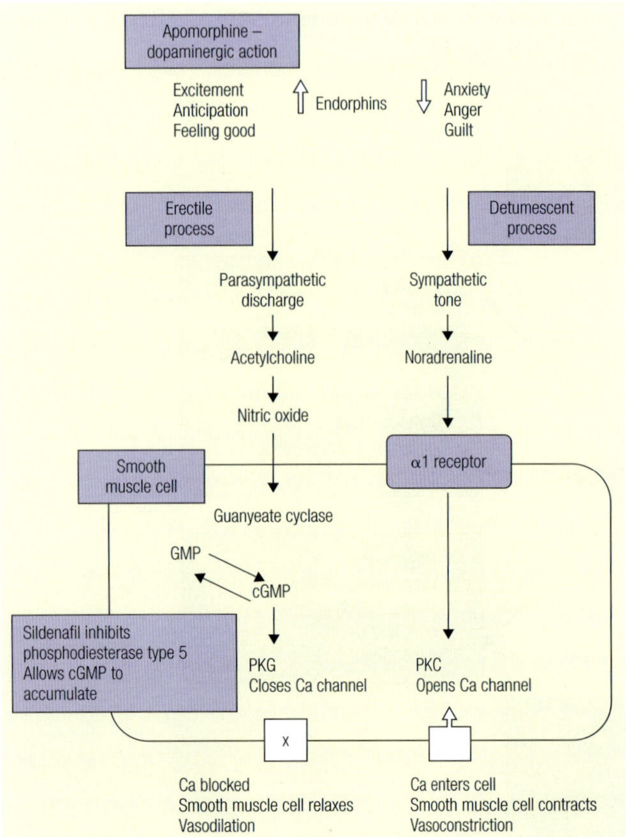

Figure 45.5 Pathophysiology of erectile dysfunction

acquired erectile dysfunction. Masters and Johnson quote significant improvement in around three-quarters of men with acquired dysfunction and around half of men with lifelong erectile dysfunction,[10] with these gains sustained in 2- to 5-year follow-up.[41]

Intracavernosal (injected) or urethral alprostadil is an effective second-line treatment where PDE5 inhibitors are contraindicated or ineffective, but it can be associated with penile pain and, occasionally, prolonged erection.[41] Numerous other prescribed and non-prescribed treatments have been used, but with weak evidence of efficacy, including the α2-adrenergic antagonist yohimbine, a centrally acting aphrodisiac used for more than a century, specific serotonin reuptake inhibitors (trazodone) and red-Korea ginseng.[41] Vascular reconstructive surgery has been shown to have poor long-term outcomes as a treatment for erectile dysfunction of vascular origin.[41]

The role of erectile dysfunction as a possible early warning sign of cardiovascular disease is increasingly clear. With a high prevalence of cardiovascular co-morbidity among men seeking treatment for erectile dysfunction, the opportunity for cardiovascular secondary prevention should not be missed, and caution should be observed in treating those at highest cardiac risk, such as men with recent myocardial infarction or unstable angina, because of the potential risks of sexual activity on the one hand and the effects of PDE5 inhibitors on cardiac smooth muscle on the other hand.[41]

Ejaculatory problems

Ejaculatory problems, of which premature ejaculation is by far the most common, are predominantly psychogenic, with only a minority caused by organic disease. Premature ejaculation, or ejaculation that occurs immediately after or even before penetration, is one of the most common forms of male sexual dysfunction, affecting 20–25 per cent of surveyed men in industrialized countries,[42,43] although prevalence data are fraught with methodological difficulties related to the subjective nature of the definition of 'prematurity'.[44] Masters and Johnson's definition was ejaculation that occurred too soon for the partner to reach orgasm, while other definitions have been based on a given length of time in the vagina before ejaculation. For practical, clinical purposes, it is the relationship between speed of ejaculation and the satisfaction of both partners that is deemed important. Although ejaculation is often thought of as the visible manifestation of orgasm, the two are neurologically distinct, and men who ejaculate very rapidly often describe a lack of orgasmic satisfaction.

The problem of premature ejaculation can be compounded by the partner's frustration and sometimes anger, with secret resentment in both partners.

Premature ejaculation can be a transient problem in adolescence or an occasional event throughout a man's sexual life course, but for many men who present to psychosexual clinics it is a primary and persistent problem, experienced continuously since the onset of sexual activity. The causes are individual, and treatment involves their careful exploration, which may include sexual shame acquired in childhood or early sexual relationships, current relationship discord, life stresses, more generalized anxiety, physical or mental illness in the patient or his partner, or unconscious hostility towards the opposite sex.

A number of behavioural techniques help some men to delay orgasm, including the 'squeeze' technique, where firm squeezing of the glans penis can delay orgasm, the 'stop–start' technique used to introduce space into the process of arousal, and local anaesthetic gels and creams.[21]

Delayed ejaculation can be partial or, rarely, complete and associated with anorgasmia. Although it is natural for sexual arousability in men to decline with increasing age, with more stimulation required over a longer period of time, and a decreased volume and forcefulness of ejaculate, and it is unhelpful to 'pathologize' this normal trend, a small minority of men have difficulty in ejaculating at all. There is no shorthand checklist of psychosexual causes, men who struggle to ejaculate may also seem highly controlled and lacking in spontaneity in the consultation, and these clues can often point towards difficulty in letting go of other emotions, or having access to their own liveliness in the presence of an intimate partner. They often come from families where the showing of emotion of any sort was not encouraged. Rarely, an inability to ejaculate is accompanied by pain, which is often investigated in a urology or genitourinary medicine clinic to exclude prostatic or seminal vesicle pathology. Even here, the pain often proves to be related to an emotional pain.

Vaginismus

Vaginismus describes an involuntary spasm of the muscles surrounding the outer third of the vagina that occurs in response to any attempt to penetrate. When severe, it can also involve the thigh adductors, preventing anyone from approaching the external genitalia. The woman may be seen retreating up the examination couch, clamping her knees together, or she may perch nervously on the edge of the couch, unwilling to adopt a reclining position to allow examination. A woman may or may not describe pain in association with penetration, but often an overriding terror of being touched is sufficiently powerful to preclude any meaningful examination or penetration. She may be well aware that her own muscular contraction is 'causing the problem' but nevertheless is unable to prevent this by means of any conscious effort. Her body and her mind are at odds in ways that defeat her, her partner and often her doctors.

Vaginismus is not a disease but a symptom, with a variety of possible physical or, more commonly, psychological causes. These are variable, individual and cannot be summarized in a simple checklist. Sometimes a woman will report an inability to use tampons, indicating an absolute aversion to penetration, whereas sometimes the problem occurs only during sex, suggesting that it is penetration outside of her own control that is the problem. A woman may present with vaginismus directly or, often, in a hidden form referred to by psychosexual doctors as a 'calling card', such as recurrent thrush, inability to have a smear test taken, or non-consummation discovered as part of infertility treatment. It is a symptom often laden with fear or shame, or both. It is not uncommon for a woman to speak of feeling guilty towards her partner, and trapped between the terror of penetration and the terror of losing him. High anxiety and a sense of 'block' are often palpable in the consulting room.

A woman's resistance to penetration may express itself in the doctor–patient relationship not only literally, in an inability to allow physical examination, but also metaphorically, in terms of an emotional recoiling or 'shutting down' in response to 'penetrative' questioning. The gentle analysis of these symbolic behaviours in the consulting room often leads to disclosure of just what or who it is that needs to be kept out, or would once have needed to be kept out but could not be. There may turn out to be connections with current feelings such as anger against the current partner, or past-traumatic experience, such as sexual abuse in childhood; but it is essential to make no assumptions and instead to stick rigorously to the narrative and behavioural evidence presented and observed in the room.

The management of vaginismus usually involves a kind of gentle persistence, in which the doctor neither colludes with the 'impossibility' of getting to the heart of things nor attempts to railroad a path through sensitive territory in pursuit of a therapeutic goal. During the course of this, the doctor may experience therapeutic frustration that mirrors the partner's sexual frustration, and perhaps the patient's frustration with herself, and may feel inclined either to bully or to give up. The doctor's capacity to observe his or her own feelings and sometimes to use this observation to make connections with the patient's or the partner's experience is an essential part of maintaining the therapeutic connection and staying on course with the diagnostic work. Discovering the mind–body connection, where possible, often affords considerable emotional relief to a woman who has seen her behaviour as 'senseless' and can allow her to take over from the doctor and attitude of gentle persistence with herself, to own her own problem, and to find her own way to symptom resolution.

Behavioural methods such as inviting a woman to attempt putting a finger or fingers in her own vagina, either alone or during the examination, can be a helpful addition or alternative to psychodynamic work, by creating a sense of possibility and 'ownership'. Similarly, graded dilators of increasing sizes can sometimes offer an opportunity to experiment with the possibility of penetration away from the complexity of sexual relating. A 2001 Cochrane review of vaginismus found only three studies, none placebo-controlled, and concluded that evidence from uncontrolled studies suggests that sex therapy may be helpful.[21,45]

Dyspareunia

Dyspareunia, or painful sex, is reported almost exclusively by women. It may be deep, felt high in the vagina or in the abdomen on deep penetration, or superficial, felt at the introitus at the onset of penetration. It can be momentary or last for hours or even days. Its primary causes can be physical or psychosomatic, but even in the minority of women in whom a biological diagnosis with a straightforward treatment is found it usually has both somatic and emotional consequences. It may present directly or more indirectly as generalized pelvic pain, dysmenorrhoea, inability to have a smear test, or recurrent complaints of vaginal discharge or vulval soreness.

Before psychosexual referral, these women will often have had multiple investigations in a gynaecology or sexual health setting. Because pain is a symptom that strongly invites a medical explanation, it can be challenging to make a psychosomatic diagnosis. The individual doctor may feel considerable pressure to find a physical diagnosis and treatment and, as a profession, we conceal our collective medical impotence in the coining of so-called functional disorders, such as vulvovestibulitis, with multiple aetiological theories, and very limited evidence for the efficacy of biological treatments such as local anaesthetic creams.[21] Although it is important, faced with pain, to remain a physical doctor and consider possible physical pathology such as ovarian or vulval disease or endometriosis, it is also important not to hide behind biological investigations and hypotheses and miss relevant emotional 'sore spots'.

Psychosomatic dyspareunia does not necessarily need long-term intervention, but it does need a careful physical and emotional history-taking, clarifying the nature and location of the pain, any signs of possible organic pathology, and the meaning and consequences of this pain for this woman. It is important to acknowledge that the pain is real and physical, whatever its aetiology, but also to suggest that feelings might be involved and to ask after these explicitly rather than to make assumptions.

Psychosomatic pain is always individual in origin. It might be a way of holding her partner at bay or expressing anger; it might express grief, loss or fear. Timing of onset can be a clue and perhaps point to pain, anger, grief or fear connected with a life event such as the traumatic delivery of a baby, an abortion, a death, an affair, sterilization, infertility or hysterectomy. In short, pelvic or vaginal pain can symbolize hurt sensitivity arising elsewhere in a woman's past or present life. At best, brief psychodynamic intervention can spare her years of fruitless and ineffective treatments.

Even dyspareunia of purely physical origin such as infection or cancer may become complicated by emotional distress, such as self-disgust, anger or terror.

Anorgasmia

Anorgasmia presents almost exclusively in women, can be lifelong or acquired, and has no single aetiology.[46] Physical causes, which include hypopituitarism, late-stage diabetic neuropathy and extensive pelvic surgery for cancer, are relatively rare, although anorgasmia can arise more commonly as a side effect of antidepressant treatment with specific serotonin reuptake inhibitors or some antipsychotic medications. Even in these cases, biological and psychological causes are often both present, and there are usually psychological sequelae.

Acquired or secondary anorgasmia may sometime relate to situational stresses such as the presence of children or parents, or relationship difficulties such as loss of trust following an affair. These often respond well to relationship counselling. Lifelong anorgasmia is likely to have a more deep-seated cause and may benefit from a psychosomatic approach, aimed at making connections with wider personality issues or experiences in early life, such as sexual abuse.

Research into adults with sexual difficulties who had been sexually abused as children showed that almost a quarter complained of inability to achieve orgasm.[47] Sexually abused individuals often develop strategies for suppressing sexual feelings that have become fused with painful feelings. The avoidance of the painful memories blocks access to sexual arousal and orgasm. Psychosexual counselling can provide a safe space in which to confront painful feelings with which sexual arousal have become linked, allowing the patient to reclaim her sexuality for her own pleasure.

However, questionnaire surveys also show that, in general, women with orgasmic difficulties tend to have more sex-related guilt,[48,49] to be less sexually assertive,[50,51] to endorse more negative attitudes around sexual activity and masturbation,[48,52] and to be less aware of physiological signs of arousal and orgasm and fear loss of control.[53] Some of these factors are suited to cognitive-behavioural intervention, such as directed masturbation for lifelong anorgasmia,[53] couples therapy for acquired anorgasmia,[54–56] or the coital alignment technique used to maximize penile/clitoral contact during male-on-top sex. Research in this area is impeded by misclassification of anorgasmia as arousal disorder.[57]

Loss of libido

Loss of libido, also known as hypoactive sexual disorder, is perhaps the most maddeningly, medically defeating of all sexual 'symptoms'. With barely an agreed working definition for libido, whether we think of it narrowly as sexual desire or more widely as life-force or creative energy, there is little hope of neatly categorized aetiologies or symptom-specific treatments for its absence. Unlike flaccid penises and tense vaginas, the libido has no bodily locus on which doctor and patient can focus medical attention. True, there are a number of potential physical causes for loss of libido, including drugs, depression and endocrine dysfunction (Table 45.2), but sometimes even treating these causes, such as switching or reducing antidepressant medication, or

Table 45.2 Endocrine causes of loss of libido

Organ			Activity	Effect on libido	
				Men	**Women**
Adrenal gland			Increased (Cushing's disease)	Can be decreased	Variable
			Decreased (Addison's disease)	Can be impaired	Can be impaired
Pituitary gland			Increased, e.g. pituitary adenoma producing hyperprolactinaemia	Can lead to erectile dysfunction and consequent loss of libido	
			Decreased	Can be impaired	Can be decreased
Thyroid			Increased	Variable	Variable
			Decreased	Usually decreased through general debility and through testosterone synthesis and androgen and oestrogen metabolism	
Pancreas			Decreased (diabetes mellitus)	Can lead to erectile dysfunction and consequent loss of libido	
Gonads			Decreased		
	Female		Congenital, e.g. Turner's syndrome		Can be decreased
			Acquired, e.g. post-bilateral oophorectomy, chemotherapy, irradiation		Can be decreased
			Postmenopause		Variable
	Male	Primary hypogonadism	Congenital, e.g. Klinefelter's syndrome	Can be decreased	
			Acquired, e.g. post-orchidectomy, infection (e.g. mumps), trauma, irradiation, chemotherapy	Can be decreased	
		Secondary hypogonadism*	Hypergonadotrophic hypergonadism (*Drug and Therapeutics Bulletin* 1999)	Can be altered	
			Congenital, e.g. Kallman's syndrome	Can be decreased	
			Acquired, e.g. pituitary tumour**	Can be decreased	
			Systemic illness, e.g. end-stage renal and respiratory disease, obesity, poor nutrition, long-term overexercise, supraphysiological doses of steroids, marijuana, ketoconazole, spironolactone		

*The symptoms of altered sex drive, decreased secondary hair and reduced shaving without changes to the voice, body proportions or penis size would alert the doctor to the possibility of secondary hypogonadism. A single measurement of the morning basal total testosterone, luteinizing hormone, follicle-stimulating hormone (FSH) and prolactin could confirm it.

**Headaches, impaired visual fields, polydipsia and an elevated serum prolactin would indicate a hypothalamic or pituitary tumour.

offering testosterone where levels are low, can leave the loss of libido unchanged.

Loss of libido has a high prevalence of around 30–35 per cent.[58] Sometimes, for example where sexual boredom or loss of creativity in lovemaking has become a problem, behavioural approaches can be helpful, such as setting aside child-free time or using sensate focus exercises in which a focus on sexual pleasure without intercourse or orgasm is designed to reawaken a sense of intimacy and pleasure for its own sake. However, evidence for these interventions is mixed and is often based on uncontrolled studies, and they carry a high relapse rate.[56–58]

Sometimes, intractable loss of libido, ossified into a kind of institutionalized 'not caring' about sex, has become the ultimate defence against intimacy in the sexual relationship, and often in the doctor–patient relationship too. Small wonder that psychosexual doctors report high non-attendance rates even in those referred,[15] and that those patients who do attend sometimes claim to be there for their 'partner's sake': loss of libido can be 'not caring', elaborated into a whole way of life, with 'heartsink' potential for both partner and doctor. On the positive side, this symptom leaves us no medical place to hide from the difficult emotional questions. Faced with a patient who is apparently 'not bothered' but nevertheless present asking for help in the consulting room, it is often possible to use our perplexity at the mismatch to discover what has made the patient's heart sink.

There are currently no evidence-based biological treatments for loss of libido in women. Although there is increasing interest from pharmaceutical companies and some clinicians in the use of testosterone, evidence to date for its efficacy, even in women with low testosterone levels, is weak.[25]

Rare disorders of sexual function

Disorders of sexual preference

There are no reliable prevalence data on disorders of sexual preference. Clear definition is in any case difficult, because the broad spectrum of 'normal' human sexual behaviours and those considered or experienced as problematic or distressing are on a continuous spectrum. There is therefore both a degree of arbitrariness and a widespread consensus about the following categories and definitions.

ICD-10 defines disorders of sexual preference, or paraphilias, as follows:

- The individual experiences recurrent intense sexual urges and fantasies involving unusual objects or activities.
- The individual either acts on the urges or is markedly distressed by them.
- The preference has been present for at least 6 months.[33]

Fetishism

Fetishism is on a spectrum ranging from common and unintrusive sexual preferences such as the desire to see a partner wear a particular item of clothing, through more minority sexual preoccupations such as with leather, rubber or metal, to more extreme fetishes that cause distress to the individual or their partner, either because they involve repulsive objects such as faeces or because they involve illegal activity such as stealing objects.

Fetishes may arise in infancy or around puberty, often in an accidental, circumstantial way, and reinforced by masturbatory conditioning. Sociobiologists emphasize the analogy with 'imprinting', such as that seen in animals, whereas psychoanalysts emphasize symbolic meaning of the fetish objects.

Culturally acceptable and essentially harmless fetishes call for reassurance rather than treatment and help in integrating the particular preference into the relationship with a partner. Fetishes serious enough to disrupt wellbeing, relationships and normal functioning may benefit from help from a specially trained psychologist, which often involves masturbatory reconditioning and response prevention. Inhumane treatments used in the past, such as presenting the stimulus along with electric shocks or emetic drugs, are no longer acceptable.

Paedophilia

DSM-IV defines paedophilia as

> a period of at least 6 months of recurrent, intense sexually arousing fantasies, sexual urges or behaviours involving sexual behaviour with a prepubescent child or children (generally aged 13 or younger).

The formal definition also specifies that this must cause clinically significant distress or functional impairment in work or social life. However, for practical purposes, anyone with such urges may be considered a paedophile, since sexual contact with children is illegal and therefore this form of sexual preference is by definition problematic. The definition also specifies that the individual must be over 16 years and 5 years older than the child or children, a measure intended to exclude innocent exploratory behaviour common in prepubescent children, but that does not integrate research showing that sexual abusers of children can often begin early in life.

Aetiological factors include a history of sexual abuse, dysfunctional relationships in the family or origin, neglect, and emotional and physical abuse. Triggering factors often include alcohol use and life stress.

Therapists working with paedophiles report 'cognitive distortions' used to justify the behaviour, such as the belief that the activity has not harmed the child, that it was mutually enjoyable, that the child invited sexual contact by seductive behaviour, and that the child was capable of giving consent. There may be a false claim that there was an isolated incident in situations where a clear pattern of 'grooming' can be identified.

Sadomasochism

Sadomasochism describes sexual arousal or activity where

the infliction of pain or humiliation or bondage plays a key role. Sadism is arousal in association with inflicting pain, while masochism is arousal in association with having pain or humiliation inflicted. Affected individuals often feel arousal in both situations.

Voyeurism and exhibitionism

Voyeurism describes a consistent sexual drive towards watching others engaged in sexual activity, or in other intimate activities, such as undressing. Exhibitionism describes the continual or repetitive desire to expose one's genitals to strangers, usually of the opposite sex, without seeking or desiring any further contact.

Other disorders of sexual preference

Other disorders of sexual preference include frotteurism (pressing or rubbing oneself against the bodies of strangers in pursuit of sexual arousal), bestiality (sexual activity with animals) and erotophonia (sexualized telephone calls to strangers).

Disorders of gender identity

DSM-IV describes gender identity disorder as:

- a strong and persistent cross gender identification (not merely a desire for any perceived cultural advantages of being the other sex);
- persistent discomfort with his or her sex, or a sense of inappropriateness in the gender role of that sex;
- the disturbance is not concurrent with a physical intersex condition;
- the disturbance causes clinically significant distress or impairment in social, occupational or other important areas of functioning.[60]

This is almost interchangeable with the ICD-10 classification (Box 45.7). It is a rare disorder with a prevalence of 1 in 40 000–50 000. It is three to six times more common in men wishing to be women than in women wishing to men.[61] Its aetiology remains the subject of scientific speculation, but it has a high psychiatric morbidity and mortality, both treated and untreated, with 60 per cent of untreated individuals giving a history of intermittent depression and up to 20 per cent suicide attempts.[61] Its management should be undertaken by specialists in this area, but it is important that other clinicians are able to encounter it with awareness and sensitivity. It is helpful to bear in mind the following:

- True gender identity disorder is by definition persistent and associated with profound distress and high psychiatric morbidity and mortality. It is important not to diminish or dismiss it.
- It must be distinguished from homosexuality, transsexualism and transient psychosis, in connection with personality disorder, and simple non-conformism with gender expectations without a disorder of gender identity.
- It is often associated with a strong wish with for hormonal or surgical gender reassignment treatment, the achievement of which is often associated with a strong self-reported improvement in wellbeing. However, reliable long-term outcome data on such procedures are lacking.
- Treatment involves careful assessment by a psychiatrist with special expertise and involves specialist psychotherapy, a 1-year observation period to establish the constancy of the transgender wish, a trial period of a

Box 45.7 *International Classification of Diseases,* 10th revision (ICD-10) and *Diagnostic and Statistical Manual of Mental Disorders,* 4th edn (DSM-IV) disorders of sexual preference/paraphilias

ICD-10 DISORDERS OF SEXUAL PREFERENCE

- F65.0 Fetishism
- F65.1 Fetishistic transvestism
- F65.2 Exhibitionism
- F65.3 Voyeurism
- F65.4 Paedophilia
- F65.5 Sadomasochism
- F65.6–8 Multiple/other/unspecified disorders

DSM-IV PARAPHILIAS

- 302.4 Exhibitionism
- 302.81 Fetishism
- 302.89 Frotteurism
- 302.2 Paedophilia
- 302.83 Sexual masochism
- 302.84 Sexual sadism
- 302.82 Voyeurism
- 302.9 Paraphilia not otherwise specified

year in which the individual lives in the desired gender role and, only if this is successful, hormonal followed by surgical gender reassignment treatment.

- Male-to-female surgery involves penectomy, castration, construction of a neoclitoris and neovagina, and possible breast reconstruction surgery. Female-to-male surgery involves mastectomy, oophorectomy, sometimes hysterectomy, and sometimes phalloscrotoplasty (implantation of testicular and penile prostheses).

Sex and illness

Sexual function can affect and be affected by mental or physical illnesses and their treatments, either in direct physical ways or in psychologically mediated ways. It is important therefore to consider past medical and psychiatric history and drug history in a psychosexual medical consultation, even if these are subsumed in a psychotherapeutic approach to history-taking. Occasionally, optimizing or adjusting the treatment of a coexisting condition such as depression, diabetes or endometriosis will be the primary or sole treatment for sexual dysfunction. More commonly, these factors will form a part of a more complex picture, in which the clinician's role is not so much to identify a single problem to treat as to find the most promising starting point in untangling a knot of problems. It may be a question of deciding whether a woman presenting with dyspareunia following traumatic childbirth has vaginal scarring, psychological scarring amenable to psychosexual treatment, or severe enough psychological disturbance to warrant a diagnosis of post-traumatic stress disorder and/or psychiatric intervention.

A particular example is depression, which is very commonly associated with sexual dysfunction, in ways that can be complex. Depression can cause sexual dysfunction, such as loss of libido; but chronic sexual dysfunction and relationship strain can also cause or worsen depression. In addition, antidepressant and antipsychotic medications can cause sexual dysfunction such as anorgasmia secondary to treatment with specific serotonin reuptake inhibitors, which may in turn worsen depression or undermine adherence to treatment. A holistic view of the patient's global situation is essential for all concerned.

Finally, although our concern as doctors is traditionally not so much with the meaning as with the elimination of disease, we cannot escape the meanings diseases have for our patients, their families, their sexual partners, ourselves as their doctors, and society at large. Experiences such as cancer, AIDS, sexually transmitted infection, menopause, hysterectomy and sterilization can impact on lives, biologically and emotionally, non-sexually and sexually.

SUMMARY

Recognition that sexual problems usually include biological, psychological and social aspects and are best addressed in a holistic or a multidisciplinary way is now widespread. Appropriate treatment may be medical and/or psychological and may include urological, gynaecological or sexual health assessment, the treatment of any coexisting physical or mental illness such as diabetes, cancer or depression, behaviourally based sexual therapies, wider psychotherapy or counselling, and psychosexual medicine, which is a British manifestation of a psychosomatic approach. The right route of referral is not always immediately obvious because it is not dictated solely by the presenting complaint; rather, it may suggest itself from more detailed sexual and psychological history-taking. Where clear relationship difficulties or unhelpful attitudes or behaviours are revealed as a likely primary problem, behaviourally based sex therapies are often helpful. Where sexual problems are part of wider, long-term psychological distress, psychotherapy, if available in a National Health Service (NHS) setting or affordable privately, may be the most useful. Where both medical and psychological assessment are needed in parallel, or where the medical and the psychological aspects cannot readily be distinguished, psychosexual medicine, with its integrative approach, can play an important part.

KEY POINTS

- Sexuality involves both mind and body, and understanding it requires an integrated approach, both clinically and academically.
- Most sexual problems have either emotional or mixed emotional and physical causes; all have both physical and emotional consequences.
- Rarely, a sexual problem is attributable solely to organic pathology. More commonly, it may be an early warning sign of physical disease (erectile dysfunction and cardiovascular disease). Although psychosexual medical work is often psychologically focused, physical pathology must always be considered.
- Physical and psychiatric co-morbidity are common, and sexual dysfunction and other illnesses and their treatments can exacerbate each other. Maintaining a holistic overview is important.
- There is a dearth of high-quality outcomes research on sexual dysfunction, particularly in women.
- Psychosexual medicine offers a psychosomatic approach to the diagnosis and treatment of sexual dysfunction and draws on both medicine and analytical psychotherapy. It addresses the mind–body connection within an individual, predominantly, although couples work can be offered. It is particularly helpful where there is a strong physical or potentially medical element to the presenting problem. Training and registration are overseen by the Institute of Psychosexual Medicine.

- Other, non-medical cognitive-behavioural sexual therapies also have a strong tradition and are particularly useful in addressing unhelpful behaviours or beliefs and relationship difficulties. Work is normally with both partners in a couple, and is overseen by the British Society for Sexual and Relationship Therapy.
- A small number of rare sexual disorders, such as gender dysphoria and paedophilia, require specialist referral.

Box 45.8 Training in psychosexual medicine

Training with the Institute of Psychosexual Medicine is open to all practising doctors who see patients with sexual difficulties. It is experientially based, involving the regular discussion of cases brought by all participants to seminar groups. A diploma may be achieved after a minimum of 2 years of training and an examination, and full membership following a minimum of 4 years' training and a further examination. For further information, see **www.ipm.org.uk**.

Box 45.9 UK resources and organizations

- *Institute of Psychosexual Medicine (IPM) (www.ipm.org.uk, tel. 020 7580 0631):* medical, psychodynamic, mind–body sexual therapy, often with individuals.
- *British Association for Sexual and Relationship Therapy (BASRT) (***www.basrt.org.uk***, tel. 020 8543 2707):* non-medical cognitive-behavioural sexual couple and relationship therapy.
- *Relate (***www.relate.org.uk***, tel. 0300 100 1234):* non-medical cognitive-behavioural therapy, principally but not exclusively couples work.
- *Tavistock Centre for Couple Relationships (***www.tccr.org.uk***, tel. 020 8938 2431):* non-medical psychodynamic sexual relationship counselling.
- *Sexual Dysfunction Association (***www.sda.uk.net***, tel. 0870 7743571):* formerly the Impotence Association, a charitable organization helping people with sexual problems and their partners and raising awareness of the extent to which sexual conditions affect the general population. Originally, the charity focused on helping individuals with erectile dysfunction (impotence), but now it covers all forms of male and female sexual problems.
- *Balint Society (***www.balint.co.uk***):* helps general practitioners towards a better understanding of the emotional content of the doctor–patient relationship.
- *Association of Psychosexual Nursing (www.wanstead.park.btinternet.co.uk):* trains nurses in understanding the emotional content of the clinician–patient relationship.

REFERENCES

1. Descartes R (2008) *Meditations on First Philosophy*. Oxford: Oxford University Press.
2. Von Krafft Ebing R (1905) *Textbook of Insanity*. Philadelphia, PA: FA Davies.
3. Von Krafft Ebing R (1902) *Psychopathia Sexualis*. New York: Physicians' and Surgeons' Books.
4. Havelock Ellis H (1897–1928) *Studies in the Psychology of Sex, Sexual Inversion*. Philadelphia, PA: FA Davies.
5. Freud S (1991) *3 Essays on the Theory of Sexuality and Other Works*. Harmondsworth: Penguin.
6. Reich W (1983) *The Function of the Orgasm*. London: Souvenir Press.
7. Kinsey A, Pomeroy W, Martin C (1948) *Sexual Behaviour in the Human Male*. Philadelphia, PA: W.B. Saunders.
8. Kinsey A, Pomeroy W, Martin C, Gebhard P (1953) *Sexual Behaviour in the Human Female*. Philadelphia, PA: W.B. Saunders.
9 Masters W, Johnson V (1966) *Human Sexual Response*. Toronto: Bantam Books.
10. Masters W, Johnson V (1970) *Human Sexual Inadequacy*. Toronto: Bantam Books.
11. Masters W, Johnson V (1974) *The Pleasure Bond*. Toronto: Bantam Books.
12. Masters W, Johnson V (1979) *Homosexuality in Perspective*. Toronto: Bantam Books.
13. Hite S (1976) *The Hite Report on Female Sexuality*. London: Talmy Franklin.
14. Hite S (1981) *The Hite Report on Men and Male Sexuality*. London: Talmy Franklin.
15. Phillips K (1996) *The Broken Mirror: Understanding and Treating Body Dysmorphic Disorder*. New York: Oxford University Press.
16. Weijmar Schultz W, Van Andel P, Sabelis I, *et al.* (1999) Magnetic resonance imaging of male and female genitals during coitus and female sexual arousal. *British Medical Journal* 319: 1596–600.
17. Abma JC, Martinez GM, Mosher WD, Dawson BS (2004) Teenagers in the United States: sexual activity, contraceptive use, and childbearing, 2002. *Vital and Health Statistics 23* (24): 1–48.
18. Guttmacher Institute (2008) U.S. Teenage Pregnancy Statistics: National and State Trends and Trends by Race and Ethnicity. www.guttmacher.org/pubs/2006/09/11/USTPstats.pdf.
19. Guttmacher Institute (2008) Estimates of U.S. Abortion

Incidence, 2001–2003. www.guttmacher.org/pubs/2006/08/03/ab_incidence.pdf.

20. Martin JA, Hamilton BE, Sutton PD, *et al.* (2003) Births: final data for 2002. National Vital Statistics Reports **52**: 1–113.
21. Skrine R, Montford H (eds) (2001) *Psychosexual Medicine: An Introduction.* London: Arnold.
22. Beckman N, Waern M, Gustafson D, *et al.* (2008) Secular trends in self reported sexual activity and satisfaction in Swedish 70 year olds: cross sectional survey of four populations, 1971–2001. *British Medical Journal* **337**: a279.
23. Greenhalgh T, Hurwitz B (1998) *Narrative Based Medicine: Dialogue and Discourse in Clinical Practice.* London: British Medical Association.
24. Derogatis LR, Burnett AL (2007) Key methodologic issues in sexual medicine research. *Journal of Sexual Medicine* **4**: 527–37.
25. Althof, S, Leiblum, S, Chevret-Measson M, *et al.* (2005) Psychological and interpersonal dimensions of sexual function and dysfunction. *Journal of Sexual Medicine* **2**: 793–800.
26. Institute of Psychosexual Medicine (2008) Training. http://ipm.org.uk/doctors/training.
27. Blumenfield M, Strain J (2006) *Psychosomatic Medicine.* Lippincott Williams & Wilkins.
28. British Association for Sexual and Relationship Therapy. About Sexual and Relationship Therapy. www.basrt.org.uk.
29. Goldbeck-Wood S, Fonagy P (2004) The future of psychotherapy in the NHS. *British Medical Journal* **329**: 245–6.
30. Beutler LE, Machado PP, Neufeldt SA (2004) Therapist variables. In AE Bergin, SL Garfield (eds) *Handbook of Psychotherapy and Behavior Change.* New York: John Wiley & Sons.
31. Ferenczi S (1988) *The Clinical Diary.* London: Harvard University Press.
32. Staunton T (ed.) (2002) *Body Psychotherapy.* Hove: Brunner-Routledge.
33. World Health Organization (1992) *International Statistical Classification of Diseases and Related Health Problems.* Geneva: World Health Organization.
34. Winnicott D (1965) *Maturational Processes and the Facilitating Environment.* London: Hogarth Press and the Institute of Psychoanalysis.
35. Malan D (1979) *Individual Psychotherapy and the Science of Psychodynamics.* London: Butterworths.
36. Savin-Williams R, Ream G (2007) Prevalence and stability of sexual orientation components during adolescence and young adulthood. *Archives of Sexual Behavior* **36**: 385–94.
37. Jorm A, Korten A, Rodgers B, *et al.* (2002) Sexual orientation and mental health. *British Journal of Psychiatry* **180**: 423–7.
38. Laumann E, Masi C, Zuckerman E (1997) National Health and Social Life Study. *Journal of the American Medical Association* **278**: 201–3.
39. Feldman H, Goldstein I, Hatzichristou DG, Krane RJ, McKinlay JB (1994) Impotence and its medical and psychosocial correlates: results of the Massachusetts Male Aging Study. *Journal of Urology* **151**: 54–61.
40. Braun M, Wassmer G, Klotz T, *et al.* (2000) Epidemiology of erectile dysfunction: results of the Cologne Male Survey. *International Journal of Impotence Research* **12**: 305–11.
41. European Association of Urology (2001) Guidelines on erectile dysfunction. *Urology* **58**: 262–6.
42. Mohr D, Bentler L (1990) Erectile dysfunction: a review of diagnostic and treatment procedures. *Clinical Psychology Review* **10**: 123–50.
43. Porst H, Montorsi F, Rosen RC, *et al.* (2007) The Premature Ejaculation Prevalence and Attitudes (PEPA) Survey: prevalence, comorbidities and professional help-seeking. *European Urology* **51**: 816–23.
44. Montorsi F (2005) Prevalence of premature ejaculation: a global and regional perspective. *Journal of Sexual Medicine* 2 (suppl. 2): 96–102.
45. McGuire H, Hawton K (2001) Interventions for vaginismus. *Cochrane Database of Systematic Reviews* **2**: CD001760.
46. Heiman JR, Grafton-Becker V (1989) Orgasmic disorders in women. In SR Leiblum, RC Rosen (eds) *Principles and Practice of Sex Therapy: An Update for the 1990s.* New York: Guilford Press.
47. Vanhegan G, Tunnadine P, Kwantes ES (1996) Treatment of psychosexual disorders in previously abused patients. *British Journal of Family Planning* **22**: 191–3.
48. Kelly MP, Strassberg DS, Kircher JR (1990) Attitudinal and experiential correlates of anorgasmia. *Archives of Sexual Behavior* **19**: 165–77.
49. Morokoff P (1985) Effects of sex guilt, repression, sexual 'arousability', and sexual experience on female sexual arousal during erotica and fantasy. *Journal of Personality and Social Psychology* **49**: 177–87.
50. Delehanty R (1982) Changes in assertiveness and changes in orgasmic response occurring with sexual therapy for preorgasmic women. *Journal of Sex and Marital Therapy* **8**: 198–208.
51. Newcomb M (1984) Sexual behavior, responsiveness, and attitudes among women: a test of two theories. *Journal of Sex and Marital Therapy* **10**: 272–86.
52. McCabe MP, Cobain MJ (1998) The impact of individual and relationship factors on sexual dysfunction among males and females. *Journal of Sex and Marital Therapy* **13**:2.
53. Heiman J, Meston C (1997) Empirically validated treatment for sexual dysfunction. *Annual Review of Sex Research* **8**: 148–94.
54. Kilmann P, Milan R, Bolan J, *et al.* (1987) Group treatment of secondary erectile dysfunction. *Journal of Sex and Marital Therapy* **13**: 168–82.

55. McGovern K, Stewart R, LoPiccolo J (1975) Secondary orgasmic dysfunction: I. Analysis and strategies for treatment. *Archives of Sexual Behavior* **4**: 265–75.
56. Kilmann P, Mills K, Caid C, *et al.* (1986) Treatment of secondary orgasmic dysfunction: an outcome study. *Archives of Sexual Behavior* **15**: 211–29.
57. Heiman J (2002) Psychologic treatments for female sexual dysfunction: are they effective and do we need them? *Archives of Sexual Behavior* **31**: 445–50.
58. Leiblum S, Koochaki P, Rodenberg C, Rosen R (2006) Hypoactive sexual desire disorder and distress in Menopausal women: US results from the Womens' International Study of Health and Sexuality (WISHeS). *Menopause* **13**: 46–56.
59. McCabe M (2001) Evaluation of a cognitive behaviour therapy program for people with sexual dysfunction. *Journal of Sex and Marital Therapy* **27**: 259–71.
60. Hawton K (1995) Treatment of sexual dysfunctions by sex therapy and other approaches. *British Journal of Psychiatry* **167**: 307–14.
61. American Psychiatric Association (1994) *Diagnostic and Statistical Manual of Mental Disorders*, 4th edn. Washington, DC: American Psychiatric Association.
62. Wålinder J (1967) *Transsexualism: A Study of Forty-Three Cases*. Gothenburg: Akademieförlaget.

Chapter 46

Gender identity disorders

James Barrett

INTRODUCTION

Throughout this chapter the terms 'male' and 'female' refer to sex assigned at birth.

Disorders of gender identity require a more multidisciplinary input than any other disorder in psychiatry. Endocrinologists, speech and language therapists and surgeons (ENT, plastic, urological) are routinely involved. Further, the field is highly politicized, attracting much public fascination and arousing strong opinions.

Disorders of gender identity have probably always existed, inside and outside Europe.[1,2] The incidence of transsexualism is very roughly one in 60 000 males and one in 100 000 females, and it seems to have remained constant.[3] There is the suggestion that there may be a raised rate in Polynesian people, possibly related to a greater incidence of partial androgen insensitivity syndromes (Dr Herbert Bower, personal communication, 2000).

CLASSIFICATION

Currently, in the International Classification of Diseases, version 10 (ICD-10), disorders of gender identity are classified as disorders of adult personality and behaviour, and comprise the following:

64.0 Transsexualism
F64.1 Dual-role transvestism
F64.2 Gender identity disorder of childhood
F64.8 Other gender identity disorders
F64.9 Gender identity disorder, unspecified.

DIFFERENTIAL DIAGNOSIS

Important differential diagnoses include fetishistic transvestism, dysmorphophobia, autogynaephilia and some of the other disorders of personality or sexual function. Occasionally, psychoses may present in such a way as to resemble a gender identity disorder and, increasingly rarely, male homosexual or lesbian people may present as transsexual.[4,5]

Whether transvestism is contiguous with transsexualism or distinct from it is a debate that has endured over the decades.[6] The current diagnostic position including dual-role transvestism but not fetishistic transvestism as a gender identity disorder reflects this uncertainty.

Transsexualism is described in ICD-10 as a desire to live and be accepted as a member of the opposite sex, usually accompanied by a sense of discomfort with one's anatomical sex. For the diagnosis to be made, transsexual identity should have been present for at least 2 years and must not be a symptom of another mental disorder, such as schizophrenia, or associated with any intersex, genetic or sex chromosome abnormality.

This last stipulation implies that there is never a genetic or hormonal element in transsexualism and that any such abnormality, if present, would always account for the cross-gender identity. Either or both of these implications may be without foundation.

AETIOLOGY

It is not clear what causes disorders of gender identity. Originally, hypotheses about causation addressed psychological factors and came mostly from a psychoanalytical perspective.[7] Over the decades, though, what evidence there is has suggested a multifactorial aetiology, with biological factors rising in importance.

It is known that there is a raised rate of disorders of gender identity in people with Kleinfelter's syndrome.[8] It is also known that males with disorders of gender identity are more likely than chance would allow to be left-handed[8] and to have particular aptitude with computers (Dr Stephen Whittle, personal communication, 2002). Their family trees show a relative lack of maternal uncles, and they are more likely to come from lower down a male birth order. One hypothesis arising from these findings supposes that, in these families, women mount an immune response to a Y chromosome in pregnancy, the titre rising with each successive male pregnancy.[8]

A single, small, postmortem brain study showed a female-sized bed nucleus of the stria terminalis in males with transsexualism. Although interesting, this study had no control group of homosexual males without gender identity disorder, and the finding might have been caused by earlier treatment with hormones.[9]

It should be noted that nearly all these curious findings do nothing to address the genesis of gender identity disorders in females. In their case, there is the clinical suspicion that polycystic ovarian syndrome rates may be raised, but this remains statistically unproven.[9]

There is still no overarching hypothesis drawing these disparate findings together. This might, of course, simply reflect a multifactorial aetiology.

PSYCHOPATHOLOGICAL ASPECTS

There is a public and to some extent a general psychiatric perception that transsexualism is the only or at least the main disorder of gender identity. This is probably illusory,[10] but the illusion persists in part because most dual-role transvestites do not come to the attention of psychiatric services. Certainly, transsexualism is the diagnosis for which most treatment evidence is available. There is little research into dual-role transvestism, nor much into dysmorphophobia or autogynaephilia presenting as or relating to a gender identity disorder,[11–15] even though these are important differential diagnoses and there is the suggestion that non-transsexual disorders of gender identity are more associated with psychopathology.[16] These differential diagnoses may require different management from transsexualism.[17]

Originally, problems with gender identity were thought to represent severe mental illness. Most of the abnormalities detected were character disorders, but a significant proportion of patients were thought to have schizophrenia.[6,18]

Larger, more recent studies show that fewer than 10 per cent have problems associated with mental illness, genital mutilation or suicide attempts.[19] Studies now generally support the view that transsexualism is usually an isolated diagnosis and not part of any general psychopathological disorder.[20] Similar results are found in adolescents, supporting the idea that major psychopathology is not required for the development of transsexualism.[21,22] It seems that the earlier findings might have represented a sampling bias.

On the other hand, though, the inference in the current diagnostic classification that other psychiatric disorders be excluded may mean that the populations actually referred to gender identity clinics have been filtered, so that there is an artificially lower rate of psychopathology in these clinic populations, falsely suggesting a low rate of psychiatric co-morbidity.

Transsexualism has important differential diagnoses, all of which may cause gender dysphoric feelings.

Some homosexual men and lesbians may present with claims of transsexualism[5,23] and have, of course, no psychiatric diagnosis. The most frequent formal differential diagnosis is of transvestism (dual-role or fetishistic), but the others include psychoses and mood disorders.[23] Autogynaephilia may also present. This is the state of being sexually aroused by the idea of having both male and female sexual attributes (usually breasts and a penis). Autogynaephilic males usually seek oestrogen treatment to elicit this effect. Such treatment diminishes the libido that gives rise to the very desire itself, and autogynaephilia may wane over time, only to be replaced by another unusual sexual drive. For these reasons, autogynaephilia is not usually an indication for oestrogen treatment.[23]

Rarely, partial androgen insensitivity syndromes may cause cross-sex identification, and males with these syndromes would qualify for a diagnosis of gender identity disorder (not otherwise specified) because there is an abnormality of endocrine function. These syndromes can be detected only with the endocrine expertise and complex pathological testing offered by a gender identity clinic. They cannot be detected if hormone treatment has already started. The presence of a partial androgen insensitivity syndrome does not greatly alter the subsequent management of the affected patient, but it is important because, as inherited conditions, they may affect the sons of the patient's sisters. Genetic counselling may be indicated.[9]

MANAGEMENT

The treatment of disorders of gender identity may be drastic and irreversible, and so treatment should be undertaken only in a setting of diagnostic certainty.

The least certain diagnosis is that made by the patient, made as it is without any training or objectivity. This uncertainty is not lessened by the patient's high degree of conviction. Neither does the support of others with gender dysphoria help, since conviction leads people to associate with like-minded others and to discount or fail to seek out discongruent views.

Local psychiatric services are only slightly better placed to make a diagnosis, having objectivity but not experience or much training. Accordingly, diagnoses should properly be made by gender identity clinics. Internationally accepted guidelines stipulate that at least two experienced diagnostic opinions are required before any patient undergoes gender reassignment surgery. It seems sensible to have the same degree of safety in the earlier stages of treatment because an initial diagnosis leading to a change of social gender role has serious social implications, and hormone treatments (particularly in females) have many irreversible effects.

People who present at a gender identity clinic usually state that they have transsexualism and seek immediate treatment with hormones or surgery, or both. They may arrive at this point from any of a number of rather distinct earlier trajectories.

Considering male patients in whom differential diagnoses have been excluded, the most common history is that of earlier dual-role transvestism, often preceded by fetishistic transvestism. Such sexual interest as there is (it is usually slight) is directed towards females. As time passes the patient begins to feel fake and unreal in a male rather than a female role.[23]

A smaller proportion of male patients would earlier have been seen by others and themselves as feminine homosexual men, again with a low libido, with a liking for wearing female clothes. As time passes their femininity grows, and they begin to feel more female than feminine, and to be regarded as such in homosexual male circles.[23]

Female patients often give a history of having earlier been viewed by others, and less often themselves, as masculine lesbians. Their sense of masculinity becomes so overwhelming that they come to identify as male. A change of social gender role may denude such patients of much of their social circle.[24]

A small number of female patients show a sexual preference for males, but they are interested in homosexual men and identify themselves as such.[24]

A small proportion of patients seem to have displayed a sense of cross-gender identification from their earliest years and either attracted or could have attracted a diagnosis of gender identity disorder of childhood. Many patients make this claim, only for documentary evidence or the testimony of relations to refute it, or alter it to a history of childhood tomboyism or unmasculinity, which is a very different matter.[24]

Children and adolescents with gender identity disorders pose particular problems. Instinctive caution has led to surgery and hormones being delayed, although all the evidence is that with carefully selected patients early surgical intervention carries a good outcome.[25] There is a trend towards postponing puberty by means of gonadotropin-releasing hormone (GnRH) analogues and introducing cross-sex hormone treatment when the child is able to give valid consent. There is the suggestion that, for males, earlier age of onset of transsexualism was associated with better outcome,[17] which may reflect 'core' transsexualism. The question is rendered more problematic by a study that followed up ten 'feminine' boys, of whom only one became transsexual and four heterosexual. Childhood gender dysphoria appears to be a necessary but not sufficient factor in a transsexual outcome. The strength, rigidity and persistence of cross-gender behaviour through latency were thought perhaps to predict transsexual outcome.[26]

It is a cardinal principle in a gender identity clinic that reversible changes should precede irreversible changes and that no step should be undertaken unless the preceding steps have been accompanied by psychological and social improvement.

It follows from this that the first step should be a change of social gender role. This involves the patient changing their name to one clearly appropriate to their preferred gender role, and altering all their associated civil and legal documentation. They should make it clear to everyone that they have changed their social gender role. People doing this are protected from discrimination in the workplace and elsewhere by UK legislation (Sex Discrimination Act, amended 1999).

There is no evidence that providing hormone treatment before a change of social gender role makes such a transition easier or more likely. Rather, it may give rise to a seemingly endless drive for ever higher doses of hormones, each increase failing to diminish the patient's anxieties about changing role. If the change of role does not occur, or the desire to change role dissipates (as it may, despite the patient's earlier certainty that this will not be the case), the patient may be left with unwanted, irreversible bodily alteration.[27] Consequently, it is reasonable to undertake treatment with cross-sex hormones only if both a proper diagnosis has been made by an appropriately trained and experienced clinic, and a change of social gender role has been achieved satisfactorily. Clearly, such treatment varies with the birth sex of the patient.

The mainstay of treatment in male patients is high-dose oestrogen therapy. This treatment is acceptably safe provided the patient is a non-smoker and has no history of thromboembolic disease, since the major risk is that of thromboembolic problems.[9,28] In younger patients, treatment may need to be augmented by a GnRH analogue to suppress native androgen production. This is preferred to cyproterone acetate, because cyproterone acetate may cause deranged liver function tests, depression, lethargy and fatigue – seemingly more commonly in the context of gender identity disorders than that of prostate cancer.[29]

The oestrogen dose should be increased progressively over about a year to maximize eventual breast size. The use of high doses from the outset is associated with rapid onset of breast growth but the eventual development of small, hard, conical breasts whose size cannot be increased by any further hormonal manipulation.[9]

This treatment requires 6-monthly monitoring of serum lipids, prolactin and liver function tests, since, rarely, these may be deranged.

There is no role for progesterone because it seems not to have any feminizing effect, and it probably serves to slightly raise the risk of breast cancer.[9]

Oestrogen treatment causes modest breast development and even more modest reduction in facial hair growth. Androgen levels almost always fall, and the already small libido further diminishes (usually a welcome effect). Appetite is increased, and so weight gain is a common problem. There is no change in vocal quality, so speech and language therapy may be indicated.[29] If this is not fully successful, it may be augmented with a cricothyroid approximation to alter vocal quality.[30] This procedure is effective only if followed up with further speech and language therapy.

Born-male patients display feminization on top of an earlier masculinization caused by puberty. Consequently, most end up looking sufficiently female that, if they present in a clearly female role, others feel inclined to treat them as women. Nearly all would be detectable as having been born male.

Female patients require treatment with androgens, either by implant or by intramuscular injection. Oral treatment is anecdotally associated with a raised rate of hepatocellular carcinoma. It is thus ethically and legally challenging to use oral agents.[9]

Androgen treatment causes marked virilization. The first effect is an increase in libido, followed by cliteromegaly and facial and body hair growth. Vocal pitch steadily decreases to that of a male. Menstruation almost always gets less, and menopause is usually achieved within the first 6 months of treatment. Androgens also increase appetite, and so weight gain may be a problem. Muscle mass increases only if there is considerable exercise.[9]

Androgen treatment is very effective, and most born-female patients end up so masculinized that others would not suspect that they were born female save, perhaps, for unusual shortness of stature.

Although it is inappropriate for hormone treatment to start without the assessment and approval of a properly established gender identity clinic, it is best for prescription and administration to occur in a primary care setting because such treatment is likely to be lifelong and is not challenging or unduly hazardous.

Surgical procedures are not contemplated unless the patient has lived and prospered in their assumed gender role, showing psychological and social function that is at least as good as in their former role, and preferably better. A useful means of determining this is noting whether the patient can undertake an occupational role (consistent with their abilities) for at least a year. This can be verified and gives a good measure of social acceptance in the new gender role. It is sometimes termed 'the real life experience'.[31]

Born-female patients may sometimes be considered for bilateral mastectomy after having lived in a male role for a year, whether or not they have been occupied, because large breasts are a significant impediment to passing successfully as male. This procedure is not 'cosmetic' in the sense that most breast surgery for non-malignant conditions is. Rather, it is more akin to surgery for severe and intractable gynaecomastia in a young male. The psychological and social benefits of bilateral mastectomy in this setting are considerable.[32]

Genital surgery varies with the birth sex of the patient. It is not contemplated until there has been a successful life in the assumed gender role for at least 2 years.

Genital surgery for born males always includes the following:

- Penectomy
- Bilateral orchidectomy
- Cliteroplasty
- Vulvoplasty.

Vaginoplasty is usually included, but patients who have no desire for penetrative sexual relations, or no desire to form any sort of sexual relationship at all (particularly if older or in less good health), may be better served by this procedure being omitted. The absence of a vagina could be detected only by the most detailed of genital inspections.[33]

These procedures are usually completed in one stage, with the occasional need for very minor revisional procedures. Hospital in-patient stay is typically 10 days, with a convalescence of 2 months.[34] The results are very effective. At least one patient has been undetected by her general practitioner (GP) and boyfriend of 9 years. Another was undetected in the course of several lesbian relationships.[35]

Genital surgery for born-female patients (phalloplasty) is much more complex and usually comprises multiple stages. The new phallus must be constructed with material harvested from another part of the same patient. Usually the abdominal or forearm skin is used. Placing a urinary conduit in the phallus is challenging. Erectile capacity can be bestowed only by means of implanted hydraulic devices, and this, too, is challenging.[36]

The results of phalloplasty are improving all the time but would still be detected as an artificial construction by any but the most brief of glimpses. Only about a third of born-female patients opt for phalloplasty, the remainder choosing to wait until techniques improve or until their life circumstances will allow the time off work that such surgery inevitably entails.

The results of genital surgery have been subject to investigation since, as patient numbers have grown, it has became possible to properly assess the psychological and social outcomes and to relate these to features of the patients' presenting histories.

The effects of a social gender role change and the timing of surgery were addressed by fully controlled studies, which established that a change of role improved psychological function, and that, once patients had been approved for surgery, those fast-tracked showed better psychological function than those who joined a standard waiting list.[37,38]

The functional results of gender reassignment surgery have been assessed in sexual and cosmetic terms. There was general satisfaction expressed over the quality of cosmetic and functional aspects, despite orgasmic capacity after gender reassignment surgery declining in male patients and increasing in female patients.[39–41] Despite the decrease in orgasm in males, satisfaction with sex and general satisfaction with the results of surgery were high in both.[42]

There have been good outcomes in very disparate settings,[43,44] and the strong suggestion from several studies that the technical success of surgery and a subsequent legal recognition of a change of sex relate strongly to good psychological and social outcome.[45,46] Indeed, in one study, technical surgical outcome accounted for nearly all the variation in postoperative psychopathology.[47,48]

It seems increasingly clear that psychological support is needed after surgery in order to optimize outcomes, since social stressors may persist despite treatment, particularly if the patient has children.[40] There is no evidence that a change of parental gender role has any effect on the sexual development of children.[49] Despite this, many patients have experienced impaired access to their children on the grounds of their change of gender role.

PROGNOSIS

Analysis suggests that female patients tend generally to fare better than do male patients. Regrets about gender-reassignment surgery are associated with poor family and friend support, a lack of an earlier history of childhood gender identity disorder, a lack of attraction to the same biological sex, personality disorder and axis II diagnoses.[50,51] Completed military service, a history of typically 'masculine', hard jobs, and a comparatively late (older than 30 years of age) first request for surgery were also found to be negative prognostic factors in sex-reassignment evaluations. It was thought that both too much and too little ambivalence may suggest a poor prognosis.[52]

LEGAL ASPECTS

The Gender Recognition Act allows people who have changed their gender role to acquire a gender recognition certificate and, if they have a UK birth certificate, a birth certificate in their assumed gender. Applicants must have the support of a recognized specialist and another registered medical practitioner (usually their GP) and need to have lived in their assumed gender role for at least 2 years. They are not absolutely required to have undergone hormone treatment or gender reassignment surgery, but there seems to be a need for a good reason for not having done so. Applications are made to the Gender Recognition Panel (PO Box 6987, Leicester LE1 6ZX; tel: 0845 355 5155; www.grp.gov.uk).

Anyone with a gender recognition certificate is legally of their new sex, just as if they had been born so. If they have children they will remain a parent in the original sex. Adoptions would be in the new sex, so it would be possible for the person to be both a father and a mother.

KEY POINTS

- Gender identity disorders are not common.
- The most frequent gender identity disorder is dual-role transvestism, but it rarely needs medical attention.
- The least frequent gender identity disorder is transsexualism. It is not indicative of serious psychopathology.
- Diagnoses should be made by a gender identity clinic and never by the patient.
- A clear change of gender role should precede any hormone treatment.
- Bilateral mastectomy might be considered after a year of life in a male role.
- The patient should must have lived and thrived entirely in their new gender role for at least 2 years before any genital surgery.
- With these selection criteria, the outcomes of surgery are generally good.
- After treatment, patients may legally change their sex.

REFERENCES

1. Heiman EM, Cao-Van-Le (1975) Transsexualism in Vietnam. *Archives of Sexual Behavior* **4**: 89–95.
2. Ball JR, Emmerson R (1978) A case of personation. *Medical Journal of Australia* **2**: 198–201.
3. Landen M, Walinder J, Lundstrom B (1996) Prevalence, incidence and sex ratio of transsexualism. *Acta Psychiatrica Scandinavica* **93**: 221–3.
4. Barrett J (ed.) (2007) *Transsexualism and Other Disorders of Gender Identity: A Practical Guide to Management*. Oxford. Radcliffe Medical Publishing.
5. Shtasel TF (1979) Behavioral treatment of transsexualism: a case report. *Journal of Sex and Marital Therapy* **5**: 362–7.
6. Buhrich N, McConaghy N (1977) The discrete syndromes of transvestism and transsexualism. *Archives of Sexual Behavior* **6**: 483–95.
7. Lothstein LM, Levine SB (1981) Expressive psychotherapy with gender dysphoric patients. *Archives of General Psychiatry* **38**: 924–9.
8. Green R, Blanchard R (1995) Gender identity disorders. In HI Kaplan, BJ Saddock (eds) *Comprehensive Textbook of Psychiatry*, 6th edn. Baltimore, MD: Williams & Wilkins.
9. Seal LJ (2007) The practical management of hormonal treatment in adults with gender dysphoria. In J Barrett (ed.) *Transsexualism and Other Disorders of Gender Identity: A Practical Guide to Management*. Oxford. Radcliffe Medical Publishing.
10. Levine SB (1980) Psychiatric diagnosis of patients requesting sex reassignment surgery. *Journal of Sex and Marital Therapy* **6**: 164–73.
11. Blanchard R (1993) Partial versus complete autogynephilia and gender dysphoria. *Journal of Sex and Marital Therapy* **19**: 301–7.
12. Blanchard R, Collins PI (1993) Men with sexual interest in transvestites, transsexuals, and she-males. *Journal of Nervous and Mental Disease* **181**: 570–75.
13. Blanchard R (1993) Varieties of autogynephilia and their relationship to gender dysphoria. *Archives of Sexual Behavior* **22**: 241–51.

14. Blanchard R (1993) The she-male phenomenon and the concept of partial autogynephilia. *Journal of Sex and Marital Therapy* **19**: 69–76.
15. Blanchard R (1991) Clinical observations and systematic studies of autogynephilia. *Journal of Sex and Marital Therapy* **17**: 235–51.
16. Miach PP, Berah EF, Butcher JN, Rouse S (2000) Utility of the MMPI-2 in assessing gender dysphoric patients. *Journal of Personality Assessment* **75**: 268–79.
17. Blanchard R, Steiner BW, Clemmensen LH, Dickey R (1989) Prediction of regrets in postoperative transsexuals. *Canadian Journal of Psychiatry* **34**: 43–5.
18. Beatrice J (1985) A psychological comparison of heterosexuals, transvestites, preoperative transsexuals, and postoperative transsexuals. *Journal of Nervous and Mental Disease* **173**: 358–65.
19. Cole CM, O'Boyle M, Emory LE, Meyer WJ 3rd (1997) Comorbidity of gender dysphoria and other major psychiatric diagnoses. *Archives of Sexual Behavior* **26**: 13–26.
20. Haraldsen IR, Dahl AA (2000) Symptom profiles of gender dysphoric patients of transsexual type compared to patients with personality disorders and healthy adults. *Acta Psychiatrica Scandinavica* **102**: 276–81.
21. Smith YL, van Goozen SH, Cohen-Kettenis PT (2001) Adolescents with gender identity disorder who were accepted or rejected for sex reassignment surgery: a prospective follow-up study. *Journal of the American Academy of Child and Adolescent Psychiatry* **40**: 472–81.
22. Cohen-Kettenis PT, Gooren LJ (1999) Transsexualism: a review of etiology, diagnosis and treatment. *Journal of Psychosomatic Research* **46**: 315–33.
23. Barrett J (2007) Dealing with the differentials. In J Barrett (ed.) *Transsexualism and Other Disorders of Gender Identity: A Practical Guide to Management.* Oxford: Radcliffe Medical Publishing.
24. Barrett J (2007) Categorization and differential diagnosis. In J Barrett (ed.) *Transsexualism and Other Disorders of Gender Identity: A Practical Guide to Management.* Oxford: Radcliffe Medical Publishing.
25. Cohen-Kettenis PT, van Goozen SH (1997) Sex reassignment of adolescent transsexuals: a follow-up study. *Journal of the American Academy of Child and Adolescent Psychiatry* **36**: 263–71.
26. Davenport CW (1986) A follow-up study of 10 feminine boys. *Archives of Sexual Behavior* **15**: 511–17.
27. Barrett J (2007) Challenging patients and circumstances. In J Barrett (ed.) *Transsexualism and Other Disorders of Gender Identity: A Practical Guide to Management.* Oxford: Radcliffe Medical Publishing.
28. Van Kesteren PJ, Asscheman H, Megens JA, Gooren LJ (1997) Mortality and morbidity in transsexual subjects treated with cross-sex hormones. *Clinical Endocrinology* **47**: 337–42.
29. Antoni C (2007) The role of the speech and language therapist. In J Barrett (ed.) *Transsexualism and Other Disorders of Gender Identity: A Practical Guide to Management.* Oxford: Radcliffe Medical Publishing.
30. Sandhu G (2007) Feminization of the larynx and voice. In J Barrett (ed.) *Transsexualism and Other Disorders of Gender Identity: A Practical Guide to Management.* Oxford: Radcliffe Medical Publishing.
31. Barrett J (2007) The Real Life Experience. In J Barrett (ed.) *Transsexualism and Other Disorders of Gender Identity: A Practical Guide to Management.* Oxford: Radcliffe Medical Publishing.
32. Davies D, Stephenson AJ (2007) Breasts. In J Barrett (ed.) *Transsexualism and Other Disorders of Gender Identity: A Practical Guide to Management.* Oxford: Radcliffe Medical Publishing.
33. Bellringer J (2007) Genital surgery. In J Barrett (ed.) *Transsexualism and Other Disorders of Gender Identity: A Practical Guide to Management.* Oxford: Radcliffe Medical Publishing.
34. Barrett J (2007) Advice for patients undergoing vaginoplasty and vulvoplasty. In J Barrett (ed.) *Transsexualism and Other Disorders of Gender Identity: A Practical Guide to Management.* Oxford: Radcliffe Medical Publishing.
35. Barrett J (2007) Relationships. In J Barrett (ed.) *Transsexualism and Other Disorders of Gender Identity: A Practical Guide to Management.* Oxford: Radcliffe Medical Publishing.
36. Ralph D, Christopher N (2007) Phalloplasty. In J Barrett (ed.) *Transsexualism and Other Disorders of Gender Identity: A Practical Guide to Management.* Oxford: Radcliffe Medical Publishing.
37. Mate-Kole C, Freschi M, Robin A (1988) Aspects of psychiatric symptoms at different stages in the treatment of transsexualism. *British Journal of Psychiatry* **152**: 550–53.
38. Mate-Kole C, Freschi M, Robin A (1991) A controlled study of psychological and social change after surgical gender reassignment in selected male transsexuals. *British Journal of Psychiatry* **158**: 132–3.
39. Green R (1998) Sexual functioning in post-operative transsexuals: male-to-female and female-to-male. *International Journal of Impotence Research* **10** (suppl. 1): S22–4.
40. Rehman J, Lazer S, Benet AE, Schaefer LC, Melman A (1999) The reported sex and surgery satisfactions of 28 postoperative male-to-female transsexual patients. *Archives of Sexual Behavior* **28**: 71–89.
41. Lief HI, Hubschman L (1993) Orgasm in the postoperative transsexual. *Archives of Sexual Behavior* **22**: 145–55.
42. Blanchard R, Legault S, Lindsay WR (1987) Vaginoplasty outcome in male-to-female transsexuals. *Journal of Sex and Marital Therapy* **13**: 265–75.
43. Rakic Z, Starcevic V, Maric J, Kelin K (1996) The outcome of sex reassignment surgery in Belgrade: 32

patients of both sexes. *Archives of Sexual Behavior* **25**: 515–25.

44. Kuiper B, Cohen-Kettenis P (1988) Sex reassignment surgery: a study of 141 Dutch transsexuals. *Archives of Sexual Behavior* **17**: 439–57.
45. Tsoi WF, Kok LP, Yeo KL, Ratnam SS (1995) Follow-up study of female transsexuals. *Annals of the Academy of Medicine, Singapore* **24**: 664–7.
46. Stein M, Tiefer L, Melman A (1990) Followup observations of operated male-to-female transsexuals. *Journal of Urology* **143**: 1188–92.
47. Ross MW, Need JA (1989) Effects of adequacy of gender reassignment surgery on psychological adjustment: a follow-up of fourteen male-to-female patients. *Archives of Sexual Behavior* **18**: 145–53.
48. Lindemalm G, Korlin D, Uddenberg N (1986) Long-term follow-up of 'sex change' in 13 male-to-female transsexuals. *Archives of Sexual Behavior* **15**: 187–210.
49. Green R (1978) Sexual identity of 37 children raised by homosexual or transsexual parents. *American Journal of Psychiatry* **135**: 692–7.
50. Landen M, Walinder J, Hambert G, Lundstrom B (1998) Factors predictive of regret in sex reassignment. *Acta Psychiatrica Scandinavica* **97**: 284–9.
51. Bodlund O, Kullgren G (1996) Transsexualism general outcome and prognostic factors: a five-year follow-up study of nineteen transsexuals in the process of changing sex. *Archives of Sexual Behavior* **25**: 303–16.
52. Lindemalm G, Korlin D, Uddenberg N (1987) Prognostic factors vs outcome in male-to-female transsexualism: a follow-up study of 13 cases. *Acta Psychiatrica Scandinavica* **75**: 268–74.

Chapter 47

Paraphilias and sexual offenders

Ian Treasaden

INTRODUCTION

The term 'paraphilia' is from the Ancient Greek for 'irregular love' – that is, an attraction or love (*philia*) of the irregular (*para*). It implies being outside the normal range in the sphere of sex. This is an emotive area; before its discussion, it is standard to issue the formal disclaimer, if not in the words of English actor Patricia Campbell in the first half of the twentieth century that 'It doesn't matter what you do in the bedroom as long as you don't do it in the street and frighten the horses', then at least that any particular sexual behaviour done in private, and not causing harm to self or others, does not necessarily constitute a psychiatric disorder and a need for psychiatric treatment. What has constituted a paraphilia has varied through history. For instance, sexual orientation towards members of one's own sex is not considered a paraphilia nowadays, but homosexuality was listed as a psychiatric disorder in the eighth revision of the *International Classification of Diseases* (ICD-8). A further consideration in this area is the difference between *psychological theories* of sexual development, such as those of Freud – who, of course, did have theories about, for instance, homosexuality, including that it was not appropriate for a psychoanalyst to be either homosexual or bisexual – and *political arguments* – for example, about non-discrimination towards individuals not causing harm to others.

NORMAL SEXUALITY

This can be defined as that approved by society, but it varies from country to country, through history and between social levels. For instance, 300 years ago it was common in the UK for 12- to 13-year-olds to become pregnant. An alternative definition is that which is statistically common. In fact, there is a far greater width of sexual activity than is usually recognized.

Alfred Kinsey, Professor of Biology at Indiana University in the USA, amazed the general public of the USA with the results of his studies commenced in 1938. In 1948 he published *Sexual Behaviour in the Human Male* after interviewing 5300 males,[1] and in 1953 *Sexual Behaviour in the Human Female* after interviewing approximately 6000 females.[2] It was these studies, although now criticized for selection bias, that highlighted high rates of premarital sexual intercourse before the age of 20 years (73% in males, 20% in females) and the high rates of infidelity within marriage (50% of males). It also highlighted that males reached a sexual peak during late adolescence while for females it was in their thirties.

Differences in sexual behaviour between cultures have been well described by anthropologists.[3] Homosexuality was accepted in Ancient Greek and Roman times, was repressed in Elizabethan times, and is still a criminal offence in some parts of the world, but, although never the norm, it has been expected of young boys with their elders before marrying in cultures such as in New Guinea, apparently not resulting in any post-traumatic stress disorder, perhaps because of its cultural acceptability. In the past, in some specific cultures, such as in Tahiti as described by Robert Louis Stevenson, and in the Arctic, it was considered hospitable for visitors to be offered the host's wife or daughter as a sleeping companion for the night.

An important milestone in the clinical literature of paraphilias was Richard von Krafft-Ebing's 1887 book *Psychopathia Sexualis*,[4] which was translated into English from the German. Krafft-Ebing, a neuropsychiatrist, provided detailed case histories of paraphilias comparable to those described in the fourth edition of the *Diagnostic and Statistical Manual of Mental Disorders* (DSM-IV), but also including flagellation, lust murder, necrophilia, bestiality and incest.

The terms 'sexual deviance' and 'deviant (perverse) sexual behaviour' now have rather pejorative and moralistic implications, akin to the terms 'imbecile' and 'idiot', which previously were legal terms for a person with learning disability. Paraphilias are also termed 'sexual minority practices', which highlights the associated psychology of being in a minority. The characteristic features include:

- deviation from a primary adult sexual drive;
- tendency to avoid procreation;
- characterized by its *persistence* and *preference* over normal adult sexual behaviour. It is not uncommon that some normal adult sexual behaviour occurs in people

with a paraphilia. On the other hand, elements such as voyeurism and exhibitionism, and even fleeing sadism, may be present to a lesser degree in normal sexuality;
- often unable to relate adequately to adults;
- often has a cathartic (emotional releasing) function such as that seen in self-harm.

It is important to distinguish paraphilias from *facultative deviation* due to unavailability, usually transiently, of normal sexual contacts, such as in institutions such as prisons.

Another useful clinical concept is that of a *latent perversion*, which is generally well compensated for and becomes apparent only under stress, for example in marital conflict, certain circumstances or disinhibition by alcohol or drugs, or is released by mental illness, such as depression. Indeed, perverse behaviours can sometimes be seen as acting as self-esteem or mood regulators. Latent perversion represents *regressed*, as opposed to a *fixed*, deviation.

Sexual behaviour is motivated by a desire for affection and a need to belong, and not merely for orgasm. A useful analogy is that of a barrier or wall due to anxiety in forming adult relationships.[5] If the wall is too big, then the individual may:

- turn away (paedophilia, fetishism);
- peek over (voyeurism) or stand on the wall (exhibitionism);
- reach over and touch (frotteurism, indecent assault);
- crash through by force (rape).

Paraphilias or disorders of sexual preference should be distinguished from *gender dysphoria*, which is varying degrees of dissatisfaction with the current sex gender, including transsexualism. The strength of sexual drive is determined by biological factors and follows androgen levels in males and females, but gender role, identity and direction of sexual interest are determined largely by psychological factors. Before 1 year of age, it is simple to reassign sex correctly, such as in cases of hypogonadism, but this is almost impossible after 5 years of age – that is, between 1 year and 5 years, gender role is established by cultural expectation, whatever the actual genetic sex.

Androgen-insensitivity syndrome (which occurs in 1 : 30 000) results in a male appearing female, while *congenital adrenal hypoplasia* (which occurs in 1 : 6000) leads to increased levels of testosterone, resulting in a female appearing male.

Sexual orientation, for example homosexuality or bisexuality, is not now regarded as a disorder in the tenth revision of the *International Classification of Diseases* (ICD-10) or DSM-IV, unless it is egodystonic (ICD-10 F.66.1).

Non-paraphilic sexual addictions

These are culturally acceptable sexual interests and behaviours but so intense or frequent that they interfere with sustained intimate relationships, for example:

- compulsive masturbation;
- repetitive promiscuity (using people as sex objects, use of prostitutes);
- dependence upon anonymous sexual outlets, e.g. pornography, including on the Internet, or telephone sex.

They have been conceptualized as:

- addictions;
- compulsions;
- hypersexuality;
- disorders of impulse control;
- depressive equivalent, especially in the presence of (i) an affective disorder, which itself causes a disorder of sexual regulation, leading to an increase in non-conventional sexual interests and an increase in desire equivalent to bulimia nervosa, which also shares co-morbidity with depression and responds to antidepressants; or (ii) an obsessive-compulsive disorder (OCD) variant. Treatment with fluoxetine (20–60 mg/day), a selective serotonin reuptake inhibitor (SSRI) antidepressant, which is also anti-obsessional, anti-impulsive and anti-aggressive, has been recommended as effective. This would theoretically be beneficial for (i) or (ii) above.

Obsessive–compulsive disorder

In contrast to paraphilias, in OCD, as defined in ICD-10, the thought of carrying out the act must not in itself be pleasurable, even if it brings temporary relief of tension and anxiety.

PARAPHILIAS

The DSM-IV defines paraphilias as recurrent, intense, sexually arousing fantasies, sexual urges or behaviours generally involving (i) non-human objects, (ii) the suffering or humiliation of oneself or one's partner or (iii) children or other non-consenting people that occur over a period of at least 6 months (criterion A) and cause clinically significant distress or impairment in social, occupational or other important areas of functioning (criterion B) – that is, not part of normative sexual arousal patterns and interfering with capacity for reciprocal affectionate activity.[6]

Paraphilias are often experienced by the individual as insistent, demanded and fixated. The person may say they will never behave sexually in that way again but then do so in spite of law involvement and the potential risk to the self or others. They often describe an inability to stop paraphilic behaviour, unless someone externally intervenes, and also a feeling of altered consciousness at the time, which perhaps reflects high sexual arousal or dissociation.

In ICD-10, 'disorders of sexual preference' is the term used in preference to 'paraphilias'.[7] Table 47.1 describes and contrasts the types identified in ICD-10 with the paraphilias described in DSM-IV.

Table 47.1 Classification of disorders of sexual preference (ICD-10) and paraphilias (DSM-IV)

ICD-10 disorders of sexual preference		DSM-IV paraphilias		Sexual preference
F65.0	Fetishism	302.81	Fetishism	Inanimate object
F65.1	Fetishistic transvestism	302.3	Transvestic fetishism	Cross-dressing
F65.2	Exhibitionism	302.4	Exhibitionism	Exposure of genitals
F65.3	Voyeurism	302.82	Voyeurism	Looking at people engaging in sexual or intimate behaviour
F65.4	Paedophilia	302.2	Paedophilia	Children
F65.5	Sadomasochism	302.84	Sexual sadism	Making or being made to suffer
		302.83	Sexual masochism	
F65.6	Multiple disorders of sexual preference			'Polymorphous perverse'

ICD-10 points out that more than one disorder of sexual preference may occur in one individual, fetishism, transvestism and sadomasochism being the most common combination.

AETIOLOGY OF HUMAN SEXUALITY

Exact aetiologies of human sexuality are unknown. Most authorities speak of a combination of constitutional and acquired characteristics, and all schools have contributed observations and theories that help our understanding. In spite of psychodynamic interest, sex is one of the most biological of human functions. As with other branches of medicine and biology, the importance attached to nature and nurture has varied over time.

Constitutional factors

Genetic factors

It appears that genetic factors do have a bearing on the development of human sexuality, as shown by work on sexual orientation. Kallman originally reported 100 per cent concordance for homosexuality in monozygotes.[8] However, as he noted, his population comprised mentally ill institutionalized men and he later considered these figures to have been statistical artefacts. Numerous discordant monozygotic pairs have been reported.

Eckert and colleagues, after studying monozygotic twins reared apart, found some concordance for male homosexuality but none for females.[9] Bailey and Pillard have found concordance rates for homosexuality of 52 per cent in monozygotes and 22 per cent for dizygotes compared with a rate of less than 10 per cent for non-twin biological brothers.[10] Such work has also been replicated on female homosexuals. Other authors have found lower concordance rates. Family studies have suggested that sexual orientation is inherited through the maternal side – that is, possibly X-chromosome-linked, expressed in men but carried by women. Hamer and colleagues found that 33 of 40 pairs of homosexual male siblings had five shared markers on the distal arm of the X-chromosome (Xq 28 locus for sexual orientation, $P = 0.00001$).[11] It is unlikely that there is one 'gay gene'. There are probably many and none absolute. Also, twin studies have shown that half or more of variability on sexual orientation is not inherited. Overall, large discordant rates for paraphilias have been found in spite of the same genes and environment.[12]

Kleinfelter's syndrome, due to the chromosomal abnormality XXY, has been associated with not only psychosexual infantilism but also increased rates of paedophilia.

Hormonal influence on the prenatal brain

Harris and Levine have shown that androgens in very young animals given at critical periods affect their normal rough-and-tumble play and their adult sexual behaviour, which leads to a similar theory for the case of humans.[13] It has been theorized that the basic human brain is female; exposure to androgens, due to the Y-chromosome, leads to the differentiation to a male brain. However, there is no clear evidence for this leading to paraphilias in humans, even for those exposed to large doses of exogenous hormones prenatally.

Hormone levels

There is no evidence for differing levels of testosterone in paraphilias or homosexuals in spite of previous claims. Hormones have more complex effects. High testosterone levels are, however, associated with aggression, which is linked to limbic pleasure centres, perhaps accounting for the association of sex and violence.

Neuroanatomical basis

Brain damage has been suggested as a possible biological basis for paraphilias,[12] perhaps by affecting perception of erogenous zones, although these themselves vary in importance across cultures. People with temporal lobe epilepsy have an excess of sexual dysfunctions, including paraphilias.

A biological basis is also suggested by the great resistance of paraphilias to change.

Environmental factors

Although often cited as aetiological factors in paraphilias, the evidence base is weak. Factors cited include the following:

- *Unsatisfactory or absent father*
- *Overprotective or close-binding intimate mother*
- *Child's temperament and health* leading to the mother being overprotective
- *Analytical theory:* paraphilias are seen as resulting from desires, real or fantasy experiences or conflicts at particular stages of psychosexual development at which the individual becomes fixed. Ego defence mechanisms are regarded as important. Paraphilias may also be seen as a solution to castration fear during the development of infantile sexuality. Although society views sexuality as a phenomenon that follows the onset of puberty in adolescence, sexuality is not only present through the so-called Freudian latent period but also is evident in the womb, where the fetuses can be seen to be masturbating
- *A solution to the problem of relating normally and forming adult social relationships:* in monkey colonies, low-dominance monkeys adopt a passive sexual position in relation to high-dominance monkeys. In humans, dominance is affected by mood and environmental stress. Maternally deprived monkeys not only develop into sexually incompetent adults but also exhibit sexual minority practices akin to paraphilias[14]
- *Behaviour theory:* paraphilias can be understood in terms of learning theory, e.g.
  - training by family;
  - conjunction of a neutral object with sexual arousal or reinforcement.

First sexual experiences can be important. Childhood sexual abuse is associated with paedophilia. US students were conditioned to develop a foot fetish by pairing slides of boots with those of nude women.[15] However, clinically, learning theory seems an insufficient total explanation for paraphilias. Cultural factors, symbolism of objects, deficiencies in normal sexual arousal, and deficits in social skills and social anxiety may all be relevant.

Paraphilias or disorders of sexual preference are more common in males. Theories why this may be so include the following:

- Male children have to separate from the mother and move to identify with the father.
- The basic template of the brain is female, from which the male brains may be unsuccessfully modified.
- Visual aspects may be more important for males compared with the overall relationship for females. Males also self-evidently have an external visual feedback organ – the penis – of sexual arousal.
- Different gender roles: males are more likely to make advances; females are more submissive. This may merely be cultural.
- Male perverse acts are aimed at external part objects. Equivalent female perverse acts are aimed at themselves, e.g. self-mutilation, anorexia nervosa, or objects of own creation (babies). Male external genitalia symbolically reflect externalizing of aggression and alcohol abuse. Female genitalia symbolically reflect the turning-in of the equivalent of female perverse acts.[16]

Interactional model

An interactional model (Figure 47.1) provides a theory to account for the multiple factors above. Genes and hormones give rise to certain temperamental and personality traits. Genes may also lead to different environmental experiences, for example through certain personality traits such as sensation-seeking. These interact with the environment and are shaped and reshaped by experience and give rise to adult sexuality, including paraphilias. Paraphilias are clearly phenotypic, not genotypic. As such, this is a biopsychosociocultural-political model of human sexuality. An example to illustrate this is given in Figure 47.2.

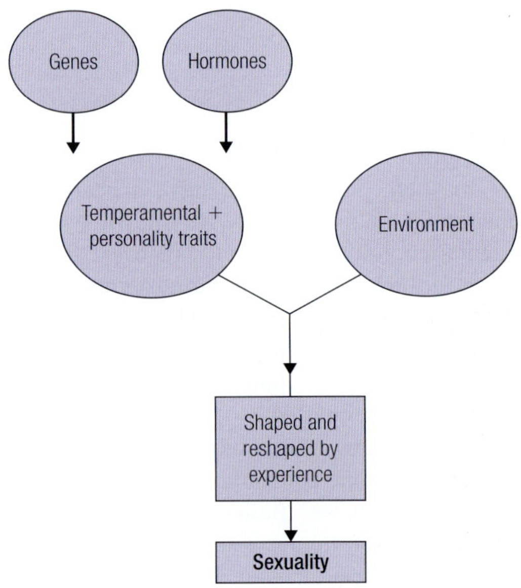

Figure 47.1 Interactional model of human sexuality: a biopsychosociocultural-political model

ASSESSMENT OF HUMAN SEXUALITY

In assessing human sexuality, it is necessary to consider the following:

- *Sexual fantasies:* these are most important and cannot be measured in animal studies.
- *Sexual activity:* human sexual activity is not predominantly a cyclical reproductive activity, as in non-humans. This is a further limitation of animal studies.
- *Sense of identity.*
- *Social role.*

TRANSVESTISM

Transvestism is the desire to wear clothing appropriate to the opposite sex (cross-dressing), often associated with sexually arousing fantasies, urges and behaviour and sexual gratification, in which case it may be regarded as a form of fetishism, referred to in ICD-10 as 'fetishistic transvestism', which is the wearing of the clothes of the opposite sex in order to obtain sexual excitement. DSM-IV confines this paraphilia to heterosexual males. Transvestism is a paraphilia or disorder of sexual preference, in contrast to transsexualism (Table 47.2).[17]

Transsexualism is a gender disorder. It is a wish to be able to function as a member of the opposite sex associated with a compulsive conviction that the person is assigned to the wrong gender. The person may wish to function as a member of the opposite sex anatomically and physiologically. Such individuals may be referred to as 'trans'.

Dual-role transvestism involves the wearing of clothes of the opposite sex in order to enjoy temporary membership of the opposite sex without the desire for permanent change of sex. Unlike transvestism, it is not associated with sexual excitement.

The term 'transgenderism' includes transvestism and transsexualism.

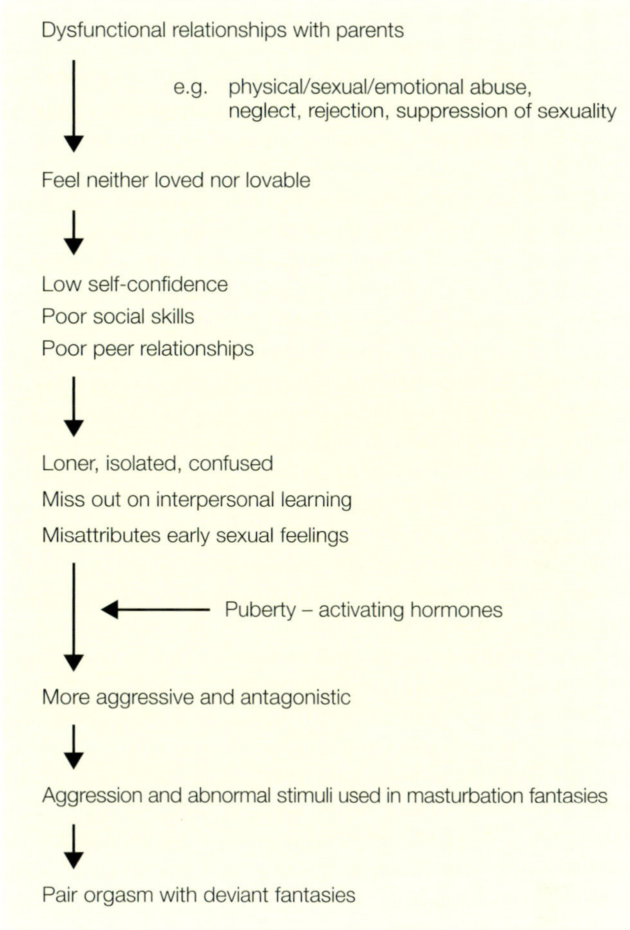

Figure 47.2 Example of interactional model of human sexuality

Incidence

The prevalence is unknown, but it is estimated that there are around 30 000 transvestites in the British Isles, most never coming to the attention of the medical or legal professions. Transvestism may be the most common paraphilia. It is not uncommon as a transient developmental phenomenon around 10 years of age in boys.

Table 47.2 Differentiating transsexualism from transvestism

	Transsexualism	Transvestism
If stop cross-dressing	Dysphoric state unassociated with sex; can forgo for period	Anxious; relieved when cross-dresses and by masturbation
After recent losses	–	Greater disorder
Sex of communal toilets used	Female only	Female only when cross-dressing
In toilet: sit/stand to urinate; touch penis during urination and masturbation	Repulsion at own genitalia	Like/value genitalia and pleasure of them

Aetiology

- *Analytical theory:* transvestism is seen as a solution to castration fears or an attempt to identify with the individual's mother through wearing female clothes to recapture the primitive sexuality of having her skin against his. Physical or emotional distance from the father is also cited.
- *Particular personality characteristics:* transvestism is seen sometimes with obsessional personalities, where the paraphilia has an obsessive characteristic. However, other personalities are clinically apparent. Some studies suggest that 50–70 per cent of transvestites can be diagnosed as having a personality disorder.
- *Abnormal conditioning.*
- *Family background:* a pattern of a rigid, uncongenial or absent father and a dominant or overprotective mother has been described.

Behaviour patterns

Most information on the clinical features is derived from surveys, for example of 504 cases in American and Australian clubs.[18] In transvestites, the impulse arises during early childhood. Cross-dressing is practised at all convenient opportunities. The condition appears to be very persistent and becomes associated with sexual arousal after puberty. Subjects are generally but not necessarily heterosexual in orientation.

Transvestism may be:

- *Compulsive:* in such cases, tension relief is apparent when the individual gives into the compulsion. There is no wish to change sex, but satisfaction from passing off the self as a member of the opposite sex may be apparent.
- *Symptomatic:* this is seen in homosexuality, lesbianism and transsexualism.

Treatment

The majority of transvestites do not request treatment or wish to be 'cured'. Some are brought for treatment by relatives or their partner. Others are referred because of brushes with the law due to personality difficulties rather than (except for the stealing of clothes) their specific paraphilia, for example soliciting or importuning in a public place for immoral purposes, or insulting behaviour likely to cause a breach of the peace. Historically, 'success' was claimed with aversion therapy, although follow-up indicates that many transvestites relapse after attempts at treatment.

EXHIBITIONISM

This is the exposing of the genitals to an unsuspecting stranger, usually a member of the opposite sex.

Indecent exposure

This is the corresponding offence in England and Wales resulting from exhibitionism of 'openly, lewdly and obscenely exposing his person with intent to insult any female' (1824 Vagrancy Act). The comparable behaviour in females, for example female streakers, is dealt with by the offence of 'behaviour likely to cause a breach of the peace'. It is a summary, non-indictable offence – that is, the individual can be tried without a jury by a magistrate's court and, as such, is not recorded in the England and Wales criminal statistics as a notifiable offence.

Incidence

There are over 3000 convictions in England and Wales for indecent exposure each year. This is the most common type of sexual offence committed by adults. The rate for adults has remained steady, but the rate for individuals under 21 years has increased since 1948. It is more common in summer. Cultural factors may be important. It is said to be rare in non-psychotic Afro-Caribbean people.

Classification (after Rooth[19])

- *Type 1 (80%):* characteristically this involves an inhibited young man of relatively normal personality and good character, who struggles against his impulse but finds it irresistible. He feels anxious, guilty and humiliated because of it. He exposes with a flaccid penis, does not masturbate, and derives little if any pleasure from the act. The behaviour is probably related to assertiveness. Such individuals value being in control, however briefly, of the transaction, whether it induces fear, annoyance or even amusement. They want a response but not the female to initiate sex. This type is said to be not physically dangerous.
- *Type 2 (20%):* these individuals are less inhibited and more psychopathic. They expose in a state of great excitement, with an erect penis and masturbation. These individuals obtain great pleasure and show little guilt. In this group, the act may be associated with a marked sadistic element, other sexual disorders and other types of offence. These individuals can be seen as trying to break a barrier to their forming a relationship and, as such, may escalate their behaviour to include accompanying indecent suggestions such as 'Kop a load of this!', touching, thoughts, and acts of indecent assault or rape.

This classification is only a guide, and many individuals show features of both categories. Exhibitionists are more likely to show two or more paraphilias, such as voyeurism and making obscene telephone calls.

Aetiology

- *Family background:* a greater relationship with the mother and a poor relationship with the father has often been described.

- *Psychoanalytical viewpoint:* the deviation is said to stand against the fear of impotence and castration.
- *Excessive inhibitions due to family attitudes:* the caricature of exhibitionists wearing dirty raincoats may be seen as hiding something viewed as dirty.
- *Behavioural theories:* these include various explanations of learning and reinforcement by perverse masturbation fantasies.

Clinical presentation

Individuals with exhibitionism have a normal distribution of intelligence and are seen in all social classes. Common personality traits described include immaturity, passivity and obsessionality. The most common age of onset is the late teens; a late onset suggests major psychiatric disorder, including depression, alcoholism and even general paralysis of the insane (GPI). Only about 5 per cent of individuals with exhibitionism are psychotic or have a learning disability. Early sexual development is usually unremarkable. A normal sexual appetite is present at puberty but, with the onset of adolescence, there is mounting anxiety about forming heterosexual relationships; indeed, such individuals tend to be less successful in establishing heterosexual relationships. Premature ejaculation and impotence are common. However, stable relationships and marriages are often subsequently made by individuals in the type 1 group.

The act is frequently on favourite 'hunting grounds'. The individual may claim that he was simply urinating because he could not wait any longer. On the other hand, the not uncommon observed behaviour of individuals urinating in public, for example not going behind a hedge, may also reflect latent exhibitionist behaviour. Discretion is often absent, with very high risk-taking. Activity may be higher in depressive moods. The witness chosen is generally a stranger. There is a desire to engage the woman's attention in a situation in which the individual, normally a passive person, is in control. The reaction most unwanted is that of indifference. This brief encounter is associated with feelings of excitement, exhilaration and achievement. Victims are commonly girls around the age of puberty or women. A preference for children is said to occur in the more immature and timid individuals, who are frightened of women. However, crime surveys show that perhaps the majority of females in the UK are exposed to at some time during their lifetime.

Prognosis

Eighty per cent of exposers do not re-offend once convicted; however, they may do so frequently before conviction. There is a small recidivist group who persist, but in this group the behaviour falls off in the forties. Generally, exhibitionists are physically harmless, non-violent people. A few may escalate to become paedophiles, and some may commit violent offences, either sexual or otherwise.[20] The more offences committed, the worse the prognosis. A good prognosis is associated with mature sexual experiences, including sustained sexual relationships and marriage, and otherwise good social relationships and work record.

Management

Management has been eclectic.[21] Anti-libidinal drugs have been used as a temporary expedient. Supportive psychotherapy may be useful by increasing the self-esteem of the often timid, anxious type 1 offenders; such therapy may offer these individuals their only emotional release. Group therapy is also used; the probation service may run groups for convicted indecent exposers, which has the advantage that all such members of the group know why they are there and are subsequently less deceiving. Cognitive-behavioural therapy (CBT) is the specific psychological treatment of choice. In the past, aversion techniques were used; there was even a recommendation for exposers to wear their trousers back-to-front.

PAEDOPHILIA

This is the sexual preference for prepubertal children or children under 13 years of age. The term 'hebephilia' refers to a sexual preference for young people of adolescent age. To meet the DSM-IV diagnostic criteria for paedophilia, the person must be at least 16 years of age and at least 5 years older than the child or children. The majority of paedophiles are male, but female paedophiles do exist. Paedophiles are subject to public outrage and viewed as monsters, and their behaviour is seen as unexplainable in spite of the way such individuals might be seen as having difficulty distinguishing affection to children and its sexualization.

Underage sex

It was not uncommon 300 years ago for females to become pregnant at the age of 12–13 years. Even in Victorian times, in England and Wales it was legal to have sexual intercourse with girls under 13 years of age. Now sex with a female under 16 years of age is always illegal, as consent at that age is considered invalid. Sex with a female under 13 years of age is equivalent to rape in seriousness; it is, however, a valid defence if the male is under 24 years of age and believes the female to be older than 16 years, provided there are no previous similar offences. If the sex is by force or against the female's will, then the offence is equivalent to rape. The age cut-off of 16 years may be seen as rather arbitrary compared with the psychologically more important stage of emotional development. In addition, individuals of the age of 10 years are criminally responsible and may receive a custodial sentence if convicted. One can legally buy a pet at 12 years of age, have sexual intercourse at 16 years of age, drive a car at 17 years of age and vote at 18 years of age in England and Wales.

Classification

Clinically, it is useful to distinguish those individuals with a fixed disorder of the sexual preference of paedophilia, estimated in numbers to be about 300–400 in the UK, compared with larger groups of people whose paedophilic behaviour represents regression, such as under stress, as a result of mental illness or following substance abuse. The evidence base regarding paedophilia is limited.[22]

Other classifications include the following:

- *By the characteristics of the offender:*
  - Adolescent – such behaviour usually represents an emotionally and sexually immature investigation. Rarely but tragically, sometimes the offender kills the victim in panic after the victim screams or in order to conceal the offence. This contributes to the average four sex murders per year of children in the UK.
  - Elderly – this group includes lonely, isolated individuals with a fear of impotence.
- *By relationship to children:*
  - The sexuality arises out of a relationship to the child. This is the most common type of paedophilia – the group represents about 80 per cent of paedophiles. The offender has an affection for the child or children and no particular wish to harm them, although clearly the act is illegal. In effect, the offender may be 'in love' with the child. Deprived children may more often be victims, as they may be more open to strangers and seeking affection. Freud pointed out that children do have sexuality and seek adult affection; however, it is an adult's responsibility not to sexualize their relationships with children.
  - The child is merely a source of sexual gratification. Here, the victim is generally a stranger and the relationship a casual one. Two groups are seen, characterized by (i) non-aggressive seduction with money or sweets (this is the group parents warn their children against) and (ii) an aggressive seduction or rape associated with violence.
- *By the sex of the victim:*
  - Heterosexual group – individuals in this group are often married, have lower reconviction rates and are less criminal.
  - Homosexual group – individuals tend to be single and more likely to re-offend. This group carries a worse prognosis.
  - Indiscriminate group – where the victims are of either sex. This group includes up to 20 per cent of paedophiles. The victims are more likely to be younger (6–11 years), perhaps because both sexes at that age are physically similar and asexual.

'Child molesters'

Research on adults who sexually abuse children ('child molesters', i.e. not simply primary paedophiles) has found that they are more indiscriminate than previously thought, often choosing victims of either sex and of a broad age range and choosing both intra- and extrafamilial victims. Up to 90 per cent of child molesting is intrafamilial. Taking offenders convicted of sexual offences against children in general, criminal statistics for England and Wales suggest that around 80 per cent of offenders know the child, of whom 13 per cent are relatives. Few such sexual offences are life-threatening, certainly compared with the average of 80 children killed in England and Wales each year by their parents or a stranger. Sexual killing of a child and abduction of a child by a paedophile occur in fewer than ten cases a year.

Aetiology

Paedophile offences are often committed for reasons of power to counter low self-esteem as much as for sex.[23] Paedophiles often abuse a child of the sex and age when they were abused themselves, which was often their first significant sexual experience. Most paedophiles do not have impulsive personalities and may 'groom' and seduce a victim over a lengthy period. One in ten abused girls and one in four abused boys are abused by women, either alone or as coerced accomplices or co-offenders with men.[24,25] Such involvement of women in offences does not necessarily reflect passivity in the face of a dominant male co-offender but may reflect the woman's own primary sexual deviance.

There is no definite evidence of an increase in sexual assaults on children by paedophiles in the UK, but their visibility and conviction rates have increased due to the greater ease of detecting the illegal use of the Internet to view indecent paedophilic images, compared with the previous pattern of viewing such images in private in magazines.

Clinical features

Paedophiles have a normal intelligence quotient (IQ), education and occupational range. They often have a poor ability to relate to adults, while being proud of their ability to relate to children, although in reality this does not differ from others. Full coitus is rare, and behaviour may be fondling or exhibiting and sometimes orgiastic. Two-thirds of the victims participate, for example by kissing and cuddling. Offending often follows alcohol abuse.

Management

Acceptance of responsibility for the sexual abuse is usually essential. However, paedophiles often admit only to those offences for which they have been caught. Success has been claimed for all forms of treatment, including psychotherapy, CBT and anti-libidinal medication. The homosexual form of paedophilia has the worst prognosis and is generally regarded as extremely difficult to treat. Most success has occurred with anti-androgen hormone therapies. Castration has never been used in the UK, but it was reported to be successful in selected cases of repetitive paedophile rape offenders who were then subject to indefinite detention at Herstedvester Prison in Denmark.[26] However, a relationship with a child may be so important that, even after an individual has been made sexually impotent, the adult may still seek out children.

Prognosis

Untreated, such individuals may abuse large numbers of victims. Recidivism rates are high, even with treatment, and do not decrease over time. Fifteen per cent are reconvicted in law in England and Wales, while up to 35–45 per cent may re-offend on the basis of self-reports. Recidivism is associated with early onset, length of history, variety of sexual offending, offending against both sexes, and deviant arousal to paedophile images on penile plethysmography. Paedophiles on sex offender registers, which are available to social services departments, are excluded from adoption and fostering by such agencies.

Studies on paedophilia include cases where there appear to have been trivial incidents, or activities involving an otherwise sexually active adolescent.[27] Parental reactions may partly determine the long-term effects of being a victim as a child, and isolated minor abuse may have minimal long-term effects. However, Mullen has shown that childhood sexual abuse can adversely affect adult functioning, resulting in intergenerational problems, including uncaring or overcontrolling parents, sexual adjustment difficulties, decrease in socioeconomic status due to disruption of a sense of effective agency and low self-esteem, and increased substance abuse, personality problems, anxiety and depression.[28]

RAPE

Definition

This is an offence, not a paraphilia, but it is covered here for convenience. Rape is anal or vaginal penetration by a penis – that is, sexual intercourse with a man or woman without his or her consent, by fear or force or fraud. Full penetration need not occur. The very rare female equivalent behaviour results in a charge of indecent assault, although females assisting males in rape may be convicted of rape themselves. An offender under the age of 14 years cannot be convicted of rape or attempted rape in the UK but can be convicted of indecent assault.

In England and Wales, a law in 1736 stated that it was not illegal to be raped by one's husband. This clearly reflected attitudes of the time, including the so-called 'rule of thumb', where it was legal for a man to hit his wife with an implement no wider than his thumb. It was not until 1990 that the Court of Appeal ruled that if a husband raped his wife and they were separated, this did constitute rape in law. In 1994, the Public Order and Criminal Justice Act included males for the first time in the definition of victims of rape.

Incidence

The true incidence is unknown because, in spite of increased reporting in recent years, only a fraction of cases are reported. Home Office estimates for England and Wales in 2000 suggested that only 10–25 per cent of victims tell the police; of these reports, only two-thirds were recorded as offences of rape. However, there has been a three-fold increase in convictions since the 1980s. The nature of the offence means that it is often one person's word against another; in England and Wales, only 6 per cent of individuals charged with rape are convicted. Most cases reported are 'date rape'.

Psychopathology

Although by definition a sexual offence, rape often represents displaced aggression,[29] possibly from a rejecting mother or a rejecting society. It may at times be a defence against homosexuality. Evolutionary theory suggests rape is a way for low-status individuals to pass on their genes.

Clinically, offenders often perceive the passivity of the victim – often induced through fear – as consent and that they enjoy the domination and denigration.[30]

Rape is not confined to humans, with examples in nature including ducks (especially in artificial ponds), gorillas, scorpions and bees.

Classification

Various classifications have been attempted, such as that of Gibbens and colleagues.[31] The following is clinically practical:

- *'Normal' rape:* this is described as occurring when normal social sanctions are removed and new group pressures and stresses are substituted, e.g. invading armies such as during the Second World War and in Bosnia, and by Hell's Angels. It may be that the combination in wartime of tension, arousal and of having already been violent makes it easier, especially in groups, to commit rape. It may bond troops together and be used to induce fear and alter the ethnicity of opposing communities. It may also lead to men not wishing to leave their families and fight.
- *Aggressive personality:* in this group, rape is one aspect of generalized aggressive behaviour. Victims are seen by the rapist as objects to be used or defiled.

- *Inhibited, frustrated men:* these men are isolated and unable, through their particular psychological difficulties, to relate normally to women. Such individuals are often aware of, and dislike, the increasing drive to attack and rape. The act may be preceded by indecent exposure. This group is less common than that of aggressive personalities.
- *Sadistic men:* these men are often isolated socially, and the behaviour is egosyntonic and enjoyed. Such individuals are often from a very disturbed background with a rejecting mother.
- *Paedophilic rapists.*
- *Mental illness or learning disability:* the association of rape with mental illness is due largely to the resulting general disinhibition of behaviour. Mania may also lead to rape through increased sex drive. For deluded rapists, one should note the sexual content of their delusions. However, most psychotic patients who rape do not do so directly due to their delusions,[32] which contrasts with violence associated with psychosis. Rarely, organic factors, such as a seminoma secreting androgens, may be important.

Epidemiology

Most male rapists are under 25 years of age, single and not mentally ill and often have convictions for non-sexual offences, often for violence. Thirty per cent of victims are neighbours or acquaintances. Twenty per cent of victims have a criminal record, often of soliciting. Prostitutes are the group most at risk of being victims. Half of rapes are committed by someone known by the victim for less than 24 h. Twelve per cent of rapes are by total strangers. The incidence is higher in the USA than in the UK, in cities, during the summer, at weekends, and in the first half of the night.

Assessment of the alleged rapist

This should include a full history from the alleged rapist, including sexual fantasies and impulses, combined with an objective account of the offence (e.g. from statements or Crown Court depositions), a list of all past offences, and details of any previous psychiatric assessments and management.

Management

This must reflect the underlying cause. Psychological treatment to improve social functioning, such as social skills training, may be necessary but is likely to be insufficient to prevent re-offending. Anti-libidinal treatment can be used where the patient feels that his sexual drive is a factor in the motivation. However, most offenders do not consider themselves in need of psychiatric help, and 80 per cent are sentenced to prison following conviction, where they are paradoxically more highly regarded than child molesters, who tend to be scapegoated. Some specialized prison regimes offering sex offender treatment programmes are available in England and Wales for serious sex offenders.

If psychiatric in-patient treatment is offered, this will usually have to be under conditions of security, such as in a medium secure unit or a maximum secure or special hospital, and will be on the basis that the individual is detained on grounds of mental disorder, on the basis of underlying mental illness or severe personality disorder, and since, but not before, the Mental Health Act 2007 of England and Wales, sexual deviancy.

Management of the victim requires specialized counselling. Victims may have problems of guilt, pregnancy, venereal disease and fear of being shunned by friends and partners, and may have to deal with the stress of court appearance. Overall, the more the victim struggles during rape, the more he or she is likely to sustain injuries, unlike the situation for other, non-sexual, violent offences. However, the less the victim struggles, the more guilt and depression he or she may experience.

Prognosis

Follow-up of men charged with rape show that 90 per cent will not commit a second rape. However, 15–20 per cent will commit a sexual assault of some sort, and 17 per cent commit violent offences. The risk of similarly dangerously re-offending, however, is apparent only over a long follow-up period (e.g. 15 years) and not in the short term (e.g. 2 years).[33] A comparison of exhibitionists and rapists is shown in Table 47.3.

OTHER PARAPHILIAS

Not all sexually deviant behaviour is against the law, but some, such as paedophilia, always is. However, a combination of paraphilic behaviour and crime creates a high newsworthiness.

Fetishism

This is sexual arousal and gratification arising primarily and preferentially from inanimate articles. It can lead to recurrent convictions for theft, for example of used underwear from clothes lines, referred to as 'snowdropping' among prisoners. It is the thought of such articles having belonged to others that is important, in contrast to the theft of unused items from stores. Fetishism may be compulsive or symptomatic. In the latter, male individuals may be impotent unless fetish objects such as black stockings, leather gear or whips are present. Fetishistic objects can be classified into three main groups: articles that are often pink, red, furry, shiny and spherical; articles representing threat, such as black leather and whips; and symbols of femininity, such as female lingerie and shoes. The term

Table 47.3 Comparison of exhibitionists and rapists

	Exhibitionists	Rapists
Age (years)	20–40	18–26
Social class	Relatively upper	Lower
Marital status	60% married	Single
Ethnic	White	–
Intelligence level	Relatively high	Lower
Time of offence	Daylight, midweek (Tuesday)	Night, weekend
Victim	85% unknown	Often known (≥50%)

mysophilia reflects the preference for smelly soiled clothes. Unusual fetishisms described have included car exhaust pipes.[34] If the desire is focused on a part of the body, such as the feet, then DSM-IV regards this as partialism rather than fetishism. Ethologically, fetishism has been viewed as possibly arising from imprinting, as seen in ducklings, reflecting a child crawling and following a mother at shoe level.

Bestiality/zoophilia

This represents a sexual desire and preference for sexual or anal intercourse with animals. The term 'formicophilia' refers to the preference for small animals such as ants touching the erogenous zones. Of note, the offence of buggery refers to anal intercourse by a man with a man or woman, or anal or vaginal intercourse by a man or a woman with an animal, and still carries a maximum sentence of life imprisonment in England and Wales. The term 'buggery' originates from reference to the Christian group Bogomils of Bosnia.

Scotophilia/voyeurism

As defined in DSM-IV, this is sexual arousal derived from observing an unsuspecting person who is naked or in the process of disrobing or engaging in sexual activity. There may be masturbation during the act. It appears exclusive to men. It is epitomized by 'Peeping Tom', a tailor who peeped at the naked Lady Godiva as she rode through Coventry in protest against her husband Leofric, Earl of Mercia, imposing a heavy tax in the first millennium AD.

Telephone scatalogia or scataphilia

This refers to the making of obscene or lewd telephone calls. Usually it is by an individual with an inadequate personality and represents a form of voyeurism. It is usually chance who the individual phones, hence the importance of not giving out one's telephone number when answering the telephone. No response is the best response to such calls. Technology now allows the police to tap and trace such calls.

Frotteurism

In DSM-IV, this refers to the pleasure from touching and rubbing against a non-consenting person. It usually occurs in crowded or confined spaces such as a busy train. The term originates from the French word *frottage*, meaning 'rubbing'.

Sadism

In DSM-IV, sexual sadism refers to recurrent, intense, sexually arousing fantasies, sexual urges or behaviours involving acts in which the psychological or physical suffering, including humiliation, of the victim is exciting to the person. Sometimes the act is with a consenting partner who has sexual masochism. It includes sexual arousal by violence, which contrasts with rapists, who are aroused by forced sexual intercourse. *Biastophilia* or *raptophilia* is the sexual preference for rape. Sadistic violence allows emotional distance but physical proximity. Such individuals find that indulging in aggressive acts bolsters their low self-esteem. Individuals with sexual sadism paraphilia should be contrasted with those attending S and M fantasy clubs, where the behaviour is not developmental. Brittain provided the classic clinical description of the sadistic murderer syndrome.[35] Such individuals may have a past history of working in positions of power over people and animals, such as in butchery, and having interests in Nazism, torture and weapons, which they collect and often store at home, reflecting the content of their mind. Such individuals may have schizoid introspective personalities and, in the absence of relationships and normal rewards, may develop sadistic fantasies to which they habituate, resulting in them proceeding to follow or stalk and later act out those fantasies towards others. Individuals with sadistic personality traits may be very resistant to specific psychological treatment and, if they violently offend, in spite of subsequently often being model prisoners, given the opportunity are likely to seriously harm or murder others in future – and they know it.[36] Compared with rapists, sexual murderers are more overcontrolled, bottling up their temper, have more past convictions for rape, and are more socially isolated and more likely to lack a sexual partner in the year before the offence.[37]

Serial killing

The first sadistic act against an individual is very reinforcing but never matches exactly the individual's fantasy. This may lead to repetition and, in its extreme form and if not caught, serial killing. Such individuals, who often feel powerless and inadequate, may seek the notoriety and power associated with serial killing. Although there has always been serial killing, the 1992 film *The Silence of the Lambs*, with its depiction of Hannibal Lecter, the cannibal psychopathic psychiatrist, has led to serial killing becoming a postmodern hyper-real spectacle of morbid public interest.

Literature on serial killing is limited by the fact that offenders often commit suicide following offending, but profiles suggest that they tend to be non-psychotic, white males, aged 20–30 years, from social classes III–IV, and who often have a history of using firearms and dramatic scenarios to express resentment and anger at frustrations in their life and personality difficulties. Some individuals may be psychotic, in which case the victims tend to be strangers. Mutilation before death is associated with psychopathy (organized), while mutilation following death (disorganized) is seen among psychotic serial killers, including those with schizophrenia.

Masochism

In DSM-IV, sexual masochism refers to recurrent, intense, sexually arousing fantasies, sexual urges or behaviours involving the act of being humiliated, beaten, bound or otherwise made to suffer. Examples given in DSM-IV include being forced to crawl, being kept in a cage, bondage, being blindfolded, and being whipped, spanked, pinched, beaten, bruised, cut, raped, stabbed or tortured.

In masochism, individuals are aroused by violence to themselves and, indeed, may make others angry with them to this end. *Algolagnia* is the love of pain alone.

Necrophilia

This involves sexual desire for corpses. Described as increased in occurrence among mortuary attendants, it is, in fact, less rare than might be apparent and sometimes occurs following homicide, perhaps in a manner akin to when elephants indulge in sexual intercourse with fellow elephants who have died, as if to bring them back to life. To protect the relatives of victims, such behaviour is often not revealed in court.

Autoerotic asphyxia (hypoxyphilia or asphyxiophilia)

This relates to the enhancement of orgasm by reducing oxygen intake, for example by using a noose around the neck. Such behaviour is associated with the risk of fatality, which in turn may be the first indication to others of such behaviour. Partial drowning has also been described.[38]

Other paraphilias

Coprophilia is the sexual gratification from the sight of or contact with (e.g. by smearing) faeces. *Coprophagia* is the ingesting of faeces. The presence of either usually reflects a very low self-esteem. *Urophilia* or *undinism* (from the Greek for 'water spirit' or 'nymph') includes being urinated on (*urolognia* – 'golden shower'), the drinking of urine and urinating during sexual relations. Such practices are referred to as 'water sports'. In *urethralism*, objects are inserted into the urethra, which may include a liking for catheterization (*catheterophilia*). In *klismaphilia*, rectal enemas are used. These paraphilias are included under the DSM-IV category 302.9 Paraphilias not otherwise specified (NOS).

Vampirism includes sexual gratification at the sight of and contact with blood. Vampirism and *cannibalism* have been reviewed.[39]

Infundibulation or *stigmatophilia* includes the boring of holes, body-piercing and the wearing of rings through the skin. An example is the insertion of the so-called 'Prince Albert ring' through the penis, which is said to intensify the effects of masturbation.

Apotemnophilia refers to sexual preference for being an amputee. It may lead to individuals, known as 'wannabes', disabling or injuring themselves. *Acrotomophobia* is a paraphilia dependent upon a partner being an amputee. This corresponds to those known as 'devotees'. These two paraphilias should be contrasted with *amputee identity disorder* (AID), in which individuals are referred to as 'needtobes'.

Pygmalionism is the sexual preference for objects in the form of people.

In *vogueing*, individuals dress up as a celebrity, such as Elvis Presley or Madonna.

Trashcanners take objects from celebrities' dustbins, including for sexual purposes.

The digital age has heralded *cybersex* and *teledildonics*.

Other paraphilias include *narratophilia* (listening to accounts of sexual activity), *gerontophilia* (sexual gratification from an elderly partner), *hybristophilia* (sexual gratification from a person who has committed a crime), and *chrematistophilia* (being charged for or forced to pay for sex, or being robbed by the sexual partner).

Some individuals are described as being *polymorphous perverse*, in that they have an infantile sexual development and may be aroused by multiple stimuli, such as the wind, and in turn may present with a history of a number of apparent paraphilic behaviours and, indeed, may sexually offend in a number of ways. King has described a case where an individual was aroused by his own sneezing and by the sneezing of others, the sneezing being conceptualized as a fetishistic interest.[40]

Hypersexuality

This is sometimes referred to as *nymphomania* or *satyriasis*. There is a much wider range of sexual drive between individuals than is acknowledged in society. However, only very rarely is hypersexuality due to high testosterone levels. It can be associated with high levels of tension and anxiety.

RELATED OFFENCES

Incest

This is when an individual has a sexual relationship with a first-degree relative and is aware of this. Sibling incest may be the most common form of incest, but father–daughter incest is most reported to authorities and may often be associated with collusion of the mother to prevent unwanted sexual advances. Such behaviour has been classified into three types: endogamic, paedophilic, and promiscuous. It is said to be associated within families where there is overcrowding and poor personal boundaries.[41–43]

Prostitution

Prostitution itself is not an offence, but soliciting and keeping a brothel are offences. Economic motives are commonly given as a rationalization for prostitution, and the financial rewards can be high. However, prostitutes as a group show an excess of mental disorder, self-harm, alcohol or drug abuse, physical disorders, personality disorders and bisexuality and are more likely to have been sexually abused.

Pornography

This is sometimes cited in court as the primary cause of a sexual offence. In reality this is rarely so, but pornography is used more often by people with personality disorder or paraphilias.

Sexual acts and aggression

Where aggression accompanies sexual acts, it can clinically be useful to conceptualize the act along a continuum, as shown in Figure 47.3. The link between sex and violence may theoretically be through the limbic system and testosterone.

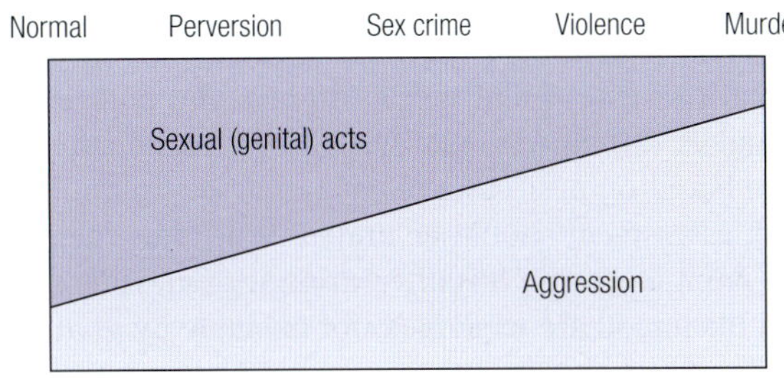

Figure 47.3 Relationship between sexual acts and aggression

ASSESSMENT OF PARAPHILIAS

Referrals for assessment may be due to the following:

- *Formal referral by authorities following law involvement:* such individuals may have limited, if any, motivation to change. They may already be serving a custodial sentence.
- *Individual's distress caused by their paraphilia:* these individuals may fear that their behaviour will impair their health, career or result in law involvement. Such individuals may vary in the degree to which they wish to develop normal sexual desires and behaviours.
- *Distress of the individual's partner caused by the paraphilic behaviour:* such individuals may, in turn, be concerned at their partner's reaction.
- *Sexual dysfunction:* e.g. erectile difficulties, secondary to paraphilias or reliance on paraphilias for arousal, e.g. fetishistic objects. The individual's partner may also be concerned at the resulting sexual dysfunction and wish for help to this end.
- *Gender identity disorder.*

Clinical risk assessment

Sexual fantasies and impulses will need to be explored, but this may not always be easy.

Freud referred to individuals not telling the truth in the area of sexuality.[44] It is important to determine whether the fantasies or impulses are egosyntonic or egodystonic. It is also important to establish whether there has been an escalation in behaviours, for example to attempt and act out the fantasies. It is important to establish whether fantasies are about specific known individuals, and whether the fantasies involve consent or force. The relationship, if any, of paraphilic behaviour to alcohol consumption, drug abuse or the use of pornography needs to be established.

Information-gathering should include talking to informants such as the person's partner. In the case of sexual offenders, depositions or statements should be considered, usually available only in the cases of serious sexual offences before a Crown Court, along with a list of previous convictions and social enquiry reports for the court prepared by probation officers. Previous psychiatric records and, when relevant, general practice records should be obtained and formal psychiatric disorder confirmed or excluded.

Clinical risk assessment is open to bias and poor consistency and is difficult to qualify. It is often inductive, for example based on past cases or cases that went wrong.

A risk assessment should be undertaken,[45] but categorizing risk from low to high is often arbitrary unless its meaning and likelihood are explained, for example by giving the immediacy, frequency or consequences of risk.

Standardized structured risk assessments

Formal psychological testing, for example with the Thorne Sex Inventory, may assist. For sex offenders, actuarial risk assessment instruments that look at static risk factors such as age, number and type of previous offences, type of victim and history of cohabitation, such as STATIC-99[46] and Risk Matrix 2000,[47] are objective, unbiased and deductive, but they are only moderately predictive and first offenders score less. The Risk Matrix 2000 categorizes sexual and violent offenders from low to very high risk. However, instruments that look at dynamic (changeable) risk factors, both relatively stable, such as personality factors (e.g. STABLE 2007), and acute (e.g. ACUTE-2007), can assist professional judgement further. Other examples include Sexual Violence Risk-20 (SVR-20),[48] Risk of Sexual Violence Protocol (RSVP)[49] and Sexual Assessment of Risk and Need (SARN).[50] The SARN is useful in developing treatment plans and measuring change.

Penile plethysmography or phallometry

Penile plethysmography or phallometry with the subject's consent may elicit deviant arousal patterns, for example to children or rape, and may counter the tendency of sex offenders to denial or self-report errors. Penile plethysmography, however, tends to be less reliable in institutions compared with in the community, where there may be more stimuli to paraphilic interests and behaviours.

Polygraph as lie detector

This has been found to be useful in countering denial among paedophiles in the community, for example revealing more high-risk behaviours such as unsupervised contact with children than is apparent from the history given by the individual.[51]

Management

The aims of management need to be realistic and, ideally, the goals agreed with the individual. Elimination of the paraphilia is often not possible, but control is more often achieved. Attempts to remove or reduce paraphilias usually require the enhancement of other outlets. In general, individuals with a stable personality, who are well motivated and who have some past adult sexual fantasies or experience, do best. However, motivation may be difficult to assess when an individual is under the stress of a forthcoming court appearance and facing custody. There are no good controlled trials of long-term as opposed to short-term treatment for people with paraphilias, particularly if they have committed sexual offences. In addition, negative countertransference among professionals may lead to rejection from treatment.

Regarding sex offenders, 80 per cent do not re-offend once first convicted, but it is the recidivist who seeks or is sent for treatment. However, if an individual has committed more than two sexual offences and has had no adult sexual experience, then one must assume that the offending will continue. The deterrent effect of the law may be more effective than treatment, although Home Office statistics suggest that recidivism rates among sexual offenders released from prison are less compared with those of other offenders during the first 2 years (16% *v.* 56%). However, long-term follow-up studies of sexual offenders indicate more pessimistic outcomes.[52]

In prison, paedophiles may be subject to more victimization compared with rapists. Sex offenders are often scapegoated, even by those who have committed rape or homicide, and this may relate to the psychodynamics of being in single-sex custodial institutions. Since the introduction of the Criminal Justice Act 1991, sex offenders may be subject to indeterminate supervision.

Any intercurrent mental illness should be treated. Coexisting problems such as social anxiety, social skills deficits, poor sex education and marital difficulties should be tackled, but it is unlikely that this alone will stop paraphilias or associated sexual offending. Individuals often present requesting to be made to stop their paraphilic behaviour, when really they need to be made to *want* to stop.

Psychodynamic approaches, as described by Zachery,[53] by both individual and group therapy (e.g. at the Portman Clinic in north London) have been attempted, but the stress of such therapy may in some individuals increase the risk in the short term of offending due to acting out and perhaps by the inducement of guilt, leading to them being more readily apprehended.

There is a stronger evidence base for cognitive-behavioural approaches. Nagayam-Hall showed that of those sexual offenders who completed a CBT programme, only 19 per cent re-offended, compared with 27 per cent among controls.[54] Cognitive-behavioural approaches include the following:

- *Reduction of deviant sexual arousal:* aversion therapy, including electrical aversion, is now almost never used. It involved repeated pairing of the stimulus for paraphilias, e.g. in the form of visual images, with unpleasant stimuli such as electric shocks. In covert sensitization, the aversion is imaginal: for example, the individual is asked to fantasize about their paraphilic behaviour and then to imagine an aversive scene, e.g. the attendance of a police officer or others observing the act.[55]
- *Increasing non-deviant sexual arousal:* this may be undertaken by masturbatory orgasmic reconditioning,[56]

in which there is reinforcement of non-paraphilic arousal and desires by asking the individual to switch to fantasies of conventional sexual stimuli when orgasm is imminent as a result of masturbating to paraphilic fantasies – that is, an attempt is made to pair arousal with normal sexuality. The point of switching to conventional fantasies is gradually brought forward. The goal is that the entire episode takes place to non-paraphilic fantasies. Another technique is *fading* or *satiational therapy*.[57] In this the individual is instructed to fantasize and masturbate to the paraphilic act for extended periods, perhaps up to an hour, as a result of which it is theorized that satiation to the paraphilia should take place. More controversially, *surrogate therapy* has been used to increase non-deviant sexual arousal.
- *Self-control training:* CBT approaches can be used to clarify and modify faulty cognitions, e.g. that the victim enjoyed it, to enhance empathy for the victims, and to learn to avoid high-risk situations.
- *Partial incorporation of paraphilia to sexual repertoire:* this is practical only if the paraphilia is acceptable and legal, as would not be the case in paedophilia, and something that the individual's partner can tolerate. Individual sessions with the partner may need to be undertaken in order to establish this; thereafter, the couple may be helped to reduce the role of the paraphilia in their sexual relationship, e.g. in a leather fetish, leather worn may be reduced to merely an armband. A negotiated timetable approach may also lead to temporal control, e.g. to certain days of the week for the paraphilia.[58] Success with such an approach has also been described in people with fetishism.[59]

Sex offender treatment programmes have been developed for both those in the community and those in prison. They involve, usually in group work, understanding offence cycles, challenging distorted cognitions (e.g. paedophiles believing that they satisfy children's natural sexual urges), understanding the harm done to the victim, fantasy modification, social skills training, anger management control and relapse prevention work. Booster programmes, for example pre-release from custody, may be required.

Evaluation of such programmes has differentiated high-risk from low-risk offenders, with high-risk offenders being characterized by social inadequacy, lack of empathy for victims, distorted thinking, increased sexual obsessions and abnormal emotional congruence, leading to distorted emotional attachment, for example to children.[60,61]

The psychological management of child sexual abusers and high-risk sexual offenders has been well detailed by Craissati.[62,63]

Anti-libidinal treatment

Anti-libidinal treatment reduces sexual drive but is not concerned with the direction of that drive. It is, therefore, most effective when sexual activity is directed towards orgasm but least effective when such activity is directed primarily to forming a relationship, for example in some paedophiles, where anti-libidinal treatment may not affect re-offending rates. Anti-libidinal treatment may suppress both 'normal' sexual drive and paraphilic interests, and individuals may fear losing their sexuality as a result of such treatment. An unspoken fear of prisoners in general is that medication may result in loss of libido.

Castration has never been used as an anti-libidinal treatment in the UK. Oestrogens have been used in the past, but these have severe feminizing effects. *Benperidol* is a major tranquillizer that may not be any more effective than other such neuroleptic medications in reducing sex drive, but it has the advantage of avoiding the need for the detailed written consent and the pretreatment work-up required with cyproterone acetate.

More recently, *selective serotonin reuptake inhibitor (SSRI) antidepressants* have been used as a first-line medication treatment where preoccupation and rumination over the paraphilic behaviour are apparent, for example with exhibitionism. The evidence base, however, is case studies and small open trials of such antidepressants. Most used and reported is fluoxetine.

Medroxyprogesterone acetate is widely used in the USA. It induces the liver enzyme testosterone A reductase, leading to increased metabolism and reduced plasma testosterone levels. There are also antigonadotropic effects.

Cyproterone acetate is used more widely in the UK, Europe and Canada. It specifically blocks androgen effects and has an antigonadotropic action. It inhibits the production of testosterone by enzyme block, competitively antagonizes testosterone, acts on the hypothalamic centre and is progestrogenic. The usual dose is 50 mg orally twice daily, but an injection is also available from Germany. Indications include hypersexuality (including for females), indecent exposure and unwanted sexual fantasies. It has also been used in aggression in severe learning disability, and as a male contraceptive in small doses. It does not work if sexual behaviour is associated with alcohol abuse. It has some effect within 48 h and reduces sexual drive after 10–14 days. There is a reduction in spermatogenesis (oligospermia) and loss of ejaculation. It reduces sexual thoughts and behaviour.[64] Unwanted effects include gynaecomastia in 10–15 per cent of patients, which often remits, especially if it is not extensive, when treatment stops. Previous concerns about inducing breast cancer have been discounted. There may be loss of body hair with prolonged treatment. Occasionally depression is seen in the third week, and sometimes there is habituation requiring an increased dose. The effects are reversible, although this takes some months. Some patients retain erections and sex drive in spite of high doses. In the testes, germinal cells are reversibly damaged (seminiferous tubular arrest – fertility is preserved) and Leydig cells are irreversibly damaged.

Before treatment, it is essential to conduct a full physical examination, obtain written consent and undertake liver function tests, sperm count and testosterone levels as baselines, including to counter any subsequent litigation, especially where the medication is blamed for infertility.

Goserelin is a luteinizing hormone releasing hormone (LHRH) analogue. It is licensed only for treatment of cancer of the prostate and breast, but it may be effective as an anti-libidinal treatment in patients resistant to cyproterone acetate.

Hormone treatments are emotive, but if psychological treatments do not work and serious sexual re-offending is certain (e.g. high-risk offenders leaving prison after a custodial sentence), then their use appears justified. However, those people most in need of treatment may not consent. Some treated individuals who re-offend blame their medical practitioners for inadequately treating them with doses that are too low. Some individuals cite the resulting lack of sex drive as a cause of increased subsequent aggression.

LEGISLATION RELEVANT TO SEX OFFENDERS IN ENGLAND AND WALES

The public and media concern that something must be done to better manage sex offenders has led to new legal initiatives in recent years in England and Wales and, indeed, elsewhere.

The *Criminal Justice Act 1991* has resulted in sex offenders receiving longer sentences and longer periods on licence than otherwise would have been the case in order to protect the public from serious harm.

The *Crime (Sentences) Act 1997* introduced a mandatory life sentence for a second serious offence, such as rape, attempted rape or sex with a girl under 13 years.

The *Sex Offenders Act 1997* specifies that offenders must notify the police of their name, date of birth and address and any changes of address, not only if they are convicted of a sexual offence but also if they are cautioned, unfit to plead or not guilty by reason of insanity, and whether the individual is in hospital or prison, on penalty of a fine or up to 6 months' imprisonment. Under this Act, a defendant can face trial even if the offence occurred abroad.

Under the *Crime and Disorder Act 1998*, the police can apply for a sex offences prevention order (SOPO) to prohibit an individual from being in certain areas at specified times (e.g. children's playgrounds), if (i) the individual has been previously convicted or cautioned for a sexual offence, or (ii) the individual is behaving in a way that suggests the public is at serious risk of harm.

Extended sentences under *Section 85 of the Powers of the Criminal Courts (Sentencing) Act 2000* have been introduced 'to protect the public from serious harm from the offender' (violent or sexual). There are two components: a standard custodial term and an extended period of licence, up to 10 years for a sexual offence and 5 years for a violent offence.

The *Criminal Justice Act 2003* introduced 'indeterminate sentences for public protection' in respect of high-risk offenders, a measure equivalent to a life sentence. This Act also described Schedule 15 offences, which supercedes the *Children and Young Persons' Act 1993* Schedule 1 offences, includes all offences against children up to the age of 17 years. The management of such offenders is covered by guidance from the Home Office for interagency cooperation.

Following the *Criminal Justice and Court Services Act 2000*, under Sections 67 and 68, multi-agency public protection arrangements (MAPPAs), in force since 2001, have placed a legal responsibility on the police and probation services to assess and manage those at risk of serious harm to others, including sex offenders, with a duty on psychiatrists to cooperate with this.

Dangerous severe personality disorder (DSPD) units in special hospitals such as Rampton and Broadmoor hospitals and in prisons such as HMP Frankland and HMP Whitmoor in England have also taken individuals who are primarily sexual offenders, such as paedophiles.

CONCLUSIONS

It is important to remember that paraphilias may be non-problematic and may not lead to sexual offending, and that only a small proportion of individuals with paraphilias are referred for psychiatric assessment and help, including because such individuals may not be motivated to change. On the other hand, individuals with paraphilias may present with sexual and marital dysfunction, depression and anxiety without acknowledging the underlying paraphilia. In addition, paraphilias may not be eliminated by treatment, and only control may be achievable – hence the importance of realistic agreed goals with a patient presenting with a paraphilia.

KEY POINTS

- Paraphilias (DSM-IV) or disorders of sexual preference are persistently preferred to normal adult sexual behaviour.
- Primary (fixed) paraphilias should be distinguished from facultative deviation due to unavailability of normal sexual outlets and from latent perversion (regressed) that follows stress (e.g. marital conflict, disinhibition by alcohol or drugs) or is released by mental illness.
- Although paraphilias can result in sexual and marital dysfunction, depression and anxiety, only a small proportion of people with paraphilias are ever referred to psychiatrists.
- Not all paraphilic behaviours are against the law, and not all sexual offenders have a disorder of sexual preference.
- The most common sexual offence is indecent exposure, which is associated with the paraphilia of exhibitionism. Most such offenders are inhibited, non-violent young men who do not re-offend once

convicted. A few are more psychopathic and become sexually aroused by exhibitionism.

- Paraphilias may not be eliminated by treatment, and only control may be achievable. Cognitive-behavioural approaches have been found to be most effective.
- Standard structured risk assessments that assess static and dynamic risk factors in sex offenders (e.g. SVR-20, RSVP, SARN) can supplement clinical risk assessment and are better than actuarial risk assessments alone (e.g. Static-99, Risk Matrix 2000).
- Penile plethysmography and the use of a polygraph as a lie detector may assist in the management of sex offenders.
- Anti-libidinal medication, for example cyproterone acetate, reduces sexual drive but is not concerned with the direction of that drive. It is most effective when sexual activity is directed towards orgasm but least effective when such activity is directed primarily to forming a relationship, such as in some paedophiles. Anti-libidinal treatment may not affect re-offending rates.

REFERENCES

1. Kinsey AC, Pomeroy WB, Martin CE (1948) *Sexual Behaviour in the Human Male*. Philadelphia, PA: W.B. Saunders.
2. Kinsey AC, Pomeroy WB, Martin CE (1953) *Sexual Behaviour in the Human Female*. Philadelphia, PA: W.B. Saunders.
3. Ford CS, Beach FA (1951) *Patterns of Sexual Behavior*. New York: Harper.
4. Von Krafft-Ebing R (1965) *Psychopathia Sexualis* (transl. FS Klaf). New York: Putnam.
5. Scott PD (1964) Definition, classification, prognosis and treatment. In I Rosen (ed.) *The Pathology and Treatment of Sexual Deviation*. Oxford: Oxford University Press.
6. American Psychiatric Association (1994) *Diagnostic and Statistical Manual of Mental Disorders*, 4th edn. Washington, DC: American Psychiatric Association.
7. World Health Organization (1992) *ICD-10 Classifications of Mental and Behavioural Disorders: Clinical Descriptions and Diagnostic Guidelines*. Geneva: World Health Organization.
8. Kallman FJ (1952) Study on the genetic effects of male homosexuality. *Journal of Nervous and Mental Disorders* **115**: 1283–98.
9. Eckert ED, Bouchard TJ, Bohlen J, Heston LL (1986) Homosexuality in monozygotic twins reared apart. *British Journal of Psychiatry* **148**: 421–5.
10. Bailey JM, Pillard RC (1991) A genetic study of male sexual orientation. *Archives of General Psychiatry* **48**: 1089–96.
11. Hamer DH, Hu S, Magnuson VL, *et al.* (1993) A linkage between DNA markers on the X chromosome and male sexual orientation. *Science* **261**: 321–7.
12. Flor-Henry P (1987) Cerebral aspects of sexual deviation. In G Wilson (ed.) *Variant Sexuality*. London: Croom Helm.
13. Harris GW, Levine S (1962) Sexual differentiation of the brain and its experimental control. *Journal of Physiology* **163**: 42–3.
14. Harlow HF (1965) Sexual behaviour in the rhesus monkey. In FA Beach (ed.) *Sex and Behaviour*. New York: John Wiley & Sons.
15. Rachman S (1966) Sexual fetishisms: an experimental analogue. *Psychological Record* **16**: 293–6.
16. Welldon E, Mother M (1988) *Whore: The Ideation and Denigration of Motherhood*. Lawson: Free Association Books.
17. Randell J (1970) Transvestism and transsexualism. *British Journal of Hospital Medicine* **3**: 211.
18. Prince V, Bentler P (1972) Survey of 504 cases of transvestism. *Psychological Reports* **31**: 903–17.
19. Rooth FG (1975) Indecent exposure and exhibitionism. In T Silverstone, B Barraclough (eds) *Contemporary Psychiatry*. Ashford: Headley Brothers.
20. Rooth FG (1973) Exhibitionism, sexual violence and paedophilia. *British Journal of Psychiatry* **122**: 105–10.
21. Rooth FG (1980) Exhibitionism: an eclectic approach to its management. *British Journal of Hospital Medicine* **49**: 366–70.
22. McConghy N (1998) Paedophilia: a review of the evidence. *Australian and New Zealand Journal of Psychiatry* **32**: 252–65.
23. Finkelhor D (1998) *A Source Book on Child Sexual Abuse*. Beverley Hills, CA: Saga Publications.
24. Wilkins R (1990) Women who sexually abuse children. *British Medical Journal* **300**: 1153–4.
25. Saradjian J (1996) *Women Who Sexually Abuse Children: From Research to Clinical Practice*. Chichester: John Wiley & Sons.
26. Sturup GK (1971) Castration: the total treatment. In RLP Resnik, ME Wolfgang (eds) *Sexual Behaviours*. Boston, MA: Little, Brown.
27. West DJ (2000) Paedophilia: plague or panic. *Journal of Forensic Psychiatry* **11**: 511–31.
28. Muller PE (1993) Child sexual abuse and mental health: the development of disorders. *Journal of Interpersonal Violence* **8**: 429.
29. Groth AN, Burgess AW, Holmstrom LL (1988) Rape, power, anger and sexuality. *American Journal of Psychiatry* **134**: 1239–43.
30. West DJ (1978) *Understanding Sexual Attacks*. London: Heinemann.
31. Gibbens TCN, Way C, Soothill KL (1977) Behavioural types of rape. *British Journal of Psychiatry* **130**: 32–42.
32. Smith AD, Taylor PJ (1999) Serious sex offending against women by men with schizophrenia: relationship of illness and psychotic symptoms to offending. *British Journal of Psychiatry* **174**: 222–37.
33. Soothill K, Gibbons T (1978) Recidivism of sexual offenders: a reappraisal. *British Journal of Criminology* **18**: 267–76.

34. Bergman P (1947) Analysis of an unusual case of fetishism. *Bulletin of the Meninger Clinic* **11**: 69–75.
35. Brittain RP (1970) The sadistic murderer. *Medicine, Science and the Law* **10**: 198–207.
36. MacCulloch MJ, Snowden P, Wood P, Mills H (1983) Sadistic fantasy, sadistic behaviour and offending. *British Journal of Psychiatry* **143**: 20–29.
37. Grubin D (1994) Sexual murder. *British Journal of Psychiatry* **165**: 624–9.
38. Sivaloganathan S (1984) Aqua-eroticum: a case of auto-erotic drowning. *Medicine, Science and the Law* **24**: 300–302.
39. Fahy T, Wessley S, David A (1998) Werewolves, vampires and cannibals. *Medicine, Science and the Law* **28**: 145–9.
40. King MB (1990) Sneezing as a fetish object. *Sex Marital Therapy* **5**: 69–72.
41. Batten DA (1983) Incest: a review of the literature. *Medicine, Science and the Law* **23**: 245–53.
42. Gibbens TCN, Soothill KL, Way CK (1978) Sibling and parent child incest offenders. *British Journal of Criminology* **18**: 40–52.
43. Lukianovicz N (1972) Incest. *British Journal of Psychiatry* **120**: 301–13.
44. Freud S (1953) Three essays on the theory of sexuality 1905. In J Strachey (ed) *The Standard Edition of the Complete Works of Sigmund Freud*, Vol. 7. London: Hogarth Press.
45. Fisher D, Thornton A (1993) Assessing risk of re-offending in sexual offenders. *Journal of Mental Health* **2**: 105–17.
46. Hanson RK, Thornton D (2000) Improving risk assessments for sex offenders: a comparison of three actuarial scales. *Law on Human Behaviour* **24**: 119–36.
47. Thornton D, Mann R, Webster S, *et al.* (2003) Distinguishing and combining risks for sexual and violent recidivism. *Annals of the New York Academy of Science* **989**: 225–35.
48. Boer D, Hart S, Kropp R, Webster C (1998) *Manual for the Sexual Violence Risk-20: Professional Guidelines for Assessing Risk of Sexual Violence.* Lutz, FL: Psychological Assessment Resources.
49. Hart S, Kropp R, Laws R, *et al.* (2003) *The Risk for Sexual Violence Protocol (RSVP): Structured Professional Guidelines for Assessing Risk for Sexual Violence.* Burnaby, BC: Mental Health, Law, and Policy Institute, Simon Fraser University.
50. Webster SD, Mann RE, Carter AJ, *et al.* (2005) Inter-rater reliability of dynamic risk assessment with sexual offenders. *Psychology and Criminal Law* **12**: 439–52.
51. Grubin D, Madsen L, Parsons S, Sosnowski D, Warberg B (2004) A prospective study of the impact of polygraphy on high risk behaviours in adult sex offenders. *Sex abuse Journal Research Treatment* **16**: 209–22.
52. Soothill K, Gibbons T (1978) Recidivism of sexual offenders: a reappraisal. *British Journal of Criminology* **18**: 267–76.
53. Zachery A (1998) Individual psychoanalytical psychotherapy with perpetrators of sexual abuse. *Advances in Psychiatric Treatment* **4**: 77–81.
54. Nagayama-Hall JC (1995) Sexual offender recidivism revisited: a metanalysis of recent treatment studies. *Journal of Consulting and Clinical Psychology* **63**: 802–9.
55. Cautela JR, Wisocki PA (1971) Covert sensitization for treatment of sexual deviations. *Psychological Record* **21**: 37–48.
56. Marquis JM (1970) Orgasmic reconditioning: changing sexual object choice through controlling masturbation fantasies. *Journal of Behavior Therapy and Experimental Psychiatry* **1**: 263–71.
57. Marshall WL (1979) Satiation therapy: a procedure for reducing deviant sexual arousal. *Journal of Applied Behavior Analysis* **12**: 10–22.
58. Crowe MJ, Ridley J (2000) *Therapy with Couples.* Oxford: Blackwell.
59. De Silva P (1995) Paraphilias and sexual dysfunction. *International Review of Psychiatry* **7**: 225–9.
60. Barker M, Morgan R (1993) *Sex Offenders: A Framework for Valuation of Community-Based Treatment.* London: HMSO.
61. Beckett R, Beech A, Fisher D, Fordham AS (1994) *Community-Based Treatment for Sex Offenders: An Evaluation of Seven Treatment Programmes.* London: HMSO.
62. Craissati J (1998) *Child Sexual Abusers: A Community Treatment Approach.* Hove: Taylor & Francis.
63. Craissati J (2004) *Managing High Risk Sexual Offenders in the Community: A Psychological Approach.* Hove: Brunner/Routledge.
64. Bancroft J, Tennent TG, Loucas K, Cass J (1974) The control of deviant sexual behaviour by drugs: behavioural change following oestrogens and antiandrogens. *British Journal of Psychiatry* **125**: 310–15.

Chapter 48

Psychiatric assessment of physical illness

Geoffrey Lloyd

INTRODUCTION

Physical and psychiatric illnesses are so inextricably interrelated[1,2] that the ability to assess the mental state of physically ill patients is an essential skill required by all clinicians.[3] The development of a physical illness, either acute or long-term, substantially increases the likelihood of a wide range of psychiatric disorders, which add considerably to the level of disability and which may worsen the prognosis of the physical condition.[4]

BACKGROUND INFORMATION

Knowledge of the nature of the physical illness, its severity, its prognosis and the response to treatment is essential. Clinicians in primary and secondary care are usually well aware of these details. For a psychiatrist who is asked to assess a physically ill patient, it is necessary to discover as much as possible about the underlying illness from the referring doctor and from other sources, such as the medical notes and correspondence from the general practitioner (GP). These may also provide evidence of previous psychiatric disorders or episodes of deliberate self-harm. It is important to know whether the patient is currently in contact with a mental health service. There may be evidence of family and social problems which could influence the patient's response to the illness and create difficulty when planning discharge from hospital. The medical diagnosis, if established, must be understood, and it is important to know the severity of the condition. For example, in cases of cancer, is there evidence of metastatic spread or is the disease localized and likely to be cured completely? In neurological disorders, it should be established whether there is cerebral involvement that could cause generalized intellectual impairment or whether there is a discrete lesion giving rise to specific neuropsychiatric disorders such as dysphasia and amnesia. It should be established with the medical team whether the patient is aware of the diagnosis and prognosis. Current practice usually involves an open discussion of the medical condition but, despite having been fully informed, some patients deny any knowledge of their condition and may use denial as a protective shield.

Investigations

The clinical findings should be reviewed in the light of results of available investigations. Laboratory results should be scrutinized for evidence of metabolic disturbance (urea, electrolytes, liver function tests), endocrine abnormalities (particularly thyroxine, thyroid-stimulating hormone (TSH) and cortisol levels) and infection (raised erythrocyte sedimentation rate (ESR) and C-reactive protein (CRP)). Elevated figures for γ-glutamyltransferase (GGT) and mean corpuscular volume (MCV) are sometimes the first indicators of hazardous alcohol consumption. Computed tomography (CT) and magnetic resonance imaging (MRI) results should be reviewed for evidence of localized cerebral pathology or diffuse changes as are seen in the dementias.

Treatment

The drug chart must be examined to establish which drugs the patient has been taking recently and is currently being prescribed. Many medically prescribed drugs have adverse psychiatric side effects,[5] which include anxiety, depression, mania, delirium and isolated psychotic experiences. Corticosteroids are among the best-recognized culprits, but other potential causes include adrenergic antagonists, anticonvulsants, antiparkinsonian drugs and anti-retrovirals. An adverse psychiatric reaction to a drug can be diagnosed with some confidence if the reaction follows closely after the administration of the drug and resolves on stopping the drug. There may be a history of a similar response when the drug was administered previously.

Other treatments should also be noted, including previous and proposed operations, radiotherapy and bone-marrow transplantation. The wider treatment environment is also important. Many people feel threatened by the high-technology environment of an intensive care unit (ICU) or high dependency unit (HDU).[6] Isolation is another source of stress and can contribute to the development of anxiety, depression and psychotic disorders in patients being treated for severe infections or following immunosuppression.

Reason for referral

The psychiatrist should establish what particular issues the referring medical team want to be addressed. These include a diagnostic opinion, assessing suicidal risk, advice on medication and adherence to treatment regimes, help in managing challenging behaviours, and establishing whether the patient has capacity to consent or withhold consent to treatment that is considered medically necessary. The psychiatrist should confirm that the patient is aware of the referral and has agreed to an assessment by a psychiatrist.

PRIVACY AND COMMUNICATION

Ideally, all psychiatric assessments should be conducted in privacy, either in the patient's home, in an out-patient office or in a side room of a medical ward. However, a single room cannot always be obtained, and in hospital the interview sometimes has to be conducted by the bedside in an open ward if the patient is too ill to be moved. If this is the case, then it is preferable for the interview to be conducted with the curtains drawn around the bed.

If the patient is not fluent in English, a translator should be arranged. Most hospital trusts now have a panel of available translators covering a wide range of languages likely to be encountered in the area. In my opinion, it is better to involve a professional translator rather than a relative, at least in the first instance. If the translator is familiar with the patient's cultural background, then the translator may be able to advise the clinician of particular cultural beliefs concerning health, illness, healthcare and treatment that may impinge on the patient's mental state and coping abilities. Several of these beliefs stem from religious teaching. In a culturally diverse society, a clinician needs to know as much as possible about the different ways in which people interpret bodily symptoms and the need for treatment.

Many illnesses are associated with communication problems, and the clinician should be aware of these so that special provision can be made. For patients with visual impairment, the interviewer should avoid sitting with a source of light behind him or her. The source of light should be on the interviewer's face, and eye contact must be established as far as possible. Written information must be given in a large font. For patients with hearing difficulties, the clinician should speak clearly but avoid shouting. The clinician should face the patient when speaking and use simple sign language where appropriate. Providing written information is very helpful. Similar considerations apply if there are communication problems due to dysphasia, dysarthria or cognitive impairment. Speech is impossible for patients who are treated in an ICU or HDU and who are being ventilated via endotracheal intubation. In these circumstances, only a limited assessment can be undertaken, and it will be necessary to use closed rather than open-ended questions, with printed cards giving the patient the opportunity to give 'yes' or 'no' answers.

THE HISTORY

In most cases, the history is taken in much the same manner as in any psychiatric assessment. This includes the family background, noting especially any family history of psychiatric and medical illnesses that may have a genetic component, and the patient's developmental and personal history. A tactful enquiry about childhood abuse should be made. Sexual abuse in childhood is now established as a predisposing factor for several psychiatric disorders in adult life, including the functional somatic syndromes that are seen so commonly in medical practice. Previous medical illnesses must be discussed, with emphasis on how the patient coped with them and whether they were associated with psychological symptoms. Frequent attendance at a GP's surgery for minor or unexplained symptoms raises the possibility of a somatization syndrome. The onset and evolution of the current physical illness should be established before proceeding to determine how the patient has coped with the symptoms, functional disability and the need for treatment.

Coping styles

Coping strategies in the face of illness usually reflect coping styles that have been developed since childhood, but it must be remembered that coping is a dynamic and flexible process, changing with time and with the varying demands of the illness. It is when the usual coping strategies break down that serious psychiatric problems emerge.[7,8] All illnesses except the very trivial involve some degree of adjustment of lifestyle, including the fundamental decisions of whether to seek medical advice, agree to treatment, take time off work and curtail leisure activities. In the case of chronic illnesses, these lifestyle changes may have to be permanent, and the illness is then perceived as involving a loss of status, income, ambition or social supports.

Some people cope with illness by finding out as much information about the illness as possible by consulting medical books and websites; they involve themselves closely with the treatment regime and are often critical of what they perceive as medical ambiguity or shortcomings. Others, in contrast, cope by distancing themselves from the emotional impact of becoming ill, tending to minimize symptoms and disability and continuing to follow existing or new leisure interests. This strategy reflects a degree of denial. In extreme cases of denial, the coping is maladaptive, in that it leads to rejection of medical advice and treatment and continuation of an unhealthy lifestyle.

Depression and anxiety

Mood changes should be elicited. Was there evidence of anxiety, depression or any other psychiatric disorder before the onset of the physical illness? If so, have the psychological symptoms been affected adversely by the illness and its treatment? If psychological symptoms have developed after the onset of the physical illness, their course and severity should be elicited, particularly whether they fluctuate in parallel with the course of the underlying illness. The patient's understanding of the illness should be discussed. There is not always a close relationship between the severity of the physical illness and the development of a psychiatric disorder. The patient's perception of the illness appears more important. It is therefore important to understand the implications of the illness for the patient's relationships, career prospects, financial circumstances and ability to pursue leisure activities. Sometimes illness is perceived as a punishment, particularly if the patient believes that some aspects of their behaviour have been responsible for causing the illness. The patient may then feel guilty, sometimes with psychotic intensity, which leads to severe depressive reactions for some people. Suicidal ideas need to be explored whenever a depressed mood has been elicited.

Not much emphasis can be placed on somatic symptoms when assessing depression in medically ill patients. Anorexia, weight change, fatigue, reduced libido, sleep disturbance and bodily pains can all be explained by the underlying condition. Diagnostic attention has therefore to be focused on the psychological symptoms that accompany depressed mood, including anhedonia, reduced interest, lack of motivation, guilt, hopelessness and self-blame.

Anxiety is commonly associated with medical illness. It is often related to the illness itself, particularly when there is uncertainty about the diagnosis, treatment or prognosis. Clarity of communication on the part of the multidisciplinary team does much to alleviate this anxiety. Anxiety is a prominent feature of hyperthyroidism, phaeochromocytoma and hypoglycaemia from any cause. In some people, anxiety is related to specific aspects of the medical treatment, such as having intravenous injections or undergoing radiotherapy, or to investigations such as bronchoscopy, colonoscopy or blood tests for human immunodeficiency virus (HIV) infection. In severe cases, the anxiety has a phobic element and leads to avoidance of the medical treatment or investigation. Sedation with a benzodiazepine or cognitive-behaviour therapy is then required to enable treatment to proceed. Episodic anxiety, which is a cardinal feature of panic attacks, is a common reason for medical referral and can create much diagnostic difficulty, particularly when associated with physical conditions such as ischaemic heart disease presenting with chest pain.

Following exceptionally threatening events, such as major accidents, physical assault or natural disasters, symptoms of post-traumatic stress disorder (PTSD) develop in up to one-third of cases. It is important to enquire about recurrent episodes of reliving the trauma through flashbacks or nightmares, together with emotional blunting, hyperarousal, hypervigilance and an avoidance of situations that evoke memories of the original stressor. PTSD is most likely to be diagnosed in patients admitted following road traffic and other major accidents and following serious assault. It has also been described as a response to medical illness[9] and following childbirth[10] when this has been a traumatic experience for the mother. Symptoms of PTSD may emerge up to 6 months after the triggering event, and so the diagnosis has to be considered in patients who have long since been discharged from hospital.

Psychotic symptoms

Psychotic symptoms should be explored. If present, they are usually related to a pre-existing schizophrenic or affective illness. It is important to establish what medication, if any, the patient is taking for these illnesses and to ensure this is maintained during a medical admission, unless there are side effects that necessitate changing to an alternative drug. This should be done in conjunction with the patient's GP or community psychiatrist. The development of psychotic symptoms during the course of a medical illness usually indicates the onset of delirium or, less commonly, an affective disorder. Visual or tactile hallucinations are the most common sensory disturbances. Secondary delusions may be superimposed on these false perceptions. The level of consciousness is impaired, but the symptoms fluctuate, and so a history from nursing staff is essential to chart the course of the delirium.

Body image

Disturbance of body image should be considered in young women when there is a history of weight loss, extreme dieting, binge eating or use of laxatives or purgatives. If associated with amenorrhoea for more than 3 months, these symptoms are indicative of anorexia nervosa. However, it must be remembered that the characteristic drive to become thin and the abnormal eating habits may be denied at a first interview and admitted only when the patient has gained confidence in her doctor. Localized disturbance of body image may be seen in people who request cosmetic surgery for minor physical abnormalities.[11] A psychiatric opinion may be requested before a decision to operate is made. The most common operations requested involve the nose (rhinoplasty), breasts (enlargement or reduction) and ears. Body dysmorphic disorder is characterized by a preoccupation with a perceived defect in appearance that, to an observer, is entirely normal or only slightly abnormal. The person's concern is highly excessive, and there are unrealistic expectations that an operation will resolve the physical problem and all the psychosocial difficulties attributed to it. Surgery is usually contraindicated in these cases.

Cognitive function

A history of progressive cognitive decline involving memory, concentration, orientation, thinking, learning capacity and judgement is highly suggestive of dementia. There may be little insight into these intellectual changes, and so it is important to take a history from a close relative or friend. Difficulty coping at work, problems with driving, and loss of social skills may all be described by the informant. Executive function involves the ability to plan, initiate and organize behaviour in general and certain tasks in particular. Loss of executive function suggests frontal lobe pathology.

In the context of an acute medical illness, reports of drowsiness, impaired concentration and disorientation indicate the possibility of delirium due to infection, drugs or metabolic upset. The patient may be unaware of these problems, and so reliance has to be placed on accounts from relatives and nursing staff who are in close contact with the patient.

Alcohol misuse

The association between alcohol misuse and medical problems is so well established that screening for problem drinking is a routine part of a medical assessment, but the psychiatrist may need to amplify what a primary care or hospital doctor has already established. Alcohol-related problems comprise a substantial proportion of the clinical work in all departments of a general hospital,[12] with accident and emergency departments having a particularly high prevalence.[13] Consumption of alcohol is increasing in the UK, and so alcohol-related medical admissions are likely to continue rising for the foreseeable future.[14,15] Early detection is crucial if permanent damage is to be avoided.[16]

The following clinical presentations are particularly likely to be associated with alcohol misuse:

- *Deliberate self-harm:* drug overdose, self-cutting, jumping from a height, attempted drowning
- *Trauma:* road traffic accidents, falls, assaults
- *Cardiovascular:* hypertension, arrhythmias, cardiomyopathy
- *Gastrointestinal:* dyspepsia, gastritis, haematemesis, diarrhoea, malabsorption, pancreatitis, fatty liver, acute hepatitis, cirrhosis
- *Neurological:* stroke, peripheral neuropathy, withdrawal fits, Wernicke–Korsakoff syndrome, cerebellar ataxia, dementia
- *Musculoskeletal:* myopathy, osteoporosis, gout
- *Malignancies:* oropharynx, oesophagus, liver, colon, breast, lung
- *Haematological:* bleeding disorders, thrombocytopenia, neutropenia
- *Dermatological:* multiple bruising, psoriasis, increased capillarization of facial skin, acne rosacea
- *Respiratory:* aspiration pneumonia, rib fractures, pneumothorax
- *Others:* impotence, infertility, obesity, diabetes.

A careful account of the patient's drinking habits should be recorded. It is useful to ask about a typical week's consumption and maximum weekly consumption. Alcohol intake is calculated in units, 1 unit being equivalent to 8 g of alcohol. This has traditionally been equated to a single measure of spirits, half a pint of beer or a 100-mL glass of table wine. However, this calculation needs to be revised for higher-strength beers and New World wines, some of the latter having an alcohol content of 15 per cent or more. Hazardous drinking is defined as an average daily consumption of over 40 g (5 units) of pure ethanol for men and over 20 g (2.5 units) for women. These are the self-reported levels of consumption above which there is an increasing risk of medical harm.

An alcohol dependence syndrome is suggested by a history of morning tremor, anxiety, insomnia, retching, morning drinking to relieve tremor, visual hallucinations, withdrawal fits and concurrent use of benzodiazepines. Withdrawal symptoms are likely to emerge following admission to hospital, where the patient no longer has access to alcohol.[17]

Drug misuse

Illicit drugs are also highly associated with medical problems and can affect every organ system.[18] Drugs greatly increase the risk of traumatic injury, and so drug users are overrepresented among accident and emergency patients following road traffic accidents and assaults. Canning and colleagues reported that 6 per cent of acute medical admissions were drug-dependent and 14 per cent were drug users.[19] The most common drugs taken by these patients were cannabis, amphetamines, ecstasy and cocaine. Polydrug use appears to be increasing in frequency. Clinical presentations associated with a particularly high prevalence of drug misuse are deliberate self-harm, HIV/acquired immunodeficiency syndrome (AIDS), hepatitis and septicaemia.

A high index of suspicion is essential. It is important that specific questions about drug use are asked. These should cover the nature and dose of the drug, the duration for which the drug has been taken, and the time of the last dose.

Sexual problems

Taking a sexual history is one of the most sensitive areas covered by a psychiatric assessment. Unless sexual problems are among the patient's presenting complaints, it is advisable not to broach the subject until a good rapport has been established. This may mean deferring until a second or subsequent interview and then discussing the subject in stages. The patient's sexual partner should not be interviewed without the explicit agreement of the patient being obtained and recorded in the medical notes.

It is well established that sexual problems are common among medical patients. The emotional impact of becoming ill, with its associated sense of loss of attractiveness, can adversely affect sexual interest, performance and desire, but an increasing amount of evidence points to the role of physical factors in the aetiology of sexual problems. Peripheral neuropathy and vascular disease are among the most common causes. Sexual problems are therefore frequently seen in association with diabetes, hypertension, arteriosclerosis and chronic alcoholism. Other neurological causes include multiple sclerosis, spinal cord lesions, Parkinson's disease and stroke. Localized diseases of the genitourinary tract are also important causes. In men, these diseases include prostatitis, sexually transmitted infections (STIs) and lesions of the penis such as Peyronie's disease; female conditions include endometriosis, pelvic inflammatory disease, and vulval infections and tumours. A wide range of medically prescribed drugs have adverse sexual side effects. Chief among these are antidepressants, antihypertensives and anti-androgens. Alcohol and illicit drugs are often taken in the hope that they will enhance desire and performance, but the reverse is usually true.

Privacy is important to enable a full history to be taken. The patient's current sexual relationship must be discussed in its widest sense; this enables a sensitive exploration of sexual orientation to take place. Frequency of sexual intercourse should be elicited with particular reference to recent loss of desire, erectile difficulties and reduced orgasmic capacity. In rare cases, a history of gender dysphoria will be uncovered, and there may be an expressed wish for surgical alteration of gender role. Such cases need to be referred to a clinic specializing in gender identity disorders.

MENTAL STATE

A full mental state examination may not be possible, and not all aspects listed below can be explored at the first assessment. It is often necessary to conduct the examination on several occasions, particularly when there is reason to suspect that any psychological changes elicited are fluctuating.

General appearance and behaviour

It is usually the case that a full physical examination has been conducted by the referring doctor, and this should not be repeated unless there are indications from the history that undetected pathology is present. However, the patient's general appearance should be described. Several clues might indicate that the medical condition could adversely affect the patient's mental state, such as weight loss, cyanosis, jaundice, a cushingoid face, and evidence of thyroid over- or underactivity. When alcohol is a problem, acne rosacea or facial reddening due to increased capillarization may be evident. Alcohol may be smelled on the breath, and there may be tremulousness and apprehension, indicative of a withdrawal state.

Withdrawal from opiate drugs occurs when drug-dependent individuals cannot get access to their usual supply, as happens when they are admitted to hospital. The characteristic signs are yawning, sneezing, rhinorrhoea, runny eyes, goose flesh, tachycardia and muscle twitching. Signs of sedative withdrawal include agitation, tremor, postural hypotension and tachycardia.

Evidence of psychomotor retardation, overactivity or agitation should be noted. The facial expression and bodily posture may give strong clues to a disturbance of mood. Disinhibited and overfamiliar behaviour are features of manic states or frontal lobe lesions.

The patient's attitude to the assessment should be recorded. Is the patient cooperative, or is there resentment or even aggressive behaviour towards the psychiatrist, medical and nursing staff and other patients?

Speech

Any problem of the articulation of words (dysarthria) should be noted. In the absence of local pathology in the oropharynx, dysarthria is suggestive of cerebellar pathology. Speech production is diminished in rate and volume in depression; it is speeded up in manic states, when speech may also indicate flight of ideas, with rapid change of content from one topic to another and with only minimal connection between them. In stuporose patients, there may be no speech production at all and there is little or no generalized motor activity.

Evidence of dysphasia should be assessed because this is a strong indicator of focal cerebral pathology. Difficulty in the production of spoken language – motor or expressive dysphasia – is associated with lesions in the posterior part of the third frontal convolution in the dominant hemisphere, Broca's area. Speech production is sparse and hesitant, words are chosen incorrectly, and the patient usually appears flustered when attempting to speak. Written language is affected similarly. Nominal dysphasia refers to difficulty in naming familiar objects, such as a pen, watch or spectacles, when the examiner points to them. This disorder can occur in widespread cerebral pathology and with focal lesions of the dominant angular gyrus.

Receptive dysphasia involves difficulty in the comprehension of speech and is associated with lesions in the first convolution of the dominant temporal lobe, known as Wernicke's area. The patient has difficulty understanding the meaning of words and therefore in responding to commands. Speech is impaired, with grammatical errors, wrong words and neologisms, but the speech is produced in a fluent rhythm and apparently without distress to the patient.

Mood disturbance

Subjective mood should be explored by asking how the patient is currently feeling in his or her spirits. Unusual sadness, hopelessness, loss of interest and anhedonia are common manifestations of depression. Less commonly, psychotic symptoms are seen in patients who are severely depressed. Delusions of guilt and punishment may involve beliefs about the causation of the physical illness. Conversely, there may be a delusional conviction of bodily organs having ceased to function or of having cancer, AIDS or some other potentially fatal illness even though medical reassurance has been given that no such illness has been found. It is important to follow the evolution of depressive symptoms. Many resolve with improvement in the medical condition and are best regarded as part of an adjustment disorder. Others are more persistent and do not improve with physical recovery; specific psychological or antidepressant treatment is then indicated.

Mania is much rarer than depression in medically ill patients and is often related to drug therapy, particularly with steroids. There are the characteristic features of elation, grandiose beliefs, overactivity and disinhibited behaviour towards staff and other patients. Not surprisingly, nurses find these patients extremely difficult to manage on a medical ward.

Interviewing terminally ill patients poses special problems. Doctors often feel uncomfortable in these situations, not knowing how far to probe into the patient's concerns. However, most patients want to be told if their condition is terminal. Psychiatric problems are common, and patients generally welcome the opportunity to discuss them. Religious and spiritual matters may be very important, and access to religious counselling should be available. For patients who deny the implications of their condition, it is important to respect defence mechanisms but also to offer the opportunity for the patient to ask questions so that they can be given as much information as they request. Not all questions will be raised at the first interview, and so follow-up interviews should be arranged.

Many patients admit to feeling anxious during treatment for a medical illness. Anxiety is most marked in the early stages of the illness, when the diagnosis may be unclear, or before stressful investigations or operations. In a few cases, anxiety is disabling and leads to signs and symptoms of autonomic arousal that cause considerable distress. Anxiety in relation to particular procedures, such as venepuncture, chemotherapy or radiotherapy, can lead to avoidance and refusal of further treatment.

Patients admitted to hospital following trauma are at risk of developing PTSD[20] and describe the characteristic symptoms of nightmares, flashbacks, sleep disturbance, hypervigilance, hyperarousal and avoidance of cues associated with the original trauma. However, these symptoms may not emerge during hospital treatment but become apparent only several weeks after the patient leaves hospital.

Assessment of suicide risk

This is a crucial aspect of the psychiatric assessment. Medically ill patients are at increased risk of committing suicide[21] and may be specifically referred by medical staff because suicidal thoughts have been expressed. But most assessments of suicidal risk are conducted on patients who have been admitted to hospital after acts of deliberate self-harm.[22] The assessment should identify patients with a significant psychiatric illness and those who are at high risk of attempting or repeating self-harm. It should enable a management plan to be devised and it can, in itself, have a therapeutic effect. The topics to be covered are as follows:

- Motivation for committing suicide
- Immediate predisposing stressful events
- Current social difficulties
- Degree of planning an attempt
- Whether there are plans anticipating death, e.g. suicide note written, personal affairs sorted
- Previous attempts
- Previous psychiatric history
- Family history of suicide and psychiatric illness
- Tendency to misuse alcohol and other drugs
- Coping resources and plans for future
- Evidence of personality disorder.

As a general principle, the following features increase the risk of suicide:

- Advancing age
- Previous episodes of self-harm
- Male sex
- Evidence of psychiatric illness, especially depression and schizophrenia
- Personality disorder
- Unemployment
- Social isolation
- Recent separation or bereavement
- Alcohol or drug misuse
- Lower social class.

Further psychiatric care should be organized on the basis of this assessment. Most patients can be discharged home safely following an episode of self-harm if adequate support and ongoing care from a community mental health team can be provided. Patients identified as being at high risk should usually be transferred to a psychiatric unit. If medical factors preclude this, then consideration should be given to arranging observation and therapeutic intervention from an experienced psychiatric nurse until transfer can be effected.

Psychotic symptoms

If there is evidence of an antecedent psychotic illness, the characteristic delusions, hallucinations and thought disorder will be apparent or revealed by appropriate questions concerning unusual beliefs or sensory experiences. An acute delusional system emerging during the course of a medical illness most commonly reflects a delirious state; abnormal sensory perceptions in response to normal stimuli (illusions) may be present, together with hallucinations, typically in the visual and tactile modalities. A less common delusional system can arise in clear consciousness without any hallucinatory experiences. The delusions nearly always involve a belief of imminent persecution or assault from the staff, and the patient may respond violently to the fear of attack. This is most likely to develop in susceptible people with paranoid personality traits who are being treated in ICU or the coronary care unit (CCU) and are surrounded by unfamiliar technological equipment. Distinction of this acute psychotic reaction from delirium is important because the symptoms may not resolve until the patient can be moved to a less threatening environment.

Cognitive function

In view of the frequency of cognitive impairment in medical patients, it is often necessary to evaluate cognitive function at an early stage in the examination. Any impairment that is elicited may influence the interpretation of other mental symptoms. Level of consciousness should be assessed according to the patient's alertness, ability to concentrate on the interview or tendency to drift off to sleep. Impaired alertness is a cardinal feature of delirium, but apparent lucidity at the time of assessment does not exclude delirium because symptoms fluctuate markedly, typically being worse at night. Importance should therefore be given to nursing reports of varying alertness and other symptoms during the course of a day.

Attention and concentration can be assessed by asking the patient to carry out some simple mental tasks, such as repeating the months of the year backwards, serially subtracting 7 from 100, and repeating a number of digits forwards and backwards.

Orientation, which involves registering and retaining information, should be checked by asking the patient to give the date, the day of the week, the month and the year (orientation for time) and to name the present location, floor of the building, name of the hospital, street address and town (orientation for place). Orientation for person is assessed by asking the patient his or her name. This information is lost in advanced cases of dementia, in some psychotic illnesses and in dissociative amnesias.

Memory involves the ability to register, retain and retrieve information.[23] Short-term memory is assessed clinically by presenting new information, such as a name and address or a series of words, asking the patient to repeat it immediately to check registration, and then asking the patient to repeat it again after an interval of 5 min or so, during which time the patient's attention is diverted to other topics. Memory for recent events such as major items of news should also be noted. Remote memories are more difficult to assess, but it is helpful to note the ability to recall memories from childhood, particularly if these can be verified from other sources. Confabulation refers to a tendency to fill in gaps in memory by inserting false memories; these are often memories of events that have taken place but that have become grossly displaced in time. Confabulation is classically seen in Korsakoff's syndrome.

Mental capacity

Mental capacity is required if patients are to understand the nature of their illness and the need for treatment and to be able to withhold or give consent to treatment. Its assessment should be an integral part of the psychiatric examination and is sometimes the specific reason why a psychiatric opinion is sought.[24,25] All medical clinicians should be able to assess capacity, but a second opinion may be requested if the decision has major consequences and if the physician believes the patient has made an unwise choice. The assessment of a patient's capacity should be undertaken specifically in relation to the decision that the patient is required to make.[26] Lack of capacity is more common than is often thought to be the case. Raymont and colleagues assessed 159 acute medical admissions and judged 31 per cent of the patients to lack capacity according to legal criteria.[27] Only a quarter of these patients were identified as such by their treating medical teams. Mental capacity has important legal implications because, in the absence of capacity, patients have to be treated under common law or the Mental Capacity Act (2005), provided that the treatment is considered to be in their best interest. The least restrictive treatment option should be used but, before deciding that the patient lacks capacity, every effort should be made to facilitate his or her ability to make a decision. The law assumes that people have the capacity to make decisions about their own treatment, even if refusing treatment may lead to permanent damage and premature death. Before the introduction of the Mental Capacity Act in England and Wales, no other person could give or withhold consent on behalf of an adult patient, but the Act has now allowed proxy decision-makers to be appointed. A person who has capacity can now grant lasting power of attorney to one or more people, who can then decide on that person's treatment, should capacity subsequently be lost. There is also provision for the court to appoint one or more deputies who can decide on treatment on behalf of a patient who already lacks capacity.

Lack of capacity exists if the patient is unable to:

- understand information relevant to the decision;
- retain the information;
- weigh up the information in order to make a decision;
- communicate a decision.

In most cases in medical practice, lack of capacity results from cognitive impairment. This may be transient, as seen in delirium, or permanent, as is the case in dementia.

Pre-existing psychiatric disorders such as schizophrenia, depression and, in certain cases, phobias can also impair capacity.[28]

The use of questionnaires

Diagnosis in psychiatry rests firmly on the basis of an interview conducted by an experienced psychiatrist. Questionnaires do not replace the clinical assessment, but they can be useful as screening instruments and in quantifying the severity of symptoms and following their temporal evolution, particularly in response to treatment. The following are some of the questionnaires that have been found to be helpful in assessing medically ill patients:

- *Hospital Anxiety and Depression Scale (HADS):* this is a short simple scale that measures anxiety and depression separately, each on a 21-point scale.[29] It has been specifically designed to exclude somatic symptoms of mood disorder, and thus it is particularly suitable for use in a medical population.
- *General Health Questionnaire:* the full questionnaire contains 60 items, but shorter versions consisting of 12, 28 or 30 items are more appropriate for medical patients. This questionnaire has been used widely as a screening instrument and is acceptable to people who do not regard themselves as mentally ill.[30] The sensitivity and specificity vary according to the population studied, and the threshold score is affected by the degree of physical illness, and so the questionnaire needs to be standardized for the group of patients with whom it is being used.
- *Beck Depression Inventory:* one of the earliest structured questionnaires, this has been used widely with medical patients.[31] It is a 21-item scale, but it contains somatic questions, so it can lead to false-positive results.
- *Mini Mental State Examination:* this is the most widely used test to assess cognitive impairment.[32] It is administered by the clinician and assesses orientation, registration, recall, attention, concentration and language. It can detect cognitive deficits in dementia and following head injury, but it lacks sensitivity to detect subtle loss of memory, particularly in well-educated people.
- *CAGE:* this brief screening test is used to detect severely affected problem drinkers.[33] It asks four questions, concerning whether the patient has: (i) attempted to *cut* back on drinking, (ii) been *annoyed* at criticism of their drinking, (iii) felt *guilty* about their drinking or (iv) used alcohol as an *eye-opener.* It does not detect hazardous drinking and can seem too confrontational for use with this group.
- *Alcohol Use Disorders Inventory (AUDIT):* this is more suitable for the detection of hazardous drinking.[34] In briefer form, it has been used successfully to identify hazardous drinkers in a maxillofacial unit[35] and in an accident and emergency department.[36]

COMMUNICATION

Once the history and mental state examination have been completed, the psychiatric opinion should be communicated immediately to the referring doctor. This is best done verbally but supplemented by a written entry in the clinical notes. A typed summary should follow later. The opinion should include a definitive psychiatric diagnosis, a review of aetiological factors, and clear advice on management. If a diagnosis cannot be reached at the first interview, a differential diagnosis should be given, together with advice on further investigations and other sources of information. The psychiatrist should review the patient once these are available. No assessment is complete without informing the patient what conclusions the psychiatrist has reached and what further treatment, if any, is being recommended.

KEY POINTS

- The development of a physical illness, either acute or long-term, substantially increases the likelihood of a wide range of psychiatric disorders, which adds considerably to the level of disability and may worsen the prognosis of the physical condition.
- Knowledge of the nature of the physical illness, its severity, its prognosis and its response to treatment is essential.
- Ideally, all psychiatric assessments should be conducted in privacy, either in the patient's home, in an out-patient office or in a side room of a medical ward.
- Many illnesses are associated with communication problems, and the clinician should be aware of these so that special provision can be made.
- In most cases, the history is taken in much the same manner as in any psychiatric assessment.
- It is often necessary to conduct the mental-state examination on several occasions, particularly when there is reason to suspect that any psychological changes elicited are fluctuating.
- Assessment of suicide risk is a crucial aspect of the psychiatric assessment.
- Questionnaires do not replace the clinical assessment but can be useful as screening instruments and in quantifying the severity of symptoms and following their temporal evolution, particularly in response to treatment.
- Once the history and mental-state examination have been completed, the psychiatric opinion should be communicated immediately to the referring doctor.

REFERENCES

1. Kisley SR, Goldberg DP (1996) Physical and psychiatric comorbidity in general practice. *British Journal of Psychiatry* **169**: 236–42.
2. Stansfeld SA, Smith GD, Marmot M (1993) Association between physical and psychological morbidity in the

Whitehall II study. *Journal of Psychosomatic Research* **37**: 227–38.
3. Royal College of Physicians, Royal College of Psychiatrists (2003) *The Psychological Care of Medical Patients: A Practical Guide*. London: Royal College of Physicians and Royal College of Psychiatrists.
4. Frasure-Smith N, Lesperance F (2003) Depression and other psychological risks following myocardial infarction. *Archives of General Psychiatry* **60**: 627–36.
5. Turjanski N, Lloyd GG (2005) Psychiatric side-effects of medications: recent developments. *Advances in Psychiatric Treatment* **11**: 58–70.
6. Gledhill J, Lloyd GG (2000) Liaison psychiatry in intensive care units. In R Peveler, E Feldman, T Friedman (eds) *Liaison Psychiatry: Planning Services for Specialist Settings*. London: Gaskell.
7. Lloyd G (2007) Understanding psychological reactions to physical illness. In GG Lloyd, E Guthrie (eds) *Handbook of Liaison Psychiatry*. Cambridge: Cambridge University Press.
8. Chochinov HM (2001) Depression in cancer patients. *Lancet Oncology* **2**: 499–505.
9. Mayou RA, Smith KA (1997) Post traumatic symptoms following medical illness and treatment. *Journal of Psychosomatic Research* **43**: 121–3.
10. Ballard CG, Stanley AK, Brockington IF (1995) Post-traumatic stress disorder (PTSD) after childbirth. *British Journal of Psychiatry* **166**: 525–8.
11. Veale D, Boocock A, Gournay K, *et al.* (1996) Body dysmorphic disorder: a survey of fifty cases. *British Journal of Psychiatry* **169**: 196–201.
12. Royal College of Physicians (2001) *Alcohol: Can the NHS Afford it? Recommendations for a Coherent Alcohol Strategy for Hospitals*. London: Royal College of Physicians.
13. Yates DW, Hadfield FM, Peters K (1987) Alcohol consumption of patients attending two accident and emergency departments in north-west England. *Journal of the Royal Society of Medicine* **80**: 486–9.
14. Smart RG, Mann RE, Suurvali H (1998) Changes in liver cirrhosis death rates in different countries in relation to per capita alcohol consumption and Alcoholics Anonymous membership. *Journal of Studies on Alcohol* **59**: 245–9.
15. Leon DA, McCambridge J (2006) Liver cirrhosis mortality rates in Britain from 1950 to 2002: an analysis of routine data. *Lancet* **367**: 52–6.
16. Parker AJ, Marshal EJ, Ball DM (2008) Diagnosis and management of alcohol use disorders. *British Medical Journal* **336**: 496–501.
17. McKeon A, Frye MA, Delanty N (2008) The alcohol withdrawal syndrome. *Journal of Neurology, Neurosurgery, and Psychiatry* **79**: 854–62.
18. Crome I, Ghodse H (2007) Drug misuse in medical patients. In GG Lloyd, E Guthrie (eds) *Handbook of Liaison Psychiatry*. Cambridge: Cambridge University Press.
19. Canning UP, Kennell-Webb SA, Marshall EJ (1999) Substance misuse in acute general medical admissions. *Quarterly Journal of Medicine* **92**: 319–26.
20. Mayou R, Bryant B (2002) Outcome three years after a road traffic accident. *Psychological Medicine* **32**: 671–5.
21. Harris EC, Barraclough B (1984) Suicide as an outcome for medical disorders. *Medicine (Baltimore)* **73**: 281–96.
22. Hawton K, Catalan J (1987) *Attempted Suicide: A Practical Guide to its Nature and Management*. Oxford: Oxford University Press.
23. Kopelman MD (2002) Disorders of memory. *Brain* **125**: 2152–90.
24. Hotopf M (2005) The assessment of mental capacity. *Clinical Medicine* **5**: 580–84.
25. Mukherjee E, Foster R (2008) The Mental Capacity Act 2007 and capacity assessments: a guide for the non-psychiatrist. *Clinical Medicine* **8**: 65–9.
26. Nicholson TRJ, Cutter W, Hotopf M (2008) Assessing mental capacity: the Mental Capacity Act. *British Medical Journal* **336**: 322–5.
27. Raymont V, Bingley W, Buchanan A, *et al.* (2004) The prevalence of mental incapacity in medical inpatients and associated risk factors. *Lancet* **364**: 1421–7.
28. Feldman E (2007) Legal and ethical issues in liaison psychiatry. In GG Lloyd, E Guthrie (eds) *Handbook of Liaison Psychiatry*. Cambridge: Cambridge University Press.
29. Zigmond AS, Snaith RP (1983) The Hospital Anxiety and Depression Scale. *Acta Psychiatrica Scandinavica* **67**: 361–70.
30. Goldberg D (1986) The use of the general health questionnaire in medical patients. *British Medical Journal* **293**: 1188–9.
31. Beck AT, Ward CH, Mendelson M, *et al.* (1961) An inventory for measuring depression. *Archives of General Psychiatry* **4**: 561–71.
32. Folstein MF, Folstein SE, McHugh PR (1975) The Mini Mental State Examination: a practical method for grading the cognitive state of patients for clinicians. *Journal of Psychiatric Research* **12**: 189–98.
33. Ewing JA (1984) Detecting alcoholism: the CAGE questionnaire. *Journal of the American Medical Association* **252**: 1905–7.
34. Saunders JB, Aasland OG, Babor TF, *et al.* (1993) Development of the Alcohol Use Disorders Identification Test (Audit): WHO collaborative project on early detection of persons with harmful alcohol consumption-II. *Addiction* **88**: 791–804.
35. Hodgson R, Alwyn T, John B, *et al.* (2002) The FAST Alcohol Screening Test. *Alcohol and Alcoholism* **37**: 61–6.
36. Smith SGT, Touquet R, Wright S, *et al.* (1996) Detection of alcohol misusing patients in accident and emergency departments: the Paddington Alcohol Test (PAT). *Journal of Accident and Emergency Medicine* **13**: 591–9.

Chapter 49

Overlapping multi-system, multi-organ illnesses/syndromes

Malcolm Hooper

GENERAL CONSIDERATIONS

These illnesses, summarized in Figure 49.1, have variously been described as 'syndromes of uncertain origin'[1] and 'unexplained illnesses'.[2] They are the subject of much controversy and not a little polemic.

It is helpful to define the term 'syndrome', which has been the subject of much, sometimes acrimonious, debate when applied to these illnesses, particularly Gulf War syndrome (GWS).

> The Greek origin of syndrome is *syn–*, together, and *–drome*, a track for running. One must determine the tracks of travel and observe the travel of the patient's syndrome components. Because research definitions define a static collection of symptom entities, they have ignored or downplayed the critical dynamic features of this syndrome, as lived by patients... It is important for the clinician to observe the dynamics of the whole cluster of symptoms in their interaction, additive effects, and the disruption to patients' lives over a period of time.[3]

A recent Congressionally-mandated American research report on Gulf War Syndrome avoids the debate on semantics that has resulted in casuistry and delay in addressing this condition and names it, Gulf War illness, GWI.[4] GWI is defined as a complex chronic multi-system illness characterized by a coherent pattern of symptoms and now shown to be causally associated with exposures to organophosphate pesticides and pyridostigmine bromide (given prophylactically to protect against the nerve agent soman) whilst other toxic exposures are not ruled out. Extensive and advanced SPECT neuroimaging studies have found changes in normalized blood flow to deep brain areas that would not be identified in routine scans. The brain structures affected include the caudate, amygdala, hippocampus, putamen and thalamus and are consistent with the multiple symptoms reported.[5]

The similarity of these symptoms in different conditions has been interpreted by some as an indication of common psychogenic origin, but this is no longer tenable in the light of the extensive biomedical studies reported in all these fields, particularly myalgic encephalomyelitis (ME)/chronic

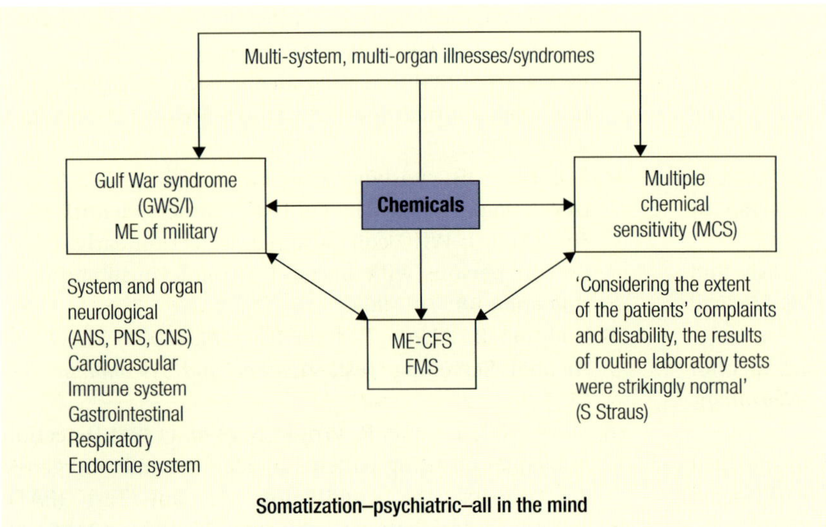

Figure 49.1 Overlapping multi-system, multi-organ illnesses/syndromes

ANS, autonomic nervous system; CNS, central nervous system; FMS, fibromyalgia syndrome; GWS/I, Gulf War syndrome/illness; ME-CFS, myalgic encephalomyelitis/chronic fatigue syndrome; PNS, peripheral nervous system.

Table 49.1 Common symptoms identified in multi-system, multi-organ syndromes/illnesses

Symptoms	Organo-phosphate poisoning	Gulf War syndrome/ illness	Multiple chemical sensitivity	Fibromyalgia syndrome	Chronic fatigue immune dysregulation syndrome	Multiple sclerosis	HIV/AIDS
Joint pain	+	+	+	Around joint area	+	+	+
Fatigue	+	+	+	+	+	+	+
Headache	+	+	+	+	+	+	+
Memory problems	+	+	+	+	+	+	+
Disturbed sleep	+	+	+	+	+	Due to medicines	+
Skin problems	+	+	+	+	+	Burning skin	+
Concentration problems	+	+	+	+	+	+	+
Depression	+	+	+	+	+	+	+
Muscle pain	+	+	+	+	+	+	+
Dizziness	+	+	+	+	+	+	+
Irritable bowel	+	+	+	+	+	+	+
Peripheral paraesthesia/tingling	+	+	+	+	+	+	+
Chemical/ environmental sensitivity	+	+	+	+	+	Reported	–
Eye problems	+	+	+	+	+	+	+
Anxiety	+	+	+	+	+	+	+
Tachycardia or chest pain	+	+	+	+	+	+	+
Breathing problems	+	+	+	Reported	+	+	+
Light sensitivity	+/–	+	+	Reported	+	+	–

+, symptoms present; –, symptoms absent.

HIV/AIDS, human immunodeficiency virus/acquired immunodeficiency syndrome.

fatigue syndrome (CFS).[6] The inclusion of multiple sclerosis (MS) and human immunodeficiency virus (HIV)/acquired immunodeficiency syndrome (AIDS) in Table 49.1 points to the involvement of both the nervous system and the immune system in these complex multi-system illnesses/ syndromes.

The challenge of these illnesses/syndromes has given rise to a stark conflict between psychiatry and biomedical science, which has been set in opposition by some psychiatrists who espouse somatization as the basis of these many other illnesses/syndromes.[7] Patients, other clinicians and scientists see them as biomedical illnesses of organic origin.[8] This debate has been particularly aggressive in the UK, but it is pursued elsewhere in the developed world and is associated with concerns about diagnosis, treatment and the care of people who suffer from the illnesses/syndromes. The latter involves the global insurance industry and national benefit systems for people disabled by these illnesses. These wider concerns reach into the heart of government and national and international policy, particularly with regard to the activities of large multinational corporations involved in the insurance industry and others responsible for the release of chemicals into the environment. Ordinary people, without the support of governments and without the necessary resources to challenge these policies, are often unable to find a voice for their concerns and those of their children.

It is no longer necessary to regard these illnesses/syndromes as of 'unexplained' or 'uncertain' origin, since we now have a much better understanding of their aetiology and the biological processes underlying them.

Figure 49.2 summarizes the major stressors that may give rise to these illnesses/syndromes and points to a way forward for the future in which science and medicine, including psychiatry, can contribute to helping those who are ill.

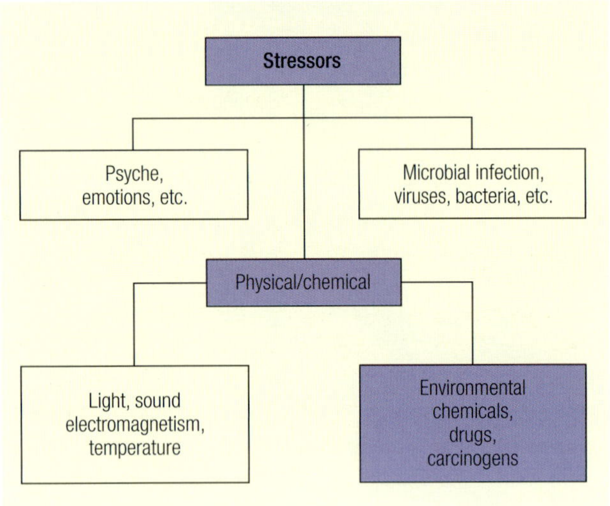

Figure 49.2 Sources of major stressors associated with multi-system, multi-organ illnesses/syndromes

Somatization has a poor track record, having been offered as an explanation of previously 'unexplained' medical conditions, including diabetes, Parkinson's disease and MS. The growth of modern science and the introduction of powerful investigatory techniques such as magnetic resonance has uncovered details of brain chemistry that clearly show damage to the areas of the brain, which in some cases can be linked to the specific clinical symptoms observed in patients.[9,10] Dalen, a psychiatrist, has published a powerful critique of the concept of somatization that shows that the use of this idea to explain previously unexplained illnesses, often in excess among women, is often founded on ignorance and a failure to investigate new clinical phenomena.[11]

An alternative view involves the biopsychosocial theory that is offered as an understanding of these multi-system illnesses. This has received short shrift from another psychiatrist,[12] who has criticized the lack of a credible intellectual basis for this concept. In contrast, the intellectual underpinnings of the biomedical studies are becoming increasingly understood (Figure 49.3).[13]

These oppositional attitudes lead to confusion in diagnosis, treatment and care and have resulted in some truly horrific cases in which people have been sectioned against their wishes, families divided and patients shown no compassion. Parents of young people have been accused of Munchausen's syndrome by proxy.[14] The result is bitterness and accusation, leaving patients and carers feeling abandoned and distressed.

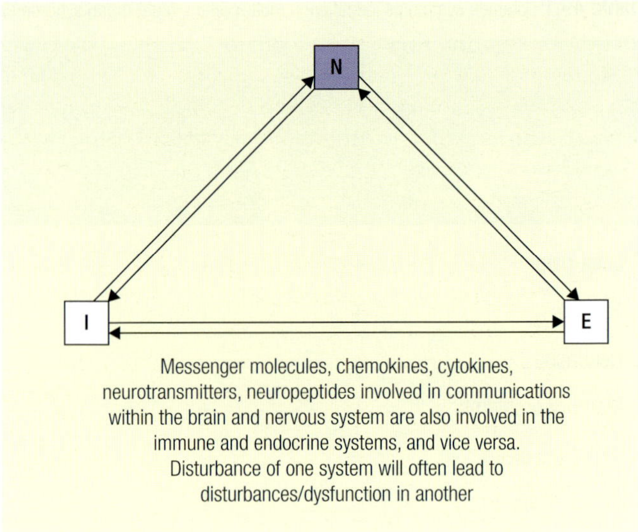

Figure 49.3 Neuroendocrine–immune paradigm that underpins complex overlapping syndromes

E, endocrine; I, immunological; N, neurological.

Diagnosis has become a major issue in relation to all these illnesses, but it is now becoming clear that the currently accepted diagnostic criteria are inadequate and lump together people with disparate conditions. Figure 49.4 summarizes the Medical Outcomes Study 36-item Short-Form health survey (SF-36) scores of three different groups that meet the most widely used Centers for Disease Control and Prevention (CDC) 1994 definition for CFS.[15] ME/CFS patients were significantly less impaired than the other two groups in terms of role emotional and mental health.

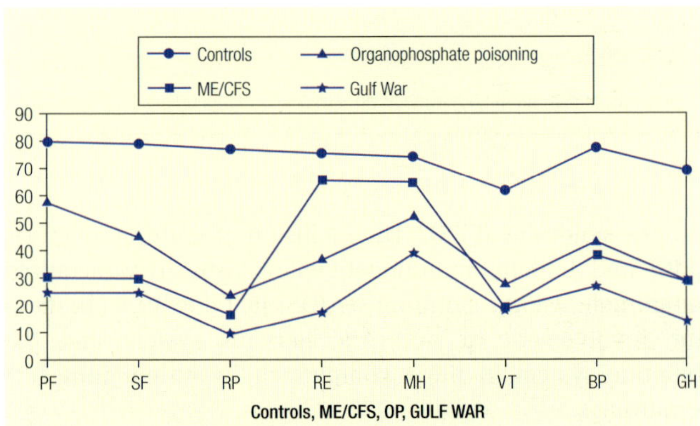

Figure 49.4 SF-36 scores among different groups with complex multi-system, multi-organ illnesses/syndromes

PF, physical functioning (10); SF, social functioning (2); RP, role limitations – physical problems (4); RE, role limitations – emotional problems (3); MH, mental health (5); VT, vitality/energy (4); BP, pain (2); GH, general health (5).

ME/CFS, Myalgic encephalomyelitis/chronic fatigue syndrome.

Organophosphate poisoned patients were significantly less impaired than the other groups as regards physical functioning and social functioning. However, GW patients reported significantly greater levels of bodily pain and had a significantly poorer general health scores. The latter is consistent with one of the seven clinical phenotypes identified in a genetics study by Kerr and colleagues.[16]

Distinctive tests that differentiate between the different groups of subjects are now being identified. In patients with ME/CFS, the delayed vascular response to acetylcholine is unique and differentiates such patients from patients with fibromyalgia. An initial genetics report identified single nucleotide polymorphisms (SNPs) characteristic of severe forms of fibromyalgia that distinguished patients with fibromyalgia from patients with severe ME/CFS.[17] Differential pathology has been reported in neutrophils obtained from Gulf War veterans (mainly necrotic) and patients with ME/CFS (mainly apoptotic).[18]

Figure 49.2 makes clear that psychiatry and psychology have a place and a role in these complex illnesses. Reactive depression is not uncommon among sick patients and needs to be treated in some cases. Other profound and long-established human activities such as meditation and prayer can also help some patients who are ill. It is of paramount importance to make clear diagnoses using the best and most appropriate investigations followed by the most effective treatments available.

Because of the dichotomy between the psychiatric and biomedical approaches to these illnesses, and the failure to provide clear diagnostic criteria, many patients are misdiagnosed and referred unnecessarily for psychiatric assessment. This places avoidable demands on the mental health services, which are already greatly overstretched,[19] and leads to inappropriate and ineffectual treatment of patients with these illnesses.

These illnesses/syndromes are a challenge to contemporary medicine and science, but above all to our common humanity, as we seek to engage with people who are ill and need our full support.

Chapters 50 and 51 consider in detail aspects of these multi-system, multi-organ illnesses/syndromes, particularly ME/CFS, fibromyalgia and multiple chemical sensitivity.

KEY POINTS

- All of these illnesses are complex, challenging, chronic organic illnesses.
- They are not primarily stress or psychiatric in origin.
- The recognition of subgroups within each illness is important for diagnosis and treatment.
- Thorough and careful physical examination and the use of judiciously selected tests are important.

REFERENCES

1. Beers MH, Berkow R, Merck Research Laboratories (1999) Syndromes of uncertain origin. In *Merck Manual of Diagnosis and Therapy*. Whitehouse Station, NJ: Merck Research Laboratories.
2. Pall ML (2007) *Explaining 'Unexplained Illnesses'*. New York: Harrington Park Press.
3. Carruthers BM and van de Sande IM (2005) *Myalgic Encephalomyelitis/Chronic Fatigue Syndrome: A Clinical Case Definition and Guideline for Medical Practitioners – An Overview of the Canadian Consensus Document*. (A summary of 'Myalgic Encephalomyelitis/ Chronic Fatigue Syndrome: Clinical Working Case Definition Diagnostic and Treatment Guidelines A consensus Document.') *J Chronic Fatigue Syndrome* 11:7–115.
4. Gulf War Illness and the Health of Gulf War Veterans; Scientific Findings and Recommendations. Research Advisory Committee on Gulf War Veterans' Illnesses, November 2008. Download, May 25th 2009. http://www1.va.gov/rac-gwvi/docs/GWIandHealthof GWVeterans_RAC-GWVIReport_2008.pdf
5. Haley RW, Spence JS, Carmack PS, Gunstb RF, Schucanyb WR, Petty F, Devous MD, Bontee FJ, Trivedic MH (2009) Abnormal brain response to cholinergic challenge in chronic encephalopathy from the 1991 Gulf War. *Psychiatry Research: Neuroimaging* **171**: 207–20.
6. Komaroff A (2006) Centers for Disease Control and Prevention. Press conference, 3 November 2006. www.cdc.gov/od/oc/media/transcripts/t061103.htm.
7. Wessely S, Nimnuan C, Sharpe M (1999) Functional somatic syndromes: one or many? *Lancet* **354**: 936–9.
8. P Englebienne, K De Meirleir (eds) (2002) *Chronic Fatigue Syndrome: A Biological Approach*. Boca Raton, FL: CRC Press.
9. Puri BK, Counsell SJ, Zaman R, *et al.* (2002) Relative increase in choline in the occipital cortex in chronic fatigue syndrome. *Acta Psychiatrica Scandinavica* **106**: 224–6.
10. Haley RW, Marshall WW, McDonald GG, *et al.* (2000) Brain abnormalities in Gulf War syndrome: evaluation with 1H MR spectroscopy. *Radiology* **215**: 807–17.
11. Dalen P (2003) Somatic medicine abuses psychiatry and neglects causal research. http://art-bin.com/art/dalen_en.html.
12. McLaren N (2001) The biopsychosocial model and scientific fraud. *Australian and New Zealand Journal of Psychiatry* **35**: 724–30.
13. Rowat SC (1998) The neuroendocrine immune comprehensive integrative defence system. *Environmental Health Perspectives* **106** (suppl. 1): S85–109.
14. Walker MJ (2003) *Skewed: Psychiatric Hegemony and the Manufacture of Mental Illness*. London: Slingshot Publications.

15. Kennedy G, Abbot NC, Spence V, *et al.* (2004) The specificity of the CDC-1994 criteria for chronic fatigue syndrome: comparison of health status in three groups of patients who fulfill the criteria. *Annals of Epidemiology* **14**: 95–100.
16. Kerr JR, Petty R, Burke B, *et al.* (2008) Gene expression subtypes in patients with chronic fatigue syndrome/myalgic encephalomyelitis. *Journal of Infectious Diseases* **197**: 1171–84.
17. Estibaliz Olano (2007) Genetic Profiles New Horizons international conference on ME/CFS biomedical research. Edinburgh, 25 May 2007. DVD available from www.meresearch.org.uk.
18. Kennedy G, Spence VA, Underwood C, *et al.* (2004) Increased neutrophil apoptosis in chronic fatigue syndrome. *Journal of Clinical Pathology* **57**: 891–3.
19. Bhugra D (2008) Quoted in Amelia Hill 'Top Psychiatrist attacks NHS over mental health'. The Observer 29th June 2008, p.1&7.

Chapter 50

Multiple chemical sensitivity

Malcolm Hooper

INTRODUCTION

Multiple chemical sensitivity (MCS) is a complex, multi-symptom, multi-system multi-organ illness that is induced by exposure to a wide variety of toxic environmental insults. It is often co-morbid with other overlapping syndromes and evokes a similar range of symptoms (Table 50.1).[1–5]

WHAT'S IN A NAME?

MCS goes under many names and overlaps with many other syndromes and conditions (see Table 50.1). The most frequently used terms recognize that chemicals and the environment are understood by the affected people to be associated with their disabling illnesses. Among the overlapping syndromes are disorders, diseases and misdiagnoses that any competent physician would be expected to identify, for example coeliac disease, carbon monoxide poisoning and hypothyroidism.

Other descriptors are drawn from particular locations, for example 'Gulf War syndrome' (GWS) from the first Gulf War (1990–91) and 'new buildings syndrome' with new furnishings. Occupations such as carpet-fitting, commercial flying and cabin crew, and shepherding are associated with the same constellation of symptoms. Other descriptors indicate the comprehensive nature of the illness and try to place it within known clinical conditions such as allergy. More specific terms seek to identify the mechanism of the illness (e.g. toxicant-induced loss of tolerance, TILT) or cause of the illness (e.g. systemic candidiasis). An interesting inclusion in the list is electromagnetic sensitivity; this often follows chemical exposure but can be a primary event.[6,7]

The bewildering number and origins of so many names reflects the problems of grappling with such a complex illness and trying to understand it in order to effectively diagnose and treat patients who have it.

The World Health Organization (WHO) classifies MCS under chapters S00–T98 – injury, poisoning and certain other consequences of external causes, specifically at T66–78 – other unspecified effects of external causes and T78.4 – allergy, unspecified; hypersensitivity not otherwise specified (NOS), idiosyncracy NOS. Among the exposures specifically listed are pesticides of various chemical types, fungicides and rodenticides, although the important chemicals polychlorinated biphenyls (PCBs) are not included (Table 50.2).[8]

This confusion is reflected in the prolonged and sometimes acrimonious debate that surrounds MCS and involves clinicians, patients and patient support groups, and demands for recognition from governments, the chemical, pharmaceutical and insurance industries, and regulatory authorities in many countries.

DEFINITION AND DIAGNOSTIC CRITERIA

Definition

The 1999 consensus is widely accepted and defines MCS as follows:[9]

- A chronic condition
- With symptoms that recur reproducibly
- In response to low levels of exposure
- To multiple unrelated chemicals
- Improves or resolves when incitants are removed
- Symptoms occur in multiple organ systems.

The major symptoms of MCS are summarized in Table 50.1, but a more extensive list is given in Table 50.3.

Objective clinical signs have been identified in a wide variety of tissues and clinical systems in MCS (Box 50.1).

Diagnosis

Diagnosis should be made in the light of the above criteria. A comprehensive paper by Heuser emphasizes the need for the following:[10]

- A very thorough history
- A thorough physical examination, with special attention to the skin, blood pressure (orthostatic hypotension), movement and coordination

Table 50.1 Names used to describe multiple chemical sensitivity (MCS) and overlapping syndromes

Aspects of environmental sensitivities	Commonly overlapping conditions
State of heightened reactivity to the environment	Fibromyalgia
Total allergy syndrome	Myalgic encephalomyelitis (ME), chronic fatigue syndrome
Universal allergy	Postviral fatigue syndrome
Toxicant-induced loss of tolerance (TILT)	Post-infectious neuromyasthenia
Multiple chemical sensitivity(ies) (MCS)	Yuppie flu
Multiple chemical hypersensitivity(ies)	Chronic pain
Chemical intolerance(s)	Migraine
Chemical acquired immunodeficiency syndrome (AIDS)	Arthritis
Gulf War illness/syndrome (GWI/S)	Allergies
Idiopathic environmental intolerance (IEI)	Rhinitis
Environmental illness (EI)	Asthma
Environmental irritant syndrome	Food intolerance syndrome
Chemical injury/allergy	Coeliac disease
Toxic injury	Irritable bowel syndrome
Tight building syndrome	Major depression
Sick building syndrome	Anxiety or panic disorder
Twentieth-century disease	Hypothyroidism
Chemically induced illness	Aerotoxic syndrome
Chemical hypersensitivity syndrome	Organophosphate poisoning
Chemophobia	Sheep-dipper's flu
Electromagnetic (hyper)sensitivities/intolerance	Disorders of porphyrin metabolism
Toxic carpet syndrome	Carbon monoxide poisoning
Systemic candidiasis	
Multiple sensory sensitivity syndrome (MUSES)	

- The use of appropriate clinical, laboratory and psychological tests.

Single-proton-emission computed tomography (SPECT), positron-emission tomography (PET), magnetic resonance imaging (MRI)[11] and quantitative electroencephalography (qEEG) all provide details of any abnormal lack of function in the central nervous system. Magnetic resonance spectroscopy (MRS) also provides a powerful tool that has identified brain damage in veterans of the first Gulf War.[12] Current perception threshold studies are especially important in investigating the peripheral nervous system, as they assess the small but important C-fibres (see below). Autonomic function needs to be assessed with regard to temperature, perspiration, vascular tone, heart rate, smooth muscle tone and other functions. The eyes are important, since dry eye syndrome is common in MCS. Ear, nose and throat complaints are also common and need to be investigated fully, as nasal and pulmonary passages are frequently damaged or dysfunctional. Gastrointestinal problems occur regularly, with malabsorption and weight loss. Liver function tests are valuable, while low salivary immunoglobulin A (IgA) levels often indicate an impaired mucosal defence mechanism. Kidneys and the urinary tract may be

Table 50.2 World Health Organization *International Classification of Diseases*, 10th revision (ICD-10) classification of various toxic chemicals

Code	Description
T60.0	Toxic effect of organophosphate and carbamate insecticides
T60.1	Toxic effect of halogenated insecticides
T60.2	Toxic effect of other insecticides
T60.3	Toxic effect of herbicides and fungicides
T60.4	Toxic effect of rodenticides
T60.8	Toxic effect of other pesticides
T60.9	Toxic effect of pesticide, unspecified
X48	Accidental poisoning by and exposure to pesticides
X68	Intentional self-poisoning by and exposure to pesticides
X-87	Assault by pesticides
Y-18	Poisoning by and exposure to pesticides

Note: ICD-10 does not have specific codes for disinfectants. To find disinfectant poisonings, try T54, X49, X69, X87 and &19, which are codes for corrosive and noxious substances.

Table 50.3 Symptom list* compiled by the JHU Multi-Center study of multiple chemical sensitivity (MCS) immunology

System	Number
Cardiovascular	9
Digestive	18
Ears/hearing	7
Eyes/vision	12
Genitourinary	10
Head	6
Mouth/taste	14
Musculoskeletal	14
Neck	3
Nervous system	43
Nose/smell	10
Systemic/others	17
Vascular	5
Reproductive	17
Respiratory	6
Skin/touch	7
Throat	5
Total symptoms	*203*

*Number of symptoms associated with the different organs/systems listed.

Box 50.1 Objective clinical signs reported in multiple chemical sensitivity

- Abnormal blood and plasma
- Impaired circulation
- Impaired heart function
- Impaired detoxification pathways
- Ear and hearing abnormalities
- Endocrine deficiencies
- Gastrointestinal impairment
- Immune system activation
- Increased mast cells
- Mineral deficiencies
- Musculoskeletal abnormalities
- Neurocognitive deficiencies
- Nose and smell abnormalities
- Porphyrin enzyme abnormalities
- Respiratory impairment
- Sensory nerve impairment
- Vestibular impairment
- Vitamin deficiencies
- Xenobiotics in fat, blood, urine and hair.

damaged; haematuria should be checked, together with other markers of kidney function. The skin is frequently affected, with rashes, itching, welts, hives, flushing, blood blisters and dermatitis. Immune function needs to be checked and investigated, with immunoglobulin E (IgE) and eosinophil measurements, and specific cells (e.g. CD3, CD26) counted. Autoimmune disease markers should be looked for, for example phospholipids and nuclear antibodies. The endocrine system is commonly disabled or dysfunctional, and so thyroid, cortisol and dehydroepiandrosterone (DHEA) tests are important.

Psychological tests of motor activity, sensory function, memory and cognition are all valuable.[13,14]

Only when all this has been done may a psychiatric or psychogenic diagnosis be considered in the light of possible co-morbid emotional problems.[15]

INTERNATIONAL RECOGNITION OF MCS

MCS is increasingly recognized by legal and medical systems. It was first officially recognized in Germany and described, using the WHO's ICD, as ICD-10-SGB-V, November 2000, under the code T78.4, 'allergy, otherwise not specified'.[16] Reports from Australia[17] and Denmark[18] have also been published. The Australian report includes a literature assessment, evidence from 22 witnesses, and 167 written submissions from Australia and overseas. It makes a recommendation for classification of MCS under its own modification of the WHO codes as ICD-10-AM. The Danish report is more limited, drawing largely on a published review assessing the situation in the UK.[19]

In North America, MCS is widely recognized. In the USA, official recognition takes the form of reports from the Department of Justice, the Department of Housing and Urban Development, and the Department of Education, which accept MCS as a legitimate condition for their purposes. Medical resistance to MCS has begun to evaporate among the American College of Physicians.[20] The American Medical Association and American Lung Association and Environmental Protection Agency state that 'Claimants should not be dismissed as psychogenic and a thorough workup is essential ...' Large population surveys report 16–33 per cent of people as being sensitive to everyday chemicals.

In 1998, 25 US federal and 28 US state authorities were listed and summaries of medical and legal/compensation papers and cases provided. Canada has recognized MCS in ten state authorities[21] and has published a major review of the evidence linking its recognition to human rights.[22]

In contrast, official sources in the UK have been resistant to any recognition of chemical sensitivity. The British Society for Allergy, Environmental and Nutritional Medicine (BSAENM; now the British Society of Ecological Medicine, BSEM) has published substantial evidence in recognition of MCS as an organic illness that can be diagnosed and treated effectively.[23,24] Although MCS does not fit comfortably into current views on allergy, the Royal College of Physicians' report *Allergy: The Unmet Need* records a huge increase in allergy in the UK.[25] Currently one person in three in the UK has some form of allergy, a total of 18 million people; of these, some 3 million have severe allergies. The Royal Commission on Environmental Pollution identified the need for a proper understanding of the health effects of novel chemicals used widely and distributed ubiquitously in the environment.[26] A further report by the Royal Commission endorsed the validity of GWS, myalgic encephalomyelitis (ME; chronic fatigue syndrome, CFS) and MCS in its appendices.[22] The Research Advisory Committee on Gulf War Veterans' Illnesses from the USA summarized epidemiological studies indicating that 28–32 per cent of veterans from the first Gulf War are now ill with symptoms, including MCS.[27]

Veterans of the first Gulf War represent large cohorts of fit, young, mainly male military personnel from the USA ($n = 697\,000$) and the UK ($n = 53\,000$) who were exposed to a wide variety of biological and chemical toxins.[28] Such large numbers of personnel allow considerable statistical analysis of their illnesses (GWS). There is extensive evidence of damage to the central, autonomic and peripheral nervous systems, to the cardiovascular system, and to other organs and bodily systems, and there is evidence of birth defects in some offspring.

In Sweden, electrosensitivity is officially recognized but is seen as a condition rather than a disease.

PREVALENCE OF MCS AND ESTIMATED COSTS IN THE USA

The confusion and lack of uniformity in trying to assess the prevalence of MCS in various communities makes any figures open to questioning; however, various large population surveys report 16–33 per cent of people being sensitive to everyday chemicals, with the best estimates coming from studies and reports in the USA (Table 50.4).[29]

Table 50.4 Prevalence of multiple chemical sensitivity (MCS)

Reference	% with MCS
Bell *et al.*[31]	15
Bell *et al.*[32]	17
Meggs *et al.*[33]	33
Voorhees[34]	17
Bell *et al.*[35]	30 (Gulf War veterans)
Kreutzer *et al.*[36]	15.9 (doctor diagnosed 6.3)
Caress and Steinemann[37]	12.6
Caress and Steinemann[38]	11.2
Caress and Steinemann[39]	11.2 (doctor diagnosed 7.4)

All studies report MCS as more common in women but not associated with socioeconomic status.

Source: Centers for Disease Control and Prevention.[30]

A surprising number of people report sensitivity to ordinary everyday chemicals. The figures range from an average of eleven to seventeen percent, with spikes as high as thirty percent of subjects who report reactions to multiple chemical incitants. The figures reveal that at least two percent, and as many as six percent, have been so bothered by chemical exposures that they sought medical care and received a doctor-diagnosis of multiple chemical sensitivity (MCS). Applying the case definition criteria to the average reported chemical sensitivity, it appears that 1.5 out of 10 people suffer from MCS. Health care utilization costs directly related to MCS have been estimated at approximately $1581 annually per patient. The United States population is estimated to be 302.8 million. Prevalence studies predict that approximately 15% of the United States population, now estimated at 302.8 million, suffers from MCS; therefore, direct health care utilization costs amount to a staggering $71.8 billion dollars per year. Estimated costs for MCS and other disorders linked to neurotoxicity amount to an additional $81.5 to $167 billion annually in lost productivity. Cumulative social and economic costs identified in four case studies of illnesses that are candidates for environmental causation totalled between $568 billion and $793 billion dollars per year.[30]

By any criteria, the impact of MCS on individual and community health and the cost to the nation (healthcare budgets) and those directly concerned with the illness (carers and dependants) is considerable.

CHEMICALS INVOLVED

The number and nature of chemicals associated with MCS is huge and covers many different chemical classes, biological activities and sources. Table 50.5 summarizes the major chemicals, their sources and their biological activities.[21,29,40–43] American national studies commenced in 1999, but so far these cover only 148 different compounds.[30,44] There are important concerns about how to interpret the data and the need to avoid a one-size-fits-all approach. It is necessary to take into account individual factors, including absorption, distribution, metabolism, excretion, genetics, age, sex, environment and nutritional status.[45]

Various studies have found extensive chemical contamination of people throughout the world.[46–48] Of particular interest is the identification of hundreds of toxic compounds in cord blood, indicating that even in utero, when cellular replication is at its greatest, there is no protection against many very toxic compounds.[49,50]

Of special note is a report that identified 287 different chemicals in cord blood from newborns. Of these chemicals, 217 were toxic to the brain and nervous system, 208 could cause developmental problems, and 108 cause cancer in humans and animals.[50] American organizations have emphasized the connection between mental retardation and other developmental disorders, including autism-spectrum disorders, and learning and developmental conditions in children,[48,51] and they stress the lack of any testing of individual chemicals and mixtures for these disorders. Chronic neurological and neuropsychiatric conditions are increasing in older people, possibly as a result of the massive increase in environmental toxins.[52]

The problem was first highlighted in Rachel Carson's groundbreaking work *Silent Spring*,[53] which was then followed by other publications.[54] Many compounds have been withdrawn but, because of their persistence in the environment and people, contamination is now widespread. For example, PCBs were banned in 1979 in America, but people born after that date are commonly contaminated with these compounds.

A comprehensive study provides considerable data on extensive biological damage to fertility, intelligence and survival as a result of the untrammelled use and irresponsible spread of numerous untested environmental chemicals.[55]

Table 50.5 Major classes of chemicals associated with multiple chemical sensitivity (MCS)

Chemical class	Known biological activities	Common sources/uses
Highly substituted, poly- or per-halogenated organic compounds with chlorine, bromine or fluorine atoms*, e.g. DDT, DDE, lindane, hexachlorobenzene, hexachlorocyclohexanes, PCBs, aldrin, dieldrin, PBDEs, perfluorooctanoic acid polymers and derivatives	Carcinogenic, mutagenic, kidney and liver damage, endocrine disruption	Household and agricultural pesticides as sprays and dusts, electrical insulation, flame-retardants, non-stick kitchen utensils, stain-resistant fabrics
Organophosphates, nerve agents	Nerve toxins, immune dysregulation, inhibition of key enzymes	Various pesticides in agriculture, fisheries, herbicides, engine oils
Phthalates, nonylphenol, bisphenol A and B*	Endocrine disruption	Polymers, plasticizers, toys, babies' pacifiers, dialysis tubing
VOCs, aliphatic and aromatic compounds*, formaldehyde, aldehydes, esters, ketones, acids, alcohols, toluene	Disruption of brain function, nerve damage, carcinogenic	Ubiquitous in fragrances, perfumes, household goods, solvents, fuels, paints, polymers
PAHs	Carcinogenic, mutagenic	Burning fuels, exhaust fumes, power stations
Heavy metals: mercury*, lead, cadmium, arsenic, organometallics, tributyltin*	Neurotoxicity, tissue damage, endocrine disruption	Anti-fouling paints, fuels, preservatives, pesticides, electrical goods, crematoria

*Bioaccumlative and biomagnified through the food chain.

DDT, dichlorodiphenyltrichloroethane; DDE, dichlorodichlorophenylethene (major metabolite of DDT); PAHs, polyaromatic hydrocarbons; PBDEs, polybromodiphenylethers; PCBs, polychlorobiphenyls; VOCs, volatile organic compounds.

The challenge is to understand:

- how such diverse chemicals can provoke very sensitive responses to chemically unrelated compounds – this raises new question about drug and chemical receptors and how they operate;
- how very low levels of exposure well below those affecting the majority of people can provoke such extensive and profound biological effects – this questions the basic understanding of toxicology, particularly the relationship between dose and response and genetics;
- how the damage to one generation can be transmitted to succeeding generations.

In response to these challenges, new mechanisms of drug and chemical action have been proposed, coupled with technologies that provide hidden details of bodily systems, particularly the brain. A further challenge is to understand:

- how so many different chemicals, which have not been evaluated for adverse biological effects, have come to be released for general use;
- how novel chemicals can be assessed effectively before release into general use.

In response to these challenges, new regulatory systems have been advocated, particularly Registration, Evaluation, Authorisation and Restriction of Chemical Substances (REACH) in Europe.[56] In the USA, action is being demanded to establish a similar regulatory authority.[57]

Estimates from various sources indicate that 80 000–100 000 compounds currently used commercially and distributed in a wide variety of products have never been assessed toxicologically or have been assessed only as single entities and not in the complex mixtures in which they are delivered in most products.[58–60]

Clearly, in addition to the concerns about health, there are important commercial, political and economic considerations around the use and development of chemicals in today's world. There is no doubt that there is considerable vested interest and even secrecy when MCS is being considered, not unlike the activities and attitudes around tobacco-smoking, nuclear power, and genetically modified (GM) crops. A big divide lies between those espousing a purely psychogenic, psychiatric or psychological understanding of the illness and those seeking to understand the illness as an organic illness with a clear biological basis.

PSYCHOGENIC, PSYCHIATRIC AND PSYCHOLOGICAL VERSUS THE BIOLOGICAL UNDERSTANDING OF MCS

This is well exemplified by the following titles:

- 'Allergic to life: psychological factors in environmental illness'[61]
- 'In search of non-disease'.[62]

In marked contrast are the following:

- *Stop the 21st Century Killing You*[63]
- *Chemical Exposures: Low Levels and High Stakes*[64]
- *Chemical Sensitivity*, a large medical publication in four volumes with an allied website.[65]

The website 'Chemical sensitivity in mainstream medical documentation' considers all aspects of the debate about MCS, with a strong emphasis on the implications for people who are affected by MCS.[66]

A major two-stage population study of MCS found that only 1.4 per cent of the population studied had emotional problems before exposures occurred, but that after the development of MCS 37.7 per cent of the population had emotional problems, indicating that MCS had a biological rather than psychogenic origin.[25] This is hardly surprising, since any chronic illness is likely to precipitate emotional problems.

THE DEBATE

MCS and other illnesses from a variety of medical specialties have been described as functional somatic syndromes[5] in order to provide a comprehensive scheme for understanding these complex and little-understood conditions/illnesses. This approach has been severely criticized as a disguise for medical ignorance that seeks to label emerging illnesses as psychiatric when they present with symptoms very different from those of established mental illnesses:

> It must be noted that there is no proof that it is justified to apply the label somatisation to such conditions as chronic fatigue syndrome and several more illnesses that established medicine has so far failed to explain scientifically... Don't hesitate to ask questions about scientific evidence behind this talk about somatisation. Be persistent, because a diagnosis of somatisation is definitely not an innocuous label. It will close various doors and lead (to) treatments that usually get nowhere.[14]

Somatization has a poor track record, being used at one time to 'explain' diabetes, Parkinson's disease, multiple sclerosis and Grave's disease. All of these now have clear, well-established biological foundations.[46–49,67]

The biopsychosocial theory is now offered as the basis for understanding these complex illnesses/conditions. However, although this appears to embrace a more holistic view, one of its major critics states: 'The biopsychosocial theory lacks an intellectually sound basis, and spells the failure and possible imminent extinction of modern psychiatry.'[15]

The intellectual basis for the biological understanding of MCS is found in the neuroendocrine–immune (NEI) paradigm (Figure 50.1). This integrated communication system includes messenger molecules that are released in response to a wide range of challenges. Since these challenges include stress, it is important that the impact of stress is recognized in patients with MCS, but not by denying the

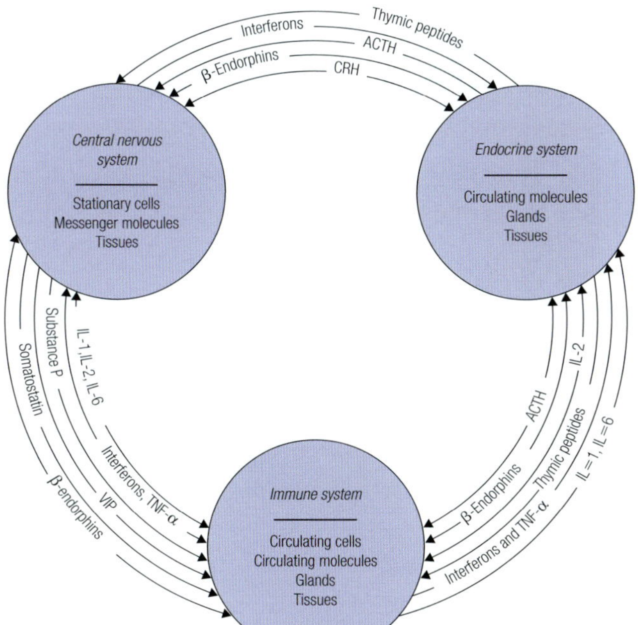

Figure 50.1 The neuroendocrine immune comprehensive integrative defence system

ACTH, adrenocortiotrophic hormone; CRH, corticotropin-releasing hormone; IL, interleukin; TNF, tumour necrosis factor; VIP, vasoactive intestinal peptide.

biological impact of chemical exposures. Many patients with MCS report high levels of stress if they are disbelieved or falsely accused when seeking medical help for this syndrome.

A German multicentre study on MCS examined 291 consecutive out-patients between 2000 and 2003 in considerable depth and concluded that:[50]

- there was no characteristic set of symptoms for MCS, although many symptoms and clinical signs were identified;
- there was no systematic connection between complaints and any triggers;
- there was no evidence for any genetic predisposition but only metabolic variations in specific alleles;
- there was no obvious disturbance of the olfactory system;
- patients with MCS suffered more often from mental disorders that had commenced 'many years before environment-related health complaints';
- 'overall the study did not support a toxicogenic-somatic basis of the MCS phenomenon'.

These serious and comprehensive conclusions contradict many other studies.[21,25,27,28,30,43] However, the same study noted some real problems when engaging with MCS:

- A lack of biomarkers, which are now being identified in specific cases[68,69]
- A lack of clear-cut parameters of dysfunction
- Case criteria were usually formulated only vaguely and were open to multiple interpretations
- '... despite all efforts of standardisation ... such attempts [were] very limited in clinical-based studies ... for each individual case completely different examination may be used which makes standardisation of diagnostic procedures much more difficult'.[50]

This final statement points to two different approaches to environmental medicine: (i) a one-size-fits-all approach when considering a patient population and (ii) an approach that sees patients as unique individuals who require individualized medicine for their effective treatment and support.

The study was restricted to volatile organic compound (VOCs) and olfaction and used the 1987 Cullen criteria rather than the more widely agreed 1999 consensus.[42] Even here, an important study involving capsaicin, a classical vanilloid receptor agonist, has been ignored; this study concluded:

> Upper and lower airway symptoms induced by chemicals and scents represent an entity of chronic disease, different from asthma or chronic obstructive pulmonary disease, with persistent symptoms, a reduced health-related quality of life and unchanged sensory hyperreactivity.[70]

Other papers conclude that the combined environmental annoyance, smells and electrical equipment is a better predictor of chemical intolerance[71] and that above-average odour discrimination ability was associated with lower ratings of odour intensity and nausea.[58,59]

There was no consideration of any possible influence of extensive and multiple contamination by xenobiotics. People from Central Europe were found to carry the highest burden of such compounds.[48]

Additive and synergistic effects of such contamination were not considered. There was no consideration of mutagenic and developmental effects of chemical exposure.[46–50,58,59,68–71]

There was no consideration of possible brain damage from other widely dispersed toxins such as pesticides.[44,72,73] No psychometric tests[45,51] appear to have been carried out. Sickness behaviour is well-known to be associated with changes in levels of important cytokines that influence the brain–immune axis,[60] but this does not appear to have been investigated.

Overall, the firm conclusions are less secure than they may at first appear.

More recent papers report that exposure to VOCs increases plasma levels of vasoactive intestinal peptide (VIP), substance P and nerve growth factors in self-reported MCS patients (sMCS).[74] Exposure to diesel fumes induced both Th-1 and Th-2 chemokines.[75]

A major conference hosted by the Chemical Injury Information Network (CIIN) provided a comprehensive survey of MCS with copies of important papers in the field.[76]

CONCEPTS AND MECHANISMS

Triggering

Many people with MCS can identify an event when they experienced a large exposure to a toxic chemical, such as a pesticide being sprayed outside or inside the house, a workplace exposure, an accidental spillage or an adventitious agricultural spraying. This is followed by an increasing sensitivity to the same or related chemicals and then to quite diverse chemicals in very different situations. Gulf War veterans show an increased incidence of chemical sensitivity and MCS.[66,77,78] More than 40 possible battlefield exposures in 1990–91 have been identified,[79] with the major ones being vaccines, pyridostigmine bromide (anti-nerve agent prophylaxis), pesticides (organophosphates, pyrethroids, lindane), nerve agents (sarin, tabun, VX), depleted uranium, oil and smoke.[67] Frequently, veterans develop chemical sensitivity to perfume worn by their partners or children and previously enjoyed by the veteran, to alcohol and to petroleum fumes, which previously was not a problem.[66,80,81] The chemistry of perfumes and petroleum products is extensive and diverse and very different from that of pesticides, vaccines and the major Gulf War exposures.

Chronic low-dose exposure to chemicals that may not be apparent to a person can also lead to MCS by a process known as 'kindling'.[79] Rowat, as part of his proposed integrative defence mechanisms, defines kindling as follows:

Kindling refers to neural processes that mediate lasting changes in brain function in response to repeated, temporally spaced application of neurobehaviorally active agents.

Partial limbic kindling is a progressive and persistent lowering of the threshold for eliciting electrical after-discharges, but not motor seizures, in certain brain structures such as amygdala and hippocampus; behavioral consequences include increased avoidant behaviors.

The range of physical action for kindling includes various brain structures, e.g. the cortex and especially the limbic brain including the olfactory bulb and amygdala. Changes in brain chemistry are found, including a decrease in acetylcholinesterase enzyme activity that parallels the increase in sensitivity. Calcium-binding protein and tyrosine hydroxylase activity are reportedly reduced, and there are changes in β-noradrenergic binding. Benzodiazepine receptor binding is modified, as are transmitter GABA [γ-aminobutyric acid] and *N*-methyl-D-aspartate [NMDA] functions. Zinc may be implicated through GABA. Superoxide dismutase may also be involved. These changes may be irreversible.[15]

The blood–brain barrier

The blood–brain barrier is the barrier of endothelial cells lining the blood vessels in the brain (Figure 50.2). The cells possess tight cell junctions that severely restrict access of compounds from the blood into the brain. This is a protective mechanism to restrict entry into the brain of biological and chemical toxins that may be ingested, inhaled or generated by infection in other parts of the body or by injury. There are selective transport mechanisms that supply neuronal and other cells with essential nutrients.

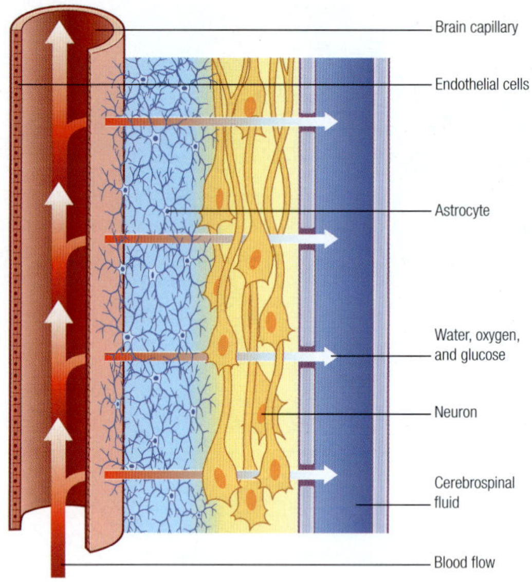

Figure 50.2 Blood–brain barrier
Reproduced with permission from ref. 82

Tight cell junctions occur in other tissues, particularly the gut and the lungs. This protection limits transport across the gut wall (e.g. toxins and infections in food and water) and the lungs (e.g. inhaled toxins), but it is known to be breached by many chemicals, including various pesticides.[83–86] The blood–testes barrier is similarly breached.[87] Microbial zona occludens toxins (ZOT) also open the tight cell junctions of the blood–brain barrier.[88,89] Inflammatory cytokines[90] and other peptide molecules are also effective.[91]

The bypassing of the blood–brain barrier by intraneuronal transport via the olfactory bulb allows toxins direct access into the brain.[79]

A study in mice found that doses of parathion or permethrin at attomolar (10^{-18} molar) concentrations opened up the blood–brain barrier and increased transport of a marker compound into the brain by about 20 per cent.[92] These tiny quantities correspond to the amount of residue that would be found on a single apple following spraying.

The blood–brain barrier is least efficient in the region of the paleolithic brain, and any leakage through the barrier will be greatest in the basal ganglia, brainstem, thalamus, hypothalamus and pituitary gland.

Essential tissue barriers can be opened or bypassed by various mechanisms that are known to be associated with MCS and related overlapping syndromes.

Toxicant-induced loss of tolerance

The concept of TILT was proposed as a useful alternative to MCS in 1998[79] and was fully developed later.[93] A common mechanism is postulated for both drug addiction and multiple chemical intolerance, but with opposite responses – addiction (a demand for regular and repeated doses) and abdiction (avoidance of a substance). In both cases, the intent is to avoid withdrawal symptoms associated with a lack or presence of the substance. The basic idea is set out in Figure 50.3, in which the normal response to a stimulant (e.g. caffeine) involves stimulation followed by recovery. Loss of tolerance leads to an increased response, which leads to alternative strategies, abdication (avoidance) or addiction (persistent reinforcing doses).

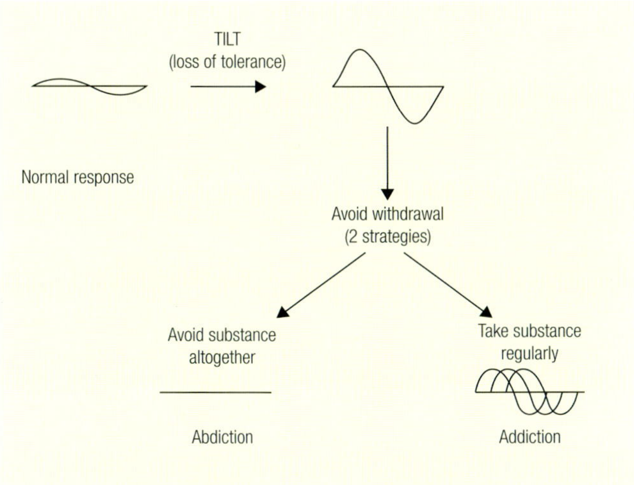

Figure 50.3 Toxicant-induced loss of tolerance (TILT): relationship between abdiction and addiction

Miller, in making a case for TILT, relies heavily on the data from various studies involving Gulf War veterans.[81] In particular, she draws attention to the concomitant development of a number of cravings for chocolate, sugar and caffeine in these veterans. This phenomenon has not been commented on previously.

Another aspect of the proposed relationship between abdiction and addiction is that dopaminergic, 5-hydroxytrypamine (5-HT) and opioid neural pathways in the brain are associated with addiction and the response to addictive drugs and food. These same pathways are damaged in Gulf War veterans.

Volatile or aerosolized inhaled substances may be carried by intraneuronal transport along the olfactory tract directly into the limbic system (Figure 50.4). This bypasses the blood–brain barrier and introduces compounds directly into deep (silent) brain structures where many basic bodily responses are controlled.

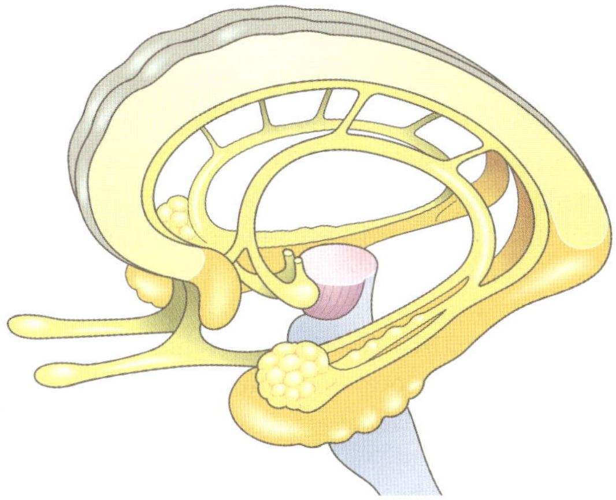

Figure 50.4 Limbic system, showing the olfactory tracts

Allergy, neurogenic inflammation and switching

The association of MCS with allergy has been the subject of considerable debate, concerned mainly with the definition of allergy. One common scheme recognizes four kinds of allergy and hypersensitivity:[94]

- *Type 1:* mediated by immunoglobulin E (IgE) and almost immediate (2–30 min). May lead to systemic anaphylaxis, which can be life-threatening, or to more localized anaphylaxis (e.g. insect bites, hay fever, asthma, hives, eczema, food allergies). IgE interacts with specific cells (basophils, mast cells), which are stimulated to release potent vasoactive mediators such as histamine and leucotrienes.
- *Type 2:* antibody-mediated. The antibodies immunoglobulin G (IgG) and immunoglobulin M (IgM) attack sites on cell walls, leading to total destruction of the cell. This process takes 2–8 h. The cell damage or loss can be very serious. Examples include blood-transfusion reactions and some types of anaemia.
- *Type 3:* involves antigen–antibody (IgG) complex formation and takes 2–8 h. The antigen–antibody complex precipitates in various tissues and induces an inflammatory reaction. Examples include a number of chronic illnesses, including glomerulonephritis, rheumatoid arthritis and systemic lupus erythematosus (SLE). A delayed response to insect bites or vaccines may operate by this mechanism.
- *Type 4:* cell-mediated. Hypersensitivity is slow (24–72 h). It involves sensitized immune cells, special T-cells that release chemical messengers (cytokines) that activate other immune cells, causing direct cell damage. Contact dermatitis, tubercular lesions and graft rejection are examples.

Not uncommonly, a single chemical or group of chemicals can induce more than one type of allergic response, for example penicillins can cause types 1–4 reactions.

Meggs and colleagues define allergy as a type 1 reaction. They regard MCS as the opposite side of the coin, sharing a similar mechanism to allergy:[95,96]

- The response to an allergen or a chemical irritant is not limited to the immediate site of application or entry. For example, about 2 per cent of people with asthma have their asthma triggered by eating certain foods or alcohol.[97] The inoculation of the gut leads to a response in the lungs: Meggs calls this 'switching'. Bee stings may cause a generalized reaction involving the whole body and not only the local area affected by the sting itself. Similarly, chemicals that are generally inhaled can cause diverse symptomatology associated with the central nervous system, headaches, pain, rashes and gastrointestinal disturbances.
- Adaptation is a key four-stage construct in chemical exposures that has been known from the 1950s. The removal of the offending chemical(s) will lead to recovery, except at stage 3:
  - *Stage 0:* exposures are tolerated without illness.
  - *Stage 1:* exposure leads to multiple complaints, e.g. headache, nausea, itching, flushing.
  - *Stage 2:* inflammation occurs in one or more organs, e.g. rhinitis, asthma, arthritis, myositis (inflammatory muscle disease). Continued low-dose exposure at this stage will propagate the inflammatory condition(s).
  - *Stage 3:* fibrosis with tissue damage, irreversible lung disease, advanced asthma, deforming arthritis, etc. All the major systems can be affected, including musculoskeletal, respiratory, cardiovascular, gastrointestinal, genitourinary and nervous.
- Conditioning is a feature of MCS. In chemical sensitivity, the most common classes of chemicals to trigger a reaction are volatile and odorous. The odour threshold is many times lower than the chemical irritancy threshold, and this may explain the large difference in exposure levels that develop in people with MCS.
- Essentially, chemical irritants bind to receptors on unmyelinated sensory nerve C-fibres, which are found in the gut, airways, eye and genitourinary system and are more numerous in patients with MCS. Binding triggers an inflammatory response via an axon reflex, leading to release of substance P and subsequently other localized mediators of inflammation by interaction with mast cells (Figures 50.5 and 50.6).

Central pathways also activate parasympathetic or sympathetic nerves with effects on more distant organs.[98]

Meggs and colleagues make much use of data from studies on Gulf War veterans; they report extensive intolerance to petrol, diesel, oils and exhaust fumes.[99] Many veterans describe their response as loss of awareness ('spaced out'), loss of motor control and ataxia. In some cases, this was so marked that driving became dangerous. Some veterans are unable to fill up their vehicle at a petrol station because this would render them incapable of driving safely. Mortality studies on Gulf War veterans show that there is an excess of deaths from motor vehicle accidents in this group.[27] Although this has been dismissed by the UK Ministry of Defence (MoD) and the US Department of Defense (DoD) as a legacy of military service resulting in extravagant and risk-taking behaviour and an inability to cope with a return to civilian life, no other explanation has been forthcoming. MCS offers another explanation that better accords with the evidence and military training, which requires that extravagant risks be avoided and makes motor control and awareness paramount.

A useful summary of the varied responses to chemical exposures is given in Figure 50.7. This includes the recognition of the importance of perception and central integration of the experience (Figure 50.8).

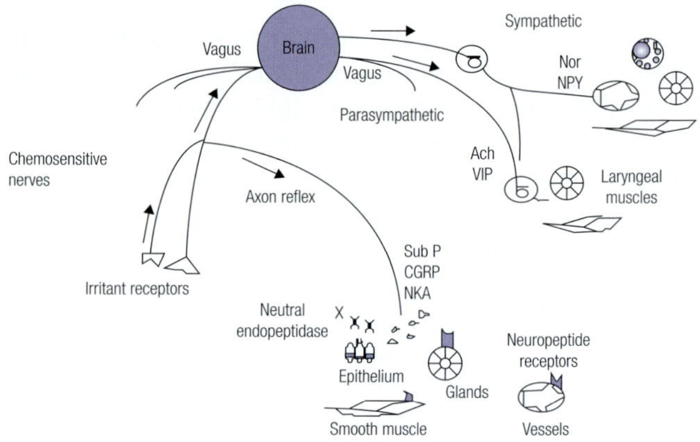

Figure 50.5 Axon and central reflexes initiated by triggering chemosensitive receptors on C-fibres

Ach, acetylcholine; CGRP, calcitonin gene-related peptide; NKA, neurokinin A; Nor, noradrenaline; NPY, neuropeptide Y; Sub P, substance P; VIP, vasoactive intestinal peptide.

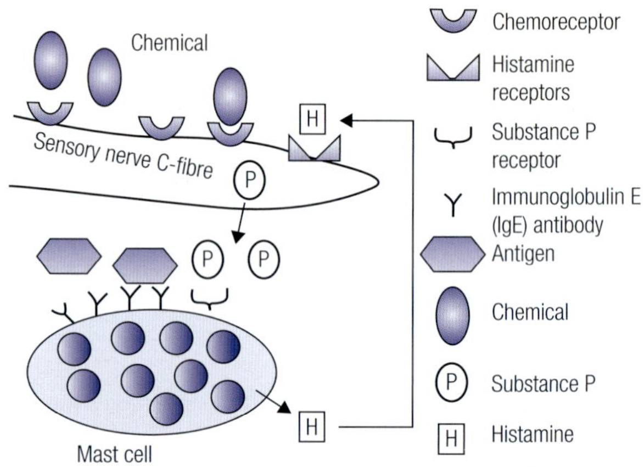

Figure 50.6 Localized release of substance P triggered by chemical activation, leading to further release of inflammatory mediators from mast cells

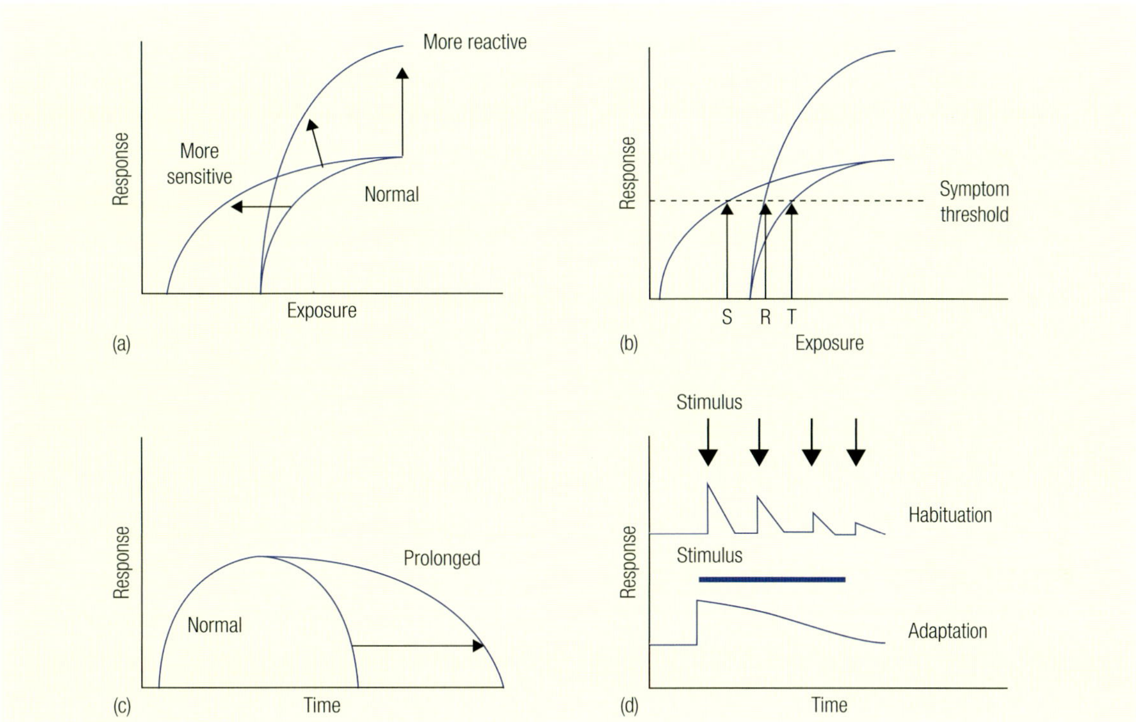

Figure 50.7 Summary of responses to chemical exposures. (a) More sensitive = a decrease in the magnitude of exposure required to initiate the response; more reactive = an increase in the slope or in the maximum level of the exposure–response curve. (b) The threshold for perceiving symptoms may occur in the mid-position of the exposure–response curve (T). As a result, the clinical report of increased sensitivity could mean that the individual has become more reactive (R) or more sensitive (S). (c) Recognition of symptoms may require the response to be present for a certain duration. The clinical report of increased sensitivity could mean that the response has become more prolonged. (d) Habituation = decreasing responses with single repeat exposures; adaptation = progressive decrease in magnitude of response with prolonged exposure

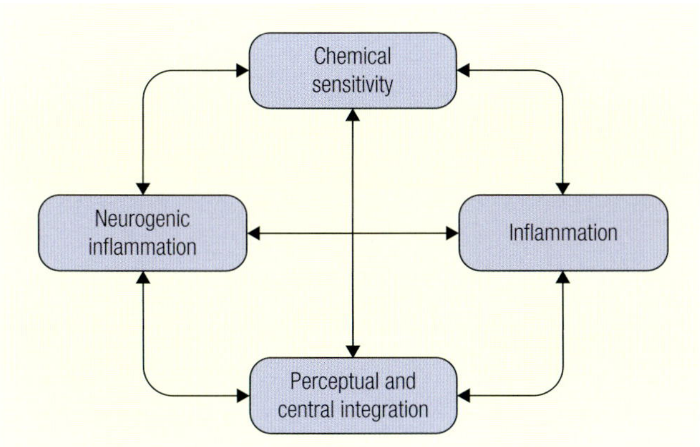

Figure 50.8 Potential interactions between chemical sensitivity and the domains of neurogenic inflammation, perceptual and central integration, and non-neurogenic inflammation

DAMAGE TO DEEP BRAIN STRUCTURES

Haley found clear evidence from MRS of cell death in the basal ganglia and brainstem of sick American veterans from the first Gulf War (Figure 50.9).[12] Later studies in animals and from historical exposures found more areas of the brain to be damaged, leading to the conclusion that 'While preliminary, such findings raise the concern that ill Gulf War veterans may have neuronal damage in multiple regions of the brain'.[27] Undoubtedly, the major chemicals involved are inhibitors of acetylcholinesterase, organophosphate insecticides, the nerve agent sarin and pyridostigmine bromide – the so-called 'cholinergic triple whammy'.[67] A useful paper analyses studies of sick veterans, agricultural workers and shepherds.[100]

Damage to the deep brain structures is consistent with penetration of the blood–brain barrier by toxic chemicals either via the bloodstream or by intraneuronal transport

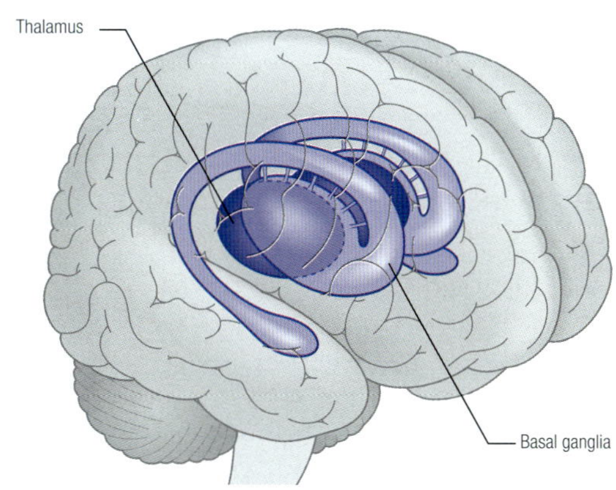

Figure 50.9 Basal ganglia wrapped round the thalamus, deep in the brain

along the olfactory tract, as suggested by Ashford and Miller.[64] Undoubtedly, veterans of the first Gulf War were exposed to a large number of diverse chemical and biological toxins and considerable electromagnetic radiation from many sources. Some 25–30 per cent of these veterans are now ill,[27] and for this to happen to healthy young people in the prime of life serves as a warning to the whole of society about taking care with the manner in which we expose even the healthiest people to novel chemicals. The counter view, that seeks to establish Gulf War illness (GWI)/GWS as a psychiatric illness,[101] is typical of the debate that rages around MCS in the face of incontrovertible and replicated evidence of significant brain damage in sick Gulf War veterans.[99] It is important to examine the implications for mental health rather than to claim that there is no such evidence.

METABOLISM AND CHEMICALS

The liver is the main but not the only organ of metabolism and is crucial in removing both endogenous and exogenous compounds/xenobiotics from the body. Metabolic processes are generally well understood and involve a range of established chemical reactions. Of particular importance is a two-stage process involving phase 1 and phase 2 metabolism. Phase 1 involves a large family of haem-containing enzymes, mono-oxygenases and cytochrome P450 enzymes (CYP450),[93,102] which introduce oxygen atoms into organic compounds that are largely lipid-soluble, creating highly reactive intermediates. In phase 2, these intermediates undergo conjugation with a variety of molecules to generate water-soluble products that can be excreted in the urine (Figure 50.10).[103] An important but secondary process involves excretion of some lipid compounds in the faeces.

Human CYPs play an important part in the transformation of many key endogenous compounds (e.g. steroidogenesis) but they have been studied most widely in connection with drug metabolism and some carcinogenic compounds (e.g. polycyclic aromatic hydrocarbons, PAHs). The metabolism and elimination of xenobiotics is now an important area of toxicology.[104,105] CYP450s are involved in the metabolism of about 75 per cent of drugs and xenobiotics and are present in many important areas in the body, including the mitochondrial membranes, the blood–brain barrier, the gastrointestinal tract and the liver. Many xenobiotics distributed widely in the environment are PAHs. Phase 1 metabolism transforms PAHs via the introduction of active oxygen species into very reactive compounds such as epoxides, which in turn undergo phase 2 conjugation into more polar compounds, which can be excreted in the urine. If oxidative phase 1 processes are not controlled carefully and coupled with phase 2 reactions, then destructive reactive oxygen species (ROS) are produced, leading to oxidative stress, which can cause considerable tissue damage – a feature of all complex multi-system illnesses.[2] Reliable data

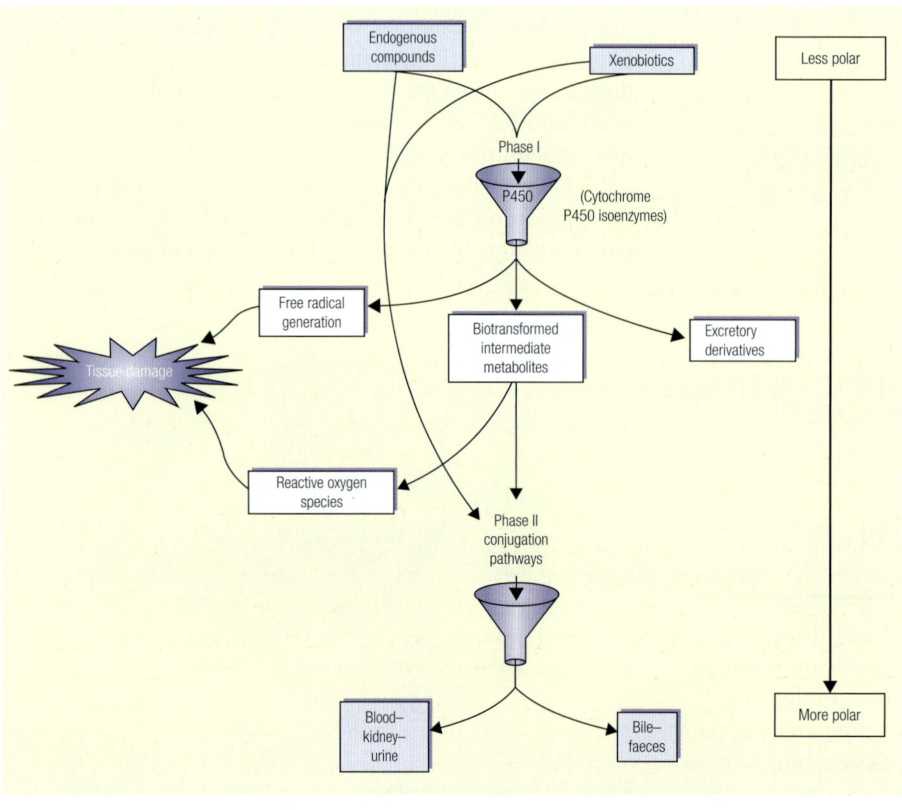

Figure 50.10 Phase 1 and phase 2 metabolism. Cytochrome P450 (CYP450) enzymes generate free radicals and reactive intermediates

are available for ME/CFS,[106,107] GWS,[99,100] organochlorine pesticides[108] and organophosphate pesticides, alone or in combination with other xenobiotics.[109,110] Both mitochondrial function and the nervous system are affected.

Oxidative stress, defined as an imbalance between reactive oxygen species and free radicals and antioxidant compounds, can also arise from other defence processes such as inflammation, which are also tightly controlled under normal circumstances.

This insight into multi-system illnesses suggests useful ways of providing treatment for patients with MCS.

Bioactivation can be a result of the metabolic conversion of xenobiotics (aflatoxins) and drugs (ethyl carbamate, troglitazone, terfenadine)[104] to more toxic compounds. In contrast, many persistent and bioaccumulative compounds possess bonds that are resistant to cleavage in metabolic reactions. This is particularly true of carbon–halogen bonds attached to aromatic or ethylenic carbon atoms. Such compounds accumulate up the food chain, leading to increasing doses in the organisms, including humans, that are at the top of the food chain. Significant contamination of fish oils with PCBs and dioxins[111] and of tuna and swordfish with mercury[112] have been reported, leading to advice to restrict the intake of these foodstuffs. Mercury is both concentrated and bioactivated to methyl mercury when it passes up the food chain, and this was the cause of the severe neurotoxic/psychiatric Minamata disease.[113,114]

Phase 2 metabolism assists the elimination of many compounds by conjugation of reactive chemical groups present in endogenous and exogenous compounds. The classical example is paracetamol. The metabolic pathway involves conjugation with sulphate or glucuronyl groups, but when these become exhausted in patient who has taken an overdose, a toxic quinoneimine is formed, which binds to glutathione, the primary cellular antioxidant molecule. The progressive removal of glutathione is responsible for the slow but often inevitable fatal effects of paracetamol.[98]

GENETICS

ME/CFS has been investigated extensively by Kerr and colleagues, who have identified some 88 genes that are mainly up-regulated in very sick patients with ME/CFS.[19,115] The larger study identified seven clinical phenotypes for ME/CFS.[19,116] Although such studies have yet to be carried out on patients with MCS, there is evidence of genetic susceptibility in some studies.

The importance of genetic variations in drug- and xenobiotic-metabolizing enzymes was recognized at the beginning of the twenty-first century:[117,118]

> The underlying genetic predisposition of each patient will reflect combinations of poor- and extensive-metabolizer phenotypes; if these enzymes cooperate in the same metabolic pathway for any given drug or environmental agent, such ecogenetic variability might be synergistic and lead to as much as 30- or >40-fold differences in activation or degradation. The end result can be large interindividual differences in risk of environmentally caused toxicity or cancer.[119]

In one study, there was an 18-fold increase in the risk of MCS when interactions between CYP2D6 and NAT2 metabolizing enzymes occurred.[120] Another study found that variations in *NAT2* and *GST* genes were linked to increased chemical sensitivity.[121] One study did not find any link with some allele frequencies, but it considered only *NAT1*, *NAT2*, *PON1* and *PON2* and did not consider *CYP2D6* or *GST* genes.[122] Because of the large number of genetic variants of the many enzymes involved in xenobiotic metabolism, this is a complex but urgent area of study that will be very fruitful in understanding the widespread variations in MCS. Analogous studies to those of Kerr and colleagues are urgently needed.

Although traditionally the major concern has been with drug metabolism (pharmacogenomics), the wider term 'toxicogenomics'[123] has been introduced, and a paper describes how exposures to arsenic in drinking water can alter the gene function in babies born to mothers exposed in this way.[124] This disturbing link of arsenic exposure to increased inflammatory responses in the succeeding generation increases the urgency to recognize and treat MCS, of which it is a part.

The enzyme paraoxonase 1 (PON1) has been particularly well studied. It plays a key role in protecting against oxidative stress associated with the oxidation of low-density lipid particles. It is now recognized as a key enzyme in removing organophosphates[104,105] and nerve agents from the body. It is important in GWS, where initially it was proposed that genetic variants Q and R, respectively involving the amino acids glutamine or arginine at position 192 in the enzyme, were important;[125] soon, however, it was found that it was the level of the enzymes and not their genetic form that was important.[126,127] The use of leaded petrol in the Gulf War may well have depressed the levels of PON1, making the troops more susceptible to the toxic effects of organophosphates and nerve agents.[128] This illustrates the complexity of MCS where two apparently independent factors have been found to impact on the same biological system. Later studies indicated that there is genetic control of the levels of the enzyme produced,[109,129,130] particularly in connection with the recognition of organophosphates in aerotoxic syndrome.[131]

Polymorphisms

Polymorphisms are defined as variations in gene structure that are too common to be due merely to new mutations. A polymorphism must have a frequency of at least 1 per cent in the population. They have become the subject of intense research, as small changes in gene structure can now be identified that have been associated with the risk of developing chronic diseases in later life and also predicting the consequences of gene–environment interactions.[132] In single-nucleotide polymorphisms (SNPs), a single nucleotide change occurs that alters the function of the gene; for example, in the *PON1* gene, the trinucleotide sequences for the key amino acids at position 192 in the enzyme are glutamine (CAG) and arginine (CGG) and involve the single exchange of adenine (A) for guanosine (G). However, it is now clear that almost 200 polymorphisms have been found in *PON1*, although not all are functional. The direct measurement of the enzyme itself is the most reliable way of investigating its role in disease:

> We, along with other authors, would strongly suggest that all further epidemiological studies into the role of PON1 and disease should include a measurement of the enzyme itself in addition to the genetic polymorphisms.[133]

This conclusion is a measure of the difficulties of investigating complex multi-system illnesses such as MCS.

Epigenetics

Epigenetics concerns changes in the phenotypic expression of inherited genes by chemical modification of DNA and chromatin, which results in changes of gene function (transcription, replication, translation, combination). Such modifications involve methylation of DNA or methylation, acetylation, phosphorylation, ribosylation or ubiquitination of chromatin. These processes result in remodelling of chromatin, with subsequent changes in gene expression. Genes may be silenced or activated by these processes, which can cause permanent and heritable, or transient, changes in the phenotype.[134] These changes can occur throughout life: preconceptually, in either parent; periconceptually; early or late gestation; and in neonates, children, young adults and older

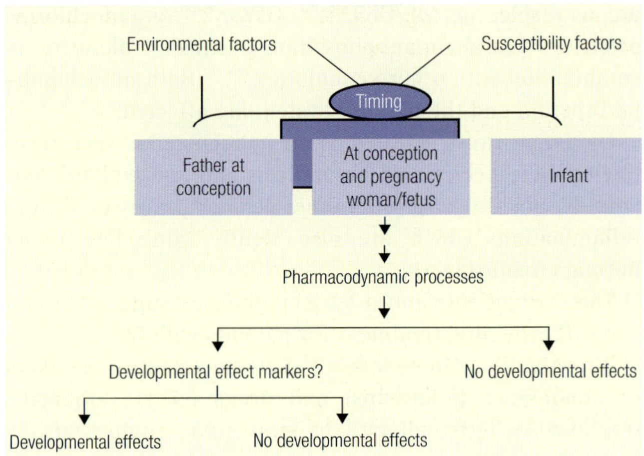

Figure 50.11 Interaction of factors potentially leading to adverse health outcomes

adults. Animal and epidemiological studies have identified changes in the reproductive organs, uterus and mammary glands, including cancers in later life (diethylstilboestrol, DES; bisphenol A, BPA), prostate problems (methoxychlor), sperm-counts, fertility problems, hypospadias (phthalates), nutritional effects, obesity (DES, tributyltin (TBT), BPA) and early-onset parkinsonism (paraquat, maneb).[135] The major factors are presented in Figure 50.11.[136]

It is a matter for concern that the nutritional status of the mother may have serious developmental outcomes for her offspring when they reach adult later life (Figure 50.12).[137] Combined with these adverse developmental effects, environmentally encountered heavy metals such as arsenic, manganese[138] and lead[119] will exacerbate the deficits imposed on children, particularly in the developing world, where parents, especially mothers, are under prolonged

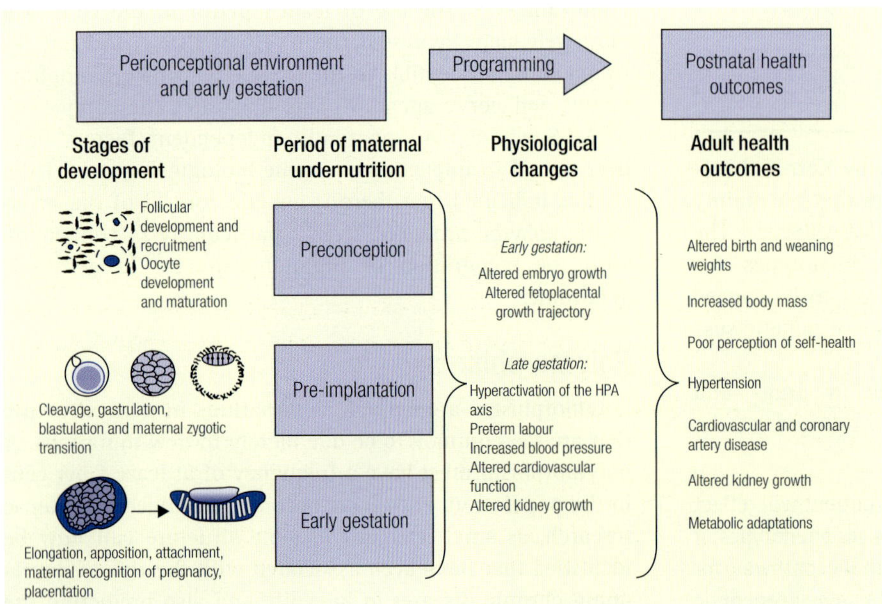

Figure 50.12 Current understanding of how maternal undernutrition during the periconceptual and early gestational windows of development may programme pathophysiology and adult disease

HPA, hypothalamus–pituitary axis.

socioeconomic stress.[139] This avoidable loss of human potential is a grievous loss to the world community.

Mitochondrial DNA

Mitochondrial DNA is derived only from the mother and is known to more readily undergo mutations and damage compared with nuclear DNA. Pathogenic mutations in mitochondrial DNA have been reported to be common.[140] The question arises as to what effects environmental toxins have in this process. Are epigenetic changes involved? Since oxidative stress, a feature of MCS, is associated with compromised mitochondrial function, these latest findings may be very important for the future.

THE NO/ONOO HYPOTHESIS

Pall brought together a long series of papers and reviews concerning the NO/ONOO (nitric oxide/peroxynitrite) hypothesis (Figure 50.13).[141] This provides a comprehensive disease paradigm for ME/CFS, MCS, fibromyalgia, post-traumatic stress disorder (PTSD), GWS and related illnesses.

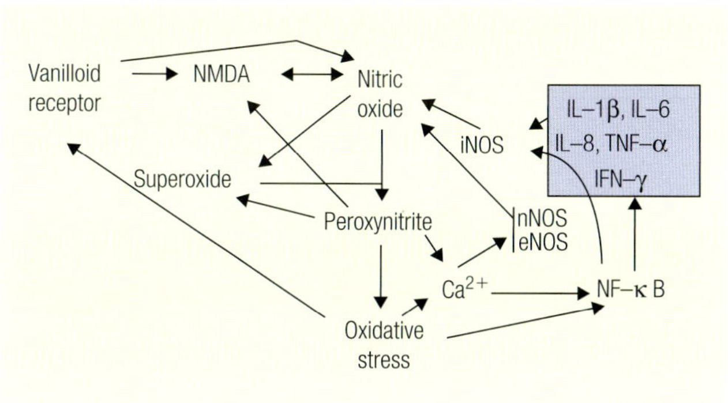

Figure 50.13 NO/ONOO (nitric oxide/peroxynitrite) cycle
eNOS, endothelial nitric oxide synthase; IFN, interferon; IL, interleukin; iNOS, inducible nitric oxide synthase; NMDA, *N*-methyl-D-aspartate; nNOS, neuronal nitric oxide synthase; TNF, tumour necrosis factor.

At the heart of this paradigm is the formation of the potent free radical and oxidant, nitric oxide (NO). NO reacts with superoxide, which is generated mainly in mitochondria in small amounts, as part of the normal synthesis of adenosine triphosphate (ATP), the body's principal energy molecule. Nitric oxide and superoxide combine to form peroxynitrite (ONOO), a very potent oxidizing molecule. This, in turn, generates oxidative stress, which is already a feature of the overlapping syndromes that include MCS. Oxidative stress activates the gene transcription factor NFκB, increasing the activity of inducible nitric oxide synthase (iNOS) and the levels of inflammatory cytokines (e.g. interleukin 6, IL-6), which also stimulate iNOS. At the same time, ionic calcium is released from intracellular stores, which stimulates the activity of neuronal nitric oxidase synthase (nNOS) and endothelial nitric oxidase synthase (eNOS). Oxidative stress and superoxide further stimulate the vanilloid receptor, VR1, which is a promiscuous chemoreceptor found on C-nerve fibres. The vanilloid receptor and NO evoke stimulation of the excitatory NMDA glutamate receptors. These interacting positive-feedback cycles provide vicious and destructive biochemical cycles that afford a comprehensive understanding of the characteristic signs and symptoms of all the overlapping syndromes, including MCS. This explanation means that the so-called 'unexplained illnesses' are to a large degree explained – the controversy is at an end. However, among the stressors for ME/CFS are severe psychological stress and trauma. In an interesting presentation, Perry described how prior brain injury or damage (e.g. in people with Alzheimer's dementia) followed by a modest systemic infection leads to a massive inflammatory response in the central nervous system in experimental animals and, from limited studies, in elderly people.[142] This work addresses one of the conundrums of MCS: how can small events provoke such large and extensive adverse effects found in patients with ME/CFS and MCS? Since organophosphates provoke significant but delayed brain damage via NO,[143] it is likely that toxicant exposure coupled with a mild systemic infection may also provoke significant inflammation in the brain.

THE CHALLENGE TO TOXICOLOGY

Table 50.6 shows some conceptual shifts in toxicology.[144]

Low-level exposure

There are many examples of low levels of exposure having significant effects on biological organisms and humans some 100-fold lower than the no observable adverse effects level (NOEAL or NOEL) or allowed daily intake (ADI). Tributyltin, with a NOEL of parts per billion (ppb), caused sterility in dog whelks at 20 parts per trillion (ppt), while permethrin with an ADI of 0.7 parts per million (ppm) killed most water invertebrates at 5–10 ppb.[145] In mammalian systems, endocrine-disrupting chemicals with oestrogenic activity evoke responses at very low doses, comparable with those found in the environment and consumed by people, but higher doses had contradictory effects, making it essential to develop biological testing systems that will be responsive to low doses of environmental toxins.[146] An important aspect of testing chemically sensitive people is the need to allow a period for adaptation before exposures in order to ensure reliable and reproducible experimental measurements.[147]

Table 50.6 Conceptual shifts in toxicology

Old concept	New concept
High-level contamination overwhelms detoxification and other defence mechanisms	Low-level contamination hijacks control of development
The dose makes the poison	Non-monotonic dose–response curves are common, in which low-level exposure causes effects that disappear at higher levels
Only high levels of exposure matter	Impacts caused at what had been assumed to be background levels
Focus on adults	Periods of rapid growth and development (prenatal through puberty) are most sensitive to exposure
A small number of 'bad actors'	Many chemicals previously thought safe are biologically active and capable of interfering with signalling systems
Immediate cause and effect	Long latencies are common; fetal programming can lead to disease and disabilities decades later
Examine chemicals one compound at a time	In real life, mixtures are the rule; they can lead to effects at much lower levels than indicated by simple experiments with single chemicals
Focus on traditional toxicological endpoints such as mutagenesis, carcinogenesis and cell death	Wide range of health endpoints, e.g. immune system dysfunction (hyper-/hypo-active), neurological/cognitive/behavioural effects, reproductive dysfunction, chronic diseases
One-to-one mapping of contaminant to disease or disability	Same contaminant can cause many different effects, depending upon when exposure occurs during development and what signals it disrupts; multiple contaminants can cause the same endpoint if they disrupt the same developmental process

Additivity, antagonism, synergism, non-monotonic dose–response curves and hormesis

Environmental toxicants are usually encountered in complex mixtures, but most are tested individually. The combined effects of such compounds might be expected to be additive, antagonistic or synergistic. The study of these relationships is complex and varied,[148] but examples of such interactions have been found experimentally in whole animals and in isolated biological in vitro systems:

- *Additivity:* using a yeast oestrogen screen, the effects of four different oestrogenic compounds (4-nonylphenol, 4-octylphenol, *o,p*-dichlorodiphenyltrichloroethane (DDT), genistein) in two to four component mixtures were found to be additive.[149]
- *Antagonism:* this was described in a study of the teratogenic effects of mixtures of PCBs.[150] It was found that the immunotoxic effects of one PCB congener were antagonized by another closely related conger.
- *Synergism:* this arises when the overall toxic effects of a mixture are greater than the sum of those of the individual components. This has been observed with acetylcholinesterase inhibitors and *N,N*-diethyl m-toluamide (DEET), an insect repellent used in the first Gulf War in 1990–91,[151] in pesticide formulations[152] and in herbicide formulations.[153] The so-called 'inerts' in product formulations can increase toxicity and should be included in routine testing of any products, which commonly involves only a single active ingredient. These effects can be very large, with increases in toxicity of more than 100- or 1000-fold. Disturbingly, commonly used food additives also show synergistic increases in developmental neurotoxicity tests.[154]
- *Non-monotonic dose–response curves:* classical toxicology uses linear dose–responses to estimate the limits for exposure to environmental toxins (Figure 50.14). This effect involves the assumption that dose–response is linear and, at a sufficiently low dose, becomes zero – the NOEL. The data, usually from animal experiments, are then adjusted arbitrarily by reducing the identified dose by one or more orders of magnitude in order to obtain the reference dose. The reference dose is chosen to accommodate possible differences between animal and human responses, and the different sensitivities of children and elderly people. The NOEL is, in this way, reduced to an estimated reference dose some 100–1000 times lower than the observed experimentally determined dose.

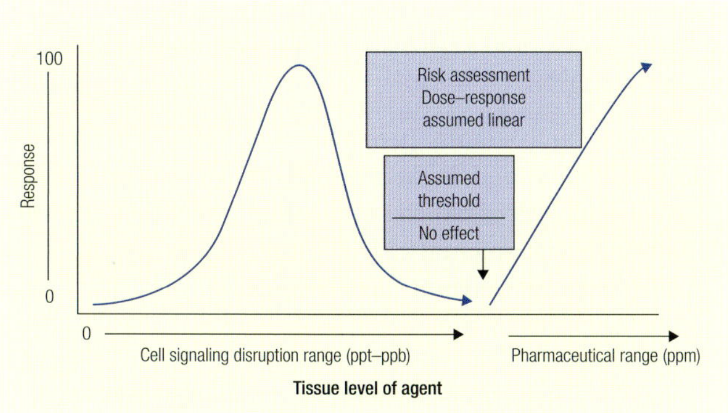

Figure 50.14 Dose–response curves found in toxicology: inverted U- curve for cell signalling disruptors

Courtesy of Professor Vyvyan Howard.

Figure 50.14 shows that at doses below the NOEL, toxic effects are found in a bell-shaped or inverted U-shaped dose–response curve. Note the large concentration differences associated with the conventional linear part of the dose–response curve and those with the non-monotonic part of the curve.

Figure 50.15 illustrates the different forms of non-monotonic curves that have been found for many environmental toxins.[155] Among the earliest investigators of this phenomenon was Frederick Vom Saal, who studied the oestrogenic effects of drugs and environmental toxins, particularly BPA, in mice.[133] In a paper published in 1997, Vom Saal and colleagues wrote (author's italics):

> Our findings show for the first time that fetal exposure to environmentally relevant parts-per-billion (ppb) doses of bisphenol A, *in the range currently being consumed by people*, can alter the adult reproductive system in mice.[156]

Endocrine disrupters have been studied widely. Doses as low 10^{-11} molar have evoked immune responses similar to those caused by oestradiol that involve the release of histamine and cytokines from mast cells in cell culture,[157]

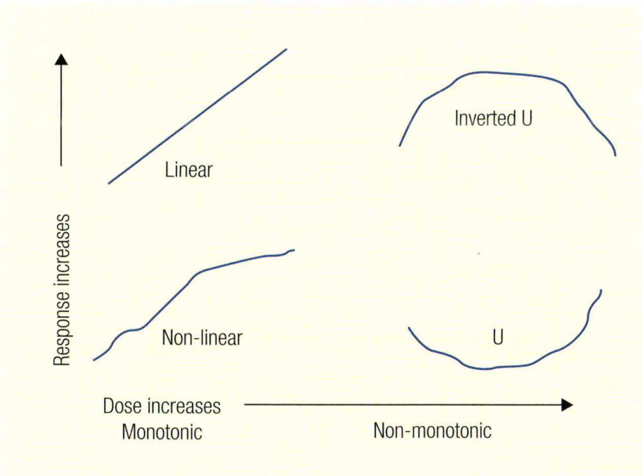

Figure 50.15 Different linear and non-monotonic dose–response curves

providing further evidence of the interrelationship between the endocrine and immune systems.[16]

The situation is complicated by the discovery of two classes of oestradiol receptors, one in the nucleus and one that is membrane-bound. The membrane-bound receptor is equally sensitive to oestradiol and bisphenol A, while the nuclear receptor is much less sensitive to bisphenol A.[158] The crucial nature of the test systems must be considered when determining the NOEL and reference doses.

Hormesis

Hormesis is defined as low-dose stimulation and high-dose inhibition and follows a non-monotonic dose–response curve. It has been used to claim that low doses of environmental toxins should be regarded as beneficial and be the default position adopted by regulators and clinically. There has been a thorough evaluation of this view, which emphasizes that:[159]

- underlying mechanisms of action, and not simply empirical data, must be considered;
- stimulatory effects are not always beneficial and may be harmful;
- all the induced effects of a toxicants, and not only the beneficial ones, must be considered;
- any health decisions based on beneficial effects must address interindividual differences, including susceptibility, genetic factors, life stage and health status;
- any health decisions based on beneficial effects must address the fact that other environmental and workplace exposures may alter the low-dose response of a single agent.

This excellent paper puts all these considerations into a generalized theoretical framework and includes many telling experimental examples. For instance, 2,3,7,8-tetrachlorodibenzodioxin (TCDD), an environmental carcinogen, has been quoted as having low-dose beneficial effects. Closer examination of the data shows this to be false, since the incidence of tumours of the liver, lung, tongue and nasal turbinates increased, while incidence of tumours of the pituitary, uterus, mammary glands, pancreas and adrenal glands decreased.

In one study claiming the hormetic effects of cadmium, a non-statistical decrease in testicular cancer in rats was accompanied by a statistical increase in prostatic hyperplasia and an increase in prostate tumours per animal in the hormetic range.

Ethanol is cited as a classic hormetic agent, since beneficial outcomes – reduced risk of coronary heart disease and a reduction in mortality – have been identified with low consumption, in contrast to increases at higher doses of, among other things, neurological disorders, cancers and liver cirrhosis. However, small amounts of alcohol (0.5 units per day) in pregnancy have been associated with adverse behavioural outcomes such as aggression in children.

Developmental effects of environmental exposures

Intergenerational effects

Diethylstilboestrol (DES) is known to cause malformation of the uterus in daughters born to women who received DES during pregnancy, predisposing the daughters to rare uterine cancers. In rats, androgen receptors were permanently raised in male offspring of females given DES during pregnancy, with an increase in the size of the prostate gland. BPA caused similar changes.[160,161] DDT lengthened the time to pregnancy (fecundability) in the daughters of mothers exposed to DDT; the probability of pregnancy fell by 32 per cent per 10 µg/L in maternal serum.[164]

Effects on the fetus and babies

The most rapid multiplication of cells and differentiation of tissues occurs during fetal growth and development within the womb. This is when key biological processes are most susceptible to disturbance by xenobiotics. The notion that the developing fetus is protected during its growth and development within the womb has been shown to be wrong. Many xenobiotics cross the placental barrier and can disrupt many crucial stages of development.

A ruling by the USA high court awarded damages of $4 million to John Castillo, who was born without eyes (anophthalmia) following his mother's exposure to the fungicide benlate when she was 6–7 weeks' pregnant with her son. The exposure occurred on a single day when Mrs Castillo was accidentally sprayed while walking. The initial case was hotly contested by DuPont, the manufacturer of benlate, but the case was upheld and then lost on appeal before the final ruling of the Florida supreme court in 2003.[163] The time of the exposure in the Castillo case corresponded to the time of maximum cellular replication and organogenesis in the developing fetus. The company had funded a 2002 study that showed benlate to be concentrated to the eyes in rats. This report was unpublished but reported by the *Guardian* newspaper.[139] Benlate has been the subject of numerous other cases and has now been withdrawn, after 33 years on the market.

Cord blood studies identified hundreds of toxins to which the fetus had been exposed, many of them developmental neurotoxins. This is of particular concern to the American Association on Mental Retardation (AAMR; now the American Association on Intellectual and Developmental Disabilities, AAIDD), which stated: 'The evidence is mounting that exposure to environmental pollutants and toxins are contributing to poorer health and significant increases in chronic disease and disabilities in our society'.[43] Some 17–18 per cent of Americans under age 18 years are claimed to be affected.[164]

A scientific consensus statement on environmental agents associated with neurodevelopmental disorders brings together the most up-to-date information of a large group of concerned scientists in the USA and emphasizes the following:[36]

- Children and young people cannot be considered as 'small adults' and show marked differences in physiology and routes of exposure. They are often more susceptible to environmental exposures.
- Low doses of toxicants can alter gene expression and affect learning and development.
- Effects can be delayed.
- Genetic polymorphisms render some subgroups more sensitive than others to certain chemicals.

Autism, attention deficit hyperactivity disorder (ADHD) dyslexia, mental retardation, lowered intelligence quotient (IQ) and other disorders of learning and behaviour are highly prevalent among American children. These conditions appear to be rising, with presently 5–15 per cent of all children under the age of 18 years in the USA affected – more than 12 million children. ADHD has been shown to be linked to food additives used in children's drinks and foods.[165] Autism-spectrum disorder appears to be ten times more prevalent now than in the 1980s. The costs of providing special educational services in the USA have been estimated at $77.3 billion, twice the cost of regular education. In addition, there is the human cost for families and communities.

Agents definitely found to be associated with learning and development disabilities (LDDs) are alcohol, lead, mercury, manganese, arsenic, PCBs, polybromodiphenylethers (PBDEs), solvents, PAHs, pesticides and nicotine in tobacco smoke. The damaging effects of these toxins have been known for many years, but the development of products containing them has been allowed to take place on economic grounds. A good example is lead. The toxic neurodevelopmental properties of lead have been known for years; however, its use in paints and in petrol was stopped only after much struggle. The failure of policy-makers to protect young children by not acting quickly in response to the science has laid waste countless young lives. The Centers for Disease Control and Prevention (CDC) has not changed the standard for acceptable blood levels of lead in children since 1985, although the most recent proposal for a level of 2 µg/dL is some 12.5 times lower than the 1985 level.

Solvents and solvent-based products (Table 50.7) are frequently involved as neurotoxins and are ubiquitous in the environment.

Effects on elderly people

The Pritchard Report examined changing patterns of adult (age 45–74 years) neurological deaths in the major Western world in the period 1979–97 and found significant increase in chronic illnesses, for which the report suggested possible environmental factors.[37]

Table 50.7 Neurotoxins: common solvents and solvent-based products

Mostly solvent-based	Partially solvent-based
Gasoline	Glues
Diesel fuel	Adhesives
Charcoal lighter fluid	Oil-based paints
Lantern fuel	Fingernail polish
Grease	Furniture polishes
Lubricating oils	Floor polishes and waxes
Degreasing agents	Spot removers
Paint strippers	Metal and wood cleaners
Paint thinner	Correction fluid
Turpentine	Computer disk cleaners
Nail-polish remover	Varnishes and shellacs
Rubbing alcohol	Wood and concrete stains

Delayed effects

One of the most worrying aspects of chemical exposures and MCS is the development of delayed neurotoxic effects years after the initial exposure, which may have been at low levels. This has been found with GWS[66] and in survivors of terrorist attacks using the nerve agent sarin.[129,166–168] Such temporal relationships are easily missed without a very thorough history.

TREATMENT

A survey of 917 people with MCS enquired about illness rating: the results were mild (7%), moderate (32%), severe (45%) or totally disabling (13%), with the respondents being mainly white (95%) and predominantly women (82%).[169] A total of 101 treatment and management techniques procedures, and their perceived efficacy, were assessed. A help/harm ratio was devised that allowed comparison of the different treatments tried by the respondents (Table 50.8). The higher the ratio, the more helpful the treatment, with a ratio of 10 indicating that ten times more people found the treatment helpful compared with those who found it harmful. The lower the ratio, the more harmful the treatment, with a ratio of 0.1 indicating that ten times more people found the treatment harmful compared with those who found it helpful. A ratio of 1 indicates that there was an equal balance between help and harm.

The three most highly rated treatments were:

- a chemical-free living space (ratio 155.2);
- avoidance of chemicals (ratio 118.6);
- prayer (ratio 48.3).

Other reports emphasize the importance of a chemical-free living space and avoidance of chemicals in health, education, legal and benefit provisions.[21,22,27,28,40,61,62] It is clearly common sense to avoid known chemicals that cause the patient problems and to avoid contact with other chemicals on the precautionary principle. Chemical-free living space is humane and less costly than attempting to provide long-term medical care for this complex condition. The inclusion of prayer is striking and indicates the need to consider

Table 50.8 Top 12 treatments tried in multiple chemical sensitivity (MCS)

Treatment tried	*n*	Harmed (%)	No effect (%)	Helped (%)	Helped/harm ratio
Chemical-free living space	820	0.6	4.5	94.8	155.2
Chemical avoidance	875	0.8	4.7	94.5	118.6
Prayer	609	1.4	34.4	64.2	48.3
Meditation	423	2.8	43.3	53.8	19.2
Acupressure	308	4.5	28.3	67.2	14.9
Touch for health	75	3.8	41.8	54.4	14.3
Air filter (to prevent exposure)	786	6.0	11.8	82.1	13.7
Rotation diet	560	5.7	22.1	72.2	12.7
Acidophilus	661	4.1	44.0	52.0	12.7
Relocation	513	7.4	6.0	86.6	11.7
Reflexology	204	4.8	38.5	56.6	11.6
Personal oxygen to cope with exposures	326	7.3	14.2	78.4	10.6

people with MCS holistically. Prayer is not defined in any specific terms but excludes meditation, hypnosis and faith healing. Cognitive-behavioural therapy (CBT) is not considered specifically, but psychotherapy as a cure is rated as of no noticeable effect (65.3%) or as very harmful (6.6%). However, as a coping procedure, 47.7 per cent of patients found psychotherapy somewhat helpful, with 24.1 per cent of patients reporting no noticeable effect. Exercise is reported as causing harm (14.7%), of no noticeable effect (23.7%) or helpful (61.6%). Exercise is reported by severely ill people with ME/CFS to be positively harmful, with only 5 per cent of patients finding it helpful.[170,171]

The interventions rated as more harmful than helpful include:

- conventional medicines, particularly all antidepressants and anxiolytics (tricyclics, selective serotonin reuptake inhibitors (SSRIs), benzodiazepines) and anti-seizure drugs (help/harm ratio 0.1–0.5);
- provocation-neutralization (P-N) testing for chemicals with preservatives (help/harm ratio 0.9).

Since MCS includes heightened sensitivity to chemicals, it is not surprising that the response to drugs is also heightened. When any drugs are given, it is imperative that the initial dose is much lower (one-quarter to one-eighth) than the starting dose recommended in the formularies in order to avoid any possible (severe) reactions. The drugs generally found harmful are those that work by modifying brain function, which is a major area of damage in MCS and part of the neuroendocrine immune paradigm.

More surprising was the inclusion of P-N among the more harmful treatments. P-N is used widely and commended among some practitioners of ecological/environmental medicine.[61,62] P-N can take different forms, but these were not specified.

Initially, saunas were three to four times more helpful than harmful and feature among the recommended treatments that offer a means of detoxification.[61,62,80] However, over a longer time, saunas proved less helpful. The type of sauna used (wet or dry) was not specified. Reducing the total toxic load is seen as a desirable goal in treatment.[61,62,80,96,172,173]

Diet was also generally helpful. Only a rotation diet was mentioned, although other exclusion diets, in which dairy and gluten are the first to be removed, using a food diary[61,62,80] or following the Stone Age diet[62] may also be helpful. Other aspects of diet modification include using acidophilus to support gut flora, which, with related probiotics, features in many diets.

Detoxification includes removal of dental fillings, with a help/harm ratio of 4.8, and the use of UltraClear®, a combination product designed to comprehensively support the gut, with a health/harm ratio of only 1.

Many people had tried a range of mineral, vitamin and co-factor formulations, but the individual help/harm ratio scores varied between 8.6 and 4.1. No specific mineral, vitamin and co-factor combinations were used. One study found that MCS was not associated with vitamin deficiency or thyroid function, but lower lymphocyte counts suggested immune dysfunction with VOCs.[160] The advent of specific tests that allow the identification of toxins permits more precision in designing treatments. Such tests identify blockade of mitochondrial function, DNA adducts[161,174–176] and analysis of needle-fat biopsies. Pesticide load has been reduced by choline and vitamin C.[177] Vitamin B2 has long been used to treat neuropsychiatric disorders where no anaemia or macrocytosis is present.

Various combinations of supplements (vitamins, minerals and other co-factors) in a wide variety of combinations have been recommended. Among the most useful is one supporting mitochondrial function – *N*-acetyl-L-carnitine, co-enzyme Q10, niacin, ribose and magnesium. A more complex mixture of potent antioxidants is being trialled in the USA.[2]

An important question about the testing of adults for environmental chemical contamination is:

> Could we be trying to correlate exposure and effect at the wrong time? If it is prenatal, or early life stage, exposure that is critical to disease susceptibility, why are we measuring environmental chemicals in people once they have developed breast cancer? The critical exposure window may have been much earlier.[178]

This underlines the urgency to recognize many chemicals as major developmental hazards, which must be addressed at the earliest possible moment in order to avoid longer-term and adverse consequences.

POLITICAL, SOCIAL AND MEDICAL ACTION

The response of governments, global corporations, industry and society to the accumulating evidence of the hazards of chemical contamination has been to minimize the observed effects, to accuse the scientists involved of poor science,[73] scare-mongering,[161,179] unrealistic attitudes[180] and, in a number of extreme cases, vilification and character assassination.[181,182] Government activities and research funding have been dictated by policy and not open, independent, transparent science. In an article that called for research, not propaganda, the reluctance of the medical establishment to embrace change was challenged. US Representative and physician Dave Weldon said:

> Mind you, half of Dr. Wakefield's theory has been proven correct and accepted in the medical community. Hundreds of children with regressive autism and GI [gastrointestinal] dysfunction have been scoped and clinicians are seeing the inflammatory bowel disease he first described. The NIH [National Institutes of Health] is finally funding an attempt to repeat Dr. O'Leary's findings of measles RNA in Wakefield's biopsy specimens, though I am disappointed it has taken this long.

A similar story is described by Arpad Pusztai, whose work upset the establishment's ideological commitment to GM crops and food.[183]

Evidence has been sought to support policy rather than to design policy in response to medical and scientific evidence. Disturbing scientific and medical studies are being denied rather than replicated in order to establish their validity.

The failure of government and regulators to act on a report on food colouring and ADHD in this matter is regrettable and symptomatic of the unwillingness to make changes in our chemical environment that are resisted by the industry, even in the light of good science.[184] Both the Food Standards Agency (FSA)[185] and the European Food Standards Agency[186] refused to endorse the precautionary principle and withdraw the products immediately.

The phthalates reveal a similar story. These were banned in some countries from 1977,[187] but in the USA the toy industry launched strong resistance to a ban in America.[188] One study reports a positive association between urinary phthalate metabolites and adult male (age 20–59 years) obesity.[189] There were other positive associations with adverse health effects among young women and elderly people, but not in children.

The attitude to xenobiotics in the environment is reminiscent of the fight against tobacco and smoking. It seems that many people and organizations are prepared to sacrifice the health of present and future generations in order to make a fast buck or allow national tax income to be protected.

GULF WAR SYNDROME/ILLNESS

In November 2008, a second report on GWI was released by the Congressionally mandated Research Advisory Committee on Gulf War Veterans' Illness (RACGWVI).[190] The 450-page report with some 1800 references validates the earlier conclusions of the 2004 report and states:

> The illnesses suffered by veterans were a result of unique circumstances in which they were exposed to a considerable number of toxic insults. The most important of these were:
>
> - receiving multiple vaccines, some experimental;
> - pyridostigmine bromide, also experimental, in Nerve Agent Pre-treatment Set (NAPS) tablets;
> - pesticides, especially organophosphates, used to keep down disease vectors;
> - exposure to low levels of chemical warfare agents in the form of nerve agents.

GWI has the following features:

- It is a chronic multi-system physical medical condition with a coherent pattern of symptoms.
- Many veterans show evidence of physical brain injury in the form of neuropsychological impairment, which cannot be detected by routine tests.
- It is not a stress-related condition.
- There is a twofold increase in motor neuron disease and brain cancer in people with GWI.

CONCLUSIONS

MCS is a medical, scientific, political, legal and social issue that needs to be addressed within our society as a matter of urgency. It is now beyond argument that xenobiotics have the potential to damage present and future generations.

The role of psychiatry is to embrace the science and medicine that provide the evidence of chemical and environmental damage and to support those people who have to cope with this condition.

The role of industry, science and medicine is to carry out comprehensive and independent chemical, toxicological, pharmacological and clinical studies to ensure that all products in the marketplace are safe for widespread use in the community. All data should be available for examination in the same way that scientific papers are scrutinized before publication by independent scientists and clinicians.[191] Vested interest should have no part in this process.

The role of politics is to protect its citizens with independent funding, coupled with robust and clear regulations, without any influence from vested interests that pay thousands of pounds in lobbying fees to exert control over the political process.

Where people are physically, chemically or biologically exposed to any hazard and develop MCS and related conditions, their welfare should be put first and every provision made to ensure that they have the resources required to cope with the environment of the twenty-first century.

KEY POINTS

- MCS is a complex, chronic multi-system condition.
- It is associated with exposure to a wide variety of novel chemicals, environmental, agricultural and dietary.
- It requires a much more responsible and careful assessment and regulation of all novel chemicals in line with the precautionary principle.
- It requires recognition of the new understanding emerging from recent studies in toxicology, metabolism, genetics, epigenetics and developmental biology.
- Recognition of the condition by clinicians, education, health authorities and government authorities is required for effective treatment, the most important of which is the removal of incitants and the provision of a clean and controlled living environment.
- Research is needed in order to establish other treatments that may help at various stages of the condition.
- There may be a need for subgrouping of people with MCS.

REFERENCES

1. Sears M (2007) *The Medical Perspective on Environmental Sensitivities. Canadian Human Rights Commission.* www.chrc-ccdp.ca/research_program_recherche/esensitivities_hypersensibilitee/page14-en.asp.
2. Lacour M, Zunder T, Schmidtke K, Vaith P, Scheidt C (2005) Multiple chemical sensitivity syndrome (MCS): suggestions for an extension of the U.S. MCS-case definition. *International Journal of Hygiene and Environmental Health* **208**: 141–51.
3. Miller CS (2001) The compelling anomaly of chemical intolerance. *Annals of the New York Academy of Sciences* **933**: 1–23.
4. Busse JW, Reid S, Lernoff A, *et al.* (2006) Managing environmental sensitivity: an overview illustrated with a case report. *Journal of the Canadian Chiropractic Association* **52**: 66–95.
5. Donnay A (2004) Multiple chemical sensitivity or MUSES syndrome? Occupational Medicine Residents' Seminar Series Environmental and Occupational Health Sciences Institute Rutgers University, Piscataway, NJ, 17 February 2004. www.mcsrr.org.
6. Johansson O (2004) Electrohypersensitivity: state-of-the-art of a functional impairment. *Electromagnetic Biology and Medicine* **25**: 245–58.
7. Tallmo K-E (2003) *A Life Redirected and Consensus and Canaries.* www.art-bin.com/pdf/red_canaries_en.pdf.
8. National Institute for Occupational Safety and Health (2006) *Pesticide-Related Illness and Injury Surveillance: A How-To Guide For State-Based Programs.* www.cdc.gov/niosh/docs/2006-102/2006-102d.html.
9. *Archives of Environmental Health* (1999) Multiple chemical sensitivity: a 1999 consensus. *Archives of Environmental Health* **54**: 147–9.
10. Heuser G (2002) Defining chemical injury: a diagnostic protocol and profile of chemically injured civilians, industrial workers and Gulf war veterans. *International Perspectives in Public Health* **13**: 1–16.
11. Salvador L (2007) *Position Statement: Multiple Chemical Sensitivity.* http://mcs-america.org/MCSPositionStatement.pdf.
12. Haley RW, Fleckenstein, JL, Bonte FJ, *et al.* (2000) Brain abnormalities in Gulf War syndrome: evaluation with ^{1}H MR spectroscopy. *Radiology* **215**: 807–17.
13. Kulig BM (1996) Comprehensive neurotoxicity assessment. *Environmental Health Perspectives* **104** (suppl. 2): 317–22.
14 Wetherell A (1997) Cognitive and psychomotor performance tests and experimental design in multiple chemical sensitivity. *Environmental Health Perspectives* **105** (suppl. 2): 495–503.
15. Davidoff AL, Fogarty L (1994) Psychogenic origins of multiple chemical sensitivities syndrome: a critical review of the research literature. *Archives of Environmental Health* **49**: 316–25.
16. Deutschen Institut für Medizinische Dokumentation und Information (DIMDI) (2000) *Internationale statistische Klassification der Krankheiten und verwandter Gesundheitprobleme,* 10th revision. Cologne: Deutschen Institut für Medizinische Dokumentation und Information.
17. Parliament of South Australia (2005) Inquiry into MCS: 2nd Report of the Social Development Committee on MCS. Adelaide: Parliament of South Australia.
18. Danish Environmental Protection Agency (2005) Multiple chemical sensitivity, MCS. Environmental project no. 988. http://www2.mst.dk/Udgiv/publications/2005/87-7614-548-4/pdf/87-7614-549-2.pdf.
19. Gravelling RA, Pilkington A, George JKP, *et al.* (1999) A review of multiple chemical sensitivity. *Occupational and Environmental Medicine* **56**: 73–85.
20. Magill MK, Suruda (1998) A multiple chemical sensitivity syndrome. *American Family Physician* **58**: 721–30.
21. WWF-UK (2004) *Contamination: The Next Generation – Results of the Family Chemical Contamination Survey.* www.wwf.org.uk/filelibrary/pdf/family_biomonitoring.pdf.
22. Royal Commission on Environmental Pollution (2005) *Crop Spraying and the Health of Residents and Bystanders.* www.rcep.org.uk/cropspraying.htm.
23. Eaton KK, Anthony HM (2000) *MCS: Recognition and Management.* Knighton: British Society for Allergy, Environmental and Nutritional Medicine.
24. Anthony H, Birtwistle S, Eaton K, Maberly J (2000) *Environmental Medicine Clinical Practice.* Knighton: British Society for Allergy, Environmental and Nutritional Medicine.
25. Royal College of Physicians (2003) *Allergy: The Unmet Need – A Blueprint for Better Patient Care.* London: Royal College of Physicians.
26. Royal Commission on Environmental Pollution (2003) *Chemicals in Products: Safeguarding the Environment and Human Health.* Cm 5827. London: HMSO.
27. Research Advisory Committee on Gulf War Veterans' Illness (2004) *RACGWVI Scientific Progress in Understanding Gulf War Veterans' Illnesses: Report and Recommendations.* http://www1.va.gov/racgwvi/docs/ReportandRecommendations_2004.pdf.
28. Hooper M (1999) The most toxic war in western military history: evidence submitted to the House of Commons Select Defence Committee, December 1999. In *7th Report of Defence Select Committee: Gulf Veterans' Illnesses – Report and Proceedings of the Committee with Minutes of Evidence and Appendices, April 19th 2000.* London: HMSO.
29. WWF-UK, The Co-operative Bank (2004) *Chemical Check Up: An Analysis of Chemicals in the Blood of*

Members of the European Parliament. http://assets.panda.org/downloads/checkupmain.pdf.
30. Centers for Disease Control and Prevention (2005) *Third National Report on Human Exposure to Environmental Chemicals.* Atlanta, GA: Centers for Disease Control and Prevention.
31. Bell IR, Schwartz GE, Peterson JM, Amend D (1993) Self-reported illness from chemical odors in young adults without clinical syndromes or occupational exposures. *Archives of Environmental Health* **48**: 6–13.
32. Bell IR, Schwartz GE, Peterson JM, Amend D, Stini WA (1993) Possible time-dependent sensitization to xenobiotics: self-reported illness from chemical odors, foods, and opiate drugs in an older adult population. *Archives of Environmental Health* **48**: 315–27.
33. Meggs WJ, Dunn KA, Bloch RM, Goodman PE, Davidoff AL (1996) Prevalence and nature of allergy and chemical sensitivity in a general population. *Archives of Environmental Health* **51**: 275–82.
34. Voorhees RE (1998) Memo from Deputy State Epidemiologist Voorhees to Joe Thompson, Special Counsel, Office of the Governor. Santa Fe, NM: New Mexico Department of Health.
35. Bell IR, Warg-Damiani L, Baldwin CM, Walsh ME, Schwartz GE (1998) Self-reported chemical sensitivity and wartime chemical exposures in Gulf War veterans with and without decreased global health ratings. *Military Medicine* **163**: 725–32.
36. Kreutzer R, Neutra RR, Lashuay N (1999) Prevalence of people reporting sensitivities to chemicals in a population-based survey. *American Journal of Epidemiology* **150**: 1–12.
37. Caress SM, Steinemann AC (2004) Prevalence of multiple chemical sensitivities: a population-based study in the southeastern United States. *American Journal of Public Health* **94**: 746–7.
38. Caress SM, Steinemann AC (2004) A national population study of the prevalence of multiple chemical sensitivity. *Archives of Environmental Health* **59**: 300–305.
39. Caress SM, Steinemann AC (2005) National prevalence of asthma and chemical hypersensitivity: an examination of potential overlap. *Journal of Occupational and Environmental Medicine* **47**: 518–22.
40. WWF-UK, The Co-operative Bank (2003) *Contamination: The Results of WWF's Biomonitoring Survey.* www.wwf.org.uk/filelibrary/pdf/biomonitoringresults.pdf.
41. Greenpeace Nederland, Greenpeace International, WWF-UK (2005) *A Present for Life: Hazardous Chemicals in Umbilical Cord Blood.* www.wwf.org.uk/filelibrary/pdf/presentforlife.pdf.
42. Environmental Working Group Report (2005) *Body Burden: The Pollution in Newborns.* http://archive.ewg.org/reports_content/bodyburden2/pdf/bodyburden2_final-r2.pdf.
43. Croser MD, Seiter M (2003) *Pollution, Toxic Chemicals, and Mental Retardation.* www.aamr.org/ehi/media/Toxic_Chemical_MR.pdf.
44. National Center for Health Statistics (2003) *National Health and Nutrition Examination Survey.* Hyattsville, MD: National Center for Health Statistics.
45. Needham LL, Barr DB, Calafat AM (2005) Characterising children's exposures: beyond NHANES. *Neurotoxicology* **26**: 547–53.
46. Daniels GE (1936) Emotional and instinctual factors in diabetes mellitus. *American Journal of Psychiatry* **93**: 711–724.
47. Booth G (1948) Psychodynamics in parkinsonism. *Psychosomatic Medicine* **10**: 1–14.
48. Philippopoulos GS, Wittkower ED, Cousineau MA (1958) The etiologic significance of emotional factors in onset and exacerbations of multiple sclerosis. *Psychosomatic Medicine* **20**: 458–74.
49. Crawford R (1897) Graves disease: an emotional disorder. *King's College Hospital Report* **3**: 45–56.
50. Eis D, Helm D, Muhlinghaus T, *et al.* (2008) A German multicentre study on multiple chemical sensitivity (MCS). *International Journal of Hygiene and Environmental Health* **211**: 658–81.
51. Gilbert SG (ed.) (2008) *Scientific Consensus Statement on Environmental Agents Associated with Neurodevelopmental Disorders.* www.iceh.org/pdfs/LDDI/LDDIStatement.pdf.
52. Pritchard C, Baldwin D, Mayers A (2004) Changing patterns of adult (45–74 years) neurological deaths in the major Western world countries 1979–1997. *Public Health* **118**: 268–83.
53. Carson R (1962) *Silent Spring.* Greenwich, CT: Fawcett.
54. Cadbury D (1998) *The Feminization of Nature: Our Future at Risk.* London: Penguin.
55. Colborn T, Dumanoski D, Myers JP (1996) *Our Stolen Future: Are We Threatening Our Fertility, Intelligence and Survival?* New York: Dutton.
56. REACH. COM 2003 0644 (2003) Proposal for a Regulation of the European Parliament and of the Council concerning the Registration, Evaluation, Authorisation and Restriction of Chemicals (REACH), establishing a European Chemicals Agency and amending Directive 1999/45/EC and Regulation (EC) on Persistent Organic Pollutants Proposal for a Directive of the European Parliament and of the Council amending Council Directive 67/548/EEC in order to adapt it to Regulation (EC) of the European Parliament and of the Council concerning the registration, evaluation, authorisation, and restriction of chemicals. Brussels: Commission of the European Communities.
57. United States Government Accountability Office (2005) *Chemical Regulation: Approaches in the United States, Canada, and the European Union.* GAO-06-217R Chemical Regulation 2005. www.gao.gov/new.items/d06217r.pdf.

58. Persson R, Carlsson Eek F, Osterberg K, *et al.* (2008) A two-week monitoring of self-reported arousal, worry and attribution among person with annoyance attributed to electrical equipment and smells. *Scandinavian Journal of Psychology* **49**: 345–56.
59. Van Thriel C, Kiesswetter E, Schaper M, *et al.* (2008) Odor annoyance of environmental chemicals: sensory and cognitive influences. *Journal of Toxicology and Environmental Health. Part A* **71**: 776–85.
60. Dantzer R, Kelley KW (2007) Twenty years research on cytokine-induced sickness behavior. *Brain, Behavior, and Immunity* **21**: 153–60.
61. Simon GE, Katon WJ, Sparks PJ (199) Allergic to life: psychological factors in environmental illness. *American Journal of Psychiatry* **147**: 901–6.
62. Smith R (2002) In search of non-disease. *British Medical Journal* **324**: 883–5, 912–13.
63. Bailey-Hamilton P (2005) *Stop the 21st Century Killing You: Toxic Chemicals Have Invaded Our Lives – Fight back! Eliminate Toxins, Tackle Illness, Get Healthy and Live Longer.* London: Vermillion.
64. Ashford AN, Miller CS (1998) *Chemical Exposures: Low Levels and High Stakes*, 2nd edn. New York: John Wiley & Sons.
65. Rea WJ (1998) *Chemical Sensitivity.* Boca Raton, FL: CRC-Lewis.
66. (2006) Chemical sensitivity in mainstream medical documentation. www.chemicalsensitivitypart1.blogspot.com.
67. Daniels GE (1936) Analysis of a case of neurosis with diabetes mellitus. *Psychoanalytical Quarterly* **5**: 513.
68. Furlong CE, Cole TB, Richter RJ, *et al.* (2005) Biomarkers for exposure and sensitivity to organophosphorus (OP) compounds. In C Winder (ed.) *Contaminated Air Protection Conference Proceedings.* Sydney: University of New South Wales.
69. Costa LG, Cole TB, Vitalone A, Furlong CE (2005) Measurement of paraoxonase (PON1) status as a potential biomarker of susceptibility to organophosphate toxicity. *Clinica Chimica Acta* **352**: 37–47.
70. Ternesten-Hasseus E, Lowhagen O, Millqvist E (2007) Quality of life and capsaicin sensitivity in patients with airway symptoms induced by chemicals and scents: a longitudinal study. *Environmental Health Perspectives* **115**: 425–9.
71. Osterberg K, Persson R, Karlson B, Orbaek P (2004) Annoyance and performance of three environmentally intolerant groups during experimental challenge with chemical odours. *Scandinavian Journal of Work, Environment and Health* **30**: 486–96.
72. Slotkin TA, Bodwell BE, Levin ED, *et al.* (2008) Low doses of diazinon affect brain development. *Environmental Health Perspectives* **116**: 340–48.
73. Hancock DB, Martin ER, Mayhew GM, *et al.* (2008) Pesticide exposure and risk of Parkinson's disease: a family-based case-control study. *BMC Neurology* **8**: 6.
74. Kimata H (2004) Effect of exposure to volatile organic compounds on plasma levels of neuropeptides, nerve growth factor and histamine in patients with self-reported multiple chemical sensitivity. *International Journal of Hygiene and Environmental Health* **207**: 159–63.
75. Senechal S, De Nadai P, Ralainirina N, *et al.* (2003) Effect of diesel on chemokines and chemokine receptors involved in helper T cell type 1/type 2 recruitment in patients with asthma. *American Journal of Respiratory and Critical Care Medicine* **168**: 215–21.
76. Chemical Injury Information Network (2006) *Multiple Chemical Sensitivity: Case Definition Workshop Workbook.* White Sulphur Springs, MT: Chemical Injury Information Network.
77. Reid S, Hotopf M, Hull L, *et al.* (2001) Multiple chemical sensitivity and chronic fatigue syndrome in British Gulf War veterans. *American Journal of Epidemiology* **153**: 604–9.
78. Proctor SP (2000) Chemical sensitivity and gulf war veterans' illnesses. *Occupational Medicine* **15**: 587–99.
79. Fulco C, Liverman CT, Sox HC, Institute of Medicine (2000) *Gulf War and Health.* Washington, DC: National Academy Press.
80. Meggs WJ (1999) Gulf War syndrome, chronic fatigue syndrome, and the multiple chemical sensitivity syndrome: stirring the cauldron of confusion. *Archives of Environmental Health* **54**: 309–11.
81. Miller CS (2000) Toxicant-induced loss of tolerance. *Addiction* **96**: 115–39.
82. Baggaley A (ed.) *Human Body.* London: Dorling Kindersley.
83. Gupta A (1999) Functional impairment of blood–brain barrier following pesticide exposure during early development in rats. *Human and Experimental Toxicology* **18**: 174–9.
84. Song X, Pope C, Murthy R, *et al.* (2004) Interactive effects of paraoxon and pyridostigmine on blood–brain barrier integrity and cholinergic toxicity. *Toxicological Sciences* **78**: 241–7.
85. Abdel-Rahman A, Shetty AK, Abou-Donia MB (2002) Disruption of the blood–brain barrier and neuronal cell death in cingulate cortex, dentate gyrus, thalamus, and hypothalamus in a rat model of Gulf-War syndrome. *Neurobiology of Disease* **10**: 306–26.
86. Abdel-Rahman A, Shetty AK, Abou-Donia MB (2001) Subchronic dermal application of N,N-diethyl m-toluamide (DEET) and permethrin to adult rats, alone or in combination, causes diffuse neuronal cell death and cytoskeletal abnormalities in the cerebral cortex and the hippocampus, and Purkinje neuron loss in the cerebellum. *Experimental Neurology* **172**: 153–71.
87. Abou-Donia M, Suliman H, Khan W, Abdel-Rahman A (2003) Testicular germ-cell apoptosis in stressed rats following combined exposure to pyridostigmine bromide, N,N-diethyl m-toluamide (DEET), and perme-

thrin. *Journal of Toxicology and Environmental Health. Part A* **66**: 57–73.

88. Di Pierro M, Lu R, Uzzau S, *et al.* (2001) Zonula occludens toxin structure–function analysis identification of the fragment biologically active on tight cell junctions and of the zonulin receptor binding domain. *Journal of Biological Chemistry* **276**: 19160–65.
89. Wang W, Uzzau S, Goldblum SE, Fasano A (2000) Human zonulin, a potential modulator of intestinal tight junctions. *Journal of Cell Science* **113**: 4435–40.
90. Walsh SV, Hopkins AM, Nusrat A (2000) Modulation of tight junction structure and function by cytokines. *Advanced Drug Delivery Reviews* **41**: 303–13.
91. Broughman JR, Brandt RM, Hastings C, *et al.* (2004) Channel-forming peptide modulates transepithelial electrical conductance and solute permeability. *American Journal of Physiology. Cell Physiology* **286**: C1312–23.
92. Vogel JS, Garrett A, Keating II, Buchholz BA (2002) Protein binding of isofluorophate *in vivo* after co-exposure to multiple chemicals. *Environmental Health Perspectives* **110** (suppl. 6): 1–7.
93. Guengerich FP (2008) Cytochrome P450 and chemical toxicology. *Chemical Research in Toxicology* **21**: 70–83.
94. Kuby J (1997) *Immunology*, 3rd edn. New York: Freeman.
95. Bascom R, Meggs WJ, Frampton M, *et al.* (1997) Neurogenic inflammation: with additional discussion of central and perceptual integration of non-neurogenic inflammation. *Environmental Health Perspectives* **105** (suppl. 2): 531–7.
96. Meggs WJ (1999) Mechanisms of allergy and chemical sensitivity. *Toxicology and Industrial Health* **15**: 331–8.
97. Medscape Today (2000) Poll Results. www.medscape.com/px/instantpollservlet/result?PollID=15&BackURL=/px/instantservlet.
98. Wikipedia (2009) *Paracetamol.* http://en.wikipedia.org/wiki/Paracetamol#cite_note-foye_medchem-21.
99. Meyerhoff DJ, Lindgren J, Hardin D, Griffis JM, Weiner MW (2001) Reduced N-acetylaspartate in the right basal ganglia of ill Gulf War veterans by magnetic resonance spectroscopy. *Proceedings of the International Society of Magnetic Resonance Medicine* **9**: 994.
100. Golomb BA (2008) Acetylcholinesterase inhibitors and Gulf War illnesses. *Proceedings of the National Academy of Sciences, USA* **105**: 4295–300.
101. Blazer D, Gray GC, Hotopf M, *et al.* (2008) Acetylcholinesterase inhibition and Gulf War illnesses: conclusions are not supported by independent reviews of the same evidence. *Proceedings of the National Academy of Sciences, USA* **105**: E20.
102. Wikipedia (2009) *Cytochrome P450.* http://en.wikipedia.org/wiki/Cytochrome_P450.
103. Bland J, Costarella L, Levin B (1999) *Clinical Nutrition: A Functional Approach.* Gig Harbour, WA: Institute for Functional Medicine.
104. Cherry N, Mackness MI, Durrington PN (2002) Paraoxonase (PON1) polymorphisms in farmers attributing ill-health to sheep dip. *Lancet* **359**: 763–4.
105. Furlong CE, Li WF, Richter RJ (2000) Genetic and temporal determinants of pesticide sensitivity: role of paraoxonase (PON1). *Neurotoxicology* **21**: 91–100.
106. Rigden S (1999) *Chronic Fatigue Syndrome (CFS).* Gig Harbour, WA: Institute for Functional Medicine.
107. Kennedy G, Spence VA, McLaren M, *et al.* (2005) Oxidative stress levels are raised in chronic fatigue syndrome and are associated with clinical symptoms. *Free Radical Biology and Medicine* **39**: 584–9.
108. Rodriguez-Ariza A, Alhama J, Diaz-Mendez FM, Lopez-Barea J (1999) Content of 8-oxodG in chromosomal and DNA of *Sparus aurata* fish as biomarker of oxidative stress and environmental pollution. *Mutation Research* **438**: 97–107.
109. Costa LG, Cole TB, Furlong CE (2006) Gene–environment interactions: paraoxonase (PON) and sensitivity to organophosphate toxicity. *Laboratory Medicine* **37**: 109–14.
110. Abou-Donia MB (2003) Organophosphorus ester-induced chronic neurotoxicity. *Archives of Environmental Health* **58**: 484–97.
111. British Dietetic Association (2009) *Fish PCBs and Dioxins.* www.bda.uk.com/Downloads/Fish_PCBs_and_Dioxins.pdf.
112. Food and Drug Administration (1994) *Mercury in Fish: Cause for Concern?* www.fda.gov/fdac/reprints/mercury.html.
113. Eto K, Takahashi H, Kakita A, *et al.* (2006) A pathological study of Minamata disease (methylmercury poisoning): special reference to Niigata Minamata disease. *Neuropathology* **26**: A14.
114. Ui J (1992) *Industrial Pollution in Japan.* Tokyo: United Nations University Press.
115. Kaushik N, Fear D, Richards SC, *et al.* (2005) Gene expression in peripheral blood mononuclear cells from patients with chronic fatigue syndrome. *Journal of Clinical Pathology* **58**: 826–32.
116. Kerr J, Burke B, Petty R, *et al.* (2008) Seven genomic subtypes of chronic fatigue syndrome/myalgic encephalomyelitis (CFS/ME): a detailed analysis of gene networks and clinical phenotypes *Journal of Clinical Pathology* **61**: 730–39.
117. Nebert DW (2000) Drug-metabolizing enzymes, polymorphisms and interindividual response to environmental toxicants. *Clinical Chemistry and Laboratory Medicine* **38**: 857–61.
118. Ma MK, Woo MH, Mcleod HL (2002) Genetic Basis of Drug Metabolism. *American Journal of Health-System Pharmacy* **59**: 2061–9.
119. Cory-Slechta DA, Virgolini MB, Rossi-George A, *et al.* (2008) Lifetime consequences of combined maternal lead and stress. *Basic and Clinical Pharmacology and Toxicology* **102**: 218–27.

120. McKeown-Eyssen G, Baines C, Cole DEC, *et al.* (2004) Case-control study of genotypes in multiple chemical sensitivity: CYP2D6, NAT1, NAT2, PON1, PON2 and MTHFR. *International Journal of Epidemiology* **33**: 971–8.
121. Schnakenberg E, Fabig K-R, Stanulla M, *et al.* (2007) A cross-sectional study of self-reported chemical-related sensitivity is associated with gene variants of drug-metabolizing enzymes. *Environmental Health* **6**: 6.
122. Wiesmuller GA, Niggemann H, Weissbach W, *et al.* (2008) Sequence variations in subjects with self-reported multiple chemical sensitivity(sMCS): a case-controlled study. *Journal of Toxicology and Environmental Health. Part A* **71**: 786–94.
123. Melton L (2008) Predictive toxicogenomics: playing the genes you're dealt. *Chemistry World* **July**: 62–6.
124. Fry RC, Navasumrit P, Valiathan C, *et al.* (2007) Activation of inflammation/NF-kappaB signaling in infants born to arsenic-exposed mothers. *PLoS Genetics* **3**: e207.
125. Haley RW, Billecke S, La Du BN (1999) Association of low PON1 type Q (type A) arylesterase activity with neurologic symptom complexes in Gulf War veterans. *Toxicology and Applied Pharmacology* **157**: 227–33.
126. Mackness B, Durrington PN, Mackness MI (2000) Low paraoxonase in Persian Gulf War veterans self-reporting Gulf War syndrome. *Biochemical and Biophysical Research Communications* **276**: 729–33.
127. Hotopf M, Mackness M, Nikolaou V, *et al.* (2003) Paraoxonase in Persian Gulf War veterans. *Journal of Occupational and Environmental Medicine* **45**: 668–75.
128. Klevay LM (2007) Lead exposure is associated with decreased serum paraoxonase (PON1) activity and genotypes. *Environmental Health Perspectives* **115**: 2–8.
129. Furlong CE (207) Genetic variability in the cytochrome P450-paraoxonase 1 (PON1) pathway for detoxication of organophosphorus compounds. *Journal of Biochemical and Molecular Toxicology* **21**: 197–205.
130. Mackness B, Davie GK, Turkie W, *et al.* (2001) Paraoxonase status in coronary heart disease: are activity and concentration more important than genotype? *Arteriosclerosis, Thrombosis, and Vascular Biology* **21**: 1451–7.
131. Michaelis S (ed.) (2007) *Aviation Contaminated Air Reference Manual*. England: S Michaelis.
132. Bellinger DC (2008) Neurodevelopmental effects of early exposures to chemical contaminants: reducing uncertainty in epidemiological studies. *Basic and Clinical Pharmacology and Toxicology* **102**: 237–44.
133. Gross L (2007) The toxic origins of disease. *Public Library of Sciences* **5**: 1392–8.
134. Heindel JJ (2008) Animal models for probing the developmental basis of disease and dysfunction paradigm. *Basic and Clinical Pharmacology and Toxicology* **102**: 76–81.
135. Grandjean P (2008) Prenatal programming and toxicity. *Basic and Clinical Pharmacology and Toxicology* **102**: 71–2.
136. Needham LL, Calafat AM, Barr DB (2008) Assessing developmental toxicant exposures via biomonitoring. *Basic and Clinical Pharmacology and Toxicology* **102**: 100–108.
137. McMillen IC, MacLaughlin SM, Muhlhausler BS, *et al.* (2008) Developmental origins of adult health and disease: the role of periconceptual and foetal nutrition. *Basic and Clinical Pharmacology and Toxicology* **102**: 82–9.
138. Wasserman GA, Liu X, Factor-Litvak P, *et al.* (2008) Developmental impacts of heavy metals and undernutrition. *Basic and Clinical Pharmacology and Toxicology* **102**: 212–17.
139. Pesticide Action Network (2003) *Court Finds DuPont Product Responsible for Birth Defects*. www.pan-uk.org/pestnews/Issue/pn62/pn62p16.htm.
140. Elliott HR, Samuels DC, Eden JA, *et al.* (2008) Pathogenic mitochondrial DNA mutations are common in the general population. *American Journal of Human Genetics* **83**: 254–60.
141. Pall ML (2007) *Explaining 'Unexplained Illnesses': Disease Paradigm for Chronic Fatigue Syndrome, Multiple Chemical Sensitivity, Fibromyalgia, Post-Traumatic Stress Disorder, Gulf War Syndrome, and Others*. New York: Harrington Park Press.
142. Perry H (2008) The effects of systemic inflammation on the brain. Presented at Solutions Colloquium on ME/CFS and Fibromyalgia, Southampton, UK, 12 February 2008.
143. Kim Y-B, Hur G-H, Shin S, *et al.* (1999) Organophosphate-induced brain injuries: delayed apoptosis mediated by nitric oxide. *Environmental Toxicology and Pharmacology* **7**: 147–52.
144. Myers JP, Guilette LJ, Palenza P *et al.* (2003) The emerging science of endocrine disruption. In RC Ragaini (ed) *Proceedings of Conference: International Seminar on Nuclear War and Planetary Emergencies. 30th Session, Ence. Sicily*. Singapore: World Scientific Publishers.
145. Pesticides Action Network (2004) *Pesticides in Your Food*. www.pan-uk.org/Projects/Food/PAN%20UK%20food%20poster%2006.pdf.
146. Welshons WV, Thayer KA, Judy BM, *et al.* (2003) Large effects from small exposures: I. Mechanisms for endocrine disrupting chemicals with estrogenic activity. *Environmental Health Perspectives* **111**: 994–1006.
147. Joffres MR, Sampalli T, Fox RA (2005) Physiologic and symptomatic responses to low-level substances in individuals with and without chemical sensitivities: a randomized controlled blinded pilot booth study. *Environmental Health Perspectives* **113**: 1178–83.
148. Christopher J. Borgert CJ, Borgert SA, Findley KC

(2005) Synergism, antagonism, or additivity of dietary supplements: application of theory to case studies. *Thrombosis Research* **117**: 123–32.

149. Rajapakse N, Silva E, Kortenkamp A (2002) Combining xenoestrogens at levels below individual no-observed-effect concentrations dramatically enhances steroid hormone action. *Environmental Health Perspectives* **110**: 917–21.
150. Zhao F, Mayura K, Harper N, Safe SH, Phillips TD (1997) Inhibition of 3,3′,4,4′,5-pentachlorobiphenyl-induced fetal cleft palate and immunotoxicity in C57BL/6 mice by 2,2′,4,4′,5,5′-hexachlorobiphenyl. *Chemosphere* **34**: 1605–13.
151. Abou-Donia MB, Wilmarth KR, Jensen KF, Oehme FW, Kurt TL (1996) Neurotoxicity resulting from coexposure to pyridostigmine bromide, DEET, and permethrin: implications of Gulf War chemical exposures. *Journal of Toxicology and Environmental Health* **48**: 35–56.
152. Axelrad JC, Howard CV, McLean WG (2002) Interactions between pesticides and components of pesticide formulations in an in vitro neurotoxicity test. *Toxicology* **173**: 259–68.
153. Richard S, Moslemi S, Sipahutar H, *et al.* (2005) Differential effects of glyphosate and roundup on human placental cells and aromatase. *Environmental Health Perspectives* **113**: 716–20.
154. Lau K, McLean WG, Williams DP, Howard CV (2006) Synergistic interactions between commonly used food additives in a developmental neurotoxicity test. *Toxicological Science* **90**: 178–87.
155. Meyer P, Hessler W (2007) Does 'the dose make the poison'? Non-monotonic dose–response curves. www.ourstolenfuture.org/NewScience/lowdose/2007/2007-04-30%20Does%20the%20Dose%20Make%20the%20Poison.pdf.
156. Nagel SC, vom Saal FS, Thayer KA, *et al.* (1997) Relative binding affinity-serum modified access (RBA-SMA) assay predicts the relative in vivo bioactivity of the xenoestrogens bisphenol A and octylphenol. *Environmental Health Perspectives* **105**: 70–76.
157. Narita S-I, Goldblum RM, Watson CS, *et al.* (2007) Environmental oestrogens induce mast cell degranulation and enhance IgE-mediated release of allergic mediators. *Environmental Health Perspectives* **115**: 48–52.
158. Wozniak AL, Bulayeva NN, Watson CS (2005) Xenoestrogens at picomolar to nanomolar concentrations trigger membrane estrogen receptor-alpha-mediated Ca^{++} fluxes and prolactin release in GH3/B6 pituitary tumour cells. *Environmental Health Perspectives* **113**: 431–9.
159. Thayer KA, Melnick R, Burns K, *et al.* (2005) Fundamental flaws of hormesis for public health decisions. *Environmental Health Perspectives* **113**: 1271–6.
160. Baines CJ, McKeown-Eyssen GE, Riley N, *et al.* (2004) Case–control study of multiple chemical sensitivity, comparing haematology, biochemistry, vitamins and serum volatile organic compound measures. *Occupational Medicine* **54**: 408–18.
161. Andre V, Le Goff J, Pottier D, *et al.* (2007) Evaluation of bulky DNA adduct levels after pesticide use: comparison between open-field farmers and fruit growers. *Toxicological and Environmental Chemistry* **89**: 125–39.
162. Cohn BA, Cirillo PM, Wolff MS, *et al.* (2003) DDT and DDE exposure in mothers and time to pregnancy in daughters. *Lancet* **361**: 2205–6.
163. John Castillo *v.* EI DuPont De Nemours & co. INC *et al.* no. SC00-490 p. 1–60, 10 July 2003.
164. American Public Health Association (2004) The Learning and Developmental Disabilities Initiative: New Research, Educational and Policy Efforts to Prevent Exposures to Neurotoxicants. Presented at Public Health and the Environment, 6–10 November, Washington, DC. http://apha.confex.com/apha/132am/techprogram/session_13649.htm.
165. McCann D, Barrett A, Cooper A, *et al.* (2007) Food additives and hyperactive behaviour in 3-year-old and 8/9-year-old children in the community: a randomised, double-blinded, placebo-controlled trial. *Lancet* **370**: 1560–67; erratum 1542.
166. Xie K, Gupta RP, Abou-Donia MB (2002) Protein levels of neurofilament subunits in the hen central nervous system following prevention and potentiation of diisopropyl phosphorofluoridate (DFP)-induced delayed neurotoxicity. *Biochemical Pharmacology* **63**: 11–19.
167. Tirupapuliyur VD, Patel AG, Greenfield ST, *et al.* (2006) Gene expression profiles of the rat brain both immediately and 3 months following acute sarin exposure. *Biochemical Pharmacology* **71**: 497–520.
168. Duffy FH, Burchfiel JL, Bartels PH, Goan M, Sim VM (1980) Long term effects of organophosphate sarin on EEG on monkeys and humans. *Neurotoxicology* **1**: 667–89.
169. Gibson PR, Elms AN-M, Ruding LA (2003) Perceived treatment efficacy for conventional and alternative therapies reported by persons with multiple chemical sensitivity. *Environmental Health Perspectives* **111**: 1498–504.
170. 25% ME Group (2004) Severely Affected ME (Myalgic Encephalomyelitis): Analysis on Report on Questionnaire Issued January 2004. www.25megroup.org/Group%20Leaflets/Group%20reports/March%202004%20Severe%20ME%20Analysis%20Report.doc.
171. Nolan R (2007) A serious lack of evidence for NICE guidelines. Rapid response to Baker R, Shaw EJ (2007) Diagnosis and management of chronic fatigue syndrome or myalgic encephalomyelitis (or encephalopathy): summary of NICE guidance. *British Medical Journal* **335**: 446–8.

172. Health and Wellness Institute of Integrative Medicine (2004) *Detoxification Fact Sheet.* www.ehealthandhealing.com/html/healthfactsheets/DetoxificationFactSheet.doc.pdf.
173. Myhill S (2008) *Chemical Poisoning and Multiple Chemical Sensitivity (MCS): How to Reduce the Body Load.* www.drmyhill.co.uk/article.cfm?id=416.
174. Novak K (2003) Cancer susceptibility: role of genes, environment, and diet: PAH/DDT DNA adducts. *Medscape General Medicine* (1).
175. McLaren-Howard J (2002) The detection of DNA adducts (risk factors for DNA damage): a method for genomic DNA, the results and some effects of nutritional intervention. *Journal of Nutrition and Environmental Medicine* **12**: 19–31.
176. Zhao S, Amarjit N, Gierthy J, Eadon G (2001) Detection and characterization of DNA adducts formed from PCB metabolites in HepG2 cell line. Presented at Changing Environmental Awareness: Societal Concerns and Scientific Responses, 22nd Society of Environmental Toxicology and Chemistry annual meeting, 14 November, Baltimore, MD.
177. Richardson J (2000) Four cases of pesticide poisoning presenting as ME, treated with choline/ascorbic acid mixture. *Journal of Chronic Fatigue* **6**: 11–21.
178. Birnbaum LS, SE Fenton (2003) Cancer and developmental exposure to endocrine disruptors. *Environmental Health Perspectives* **111**: 389–94.
179. Van Noorden R (2006) Neurotoxicology fears branded alarmist. *Chemistry World* **December**: 10.
180. Meikle J (2008) EU plans warning labels on artificial colours. *Guardian*, 1 August.
181. United Kingdom Ombudsman Network (2004) Government & Health Care Ombudsmen. http://ombudsman.co.uk/_wsn/page3.html.
182. Yazbak FE (2004) Response to Gottlieb S (2004) Study finds no connection between MMR vaccine and autism. *British Medical Journal* **328**: 421a. www.bmj.com/cgi/eletters/328/7437/421-a.
183. Pusztai A (2000) Scientific results in conflict with business and state interests. Presented at Stockholm conference 14 June. www.psrast.org/pusztai.htm.
184. Bateman B, Warner JO, Hutchinson E, *et al.* (2004) The effects of a double blind, placebo controlled, artificial food colourings and benzoate preservative challenge on hyperactivity in a general population sample of preschool children. *Archives of Disease in Childhood* **89**: 506–11.
185. Food Standards Agency (2008) Update on artificial food colours. www.food.gov.uk/multimedia/pdfs/coloursletter.pdf.
186. University of Southampton (2008) *Southampton Response to EFSA Evaluation of Study on Food Additives and Children's Behaviour.* www.southampton.ac.uk/mediacentre/news/2008/mar/08_50.shtml.
187. American Chemistry Council (2008) *American Chemistry Council has Mixed Response to Passage of Consumer Product Safety Modernization Act.* www.phthalates.org/mediacenter/panelstatement.asp?ID=87.
188. Greenpeace (1998) *Greenpeace Refutes Claims by the International Council of Toy Industries (ICTI) May, 1998.* http://archive.greenpeace.org/comms/97/pvctoys/documents/icti.html.
189. Hatch EE, Nelson JW, Qureshi MM, et al. (2008) Association of urinary phthalate metabolite concentrations with body mass index and waist circumference: a cross-sectional study of NHANES data, 1999–2002. *Environmental Health* **7**: 27.
190. Research Advisory Committee on Gulf War Veterans' Illnesses (2008) *Gulf War Illness and the Health of Gulf War Veterans: Scientific Findings and Recommendations.* http://www1.va.gov/rac-gwvi/docs/GWIandHealthofGWVeterans_RAC-GWVIReport_2008.pdf.
191. Charlton BG (2008) Zombie science: a sinister consequence of evaluating scientific theories purely on the basis of enlightened self-interest. *Medical Hypotheses* **71**: 327–9.

Chapter 51

Mental health problems in patients with myalgic encephalomyelitis and fibromyalgia syndrome

Byron Hyde

INTRODUCTION

Since 1934 at least 70 myalgic encephalomyelitis (ME)-type epidemics have occurred around the world.[1] Yet most physicians and the public remain unclear as to the cause and characteristics of ME. Many physicians debate the existence of ME as a valid medical entity. To put it kindly, many physicians simply find ME and patients with ME an unwanted bother. Since 1934, when the first well-documented ME epidemic ravaged the Los Angeles County Hospital,[2] ME as a diagnosis has refused to go away and the mental health aspects of ME and chronic fatigue syndrome (CFS) not only remain but also appear to increase. We require a better understanding of ME and CFS. Even with knowledge, treating the mental health problems of the patient with ME will remain a formidable task.

Since 1984, I have been asking the question, 'What is ME?' First I sought out the few original ME experts in various countries who had examined patients with ME and the ME epidemics since 1934. I examined patients and questioned physicians from the 1934 Los Angeles epidemic, the 1947–48 Iceland epidemic,[3] and the various UK, New Zealand, Australian and Canadian epidemics, and I visited each of these epidemic sites. For the next 24 years, I have intensively investigated patients with ME and asked: 'What are the pathologies of the patient with ME that cause them to remain ill and unable to carry out the tasks that they were so good at before their illness onset?'

During the past 24 years, I have confined my practice to patients with ME and CFS. As much as possible, I have examined every organ and system of each of thousands of patients with ME, thanks to the totally free access that patients and physicians have to all tests and specialists in the Canadian health system.[4] The following chapter represents a small amount of what I have discovered during the years that I have questioned ME experts, studied the considerable ME literature, and examined thousands of patients with ME and CFS. What became obvious to me is that we cannot understand the patient with ME without examining the patient in great detail, along with his or her environment, social system and belief structure. We must also examine the limitations, usually imposed by government bureaucracy, that prevent physicians from adequately examining patients with ME.

THE WRITER'S PREJUDICE

Allow me to start by first acquainting you with my prejudice of what I believe constitutes a patient with ME, since it may interfere with any preconceived perceptions that you bring to this discussion. My prejudice is this: the patient with ME has been with us a very long time, undoubtedly many centuries, but it was only in the twentieth century that we had the technology and medical organization to distinguish ME as a specific illness category and a communication system (the Internet) that enabled these patients to find each other and group together, often much to the regret of the physicians and often with an inaccurate diagnosis not based upon scientific evidence.

A succinct definition of ME is this:

ME is an acute-onset, diffuse injury of the central nervous system (CNS) that in turn either provokes or is associated with organ, system and social pathologies that prevent the patient from effectively competing in their previous work and social culture.

Classically, ME occurs in epidemic and endemic periods, as in the 1934 Los Angeles, the 1947–48 Akureyri or the various UK epidemics. The onset of illness in both the historical and today's patients is often associated with an apparent infectious disease, immunization, and traumatic or toxic exposure in the immediate previous days or by repeated traumas in the prior weeks and months.

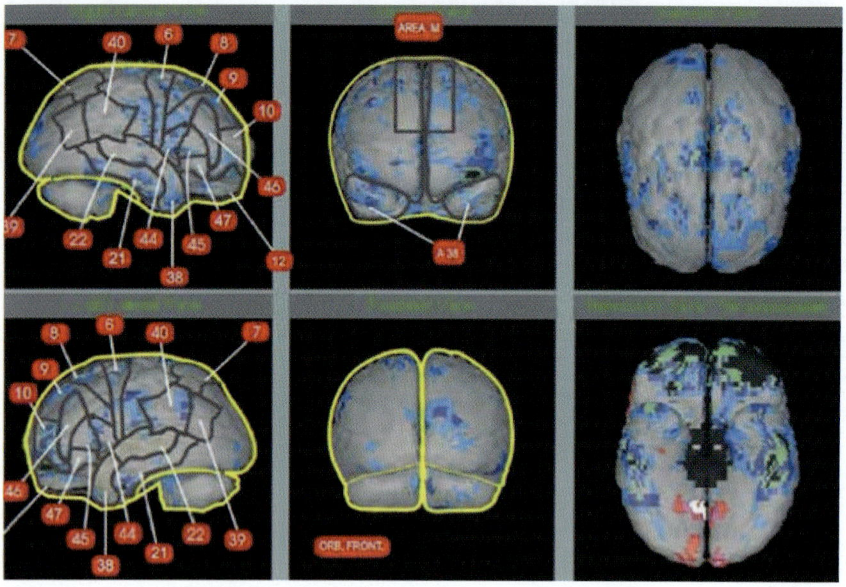

Figure 51.1 Brain single-photon-emission computed tomography (SPECT) of typical patient with myalgic encephalomyelitis (ME). This is a typical severe ME brain, as visualized by SPECT at illness onset, with Brodmann areas indicated. Blue areas represent the significant typical hypoperfused areas of this dysfunctional brain. This schoolteacher fell ill following a severe influenza-like infectious episode 1 week after return to school. The patient went on to develop thyroid malignancy and *Clostridium difficile* infection several years later. Typical ME features: teacher, female, age 40 years at illness onset, post-infectious, no significant recovery during 15-year follow-up

The key terms in this definition are:

- acute-onset;
- diffuse CNS injury;
- complex organ, system and social pathologies.

Figure 51.1 shows a single-photon-emission computed tomography (SPECT) brain scan of a typical patient with ME.

In the clinical situation, both the physician and the patient are confronted with another problem. Which patient has ME? Which patient is misdiagnosed as having ME? Possibilities include the following:

- Chronic patients with ME and its associated organ, system and social pathologies
- Chronic patients with undiagnosed or missed single or cumulative major medical illness or pathology diagnosed as ME but suggesting low-grade or slowly progressive injury
- Patients with classical psychiatric disease that may or may not be complicated by organ or system pathology
- Acutely ill patients misdiagnosed as ME but with a potentially treatable progressive illness.

The first three patient categories above tend to have similar mental and social health issues and can be discussed as a group. By definition, the referring physician never diagnoses any of the missed major pathologies. If they did, then probably the patient would not be referred to as having ME or CFS. The big danger, the veritable mine in the minefield, is the last – the patient who, either diagnosed by a physician or self-diagnosed, has recent-onset ME. Too often have I seen fellow physicians who tell me they have ME, laugh and then say they do not require an examination, only to find that had they been examined properly an undiagnosed malignancy would have been discovered when it was still treatable. The greatest tragedy is to miss a diagnosis that could have been treated, and perhaps cured, by the physician who had taken the patient's symptoms not as a diagnosis but as a medical mystery to be solved by scientific testing. This also represents my major criticism of the diagnosis of ME, either by the physician or by the patient. My criticism is not directed toward the psychiatrist but to the physicians who, for whatever reason, have failed to properly investigate and follow these reputed patients with ME before referring them to psychiatry.

THE PATIENT WITH M.E. AND HER MYTHOLOGIES

For the clinical psychiatrist and clinical medicine physician, it is the patient's complex mythologies, perhaps more than scientific understanding, that overwhelm both the patient and the physician. It is essential to understand these patient mythologies in order to help the patient with ME. Our patient is more than an injured body and brain: she is an integrated part of a complex belief and social structure with all of its values and prejudices.

If you were to be referred four real patients with ME, on average three would be girls or women and one would be a boy or a man. This 75 per cent percentage of females corresponds approximately to many autoimmune illnesses, such as multiple sclerosis and rheumatoid disease, but this of course does not validate ME as an autoimmune disease.

The child and adult sex distribution charts shown in Figures 51.2 and 51.3 were developed from an epidemiological study of approximately 2000 patients with ME or CFS investigated by the Nightingale Research Foundation during the epidemic period 1984–92. Note the significant divergence of females from males at puberty and the rapid drop in adult women new cases at menopause.

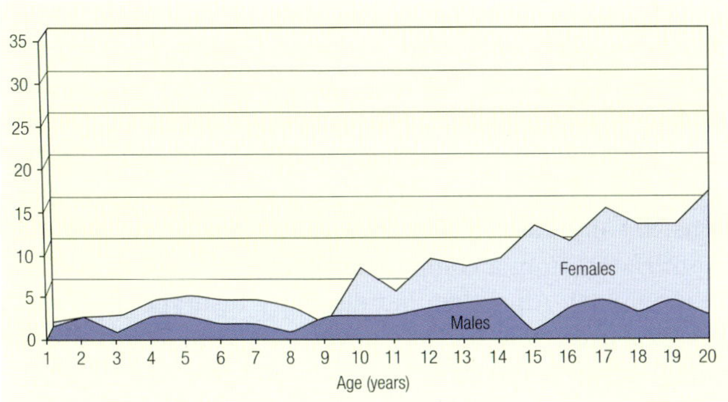

Figure 51.2 Sex and age of patients with myalgic encephalomyelitis (ME)/chronic fatigue syndrome (CFS) seen between 1984 and 1992 at the Nightingale Research Clinic: children and youths (age 0–21 years)

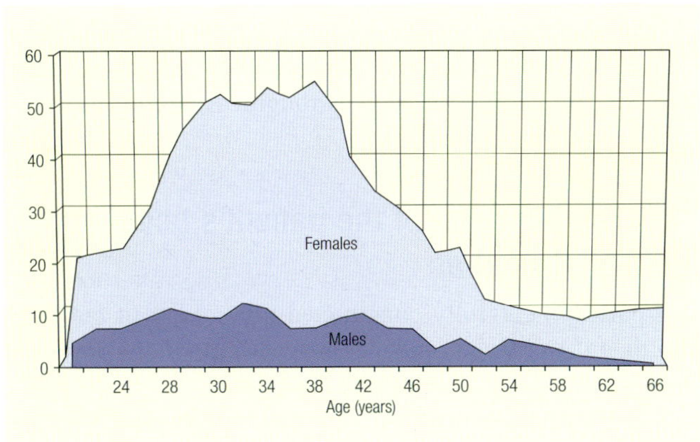

Figure 51.3 Sex and age of patients with myalgic encephalomyelitis (ME)/chronic fatigue syndrome (CFS) seen between 1984 and 1992 at the Nightingale Research Clinic: adults (age 22–70 years)

The patient before falling ill

From a mental health aspect, our patient with ME has a health history in addition to her present illness. Perhaps even more importantly, she has a vision of the future. The patient's past truly is prologue and the future is an existential necessity, both of which are capable of being destroyed. If you were to describe this young woman before the time when she fell ill, you would have acknowledged that she was a hard-working woman with many prior achievements and who contemplates realistic future goals. If she is a parent, then in most cases she would have aspirations for her children, real or imagined, to do even better than herself. If our patient is a student, in most cases she will have all of the uncertainties, fears of youth, physical vigour and boundless energy, but also wonderful potential aspirations. Like Goethe's Faust, she has yet to learn that her existence is defined not by the goals but the very striving necessary to reach these goals.

Our patient before becoming ill will have already achieved a lot, including a higher education. Most often she will be a teacher or healthcare worker with one or more degrees. You will note a strong school and healthcare bias to this illness, suggesting an increased exposure to infectious diseases and with long hours of exhausting work. To a lesser degree, the patient's occupation will mirror the local employment population bias, but the school and healthcare bias will be paramount.

The occupations of 2000 consecutive patients with ME were tabulated during the epidemic period of 1984–92 (Figure 51.4). These patients came from across Canada, the USA and, to a lesser extent, the UK. Consequently, the figures are not prejudiced by local employment. By percentage, the single largest occupation was among respiratory technologies, followed by healthcare workers, including physicians, nurses and technicians in residential institutions for disabled people, who may have an increased infectious rate.

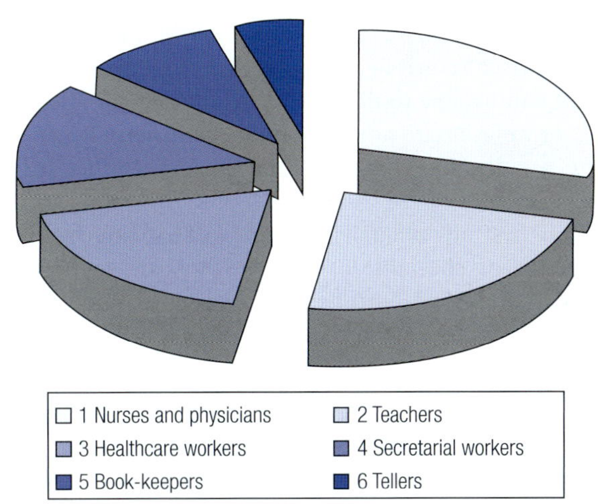

Figure 51.4 Occupation of patients with myalgic encephalomyelitis (ME) at illness onset

Often our patient will have been active in sports, with repeat associated minor and moderate physical traumas, often to the head and neck region. If you check her school record from kindergarten to the present, she will have missed a negligible amount of school. In most cases, before falling ill she will have had a history of excellent health, with no psychiatric associations. In my experience, except for those patients with a significant psychiatric family history, few of these patients with ME will be psychiatric patients. If you are an old physician like me, then our patient before falling ill will have been a person you would be proud to call your daughter. She will have an identity, courage, achievements and a belief structure with which you can associate. However, it is this belief structure as much as her illness that will provoke a significant part of what you perceive to be her illness. Thus, understanding her belief structure and her identity is important.

The patient's pre-illness identity and health belief structure

Our patient simply does not think about illness. If she is a parent, perhaps she has the natural concerns of any mother for her children, obtaining the right immunizations and paying occasional visits to the general practitioner (GP). She has never been significantly ill herself. Why think about illness? Visits to the doctor are for her pregnancies, routine Pap smear tests and breast examinations.

If you ask her about falling ill, she will dismiss the subject; illness is something short-term, a cold, perhaps off for a day or two and then back to school or work again. As a worker, she enjoys her job, the camaraderie, the striving; she loves her paycheque, even if it is too small – and it always is too small. She could be your daughter, your best friend's daughter or your granddaughter.

Life is simple for her. Should she fall ill and not recover sufficiently to return to work within a few days, she knows her GP will be able to diagnose and solve the problem with a pill or appropriate advice. Failing that, her GP will refer her to a colleague who will cure her and get her back to work.

If this first attempt fails, she knows that there will be a consultant or specialist out there who can appropriately diagnose, treat and cure her, but she never really gets to that concept, since the thought that her GP cannot treat and cure her simply never comes into her head.

Our patient has been working professionally or semi-professionally for over 15 years without ever falling ill. Let us assume our patient is North American. She believes she has taken adequate steps to ensure access to good and prompt healthcare. She has both short- and long-term insurance coverage deducted from her paycheque. She will have a mortgage, but she may not have taken out mortgage insurance, skimping on this to pay for her child's piano lessons. In any case, if she does fall ill for a few weeks or months, say from a compound fracture in a skiing accident in the French Alps, then her disability insurance will cover her expenses. No, she has never looked at her insurance policy. Why should she?

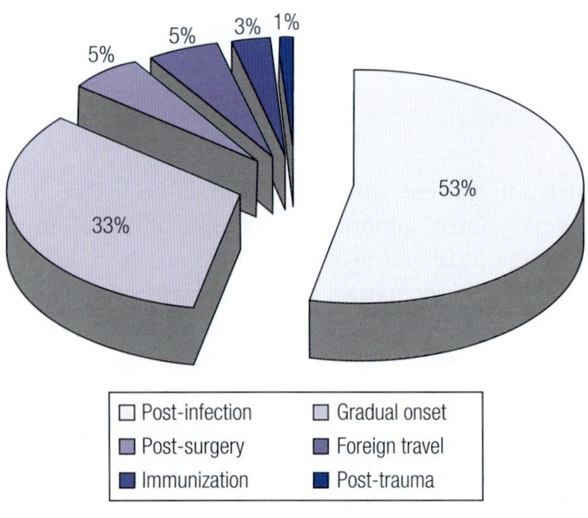

Figure 51.5 Triggers ascribed by the patient as a possible cause of their present illness in 2000 cases of myalgic encephalomyelitis (ME)/chronic fatigue syndrome (CFS), 1984–1992. The gradual-onset patients tended to have no apparent associated triggers

In the more than 2000 or 3000 patients with ME and CFS who have consulted me during the past 25 years in Canada, the UK and the USA, before their illness the majority had a long history of health, free of any serious medical or psychiatric illness; very few ever imagined themselves becoming ill with a chronic illness. Illness triggers are not always reliable as a cause of illness in all cases, but the data in Figure 51.5, taken from a large survey of almost 2000 patients, are perhaps reliable as rough casual indicators.

The disintegration of the patient's belief and identity structures

Our patient's carefully constructed mythology of enduring health until old age, and her perceptions of the infallible medical world, are about to be destroyed.

What will now confront our previous worker bee and future patient amounts not only to a total destruction of her most important belief structures but also to the ultimate loss of her identity, an identity carefully constructed since youth.

The young woman falls ill. Her illness usually has an acute onset, but it is not short-term. From then on, nothing works, nothing unfolds in the manner she might have perceived it before the onset of this strange illness.

She does not become better in 2–3 days. In almost all cases, her doctor does not appreciate that he or she is dealing with the onset of a chronic illness. Since most acute illnesses tend to resolve on their own, her GP tells her that she will be fine in another week. That does not happen: her illness persists. Then or at the next appointment, her GP may prescribe a medication or treatment and may send her for a few tests, usually a complete blood count and a urinalysis and not much else. The tests tell her GP nothing because he or she does not know what tests to order; nor does the GP know at this point what he or she is dealing with. Sooner or later her GP will refer her to a consultant.

'No findings of note,' the reply comes back. 'Perhaps your patient is depressed?'

If her GP has not made the diagnosis by now, he or she soon will. It is likely to be anxiety neurosis, depression, work avoidance or family dispute – all diagnoses that are safe to make, all of which have no proof. Often notations in the history are not told to the patient; these notations, when sent on to the next doctor or other agencies, may undermine the patient's later chance for insurance benefits or state incapacity or disability allowances. The doctor is thus protected, but not necessarily the patient. Our patient may even be given an antidepressant that, over time, succeeds only in significantly increasing her weight. Usually the patient is given a psychiatric diagnosis by the GP and referred to a psychiatrist, although there has been no previous psychiatric history. At times she may believe her GP that she is depressed; more often she does not. Even if the doctor diagnoses ME, he or she is unable to treat ME adequately. There simply is no magic pill and no remedy, and there is very little valid knowledge about the significance of the diagnosis. The psychiatrist immediately is at a disadvantage: he or she believes that physical disease has been ruled out. Yet physical disease has not been ruled out, and in most cases it has not even been seriously investigated. Our patient is now labelled 'ME or CFS', but often the doctor thinks anxiety neurosis, depression or conversion disorder. If the doctor thinks CFS, then this is no more than a poorly defined label; if he or she thinks ME, then this may be the least properly investigated epidemic and endemic illness in existence. In the UK, very few of these patients so diagnosed have ever been subjected to any significant scientific investigation; many have not even had a serious physical examination.

Weeks and even months go by. No medication and no treatment works. Nothing works and the illness persists.

Within 2 months, her disability insurance raises its head. Since there is no documented evidence for any significant illness, her insurer does not bother paying. Sweet soul that she is, she honestly believes that if the insurance company only knew how ill she were, then it would send her a disability cheque. The insurance company has a good cop who pretends to be the patient's friend, talks her into going back to work or tells her the company is just waiting for a few more results to be sent in. She tries to go back to work and falls flat on her face. Before long, a year has gone by and in many cases the insurance company still has not honoured the disability pension. Some insurance companies actually guide the patient along until it is outside the time limits for her to make a qualified application for benefits. By now, much if not all of her savings have been dissipated. All ballast, including her child's music lessons and the piano, have gone. Rapidly she is stripped to the economic bone. If she has not been frantic up to now, she soon will be.

The search

Our patient, worker bee that she is, after months and possibly a year or two, having failed to find a helpful doctor and failed to have been awarded her disability pension, searches the Internet for an expert who will treat her. Her GP and often her family and friends have given up on her. Yet she cannot believe that there is not someone out there who can diagnose and treat her and get her back to work, give her back her family, paycheque and friends, and restore her identity. She amasses reams of garbled information, which is often misinformation – but she does not believe this. She is going to educate her doctor about the 'true facts' about ME. However, on the Internet, she also encounters mixed in with the facts some of the most incredible hogwash imaginable; she will meet some of the slickest charlatans in the business, the penny-and-pound thieves who sell her miraculous alternative medications that do not work and sometimes kill. Before long, our disabled patient is paying out, in effect gambling, incredible sums of her much-needed money in the vain hope that these miracle cures will soon make her better and get her back to work. They do not work.

Some of the more brilliant charlatans, the highwaymen of the twenty-first century, will guarantee to restore her health: 'Our treatment has saved thousands of people, but this treatment is expensive, very expensive, but isn't your health worth it?' She bites! If she or her family are desperate enough, they will sell their house, invest their life's income in a desperate gamble not to lose all. They lose all! Sometimes she will lose her family; but worse, she will lose her carefully crafted identity as a proud member of her community, a successful worker and a student of life. She loses all that she was and intended to be. She cannot even be a good mother. She thinks about the piano lessons that have stopped and the piano that has moved out, and she feels that she is now failing as a parent. Nothing works.

Several times she tries to go back to work but simply cannot endure. Since she has no adequate psychiatric or physical diagnosis, her long-term insurance policy has either stopped after a short while or in many cases has never begun. The insurance companies know these patients well. They know their client has no funds, no physical energy and no resources to fight back. Our patient's partner may have left her; he can no longer take the expense or handle chronic illness, the lack of sex, his wife's inability to even go out for a show. Alone, or with her children, she may return to live with her ageing parents. Without supportive parents, she may fall into a life of welfare benefits and despair, barely eking out an existence. She may kill herself. Only if she is one of the wealthy few, one with funds that are not wasted, or who succeeds in obtaining her disability pension, is our patient able to survive with any integrity. Many patients become bitter, writing diatribes, attacking authorities, doctors included. Many doctors simply lump them all into one more group of nutters.

She will have been referred to you, a psychiatrist. You are kind to her. You speak in a soothing manner. Having lost everything, at last she has found a friendly ear, someone who will believe her. She cries – a sure sign of depression – and out comes the prescription pad for the first of an endless series of antidepressive medications that succeed only in propelling this normal-looking athletic woman into a state of obesity, still unable to return to work. If our patient resists this treatment, she is written off as 'not complying'.

DOCTORS: THEIR FEAR OF EMBARRASSMENT AND THE ECONOMIC REALITY

Let me introduce you to a few of the doctors that this woman has consulted. Like our patient, these doctors have their own history and mythologies.

Most doctors were some of the top students in their primary and secondary school systems. Then they were enrolled in medicine, where they met hundreds of other medical students with a history of being at the top of their class. Only a few of the hundreds of these medical students can ever expect to be at the top. Only a handful would be considered to be the most brilliant and have honours bestowed upon them. No one doubts that the top students would be truly brilliant. But, depending upon the school and the teacher, their brilliance may in large part be the ability to give back a wide range of accepted facts in a clear, concise, organized manner. It is a curious thing that many of the very top students do not continue in clinical medicine. They are not always interested in people as much as they are in excellence. The majority of the other graduating doctors in their class fall into other groups, and those who have not lost their curiosity may become some of the very best clinical physicians and researchers. Yet others who have always been first, the best in their class, have been needlessly embarrassed at not being one of the exalted top few. For many such students of medicine, this may be the end of independent thinking, of exploring, of challenging the accepted wisdom. It is precisely this need not to be embarrassed further that caused doctors for centuries not to discover circulation or the concept of infectious disease and almost every modern aspect of medicine. For centuries, they survived by embracing the accepted wisdom.

There is another problem concerning the referring GPs who will refer the patient with ME to you. During the past 40 years, except for a few subspecialties, most doctors' real taxable incomes in North America, the UK and Western Europe have fallen from one of the highest in the community to that of a modest middle-income person. You may be earning less than your patient with ME was earning before she became too ill to work. The doctor starts in practice with debts. Without help from their parents, in most cases there is no way that doctors in North America can afford to buy the house that any doctor purchased 40 years ago or even 20 years ago. The medical magazines talk about making your practice more efficient, which essentially means seeing more patients for less and less time. Essentially, that means getting the patient out of the clinic by giving them a pill, sometimes any pill. They and you pretend this is not so, but you too have a mortgage and your partner expects you to buy that magical piano, pay for your child's piano lessons and the family trips to ski in France this winter, or simply take that cruise advertised in the doctors' magazines. Unless you take a government, pharmaceutical industry or insurance company job as a doctor, or you succeed in getting one of the senior positions in the hospital on a salary, unless you work a 60-h week or see patients outside the National Health Service (NHS), not only will your income be modest but also you will be judging yourself against an unrealistic measuring stick of those doctors who have come before you and a few of your colleagues who appear to be wealthy. You simply do not need a troublesome, complicated patient with ME who will take up your valuable time.

I am still talking here primarily about the non-psychiatrist physician. Money is status. Time is money, and few can take the time to explore the incredible significance of the relatively young chronic patient with diffuse brain injury. These patients with ME simply take too much time. Consequence? The primary care doctor simply sends the patient with ME to the psychiatrist, who they believe has all the time in the world. The psychiatrist in turn will assume that, as in all reputed psychiatric patients, the primary care doctor and the consultant have adequately investigated the referred patient who now sits in front of them. Yet you, as a doctor, should know better – and many do. The system in the UK prevents most primary care doctors from even ordering a full technological evaluation of their patient. The system in the UK, North America and much of Europe does not give the doctor time or money to explore this fascinating patient. Worse, there are no specialty clinics working inside the NHS that have the time, authority or financing to properly investigate these patients with ME for physical cause of disease. This total chronic failure to systematically examine the patient with ME has not been helpful, either to the patient with ME or to the psychiatrist.

The relatively young, chronically physically ill public in the UK tend to be very critical of the psychiatrist, and often needlessly so. Yet, as a psychiatrist, you have both a disadvantage and an advantage over the regular non-psychiatrist. The disadvantage is that your income may be one of the lowest in the medical community. The advantage is that your expenses are less and you alone among your colleagues will be able to listen to your patient for a considerable time. Perhaps you will be the first doctor who has the time to listen to her and who can get to the physical root of her anxiety, even if you cannot improve her material life. It is here where your difficulty becomes even more complicated.

Like many of your medical and psychiatrist colleagues, you will not want this patient. She simply takes up too much time in the clinic, and you wish to see her depart so that you may get on to a treatable patient. Many of your own psychiatrist colleagues will believe that any patient with ME is simply expressing some form of hysterical behaviour, is a whiner, is someone who does not want to work, or, worse, is boringly uninteresting. The patient will believe she knows much more about ME than you do; perhaps she does, but that is irritating to you and often her information is as highly inaccurate as yours has been. We are now looking at a major treatment impasse, including hostility, which may be mutual, and poorly organized information on both sides.

There is one final aspect to these patients with ME. Few patients realize the two-way nature of medicine, the great joy of being a doctor, of making a clear diagnosis of the patient and getting that ill patient either back to health or at least to a position where they can manage. Yet this patient with ME is not some fascinating patient with bipolar disorder from the Bank of England who has just ripped through a few billion pounds of your country's money. She is not a schizophrenic poet of immense talent and immense self-destructive powers. This is not a case where there is a good chance you can bring banker or poet back to reality. It is so easy to tell yourself that this is one more case of ME hysteria.

How can you, the psychiatrist or for that matter any doctor, help this young woman?

If you catch the patient in time, you can attempt to help this unbelieving patient to stop wasting her valuable and decreasing funds on bogus care and treatments, usually from non-doctors. If you believe that the patient is significantly disabled, and in my experience few patients in this category ever lie and most are more disabled than even they realize, then you can help her obtain appropriate state benefits or her entitlement to disability insurance. More than any other assistance you can provide, this may help her save part of her identity and perhaps her life, and she will bless you for it forever. This may take work, and it would be good to have a psychiatrist colleague or ombudsman whose work is limited to handling these matters to whom you can refer this patient. It takes both significant time and skill in assisting these patients with the insurance industry and benefits systems.

It is not only the uninformed doctor who represents a problem but also the reputedly informed patient. Both doctors and patients have bought into the nineteenth-century Oslerian principle that the best way to treat and possibly cure a patient is to diagnose the illness as to the cause, treat the cause and, with knowledge and luck, cure the patient. The problem is the phrase 'the cause', since many of these patients have multiple causes giving rise to their disability. This unicausal theory of medical pathology worked for pulmonary tuberculosis, for syphilis, so why not ME? Well, what if there is not a single cause of the illness? What if the patient with ME is disabled due to multiple cumulative pathologies?

MULTIPLE PATHOLOGY PATIENTS

My clinic is in the process of an in-depth study of the last 53 consecutive patients referred to us with a diagnosis of ME or CFS. In this group:

- 100 per cent had missed measurable brain dysfunction;
- 98 per cent had measurable significant sleep dysfunctions that included (i) lack of type 3 and 4 sleep, (ii) abnormal, absent or significantly delayed rapid eye movement (REM), (iii) central and peripheral apnoea, (iv) restless legs syndrome and (v) oxygen saturation that fell below 88 per cent (interestingly, oxygen saturation below 88% caused loss of consciousness in an aircraft pilot);
- 74 per cent had measurable thyroid dysfunction;
- 47 per cent had measurable significant arthritic, rheumatoid changes or other indicators that were previously diagnosed as fibromyalgia;
- 47 per cent had other missed major disease, including cardiac disease, malignant disease, vascular injuries and autonomic nervous system dysfunction;
- at least 16 per cent had typical psychiatric illness but, in addition, missed physical disease.

The problem here is not the multiple pathologies but the fact that the primary or consulting doctors missed these multiple diagnoses.

We subdivided the 53 patients in this study under occupations. This is what we found:

- Nineteen patients (37%) were school-associated professors, teachers or students.
- Nine patients (17%) were civil servants, the majority with young children in school.
- Five patients (10%) were healthcare workers.

This study of a group of 53 patients with ME/CFS was biased due to the fact that in Ottawa, Canada, a large percentage of the inhabitants are government workers. In an earlier study that looked at 2000 patients from across Canada and the USA, school and healthcare workers represented over 70 per cent of the 2000 patients. This suggested that ME was usually associated with a high exposure to infections.

As noted in the group of 53 patients, the single largest group was 19 (37%) of the total. These were students and teaching staff at primary, secondary and university educational institutions. For brevity, I will confine this discussion regarding pathological findings to these 19 patients referred to me as patients with ME who were teachers and students. This dominant group also contained the largest number of youths and children.

Collectively, these 19 school-associated patients had been seen by over 200 doctors. All had missed the following pathologies, which were found by extensive history, physical and technological examinations:

Dysautanomia and postural orthostatic tachycardia

Check your patient's arterial blood pressure, pulse pressure and heart rate when they are lying, sitting and standing. Have your patient stand without moving and check their blood pressure every minute for 10–15 min, stopping if their pressure drops precipitously or their heart rate accelerates above 120 bpm. If you find the blood pressure falling or the pulse pressure narrowing significantly, immediately stop the test and ask the patient to sit down. Make one of your first patient visits a 2- to 3-h visit in order to obtain a full life history. Note how many times the patient has to go to the toilet during this visit, suggesting possible pituitary or other endocrine disease. Do not allow the patient to have a water bottle with her during this time.

Measurable brain disease in patients with ME

A surprising 100 per cent of the 19 teachers and students had significant brain changes or anomalies by one or all of technical examination, measurement or history. If you can, order or have your medical colleagues order a brain SPECT, a magnetic resonance imaging (MRI) scan with contrast of the brain that includes pituitary, cerebellar tonsils and cervical spine area.

As mentioned earlier, the following pathologies were missed by over 200 examining doctors, who possibly did not believe they were dealing with significant physical disease and so did not do an extensive examination of these patients. We found the following:

- A patient with tertiary CNS syphilis and who was also positive for hepatitis B diagnosed as having simple major depression
- Leucoencephalopathy with ventricular hypertrophy in a youth
- One adult with significantly abnormal electroencephalograms (EEGs)
- One youth with missed nocturnal seizures and seizure-associated episodic complete heart block, causing syncope, significant hypoglycaemia and obstructive chronic tonsillitis that occluded his pharynx when sleeping on his back
- A youth with Chiari syndrome with ventriculomegaly
- An older patient with significant generalized brain atrophy and ventricular hypertrophy
- A patient who had been in the area of the Chernobyl disaster as a 1-year-old child and who had a subarachnoid cyst that had displaced two-thirds of the left hemisphere, including the entire left frontal lobe, the entire left temporal lobe and the anterior part of the left parietal lobe, but who had no observed neurological examination abnormalities either on neuromuscular examination or in gross intelligence. He simply had overwhelming exhaustion. He had graduated with a master's degree
- A patient with complete atresia of the middle cerebral artery
- A patient with multiple CNS vascular changes.

In addition to these findings, many patients had major SPECT brain changes in both hemispheres, the midbrain and the brainstem.

The average age of these 19 students and teachers was 33 years.

Two of the 19 patients had incapacitating autonomic nervous system dysfunction. One, a master's student who fell ill immediately following recombinant hepatitis B immunization and is now house-confined, has a highly positive tilt table test and is unable to maintain her blood pressure at a physiologically normal level while standing or on movement.

The rewards in properly investigating this group of patients are significant. Although we did not find any patients with multiple sclerosis (MS) in this group of 19, we did pick up a missed case of MS in the total group of 53 consecutive patients and a surprising number of single large (diameter ≤ 2 cm) CNS demyelinating lesions that do not qualify as diagnostic of MS. Each of the patients with non-MS single-lesion demyelination was associated with markedly abnormal SPECT brain scans. Also in the group of 53 consecutive patients, but not in the school-associated group, we found a missed significant brain aneurysm in addition to numerous other organ pathologies in the same patient. The aneurysm has since been repaired. Another patient had a right lenticular haemorrhage, which the neurologist then dismissed as minor; on SPECT we were able to demonstrate a 3- to 4-cm halo of abnormal activity around the lenticular lesion consisting of highly significantly hypoperfused brain tissue. In addition, we observed a decrease in perfusion in the entire right lobe of this patient, but with a normal left hemisphere perfusion. Clearly some localized non-motor cerebral accidents may provoke profound generalized CNS changes.

Are these all patients with ME? No, of course not; but in real terms, it does not matter. These individuals were all diagnosed as having ME or CFS by otherwise competent doctors who dismissed the patient when they came with a diagnosis of ME. These will be the same people who are referred to you as patients with ME by GPs and internists who simply think these patients complaining of acute or gradual-onset fatigue and cognitive dysfunction have ME or CFS and either have no idea how to investigate them or simply are unwilling to take the time to do so.

Thyroid disease in patients with ME

For some reason, the centuries-old medical knowledge of the physiological association of thyroid disease and intellectual, emotional, psychiatric, cardiac and other endocrine pathology seems to have escaped the 7 min-per-patient visits of many primary care and specialist doctors. Most non-psychiatrist doctors limit their examination of the thyroid to a cursory palpation of the gland for nodules and perhaps order thyroid-stimulating hormone (TSH) and free thyroxine (T4) tests. In most cases these doctors will not find disease. It is essential to request a thyroid ultrasound on all patients with ME. In addition, the doctor must ask the ultrasound technician to give the measurement of each thyroid lobe; if you do not, the technician or the doctor reading the ultrasound result will often just say 'normal' if there are no nodules or the gland is homogeneous. Why the measurements? Simple: the Mayo Clinic normal thyroid sizes are 13–21 cm^3 for females and 15–23 cm^3 for males. They arrive at these figures by multiplying together the three dimensions of each lobe and adding the left and right lobe measurements as though the thyroid were a regular rectangle. This is not the actual size of the thyroid. If you have access only to an old ultrasound device, then the radiologist may give you these crude rectangular volumes. It is necessary to multiply these volumes by a factor of 0.51. This will give you the approximate normal thyroid volumes of two irregular solid spheres. The real volumes are then half the Mayo suggested volumes, or 6.5–10.5 cm^3 for females and 7.5–11.5 cm^3 for males. It is important to know this, since modern ultrasound machines give this calculation in terms of the 6.5–10.5 cm^3 female thyroid volume scales. These are not gold standards, but if you bring in a thyroid at less than 4 cm^3 or over 15 cm^3 you know you are dealing with an atrophic or hypertrophic thyroid, respectively, with possible intellectual, emotional and psychiatric consequences. Sometimes, simply by appropriately treating these patients with T4 or tri-iodothyronine (T3), you can cure their fatigue and cognitive dysfunctions. (Note: patients on previously prescribed or over-the-counter thyroid medications may have a hypotrophic thyroid.)

Nor can you count simply on the usual TSH, free T4 (FT4) and free T3 (FT3) thyroid tests that are stated as normal or slightly abnormal. If the basic injury to the thyroid is vascular, as I believe it to be in most ME brains, then often the parathyroid hormone (PTH) and the ionized calcium will become abnormal before the usual thyroid tests. I do all of these tests, including thyroglobulin, thyroglobulin antibodies and microsomal antibodies, as well as an ultrasound, on each and every patient with ME that I see. In the group of 19 teachers and students in our group of 53 referred patients with ME, we found 14 patients (74%) with abnormal thyroid activity. I have also found several patients with new-onset ME with normal initial thyroid chemistry but with a significantly shrinking thyroid when the ultrasound was repeated in 1–2 years, which may suggest a vascular problem.

In the last 100 patients with ME/CFS, we also have found missed thyroid malignancies in 6 per cent. Some doctors discount this figure, since thyroid malignancies are considered to be common and not particularly dangerous, but that is not true for a young population. In one of the group of 53 patients, we discovered a thyroid malignancy that had already disseminated.

There is one more thing you must know before we leave the thyroid. T4 does very little on its own: T4 must first be discharged into the bloodstream and then transported to the liver and kidneys, where one of the iodines is removed to make T3. If there is pathology in this conversion, then an isomer called reverse T3 is made. In simple terms, the importance of this is paramount. T3 is one of the keys that turn on each body cell. If your patient is producing too much reverse T3, then this reverse T3 fits into the cell's energy receptor and breaks off, and the cell energy cycle cannot function normally. All the T4 in the world will not help this patient: she requires T3. Is it enough to ask for a reverse T3 level? No! Often the laboratory will give you a reverse T3 level in the normal or high normal range. You need also to order an FT3 at the same time and then divide the reverse T3 level by the normal T3 level; if the result reaches 10 per cent or more, your patient probably requires exogenous T3. But be careful; these patients with ME tend to be very medication-sensitive, so you should start at 5 μg daily, increasing every 2–4 weeks until you reach 25 μg and then stay at that dosage for some months before considering raising it to a normal dosage or subnormal dosage. If the patient has a heart condition as well, take advice from a cardiologist on the safety of giving T3 to this patient. All of these patients want to get back to normal in 5 min, but this is dangerous if part of the problem is thyroid dysfunction. Starting T3 at too high a dosage or increasing the dosage too rapidly may provoke seriously irregular heart rates, irregular cardiac rhythm and rapidly altering blood pressures. It may take up to a year or longer to slowly restore the patient with ME to normal thyroid levels.

Sleep dysfunction

All patients with ME should have at least one sleep study and some sleep studies with film monitoring to observe the presence of nocturnal seizures missed in daytime EEGs. In our group of 53 patients, we found only one patient with a normal sleep study; her dysautanomia was so severe that she was in a state of vascular collapse. Some authorities state that the abnormal sleep study can be blamed on the way the study is done, or the hospital environment in which these tests are performed, but generally these patients have non-restorative sleep. In our studies, 70 per cent of the 53 patients had no stage 3 or stage 4 sleep. This is the sleep phase where short-term memory is laid down. In addition, 77 per cent had grossly insufficient REM and very long REM latency. Among other functions that occur during REM is the burning into the neuron system of short-term memory: it is no wonder, then, that these patients describe short-term memory loss.

Interestingly, if the oxygen saturation falls below 92 per cent, commercial pilots become both colour- and night-blind and have difficulty landing their planes during the night. If the oxygen saturation in the cockpit falls below 88 per cent, the pilot has a good chance of losing consciousness and crashing the plane. Accordingly, oxygen saturation is monitored carefully in the cockpit, although less so in the passenger compartment. In our study of 53 patients, the oxygen saturation in 25 patients (53%) fell below 92 per cent during the sleep study; the oxygen saturation in 17 patients (30%) fell to 88 per cent or below. In other words, they were not sleeping: they were unconscious. The oxygen levels at least are potentially correctable pathologies.

Respiratory dysfunction

In our group of 19 students and teachers, ten patients (53%) had some measurable respiratory dysfunction. We did not count a history of asthma in this group, although in many patients there was an obvious overlap. Had we included a history of asthma, it is possible that even more patients would have had measurable respiratory dysfunction.

Missed miscellaneous disease

In our group, 47 per cent of patients had major missed illness, including the following:

- A case of tertiary syphilis and hepatitis B
- Four patients with significant heart disease
- A patient with respiratory dysfunction with significant pulmonary valve disease
- One juvenile and two type II cases of missed diabetes
- One patient with Ehlers–Danlos syndrome
- Numerous rheumatoid and significant spinal anomalies.

Although two patients had significant incapacitating autonomic nervous system dysfunction, several had lesser degrees of measurable dysfunction.

One patient in the group of 53 patients was a young lawyer and Olympic runner. He was referred to me as a patient with ME due to extreme fatigue and had Marfan-like anatomical changes. He had a missed hyperelastic distended thoracic aorta picked up on echocardiogram. In addition, he had lumbar dural ectasia on computed tomography (CT) scanning (seen in 65–92% of patients with Marfan's syndrome). At least seven doctors had each missed this diagnosis. The patient denied any family history of Marfan's syndrome until he was asked to enquire of his remote cousins. Three of his second cousins had a family history of ascending aorta surgical replacement in their twenties. The cause of his thoracic aorta pathology was complicated by the fact that he had been infected with brucellosis while training in South Africa. Brucellosis can also cause aortic aneurysm. A detailed extended family history is essential in investigating ME-type patients.

Psychiatric disease

Patients with ME like to believe that there is no psychiatric disease associated with ME. Some psychiatrists and primary care and specialist doctors like to believe that 100 per cent of patients with ME have psychiatric disease. What did we find? Many of these patients with ME had been referred to psychiatrists before our examination of them; six patients (32%) were diagnosed with primary psychiatric disease. After we had finished our investigation, we found only three patients (16%) with treatable psychiatric disease. There are several reasons for this discrepancy. We believe that some psychiatrists, to assist a destitute patient with ME, may give a psychiatric diagnosis simply to assist the patient in obtaining their disability pension.

Let me give you a brief review of some of these psychiatric patients.

The patient with tertiary syphilis was first diagnosed with unipolar or major depressive disease. This patient also had hepatitis B.

Another patient had major childhood abuse, during which time she was placed in a reformatory and also various psychiatric hospitals in Switzerland by the woman who had adopted her as an infant. This incarceration first occurred when the patient reached puberty and may have been due to the mother's sexual jealousy of having another female sharing her ambassador husband's innocent affections. On her own resources, my patient obtained her master's degree, became a secondary school teacher, and is fluent in English, French, German, Italian, Spanish and Latin. There was obvious trauma. Today, aged 53 years, she is exhausted, perhaps simply worn out, and she certainly has anxiety and depression.

A third teacher, also adopted, initially diagnosed as having depression, has serious food addiction, which in itself has caused multiple medical problems. He certainly has no overt psychiatric illness, but he does have brain dysfunction and memory disorder. He also had missed generalized vascular disease, missed diabetes and missed myocardial infarction and is one of the two patients in the school group with generalized atrophic brain syndrome.

The husband of another patient, also a teacher, committed suicide; the patient has made two attempts on her own life and was reasonably diagnosed as having unipolar or major depressive disease.

Two other patients were diagnosed as having unipolar depression. Both had seronegative rheumatoid arthritis and both had measurable significant heart disease.

Each of these six patients also had other major physical pathology. How many of the six were truly classical psychiatric diseases? Probably three, or four if you count the teacher with brain atrophy and cognitive dysfunction. What is most incredible is the truly remarkable resilience of some of these patients despite their multiple organ and system disease.

Do these 53 consecutive chronically ill patients have ME? Is that important? Doctors who believed that the patients had ME or CFS referred all these patients to me. The same patients will be referred to you with the same bewildering array of pathologies. Can you afford to dismiss them as psychiatric patients if they have not been properly investigated first? Since all of the definitions of CFS and to a lesser extent those of ME are based upon symptoms common to a multitude of serious pathophysiological illnesses, under the present understanding of ME and CFS, doctors, whether primary care, consultant or psychiatrists, cannot simply dismiss these patients without first documenting an extensive investigation of the individual patient. A thorough investigation of the chronically ill younger patient is fundamental to good medicine.

DEFINITIONS OF M.E. AND C.F.S.

You may remember the lines of Mathew Arnold's poem 'Dover Beach'. ME and CFS definitions are a bit like that.

And we are here as on a darkling plain
Swept with confused alarms of struggle and flight
Where ignorant armies clash by night.

The reason that I did not start this chapter with a definition of ME is that there is no general accepted agreement on the definition of ME, or the pathophysiology of ME, or an accepted understanding of ME chronicity. Many doctors simply do not believe that ME exists except as one of various psychiatric or social disorders or as an Internet-constructed example of mass hysteria. One would think that this was bad enough, but it gets worse. There is disagreement as to whether ME and CFS represent the same disease spectrum. There are now thousands of scientific publications on ME and CFS, but those publications on physical dysfunction are much like the parable of the six blind wise men of Hindustan, who individually described the elephant as a wall, a spear, a snake, a tree, a rope and a fan. To my knowledge, since and including the 1932 ME epidemic in the LA County Hospital and the first excellent publication of that epidemic by AG Gilliam, no one has ever done a complete long-term systematic scientific study on any significant number or patients with ME or CFS. No wonder, then, that doctors and scientists are in disarray on ME and CFS. It is also obvious that many people diagnosed with ME and CFS are missed patients with multi-system, multi-organ pathology. Are these pathologies due to a specific CNS injury or generalized injuries acquired during the initial infectious, immunological, chemical or traumatic injuries, or are they genetically related illnesses? We simply do not know.

Nor is there any agreement as to whether ME[5] represents the same disability as CFS.[6,7] In the USA, the conflicting name for CFS is 'chronic fatigue and immune dysfunction syndrome' (CFIDS). In the UK, some doctors have used the term 'postviral syndrome' to describe ME. In addition to the above definitions, there are possibly better, more recent definitions, including the so-called 'Canadian definition'[8] and the 'children's definitions' by Jason and colleagues.[9,10] Unlike any other medical condition, real or imagined, I know of no other where there are two warring armies of very well-educated doctors who are so critical of the others' views on the subject as to whether this is a real or imagined illness or whether ME is the same as CFS. There should be no surprise when I tell you that there is no accepted agreement on the treatment of ME or CFS either. This treatment quandary is particularly true if you examine the complexity of the pathologies hidden within the group of patients I have discussed above and whom well-educated doctors refer to as having ME and CFS. Let us briefly discuss the definitions.

Definitions of reputed infectious and other diseases come in various sizes and constructions, but essentially there are two types of definitions:

- *Epidemic-based definitions:* these are from the bottom up and are based upon epidemic findings when large groups of individuals fall ill at the same time, usually in confined quarters. The clarity of such a definition changes with technological and clinical advancements, particularly if a single causative agent is found. Physicians and researchers who investigate the epidemics always construct these definitions. These definitions, often faulty, at least have the benefit of being based on physical findings and follow-up of actual patient illness by doctors and scientists who investigate the actual patients over a period of time.
- *Theoretical-based definitions:* these are based on a theory of preconceived limits of what an illness is supposed to be and what is supposed to happen in the illness. They are often based upon symptoms rather than pathological findings. The Centers for Disease Control and Prevention (CDC) definitions of CFS are typical of this type of bureaucratic definition. This type of definition excludes all patients who do not follow this hypothetically derived definition. This type of definition is often bureaucratic, dictated from the top down, and those that direct this definitional process at times tend to have little and often no experience in primary patient investigation of the illness process that they are attempting to describe. Unfortunately, this is not unusual in medicine today. Since the same symptoms are often common to a multitude of different illnesses, these definitions tend to be misleading.

Why is the derivation of a definition important? Before Pierre Marie and Ivan Wickman's description of epidemic poliomyelitis based upon the first major poliomyelitis epidemics in 1887 and 1895 in Stockholm,[11,12] what we now know as poliomyelitis was described under a multitude of different diseases, with multiple different names and different causes. Epidemic descriptions by clinical investigators with careful follow-up have the advantage of bringing together the multiple and varied aspects of a single illness. One eminent French neurologist in the 1890s described the Scandinavian polio epidemics discussed by Wickman as examples of mass hysteria, although he had never been to Scandinavia or examined any patient. It was only when doctors such as Wickman studied the outcome of the late nineteenth-century Scandinavian poliomyelitis epidemics that doctors and scientists were able to bring these previously multiple disease phenomena together under one classification. Unfortunately, in none of the more than 60 epidemics of ME has anyone thought to do a funded systematic pathophysiological investigation and long-term follow-up of these epidemic patients. This itself is perhaps the biggest tragedy.

Definitions of ME

Doctors and workers who studied patients during epidemics of ME developed the following definitions. The definitions were not good, since most were developed at a time when virology was in its infancy or later when scientific research was largely underfunded:

- *Onset and location:* these were acute, epidemic and concurrent endemic episodes that occurred in both children and adults starting in late summer and early autumn in the north temperate zone. Onset of new disease tended to decrease rapidly after October, finally trailing off during the Christmas–New Year period. Most frequently described epidemics occurred in schools, hospitals and military camps, particularly when associated with institutional residences and crowding. Increased endemic infection was often noted at the same time.
- *Symptoms:* the symptom picture is characterized by its acute explosive onset, the severity of the CNS, autonomic and vascular symptoms, the associated malaise, and the often fleeting muscle and joint pains, but with a paucity of physical signs on physical examination and very low death rate. Little is said about duration and long-term findings. In my experience, depending upon the individual case, after weeks, months or sometimes years, this acute symptom picture gradually decreases in intensity. However, the average patient's intellectual, physical and emotional stamina, whose decrease tended to be noticed within 2–4 weeks of illness onset, rarely recovers sufficiently for the patient to manage in the competitive world if the illness continues beyond 2 years. As in any true disease, there is variable severity and simply misdiagnosis.
- *Pathology:* the few deaths that went to autopsy demonstrated CNS injuries to the basal ganglia and other brain areas, and injuries to the anterior horn cells and dorsal root ganglia (A Chaudhuri, personal communication, February 2009). Unlike in paralytic poliomyelitis, the anterior horn cells tend to be injured rather than destroyed. Deaths occurred during and following the epidemics, including three children under 12 years of age who died of Parkinson's disease within 2 years of falling ill during the 1947 Iceland epidemic.
- *Clinical tests:* abnormal EEGs were found in the Royal Free epidemics.[13,14] Abnormal electromyography (EMG) was found in the LA, Copenhagen, Royal Free and Coventry epidemics. Neurologist Charles Poser found oligoclonal banding in some sporadic cases in referred patients at Harvard's Mount Sinai Hospital,[15] but he is perhaps the only doctor to have taken routine spinal fluids. Oligoclonal banding suggests CNS injury. These were all earlier epidemics. Outside of our own work, to my knowledge little if any systematic investigation has been done of significant groups of patients in the multitude of post-1984 cluster, epidemic and endemic cases.
- *Cause:* in the more than 60 epidemics and clusters described, only in four was an infectious source actually recovered and described. In four of the instances, this virus was an enterovirus or ECHO enterovirus, which were recovered in the later Akureyri episodes,[16] the Coventry epidemic[17] and the Ottawa 1984 clusters by DN Galbraith and C Nairn of Ruckhill Hospital, Glasgow (unpublished investigations). In Ontario, the provincial virologists also observed an association only with enteroviruses during the 1984–90 epidemic periods[18] and a negative association with Epstein–Barr virus (EBV). Concomitant gastrointestinal bacterial infection with Bethesda Ballerup paracolon group[19] was isolated in some of the patients in the Bethesda outbreak. It was not believed to be a cause. John Chia in California has recovered enterovirus from the gastric mucosa in multiple sporadic ME patients whom he has investigated.[20] The great difficulty in recovering polio enteroviruses in living patients should be remembered; almost all polioviruses in patients with polio were recovered from autopsy cases.
- *Incubation period:* in the 60 or so described epidemics, when an observed incubation period was noted, in most cases they were stated as 3–6 days.[21] Except for the 1934 LA epidemic, which was associated within days of immunization of the hospital staff, no other incidence of immunization association was specifically recorded. Most enteroviruses have an incubation period of 8–40 days, making EBV virus with a 40-day incubation period a highly unlike cause of epidemic ME.

Definitions of CFS

These are definitions that started with the 1988 National Institutes of Health (NIH)/CDC Holmes definition.[6] The important fact with regard to this definition is that only 2 of the 16 authors had routinely investigated patients with ME and published on ME or CFS before or after the publication. The 1988 definition was followed up by the 1991 Oxford Guidelines[22] and the 1992 NIH/CDC Fuckuda definitions, which at best were copies of the 1988 definition. These three definitions are examples of theoretical definitions and are not based upon significant patient examination. If anything, they served to confuse the severity of ME that was associated with the term CFS. The later, so-called Canadian definition[8] is unique in the fact that the majority of the authors had long-term experience of examining patients with ME. This definition discusses many of the findings in this chapter. The definition is lacking in that it was not based significantly upon actual organ and system pathophysiology and examination. It does not distinguish between ME and CFS. This definition is also much too long and complex; however, it remains the closest among the published definitions in describing the actual disease known as ME.

The fault is not in our stars nor among the doctors or the patients, but in the system in which these two often apposing forces, the doctor and patient, theory and scientific investigation, exist. Until we conduct systematic long-term and in-depth scientific investigation of these patients, we will see no progress. Until then, I can only recommend that the doctor offers kindness to and toleration of these chronically disabled largely mistreated patients with ME and CFS. To the government of the UK, I can only recommend the nationwide funding of a serious scientific approach to the long-term pathophysiological investigation of these chronically disabled citizens. And until then, to paraphrase Arnold, we **remain** 'on a darkling plain ...'

Swept with confused alarms of struggle and flight,
Where ignorant armies clash by night.

KEY POINTS

- ME occurs as an epidemic and endemic disease. The injured patients as a group have rarely been investigated systematically during the past 50 years with the force of modern scientific and clinical investigational tools. Doctors investigating the patient with ME have rarely if ever received any significant funds for in-depth scientific investigation of organ and system pathologies.
- ME epidemic patients as a group have never been subjected to any long-term follow-up. Grufferman has suggested the possibility of increased cancer risk in the cohorts of epidemic ME-type patients.[23]
- ME and CFS are symptom-based definitions that have become simple garbage-bag terms for large numbers of patients with acute or gradual-onset physical and cognitive diseases affecting stamina, work and school ability. Thus, the terms ME and CFS have acted as an excuse to downplay the importance of these chronically ill patients and to not properly investigate these patients.
- The patient with ME has been largely disenfranchised from modern medical investigation and suitable medical assistance. Since most of these individuals tend to be relatively young, highly educated individuals in the medical and teaching professions, their loss of tax income to the government would more than offset their in-depth investigational costs.
- The majority of patients with ME or CFS that we have investigated in the UK, the USA or Canada represent multiple missed pathologies rather than any single disease entity. Whether these pathologies are caused by an initial CNS injury that deregulates the complex neuroimmune and neurochemical system and organ physiology of the patient or are simply co-morbidities is simply not known.
- There will never be a single treatment, whether pharmaceutical, physical, psychological or psychiatric, that will have any significant effect in the treatment of the majority of patients with ME and CFS, since they do not have a common trigger or common organ and system pathologies. It is necessary to first investigate the pathophysiological injuries and then treat them where possible to obtain a reasonable chance of a cure or treatment.
- The ME community continues to be a growing concern to many doctors and the state. This community is unlikely to disappear.
- Both patient and doctor mythologies continue to form a major part in the failure to assist the patient with ME.
- One group of patients with ME and CFS for whom we know their pathology – the patients with dysautanomia – have seen no advance in funding or investigation of treatment in the past 30 years, to such an extent that most major cities and university medical schools in the UK, Europe and North America simply have no investigational ability in this area.
- The major problems in understanding the illness and disability of patients with ME and CFS lie in the following areas: (i) the Oslerian concept of a single pathology causing a single disease spectrum; (ii) the misguided notion that patients with ME and CFS are people who can 'think themselves sick'; (iii) the lack of funding and resources in the physical investigation into the pathologies and pathophysiologies of these patients; (iv) the failure to do any long-term follow-up study of this group of chronically ill patients; (v) the patient mythologies that magic treatments can cure the patient; and (vi) the erroneous and facile belief that patients with ME and CFS simply have variations of hysteria, somatization disorders or somatoform disorders in general.

REFERENCES

1. Parish JG (1992) A bibliography of ME/CFS epidemics. In BM Hyde (ed.) *The Clinical and Scientific Basis of Myalgic Encephalomyelitis/Chronic Fatigue Syndrome.* Ottawa: Nightingale Research Foundation.
2. Gilliam AG (1938) Epidemiological study of an epidemic, diagnosed as poliomyelitis, occurring among the personnel of the Los Angeles County General Hospital during the summer of 1934. *Public Health Bulletin* **240**.
3. Sigurdsson B (1990) *Ritverk: Collected Scientific Papers, 1936–1962.* Reykjavik.
4. Hyde B (2003) The complexities of diagnosis. In LA Jason (ed.) *Handbook of Chronic Fatigue Syndrome.* Hoboken, NJ: John Wiley & Sons.
5. Hyde BM (1992) The definitions of ME/CFS: a review. In BM Hyde (ed.) *The Clinical and Scientific Basis of Myalgic Encephalomyelitis/Chronic Fatigue Syndrome.* Ottawa: Nightingale Research Foundation.
6. Holmes GP, Kaplan JE, Gantz NM, *et al* (1888) Chronic fatigue syndrome: a working case definition. *Annals of Internal Medicine* **108**: 387–9.
7. Fukuda K, Stephen E, Straus SE, *et al.* (1994) The chronic fatigue syndrome: a comprehensive approach to its definition and study. *Annals of Internal Medicine* **121**: 953–9.

8. Carruthers BM, Jain A, De Meirleir Kl, *et al.* (2003) Myalgic encephalomyelitis/chronic fatigue syndrome: clinical working case definition, diagnostic and treatment protocols. *Journal of Chronic Fatigue Syndrome* **11**: 7–116.
9. Jason LA, Bell DS, De Meirleir K, *et al.* (2006) A pediatric case definition for myalgic encephalomyelitis and chronic fatigue syndrome. *Journal of Chronic Fatigue Syndrome* **13**: 1–44.
10. Jason LA, Porter N, Shelleby E, *et al.* (2008) A case definition for children with myalgic encephalomyelitis/ chronic fatigue syndrome. *Clinical Medicine: Pediatrics* **1**: 53–7.
11. Wickman I (1911) *Die akute Poliomyelitis bzw: Heine-Medinsche Krankheit.* Berlin: Springer.
12. Wickman I (1913) *Acute Poliomyelitis: Heine-Medin's Disease* (transl. J Maloney). New York: Journal of Nervous and Mental Disease Publishing Co.
13. Pampiglione G, Harris R, Kennedy J (1978) Neurological and electroencephalographic investigations in myalgic encephalomyelitis. *Postgraduate Medical Journal* **54**: 752–4.
14. Warner C, Cookfiar D, Heffner R, *et al.* (1989) Neurological abnormalities in chronic fatigue syndrome. *Neurology* **39** (suppl. 1): 420.
15. Poser C (1992) The differential diagnosis between multiple sclerosis and chronic fatigue postviral syndrome. In BM Hyde (ed.) In BM Hyde (ed.) *The Clinical and Scientific Basis of Myalgic Encephalomyelitis/Chronic Fatigue Syndrome.* Ottawa: Nightingale Research Foundation.
16. Hyde B (1991) The Akureyi epidemic. In R Jenkins, JF Mowbray (eds) *Post-Viral Fatigue Syndrome.* Chichester: John Wiley & Sons.
17. Lyle WH (1959) An outbreak of disease believed to have been caused by ECHO 9 virus. *Annals of Internal Medicine* **51**: 248–9.
18. McLaughlin MD (1991) Health and Welfare Canada: Proceedings of a Workshop. Ontario: Laboratory Services Branch, Ontario Ministry of Health.
19. Shelokov A, Habel K, Verder E, *et al.* (1957) Epidemic neuromyasthenia: an outbreak of poliomyelitis-like illness in student nurses. *New England Journal of Medicine* **257**: 345–55.
20. Chia JK, Chia AW (2008) Chronic fatigue syndrome is associated with chronic enterovirus infection of the stomach. *Journal of Clinical Pathology* **61**: 43–8.
21. Hyde B, Bastien S, Jain A (1992) Patterns of neuropsychological abnormalities and cognitive impairment in adults and children. In BM Hyde (ed.) *The Clinical and Scientific Basis of Myalgic Encephalomyelitis/Chronic Fatigue Syndrome.* Ottawa: Nightingale Research Foundation.
22. Sharpe MC, Archard LC, Banatvale JE, *et al.* (1991) A report: chronic fatigue syndrome – guidelines for research. *Journal of the Royal Society of Medicine* **84**: 118–21.
23. Grufferman S (1992) Epidemiologic and immunologic findings in clusters of chronic fatigue syndrome. In BM Hyde (ed.) *The Clinical and Scientific Basis of Myalgic Encephalomyelitis/Chronic Fatigue Syndrome.* Ottawa: Nightingale Research Foundation.

Chapter 52

Pain and psychiatry

Stephen Tyrer

INTRODUCTION

It is now well established that psychological and psychiatric factors are of considerable importance in the evaluation of pain. The subject of pain used to be considered the province of the physiologist, physician and surgeon. In a prominent medical textbook written in 1968, pain was simply defined as 'A sensory experience evoked by stimuli that injure'.[1] This explanation of tissue damage that posits the generation of nervous impulses along recognized pain pathways is appropriate for most, although not all, pains arising from an acute injury. But if pain persists beyond the normal time of healing, which is normally less than 3 months but can be as long as 6 months, the correspondence between extent of injury and pain sensation is much less precise.

A measurable number of people with chronic pain show no demonstrable evidence of nerve or tissue damage, although many of these individuals will have sustained injury in the past. Other people sustain major injuries during intense physical activity or in highly emotionally charged situations such as the heat of battle and realize only subsequently that damage has occurred. It is for this reason that in 1979 the Taxonomy Committee of the newly formed International Association for the Study of Pain defined pain as 'an unpleasant sensory and emotional experience associated with actual or potential tissue damage, or described in terms of such damage'. The Committee amplified this definition further by stating that 'activity induced in the nociceptor and nociceptive pathways by a noxious stimulus is not pain, which is always a psychological state'.[2]

HISTORICAL BACKGROUND

The word 'pain' comes from the Latin *poena*, which means punishment or penalty, after the Roman goddess of punishment. The term was originally used for the punishment of an offence against the law. Over time, the word was increasingly used to denote suffering, particularly if this had resulted from a blameworthy act.

Early writers equated emotional suffering with pain, and the words were used interchangeably. Aristotle argued that suffering, which included pain, was perceived as a non-material form. He stated that if the intellect were a specific material organ (or part of one), then it would be restricted to receiving only certain kinds of information, as the eye is restricted to receiving visual data and the ear is restricted to receiving auditory data. This reasoning is often referred to as 'monistic' or 'monism' and essentially derives all phenomena from a single origin – that is, body and mind are both aspects of the same underlying substance

This view was challenged by Descartes in his *Meditations on First Philosophy* in 1641 (see www.iep.utm.edu/d/descarte.htm#h2). In this work, Descartes explained that he could doubt whether he had a body (it could be that he was dreaming of it or that it was an illusion created by an evil demon), but he could not doubt whether he had a mind. He reasoned, therefore, that the mind and body were different things. The essential distinction between what is now termed 'Cartesian dualism', in honour of Descartes, is that the immaterial mind and the material body, while being distinct substances, causally interact. Descartes identified the mind with consciousness and self-awareness, and clearly distinguished this from the brain, which was the seat of intelligence. There continues to be debate about this issue.[3]

Shortly after developing this philosophy, and derived *pari passu* from it, Descartes showed that the experience of pain depended upon the integrity of the sensory nerve pathway from the periphery to the brain:

> When I feel pain in the foot, this feeling is communicated by means of nerves in the foot, which are then carried in cords to the brain, where feelings are represented. The feeling of pain arises from the brain as though this pain was in the foot.[4,5]

For over 250 years after this work, pain was largely described as an organic phenomenon. The experimental work then conducted supported the contention that, in people complaining of pain, there must be a source of injury. Non-organic pain was not considered. It was not until Breuer and Freud described in detailed case histories,[6] originally published in 1895, that pain could be a manifestation of a psychological problem that the role of psychological factors in leading to pain was reconsidered.

The concept of 'emotional pain' occupied a select group of British psychiatrists in the 1960s. Erwin Stengel saw a parallel of alteration in pain perception as a result of parietal lobe dysfunction in patients with vascular damage with the pain responses of people with schizophrenia and in people with intellectual disability.[7] He recognized that people who deliberately inflict pain on themselves are often impervious to the pain arising from the consequent tissue damage. In work in Stengel's department, the activation of pain by arousal and apprehension was recognized. Above all, Stengel was intrigued that no doctor had defined pain in a way that recognized that it was a subjective phenomenon.[7] The controversy between Stengel and Eliot Slater about this issue, published in the *British Journal of Psychiatry* in 1966, illustrates the differences between Cartesian and modified monistic views of practitioners about the origin of pain.[8]

Stengel's work in this area led to a sprouting of interest in Sheffield, where he was the first head of the university's Department of Psychiatry at this time. Three junior psychiatrists in his department have since become prominent researchers in this area – Harold Merskey, Izzy Pilowsky and Sir Michael Bond. All have contributed an extraordinary amount to the contribution of psychiatric and physical features to the perception of pain. Few UK psychiatrists now enter this area, illustrating perhaps the lack of resources allocated to liaison psychiatry at this time.

Shortly before the time when Stengel was articulating his views in England, psychiatrists in the USA were aware of the fact that many people with pain referred to physicians did not have sufficient physical factors to explain their symptoms. An esteemed medical physician and psychiatrist, George Engel, believed that, although pain may originally develop from an external source, it often becomes a psychological phenomenon. He described risk factors for developing chronic pain, including a history of defeat, significant guilt, unsatisfied aggressive impulses and a history of real or imagined loss.[9] His work in this area convinced him that medicine had to assess the contribution of emotional and environmental factors in the development of disease, and he later elaborated his ideas in a seminal paper in *Science*, in which he was the first to posit the notion of a biopsychosocial model of illness.[10]

Around the time Engel was proposing that psychological factors influenced the presentation of pain, a new model was developed by a physiologist and a psychologist. This model was termed the 'gate theory', as an integral part of the model was that cells in the dorsal horn of the sensory ganglia in the spinal cord acted as a 'gate' that allowed pain impulses to pass up to the cerebral cortex when open but restricted these when closed.[11] The theory proposed that transmission of information about pain to the brain depends upon activation of cells in the dorsal horn of the spinal cord called transmission (T) cells (Figure 52.1). These cells are influenced by both myelinated and unmyelinated fibres; the larger myelinated A fibres inhibit T-cell transmission, whereas the smaller unmyelinated C fibres facilitate it. Activity in these nerve fibres depends in turn on the

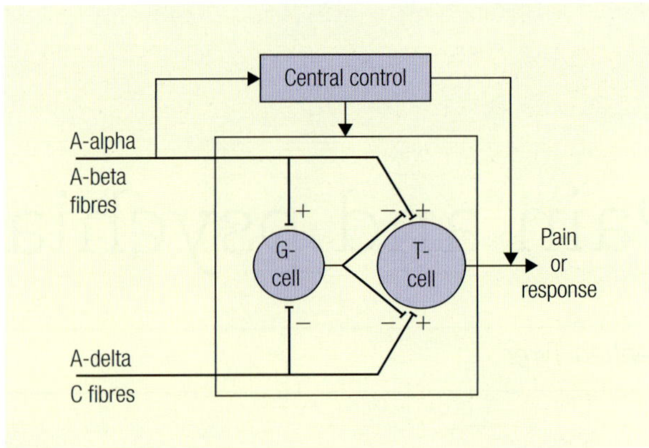

Figure 52.1 Circuit diagram of the gate-control theory of pain perception proposed by Melzack and Wall in 1965

action of a further cell in the dorsal horn close to the T-cell. This cell, called the gate or gelatinosa cell (G-cell), is situated in the substantia gelatinosa of the dorsal horn; it is activated by branches from large myelinated fibres concerned with touch and proprioception and is inhibited by action of the C fibres. The greater the activation of the G-cell, the more T-cell transmission rostrally to the brain is inhibited. In other words, the greater the A nerve fibre activity, the fewer pain impulses reach the brain.

In addition to this peripheral modification of nervous impulses that have the potential to give rise to pain, there is also central control from the brain itself. This is achieved by both neurochemical and neurophysiological methods. Stimulation of encephalinergic neurons in certain regions of the midbrain (periaqueductal grey, hypothalamus), frequently using serotonin as the relevant neurotransmitter, reduces the intensity of the nervous traffic ascending up the spinal cord from the T-cell. Originally it was thought that there was a direct link between these descending pathways and the G-cell but, although this is probably the case, it is now recognized that control of this pathway also involves other mechanisms. Central influences can also increase pain perception and frequently do so. Increased anxiety and focusing attention on pain have been shown clearly to accentuate painful feelings.

PSYCHIATRIC DISORDERS AND PAIN

Psychiatric disorders are more frequently manifest in patients with chronic pain than in the standard population. This has been found in patients complaining of pain who attend general medical clinics, general practices and pain clinics.[12] In some cases, psychiatric disorders may present with pain as the prime symptom. This is certainly known for chest pain in adolescents,[13] abdominal pain in childhood,[14] panic disorder,[15] post-traumatic stress disorder (PTSD),[16] and the rare presentation of psychotic disorders with delusional pain.[17] However, even in these patients,

Table 52.1 Mechanisms by which pain is experienced despite apparent insufficient sensory stimuli

Condition	Mechanism
Undiagnosed medical condition	The disease may be at an early stage or the biochemical or radiological markers may not show abnormality
Painful conditions about which there is debate over their origin because of difficulty in diagnosis	There is debate about whether some well-recognized painful conditions have an organic basis; this applies in particular to chronic regional pain syndrome, originally thought to be due to sympathetic nerve damage, but where sympathetic blockade is often unhelpful
Exaggeration of an existing trivial painful condition	This is frequent and occurs in people who are worried about what the pain means and its impact; these individuals tend to have a low pain tolerance
Pain arising due to muscle tension, which may be concerned directly with worries about pain	Anxiety and worries lead to bracing and guarding of muscles, which gives rise to pain; these may be related to factors other than the pain itself, but there may be concerns that the pain itself can accentuate the condition
Hypochondriacal disorder	The patient believes that he or she has a serious or progressive physical disorder that persists despite negative investigations and reassurance; this may occur in a patient who has previously experienced an organic pain but has had apparently successful treatment, e.g. angina pain because of anxiety
Fear of pain	In some patients the perception of pain is interpreted in a malign way and there is further rumination and worry about effects on the body, leading to a reduction in function; in others, fear of pain occurs because of fear of anxiety-related sensations associated with painful episodes
Dissociative conditions, e.g. guilt	Occurs rarely when people have a need to express grief and distress as pain as a result of grief or self-punishment; pain is an expression of atonement; phantom limb pain used to be placed in this category, but it is now known to have a sound organic basis
Identification with the sufferer, e.g. couvade	Occurs when there is strong emotional attachment between a relative or friend and someone who is in pain
Delusional pain	Rare, but when it does occur the reason is readily apparent; e.g. a patient who believes he is Jesus Christ may complain of pain in his wrists and ankles because of the nails that have been inserted

who have an apparent non-organic pain, it cannot be said categorically that the psychiatric disorder has *caused* the pain. The mechanisms by which pain is experienced in the absence of sufficient sensory stimuli to account for the intensity of the feeling are indicated in Table 52.1. The psychological processes involved in these include:

- anxiety and arousal;
- fear of pain;
- modelling;
- dissociation and guilt;
- identification;
- delusions.

Anxiety

Anxiety disorders have been found to be correlated more closely than depression with chronic painful conditions in a large US sample of patients with chronic pain.[18] In particular, people who are fearful of anxiety-related sensations, who interpret somatic symptoms as harmful and who avoid situations where these feelings are likely to arise have greater disability.[19] The term 'anxiety sensitivity' has been used to describe this condition in these individuals.[20] Such patients are on the lookout for any potential problem in their environment and show increased evidence of somatic anxiety symptoms and fear in situations that may give rise to pain.

Fear of pain

Fear of pain explains the mechanism of psychological distress in vulnerable patients who become disabled with chronic pain. In predisposed patients, the perception of pain is interpreted in a malign way through a process of what has been described as catastrophization.[19] The cause of the pain is viewed in a horrific light, and there is further rumination and worry about the effects of this on the body. This process may occur because of previous life experiences, particularly those of episodes of situations involving pain, anxiety and perceived threats to physical integrity. The symptoms of distress persuade the patient to avoid activities that give rise to further pain. This reduction in mobility limits the process of re-establishment of physical routines that are essential in enabling recovery from injury, and the painful state is reinforced.[21]

Modelling

It is frequently found that people with chronic pain have relatives with a similar condition. It is reasonable to posit, under these circumstances, that there is an expectation to follow the path of invalidism, which may be acquired through the patient modelling themselves on the affected relative.

Dissociation and guilt

There may be an aetiological association between the development of dissociation episodes and the development of chronic pain, but this is a very rare event. Dissociation fugue occurring at the time of chronic pain was found to occur in 0.16 per cent of referrals to a comprehensive pain facility.[22] Engel found that a number of his patients were pain-prone because of guilt about a previous minor misdemeanour, usually involving a member of the family. He proposed that these people had aggressive feelings that they were unable to express.[9] In practice, few patients seen in practice fit this description.

Identification

The incidence of dissociative identity disorder was found to be low in a major facility in Florida, at 0.08 per cent.[22] Stengel describes a number of examples in his Maudsley lecture,[7] but in practice this is a rare event.

Delusional disorders

Rarely, delusions of pain occur. When they do occur, they are usually found in people with delusional disorders or schizophrenia.

EFFECT OF PAIN ON PRESENTATION OF ILLNESS

In the majority of patients with chronic pain, it is much more common for psychiatric disorders to develop because of widespread pain.[23,24] Pain affects enjoyment, reduces the opportunity to take part in pleasurable activities, and fundamentally changes the whole direction of a person's life. The most common psychiatric diagnoses found in patients with chronic pain are described in the following sections.

Depression

According to standard psychiatric schedules, depressive illness is the most common associated psychiatric disorder found in patients with chronic pain. Between 20 per cent and 50 per cent of patients attending chronic pain clinics fulfil the criteria for this diagnosis.[12,25,26] Some studies have challenged these findings, and it is now generally recognized that anxiety has more impact in determining the intensity and expression of pain. Depression is found so frequently in a population of people with chronic pain because loss of appetite or weight, changes in sleep pattern and poor concentration are found in patients with chronic pain who are not necessarily depressed. It has, therefore, been recommended in physically unwell patients that these somatic symptoms be replaced with non-somatic alternatives.[27] If changes in appetite or weight are replaced by a depressed appearance, sleep disturbances by social withdrawal, fatigue by brooding, and diminished concentration by lack of reactivity to pleasant events, then the diagnostic confidence of depression in patients with chronic pain is increased.[28]

The risk of death by suicide is increased in patients with chronic pain. In a systematic review, it was found that, relative to controls, risk of death by suicide was doubled in patients with chronic pain.[29] A number of risk factors for suicidal intent in chronic pain were identified in this review, including:

- the type, intensity and duration of pain;
- sleep-onset insomnia co-occurring with pain;
- hopelessness about pain;
- desire for escape from pain;
- pain catastrophizing – negative thoughts in which pain is seen in terms of extremes, e.g. 'I worry that it will never end', which is highly related to hopelessness about pain.

There is debate about how far to treat depression in people with chronic pain. Cognitive-behavioural therapy (CBT) is sometimes utilized, but usually in the context of treatment aimed at altering attributions arising from the chronic painful state. Although there is a belief by some that standard antidepressant drugs are not effective in such patients,[30] based in part on limited evidence that these agents are no more effective in depressed compared with non-depressed patients,[31] studies have shown that depression is ameliorated in such patients[32] and that these drugs also reduce pain.[33–35] The serotonin and noradrenaline reuptake inhibitors (SNRIs) are more effective than the selective serotonin reuptake inhibitors (SSRIs) in reducing one type of pain, neuropathic pain.[36]

Anxiety and stress-related disorders

The diagnoses included under this rubric comprise generalized anxiety disorder, panic disorder, phobias, PTSD, adjustment disorders and obsessive–compulsive disorder.

Early work suggested that female patients with chronic pain and who were not seeking compensation had a higher frequency of generalized anxiety disorder (GAD) than expected,[37] although women with anxiety were not found to have a poorer prognosis compared with men in a more recent investigation.[38] Higher degrees of anxiety were related to greater intensity of pain in this study.[38] It has been suggested that patients with chronic pain may use worry to reduce the physical sensations associated with pain and thus fulfil the diagnostic criteria for GAD.[39] This hypothesis does not have experimental proof.

CBT has been shown to be effective in chronic painful conditions.[40] This treatment is also used in GAD associated with pain.[41] It has been shown that in patients with low back pain who have pain-related anxiety and are receiving CBT combined with physical therapy, improvement in anxiety was more important than changes in physical capacity in predicting outcome.[42] In a World Health Organization (WHO) survey, people with back and neck pain were over two and a half times more likely to have GAD than controls without such pain.[43] This survey was not able to show the temporal relationship between pain and anxiety, but other studies have strongly suggested that anxiety sensitivity is a feature in this population.[19,42]

Panic disorder

Although the pain sensitivity of patients with panic disorder has been reported to be no different from that of controls,[44] patients with chronic painful conditions are more likely than average to have panic.[18] People with migraine attacks may be particularly prone.[45] These findings suggest that panic and migraine may be related directly through a single mechanism.

Phobias

A phobia may develop because of the experience of the event leading to the pain, for example travel phobia following a road traffic accident.[46] The condition known as social phobia, in which the patient feels anxious in social situations and avoids such engagements, has been found to be overrepresented in disabled workers with chronic musculoskeletal pain.[47]

Stress disorders

The only relevant stress disorder in this context is PTSD. There is clear evidence that the experience and management of pain can be aggravated by PTSD. One of the main reasons for this is because PTSD is associated with high anxiety, and we have seen that anxiety is associated comorbidly with chronic pain.[18] Furthermore, the presence of PTSD is a poor prognostic sign.[48,49] Hyperarousal, excessive attention to changes in the environment, and an inclination to focus on bodily symptoms are frequent accompaniments of both PTSD and chronic pain, which may explain these findings.[50]

If PTSD is identified, treatment should be carried out by a specialized team familiar with treatment procedures in this condition. Debriefing and superficial treatments of this type are not valuable and have been found to worsen the prognosis in patients with more intense symptoms.[51] Trauma-focused CBT and eye movement desensitization and reprocessing (EMDR), a technique that involves movement of the patient's eyes in a systematic way while recalling disturbing memories, have been found to be effective in treating PTSD in a meta-analysis.[52] Either of these treatments is recommended as first-line in the treatment of PTSD according to national guidelines.[53] If facilities for such treatment are not available, or if these therapies are not successful, then treatment with the antidepressant drugs amitriptyline, mirtazapine or phenelzine has been shown to be effective.[53]

Personality disorders

Although it has been said that personality disorders are more common in patients with chronic pain,[54] there has been a dearth of good research in this area. People without any previous history of personality disorders may appear to have such a condition because of the exacerbation of premorbid personality characteristics resulting from pain and subsequent stresses.[55] Originally it was thought that some patients who developed chronic pain had a 'pain-prone personality', but there is very little evidence for such a label.[56]

A study of out-patients attending a chronic pain clinic in Germany showed that more than one in ten subjects had a paranoid or a borderline personality disorder, with passive–aggressive, avoidant and obsessive–compulsive personality disorders being significantly overrepresented compared with a control group.[57]

Individuals with borderline personality disorder and other cluster B personality disorders are at greater risk of misusing medication, and benzodiazepines and opioid drugs should be prescribed very carefully in this group. There is very limited evidence that antidepressants, particularly the SSRIs and the monoamine oxidase inhibitors (MAOIs), have some benefits in the management of this condition; there is lesser evidence for the advantages of antipsychotic drugs and mood stabilizers.[58] There is no basis to recommend different treatments for the different personality disorders.

A structured evidence-based review warns all pain clinicians to be sceptical about the assessment of personality in patients who are in pain.[59] Personality profiles of patients who have chronic pain usually alter considerably if the pain is reduced. This was shown in 1975 but is not generally realized.[60] This change has been shown convincingly for the widely quoted Minnesota Multiphasic Personality Inventory schedule (MMPI).[61] These findings illustrate that many personality questionnaires are influenced by the current state of the individual, including physical and mental health.

Somatoform disorders

For a diagnosis of a somatoform disorder to be made, there should be continued presentation of physical symptoms together with persistent requests for medical investigations despite negative findings of organic illness and reassurance by doctors that the symptoms have no physical basis. In some patients, physical disorders may have been present but they do not explain the nature and extent of the present symptoms or the distress and preoccupation of the patient.

These disorders are frequent. In a survey of patients attending a general practice clinic in Holland, the prevalence of somatoform disorders was as high as 21.9 per cent.[62] Many of these patients are severely disabled, but it is only the minority that are likely to be assessed by clinical psychologists or psychiatrists, despite a recommendation advocating joint working between liaison psychiatrists and pain physicians.[63]

The value of the present classifications of these syndromes has been brought into question because of the imprecise categorization of such disorders and the fact that many patients fall into the category of undifferentiated somatoform disorder, a watered-down version of somatization disorder. Pain is only one of the symptoms that can occur in a somatoform disorder. Those somatoform disorders that are concerned with painful conditions are described in the following sections, together with their *International Classification of Diseases*, 10th revision (ICD-10) codes.

Persistent somatoform pain disorder (F45.4)

The main complaint in this disorder is of persistent, severe and distressing pain that cannot be explained fully by any bodily process or physical disorder. Furthermore, this occurs in association with emotional conflict or psychosocial problems that are considered to be the main cause.[64] The threshold for a diagnosis of pain disorder in the *Diagnostic and Statistical Manual*, 4th edition (DSM-IV) is lower than in ICD-10.

There are two established treatments for this condition, antidepressants and CBT. Antidepressants that inhibit both serotonin and noradrenaline uptake, such as amitriptyline and venlafaxine, are more effective than the SSRIs.[32,65] CBT has been shown to be of definite value in patients who have reached the stage of accepting that medical or surgical interventions are not indicated.[40]

Hypochondriacal disorder (F45.2)

In this condition, the patient believes that he or she has a serious or progressive physical disorder that persists, despite negative investigations and reassurance. Some 1–2 per cent of the patients in the general population have been found to have hypochondriacal features; these features are more evident in older people.[66] Fear of disease (disease phobia) is associated with anxiety, whereas a false belief of having a disease (disease conviction) is associated more with somatic symptoms. Although this condition may seem to be more frequent in patients with chronic pain, there has been no recent survey of this condition in a pain clinic.

Somatization disorder (F45.0)

Somatization disorder, formerly known as Briquet's syndrome, is by far the most crippling somatoform disorder. Its main features are multiple, recurrent and frequently changing physical symptoms, which have been present for many years. Most patients have a long and complicated history of contact with both primary and specialist medical care services, during which time many negative investigations have been carried out. Personality disorders, particularly of the passive-dependent and histrionic types, are considerably overrepresented compared with control subjects with anxiety and depression.[67] The female/male ratio of patients with this condition is 5 : 1. The prevalence rate has been estimated to be 0.5 per cent, but this is probably an underestimate and the true rate is probably higher.[68]

In practice, the diagnosis of undifferentiated somatoform disorder (F45.1), which has a lower criterion for diagnosis, is found to be much the most frequent diagnosis in standard populations.[69,70] This category comprises a raft of heterogeneous conditions in which physical and psychiatric disorders intermingle.

Psychoactive substance use

There is a higher rate of alcohol and analgesic misuse in patients with chronic pain. Between 12 per cent and 28 per cent of patients attending specialized pain clinic facilities reach the criterion for diagnosis under this category.[25] High average alcohol consumption before developing a chronic painful state was found to be a poor prognostic sign in a large follow-up study of patients with lower limb pain.[71]

Despite these findings of an increased prevalence of substance misuse, generally there has been a change in attitude about the use of opioid medication for patients with chronic non-malignant pain. Although it has been argued that long-term opioid use leads to increased drug dependency and further functional impairment in patients who have disproportionate pain and disability,[72] studies have not found clear evidence that this is the case. In a large study of patients with chronic pain comparing opioid users with non-users, there was no increase in illness behaviour exhibited by the opioid users after controlling for other variables.[73] Benzodiazepine use, on the other hand, was associated with reduced activity and disability.

Brief psychosocial interventions and contingency management (which consists of payment of money or tokens to patients if they succeed in reducing opiate use) have been found to improve compliance with therapy.[74]

Factitious disorder

In factitious disorder, patients consciously fabricate symptoms and may even physically injure themselves in order to produce symptoms and signs that are typical of an organic illness. The motivation for exhibiting such symptoms in factitious disorder is to obtain medical care. Abdominal pain, often suspected to be due to renal or biliary colic, is the most frequent presentation of a painful factitious disorder. Most people encountered in clinical practice with this disorder are healthcare professionals, with a considerable female preponderance.[75] They are often found to have a number of different diagnoses at different times. Their families are closely involved and are convinced of an organic aetiology. Frequent attendance at emergency departments, coupled with negative investigations, raises suspicions that this disorder may be present.

Malingering

In malingering there is a conscious wish to fabricate symptoms. However, malingerers behave in this way in order to obtain financial gain or to avoid situations for certain responsibilities.

CONCLUSIONS

When examining patients with long-standing pain, distress should be distinguished from illness. In the majority of cases, all avenues in alleviating the pain should be explored first, although treatment for any psychiatric illness should not be delayed.

KEY POINTS

- Until the middle of the twentieth century, the mind–body dualistic philosophy drove the interpretation of painful states. There is now recognition that a modified monistic view may be more valid.
- Patients in pain who develop a psychiatric disorder do so usually as a consequence of their chronic painful illness. Depression is common.
- Anxiety is the driving affect that affects the perception of pain.
- In many cases, it is appropriate to treat depression with antidepressant drugs, particularly if there is pervasive loss of pleasure. The SSRIs are usually employed first, but tricyclic antidepressants and SNRIs are more appropriate if there is evidence of a neuropathic pain state.
- PTSD is a poor prognostic sign in people with chronic pain who have developed pain following an injury.
- People with borderline and dependent personality disorders require a contract to be established early in therapy, applying particular care to the administration of drugs.
- Substance misuse, which includes both alcohol and drugs, occurs in one in between four and eight people with chronic pain attending pain clinics.

REFERENCES

1. Mountcastle VB (ed.) (1968) *Medical Physiology*, 12th edn. St Louis, MO: Mosby.
2. Merskey H (1979) Pain terms: a list with definitions and notes on the usage. *Pain* **6**: 249–52.
3. Williamson OD, Buchanan DA, Quintner JL, Cohen ML (2005) Pain beyond monism and dualism. *Pain* **116**: 169–70.
4. Descartes R (1647) *Meditations Touchant la Première Philosophie*. Geneva: Athena. http://un2sg4.unige.ch/athena/descartes/desc_med_frame0.html.
5. Khodoss F (1986) *Méditations métaphysiques/René Descartes; texte, trad., Objections et Réponses*, 9th edn. Paris: Presses Universitaires de France.
6. Breuer J, Freud S (1957) *Studies on Hysteria* (trans. J Strachey). New York: Basic Books.
7. Stengel E (1965) Pain and the psychiatrist. *British Journal of Psychiatry* **111**: 795–802.
8. Slater E (1966) Pain and the psychiatrist. *British Journal of Psychiatry* **112**: 329–31.
9. Engel G (1959) 'Psychogenic' pain and the pain-prone patient. *American Journal of Medicine* **26**: 899–918.
10. Engel G (1977) The need for a new medical model: a challenge for biomedical science. *Science* **196**: 129–36.
11. Melzack R, Wall PD (1965) Pain mechanisms: a new theory. *Science* **150**: 971–9.
12. Tyrer SP, Capon N, Peterson DN, *et al.* (1989) The detection of psychiatric illness and psychological handicaps in a British pain clinic population. *Pain* **36**: 63–74.
13. Hotopf M, Mayou R, Wadsworth M, Wessely S (1999) Psychosocial and developmental antecedents of chest pain in young adults. *Psychosomatic Medicine* **61**: 861–7.
14. Garber J, Zeman J, Walker LS (1990) Recurrent abdominal pain in children: psychiatric diagnoses and parental psychopathology. *Journal of the American Academy of Child and Adolescent Psychiatry* **29**: 648–56.
15. Meuret A, White KS, Ritz T, *et al.* (2006) Panic attack symptom dimensions and their relationship to illness characteristics in panic disorder. *Journal of Psychiatric Research* **40**: 520–27.
16. Palyo S, Beck JG (2005) Post-traumatic stress disorder symptoms, pain, and perceived life control: associations with psychosocial and physical functioning. *Pain* **117**: 121–7.
17. Fisher C (2003) The reach of neurology. *Archives of Neurology* **60**: 173–7.
18. McWilliams L, Goodwin RD, Cox BJ (2004) Depression and anxiety associated with three pain conditions: results from a nationally representative sample. *Pain* **111**: 77–83.
19. Asmundson GJG, Vlaeyen JWS, Crombez G (2004) *Understanding and Treating Fear of Pain*. Oxford: Oxford University Press.

20. Reiss S, Peterson RA, Gursky DM, McNally RJ (1986) Anxiety sensitivity, anxiety frequency and the prediction of fearfulness. *Behaviour Research and Therapy* **24**: 1–8.
21. Peters ML, Vlaeyen JWS, Weber WEJ (2005) The joint contribution of physical pathology, pain-related fear and catastrophizing to chronic back pain disability. *Pain* **113**: 45–50.
22. Fishbain DA, Cutler RB, Rosomoff HL, Rosomoff RS (2001) Pain-determined dissociation episodes. *Pain Medicine* **2**: 216–24.
23. Gamsa A (1990) Is emotional disturbance a precipitator or a consequence of chronic pain? *Pain* **42**: 183–95.
24. Tyrer S (2006) Psychosomatic pain. *British Journal of Psychiatry* **188**: 91–3.
25. Polatin P, Kinney RK, Gatchel RJ, *et al.* (1993) Psychiatric illness and chronic low back pain: the mind and the spine – which goes first? *Spine* **18**: 66–71.
26. Fishbain D, Cutler R Rosomoff HL, Rosomoff RS (1997) Chronic pain-associated depression: antecedent or consequence of chronic pain? A review. *Clinical Journal of Pain* **13**: 116–37.
27. Endicott J (1984) Measurement of depression in patients with cancer. *Cancer* **53**: 2243–8.
28. Wilson K, Mikail SF, D'Eon JL, Minns JE (2001) Alternative diagnostic criteria for major depressive disorder in patients with chronic pain. *Pain* **91**: 227–34.
29. Tang N, Crane C (2006) Suicidality in chronic pain: a review of the prevalence, risk factors and psychological links. *Psychological Medicine* **36**: 575–86.
30. Stimmel G, Escobar JI (1986) Antidepressants in chronic pain: a review of efficacy. *Pharmacotherapy* **6**: 262–7.
31. Richeimer S, Bajwa ZH, Kahraman SS, *et al.* (1997) Utilization patterns of tricyclic antidepressants in a multidisciplinary pain clinic: a survey. *Clinical Journal of Pain* **13**: 324–9.
32. Fishbain D (2000) Evidence-based data on pain relief with antidepressants. *Annals of Medicine* **32**: 305–16.
33. Sullivan M, Robinson JP (2006) Antidepressant and anticonvulsant medication for chronic pain. *Physical Medicine and Rehabilitation Clinics of North America* **17**: 381–400.
34. Onghena P, Van Houdenhove B (1992) Antidepressant-induced analgesia in chronic non-malignant pain: a meta-analysis of 39 placebo-controlled studies. *Pain* **49**: 205–19.
35. McQuay H, Moore RA (1997) Antidepressants and chronic pain. *British Medical Journal* **314**: 763–4.
36. Barkin R, Barkin S (2005) The role of venlafaxine and duloxetine in the treatment of depression with decremental changes in somatic symptoms of pain, chronic pain, and the pharmacokinetics and clinical considerations of duloxetine pharmacotherapy. *American Journal of Therapeutics* **12**: 431–8.
37. Fishbain DA, Goldberg M, Labbe E, Steele R, Rosomoff F (1988) Compensation and non-compensation chronic pain patients compared for DSM-III operational diagnoses. *Pain* **32**: 197–206.
38. Keogh E, McCracken LM, Eccleston C (2006) Gender moderates the association between depression and disability in chronic pain patients. *European Journal of Pain* **10**: 413–22.
39. Borkovec TD, Alcaine O, Behar E (2004) Avoidance theory of worry and generalized anxiety disorder. In RG Heimberg, CL Turk, DS Mennin (eds) *Generalized Anxiety Disorder in Research and Practice*. New York: Guilford Press.
40. Morley S, Eccleston C, Williams A (1999) Systematic review and meta-analysis of randomized controlled trials of cognitive behaviour therapy and behaviour therapy for chronic pain in adults, excluding headache. *Pain* **80**: 1–13.
41. Raudenska J, Javurkova A (2003) Cognitive-behavioral therapy of depression, generalized anxiety disorder and panic disorder in chronic pain. *Bolest* **6**: 8–16.
42. McCracken LM, Gross RT, Eccleston C (2002) Multimethod assessment of treatment process in chronic low back pain: comparison of reported pain-related anxiety with directly measured physical capacity. *Behaviour Research and Therapy* **40**: 585–94.
43. Demyttenaere K, Bruffaerts R, Lee S, *et al.* (2007) Mental disorders among persons with chronic back or neck pain: results from the world mental health surveys. *Pain* **129**: 332–42.
44. Roy-Byrne P, Uhde TW, Post RM, *et al.* (1985) Normal pain sensitivity in patients with panic disorder. *Psychiatry Research* **14**: 77–84.
45. Breslau N, Davis GC (1993) Migraine, physical health and psychiatric disorder: a prospective epidemiologic study in young adults. *Journal of Psychiatric Research* **27**: 211–21.
46. Mayou R, Bryant BM (1994) Effects of road traffic accidents on travel. *Injury* **25**: 457–60.
47. Asmundson G, Jacobson SJ, Allerdings MD, Norton GR (1996) Social phobia in disabled workers with chronic musculoskeletal pain. *Behaviour Research and Therapy* **34**: 939–43.
48. Mason S, Turpin G, Woods D, *et al.* (2006) Risk factors for psychological distress following injury. *British Journal of Clinical Psychology* **45**: 217–30.
49. Geisser ME, Roth RS, Bachman JE, Eckert TA (1996) The relationship between symptoms of post-traumatic stress disorder and pain, affective disturbance and disability among patients with accident and non-accident related pain. *Pain* **66**: 207–14.
50. Asmundson G, Coons MJ, Taylor S, Katz J (2002) PTSD and the experience of pain: research and clinical implications of shared vulnerability and mutual maintenance models. *Canadian Journal of Psychiatry* **47**: 930–37.
51. Mayou R, Ehlers A, Hobbs M (2000) Psychological debriefing for road traffic accident victims: three-year follow-up of a randomized controlled trial. *British Journal of Psychiatry* **176**: 589–93.

52. Bradley R, Greene J, Russ E, *et al.* (2005) A multidimensional meta-analysis of psychotherapy for PTSD. *American Journal of Psychiatry* **162**: 214–27.
53. National Institute of Health and Clinical Excellence (2005) *Management of Post-Traumatic Stress Disorder in Adults in Primary, Secondary and Community Care.* Clinical guideline 26. London: National Institute of Health and Clinical Excellence.
54. Weisberg JN (2000) Personality and personality disorders in chronic pain. *Current Review of Pain* **4**: 60–70.
55. Polatin P, Gatchel RJ, Fishbain DA, Weisberg JN, Keefe FJ (1997) Personality disorders in the chronic pain population: basic concepts, empirical findings, and clinical implications. *Pain Forum* **6**: 1–21.
56. Turk D, Salovey P (1984) 'Chronic pain as a variant of depressive disease': a critical reappraisal. *Journal of Nervous and Mental Disease* **172**: 398–404.
57. Conrad R, Schilling R, Bausch C, *et al.* (2007) Temperament and character personality profiles and personality disorders in chronic pain patients. *Pain* **130**: 144–56.
58. Tyrer P, Bateman AW (2004) Drug treatment for personality disorders. *Advances in Psychiatric Treatment* **10**: 389–98.
59. Fishbain DA, Cole B, Cutler RB, *et al.* (2006) Chronic pain and the measurement of personality: do states influence traits? *Pain Medicine* **7**: 509–29.
60. Sternbach R, Timmermans G (1975) Personality changes associated with reduction of pain. *Pain* **1**: 177–81.
61. Love PW, Peck CL (1987) The MMPI and psychological factors in chronic low back pain: a review. *Pain* **28**: 1–12.
62. De Waal M, Arnold, IA, Eekhof JAH (2004) Somatoform disorders in general practice: prevalence, functional impairment and comorbidity with anxiety and depressive disorders. *British Journal of Psychiatry* **184**: 470–76.
63. Dolin S, Stephens J (1998) Pain clinics and liaison psychiatry. *Anaesthesia* **53**: 317–19.
64. World Health Organization (1992) *The ICD-10 Classification of Mental and Behavioural Disorders: Clinical Descriptions and Diagnostic Guidelines.* Geneva: World Health Organization.
65. McAllister-Williams RH, Tyrer SP (2003) Antidepressants for the treatment of depression and anxiety disorders: the same mechanism of action? In S Kasper, JA den Boer, JMA Sitsen (eds) *Handbook of Depression and Anxiety.* New York: M. Dekker.
66. Kellner R, Hernandez J, Pathak D (1992) Hypochondriacal fears and beliefs, anxiety, and somatization. *British Journal of Psychiatry* **160**: 525–32.
67. Stern J, Murphy M, Bass C (1993) Personality disorders in patients with somatization disorder: a controlled study. *British Journal of Psychiatry* **163**: 785–9.
68. Bhui K, Hotopf M (1997) Somatization disorder. *British Journal of Hospital Medicine* **58**: 145–9.
69. Bass C, Peveler R, House A (2001) Somatoform disorders: severe psychiatric illnesses neglected by psychiatrists. *British Journal of Psychiatry* **179**: 11–14.
70. Sharpe M, Mayou R (2004) Somatoform disorders: a help or hindrance to good patient care? *British Journal of Psychiatry* **184**: 465–7.
71. Castillo R, MacKenzie EJ, Wegener ST, Bosse MJ (2006) Prevalence of chronic pain seven years following limb threatening lower extremity trauma. *Pain* **124**: 321–9.
72. Schofferman J (1993) Long-term use of opioid analgesics for the treatment of chronic pain of nonmalignant origin. *Journal of Pain and Symptom Management* **8**: 279–88.
73. Ciccone D, Just N, Bandilla EB, *et al.* (2000) Psychological correlates of opioid use in patients with chronic nonmalignant pain: a preliminary test of the downhill spiral hypothesis. *Journal of Pain and Symptom Management* **20**: 180–92.
74. National Institute for Health and Clinical Excellence (2007) *Interventions to Reduce Substance Misuse Among Vulnerable Young People.* London: National Institute for Health and Clinical Excellence.
75. Allanson J, Bass C, Wade DT (2002) Characteristics of patients with persistent severe disability and medically unexplained neurological symptoms: a pilot study. *Journal of Neurology, Neurosurgery and Psychiatry* **73**: 307–9.

Chapter 53

Sleep disorders

John Shneerson

ASSESSMENT OF SLEEP DISORDERS

History and examination

It is often more difficult to take a history of a sleep disorder than to ask about complaints occurring during wakefulness. The patient may have little or no awareness of the problem. It may be only the patient's partner who can describe the events. After establishing the nature and timing, relative to both the clock and the onset of sleep, it is important to establish the time that the patient goes to bed, how long it takes to fall asleep, how often and why the patient awakens during the night, and what time the patient wakes up and gets out of bed. Feeling unrefreshed on waking may be due simply to sleep inertia, but if it persists during the day it should trigger enquiry into the cause of excessive sleepiness. If enough sleep is being obtained at night, then causes of disturbed sleep, such as an adverse sleeping environment, sleep apnoeas or restless legs syndrome, should be asked for, together with specific symptoms for other conditions that may cause excessive sleepiness, such as narcolepsy.

If the main complaint is lack of sleep at night, it is worth establishing whether this is difficulty in initiating sleep, maintaining sleep or waking early in the morning, since these three types of insomnia tend to have different causes. The cause of the difficulty in sleeping may be sensed by the patient to be primarily mental or physical, and the details should be obtained. Many patients with insomnia feel physically and mentally fatigued during the day. This should be distinguished from true excessive sleepiness.

If the primary complaint is of abnormal behaviours during sleep, then the patient's recall should be distinguished from the descriptions of the observer or partner. In contrast, with vivid dreams or nightmares, it is usually the patient who is able to give the most information, but occasionally, as in REM sleep behaviour disorder, the subject may forget the content of the abnormal dreams and the partner may be able to give useful information.

With patients who are excessively sleepy, the details of any naps or tendency to fall asleep during the day should be obtained. A simple measure of the severity of sleepiness is the Epworth Sleepiness Scale (Table 53.1). Details of the patient's activities during the day, and particularly in the hours before sleep, together with the patient's attitudes and beliefs about sleep, may give useful insights into the causes of difficulty in sleeping and excessive daytime sleepiness.

A careful medical and psychiatric history is required. A family history is particularly important in sleep walking and restless legs syndrome. Many drugs influence sleep and wakefulness, and details of drugs taken both currently and in the past should be obtained.

Physical examination is usually less helpful than a careful history. It can, however, show enlarged tonsils in patients who snore or have sleep apnoeas, and reveal psychiatric abnormalities in a wide range of sleep disorders. A neurological examination may be required, particularly to assess the cause of daytime sleepiness or motor disorders during sleep.

Polysomnography

Polysomnography is the simultaneous acquisition of several physiological signals during sleep. The most important of these are the electroencephalogram (EEG), electro-oculogram (EOG) and electromyogram (EMG), which enable sleep to be distinguished from wakefulness, the states of NREM and REM sleep to be identified, and the stages of NREM sleep to be distinguished.[1] The EEG electrodes sample cerebral cortical activity, which is very different in NREM sleep compared with REM sleep and wakefulness. As the stages of NREM sleep deepen, the frequency of the EEG falls and its amplitude increases. Delta waves are a feature, particularly of the deeper stages (3 and 4) of NREM sleep, which are often known together as 'slow-wave sleep'. Other variables that are commonly recorded in polysomnography include respiratory sounds, air flow, chest wall and abdominal movement, oxygen saturation, heart rate, EMG from a limb (usually the anterior tibialis muscle in the leg) and sometimes oesophageal pH and pressure monitoring.

Assessment of daytime sleepiness can be aided by completion of sleep diaries and self-assessment scales such as the Epworth Sleepiness Scale.[2,3] Behavioural performance tests such as reaction time tests[4] and driving simulators are

Table 53.1 Epworth sleepiness scale

How likely are you to fall asleep in the following situations, in contrast to just feeling tired? This refers to your usual way of life in the past few weeks. Even if you have not done some of these things recently, try to work out how they would have affected you. Use the following scale to choose the most appropriate number for each situation:

0 = would never doze
1 = slight chance of dozing
2 = moderate chance of dozing
3 = high chance of dozing

Situation	0	1	2	3
Sitting and reading				
Watching television				
Sitting inactive in a public place (e.g. a theatre or a meeting)				
As a passenger in a car for an hour without a break				
Lying down in the afternoon, when circumstances allow				
Sittting and talking to someone				
Sitting quietly after lunch without alcohol				
In a car, while stopped for a few minutes in traffic				

not used routinely, but they can be helpful in specific circumstances. Tracking tests and tests of higher cognitive function, such as planning and decision-making, can help to assess the degree of sleepiness, the ability to maintain attention and other aspects of cortical function.

The multiple sleep latency test (MSLT), in which the subject is asked to try to fall asleep in a darkened room four times during the day, is an objective test of daytime sleepiness.[5] It requires EEG, EOG and EMG signals to assess whether the subject is awake or asleep. In narcolepsy, not only is the MSLT shorter than normal, but also REM sleep is characteristically seen on at least two of the tests. The maintenance of wakefulness test (MWT) requires the same EEG, EOG and EMG monitoring, but the subject is asked to stay awake in a darkened room for as long as possible rather than to fall asleep.[6,7]

SLEEP, DRUGS AND PSYCHIATRIC DISORDERS

There are a variety of drugs used in psychiatric disorders that may affect sleep. Conversely, there are a large range of medical and social and recreational drugs that influence both sleep and psychiatric conditions.

Medical drugs

Hypnotics

Most of the hypnotics affect the functioning of γ-aminobutyric acid (GABA), which is a widely distributed inhibitory amino acid transmitter.[8] $GABA_A$ rather than $GABA_B$ receptors are affected. The benzodiazepines, zopiclone, eszopiclone, zolpidem, zaleplon and indiplon fall into this group. Barbiturates and alcohol bind directly to the GABA receptors and to their own receptors.

Most of these hypnotics have a rapid onset, but they have a variable half-life. They may increase the total sleep time and shorten the sleep latency, but most of them have little effect on stages 3 and 4 of NREM sleep. They tend to increase the duration of stage 2 of NREM sleep. The exception is sodium oxybate, which increases the duration of stages 3 and 4 of NREM sleep; possibly through this mechanism, it improves daytime alertness in narcolepsy, consolidates night-time sleep and relieves cataplexy.

Antidepressants

Depression may be related to overactivity of cholinergic relative to monoaminergic systems in the central nervous system (Table 53.2). Most antidepressants tend to restore the balance of these two neurotransmitters. Almost all

Table 53.2 Effects of psychoactive drugs on sleep

Drug	Total sleep time	Sleep latency	Arousals	Stages 1 and 2 NREM sleep	Stages 3 and 4 NREM sleep	REM sleep latency	REM sleep
Antipsychotics	↑	↓	–	–	Slight ↑	–	Variable
Antidepressants	–	–	↓	–	↑	↑	↑
Lithium	–	–	↓	–	↑	↑	↓

NREM, non-rapid eye movement; REM, rapid eye movement.

antidepressants increase the latency until the first REM sleep episode, reduce the total duration of REM sleep and increase the duration of stages 3 and 4 NREM sleep. The exceptions are moclobemide, bupropion and mirtazapine.[9] Lithium has similar effects to conventional antidepressants but also delays the circadian rhythms slightly.

Antipsychotics

The older antipsychotics antagonize the dopamine receptors D2 and D3 in particular and inhibit the ascending the reticular activating system, limbic system and cerebral cortex. Atypical antipsychotics antagonize 5-hydroxytryptamine 2 (5-HT2) receptors in particular. The older drugs increase total sleep time, reduce sleep latency and usually increase the duration of stages 2, 3 and 4 of NREM sleep (see Table 53.2). Atypical antipsychotics, particularly olanzapine, increase the duration of stages 3 and 4 of NREM sleep and often cause daytime sleepiness.

Cholinesterase inhibitors

These drugs, which are used in dementia, increase the duration of REM sleep and often cause insomnia, intense dreams and nightmares.

Social and recreational drugs

Alcohol

Alcohol has a similar effect on GABA receptors to the hypnotics, but it also has its own receptor and acts as a glutamate inhibitor. Low doses of alcohol increase the total sleep time, reduce sleep latency, reduce latency before stages 3 and 4 of NREM sleep, and suppress REM sleep. After larger intakes, stages 3 and 4 of NREM sleep are reduced and its diuretic effect causes awakenings from sleep. Chronic alcohol ingestion can severely disrupt the sleep–wake cycle, and even after abstinence abnormal sleep architecture often persists for a prolonged period.

Caffeine

Caffeine acts as an antagonist at adenosine receptors and tends to increase wakefulness. It reduces total sleep time, increases the sleep latency and reduces the duration of stages 3 and 4 of NREM sleep and of REM sleep. It commonly causes insomnia if taken later in the evening or in large doses.

Nicotine

Nicotine acts on nicotinic cholinergic receptors. In low doses it is excitatory, but in high doses it is inhibitory. It appears to reduce the total sleep time, increase sleep latency and reduce the duration of REM sleep in higher doses.

Amphetamines

Amphetamines increase activity at dopamine, noradrenaline and 5-HT synapses, particularly in the brainstem and cerebral cortex. They have an alerting effect, reduce total sleep time and reduce the duration of stages 3 and 4 of NREM sleep and of REM sleep.

Chronic use of cocaine leads to sleep deprivation, and abrupt withdrawal leads to depression and prolonged sleep, with REM sleep rebound. Ecstasy is both a stimulant and a hallucinogenic drug that reduces REM sleep duration.

Cannabinoids

These drugs act at CB1 and CB2 receptors. They reduce the duration of REM sleep and slightly increase the duration of stages 3 and 4 of NREM sleep. Withdrawal leads to REM sleep rebound.[10,11]

EXCESSIVE DAYTIME SLEEPINESS

Excessive daytime sleepiness should be distinguished from physical fatigue or weariness and mental fatigue, which is characterized by the inability to sustain concentration, for instance on a conversation or while reading. The nature of sleepiness is probably similar whatever its cause, and the subject is usually aware of feeling sleepy before sleep is entered. Rapidly developing sleepiness with very little warning beforehand may, however, occur in narcolepsy and parkinsonism.

Effects of sleepiness

With increasing sleepiness, the level of alertness falls, concentration deteriorates and attention, particularly for prolonged monotonous tasks, is impaired. Mood changes, particularly irritability and paranoia, are common.[12] Stereotyped behaviour, with the loss of innovative responses, verbal fluency[13] and mental flexibility, is characteristic. Working memory deteriorates, and planning and executive functions are impaired.[14]

There is deterioration in physical performance, particularly for prolonged or monotonous tasks, with a sense of fatigue and even episodes of automatic behaviour, in which inappropriate actions are carried out with reduced vigilance and subsequent amnesia.

Excessive daytime sleepiness impacts on family and social life and recreational activities. In children it often leads to poor school performance and impaired concentration, which may be interpreted as attention deficit hyperactivity disorder (ADHD). In adults there is a fall in productivity at work, with an increased number of errors and a risk of occupational accidents, particularly with moving machinery.[15]

Sleepiness and driving

It has been estimated that around 1–3 per cent of all road traffic accidents, perhaps 10 per cent of serious accidents and 20 per cent of motorway accidents are related to driver drowsiness. These particularly involve males under the age of 30 years who are driving alone and who appear to be unable to recognize their degree of sleepiness.[16] Sleep-related accidents occur particularly between 2 a.m. and 6 a.m. and between 2 p.m. and 4 p.m., when the circadian rhythms most strongly promote sleepiness.[17] Pre-accident behaviour includes fluctuating vehicle speed due to intermittent loss of muscle activity in the leg controlling the accelerator at the transition into sleep, shunting accidents at traffic lights and roundabouts, and weaving from lane to lane. At the time of the accident, there is often no evidence for braking or taking avoiding action.

Causes of excessive daytime sleepiness

Insufficient duration of sleep (sleep restriction)

This is the most common cause of sleepiness and is usually the result of social or work pressures or shift work, which also reduces the quality of sleep through altering its timing and regularity. A careful history should detect sleep restriction. It is important to discuss with the patient how other competing priorities can be managed so that adequate sleep is obtained.

Impaired quality of sleep (sleep fragmentation)

Poor quality of sleep may be due to an adverse sleep environment, which may be noisy, light, too hot or too cold, or uncomfortable. It may also be due to medical disorders that disrupt sleep, such as pain and discomfort, drugs such as caffeine or excessive alcohol, and conditions appearing during sleep, particularly obstructive sleep apnoeas and periodic limb movements as part of restless legs syndrome.

Hypersomnias

In these conditions, although sleep may be of normal duration, it is unrefreshing and the subject remains sleepy or naps during the day. Narcolepsy is usually regarded as a hypersomnia, but the total sleep time during the day and night is increased only slightly. In idiopathic hypersomnia, however, there is prolonged nocturnal sleep, with difficulty in waking in the morning associated with prolonged unrefreshing naps during the day. Sedative drugs may produce a similar clinical picture.

Individual disorders causing excessive daytime sleepiness

Narcolepsy

Narcolepsy is a disorder of REM sleep in which fragments of this intrude into wakefulness. Sleep itself is destabilized, with frequent nocturnal awakenings.[18] Its prevalence is around 1 in 2000–3000. It usually arises in adolescents or young adults. Insomnia at night is combined with severe sleepiness during the day. The physiological loss of muscle tone in REM sleep is manifested as sleep paralysis, often at the onset of sleep, and cataplexy, which is a loss of muscle tone in response to sudden or intense emotion, usually laughter. The intensity of dream mentation is increased, leading to hypnagogic and hypnopompic hallucinations and vivid dreams at night.

Narcolepsy may be triggered by environmental factors,[19] but it also has a genetic component.[20] Lack of functioning of orexin-producing neurons in the perifornical hypothalamus appears to be a common factor in classical narcolepsy.[21,22]

The presence of cataplexy is virtually specific to narcolepsy,[23] but if there is diagnostic doubt polysomnography with multiple sleep latency tests are usually helpful (Box 53.1). Sleep-onset REM sleep during the overnight study with a short sleep latency and two or more episodes of sleep-onset REM sleep during the MSLTs are characteristic of narcolepsy. HLA DQB*01602 is present in over 90 per

Box 53.1 Differential diagnosis of cataplexy

- Sleep 'attack'
- Epilepsy, especially gelastic and atonic
- Vertebrobasilar insufficiency
- Cardiac dysrhythmias
- Myasthenia gravis
- Periodic paralysis
- Faints
- Gelastic syncope
- Hysteria.

cent of white people with narcolepsy. It is also present in around 25 per cent of the normal population, but its absence makes narcolepsy unlikely. Estimation of cerebrospinal fluid orexin concentration is currently a research procedure, but low values are typical of narcolepsy.

Explanation of the nature and prognosis of the symptoms and advice about lifestyle factors to manage their impact is important. The first-line medication for excessive daytime sleepiness is modafinil,[24,25] but if this is poorly tolerated or ineffective dexamphetamine and methylphenidate are alternatives. Cataplexy is usually treated with an antidepressant[26] such as venlafaxine, but if this or daytime sleepiness remain troublesome sodium oxybate is usually effective.[27]

Obstructive sleep apnoeas

These are characterized by transient obstruction of the upper airway, usually at pharyngeal level.[28] They may occur up to 500 times each night, and each is associated with a micro-arousal from sleep. These fragment sleep and lead to daytime sleepiness. The condition is most common in middle-aged males, particularly if they are obese, but it can occur at any age in both sexes.[29]

The characteristic clinical features are a combination of snoring with apnoeas witnessed by the partner and excessive daytime sleepiness. Diagnosis can be confirmed by sleep studies, including domiciliary oximetry studies.[30,31] Attention to lifestyle factors, particularly weight loss, is important; particularly in children, tonsillectomy may be effective.[32] Mandibular advancement devices that protrude the lower jaw and tongue and thereby increase the dimensions of the pharyngeal airway are often effective in mild sleep apnoeas, but they may be tolerated poorly.[33] The most effective treatment is a nasal continuous-positive airway pressure (CPAP) system, which inflates the airway.[34] This prevents the airway obstructing and relieves both the symptoms and the consequences of sleep apnoeas,[35] including the increased risk of myocardial infarction, stroke, hypertension and road traffic accidents.[36]

Idiopathic hypersomnia

This condition usually affects young adults and is characterized by prolonged unrefreshing sleep, difficulty in waking in the mornings, and prolonged unrefreshing naps.[37] None of the other features of narcolepsy are present. No cause is found, although a similar condition may appear after brain injury. Treatment with modafinil, or if necessary dexamphetamine, is usually effective.

Psychiatric disorders

Excessive daytime sleepiness is caused only occasionally by psychiatric problems, although it is a feature of depression, particularly in adolescents and young adults. It can develop as a protective psychological reaction to circumstances that are difficult to cope with. This may be difficult to distinguish from idiopathic hypersomnia. Daytime sleepiness in schizophrenia is usually due to sedative medication or sleep apnoeas associated with obesity rather than the disorder itself.

INSOMNIA

Insomnia is the most common sleep disorder, and at any one time 10–15 per cent of the population has this problem. It is more common in females and in older people.[38] Insomnia is not a diagnosis but a symptom complex of the perception of insufficient or poor-quality sleep, despite an adequate opportunity to sleep, together with a feeling of being unrefreshed or fatigued on waking and during the day. Insomnia may be transient (adjustment sleep disorder), when it is usually a response to a stressful event.[39] The pattern of insomnia may be primarily a difficulty in initiating sleep (DIS; sleep-onset insomnia), difficulty in maintaining sleep (DMS; sleep-maintenance insomnia) or early-morning wakening (EMW).

Effects of insomnia

Insomnia is associated with a lower delta power on the EEG during sleep and intrusion of alpha waves, suggesting a lower threshold for arousal to stimuli such as pain or noise. The heart rate is faster in all stages of sleep, as in wakefulness, and hypertension is more common in people with insomnia than in the normal population.

The psychological consequences of insomnia are loss of concentration and deterioration of memory, irritability, mood disturbance, loss of motivation, and increased risk of anxiety and depression. There is also a sensation of physical weariness, fatigue and muscle aches, which are usually worst in the limbs but may be associated with headaches.

Causes of insomnia

Primary insomnia (hyperarousal states)

The hyperarousal state that underlies primary insomnia is also present during wakefulness.[40] There may be a genetic predisposition, exacerbated by, for instance, shift work or age.[41] Precipitating factors can be detected in 75 per cent of people with chronic insomnia and include a wide range of stressful situations, which lead to an increase in both physiological and psychological arousal. Once insomnia has been established, it is often perpetuated by maladaptive attitudes, beliefs and behaviours that lead to poor sleep hygiene.

There are several clinical types of primary insomnia, including the following:

- *Sleep state misperception:* in this condition, the duration of sleep may be normal, but it is perceived to be short despite the absence of any physiological abnormalities during sleep. The risks of hypertension and depression appear to be similar to those in people with true primary insomnia.

- *Psychophysiological (conditioned) insomnia:* this is an apprehensive concern about difficulties in sleeping, which perpetuates insomnia. It is in effect a focal anxiety state centred on the inability to sleep adequately. The sleep difficulty may become a major concern during wakefulness.[42]
- *Anxiety states:* these are often associated with poor sleep at night and waking with panic attacks.
- *Chronic fatigue syndrome:* there is often hypersomnia initially, followed by a prolonged period of insomnia, which is usually related to poor sleep hygiene secondary to the fatigue, associated with anxiety about obtaining sufficient sleep.
- *Fibromyalgia:* sleep is usually considered to be unrefreshing and light. Polysomnography often shows alpha intrusion. The sleep problems of fibromyalgia overlap with those of chronic fatigue syndrome.

Co-morbid (secondary) insomnia

It is now recognized that insomnia associated with a wide variety of psychiatric and physical disorders is not simply the result of these disorders but one of their causes. It often requires treatment in addition to the treatment of the associated co-morbidity.

Depression

Insomnia is a common and often initial symptom of depression. There is difficulty maintaining sleep and early-morning awakening rather than difficulty initiating sleep. Excessive sleepiness during the day is a feature of depression in younger patients.[43]

There appears to be an increase in drive to enter REM sleep combined with a weakened drive for NREM sleep (Figure 53.1). As a result, there is characteristically a short total sleep time, with short latency until the first REM sleep episode, and an increase in the duration of REM sleep, with reduction in stages 3 and 4 of NREM sleep. There is an increase in sleep stages 1 and 2 and frequent awakenings. These features are seen particularly during an episode of depression, but they may persist after treatment; in particular, the REM sleep latency often remains short. There is also a tendency towards an advanced sleep phase, which probably contributes to early-morning wakening.

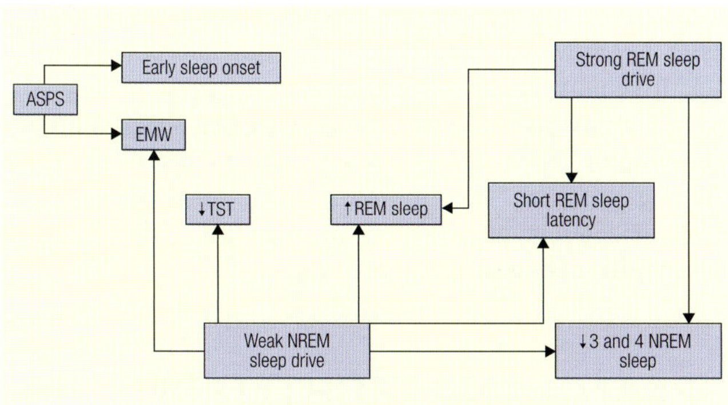

Figure 53.1 Abnormalities of sleep control in depression

ASPS, advanced sleep phase syndrome; EMW, early-morning awakening; NREM, non-rapid eye movement; REM, rapid eye movement; TST, total sleep time.

Sleep deprivation may elevate the mood in depression and even lead to mania in bipolar disorders.[44] Sleep deprivation increases the drive to NREM sleep and, particularly if sleep is lost during the latter part of the night, the duration of REM sleep will be curtailed. Reduction in duration of REM sleep is also a feature of most antidepressant drugs and of electroconvulsive treatment. Sedative antidepressants such as tricyclics and mirtazapine are usually effective in relieving insomnia due to depression, but an alternative is a selective serotonin reuptake inhibitor (SSRI) antidepressant with a short course of a hypnotic.[45]

Bipolar disorder

The manic phase of bipolar disorder is usually associated with around 3–4 h sleep each night. There may also be abnormalities in circadian rhythms, including cortisol secretion.

Post-traumatic stress disorder

Post-traumatic stress disorder (PTSD) may follow a military or civilian traumatic event and is characterized by insomnia, intrusive thoughts, flashbacks, nightmares and avoidance behaviour. The nightmares occur especially between midnight and 3 a.m. They may arise from stages 1 and 2 of NREM sleep as well as from REM sleep, in contrast to the usual type of nightmare. Their content relates to the precipitating event, although it may be generalized and hardly recognizable.

PTSD leads to a hyperarousal state both while awake while and asleep. As a result, there is insomnia, with difficulty in initiating and maintaining sleep. Panic attacks may occur, both during the day and at night, and insomnia may be exacerbated by depression.

Antidepressants, particularly SSRIs or venlafaxine, combined with behavioural therapy and psychotherapy may help to relieve the sleep-related symptoms. The nightmares and associated motor abnormalities often respond to prazosin.

Schizophrenia

Schizophrenia characteristically causes difficulty in initiating and maintaining sleep.[46] These are particularly problems during and before acute exacerbations. The dreams of people with schizophrenia often feature strangers in an environment that is hostile to the patient. These dreams should be distinguished from hallucinations during wakefulness. Daytime sleepiness in schizophrenia is usually related to psychotropic drugs rather than to the schizophrenia itself.

Dementia

Insomnia is a common problem in dementia, particularly Alzheimer's disease and multi-infarct dementia.[47] The normal sleep architecture disintegrates, with loss of the sleep cycles of NREM and REM sleep. Daytime naps are taken frequently, and an advanced sleep phase with an early sleep onset and early waking time is common. 'Sundowning' is a problem particularly with Alzheimer's disease and is characterized by agitation, particularly in the afternoon and early evening, associated with wandering and confused behaviour. It improves with light therapy and is more common in the winter, when there is less light exposure.

The duration of stages 3 and 4 of NREM sleep is shortened, and there is an increase in REM sleep latency and a shorter duration of REM sleep.

The sleep-related symptoms may improve with sleep hygiene advice, particularly regular sleep–wake patterns, increased exposure to light in the day, more physical activity during the day, and the avoidance of stimulants such as caffeine and disturbance from attendants at night.[48,49] Long-acting hypnotics that induce daytime sedation are best avoided.[50]

Treatment of insomnia

The most important aspect of the treatment of insomnia is attention to sleep hygiene.[51] Any underlying cause should be recognized and treated, whether this is physical or psychiatric. Attention to drugs that may contribute to insomnia, such as caffeine and nicotine, is important. Advice should be given about shift work.

Hypnotics may be effective in the short term,[52] but it is usually recommended that their use is restricted to less than 1 month.[53] Cognitive-behavioural therapy (CBT) may have long-term benefits, but its availability is limited.[54,55]

PARASOMNIAS

This unsatisfactory term is conventionally used to describe unusual, undesirable and episodic events in sleep that are not due primarily to another sleep disorder. It is, however difficult, to separate sleep disorders from the motor behaviours during sleep. Including the undesirable component also leads to a subjective assessment of what is a parasomnia. The range of unusual events during sleep is so broad that the term 'parasomnia' includes a very heterogeneous collection of conditions. In addition, some of these conditions are so common that they merge into normality.

Abnormal behaviour during sleep falls into three main categories.

NREM sleep disorders

These include sleeptalking, sleepwalking, sleep terrors, sleep-eating and sexual activity in sleep. The first three are most common in childhood, have a familial, probably genetic background, and can be precipitated by factors that increase the depth or duration of stages 3 and 4 of NREM sleep. These factors include sleep deprivation, hypnotics, alcohol, and factors that tend to cause arousal from sleep, such as a noisy environment, stress, and sleep fragmentation due to sleep apnoeas or restless legs syndrome. A primary psychiatric cause is unusual. Polysomnography is not diagnostic but excludes other causes for the episodes. Explanation and reassurance may be sufficient, but advice about safety issues, avoidance of precipitating factors, and occasionally drug treatment, including hypnotics and antidepressants, may be of help.

Sleep-eating and sexual activity during sleep tend to occur in young adults with a previous history of sleepwalking or sleep terrors. They should be distinguished from these activities occurring during wakefulness at night that are not recognized or are denied by the patient.

REM sleep abnormalities

The most important condition is the REM sleep behaviour disorder (RBD).[56] This occurs in elderly males and is often the first feature of degenerative neurological conditions, particularly parkinsonism, but also multiple system atrophy and Lewy body disease.[57] It is characterized by dreams with an aggressive content in which the patient is attacked or chased by strangers. The normal inhibition of motor activity ('atonia') in REM sleep is lost,[58,59] so that these dreams are physically enacted, often with resulting injuries to the patient or their partner. Polysomnography shows retention of muscle tone during REM sleep and the nature of the physical activity. Clonazepam, zopiclone and melatonin are usually effective.

Restless legs syndrome (Ekbom's syndrome)

This condition may affect up to 10 per cent of the adult population mildly and is troublesome in around 2 per cent of people. It is often familial, but it may be secondary to factors such as iron deficiency, renal failure and drugs, including antidepressants, antihistamines, antipsychotics and lithium. It is also a feature of normal pregnancy. It is characterized by an unpleasant sensation inside the legs occurring in the evenings, an urge to move the legs, and relief by movement (Box 53.2). During sleep it leads to repetitive movements of the legs, which fragment sleep. The main complaints are difficulty in initiating sleep and daytime fatigue. The most effective treatment is a dopaminergic agent such as ropinirole or pramipexole, but benzodiazepines, opiates and anti-epileptic drugs such as gabapentin may also be useful.

DREAMS AND NIGHTMARES

Dreams that include a complex narrative with visual and other images are usually associated with REM sleep. They appear to be initiated by the pontine centres responsible for this. The bizarre nature of dreams is related to partial loss of frontal lobe function in REM sleep and to the loose mental associations that are characteristic of REM sleep.[60]

In pure NREM sleep there may be dreams with a simple content and that typically involve problem-solving,[61] whereas REM sleep dreams have more narrative and emotional content.[62] Similar processes can occur before the onset of sleep (hypnagogic hallucinations) and after waking (hypnopompic hallucinations); they are particularly characteristic of narcolepsy. The content of dreams differs according to age, culture and gender, and they vary considerably in their emotional content, vividness, timing during the night, and the extent of recall afterwards.

Nightmares are most common between the ages of 6 years and 10 years, but they occur occasionally in 40–50 per cent of adults. Nightmares are dreams that are terrifying and lead to an intense anxiety or fear on arousal from sleep, although there is little physical or autonomic overactivity.[63] There is no confusion on wakening, and they occur particularly during the last third of the night, when REM sleep is most prolonged. Polysomnography is rarely required, but nightmares should be distinguished from REM sleep behaviour disorder, nocturnal panic attacks and sleep terrors, which have little dream imagery and occur early in the night, and epilepsy. They may respond to antidepressants, which reduce the duration of REM sleep, and CBT, including imagery rehearsal therapy, in which the content of the nightmares can be modified into a non-frightening narrative.

Box 53.2 Descriptions of abnormal sensations in the restless legs syndrome

- Unpleasant
- Uncomfortable
- Creeping
- Crawling
- Wriggling
- Alive
- Irritating
- Pulling
- Stretching
- Heavy
- Tired
- Tingling
- Pins and needles
- Electric
- Burning
- Aching
- Itching
- Cramping
- Painful
- Like insects or worms inside the legs.

KEY POINTS

- A diagnosis can often be reached from a careful sleep history, but sleep studies, particularly limited respiratory studies or polysomnography, are often required.
- A wide range of medications can profoundly affect sleep and its disorders.
- Excessive daytime sleepiness may be due to insufficient sleep, poor quality of sleep, or neurological disorders such as narcolepsy.
- Insomnia is a feature of several psychiatric disorders, and both the insomnia and the underlying condition require treatment.
- Normal motor and sensory events during sleep should be distinguished from pathological conditions.

REFERENCES

1. Rechtschaffen A, Kales A (eds) (1968) *A Manual of Standardized Terminology, Techniques and Scoring System for Sleep Stages of Human Subjects.* Los Angeles, CA: Brain Information Service/Brain Research Institute.
2. Olson LG, Cole MF, Ambrogetti A (1998) Correlations among Epworth Sleepiness Scale scores, multiple sleep latency tests and psychological symptoms. *Journal of Sleep Research* **7**: 248–53.
3. Johns MW (1991) A new method for measuring daytime sleepiness: the Epworth Sleepiness Scale. *Sleep* **14**: 540–45.
4. Balkin TJ, Bliese PD, Belenky G, *et al.* (2004) Comparative utility of instruments for monitoring sleepiness-related performance decrements in the operational environment. *Journal of Sleep Research* **13**: 219–27.
5. Arand D, Bonnet M, Hurwitz T, *et al.* (2005) The clinical use of the MSLT and MWT. *Sleep* **28**: 123–44.
6. Sangal RB, Thomas L, Mitler MM (1992) Maintenance of Wakefulness Test and Multiple Sleep Latency Test: measurement of different abilities in patients with sleep disorders. *Chest* **101**: 898–902.
7. Doghramji K, Mitler MM, Sangal RB, *et al.* (1997) A normative study of the maintenance of wakefulness test (MWT). *Electroencephalography and Clinical Neurophysiology* **103**: 554–62.
8. Gillin JC (1991) The long and the short of sleeping pills. *New England Journal of Medicine* **324**: 1735–6.
9. Aslan S, Isik E, Cosar B (2002) The effects of mirtazapine on sleep: a placebo controlled, double-blind study in young healthy volunteers. *Sleep* **25**: 677–9.
10. Hall W, Solowij N (1998) Adverse effects of cannabis. *Lancet* **352**: 1611–16.
11. Bolla KI, Lesage SR, Gamaldo CE, *et al.* (2008) Sleep disturbance in heavy marijuana users. *Sleep* **31**: 901–8.

12. Jones K, Harrison Y (2001) Frontal lobe function, sleep loss and fragmented sleep. *Sleep Medicine Reviews* **5**: 463–75.
13. Harrison Y, Horne JA (1998) Sleep loss impairs short and novel language tasks having a prefrontal focus. *Journal of Sleep Research* **7**: 95–100.
14. Fulda S, Schulz H (2001) Cognitive dysfunction in sleep disorders. *Sleep Medicine Reviews* **5**: 423–45.
15. Melamed S, Oksenberg A (2002) Excessive daytime sleepiness and risk of occupational injuries in non-shift daytime workers. *Sleep* **25**: 315–22.
16. Akerstedt T, Kecklund G (2001) Age, gender and early morning highway accidents. *Journal of Sleep Research* **10**: 105–10.
17. Mitler MM, Miller JC, Lipsitz JJ, Walsh JK, Wylie CD (1997) The sleep of long-haul truck drivers. *New England Journal of Medicine* **337**: 755–61.
18. Plazzi G, Serra L, Ferri R (2008) Nocturnal aspects of narcolepsy with cataplexy. *Sleep Medicine Reviews* **12**: 109–28.
19. Picchioni D, Mignot EJ, Harsh JR (2004) The month-of-birth pattern in narcolepsy is moderated by cataplexy severity and may be independent of HLA-DQB1*0602. *Sleep* **27**: 1471–5.
20. Mignot E (1998) Genetic and familial aspects of narcolepsy. *Neurology* **50** (suppl. 1): S16–22.
21. Krahn LE, Pankratz VS, Oliver L, Boeve BF, Silber MH (2002) Hypocretin (orexin) levels in cerebrospinal fluid of patients with narcolepsy: relationship to cataplexy and HLA DQB1*0602 status. *Sleep* **25**: 733–6.
22. Hungs M, Mignot E (2001) Hypocretin/orexin, sleep and narcolepsy. *BioEssays* **23**: 397–408.
23. Parkes JD, Chen SY, Clift SJ, Dahlitz MJ, Dunn G (1998) The clinical diagnosis of the narcoleptic syndrome. *Journal of Sleep Research* **7**: 41–52.
24. Schwartz JRL, Schwartz ER, Veit CA, Blakely EA (1998) Modafinil for the treatment of excessive day-time sleepiness associated with narcolepsy. *Today's Therapeutic Trends* **16**: 287–308.
25. US Modafinil in Narcolepsy Multicenter Study Group (1998) Randomized trial of modafinil for the treatment of pathological somnolence in narcolepsy. *Annals of Neurology* **43**: 88–97.
26. Larrosa O, Llave Y de la, Barrio S, Granizo JJ, Garcia-Borreguero D (2001) Stimulant and anticataplectic effects of reboxetine in patients with narcolepsy: a pilot study. *Sleep* **24**: 282–5.
27. The US Xyrem[R] Multicenter Study Group (2002) A randomized, double blind, placebo-controlled multicenter trial comparing the effects of three doses of orally administered sodium oxybate with placebo for the treatment of narcolepsy. *Sleep* **25**: 42–8.
28. Stradling JR, Davies RJO (2004) Sleep 1: obstructive sleep apnoea/hypopnoea syndrome: definitions, epidemiology, and natural history. *Thorax* **59**: 73–8.
29. Stradling JR, Crosby JH (1991) Predictors and prevalence of obstructive sleep apnoea and snoring in 1001 middle aged men. *Thorax* **46**: 85–90.
30. Raymond B, Cayton RM, Chappell MJ (2003) Combined index of heart rate variability and oximetry in screening for the sleep apnoea/hypopnoea syndrome. *Journal of Sleep Research* **12**: 53–61.
31. Flemons WW, Littner MR, Rowley JA, *et al.* (2003) Home diagnosis of sleep apnea: a systematic review of the literature. *Chest* **124**: 1543–79.
32. De Backer W (1998) Non-CPAP treatment of obstructive sleep apnoea. *Monaldi Archives for Chest Disease* **53**: 625–9.
33. Marklund M, Persson M, Franklin KA (1998) Treatment success with a mandibular advancement device is related to supine-dependent sleep apnea. *Chest* **114**: 1630–35.
34. Loube DI, Gay PC, Strohl KP, *et al.* (1999) Indications for positive airway pressure treatment of adult obstructive sleep apnea patients. *Chest* **115**: 863–6.
35. Ballester E, Badia JR, Hernandez L, *et al.* (1999) Evidence of the effectiveness of continuous positive airway pressure in the treatment of sleep apnea/hypopnea syndrome. *American Journal of Respiratory and Critical Care Medicine* **159**: 495–501.
36. George CFP (2001) Reduction in motor vehicle collisions following treatment of sleep apnoea with nasal CPAP. *Thorax* **56**: 508–12.
37. Billiard M, Dauvilliers Y (2001) Idiopathic hypersomnia. *Sleep Medicine Reviews* **5**: 351–60.
38. Jensen E, Dehlin O, Hagberg B, Samuelsson G, Svensson T (1998) Insomnia in an 80-year-old population: relationship to medical, psychological and social factors. *Journal of Sleep Research* **7**: 183–9.
39. Jansson-Frojmark M, Linton SJ (2008) The course of insomnia over one year: a longitudinal study in the general population in Sweden. *Sleep* **31**: 881–6.
40. Bonnet MH, Arand DL (1997) Hyperarousal and insomnia. *Sleep Medicine Reviews* **1**: 97–108.
41. Vahtera J, Kivimaki M, Hublin C, *et al.* (2007) Liability to anxiety and severe life events as predictors of new-onset sleep disturbances. *Sleep* **30**: 1537–46.
42. Bastien CH, St Jean G, Morin CM, Turcotte I, Carrier J (2008) Chronic psychophysiological insomnia: hyperarousal and/or inhibition deficits? An ERPs investigation. *Sleep* **31**: 887–98.
43. Adrien J (2002) Neurobiological bases for the relation between sleep and depression. *Sleep Medicine Reviews* **6**: 341–51.
44. Giedke H, Schwarzler F (2002) Therapeutic use of sleep deprivation in depression. *Sleep Medicine Reviews* **6**: 361–77.
45. Jindal RD, Thase ME (2004) Treatment of insomnia associated with clinical depression. *Sleep Medicine Reviews* **8**: 19–30.
46. Monti JM, Monti D (2004) Sleep in schizophrenia patients and the effects of antipsychotic drugs. *Sleep Medicine Reviews* **8**: 133–48.

47. Reynolds CF, Hoch CC, Stack J, Campbell D (1988) The nature and management of sleep/wake disturbance in Alzheimer's dementia. *Psychopharmacology Bulletin* **24**: 43–8.
48. Benedetti F, Barbini B, Colombo C, Smeraldi E (2007) Chronotherapeutics in a psychiatric ward. *Sleep Medicine Reviews* **11**: 509–22.
49. Terman M (2007) Evolving applications of light therapy. *Sleep Medicine Reviews* **11**: 497–507.
50. McCurry SM, Reynolds CF III, Ancoli-Israel S, Teri L, Vitiello MV (2000) Treatment of sleep disturbance in Alzheimer's disease. *Sleep Medicine Reviews* **4**: 603–28.
51. Stepanski EJ, Wyatt JK (2003) Use of sleep hygiene in the treatment of insomnia. *Sleep Medicine Reviews* **7**: 215–25.
52. Wagner J, Wagner ML (2000) Non-benzodiazepines for the treatment of insomnia. *Sleep Medicine Reviews* **4**: 551–81.
53. Mendelson WB, Roth T, Cassella J, *et al.* (2004) The treatment of chronic insomnia: drug indications, chronic use and abuse liability – summary of a 2001 new clinical drug evaluation unit meeting symposium. *Sleep Medicine Reviews* **8**: 7–17.
54. Edinger JD, Wohlgemuth WK, Radtke RA, Marsh GR, Quillian RE (2001) Does cognitive-behavioral insomnia therapy alter dysfunctional beliefs about sleep? *Sleep* **24**: 591–8.
55. Montgomery P, Dennis J (2004) A systematic review of non-pharmacological therapies for sleep problems in later life. *Sleep Medicine Reviews* **8**: 47–62.
56. Schenck CH, Mahowald MW (2002) REM Sleep behavior disorder: clinical, developmental, and neuroscience perspectives 16 years after its formal identification in SLEEP. *Sleep* **25**: 120–38.
57. Schenck CH, Bundlie SR, Mahowald MW (1996) Delayed emergence of a parkinsonian disorder in 38% of 29 older men initially diagnosed with idiopathic rapid eye movement sleep behavior disorder. *Neurology* **46**: 388–93.
58. Sforza E, Krieger J, Petiau C (1997) REM sleep behavior disorder: clinical and physiopathological findings. *Sleep Medicine Reviews* **1**: 57–69.
59. Desseilles M, Dang-Vu T, Schabus M, *et al.* (2008) Neuroimaging insights into the pathophysiology of sleep disorders. *Sleep* **31**: 777–94.
60. Hobson JA, Pace-Schott EF (2002) The cognitive neuroscience of sleep: neuronal systems, consciousness and learning. *Neuroscience* **3**: 679–93.
61. Suzuki H, Uchiyama M, Tagaya H, *et al.* (2004) Dreaming during non-rapid eye movement sleep in the absence of prior rapid eye movement sleep. *Sleep* **27**: 1486–90.
62. Takeuchi T, Miyasita A, Inugami M, Yamamoto Y (2001) Intrinsic dreams are not produced without REM sleep mechanisms: evidence through elicitation of sleep onset REM periods. *Journal of Sleep Research* **10**: 43–52.
63. Blagrove M, Farmer L, Williams E (2004) The relationship of nightmare frequency and nightmare distress to well-being. *Journal of Sleep Research* **13**: 129–36.

Chapter 54

Suicide and deliberate self-harm

Chris Hawley, Paul St John Smith and Ash Padhi

SUICIDE

Introduction

Suicide has been common throughout human history. The Romans regarded suicide as permissible, provided one was not a soldier or a slave (i.e. of economic value to the State). Socrates regarded suicide as against God's will but permissible if God sent 'necessity' on a man. Christian clerics condemned suicide at the Council of Arles in AD452, and Islamic texts specifically proscribe suicide. At times, suicide has been considered either appropriate or noble; death by *seppuku* was preferred to dishonour by Samurai, and insurgent Jews, rather than face enslavement by the Romans, died in a mass suicide at Masada in AD74.

Any account of suicide is influenced by a society's prevailing philosophical values. Emile Durkheim viewed suicide as a social phenomenon occurring under four conditions: (i) *anomic* (anomie – a social environment lacking norms), (ii) *egoistic* (an individual detached from society), (iii) *altruistic* (suicide for the greater social good) and (iv) *fatalistic* (to die rather than to endure oppression).[1] The prevailing ideological account in Western society regards suicide as the pathological outcome of a diseased state of mind and successful suicidants as victims rather than perpetrators.

Statutory considerations

Suicides are regarded in English law as a mode of death that is unnatural, self-inflicted, deliberate and intended. A verdict of suicide is returned by the Coroner's court only if suicide intent can be demonstrated beyond reasonable doubt; if not, then an open or other verdict will be returned (Box 54.1).[2]

Box 54.1 Possible verdicts that may be returned by a Coroner in England

- Natural causes
- Industrial disease
- Want of attention at birth
- Stillbirth
- Death by abuse of drugs
- Suicide
- Accidental death
- Misadventure
- Neglect
- Unlawful killing
- Lawful killing
- Open verdict.

Two-thirds of open verdicts would be considered probable suicides when judged by clinical standards. Of clinically probable suicides, half of men and a quarter of women receive Coroners' verdicts other than suicide. Thus, the legal determination of suicide is not a reliable indicator of its true incidence. Furthermore, the threshold at which a suicide verdict is returned varies between Coroners.[3] Apparent variations in the suicide rates between countries are attributable partly to differences in legal criteria and sociocultural factors affecting reporting.

Suicide researchers use either an exclusive or an inclusive framework for case ascertainment. The exclusive framework includes only cases that have received a Coroner's verdict of suicide. The inclusive framework includes cases where a Coroner returned a verdict of suicide and cases where the intent to die is undetermined. The, usually preferred, inclusive method estimates the incidence of suicide as one-third higher than the exclusive method.

The Suicide Act abrogated the previous law whereby it was a crime for a person to commit suicide.[4] However, complicity in the suicide of another person by having 'aided, abetted, counseled or procured the suicide' became a criminal offence punishable by imprisonment. The Suicide Act is therefore relevant to the continuing moral debate about end-of-life decisions and assisted dying.

Incidence and method of suicide

The current suicide rate in England is $10.5/10^5$ population/year and is declining (Figure 54.1).[5] This is in contrast to the worldwide picture of a 50 per cent increase in the incidence of suicide over the past five decades and projections that this will to continue to rise. The current global

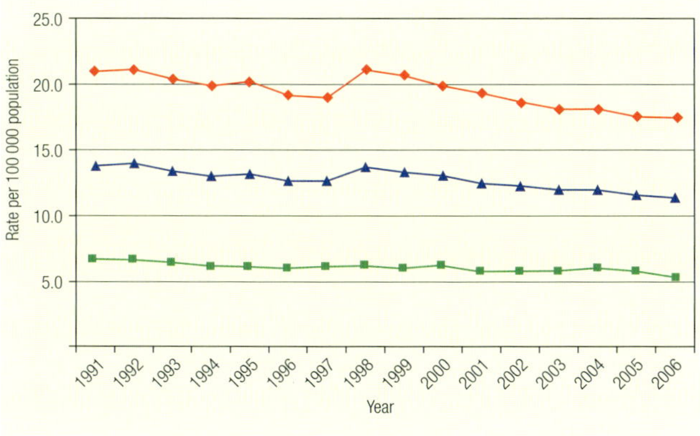

Figure 54.1 UK suicide rates 1991–2006 (rate per 100 000 population)

Source: Office for National Statistics (2008).

suicide rate is estimated to be $17/10^5$/year, and suicide accounts for 1 per cent of female deaths and 2 per cent of male deaths.[6]

The highest suicide rates are found in Russia, Belarus and Lithuania ($36–42/10^5$/year) (Table 54.1).[7] In the USA the suicide rate varies by state; for example, in Washington, DC, it is $7/10^5$/year but in Nevada it is $23/10^5$/year (the national average is $11/10^5$/year).[8] The differences in the suicide rates across European countries cannot be explained solely by sociocultural differences, and population genetics may be a relevant factor; for example, Hungary and Finland have populations with a common genetic origin and a high rate of suicide, but they differ greatly in their economic, cultural and political histories.[9]

In England, the most common methods of suicide are hanging for men and drug poisoning for women (Table 54.2).[10] The preferred methods of suicide appear to be influenced by the available means. There are four notable examples:

- *Coal gas:* until 1965, poisoning with domestic coal gas accounted for half of all suicides. Natural gas was introduced in 1965 and in the following years the suicide rate declined without any evidence of method substitution.[11]
- *Firearms:* in North America, firearms are involved in 60 per cent of male suicides and 30 per cent of female suicides. States with the most restrictive gun laws have the fewest suicides involving firearms and lower suicide rates overall.[12]
- *Vehicle exhaust:* in England, from 1993 onwards, it was required that new cars should be fitted with catalytic converters, which oxidize carbon monoxide (CO) to carbon dioxide (CO_2). Suicide by exhaust inhalation, once the most popular male method, declined by 90 per cent over the following decade.[13] However, over the same period, there was an increase in male suicide by hanging, suggesting method substitution.[14]
- *Analgesics:* from 1998, the size of packets of analgesics that could be sold over the counter at retail outlets was restricted by English law to 32 tablets. Subsequently, suicide deaths from paracetamol and salicylates reduced by 22 per cent.[15,16]

Table 54.1 Reported suicide rates by country per 100 000 population: representative data

$0–3/10^5$	$4–7/10^5$	$8–13/10^5$	$14–20/10^5$	$21–42/10^5$
Greece	Italy	Australia	France	Lithuania
Paraguay	UK	Ireland	Switzerland	Belarus
Philippines	Argentina	Portugal	Poland	Russia
Azerbaijan	Israel	Norway	China	Kazakhstan
Bahamas	Brazil	India	Denmark	Japan
Egypt	Thailand	Netherlands	Sweden	Finland

Source: World Health Organization (2003).

Table 54.2 Method of suicide: England and Wales, 1979–2001

Method	Males (%)	Females (%)
Hanging	44	27
Drug-related poisoning	20	46
Other poisoning*	10	3
Other and unspecified	9	9
Drowning	5	7
Moving object (e.g. train)	4	3
Firearms and explosives	3	1
Sharp objects	2	1
Jumping/falling from high place	3	3

*Mainly vehicle exhaust.

Source: Office for National Statistics (2003).

The choice of method is influenced by sociodemographic factors. Jumping from high places is preferred by youths, compared with drowning, which is a choice of older people. In Asia, ingestion of pesticides in rural areas is common and self-immolation is commonly observed in Asian women.

Sociodemographic factors associating with suicide

Gender

Annual suicide rates are higher for men than for women in all countries, except China, where the obverse applies. In England, the male/female ratio is 3 : 1 (see Figure 54.1).

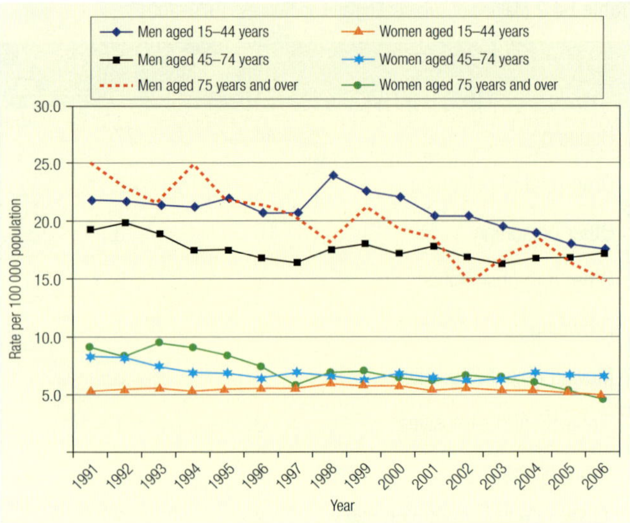

Figure 54.2 UK age-standardized suicide rate per 100 000 population, 1991–2006

Source: Office for National Statistics (2008).

Age

In children under 10 years of age, the suicide rate is near zero. In 10- to 14-year-olds, the rate is approximately $1/10^5$/year. From age 15 years, the rate approximates that of the adult population.[17] In adults, there is not a consistent association between suicide rate and age. For example, in 1991 elderly people (≥75 years) had higher rates of suicide than young adults, but from 1998 the suicide rate in elderly people has been lower (Figure 54.2).[13,18]

Occupation and social class

In the UK, the standardized mortality ratio (SMR) for suicide is four times higher for men from social class V compared with those in social class I.[19] However, proportional mortality ratios (PMR) show minimal class differences.[20] An unemployed man has a two to three times greater probability of suicide than his employed counterparts (Figure 54.3).

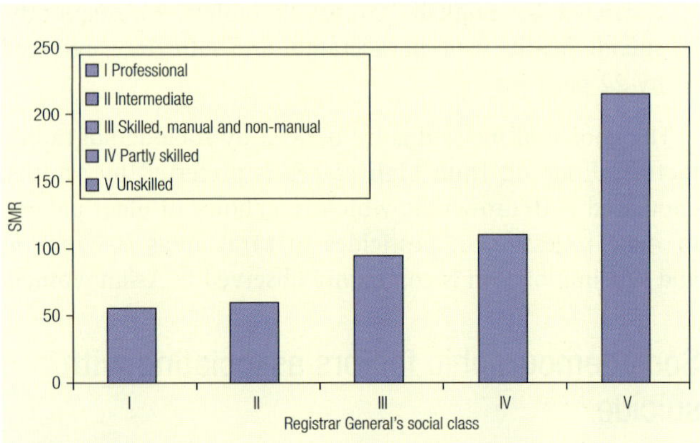

Figure 54.3 Social class and suicide: representative UK data

SMR, standardized mortality ratio.

Source: Office for National Statistics (2008).

Suicide rates are higher in certain professionals, such as veterinarians, dentists, pharmacists, doctors, salespeople, farmers, publicans, drivers and nurses.[21] Access to means may be a relevant factor – for example, drugs for healthcare practitioners and pesticides and guns for farmers. Students are not at special risk of suicide.

Marital status and sexuality

Marital status shows a weak or inconsistent association with suicide. Among women, there are no statistically significant differentials in the risk of suicide by marital status categories. The relative risk (RR) of suicide is about 2 in divorced or separated men, but the association with bachelor or widower status is variable between studies.[22] Young homosexual men and women are two to three times more likely to attempt suicide than other young people.

Ethnicity

The data on ethnic or racial group and suicide are inconsistent and hard to interpret.[23] For example, the rate of suicide in minority ethnic groups is higher where such groups are in a small minority, but lower where they form a large minority of the population.[24]

Temporal patterns

In both hemispheres, the rate of suicide in winter months is half that of the rest of the year, but such seasonal variations are now diminishing.[25,26] Data from the UK and Japan indicate that 15 per cent more suicides occur on Mondays than on other days of the week.[27,28] The cause or significance of these temporal associations is not known.

Criminality

A history of criminal or violent behaviour is associated with suicide. The SMR for suicide in prison inmates is 5, with a particular excess in boys aged 15–17 years (SMR 18).[29] Ninety per cent of prisoner suicides are by hanging. A third of cases have a past psychiatric history and half have a history of parasuicide.

Intelligence

Gunnell and colleagues found that the level of performance on a logic test was inversely correlated with the suicide rate (Figure 54.4).[30] In these Swedish male conscripts, the risk of suicide was three times higher in those with low, rather than high, logic test performance.

Psychobiology of suicide

Inheritance

A seminal study of the Old Order Amish community found that 26 suicides over a century occurred predominantly in four families in which mood disorder was also common. Other families with a similarly high prevalence of mood disorder did not contain any cases of suicide.[31]

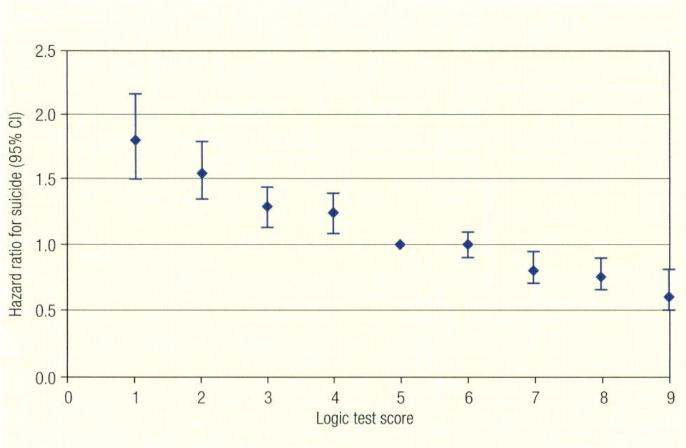

Figure 54.4 Fully adjusted suicide hazard ratios by categories of logic intelligence test score (category 5 is reference)

CI, confidence interval.

Reproduced from Gunnell *et al.* (2005).[30]

Roy and Segal examined the surviving twin of 28 twin pairs who had died by suicide. Four of 13 monozygotic (MZ) twins had attempted suicide compared with 0 of 15 dizygotic (DZ) twins.[32] This finding is consistent with a previous study of 176 twin pairs in each of which at least 1 twin had committed suicide: in 9 of these twin pairs, both had committed suicide; of these 9, 7 were among 62 MZ pairs and 2 among 114 DZ pairs ($P<0.01$).[33]

After adjustment for psychological, psychiatric and social factors, the heritability of suicidal behaviours is estimated to be 30–50 per cent.[34–36] However, many human behavioural traits have similar levels of heritability, for example extroversion.[37,38]

A number of genes have been proposed as candidates for transmission of suicidal propensities, but these associations are not replicated consistently (Table 54.3).[39]

Neurobiology

Elevated plasma and urinary levels of cortisol, and decreased output of urinary homovanillic acid (HVA), have been found in patients who attempt suicide in comparison with non-suicidal patient controls.[40–42]

Many studies of 5-hydoxyindoleacetic acid (5-HIAA; a major metabolite of serotonin) in the cerebrospinal fluid (CSF) have produced convergent results, including:[43]

- lower 5-HIAA levels in suicide attempters and completers than in controls;
- levels of CSF 5-HIAA are significantly lower in high-lethality compared with low-lethality attempters;
- low 5-HIAA also associates with greater impulsivity and likelihood of repetition;
- studies of the association between CSF 5-HIAA levels and the tryptophan hydroxylase (*TPH*) gene reveal that carriers of the 779C allele for the *TPH* gene are more likely to have low CSF 5-HIAA concentrations.[44] Impulsive offenders with a suicidal history are also more likely to carry the 779C allele, suggesting a common link between low 5-HIAA, impulsivity and suicidality.[45] The A218C polymorphism in intron 7 of the *TPH* gene does not show any association with suicidal behaviours.[46]

Other data implicating brain serotonin function in suicide include evidence of a blunted prolactin response to fenfluramine in suicide attempters, and reduced 5-hydroxytryptamine (5-HT) uptake, fewer serotonin transporter (5-HTT) sites, and increased density of 5-HT2A receptors in the platelets of suicide attempters.[47–49]

Findings from postmortem brain studies of suicide cases include:

- reduced binding sites for corticotropin-releasing hormone (CRH);[50]
- decreased presynaptic serotonergic binding sites;

Table 54.3 Association analyses of genes predisposing to suicide or suicidal behaviour

Gene	Locus	Association evidence
Serotonin transporter	17q11.2	7 positive and 7 negative studies; 2 positive meta-analyses
Tryptophan hydroxylase	11p15–14	5 positive and 7 negative studies; 2 positive meta-analyses; 1 negative meta-analysis
Monoamine oxidase A	Xp11.23	3 positive and 2 negative studies
Serotonin receptor 1A (*5-HT1A*)	5q11.2–q13	1 positive and 2 negative studies
Serotonin receptor 1B (*5-HT1B*)	6q13	1 positive and 5 negative studies
Serotonin receptor 2A (*5-HT2A*)	13q14.2	3 positive and 9 negative studies; 1 negative meta-analysis
Catechol-O-methyltransferase (*COMT*)	22q11.21	3 positive and 2 negative studies
Dopamine receptor 2 (*DRD2*)	11q23	1 positive and 1 negative studies
Dopamine receptor 4 (*DRD4*)	11p15.5	2 negative studies

Source: Savitz *et al.* (2006).[39]

- increased gene expression of 5-HT2A receptors;[51]
- an association between completed suicide and alterations in both the phosphoinositide and adenylyl cyclase/cyclic adenosine monophosphate (cAMP) signalling systems;[52,53]
- decreased binding of [3H]phorbol dibutyrate to protein kinase C.[54]

Abnormalities have also been described in noradrenaline function, for example fewer noradrenergic neurons in the locus coeruleus of suicide cases, increased brainstem levels of tyrosine hydroxylase and lower levels of postsynaptic adrenergic receptors in the cortex.[20]

Notwithstanding the interesting nature of many of the neurobiological findings, considerable caution must be applied in interpreting them. A complete theory of how the neurobiological associations might relate to psychological functions and to the ultimate choice to kill oneself has yet to emerge.

Suicide and mental disorders

Overview

In Barraclough and colleagues' historic study of 100 cases of suicide, the antemortem psychiatric state was considered to be depression in 70 per cent of cases, alcoholism in 15 per cent, schizophrenia in 3 per cent, anxiety disorder in 3 per cent, other diagnoses in 2 per cent and 'not mentally ill' in 7 per cent.[55] This study was pivotal in portraying suicide as consequent on mental illness, and subsequent studies have produced convergent findings (Table 54.4).[56–59]

Table 54.4 Diagnoses in cases of completed suicide

Principal diagnosis	%
Depressive disorder	32
Substance-related disorder	20
Personality disorder	10
Anxiety disorders	10
Schizophrenia	9
Other DSM axis I diagnosis	5
No mental disorder	5
Insufficient information	5
Bipolar disorder	3
Organic disorder	1
Schizoaffective and other psychoses	<1

DSM, *Diagnostic and Statistical Manual of Mental Disorders.*

Cases of suicide with any axis I diagnosis constituted 80–90 per cent of the total suicides in most studies.

Bipolar disorder

The annual incidence of suicide in people with bipolar disorder is about 0.15 per cent, with a case fatality index (CFI; the percentage of patients who end life by suicide) of 3 per cent over 20 years.[60] Suicide attempts occur at a rate of 1 per cent per year. The lifetime rate for suicide attempts is 52 per cent versus 26 per cent, respectively, for patients with and without a family history of suicide.[61]

Schizophrenia

Estimates of the CFI in schizophrenia based upon individual studies of up to 22 years' follow-up range from 2 per cent to 30 per cent. A meta-analysis found a CFI of 5.6 per cent, with a preponderance of suicide occurring early in the course of the disorder.[62] The SMR for suicide in schizophrenia is about 12.[63] The associations of suicide within schizophrenia (i.e. comparing living people with schizophrenia versus people with schizophrenia who died by suicide) are summarized in Table 54.5.[64] The associations of suicide within schizophrenia are different from those that apply in the general population. For example, family history of suicide, alcohol misuse, gender and living alone show a weak or absent association in schizophrenia in contrast to suicides generally.

Table 54.5 Associations of suicide within schizophrenia

Risk factor	Relative risk
Recent suicide ideation	12
Fear of mental disintegration	6
Drug misuse or dependence	2.5
Recent depression	2.5
Recent loss	2.5
History of suicide attempt	2
Past depression	2
Poor compliance with treatment	2
Past suicidal ideation	2
Hallucinations	0.5

Source: Hawton *et al.* (2005).[64]

Depression

In an epidemiological study of depressed cases, Simon and VonKorff found that the standardized incidence rate for suicide in depression was related to greater severity and morbidity: 224 suicides/10^5 person-years in ever-hospitalized patients, 43/10^5 person-years in general practice (GP) cases, and 0/10^5 person-years in cases not judged to be in need of antidepressants.[65] Thus, alarmist assertions that 'up to 15 per cent of patients with unipolar depression eventually commit suicide' apply only to an extremely ill minority of patients with depression.[66]

Alcohol use

Suicide occurs in 2–3 per cent of patients with hospital-treated alcoholism. This represents an SMR of 60–120 times the risk of suicide compared with those without psychiatric illness in the general population.[67] Co-morbid alcohol misuse is found in 20 per cent of all suicides.[68] Heavier drinking (≥414 g/week = 52 units/week) is associated with a RR of 2.3 for suicide compared with occasional drinkers. Alcohol abstainers also have a RR of 2.3 for suicide compared WITH occasional drinkers.[69] This may be because former alcoholics are a part of the group of current abstainers.

Cannabis

Beautrais and colleagues concluded that much of the association between cannabis misuse and suicide attempts arises because cannabis misusers tend to come from disadvantaged backgrounds and have co-morbid mental disorders.[70] Nevertheless, cannabis misuse may make an independent contribution to risk of suicide attempts.

Personality disorders

There is an unequivocal association between personality and suicidal behaviour, most evident in young people and in people with cluster B personality disorders. Seventeen per cent of adolescent suicides meet criteria for conduct disorder or antisocial personality disorder (APD).[71] People with borderline personality disorder represent 9–33 per cent of all suicides, and the CFI is 3–10 per cent.[72] The RR of suicide in APD is about 9 and the CFI is 5 per cent.

There is a strong association between an adult's suicidal propensities and having experienced brutality, humiliation and abuse in childhood.[73] A person's upbringing shapes their adult personality, and Harlow's experiments on primates remain an easily understood analogue for the effects of abuse and deprivation on human personality adjustment.[74]

Other clinical groups

The suicide rate in admitted psychiatric patients is 13 per 10 000 admissions, equal in males and females. This implies a RR of 100–200 compared with the population base rate. Three-quarters of these suicides occur while the patient is on leave from hospital. The most common method is drowning (30%). Hanging, being hit by a train, jumping and self-poisoning each account for 10–15 per cent of cases.[75] The peaks of suicide in relation to hospitalization are in the first week after admission and the first week after discharge.[76] Seven in 10 000 patients kill themselves within 28 days of discharge from psychiatric hospital.[77]

The RR of suicide in the postnatal period is low (SMR 1.14), and suicide is a leading cause of maternal deaths in this period only because other causes of death are even rarer. However, suicide occurs in 1 in 500 cases of postnatal psychosis, and in these cases the utmost clinical vigilance is required.[78]

Treatment factors

Some medicines may be pro-suicidal and others anti-suicidal.

Antidepressants

The current balance of evidence regarding the pro-suicidal effects of selective serotonin reuptake inhibitors (SSRIs) is as follows:

- In adults aged 19–64 years, SSRI use is not associated with suicide attempts or suicide deaths (odds ratio (OR) about 0.85).[79]
- In children and young people aged 6–18 years, SSRI use is associated with suicide attempts (OR = 1.52) and suicide deaths (OR = 15.62; 95% confidence interval (CI) 1.65 to infinity).[80]
- In elderly people, there is an association between violent suicide and SSRIs (OR = 4.8), but not with other antidepressants.[81]

Atomoxetine

Six suicide-related events, but no actual suicides, were identified in 1357 paediatric patients with attention deficit hyperactivity disorder (ADHD) receiving atomoxetine, while no events were seen in the 851 patients taking placebo.[82]

Anti-epileptics

In clinical trials of anti-epileptics, the rate of suicide was 4/28 000 in subjects receiving anti-epileptics and 0/16 000 on placebo. Emergent suicidal ideation occurred in 105 and 35 subjects, respectively.[83] Epilepsy itself confers a threefold increase in the probability for suicide over the population base rate.[84]

Other agents

The *British National Formulary* (BNF) lists suicide attempts as a side effect of interferon-beta and systemic corticosteroids, suicide risk as a contraindication to disulfiram, and suicidal ideation as a caution in the use of the CB1 inverse agonist rimonabant.[85] A supposed association between isotretinoin and suicide is not supported by the available data.[86]

Lithium

The current data support the view that lithium is specifically anti-suicidal in comparison with placebo and other mood stabilizers in bipolar disorder, and its use would be associated with 50 per cent fewer suicides than might otherwise be the case.[87]

Clozapine

Clozapine may be anti-suicidal in schizophrenia.[88,89] The InterSePT study compared clozapine and olanzapine (n = 980).[90] Over 2 years, 7 per cent of clozapine-treated patients attempted suicide compared with 11 per cent of patients taking olanzapine (P = 0.03). There was no significant difference in the frequency of completed suicide (5 clozapine-treated patients *v.* 3 olanzapine-treated patients; P = 0.73).

Suicide prevention

Approaches to suicide prevention can be grouped as follows:[91]

- *Whole-population strategies:* at a whole-population level, suicide rates are probably amenable to influence. Proposed approaches include improving social welfare (e.g. employment, housing), school and workplace mental-health promotion, public education, action on alcohol and drugs, and controlling access to means of suicide (e.g. plastic-bag design, firearms).
- *High-risk subgroups strategies:* approaches to high-risk subgroups include providing counselling services for socially dislocated young males, offering assistance for children leaving care, improving the assessment of parasuicide cases in accident and emergency departments, and improving the recognition of depression in GP populations. The Gotland Study demonstrated that educating GPs in the treatment of depression reduced that island's suicide rate, although some authors have disputed the generalizability of the findings.[92]
- *Mental health services:* substantial investment in National Health Service (NHS) mental health services in England has been accompanied by changes in service delivery aimed in part at reducing suicide rates. Initiatives include crisis intervention teams, 24-h access to services, and removing ligature points from in-patient environments. The unifying theme is that by effecting overall improvements in mental health services, fewer suicides will occur.
- *Case-by-case intervention:* the optimistic account of suicide prevention at a policy level appears discordant with the views of many clinical practitioners that suicide is hardly preventable in an individual patient. Such latter views are not irrational. Obtaining even minimal sensitivity (i.e. true positives) in predicting suicide is at the expense of an overwhelming number of false-positive predictions, for example a ratio of about 1 : 50 reported by Powell and colleagues.[75] Nonetheless, clinicians will reasonably strive to minimize the potential for suicide in their patients. A conventional account is to view the relevant risk factors as (i) static, (ii) stable, (iii) dynamic and (iv) future.[93] Although the format provides no calculus of risk (e.g. if a person got married but lost their job, would there be a net increase or net decrease in their suicide potential?), it is nevertheless a suitable one for articulating the evaluation of a patient. However, whether any specific clinical action with any individual patient at any particular point in time alters the overall trajectory of that patient towards, or away from, suicide, is very hard to test empirically (Table 54.6).

An aim of the National Suicide Prevention Strategy for England was to achieve a 15 per cent reduction in the rate of suicide by 2010.[94] Key points from this strategy and other related documents are summarized in Box 54.2.[95–97]

Trends have been favourable (see Figures 54.1 and 54.2), although establishing a causal association between policy intention and observed outcome cannot be asserted unequivocally. Supporting the strategy is the National Confidential Inquiry into Suicide and Homicide by People with Mental Illness.[96,97] This inquiry collects clinical data on all cases of suicide by people in contact with mental health services in the UK and makes periodic recommendations that carry considerable political weight (see Box 54.2).

PARASUICIDE

Definition and terminology

There is no completely satisfactory terminology covering the behaviours of people who injure or poison themselves

Table 54.6 Static, stable, dynamic and future factors in suicide

Static factors (permanent or now immutable features)	Stable factors (long-term, likely to persist, but not fixed)	Dynamic factors (highly variable in extent or persistence)	Future factors (unknown future state of affairs)
Gender	Age	Substance abuse	Response to treatment
Family background	Enduring mental illness	Anxiety symptoms	Bereavement
History of overdose	Personality	Relationship conflict	Onset of physical disease
Childhood deprivation	Marital/parenting status	Cognitions	
	Life skills	Compliance with treatment	

Source: Bouch and Marshall (2005).[93]

Box 54.2 Governmental recommendations for suicide prevention

STRATEGIES FOR SUICIDE PREVENTION (1999–2002)[94]

- Staff training in the management of risk
- Highest level of care programme approach (CPA) for in-patients with severe mental illness and self-harm
- Care plans to specify to deal with non-compliance with pharmacotherapy
- Prompt access to services for people in crisis and their families
- Assertive outreach teams
- Promote use of atypical antipsychotic drugs
- Special services for co-morbid substance misuse with mental illness
- In-patient wards to remove or cover all likely ligature points
- 7-day follow-up of discharged in-patients
- Prescribe only small quantities of medication to patients who self-harm
- Post-incident case reviews.

NATIONAL INSTITUTE FOR HEALTH AND CLINICAL EXCELLENCE (2004)[98]

- Assessment of needs and risks
- Sharing the written assessment with the service user
- Including social, psychological and motivational factors specific to the act in the assessment of self-harm
- Using a standardized risk assessment scale to identify patients at high risk of repetition of self-harm or suicide but not to use it to identify patients at low risk who are not then offered services
- Providing the service user with relevant written information about treatments and services.

MEASURES TO REDUCE SUICIDES (2006)[97]

- Improved observation and physical environment in psychiatric wards
- Strengthen the transition from ward to community.

with a non-fatal outcome. Various terms that are commonly used to describe these are set out in Box 54.3.[98] Kreitman and colleagues rejected the term 'attempted suicide' on the grounds that the great majority of patients so designated were not, in fact, attempting suicide.[99] Instead, the term 'parasuicide' was proposed to represent 'an act which is like suicide, yet is something other than suicide'. The definition adopted by the World Health Organization (WHO)/EURO Multicentre Study on Parasuicide was:

Box 54.3 Commonly applied terms to describe the behaviours of people who injure or poison themselves with a non-fatal outcome

- Self-harm
- Deliberate self-harm
- Intentional self-harm
- Parasuicide
- Attempted suicide
- Failed suicide
- Non-fatal suicidal behaviour
- Self-inflicted violence
- Self-poisoning
- Self-injury
- Self-mutilation.

> An act with non-fatal outcome in which an individual deliberately initiates a non-habitual behavior, that without intervention from others will cause self-harm, or deliberately ingests a substance in excess of the prescribed or generally recognized dosage, and which is aimed at realizing changes that the person desires via the actual or expected physical consequences.[100]

It may be that standardization of the terminology can never be achieved because the cases being referred to are diverse with respect to both the intention behind the act and the degree of medical seriousness that results. Thus, clinically, the preferred term will be the one that best describes the patient under consideration at the time.

Epidemiology

Incidence

The person-based incidence of parasuicide is approximately $170/10^5$ population/year in Europe, with regional averages concealing local variations, for example Cergy-Pontoise (France) – $440/10^5$/year, Guipuzcoa (Spain) – $60/10^5$/year.[101] In the USA and Canada, the figures are $225/10^5$/year and $304/10^5$/year, respectively.[102,103]

England, in the uppermost quartile for Europe, has a presentation rate of parasuicide of above $300/10^5$/year and an admission rate of about $130/10^5$/year. Within England, adjacent postal districts show up to a seven-fold difference in the rate of parasuicide. In England, as elsewhere, there is an association with social deprivation and average income; the rate of parasuicide in the most disadvantaged quintile of the population is three to four times that of the least disadvantaged quintile.[104,105]

Changes over time

In England, rates of parasuicide increased in the 1960s and 1970s and have thereafter fluctuated in the range 250–$350/10^5$/year (Figure 54.5). Data from both Belgian and English studies found an increasing rate of parasuicide among young males (aged 15–42 years) in the 1980s to 1990s, but this increase has not been sustained.[106]

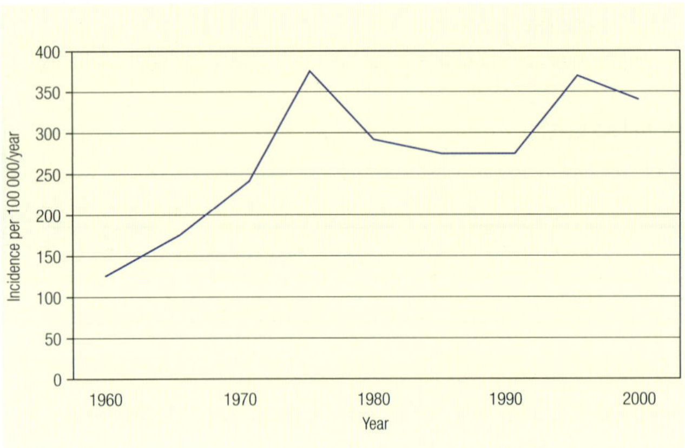

Figure 54.5 Parasuicide rates in the UK: representative data

Age and gender

People aged 15–24 years account for 40 per cent of cases, 25- to 34-year-olds for 25 per cent of cases, 35- to 44-year-olds for 15 per cent of cases, 45- to 54-year-olds for 10 per cent of cases, and people aged 55 years and older for 10 per cent of cases.[107,108] Some 60 per cent of parasuicide cases are females.

Method

Self-poisoning accounts for 80–90 per cent of presentations. Paracetamol is employed in some 40 per cent of overdoses, antidepressants (mainly SSRIs) in 30 per cent, minor tranquillizers in 20 per cent, non-opiate analgesics other than paracetamol in 10 per cent, and other diverse substances in 30 per cent; overdoses commonly involve more than one substance, and hence the sum is greater than 100 per cent. Self-injury accounts for 10–15 per cent of presentations; of these, three-quarters involve cutting to the arm or wrist.[109]

Non-clinical populations

Klonsky and colleagues found that 4 per cent of young male and female air force recruits engaged in recurrent self-harm.[110] In this population, a history of self-harm was correlated with features of nearly all the *Diagnostic and Statistical Manual*, 4th edition (DSM-IV) personality types, schizotypal, borderline, dependent and avoidant in particular. In the general population, 3–5 per cent of people have had some degree of suicidal thinking in the past year and 1 per cent in the past week.[111,112]

Psychosocial factors

Diagnostic associations

Some 30–70 per cent of people who present with parasuicide are depressed at the point of presentation. Around the time of parasuicide, the average score on the Montgomery Åsberg Depression Rating Scale is 25 points.[108,113–115] However, using the Personality Assessment Schedule,[116] Haw and colleagues found that 46 per cent of cases have personality disorder and an additional 33 per cent have 'accentuated personality traits'.[108] This observation, and the fact that a quarter of cases exhibit harmful use of alcohol, suggests that the concept of 'depression' in this group is a broad one. Diagnoses of distinct and severe mental illness (e.g. bipolar disorder, schizophrenia) are found in no more than 5 per cent of parasuicide cases.[108,113] Anxiety, stress-related and somatoform disorders are found in approximately 25 per cent of cases and eating disorders in 10 per cent. A single-term diagnosis is an inadequate characterization of most parasuicide cases who commonly exhibit multiple and overlapping psychopathologies.

Personality genetics

Many studies have described strong associations between personality traits and parasuicide. These traits include aggression, anxiety, neuroticism, impulsivity, hostility and psychoticism.[117] Personality traits are influenced by genetics and polymorphisms coding for the serotonin transporter, 5-HT1A, 5-HT2A, 5-HT1B and 5-HT3B receptors, have been variously associated with traits such as neuroticism, anger and impulsivity. These same polymorphisms have also shown an association with suicidal thoughts and behaviour.[117,118] It is plausible that the effect of 'parasuicide genes' is mediated through an intermediate effect on personality.

Social problems

Common clinical experience is that there has usually been some emotional problem preceding parasuicide. Hawton and colleagues found these problems to be with partners (in 50% of cases), family members (40%), employment (30%) and finances (20%).[109] Alcohol had been consumed in the 6 h preceding parasuicide by 45 per cent of women and 55 per cent of men.

Problem-solving

One tenable psychological model of parasuicide proposes that what such cases have in common are deficient strategies for problem-solving; for example, having a passive rather than an active response to problems and perceiving the negative outcomes as more likely than possible positive outcomes. Thus, 'hopelessness', historically given great emphasis as a mediating variable in suicidal behaviour, may have a complex relationship with other variables such as deficient problem-solving, cognitive rigidity and dichotomous thinking.[101]

Assessment

Repetition or progression

In clinical populations, 16 per cent of parasuicide cases repeat self-harm within 6 months and 25 per cent over 10 years.[119–123] Completed suicide occurs in 1–2 per cent of cases in the first year after parasuicide and in 3–7 per cent over 10 years. [119–123] In the most disturbed cases (e.g. people with schizophrenia or severe borderline personality disorder), completed suicide occurs in 10–15 per cent over 10–20 years.[124]

Assessment

In England it is NHS policy that all patients presenting with parasuicide should be subject to an assessment by a suitably skilled professional.[98,125] The content of such an assessment has been described in various ways, but for the psychiatrist it amounts to obtaining a full psychiatric history and mental state examination, leading to a working diagnosis or formulation as a basis for further action.

It is conventional when assessing parasuicide cases to take account of risk factors for repetition and subsequent progression to completed suicide. The factors mentioned in the National Institute of Health and Clinical Excellence (NICE) Clinical guideline 16 (Table 54.7) are those most commonly cited.[98]

However, the limitations of the conventional account of risk factors are readily apparent. For example, the weight that should be accorded to particular features is undefined, many features are matters of degree rather than category, and co-linear relationships between certain items would be expected. Thus, although it is easy to say *what* factors should be taken into account, meaningful proposals about *how* they should be taken into account have yet to be made.

Screening

It might be that structured screening and assessment instruments would offer some assistance, but the findings are not encouraging. A meta-analysis of the Beck Hopelessness Scale (BHS) found a sensitivity of 80 per cent and a specificity of 40 per cent for detecting completed suicide.[126,127] In a typical clinical environment, this would yield a positive predictive value (PPV) of little more than 1 per cent. Furthermore, with the Suicide Intent Scale (SIS),[128] there have been counterintuitive findings; for example, among male patients, 12.4 per cent of those with high SIS scores harmed themselves again within 12 months compared with 22.3 per cent of those with low SIS scores ($\chi^2 = 18.26$, $P < 0.0001$).[129] Although the BHS, SIS or SAD PERSONS scales may aid the clinician in the process of assessment, they do not form a valid basis for clinical decisions.[130]

Mental capacity

It is common for people presenting with parasuicide to be uncooperative with assessment and to discharge themselves prematurely from accident and emergency (A&E)

Table 54.7 Risk factors for repetition of non-fatal self-harm and for completed suicide, as described in National Institute of Health and Clinical Excellence (NICE) Clinical guideline 16

Non-fatal repetition of self-harm	Completed suicide
History of self-harm before the current episode	Older age
Psychiatric history, especially as an in-patient	Male
Current unemployment	Previous attempts
Lower social class	Psychiatric history (especially in-patient treatment)
Alcohol- or drug-related problems	Unemployment
Criminal record	Poor physical health
Antisocial personality	Living alone
Uncooperative with general hospital treatment	Medical severity of the act, especially near-fatal self-harm
Hopelessness	Hopelessness
High suicidal intent	Continuing high suicidal intent

departments. Where a patient is refusing essential clinical attention, their mental capacity should be evaluated. If a patient lacks mental capacity (even temporarily), then they may be prevented from leaving an A&E department without the use of the Mental Health Act.[98,131]

Management following parasuicide

Where a presentation with parasuicide reveals a distinct psychiatric diagnosis, then the management will be that of the condition in question. It is more difficult to decide on the appropriate attention for the broader group of parasuicide cases characterized by marginal depressive symptoms, situational problems, aberrant personality features and an absence of distinct mental illness. Psychiatric admission is seldom productive, and compliance with out-patient or community follow-up is poor even when waiting times are minimal.[132]

Studies of psychosocial or psychotherapeutic interventions aimed at reducing the repetition rate for self-harm have produced inconclusive results.[133] The POPMACT study compared brief, manual-assisted cognitive-behavioural therapy (CBT) with treatment-as-usual (TAU) in 400 people.[114] The 12-month repetition rate did not differ between CBT and TAU (39% *v*. 46%, $P = 0.20$). Conversely, Guthrie and colleagues found that brief psychodynamic therapy was associated with a reduced recurrence of self-harm compared with TAU (9% *v*. 28%, $n = 119$, $P = 0.015$).[134] Dialectical behaviour therapy (DBT) is commonly cited as being of special benefit for prevention of repeated parasuicide.[135] The repetition rate at 1 year was found to be 59 per cent for DBT versus 95 per cent for usual psychotherapy ($n = 50$, $P < 0.01$). Tarrier and colleagues concluded that, although many studies produce favourable results, optimism is tempered by evidence of publication bias.[136]

Providing patients with contact cards permitting on-demand access to care has not been shown to have an effect on repetition rate (3 studies; $n = 1144$, RR = 0.79, 95% CI 0.39 to 1.57).[137–139]

It is doubtful whether pharmacotherapy has a role in the management of repeated parasuicide. Montgomery and colleagues demonstrated a clinically significant effect of low-dose (20 mg) depot flupentixol in reducing repetition of self-harm.[140]A study versus placebo showed equivocal benefit for paroxetine on the repetition of self-harm over 1 year ($n = 91$, 47% *v*. 33%, $P = 0.12$).[141] Studies specifically in borderline personality disorder (taking these to be likely cases for parasuicide) have shown benefits for patients taking olanzapine but not ziprasidone on psychopathology.[141–143] On balance, although there are sufficient data to support the use of pharmacotherapy where a clinician feels so inclined, general recommendations cannot be made.

Ultimately, there is no management of parasuicide per se because parasuicide is a behaviour rather than a disease or disorder and marks the presence of many social, psychological, personality and psychiatric dysfunctions. Until such time as there are major research advances, management remains a matter of clinical judgement on a case-by-case basis.

CONCLUSION

The biomedical literature on suicide emphasizes the search for deterministic causes of suicide, but the most that can be said at present is that it is multifactorial. There are many philosophical and ethical questions that could be raised. For example, can suicide be considered a choice that people make? If so, is it rational or irrational, and what standard of rationality would apply? How is it that deaths by suicide become referred to as 'tragedies' but deaths by motor vehicle as 'accidents'? Such questions, although beyond the scope of this text, invite considerable reflection.

KEY POINTS

- In England, the current annual suicide rate is about $10.5/10^5$ population and the parasuicide rate is about $300/10^5$/year.
- Although many social, clinical and biological associations have been identified, a satisfactory explanatory model of suicide has yet to be proposed.
- Population-based or public health measures to reduce suicide can be effective.
- The ability of clinicians to predict suicide in individual clinical cases is minimal.
- Suicide and parasuicide cases differ substantially in their clinical and sociodemographic characteristics.
- Mental illness is common in cases of suicide but uncommon in cases of parasuicide.
- The essence of assessing a parasuicide case is to take the psychiatric history and examine the mental state, from which formulation and management will follow.
- The evidence that psychotherapies reduce the repetition rates for parasuicide is inconclusive.

REFERENCES

1. Durkheim E (2001) *Le suicide: étude de sociologie.* Boston, MA: Adamant Media Corporation.
2. O'Donnell I, Farmer R (1995) The limitations of official suicide statistics. *British Journal of Psychiatry* **166**: 458–61.
3. Neeleman J, Wessely S (1997) Changes in classification of suicide in England and Wales: time trends and associations with coroners' professional backgrounds. *Psychological Medicine* **27**: 467–72.
4. (1961) *The Suicide Act (c.60).* London: The Stationery Office.
5. Baker A, Brock A, Fegan G, *et al.* (2006) Suicide trends

and geographical variations in the United Kingdom, 1991–2004. *Health Statistics Quarterly* **31**: 6–22.
6. Bertolote JM, Fleischmann A (2002) Suicide and psychiatric diagnosis: a worldwide perspective. *World Psychiatry* **1**: 181–5.
7. World Health Organization (1999) *Figures and Facts About Suicide*. Geneva: World Health Organization.
8. American Association of Suicidology (2005) *National Suicide Statistics*. New York: American Association of Suicidology. www.suicidology.org/web/guest/stats-and-tools/statistics.
9. Marusic A, Farmer A (2001) Genetic risk factors as possible causes of the variation in European suicide rates. *British Journal of Psychiatry* **179**: 194–6.
10. Brock A, Griffiths C (2003) Trends in suicide by method in England and Wales, 1979 to 2001. *Health Statistics Quarterly* **20**: 7–18.
11. Kreitman N (1976) The coal gas story: United Kingdom suicide rates, 1960–1971. *British Journal of Preventative and Social Medicine* **30**: 86–93.
12. Connor KR, Zhong Y (2003) State firearm laws and rates of suicide in men and women. *American Journal of Preventive Medicine* **25**: 320–24.
13. Biddle L, Brock A, Brookes S, Gunnell D (2008) Suicide rates in young men in England and Wales in the 21st century: time trend study. *British Medical Journal* **336**: 539–42.
14. Amos T, Appleby L, Kiernan K (2001) Changes in rates of suicide by car exhaust asphyxiation in England and Wales. *Psychological Medicine* **31**: 935–9.
15. Hawton K, Townsend E, Deeks J, *et al.* (2001) Effects of legislation restricting pack sizes of paracetamol and salicylate on self poisoning in the United Kingdom: before and after study. *British Medical Journal* **322**: 1–7.
16. Morgan O, Griffiths C (2005) Impact of paracetamol pack size restrictions on poisoning from paracetamol in England and Wales: an observational study. *Journal of Public Health* **27**: 19–24.
17. McClure GMG (2001) Suicide in children and adolescents in England and Wales 1970–1998. *British Journal of Psychiatry* **178**: 469–74.
18. Office for National Statistics (2009) UK Suicide Rates Continue to Fall. London: Office for National Statistics. www.statistics.gov.uk/cci/nugget.asp?id=1092.
19. Kreitman N, Carstairs V, Duffy J (1991) Association of age and social class with suicide among men in Great Britain. *Journal of Epidemiology and Community Health* **45**: 195–202.
20. Griffiths C, Ladva G, Brock A, Baker A (2003) Trends in suicide by marital status in England and Wales, 1982–2005. *Health Statistics Quarterly* **20**: 25–37.
21. Belbin A, Gibbs D, Gunnell D, *et al.* (2006) Male suicide and occupation in Scotland provides information on proportional mortality ratios by occupation in men in Scotland for 1981–1999. *Health Statistics Quarterly* **29**: 26–9.
22. Kposowa AJ (2000) Marital status and suicide in the National Longitudinal Mortality Study. *Journal of Epidemiology and Community Health* **54**: 254–61.
23. McKenzie K, Crawford M (2003) Suicide in ethnic minority groups. *British Journal of Psychiatry* **183**: 100–101.
24. Neeleman J, Wilson-Jones C, Wessely S (2001) Ethnic density and deliberate self harm: a small area study in south east London. *Journal of Epidemiology and Community Health* **55**: 85–90.
25. Lambert G, Reid C, Kaye D, *et al.* (2003) Increased suicide rate in the middle-aged and its association with hours of sunlight. *American Journal of Psychiatry* **160**: 793–5.
26. Yip P, Chao A, Chiu C (2000) Seasonal variation in suicides: diminished or vanished: experience from England and Wales 1982–1996. *British Journal of Psychiatry* **177**: 366–9.
27. Johnson H, Brock A, Griffiths C, Rooney C (2005) Mortality from suicide and drug-related poisoning by day of the week in England and Wales, 1993–2002. *Health Statistics Quarterly* **27**: 13–16.
28. Nishi M, Miyake H, Okamoto H, *et al.* (2000) Relationship between suicide and holidays. *Journal of Epidemiology* **10**: 317–20.
29. Fazel S, Benning R, Danesh J (2005) Suicides in male prisoners in England and Wales, 1978–2003. *Lancet* **366**: 1301–2.
30. Gunnell D, Magnusson PKE, Rasmussen F (2005) Low intelligence test scores in 18 year old men and risk of suicide: cohort study. *British Medical Journal* **330**: 167–70.
31. Egeland JA, Sussex JN (1985) Suicide and family loading for affective disorders. *Journal of the American Medical Association* **254**: 915–18.
32. Roy A, Segal N (2001) Suicidal behavior in twins: a replication. *Journal of Affective Disorders* **66**: 71–4.
33. Roy A, Segal N, Centerwall B, Robinette D (1991) Suicide in twins. *Archives of General Psychiatry* **48**: 29–32.
34. Statham D, Statham J, Heath AC, *et al.* (1998) Suicidal behaviour: an epidemiological and genetic study. *Psychological Medicine* **28**: 839–55.
35. Glowinski AL, Bucholz KK, Nelson EC, *et al.* (2001) Suicide attempts in an adolescent female twin sample. *Journal of the American Academy of Child and Adolescent Psychiatry* **40**: 1300–307.
36. Fu Q, Heath AC, Bucholz KK, *et al.* (2002) A twin study of genetic and environmental influences on suicidability in men. *Psychology Medicine* **32**: 11–24.
37. Floderus-Myrhed B, Pedersen N, Rasmuson I (1980) Assessment of heritability for personality, based on a short-form of the Eysenck personality inventory: a study of 12,898 twin pairs. *Behavior Genetics* **10**: 153–62.
38. Kerry L, Jang W, Livesley J, Vemon PA (1996) Heritability of the big five personality dimensions and

their facets: a twin study. *Journal of Personality* **64**: 577–92.

39. Savitz JB, Cupido CL, Ramesar RS (2006) Trends in suicidology: personality as an endophenotype for molecular genetic investigations. *PLoS Medicine* **3**: e107.
40. Coryell W, Schlesser M (2001) The dexamethasone suppression test and suicide prediction. *American Journal of Psychiatry* **158**: 748–53.
41. Norman WH, Brown WA, Miller IW, *et al.* (1990) The dexamethasone suppression test and completed suicide. *Acta Psychiatrica Scandinavica* **81**: 120–25.
42. Roy A, Karoum F, Pollack S (1992) Marked reduction in indexes of dopamine metabolism among patients with depression who attempt suicide. *Archives of General Psychiatry* **49**: 447–50.
43. Roggenbach J, Müller-Oerlinghausen B, Franke L (2002) Suicidality, impulsivity and aggression: is there a link to 5HIAA concentration in the cerebrospinal fluid? *Psychiatry Research* **113**: 193–206.
44. Joiner TE, Brown JS, Wingate LR (2005) The psychology and neurobiology of suicidal behavior. *Annual Review of Psychology* **56**: 287–314.
45. Nielsen DA, Virkkunen M, Lappalainen J, *et al.* (1998) A tryptophan hydroxylase gene marker for suicidality and alcoholism. *Archives of General Psychiatry* **55**: 593–602.
46. Viana MM, de Marco LA, Boson WL, *et al.* (2006) Investigation of A218C tryptophan hydroxylase polymorphism: association with familial suicide behavior and proband's suicide attempt characteristics. *Genes, Brain and Behavior* **5**: 340–45.
47. Pandey GN, Pandey SC, Dwivedi Y, *et al.* (1995) Platelet serotonin-2 receptors: a potential biological marker for suicidal behavior. *American Journal of Psychiatry* **152**: 850–55.
48. Pandey GN, Pandey SC, Janicak PG, *et al.* (1990) Platelet serotonin-2 receptor binding sites in depression and suicide. *Biological Psychiatry* **28**: 215–22.
49. Mann JJ, Malone KM (1997) Cerebrospinal fluid amines and higher lethality suicide attempts in depressed patients. *Biological Psychiatry* **41**: 162–71.
50. Nemeroff CB, Owens MJ, Bissette G, *et al.* (1988) Reduced corticotropin-releasing factor binding sites in the frontal cortex of suicide victims. *Archives of General Psychiatry* **45**: 577–9.
51. Mann JJ (2002) A current perspective of suicide and attempted suicide. *Annals of Internal Medicine* **136**: 302–11.
52. Dwivedi Y, Conley R, Roberts RC, *et al.* (2002) [3H]cAMP binding sites and protein kinase A activity in the prefrontal cortex of suicide victims. *American Journal of Psychiatry* **159**: 66–73.
53. Dwivedi Y, Rizavi HS, Conley RR, *et al.* (2002) mRNA and protein expression of selective alpha subunits of G proteins are abnormal in prefrontal cortex of suicide victims. *Neuropsychopharmacology* **27**: 499–517.
54. Pandey GN, Dwivedi Y, Pandey SC, *et al.* (1997) Protein kinase C in the postmortem brain of teenage suicide victims. *Neuroscience Letters* **228**: 111–14.
55. Barraclough B, Bunch J, Nelson B, Sainsbury P (1974) A hundred cases of suicide: clinical aspects. *British Journal of Psychiatry* **125**: 355–73.
56. Rich CL, Young D, Fowler RC (1986) San Diego suicide study I: young vs. old subjects. *Archives of General Psychiatry* **43**: 577–82.
57. Isometsä E, Henriksson M, Marttunen M, *et al.* (1995) Mental disorders in young and middle aged men who commit suicide. *British Medical Journal* **310**: 1366–7.
58. Cheng AT (1995) Mental illness and suicide: a case–control study in east Taiwan. *Archives of General Psychiatry* **52**: 594–603.
59. Conwell Y, Duberstein PR, Cox C, *et al.* (1996) Relationships of age and axis I diagnoses in victims of completed suicide: a psychological autopsy study. *American Journal of Psychiatry* **153**: 1001–8.
60. Dutta R, Boydell J, Kennedy N, *et al.* (2007) Suicide and other causes of mortality in bipolar disorder: a longitudinal study. *Psychological Medicine* **37**: 839–47.
61. Romero S, Colom F, Iosif AM, *et al.* (2007) Relevance of family history of suicide in the long-term outcome of bipolar disorders. *Journal of Clinical Psychiatry* **68**: 1517–21.
62. Palmer BA, Pankratz VS, Bostwick JM (2005) The lifetime risk of suicide in schizophrenia. *Archives of General Psychiatry* **62**: 247–53.
63. Brown S, Barraclough B (2000) Causes of the excess mortality of schizophrenia. *British Journal of Psychiatry* **177**: 212–17.
64. Hawton K, Haw C, Sinclair J, Deeks JJ (2005) Schizophrenia and suicide: systematic review of risk factors. *British Journal of Psychiatry* **187**: 9–20.
65. Simon GE, VonKorff M (1998) Suicide mortality among patients treated for depression in an insured population. *American Journal of Epidemiology* **147**: 155–60.
66. Cipriani A, Barbui C, Geddes JR (2005) Suicide, depression, and antidepressants: patients and clinicians need to balance benefits and harms. *British Medical Journal* **330**: 373–4.
67. Murphy GE, Wetzel RD (1990) The lifetime risk of suicide in alcoholism. *Archives of General Psychiatry* **47**: 383–92.
68. Sher L (2006) Alcohol consumption and suicide. *Quarterly Journal of Medicine* **99**: 57–61.
69. Akechi T, Iwasaki M, Uchitomi Y, Tsugane S (2006) Alcohol consumption and suicide among middle-aged men in Japan. *British Journal of Psychiatry* **188**: 231–6.
70. Beautrais AL, Joyce PR, Mulder RT (1999) Cannabis abuse and serious suicide attempts. *Addiction* **94**: 1155–64.

71. Marttunen MJ, Aro HM, Henriksson MM, Lönnqvist JK (1994) Antisocial behaviour in adolescent suicide. *Acta Psychiatrica Scandinavica* **89**: 167.
72. Paris J (2002) Chronic suicidality among patients with borderline personality disorder. *Psychiatric Services* **53**: 738–42.
73. Stone MH (1992) Suicide in borderline and other adolescents. *Adolescent Psychiatry* **18**: 289–305.
74. Young LD, Suome SS, Harlow HF, McKinney WT (1973) Early stress and later response to separation in rhesus monkey. *American Journal of Psychiatry* **130**: 400–405.
75. Powell J, Geddes J, Deeks J, *et al.* (2000) Suicide in psychiatric hospital in-patients: risk factors and their predictive power. *British Journal of Psychiatry* **176**: 266–72.
76. Qin P, Nordentoft M (2005) Suicide risk in relation to psychiatric hospitalization. *Archives of General Psychiatry* **62**: 427–32.
77. Geddes JR, Juszczak E (1995) Period trends in rate of suicide in first 28 days after discharge from psychiatric hospital in Scotland, 1968–92. *British Medical Journal* **311**: 1368–9.
78. Oates M (2003) Perinatal psychiatric disorders: a leading cause of maternal morbidity and mortality. *British Medical Bulletin* **67**: 219–29.
79. Gunnell D, Saperia J, Ashby D (2005) Selective serotonin reuptake inhibitors (SSRIs) and suicide in adults: meta-analysis of drug company data from placebo controlled, randomised controlled trials submitted to the MHRA's safety review. *British Medical Journal* **330**: 385–9.
80. Olfson M, Marcus SC, Shaffer D (2006) Antidepressant drug therapy and suicide in severely depressed children and adults: a case–control study. *Archives of General Psychiatry* **63**: 865–72.
81. Juurlink DN, Mamdani MM, Kopp A, Redelmeier DA (2006) The risk of suicide with selective serotonin reuptake inhibitors in the elderly. *American Journal of Psychiatry* **163**: 813–21.
82. Virani A (2005) Perspectives in psychopharmacology: spotlight on atomoxetine. *Canadian Child and Adolescent Psychiatry Review* **14**: 96–8.
83. Food and Drug Administration (2008) *Suicidal Behavior and Ideation and Antiepileptic Drugs*. Silver Spring, MD: Food and Drug Administration. www.fda.gov/CDER/Drug/infopage/antiepileptics/default.htm.
84. Christensen J, Vestergaard M, Mortensen PB, *et al.* (2007) Epilepsy and risk of suicide: a population-based case–control study. *Lancet Neurology* **6**: 693–8.
85. Joint Formulary Committee (2008) *British National Formulary 55*. London: Pharmaceutical Press.
86. Magin P, Pond D, Smith W (2005) Isotretinoin, depression and suicide: a review of the evidence. *British Journal of General Practice* **55**:134–8.
87. Cipriani A, Pretty H, Hawton K, Geddes JR (2005) Lithium in the prevention of suicidal behavior and all-cause mortality in patients with mood disorders: a systematic review of randomized trials. *American Journal of Psychiatry* **162**: 1805–19.
88. Walker AM, Lanza LL, Arellano F, Rothman KJ (1997) Mortality in current and former users of clozapine. *Epidemiology* **8**: 671–7.
89. Kerwin R (2003) Clozapine and prevention of suicide in schizophrenia: a viewpoint by Robert Kerwin. *CNS Drugs* **17**: 281–3.
90. Meltzer HY, Alphs L, Green AI, *et al.* (2003) Clozapine treatment for suicidality in schizophrenia: International Suicide Prevention Trial (InterSePT). *Archives of General Psychiatry* **60**: 82–91.
91. Mann JJ, Apter A, Bertolote J, *et al.* (2005) Suicide prevention strategies. *Journal of the American Medical Association* **294**: 2064–74.
92. Rutz W, von Knorring L, Wålinder J (1989) Frequency of suicide on Gotland after systematic postgraduate education of general practitioners. *Acta Psychiatrica Scandinavica* **80**: 151–4.
93. Bouch J, Marshall JJ (2005) Suicide risk: structured professional judgement. *Advances in Psychiatric Treatment* **11**: 84–91.
94. Department of Health (2002) *National Suicide Prevention Strategy for England*. London: Department of Health.
95. Department of Health (2001) *Safety First: Five-Year Report of the National Confidential Inquiry into Suicide and Homicide by People with Mental Illness*. London: Department of Health.
96. Department of Health (1999) *Saving Lives: Our Healthier Nation*. London: Department of Health.
97. National Confidential Inquiry into Suicide and Homicide by People with Mental Illness (2006) *Avoidable Deaths: Five Year Report of the National Confidential Inquiry into Suicide and Homicide by People with Mental Illness*. Manchester: National Confidential Inquiry into Suicide and Homicide by People with Mental Illness.
98. National Collaborating Centre for Mental Health (2004) *Self-Harm: The Short-Term Physical and Psychological Management and Secondary Prevention of Self-Harm in Primary and Secondary Care*. National Clinical Practice guideline no. 16. Leicester: British Psychological Society.
99. Kreitman N, Philip AE, Greer S, Bagley CR (1969) Parasuicide. *British Journal of Psychiatry* **115**: 746–7.
100. Platt S, Bille-Brahe U, Kerkhof A, *et al.* (1992) Parasuicide in Europe: the WHO/EURO multicentre study on parasuicide. I: Introduction and preliminary analysis for 1989. *Acta Psychiatrica Scandinavica* **85**: 97–104.
101. Hawton K, van Heeringen (eds) (2000) *The International Handbook of Suicide and Attempted Suicide*. Chichester: John Wiley & Sons.

102. Olfson M, Gameroff MJ, Marcus SC, *et al.* (2005) Emergency treatment of young people following deliberate self-harm. *Archives of General Psychiatry* **62**: 1122–8.
103. Leenaars AA (ed.) (1998) *Suicide in Canada*. Toronto: University of Toronto Press.
104. North West Public Health Observatory. *Mental Health, Self-Harm and Alcohol Specific Conditions*. www.nwph.net/nwpho/inequalities/health_wealth_ch17_(2).pdf. Liverpool: North West Public Health Observatory.
105. Newman SC, Stuart H (2005) An ecologic study of parasuicide in Edmonton and Calgary. *Canadian Journal of Psychiatry* **50**: 275–80.
106. Van Heeringen K, De Volder V (2002) Trends in attempted suicide in adolescents and young adults in Gent, 1986–1995. *Archives of Suicide Research* **6**: 135–41.
107. Cooper J, Kapur N, Mackway-Jones K (2007) A comparison between clinicians' assessment and the Manchester Self-Harm Rule: a cohort study. *Emergency Medicine Journal* **24**: 720–21.
108. Haw C, Hawton K, Houston K, Townend E (2001) Psychiatric and personality disorders in deliberate self-harm patients. *British Journal of Psychiatry* **178**: 48–54.
109. Hawton K, Harriss S, Hall S, *et al.* (2003) Deliberate self-harm in Oxford, 1990–2000: a time of change in patient characteristics. *Psychological Medicine* **33**: 987–95.
110. Klonsky ED, Oltmanns TF, Turkheimer E (2003) Deliberate self-harm in a non-clinical population: prevalence and psychological correlates. *American Journal of Psychiatry* **160**: 1501–8.
111. Dennis M, Baillon S, Brugha T, *et al.* (2007) The spectrum of suicidal ideation in Great Britain: comparisons across a 16–74 years age range. *Psychological Medicine* **37**: 795–805.
112. Thomas HV, Crawford M, Meltzer H, Lewis G (2002) Thinking life is not worth living: a population survey of Great Britain. *Social Psychiatry and Psychiatric Epidemiology* **37**: 351–6.
113. McCauley M, Russell V, Bedford D, *et al.* (2001) Assessment following deliberate self-harm: who are we seeing and are we following the guidelines? *Irish Journal of Psychological Medicine* **18**: 116–19.
114. Tyrer P, Thompson S, Schmidt U, *et al.* (2003) Randomized controlled trial of brief cognitive behaviour therapy versus treatment as usual in recurrent deliberate self-harm: the POPMACT study. *Psychological Medicine* **33**: 969–76.
115. Montgomery SA, Åsberg M (1979) A new depression scale designed to be sensitive to change. *British Journal of Psychiatry* **134**: 382–9.
116. Tyrer P, Alexander J (1979) Classification of personality disorder. *British Journal of Psychiatry* **135**: 163–7.
117. Brezo J, Paris J, Turecki G (2006) Personality traits as correlates of suicidal ideation, suicide attempts, and suicide completions: a systematic review. *Acta Psychiatrica Scandinavica* **113**: 180–206.
118. Du L, Bakish D, Lapierre YD, *et al.* (2000) Association of polymorphism of serotonin 2A receptor gene with suicidal ideation in major depressive disorder. *American Journal of Medical Genetics* **96**: 56–60.
119. Cooper J, Kapur N, Mackway-Jones K (2007) A comparison between clinicians' assessment and the Manchester Self-Harm Rule: a cohort study. *Emergency Medicine Journal* **24**: 720–21.
120. Zahl DL, Hawton K (2004) Repetition of deliberate self-harm and subsequent suicide risk: long-term follow-up study of 11 583 patients. *British Journal of Psychiatry* **185**: 70–75.
121. Hall DJ, O'Brien F, C Stark, *et al.* (1998) Thirteen-year follow-up of deliberate self-harm, using linked data. *British Journal of Psychiatry* **172**: 239–42.
122. Owens D, Horrocks J, House A (2002) Fatal and non-fatal repetition of self-harm: Systematic Review. *British Journal of Psychiatry* **181**: 193–9.
123. Johnsson Fridell E, Ojehagen A, Träskman-Bendz L (1996) A 5-year follow-up study of suicide attempts. *Acta Psychiatrica Scandinavica* **93**:151–7.
124. Paris J, Zweig-Frank H (2001) A 27-year follow-up of patients with borderline personality disorder. *Comprehensive Psychiatry* **42**: 482–7.
125. Department of Health and Social Security (1984) *The Management of Deliberate Self Harm*. London: Department of Health and Social Security.
126. McMillan D, Gilbody S, Beresford E, Neilly L (2007) Can we predict suicide and non-fatal self-harm with the Beck Hopelessness Scale? A meta-analysis. *Psychological Medicine* **37**: 769–78.
127. Beck AT, Weissman A, Lester D, Trexler L (1974) The measurement of pessimism: the Hopelessness Scale. *Journal of Consulting and Clinical Psychology* **42**: 861–5.
128. Pierce DW (1977) Suicidal intent in self-injury. *British Journal of Psychiatry* **130**: 377–8.
129. Harriss L, Hawton K, Zahl D (2005) Value of measuring suicidal intent in the assessment of people attending hospital following self-poisoning or self-injury. *British Journal of Psychiatry* **186**: 60–66.
130. Patterson WM, Dohn HH, Bird J, Patterson GA (1983) Evaluation of suicidal patients: the SADPERSONS scale. *Psychosomatics* **24**: 343–9.
131. HMSO (2005) *The Mental Capacity Act*. London: HMSO.
132. Owens D, Dennis M, Jones S, *et al.* (1991) Self-poisoning patients discharged from accident and emergency: risk factors and outcome. *Journal of the Royal College of Physicians of London* **25**: 218–22.
133. Hawton K, Arensman E, Townsend E, *et al.* (1998) Deliberate self harm: systematic review of efficacy of

psychosocial and pharmacological treatments in preventing repetition. *British Medical Journal* **317**: 441–7.

134. Guthrie E, Kapur N, Mackway-Jones K, *at al.* (2001) Randomised controlled trial of brief psychological intervention after deliberate self poisoning. *British Medical Journal* **323**: 1–5.
135. Linehan MM, Armstrong HE, Suarez A, *et al.* (1991) Cognitive-behavioral treatment of chronically parasuicidal borderline patients. *Archives of General Psychiatry* **48**: 1060–64.
136. Tarrier N, Taylor K, Gooding P (2008) Cognitive-behavioral interventions to reduce suicide behavior. *Behavior Modification* **32**: 77–108.
137. Cotgrove A, Zirinsky L, Black D, Weston D (1995) Secondary prevention of attempted suicide in adolescence. *Journal of Adolescence* **18**: 569–77.
138. Morgan HG, Jones EM, Owen, JH (1993) Secondary prevention of non-fatal deliberate self-harm: the green card study. *British Journal of Psychiatry* **163**: 111–12.
139. Evans M, Morgan H, Hayward A, Gunnell D (1999) Crisis telephone consultation for deliberate self-harm patients; effects on repetition. *British Journal of Psychiatry* **175**: 23–7.
140. Montgomery SA, Montgomery DB, Jayanthi-Rani S, *et al.* (1979) Maintenance therapy in repeat suicidal behaviour: a placebo controlled trial. In International Association for Suicide Prevention (Canada), Canadian Mental Health Association (eds). *Proceedings of the 10th International Congress for Suicide Prevention and Crisis Intervention.* Ottawa: International Association for Suicide Prevention (Canada).
141. Verkes RJ, Van der Mast RC, Hengeveld MW, *et al.* (1998) Reduction by paroxetine of suicidal behavior in patients with repeated suicide attempts but not major depression. *American Journal of Psychiatry* **155**: 543–7.
142. Bogenschutz MP, Nurnberg H (2004) Olanzapine versus placebo in the treatment of borderline personality disorder. *Journal of Clinical Psychiatry* **65**: 104–9.
143. Pascual JC, Soler J, Puigdemont D, *et al.* (2008) Ziprasidone in the treatment of borderline personality disorder: a double-blind, placebo controlled, randomized study. *Journal of Clinical Psychiatry* **69**: 603–8.

Chapter 55

Emergency psychiatry

Basant K Puri and Ian Treasaden

INTRODUCTION

In this chapter we primarily discuss emergencies in psychiatry that fall into the following areas: acute behavioural disturbances; acute alcohol withdrawal; and medication-induced psychiatric emergencies. Other psychiatric emergencies are dealt with elsewhere in this book. A comprehensive account of practical details on cardiopulmonary resuscitation is to be found in Puri and Treasaden.[1]

GENERAL POINTS

It is useful to bear in mind the following general points when dealing with emergencies in psychiatry:[1]

- Ensure your own safety as well as that of the staff and, indeed, the patient.
- Always consider an organic cause and manage this.
- Patient confidentiality is not absolute. (For example, in the UK, the General Medical Council (GMC) accepts that doctors can reveal information if there is an immediate grave risk to the patient or others.)
- Always seek corroborative information, e.g. previous medical records, third-party information.
- Consult senior colleagues and other members of a multidisciplinary team, with whom you can also share responsibility for difficult decisions.
- Maintain good contemporaneous records of assessment and management decisions.
- 'If it's not recorded, it didn't happen' is a good precautionary principle.
- At the least, records are evidence of what may have happened, but in reviews, enquiries and, indeed, courts, doctors will always have the opportunity to expand on their records.

ACUTE BEHAVIOURAL DISTURBANCES

It is important to ensure that adequate numbers of appropriate staff are present to manage the situation. If necessary, police assistance should be sought, including helping to disarm the patient. Rocca and colleagues have suggested that the initial behavioural and environmental interventions shown in Box 55.1 should be considered.[2]

Before physical interventions are considered, an attempt to verbally talk down an aggressive or otherwise behaviourally disturbed patient should be made. Approaches on how to do this are detailed in Box 55.2, while Box 55.3 describes guidance on how to manage the patient–therapist interaction.[3] Sufficient time should be given to allow the patient to be verbally talked down in spite of the fact that in an acute situation there is often staff pressure to resolve the situation by restraint and medication.

Box 55.1 Behavioural and environmental interventions

- Use a room or an area big and calm enough, and not isolated, to allow others to come quickly if help is needed.
- You and the patient should be in such a position to allow both of you to easily reach the door, which must be open.
- Choose an environment as calm as possible and without intense stimulations or triggers.
- The environment must be safe, without objects that can be potentially dangerous.
- If a suitable room is not available choose an open space.
- Keep distance: do not be too close. The violent patient needs more room than others. Never approach the patient from behind or in a rough manner.
- Never turn your back to the patient.
- Do not be confrontational, and do not look the patient in the eyes. Try to assume a neutral facial expression and voice tone, and a relaxed body posture. Try to avoid positions with crossed arms or hands behind the back.
- The patient should not be left alone.
- If others represent a trigger for the patient's violence, ask them to leave the area.
- Give information and support to relatives and significant others.
- Perform a debriefing with the staff and, if possible, also with the patient.

Reproduced from Rocca *et al.*[2]

Box 55.2 Verbal approach

- Introduce yourself and explain what are you going to do.
- Use easy words, short and clear sentences, and a calm manner.
- Use a confidential but formal tone.
- Help the patient to understand what is happening and reassure him or her about the diagnostic and therapeutic procedures to be undertaken.
- Help the patient to restore their orientation.
- Use, at least at the beginning, alliance-oriented questions and wait before querying delicate issues.
- When possible, try to talk about the real motivations of the violence.
- Set limits of acceptable behavior and tell the patient that violations will not be allowed.
- Encourage the verbal expression of feeelings, states of mind and fantasies.
- Discourage acting out. Make it clear that the patient will be held responsible for his or her actions.
- When you have to communicate your decision, do it in a clear and simple way.

Reproduced from Rocca *et al.*[2]

Box 55.3 Patient–therapist relationship variables

- Try to make procedures as flexible as possible.
- If possible, prioritize the patient's requests.
- Show empathy and talk about the negative asects of the present situation ('I understand that this is not a good period for you; it seems to me that you feel bad – you look afraid of something').
- Engage a therapeutic alliance ('in such a difficult situation you need help; allow me to help you').
- Don't lie or betray the patient's trust.
- Do not challenge the patient; do not be confrontational; do not look the patient in the eyes.
- Offer your help to discuss therapeutic aspects of mental disorder.
- Give help for problem-solving, especially with low copers. Give alternatives to violent behaviour.
- Evaluate the presence of acute and chronic stressors, especially if active, as violence triggers are related to past violence and victimization.
- Give reassurance for present or past paranoid features.
- Be careful with gender issues.
- If needed, give the patient an opportunity for time out, offer food and drinks, and if desired and possible allow the patient to smoke a cigarette or to make a phone call.

Reproduced from Rocca *et al.*[2]

Ryan and colleagues, for the Royal College of Psychiatrists, have put forward practical guidelines for the use of sedative medication in emergency situations.[3] Guidelines for non-elderly adults are shown in Figure 55.1, while Figure 55.2 gives guidelines for elderly people.[3] These guidelines also give an example of a monitoring schedule to be used after administering an injection (Box 55.4).[3] One should always be familiar with the local policies and

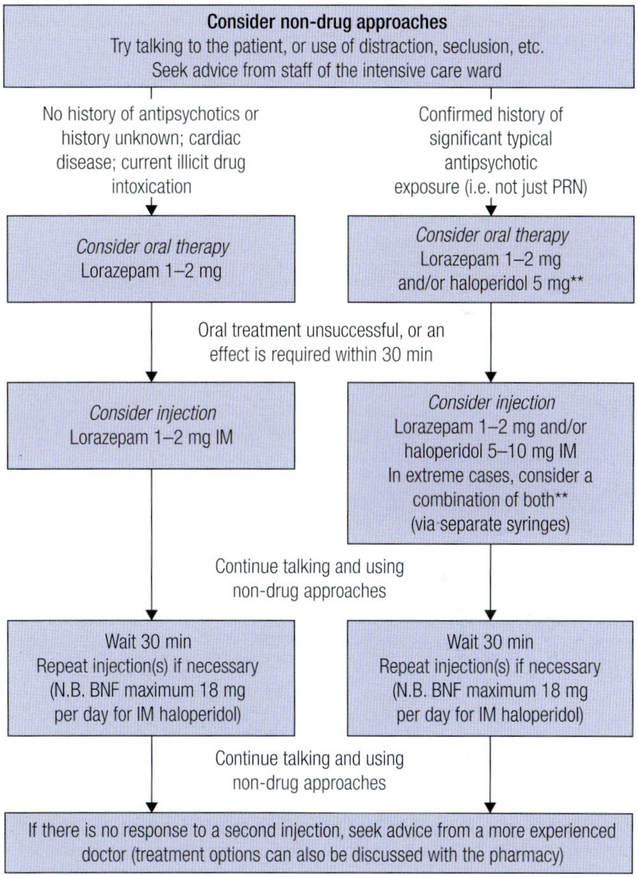

Notes

** Combination treatment may be considered on the basis of either previous knowledge of the patient that predicts poor response to a single agent, or if the level of arousal of the patient is such that forced restraint is required and will be very difficult to repeat in 30 min.

Emergency resuscitation equipment, procyclidine injection and flumazenil injection must be available before treatment.

Monitoring of the patient must be performed and recorded according to the further guidelines provided after any injection is given.

Procyclidine injection 3–10 mg can be given IV or IM for acute dystonic or parkinsonian reactions.

Flumazenil (a benzodiazepine antagonist) must be given if the respiration rate falls to <10 breaths/min after lorazepam has been used (see panel below).

Give flumazenil 200 μg IV over 15 s. If desired level of consciousness is not obtained within 60 s, a further 100 μg can be injected and repeated at 60-s intervals to a maximum total dose of 1 mg (1000 μg) in 24 h (initial + 8 additional doses). Monitor respiration rate continuously until it returns to baseline level. N.B. The effect of flumazenil may wear off and respiratory depression can return – monitoring must therefore continue beyond initial recovery of respiratory function

Figure 55.1 Royal College of Psychiatrists' sedation guidelines for non-elderly adults

BNF, British National Formulary; IM, intramuscular; IV, intravenous; PRN, when required.

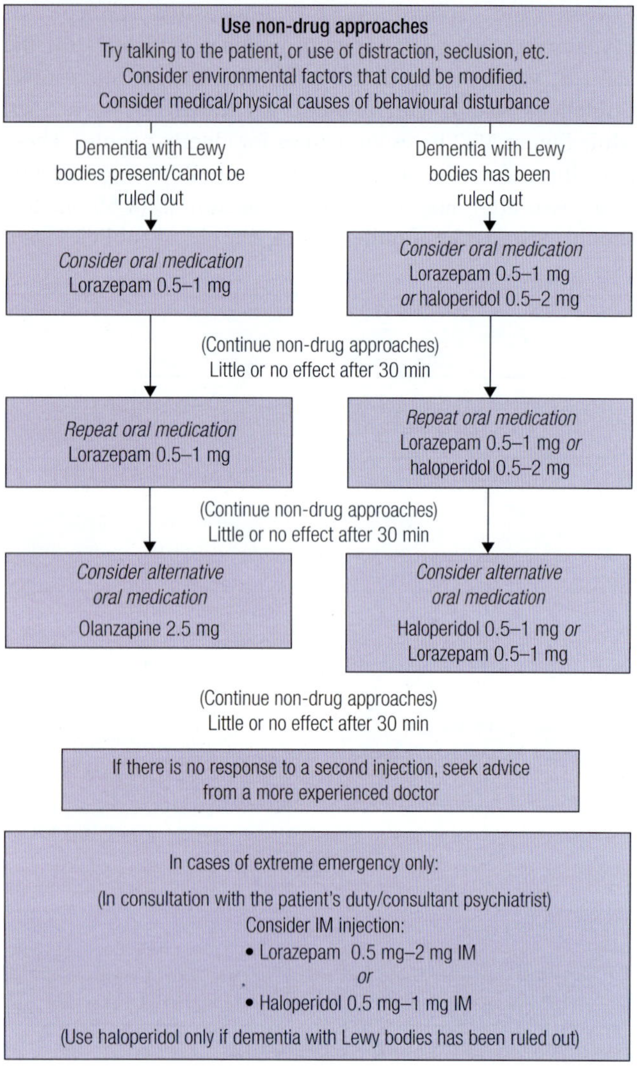

These guidelines apply where a frail patient over 65 years of age is behaving in a disturbed or violent manner that is unusual for him or her and that cannot be modified by interventions already in their care-plan. For physically fit patients and those currently or previously treated with higher doses of antipsychotics, the protocol for younger adults may be more appropriate. Details of the clinical situation and all interventions must be recorded in the patient's medical notes.

Emergency resuscitation equipment, procyclidine injection and flumazenil injection must be available before treatment

Medication should be the last resort in older people. If required, medication must be used cautiously and only by the oral route (except in very extreme emergencies – see lower panel). (Note the Mental Health Act 1983 status of the patient.)

Monitoring of the patient must be performed and recorded according to the further guidelines provided after any injection is given.

Procyclidine injection 2.5–5 mg can be given IV or IM for acute dystonic or parkinsonian reactions.

Flumazenil (a benzodiazepine antagonist) must be given if the respiration rate falls to <10 breaths/min after lorazepam has been used (see panel below).

> Give flumazenil 200 µg IV over 15 s. If desired level of consciousness is not obtained within 60 s, a further 100 µg can be injected and repeated at 60-s intervals to a maximum total dose of 1 mg (1000 µg) in 24 h (initial + 8 additional doses). Monitor respiration rate continuously until it returns to baseline level. N.B. The effect of flumazenil may wear off and respiratory depression return – monitoring must continue beyond initial recovery of respiration.

Figure 55.2 Royal College of Psychiatrists' sedation guidelines for elderly adults BNF, British National Formulary; IM, intramuscular; IV, intravenous.

> **Box 55.4 Example of a monitoring schedule from the Royal College of Psychiatrists**
>
> After injections, this monitoring schedule must be followed, unless there are compelling reasons for doing otherwise, and must be recorded in all cases:
>
> - Pulse and respiration as soon as possible after injection, then every 5 min for 1 hr.
> - Temperature (using Tempadots) as soon as possible after injection as a baseline then at 5, 10, 15 and 60 min.
> - Blood pressure at 30 and 60 min after injection.
> - Monitor for signs of neurological reactions (e.g. acute dystonia, acute parkinsonism).
>
> Reproduced from Ryan *et al.*[3]

procedures for the management of acute aggression and other behavioural disturbance. One would need to be able to justify and fully document any deviation from such guidelines, including countering any future litigation.

Following any serious untoward incident, it is useful to have a staff debriefing meeting. In a psychiatric in-patient setting, other patients may be reassured in community meetings. Carers may also need reassurance.

After the acute situation is stabilized, consideration needs to be given to the medium- and longer-term management to prevent re-occurrence. This may include treatment to control any underlying mental disorder. Such treatment may include psychotropic medication, cognitive-behavioural approaches (including anger management) and possibly long-term psychotherapy.

ACUTE ALCOHOL WITHDRAWAL

Alcohol withdrawal can be considered not to be a psychiatric emergency in the sense that its primary management requires close liaison with a general medical team, who nowadays often undertake such treatment. Detoxification is the medical management of withdrawal symptomatology in individuals who have psychoactive substance dependence. It involves medication to reduce withdrawal symptomatology, close monitoring and nutritional supplementation. Alcohol withdrawal can arise as an emergency in general medical or surgical wards, for instance, or in police custody or prisons. Planned detoxification may be carried out on an in- or out-patient basis. The latter depends on the availability of adequate support. In-patient detoxification will be required if there is evidence of acute organic mental disorder, including delirium, significant co-morbid physical illness, seizures, and lack of available support in the community.

Benzodiazepines are used to ameliorate withdrawal symptomatology and to reduce the risk of seizures.

Chlordiazepoxide is often preferred in out-patient detoxification for its lower abuse potential, while diazepam is favoured for in-patient detoxification as it is faster-acting, allows for better dose titration and can be administered gradually. A benzodiazepine withdrawal regime is indicated where there are current symptoms or signs of withdrawal, a diagnosis of alcohol-dependent syndrome or a consumption of at least 10 units of alcohol daily over the previous fortnight. A possible out-patient reducing regime with chlordiazepoxide for a male adult is to commence with 90 mg (divided into three or four doses) on day 1, reducing to a total of 80 mg on day 2 (in four divided doses), a total of 50 mg on day 3, a total of 40 mg on day 4, and finally a total of 20 mg on day 5.

Benzodiazepines are usually sufficient as anticonvulsants in the above dosages, especially as other anticonvulsants do not reach therapeutic levels within this period of risk. Similarly, a benzodiazepine will usually control hallucinations or delusions that develop, but antipsychotic medication can be used if the benzodiazepine is insufficient. However, one should bear in mind that antipsychotics reduce the seizure threshold.

High-potency parenteral thiamine (vitamin B1) should be given if there is evidence of developing Wernicke-Korsakoff syndrome; in the UK, injections of Pabrinex® are generally used, which contain ascorbic acid, nicotinamide, pyridoxine, riboflavin and thiamine. In view of the fact that anaphylaxis has been reported with such treatment, facilities should be available for resuscitation. The parenteral treatment can be followed by a course of oral thiamine. Other psychotropic medications, such as those for associated anxiety or depression, should generally be avoided until such symptoms can be assessed in the absence of the effects of alcohol or its withdrawal.

MEDICATION-INDUCED EMERGENCIES

Acute dystonic reactions

Dystonic reactions can be painful and frightening and can occur on starting, increasing or withdrawing antipsychotic medication, particularly older typical drugs. They are more common in young men and are seen in approximately 10 per cent of patients exposed to older typical drugs (phenothiazines, butyrophenones).[4]

The most common features are torticollis, oculogyric crisis, tongue protrusion, grimacing and opisthotonos. Other features include retrocollis, dysarthria and dysphagia. Affected individuals may be unable to swallow or speak clearly and, in severe cases, the back may arch or the jaw dislocate.

The immediate treatment is parenteral antimuscarinic (anticholinergic) medication, such as procyclidine 5 mg intravenously or intramuscularly, or benzatropine (benztropine) 2 mg intravenously, which can be effective in minutes.

Subsequent management may include reduction in dose or changes in antipsychotic medication or oral antimuscarinic medication, for example procyclidine 5 mg every 8 h; note, however, that procyclidine, particularly at high doses, may produce euphoria and mydriasis and is associated with an abuse potential. Diazepam may also help but is less specific.

Oculogyric crisis

This acute dystonic reaction has become less common where newer atypical antipsychotics are used in preference to the older typical antipsychotics. After an initial phase of restlessness or agitation, during which the patient might develop a fixed stare, the full-blown oculogyric crisis characteristically manifests with arching of the neck and ocular involuntary movement superiorly and possibly laterally, although ocular convergence and downward movement may occur. The tongue may be protruded and the mouth opened widely. Rapid blinking, lacrimation, mutism or palilalia, and tachycardia may also occur.

Antipsychotic-induced oculogyric crises have been found to occur late in the day and at regular intervals, and to be associated with autonomic symptoms such as profuse sweating, facial flushing, transitory hypertension and difficulty in micturition; they have also been reported to be associated with transient psychiatric symptoms.[5]

Other medical causes of oculogyric crisis include:[1]

- post-encephalitic Parkinson's disease;
- herpes encephalitis;
- juvenile Parkinson's disease;
- non-antipsychotic psychotropic drugs, e.g. benzodiazepines, lithium salts, carbamazepine, tricyclic antidepressants, reserpine;
- other drugs, e.g. metoclopramide (a substituted benzamide), cisplatin, levodopa, nifedipine, chloroquine;
- influenza immunization;
- head injury;
- neurosyphilis;
- multiple sclerosis;
- Tourette's (Gilles de la Tourette's) syndrome;
- bilateral thalamic infarction;
- cystic glioma of the third ventricle;
- fourth-ventricle lesions.

In terms of management, it is important to review the current medication regime, particularly as it relates to the past 24 h. If the cause appears to be antipsychotic medication, then the patient should be reassured and an antimuscarinic drug administered parenterally. Regular oral antimuscarinic treatment may be needed in the short term.

Consideration may need to be given to changing the antipsychotic drug that caused the reaction.

In the absence of the patient receiving antipsychotic medication, a full history, careful perusal of the case notes, a physical examination and appropriate investigations may be required in order to detect other medical causes.

Neuroleptic malignant syndrome

This life-threatening medical emergency requires immediate treatment. Although neuroleptic malignant syndrome usually occurs with drugs that directly act on central dopaminergic systems, such as antipsychotic medication, it has also been reported with other drugs, including tricyclic antidepressants. Neuroleptic malignant syndrome is likely to be an idiosyncratic reaction; some patients have been cautiously re-challenged with the same agent without recurrence. High-potency typical antipsychotics such as haloperidol are more likely to cause the reaction.

The clinical features include the following:[1]

- Autonomic dysfunction:
  - Hyperthermia
  - Labile blood pressure
  - Pallor
  - Sweating
  - Tachycardia
- Fluctuating level of consciousness (stupor)
- Muscular rigidity
- Urinary incontinence.

The condition may last for longer than a week after stopping the antipsychotic drug.

Characteristically, the serum creatine kinase is raised and there is a leucocytosis. Raised urinary myoglobin may also be detected.

Antipsychotic medication should be stopped immediately. The patient should be admitted as an in-patient to a medical ward, where maximal supportive care should be instituted. Sometimes dantrolene or bromocriptine (a dopamine agonist) may be required.

After recovery, the issue of reintroduction of the antipsychotic drug is likely to arise. A period of at least 2 weeks should elapse in the case of oral medication and a period of at least 6 weeks in the case of parenteral medication. The patient should be monitored carefully at this time for any signs of re-emergence of the syndrome before an attempt is made to reintroduce antipsychotic medication. It may be sensible to use a different, low-potency antipsychotic instead of the drug that was associated with the occurrence of neuroleptic malignant syndrome.

Complications such as respiratory, cardiovascular and renal failure contribute to an overall mortality of higher than 10 per cent.

Clozapine

Pharmacotherapy with clozapine may be associated with fatal agranulocytosis, fatal myocarditis and cardiomyopathy, fatal pulmonary embolism and life-threatening constipation.

Agranulocytosis occurs in around 3 per cent of patients on clozapine. All patients must receive regular haematological investigations to check for the development of neutropenia.

Fatal myocarditis is most common during the first 2 months of treatment. The UK Committee on Safety of Medicines has recommended the following:[1]

- Take a physical examination and medical history before starting clozapine.
- The patient should have a specialist examination if cardiac abnormalities or history of heart disease are found. Clozapine should be initiated only in the absence of severe heart disease and if benefit outweighs risk.
- Persistent tachycardia, especially in the first 2 months, should prompt observation for other indicators for myocarditis or cardiomyopathy.
- If myocarditis or cardiomyopathy is suspected, clozapine should be stopped and the patient evaluated urgently by a cardiologist.
- Clozapine should be discontinued permanently if there is clozapine-induced myocarditis or cardiomyopathy.

Sudden clozapine withdrawal may be associated with rebound psychosis.

Serotonin syndrome

Serotonin syndrome may follow the administration of selective serotonin reuptake inhibitors (SSRIs) and also lithium salts and is characterized by:[1]

- confusion;
- pyrexia and shivering;
- sweating;
- hyperreflexia;
- ataxia;
- myoclonus;
- akathisia;
- tremor;
- diarrhoea;
- poor coordination.

Cyproheptadine, which is an antihistaminic, antiserotonin and anticholinergic medication, has been used as a treatment.

Others

Lithium toxicity, paradoxical reactions to benzodiazepines, hyponatraemia associated with antidepressants, monoamine oxidase inhibitor (MAOI) reactions with tyramine-rich foods (the 'cheese reaction') and poisoning with psychotropic medication are discussed in Chapter 57.

KEY POINTS

- Ensuring the safety of staff and patients in psychiatric emergencies is paramount.
- Always consider the possibility of organic aetiology.
- Before physical interventions are considered, an attempt verbally to talk down an aggressive or otherwise behaviourally disturbed patient should be made.
- One should be familiar with local policies and procedures for the use of, and monitoring following, sedative medication to control behavioural disturbance.
- Following any serious untoward incident, it is useful to have a staff debriefing meeting, including learning any lessons.
- Benzodiazepines are usually sufficient on their own to ameliorate alcohol-withdrawal symptomatology and to reduce the risk of seizures.
- High-potency parenteral thiamine (vitamin B1) is usually given if there is evidence of developing Wernicke–Korsakoff syndrome, but this carries the risk of anaphylaxis.
- Oculogyric crises are painful and frightening; if the cause appears to be antipsychotic medication, then the patient should be reassured and an antimuscarinic drug administered parenterally.
- Neuroleptic malignant syndrome is a life-threatening medical emergency requiring immediate treatment and carries a mortality rate of over 10 per cent.
- Pharmacotherapy with clozapine may be associated with fatal agranulocytosis, fatal myocarditis and cardiomyopathy, fatal pulmonary embolism and life-threatening constipation.

FURTHER READING

Puri BK, Treasaden IH (2008) *Emergencies in Psychiatry*. Oxford: Oxford University Press.

REFERENCES

1. Puri BK, Treasaden IH (2008) *Emergencies in Psychiatry*. Oxford: Oxford University Press.
2. Rocca P, Villari V, Bogetto F (2006) Managing the aggressive and violent patient in the psychiatric emergency. *Progress in Neuro-psychopharmacology and Biological Psychiatry* **30**: 586–98.
3. Ryan J, Bolton JGF, Gill PV (2004) *Psychiatric Services to Accident and Emergency Departments*. London: Royal College of Psychiatrists.
4. American Psychiatric Association (1997) Practice guideline for the treatment of patients with schizophrenia. *American Journal of Psychiatry* **154** (4 suppl.): 1–63.
5. Abe K (2006) Psychiatric symptoms associated with oculogyric crisis: a review of literature for the characterization of antipsychotic-induced episodes. *World Journal of Biological Psychiatry* **7**: 70–74.

Chapter 56

Care of the dying and bereaved

Hilary Pavis and Maelie Swanwick

PALLIATIVE CARE

The World Health Organization (WHO) has defined palliative care as:

The active holistic care of patients with advanced progressive illness. Management of pain and other symptoms and provision of psychological, social and spiritual care is paramount. The goal of palliative care is achievement of the best quality of life for patients and their families. Many aspects of palliative care are also applicable earlier in the course of the illness in conjunction with other treatments.[1]

Core principles of palliative care are:

- affirming life and regarding death as a normal process;
- neither hastening nor postponing death;
- providing relief from pain and other symptoms;
- integrating the psychological and spiritual aspects of care;
- offering a support system to help patients live as actively as possible until death;
- offering a support system to help the family cope during the patient's illness and in their own bereavement.

The principles of palliative care should not be restricted to patients with cancer or to the last few days of life. Figures released by the Office of National Statistics show that in 2005 malignant neoplasm was reported as the cause of a quarter of all deaths; at least another quarter of patients died from a chronic progressive disorder such as heart failure, renal failure, chronic obstructive pulmonary disease or Parkinson's disease. Alzheimer's disease, senility and vascular and unspecified dementia account for 5 per cent of all deaths.[2] The time course of non-malignant illnesses is typically longer and death less predictable, but disability and the range of symptoms endured, both physical and psychological, are remarkably similar. In their comparison of symptom prevalence in advanced disease, Solano and colleagues reviewed 64 original studies to find that pain, fatigue and breathlessness were experienced by a substantial number of patients with cancer, acquired immunodeficiency syndrome (AIDS), heart disease, chronic obstructive pulmonary disease and renal disease.[3] Patients with chronic lung disease and lung cancer have a comparable number of symptoms in the last year of life, although patients with chronic lung disease may have symptoms for longer and, perhaps surprisingly, experience more breathlessness.[4] Similarly, patients with advanced renal failure have impaired quality of life and symptom burden at least as severe as terminal cancer patients.[5] More than half of the patients admitted to hospital with heart disease complain of pain and dyspnoea, although only around a third have adequate treatment.[6]

Patients with non-malignant disease often have a stormy course towards the end of their life, with frequent relapses that may require hospital admission. Identifying the terminal phase of an illness such as heart failure can be difficult. Palliative care should be considered on the basis of the individual's holistically assessed needs rather than prognosis. When deciding whether palliative care is appropriate for the patient with a chronic progressive disease, a useful question to ask oneself is 'Would I be surprised if this patient were to die in the next 6–12 months?'[7]

The perception and severity of symptoms experienced at the end of life depend not only on the impact of the physical illness itself but also on the emotional state of the patient.

Pain

Pain is a subjective experience and, although the physical insult may determine the site of the pain, social, psychological and spiritual factors also influence the severity of the pain and the disability caused. The concept of 'total pain' was proposed by Cecily Saunders to acknowledge the multidimensional aspect of pain (Figure 56.1).[8]

Patients with cancer frequently believe, and fear, that they will experience pain at some point in their illness, but the reality is that a quarter of patients with cancer will have no pain.[9] Conversely, pain in non-malignant disease is often overlooked and treated poorly.[6] Staff in nursing homes judged pain to be significantly less in cognitively impaired residents compared with in cognitively intact residents; consequently, cognitively impaired patients received less analgesia.[10] In patients unable to communicate, changes in behaviour, such as becoming agitated or

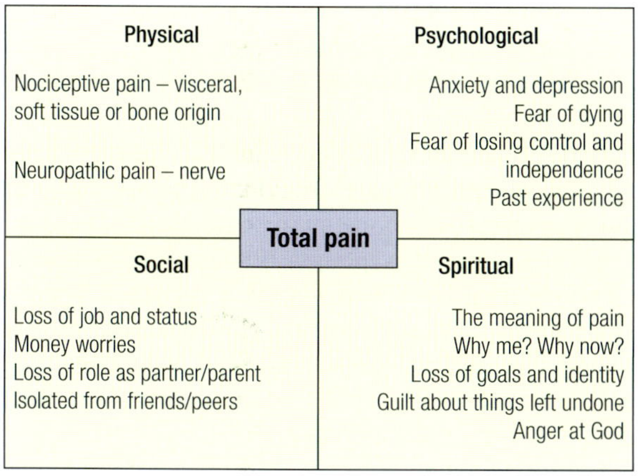

Figure 56.1 Total pain

withdrawn, shouting out, grimacing, refusing food or reduced mobility, may be the first signs that there is discomfort.

Pain may be caused by:

- the illness itself, e.g. cancer tumour pressure pain or nerve infiltration, muscle spasm and contractures;
- debility as a consequence of advanced disease, e.g. pressure sores and constipation;
- adverse effects of treatment, e.g. mucositis following radiotherapy and gout triggered by high-dose diuretics in patients with heart failure;
- concurrent problems such as arthritis.

Identifying the cause of the pain will influence the choice of treatment or analgesic; for example, colicky abdominal pain due to constipation may be best treated with laxatives, whereas liver capsular pain may respond better to a non-steroidal anti-inflammatory drug (NSAID).

The WHO devised the analgesic ladder as a stepwise approach to increasing pain (Figure 56.2).[11] Wherever possible, analgesia should be given orally and on a regular basis.

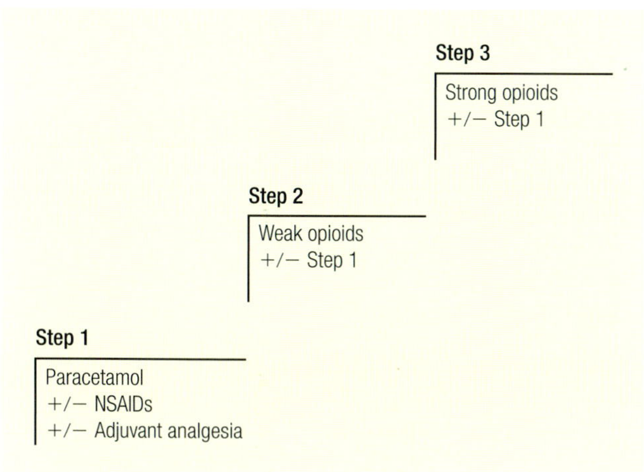

Figure 56.2 World Health Organization analgesic ladder
NSAIDs, non-steroidal anti-inflammatory drugs.

The analgesic ladder advocates the initial use of simple analgesia such as paracetamol or an NSAID with an adjuvant drug, depending on the cause of the pain. If this pain relief is insufficient, then a weak opioid such as codeine is added to the regime, or a strong opioid replaces the weak and the dose is titrated upwards until adequate pain relief is achieved. (See Table 56.1 for strong and weak opioids.) Wherever possible, analgesia should be given by mouth. Alternative routes of administration need to be considered if the patient is too unwell to swallow or is unable to keep medication down due to vomiting.[12] The strong opioid of choice in the UK is morphine, which is available in both immediate- and modified-release preparations.

Table 56.1 Strong and weak opioids[13]

Opioid	Approximate potency ratio compared with morphine
Morphine	1
Diamorphine	2–3
Fentanyl	100–150
Oxycodone	1.5–2
Methadone	5–10
Codeine	1/10

Other strong opioids commonly used for pain control include diamorphine, fentanyl, oxycodone and methadone. Fentanyl can be absorbed both transdermally (as a patch applied to the skin) and transmucosally (as a lozenge rubbed against the buccal mucosa). A strong opioid may be needed at any stage of the illness if the pain is severe and should not be withheld or given in an inadequate dose for fear of dependence. Opiate addiction is seen rarely in the clinical management of pain in patients with cancer.[14,15] Adjuvant drugs often provide additional analgesic relief in difficult pain conditions such as neuropathic pain, despite their primary indication being other than pain. Examples include antidepressants (e.g. amitriptyline, dosulepin (dothiepin)), anticonvulsants (e.g. carbamazepine, gabapentin), anti-arrhythmics (e.g. mexiletine, flecainide) and dexamethasone.

Adverse effects of opioids

Side effects may be seen when the opioid is initially taken in opioid-naive patients or when the dose is escalated rapidly. They include the following:[14]

- Sedation
- Confusion and hallucinations
- Nausea and vomiting

- Constipation
- Dry mouth
- Myoclonus.

These side effects are common to all opioids, although some patients may tolerate one opioid better than another. Sedation and nausea often resolve within a few days, and it is worth warning patients of the side effects in order to encourage compliance. Nausea and vomiting can be controlled with anti-emetics such as metoclopramide or haloperidol. Constipation should be pre-empted and laxatives prescribed.

Opiate toxicity occurs when the intake of opioid exceeds the body's ability to excrete the active metabolites, for example accumulation of morphine metabolites in renal failure. In such circumstances, a previously pain-controlled patient on a stable dose of morphine may present as confused, agitated and hallucinating, or with reduced conscious state and myoclonic jerks. If appropriate, decreasing the dose of morphine and rehydrating the patient reduces the active metabolites and may improve the toxicity. Switching to an alternative opioid or another route of administration may also reduce the side effects.[16] Low-dose haloperidol (1.5–3 mg orally or subcutaneously) may be used in the interim to settle the agitation and hallucinations.

It is a great concern to many patients that they may have to give up driving while taking opioids, but this is generally not the case. A review of the psychomotor skills of patients taking long-term opioids concluded that the evidence supported no impairment of driving-related skills and that patients taking opioids were no more likely to be involved in motor accidents.[15] Patients may be advised not to drive or operate machinery when opioids are first initiated or the dose is increased due to the risk of increased sedation. Once the sedation has resolved and the patient feels back to their usual level of alertness, they may resume driving.

The fear of addiction to opioids is also exaggerated. Very few patients with cancer and with pain, without a previous history of addiction, become addicted.[17,18] This fear restricts adequate opioid prescribing by some physicians and reduces patient compliance. Some physical tolerance to the opioid may develop, although this does not result in the escalating need for opioids. Withdrawal symptoms such as diarrhoea, abdominal cramps, anxiety, sweating, hypersalivation and rhinorrhoea may occur if the opioid is stopped suddenly or an opioid antagonist such as naloxone is administered. For this reason, opioids should be reduced gradually after a successful intervention to reduce pain such as radiotherapy.

Bisphosphonates, both orally and intravenously, have been shown to relieve metastatic bone pain.[19–21] Zoledronate 4 mg is given intravenously in 100 ml 0.9% saline over 15 min and repeated at 4- to 6-week intervals. The dose is reduced according to creatinine clearance. Daily oral calcium supplements are given to prevent hypocalcaemia. Common side effects from intravenous bisphosphonates include flu-like symptoms; more rarely, intravenous bisphosphonates have been linked with osteonecrosis of the jaw.

Palliative chemotherapy and radiotherapy can provide significant symptom relief, the latter being particularly useful for metastatic bone pain. Orthopaedic procedures such as bone-pinning, kyphoplasty and spinal stabilization can provide pain relief and maintain function. Neurolytic blocks with local anaesthetic and corticosteroid may provide local and regional pain relief; such techniques include spinal blockade, intercostal blocks and coeliac plexus blocks.

Non-drug methods such as heat pads, transcutaneous electrical nerve stimulation (TENS) and acupuncture may be helpful to some patients, particularly those who shun tablets. There is no strong evidence base to support the use of complementary therapies for pain relief, but anecdotally patients frequently report benefit from treatments such as aromatherapy massage, reiki and reflexology. Relaxation can significantly improve treatment-related symptoms such as nausea and pain in patients with cancer.[22]

Pain occasionally fails to respond to analgesia, and at times it may be appropriate to return to the total pain model and consider the other factors that may be affecting the patient's perception of the pain.

Nausea and vomiting

Nausea and vomiting are common and distressing symptoms often associated with anorexia and weight loss. The causes are multiple and may often be multifactorial. Some of the common causes include the following:

- *Gastrointestinal:*
  - Carcinoma of the stomach or head of pancreas causing gastric outlet obstruction
  - Gastritis
  - Infection
  - Bowel obstruction
  - Constipation
  - Radiotherapy
- *Drugs:*
  - Chemotherapy
  - Opioids
- *Metabolic:*
  - Uraemia
  - Hypercalcaemia of malignancy
- Raised intracranial pressure
- Anxiety, fear, severe pain.

Numerous anti-emetics are available, but the choice of a specific drug depends on the presumed cause of the vomiting; for example, nausea caused by constipation or hypercalcaemia would be best dealt with by treating the constipation with laxatives and the hypercalcaemia with a bisphosphonate. A prokinetic drug such as metoclopramide

10–20 mg three times a day may relieve the nausea due to gastric outlet obstruction but may aggravate colicky abdominal pain in bowel obstruction, where cyclizine 50 mg three times a day may be a better anti-emetic. The 5-HT_3 receptor agonists ondansetron and granisetron provide good relief for the nausea induced by chemotherapy, while dopamine antagonists may relieve biochemical or drug-induced nausea by blocking the dopamine receptors at the chemoreceptor trigger zone. High-dose dexamethasone up to 16 mg per day may be given to reduce raised intracranial pressure. Anti-emetics can be given by mouth, but if vomiting is severe absorption can be unpredictable. In such instances, medication can be given subcutaneously.

Breathlessness

The unpleasant awareness of struggling to breathe is a symptom common to the advanced stage of many illnesses and occurs in up to 75 per cent of patients. Like pain and nausea, breathlessness can have many origins:

- *Lung disease:*
  - Chronic, e.g. chronic obstructive pulmonary disease (COPD)
  - Infection, e.g. pneumonia, pleurisy
  - Pulmonary embolus
  - Malignant, e.g. lung cancer, pulmonary metastases and mesothelioma, all of which may cause a malignant effusion
- *Cardiac:*
  - Acute left ventricular failure with lung congestion
  - Chronic heart failure
- Anaemia
- *Ascites:*
  - Splinting the diaphragm
- *Neuromuscular degeneration:*
  - Motor neuron disease
- *Treatment-induced:*
  - Pneumonectomy
  - Radiation- or chemotherapy-induced pneumonitis
- Anxiety, panic and severe pain.

Wherever possible, the underlying cause of breathlessness should be treated, namely antibiotics for pneumonia, furosemide for acute left ventricular failure, blood transfusion to correct anaemia, and paracentesis to drain ascites. If this is not possible or if breathlessness persists despite attempts to correct the cause, then the following drug and non-drug measures should be tried.

Drug measures

- Low-dose immediate-release opioids have been demonstrated to be beneficial for breathlessness associated with both malignant and non-malignant disease.[23,24] A typical regime may initially start with oral morphine 2.5–5 mg as required, up to every 4 h, and titrating upwards until the desired effect is achieved. Sustained release preparations of morphine given to patients with COPD improved breathlessness and sleep.[25]
- Low-dose benzodiazepines may be helpful for the anxious dyspnoeic patient. Benzodiazepines may enhance the benefit of opiates in relieving breathlessness.[26] Benzodiazepines alone in the non-anxious patient may not improve the sensation of dyspnoea or improve exercise tolerance.[27] For the anxious breathless patient, low-dose diazepam may be taken on a regular basis. Lorazepam 1 mg can be used sublingually for panic attacks and any remaining medication may be removed when the attack has subsided.
- Oxygen therapy via cylinders or concentrators may be helpful for a few patients, although care needs to be taken in patients with COPD, who rely on their hypoxia to drive ventilation. Appropriate assessment is important. For patients with mild hypoxia, non-drug measures may be more beneficial.[28] In a small group of patients with COPD, Liss and Grant found no improvement in reported breathlessness with increasing inspired nasal oxygen concentration, but they did demonstrate an increase in breathlessness after anaesthetizing the nasal passages with topical lidocaine, which suggests that oxygen had a placebo effect.[29]

Non-drug measures

- Reassurance
- For some patients, fans can be as effective as oxygen for symptom relief
- Breathing exercises and relaxation
- Repositioning.

Psychological problems

Much of the evidence for psychiatric disorders at the end of life comes from the adult cancer population.[30] The prevalence of psychiatric morbidity in patients with cancer is high. Derogatis and colleagues assessed 215 patients with cancer and found that 44 per cent had a psychiatric diagnosis, of which 68 per cent had an adjustment disorder, 13 per cent a major affective disorder and 4 per cent anxiety disorders.[31] In a systematic review of patients with advanced disease in a palliative care setting, a prevalence of definite depression ranged from 19 per cent to 34 per cent, with a prevalence of major depression ranging from 5 per cent to 26 per cent.[32] Psychiatric disorder is poorly detected in patients with cancer, and only a minority of patients receive adequate treatment.[30] Diagnosis of an affective disorder can be difficult due to the overlap of symptoms encountered in terminal illness and depression, such as pain, poor appetite, fatigue and poor concentration; the symptom 'loss of interest' may help to identify the depressed patient with cancer.[33] Depressed patients with cancer exhibit more symptoms, particularly pain, insomnia and fatigue, than non-depressed patients and tend to rate their symptoms as more severe.[34,35] Patients' concerns about their illness are an indicator of psychological distress: those with four or more concerns (particularly concerns about sexuality, feeling upset or feeling different) had significantly more anxiety or depression.[36,37]

After a diagnosis of a life-threatening illness, a patient will experience a range of emotions. Massie and Holland proposed a model of phases of normal adjustment.[38] Phase 1, or the initial response, is characterized by disbelief and denial, which they suggest allows a 'temporary emotional distancing' from the crisis, for some the response may be one of despair. After a few days, the patient may enter second phase of dysphoria, where they may exhibit anxiety, depression and poor concentration. This phase may last a couple of weeks, before the third phase of adaptation is reached.

Elizabeth Kübler-Ross interviewed patients with cancer during the 1960s and identified five common stages through which patients may pass from diagnosis to death:[39]

1. *Denial:* a transient stage while the bad news sinks in. Some patients may use denial during later stages of their illness, for example when diagnosed with metastases. Denial is rarely maintained throughout the course of the illness but is a defence mechanism for some patients protecting them from distress.
2. *Anger:* feelings of resentment and frustration may be directed in all directions, towards family and friends, healthcare professionals, God or the patient themselves. Family members may find these emotions difficult to cope with and require support themselves.
3. *Bargaining:* patients may make promises with themselves, their doctors or God in order to maintain hope and extend life.
4. *Depression:* when the impact of the diagnosis has subsided, the patient then has to face the losses, whether real or imaginary, ahead. It may be the loss of health and independence or the loss of role in society and among peers and family. There may also be the fear of disfigurement, abandonment and uncontrolled symptoms such as pain leading to despair and depression.
5. *Acceptance:* patients may accept their impending death at varying stages in their illness. Some put their affairs in order, make peace with estranged family and friends, and arrange their funeral while still active; others, however, may appear to accept their fate only when fatigue increases and they are too weak to resist.

Some patients may not pass through Kübler-Ross's five stages neatly, and instead may skip stages or oscillate back and forth; some patients may exhibit several stages at the same time. The five-stage model has been adapted by other authors acknowledging that the patient may have a mixture of reactions characteristic of the age and personality of the patient and the social context in which they find themselves, rather than the stage of dying.[40]

Clinical staff may lack the skills and knowledge to recognize a normal reaction to a cancer diagnosis and to distinguish this from a psychiatric disorder, some even believing that the latter is inevitable in cancer.[41] For staff with no specialist psychiatry training, screening tools for detecting psychiatric disorder may be valuable. The single question 'Are you depressed?' asked of a group of terminally ill North Americans correctly identified depressed patients,[42] but the results were not repeated when the same question was asked of British patients.[43] The Hospital Anxiety and Depression Scale (HADS) and Edinburgh Post-Natal Depression Scale (EPDS) have both been shown to be effective in screening for depression in a palliative population and acceptable to the patients.[44] There has been little research into the use of antidepressants at the end of life, although review of the few studies available does suggest that antidepressants are effective.[45,46] For some patients with a prognosis of a few weeks, the time for a therapeutic response to standard antidepressants may be unacceptable.

Delirium

Delirium is an acute confusional state associated with clouding of consciousness, in contrast to dementia where there is no drowsiness unless compounded by delirium. Delirium is often encountered at the end of life and frequently seen in patients with cancer. The patient may present as agitated, aggressive, confused and hallucinating, with a disrupted sleep–wake cycle (hyperactive), or they may be withdrawn, drowsy and confused (hypoactive). Hypoactive delirium can frequently be missed in patients and undertreated. There are many possible causes of delirium; the more common ones at the end of life include the following:

- Infection
- *Drugs:*
  - Opiates
  - Anticholinergics
  - Steroids
- *Metabolic:*
  - Encephalopathy secondary to liver or kidney failure
  - Hypercalcaemia
  - Hyponatraemia
- *Withdrawal states:*
  - Alcohol
  - Nicotine

Delirium is very distressing for both the patient and their family, and early identification is important. Reversible causes should be corrected if possible, and the patient should be nursed in a calm, non-confrontational environment. The patient should be communicated with clearly, using and often repeating simple explanations. Low lighting at night can help to reduce misinterpretation of objects or people around the patient. Centrally acting drugs thought to be causing delirium should be reduced or stopped. Low-dose haloperidol 1.5–3 mg at night may be effective for the distressed, agitated or withdrawn patient.

Delirium at the end of life is frequently referred to as 'terminal agitation'. It is irreversible and often multifactorial, although due to the inappropriateness of investigations at the end of life specific causes are commonly not identified. Speculated factors include biochemical derangement and dehydration, multi-organ failure with accumulation of metabolites and drugs, direct metastatic or paraneoplastic effects, hypoxia and possibly spiritual distress.

Dying

The dying phase is all too commonly unrecognized in the acute hospital, especially by junior staff. As end of-life care becomes increasing medicalized, there is a danger that death too is becoming medicalized, with patients being subjected to futile treatments.[47] There is considerable debate as to what makes a 'good death', although there are some consistent themes:[48–51]

- Maintaining dignity
- Physical comfort and without emotional distress
- Being with family and loved ones
- Dying in one's place of choice
- Awareness of death and acceptance of death.

In order to help a patient achieve a 'good death', the recognition of impending death is important. Functional decline at the end of life is very variable and may depend on age and the disease. Patients dying of a sudden, unexpected death may have been very active and independent in the previous months. Patients with cancer have a gradual deterioration in functional status in the last 3 months of life. Patients with chronic disease such as lung or heart failure have a fluctuating course with acute exacerbations, but they may have frequent hospital admissions and become more dependent in their final 3 months.[52] As death approaches and the patient becomes more fatigued, there are several features that indicate that death may be only days away:[53]

- Poor oral intake and struggling to take more than sips of fluid
- Difficulty swallowing tablets
- Profound weakness
- Bed-bound
- Semi-comatose.

Ellershaw and colleagues recognized that a majority of patients were dying in the acute hospital setting and developed a multidisciplinary care pathway to help identify the dying patient and promote a good death. The Liverpool Care Pathway (LCP) aims to improve dying by promoting review of symptoms, psychological and spiritual issues, and prompting good communication between professionals and family members. It reminds staff to review existing medication and discontinue unnecessary medical interventions while prescribing anticipatory drugs for the patient's comfort.[54–56] Anticipatory drugs are prescribed subcutaneously for ease of administration and may include the following:

- Morphine or diamorphine for pain
- Anti-emetics such as cyclizine or haloperidol
- Hyoscine butylbromide for noisy respiratory tract secretions
- Midazolam for agitation.

The dose of opiate or benzodiazepine will often depend on whether the patient has been on regular doses before. Advice can be obtained from the local specialist palliative care team. If the patient requires frequent doses of medication, it can be given by continuous subcutaneous infusion via a syringe driver over a 24-h period.

Personal experience of the death of a loved one can have a profound and lasting effect on the individual.[57] A 'good death' does not diminish the pain of the loss but may help that individual through their own bereavement period and when facing their own mortality.

BEREAVEMENT

Grief is a normal response to loss and will be experienced by most people at some point in their lives. It has a recognized aetiology and phases, but in any individual its course is very personal and influenced by age, social and cultural factors.

Bereavement is well known to be a causal factor in a number of psychiatric conditions. Grief may also coexist with anxiety states or depression, and differentiation is important if unnecessary suffering is to be prevented. Psychiatrists may be asked to supervise bereavement counsellors when knowledge of complicated grief and its management may be needed. Bereavement, however, is not always a negative experience, and it can sometimes be a time of personal growth.

Definitions

- *Bereavement:* the objective situation of having lost someone significant.
- *Grief:* the primarily emotional (affective) reaction to the loss of a loved one through death.
- *Mourning:* the social expressions or acts expressive of grief that are shaped by the practices of a given society or culture group.[58]

The concept of anticipatory grief is described by Parkes as the psychological and emotional reaction to anticipation of bereavement.[59]

Theoretical models of loss and bereavement

Theoretical models can be helpful in understanding the phenomena and course of normal bereavement and can assist our clinical work with bereaved people. There is no single explanatory model of loss and bereavement, and many different models and theories are described in the literature. Parkes considers that it is helpful to view the theories as complementary rather than conflicting with each other in their approaches.[60]

Freud pioneered early work on bereavement and in his classic text *Mourning and Melancholia* recorded both the similarities and the differences between grief and depression and normal and pathological grief.[61]

Bowlby's early work, in association with James Robertson and Mary Ainsworth, focused on the behaviour and attachments of children separated from their mothers under traumatic conditions.[62] He identified a constant sequence of behaviours in these children, namely protest, despair, yearning and detachment. He adopted attachment theory as a way of understanding the emotional response to the severing of a close bond. John Bowlby was joined by Colin Murray Parkes in 1962 at the Tavistock Clinic, and they collaborated closely until Bowlby's death in 1992. Their work continues to remain central to our understanding of the grief process.

Bowlby and Parkes noticed similarities in the grief of adults and young children following the loss of close and significant individuals. They conceptualized grief following bereavement to be a form of separation anxiety, originally in a three-phase model.[63] They later jointly developed this into a four-phase model (see below). Phase theory originally required the bond to the deceased to be broken in order for resolution of grief to have occurred, but more recently this idea has been challenged.

Parkes developed a theory of bereavement as a psychosocial transition (PST). Such an event is relatively sudden, has lasting implications and invalidates a person's set of expectations and assumptions about their world. This necessitates adjustment and revision of the person's 'assumptive world.'[64]

Worden, in the 1980s, proposed a model of grieving with some different features.[65] He considers that the grieving person must accomplish four tasks before mourning can be completed and a healthy adjustment made. These tasks are to accept the reality of the loss; to work through the pain of grief; to adjust to an environment in which the deceased is missing; and emotionally to relocate the deceased and move on with life.

A newer model is that of the dual-process model of coping with bereavement, described by Stroebe and Schut.[66] They propose that, in grieving, people undertake, in varying proportions, what could be called loss- and restoration-oriented coping activities. Both categories of stressor require coping effort during bereavement, although this coping is of necessity a part of everyday life. The loss-orientation refers to dealing with part of the loss experience (and has some similarities to the grief work process), whereas the restoration-orientation component refers to coping with the stressors that arise as a consequence of the bereavement. The central component of the model is that oscillation occurs between these two states and that this is necessary for optimal adjustment. In addition, they also argue the need for 'dosage' of grieving when respite is taken from either loss- or restoration-oriented coping activities as an adaptive means of coping.

Klass and colleagues have proposed a 'continuing bonds model of grief.'[67] They propose that bereaved people remain involved and connected to the deceased and that they actively construct an inner representation of the deceased that is part of the grieving.[67] They suggest that, although the intensity of the relationship may diminish with time, the relationship does not disappear and can help to inform their future. Their model is supported by some eastern cultures and the grief process of children.

Rubin has described the Two-Track Model of Bereavement, in which the loss is conceptualized as two interactive axes or tracks.[68] Track I is concerned with biopsychosocial functioning, whereas track II relates to the bereaved person's ongoing emotional attachment and relationship to the deceased.

The nature of normal grief

The first systematic study of acute grief was carried out by Lindemann in 1944.[69] He studied the bereaved survivors of a nightclub fire, along with other groups, and established grief as a distinct syndrome with recognizable symptoms and a defined course. The following were common to all people in acute grief:

- Waves of somatic distress, for example sighing respiration, lack of strength
- Intense preoccupation with the image of the deceased
- Guilt
- Irritability and anger
- Restlessness and aimlessness.

The phases or stages of grief

Parkes and Bowlby have described phases of grief or bereavement.[60] They describe grief as a process and not a state.[60] It involves a succession of clinical symptoms that blend into and replace one another. They emphasize that these phases or stages are guidelines only and are not intended to dictate where a bereaved individual ought to be at a particular time in the course of their grief. It is well recognized that an individual may pass back and forth in a fluid way between phases.

The following phases are described:[59]

- *Phase of numbness:* this is the immediate reaction to the shock of death. There is numbness or a feeling of unreality: 'I can't take it in – it doesn't seem real.' This may last for hours or weeks.
- *Phase of pining:* as the death is acknowledged, there may be periods of intense pining and yearning for the

lost person. There is a tendency to weep, interspersed with quiet periods of anxiety and tension. Preoccupation with images of the deceased occurs. There may be anger and somatic distress, and anxiety may escalate to hyperventilation and panic attacks. Short-term memory is poor, and there may be irritability and depression.

- *Phase of disorganization and despair:* the pangs of grief reduce in intensity, interspersed with longer periods of apathy and despair. Ruminations over events leading up to the death may persist. A sense of the presence of the dead person, illusions, misinterpretations and hypnogogic hallucinations may occur.
- *Phase of reorganization and recovery:* Most people are aware of recovery in the second year after loss and can engage in activities directed to the future. Anniversaries, however, are often times of renewed grieving, following which energy usually returns.

It is difficult to demarcate a normal end point of grief, as studies have shown significant distress at 13 months and longer after bereavement.[70]

Although the stage theory of grief is widely accepted, the first empirical study of the sequence was carried out in 2007 by Maciejewski and colleagues.[71] They carried out a longitudinal cohort study, the Yale Bereavement Study, assessing five grief indicators (disbelief, yearning, anger, depression, and acceptance) from 1 month to 24 months after loss. Contrary to the traditional stage theory of grief in which disbelief predominates first and acceptance is reached slowly, they found acceptance and yearning for the deceased the most frequently endorsed items. However, each negative grief indicator peaked in the sequence proposed by the stage theory, within 6 months after loss.

Shuchter and Zisook have described a multidimensional approach to the grief experiences of newly bereaved spouses.[72] The following dimensions are involved:

- Emotional and cognitive states
- Coping strategies
- Continuing relationship with the deceased
- Health and social functioning
- Changes in relationships
- Changes in identity.

Although many of the bereavement studies involve white, English-speaking groups, cultural rituals and practices strongly influence grief in different cultures and different parts of the world.[73]

Functional neuroanatomy of grief

Gundel and colleagues carried out the first functional magnetic resonance imaging (fMRI) study of grief.[74] Symptoms of grief were elicited in eight bereaved women by means of photographs of their deceased relative and words specific to the death event. They were also asked to view photographs of a stranger and 'neutral words'. These were put together as 60 composites in total, such as 'deceased and grief word' and 'stranger and grief word', and were presented to the study subjects during scanning. Three brain regions were activated independently by the picture and word factors: posterior cingulate cortex, medial/superior frontal gyrus and cerebellum. When the picture of the deceased was shown, distinct activity was also seen in the cuneus, superior lingual gyrus, insula, dorsal anterior cingulate cortex, inferior temporal gyrus and fusiform gyrus. When the death-related words were shown, distinct activity was seen in the precuneus, precentral gyrus, midbrain and vermis. The authors concluded that grief is mediated by a distributed neural network that subserves affect processing, memory retrieval, processing of familiar faces, visual imagery, autonomic regulation and modulation/coordination of these functions.

O'Connor, one of the authors of the study above, provides further background to this area and describes how neuroimaging may contribute to current debates in the bereavement literature.[75]

Assessing the risk of bereavement

Grief affects some people more adversely than others, and in most cases several factors may contribute. The factors that research has shown to contribute to a poor bereavement outcome are summarized in Table 56.2.[76,77]

Stroebe and colleagues have also described factors that promote 'resilience' and are protective, such as a secure attachment style in relations with others and perceived control over daily activities.[77]

Although many risk factors have been described, little is known about the way in which individual factors interact to cause a particular outcome. Stroebe and colleagues have developed an integrative risk factor framework for predicting bereavement outcome, which they hope will stimulate research in this area. Their framework includes five variables: the nature of the stressor; interpersonal resources; intrapersonal resources; appraisal; and coping processes and outcomes.[78]

The complications of bereavement

Mortality

Bereavement can be associated with increased mortality. The evidence for this comes predominantly from longitudinal studies in which bereaved people are matched with non-bereaved subjects for age, sex and other variables. An early study in 1963 by Young and colleagues followed a cohort of 4486 widowers aged 55 years and older over 5 years.[79] They found that, during the first 6 months of bereavement, widowers had an increased mortality rate of 40 per cent greater than for married men of the same age. After the first 6 months of bereavement, the mortality fell back to that of married men. A longer follow-up period of 9 years by Parkes and colleagues provided additional information on cause of death. Cardiovascular disorders

Table 56.2 Factors associated with a poor bereavement outcome

Circumstances of death	Untimely, e.g. death of a child
	Traumatic, sudden or unexpected
	Stigmatized, e.g. suicide
	Painful, horrifying or mismanaged
	Severe distress in the terminal phase of life
	Multiple deaths
Characteristics of survivor	Excessively dependent or ambivalent relationship with the deceased, or one lacking in harmony
	Personality: 'grief-prone' or insecure and over-anxious
	Previous psychiatric illness
	Childhood loss
	Physically disabled or ill
Social circumstances	Absent or unsupportive family
	Detached from traditional cultural and religious support systems
	Social isolation
	Caring for dependants

('coronary thrombosis and other arteriosclerotic and degenerative heart diseases') accounted for two-thirds of the excess mortality, 67 per cent greater than the expected number.[80]

Helsing and colleagues carried out a sizeable retrospective cohort study between 1963 and 1974 of 4032 bereaved men and women.[81] The group was followed until 1975. They added a range of control factors, including race, education, church attendance, number in a household, and smoking, making their study highly comprehensive and controlled. In contrast to previous studies, they did not find an increased risk immediately after bereavement. Their results indicated a significantly higher mortality rate (based on person-years at risk) for widowers than for married males. Such a difference was not observed between widows and married females. Younger people were at higher risk than older people after death of a spouse. Mortality rates among widowed males who remarried were very much lower than in those who did not remarry, although no effect on mortality was noted for females who remarried. After 3 years' follow-up, however, those who had not remarried had a higher mortality than the remarried or married people.

Martikainen and Valkonen examined excess mortality and its cause in a large Finnish study of 1 580 000 married people.[82] They found that excess mortality among bereaved people was high for accidental, violent and alcohol-related causes (50–150%), moderate for chronic ischaemic heart disease and lung cancer (20–35%) and low for other causes (5–15%). The excess mortality was greater in the first 6 months for all causes and among younger men.

A large number of studies predominantly of spousal bereavement have been reviewed by Stroebe and colleagues.[77] The majority have shown an early excess risk of mortality among bereaved people. This extends to non-conjugal relationships and across cultures and countries. The relative risk of mortality is higher for widowers than for widows and higher in younger age groups than older age groups.

The mortality associated with bereavement must, however, be assessed in terms of the absolute number of people who die. Stroebe and colleagues suggest that the figure is low, with approximately 5 per cent of widowers versus 3 per cent of married men aged 55 years and older dying in the first 6 months after bereavement.[77]

Physical ill-health

People who have been bereaved are more likely to have physical health problems, especially if the bereavement is recent.

In an early study, Parkes studied the medical records of 44 unselected widows before and after bereavement.[83] The consultation rate for physical symptoms was increased by 50 per cent in both older and younger widows. The change was most pronounced for the subgroup diagnosed 'osteoarthritis'. In a subsequent study by Parkes and Brown in Boston, MA, USA, 68 widows and widowers under age 45 years, who had been bereaved 14 months previously, were compared with 68 matched controls by questionnaire interviews on health matters.[84] They found that the hospitalization rate was higher in the bereaved group than in matched married controls. They also reported more changes in sleep, appetite and weight. Increased psychological and somatic symptoms commonly associated with anxiety were found in the bereaved group. Autonomic symptoms such as chest pains, dizziness and headaches were also more common in the bereaved people.

Other studies have also found more disability and higher use of medications. Thompson and colleagues found older bereaved spouses to be at greater risk of a new or worsened illness, and their self-reported use of medication was higher.[85]

Various mechanisms have been proposed to explain why some individuals are more vulnerable following bereavement:[86]

- *Behavioural changes:*
  - In social ties and living arrangements
  - For widowers, increased alcohol consumption and the loss of the sole confidante
- *Neuroendocrine and immunological changes:*[86]
  - Increased urinary free cortisol excretion
  - Raised plasma cortisol levels
  - Positive dexamethasone suppression test
  - Elevated serum growth hormone in response to stress
  - Increase in growth hormone secretion
- Reduced lymphocyte response to mitogens in widows and widowers 2 months after the loss, and reduced T-cell subpopulation and natural killer cell activity.

Psychiatric disorders

The most frequently reported psychiatric complications of bereavement are major depression, anxiety disorders and post-traumatic stress disorder (PTSD). Pre-existing conditions such as alcohol and substance misuse may be exacerbated. Importantly, any psychiatric condition may coexist with complicated grief. Treatment of any psychiatric disorder must run in parallel with facilitation of the grief process.

A study of depressive syndromes in the first year after the death of a spouse found that 24 per cent of 350 widows and widowers met criteria for depressive episodes at 2 months, 23 per cent did so at 7 months and 16 per cent did so at 13 months.[87] The rate was 4 per cent in a group whose spouses were still living. At 13 months, those at particular risk were younger widows and widowers and people with a past history of depression. Sub-syndromal symptomatic depression is also prevalent through the first 2 years of widowhood and is responsible for significant morbidity.[88] According to the *Diagnostic and Statistical Manual*, 4th edition (DSM-IV), the diagnosis of a major depressive episode should not be made if a recent bereavement could account for the symptoms and the symptoms do not persist beyond 2 months. This is currently the subject of considerable debate.[89] Recent investigators, however, have found that by 2 months after bereavement, depression may already be chronic and a cause of considerable morbidity.[90] Evaluation of all major depressive syndromes 2 months after bereavement should be performed and appropriate treatment considered.

The suicide risk of widows and widowers is increased particularly in the first week after bereavement but falls in the first month.[91]

Anxiety disorders can occur in bereavement.[92,93] Jacobs and colleagues found a large overlap between anxiety disorders and major depression.[92]

PTSD and bereavement phenomena may become closely mixed together, particularly when the death has been very traumatic, such as suicide or murder. The PTSD-type symptoms may interfere with the capacity to grieve and often require treatment first before the grief can be facilitated.[94]

Complicated grief disorder

A number of researchers have moved to the position that complicated grief represents a distinct syndrome.[95,96] Many different terms have been used to describe this disorder in the literature, including pathological grief, abnormal grief, atypical grief, traumatic grief and chronic grief.[97]

Parkes and Weiss developed a classification of pathological grief[98] based on a study of American widowers and widows. They identified delayed or repressed grief, often in response to an unexpected loss; conflicted grief, occurring when the survivor has ambivalent feelings toward the deceased; and chronic grief, often occurring in a relationship where one partner was dependent on the other.

However, some researchers now feel that complicated grief disorder (CGD) is a single disorder that may display features of the original subtypes in varying amounts. Bereaved people with CGD typically appear stuck in a state of chronic mourning.[97] Studies have shown complicated grief to be distinct from normal grief, major depression[99] and PTSD.

Complicated grief disorder has been proposed as a syndrome for inclusion in the next edition of the DSM.[97] A diagnosis of CGD requires that the bereaved person must have persistent and disruptive yearning, pining and longing for the deceased. Diagnostic criteria specify that the person must also experience four of the following eight symptoms as marked, overwhelming or extreme:

- Trouble accepting the death
- Inability to trust others since the death
- Excessive bitterness related to the death
- Feeling uneasy about moving on
- Detachment from formerly close others
- Feeling life is meaningless without the deceased
- Feeling that the future holds no prospect for fulfilment without the deceased
- Feeling agitated since the death.

The symptoms must have been present for at least 6 months and must cause marked dysfunction in social, occupational or other important domains of functioning.

It is important to note that CGD is diagnosed only at a minimum of 6 months after loss. This is because many of the symptoms are present in normal grief early on but can be expected to have declined by 6 months and not be a cause of significant functional impairment. The disorder may often occur alongside major depressive disorder and PTSD.

Bereaved people with CGD symptoms have been shown to have an increased risk of cancer, hypertension, cardiac events and suicidal ideation.[97] They have also been associated with functional impairments, adverse health behaviours and depressive disorders.[90]

Particular risk factors for CGD include the following:[96,97]

- Sudden unexpected deaths
- A dependent relationship with the deceased person
- Childhood abuse and serious neglect
- Childhood separation anxiety
- Lack of preparation before the death and lack of support after it.

Evidence supporting interventions to help bereaved people

General principles

The majority of bereaved people neither need nor benefit from professional help. They are able to grieve their loss with support from family and friends in the context of their own particular social, spiritual and cultural background. Others derive support from their general practitioner (GP) or religious minister. For some people who remain socially isolated, voluntary organizations such as CRUSE may be helpful.

Before death, attention to the way in which 'bad news' is broken, anticipatory grief and overall care of the family unit have also been shown to positively affect the course of bereavement.

Schut and colleagues have categorized grief interventions as follows:[100]

- *General or primary preventive interventions:* open to all bereaved people.
- *Secondary preventive interventions:* screen for high-risk bereaved individuals;
- *Tertiary preventive interventions:* usually psychotherapeutic or psychological treatments for bereaved people with, for example, complicated grief or bereavement-associated depression.

Despite the widespread proliferation of grief interventions ranging from counselling to different types of psychotherapy, two reviews suggest that some do not show significant benefit and highlight limitations in aspects of the methodology of many studies.[77,100]

Primary preventive interventions

Schut and colleagues reviewed the studies of primary prevention.[100] They found a range of studies, some with methodological flaws, and others with interventions that did not show positive effects or benefits that were only short-lived and not sustained. They concluded that none of the primary intervention studies could be described as 'evidence-based'. However, the studies aimed at helping bereaved children to cope with the loss of a parent or sibling appeared to show positive results.

Secondary preventive interventions

The effects of secondary preventive interventions are more promising. The first study to show the benefit of offering intervention to high risk bereaved individuals was carried out by Raphael.[101] She assessed a group at high risk of complicated grief selected with particular risk factors: the traumatic sudden death of their partner, low social support, an ambivalent relationship with the deceased, and multiple concurrent stressful life events. The treatment group received specific support for grief in the first 3 months of bereavement, whereas the control group received no intervention. A significant benefit as seen by reduction in symptoms was seen in the intervention group compared with the control group.

Schut and colleagues have reviewed other studies and concluded that the effects of intervention were modest and not always long-lasting.[100]

Bereavement by suicide, although not necessarily more severe, can present specific difficulties for the surviving relatives. One case–control study found that inquest procedures and media reporting were a frequent source of distress for bereaved relatives, and feelings of stigma, shame and rejection were more common than in other bereavements.[102] These problems make coping more difficult and many people will require specialist help.[103]

Most specialist palliative care units and hospices in the UK have well-developed bereavement services available to any grieving relatives known to the service. They are proactive in screening for individuals at high risk of poor bereavement outcomes and offering appropriate support.

Tertiary preventive interventions

Most studies conclude that tertiary preventive interventions for people with complicated grief are generally helpful.[100] This includes interventions for bereavement-related major depressive disorder[104] and PTSD. Complicated grief can be differentiated from major depression and PTSD, and this is important, because studies so far show that treatment of the depressive disorder has little effect on the complicated grief symptoms, which require a different approach.

A variety of therapies have been tried for complicated grief, which may be individual-, group- or family-oriented and include guided mourning, interpersonal or psychodynamic therapy, cognitive-behaviour therapy and family-focused grief therapy. Two factors considered important to the outcome of treatment are whether the bereaved person asks for help directly and the timing of the intervention.[100]

Shear and colleagues were the first to target the symptoms of complicated grief directly.[105] They developed a targeted complicated grief treatment involving interpersonal psychotherapy (IPT) for grief-related depression to address the depressive symptoms and IPT techniques modified to include cognitive-behavioural therapy for addressing PTSD symptoms, for example intrusive images. Patients were randomized to receive IPT ($n = 46$) or complicated grief treatment ($n = 49$). The response rate was greater for complicated grief treatment (51%) than for IPT (28%), and the time to response was faster for complicated grief treatment.

Other studies have also shown interesting results. One controlled trial of brief psychotherapy and mutual-help group treatment for widows with unresolved grief reactions found that both treatments were equally efficacious at the end of treatment.[106] Another, Internet-based cognitive-behavioural therapy programme targeted at bereaved people suffering from complicated grief found that the treatment group showed significant improvement compared with the control group.[107]

Kissane and Bloch have described in detail the use of family-focused grief therapy in palliative care and bereavement.[108,109] They carried out a randomized trial with 81 families participating. Significant improvements were seen in distress and depression in certain groups and in 'intermediate' and 'sullen' families, and the authors concluded that the therapy had the potential to prevent pathological grief.

However, although there are many different types of intervention for bereavement-related difficulties described in the literature, it is apparent that more research is needed to establish which types are effective and for whom.

KEY POINTS

- Patients with malignant and non-malignant disease have a similar symptom burden at the end of life. Palliative care is available to all, depending on the need rather than the diagnosis.
- Symptoms such as pain, nausea and breathlessness may be multi-factorial in cause and have a psychological, social, spiritual and physical basis.
- The prevalence of psychiatric disorder in patients with cancer is high, although depression is frequently undiagnosed and untreated.
- A 'good death' can be achieved by early recognition of the dying phase, good communication with all involved, anticipation of symptoms and their timely management.
- Models of bereavement can assist in our clinical work with the bereaved.
- Bereavement can be associated with significant morbidity and mortality.
- Identifiable risk factors may be associated with a poor bereavement outcome.
- Complicated grief is distinct from other bereavement-associated psychiatric conditions. Particular types of therapy appear specific for complicated grief.
- A strong proposal has been made for CGD to be recognized as a separate diagnosis in the future DSM-V.
- More research needs to done on interventions for bereavement related difficulties and on resilience, or the factors that enable some people to cope better than others after bereavement.

REFERENCES

1. World Health Organization (1990) *Cancer Pain Relief and Palliative Care.* Geneva: World Health Organization.
2. Office of National Statistics (2005) *Review of the Registrar General on Deaths by Cause, Sex and Age in England and Wales.* www.statistics.gov.uk/downloads/theme_health/Dh2_32/Table2.1.xls.
3. Solano JP, Gomes B, Higginson IJ (2006) A comparison of symptom prevalence in far advanced cancer, AIDS, heart disease, chronic obstructive pulmonary disease and renal disease. *Journal of Pain and Symptom Management* **31**: 58–69.
4. Edmonds P, Karlsen S, Khan S, Addington-Hall J (2001) A comparison of the palliative care needs of patients dying from chronic respiratory disease and lung cancer. *Palliative Medicine* **15**: 287–95.
5. Saini T, Murtagh FEM, Dupont PJ, *et al.* (2006) Comparative pilot study of symptoms and quality of life in cancer patients and patients with end stage renal disease. *Palliative Medicine* **20**: 631–6.
6. McCarthy M, Lay M, Addington-Hall J (1996) Dying from heart disease. *Journal of the Royal College of Physicians* **30**: 325–8.
7. Murray SA, Boyd K, Sheikh A (2005) Palliative care in chronic illness. *British Medical Journal* **330**: 611–12.
8. Saunders C (1967) *The Management of Terminal Illness.* London: Edward Arnold.
9. Bonica J (1990) Cancer pain: current status and future needs. In J Bonica (ed.) *The Management of Pain.* Philadelphia, PA: Lea & Febiger.
10. Reynolds KS, Hanson LC, DeVellis RF, *et al.* (2008) Disparities in pain management between cognitively intact and cognitively impaired nursing home residents. *Journal of Pain and Symptom Management* **35**: 388–96.
11. World Health Organization (1986) *Cancer Pain Relief.* Geneva: World Health Organization.
12. Hanks GW, de Conno F, Cherny N, *et al.* (2001) Expert working group of the Research Network of the European Association for Palliative Care. Morphine and alternative opioids in cancer pain: the EAPC recommendations. *British Journal of Cancer* **84**: 587–93.

13. Twycross R, Wilcock A (2007) *Palliative Care Formulary*, 3rd edn. www.palliativedrugs.com.
14. British Medical Association, Royal Pharmaceutical Society of Great Britain *British National Forumlary.* www.bnf.org.
15. Fishbain DA, Cutler RB, Rosomoff HL, *et al.* (2003) Are opioid-dependent/tolerant patients impaired in driving-related skills: a structures evidence-based review. *Journal of Pain and Symptom Management* **25**: 559–77.
16. Cherny N, Ripamonti C, Pereira J, *et al.* (2001) Expert working group of the European Association for Palliative Care. Strategies to manage the adverse effects of oral morphine: an evidence-based report. *Journal of Clinical Oncology* **19**: 2542–54.
17. Aronoff GM (2000) Opioids in chronic pain management: is there a significant risk of addiction? *Current Review of Pain* **4**: 112–21.
18. Hojsted J, Sjogren P (2007) Addiction to opioids in chronic pain: a literature review. *European Journal of Pain* **11**: 490–518.
19. Mannix K, Ahmedzai SH, Anderson H, *et al.* (2000) Using bisphosphonates to control the pain of bone metastases: evidence-based guidelines for palliative care. *Palliative Medicine* **14**: 455–61.
20. Ross JR, Saunders Y, Edmonds PM, *et al.* (2003) Systematic review of role of bisphosphonates on skeletal morbidity in metastatic cancer. *British Medical Journal* **327**: 469–72.
21. Body J-J (2006) Bisphosphonates for malignancy-related bone disease: current status, future developments. *Supportive Care in Cancer* **14**: 408–18.
22. Leubbert K, Dahme B, Hasenbring M (2001) The effectiveness of relaxation training in reducing treatment-related symptoms and improving emotional adjustment in acute non-surgical cancer treatment: a meta-analytical review. *Psycho-oncology* **10**: 409–502.
23. Chua TP, Harrington D, Ponikowski P, *et al.* (1997) Effects of dihydrocodeine on chemosensitivity and exercise tolerance in patients with chronic heart failure. *Journal of the American College of Cardiology* **29**: 147–52.
24. Johnson MJ, McDonagh TA, Harkness A, *et al.* (2002) Morphine for the relief of breathlessness in patients with chronic heart failure: a pilot study. *European Journal of Heart Failure* **4**: 753–6.
25. Abernethy AP, Currow DC, Frith P, *et al.* (2003) Randomised, double blind, placebo controlled crossover trial of sustained release morphine for the management of refractory dyspnoea. *British Medical Journal* **327**: 523–6.
26. Navigante AH, Cerchietti LC, Castro MA, *et al.* (2006) Midazolam as adjunct therapy to morphine in the alleviation of severe dyspnoea perception in patients with advanced cancer. *Journal of Pain and Symptom Management* **31**: 38–47.
27. Man GCW, Hsu K, Sproule BJ (1986) Effects of alprazolam on exercise and dyspnoea in patients with chronic obstructive pulmonary disease. *Chest* **90**: 832–6.
28. Booth S, Wade R, Johnson MJ, *et al.* (2004) The use of oxygen in the palliation of breathlessness: a report of the expert working group of the Scientific Committee of the Association of Palliative Medicine. *Respiratory Medicine* **98**: 66–77.
29. Liss HP, Grant BJ (1988) The effect of nasal flow on breathlessness in patients with chronic obstructive pulmonary disease. *American Review of Respiratory Disease* **137**: 1285–8.
30. Stiefel F, Trill MD, Berney A, *et al.* (2001) Depression in palliative care: a pragmatic report from the Expert Working Group of the European Association for Palliative Care. *Supportive Care in Cancer* **9**: 477–88.
31. Derogatis LR, Morrow GR, Fetting J, *et al.* (1983) The prevalence of psychiatric disorders among cancer patients. *Journal of the American Medical Association* **249**: 751–7.
32. Hotopf M, Chidgey J, Addington-Hall J, Lan Ly K (2002) Depression in advanced disease: a systematic review. Part 1: prevalence and case finding. *Palliative Medicine* **16**: 81–97.
33. Reuter K, Raugust S, Bengel J, Härter M (2004) Depressive symptom patterns and their consequence for diagnosis of affective disorders in cancer patients. *Supportive Care in Cancer* **12**: 864–70.
34. Lloyd-Williams M, Dennis M, Taylor F (2004) A prospective study to determine the association between physical symptoms and depression in patients with advanced cancer. *Palliative Medicine* **18**: 558–63.
35. Chen M-L, Chang H-K (2004) Physical symptom profiles of depressed and non-depressed patient with cancer. *Palliative Medicine* **18**: 712–18.
36. Harrison J, Maguire P, Ibbotson T, *et al.* (1994) Concerns, confiding and psychiatric disorder in newly diagnosed cancer patients: a descriptive study. *Psycho-oncology* **3**: 173–9.
37. Heaven CM, Maguire P (1998) The relationship between patients' concerns and psychological distress in a hospice setting. *Psycho-oncology* **7**: 502–7.
38. Massie MJ, Holland JC (1989) Overview of normal reactions and prevalence of psychiatric disorder. In J Rowland, JC Holland (eds) *Handbook of Psycho-Oncology*. New York: Oxford University Press.
39. Kübler-Ross E (1970) *On Death and Dying*. London: Tavistock/Routledge.
40. Rowland JH (1989) Developmental stage and adaptation: adult model. In J Rowland, JC Holland (eds) *Handbook of Psycho-Oncology*. New York: Oxford University Press.
41. Block SD (2000) Assessing and managing depression in the terminally ill patient. *Annals of Internal Medicine* **132**: 209–18.

42. Chochinov HM, Wilson KG, Enns M, Lander S (1997) 'Are you depressed?': screening for depression in the terminally ill. *American Journal of Psychiatry* **154**: 674–6.
43. Lloyd-Williams M, Dennis M, Taylor F, Baker I (2003) Is asking patients in palliative care, 'Are you depressed?' appropriate? Prospective study. *British Medical Journal* **327**: 372–3.
44. Lloyd-Williams M, Spiller, Ward J (2003) Which depression screening tools should be used in palliative care? *Palliative Medicine* **17**: 40–43.
45. Lan Ly K, Chidgey J, Addington-Hall J, Hotopf M (2002) Depression in palliative care: a systematic review. Part 2: treatment. *Palliative Medicine* **16**: 279–84.
46. Lloyd-Williams M (2004) Are antidepressants effective in cancer patients? *Progress in Palliative Care* **12**: 217–19.
47. Clark D (2002) Between hope and acceptance: the medicalisation of dying. *British Medical Journal* **321**: 905–7.
48. Payne S, Langley-Evans A, Hillier R (1996) Perceptions of a 'good' death: a comparative study of the views of hospice staff and patients. *Palliative Medicine* **10**: 307–12.
49. Miyashita M, Sanjo M, Morita T, *et al.* (2007) Good death in cancer: a nationwide quantitative study. *Annals of Oncology* **18**: 1090–97.
50. Kehl K (2006) Moving towards peace: an analysis of the concept of a good death. *American Journal of Hospice and Palliative Care* **23**: 277–86.
51. Goldsteen M, Houtepen R, Proot IM, *et al.* (2006) What is a good death? Terminally ill patients dealing with normative expectations around death and dying. *Patient Education and Counselling* **64**: 378–86.
52. Lunney JR, Lynn J, Foley DJ, *et al.* (2003) Patterns of functional decline at the end of life. *Journal of the American Medical Association* **289**: 2387–92.
53. Higgs R (1999) The diagnosis of dying. *Journal of the Royal College of Physicians* **33**: 110–12.
54. Ellershaw J, Foster A, Murphy D, *et al.* (1997) Developing an integrated care pathway for the dying patient. *European Journal of Palliative Care* **4**: 203–7.
55. Ellershaw J, Smith C, Overill S, *et al.* (2001) Care of the dying: setting standards for symptom control in the last 48 hours of life. *Journal of Pain and Symptom Management* **21**:12–17.
56. Ellershaw J, Ward C (2003) Care of the dying patient: the last hours or days of life. *British Medical Journal* **326**: 30–34.
57. Neuberger J (2003) Commentary: a 'good death' is possible in the NHS. *British Medical Journal* **326**: 34.
58. Stroebe MS, Hansson RO, Stroebe W, Schut H (2001) Introduction: concepts and issues in bereavement research. In MS Stroebe, RO Hansson, W Stroebe, H Schut (eds) *Handbook of Bereavement Research: Consequences, Coping and Care*. Washington, DC: American Psychological Association.
59. Parkes CM (1998) Bereavement. In D Doyle, GWC Hanks, N MacDonald (eds) *Oxford Textbook of Palliative Medicine*. Oxford: Oxford University Press.
60. Parkes CM (1996) *Bereavement: Studies of Grief in Adult Life*. London: Penguin.
61. Freud S (1917) *Mourning and Melancholia*. London: Hogarth.
62. Bowlby J (1969) *Attachment and Loss*, Vol. 1: Attachment. London: Hogarth Press.
63. Bowlby J (1980) *Attachment and Loss*, Vol. 3: Loss – sadness and depression. London: Hogarth Press.
64. Parkes CM (1993) Bereavement as a psychosocial transition: processes of adaptation to change. In MS Stroebe, W Stroebe, RO Hansson (eds) *Handbook of Bereavement: Theory, Research and Intervention*. Cambridge: Cambridge University Press.
65. Worden JW (1983) *Grief Counselling and Grief Therapy: A Handbook for the Mental Health Practitioner*. London: Tavistock.
66. Stroebe M, Schut H (1999) The dual process model of coping with bereavement: rationale and description. *Death Studies* **23**: 197–224.
67. Klass D, Silverman PR, Nickman SL (eds) (1996) *Continuing Bonds: New Understandings of Grief*. Philadelphia, PA: Taylor & Francis.
68. Rubin S (1981) A two-track model of bereavement: theory and application in research. *American Journal of Orthopsychiatry* **51**: 101–9.
69. Lindemann E (1944) The symptomatology and management of acute grief. *American Journal of Psychiatry* **101**: 141.
70. Bornstein PE, Clayton PJ, Halikas JA, *et al.* (1973) The depression of widowhood after thirteen months. *British Journal of Psychiatry* **122**: 561–6.
71. Maciejewski PK, Zhang B, Block SD, *et al.* (2007) An empirical examination of the stage theory of grief. *Journal of the American Medical Association* **7**: 716–23.
72. Shuchter SR, Zisook S (1993) The course of normal grief. In MS Stroebe, W Stroebe, RO Hansson (eds) *Handbook of Bereavement, Theory, Research and Intervention*. Cambridge: Cambridge University Press.
73. Parkes CM, Laungani P, Young B (eds) (1977) *Death and Bereavement Across Cultures*. London: Routledge.
74. Gundel H, O'Connor M-F, Littrel L, *et al.* (2003) Functional neuroanatomy of grief: an fMRI study. *American Journal of Psychiatry* **160**: 1946–53.
75. O'Connor M-F (2005) Bereavement and the brain: invitation to a conversation between bereavement researchers and neuroscientists. *Death Studies* **29**: 905–22.
76. Parkes CM (1985) Bereavement. *British Journal of Psychiatry* **146**: 11–17.
77. Stroebe M, Schut H, Stroebe W (2007) Health outcomes of bereavement. *Lancet* **370**: 1960–73).

78. Stroebe MS, Folkman S, Hansson RO, Schut H (2006) The prediction of bereavement outcome: development of an integrative risk factor framework. *Social Science and Medicine* **63**: 2440–51.
79. Young M, Benjamin B, Wallis C (1963) The mortality of widowers. *Lancet* **2**: 454–6.
80. Parkes CM, Benjamin B, Fitzgerald RG (1969) Broken heart: a statistical study of increased mortality among widowers. *British Medical Journal* **1**: 740–43.
81. Helsing KJ, Szklo M, Comstock GW (1981) Factors associated with mortality after widowhood. *American Journal of Public Health* **71**:802–9.
82. Martikainen P,Valkonen T (1996) Mortality after the death of a spouse: rates and causes of death in a large Finnish cohort. *American Journal of Public Health* **86**: 1087–93.
83. Parkes CM (1964) Effect of bereavement on physical and mental health: a study of the medical records of widows. *British Medical Journal* **2**: 274–9.
84. Parkes CM, Brown RJ (1972) Health after bereavement: a controlled study of young Boston widows and widowers. *Psychosomatic Medicine* **34**: 449–61.
85. Thompson LW, Breckenridge JN, Gallagher D, Peterson JA (1984) Effects of bereavement on self-perceptions of physical health in elderly widows and widowers. *Journal of Gerontology* **39**: 309–14.
86. Biondi M, Picardi A (1996) Clinical and biological aspects of bereavement and loss-induced depression: a reappraisal. *Psychotherapy and Psychosomatics* **65**: 229–45.
87. Zisook S, Shuchter SR (1991) Depression through the first year after the death of a spouse. *American Journal of Psychiatry* **148**: 346–52.
88. Zisook S, Shuchter SR, Sledge PA, *et al.* (1994) The spectrum of depressive phenomena after spousal bereavement. *Journal of Clinical Psychiatry* **55** (suppl.): 29–36.
89. Zisook S, Shear K, Kendler KS (2007) Validity of the bereavement exclusion criterion for the diagnosis of major depressive episode. *World Psychiatry* **6**: 102–7.
90. Zisook S, Shuchter SR (1993) Uncomplicated bereavement. *Journal of Clinical Psychiatry* **54**: 365–72.
91. Ajdacic-Gross V, Ring M, Gadola E (2008) Suicide after bereavement: an overlooked problem. *Psychological Medicine* **29**: 1–4.
92. Jacobs S, Hansen F, Kasl S, *et al.* (1990) Anxiety disorders during acute bereavement: risk and risk factors. *Journal of Clinical Psychiatry* **51**:269–74.
93. Zisook S, Schneider D, Shuchter SR (1990) Anxiety and bereavement. *Psychiatric Medicine* **8**: 83–96.
94. Raphael B, Minkov C, Dobson M (2001) Psychotherapeutic and pharmacological intervention for bereaved persons. In MS Stroebe, RO Hansson, W Stroebe, H Schut (eds) *Handbook of Bereavement Research: Consequences, Coping and Care.* Washington, DC: American Psychological Association.
95. Horowitz MJ, Siegel B, Holen A, *et al.* (1997) Diagnostic criteria for complicated grief disorder. *American Journal of Psychiatry* **154**: 904–10.
96. Prigerson HG, Shear MK, Jacobs SC, *et al.* (1999) Consensus criteria for traumatic grief: a preliminary empirical test. *British Journal of Psychiatry* **174**: 67–73.
97. Zhang BMS, El-Jawari ABS, Prigerson HG (2006) Update on bereavement research: evidence-based guidelines for the diagnosis and treatment of complicated bereavement. *Journal of Palliative Medicine* **9**: 1188–203.
98. Parkes CM, Weiss RS (1983) *Recovery from Bereavement.* New York: Basic Books.
99. Boelen PA, van den Bout J, de Keijser J (2003) Traumatic grief as a disorder distinct from bereavement-related depression and anxiety: a replication study with bereaved mental health care patients. *American Journal of Psychiatry* **160**: 1339–41.
100. Schut H, Stroebe MS, Van Den Bout J, Terheggen M (2001) The efficacy of bereavement interventions: determining who benefits. In MS Stroebe, RO Hansson, W Stroebe, H Schut (eds) *Handbook of Bereavement Research: Consequences, Coping and Care.* Washington, DC: American Psychological Association.
101. Raphael B (1977) Preventive intervention with the recently bereaved. *Archives of General Psychiatry* **34**: 1450–54.
102. Harwood D, Hawton K, Hope T, Jacoby R (2002) The grief experiences and needs of bereaved relatives and friends of older people dying through suicide: a descriptive and case-control study. *Journal of Affective Disorders* **72**: 185–94.
103. Hawton K, Simkin S (2003) Helping people bereaved by suicide. *British Medical Journal* **327**: 177–8.
104. Reynolds III CF, Miller MD, Pasternak RE, *et al.* (1999) Treatment of bereavement-related major depressive episodes in later life: a controlled study of acute and continuation treatment with nortriptyline and interpersonal psychotherapy. *American Journal of Psychiatry* **156**: 202–8.
105. Shear S, Frank E, Houck PR, Reynolds CF (2005) Treatment of complicated grief: a randomized controlled trial. *Journal of the American Medical Association* **293**: 2601–8.
106. Marmar CR, Horowitz MJ, Weiss DS, *et al.* (1988) A controlled trial of brief psychotherapy and mutual-help group treatment of conjugal bereavement. *American Journal of Psychiatry* **145**: 203–9.
107. Wagner B, Knaevelsrud C, Maercker A (2006) Internet-based cognitive-behavioural therapy for complicated grief: a randomized controlled trial. *Death Studies* **30**: 429–53.
108. Kissane DW, Bloch S (2002) *Family Focused Grief Therapy.* Buckingham: Open University Press.
109. Kissane DW, McKenzie M, Bloch S (2006) *American Journal of Psychiatry* **163**: 1208–18.

PART 5

Approaches to treatment

Chapter 57

Clinical psychopharmacology

Malcolm Lader and David Taylor

HISTORICAL OVERVIEW

Psychopharmacology – the study of medicines with effects on brain functions – is both an old subject and a new topic. Humans have exploited mind-altering substances for thousands of years, and ancient texts have numerous references to these drugs. But in the past 50 years, dating from the discovery and introduction of the antipsychotics, antidepressants, lithium and anxiolytics, psychiatry has benefited from the discovery of numerous psychotropic substances. Continuity has been maintained between the old and the new as many of these substances date back thousands of years but are still in use, alcohol and opium derivates being prime examples.

The history of psychopharmacology and psychopharmacologists has been reviewed extensively.[1–3] For the current observer, the intriguing paradox is the general acceptance of numerous therapeutic agents by practising psychiatrists but the reluctance, if not downright opposition, by both a minority of practitioners and numerous patient and client groups to use these agents. Polemical arguments persist over whether the risks of various medications outweigh their benefits.[4] The recent hardening of lay attitudes against psychotropic medication and medication in general can be set against a scepticism regarding scientific claims and a concern that scientists are insufficiently critical and inadequately aware of moral and ethical issues concerning therapeutic drug use. For these reasons, it is important that the prescriber sets their usage into the context of historical background and current mores.

The earlier psychotropic substances included alcohol and opioid compounds, but a large number of names are cited in recorded texts and an extensive oral tradition. Some of these medications such as 'soma' have not been identified fully. Use of such psychoactive drugs could occur in a religious context, some of which survive. Examples include mescaline and toxic mushrooms.[5]

For centuries, very few psychotropic drugs were available. Psychotropic treatment remained inchoate, with restraints and punishments substituting for any humane measures. By the Age of Enlightenment in the eighteenth century, more sympathetic methods of management were adopted and psychiatric patients were less frequently regarded as objects of derision, as in the well-documented Bethlem visits.[6] But right into the nineteenth century, pharmacological treatments were restricted to crude sedatives such as the opioids and then bromide, chloral hydrate and paraldehyde.

By the beginning of the twentieth century, other agents, particularly the barbiturates, were being introduced as powerful sedatives. The 1930s saw the start of usage of amphetamines, but their antidepressant effects were unimpressive. Two other physical treatments were tried: first, the induction of fits, first chemically and then electrically, and electroconvulsive therapy (ECT) still survives; second, brain surgery – lobotomy – which was the subject of a horrendous, indiscriminate overuse, echoes of which persist.

The modern revolution in psychopharmacology dates from the 1950s. By that time, the numbers of occupants of mental hospitals had peaked, but there was little if anything in the way of specific remedies. The discovery of the powerful sedative and antipsychotic effects of chlorpromazine, an antihistamine derivative, was greeted with enthusiasm by some, but by no means all, psychiatrists. Those working in mental hospitals – the 'alienists' – regarded chlorpromazine as a wonder drug that would empty their overcrowded wards. Others relied on social measures to reintegrate their patients into the community. Slowly the two sides came together, and combined measures were adopted.

Following soon after, imipramine was tried as an antipsychotic but was found rather serendipitously to have undoubted antidepressant properties, particularly in the more severe patients with biological features such as sleep and appetite impairment.[7] About the same time, another serendipitous discovery, that iproniazid raised the mood of patients with tuberculosis, led to the introduction of the less popular monoamine oxidase inhibitors (MAOIs). Lithium's effects on regulating mood were also described, but its exploitation proved more contentious.

Sedatives used to lessen anxiety and induce sleep were also refined with the discovery and enormous popularity of the benzodiazepines. Unfortunately, unwanted effects such as oversedation, paradoxical excitement and withdrawal problems caused a reaction, both within the medical profession and among lay people, that still reverberates.

The problem of dementia had always been neglected, but demographic trends with ageing populations in Western countries led to the development of various drugs to help manage cognitive deficits.

Over the intervening years, numerous developments have refined our psychotropic substances. The most noticeable examples have been the introduction of a heterogeneous assortment of atypical antipsychotic drugs and of more selective antidepressants, the selective serotonin reuptake inhibitors (SSRIs) and the serotonin and noradrenaline reuptake inhibitors (SNRIs).

Throughout all this time, the mechanisms of action of psychotropic agents have been elucidated only slowly. This is not surprising. Classical neurotransmitters such as serotonin in the brain were discovered only at about the time the drugs were introduced. Perusal of texts from the 1950s shows how primitive our neuropharmacological knowledge was then. The revolution in our understanding of the anatomy, physiology and biochemistry of the brain has proceeded apace, facilitated by major developments in our chemical and behavioural techniques. But we still have gaps in our understanding: for example, why is clozapine, originally developed in the 1960s and 1970s, still the only atypical antipsychotic drug with enhanced efficacy? The advances in neuropharmacology have also led to the evaluation of novel agents acting selectively on subgroups of receptors. Psychopharmacology has got its second wind, and real advances rather than molecular refinements may be in the offing.

On the clinical level, our techniques have become more refined and sensitive. Clinical trial methodology has been revolutionized, partly at the behest of the regulatory authorities. Clinical trials involve vastly greater numbers of subjects, and statistical analyses are substantially more sophisticated.[8] Data are scrutinized and ranked in quality. This has culminated in the Cochrane initiative, with standardized reviews and meta-analyses of an exhaustive range of topics.[9] Other useful sources of information include comprehensive reviews in refereed journals. These can be compendious (e.g. Thornley and Adams[10]). The need for evidence-based decisions has been voiced repeatedly (e.g. Geddes *et al.*[11]).

The classification of psychotropic drugs still reflects our classification of psychiatric symptoms, together with some use of putative biochemical mechanisms. Thus, the *British National Formulary* (BNF) contains Section 4, headed 'Central nervous system' (Table 57.1).

Subsections 4.1–4.4 and 4.10–4.11 would be regarded as 'core' psychotropic drugs. Nevertheless, the remainder have central nervous system (CNS) effects, and drugs used primarily for non-CNS indications can also have CNS effects, usually unwanted (e.g. sedation with the older antihistamines, stimulation with bronchodilators). Most of the headings are symptomatic or syndromal, for example 'antipsychotic'; a few are biochemical, for example 'monoamine-oxidase inhibitors'. Sometimes the rubric has become too limited; for example, the SSRIs are classified as antidepressants but are widely licensed and prescribed for the anxiety disorders.

Table 57.1 *British National Formulary* headings

Central nervous system	
4.1	**Hypnotics and anxiolytics**
	4.1.1 Hypnotics
	4.1.2 Anxiolytics
	4.1.3 Barbiturates
4.2	**Drugs used in psychoses and related disorders**
	4.2.1 Antipsychotic drugs
	4.2.2 Antipsychotic depot injections
	4.2.3 Antimanic drugs
4.3	**Antidepressant drugs**
	4.3.1 Tricyclic and related antidepressant drugs
	4.3.2 Monoamine-oxidase inhibitors
	4.3.3 Selective serotonin re-uptake inhibitors
	4.3.4 Other antidepressant drugs
4.4	**Central nervous system stimulants**
4.5	**Drugs used in the treatment of obesity**
	4.5.1 Anti-obesity drugs acting on the gastro-intestinal tract
	4.5.2 Centrally acting appetite suppressants
4.6	**Drugs used in nausea and vertigo**
4.7	**Analgesics**
	4.7.1 Non-opioid analgesics
	4.7.2 Opioid analgesics
	4.7.3 Neuropathic pain
	4.7.4 Antimigraine drugs
	4.7.4.1 Treatment of the acute migraine attack
	4.7.4.2 Prophylaxis of migraine
	4.7.4.3 Cluster headache
4.8	**Antiepileptic**
	4.8.1 Control of epilepsy
	4.8.2 Drugs used in status epilepticus
	4.8.3 Febrile convulsions
4.9	**Drugs used in parkinsonism and related disorders**
	4.9.1 Dopaminergic drugs used in parkinsonism
	4.9.2 Antimuscarinic drugs used in parkinsonism
	4.9.3 Drugs used in essential tremor, chorea, tics and related disorders
4.10	**Drugs used in substance dependence**
4.11	**Drugs for dementia**

PHARMACOKINETICS

The study of pharmacokinetics involves observations of what happens to drugs once administered. As such, it involves the study of what the body does to drugs, as opposed to pharmacodynamics, the study of what drugs do to the body.

All pharmacokinetic processes can be expressed mathematically, and this is of considerable value in determining and predicting the pharmacokinetic properties of drugs. Clinically, however, mathematical modelling of pharmacokinetic processes is of very limited utility. Much more important is an understanding of the basic principles of what happens to drugs when administered by different routes, and how single and multiple dosing of different formulations affect plasma concentration–time relationships (Figure 57.1).

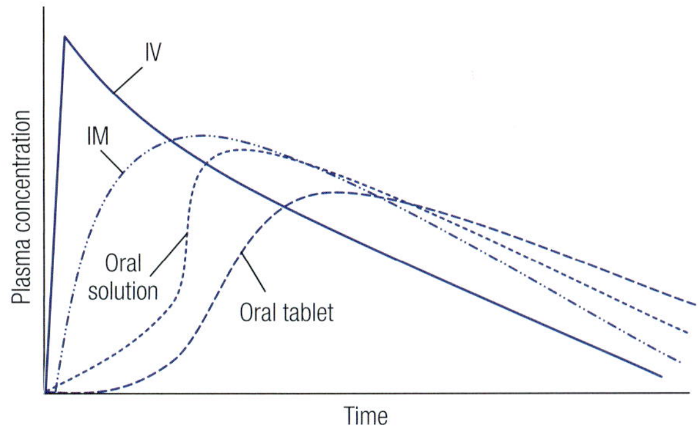

Figure 57.1 Plasma concentration versus time – routes of administration IM, intramuscular; IV, intravenous.

Pharmacokinetics is traditionally divided into absorption, distribution, metabolism and elimination. Although this is a useful division, not all processes occur with all drugs, and additional processes occur with some formulations of drugs. Note also that, although these processes do take place in this sequence, it is usual for two, three or even all four processes to overlap.

Absorption

Absorption describes the process of the passage of a drug from the gut or the drug's site of administration into the bloodstream.

Oral administration

The most commonly used formulation for oral administration is the tablet, a ubiquitous but surprisingly complicated dosage form. Tablets contain not only drug but also a variety of other substances incorporated for various functions. These include lubricants (to allow passage through tabletting machines), fillers (to bulk tablets of minute drug dosage), binding agents and so-called bursters (to allow water to penetrate the tablet once exposed to an aqueous environment). Once taken, tablets cannot be absorbed as a whole but first need to disintegrate in order to allow dissolution in the stomach and bowel fluids. Only dissolved substances can be absorbed, usually by passive diffusion along the concentration gradient but occasionally by active transport mechanisms.

The necessity for disintegration and dissolution delays absorption and therefore delays drug action – tablets do not have a rapid therapeutic effect. The disintegration process can be manipulated to produce modified-release or controlled-release tablets. Here, disintegration is slowed by physical means (e.g. incorporating drug into a wax matrix) and becomes the rate-limiting step in absorption. The rate of absorption is slowed and the duration of drug action usually prolonged. Many tablets are film- or sugar-coated to improve taste or appearance. These coatings may delay absorption to a small extent.

Capsules incorporate powdered or liquid drug into a gelatine sheath. There is no need for disintegration, but absorption is slowed by the dissolution of the gelatine capsules and by wetting of the drug powder (clumps of dry powder often resist water entry). Absorption from capsules is generally similar to that of tablets, although liquid-filled capsules allow fairly prompt absorption.

Liquid oral formulations show slightly different absorption characteristics. Suspensions contain undissolved drug particles suspended in a vehicle, usually water or syrup. When the liquid is taken, absorption is fairly brisk because disintegration need not take place, although dissolution is still necessary. With solutions (dissolved drug in a vehicle), absorption is very prompt as the drug is actually given in an absorbable form.

Once absorbed, orally administered drug is carried in the hepatic portal vein to the liver. The liver is presented with the entire drug absorbed often at high concentration and so substantial hepatic metabolism may take place. This is the well-known first-pass effect. The amount of drug reaching the general circulation after oral administration is known as the oral bioavailability. This quality is expressed as a percentage or fraction and incorporates in its value the extent of absorption and the effect of first-pass hepatic metabolism.

Sublingual, buccal and rectal administration

Some drugs (buprenorphine, midazolam, lorazepam) may be given sublingually or via the buccal route. Sublingual tablets usually disintegrate within seconds, allowing dissolution and absorption. Liquid drugs given in this way are absorbed within a few minutes. First-pass metabolism is avoided and so bioavailability is often very much higher than when given orally. Rectal administration also allows very prompt absorption and mostly avoids first-pass metabolism. None of these routes allows release of drug to be modified in any meaningful way, and so administration by these routes is usually reserved for drugs with poor oral availability (buprenorphine) or where a rapid effect is required (midazolam).

Parenteral administration

Subcutaneous administration of drugs or drugs in solution usually provides a rapid onset of action. Injected drug diffuses fairly rapidly into local blood vessels and is carried into the general circulation. Intramuscular (IM) injection is usually more rapidly effective because of the relatively greater blood flow in muscles. IM injections are usually of drugs in aqueous solution, but drug release can be controlled by the use of injectable suspensions (e.g. some corticosteroids) or by the use of drug dissolved in vegetable oil (e.g. antipsychotic depot injections). Both methods provide slow release of drug over days or weeks. Intravenous (IV) injections are usually effective within a few seconds – the drug is injected directly into the general circulation.

Distribution

Once a drug reaches the general circulation, it is said to undergo the process of distribution. That is, the drug equilibrates between the blood and the tissues according to various factors. These include plasma protein binding, water and lipid solubility, molecular size, pH partition and tissue binding. The apparent volume of distribution (V_d) is a measure used to indicate the extent to which a drug equilibrates outside the blood compartment. Small values indicate that the drug is held in the blood compartment, larger values (some several hundred litres – hence 'apparent') indicate that much of the drug is held in the tissues. The volume of distribution is easy to calculate. Say we give 200 mg of a drug that shows 50 per cent bioavailability, and we find that the resultant plasma level is 20 mg/L. The volume of distribution is the volume that is required to account for the entire drug reaching the circulation – in this case, 100 mg/20 mg = 5 L (i.e. most or all of the drug is in the blood compartment).

Psychoactive drugs are usually highly lipid-soluble and show a large or very large volume of distribution. Lipid solubility is required to allow the drug to pass the blood–brain barrier (the barrier presented to chemical entities by endothelial cells of cerebral capillaries). The absence of fenestrations (gaps or windows) between endothelial cells in brain capillaries means that chemicals must pass through the cells to enter the brain. This factor limits transit to lipid-soluble chemicals and chemicals subject to active transport mechanism (some simple sugars and amino acids). This high lipid solubility shown by most psychoactive drugs also means that they are subject to extensive metabolism (water-soluble drugs can be excreted unchanged).

Metabolism

Drug metabolism involves chemical modification of the drug, usually to render it less toxic or active (sometimes more toxic or active – a 'pro-drug') and more polar and water-soluble to facilitate urinary excretion. Phase I metabolism generally involves minor chemical reactions (hydroxylation, demethylation) catalysed by cytochrome p450 (CYP) and other enzymes in the liver and sometimes in the gut and elsewhere. Phase II reactions are those that involve the combination (conjugation) of the drug or primary metabolite with another molecule to form a complex such as a glucuronide. These compounds are polar and invariably inactive and are readily removed by the kidney (morphine-6-glucuronide is a rare active glucuronide).

Metabolic enzymes

Phase I drug metabolism is performed by a range of hepatic and extra-hepatic enzymes. These include the cytochrome enzymes (CYP), flavin-containing mono-oxygenases (FMO), monoamine oxidase and alcohol dehydrogenase. The CYP enzymes are most important in respect to drug metabolism.

CYP enzymes catalyse oxidative reactions and are subcategorized according to their encoding genes. Drug metabolism is catalysed mainly by CYP1A2, CYP3A4, CYP2C9/19 and CYP2D6 (CYP2E1 has a role in alcohol metabolism). There are a great many other CYP enzymes involved in the metabolism of endogenous steroids, fatty acids, cholesterol and certain vitamins.

CYP enzymes show some genetic variations, and their function can be suppressed (enzyme inhibition) or increased (enzyme induction) by other substances (drugs, foodstuffs, polyaromatic hydrocarbons contained in cigarette smoke). Table 57.2 shows the CYP enzymes commonly involved in psychoactive drug metabolism.

Excretion

Drugs are eliminated from the body either unchanged or as metabolites. Lipid-soluble drugs are usually metabolized to polar conjugates to allow excretion. Typically, most drugs are excreted by the kidney, although biliary, faecal and pulmonary excretion occurs with some drugs.

Renal excretion may involve glomerular filtration, active tubular secretion and passive tubular re-absorption. All three processes are dependent on glomerular filtration rate. Only free (i.e. unbound) drug can be excreted. Hepatocytes also excrete drugs, even lipid-soluble parent drugs and metabolites. Active transport mechanisms are usually involved. Drug passes into the bile and then may be re-absorbed (enterohepatic recycling) or eliminated in the faeces. Pulmonary excretion is seen only with volatile anaesthetic gases and vapours and, to a small extent, with compounds such as ethanol.

Because of their lipophilicity, psychoactive drugs are usually metabolized, often extensively and by a variety of pathways, before being eliminated. A very few psychotropics are excreted unchanged; these include lithium, sulpiride and amisulpride. The clinical doses of these drugs (up to

Table 57.2 Cytochrome P450 enzymes and psychotropic drugs

Enzyme	CYP1A2	CYP2C19	CYP2C9	CYP2D6	CYP3A4
Genetic variation	Individual variation in activity	3% of Caucasians are poor metabolizers	5–10% Caucasians are poor metabolizers	5–10% Caucasians are poor metabolizers	Individual variation in activity
Substrates	Amitriptyline, caffeine, clozapine, fluvoxamine, haloperidol, olanzapine	Amitriptyline, citalopram, clomipramine, diazepam, imipramine, moclobemide	Amitriptyline, fluoxetine	Amphetamine, amitriptyline, aripiprazole, atomoxetine, chlorpromazine, clomipramine, duloxetine, fluoxetine, haloperidol, imipramine, paroxetine, perphenazine, promethazine, venlafaxine, zuclopenthixol	Alprazolam, aripiprazole, buspirone, cocaine, diazepam, haloperidol, methadone, midazolam, quetiapine, risperidone, trazodone, zaleplon, zolpidem
Inhibitors	Fluvoxamine	Fluoxetine, fluvoxamine, modafinil, topiramate	Fluvoxamine, sertraline	Bupropion, fluoxetine, duloxetine, paroxetine, sertraline	Fluvoxamine, fluoxetine
Inducers	Chargrilled meat, cigarette smoke, modafinil	Carbamazepine	Secobarbital	Dexamethasone	Barbiturates, carbamazepine, St John's wort

and over 1 g a day) are an indirect indication of the poor lipid solubility: high doses are needed to ensure that sufficient quantities enter the brain.

Clearance

Clearance (CL) is the term used to define the rate of elimination of a drug. Mathematically, it is a product of the elimination rate constant (K_e) and the volume of distribution (V_d).

$$CL = K_e V_d$$

Clearance is expressed in litres/hour, and so rate of drug removal from the body can be seen as a function of drug concentration, assuming clearance remains constant. For example, if clearance of drug X is 5 L/h, then when the concentration of X is 100 mg/L the amount eliminated per hour will be 5×100 mg = 500 mg. When the plasma concentration is 10 mg/L, then the amount removed will be 5×10 mg = 50 mg/h. This aptly demonstrates the nature of so-called first-order kinetics of drug elimination – the rate of drug elimination is dependent on plasma concentration (the higher the concentration, the faster the elimination).

The nature of first-order kinetics can also be seen in the measure of drug persistence in the body – the plasma half-life ($t_{1/2}$). This measure gives the time for plasma concentration to fall by a half. The time taken for plasma concentration to fall from 100 mg/L to 50 mg/L will be the same as the time for the concentration to fall from 10 mg/L to 5 mg/L. This exponential decay can be seen in plasma concentration–time graphs, particularly those following IV administration.

Multiple dosing and steady state

Most psychoactive drugs are given in repeated, regular dosing to treat enduring conditions. In multiple dosing, absorbed drug is added to drug already in the system. The plasma level obtained after the second dose will therefore be higher than that seen after the first dose. Plasma levels continue to rise until a steady state is achieved, when rate of drug availability equals rate of drug removal (another result of first-order kinetic processes). Attainment of steady state usually takes four to five half-lives to achieve in regular dosing (the frequency of dosing does not affect the time to attainment of steady state, unless the intervals are so long that all previously administered drug has been removed).

Knowledge of steady-state kinetics has two important implications. First, it should be understood that plasma levels are usually much higher at steady state than after the first or second dose (Figure 57.2) and so assessment of drug effect or tolerability should be delayed until steady state is achieved. Second, the use of plasma levels to ensure response or safety will usually be appropriate only once steady-state levels are achieved.

Plasma drug levels and therapeutic response

The action of all drugs is dependent on their concentration at the site of action. This, in turn, is proportional to drug plasma level. Plasma level is related directly to dose and

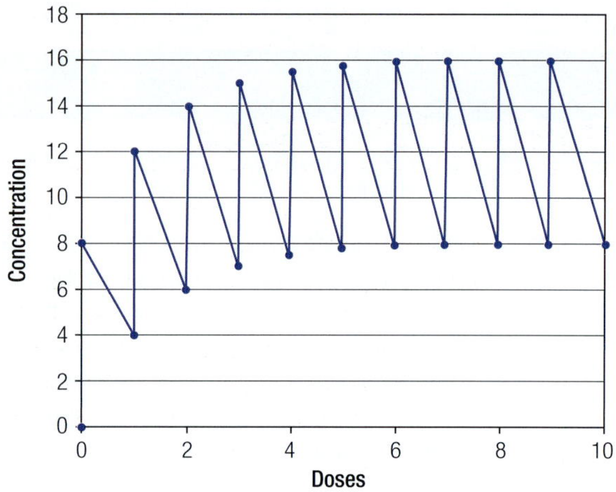

Figure 57.2 Attainment of steady state (intravenous example)

frequency of dosing. However, because of individual and genetic variation in absorption, metabolism and excretion, drug plasma level is sometimes difficult to predict from dose alone. So, for some drugs, plasma level monitoring (or therapeutic drug monitoring, TDM) is essential to ensure their safe and effective use. In psychiatry, TDM is mandatory for lithium, very useful for clozapine, carbamazepine and valproate, and sometimes beneficial for olanzapine, risperidone and tricyclic antidepressants (TCAs).

A prerequisite for the use of TDM with a particular drug is that its plasma levels should be related clearly to its therapeutic or adverse effects. In fact, plasma level is always related to these outcomes – a plasma level of zero produces no effect, certain concentrations slightly above zero will also produce no effect, higher levels will give rise to therapeutic and/or adverse effects, and higher levels still will probably produce no further therapeutic effect but more severe or frequent adverse effects. For most psychotropics, the precise relationship between dose or plasma level and therapeutics has not been defined clearly. The main reason for this is that not all patients show a response, and so in some individuals no therapeutic effect will be seen, no matter what dose or plasma level is attained. This makes difficult the process of establishing exact dose– (or plasma level–) response relationships.

For TDM to be clinically useful, the measured drug plasma level must have some inherent meaning – it should indicate the likelihood of therapeutic or adverse effects. For the psychotropics listed above, a target range (sometimes misleadingly termed 'therapeutic' or even 'normal' range) has been defined. This is a range of plasma levels where clinical effectiveness can be expected while adverse effects are minimized. The lower limit is usually the lowest plasma level at which effect might be seen, and the upper limit is that at which adverse effects become unacceptable. The target range is inevitably something of an approximation, and so it should not be taken as holy writ. Moreover, where therapeutic or adverse effects are obvious, plasma level becomes immaterial. This is a frequent occurrence in practice: some patients will respond at apparently subtherapeutic plasma levels, while others will suffer severe adverse effects with plasma levels in the target range. In such cases, it always pays to treat the patient (i.e. what you see before you) rather than to be concerned obsessively about achieving the 'right' plasma level.

Sampling

Appropriate blood sampling is crucial to effective TDM. Plasma levels vary over time, sometimes showing substantial peak-to-trough variation within the dosing interval. Target ranges are generally set for plasma samples taken at a particular time in respect to the previous dose and may be less useful or even meaningless for samples taken at other times. It is essential, therefore, to make the effort to sample at the appropriate time, and it is imperative that the times of sampling and of the previous dose are recorded on the pathology request slip. Changes in reported plasma levels in individual patients may well be a result of changes in sampling times rather than, say, a change in compliance.

Lithium

TDM is essential when prescribing lithium because it has a narrow therapeutic index (toxic levels are only slightly above therapeutic levels), because plasma level is difficult to predict from the dose alone, and because its prophylactic effect in bipolar disorder is difficult to discern clinically. Various studies have suggested a target range of around 0.8–1.2 mmol/L (12-h post-dose sampling) for bipolar prophylaxis.[12,13] However, possibly the most reliable predictor of effect is the reduction in plasma level: abrupt changes seem to provoke increased frequency of relapse.[14] In acute mania, there is some evidence that plasma levels of 1.0–1.2 mmol/L are necessary for an adequate effect.[15]

Clozapine

With clozapine, TDM is useful principally because plasma level attained varies considerably in individuals given the same dose (gender and smoking status have a profound influence on clozapine metabolism).[16,17] The threshold for therapeutic effect is around 0.35 mg/L,[17] and important adverse effects such as seizures tend to occur at plasma levels above 1.0 mg/L.[18] The recommended target range is 0.35–0.6 mg/L.[19] Blood samples are usually drawn at the end of the dosing interval (i.e. trough sample).

Carbamazepine

The target range for carbamazepine in bipolar disorder has not been established clearly, but TDM is useful nonetheless because of the drug's ability to induce its own metabolism and the variation in plasma levels that results from this. Trough plasma levels above 7 mg/L seem to be associated with response.[20] Adverse effects such as diplopia and dizziness usually become intolerable at plasma levels of around 10 mg/L.[21] Modified-release carbamazepine tablets are generally tolerated better because they result in lower peak plasma levels than conventional tablets.[22]

Valproate

In epilepsy, the target range for valproate is 50–100 mg/L. Most trials establishing valproate's utility in mania and bipolar prophylaxis have utilized this range as a guide to dosing. In mania, response seems to improve as trough plasma levels increase from 50 mg/L to 125 mg/L,[23] so TDM is probably useful. At the very least, TDM should prevent underdosing of valproate.

Olanzapine

Dose–response relationships for olanzapine are not defined clearly, largely because of the absence of fixed-dose studies in the literature. Plasma level–response relationships are better understood, and a threshold for response has been discerned at around 20 μg/L (12-h post-dose).[24,25] Levels above 40 μg/L seem to offer no additional benefit.[26] A target range of 20–40 μg/L has been suggested.[27] In practice, olanzapine TDM is helpful only where response is not seen at the highest licensed dose or where compliance is in doubt.

Risperidone

Few UK laboratories measure risperidone plasma levels. A target range of 20–60 μg/L has been suggested.[19] Dose–response relationships for oral risperidone are well understood,[28] and so risperidone TDM is perhaps only of value with risperidone long-acting injection where appropriate dosing is difficult because of its delayed release characteristics and uncertainty over appropriate dosing.[29]

Tricyclic antidepressants

TDM of tricyclics is now undertaken rarely, but it is occasionally helpful. Therapeutic plasma levels are usually around 100 μg/L (target ranges vary according to drug).[30] Plasma levels are useful in cases of non-response or suspected non-compliance. Tricyclic toxicity is best assessed by electrocardiogram (ECG) rather than drug plasma level.

Other drugs

In the UK, TDM practices leave a lot to be desired. Often, a prescriber will send off a blood sample for drug plasma level determination with little knowledge of its likely value. The analyst assumes that the prescriber would not request a drug assay without good reason, determines the plasma level, and reports this to the prescriber. The prescriber assumes that if the laboratory undertakes the assay, then it must be of some use, and so it goes on. In fact, TDM is entirely inappropriate for the large majority of psychotropic drugs (SSRIs, most antipsychotics, benzodiazepines), either because the effect or plasma level is predicted readily from the dose given or because no reliable target range has been defined. Even plasma level requests aimed at ruling out non-compliance have limited utility: a plasma level of zero or close to zero indicates recent non-compliance, but any other value is impossible to interpret.

PHARMACODYNAMICS

The background to this section is set out in detail in Chapters 23 and 24. See also Leonard.[31]

The term 'pharmacodynamics' refers to the effect of a drug on biological mechanisms – in psychopharmacology, specifically in the brain. The key structure is the synapse, which is the gap between one neuron (presynaptic) and the next (postsynaptic). The key substance is the neurotransmitter that is released from the presynaptic axon and diffuses to the postsynaptic dendrites of the next neuron. Thus, an electrical signal is converted into a chemical one and then back into another electrical signal (excitation), or prevents the electrical signal (inhibition). Several neurotransmitters can act in the same synapse, allowing for subtle multiple influences, in contrast to the axonal transmission, which is all-or-none. The mammalian CNS contains over 50 neurotransmitters, of which the most relevant to psychopharmacology are acetylcholine, dopamine, noradrenaline (norepinephrine), serotonin (5-hydroxytryptamine, 5-HT), glutamate, histamine, the encephalins, γ-aminobutyric acid (GABA) and glycine. The release of the small molecule transmitter is often accompanied by the release of larger molecule peptides as co-transmitters. The effect of the neurotransmitter will also depend on the characteristics of the receptor to which it binds, and can stimulate or inhibit neuronal activity.

The schema of axonal impulse → neurotransmitter → neuron is now known to be oversimplified, and dendritic release can also occur. Axons can be branched, which increases the complexity. Further, neurons can be plastic and alter their properties with use and disuse. The anatomical organization of the 10^{12} neurons in the brain is exceedingly complex, and drug actions are accordingly complicated.

Neurotransmitter function

The elucidation of neurotransmitter and drug functions has been two-way traffic – the discovery of a putative transmitter led to examination of psychotropic drug effects on that transmitter's mechanisms, and the drug could be used in the search to establish the physiological function of that transmitter. For example, serotonin was found in the brain and then lysergic acid diethylamide (LSD) was found to exert its hallucinogenic properties by interacting with it. Criteria have been generally adopted as necessary requirements to establish a substance as a transmitter (Box 57.1).

Receptors

Receptors are complex protein structures, often with different types of subunit. They surround and control an ion

Box 57.1 Criteria necessary for a neurotransmitter

- It should be present in nerve terminals and their vicinity.
- The passage of a nerve impulse should release the transmitter.
- Enzymes for the synthesis and breakdown of the substance should be present in the nerve ending and synapse.
- A physiological response (excitation, inhibition or modulation) should follow its release.
- This response can be mimicked by local application to the postsynaptic receptor site.
- The response should be blocked selectively by an antagonist and potentiated by an agonist.

channel across the nerve membrane that governs the entry of various ions into the neuron, altering its excitability. Sodium, potassium and calcium are the most common cations involved. The effects of the transmitter can be fast (inotropic) or slow (metabotropic); both are important in psychopharmacology. The latter receptors are linked to intracellular second messengers.

Presynaptic activity can be altered by auto-inhibition, thus providing a negative feedback system. The neurotransmitters are typically stored in vesicles, which can be altered by drugs; for example, reserpine depletes neurons of dopamine.

Postsynaptic mechanisms can involve an increase (up-regulation) or decrease (down-regulation) of receptor numbers, according to activity across the synapse, another feedback mechanism. Long-term use may be associated with a change in the receptor itself; for example, it has been suggested that benzodiazepine tolerance and dependence involve the synthesis of a different balance of receptor subunits.

A drug may change the balance postsynaptically, but its effects will then be opposed by a change in the receptor numbers in an attempt to overcome its effects. SSRIs prevent the reuptake of serotonin back into the presynaptic neurons, increasing the drug's availability and action on the postsynaptic receptors. These and other receptors further down the neuronal cascade then become reduced in number ('down-regulated') to overcome the stimulation.

Complex mechanisms exist to terminate the actions of the neurotransmitter. Enzymes can be found in the synapse and its vicinity. Some transmitters are re-absorbed back into the presynaptic neurons, where they may re-enter the storage vesicles or be metabolized intracellularly. These disposal mechanisms are a prime target for psychotropic drug action, such as MAOIs and SSRIs. Most other psychotropics act on the receptors themselves, both pre- and postsynaptic. Although neurotransmitters can be widespread in the brain (e.g. GABA, glutamate), others are found in fairly well-defined systems, such as the dopaminergic system. However, although the cell bodies may be found in circumscribed areas, their projections may be very diffuse in the brain, particularly the cortex.

Individual neurotransmitters

The large number of neurotransmitters precludes any detailed discussion. The main features of those most relevant to psychopharmacology are listed in Table 57.3.

Table 57.3 Features of the main neurotransmitters involved in the action of psychotropic drugs

Transmitter	Precursor	Metabolites	Receptors	Drug actions	Psychiatric disease
Serotonin (5-HT)	L-Tryptophan	5-HIAA (melatonin in the pineal)	About 15 subtypes	Tricyclics, SSRIs, SNRIs, MAOIs	Depression, mania
Dopamine	L-Tyrosine	Several	D_1, D_5, D_2, D_3, D_4	Antipsychotics, amphetamines, cocaine	Schizophrenia, ADHD, OCD, (Parkinson's disease)
Noradrenaline	L-Tyrosine	Several	$\alpha1$, $\alpha2$, $\beta1$, $\beta2$	Agonists, antagonists	Depression, mania, anxiety
Acetylcholine	Choline	Choline	Muscarinic, nicotinic	Acetylcholinesterase inhibitors, nicotine	Dementia, ?mania
GABA	Glutamate	Succinic, semi-aldehyde	A, B, C	Benzodiazepines, baclofen	Anxiety, epilepsy
Glutamate	–	Several	NMDA/kainate	Memantine, lamotrigine, phencyclidine	Dementia, epilepsy, ?schizophrenia

ADHD, attention deficit hyperactivity disorder; GABA, γ-aminobutyric acid; 5-HIAA, 5-hydroxyindoleacetic acid; 5-HT, 5-hydroxytryptamine; MAOI, monoamine oxidase inhibitor; NMDA, *N*-methyl-D-aspartate; OCD, obsessive–compulsive disorder; SNRI, serotonin and noradrenaline reuptake inhibitor; SSRI, selective serotonin reuptake inhibitor.

Electroconvulsive therapy

This treatment has established efficacy in severe depression, but it may induce cognitive defects. Numerous changes occur in the brain. Those most likely to be associated with the therapeutic response include increases in serotonin and noradrenaline, enhanced postsynaptic 5-HT$_2$ activity and decreased postsynaptic beta-adrenergic activity. The memory deficit may be an expression of decreased function of central muscarinic receptors.

FACTORS INFLUENCING TREATMENT

Initial level effects

The response of an individual to a drug treatment will often be partly dependent on the initial level of activity. For example, very depressed patients tend to be more responsive than mildly depressed individuals to antidepressants. Indeed, it has been asserted that SSRIs have no demonstrable efficacy in mildly ill patients, so that antidepressants are not indicated.[32] In patients with dementia, some cognitive enhancers are not recommended in the early stages of the condition but are reserved for later stages (Mini Mental State Examination (MMSE) 10–20).[33]

Dose effects

The effect of a drug varies with dose. The classic dose–effect curve is sigmoid, with a slow increase in effect at the lowest doses, a steady increase in effect, and then a flattening off at higher levels. The maximum effect can vary greatly from drug to drug. A good example concerns the analgesics. Non-opioid agents, no matter how high the dose, cannot achieve the degree of effective analgesia of an opioid.

The dose–effect relationship is important in influencing the way a drug is administered in practice. Some drugs have unwanted effects at dose levels close to those needed for a therapeutic effect. For example, extrapyramidal side effects (EPSEs) occur at doses of typical antipsychotics only just above those inducing a worthwhile therapeutic effect. Lithium has such a narrow therapeutic margin between risk and benefit doses that routine serum drug estimations are used to optimize dosages.

Doses of drugs are often recommended as a range. Generally speaking, treatment is initiated at the lower end of the range and the dose is increased if no response is forthcoming after a reasonable trial period. However, there have been very few studies in which this strategy has been tested adequately. The appropriate trial design is to select a group of predefined non-responders and randomize them to continue double-blind on their dose plus placebo or the extra dose. There are few trials of this nature. Fixed-dose studies of antipsychotics suggest a fixed threshold for therapeutic effect above which dose increases show no benefit,[28,34] and the National Institute for Health and Clinical Excellence (NICE) suggests that lowest licensed doses of SSRI antidepressants are sufficient for most people.[32] Nevertheless, dosage increase is usually routine.

Time effects

Drug effects change over time. Repeated doses may induce effects not discernible with single-dose administration. Two main processes are relevant. With long-acting compounds, accumulation must occur in order for a therapeutic level to be attained. An opposing process is that of tolerance, wherein repeated doses result in tolerance, so that effects wane or the dose has to be increased to maintain the effect. Some drugs of misuse, such as the stimulants and sedative hypnotics, are prone to show tolerance with marked escalation of dosage.

One phenomenon that has prompted much debate is the delay of onset of detectable response to the antidepressants and the antipsychotics. The conventional view is that the initial week or two of administration is characterized by unwanted effects such as sedation and nausea, without any clear signs of improvement. Then the side effects wane and remission begins. This time sequence has been challenged by others, who point out that controlled trial data with both classes of medication show some improvement from early on but that this does not reach statistical let alone clinical significance until 2 weeks or more.

Individual variation

As with almost all biological responses, much individual variation can be discerned. Factors such as ethnicity and genetic heterogeneity have been elucidated, but much of this patient-to-patient variation remains unexplained. Pharmacokinetic differences between people are also important, and many studies have investigated this. Despite all this endeavour, lithium and some other mood-regulators remain the only psychotropic medications in which estimation of bodily concentrations is routine.

Variation in response can also occur in the same individual at different times or even within the 24-h diurnal cycle. The severity of the illness may also govern the response, with higher doses needed when a patient relapses than when on maintenance treatment. Some patients can be taught to self-monitor their psychiatric symptoms with a view to increasing the dose if they sense that relapse is imminent.

Milieu effects

Drugs are given to individuals in specific social situations, such as the home or a ward in the hospital. Drug responses may be modified accordingly. The classic example was the introduction of chlorpromazine in the 1960s. Some sceptics regarded the undoubted subsequent benefits, including enhanced discharge rates, as reflecting the greater confidence and optimism of the nursing staff, rather than a specific pharmacological effect. In turn, this facilitated a more liberal mental health policy, which increased the beneficial effects, thus setting up a 'virtuous cycle'.

Another interpretation was that the drug and non-drug effects were not interacting positively but that either could be effective on their own, and there was no gain in combining them. The most extreme view was that one treatment could interfere with the other, a negative interaction. Over time, it has become accepted that a positive interaction occurs even when both components of treatment are already optimal.

Therapist effects are also operating. A prescriber with a positive but still critical attitude to drug therapy tends to have better results than the sceptic.

Placebo effects

Placebo effects have become a large topic in pharmacology. They are often particularly noticeable with respect to psychotropic medication and psychiatric patients. In trial after trial, in a range of disorders, 30–50 per cent of patients show a clinically useful improvement on placebo. Many factors are involved. One is the panoply of attention and optimism that surrounds the participant in a clinical trial. This response occurs even though the patient is aware that he or she is taking an inert substance. The hopes, fears and expectancies of the individual operate to good effect.

Another feature that may masquerade as a placebo effect is natural remission. A proportion of patients will improve because that is the natural progression of that type of illness. But even in chronic non-remitting disorders, the placebo effect may be appreciable.

Controlled trials

The methodology involved in the evaluation of a treatment has proceeded apace over the past few decades. No longer is it acceptable to give a few specialists a new drug to try out and to take their opinions as worthwhile. Under pressure from drug regulatory authorities and academic experts, strict guidelines have evolved for the controlled assessment of medications, new and old. This type of trial is the accepted gold standard to evaluate both efficacy and risk. The following are the main components:[8]

- Careful selection of the target population using standard diagnostic criteria, usually from the *Diagnostic and Statistical Manual*, version 4 (DSM-IV) or the *International Classification of Diseases*, version 10 (ICD-10). A screening instrument may be used.
- Exclusion of patients who are inappropriate or may be at particular risk of adverse effects, e.g. women of child-bearing potential not using effective contraception, or patients taking other medications or illicit drugs.
- Use of appropriate, sensitive and validated outcome criteria, usually employing a rating scale or an objective measure like the polysomnogram. Investigators should be trained in their use.
- Allocation using a randomization procedure to the test drug and a placebo, often with a standard medication as a comparator. The comparator allows a post-hoc estimate of the sensitivity of the trial because it should separate from placebo. If it does not, then no conclusions can be drawn, as the study seems insensitive. The placebo should match the test drug in every way possible.
- Neither the patients nor the investigators should be aware of which medication any individual patient is taking (double-blind). Ideally, one investigator should question the patient about adverse effects, and the efficacy should be assessed by a separate observer. This was a particular problem with older medications, which were very likely to induce unwanted effects that the patient would report, thus invalidating the double-blind procedures.
- The design of the study should be rigorous and the proposed statistical analyses set out unequivocally in the protocol. An experienced statistician should be involved from the start.
- The outcome variables should be predesignated as 'primary', upon which the outcome of the trial depends, and 'secondary'. This prevents cherry-picking of significant variables post hoc. More general measures such as quality of life may be helpful.
- A clear distinction should be maintained conceptually between statistical significance with a preset level, usually 0.05, and clinical significance, which is the investigator's clinical judgement as to whether the statistical difference has any real meaning in practice. Variables such as response and remission rates are often more apposite than changes on the rating scale.
- Careful records are kept of adverse effects. These can be objective such as QT_c prolongation of the ECG, or subjective complaints volunteered spontaneously by the patient or elicited by the investigator, perhaps using a standard scale.
- Dosage schedules must be chosen carefully. Are patients going to be allocated to fixed doses throughout the duration of the study, or can the dose be varied according to the patients' response and tolerability? Are several fixed doses to be used, thus providing a dose–effect curve? How are the doses chosen, and is the dose of the comparator a fair one? There are numerous quite complex considerations here.
- The duration of the trial must also be chosen judiciously. If the duration is too short, then the therapeutic effects may not be sufficiently evident to reach statistical significance. If the duration is too long, then in some conditions natural remission in both groups may obscure any effect. Longer-term assessment usually takes the form of relapse-prevention, whereby responders to a test

medication are allocated randomly to continue on the medication or to switch to placebo: relapse rates are then calculated.

- The number of patients entered into the trial should be sufficient to allow a conclusion to be obtained with a reasonable degree of probability. It is pointless and unethical to enter so few patients that significant differences are unlikely to accrue. The number can be computed in advance (power calculations).
- Compliance with medication can be monitored with tablet counts or random urine or blood tests. Best of all is to retain the patient's confidence.
- The protocol for the study should be submitted to the appropriate ethical committee and the patient should give informed consent, preferably written. Serious adverse events should be referred immediately to the ethical committee and, where necessary, to the relevant regulatory authority.

PRINCIPLES OF RATIONAL PRESCRIBING

This is a huge topic that has been revolutionized by the advent of numerous guidelines for prescribing. Such guidelines can be promulgated by a variety of agencies, both national and international. In the UK, the British Association for Psychopharmacology and the Royal College of Psychiatrists have been active in setting out advice on treating various disorders and problems. Official bodies such as the Committee on Safety of Medicines have issued warnings on particular adverse effects. NICE has produced influential but sometimes contentious guidelines on a range of disorders; the guidelines tend to emphasize non-drug treatments, especially for less seriously ill patients.

The topic of severity of the presenting complaint has tended to dominate this area. Most conditions form a pyramid of frequency, with many mildly ill people only just attaining 'caseness', and some moderately ill individuals above them, and culminating in a peak of a few severely ill patients. The first decision is whether to treat at all or to resort to 'watchful waiting' and reassurance, non-drug methods such as sleep hygiene with insomnia, or lifestyle advice. More elaborate psychological techniques such as cognitive-behavioural therapy (CBT) may be recommended.

If a drug is deemed appropriate, a low dose should be tried initially, particularly in elderly patients and patients with physical illness. The patient should be informed fully about the medication, its effectiveness and its more common adverse effects. Appropriate tests should be carried out, such as renal function in patients being considered for lithium therapy and blood counts in candidates for clozapine.

An adequate time should elapse before an increase in dose is contemplated. The dose can be increased up to the recommended maximum in the BNF. Beyond that, any increases should be very circumspect and the reasons documented carefully and legibly in the notes. This is particularly necessary with antipsychotic medication, where dosage ranges tend to be wide.[35]

The duration of treatment is an important consideration. With some, such as the benzodiazepines, duration should be minimal; with others, such as the SSRIs, the treatment should not be curtailed prematurely.

The choice of medication will reflect the information contained in the reviews but also the individual prescriber's experience and predilections. If the first treatment proves unsuccessful, then guidelines for resistant or refractory patients should be followed for the second and even third choices. Ancillary symptomatic treatment may be needed, for example hypnotic medication in the unresponsive depressive patient plagued by severe insomnia. Side effects of the primary medication may need symptomatic treatment, but the number of concomitant medications must be monitored and minimized. Too often, even now, some patients end up on multiple drugs with the high risk of drug interactions.

Prescribers should be very clear as to whether their prescription is for a licensed indication for that medication or whether it is unlicensed ('ex-label'). The medicolegal implications are vastly different.[36] If such a usage is resorted to, the notes should state very clearly why, and the reasons discussed with the patient and/or the carers.

DRUG CLASSES

Antipsychotics

The earliest true antipsychotic, chlorpromazine, is a derivative of phenothiazine compounds originally developed as commercial dyes in the 1880s. Chlorpromazine was found, by chance, to have antipsychotic activity in the early 1950s. Early developments involved minor modifications of the phenothiazine structure to produce compounds such as thioridazine (now withdrawn) and prochlorperazine (used as an anti-emetic). In the 1960s Paul Janssen developed haloperidol, a butyrophenone compound, from pethidine. Further phenothiazines (fluphenazine, trifluoperazine) were also developed, along with closely related thioxanthine compounds such as flupentixol. Also in the 1960s, antipsychotics were shown to share antagonist properties at dopamine receptors. For a while, development centred on producing drugs whose pharmacological activity was limited to dopamine antagonism. Examples include pimozide (a diphenylbutylpiperidine) and sulpiride (a substituted benzamide).

All of these drugs were effective antipsychotics, with little to choose between them in terms of efficacy, and all caused parkinsonian symptoms and tardive dyskinesia as a result of their dopamine antagonist effects. Clozapine, a drug first used in the 1960s, was seen to be effective without causing extrapyramidal symptoms. Clozapine became known as an atypical antipsychotic because it did not cause typical adverse effects. In the 1990s, clozapine was reintroduced as an antipsychotic, having earlier been withdrawn because of its association with agranulocytosis. Other atypical antipsychotics followed: risperidone, olanzapine, sertindole, quetiapine and amisulpride. These drugs are classified by their atypical nature (although some are atypical only at low doses) and not by their chemistry. Clozapine, olanzapine and quetiapine share a similar chemical structure, but the others are more diverse. Aripiprazole is also atypical but, unlike other antipsychotics, both conventional and atypical, it is a dopamine partial agonist rather than an antagonist. Bifeprunox is similar.

There are thus two broad groups of antipsychotics, conventional (typical) or first-generation drugs, and atypical or second-generation drugs. Conventional drugs are subdivided according to their chemistry, and atypical drugs according to their pharmacology (Table 57.4).

All antipsychotics are active orally, and some are used parenterally (e.g. haloperidol) as simple IM or IV injections. Some phenothiazines and thioxanthines have a terminal -OH group, which allows reaction (esterification) with long-chain carboxylic acids to form oil soluble esters (e.g. decanoate, enanthate, palmitate). These drug esters are highly lipid-soluble and are given in vegetable oils as IM depot injections. Slow release from the oily depot affords stable plasma levels over several weeks. Examples include pipotiazine palmitate, fluphenazine decanoate and flupentixol decanoate. Some atypical drugs are also given as depot injections, although their formulations differ. Risperidone, for example, is given as a suspension of microcrystalline particles in which risperidone is incorporated. The drug is released slowly as the particle breaks down.

Efficacy

The efficacy of antipsychotics is usually assessed in randomized, placebo-controlled trials lasting 4, 6 or 8 weeks. Symptomatic change is evaluated using the Positive and Negative Symptom Scale (PANSS)[37] or the Brief Psychiatric Rating Scale (BPRS).[38] A reduction of 20 per cent in either scale is usually defined as a response. In first-episode schizophrenia, response is usually seen in more than 80 per cent of patients treated,[39] depending on the trial conditions and drugs used. In so-called refractory schizophrenia, responders usually number less than 10 per cent when standard treatments are used.[40]

Efficacy studies have largely revealed a wide range of antipsychotics to have very similar effects on psychotic symptoms in schizophrenia. In refractory schizophrenia, clozapine is substantially more effective than conventional and some atypical antipsychotics.[40] High-dose olanzapine may have similar properties.[41,42] A large meta-analysis of efficacy studies suggested that clozapine, olanzapine,

Table 57.4 Classification of antipsychotics

Group	Subgroup	Examples	Properties
Typical	Phenothiazines – aliphatic	Chlorpromazine, promazine	Sedative, low potency, antimuscarinic
	Phenothiazines – piperidine	Thioridazine*, pipotiazine	Sedative, low potency, very antimuscarinic, lower risk of EPSE
	Phenothiazines– piperazine	Fluphenazine, trifluoperazine, prochlorperazine, perphenazine	Less sedative, high potency, less antimuscarinic, higher rate of EPSE
	Thioxanthines	Flupentixol, zuclopenthixol, thiothixene*	As aliphatic phenothiazines
	Butyrophenones	Haloperidol, droperidol*, benperidol	As piperazine phenothiazines
	Diphenylbutylpiperidines	Pimozide	As piperazine phenothiazines
	Substituted benzamide	Sulpiride, amisulpride**	Low sedation, low EPSE, renally excreted,
Atypical	Multi-receptor antagonists	Clozapine, olanzapine, quetiapine	Sedative, high risk of weight gain
	D_2/5-HT_2 antagonists	Risperidone, sertindole, asenapine, ziprasidone, zotepine, paliperidone	Less sedative, lower risk of weight gain
	Dopamine partial antagonists	Aripiprazole, bifeprunox	No sedation, very low risk of weight gain

NB: potency is not related to efficacy. Low-potency drugs require higher doses to be effective (e.g. 100 mg/day); high-potency drugs are given in lower doses (e.g. < 20 mg/day).

*No longer used.

**Usually classified as atypical.

EPSE, extrapyramidal side effects; 5-HT, 5-hydroxytryptamine.

risperidone and amisulpride were significantly more efficacious than conventional antipsychotics.[43] This perhaps reflects these drugs' reduced propensity to produce extrapyramidal effects and the resulting improvement in negative symptoms of schizophrenia.

Effectiveness studies, which study a more diverse range of patients under more naturalistic clinic conditions, have suggested differences between antipsychotics. Clozapine is clearly supremely effective in refractory schizophrenia, and olanzapine may have some useful effectiveness.[44] Olanzapine and risperidone also appear to have advantages in patients intolerant of other drugs.[45] Quetiapine appears to have relatively weak antipsychotic effectiveness.[44–46]

Rational prescribing of antipsychotics involves the use of a single antipsychotic drug at a licensed dose. In the UK and elsewhere, antipsychotic polypharmacy and high-dose prescribing are very common.[47,48] A major factor in both practices is the use of 'when necessary' (PRN) prescribing of antipsychotics.[49] In such cases, antipsychotics are generally prescribed for their sedative effects; sedatives such as promethazine and benzodiazepines are thus better choices.

Antipsychotic polypharmacy appears to offer no therapeutic benefits over single-dose treatment and may worsen outcome and increase mortality.[50,51] Polypharmacy with clozapine is often recommended where clozapine alone has failed,[19] but even this strategy has only a minimal evidence base to support it.[52] Similarly, high-dose antipsychotics offer no advantages.[53] In fact, most if not all antipsychotics show a threshold-type dose–response relationship, with optimal doses often shown to be at the lower end of the licensed dose range.[28,34]

In organic psychosis, the same principles of rational prescribing apply. Choice of antipsychotic is based on individual characteristics, in the absence of a body of controlled trials of different agents. In psychosis of dementia, antipsychotics have only a limited effect,[54] a fact not reflected in their widespread use in elderly patients.

Anticonvulsants

Anticonvulsant drugs show an extremely wide range of chemical structures and have a correspondingly wide range of actions and adverse effects. Their modes of action often involve either enhancing the activity of the inhibitory transmitter GABA or antagonizing the effects of the excitatory transmitter glutamate. Classification is usually by chemistry, but clinical use and pharmacological mechanisms are sometimes used. In this chapter, anticonvulsants are classified primarily according to their chemistry.

Aldehydes

Paraldehyde is still used occasionally, either by the IM route or rectally. It is usually reserved for refractory status epileptics. Glass syringes should be used, as paraldehyde dissolves some plastics. Its mode of action is unknown. Paraldehyde undergoes significant pulmonary excretion.

Barbiturates

These were once the mainstay of the treatment of epilepsy but they are now rarely used because of their adverse cognitive effects and enzyme-inducing properties. Phenobarbital and primidone (a pro-drug of phenobarbital) are the only products still licensed for epilepsy in the UK. TDM may be helpful for both products: the target range for plasma levels is 15–40 mg/L. Phenobarbital injection is still used occasionally in status epilepticus.

Benzodiazepines

Most benzodiazepines have anticonvulsant properties (they enhance GABA activity). Clobazam, clonazepam and clorazepate are used orally in the prophylaxis of seizures. Tolerance can develop. Diazepam (IV or rectally), lorazepam (IV or IM) and midazolam (IV, IM or via buccal mucosa) are used in status epilepticus.

Carboxamides

Carbamazepine is used extensively in a variety of seizure disorders and in trigeminal neuralgia and bipolar disorder. Oxcarbazepine is similar to carbamazepine (its structure has an additional oxygen atom) but seems to be tolerated better and less prone to drug interactions.[55] Both drugs act by stabilizing voltage-gated sodium channels, thus suppressing repeated neuronal firing. TDM is useful with carbamazepine, both in epilepsy and in bipolar disorder. The target range is usually 8–12 mg/L.

Fatty acids

Valproate, vigabatrin and tiagabine are fatty acids. The mode of action of valproate is poorly understood.[56] Vigabatrin inhibits GABA metabolism, and tiagabine is a GABA reuptake inhibitor. Valproate is the most widely used. TDM is helpful with valproate. The target range is 50–100 mg/L in epilepsy.

Fructose derivatives

Topiramate is a fructose derivative licensed for the treatment of a range of seizure disorders and for migraine prophylaxis. It has multiple actions, including enhancement of GABA and inhibition of glutamate. It is one of the few drugs used in psychiatry that reliably causes weight loss. Impairment of memory and concentration can be problematic.

GABA analogues

This group includes gabapentin, pregabalin and vigabatrin. The mode of action seems to include binding to voltage-gated calcium channels (gabapentin, pregabalin). Gabapentin was once used in mania. Pregabalin is effective in anxiety.[57]

Hydantoins

Phenytoin and fosphenytoin (a phenytoin pro-drug used parenterally) are used widely in epilepsy. The mode of action is similar to that of carbamazepine. Phenytoin famously shows capacity-limited or zero-order metabolism. Small changes in dose can give rise to extensive changes in plasma level. The target range is 10–20 mg/L.

Pyrrolidines

Levetiracetam is a relatively new anticonvulsant given orally and IV. Its mode of action is complex and poorly understood.

Succinimides

Ethosuximide was once in widespread use, but it is now used rarely. Its main use is in absence seizures, but blood dyscrasias can be problematic. Its mode of action is unknown.

Sulfonamides

Acetazolamide is no longer used in epilepsy, except in that associated with menstruation, but zonisamide is licensed for refractory partial seizures with or without secondary generalization. Zonisamide may act by binding to voltage-gated sodium and calcium channels.

Triazines

Lamotrigine is an effective anticonvulsant that also shows efficacy in bipolar depression and as a prophylaxis against bipolar depression.[58] Lamotrigine inhibits glutamate release. Its use is made complicated by the need for slow titration (because of the risk of rash, which can be life-threatening) and by interaction with valproate (a common co-therapy). TDM is sometimes undertaken, but a target range has not been defined.

Drugs for Alzheimer's disease

Alzheimer's disease involves numerous structural and neurochemical changes that pharmacotherapy attempts to correct at least partly. The function of acetylcholine is known to be reduced in Alzheimer's disease, and drugs that inhibit acetylcholine metabolism (acetylcholinesterase inhibitors, ACHIs) afford some symptomatic improvement. Three acetylcholinesterase inhibitors are in widespread use in the UK, as is a drug with multiple actions, memantine.

Acetylcholinesterase inhibitors

Donepezil was the first ACHI to be marketed in the UK for use in Alzheimer's disease,[59] although its use had been preceded by tacrine, a similar, but unlicensed drug with problematic hepatic adverse effects and a short plasma half-life. Donepezil is usually tolerated well (nausea and diarrhoea are the most common adverse effects) and can be given once daily. It is subject to hepatic metabolism catalysed by CYP2D6 and CYP3A4. It has a robust but small effect on cognitive symptoms of Alzheimer's disease.

Rivastigmine has a similar mode of action to donepezil, except that its action on acetylcholinesterase is more prolonged (pseudo-irreversible inhibition).[60] It is metabolized at the site of action, with a plasma half-life of around 2 h; there is no hepatic metabolism. Rivastigmine is usually given orally twice daily or via a once-daily transdermal patch. Efficacy and tolerability are similar to those of donepezil. Galantamine, the third ACHI, is derived from bulbs and flowers of snowdrops and related species.[61] It may also possess nicotinic receptor agonist activity. Galantamine has a plasma half-life of around 7 h, but modified-release preparations allow once-daily dosing. It is metabolised by CYP2D6 and CYP3A4. Galantamine has similar efficacy and tolerability to donepezil.

Memantine

One theory for the loss of neurons in Alzheimer's disease is that neurons are damaged by excitotoxic injury induced by excess glutamate and overstimulation of *N*-methyl-D-aspartate (NMDA) receptors.[62] Memantine is an NMDA receptor antagonist thought to have neuroprotective activity.[63] It has a measurable but small effect on change in symptom severity, either when used alone or when given with an ACHI. Adverse effects include dizziness, confusion and constipation. Memantine is metabolized in the liver to inactive compounds. Cytochrome p450 enzymes are not involved.

Cognitive enhancers

There are four licensed drugs that might be considered cognitive enhancers, all of which are licensed for the treatment of Alzheimer's disease. The ACHIs donepezil, rivastigmine and galantamine have remarkably similar therapeutic effects, all delaying deterioration by around 9 months.[64–66] Memantine has similar efficacy.[67] Rational prescribing involves using the highest tolerated dose and avoiding the concomitant use of anticholinergic drugs.

Delirium

Delirium is a common event in hospitals and is a frequent cause of confusion in elderly patients. Effective treatments include benzodiazepines, conventional antipsychotics, and newer antipsychotics such as risperidone and olanzapine.[68] The benzodiazepine lorazepam is probably the drug of choice owing to its rapid onset and relatively short duration of action.

Antidepressants

These are medications effective in the treatment of major depressive disorders of moderate and severe degree, including depressive syndromes associated with physical illnesses. Patients with dysthymic disorder may also respond. The main classes include the TCAs and related compounds, the SSRIs, the SNRIs and the MAOIs (both selective and non-selective).[69] Stimulants such as the amphetamines are not antidepressants but can elevate mood in normal subjects. St

John's wort (*Hypericum perforatum*) is a widely used herbal remedy, with some MAOI activity, with efficacy in mild depression.[70]

The antidepressant actions of the MAOIs were discovered when patients with tuberculosis treated with iproniazid (related to isoniazid) became euphoric. The MAOIs are used infrequently and currently comprise phenelzine, isocarboxazid and tranylcypromine. They act by irreversibly blocking the enzyme monoamine oxidase in the brain and elsewhere. Tranylcypromine is closely related to the amphetamines and shares their stimulant properties. The blockade of MAO raises amine-type neurotransmitter levels in the brain and underlies the antidepressant and anti-anxiety actions, especially against phobic symptoms. The blockade also raises amine levels in the bowel. The well-known interactions with other amines and similar substances result from the MAO inhibition that prevents the breakdown of tyramine in ingested food such as cheese, broad-bean pods, pickled herring, and soya and meat extracts.[71] This results in tyramine passing into the bloodstream and causing dangerous hypertensive crises. The other problem is interaction with indirect-acting sympathomimetics in cough and decongestant preparations, and with pethidine. These hazards can persist for 2–3 weeks after the MAOI is discontinued, as the inhibition is irreversible and new enzyme has to be synthesized.

To overcome this problem, reversible MAOIs have been developed. The only one extant is moclobemide, which is selective on only one form of the enzyme, MAO type A. It is much less likely to be associated with pressor responses, but it is not regarded as efficacious as the classic MAOIs.

The TCAs were also discovered serendipitously, this time in the search for antipsychotics following the advent of chlorpromazine. Imipramine, chemically similar to chlorpromazine, had no appreciable antipsychotic activity but helped patients with depression, particularly those with biological features. A whole range of similar compounds were then developed, including amitriptyline, amoxapine, clomipramine, dosulepin (dothiepin), doxepin, lofepramine, and trimipramine. Related but non-tricyclic compounds are maprotiline, mianserin and trazodone. Their usage differs substantially between countries, and each prescriber has her or his favourite among the TCAs.

The mechanism of action was elucidated after the empirical clinical demonstration of efficacy.[72] The main action of TCAs is to inhibit the reuptake of serotonin and noradrenaline (and, to a lesser extent, dopamine) from the synaptic cleft, back into the presynaptic neurons. Most TCAs affect serotonin disposition either on its own or in conjunction with noradrenaline. Sometimes, as with amitriptyline and clomipramine, the demethylated metabolite primarily blocks noradrenaline reuptake. Others, such as maprotiline, affect noradrenaline uptake alone. Buproprion (amfebutamone), licensed as an antidepressant in the USA but not in the UK, affects mainly noradrenaline and dopamine.

The TCAs are 'dirty drugs':[73] they also have actions on cholinergic, alpha-adrenergic and histaminergic receptors, believed to be unnecessary for the antidepressant response. This results in anticholinergic side effects such as dry mouth, blurred vision, constipation and urinary retention; alpha-blocking effects with hypotension and dizziness, particularly in elderly patients (and priapism, especially with trazodone); and antihistaminergic effects, with sedation, sometimes profound. Other unwanted effects include sweating, hyponatraemia and ECG changes. TCAs are dangerous in overdose: lofepramine is probably the safest of the group.[74]

The SSRIs and the SNRIs are direct descendants of the TCAs. When it became apparent that only the reuptake blockades were associated with antidepressant activity, the race was on for pharmaceutical companies to develop more selective compounds, thereby reducing side effects. The first group were SSRIs, starting with zimeldine (withdrawn because of neurotoxicity), followed by (in alphabetical order) citalopram, escitalopram, fluoxetine, fluvoxamine, paroxetine and sertraline. They are less sedating, have fewer or no anticholinergic effects and are less cardiotoxic than the TCAs.[75] They can induce side effects such as nausea and diarrhoea, anorexia with weight loss, and heightened anxiety and sexual problems. As with other antidepressants, hypomania can be induced in susceptible patients. Because of changes in serotonin peripherally, platelet adhesion is decreased and bleeding may occur. The more common side effects such as nausea are clearly dose-related but tend to wane with continued use.

The SNRIs were developed with a similar rationale to the SSRIs, but with an additional claim that, as they acted selectively on two neurotransmitters, they would prove more effective than the SSRIs. This claim is still debated. The first introduction was venlafaxine, followed more recently by duloxetine.[76] The side-effect profiles are similar to those of SSRIs, but the noradrenaline reuptake inhibition is associated at higher doses with a clinically significant rise in blood pressure. Concerns about the arrhythmogenic properties led to a temporary restriction on prescribing venlafaxine.[77] Blood pressure should be monitored in all patients receiving SNRIs.

Reboxetine is a selective noradrenaline reuptake inhibitor with some anticholinergic-type side effects[78] and may also increase blood pressure. Mirtazapine acts in a complex way and resembles mianserin; it is sedative and associated with definite weight gain.

Finally, the amino acid L-tryptophan, the precursor of serotonin, appears to benefit a few patients when given adjunctively to patients with treatment-resistant severe depression.[79]

It can be seen that the pharmacology of the antidepressants focuses on their actions on serotonin, noradrenaline and, to a minor extent, dopamine. Nevertheless, despite the establishment of efficacy in a range of disorders, the mode of action of these compounds remains unclear. Add to that the demonstration of efficacy in other disorders such as anxiety, and our limited understanding becomes apparent. It is hardly surprising that a range of other biochemical mechanisms are constantly being explored to seek targets for novel drug actions – so far, with only limited success. Too often, a promising compound with an unusual putative mechanism of action fails to fulfil its promise in the clinic.

Therapeutic issues

The treatment of depression and other mood disorders is discussed in other chapters. We have selected some aspects that have particular relevance to the psychopharmacology of the antidepressants.

Basic principles

It is important to discuss at some length with the patient the diagnosis of depression and its implications, and the need for medication. The reasons for the particular choice of antidepressant should be explained. The likely outcome of the treatment should be estimated, without exaggerating the probability of a rapid and complete response. The possibility and type of unwanted effects should be outlined carefully without unduly alarming the patient.

The initial dose of a TCA should be such as to minimize unwanted effects and will usually need increasing as side effects wane. The SSRI dosage is usually an efficacious one from the start but may need increasing if the response is unsatisfactory. For a single episode, continue treatment for at least 4–6 months after apparent remission. For repeated relapse, longer-term or maintenance treatment may need to be considered. The early stages of drug administration need careful monitoring, especially in patients under the age of 30 years. Restlessness, agitation (a form of akathisia) and suicidality may ensue or increase.[80] Dosage adjustments are then necessary. Dosages, particularly of paroxetine and venlafaxine, should be tapered off carefully. Even so, some withdrawal symptoms may supervene, so the patient should be forewarned.[81]

Children and adolescents

This is a complex topic dealt with elsewhere.

Elderly people

Depression is particularly common in elderly people.[82] Suicide is an especial risk and is a danger in socially isolated or recently widowed people. Most physical illnesses are more common in elderly people and are associated with an increased risk of depression. Examples include Parkinson's disease, cardiovascular and respiratory diseases, and chronic pain, particularly joint pain, with its association of restricted movement. Elderly people are likely to be taking medication for their physical illnesses, with the consequent risk of increased adverse reactions and complex drug interactions.

The TCAs are often poorly tolerated in elderly patients, who are prone to develop troublesome symptoms such as dry mouth, blurring of vision, constipation, urinary retention and postural hypotension. SSRIs are tolerated better.[82] Treatment should be initiated at half the dose, but full doses may be needed. The risk of gastrointestinal or cutaneous bleeding may be increased, particularly in very elderly people. Sedative antidepressants should be monitored carefully, as confusion may ensue. Response often seems slower in elderly patients than in younger adults. Patients who have suffered repeated episodes may need indefinite treatment.[83] Because of the likelihood of drug interactions in patients with physical disorders and treatments, reference should be made to the BNF drug interaction tables in order to avoid any complications of combined treatments.

Refractory depression

Refractory depression is a common problem in secondary care.[84] A fair proportion of patients referred by general practitioners (GPs) to psychiatrists have failed to respond to the antidepressant initially prescribed. The choice of an alternative is already limited. Various protocols have been drawn up, some based on clinical experience, and a few based on the scant data that are available. Either switch or augmentation regimens can be used.

The switch protocols are essentially trial-and-error. On theoretical grounds, it should be advantageous to move to a different class of drug. The most common stratagem has been to switch to venlafaxine from an SSRI, with the rationale that it is better to influence two neurotransmitters rather than one. The evidence is by no means consistent.

Direct comparisons of the SSRIs and the SNRIs show very few significant differences. A few studies suggest that escitalopram is superior to citalopram and venlafaxine. Even fewer studies establish the superior efficacy of venlafaxine to the SSRIs. Dosage considerations may affect such comparisons.

Augmentation procedures have been available for a long time. They are sometimes based on animal studies, and the results in the clinic are less impressive. The best established is the addition of lithium, aiming for a serum level of 0.4–1.0 mmol/L.[85] This is recommended by NICE,[32] which also advocates ECG monitoring. Lithium needs careful monitoring of renal and thyroid function. Other augmentation regimens with some evidence to support them include triiodothyronine, bupropion, buspirone and mirtazapine. Non-drug treatments such as CBT are also worth considering.

Long-term prevention (prophylaxis)

Depression is a recurrent, episodic disorder. Over half of patients having a first episode will have a second attack, and most of those will go on to have a third and subsequent attacks. The risk of recurrence is increased in people with marked social problems and a family history. Chronic medical illness also increases the risk of recurrence.

Continued treatment with an antidepressant reduces the risk of recurrence by up to two-thirds.[86] NICE has recommended that patients who have suffered two or more episodes of depression in the recent past, accompanied by significant functional impairment, should be kept on antidepressants for at least 2 years.[32] Re-assessment may then lead to even longer maintenance. The dosage used should be the same as that effective in the acute episode, unless there are troublesome unwanted effects such as sexual dysfunction.

Lithium has proven efficacy in preventing episodes of depression in patients with bipolar disorder but apparently less efficacy in patients with unipolar disorder.

Patients should be reassured that antidepressants are not addictive and maintain their efficacy over time. When the antidepressant is discontinued, a slow taper is recommended, although withdrawal symptoms may still occur.

Psychotic depression

Response rates to antidepressants alone in psychotically depressed patients are poor.[87] It is generally recommended that a combination of an antipsychotic and an antidepressant be used. An atypical antipsychotic such as olanzapine or quetiapine is often preferred. ECT may be needed. Whatever combination is used, care must be taken to avoid hazardous drug interactions.

Conclusions

The treatment of the more severe forms of depressive illness is a major part of the responsibilities of the psychiatrist. Although numerous medications have been developed and introduced since the MAOIs and TCAs were discovered over 50 years ago, the choices available are variations on the theme of increasing brain availability of serotonin, noradrenaline and perhaps dopamine. Although the newer drugs are generally tolerated better, there is no evidence that any material improvement in the efficacy of the antidepressants has occurred.

Mood stabilizers

This name is given to a group of drugs that comprise lithium and several agents used primarily as anticonvulsants. Their main use in psychiatry is to prevent both upswings and down-swings of mood in patients with bipolar disorder.

Historical aspects

Lithium was used as a panacea in the nineteenth century but was rediscovered in the 1940s by Cade for use in psychotic disorders. Because of difficulties in establishing its efficacy in long-term prophylaxis of mania and its undoubted toxicity, it was slow in being accepted by prescribers. Eventually schedules for its use were introduced, and it is now regarded as a useful but problematic drug.

A series of anticonvulsants were introduced into psychiatric practice, including carbamazepine, valproate compounds, lamotrigine and topiramate. Antipsychotic drugs are also used in acute mania.

Lithium

This simple cation is used to prevent and to treat mania and hypomania, recurrent depression and bipolar disorder in general. Its use in mania is limited by the slow onset of action[15] and by the possibility of potentiating the EPSEs of antipsychotic medication. Lithium is also used to augment antidepressant medication in patients with depression who appear refractory.

The most firmly established indication for lithium is in the prophylaxis of bipolar affective disorder, where it reduces both the frequency and the severity of relapses, particularly into mania.[88,89] The number needed to treat (NNT) in order to prevent relapse into mania has been estimated as 10 and into depression as 14.

A set of tests is essential before prescribing lithium – renal, thyroid and cardiac function. Reliable contraception is essential in women of childbearing potential. Patients should be prepared carefully for lithium therapy and should be told about the need for regular therapy, the signs and symptoms of incipient toxicity, the necessity of avoiding dehydration, and the need to keep constant the salt intake in the diet. Potential drug interactions should be outlined.

The efficacy of lithium has been the subject of numerous studies, including an appraisal by NICE.[90] As well as reducing the risk of relapse into an affective episode, lithium reduces the likelihood of a hypomanic upsurge with antidepressant medication. In combination with valproate, it may reduce the frequency of rapid cycling, which is usually defined as a bipolar disorder in which four or more episodes of mania or hypomania occur in a year. It can be difficult to manage and may necessitate change of the antidepressant as well as a trial of mood stabilizers. NICE recommends that a mood stabilizer should be prescribed prophylactically:

- after a single severe manic episode;
- after two or more episodes of mania;
- in recurrent hypomania characterized by significant risk of suicide, functional impairment or high rate of relapse.

Lithium is generally recommended as a first-line measure. It is not possible to predict responders with any degree of accuracy, so trial of therapy with careful monitoring must be resorted to. Patients with mania rather than depression as the dominant feature tend to respond better than those with the reverse pattern.

Abrupt discontinuation of lithium may be followed by an increased rate of relapses during the ensuing few months.[91] Tapering over a month has been clearly shown to help. Accordingly, instituting of lithium therapy should not be undertaken without careful consideration of the risk/benefit ratio right through to eventual discontinuation. Perhaps the main benefit in bipolar illness is the reduction of suicide risk to the general population level.[92]

Lithium is the main psychotropic drug that is monitored routinely. Blood is taken 12 h after the last dose. After lithium is started, a plasma level should be estimated after 4–7 days and then weekly, until a stable level has been attained. It should then be checked every 3 months. If the dose has to be adjusted, more frequent estimations should be carried out. Plasma levels of 0.6–1.0 mmol/L are usually recommended. The purpose of the monitoring is both to keep the level in the therapeutic range and to avoid toxicity.

Adverse effects are related to bodily levels and increase rapidly above 1 mmol/L. The most common milder symptoms are thirst, polyuria day and night, and fine hand tremor. Psoriasis may be aggravated. In long-term use, thyroid function may be depressed. Hyperparathyroidism may also ensue, so that monitoring of calcium may be advisable. A subjective complaint in patients taking lithium is that they feel dulled: objective impairment of memory can be demonstrated.

The relationship of renal impairment to long-term lithium therapy remains controversial. A small number of such patients develop interstitial nephritis, with reduction in renal function of clinical significance. The nephrogenic diabetes insipidus with polyuria that develops early in treatment may later become irreversible.[93]

Lithium toxicity is often overlooked, as it can ensue insidiously. There is increasing anorexia and diarrhoea, muscle twitching, drowsiness and ataxia. If the level exceeds 2 mmol/L, seizures may occur and forced diuresis may be indicated. Neurotoxicity with memory disturbance may become irreversible.[94]

Carbamazepine

This compound is an anticonvulsant and is also used to treat trigeminal neuralgia. In psychiatry it is licensed as a second-line prophylactic in bipolar illness. It has also shown efficacy against the acute symptoms of mania. It is generally considered to be less effective than lithium, and NICE considers it to be a third-line treatment.[90] Occasional use in a range of disorders such as aggressive symptoms and borderline personality disorder is based on anecdotal reports.

Plasma levels are used to monitor its administration, and a level of at least 7 mg/L is generally required in bipolar illness. Because of its complex pharmacokinetics with auto-induction, monitoring is advisable after a dose adjustment.

The main unwanted effects are drowsiness, nausea, dizziness, diplopia and ataxia. A few patients develop a generalized erythematous rash, occasionally a severe toxic epidermal necrolysis. Other complications are chronic low white blood cell count and liver problems. Full blood count and liver function tests should be monitored in long-term users.

Because of its limited efficacy, potent hepatic enzyme-inducing properties and appreciable toxicity, carbamazepine is generally kept in reserve or used in conjunction with other mood stabilizers.

Valproate

Various forms are available – sodium valproate, valproic acid and semi-sodium valproate (Depakote™). The last is licensed for the treatment of acute mania but is widely used prophylactically in bipolar affective disorder, for which the evidence is less compelling.

Adverse effects are common. Gastric irritation and intense nausea can be a problem; higher doses may be associated with confusion and lassitude. Weight gain may be a nuisance. Women complain of hair loss, but the regrowth is curly! Children on complex regimens that include valproate are at remote risk of fulminating hepatic failure. Blood dyscrasias and pancreatitis have also been documented. Keeping plasma levels below 100 mg/L has been recommended to minimize side effects, and some formulations have smoother plasma level curves after ingestion than do others.

Valproate is regarded as a teratogen. NICE recommends that it should not be used routinely in women of childbearing age.[90] If its use is imperative, women should be counselled before valproate is prescribed. Adequate contraception should be used and folate prescribed as a precaution. Unfortunately, if treatment of recurrent mania is ineffective, sexual disinhibition can be one of the first signs of relapse.

Other treatments

It seems that every new anticonvulsant sooner or later is tried in affective disorder. Lamotrigine is an example, but intriguingly it seems better in preventing relapse of bipolar depression than of mania.[95]

Topiramate[96] and oxcarbazepine[97] are also tried on occasion, usually as add-on therapy. There are limited trial data to support their efficacy.

Some patients are maintained long term on more than one mood stabilizer. Such a regimen can be established only empirically. Antipsychotic drugs are used routinely both to treat acute phases and in the long term. Clozapine is established as a treatment for refractory mania.[98]

Anxiolytics and hypnotics

These groups of drugs are discussed together as their use is dictated by custom rather than by their pharmacology. However, differences in pharmacokinetic properties do play some part.

The term 'sedative' originally meant allaying anxiety, but it now has the connotation of causing unwanted drowsiness. Instead, the terms 'anxiolytic' and '(minor) tranquillizer' are now used to describe drugs that lessen anxiety, and the term 'hypnotic' is applied to medications taken at night to induce sleep. A range of substances, including alcohol, bromides, chloral hydrate and paraldehyde were used in the nineteenth century as both sedatives and hypnotics, but they were supplanted by a range of barbiturates in the twentieth century. These were effective but caused oversedation and confusion, were prone to be abused and were dangerous in overdosage. In turn, they were replaced by first meprobamate and then by numerous benzodiazepines from the 1960s onwards. Very popular at first, the benzodiazepines were found to be associated with cognitive and psychomotor impairment, particularly in elderly patients. Their use was curtailed, but they are still used extensively.

The mode of action of the benzodiazepines is to potentiate the inhibitory neurotransmitter GABA by binding to specific receptors.[99] This can reduce the turnover of several neurotransmitters such as noradrenaline and serotonin. The main sites of action of the benzodiazepines are in the spinal cord, where they mediate muscle relaxation, the brainstem, the cerebellum, causing ataxia, and the limbic and cortical areas involved in emotional experience and behaviour. The benzodiazepines vary in their profile and activity; for example, clonazepam has more anticonvulsant properties than most.

A benzodiazepine antagonist, flumazenil, is available. It binds to benzodiazepine receptors and prevents the actions of benzodiazepines. It can be used to reverse benzodiazepine overdosage. Finally, benzodiazepine inverse agonists have been described that have the opposite effects from those seen in benzodiazepines, being pro-convulsant and anxiogenic.

In normal individuals, the depressant effects of single and repeated doses of benzodiazepines can be detected easily, as they cause dose- and time-related cognitive and psychomotor impairment. Saccadic eye movements are disrupted and short-term memory is disorganized.

It would seem logical to use long-acting benzodiazepines as anxiolytics, reserving shorter-acting ones for hypnotic use. For complex historical reasons, however, this is not so, and anxiolytic benzodiazepines vary greatly in their duration of action. In the clinic, benzodiazepines reduce generalized anxiety and muscle tension and induce sleep. They also cause detectible cognitive and psychomotor impairment and subjective sedation. Careful testing shows that, although the subjective sedation subsides as tolerance sets in after a few days, the objective impairments may persist into the longer term, showing that tolerance is system-specific. In parallel, the electroencephalogram (EEG) fast beta activity that is increased by benzodiazepines persists. An additional complexity is that anxious and insomniac patients tend to perform poorly anyway. Anxiolytic/hypnotic treatment will improve that performance, so the depressant effects of the benzodiazepines will tend to be obscured by their beneficial effects. As the benefit wanes when tolerance sets in, only the impairments remain.

Because of these changes over time, it is widely recommended that the use of benzodiazepines be restricted to 4 weeks as anxiolytics and 2 weeks as hypnotics. These injunctions are largely ignored by some prescribers, who advertently or inadvertently allow the usage to become chronic, with the risk of withdrawal and dependence problems. Benzodiazepines do not have antidepressant properties. Concern that they may even induce depression is probably misplaced; however, as they lessen anxious symptoms in patients with both anxiety and depression, the depressive symptoms come to the fore. Concerns that benzodiazepines interfere with psychological processes such as bereavement or impede CBT are not supported by evidence.

NICE recommends that the benzodiazepines should not be used in panic disorder and found no evidence for their short-term use as adjunctive treatment with antidepressants in managing depression.[100] Benzodiazepines such as lorazepam are used in conjunction with antipsychotic medication to sedate acutely disturbed psychotic patients and appear to have a potentiating action. Longer-term usage in psychotic disorders is not established.

Unwanted effects

As well as the sedative effects outlined above, ataxia, dysarthria, blurred vision, headache and gastrointestinal upset can occur. Psychiatric side effects include memory disturbances, which are strongly dose-related.[101] Elderly people are particularly at risk, and the effects can be so profound as to lead to the apparent worsening of cognitive decline.[102] Withdrawal of the medication leads to resolution of the effects. One particular concern is impairment of driving performance, which can have legal implications.[103] Another concern is that the risk of hip fractures in old people taking benzodiazepines is increased by at least 50 per cent.[104]

Another unwanted effect with possible legal complications is paradoxical excitement.[105] This disinhibitory effect of the benzodiazepines can cause increased anxiety, acute excitement and hyperactivity. Aggressive impulses may be released with hostility and rage; criminal acts such as assault and rape have been documented. Estimates of incidence range from less than 1 per cent to at least 20 per cent, depending on the patient sample. High-risk patients include those with borderline personality disorders, impulse control disorder and alcohol problems. The combination of a benzodiazepine and alcohol is particularly prone to lead to paradoxical reactions. The patient may have complete or partial amnesia for the event, such as an episode of 'air-rage'. Intravenous administration of high doses of high-potency benzodiazepines poses an enhanced risk.

Dependence and withdrawal

Withdrawal symptoms from the benzodiazepines can ensue after 4–6 weeks of use, but only in about 20–30 per cent of patients.[106] The reasons why some patients can withdraw with impunity after even years of continuous use while others undergo agonies remains unclear. Dosage reduction and complete withdrawal can result in withdrawal symptoms. These include physical symptoms such as muscle tension, spasm and weakness, 'pins and needles' and flu-like symptoms. Perceptual hypersensitivity and depersonalization are common. Anxiety and insomnia may increase, nightmares may wake the patient, memory and concentration may be impaired, and depressive symptoms may ensue. Occasionally, fits or a paranoid psychosis may occur. The symptoms come on within two to three half-lives of the particular benzodiazepine and subside within a few weeks. Some patients claim that their symptoms have persisted for months or indefinitely.

Simple advice given by the GP can be quite effective.[107] Withdrawal schedules are available widely and involve tapering, usually after substituting diazepam.[108] The rate of taper is based not on good evidence but on the clinical experience of the prescriber. Psychological therapies or support groups should be used during the period of withdrawal. Once the patient has experienced withdrawal problems, they should not be prescribed a benzodiazepine again.

Dependence and withdrawal should be distinguished from addiction and abuse, in which the individual ingests large amounts of benzodiazepines. This can be part of polydrug abuse or an extension of prescribed sedative medication that has got out of hand.

Overdosage is common but not usually dangerous.

Other anxiolytics

Buspirone is the only available member of the azapirone compounds and is a partial 5-HT_{IA} agonist. It is a reasonably effective anxiolytic in general, but its onset of action is delayed.[109] It is relatively ineffective in patients with extensive prior experience of benzodiazepine treatment. Side effects include headache, dizziness and nausea. It is not associated with sedation, tolerance or withdrawal problems.

Hydroxyzine is an antihistamine/anticholinergic drug with some anxiolytic properties.[110]

A recent introduction is pregabalin. This compound was already licensed to treat neuropathic pain and some forms of epilepsy. It binds to the alpha-2-lambda subunit of voltage-gated calcium channels in the CNS. It has proven efficacy in generalized anxiety disorder in clinical trials.[57] It has a low incidence of side effects such as dizziness, somnolence and dry mouth. Tolerance, dependence and addiction potential are low. It reduces neurotransmitter release.

The drug treatment of choice in the anxiety disorders is the SSRI/SNRI group of drugs.[100] Antipsychotic drugs are favoured by some, but no firm evidence backs their use. Beta-blockers are still used by some primary care practitioners, but this use is not evidence-based.

Hypnotic treatments

Before prescribing a hypnotic short-term, 'sleep hygiene' measures should be recommended to the patient. These include daily exercising (afternoon is optimal), avoiding napping during the day, reducing alcohol and caffeine intake, ensuring regular sleep habits, and instituting anxiety-management/relaxation techniques.

A range of hypnotic benzodiazepines are available. The 'Z-drugs' – zopiclone, zolpidem and zaleplon – are essentially short- or very short-acting benzodiazepine-like drugs.[111] The short duration of action confers some advantages, such as lack of daytime sedation, but they are inappropriate for patients with early-morning awakening.[112] They probably have less propensity to rebound and withdrawal problems than benzodiazepines of equivalent duration of action. Addiction has been documented on occasion.[113]

Whatever hypnotic is chosen, it should be given at the lowest effective dose for no more than 2 weeks. Usage on an intermittent basis is desirable. Withdrawal should be slow. It is doubtful whether the risk/benefit ratio is favourable in elderly patients.[114]

Melatonin has a long tradition of being used to induce sleep. A sustained-release preparation (Circadin™) is available for use in insomniac people aged over 55 years.[115]

Sedative antidepressants such as amitriptyline and trazodone are prescribed to help induce sleep.[116] Sedative antihistamines are also available over the counter but can cause troublesome residual sedation the next morning. Other over-the-counter herbal remedies include valerian and hops.[117]

Finally, as with treatment of anxiety, CBT has been adapted to treat insomnia but is not widely available.

Stimulants

These drugs have few recognized indications and should not be used to treat depression, obesity, debility or fatigue. The amphetamines such as dexamfetamine can cause dependence and psychoses and are widely abused. Some patients with narcolepsy may derive benefit. The amphetamines and methylphenidate can be used as first-line treatment in attention deficit hyperactivity disorder (ADHD). Atomoxetine is also recommended by NICE as part of a comprehensive treatment programme in children.[118] Side effects include insomnia, restlessness and excitability. Anorexia and growth retardation can occur. Other side effects include dry mouth, sweating, tachycardia, palpitations and hypertension. Methylphenidate has been linked to allergic reactions and blood dyscrasias.

Adult ADHD remains a controversial diagnosis, but some children with ADHD continue to show symptoms into adulthood. The efficacy of stimulants has not been established in adults, so their use should be circumspect, especially in patients with a history of drug problems.

Modafinil is used to treat patients with narcolepsy, but its use in other indications such as depression remains experimental.[119]

Caffeine is a weak stimulant that is an ingredient of many analgesic preparations. Withdrawal can be followed by a headache, which can be severe.

Drugs used in substance dependence

Disulfiram is indicated as an adjunct in the treatment of chronic alcohol dependence.[120] It inhibits aldehyde dehydrogenase, leading to interruption of alcohol metabolism at the acetaldehyde stage. This causes unpleasant symptoms such as facial flushing, throbbing headache, palpitations, nausea and vomiting. After large amounts of alcohol, the reaction can be severe, with collapse. Disulfiram reduces the number of drinking days but does not increase total abstinence.

Acamprosate is a taurine derivative that interacts with GABA systems. It somewhat reduces relapse to alcohol reuse.[121] It is contraindicated in renal and hepatic failure. Side effects mainly involve the gastrointestinal system, with diarrhoea, nausea and vomiting.

Alcohol withdrawal can be facilitated by substitution and then tapering of a benzodiazepine such as chlordiazepoxide or with clomethiazole.[122]

Bupropion is licensed as an adjunct to smoking cessation. It is a tricyclic-type antidepressant primarily affecting the reuptake of dopamine. It approximately doubles the success rate in people trying to cease smoking and lessens significantly the severity of withdrawal symptoms.[123] It is contraindicated in patients with a history of seizures. Insomnia, dry mouth and headache are common side effects.

Varenicline is a partial agonist at the nicotinic acetylcholine receptor. It is more effective than bupropion, but it also causes nausea.[124] It has recently been licensed in Europe and introduced into the UK.

Nicotine-replacement therapy is available over the counter, and a range of preparations are available. It increases the rate of achieving smoking cessation by up to two-fold.[125] Dosage is self-adjusted and varies according to the degree of dependence.

Opioid dependence

Treatment of this condition is usually initiated by specialist staff after a comprehensive assessment. Methadone (full agonist) or buprenorphine (partial agonist) can be substituted for the illicit opioid, usually diamorphine (heroin).[126] Maintenance regimens need careful monitoring and may go on for long periods of time. Overdoses, deliberate or accidental, are frequent, and naloxone is indicated in short-term management. Monitoring should be continued for some time and doses repeated as necessary. Naltrexone has been advocated as an opioid antagonist for long-term use, but debate continues as to its effectiveness.[127] It can cause severe withdrawal reactions in current opioid users, who must be detoxified first.

The problem common to management of these conditions is that patients inform doctors of their usage of alcohol and opioids, and their estimates are notoriously unreliable and misleading. The prescriber should always err on the side of caution in evaluating both the misuse of the drug involved and the patient's report of the effectiveness of any treatment. For example, a misuser may exaggerate opioid usage when methadone is being substituted, which can lead the unwary prescriber into prescribing potentially harmful amounts.

PRESCRIBING IN PREGNANCY

The prescribing of psychotropics in pregnancy presents numerous difficulties.[128] Investigation of the teratogenic effects of drugs is limited to experiments in laboratory animals. For ethical reasons, trials are not conducted in humans. Thus, assessment of teratogenic potential is based on animal studies of dubious benefit and informal observations of pregnancy outcomes in women taking drugs in clinical practice. For many older drugs, teratogenic potential is reasonably well defined: valproate and carbamazepine are highly teratogenic, whereas older antipsychotics and antidepressants appear to have very limited or no effect on the developing fetus. Despite this knowledge, prescribers in the UK have been shown to take few precautions when prescribing potentially teratogenic drugs to women of childbearing age.[129]

When prescribing in pregnancy, the balance of risks needs to be considered and discussed with the patient. On one side, there is the risk of harm to the fetus (often poorly quantified) caused by the use of effective drugs; on the other side, there is the risk of relapse presented by cessation of drug treatment or by switching to alternative treatments. No general guidelines can be given, and each individual case should be treated as such. Always consult the latest information regarding pregnancy risk, as this changes very rapidly. It should be remembered that no drug is proven to be safe in pregnancy.

ADVERSE DRUG REACTIONS

Adverse drug reactions are classified as augmented or predictable (type A) or qualitatively bizarre or unpredictable (type B).

Type A reactions are predicted by a drug's pharmacology and are usually the result of an exaggerated but otherwise normal pharmacological action. Examples in psychiatry include sedation seen with benzodiazepines and some antipsychotics, extrapyramidal reactions to conventional antipsychotics, and nausea and diarrhoea seen with cholinesterase inhibitors. Note that type A reactions can occur as a result of both the therapeutic pharmacological action and other pharmacodynamic actions (e.g. H_1 antagonism, antimuscarinic activity). Type A reactions are dose-dependent, their incidence is high (relative to type B reactions) and mortality is low.

Type B reactions cannot, at least initially, be predicted from a drug's known pharmacological actions. These reactions are usually not dose-related and occur within the recommended dose range. Type B reactions may involve genetic causes (e.g. glucose-6-phosphate dehydrogenase (G6PD) deficiency) or immunological mechanisms and are said to be idiosyncratic. The frequency of type B reactions is usually so low that their possibility may not be detected during pre-marketing screening tests and trials. Morbidity and mortality are relatively high. Examples in psychiatry include agranulocytosis with clozapine, toxic epidermal necrolysis with carbamazepine, and neutropenia with mianserin.

Reporting adverse drug reactions

In the UK, the Medicines and Healthcare Products Regulatory Agency (MHRA) organizes the Yellow Card Reporting Scheme. The MHRA monitors the safety of licensed drugs by collecting and collating spontaneous reports of suspected adverse reactions submitted by health professionals and members of the public. Reporting may be completed online at http://yellowcard.mhra.gov.uk or by using yellow cards available in all editions of the BNF. For new drugs (signified in the BNF by the black triangle symbol ▼), all suspected adverse reactions should be reported. For older drugs, only serious adverse effects should be reported. In this context, 'serious' is defined as reactions that are fatal, life-threatening, disabling, incapacitating, resulting in or prolonging hospitalization, or otherwise medically significant.

MEDICATION ERRORS

Medication errors occur in the prescribing, dispensing and administration of drugs. They are a source of considerable patient morbidity and mortality. Prescribing errors are broadly divided into two categories: errors in the decision-making process and errors in writing the prescription. Decision-making errors include prescribing a drug to which the patient is allergic, prescribing two drugs for the same indication, and prescribing too low or too high a dose. Prescription-writing errors are usually 'slips of the pen', such as mistranscribing from previous charts, prescribing without stating dose or frequency, and omitting other data such as start date or patient name. Both types of error are fairly common in psychiatry in the UK: one study found errors in almost 1 in 40 prescriptions written.[130]

Decision-making errors can be reduced by ensuring thorough knowledge of each prescribed drug's dosage regimen, therapeutic indication, adverse effects and drug interactions. Many prescribing errors relate to drugs with which the prescriber is unfamiliar (e.g. general medical drugs prescribed by psychiatrists). Prescription-writing errors are avoided or reduced in number by careful checking for accuracy and completeness of the prescription. Both types of error can be made less likely by the use of electronic prescribing systems, which prevent the use of unlicensed doses and automatically ensure completion of the prescription.

POISONING WITH PSYCHOTROPIC DRUGS

Assessing the possibility that an individual has been poisoned, and identifying that poison, requires systematic detective work by the practitioner. Poisoning can be accidental or deliberate, either self-poisoning or with criminal intent. Clues include suicide notes and the circumstances in which the individual presents; clinical clues are often non-specific. The latter is quite important, as some psychotropic drugs have antidotes, such as naloxone for opioid poisoning and flumazenil for counteracting benzodiazepines. These can also be used as diagnostic tests.

All patients in which poisoning is suspected should be examined in hospital and usually admitted. This applies particularly to drugs with delayed action such as aspirin, paracetamol and TCAs. These are often resorted to by suicidal patients, as they are easily obtainable or at hand.

Most patients can be treated only symptomatically. Respiration may be depressed, for example with barbiturates, benzodiazepines and TCAs. Assisted ventilation may be necessary, but respiratory stimulants are potentially dangerous.

CNS depressants can lower blood pressure, so the patient should be given oxygen to correct any hypoxia and fluid replacement initiated. Some stimulants, such as amphetamines, cocaine and MAOI interactions, may induce a rise in blood pressure. Cardiac conduction defects may follow TCA or phenothiazine antipsychotic overdoses; specialist advice may be needed. These drugs can also induce hypothermia. Conversely, rises in temperature may follow stimulant overdose or occur in neuroleptic malignant syndrome. Appropriate vigorous remedial measures are required.

Convulsions may occur in TCA overdoses or following bupropion. Lorazepam or diazepam should be given intravenously if the fits persist.

Removal of the poison from the stomach is not useful if the drug has been ingested an hour or more earlier. CNS drug overdoses cause drowsiness or coma, so the airway must be protected. Induction of vomiting should not be attempted. Activated charcoal can bind many drugs in the stomach, preventing their absorption.

Many psychotropic drugs are formulated in delayed- or prolonged-release versions. This can pose particular problems, as drug concentrations in the body can remain high for some time.

Active elimination specialist techniques include haemodialysis for lithium poisoning and haemoperfusion for barbiturate overdoses.

Specific psychotropic drugs

Opioids cause coma and respiratory depression.[131] Pinpoint pupils are the give-away. Naloxone is a specific antidote but will need to be repeated as it has a short half-life relative to most opioids. Compound analgesics often contain paracetamol, which may cause delayed hepatotoxicity.

Antidepressants in overdose cause a range of serious effects, including coma, respiratory depression, cardiac conduction defects with arrhythmia, and fits. The TCAs are much more likely to induce such effects than the SSRIs.[132] Metabolic acidosis may complicate the picture. Symptomatic management in hospital is advisable. Diazepam may calm the delirious patient. MAOI overdose is uncommon, but tranylcypromine acts like an amphetamine-type stimulant.

Anxiolytics and hypnotics can cause drowsiness, coma, respiratory impairment, hypotension and hypothermia. Barbiturates and meprobamate are much more dangerous than the benzodiazepines. The combination with alcohol is particularly hazardous. Flumazenil can be used to reverse benzodiazepine poisoning, but it may induce fits in physically dependent patients.

Lithium poisoning is usually seen in long-term therapy, where the excretion of the drug is reduced because of dehydration (e.g. in exceptionally hot weather) or impairment of renal function and co-administration of diuretics (or other drugs that interact). Acute lithium overdoses are actually less dangerous. Severe poisoning is associated with vomiting, diarrhoea, ataxia, convulsions, coma and renal failure.[133] The last in particular is an indication for haemodialysis. Irreversible neurotoxicity can occur otherwise.

Phenothiazines and other antipsychotics may cause some depression of consciousness and respiration.[134] Dystonic reactions may ensue and respond to anticholinergic drugs. Arrhythmias need specialist evaluation.

LEGAL ASPECTS OF PRESCRIBING DRUGS

Classes of medicinal product

The Medicines Act 1968 defines three classes of medicines:

- General Sales List (GSL) medicines
- Pharmacy (P) medicines
- Prescription-only medicines (POM).

GSL medicines may be bought from a wide range of retail outlets under certain conditions. GSL products are usually small quantities of oral medicines such as paracetamol and ibuprofen. Pharmacy medicines may be sold only in a registered pharmacy under the supervision or personal control of a registered pharmacist. Prescription-only medicines may be supplied only in accordance with a prescription by an appropriate prescriber (e.g. registered medical practitioner, veterinary surgeon, dentist, nurse prescriber, pharmacist prescriber).

Controlled drugs

The Misuse of Drugs Act 1971 (as amended) controls the use of controlled drugs. The use of controlled drugs in medicine is governed by the Misuse of Drugs Regulations 2001. Individual controlled drugs or drug preparations are classified by five schedules, outlined below.

Schedule 1 (CD Lic)

Schedule 1 drugs are those that have virtually no clinical utility and for which a Home Office licence is required in order to be lawfully in possession. Examples include LSD, ecstasy and cannabis. Doctors, nurses and pharmacists are not permitted to possess these drugs unless properly licensed by the Home Office.

Schedule 2 (CD POM)

This includes most opiates (morphine, methadone), stimulants (amphetamine) and some barbiturates. These drugs may be supplied only against a properly written prescription (see below).

Schedule 3 (CD No register POM)

These are similar to Schedule 2 drugs but are considered less harmful or less likely to be misused (e.g. buprenorphine, midazolam, temazepam, phenobarbital). Storage and record-keeping requirements differ, but prescription requirements are the same as for Schedule 2 drugs.

Schedule 4 (CD Benz POM and CD Anab POM)

Schedule 4 includes most benzodiazepines, anabolic steroids and growth hormones. Controlled drug prescription handwriting regulations do not apply.

Schedule 5 (CD Inv or CD Inv POM)

These are preparations containing small quantities of certain opiates (e.g. co-codamol; co-codaprin). Many are P medicines. CD Inv POM preparations are exempt from controlled drug prescription-writing regulations.

Controlled drug prescriptions

Prescriptions for Schedule 2 and 3 controlled drugs must be written in a certain way. In fact, it is unlawful even to issue a prescription for a controlled drug unless the following requirements are met. The prescription must:

- be signed by the prescriber;
- be dated;
- be indelibly written or printed;
- include the prescriber's address (unless to-take-away (TTA) medication);
- specify the dose to be taken;
- specify the form and strength of preparation;
- specify the total quantity or number of dosage units in both words and figures;
- specify the name and address of the intended recipient;
- in the case of a quantity intended to be dispensed in instalments, contain a direction regarding the amount and frequency of intended dispensing.

There is now no longer a requirement for the prescription to be in the prescriber's handwriting, but it must be signed clearly by the prescriber.

Prescriptions for controlled drugs (including temazepam, midazolam and Schedule 4 drugs) are valid for 28 days from the date of issue. Although not a legal requirement, it is strongly recommended that the quantity prescribed should not exceed 30 days' supply.

USE OF UNLICENSED MEDICINES

Regulatory authorities issue marketing authorization and a product licence to a drug formulation after consideration of evidence relating to efficacy and safety. The product licence stipulates the conditions to be treated and the doses allowed. The prescribing of a licensed drug for conditions other than those stated, or at doses beyond those stipulated, is known as 'off-licence' or 'off-label' prescribing.

Some medicines used in the UK do not have a formal UK product licence. Examples include drugs licensed outside the UK (ziprasidone, melperone) and UK-licensed drugs available in formulations without a product licence (e.g. buccal midazolam, certain liquid preparations of methadone, sulpiride). These are unlicensed medicines. The prescribing of unlicensed medicines and off-label prescribing require special consideration, not least because accountability for any adverse consequences may lie with the prescriber rather than the manufacturer in such cases.

Prescribing unlicensed medicines

When prescribing an unlicensed medicine, the prescriber should:

- be satisfied that there is no alternative licensed medicine that would meet the patient's needs;
- be satisfied that there is a sufficient evidence base or experience of using the medicine to assure its safety and efficacy;
- take responsibility for prescribing the unlicensed medicine and for overseeing the patient's care, including monitoring and follow-up;
- record the medicine prescribed and the reasons for doing so.

When prescribing off-label, the prescriber should:

- be satisfied that it would better serve the patient's needs than an appropriately prescribed licensed medicine;
- be satisfied that there is sufficient evidence base or experience in using to assure efficacy and safety (this is likely to involve sources other than the manufacturer's information);
- take responsibility for prescribing the medicine and for overseeing the patient's care, monitoring and follow-up or arrange for another doctor or prescriber to do so;
- make a clear, accurate and legible record of medicines prescribed and the reasons for prescribing.

When prescribing unlicensed drugs or off-label, patients should be provided with sufficient information to enable them to make an informed decision. This information would normally include an explanation for off-label prescribing or for prescribing an unlicensed preparation. However, where current practice clearly supports the use of a medicine, it may not be necessary to draw attention to the licence. Examples include the use of sodium valproate in bipolar disorder and the use of certain antipsychotics in non-schizophrenic psychosis or mania.

CONCLUSIONS

This chapter has concentrated on the pharmacological attributes of the numerous drugs used in psychiatry that have their action on the brain. The prescriber should ask the questions set out in Box 57.2; if the prescriber does not know the answers, then they should find out from a larger textbook or the BNF.

Box 57.2 Basic knowledge about a drug

- Drug name: generic or brand (trade, proprietary) name?
- Drug class: e.g. antidepressant
- Drug subclass: e.g. SSRI, dopamine antagonist
- What is its broad mechanism of action?
- Indication: why is the drug being prescribed?
- Is this a licensed indication?
- Is this a scheduled drug?
- Route: e.g. oral, parenteral. Is the drug absorbed efficiently in this modality?
- Elimination: how is the drug eliminated? Are there any active metabolites?
- Are the pharmacokinetics influenced by age or ethnicity?
- Dose: especially dosing intervals and factors that might influence this, such as age and coexistent physical conditions
- Monitoring: does the drug need regular monitoring to optimize the risk/benefit profile? Can it aid compliance?
- Duration of treatment: what is the minimum? What is the maximum?
- Could long-term use risk dependence?
- Adverse effects: what are the most common? Which are serious?
- Interactions: does the drug interact with other drugs?
- Patient factors: what should I tell the patient or carers?
- Patient information: are there dependable leaflets available?

Actual management of various disorders lies outside our remit. Reference should be made to other chapters in this book, to NICE guidelines, and to treatment guidelines drawn up by the British Association for Psychopharmacology.[135] The last deal with the drug treatment of depression, bipolar disorder, substance misuse, anxiety disorders, dementia and ADHD.

KEY POINTS

- The study of pharmacokinetics involves observations of what happens to drugs once administered.

- The use of therapeutic drug monitoring of a particular drug requires that its plasma levels should be clearly related to its therapeutic or adverse effects.
- Pharmacodynamics refers to the effect of a drug on biological mechanisms. In psychopharmacology it is specifically to the brain.
- Receptors are complex protein structures, often with different types of sub-units upon which act a large number of neurotransmitters.
- There are two broad groups of antipsychotics: conventional (typical) or first generation drugs; and those termed atypical or second generation.
- Anticonvulsant drugs have an extremely wide range of chemical structures and have a correspondingly wide range of actions and adverse effects.
- Three acetylcholinesterase inhibitors are in widespread use in the UK, as is a drug with multiple actions memantine.
- The main classes of antidepressants include the tricyclic antidepressants (TCAs) and related compounds; the selective serotonin re-uptake inhibitors (SSRIs); the serotonin norepinephrine re-uptake inhibitors (SNRIs); and the monoamine oxidase inhibitors (MAOIs), both selective and non-selective.
- Mood stabilizers are a group of drugs that comprise lithium and several agents used primarily as antidepressants: they prevent both upswings and downswings of mood in bipolar patients.
- Long-acting benzodiazepines are appropriate as anxiolytics, shorter-acting ones as hypnotics: short-term use lessens the risk of dependence.

REFERENCES

1. Healy D (1997) *The Psychopharmacologists I: Interviews*. New York: Chapman & Hall.
2. Healy D (1998) *The Psychopharmacologists II: Interviews*. Philadelphia, PA: Lippincott Williams & Wilkins.
3. Healy D (2000) *The Psychopharmacologists III: Interviews*. London: Oxford University Press.
4. Breggin P (2008) *Brain-Disabling Treatments in Psychiatry. Drugs, Electroshock, and the Psychopharmaceutical Complex*. New York: Springer.
5. Wasson RG (1968) *Soma: Divine Mushroom of Immortality, (Ethno-Mycological Studies)*. New York: Harcourt Brace Jovanovich.
6. O'Donoghue EG (1914) *The Story of Bethlehem Hospital from its Foundation in 1247*. London: Fisher Unwin.
7. Kuhn R (1958) The treatment of depressive states with G 22355 (imipramine hydrochloride). *American Journal of Psychiatry* **115**: 459–64.
8. Everitt B, Wessely S (2008) *Clinical Trials in Psychiatry*, 2nd edn. Chichester: John Wiley & Sons.
9. Cochrane Schizophrenia Group (2008) http://szg.cochrane.org/en/index.html.
10. Thornley B, Adams C (1998) Content and quality of 2000 controlled trials in schizophrenia over 50 years. *British Medical Journal* **317**: 1181–4.
11. Geddes JR, Game D, Jenkins NE, *et al.* (1996) What proportion of primary psychiatric interventions are based on evidence from randomised controlled trials? *Quality in Health Care* **5**: 215–17.
12. Prien RF, Caffey EM, Jr (1976) Relationship between dosage and response to lithium prophylaxis in recurrent depression. *American Journal of Psychiatry* **133**: 567–70.
13. Gelenberg AJ, Kane JM, Keller MB, *et al.* (1989) Comparison of standard and low serum levels of lithium for maintenance treatment of bipolar disorder. *New England Journal of Medicine* **321**: 1489–93.
14. Perlis RH, Sachs GS, Lafer B, *et al.* (2002) Effect of abrupt change from standard to low serum levels of lithium: a reanalysis of double-blind lithium maintenance data. *American Journal of Psychiatry* **159**: 1155–9.
15. Poolsup N, Li Wan PA, de Oliveira IR (2000) Systematic overview of lithium treatment in acute mania. *Journal of Clinical Pharmacy and Therapeutics* **25**: 139–56.
16. Haring C, Meise U, Humpel C, *et al.* (1989) Dose-related plasma levels of clozapine: influence of smoking behaviour, sex and age. *Psychopharmacology* **99** (suppl.): S38–40.
17. Perry PJ, Miller DD, Arndt SV, Cadoret RJ (1991) Clozapine and norclozapine plasma concentrations and clinical response of treatment refractory schizophrenic patients. *American Journal of Psychiatry* **148**: 231–5.
18. Greenwood-Smith C, Lubman DI, Castle DJ (2003) Serum clozapine levels: a review of their clinical utility. *Journal of Psychopharmacology* **17**: 234–8.
19. Taylor D, Paton C, Kerwin R (2007) *The Maudsley Prescribing Guidelines*, 9th edn. London: Informa Healthcare.
20. Taylor D, Duncan D (1997) Doses of carbamazepine and valproate in bipolar affective disorder. *Psychiatric Bulletin* **21**: 221–3.
21. Eadie MJ (2001) Therapeutic drug monitoring: antiepileptic drugs. *British Journal of Clinical Pharmacology* **52** (suppl 1): 11–20S.
22. Bialer M (2007) Extended-release formulations for the treatment of epilepsy. *CNS Drugs* **21**: 765–74.
23. Allen MH, Hirschfeld RM, Wozniak PJ, *et al.* (2006) Linear relationship of valproate serum concentration to response and optimal serum levels for acute mania. *American Journal of Psychiatry* **163**: 272–5.
24. Perry PJ (2001) Therapeutic drug monitoring of antipsychotics. *Psychopharmacology Bulletin* **35**: 19–29.
25. Fellows L, Ahmad F, Castle DJ, *et al.* (2003) Investigation of target plasma concentration–effect relationships for olanzapine in schizophrenia. *Therapeutic Drug Monitoring* **25**: 682–9.
26. Mauri MC, Steinhilber CP, Marino R, *et al.* (2005) Clinical outcome and olanzapine plasma levels in acute schizophrenia. *European Psychiatry* **20**: 55–60.

27. Robertson MD, McMullin MM (2000) Olanzapine concentrations in clinical serum and postmortem blood specimens: when does therapeutic become toxic? *Journal of Forensic Sciences* **45**: 418–21.
28. Ezewuzie N, Taylor D (2006) Establishing a dose-response relationship for oral risperidone in relapsed schizophrenia. *Journal of Psychopharmacology* **20**: 86–90.
29. Taylor D (2006) Risperidone long-acting injection in practice: more questions than answers? *Acta Psychiatrica Scandinavica* **114**: 1–2.
30. Taylor D, Duncan D (1995) Plasma levels of tricyclics and related antidepressants: are they necessary or useful? *Psychiatric Bulletin* **19**: 548–50.
31. Leonard BE (2003) *Fundamentals of Psychopharmacology*, 3rd edn. Chichester: John Wiley & Sons.
32. National Institute for Health and Clinical Excellence (2007) *Depression (Amended): Management of Depression in Primary and Secondary Care.* London: National Institute for Health and Clinical Excellence.
33. National Institute for Clinical Excellence (2006) *Dementia: Supporting People with Dementia and Their Carers in Health and Social Care.* London: National Institute for Health and Clinical Excellence.
34. Sparshatt A, Jones S, Taylor D (2008) Quetiapine: dose-response relationship in schizophrenia. *CNS Drugs* **22**: 49–68.
35. Royal College of Psychiatrists (2006) Consensus Statement on High-Dose Antipsychotic Medication. Council report 138. London: Royal College of Psychiatrists.
36. Royal College of Psychiatrists (2007) Use of Licensed Medicines for Unlicensed Applications in Psychiatric Practice. College report 142. London, Royal College of Psychiatrists.
37. Kay SR, Fiszbein A, Opler LA (1987) The positive and negative syndrome scale (PANSS) for schizophrenia. *Schizophrenia Bulletin* **13**: 261–76.
38. Overall JE, Gorham DR (1962) The Brief Psychiatric Rating Scale. *Psychological Reports* **10**: 812.
39. Lieberman J, Jody D, Geisler S, *et al.* (1993) Time course and biologic correlates of treatment response in first-episode schizophrenia. *Archives of General Psychiatry* **50**: 369–76.
40. Kane J, Honigfeld G, Singer J, Meltzer H (1988) Clozapine for the treatment-resistant schizophrenic: a double-blind comparison with chlorpromazine. *Archives of General Psychiatry* **45**: 789–96.
41. Conley RR, Kelly DL, Richardson CM, *et al.* (2003) The efficacy of high-dose olanzapine versus clozapine in treatment-resistant schizophrenia: a double-blind crossover study. *Journal of Clinical Psychopharmacology* **23**: 668–71.
42. Meltzer HY, Bobo WV, Roy A, *et al.* (2008) A randomized, double-blind comparison of clozapine and high-dose olanzapine in treatment-resistant patients with schizophrenia. *Journal of Clinical Psychiatry* **69**: 274–85.
43. Davis JM, Chen N, Glick ID (2003) A meta-analysis of the efficacy of second-generation antipsychotics. *Archives of General Psychiatry* **60**: 553–64.
44. McEvoy JP, Lieberman JA, Stroup TS, *et al.* (2006) Effectiveness of clozapine versus olanzapine, quetiapine, and risperidone in patients with chronic schizophrenia who did not respond to prior atypical antipsychotic treatment. *American Journal of Psychiatry* **163**: 600–610.
45. Stroup TS, Lieberman JA, McEvoy JP, *et al.* (2006) Effectiveness of olanzapine, quetiapine, risperidone, and ziprasidone in patients with chronic schizophrenia following discontinuation of a previous atypical antipsychotic. *American Journal of Psychiatry* **163**: 611–22.
46. Kahn RS, Fleischhacker WW, Boter H, *et al.* (2008) Effectiveness of antipsychotic drugs in first-episode schizophrenia and schizophreniform disorder: an open randomised clinical trial. *Lancet* **371**: 1085–97.
47. Paton C, Barnes TR, Cavanagh MR, *et al.* (2008) High-dose and combination antipsychotic prescribing in acute adult wards in the UK: the challenges posed by p.r.n. prescribing. *British Journal of Psychiatry* **192**: 435–9.
48. Taylor D, Mace S, Mir S, Kerwin R (2000) A prescription survey of the use of atypical antipsychotics for hospital inpatients in the United Kingdom. *International Journal of Psychiatry in Clinical Practice* **4**: 41–6.
49. Paton C, Barnes TR, Cavanagh MR, *et al.* (2008) High-dose and combination antipsychotic prescribing in acute adult wards in the UK: the challenges posed by p.r.n. prescribing. *British Journal of Psychiatry* **192**: 435–9.
50. Centorrino F, Goren JL, Hennen J, *et al.* (2004) Multiple versus single antipsychotic agents for hospitalized psychiatric patients: case-control study of risks versus benefits. *American Journal of Psychiatry* **161**: 700–706.
51. Waddington JL, Youssef HA, Kinsella A (1998) Mortality in schizophrenia: antipsychotic polypharmacy and absence of adjunctive anticholinergics over the course of a 10-year prospective study. *British Journal of Psychiatry* **173**: 1169–73.
52. Paton C, Whittington C, Barnes TR (2007) Augmentation with a second antipsychotic in patients with schizophrenia who partially respond to clozapine: a meta-analysis. *Journal of Clinical Psychopharmacology* **27**: 198–204.
53. Van PT, Marder SR, Mintz J (1990) A controlled dose comparison of haloperidol in newly admitted schizophrenic patients. *Archives of General Psychiatry* **47**: 754–8.
54. Sultzer DL, Davis SM, Tariot PN, *et al.* (2008) Clinical symptom responses to atypical antipsychotic medications in Alzheimer's disease: phase 1 outcomes from

the CATIE-AD effectiveness trial. *American Journal of Psychiatry* **165**: 844–54.
55. Bang LM, Goa KL (2004) Spotlight on oxcarbazepine in epilepsy. *CNS Drugs* **18**: 57–61.
56. Perucca E (2002) Pharmacological and therapeutic properties of valproate. *CNS Drugs* **16**: 695–714.
57. Montgomery SA (2006) Pregabalin for the treatment of generalised anxiety disorder. *Expert Opinion on Pharmacotherapy* **7**: 2139–54.
58. Goldsmith DR, Wagstaff AJ, Ibbotson T, Perry CM (2003) Lamotrigine: a review of its use in bipolar disorder. *Drugs* **63**: 2029–50.
59. Shigeta M, Homma A (2001) Donepezil for Alzheimer's disease: pharmacodynamic, pharmacokinetic, and clinical profiles. *CNS Drug Reviews* **7**: 353–68.
60. Jann MW (2000) Rivastigmine, a new-generation cholinesterase inhibitor for the treatment of Alzheimer's disease. *Pharmacotherapy* **20**: 1–12.
61. Scott LJ, Goa KL (2000) Galantamine: a review of its use in Alzheimer's disease. *Drugs* **60**: 1095–122.
62. Cacabelos R, Takeda M, Winblad B (1999) The glutamatergic system and neurodegeneration in dementia: preventive strategies in Alzheimer's disease. *International Journal of Geriatric Psychiatry* **14**: 3–47.
63. Robinson DM, Keating GM (2006) Memantine: a review of its use in Alzheimer's disease. *Drugs* **66**: 1515–34.
64. Rogers SL, Farlow MR, Doody RS, *et al.* (1998) A 24-week, double-blind, placebo-controlled trial of donepezil in patients with Alzheimer's disease. Donepezil Study Group. *Neurology* **50**: 136–45.
65. Rosler M, Anand R, Cicin-Sain A, *et al.* (1999) Efficacy and safety of rivastigmine in patients with Alzheimer's disease: international randomised controlled trial. *British Medical Journal* **318**: 633–8.
66. Jones RW, Soininen H, Hager K, *et al.* (2004) A multinational, randomised, 12-week study comparing the effects of donepezil and galantamine in patients with mild to moderate Alzheimer's disease. *International Journal of Geriatric Psychiatry* **19**: 58–67.
67. Reisberg B, Doody R, Stoffler A, *et al.* (2003) Memantine in moderate-to-severe Alzheimer's disease. *New England Journal of Medicine* **348**: 1333–41.
68. Attard A, Ranjith G, Taylor D (2008) Delirium and its treatment. *CNS Drugs* **22**: 631–44.
69. Fangmann P, Assion HJ, Juckel G, *et al.* (2008) Half a century of antidepressant drugs: on the clinical introduction of monoamine oxidase inhibitors, tricyclics, and tetracyclics: part II. Tricyclics and tetracyclics. *Journal of Clinical Psychopharmacology* **28**: 1–4.
70. Linde K, Berner M, Egger M, Mulrow C (2005) St John's wort for depression: meta-analysis of randomised controlled trials. *British Journal of Psychiatry* **186**: 99–107.
71. Livingston MG, Livingston HM (1996) Monoamine oxidase inhibitors: an update on drug interactions. *Drug Safety* **14**: 219–27.
72. Stahl SM, Palazidou L (1986) The pharmacology of depression: studies of neurotransmitter receptors lead the search for biochemical lesions and new drug therapies. *Trends in Pharmacological Sciences* **7**: 349–54.
73. Blackwell B (1981) Adverse effects of antidepressant drugs: part 1. Monoamine oxidase inhibitors and tricyclics. *Drugs* **21**: 201–19.
74. Morgan O, Griffiths C, Baker A, Majeed A (2004) Fatal toxicity of antidepressants in England and Wales 1993–2002. *Health Statistics Quarterly* 18–24.
75. Trindade E, Menon D (1998) Selective Serotonin Reuptake Inhibitors (SSRIs) for Major Depression: part 1. Evaluation of the Clinical Literature. Ottawa: Canadian Coordinating Office for Health Technology Assessment.
76. Smith D, Dempster C, Glanville J, *et al.* (2002) Efficacy and tolerability of venlafaxine compared with selective serotonin reuptake inhibitors and other antidepressants: a meta-analysis. *British Journal of Psychiatry* **180**: 396–404.
77. Taylor D, Scott JR (2006) Volte-face on venlafaxine: reasons and reflections. *Journal of Psychopharmacology* **20**: 597–601.
78. Schatzberg AF (2000) Clinical efficacy of reboxetine in major depression. *Journal of Clinical Psychiatry* **61** (suppl. 10): 31–8.
79. Young SN (1991) Use of tryptophan in combination with other antidepressant treatments: a review. *Journal of Psychiatry and Neuroscience* **16**: 241–6.
80. Lader M (2007) Antidepressants and suicidality. *Clinical Risk* **13**: 85–8.
81. Lader M (2006) Discontinuing SSRI antidepressants: prediction, assessment and management of symptoms. *Neuropsychiatric Disease and Treatment* **2** (suppl. 1): 13–20.
82. Mottram P, Wilson K, Strobl J (2006) Antidepressants for depressed elderly. *Cochrane Database of Systematic Reviews* (1): CD003491.
83. Heeren TJ, Derksen P, van Heycop Ten Ham BF, van Gent PP (1997) Treatment, outcome and predictors of response in elderly depressed in-patients. *British Journal of Psychiatry* **170**: 436–40.
84. Dunner DL, Rush AJ, Russell JM, *et al.* (2006) Prospective, long-term, multicenter study of the naturalistic outcomes of patients with treatment-resistant depression. *Journal of Clinical Psychiatry* **67**: 688–95.
85. Bauer M, Dopfmer S (1999) Lithium augmentation in treatment-resistant depression: meta-analysis of placebo-controlled studies. *Journal of Clinical Psychopharmacology* **19**: 427–34.
86. Geddes JR, Carney SM, Davies C, *et al.* (2003) Relapse prevention with antidepressant drug treatment in depressive disorders: a systematic review. *Lancet* **361**: 653–61.
87. Wijkstra JAAP, Lijmer J, Balk Ferdi J, *et al.* (2006) Pharmacological treatment for unipolar psychotic

depression: systematic review and meta-analysis. *British Journal of Psychiatry* **188**: 410–15.
88. Geddes JR, Burgess S, Hawton K, *et al.* (2004) Long-term lithium therapy for bipolar disorder: systematic review and meta-analysis of randomized controlled trials. *American Journal of Psychiatry* **161**: 217–22.
89. Muzina DJ, Calabrese JR (2005) Maintenance therapies in bipolar disorder: focus on randomized controlled trials. *Australian and New Zealand Journal of Psychiatry* **39**: 652–61.
90. National Institute for Health and Clinical Excellence (2006) *Bipolar Disorder: The Management of Bipolar Disorder in Adults, Children and Adolescents, in Primary and Secondary Care*. Clinical guideline 38. London: National Institute for Health and Clinical Excellence.
91. Cavanagh J, Smyth R, Goodwin GM (2004) Relapse into mania or depression following lithium discontinuation: a 7-year follow-up. *Acta Psychiatrica Scandinavica* **109**: 91–5.
92. Tondo L, Hennen J, Baldessarini RJ (2001) Lower suicide risk with long-term lithium treatment in major affective illness: a meta-analysis. *Acta Psychiatrica Scandinavica* **104**: 163–72.
93. Gitlin M (1999) Lithium and the kidney: an updated review. *Drug Safety* **20**: 231–43.
94. Adityanjee, Munshi KR, Thampy A (2005) The syndrome of irreversible lithium-effectuated neurotoxicity. *Clinical Neuropharmacology* **28**: 38–49.
95. Bowden CL, Calabrese JR, Sachs G, *et al.* (2003) A placebo-controlled 18-month trial of lamotrigine and lithium maintenance treatment in recently manic or hypomanic patients with bipolar I disorder. *Archives of General Psychiatry* **60**: 392–400.
96. Vieta E, Torrent C, Garcia-Ribas G, *et al.* (2002) Use of topiramate in treatment-resistant bipolar spectrum disorders. *Journal of Clinical Psychopharmacology* **22**: 431–5.
97. Lande RG (2004) Oxcarbazepine: efficacy, safety, and tolerability in the treatment of mania. *International Journal of Psychiatry in Clinical Practice* **8**: 37–40.
98. Green AI, Tohen M, Patel JK, *et al.* (2000) Clozapine in the treatment of refractory psychotic mania. *American Journal of Psychiatry* **157**: 982–6.
99. Kerr DI, Ong J (1995) GABA-B receptors. *Pharmacology and Therapeutics* **67**: 187–246.
100. National Institute for Health and Clinical Excellence (2004) *Anxiety: Management of Anxiety (Panic Disorder, with or without Agoraphobia, and Generalised Anxiety Disorder) in Adults in Primary, Secondary and Community Care*. Clinical guideline 22. London: National Institute for Health and Clinical Excellence.
101. Barker MJ, Greenwood KM, Jackson M, Crowe SF (2004) Cognitive effects of long-term benzodiazepine use: a meta-analysis. *CNS Drugs* **18**: 37–48.
102. Paterniti S, Dufouil C, Alperovitch A (2002) Long-term benzodiazepine use and cognitive decline in the elderly: the Epidemiology of Vascular Aging Study. *Journal of Clinical Psychopharmacology* **22**: 285–93.
103. Barbone F, McMahon AD, Davey PG, *et al.* (1998) Association of road-traffic accidents with benzodiazepine use. *Lancet* **352**: 1331–6.
104. Cumming RG, Le Couteur DG (2003) Benzodiazepines and risk of hip fractures in older people: a review of the evidence. *CNS Drugs* **17**: 825–37.
105. Paton C (2002) Benzodiazepines and disinhibition: a review. *Psychiatric Bulletin* **26**: 460–62.
106. Lader M (1998) Withdrawal reactions after stopping hypnotics in patients with insomnia. *CNS Drugs* **10**: 425–40.
107. Lader M, Tylee A, Donoghue J (2009) Withdrawing benzodiazepines in primary care. *CNS Drugs* **23**: 19–34.
108. Voshaar RCO, Couvee JE, Van Balkom AJLM, *et al.* (2006) Strategies for discontinuing long-term benzodiazepine use: meta-analysis. *British Journal of Psychiatry* **189**: 213–20.
109. Sramek JJ, Tansman M, Suri A, *et al.* (1996) Efficacy of buspirone in generalized anxiety disorder with coexisting mild depressive symptoms. *Journal of Clinical Psychiatry* **57**: 287–91.
110. Lader M (1999) Anxiolytic effect of hydroxyzine: a double-blind trial versus placebo and buspirone. *Human Psychopharmacology* **14** (suppl. 1): S94–102.
111. National Institute for Health and Clinical Excellence (2004) *Insomnia: Newer Hypnotic Drugs – Zaleplon, Zolpidem and Zopiclone for the Management of Insomnia*. Technology appraisal 77. London: National Institute for Health and Clinical Excellence.
112. Benca RM (2005) Diagnosis and treatment of chronic insomnia: a review. *Psychiatric Services* **56**: 332–43.
113. Sikdar S, Ruben SM (1996) Zopiclone abuse among polydrug users. *Addiction* **91**: 285–6.
114. Glass J, Lanctot KL, Herrmann N, *et al.* (2005) Sedative hypnotics in older people with insomnia: meta-analysis of risks and benefits. *British Medical Journal* **331**: 1169.
115. Zisapel N (2000) Development of a melatonin-based formulation for the treatment of insomnia in the elderly. *Drug Development Research* **50**: 226–34.
116. James SP, Mendelson WB (2004) The use of trazodone as a hypnotic: a critical review. *Journal of Clinical Psychiatry* **65**: 752–5.
117. Morin CM, Koetter U, Bastien C, *et al.* (2005) Valerian-hops combination and diphenhydramine for treating insomnia: a randomized placebo-controlled clinical trial. *Sleep* **28**: 1465–71.
118. National Institute for Health and Clinical Excellence (2006) *Methylphenidate, Atomoxetine and Dexamfetamine for Attention Deficit Hyperactivity Disorder (ADHD) in Children and Adolescents: Guidance*. Technology appraisal 98. London: National Institute for Health and Clinical Excellence.

119. Menza MA, Kaufman KR, Castellanos A (2000) Modafinil augmentation of antidepressant treatment in depression. *Journal of Clinical Psychiatry* **61**: 378–81.

120. Hughes JC, Cook CC (1997) The efficacy of disulfiram: a review of outcome studies. *Addiction* **92**: 381–95.

121. Boothby LA, Doering PL (2005) Acamprosate for the treatment of alcohol dependence. *Clinical Therapeutics* **27**: 695–714.

122. Duncan D, Taylor D (1996) Chlormethiazole or chlordiazepoxide in alcohol detoxification. *Psychiatric Bulletin* **20**: 599–601.

123. National Institute for Health and Clinical Excellence (2002) *The Clinical Effectiveness and Cost Effectiveness of Bupropion (Zyban) and Nicotine Replacement Therapy for Smoking Cessation.* Technology appraisal 39. London: National Institute for Health and Clinical Excellence.

124. Gonzales D, Rennard SI, Nides M, *et al.* (2006) Varenicline, an alpha4beta2 nicotinic acetylcholine receptor partial agonist, vs sustained-release bupropion and placebo for smoking cessation: a randomized controlled trial. *Journal of the American Medical Association* **296**: 47–55.

125. Silagy C, Lancaster T, Stead L, *et al.* (2004) Nicotine replacement therapy for smoking cessation. *Cochrane Database of Systematic Reviews* (3): CD000146.

126. National Institute for Health and Clinical Excellence (2007) *Methadone and Buprenorphine for the Management of Opioid Dependence.* Technology appraisal 114. London: National Institute for Health and Clinical Excellence.

127. National Institute for Health and Clinical Excellence (2007) *Naltrexone for the Management of Opioid Dependence.* Technology appraisal 115. London: National Institute for Health and Clinical Excellence.

128. Paton C (2008) Prescribing in pregnancy. *British Journal of Psychiatry* **192**: 321–2.

129. James L, Barnes TRE, Lelliott P, Paton C (2007) Informing patients of the teratogenic potential of mood stabilising drugs: a case notes review of the practice of psychiatrists. *Journal of Psychopharmacology* **21**: 815–19.

130. Stubbs J, Haw C, Taylor D (2006) Prescription errors in psychiatry: a multi-centre study. *Journal of Psychopharmacology* **20**: 553–61.

131. Caplehorn JR, Drummer OH (2002) Fatal methadone toxicity: signs and circumstances, and the role of benzodiazepines. *Australian and New Zealand Journal of Public Health* **26**: 358–62.

132. Henry JA (1997) Epidemiology and relative toxicity of antidepressant drugs in overdose. *Drug Safety* **16**: 374–90.

133. Tuohy K, Shemin D (2003) Acute lithium intoxication. *Dialysis and Transplantation* **32**: 478–81.

134. Trenton A, Currier G, Zwemer F (2003) Fatalities associated with therapeutic use and overdose of atypical antipsychotics. *CNS Drugs* **17**: 307–24.

135. Anderson IM, Nutt DJ, Deakin JF (2000) Evidence-based guidelines for treating depressive disorders with antidepressants: a revision of the 1993 British Association for Psychopharmacology guidelines. British Association for Psychopharmacology. *Journal of Psychopharmacology* **14**: 3–20.

Chapter 58

Electroconvulsive therapy

Allan Scott

INTRODUCTION

Electroconvulsive therapy (ECT) is the electrical induction of the type of generalized cerebral seizure associated with a tonic–clonic convulsion, with the aim of treating an abnormal mental state or neurological disorder. Efficacious treatment requires a series of inductions given two or three times a week. The history of convulsive therapies in psychiatry is not to be confused with the history of the use of electricity in medicine.[1] It was Cerletti, later aided by Bini, who developed the means of electrical induction that proved both safer and more reliable than chemical methods of inducing convulsions; the first patient, a man suffering from schizophrenia, was treated in Rome in 1938 and was eventually discharged from hospital in remission.[2] Modern ECT is now modified: it is given under general anaesthesia and with drug treatment to reduce the extent of the convulsion.

MODE OF ACTION

Seminal studies

Almost three decades ago, Kendell reviewed the seminal studies on the mode of action of ECT and concluded that there was compelling evidence that the induction of generalized seizure activity in the brain was the crucial therapeutic element.[3] He acknowledged that several studies had flaws in design that were typical of studies of that time, but two studies still merit particular mention. The first is important in the history of convulsive therapies. Laurell conducted a randomized controlled trial of two different types of convulsive therapy in endogenous depression. One of the convulsive therapies was ECT, and the other fluorothyl convulsive therapy, where induction was by inhalation of a convulsant gas.[4] ECT and fluorothyl convulsive therapy were equally efficacious.

Ottosson conducted an ingenious experiment to investigate how a modification to the extent of cerebral seizure activity affected the clinical efficacy of ECT in the treatment of endogenous depression.[5] One group of patients with depression was treated with orthodox ECT. In a second group, the electrical stimulus was only just sufficient to induce generalized seizure activity (liminal stimulation). In a third group, a liminal stimulus was preceded by the intravenous administration of lidocaine, which reduced the duration of seizure activity in the brain. Pretreatment with lidocaine considerably reduced the clinical efficacy of ECT. Nearly 50 years after this study was conducted, it can be criticized because the patients were not allocated randomly to the three experimental groups and Ottosson did not measure the effect of lidocaine on the seizure threshold. This study was important in its time because it showed that the antidepressant effect of ECT depended on the extent of cerebral seizure activity.

Refinements to original theory

A series of studies at the New York State Psychiatric Institute from 1987 led to a refinement of the original theory. The first was a clinical trial of the efficacy of liminal ECT in the treatment of major depression, although Sackeim and colleagues referred to this technique as 'threshold ECT'.[6] The novel aspect was a randomized controlled comparison of threshold ECT given with either a bilateral or a right unilateral electrode placement (see Electrode placement, below). Only 28 per cent of the patients with depression responded to threshold unilateral ECT, in contrast to a response rate of 70 per cent in the patients treated with threshold bilateral ECT. Treatment was monitored by electroencephalogram (EEG), and there was no significant difference in the length of seizure activity between the two types of ECT. Subsequent studies have shown that when right unilateral ECT is given with a dose of electricity at least six times the seizure threshold – that is, 500 per cent above the seizure threshold – then right unilateral ECT approximates to the clinical efficacy of bilateral ECT.[7,8] Although generalized cerebral seizure activity is still a necessary ingredient for the clinical efficacy of ECT, it turns out that how the cerebral seizure is induced has substantial bearing on the clinical outcome of a course of ECT.

Insights from brain imaging studies

A collaboration among neurologists and psychiatrists at Yale University School of Medicine has been important in understanding why it is that how cerebral seizure activity is induced has a bearing on the therapeutic efficacy of ECT. Single-photon-emission computed tomography (SPECT) was used to study the initiation and propagation of generalized seizures during ECT.[9] The findings challenged the belief that generalized seizures involve the entire brain homogeneously. The regions of the brain where increased blood flow was found during seizures differed, depending on how the seizures were initiated: right unilateral ECT, given with an electrical dose 2.5 times the seizure threshold, caused asymmetrical increases in both cortical and subcortical regions, with relative sparing of the left temporal lobe and left medial thalamus; in contrast, bilateral ECT caused symmetrical increases in blood flow in both the cortex and subcortical networks. Although both bilateral and right unilateral ECT produced generalized cerebral seizures associated with tonic–clonic convulsions, increases in regional cerebral blood flow differed substantially between the two types of treatment. An understanding of the significance in these differences between the two types of ECT will require greater knowledge of the functional neuroanatomy of mood and the pathophysiology of depressive illness. Preliminary studies are already under way with positron emission tomography (PET).

PET, unlike SPECT, can make direct measurements of cerebral metabolism in terms of the utilization of either oxygen or glucose. PET also has a much higher spatial resolution than SPECT. Ten patients with major depression of psychotic subtype were studied with PET using labelled fluorodeoxyglucose before and at least 2 weeks after a course of ECT.[10] Statistical parametric mapping and region of interest analysis revealed a significant increase in function in the left subgenual anterior cingulate cortex and hippocampus; the extent of the increases correlated with the extent of clinical improvement in depressive symptoms over the course of ECT. Treatment was given with either high-dose right unilateral ECT or bilateral ECT. Earlier work with PET found that cerebral blood flow was significantly reduced in the anterior cingulate cortex 10 min after an individual treatment with bilateral ECT.[11] These findings are of interest because decreased function in the anterior cingulate cortex has been described in the resting state in patients with major depression of the psychotic subtype. The subgenual anterior cingulate cortex (Figure 58.1) has also been identified as a putative target for deep brain stimulation in the management of chronic and treatment-resistant depressive illness. Clearly, such small-scale studies will require to be replicated, and several confounding factors may be at work: concomitant psychotropic drug treatment may affect regional cerebral metabolism, and the uptake of tracers may be affected by the amount of cerebral tissue in a region of interest, which in turn may be affected by factors such as age and chronicity of illness. Nevertheless, these preliminary studies point to at least one possible neuroanatomical substrate for the mode of action of ECT.

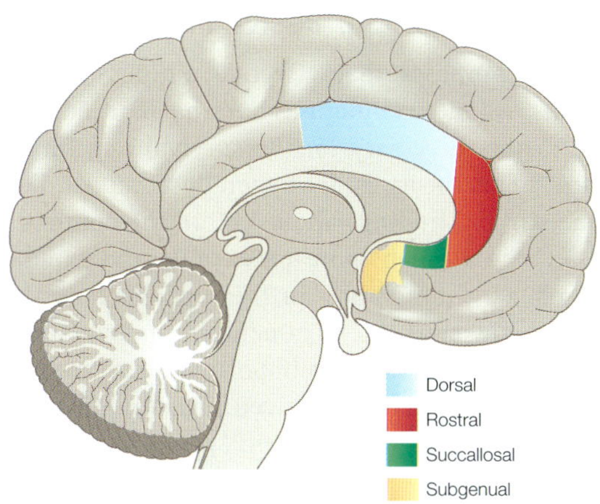

Figure 58.1 Neuroanatomy of the anterior cingulate nucleus
Redrawn with permission from ref. 10.

Neurochemical effects

There is a laboratory model of ECT called electroconvulsive shock (ECS) in which electricity is used to induce seizures in anaesthetised animals. Repeated ECS, in contrast to a single seizure, has several defined and reproducible neurochemical effects with behavioural correlates that emerge in a comparable time course to how ECT is used in patients with depression. ECT need not have a single mode of action nor work in a way similar to antidepressant drugs. Nevertheless, it is highly relevant that repeated ECS has been shown to increase functional measures of noradrenaline, serotonin and dopamine in the normal rodent brain;[12] functional measures of acetylcholine decrease, which is one plausible explanation for some of the cognitive adverse effects of ECT.[13] The neurochemical effects of repeated ECS include the down-regulation of the number of β adrenoceptors in the cortex and hippocampus, and this is accompanied by behavioural change that lasts for about 7 days after the last ECS.[12] This is an effect of interest also seen after the chronic administration of effective antidepressant drugs in animals.

The anticonvulsant hypothesis

The development of this hypothesis occurred around the time when there was increasing interest in the use of antiepileptic drugs as mood stabilizers. Effective ECT has anticonvulsant effects, and these may include a gradual rise in the seizure threshold during a course of ECT. It has been suggested that the magnitude of this rise is related to the eventual clinical outcome of a course of ECT and that it is essential for successful treatment with right unilateral ECT.[14] A study of 80 patients who recovered from an episode of unipolar major depression after a course of bilateral ECT found that the seizure threshold did not in fact change at all in 70 per cent of the patients.[15] These findings do not support the anticonvulsant hypothesis of the mode of action of ECT.

Cellular theory of depressive illness

This theory proposes that effective antidepressant treatments work via intracellular mechanisms that increase neurotropic factors necessary for the survival and function of neurones.[16] This theory is not generally accepted, but there are some striking findings about ECS in the context of this theory. ECS is a much more efficacious and rapid-acting inducer of cell proliferation in the hippocampus than are chemical antidepressant treatments.[17] It has also been shown that ECS increases two important neurotropic factors in the hippocampus, brain-derived neurotropic factor and vascular endothelial growth factor.[17]

INDICATIONS

Major depression

In 2001 the Department of Health in England commissioned a systematic review of the efficacy of ECT using modern methods of evidence-based medicine; the results for the indication of major depression were later published.[18] The UK ECT Review Group found that real ECT was substantially more efficacious than sham ECT (standardized effect size 0.91) and more efficacious than pharmacotherapy (standardized effect size 0.80) in the short-term treatment of depressive illness.

The Royal College of Psychiatrists publishes guidelines on the use of ECT;[19] Box 58.1 shows the recommended indications for ECT in major depression.

It has to be noted that the College recommendations were not consistent with guidance from the National Institute for Health and Clinical Excellence (NICE). This body conducted one of its technology appraisals on ECT and heard evidence from patients that sometimes the cognitive adverse effects of ECT outweighed its clinical benefits. NICE intended to restrict indications for ECT, and the recommendations were that ECT was to be used only to achieve rapid and short-term improvement of severe symptoms after an adequate trial of other treatment options had proved ineffective or when the condition was considered to be potentially life-threatening.[20] A dilemma for clinicians remains, and the extant recommendations from the College also include advice for prescribers to help them accommodate their practice to this discrepancy between the College and NICE. The heart of the advice is that a documented assessment of valid consent after full information about the risks and benefits of treatment would be essential to support any variance from the NICE guidance.[19]

Treatment-resistant depressive illness

The traditional view is that a history of non-response to antidepressant drug treatment during the index episode of depression has no bearing on the clinical outcome of ECT. This view has been supported by studies in the Netherlands[21] and Scotland[22] that have included representative samples of patients with depression referred for ECT – that is, patients with both unipolar and bipolar illnesses and both psychotic and non-psychotic subtypes. The traditional review has been challenged, however, by an open, well-conducted multicentre study in the USA.[23] This study included only patients with unipolar, non-psychotic depressive illness. Adequate antidepressant drug treatment was defined as at least 200 mg per day of imipramine (or equivalent) for at least 4 weeks. The probability of recovery among the patients with depression who had already failed to recover with adequate antidepressant drug treatment was only about 50 per cent, significantly lower than in the patients who had not been treated adequately. A subsequent multicentre observational study in the USA did not find a significant difference in the likelihood of remission between those patients who had and who had not already received adequate antidepressant drug treatment.[24] In fact, the observed probability of remission among the patients who

Box 58.1 Indications for electroconvulsive therapy (ECT) in major depression[19]

- *Potential treatment of choice – severe depressive illness when the illness is associated with:*
  - attempted suicide;
  - strong suicidal ideas or plans;
  - life-threatening illness because of refusal of food or fluids.
- *Treatment to be considered – severe depressive illness associated with:*
  - stupor;
  - marked psychomotor retardation;
  - depressive delusions or hallucinations.
- *Second- or third-line treatment:*
  - depressive illness that has not been treated adequately by antidepressant treatment and where social recovery has not been achieved.

The selection of ECT may be affected by:

- patient choice;
- previous experience of ineffective or intolerable medical treatment;
- previous recovery with ECT.

had already failed to recover with antidepressant drug treatment was lower than in those patients who had not received adequate antidepressant drug treatment; the difference was not, however, statistically significant. Although there may be debate about the impact of treatment resistance on the probability of remission in unipolar, non-psychotic major depression, these two studies were consistent in two points. Neither study found any suggestion that a failure to respond to a selective serotonin reuptake inhibitor (SSRI) or a monoamine oxidase inhibitor (MAOI) affected the probability of remission. It should also be noted that, even with the more conservative estimate, there is a 50 per cent chance of remission with ECT after non-response to a tricyclic (or similar) antidepressant drug, even when it has been augmented by lithium carbonate.

Bipolar disorder

Box 58.2 shows the College recommendations about the place of ECT in the treatment of patients with mania.

Box 58.2 The place of electroconvulsive therapy (ECT) in the treatment of mania[19]

- The treatment of choice for mania is a mood-stabilizing drug plus an antipsychotic drug.
- ECT may be considered for severe mania associated with:
  - life-threatening physical exhaustion;
  - treatment resistance, i.e. mania that has not responded to the treatment of choice.
- Selection of ECT may be affected by:
  - patient choice;
  - previous experience of ineffective or intolerable medical treatment;
  - previous recovery with ECT.

Schizophrenia

Box 58.3 shows the College recommendations about the place of ECT in the treatment of patients with acute schizophrenia.

Box 58.3 The place of electroconvulsive therapy (ECT) in the treatment of acute schizophrenia[19]

- The treatment of choice for acute schizophrenia is antipsychotic drug treatment.
- ECT may be considered as a fourth-line treatment, where clozapine has already proven ineffective or intolerable.

Catatonia

Box 58.4 shows the College recommendations about the place of ECT in the treatment of patients with catatonia.

Box 58.4 The place of electroconvulsive therapy (ECT) in the treatment of catatonia[19]

- Catatonia is a syndrome that may complicate several psychiatric and medical conditions.
- The treatment of choice is a benzodiazepine drug; most experience is with lorazepam.
- ECT may be indicated when treatment with lorazepam has been ineffective.

Neuropsychiatric disorders

ECT is a safe adjunctive treatment for both motor and affective symptoms in patients with Parkinson's disease with severe disability despite medical treatment.[25] ECT is also an experimental treatment for neuropsychiatric movement disorders such as neuroleptic malignant syndrome.[26] ECT has been shown to be effective in treatment-resistant status epilepticus.[27]

CONTRAINDICATIONS

ECT can be life-saving in severe psychiatric illness and may therefore have no absolute contraindications.[28] The physiology of ECT has been well described.[29] During and immediately after electrical stimulation, there is a reduction in heart rate, which may lead to bradycardia and occasionally brief asystole. Once cerebral seizure has been induced, a tachycardia ensues. Blood pressure generally parallels the heart rate during electrical stimulation and cerebral seizure activity. Patients with pre-existing hypertension do not experience more marked cardiovascular changes.[30] The cerebral utilization of oxygen and glucose and therefore cerebral blood flow doubles during cerebral seizure activity. Box 58.5 lists coexisting medical conditions that may increase the risk of ECT and are understandable in the context of the physiological changes that accompany ECT. It is important that the treatment of any coexisting medical conditions is optimized before elective treatment with ECT.

Box 58.5 Coexisting medical conditions that may increase the risk of electroconvulsive therapy (ECT)

- Increased intracranial pressure
- Recent cerebral infarction
- Severe cardiovascular or pulmonary disease
- Aneurysms or vascular malformations that might be susceptible to rupture with increased blood pressure.

SPECIAL POPULATIONS

Young people

The use of ECT in people under the age of 18 years is now very rare in developed countries.[31] In contrast to adults, the indication in young people is usually the treatment of a severe and treatment-resistant psychotic illness.[32] ECT is still an important treatment for schizophrenia in developing countries, and this may be one important reason that young people still constitute a small proportion of patients treated by ECT in such healthcare systems.[33]

Modern brief-pulse ECT machines deliver an adjustable dose of electrical energy, and it is known that only a small dose is necessary to induce cerebral seizure activity in young people.[34] Stimulus dosing must therefore take into account the lower seizure thresholds in young people,[19] and monitoring of treatment by simultaneous EEG is recommended to detect and manage any resultant prolonged cerebral seizure activity.[35] It is also advisable to try to avoid the concurrent prescription of psychotropic drug treatment that might itself lower the seizure threshold.[36]

People with learning disability

The prevalence of psychiatric illness is higher among people with learning disability than it is in the general population, but it seems that ECT is a treatment of last resort in this special population.[37] It must be acknowledged that there has never been a randomized controlled trial of ECT specifically within this special population, but observational studies have found no evidence for restricted indications or additional contraindications for people who have both a psychiatric illness and learning disability.[37]

Older adults

In contrast to general adult psychiatry, the rate of usage of ECT has only recently started to fall in the practice of old-age psychiatry.[38] Given the importance of ECT in this special population, it is disappointing that there has never been a randomized comparison of real and sham ECT. A small subanalysis of the Nottingham ECT trial was published in which efficacy was assessed specifically in patients with depression aged over 60 years; real ECT was significantly more efficacious than simulated ECT.[39]

Advancing age itself is not a contraindication to ECT. There is a higher prevalence of coexisting physical illness in older adults, but an observational study of patients with depression who were at least 75 years old found that these older adults tolerated ECT in a manner similar to younger people and experienced an improvement at least as great.[40] It is important that the treatment of any coexisting medical conditions is optimized before elective treatment. Cognitive impairment is also more prevalent in older adults referred for ECT,[40] and it is essential to monitor cognitive function carefully during a course of ECT.[19] Pre-existing cognitive impairment or the development of significant cognitive adverse effects during a course of treatment would both be an indication for the use of unilateral ECT.

THE PRESCRIBING CYCLE

Electrode placement

Electrical induction of the cerebral seizure can be undertaken with electrodes over both cerebral hemispheres – bilateral electrode placement – or over the non-dominant hemisphere only – unilateral ECT. The electrodes are applied to both temples in bilateral ECT (Figure 58.2), and to the temple and to the parietal surface in unilateral ECT (Figure 58.3).[19]

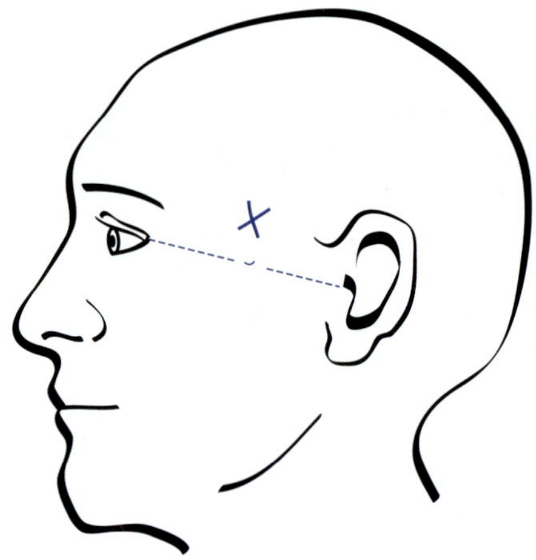

Figure 58.2 In bilateral electroconvulsive therapy (ECT), the centre of the electrode (marked with an X) should be 4 cm above, and perpendicular to, the midpoint of a line between the lateral angle of the eye and the external auditory meatus

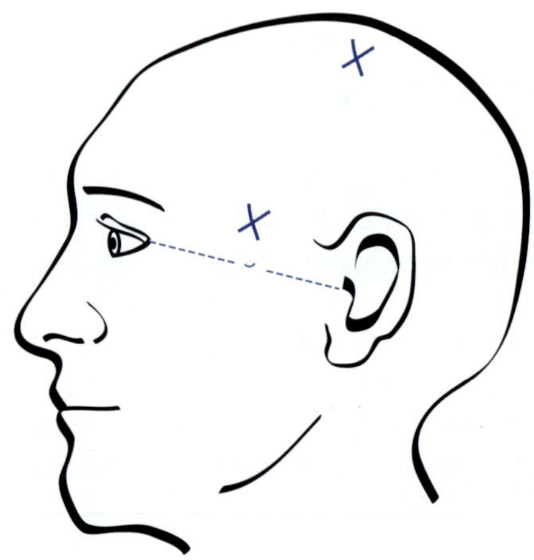

Figure 58.3 In unilateral electroconvulsive therapy (ECT), the centre of one electrode is in the same position as in bilateral ECT. The other electrode is applied over the parietal surface of the scalp over the non-dominant hemisphere, close to the vertex of the skull

It is the selection of electrode placement that has the single greatest impact both on the efficacy of treatment and on the cognitive adverse effects attributable to treatment. The UK ECT Review Group found that bilateral ECT was more efficacious than unilateral ECT (standardized effect size 0.32).[18] Electrical dose in unilateral ECT does, however, have a substantial impact on efficacy, and it could be argued that the comparison is confounded by electrical dose; nevertheless, in direct random allocation comparison of bilateral ECT with high-dose unilateral ECT – that is, an electrical dose six times the seizure threshold – it is still the case that high-dose unilateral ECT only approximates to the efficacy of bilateral ECT.[7,8] Moreover, there are patients with depression who do not experience remission with high-dose right unilateral ECT but who subsequently do experience remission with bilateral ECT.[7,8]

The cognitive adverse effects, both acute and longer-term, attributable to ECT are also more marked with bilateral ECT. Patients treated with bilateral ECT take longer to become reoriented after an individual treatment and are at substantially higher risk of prolonged disorientation after treatment.[7,8,41] The longer-term adverse effect of most concern to patients is the risk of retrograde amnesia – the realization of gaps in episodic memory for the period of weeks or months before admission to hospital. The risk of enduring retrograde amnesia is also substantially greater in patients treated with bilateral ECT.[42]

The Royal College of Psychiatrists has recommended that, where the rate of clinical improvement and completeness of response have priority, then bilateral electrode placement is preferable.[19] Where minimizing the cognitive adverse effects has priority, then unilateral electrode placement is preferable.[19] Neither unilateral nor bilateral electrode placement is therefore the treatment of choice in all indications for ECT, and, where possible, the selection of electrode placement should be part of the process of informed consent for treatment.

Frequency of treatments

The UK ECT Review Group found that treatments three times each week brought about no greater clinical improvement in depressive symptoms than treatment twice a week.[18] A meta-analysis of the comparative effects on cognitive function was not possible. Individual randomized controlled trials find that the outcome of a course of treatment is no different but that the rate of improvement may be greater in treatment three times a week; the increased rate of improvement is at the cost of more marked memory impairment during the course of treatment and up to 1 month after treatment.[43] Twice-weekly treatment is therefore optimal.

The rate of improvement may be crucial for some patients, as in treatment to save life. In this case, an evidence-based strategy to maximize the rate of clinical improvement would be to use a bilateral electrode placement with a high dose – that is, an electrical dose 2–2.5 times the seizure threshold (100–150 per cent above the seizure threshold).[19]

Number of treatments

It is remarkable that observational studies at different times and in different countries find that the average number of treatments in a course of ECT is approximately seven. Nevertheless, it is not possible to predict reliably the total number of treatments that an individual patient will require. A set course of treatment should therefore never be prescribed, and the need for further treatment should be assessed after each individual treatment. If no clinical improvement at all is seen over the first six bilateral treatments that have been administered properly, then it is highly unlikely that more treatments will bring about either significant clinical improvement or eventual recovery.[44] The management of patients who display slight or temporary improvement over the first few treatments is more problematic. It has been shown that a small but significant minority of patients with depression respond fully to treatments only beyond the eighth treatment in a course, having shown only modest improvement with earlier treatments.[44] It may therefore be perfectly reasonable to give up to 12 treatments to patients who display slight or temporary improvement over the first few treatments.

TREATMENT OUTCOME

The most comprehensive survey is from a multicentre study conducted in the USA.[45] The study involved 253 patients with a unipolar depressive illness and who were treated with bilateral ECT, given with an electrical dose 50 per cent above the seizure threshold. A total of 86 per cent of the patients completed the full course of treatment (6% dropped out because of intolerable adverse effects). Among those who completed the full course of bilateral ECT, 83 per cent of the patients with an illness of the non-psychotic subtype remitted, and 95 per cent of the patients with an illness of the psychotic subtype remitted (Figure 58.4). Remission was defined as a score of 10 or less on the Hamilton Rating Scale for Depression after two consecutive treatments, and also a fall of at least 60 per cent in depression rating from the pretreatment score. The final outcome of a course of ECT is similar in patients with a depressive episode in the context of a bipolar disorder but may be achieved with slightly fewer treatments.[46]

ADVERSE EFFECTS

It is disappointing that none of the randomized comparisons of real and sham ECT included a survey of adverse effects. It would have been informative to know which

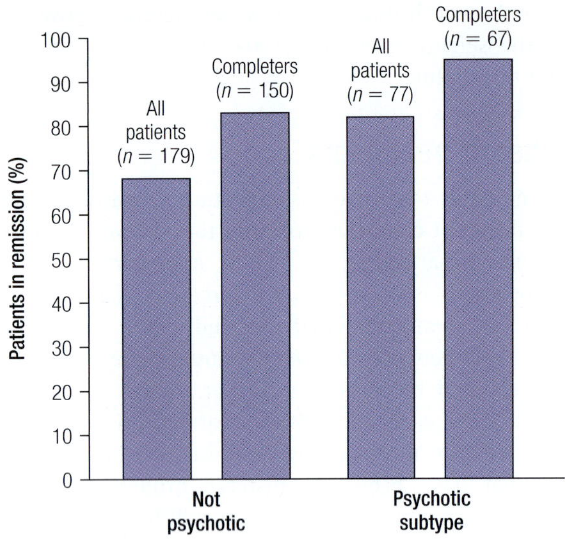

Figure 58.4 Efficacy and effectiveness of bilateral electroconvulsive therapy (ECT) in unipolar major depression. The definition of remission is given in the text

particular complaints related to the induction of cerebral seizure activity itself as opposed to the effects of anaesthesia and related interventions in a sample of depressed patients. Reported prevalences of specific adverse effects vary among surveys, presumably reflecting differences among samples in age and coexisting medical conditions. Muscle aches, headache, nausea (vomiting is less common) and memory problems are commonly reported adverse effects. Some patients experience repeated headache, and this may be an indication for prophylactic analgesia.

The temporary uncoordination and disorientation after individual treatments is characteristic of the postictal state and usually resolves spontaneously by the time the patient has returned to the ward. The prevalence of prolonged disorientation is much higher after bilateral ECT than after unilateral ECT (see Electrode placement, above). Prolonged disorientation may be an indication for a switch to unilateral ECT.

Prolonged cerebral seizure activity that requires medical treatment complicates 1–2 per cent of courses of treatment and is most likely at the first treatment.[35] It is more likely in young patients and patients with coexisting organic brain disease. The Royal College of Psychiatrists has recommended that EEG monitoring be carried out routinely, at least in the first treatment in a course of ECT.[19]

There is no credible evidence that ECT causes any kind of structural brain damage.[47] Indeed, the animal model of ECT is the most potent known inducer of hippocampal neurogenesis in rodents and non-human primates. Nevertheless, gaps in episodic memory are inevitable during a course of ECT because each individual treatment is followed by a postictal state associated with a temporary period of impaired consciousness. The most important risk factor for the persistence of retrograde amnesia is the use and number of bilateral treatments in the index course.[42]

The calculated mortality rate associated with the induction of cerebral seizure activity is fewer than two deaths per 100 000 treatments; adding deaths plausibly associated with anaesthesia, the rate is 2–10 deaths per 100 000 treatments.[48]

COMPARISON WITH OTHER PHYSICAL TREATMENTS

An experimental physical treatment for major depression is repetitive transcranial magnetic stimulation (rTMS); this involves the delivery of intense, ultra-brief magnetic pulses that pass unimpeded through the scalp and skull to induce focal electrical stimulation of the cortex of the brain. rTMS is not a convulsive therapy. A stimulating coil is held over the skull of the conscious patient and is usually tolerated well. A randomized controlled trial has compared the efficacy of ECT with rTMS of the left dorsolateral prefrontal cortex in the context of the National Health Service (NHS).[49] More than four times as many patients treated with ECT attained the a priori criteria for remission after ECT compared with those treated with rTMS. Although it must be acknowledged that rTMS is still in development, ECT proved much more efficacious among the patients with depression presently referred to ECT clinics.

KEY POINTS

- ECT is the most efficacious treatment for major depression in the short term.
- Generalized cerebral seizure activity is a necessary ingredient for clinical efficacy, but how the seizure is induced has substantial bearing on the outcome.
- The selection of electrode placement has the single greatest impact both on the efficacy of treatment and its cognitive adverse effects.
- The selection of electrode placement should, where possible, be part of the process of informed consent for treatment.
- Twice-weekly treatment is the optimal frequency.
- There is no credible evidence that ECT causes any kind of structural brain damage.
- The most robust predictor for the persistence of retrograde amnesia is the use and number of bilateral treatments.

REFERENCES

1. Fink M (1979) *Convulsive Therapy: Theory and Practice.* New York: Raven Press.
2. Endler NS (1988) The origins of electroconvulsive therapy (ECT). *Convulsive Therapy* 4: 5–23.
3. Kendell RE (1981) The present status of electroconvulsive therapy. *British Journal of Psychiatry* 139: 265–83.
4. Laurell B (1970) Flurothyl convulsive therapy. *Acta Psychiatrica Scandinavica Supplementum* 213: 1–79.

5. Ottosson JO (1960) Experimental studies of the mode of action of electroconvulsive therapy. *Acta Psychiatrica Scandinavica Supplementum* **35**: 5–6
6. Sackeim HA, Decina P, Kanzler M, *et al.* (1987) Effects of electrode placement on the efficacy of titrated, low-dose ECT. *American Journal of Psychiatry* **144**: 1449–55.
7. Sackeim HA, Prudic J, Devanand DP, *et al.* (2000) A prospective, randomized, double-blind comparison of bilateral and right unilateral ECT at different stimulus intensities. *Archives of General Psychiatry* **57**: 425–34.
8. Sackeim HA, Prudic J, Nobler MS, *et al.* (2008) Effects of pulse width and electrode placement on the efficacy and cognitive effects of electroconvulsive therapy. *Brain Stimulation* **1**: 71–83.
9. McNally KA, Blumenfeld H (2004) Focal network involvement in generalized seizures: new insights from electroconvulsive therapy. *Epilepsy and Behavior* **5**: 3–12.
10. McCormick LM, Ponto LLB, Pierson RK, *et al.* (2007) Metabolic correlates of antidepressant and antipsychotic response in patients with psychotic depression undergoing electroconvulsive therapy. *Journal of ECT* **23**: 265–73.
11. Takano H, Motohashi N, Uema T, *et al.* (2007) Changes in regional cerebral blood flow during acute electroconvulsive therapy in patients with depression. *British Journal of Psychiatry* **190**: 63–8.
12. Gleiter CH, Nutt DJ (1989) Chronic electroconvulsive shock and neurotransmitter receptors: an update. *Life Sciences* **44**: 985–1006.
13. Lerer B, Stanley M, McIntrye I, Altman H (1984) Electroconvulsive shock and brain muscarinic recpetors: relationship to anterograde amnesia. *Life Sciences* **35**: 2659–64.
14. Sackeim HA (1999) The anticonvulsant hypothesis of the mechanisms of action of ECT: current status. *Journal of ECT* **15**: 5–26.
15. Fink M, Petrides G, Kellner C, *et al.* (2008) Change in seizure threshold during electroconvulsive therapy. *Journal of ECT* **24**: 114–16.
16. Duman RS, Heninger GR, Nestler EJ (1997) A molecular and cellular theory of depression. *Archives of General Psychiatry* **54**: 597–606.
17. Warner-Schmitt JL, Duman RS (2008) VEGF as a potential target for therapeutic intervention in depression. *Current Opinion in Pharmacology* **8**: 14–19.
18. The UK ECT Review Group (2003) Efficacy and safety of electroconvulsive therapy in depressive disorder: a systematic review and meta-analysis. *Lancet* **361**: 799–808.
19. Special Committee on ECT (2005) *The ECT Handbook*, 2nd edn. London: Royal College of Psychiatrists.
20. National Institute for Health and Clinical Excellence (2003) *Electroconvulsive Therapy (ECT)*. London: National Institute for Health and Clinical Excellence.
21. Van den Broek WW, de Ley A, Mulder PGH, *et al.* (2004) Effect of antidepressant medication resistance on short-term response to electroconvulsive therapy. *Journal of Clinical Psychopharmacology* **24**: 400–403.
22. Husain S, Kevan IM, Linnell R, *et al.* (2004) Electroconvulsive therapy in depressive illness that has not responded to drug treatment. *Journal of Affective Disorders* **86**: 121–6.
23. Prudic J, Haskett RF, Mulsant B, *et al.* (1996) Resistance to antidepressant medications and short-term clinical response to ECT. *American Journal of Psychiatry* **153**: 985–92.
24. Rasmussen KG, Mueller M, Knapp RG, *et al.* (2007) Antidepressant medication treatment failure does not predict lower remission with ECT for major depressive disorder. *Journal of Clinical Psychiatry* **68**: 1701–6.
25. Faber R, Trimble MR (1991) Electroconvulsive therapy in Parkinson's disease and other movement disorders. *Movement Disorders* **6**: 293–303.
26. Davis JM, Janicak PG, Sakkas P, *et al.* (1991) Electroconvulsive therapy in the treatment of neuroleptic malignant syndrome. *Convulsive Therapies* **7**: 111–20.
27. Cline JS, Roos K (2007) Treatment of status epilepticus with electroconvulsive therapy. *Journal of ECT* **23**: 30–32.
28. Kelly KG, Zisselman M (2000) Update on electroconvulsive therapy (ECT) in older adults. *Journal of the American Geriatric Society* **48**: 560–66.
29. Abrams R (2002) *Electroconvulsive Therapy*, 4th edn. Oxford: Oxford University Press.
30. Prudic J, Sackeim HA, Decina P, *et al.* (1987) Acute effects of ECT on cardiovascular functioning: relations to patient in treatment variables. *Acta Psychiatrica Scandinavica* **75**: 344–51.
31. Scott AIF, Gardner M, Good R (2005) Fall in ECT use in young people in Edinburgh. *Journal of ECT* **21**: 50.
32. Cook A, Scott A (1992) ECT for young people. *British Journal of Psychiatry* **161**: 718–19.
33. Chanpattana W, Kunigiri G, Kramer BA, Gangadahar BN (2005) Survey of ECT practice in teaching hospitals in India. *Journal of ECT* **21**: 100–104.
34. Cohen D, Paillere-Narmot M, Basquin M (1997) Use of electroconvulsive therapy in adolescence. *Convulsive Therapies* **13**:25–31.
35. Whittaker R, Scott A, Gardner M (2007) The prevalence of prolonged cerebral seizures at the first treatment in a course of electroconvulsive therapy. *Journal of ECT* **23**: 11–13.
36. Rey JM, Walter G (1997) Half a century of ECT use in young people. *American Journal of Psychiatry* **154**: 595–602.
37. Reinblatt SP, Rifkin A, Freeman J (2004) The efficacy of ECT in adults with mental retardation experiencing psychiatric disorders. *Journal of ECT* **20**: 208–12.
38. Okagbue N, McIntosh A, Gardiner M, Scott AIF (2008) The rate of usage of electroconvulsive therapy in the city of Edinburgh, 1993–2005. *Journal of ECT* **24**: 229–31.
39. O'Leary D, Gill D, Gregor S, Shawcross C (1974) The effectiveness of real versus simulated electroconvulsive therapy in depressed elderly patients. *International Journal of Geriatric Psychiatry* **9**: 567–71.

40. Tew JD, Mulsant BH, Haskett RF, *et al.* (1999) Acute efficacy of ECT in the treatment of major depression in the old-old. *American Journal of Psychiatry* **156**: 1865–70.
41. Sackeim HA, Prudic J, Devanand DP, *et al.* (1993) Effects of stimulus intensity and electrode placement on the efficacy and cognitive effects of electroconvulsive therapy. *New England Journal of Medicine* **328**: 839–46.
42. Sackeim HA, Prudic J, Fuller R, *et al.* (2007) The cognitive effects of electroconvulsive therapy in community settings. *Neuropsychopharmacology* **32**: 244–54.
43. Shapira B, Tubi N, Drexler H, *et al.* (1998) Cost and benefit in the choice of ECT schedule: twice versus three times weekly ECT. *British Journal of Psychiatry* **172**: 44–8.
44. Segman R H, Shapira B, Gorfin M, *et al.* (1995) Onset and time course of antidepressant action: psychopharmacological implications of a controlled trial of electroconvulsive therapy. *Psychopharmacology* **119**: 440–48.
45. Petrides G, Fink M, Husain MM, *et al.* (2003) ECT remission rates in psychotic versus non-psychotic depressed patients. *Journal of ECT* **19**: 151–7.
46. Sackeim HA, Prudic J (2005) Length of ECT course in bipolar and unipolar depression. *Journal of ECT* **21**: 195–7.
47. Devanand DP, Dwork AJ, Hutchinson ER, *et al.* (1994) Does ECT alter brain structure? *American Journal of Psychiatry* **151**: 957–70.
48. Shiwach RS, Reid WH, Carmody TJ (2001) An analysis of reported deaths following electroconvulsive therapy in Texas, 1993–1998. *Psychiatric Services* **52**: 1095–7.
49. Eranti S, Mogg A, Pluck G, *et al.* (2007) A randomized, controlled trial with six-month follow-up of repetitive transcranial magnetic stimulation and electroconvulsive therapy for severe depression. *American Journal of Psychiatry* **164**: 73–81.

Chapter 59

Transcranial magnetic stimulation and vagus nerve stimulation

RH Belmaker

TRANSCRANIAL MAGNETIC STIMULATION

Transcranial magnetic stimulation (TMS) of the brain is a somatic treatment in psychiatry approved by the US Food and Drug Administration (FDA) in October 2008 for the treatment of depression under certain conditions. The potential for further development of TMS is great, and psychiatrists should be familiar with its basic principles.

The idea that a rapidly alternating magnetic field induces an electric current was described by Maxwell's equations in physics in the 1800s, and the idea that nerves work electrically, as illustrated early on by the contraction of a frog's leg upon the application of a small electric current, was demonstrated by Galvani in the 1700s. It was therefore a short conceptual step to propose that the brain could be stimulated with a rapidly alternating magnetic field and that this could affect various brain functions. Indeed, Thompson patented an idea such as this in 1910 and implied that a magnet applied to the visual areas of the occipital cortex could induce spots of light.

In actuality, the coils required to carry an electric current that is powerful enough to create a magnetic field strong enough to stimulate the brain were not available until 1985. In the first TMS machine such coils depended on metals that were developed for completely different areas of modern technology but became available in the 1980s for electromagnetic coils. The first coil able to stimulate the brain was demonstrated in 1985 by Barker in England. The easy accessibility and large amount of knowledge of the motor cortex of the human brain made this the obvious first choice for demonstration, and it is still most convincing for students of psychiatry and neurology.

The appropriate coil placed over different parts of the homunculus of the human motor cortex can induce a contraction of the appropriate peripheral muscle. For instance, a stimulus above the area of the thumb will give a slight twitch in the thumb that is visible above a certain threshold. Twitches below such a threshold can often be identified by placing an electromyographic electrode on the thumb or other peripheral muscle involved. The homunculus on the brain of the motor cortex is represented such that if one moves on the human brain closer to the midline, one can stimulate the areas of leg and cause the subject's leg to jerk. Subjects who have had such a TMS stimulus find the movement of the thumb or leg surprising and completely involuntary and do not feel a sense of conscious desire to move the stimulated part of the body. Therefore, it seems that the TMS stimulation of the motor cortex is taking a rather direct route through the descending pathways leading to the motor output.

The first uses of TMS were in neurology and developed rapidly. The progress in neurology was rapid and dramatic and was reviewed by Hallett and Cohen in the *Journal of the American Medical Association* in 1989.[1] The combination of a magnetic stimulus to the motor cortex and an electromyelogram of the peripheral muscle, say the finger, could allow the time in milliseconds from the stimulation of motor cortex to the muscle to be calculated. The magnetic coil could then be placed on the neck at the output of the motor nerve to the arm, the stimulation repeated, and the conduction time from the neck to the peripheral muscle calculated. The difference between those two times, the central conduction time, gives a measure of the amount of time from the stimulation of the motor cortex to the output of the motor nerve in the spinal cord. Many types of brain lesions increase this conduction time, and it is studied extensively in neurology. Of course, the peripheral conduction time (the length of time from the stimulus of the motor nerve in the neck to the arm or leg) could also be lengthened in various diseases of peripheral nerves, and this is an important diagnostic tool in peripheral nerve disease.

If the brain works electrically, then why not stimulate the brain with external electrical stimulation to the skull? The skull is highly resistant to electrical current, and a high current is necessary on the skin to achieve only small current passage through the brain. This voltage drop across the skull causes local heat and pain. By contrast, magnetic fields pass through the skull and other tissues as if they were transparent and convert to local electrical currents only when ions or electrically charged particles are encountered. Therefore, magnetic stimulation can induce small electrical currents deeper in the brain and with fewer side effects than external electrical stimulation.

In 1995, two groups independently conceived the notion that if the motor cortex could be stimulated directly by a magnetic field and lead to a definite measurable output, then stimulation of the 'silent' areas of the brain such as the prefrontal cortex might affect emotion, thinking or behaviour.[2] These two early papers suggested an antidepressant effect. The idea of an antidepressant effect was also perhaps inspired by a paper that came out in the same year by Sackeim and colleagues in the *New England Journal of Medicine* showing that differences in the current strength in electroconvulsive therapy (ECT) affected the treatment outcome. Until that time, clinicians using ECT tended to believe that 'a convulsion is a convulsion' and that, since a convulsion seemed to be the essential therapeutic element of ECT, it did not matter for therapeutic purposes whether this convulsion was induced unilaterally or bilaterally, barely super-threshold or highly super-threshold. Sackeim found that unilateral barely super-threshold stimulation induced convulsions that were much less therapeutic.

Subsequent research in ECT over the past 15 years has tended to confirm the idea that the nature of the ECT electrical stimulus can affect the therapeutic outcome. The idea that the nature of the electrical stimulus could affect the therapeutic outcome and that the convulsion itself was not critical may have been an essential insight that allowed the early development of TMS. However, it is unclear today whether TMS is in any sense analogous to ECT merely because both of them involve electromagnetic stimulation of the brain. It is quite possible that TMS affects depression via an entirely different mechanism. It is also possible that TMS in different parameters and of different areas of the brain may have differing effects in depression and in other psychiatric syndromes.

TMS has been studied extensively for safety in normal volunteers and in patients with different diagnoses. It apparently has no consistent neuropathological, neuroendocrine or cognitive side effects. Massively repetitive TMS stimulation in animal studies has not led to any clear histological changes. In humans, one main side effect is headache, because of muscle contraction under the site of the TMS electrode. If TMS is repeated rapidly over 20–25 times/s (hertz, Hz) and for more than 2–5 s (train length), there is a danger of seizure. Thus, in ECT a seizure is the goal of the electrical stimulation, but in TMS a seizure is a side effect. During TMS treatment, clinicians should be aware of the possibility of this side effect and should have appropriate equipment such as a respiratory bag and intravenous diazepam available if necessary. Such seizures are extremely rare during usual clinical conditions. To reduce the incidence even more, a TMS safety checklist is recommended before TMS treatment.

The site of TMS stimulation was, for most depression studies, chosen to be 5 cm anterior to the motor cortex area on the left side that leads to stimulation of the thumb. This area in studies combining TMS with magnetic resonance imaging (MRI) is in most patients the lateral prefrontal cortex. However, there is variation in skull and brain anatomy and, particularly in elderly patients with some brain atrophy, it may be that this is not the optimal coil placement. Early studies of TMS in volunteers found that stimulation of the left cortex induced sadness and of the right cortex induced happiness. This is opposite to the effects reported by most investigators for patients with depression or mania. There has been some evidence that in brain stimulation the neurophysiological effects are different if a magnetic stimulus of milliseconds in length is given once per second or less or whether it is given more frequently – rapid or repetitive TMS (rTMS). In some neurophysiological studies, the repetitive TMS is stimulatory and the single TMS inhibitory. These schemes are still theoretical and not consistent between animal in vivo and in vitro models. Human antidepressant studies have been based mostly on a heuristic or arbitrary choice of stimulation parameter and location.

Although a particular stimulation site and parameters and TMS machine were approved by the US FDA in October 2008, the well-trained clinician should realize that these parameters are not set in stone and that future developments might lead to treatments of entirely different areas of the brain with TMS or entirely different parameters of nerve stimulation and certainly other commercial machines.

TMS is usually given daily, except weekends, for 2–3 weeks in the treatment of a depressive episode. Response rates and remission rates are far below those of ECT. It is difficult to compare TMS with pharmacological antidepressant treatment. It is much more expensive, and the FDA approval was for patients who had failed one antidepressant. However, TMS is not indicated for resistant depression, and psychotic patients, suicidal patients and patients who have failed on multiple antidepressants have little chance of success with TMS.

Several companies make TMS devices, but only the Neuronetics® coil was tested, found effective in a multicentre clinical trial and approved by the FDA. There is little reason to think that it is uniquely effective in depression, however, and several similar devices are available in almost every country that are used for evaluation of peripheral nerve conduction and central nerve conduction in neurology. In some countries, it is permissible to use these devices in an off-label manner for the treatment of depression.[3]

VAGUS NERVE STIMULATION

Vagus nerve stimulation (VNS) derives from an entirely different conceptual tradition than TMS. Many anticonvulsants are effective in bipolar disorder as mood stabilizers, and antiepileptic neuropharmacology has been a steady source of new treatments for the somatic treatment of affective disorders. The vagus nerve, the tenth cranial nerve, emerges from the brain and follows a meandering pathway with numerous branches that lead to almost every organ in the body. It has been classically conceived as a parasympathetic efferent nerve, whose fibres secrete acetylcholine at multiple visceral muscarinic receptor innervated end organs, such as the heart, intestines, small blood vessels and sweat glands. However, the vagus nerve has also been found to have numerous afferent fibres that are enteroreceptive and carry information about the state of the peripheral internal organs to the brain. This afferent stimulation affects brain function and was found to have anticonvulsant properties that have been demonstrated in both human and animal studies beyond any doubt. The distance was therefore short until the trial of vagus nerve stimulation in depression.

VNS in the clinical setting involves a small operation. An electrical stimulator that can be turned on and off via remote control from outside the patient's body is placed underneath the skin. The rate and intensity of the electrical stimulation emitted by the device can also be modified. The device is connected via an electrode to the vagus nerve. The VNS once implanted remains on continuously, but clinical relief of depression is often slow. The studies resulting in FDA approval of VNS showed better results after 1 year than after 1 month. Side effects have been few, although some patients report hoarseness of their voice due to simulation of the recurrent fibres leading to the larynx. The operation, implantation and device are expensive, and the effect size of the key studies suggests that, among treatment-resistant patients, only a small number will achieve response or remission with VNS. Thus, like TMS, VNS is not a miracle treatment, although there is almost certainly a subgroup of patients for whom this may be very helpful.[4]

KEY POINTS

- Neuronal communication involves neurophysiological ion currents.
- Rapidly moving magnetic fields can generate electric currents and move ions at a distance.
- It has long been obvious that rapidly alternating magnetic fields can affect nerve and brain function.
- Magnetic stimulators exist that, when placed over the motor cortex, can induce movements of peripheral muscles given defined rates and length of pulse stimulation.
- Stimulation of certain prefrontal areas has specific effects on mood in controlled double-blind studies.
- These clinical effects are not of the magnitude of ECT and are probably unrelated in mechanism to ECT.

REFERENCES

1. Hallett M, Cohen LG (1989) Magnetism: a new method for stimulation of nerve and brain. *Journal of the American Medical Association* 262: 538–41.
2. Belmaker RH, Fleischmann A (1995) Transcranial magnetic stimulation: a potential new frontier in psychiatry. *Biological Psychiatry* 38: 419–21.
3. George MS, Belmaker RH (2007) *Transcranial Magnetic Stimulation in Clinical Psychiatry*. Washington, DC: American Psychiatric Publishing.
4. Nemeroff CB, Mayberg HS, Krahl SE, *et al.* (2006) VNS therapy in treatment-resistant depression: clinical evidence and putative neurobiological mechanisms. *Neuropsychopharmacology* 31: 1345–55.

Chapter 60

Psychotherapy: an introduction

C Susan Mizen

INTRODUCTION

There has been a dichotomy, long-standing within psychiatry, between psychological and physical approaches to treatment. Enlightened psychiatric practice has looked upon these two modalities as equal in value and bemoaned the relative predominance and availability of physical over psychological treatments

A number of recent developments, most fundamentally in neuroscience, call the basis of this dichotomy into question. Historically, there has been difficulty translating observations of the 'objective' anatomical, physiological brain, and the 'subjective' brain, the mind. More recently, researchers in the field of cognitive neuroscience have addressed themselves to such subjects as affect[1,2] and the origins of the experience of self and other,[3] which would previously have been considered to be too 'subjective' to be available to rigorous scientific methodology. Researchers in developmental neuroscience have examined the neurobiological consequences of relational trauma in infancy and the impact of the emotional environment upon brain development. Links have been established between such environmental factors and the development of psychological and psychiatric symptoms in later life.[4] Other studies have provided neuroscientific evidence for the presence of psychological defences.[5,6] Finally, functional imaging has demonstrated neurological changes occurring following both psychological and physical treatments.[7] An early study undertaken by Baxter and colleagues demonstrated a similar reduction in the metabolic rate to the head of the right caudate nucleus brought about by fluoxetine and cognitive-behavioural therapy (CBT) in patients with obsessive–compulsive disorder who responded to treatment.[8]

As neuroscience addresses itself to relevant aspects of psychological function, some of the difficulties translating from the 'neurological' to the 'psychological' become more negotiable. However, there remain dangers in prematurely and simplistically applying neurobiological findings to psychotherapeutic practice.

Alongside these developments, as evidence for the effectiveness of psychotherapeutic treatments has grown, they increasingly feature in National Institute for Health and Clinical Excellence (NICE) guidelines. This in turn has stimulated investment of public funds in psychotherapy, which is seen as a solution to the problems arising from common mental disorders such as anxiety and depression.[9] The introduction of the Improving Access to Psychological Therapies (IAPT) initiative[10] is perhaps the most striking illustration of the paradigm shift that has occurred in the perception of the psychological therapies as an agent of change. Where does this leave us with the old debates about the relative importance of medication or psychological treatments in mental health services?

Nobel Laureate Kandel has proposed a 'new intellectual framework for psychiatry'.[11] He makes the case for a rapprochement between neuroscience, psychiatry and psychoanalysis. Neuroscience can help to elucidate the diagnosis and treatment of mental disorders, but reciprocally neuroscientists benefit as psychiatrists pose some of the behavioural questions that biology needs to answer in order to advance understanding of higher mental processes. Kandel's framework is summarized in Box 60.1.

Kandel made the case for the dissolution of old divisions between:

- functional and organic mental illness;
- dichotomous thinking about the influence of nature and nurture upon higher psychological functions and psychopathology;
- physical and psychological treatments.

For the psychiatrist, the integration of psychological understanding into psychiatric practice has a developing evidence base and forms a scientific basis for clinical work. It is in this context that the Royal College of Psychiatrists has developed its new curriculum for psychotherapy training, with an emphasis on applying psychological principles and skills in psychiatric practice. The competencies required of trainees are shown in Box 60.2.

Although the formal psychological therapies themselves are dealt with in subsequent chapters, this chapter will address various aspects of psychologically informed psychiatric practice.

Box 60.1 Kandel's 'new intellectual framework for psychiatry'

- *Principle 1:* All mental processes derive from the operations of the brain, even where the causes of disturbance are clearly environmental.
- *Principle 2:* Genes and their protein products are important determinants of the interconnectedness of neurons in the brain, and their functioning exerts significant control over behaviour.
- *Principle 3:* Genes do not by themselves explain all of the variance of a given mental illness: behaviour and social factors act on the brain by modifying the expression of genes and function of nerve cells. Thus, nurture is ultimately expressed as nature.
- *Principle 4:* Alterations in gene expression induced by learning give rise to changes in neuronal connections. These form the basis for individuality and initiate and maintain abnormalities of behaviour induced by social contingencies.
- *Principle 5:* If psychotherapy is effective in bringing about long-term changes in behaviour, then it presumably does so through learning, changing gene expression, altering the strength of synaptic connections and bringing about structural changes.

Box 60.2 Royal College of Psychiatrists' psychotherapy competencies required for basic training in psychiatry

GENERAL

- Account for clinical phenomena in psychological terms
- Deploy advanced communication skills
- Display advanced emotional intelligence in dealings with patients and colleagues.

SPECIFIC

- Refer appropriately for formal psychological therapies
- Jointly manage patients receiving psychotherapy
- Deliver basic psychotherapeutic treatments in at least two modalities.

MAKING A REFERRAL TO PSYCHOLOGICAL THERAPIES

Assessing suitability for therapy

A number of factors may weigh upon the mind of the psychiatrist considering the appropriateness of referral for therapy. Among these is the context within which the patient is assessed. Assessing an acutely distressed patient while on call, the psychiatrist may be anxious about discharge without offering further help. Referral for therapy under such circumstances may reflect the psychiatrist's immediate anxiety rather than being a thought-through decision about a potentially long-term commitment, there being no such thing as 'emergency psychotherapy'. Again, referral might be made when the psychiatrist is about to move post, when patient and doctor are facing an imminent loss. Such referrals are unlikely to lead to successful engagement in therapy. Decisions about referral are best made in circumstances in which the patient is free to discuss their mixed feelings about therapy and to arrive at their own conclusions about whether to proceed. The clinician's job is to ensure that the patient is aware of the options and what therapy is likely to involve and to be realistic about the likely outcome so that the patient can come to an informed decision.

The evidence for the effectiveness of psychological therapies is set out comprehensively in a critical review of psychotherapy research undertaken by Roth and Fonagy.[12] Although in some instances referral is a simple matter of directing a patient to the appropriate evidence-based intervention, factors aside from diagnosis determine whether a patient is likely to benefit from psychological intervention or not. Table 60.1 provides a list of indications and contraindications for therapy set out in the terms used by therapists undertaking an assessment.

Table 60.2 provides a summary of the evidence base derived from Roth and Fonagy's review,[12] the Department of Health's Treatment Choice in Psychological Therapies and Counselling,[13] information from Cochrane Reviews, NICE guidelines, and manualized therapies that have been subjected to randomiszed controlled trails. The table has been adapted from the Royal College of Psychiatrists' *Psychological Therapies in Psychiatry and Primary Care.*[14]

It is important that the referring clinician has an idea of the level of therapeutic intervention required and where it can be obtained. Figure 60.1 sets out the stepped care model proposed in the IAPT practice guide.

Writing a referral to psychological therapies

Once the psychiatrist and patient have decided upon referral for psychotherapy, the written referral should include a full psychiatric assessment, including risk to self and others, with particular attention paid to the personal history, including major events of childhood and family relationships. It is useful to describe the discussion that took place about therapy so that the assessing psychotherapist is forewarned about the patient's expectations.

Jointly managing patients receiving psychotherapy

In many cases it is a good idea for patients with severe and enduring mental health problems in psychotherapy to continue to see a psychiatrist for outpatient appointments. However, the psychiatrist who is not well informed about

Table 60.1 Indications and contraindications for psychological treatments

Model	Indications	Contraindications
Psychodynamic long-term	*General:* History of 'one good relationship' Capacity to tolerate frustration Thoughtful or positive response to trial interpretation at assessment Capacity to engage emotionally with the therapist Sufficient motivation to face unwanted feelings or disavowed aspects of the self	*Specific:* Schizophrenia or history of severe psychotic breakdown Severe obsessional states Somatization Physical dependence upon alcohol or other substances *General:* History of violence likely to be enacted towards the therapist Likely decompensation leading to unmanageable increased risk to self or others, especially children or other dependants
Short-term dynamic psychotherapy	*As above plus:* Therapist able to identify focus High ego strength High motivation Psychological mindedness Able to engage and disengage	*Specific:* Serious depression Acute psychosis Borderline personality organization[15] *General:* Therapist unable to make effective contact Evidence of need for extended work[16]
Group analysis	*Specific:* alcoholism, anxiety disorders, bereavement, bulimia, depression, schizophrenia, sexual abuse *General:* Motivation to participate and get emotionally involved Positive experiences of relating to others in groups in childhood or at present Interest in exploring oneself or others Some ability to sympathize or empathize	*Specific:* Paranoid disorders with little insight Current addictive substance misuse History of violence to others without insight or regret *General:* Major problems with self-disclosure Difficulties with intimacy General personal distrust Excessive use of denial[17]
Cognitive-behavioural therapy	See evidence base	*General:* Low patient motivation Patients with positive beliefs about dysfunctional aspects of their behaviour Severe learning disability Antisocial personality (less able to attend to peripheral information and self-regulate) Poorly addressed cultural differences[18]

continued

Table 60.1 *continued*

Model	Indications	Contraindications
Interpersonal therapy	Depression, bulimia nervosa*, bipolar disorder*, social phobia*, some evidence of effectiveness*	Substance abuse
Family therapy	*General:* Family evidently dysfunctional resulting in stress Family has suffered a life event Continuing demanding circumstances, e.g. enduring mental or physical illness Identified patient symptomatic in the context of poorly functioning family Maladaptive responses to mental illness Disorganized families	*General:* Family unavailable No shared motivation for change Severe long-standing family disturbance Family equilibrium likely to decompensate A member of the family too incapacitated by psychiatric disorder Family member wishes for the privacy of individual work (in process of separation)
Arts therapies	*Specific:* psychotic illness, eating disorders, learning disability *General:* conditions not immediately amenable to verbal expression	
Integrative therapy (supportive, eclectic and integrated therapies, e.g. IPT, CAT)	Traditional 'monotherapies' have failed Presenting problem and developmental background are uncertain Therapist has generic psychotherapeutic skills but not specific skills Patient is too disturbed for 'monotherapy' Patient has a number of different problems that need to be tackled sequentially by the same therapist using a range of approaches	

CAT, cognitive analytical therapy; IPT, interpersonal therapy.

Table 60.2 Table of evidence for psychological therapies

Therapeutic modality	Depression	Postpartum depression	Bipolar disorder	Phobias	Panic disorder and agoraphobia	GAD	OCD	PTSD	Schizophrenia
CBT	Clear: Including mindfulness-based CBT	Some	Some	Clear: Social + exposure	Clear	Clear	Clear: With SSRI / Some	Clear	Some
IPT	Clear	Some	Some						
Structured/focused psychodynamic	Some				Clear			Some	
DBT									
MBT									
CAT									
Behavioural treatments	Some			Clear	Clear	Clear	Clear		
EMDR								Clear	
Family and couple interventions	Some		Some						Clear / Some: MFG
Community reinforcement approaches									
Motivational interviewing									
Social skills training/ psychoeducation			Some						Some
Supportive expressive Therapy									
Multimodal/ multisystemic									
Problem-solving therapy	Clear: Primary care					Some			Some: EI
Primary care counselling	Some: Adjustment disorders and short term only, depression	Some	Some	Some	Some	Some	Some	Some	Some

Key: Clear = clear evidence of effectiveness (orange); Some = some evidence of effectiveness (yellow)

BED, binge eating disorder; CAT, cognitive analytical therapy; CBT, cognitive-behavioural therapy; DBT, dialectical behaviour therapy; EI, early intervention; EMDR, eye movement desensitization and reprocessing; GAD, generalized anxiety disorder; IPT, interpersonal therapy; MBT, mentalization-based therapy; MFG, multiple family groups; OCD, obsessive–compulsive disorder; PTSD, post-traumatic stress disorder; SSRI, selective serotonin reuptake inhibitor.

Alcohol misuse	Drug misuse	Anorexia	Bulimia	BED	Personality disorder	Sexual dysfunction	Physical symptoms	Childhood disorders	Disorders of older people
	Cocaine						Chronic fatigue, chronic pain, hypochondriasis, multiple sclerosis, epilepsy, irritable bowel syndrome, hypertension	Depression, OCD, general anxiety disorder, conduct disorder, obesity	Depression Anxiety, sleep, dementia
								Depression	
					Borderline personality disorder, transference, focused therapy		Irritable bowel syndrome, hypochondriasis	Mixed anxiety and depression	Depression
					Self-harm in borderline personality disorder				
	Cocaine, opiates						Chronic pain	Behavioural problems in autism	Depression
	Cocaine						Type 1 diabetes in children and adults	Conduct disorder, depression	
	Cocaine								
					Avoidant self-harm		Chronic fatigue		Dementia
	Opiates								
								Adolescent conduct disorder Attention deficit hyperactivity disorder	

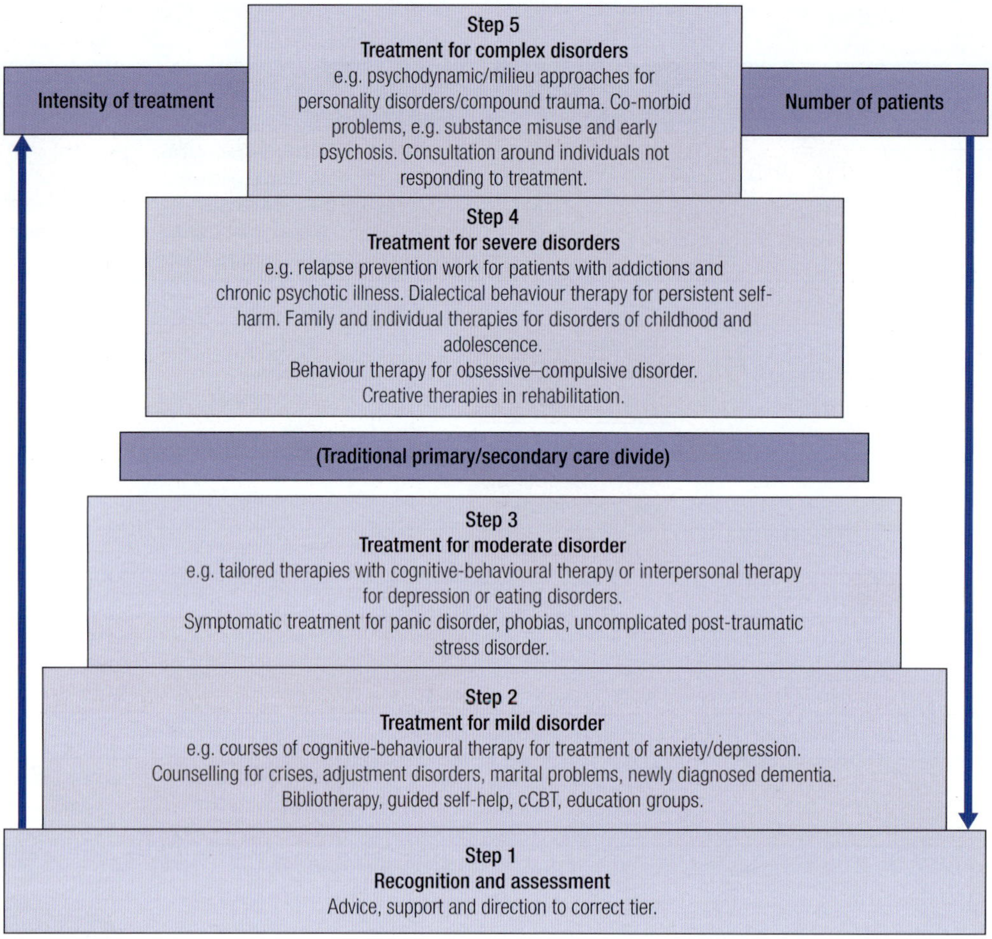

Figure 60.1 Model of stepped care
cCBT, computerized cognitive-behavioural therapy

the ethos of the therapeutic model being followed may unwittingly undermine the therapeutic work. Different models require different approaches from the psychiatrist.

The following recommendations apply to psychiatrists working alongside psychodynamic therapists:

- The patient may discuss their therapy with their psychiatrist because they are anxious and ambivalent about or disturbed by their sessions. It is important to listen and let the patient know that people are often disturbed by the process of change in therapy. It is important to encourage the patient to tell their therapist, especially when doubtful about continuing.
- The patient may, for example, think their therapist is useless, abusive, silent or intrusive. Although it is important to be alert to bad practice by the therapist, it is also important to recognize that the patient's feelings may be transference-driven or an indirect expression of anger with the therapist through the psychiatrist. The patient should be encouraged to be honest with their therapist about what they think, this being part of the therapeutic work.
- Periods of disturbance in therapy are often crisis points. A psychiatrist who supports the patient through such crises can make the difference between change occurring or not. For example, if in doubt about whether medication is likely to be helpful, contact the psychotherapist (with the patient's permission, if this has not already been granted) to discuss the way forward.
- Patients may seek a therapeutic relationship with their psychiatrist while in therapy. It is important to stay within the psychiatric role, since this may well be a part of 'acting out' of underlying psychopathology, for example playing one caregiver off against another, without being able fully to trust either.

PRESCRIBING FOR PATIENTS WHO ARE IN THERAPY

CBT has successfully established its evidence base, in part through the ways in which therapy is an analogue of medication. CBT models are manualized and can be administered with a comparable degree of confidence about the exact nature of the treatment being delivered and in what 'dosage'. This has permitted direct comparisons of the effectiveness of medication and CBT, and comparisons between the use of CBT and medication together with either treatment alone. CBT and medication augment one another's actions, and combinations of CBT and medication are therefore recommended in NICE guidelines. Aside from the possibility of synergistic neurological action, there are other reasons that therapy and medication may facilitate or confound the other's actions (Table 60.3).

Table 60.3 Advantages and disadvantages of combining cognitive-behavioural therapy (CBT) and medication

Advantages	Disadvantages
Medication may:	*Medication may:*
Increase the speed and magnitude of response to psychotherapy	Suppress feelings and impede progress in therapy
Reduce symptoms and make treatment more acceptable	Convey a message that the patient's feelings are too difficult to be dealt with in therapy
Improve ego function so the patient can make better use of therapy	Lead the patient to believe that improvement is due to medication rather that their own efforts
Psychotherapy may:	Lead to devaluation of the therapeutic relationship
Promote adaptive behaviour and improve compliance with medication	Be disadvantageous in treating PTSD, where exposure to affect is important
Decrease the likelihood of recurrence	
Provide a more comprehensive understanding of the patient's difficulties than medication alone	

PTSD, post-traumatic stress disorder.

The meaning of medication

Transference and countertransference are at work in prescribing in relation to the doctor and the medication itself. Ambivalence towards the doctor and the treatment may be partly responsible for high rates of non-compliance with psychotropic medication. It is important to understand the significance of the medication to the patient and their beliefs about it, often tied up with feelings about dependency and illness, if compliance is to be improved. The therapeutic alliance is therefore as important in prescribing as it is in psychotherapy. Conversely, understanding the patient's anxieties about taking medication can elucidate aspects of the transference to the psychiatrist.

There is strong evidence for the effectiveness of combined medication and psychotherapeutic treatments in schizophrenia and depression, and more limited data in the treatment of personality disorders, substance misuse, eating disorders, anxiety disorders and bipolar disorder.[21]

Integrated practice (therapy and medication managed by the same person)

Principles of integrated treatment include the following:

- Obtain informed consent at the outset.
- Make a formulation and set treatment goals at the outset of whatever the modality of treatment.
- Focus on alliance rather than compliance.
- Address medication issues at the beginning or end of the session.
- Symptoms are likely to increase at the end of therapy: giving extra medication is not likely to be helpful.

The problems with integrated treatment arise in mastering two complicated approaches and the need to monitor the complexities of the situation moment by moment, which make this a demanding model to deliver.

Combined, split or collaborative practice (separate practitioners offering therapy and medication)

Split treatment, which is the most usually practised model, requires good communication, especially when working with patients with personality disorder. The treating pair may not arrive at a formulation that covers both aspects of treatment and may give mixed messages to the patient. Collaboration requires commitment from both parties, meeting at the beginning to discuss the treatment plan and to clarify roles. Respective responsibilities in a crisis should be established. A further meeting should be arranged if treatment is not working or tensions arise.

Prescribing for patients attending psychodynamic therapy

There is perhaps an inherent tension between psychopharmacological and psychotherapeutic practice. Psychodynamic therapy places emphasis on affects and conflicts being made conscious, which might previously have been repressed. Medication can be characterized as opposing this and may indeed do so. A patient may approach their psychiatrist for help when they find the therapy disturbing or having attained a new-found capacity to tolerate depression rather than resorting to symptomatic ways of avoiding it, such as substance abuse or self-harm, which may be a sign of increasing psychological maturity, being unsure if they will be able to cope with such feelings.

If the psychiatrist understands the differing perspectives of psychiatry and psychotherapy, then the need for communication with the therapist when taking action or prescribing should become apparent. Without this, there is the possibility of destructive enactments – at worst, medication becoming a means of transacting a battle between the therapist and the psychiatrist.

PSYCHOTHERAPEUTIC ASPECTS OF PSYCHIATRIC PRACTICE

The role of the psychiatrist in the mental health team is shifting away from direct involvement with large caseloads, towards a consultative and leadership role in teams. Psychiatrist will be required to have expertise to carry out this role.[22]

The role of the psychiatrist

- Treating complex cases
- Consulting to teams
- Managing and leading teams
- Developing services
- Offering psychologically informed management.

An understanding of the broader implications of psychological models beyond their application in the formal therapies is essential to undertaking these tasks. Being able to make a psychological formulation is helpful in the management of all cases, especially the most complex.

FORMULATION

Psychological formulation is a hypothesis about how the diverse experiences of distress, behaviour, history, and 'here and now' interactions can be summarized into a theoretically coherent synopsis of the underlying difficulty and the factors that sustain it. Those aspects of the patient's difficulty that are remediable are identified, and the means of bringing about change are clarified.

The framework of formulation varies from one model to another. In cognitive analytical therapy (CAT), arriving at the sequential diagrammatic reformulation (SDR) is a major task of the therapy. This diagram identifies reciprocal roles described in terms of the 'inner parent' and 'inner child' and traces how target problem procedures are executed and how their consequences are self-reinforcing. The diagram provides patients with an overview of their internal world, upon which they can reflect, and is the basis for taking action to shift entrenched patterns of relating.

This demonstrates the power of a well-constructed, collaborative formulation in helping the patient to gain insight, a capacity for self-reflection and a sense of agency in being able to change their ways of relating and their symptoms.

Psychodynamic formulation

Psychodynamic theory has its own diagnostic system that parallels but does not correspond directly with psychiatric diagnosis. Diagnosis is made not on the basis of behaviour or symptoms but on the basis of theoretical constructs, as follows:

- The quality of 'internal object relationships'
- The nature of defences and conflicts
- Psychological structures and syndromes.

The term 'object' is used in psychoanalytical theory to refer to relationships with others, in the first place parents seen through the lens of infantile phantasy life, which have been internalized and form a template of unconscious assumptions, which are then projected on to others in later life.

Symptomatology is seen as secondary to these underlying and largely unconscious forces. A system for diagnostic formulation has been operationalized for research purposes.[23]

In clinical practice, psychodynamic formulation can be undertaken during psychiatric or psychotherapeutic assessment. In psychotherapy assessments, the formulation is the basis of a trial interpretation, the patient's response providing a useful indication of the likely to response to therapy. In psychiatric assessment, formulation can inform the management of the patient.

Hinshelwood described a framework for psychodynamic formulation in which the clinician hears what the patient is saying as 'pictures of relationships with objects', bearing three areas of relationships in mind.[24] These can be described in the form described by Malan as the 'triangle of person' (Figure 60.2).[16]

In order to arrive at a formulation, it is important to provide the patient with opportunities to talk without interruption for some portion of the interview in order to observe the way they relate the transference and unconscious themes. A detailed personal history should be taken, including important events such as significant separations and traumas and also the quality of relationships with important figures. The triangle is a tool to assist clear thinking in connecting aspects of the patient's presentation into a

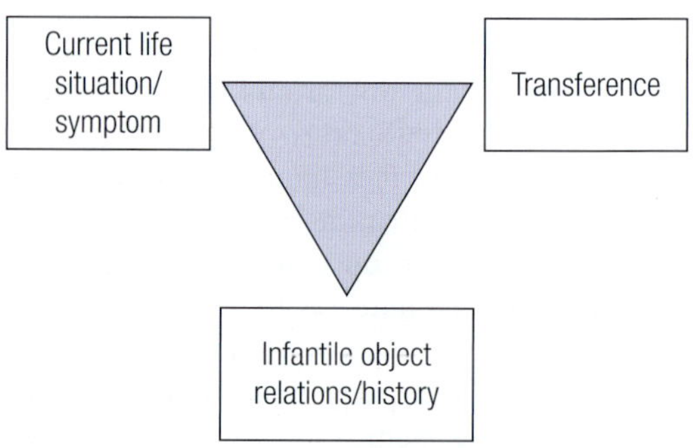

Figure 60.2 Triangle of person

coherent narrative. The coherence is brought about through finding a pattern that is repeated across all three domains.

Undrill describes a helpful list of defences to look for under diagnostic categories (Table 60.4).[25]

Case example

A community mental health team is working with a patient with a diagnosis of personality disorder who is self-harming and has a history of sexual abuse in childhood. One part of the team identifies with the patient as the victim of abuse and seeks to provide the patient with the care and protection the patient is believed to have missed. The patient confides selectively in these members of staff. The rest of the team believe that the patient is seeking attention and that the staff who are favoured by the patient are collusive, encouraging self-harm. Tensions arise in the team, and the patient's acting out becomes more severe. The team seeks advice from the psychological therapies service. Having assessed the patient, the therapist makes a formulation as follows:

Infantile object relations

In accordance with Kleinian psychoanalytical theory, the patient is anxious about the destructive effects of their aggression on the people they love and upon whom they depend, in this instance the mental health team. The patient divides/splits their emotional world into two halves/parts, others who are loved for being present who in the patient's mind are kept apart from others who are hated for being absent. The patient is defending against the possibility of losing those they are attached to by keeping these two emotional worlds apart.

Table 60.4 Defence and diagnosis

Diagnosis	Defences
Depression	Object losses in remote or recent past; ambivalence towards lost object; identification with lost object; excessive superego activity
Obsessive–compulsive disorder	Defences of isolation, undoing and reaction formation; ambivalence in object relations; anxiety about aggression; magical thinking
Anxiety disorder	Anxiety signals an unsuccessful defence; agoraphobia sometimes fear of abandonment/separation anxiety; panic disorder – onset often associated with loss; simple phobia – classically associated with symbolic significance of the phobic object
Anorexia nervosa	Difficulty separating from mother; body unconsciously perceived as occupied by introject of 'intrusive' mother, hence starved; need projected into others who are looked after; projective identification in family relations
Alcohol dependency	Associated with harsh punitive superego; alcohol acting as a 'superego solvent'; consider primary and secondary gain

Current life situation/symptom

This way of relating takes the form of alternating idealization and denigration of others, leading to short-term and unstable relationships and decompensation in the form of escalating self-harm when faced with separation.

Transference

With the team, this is played out between two factions in the staff group, one idealized/idealizing and one denigrated/denigrating.

Intervention

This situation is described to the team and their reactions framed as countertransference. The psychotherapist points out that the truth about the patient lies somewhere between the victim and perpetrator, this being a representation of an internal relationship between abuser and abused, both aspects being part of the patient's mental life. The team is advised to collude with neither position but to arrange to see the patient at a regular pre-arranged time and to take the patient's angriness about their non-availability between meetings on the chin, neither retaliating nor giving in to the demand to provide more. After a few angry and disturbed weeks, the patient's behaviour begins to settle.

THE UNCONSCIOUS IN TEAMS AND ORGANIZATIONS

Psychiatrists, particularly at senior level, are called upon to help teams work with their most complex patients, to support reflective functioning, to provide leadership and to identify aspects of the team's work that are dysfunctional. A psychological viewpoint is essential to undertaking this work, providing concepts with which to understand complex interpersonal systems.

After the First World War, psychoanalysts began to conceive of object relations theory as relevant to the social as well as the clinical field. In the 1940s and 1950s, the Tavistock Institute of Human Relations collaborated with industry to understand unconscious processes in the workplace, with a view to improving efficiency. These researchers observed that differences in the ways groups organized their work could be better understood if unconscious motives were taken into account.[26] Isabelle Menzies studied the dropout rate from nurse training.[27] She discovered that nurses organized themselves in ways that protected them from the unconscious anxieties implicit in their work and that broke up the human aspects of contact with patients. The cost of this defence was limited job satisfaction, resulting in many talented trainees leaving. Such defensive systems are rigid and uncomfortable, but because of their role in defending against anxiety they are difficult to change.

Systems theory has been added to this largely psychodynamic school of thought. In open systems theory, institutions are conceptualized as having a boundary across which inputs are drawn in, processed in accordance with the primary task, and then passed out as outputs, as would be the case in manufacturing processes.[28] Problems often arise in teams and organizations in identifying outputs and managing boundaries. An organizational consultant would take up the position of 'participant observer' to observe dynamic and systemic factors contributing to the dysfunction. The purpose of the consultation process is not necessarily to develop the team's sensitivity to their unconscious processes that might lead to greater frustration and inability to do the task, but rather to help identify the unconscious and structural obstacles to accomplishment of the task.

Unconscious aspects of organizational life

The study of unconscious processes in groups began with Freud's work *Group Psychology and the Analysis of the Ego.*[29] He described a process in which the crowd follows the leader who personifies their own ideals. In doing so, the capacity for thinking and decision-making is projected into the leader, on whom the group becomes pathologically dependent; at this point, criticizing the leader becomes impossible.

Bion's basic assumption groups

Wilfred Bion, a Kleinian psychoanalyst, defined the tendency of a group towards work on the primary task as 'the workgroup' and the unconscious tendency to avoid work on the primary task as 'basic assumption mentality'. Basic assumption mentality is a means of avoiding work when it is painful or causes conflict within the group.

Bion described three basic assumptions that occur in groups:[30]

- *Basic assumption – dependency:* the group behaves as though its primary task is to satisfy the needs and wishes of its members. The leader is expected to look after, protect and sustain the members of the group in order to make them feel good and not face them with the real demands of the task.
- *Basic assumption – fight/flight:* the group behaves as though there is a danger or enemy, which should either be attacked or fled from. The group follows the leader who is its most paranoid member. Such groups are identified by the lack of an effective response to deal with real threats.
- *Basic assumption – pairing:* the group functions in the grip of a phantasy that a future event will solve whatever the group's problem is. Some imagined coupling will bring about salvation. On the basis of this phantasy, no practical steps are taken to improve matters.

Leaders of all three groups will be followed only so long as they fulfil the basic assumptions of the group.

Different professions may mobilize the emotions of one basic assumption in the pursuit of the primary task. For example, the dependent basic assumption may be a functional adaptation on a hospital ward, where patients are asked to relinquish autonomy in order to contribute to efficient organization. The fight/flight basic assumption may be entirely appropriate to an organization such as the army, where a clear idea of fighting for a good cause against a common enemy and minimization of doubt may be highly functional.

Common problems in multidisciplinary teams

Each profession within a multidisciplinary team may have a different valency for one sort of basic assumption or another. The resulting conflict does not necessarily prevent collaboration but can result in breakdown in the functioning of the team.

Multidisciplinary teams often have difficulty developing a sense of shared purpose. The team may not have the authority to make a decision. It may behave like a band of individuals who get together when it suits them and disband when it does not, rather than functioning as a group unified around achieving a specific task.[31]

CONCLUSION

The majority of psychiatrists do not practise as psychotherapists. However, psychological thinking has applications far beyond the formal psychological therapies. In fact, psychotherapeutic skills are fundamental to psychiatric practice. These applications take many forms, including well-informed practice in referring patients to appropriate evidence-based therapies, preparing patients for assessment, and providing thoughtful support while therapy is in progress, all of which can improve therapeutic outcomes, including applying psychological understanding to prescribing and knowing how to optimize the use of medication and therapy together. Psychological thinking is also essential to the psychiatrist in their role in teams, both in planning the management of complex patients through the use of formulation and in identifying when a team is not functioning well and making appropriate use of consultation in resolving such difficulties.

KEY POINTS

- The developments in neuroscience, genetics and the changing social standing of the psychological therapies bring with them the opportunity to re-evaluate old distinctions between biological and psychological perspectives upon the aetiology of mental health disorders. This holds out the possibility of new approaches to treatment.
- The new MRCPsych curriculum recognizes that competence in the provision of psychological therapies and an understanding of their application to psychiatric practice are fundamental to good psychiatric practice.
- Assessing suitability for therapy referral requires consideration of the following factors:
  - Factors belonging to the context of the assessment which might affect treatment and referral decisions.
  - The importance of facilitating the patient in arriving at their own informed decision, providing sufficient information about the evidence and adapting the use of the evidence base to the clinical situation.
  - The psychiatrist must be aware of the level of intervention required and local therapy resources in deciding which service to refer to.
- When working as a psychiatrist alongside a psychodynamic therapist it is important to:
  - Support the patient through difficult periods and crises in therapy.
  - Recognize that negative transference can be fundamental to therapeutic change.
  - Encourage discussion of doubts about and problems with the process with the therapist.
  - Avoid splitting.
  - Refrain from embarking on therapeutic work in parallel with the therapist.
- An understanding of the complexities of the doctor–patient relationship is fundamental to effective prescribing. The potentially synergistic effects of medication and therapy can be optimized by integrated or collaborative practice, the relative merits of which are discussed.
- As the psychiatrist's role in psychiatric teams moves towards a consultation role with the most complex patients, team leadership and management, the application of psychological thinking to psychiatric practice becomes increasingly important. The ability to make a psychological formulation is essential to this work.
- Psychological understanding can be applied to the functioning of mental health teams. Unconscious defensive structures within teams can influence their work, serving to relieve the team of anxiety rather than resulting in the efficient accomplishment of the team's task. Such forces also affect the way the team selects and relates to its leader.
- Bion identified three types of basic assumption group – dependency, fight–flight and pairing – basic assumptions which may serve as functional adaptation to a teams task or may prevent functioning of the work group towards achievement of the primary task.

ACKNOWLEDGEMENT

Jeremy Holmes is thanked for useful comments on the text.

REFERENCES

1. Le Doux J (1996) *The Emotional Brain*. London, Weidenfeld & Nicholson.
2. Panksepp J (1998) *Affective Neuroscience: The Foundations of Human and Animal Emotions*. New York: Oxford University Press.
3. Damasio A (1999 *The Feeling of What Happens*. London: Heinemann.
4. Schore A (1994) *Affect Regulation and the Origin of the Self*. Mahwah, NJ: Lawrence Erlbaum Associates.
5. Kaplan-Solms K, Solms M (2000) *Clinical Studies in Neuro-Psychoanalysis*. London: Karnac Books.
6. Shevrin H, Bond J, Brakel L, Hertel HK, Williams WJ (1996) *Conscious and Unconscious Processes: Psychodynamic, Cognitive and Neurophysiological Convergences*. New York; Guilford Press.
7. Beutel ME, Huber M (2008) Functional neuroimaging: can it contribute to our understanding of processes of change? *Neuro-Psychoanalysis* **10** (1): 5–16.
8. Baxter LR, Schwartz JM, Bergman KS, *et al.* (1992) Caudate glucose metabolic rate changes with both drug and behaviour therapy for obsessive compulsive disorder. *Archives of General Psychiatry* **49**: 681–9.
9. Layard R (2005) *The Depression Report: A New Deal for Depression and Anxiety Disorders*. London: London School of Economics Centre for Economic Performance Mental Health Policy Group.
10. Department of Health (2007) *Commissioning for a Brighter Future: Improving Access to Psychological Therapies. Positive Practice Guide*. London: Department of Health.
11. Kandel ER (1998) A new intellectual framework for psychiatry. *American Journal of Psychiatry* **155**: 457–69.
12. Roth AD, Fonagy P (2004). *What Works for Whom? A Critical Review of Psychotherapy Research*, 2nd edn. New York: Guilford.
13. Department of Health (2001) *Treatment Choice in Psychological Therapies and Counselling*. London: Department of Health.
14. Royal College of Psychiatrists, Royal College of General Practitioners (2008) *Psychological Therapies in Psychiatry and Primary Care*. Document CR151. London: Royal College of Psychiatrists.
15. Mann J (1978) *Time-limited Psychotherapy*. Cambridge, MA: Harvard University Press.
16. Malan D (1979) *Individual Psychotherapy and the Science of Psychodynamics*. London: Butterworths.
17. Knauss W (1985) The treatment of psychosomatic illnesses in group-analytic psychotherapy–indications and contraindications. *Group Analysis* **XVIII**: 177–90.

18. Grant P, Young PR, De Rubeis RJ (2005) Cognitive and behavioural therapies. In GO Gabbard, JS Beck, J Holmes (eds) *Oxford Textbook of Psychotherapy*. Oxford: Oxford University Press.
19. Westra HA, Stewart SH, Conrad BE (2002) Naturalistic manner of benzodiazepine use and cognitive behaviour therapy outcome in panic disorder with agoraphobia. *Journal of Anxiety Disorders* **16**: 233–46.
20. Collins KA, Westra HA, Dozois DJA, Stewart SH (2004) The validity of the brief version of the Fear of Negative Evaluation Scale. *Journal of Anxiety Disorders* **19**: 345–59.
21. Kay J (2001) Integrated treatment: an overview. In J Kay (ed.) *Integrated Treatment for Psychiatric Disorders: Review of Psychiatry*, Vol. 20. Washington, DC: American Psychiatric Press.
22. Department of Health (2005) *New Ways of Working for Psychiatrists*. London: Department of Health.
23. Cierpka M, Grande T, Rudolf G, von der Tann M, Stasch M (2007) The operationalized psychodynamic diagnostic system: clinical relevance, reliability and validity. *Psychopathology* **40**: 209–20.
24. Hinshelwood RD (1991) Psychodynamic formulation in assessment for psychotherapy. *British Journal of Psychotherapy* **8**: 166–74.
25. Undrill G (2007) Psychoanalysis and Psychodynamics 2: The Formulation. www.guyundrill.com.
26. Trist E, Higgin G, Murray H, Pollock A (1963) *Organizational Choice*. London: Tavistock Publications.
27. Menzies Lyth IEP (1979) Social systems as a defence against anxiety: an empirical study of the nursing service of a general hospital. In E Trist, H Murray (eds) *The Social Engagement of Social Science*, Vol. 1. London: Free Association Books.
28. Miller EJ, Rice AK (1967) *Systems of Organization: The Control of Task and Sentient Boundaries*. London: Tavistock Publications.
29. Freud S (1921 [1984]) *Group Psychology and the Analysis of the Ego*. Harmondsworth: Penguin Books.
30. Bion W (1961) *Experiences in Groups*. New York: Basic Books.
31. Obholzer A, Roberts V (1994) *The Unconscious at Work*. London: Routledge.

Chapter 61

Dynamic psychotherapy

Chris Mace

INTRODUCTION

Psychodynamic psychotherapy is the oldest established form of psychological therapy that is currently in use. The attention it pays to the relationship between therapist and patient in treatment, and the theory of mental functioning on which it is based, are reasons why all psychiatrists need to be familiar with its principles. For clarity, I refer to any unnamed therapist as 'she' and any unnamed patient as 'he' throughout this chapter.

ORIGINS OF PSYCHODYNAMIC PSYCHOTHERAPY

Psychodynamic psychotherapy represents the tradition in psychotherapy derived from psychoanalysis. Psychoanalysis was developed by a Viennese neurologist, Sigmund Freud, as a 'talking cure' for people with what were then termed 'psychoneuroses'. These included the somatic presentations of 'hysteria' as well as obsessive–compulsive syndromes. The guiding principle was that symptoms arose as a consequence of active suppression of feelings and memories that the patient did not wish to experience. In order for these to remain unconscious, the conscious 'I' was protected by a variety of mechanisms of defence (see below). (Translators have used the term 'ego' for the 'I' when rendering Freud's work in English. This not only distorts his meaning but also conceals the dynamism of his language.[1]) Different kinds of defence operated in a neurosis such as hysteria compared with in obsessional–compulsive disorder. Remedying this through psychoanalysis meant 'rendering the unconscious conscious'. As Freud's own understanding of the scope and operation of unconscious mental processes grew, this could involve the retrieval of suppressed memories, understanding of meaningful but consciously unintended actions (hence the 'Freudian slip'), and the interpretation of hidden motives from the analysis of dreams. The sorts of hidden motive that Freud emphasized were those in which loving feelings were mixed with sexual excitement. He referred to a distinct kind of energy, the *libido*, to explain this. The natural expression of libido could become fixated at various points during the early years of life. Unconscious mental life was dominated by the satisfaction of libidinal wishes, the so-called *pleasure principle*. The rational everyday 'I', however, was governed by the *reality principle* in its efforts to ensure that internal representations reflected what the world beyond the 'I' actually was like.

Libidinal fixations could reflect parental behaviour or events that were experienced as highly threatening. Freud was especially interested in how libidinal longings for the parent of the opposite sex were resolved. The same-sex parent needed to prevent unrealistic hopes continuing, without crippling their young child's capacity to express affection and sexuality in their later relationships, through a prohibition that could be experienced as castrating. This was the basis of the *Oedipus complex*, played out between the child and both parents. Towards the end of his career, as he attempted to explain phenomena associated with depression, destructiveness and morbid guilt, Freud believed that a *death instinct* afforded an additional source of unconscious motivation. The death instinct became associated with the censorious part of the personality known as the 'over-I' (usually translated as 'super-ego'), whereas the pleasure principle continued to dominate the unconscious mind that he referred to as the 'it' (commonly translated as 'id').

Once he had moved beyond hypnotism and established a distinctive psychoanalytic method, Freud's clinical procedures were demanding of both the patient and the analyst. Continuity was prized, with sessions being held daily for 5 or 6 days per week. Patients were expected to avoid being distracted by their surroundings and to verbalize whatever came into their mind, without censorship or selection. This is the process of *free association*, and the basis of having patients lie back on a couch from which they do not see their analyst. The analyst was also expected to clear her mind and adopt 'evenly hovering attention' towards the patient's associations, so that she did not listen too selectively or jump to premature conclusions about their ultimate meaning. However, as the analyst became familiar with the nature of the patient's unconscious material, and the ways in which he defended against it, the analyst would assist the process of conscious recognition by *interpreta-*

tion. Interpretations were statements designed to deepen the patient's conscious understanding of their situation, based on hypotheses that form in the analyst's mind. They serve to increase the range of the patient's emotional experience and to link events and meanings that had not previously been associated.

In the early days of psychoanalytic practice, it became clear that analysts would be objects of their patients' feelings, fantasies and wishes, and that patients commonly projected wishes and expectations derived from their relationships with their parents on to the analyst. This phenomenon was recognized as *transference*. If ignored, transference could obstruct the analysis as a patient's desire to act towards the analyst on the basis of such wishes and distortions grew. However, by making transference itself the subject of interpretation, it became a valued tool in the process of making the unconscious conscious within psychotherapy. Transference has remained one of the cornerstones of psychodynamic thinking ever since. It has also received support from independent empirical research. Studies in the 1980s by Paul Crits Christoph and colleagues that looked at episodes during which people in therapy discuss key relationships confirmed that patients tend to frame their experiences of other people in terms of a very limited set of templates.[2] These templates are personal to them, and not only are repeated across their reports of current relationships but also mirror the patterns of interaction they will report having had with their own parents.

SOME KEY CONCEPTS IN PSYCHODYNAMIC PSYCHOTHERAPY

Defence

The concept of defence is central to psychodynamic thinking. It can refer to attempts to mitigate the impact of external events were we to become fully aware of them (*perceptual defence*) or from other people (*social defence*). However, psychodynamic psychotherapists tend to be most concerned about defence mechanisms that operate in reaction to threats from within. Once the mind is understood as being differentiated, with a central, aware part sitting alongside parts having operations and contents of which we are not aware, then the latter can pose a threat in themselves that may be defended against. Although there are different ways of describing and labelling the psychological defences, some are more adaptive than others; that is, they act to allow the conscious self to carry on integrating our experiences and responses in a relatively consistent way without unduly compromising the ability to function. However, other defences, although they may serve to reduce the anxiety that would otherwise be felt if uncomfortable feelings and impulses were not warded off, do so only by impairing the ability to cope in other ways. Defences of this kind either compromise the individual's ability to discern what is external reality (as in denial) or disrupt the experienced self's internal cohesion (as in splitting or dissociation). The distinction between adaptive (or *mature*) and dysfunctional (or *immature*) defences has often been upheld by psychotherapy researchers, who have linked reliance on the latter to poor long-term adaptation and risk of psychiatric illness.[3]

Working alliance

Although the term 'working alliance' was developed in psychoanalysis, it is frequently encountered in psychology, where it has been strictly defined and investigated. Three components are often defined: agreement on the goals of treatment, agreement on the method of treatment, and the empathic bond between a therapist and her patient.[4] The concept has been extremely influential because studies of factors predicting the success of psychotherapeutic interventions (irrespective of method) have consistently highlighted the importance of a good therapeutic alliance. In psychodynamic therapies, particular emphasis is placed on the quality of the felt bond within the working alliance, which reflects the therapist's sensitivity to the patient's internal state and the patient's responsiveness to the therapist's attention. Other terms that have been used to articulate this felt sense of responsiveness are 'rapport', 'mutuality' and 'attunement'.

Countertransference

Countertransference, like its complement transference, is an important influence on the working alliance in psychodynamic therapies. It refers to responses that an analyst can have to a patient that appear to be irrational or exaggerated and that may also carry a strong emotional charge. Countertransference may reflect projection on the therapist's part of her own tendency to construe present relationships on the basis of her own past experience. Or it can represent a response to affects that belong to the patient's transference that are projected into the therapist. In practice, it is usually a complex mixture of the two.

Resistance

Freud used the term 'resistance' to describe how patients would obstruct the therapy they were receiving. Although the patient may say he wants the treatment to work, the treatment represents a threat to the patient's present internal organization. Resistance represents a kind of retaliation in favour of the status quo and may take many forms both inside the therapeutic sessions and between them. Negative therapeutic reactions are a particular form of resistance. They are recognized when a patient has been making evident progress, before a sudden reversal sees him deteriorating, even though he may appear to be cooperating. Acting out is a less subtle form of resistance. Patients are said to *act out* when, instead of disclosing their thoughts and feelings to their therapist, they respond to invitations to contact their inner feelings by enacting their conflicts and distress outside of therapeutic sessions. Acting out may take the form of dramatic appeals for help from other people and incidents of self-harm. It is also possible to enact distress, rather than articulating it, during therapeutic sessions, behaviour that is sometimes referred to as *acting in*.

Regression

Regression refers to the tendency, when placed under stress, to revert to ways of coping belonging to an earlier stage of life. Some of the theoretical models of development discussed in the next session describe forms that regression can take in pathological states. Regression is to be expected, and may be encouraged, in the course of exploratory psychotherapy. During therapeutic regression, patients may become more child-like and dependent on the therapist. Indeed, failure to understand and to work with regression is a common cause of worsening, and even loss, of the working alliance. Patients differ significantly in the ease with which they regress in or out of therapy. Some, having an unstable personality structure or a tendency to dissociate, can regress with alarming ease but may also have considerable difficulty in reverting to adult ways of coping afterwards.

Interpretation

Interpretation is a key form of intervention in psychodynamic psychotherapy, being a verbal statement by the therapist designed to deepen the patient's understanding of his difficulties. While transference interpretations, which make explicit links between a patient's expectations and feelings in relation to their therapist, current significant others in their present life, and parental figures, are frequently cited, interpretation can take many other forms.

Insight

Insight refers to the discovery of psychological truths about oneself. It is an emotional as well as a cognitive accomplishment. Real insight therefore is not simply accepting such and such a piece of accurate information. It occurs when a new understanding not only feels right but also opens up new ways of feeling about things for a patient.

Working through

Psychodynamic psychotherapy is a process by which, through the modification of defences and the emergence and acceptance of relatively hidden aspects of their personalities, people can find fulfilment in love, work and play. To achieve this, those parts of the personality that are dominated by rigid defences are likely to resist such developments. Help is likely to be needed for them to soften. In practice, this is not a one-battle campaign. Advances are followed by retreats, and insights gained can even seem to disappear. Ground therefore needs to be retrodden within the therapy itself to ensure that more and more of the patient's resources are recruited to the forces of health. Working through in this way also ensures that internal change translates itself into successful adaptation in the patient's life.

Mentalization

The security of a person's attachment has been linked to their capacity to appreciate the independence of other people's minds, or to experience themselves as having a mind in which the ways they feel, think and try to act are interlinked. When attachment is disorganized, as in many people diagnosed with borderline personality disorder, this capacity is severely limited. In response to this, *mentalization* has become not only a psychological capacity, but also a therapeutic goal. *Mentalization-based therapy* (MBT) has become a significant offshoot of traditional psychodynamic psychotherapy in which the patient learns to appreciate themselves and others as having minds, with the capacity to interpret things that happen in very different ways and to have quite independent feelings and priorities.[5]

MAJOR INNOVATORS AFTER FREUD

Melanie Klein

Unlike Freud, Melanie Klein worked extensively with children as patients and drew on her experience as a mother. Her thinking about early development emphasized links between adult psychopathology and failures in the bond between mother and child. Although not jettisoning the idea of psychosexual fixation, Klein emphasized the influence of fantasy in psychological development and the importance of organizers of internal experience that were highly sensitive to experiences of mothering. These were termed 'objects', with Klein making two important and closely related distinctions. These are between the experience of *part objects* as opposed to *whole objects*, and the capacity of adults to function in either a *paranoid schizoid position* or a *depressive position*. Part objects are experienced as essentially good or bad and are associated with very strong, unprocessed feelings of love or hate. They are characteristic of a primitive and developmentally early kind of functioning that Klein inferred from her clinical work. She referred to this as the 'paranoid-schizoid position' because of its prominence in these kinds of adult psychopathology. Paranoid-schizoid functioning was associated with particular defence mechanisms, including splitting and what Klein called 'projective identification'. The latter has continued to be elaborated in various ways. It is a particularly complex form of psychological defence that implicates the analyst (or mother) as well as the patient, and it is clinically associated with states of mind found in people prone to psychosis or borderline personality.

By contrast, Klein's whole objects are experienced as embodying both desired and feared or hated aspects. Appreciating that the mother has both of these aspects is seen as a major psychological achievement, and one associated with considerable guilt on the infant's part for the attacks the mother has been subjected to by the infant when experienced as 'bad'. The capacity to appreciate and relate to whole objects is characteristic of the developmentally later depressive position. Klein attributed both depressive and manic states to difficulties in negotiating this phase successfully. (For a cogent illustrated summary, see Hinshelwood and Zarate.[6])

Klein's thinking has given rise to a whole school of psychoanalytic thinking that has been particularly influential in Britain within the psychotherapy of children and adults. Her most important successor has been Wilfrid Bion, whose impact has been worldwide. Bion developed Klein's interest in severe psychopathology to reformulate the dynamics of psychotic states. His theory of how thinking develops, which makes sense of how it can become disordered during psychotic breakdowns, has been particularly influential. It identifies the psychoanalyst as someone who shares a capacity (which Bion calls 'alpha function') with any emotionally competent mother as she interacts with her infant. Alpha function allows either of them to metabolize unbearable feelings on behalf of the patient/infant, so that they can be fed back in a form that the patient/infant can assimilate and thereby link feelings with thoughts for himself. This is the basis of the analytical action that Bion referred to as 'containment' – a term that has become very widely used, even if its original meaning has been broadened to refer to a capacity to hold all kinds of anxiety on a patient's behalf. (A useful summary of Bion's contributions can be found in Stein.[7])

Donald Winnicott

This paediatrician was well placed to observe the differences between successful and unsuccessful parenting. He emphasized the importance of play within healthy emotional development, including the healthy expression of aggression. Winnicott identified the importance of *transitional objects* (e.g. teddy bears) to provide a sense of psychological support as the infant engaged more with the world away from mother. His ideal of the 'good-enough mother' was intended to counter anxiety-driven perfectionism that otherwise prevented healthy development, leading to compensatory development of what Winnicott termed the 'false self' (for further description, see Phillips[8]).

Although Klein and Winnicott both recognized that we have a fundamental motivation to relate to others that cannot be reduced to other instincts, their thinking continued to combine references to sexual and destructive instincts alongside object-seeking. In Scotland, the philosophically talented psychoanalyst Ronald Fairbairn developed a theory in which object-seeking was primary to any other kind of motivation. A general practitioner (GP)-psychoanalyst, Michael Balint, developed the theory of regression and pioneered the application of psychoanalytic thinking within case discussion groups. These helped non-psychotherapists such as GPs to reflect on the emotional nuances of their clinical interviews, becoming known as 'Balint groups'.

Sir John Bowlby

Bowlby referred to attachments to other people as 'affectional bonds' that are just as biologically based as Freud's 'instincts'. He cited evidence drawn from ethological studies of other primates concerning critical development periods and the instinctual responses to separation and loss. The *attachment theory* that resulted has differentiated the forms or *styles* that 'insecure' attachment can take and linked their occurrence in childhood with vulnerability to psychiatric problems in adulthood. Attachment theory has emphasized the importance of actual parenting experiences (rather than fantasized ones) early in life, and provided a model for the psychodynamic therapist to provide a secure base from which a patient, like a securely attached baby, might find confidence to explore.[9] Attachment theory has emphasized the developmental importance of learning to recognize and moderate strong emotions ('affect regulation'), a function that has come to be seen as key to much subsequent psychotherapy.

Heinz Kohut

The USA has had a strong psychoanalytic tradition in which both Freudian and object relations traditions have been adopted and adapted. Like Fairbairn, the USA's most original thinker, Heinz Kohut, developed his ideas in relative isolation. Kohut's focus has been the psychopathology of narcissism, which he regarded as widely prevalent. He used the theory of the 'self object' to describe how different forms of internal transference within the self were associated with different forms of character pathology. In practice, rather than advocating a challenging, interpretative approach, Kohut championed a gentle, empathic stance towards patients whose narcissism was perceived to be the consequence of poorly attuned caregiving in the past. (For a manageable resume of Kohut's ideas, see Mitchell *et al.*[10])

Carl Jung

Jung was a Swiss psychiatrist who, as a protégé of Manfred Bleuler as well as Freud, worked extensively with people hospitalized for psychotic illnesses. He saw the frustration

of people's search for meaning as a greater psychological problem than the frustration of sexual expression and drew on studies of ancient symbols and myths, as well as his own and his patients' experiences, to argue that the individual mind is not a blank sheet at birth but is already primed by a 'collective unconscious'. Jung elaborated on the concepts of the 'complex' and the 'archetype', the exploration of these being key to his clinical method. This aims at a rebalancing of the personality through *individuation*. Although Jungian analysis is often as intensive and prolonged as psychoanalysis in practice, its basis is properly referred to as 'analytical psychology'.[11]

Jacques Lacan

In continental Europe, the most significant recent figure in developing psychodynamic ideas has been Jacques Lacan. Lacan achieved notoriety early in his career by unpredictably varying the length of his therapeutic sessions. However, his work has represented a highly original reworking of Freud's ideas that is sensitive to a postmodern world in which the personal self has become deconstructed or reduced to a set of actions, rather than having a knowable centre. Lacan turns to language in an attempt to identify key developmental processes, emphasizing the importance of a paternal function as infants learn to structure their experience of the world, and of themselves, by the way they learn to use words during a 'mirror phase' of development. Freud had acknowledged the importance of paternal functions in his conceptualization of the Oedipus complex. Lacan's reinterpretations counteract a trend in both the Kleinian and attachment-based traditions to emphasize maternal functions in the understanding of early life.

Psychoanalysis and dynamic psychotherapy

Although psychodynamic psychotherapy has continued to be indebted to psychoanalytic innovators for important theoretical ideas, the practice and spread of modern dynamic psychotherapy has depended heavily on the development of relatively brief, structured models of treatment. These have taken many forms, while continuing to emphasize the importance of early development, psychological conflict, exploration, and expression of feelings and transference within the therapeutic setting. Three key figures in the development of short-term dynamic therapies, whose influence has been lasting, are James Mann in the USA, David Malan in the UK and Habib Davanloo in Canada.

GROUP PSYCHODYNAMIC THERAPY

Psychoanalytical and psychodynamic principles have been applied successfully to working with patients in groups for over 80 years, in both out-patient and in-patient settings. Apart from the perceived benefits of providing any psychological therapy in groups in terms of efficient use of the therapist, psychodynamic group therapies afford experiences during therapy that are not available in individual work and that can be particularly helpful for some patients. For example, being in therapy alongside others can reduce the pressure to talk, or to be consistently intimate, which can make groups less daunting for some avoidant patients. Conversely, some patients who form extremely intense attachments to others, fearing abandonment in every gesture a therapist makes, can be reassured by the secure sense of others' presence that a group affords. Other individuals, normally distrustful of authority and professionals in general, can find it harder to ignore home truths that are spoken by fellow patients.

Therapeutic factors in groups

Other aspects of the group situation are likely to be experienced as helpful by most people who participate in group psychotherapy. These have been labelled by Yalom as 'curative' (later 'therapeutic') factors.[12] They include the opportunities for what has been termed 'social learning' that exposes the gaps between their self-impressions and what others actually see; the quality of support that group members can provide one another as they work through challenging situations, both internal and external; and the realization that their problems are not as unique (and they themselves not as abnormal or unforgivable) as they thought. In sum, Yalom's therapeutic factors are:

- Instillation of hope
- Universality
- Imparting information
- Altruism
- Corrective recapitulation of the primary family group
- Development of socializing techniques
- Imitative behaviour
- Interpersonal learning
- Group cohesiveness
- Catharsis
- Existential factors.

Transference in groups

The growing importance of models founded on object relationships within psychodynamic theory has highlighted the potential of groups as a therapeutic arena where patients' patterns of relating in the group can be observed and related to hypotheses about their internal world in terms of object relations and attachment patterns. In a group, patients are likely to experience the distortions of transference in relation to other patients as well as in interactions with the group's conductor. Experimenting with alternative ways of relating with others within the group can then lead to lasting changes in relationships beyond the group.

Principal group therapy theorists

Irving Yalom

In practice, different elements of groups have been emphasized by different authors. Among the 'curative' or 'therapeutic' factors outlined above, Irving Yalom has emphasized the importance of *cohesion* to a group's success. Cohesion is a measure of the positive bonds felt between members. It is reinforced by the group developing values and norms that its members subscribe to. Accordingly, the group leader is expected to assist the group's moves towards cohesion, as this will allow its members to take more risks in learning from one another.

Wilfrid Bion

Yalom's approach is antithetical to that of Wilfrid Bion, a Kleinian psychoanalyst who, with Tom Main and others, developed group-based therapeutic programmes in UK military hospitals during the Second World War. Bion felt that people very rarely actually listened or communicated with one another and that claims of agreement were usually illusory and placatory. In group situations, people would try to protect themselves from this unsettling reality by a small number of predictable shared defensive manoeuvres, which he termed 'basic assumptions'. These were *fight or flight* (in which members would act from a compulsion to either attack or retreat from the conductor); *pairing* (in which they would try to form exclusive links within the group, as if the others were not there); and *dependency* (in which members develop unrealistic expectations that the group leader will rescue them from their discomfort).[13] In carrying out the task of what was seen as necessary disillusionment, the group leader would concentrate on interpreting the actions of individuals in relation to herself and the group, to the relative exclusion of the group members' individual needs.

SH Foulkes

Something of a middle position is represented by SH Foulkes, the founder of *group analysis*. Like Bion, Foulkes saw the group as an exploratory analytical setting, where dynamics operated at group as well as individual levels. Like Yalom, Foulkes believed that groups needed active help from the conductor if the optimum environment for exploration was to be established. However, this did not necessarily involve cohesion, as Foulkes believed that differences within the group should flourish, necessarily reflecting differences in the social world of which its members were part. For Foulkes, the group conductor's task was to be a 'dynamic administrator', paying particular attention to the group's boundaries so that the group was at the same time a safe, reflective space protected from the outside world and also one where external matters that contributed to members' conflicts and difficulties could be admitted and made the subject of dialogue between the group's members.[14]

INDICATIONS FOR BRIEF, LONG-TERM AND SUPPORTIVE PSYCHOTHERAPY

Traditionally, suitability for psychodynamic psychotherapies has been assessed in terms of the person's ability to engage with and use this kind of therapy, rather than the kind of clinical problem they presented with. Capacity to work psychodynamically was therefore judged by whether the person was 'psychologically minded' and whether they had 'ego-strength'. Psychological mindedness is many faceted, but a simple definition includes being aware of and interested in emotions, motivations and potential for change in oneself and in others.[15] Ego-strength is a less widely accepted concept, which referred to the person's psychological resilience as evidenced by their capacity to withstand emotional challenges and to achieve short- and long-term goals despite hindrances. Although these ideas continue to be taught, and to have predictive validity, they can be misleading. Developed at a time when psychodynamic psychotherapies were dominant, the ideas are associated with a greater likelihood of success in almost any of the psychological therapies that are now available. Additionally, although they can appear to be traits that are either present or not, in practice they can each be enhanced as a result of psychotherapy, with the possibility that suitable preparatory work could help a person who might be thought of as unsuitable for therapy to reach and cross the traditional threshold for suitability for psychodynamic work. This may be evident from the description of mentalization already given, with MBT effectively enhancing the person's psychological mindedness. Similarly, preparatory work aimed at helping the person with 'affect regulation' and 'problem-solving' is enhancing 'ego-strength' when it is successful.

The US psychotherapist Lester Luborsky made a helpful distinction between 'supportive' and 'expressive' aspects of psychodynamic psychotherapies, recognizing that any therapy contains a combination of both components.[16] In supportive mode, coping mechanisms are consolidated. In expressive mode, exploration is facilitated and regression encouraged. The actual mixture can vary from therapy to therapy and within a therapy. Engaging a patient at a point where further consolidation of psychological mindedness and ego-strength is required means that an emphasis on supportive over expressive components would be needed before consistently exploratory work was undertaken. Starting there sets a lower threshold for potential patients to start therapeutic work. It can also render the outcome of psychotherapy even more sensitive to external factors, such as the patient's current social and family situation.

Alongside the patient's capacity to engage with a therapy, the evidence-based practice movement has emphasized considerations of presenting problems in treatment choice. There is probably more justification for this stance in the case of physical treatments than psychological ones.

Nevertheless, when the results of formal comparative clinical trials are taken into account, the evidence for the efficacy of psychodynamic psychotherapies is strongest in people with personality disorders, with clear evidence of usefulness in cases of trauma, depression, eating disorders and some kinds of medically unexplained symptoms. This should be taken into account when advising, referring and assessing new patients. (See Appendix 2 in Royal College of Psychiatrists[17] for a table comparing the evidence base for different psychological therapies. For a fuller treatment of this evidence base, see Roth and Fonagy.[18])

An important practical consideration is the quantity of therapy that the patient should be given. Time-limited therapies are favoured when patients have relatively circumscribed difficulties and where areas of weakness are offset by personal strengths. Patients need to be motivated and able to use the approach without lengthy preparation, while youth is a definite advantage when significant change is sought. Aveline has described time-limited therapy as contraindicated with people who have marked difficulties over trust and those who have a great deal of pain to gradually uncover and disclose.[19]

LEARNING PSYCHODYNAMIC PSYCHOTHERAPY

This brief summary should help to make sense of a number of the key ideas that inform current practice. When undertaking a psychodynamic psychotherapy, the therapist needs to have a working theoretical framework that equips him or her to assess patients and to initiate, carry out and successfully conclude treatments. This can be summarized as a framework of the necessary skills or competencies. Although these will be indebted to the ideas discussed here, they also stand as a body of procedural knowledge in their own right. In the past, these therapeutic skills have been largely implicit, learned by practitioners through a long and sometimes uncertain process of learning by example or osmosis. Undergoing personal therapy, an essential element of training for all forms of psychodynamic therapy, can encourage this as trainees learn to imitate their own therapists. However, the publication of formal curricula for trainee therapists can be invaluable in clarifying the practical as well as the conceptual framework of psychotherapies of all kinds. Useful examples can be found at www.skillsforhealth.org.uk.

KEY POINTS

- Psychodynamic therapies are derived from psychoanalysis.
- They emphasize the influence of early development and the relationship with the therapist during treatment.
- Therapies are provided in individual and group settings.
- There are many theoretical schools with considerable variations in practice between them.
- Psychodynamic therapies are especially suited to the treatment of recurrent difficulties and personality problems.

FURTHER READING

Bateman A, Holmes J (1995) *Introduction to Psychoanalysis*. London: Routledge.

Bernard HS, MacKenzie KR (eds) (1994) *Basics of Group Psychotherapy*. New York: Guilford Press.

Hughes P, Riordan D (2006) *Psychodynamic Psychotherapy Explained*, 2nd edn. Oxford: Radcliffe.

Malan D (1995) *Individual Psychotherapy and the Science of Psychodynamics*. London: Hodder Arnold.

Rycroft C (2005) *A Critical Dictionary of Psychoanalysis* (rev. edn). Harmondsworth: Penguin

REFERENCES

1. Bettelheim B (1984) *Freud and Man's Soul*. New York: Vintage.
2. Luborsky L, Crits-Cristoph P (1990) *Understanding Transference: The Core Conflictual Relationship Theme Method*. New York: Basic Books.
3. Vaillant G, Bond M, Vaillant C (1986) An empirically validated hierarchy of defense mechanisms. *Archives of General Psychiatry* **43**: 786–94.
4. Bordin E (1976) The generalizability of the psychoanalytic concept of the working alliance. *Psychotherapy: Theory, Research and Practice* **16**: 252–60.
5. Allen J, Fonagy P, Bateman A (2008) *Mentalizing in Clinical Practice*. Washington, DC: American Psychiatric Association.
6. Hinshelwood R, Zarate O (2006) *Introducing Melanie Klein*. London: Icon Books.
7. Stein S (1999) Bion. In S Stein (ed.) *Essentials of Psychotherapy*. Oxford: Butterworth-Heinemann.
8. Phillips A (2007) *Winnicott*. Harmonsworth: Penguin.
9. Bowlby J (2005) *A Secure Base: Parent–Child Attachment and Healthy Human Development*. Hove: Routledge.
10. Mitchell S, Black M (1995) *Freud and Beyond: A History of Modern Psychoanalytic Thought*. New York: Basic Books.
11. Stevens A (2001) *Jung: A Very Short Introduction*. Oxford: Oxford University Press.
12. Yalom I (2005) *Principles and Practice of Group Psychotherapy*, 5th edn. New York: Basic Books.
13. Bion W (1961) *Experiences in Groups*. London: Tavistock.

14. Pines M, Hearst L (1993) Group analysis. In H Kaplan, B Sadock (eds) *Comprehensive Group Psychotherapy*, 3rd edn. Baltimore, MD: Williams & Wilkins.
15. Conte H, Ratto R, Karusa T (1996) The Psychological Mindedness Scale: factor structure and relationship to outcome of psychotherapy. *Journal of Psychotherapy Practice and Research* 5: 250–59.
16. Luborsky L (1984) *Principles of Psychoanalytic Psychotherapy: A Manual for Supportive Expressive Treatment*. New York: Basic Books.
17. Royal College of Psychiatrists (2008) *CR151: Psychological Therapies in Psychiatry and Primary Care*. London: Royal College of Psychiatrists.
18. Roth A, Fonagy P (2005) *What Works for Whom?*, 2nd edn. New York: Guilford.
19. Aveline M (1995) How I assess for focal therapy. In C Mace (ed.) *The Art and Science of Assessment in Psychotherapy*. London: Routledge.

Chapter 62

Family therapy

Rudi Dallos

INTRODUCTION

The word 'systemic' has entered popular discourse in a similar way to Freudian concepts, such as unconscious drives and catharsis. It derives from general systems theory, which became one of the guiding conceptual frameworks for family therapy. However, it has a wider range of application than families and is increasingly been used to consider patterns and processes within organizations such as the National Health Service (NHS) in terms of the interactions and problems within and between different services and professional groups. For the medical professions and psychiatry, there are significant issues regarding their power relationships to other professionals and referrers. Interestingly, many of the pioneers of family therapy were medically trained and specialists in psychiatry.[1–5] It is perhaps worth speculating from the outset that the type of family therapy models they developed had a tendency to use more directive approaches to family therapy, which utilized their high status and power as physicians and psychiatrists. Later waves of family therapy that advocate more narrative, collaborative and non-directive approaches were developed by social workers.[6,7]

Family therapy has existed as a form of clinical intervention for a variety of conditions for about 50 years.[8–10] Alongside the development of a variety of forms of therapeutic techniques and orientations, 'the family' has also continually been a source of social and political debate and intervention.[11] More specifically, the concept of 'the family' has shifted and been the centre of great controversies over its desired nature and function. There have been dramatic changes in the structure and nature of family life, such that many children no longer grow up in the traditional nuclear family but live in reconstituted families with step-parents or homosexual parents or in adoptive or foster-care situations.[11,12] There have even been dramatic attempts to remove the family and replace it with structures such as communes, collectives and kibbutzim.[11] Although the debates and issues are complex and controversial, one important dimension has been the extent to which families are seen as the cause of problems – the family to blame – as opposed to the extent to which families are seen as a positive resource. These two aspects are not distinct, but social policy and political rhetoric seem to revolve in cycles between the two extremes, for example increasing attempts to control families and their functioning. Some examples include the development of antisocial behaviour orders (ASBOs), parenting orders in the criminal justice systems, and forms of early intervention such as the Sure Start parenting and child programmes designed to help correct ineffective or destructive parenting. Sure Start and similar programmes attempt to help families to become a positive resource, but possibly they also carry an assumption that something is currently awry and needs repair. The alternative stance emphasizes potential and resources that families may hold and looks to factors that may block or impede this, for example social conditions, housing, ill-health, poverty and crime. This view fosters an orientation of working alongside families to help ameliorate these conditions and free them up to function well.

Where does family therapy fit within these two broad orientations? For professionals such as general practitioners (GPs), who make decisions about referrals, this is an important question. In making referral decisions, they can set in motion pathways that potentially start to label and designate families and their members as ill or as responsible for the problems. Some family therapists have argued that the very term 'family therapy' constructs an unhelpful framework in that it implies the position of there being something wrong with the family that needs to be corrected. However politely and diplomatically the referrer tries to reassure clients that family therapy is a non-blaming approach, there is still considerable potential for family members, especially the parents, to feel blamed for the problems that one or more of them is experiencing. For these reasons, the family therapy movement has argued that it would be better to use the term 'systemic therapy'. Unfortunately, this term, as well as being less blaming, is also incomprehensible to most families and many professionals outside of the family therapy movement.

The above distinction contains some of the core variations in the different models of family therapy and their evolution.[9] Specifically, this is the distinction between *problem-* as opposed to *solution*-oriented versions of family therapy. In the former, the therapist and the team start with an exploration of the problems – what is going wrong and what the underlying cause may be. Various approaches will then be attempted to assist the family with these, such as assisting with communication, using behaviour interventions or developing insights.[1,2] In contrast, in the solution-oriented approach, the therapist may barely refer to problems and will move the discussion rapidly to the family's strengths – what is going well, and how the family can build on any positives to resist the difficulties further.[13] In practice, many family therapists combine features of both approaches, showing that they are aware of the distressing nature of the problems but not encouraging an overly negative or failing framework.

SYSTEMIC FAMILY THERAPY

Not all family therapy approaches derive from general systems theory, but arguably general systems theory has been the greatest influence on the development of family therapy theory and practice.[8–10] The most obvious difference between family therapy and other forms of therapy is that the target interventions are aimed predominantly at altering families rather than individuals. Consistent with this, family therapists spend most of their time working with groups of people rather than individuals. Of course, some other forms of therapy, such as group therapies, also involve working with groups of people; however, family therapy aims to focus on natural groups of people, such as families, who have spent considerable time with each other. This exposure to each other over time is seen as leading to the development of patterned, repetitive and predictable forms of interaction, and it is these patterns – what goes on *between* rather than what goes on *within* people – that are the focus of interest. This distinction between the individual and an interacting system is not a simple one, and it is recognized that drawing the distinction biologically between the boundaries of a person's body – the perimeter of their skin – and another's is not as straightforward as it may intuitively seem at first.[14] Certainly there is much indication that infants do not arrive in the world with such a simple distinction. For example, infants are intimately connected to the mother in the womb and are highly physiologically responsive after birth to her heartbeat, milk and voice.[15] Children differ in how much and how rapidly they separate from their parents to become autonomous, and too extreme separation or lack of it appears to be problematic.[5,8]

An early and dramatic illustration of some core systemic ideas can be seen in a piece of research conducted by Salvador Minuchin and colleagues.[2,16] In an attempt to explore the interconnections between family dynamics and internal states in individual family members, measures were taken of some physiological changes associated with levels of stress. (Ways of measuring stress levels have advanced since this study, but it is presented here since it was a pioneering study and approach to working with families.) The Collins family had two daughters, Dede (17 years) and Violet (12 years), who both had diabetes. There was no obvious difference in the girls' individual responsiveness to stress, but Dede suffered much more severely from diabetes and had been admitted to hospital for emergency treatment 23 times. Violet had some behavioural problems that her parents complained of, but her diabetes was under good control. Minuchin interviewed the parents for an hour (9–10 a.m.) while the girls watched from behind a one-way mirror. From 9.30 a.m., Minuchin deliberately encouraged the parents to discuss issues of conflict (a structural technique called intensification), which led to some experience of stress, in order to see how this affected the children. Although the children were only observing from behind the screen and could not take part in the conflict, their free fatty acid (FFA) levels rose as they observed their stressed parents. At 10 a.m., the children joined their parents, and their different roles in the family became apparent: Dede physically sat between her parents, and each parent attempted to get her support against the other so that she was in a no-win situation. Violet's allegiance was not sought in this way, and she could respond to her parents' conflict without being caught in the middle. The effects of these two roles are indicated by the changes in the girls' FFA levels (Figure 62.1).

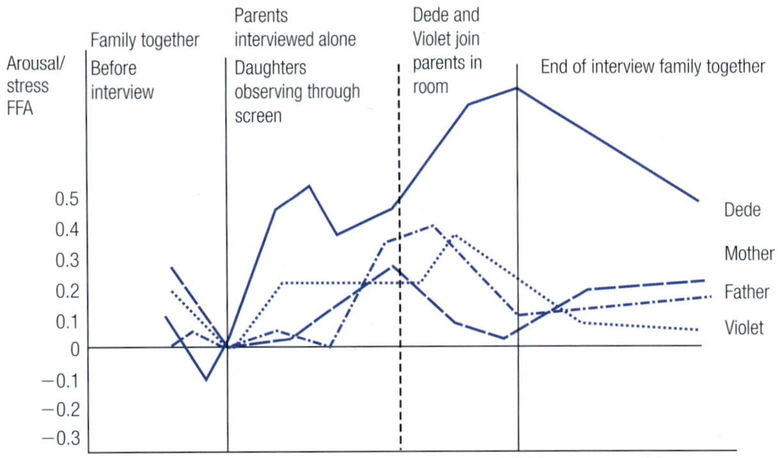

Figure 62.1 Stress and family structure
FFA, free fatty acid.

Both of the children showed an increase in their stress levels when watching the parents from behind the screen, although Dede showed a much higher increase; most interestingly, Dede then demonstrated a dramatic increase when the girls joined their parents in the room. In contrast, her sister Violet showed an initial increase and then a decrease in her stress level. Minuchin's hypothesis was that Dede acted as a conduit for the conflict in the family; as Violet saw Dede being drawn into this role, it allowed Violet to feel less stressed. Importantly, after the interview, it took much longer for Dede's stress level to settle back down in contrast with that of the other family members.

CORE SYSTEMIC CONCEPTS

This study exemplifies some core concepts underlying systemic family therapy. Individual experiences, including physiological states, are related intimately to family dynamics. Since family processes are continual, each member of the family is also continually influenced by these dynamics. Even when physically by themselves, the children may continue (as Dede so clearly shows in the study above) to be influenced by the physiological after-effects and of their memories of relationships. The example given above also demonstrates the concept of triangulation – how the parents pull Dede into their own conflict, for example by changing the topic of the conversation from their marital conflicts to Dede's diabetes when the discussion becomes too uncomfortable for them.[2,5] This shift to looking at processes between not only two but three or more people is one of the critical contributions of systemic family therapy approaches.

Symptoms as relational

The early pioneers of family therapy drew on ideas from general systems to propose that families, especially those that can come to display serious difficulties, could be seen as similar to mechanical and biological systems. Jackson proposed the concept of 'family homeostasis' to suggest that a symptom in one or more of the family members develops and functions as a response to the actions of the others in a family and becomes part of the patterning of the system.[4] Attempts to change the symptom were seen to encounter 'resistance', since the system operated as an integrated whole and strove to maintain the homeostasis. By 'resistance', Jackson implied not a conscious but a largely unconscious pattern of emotional responses to change in one or other family members. As an example, if an angry disruptive child starts to behave in a more acceptable way, then it may be that the unresolved conflicts between the parents start to surface or that another sibling starts to display difficulties or to aggravate their reformed sibling to re-engage in problems. Jackson argued that family systems containing problems or 'pathology' could be seen to operate as 'closed systems'. These operated so that any change in the symptomatic member would be met by actions in the others, which would have the sum of reducing, rather than encouraging, change. Despite family members expressing a desire to change, it was argued that the symptoms had been incorporated into the relationship dynamics and served a positive function for the family. Jackson elaborated on this idea by suggesting that families acted as if they were regulated by a set of largely unconscious rules.

This view of problems has had significant implications for our view of problems and for the relationship that systemic family therapy has with diagnostic systems, such as the *Diagnostic and Statistical Manual of Mental Disorders* (DSM). At the extreme, some systemic family therapists have questioned the value of diagnosis and suggested that it could lead to families becoming stuck around a definition of the problems as existing in one person, possibly serving to aggravate or make a condition chronic.[6,17] In contrast, some family approaches, especially the expressed-emotion, psychoeducation-based family interventions, have worked alongside diagnosis to look at how families members can be helped to live with conditions such as schizophrenia, depression autism and attention deficit hyperactivity disorder (ADHD).[18]

It is probably fair to summarize the current practice in family therapy as a hybrid between an acceptance of diagnostic categories and a fully systemic view of problems. It is recognized that many parents gain a sense of relief and feel the burden of blame lifting when they hear, for instance, that their child has ADHD. Such a diagnosis can offer a window of therapeutic opportunity while the family is less anxious to explore other explanations and to think of ways in which their interactions may make the situation better or worse. On some occasions, the consequence of such a strategy seems to be that, as the family becomes more aware of some of their processes and comes to feel safe with and trust that the therapist and the team are not blaming them, medical diagnostic considerations become less salient. However, here it is especially important to note that families live in different contexts; outside systemic therapy, they may be exposed to perspectives that continue to emphasize medical explanations. Drawing a map of the professionals with whom they are involved can help to create some clarity for the family members so that they do not rattle between competing explanations in unhelpful and confusing ways. One helpful stance can be to suggest that, for some conditions, 'the jury is still out' – for example, 'We are still not absolutely sure what the causes are, but to explore how the condition, whether or not it is an illness, may be ameliorated by the family dynamics and the support possible may be a useful activity to undertake together.'

Power

The question of power has been hotly debated in systemic family therapy. It has been argued that a central issue in a family is the need for clarity of the hierarchy and decision-making process.[2,17,19] Specifically, at significant times the parents need to be clearly in charge of the children and able to exert control and influence over them when necessary. Further to this, it was seen as essential that the parents were able to work together in a consistent way in order to exercise control to ensure the safety and social behaviour of their children. More theoretically, the concept is central to systems theory, as systems are seen as having mechanisms that exert control over, or regulate the dynamics of, a system. However, exerting control is not simply equivalent to power: Bateson criticized a simple conceptualizing of power in human relationships, arguing that one person cannot control another except in the most basic physical ways.[14] Instead, we exert influence over each other through a variety of forms of communication and interaction, such as persuasion, humour, bribery and seduction.

Context

Again drawing on biological metaphors, systemic perspectives emphasize that families and other relationships need to be understood in terms of the environment or context in which they are located. For example, a family may act differently at home, in a supermarket, in the GP's surgery and in a family therapy session. Likewise, the children may act differently at home, at school and out on the street with their friends. Each situation in effect carries different rules about what is seen as appropriate behaviour and how we ought to behave. Within the family, there can also be seen to be a variety of contexts, for example the parents alone together, the siblings with each other, the parents with the oldest or youngest child, the family with the grandparents, and so on. It is argued that such contexts are in part guided externally, for example what is or is not appropriate for parents to do in front of the children. However, families also improvise and develop their own local contexts; for example, being with the grandparents may be a context for not swearing or being too rowdy, or the grandparents may be considered fun and liked for handing out sweets.

Patterns and process

Systems theory stresses the interdependence of action in families and other relationships. Each person is seen as influencing the others, and their responses in turn influence them, which influences the first person's responses, and so on. Any action is therefore also seen as a response, and a response also as an action. Paul Watzlawick and colleagues coined the term 'circularities' to capture these essentially repetitive patterns of interaction.[20,21] This represented a fundamental shift from how relationship difficulties had been explained previously. In effect, the question of looking for a starting point – who started it – is seen as unproductive. Even if we can identify who appeared to start a particular family sequence, such as an argument, this may in turn have been a response to a previous episode.

An extremely influential idea that emerged was that problems could be seen in terms of circular patterns, whereby the family has attempted solutions to the difficulties, which instead of improving things have made matters worse.[21] To take an example, parents may decide to take a tougher line and impose firmer rules on a teenager who has shown an angry outburst at school. However, the teenager may feel that his parents, like everyone else, are 'ganging up' on him and that this is 'not fair', so he becomes increasingly angry and distrustful and engages in another angry outburst. This may propel the parents to believe that they need to do more of the same and that even harsher measures will do the trick. These early ideas led the way to the influential brief therapy and solution-focused therapies that have developed alongside the systemic therapies.[13,22]

Punctuation

Experience is not what happens to you. It is what you do with what happens to you – Aldous Huxley

The term 'punctuation' perhaps captures more than any other some of the key contributions of systemic thinking in offering an important bridge between beliefs and patterns of actions as mutually self-maintaining each other (Figure 62.2). It suggests that family members are always trying to make sense of each others' actions. Watzlawick and colleagues suggested that the flow of communication and actions in relationships is divided up into meaningful units, or chunks.[20] The term 'punctuation' was coined to describe how people develop a set of self-fulfilling perceptions or beliefs about their relationship, which can interlock, like the pieces of a jigsaw puzzle, to produce repetitive patterns. The concept of punctuation introduces the idea of systems as not simply mechanistic but as governed by patterns of beliefs or constructs. Over time, members of a family come to form predictions not only of each others' actions but also of each others' thoughts, beliefs and feelings. Since they spend a considerable amount of time together, share similar experiences and communicate continually with each other,

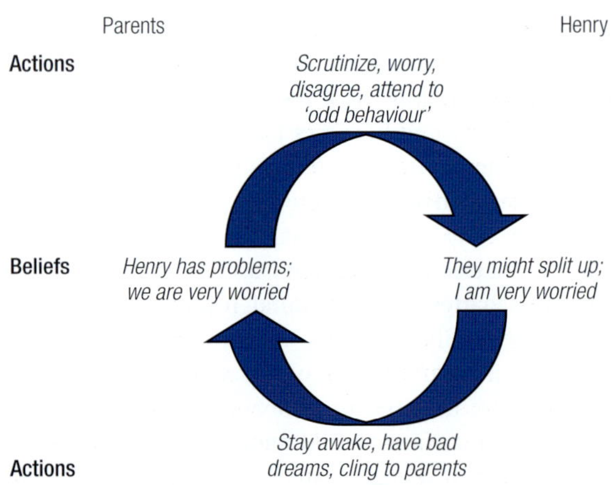

Figure 62.2 Punctuation in a family

Source: Dallos and Draper.[9]

the family members come to form a web of mutual anticipation. This serves both to explain and to predict each person's behaviour and thoughts, but also to construct and maintain them. Members of a family might be surprised if, for example, one of them expresses beliefs or shows emotions that they regard as unusual; these signs of surprise will serve to attenuate such deviations.

The concept of punctuation suggests that although two or more members of a family may appear to be acting autonomously, their choices can become interwoven, such that they become caught in repetitive patterns of action. A relatively unexplored idea that follows from this is that choice in families can be seen to be contingent – what each person decides to do is shaped and constrained by what the others do and by what they think they will do. Specifically, each member may be involved in making conscious or semi-conscious calculations about the likely consequences of a possible line of action – whether it will produce a rebuke, admiration, agreement and so on. We develop this idea of shared action in the next section. In the example in Figure 62.2, the parents were extremely concerned that Henry was showing signs of 'childhood schizophrenia', a concern that was articulated by health visitors and other medical professionals they had consulted regarding Henry's nightmares and 'bizarre' imagination. The more they watched and scrutinized Henry's behaviour, the more anxious Henry seemed to become about why his parents were so worried and about their disagreement about him. This anxiety led him to tell them more about his scary thoughts and in turn fuelled the parents' anxiety.

Family lifecycle

Family therapy has emphasized the importance of time and development in family life and the nature of problems. A key feature of this is an interest in thinking about families from a transgenerational perspective. Haley made the observation that humans, unlike any other species, are the only species to have in-laws.[17] Of course, there are wide variations in human cultures, with some societies having very close relationships – for example, three generations living in one household – and others having a nuclear family configuration, with children moving far away from their parents as they start their own families. The complex connections across the generations were one of the focal points of early system therapy. Haley described pathological triangles, whereby a grandparent could seriously undermine and disempower their child (parent) by giving contradictory instructions to their grandchild.[17] An anxious parent could, for example, become angry or withdrawn, giving over power to the grandparent and thus making their own ability to parent impossible, leading to their own depression and sense of inadequacy and confusion for the grandchild.

An influential model of problem development and change was proposed in the concept of the family lifecycle (Figure 62.3).[17,23,24] This emphasized how families may at times be

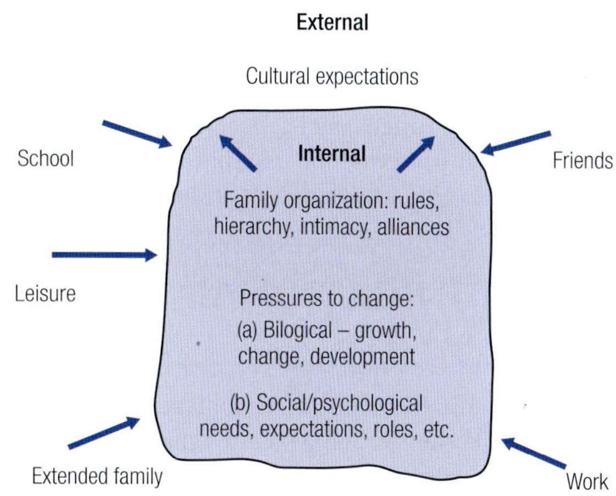

Figure 62.3 Family lifecycle: external and internal demands for change
Adapted from Dallos.[24]

faced with massive demands for change and adaptation, for example the birth of a child, divorce or remarriage, death or – perhaps due to changes in autonomy within the family – children becoming adolescents, a woman going back to work after childrearing, or retirement. It was observed that the emergence of serious problems was associated with these lifecycle transitions and their inherent demands, anxieties and stresses. Milton Erickson noted, for example, that psychotic episodes in late adolescence were seen to be related to difficulties for the family over the departure of the young person about to leave and set up his or her own home.[17] In response to the anxieties generated by the demands for change, some families appear to attempt to avoid facing these by delaying the transition. One significant way of doing this is for someone – often the person at the centre of the stage, such as the young person leaving home – to become ill in some way such that they are 'unable' to leave, which serves to disguise the complex emotional issues and anxieties. There may also be community demands such as local social upheavals and major cultural changes. In this sense, the lifecycle perspective adds to homeostasis the idea that families are not simply stuck but may in fact have to work quite hard to keep things the same, since their environment is continually shifting.

It is also possible that such patterns represent wider cultural factors, such as expectations about gender roles and opportunities for work outside the family. Attempts to simply fix such patterns in families without due recognition of the cultural factors were seen as potentially oppressive and as implicitly endorsing such inequalities. It was argued that this model could contain, in a concealed form, a range of normative, patriarchal, middle-class, white assumptions about healthy family functioning.[25]

One of the most frequently used and powerful techniques in family therapy is the use of family genograms. This is employed to trace transgenerational patterns, relationships between the generations, beliefs about the family, and traditions of dealing with problems and distress. It is often conducted as a visual activity, with the children doing the drawing, listening and commenting while the parents describe the family contexts. As well as eliciting information, this activity often elicits recognition of powerful transgenerational patterns, for example of divorce, use of drugs or alcohol, separations, gender roles and so on.

A COMMUNICATIONAL PERSPECTIVE

Therapy is essentially about communication between the therapist and the family. For systemic family therapy, communication was also a guiding concept in terms of how families learn to live together and of how problems develop. Bateson and colleagues inverted the typical explanations regarding schizophrenia by asked the question, 'In what context would schizophrenic behaviour make sense?' Their observations were that it occurred in relationships characterized by repeated contradictory and confusing communications:[26]

> A young man who had fairly well recovered from his acute schizophrenic episode was visited in the hospital by his mother. He was glad to see her and impulsively put his arms around her shoulders, whereupon she stiffened. He withdrew his arm and she asked, 'Don't you love me any more?' He then blushed, and she said, 'Dear, you must not be so easily embarrassed and afraid of your feelings.' The patient was able to stay with her only a few minutes more and following her departure he assaulted an aide and was put in the tubs [restrained].[14]

Relationships are seen to proceed through successive attempts to make sense of what is happening. At times, people communicate directly about this by phrases such as 'What do you mean?' or 'You don't seem too happy about that'. A feature of the double-bind phenomenon is that such meta-communication is not allowed, apparently due to unconscious fears of provoking anxiety. Bateson subsequently revised the double-bind theory to suggest that the process is a reciprocal one, with the child also engaged in double-binding communication. Weakland further suggested that double-binding can be seen as a three-person process.[27,28] For example, a mother with whom I worked stated that she was sometimes frightened of her son (who had schizophrenia) but also frightened to show her disapproval of some of his behaviours because of fear of rebuke from her husband. Hence, she continually displayed a pleasant smile while she spoke at times of a 'fear for her life', which was intended to disguise her anxiety and anger but also communicated a confusing and mixed message to her son. Interestingly, more recent research,[29,30] and much earlier research by Bowlby,[3] adds support to Bateson's ideas, indicating that many people with a diagnosis of psychosis have experienced profound episodes of emotional, sexual and physical abuse, which has been disguised and concealed and distorted by parents or other carers.

Family therapists attempt to clarify communication in families in a variety of ways. The therapist typically invites each member of the family to talk about their perspectives; the therapist may also intervene if one member of the family dominates the conversation or constantly interrupts the others. This may allow for more information and points of view to be expressed, but it also starts to give the family experience and practice of different ways of communicating. The observing team also pays attention to possible incongruities in communication between the verbal and non-verbal content and may help the therapist to draw attention to these with the family. Some families describe this as having a 'referee' who allows everyone to talk and ensures fair play. An interesting approach is to invite families to take home a DVD of their family therapy sessions and to discuss and comment on their interactions and communication processes in the following session.

THERAPEUTIC ASSUMPTIONS AND PRACTICE

Systemic family therapy was one of the first of the therapeutic approaches, and arguably it is still the major one to employ live supervision of the therapeutic work. Originally this was done in various ways, for example with a team observing the session from behind an observation screen or on video. Alternatively, there could be consultation with a colleague regularly offering advice. This emphasis on live supervision was based on a recognition of the complexity of working with the whole family at the same time and also on the idea that there needed to be some removal from the interaction in the room to be able to detect some of the family pattern maintaining the problems. The therapist would be consulted regularly by the team via telephone or an earpiece and given suggestions – for example, to ask the family to enact how the problems occur at home, to change seats, to engage in role-play or sculpt, for one person to speak more or less, to explore certain areas such as their attempted solutions to the problems more, and so on. After about 40 minutes, the therapist generally took a break to talk with the team and then returned with some substantive intervention, such as a reframe or paradoxical 'homework' task.

Early systemic family therapy contained some assumptions about 'healthy' family functioning along with the view that alterations made to the organizational structure of a family will change the symptomatic behaviours. Once the rules of the family system alter, so too will the behaviours; for example, if instead of enlisting a child into coalitions against each other the parents start to work together, then the child will no longer display various symptoms. Structural approaches assume that families have an objective structure, and it follows that therapy involves a process of assessment and mapping of this structure, followed by clear attempts to alter it where necessary. The therapist therefore adopts a sympathetic but nevertheless expert role in which he or she takes on the responsibility of initiating changes. Typically, the approach was to encourage different ways of interacting in the actual family sessions, sometimes with associated 'homework' tasks. As in the earlier example from the study on diabetes, Minuchin would utilize feelings in the room, for example to disrupt a triangular process involving the children at the point where the couple's conflicts were becoming too uncomfortable.[2]

In addition, early family therapy approaches included strategic techniques. These were designed not to change not only the family organization but also the interactional patterns that were maintaining the problems. Furthermore, therapists adopted a more covert and strategic approach, in the view that in many cases families were not able or were unwilling at some level to follow advice and suggestions from the therapist. The idea here was that if a family repeatedly did the opposite of what the therapist suggested – resisted the therapist's advice – then perhaps by offering the opposite of what the therapist wanted the family to do this could paradoxically produce the desired result. These interventions often required some humour and a sense of fun and trust between the therapist and the family. In one example, a family complained about how they were continually bickering and sniping at each other. Repeated attempts to explore the reasons for this and to suggest some changes did not work. Instead, the therapist suggested that they buy half a dozen water pistols; every time someone sniped or bickered, they were to be shot with a burst of cold water. The family returned, saying they had found this activity so ridiculous that they broke out in laughter whenever they started to bicker, and the problem had decreased. Other, more gentle techniques, such as suggesting that the family observe and in order to do this accurately they do not try to alter the problems, could also be effective in breaking up futile cycles of attempting to solve their problems in ways that lead to an increase rather than a decrease in the problems.

FROM PATTERNS AND PROCESSES TO BELIEFS AND NARRATIVES

During the 1980s, there was a gradual shift from an emphasis on patterns of actions to an emphasis on the construction of meanings and their creation in families and between the family and the therapist.[7] Inherent in this was a change in the perceived role of the therapist as less of an expert and more of a collaborative explorer who works alongside a family to co-create some new, more productive ways of the family seeing their situation. Furthermore, this represented a move towards an increased sensitivity to therapeutic relationships. Rather than trying to adopt an 'objective' stance, the therapist is encouraged to be continually reflective – to monitor his or her perceptions, beliefs, expectations, needs and feelings, especially in terms of how these may in turn have an influence on the family.

Earlier approaches largely adopted a functionalist view of problems: families were seen as interacting systems in which symptoms functioned to preserve stability. In a perverse way, painful and distressing symptoms rather than threatening family life and stability were often seen as holding families together: symptoms were seen as distracting from or diverting conflicts, anxieties and fears (often unconsciously held) from other areas of the family's experience. This view was challenged on the grounds that the function of a symptom was not there to be 'discovered' but was the therapist's hypothesis. In turn, how difficulties were handled – the attempted solutions – was seen as linked to the wider belief system of the family.[24,31,32]

A typical view in families is that the source of their problems lies in one member rather than in their relationships with each other. Once established, this myth can become increasingly painful to confront. For example, if the child's symptoms become severe, the parents may feel guilty and blameworthy, by the implication that their conflicts have in a sense been the cause. Young children tend to discover the power that a symptom of illness confers, such as being able to avoid school and unpleasant duties, and gaining sympathy and attention. Therefore, a child may start to collude with this state of affairs and continue to display symptoms, in part because of the apparent advantages he or she gains. This in turn can serve to confirm for the whole family, including the child, the beliefs or myths that the child is the source of the problems.

The parents may hold different beliefs and disagree on how to treat the child (e.g. discipline *v.* sympathy) and may shift positions, taking turns to side with the child – 'shifting coalitions'.[1] Psychiatric and other agencies may also perpetuate conflicting views about such conditions, which families then come to internalize and act out in their internal dynamics.

OBSERVING SYSTEMS

The process of therapy involves an interaction between two systems – the family and the therapist – and can be seen as a new third system – the therapist/family system. Rather than thinking that we could observe and analyse families in any detached and objective manner, it became increasingly clear that the therapist or observer inevitably perturbed or changed the family system by the very act of observing it. A therapist in effect came to be seen as partly seeing his or her own reflections or the ripples he or she had made in the new family/therapist system. Another therapist with the same family might see quite different things, partly because the therapist was having a different kind of effect on the family. Taken to its extreme, this suggested that there was no such thing as the real family dynamics, only our various perceptions of it.

As therapists, our perceptions and explanations of a family were invariably seen as our own constructions and a punctuation of the process between the therapist and the family. This view also gave additional emphasis to the importance of live supervision in family therapy. The therapist needed the supervision team to enable him or her to gain some ability to reflect on their joint dynamics. In turn, it was argued that the supervision team could offer only their punctuation of the therapist/family system, and attempts needed to be made to reflect on this in turn. Regular external consultation was therefore also seen as necessary to reflect on these various levels of interacting systems.

HYPOTHESIZING

A family therapy team in Milan, consisting of four psychiatrists, developed the idea of family therapy as a involving a process of progressive hypothesizing.[1] There could be no objective truth about a family, simply our subjective perceptions as observers. The best we could achieve was to formulate hypotheses ('hunches') about what was going on, which could be more or less helpful in our ways of working. A hypothesis was to be judged not in terms of its ultimate truth or falseness but in terms of how effective it was in facilitating some positive change. In part, this hypothesizing came to centre on attempts to understand each family member's own explanations and stories. Family members may disagree, sometimes violently, about their explanations and competing stories about each other, the reasons for the problems and what to do.

CIRCULAR QUESTIONING

A related idea that emerged from the Milan group was that therapy should proceed on the basis of the therapist asking the family questions in order both to explore their understanding and to trigger new ways of thinking through the questions that are asked. This is one of the most striking features of contemporary family therapy, namely that therapists ask a lot of questions. The Milan team added to this the idea that the questions were systemic in the sense that they invited family members to think about relationships – 'What does Father do when Johnny and Mother argue?' – rather than about individual causes in order to help move families away from the frequent cataloguing of complaints about a family member. Furthermore, the questions were not predetermined but were shaped in a circular way by what and how the family had previously responded. Exploration and intervention are seen not as distinct stages but as continually interwoven in systemic therapy.

REFRAMING AND RE-STORYING

Contemporary family therapy has come to emphasize as central the stories that family members tell about each other and their lives. Problems are seen to result when these stories become 'problem-saturated' – overly focused and preoccupied with their difficulties and failings. From the outset, family therapists employed the technique of reframing, which attempted to offer a new or different way of seeing a problem as an intervention.[31,32] For example, conflict in a couple could be discussed as showing a fiery passion and as something that could eventually make their relationship stronger. An important ingredient of reframing or re-storying is that the problem may be cast in a less negative and destructive light, and the actions of the family members as having positive intent, even if the outcomes appear to be problematic.

For example, Henry, aged 7 years (see Figure 62.2), was referred with worries about his strange thoughts, nightmares, bizarre images and refusal to get to sleep at night on his own. There were some concerns that he might be displaying some form of childhood schizophrenia. His mother had recently started a training course and was spending more time away from the home, possibly leading Henry to worry that the family was disintegrating. It appeared that both parents had experienced nightmares when they were children and continued to be worried, especially the father, about any indications of unusual internal states.

As a reframe, it was suggested that, rather than seeing Henry as potentially ill, he was in fact a very imaginative and sensitive boy and that he was also following in his parents' footsteps in being sensitive in this way. Furthermore, perhaps this sensitivity made him concerned about the changes that had occurred in the family, and his thoughts symbolized these. Perhaps Henry also hoped that his symptoms might ensure that his parents stayed together in order to look after him, rather than fulfil his fears that they might be going their separate ways. The reframe of Henry as creative and sensitive rather than odd and ill was accepted by the family, and they started to notice confirming comments, for example when one of his teachers had commented that she thought Henry was an imaginative boy.

SOLUTION-FOCUS

Based on the original systemic concept of circularity and failing attempted solutions, this approach attempts to divert families away from these failing patterns to areas of competence and success. As such, the approach challenges prevailing discourses of illness, pathology and dysfunction and, by focusing on competence, the family is encouraged to change how they talk and think about their difficulties. The emphasis of the approach is to move to a focus on solutions rather than only on the problems. For example, parents might describe a child who 'fights all the time' or 'lies all the time'. However, the parents may also be able, if prompted, to recall some examples of when the child has been 'cooperative' or 'honest'. Often these exceptions are seen by the family as insignificant and unimportant. From a detailed exploration of the exceptions, some clues may emerge suggesting what the family could do more of in order to encourage the exceptional behaviour. There is a related focus on changes that families may already have started to make before commencing therapy – spontaneous recovery. Rather than ignoring such changes, which are said to be common, the therapist draws the family's attentions to such changes and works with them to maintain and build on such changes. Where families find it hard to think of exceptions or changes before the sessions started, they can be invited to imagine possible solutions or to use solutions that they have seen work in their families of origin and elsewhere.

NARRATIVE THERAPY

Some therapists also engage in more or less open discussion of political issues, such as the potentially damaging effects of diagnostic labelling and sense of failure.[33] Narrative therapies recognize the natural ability that people possess to generate and evolve new narratives and stories to make sense of their experiences. In doing this, we draw on culturally shared narratives or ways of interpreting events and also our own family traditions.[6,34] The narrative therapies draw on many sources, including children's literature and folk stories, to develop ways of talking about problems and that connect with culturally shared experiences and dilemmas of life.

EXTERNALIZING PROBLEMS

White and Epston suggest that problems are derived from the internalization of oppressive 'problem saturated' ways of seeing ourselves.[6] Part of the process of problem formation and maintenance is a process of internalization, so that difficulties are seen in terms of individual or family 'faults', something deficient in individual personalities and their relationships.

The techniques for doing this include treating or speaking about the problem as an object or entity outside of the person or the family.[6] As an example, White and Epston cite how a person supposedly with schizophrenia is living an 'in the corner lifestyle' and may be encouraged to resist the all-embracing, 'totalizing' nature of such a definition of their identity by discussing how she could combat or resist the 'voices' that were harassing her. Discussions may also focus on some unique outcomes – exceptions or successful instances of how she had been able to 'defy the voices' influence'. White and Epston's approach appears to have the effect of reducing the all-pervasive nature of the labelling associated with problem, for example that 'Jim *is* a schizophrenic' or Debbie *is* an anorexic', and instead considers that the problems may be seen as just one part of the whole of their total identity. Therapeutic discussion invites people to look at the ways that they may have been drawn into accepting such views of themselves and how they have learned to engage in self-criticism, self-blame and self-accusation. More widely, discussions are encouraged about how the whole family has come to consider themselves as pathological, for example seeing themselves as a 'problem family'.

In externalizing problems, the therapist proceeds not so much by simply identifying this process but by raising questions that invite the person and family members to explore it and to create ways of resisting it. An example is Paul, aged 7 years, who was constantly and apparently uncontrollably soiling himself. Through playful conversations with the therapist, he coined a name for the problem – 'Sneaky Poo'. Subsequently, he explored how and where 'Sneaky Poo' caught him and then discovered ways that he could outwit and resist it. For example, Paul described that he was most likely to be caught when he was distracted, playing or on his computer: 'I think how I tricked him was when I rushed to the toilet, he thought I was still standing there playing.'[34]

Discussions ensued about the power of mind Paul possessed that he could use to resist 'Sneaky Poo' and use the knowledge he was coming to gather about its deceptive tactics.

CONTEMPORARY PRACTICE OF FAMILY THERAPY

Most family therapists and teams now adopt a less directive and expert stance to the early pioneers. Although teams and observation screens are still used, there are attempts to be much more transparent in the process of family therapy. Perhaps the most significant indicator of the changes is the widespread use of reflecting teams.[35]

Instead of consulting in relative secret with an anonymous supervision team, the discussions between the therapist and the team are held openly in front of the family, so that the team members share their thoughts and concerns with the family and also voice any personal connections that team members have with that they have heard about the family. Through the team's discussion, the family is invited to consider alternative stories and explanations, regarding their lives together. This may allow different family members who are holding opposing views to feel understood and perhaps enable them to move on to more constructive stories. Importantly, the reflecting team enables family members to hear and perhaps internalize a different conversation rather than simply different explanations.

In turn, the family members are invited to reflect back on the reflecting team discussion regarding what they found helpful, interesting, useful and less helpful. The guiding idea is that family members may connect with the stories in different ways and be able to choose what they found to be helpful. More implicitly, it communicates the idea that there are multiple ways of seeing events, helping to free up some of the family's more rigid ways of thinking that they may have developed as a result of their sense of anxiety, failure and desperation.

CASE EXAMPLE

The following is a section of a family therapy interview with Dorothy (age 9 years), her step-mother Anne, her father Brian and her older sister Lucy. Dorothy had been self-referred by her step-mother and her father, via their GP, for therapy because she was very angry, showed some violence towards her older sister and anger towards her step-mother, and was not complying with her medication for diabetes. Her father also had diabetes, and this made him especially sensitive to the negative consequences of this non-compliance on Dorothy's health. The case also gives an indication of the complex family relationships in which many young people who come for assistance are involved.

The following is taken from early in the first interview with Dorothy and her family. The parents had been discussing how angry Dorothy often is after a visit to her natural mother's (Liz) house. Some links are tentatively made abut how these visits may distress her, and then the conversation revolves around a discussion of the inadequacies of Liz as a responsible parent:

- *Anne:* She [Liz] has her own problems; she has a problem with alcohol ...
- *Dorothy:* No, she doesn't. She never used to ...
- *Brian:* When she drinks ... her personality changes ... that's all, Dorothy.
- *Lucy:* When she looks after us, she'll often make us stay up late and drink quite a lot. It's quite scary.
- *Dorothy:* Yeah, it's scary, but you can't ...
- *Therapist:* [to Dorothy] What does that feel like? When other people say she lets you down?
- *Dorothy:* It makes me feel quite sad sometimes ... 'cos people say things like ... it's hard to explain.
- *Therapist:* What happens to that sadness? Does it turn into something else? Does it turn into other feelings?
- *Dorothy:* It turns into anger ... Sometimes if I get angry it turns into ... like, last few times I have been in my room and I get a bit claustrophobic sometimes. I'm not really a room girl.
- *Therapist:* What helps you sort those feelings out? Can Anne help? Can Dad help? Can Lucy help?
- *Dorothy:* Lucy can help.
- *Anne:* Sometimes, when she's like that, if you go near her she just says it's your fault. She's quite violent towards her, towards Lucy ... and it's partly my fault 'cos I'm here and I'm not her mum. She'll never say anything down the phone to her mum she will just ... come off the phone and then go mad ...
- *Therapist:* [to Anne] It must be really hard for you... It can be a no-win situation because you're not Mum and if you try and be Mum ... and whichever way you try to do it you can get pushed away?

Comment

Dorothy appears to want to defend her mother, who is accused by the rest of her family of having alcoholism and being unsafe to be around. Anne, her step-mother, seems to initiate this conversation. Dorothy's father Brian steps in to support Anne but seems to try to qualify his criticism by saying 'that's all' to reassure Dorothy. Possibly Brian feels caught between a loyalty to his daughter, to his new wife, and perhaps even to his ex-wife, Dorothy's mother. Also, Dorothy's sister Lucy supports and in fact elaborates her step-mother's criticism of her mother; perhaps she has decided to replace her own mother with Anne? Above all, one feature of this short passage is that young people such as Dorothy, who may initially be seen to be causing problems for the family, are typically in a paradoxical way also the same people who are most loyal to both of their parents and trying their best to help.

Interestingly, Dorothy came into this session holding two soft toys: one was a vibrant red and orange tiger and the other was a soft, cool, blue seahorse. As the interview progressed, she started to describe these two sides to her experience – sadness that can turn into anger and no doubt back again. She also says poignantly that she is not a 'room girl', perhaps meaning that she wants to be alive and doing things rather than sad and shut away from life.

A little later in the session, the therapist felt it might be helpful to turn the discussion towards an exploration of whether there had been similar experiences in Anne and Brian's own childhoods. This can often reveal important unexpressed feelings and ideas that are shaping how they are interacting with their own children. The following interesting material emerged from the invitation to consider their past:

- *Therapist:* [to Brian and Anne] Can you say a little bit about your family backgrounds?
- *Brian:* Nasty... With my own children I've always wanted to be a full-on parent because I never got it. My parents were never interested in anything I did ... my mum and dad just fell out ... I went to live with my dad.
- *Therapist:* So it's a bit similar to what happened to your own children?
- *Brian:* Yeah, but then my dad just dropped me at my grandparents and my grandparents brought me up ...
- *Dorothy:* That's not very nice [gently touching her dad's knee, and then walking away to get on with some drawing].

In thinking about why it might have been that in this family the decision was made that the children would go with their father rather than the more typical arrangement, it might have been concluded that it was because of their mother's alcoholism. Of course there are other important issues here regarding gender roles and how easy it is to make contested assumptions that it is 'natural' for children to be with their mothers rather than their fathers. However, we also get a glimpse into what has been called a 'corrective script',[36] in that the father wants things to be different from how they were for him in his childhood. He wants to be a 'full-on' father. Yet we can also see a pattern repeating itself, in that his daughters, like him, left to live with their father after a divorce. Importantly, we can start to see that, in working with Dorothy and 'her problems', we are moving between events in the past, how things are now and people's hopes for the future. We also get a poignant glimpse of how this little girl Dorothy is listening intently to what her father has to say and provides him with comfort as she senses his sadness as he remembers his childhood. Children not only are cared for but also care for their parents. For example, in families with parents with addictions or who are depressed, disabled or ill in some other way, the children may from a very young age be conscripted in the role of carers – providers rather than receivers of physical and emotional comfort.

OVERVIEW AND SUMMARY

There are many schools of, and recent developments in, family therapy. This chapter can aim to offer only a flavour of some of the main ideas and techniques employed. There are significant debates within systemic therapy, in that some practitioners are very uncomfortable with the concept of 'technique'. Above all, there has been a move towards flexibility and diversity in how therapists operate, in particular that therapists will work with families, couples or even individuals, as seems expedient. There is also flexibility in working alongside other models, for example that some family members may be receiving medication or individual therapy, such as cognitive-behavioural therapy (CBT). This is still controversial, and there are concerns that the different conceptualizations of problems can cause confusion for families. At the same time, it is evident there has been considerable integration and assimilation across various forms of therapy, so, for example, systemic ideas are included in some individual therapies and likewise systemic therapy has continually drawn on ideas from attachment theory and psychodynamic theory.[36] We have touched on the idea that systemic therapy has expanded to consider not only family dynamics but also the relationships between and within services. Not infrequently, work with families has shown that confusions and conflicts between the professionals with whom they are involved can contribute significantly to 'stuckness' or even escalation of their problems. Thinking about problems in such a multilevel way in terms of complex interacting systems continues to be an important area of development in systemic family therapy.[9,37]

KEY POINTS

- Problems are seen as relational, arising from the interactions between members as opposed to located within individuals.
- Family therapy aims to utilize the potential in families to help resolve problems.
- Problems are seen as related to different contexts, such as grouping within the family and social and cultural factors.
- Families are seen to display repetitive patterns, which can encapsulate and maintain problems.
- Families develop patterns of meanings or punctuations, which can shape and maintain their problems.
- Cycle transitions can involve stress and demands for change, which can trigger problems and also positive changes.
- Family therapy attempts to adopt a non-expert approach in order to invite consideration of new ways of seeing the problems.
- Tasks and family experiments are employed to try out new ways of interacting.
- Family therapy is frequently conducted in teams to allow multiple perspectives to be offered to families.

REFERENCES

1. Palazzoli MS, Cecchin G, Prata G, Boscolo L (1978) *Paradox and Counter Paradox: A New Model in the Therapy of the Family in Schizophrenic Transaction.* New York: Jason Aronson.
2. Minuchin S (1974) *Families and Family Therapy.* Cambridge, MA: Harvard University Press.
3. Bowlby J (1969) *Attachment and Loss*, Vol. 1. London: Hogarth Press.
4. Jackson D (1957) The question of family homeostasis. *Psychiatry Quarterly Supplement* **31**: 79–99.
5. Bowen M (1978) *Family Therapy in Clinical Practice.* Lanham, MD: Jason Aronson.
6. White M, Epston D (1990) *Narrative Means to Therapeutic Ends.* New York: W.W. Norton.
7. Hoffman L (1993) *Exchanging Voices: A Collaborative Approach to Family Therapy.* London: Karnac.
8. Hoffman L (1981) *Foundations of Family Therapy.* New York: Basic Books.
9. Dallos R, Draper R (2005) *An Introduction to Family Therapy*, 2nd edn. Maidenhead: McGraw-Hill/Open University Press.
10. Carr A (2006) *Family Therapy: Concepts, Process and Practice*, 2nd edn. Chichester: John Wiley & Sons.
11. Muncie J, Wetherell M, Dallos R, Cochrane A (eds) (1997) *Understanding the Family.* London: Sage.
12. Perelberg RJ, Miller A (1990) *Gender and Power in Families.* London: Tavistock Routledge.
13. De Shazer S (1982) *Patterns of Brief Therapy: An Ecosystemic Approach.* New York: Guilford Press.
14. Bateson G (1972) *Steps to an Ecology of Mind: Mind and Nature.* New York: Ballantine Books.

15. Trevarthen C, Aitken KJ (2001) Infant intersubjectivity: research, theory and clinical applications. *Journal of Child Psychology and Psychiatry, and Allied Disciplines* 42: 3–48.
16. Minuchin S, Rosman B, Baker L (1978) *Psychosomatic Families: Anorexia Nervosa in Context*. Cambridge, MA: Harvard University Press.
17. Haley J (1973) *Uncommon Therapy: Psychiatric Techniques of Milton H. Erickson, M.D.* New York: W.W. Norton.
18. Leff J, Vaughn C (1985) *Expressed Emotions in Families: Its Significance for Mental Illness*. New York: Guilford Press.
19. Minuchin S, Montalvo B, Guerney BG, Jr, Rosman BL, Schumer F (1967) *Families of the Slums: An Exploration of their Structure and Treatment*. New York: Basic Books.
20. Watzlawick P, Beavin J, Jackson DD (1967) *Pragmatics of Human Communication*. New York: W.W. Norton.
21. Watzlawick P, Weakland JH, Fisch R (1974) *Change: Principles of Problem Formation and Problem Resolution*. New York: W.W. Norton.
22. Berg IM (1991) *Family Preservation: A Brief Therapy Workbook*. London: BT Press.
23. Carter E, McGoldrick M (eds) (1989) *The Changing Family Life Cycle*, 2nd edn. Boston, MA: Allyn & Bacon.
24. Dallos R (1991) *Family Belief Systems, Therapy and Change*. Buckingham: Open University Press.
25. McKinnon L, Miller D (1987) The new epistemology and the Milan approach: feminist and socio-political consideration. *Journal of Marital and Family Therapy* 13: 139–55.
26. Bateson G, Jackson DD, Haley J, Weakland JH (1956) Towards a theory of schizophrenia. *Behavioural Science* 1 (suppl. 4): 251–64.
27. Weakland J (1976) Toward a theory of schizophrenia. In CE Sluzki, DD Ransom (eds) *Double Bind: The Foundation of the Communicational Approach to the Family*. New York: Grune & Stratton.
28. Weakland J (1982) *The Tactics of Change*. San Francisco, CA: Jossey-Bass.
29. Reid J (2005) Child sexual abuse and schizophrenia. *British Journal of Psychiatry* 186: 76.
30. Crittenden P (1997) Truth, error, omission, distortion, and deception: an application of attachment theory to the assessment and treatment of psychological disorder. In SM Clancy Dollinger, LF DiLalla (eds) *Assessment and Intervention Issues Across the Life Span*. London: Lawrence Erlbaum Associates.
31. Reiss D (1980) *The Family's Construction of Reality*. London: RKP.
32. Procter HG (1996) The family construct system. In DC Kalekin-Fishman, BM Walker (eds) *The Construction of Group Realities: Culture, Society and Personal Construct Theory*. London: Krieger Publishing Company.
33. White M (1995) *Re-Authoring Lives: Interviews and Essays*. Adelaide: Dulwich Centre Publications.
34. Freeman J, Epston D, Lobovits D (1997) *Playful Approaches to Serious Problems: Narrative Therapy with Children and Their Families*. New York: W.W. Norton.
35. Andersen T (1987) The reflecting team: dialogue and meta-dialogue in clinical work. *Family Process* 26: 415–28.
36. Byng-Hall J (1995) *Rewriting Family Scripts: Improvisation and Systems Change*. New York: Guilford Press.
37. Bentovim A (1992) *Trauma Organised System: Physical and Sexual Abuse in Families*. London: Karnac.

Chapter 63

Marital therapy

David Hewison

INTRODUCTION

Marital therapy is an overall term for the treatment for dysfunctional or distressed adult couple relationships. Although the term 'marital' is used in this chapter, the theories and techniques addressed are applicable to all adult couples, whether married, in civil partnerships or not, and whether heterosexual, gay or lesbian. The treatment group is adults in a committed emotional and sexual relationship, and in this sense is both societally and self-defined. It is clear that there are overlaps between the target patient group of marital therapy and those of family therapy, parent–infant therapy and relationship therapy for individuals. One of the consistent themes in surveys of the field is the lack of a clear definition of the patient group, the aims and targets of treatment, the criteria for efficacy, and the correct methodologies for gathering a useful evidence base.[1–6] Despite this, it is also clear from a number of articles in the *British Journal of Psychiatry* and other journals that marital therapy has considerable scope for intervention in depression, as recognized by the National Institute for Health and Clinical Excellence (NICE).[7–11] In addition, marital therapy not only is valuable in reducing distress in relationships but may also be a highly cost-effective treatment.[12] The book by Snyder and Whisman is of particular relevance in addressing patients where there are coexisting mental health and relationship difficulties.[13]

This chapter aims to introduce the most common ways of treating the couple relationship psychotherapeutically in the UK, giving their characteristics and techniques and when they may be particularly indicated as a treatment. These techniques, in alphabetical order, are:

- Cognitive-behavioural marital therapy
- Emotionally focused marital therapy
- Psychodynamic/psychoanalytical marital therapy
- Systemic marital therapy.

COGNITIVE-BEHAVIOURAL MARITAL THERAPY

Key texts include Baucom *et al.*[14] and Rathus and Sanderson.[15]

Characteristics

Cognitive-behavioural marital therapy is an overall term for a range of different treatments that share key elements. It emphasizes the importance of interactions with the environment, and the feedback loop between the individual (with their own ways of perceiving the world and their own set of skills in influencing it) and others around them (who respond positively to some behaviours, so encouraging them, and negatively to others, so discouraging them). Cognitive-behavioural marital therapy addresses the role of individual cognitions and attributions of meaning to behaviours. It recognizes that patterns of interaction and response to relationship demands are ingrained from past experiences ('overlearned') and that they may result in extremely anachronistic interpretations of the current relationship, giving rise to disturbing behaviours, thoughts and feelings in one or both of the couple that are difficult to shift.

Problems in couples arise when the balance between behaviours and how they are interpreted is felt to move from largely pleasing and rewarding to largely displeasing and punishing; the way in which they do so is unique to the couple. Couples may suffer from a lack of relationship and communication skills, or they may be poor or patchy at putting into use the skills they do have. Similarly, couples will bring a set of pre-existing assumptions and beliefs about what a relationship is, which they will make use of in an automatic way to interpret the behaviours of their partner. The theory holds that changing the nature of these automatic cognitions and ways of processing the information received will lead directly to positive changes in both emotion and behaviour. As a result, this therapy focuses on relatively small behavioural interactions between the couple, examining how they are received and categorized by each partner, and aiming to minimize those that are negative and to maximize those that are positive. Problem-solving skills are developed or enhanced. Some cognitive-behavioural therapists also use elements of emotionally focused therapy in order to give the couple greater abilities to manage their affective responses to each other.

Techniques

Cognitive-behavioural therapy (CBT) is a short-term therapy of up to 25 sessions, which may begin weekly and then reduce in frequency once the therapist has understood the nature of the maladaptive interactions and goals have been set for change. It tends to be highly structured, with the therapist taking the role of collaborator, seeking the couple's agreement with their evaluation of the nature of the couple relationship and the steps that will be taken to bring about change. Attention is paid to ensuring a balance between identifying areas of conflict where things have gone wrong and areas of harmony where the couple have the experience of positively relating with each other. This keeps optimism alive in the couple relationship in the face of pessimism stemming from their difficulties.

Assessment of the couple relationship is seen as an ongoing task, clarifying unwanted target behaviours and cognitions, and setting new goals and strategies to achieve them. Goals are specific, targeted and achievable, and are sequenced in five ways:

- Goals that are more likely to be achieved are set first, as this gives the couple a positive reinforcement that change is possible and that it is achievable through the therapy process.
- Goals that are less central to the couple's sense of their difficulties are aimed for first, as this is less likely to evoke strong negative responses based on raised anxiety.
- Goals are set that increase positive interactions between the couple.
- Goals that do not impinge upon the core values of either of the couple are set before those that require more work and mutual understanding.
- Those things that simply have to be dealt with first, such as reducing the risk of violence, come before those that are important but can wait a little.

The techniques for achieving goals vary from didactic input from the therapist, informing and teaching the couple about a particular element in their relationship, through to role-play in the session, coaching and advising, and homework and exercises to do between sessions and reviewed at the next. In general, the therapist will, where necessary, train couples in basic skills of communication, such as taking responsibility for their own statements and active listening to the other; identifying faulty or dysfunctional attributions to each other's behaviour; and utilizing strategies to replace displeasing behaviours with pleasing ones.

The therapist needs to be able to de-escalate heightened levels of negative emotion and inappropriate behaviours, intervening directly where necessary to bring the couple back to the programme of work. This means that the therapist is highly active in initial sessions, tapering off as the couple are able to identify the skills they need and put them into practice.

Indications

- Where both partners are prepared to work on their relationship, and are willing to do so with a cognitive-behavioural approach
- Where there is a clear communication problem between the couple
- Where there is not an ongoing affair
- Where there is not simultaneous substance abuse
- Where neither partner is suffering from overwhelming individual difficulties stemming from their own psychopathology (although some cognitive-behavioural work may help the other partner cope with them, e.g. in maintaining social skills).

EMOTIONALLY FOCUSED MARITAL THERAPY

Key texts include those by Johnson.[16,17]

Characteristics

This marital therapy has its roots in attachment theory,[18] which puts relating at the heart of human survival. Attachment theory has investigated the kinds of attachment relationship that infants and children make and has shown how they lead to either secure or insecure dependency on another. An inner sense of secure attachment enables continual adjustment to the world and to the challenges of relating; this sense of security comes from the repeated experience of emotional responsiveness and recognition from the primary caregiver, which includes the expression and recognition of anger and distress as well as concern and love. It is the engagement with emotional life that is important, as it allows the young child to know that the other is a person like themselves, with a mind that registers feelings and that can manage the difficulties and joys of emotional awareness (an 'internal working model'). Where dependency needs have been met insufficiently or in an inconsistent way, the child will grow up with an insecure attachment, uncertain whether they are existentially safe in the world or whether another person can truly be relied upon.

Attachment theory suggests that we utilize an attachment system of alert and response whenever we come across anything that impacts upon our connection with an attachment figure, such as a parent or a partner. This will happen inevitably and may be triggered by a substantial period of absence or indeed merely a sense that the person's attention is elsewhere at the point when we are trying to be in contact with them. Its manifestations vary. With secure attachment, things such as separations will have a typical pattern: a degree of protest, a wish to cling, followed by more depressed feelings and then a kind of detachment, which is based on knowing that we are still in touch, internally, with our attachment figure. With insecure attachment, these feelings will arise more swiftly and will be far less moderated: the protest may be fury, the clinging highly intrusive, the depression turning to an inconsolable despair, and the detachment either an empty, lost hopelessness or a cold, indifferent turning-away. These feelings tend to manifest themselves either as states of anxiety or as a push to avoid an unwanted emotional experience. In adult couple relationships, the anxiety may well manifest itself as anger and rage, and the avoidance may well be seen in hostility (and the attribution of this to the partner), which even gets triggered when the partner themselves shows distress or their own dependency needs, making for stormy and difficult relationships.

Emotionally focused marital therapy seeks to enhance secure attachment ways of experiencing emotion and to reduce the anxiety or avoidance that comes with insecure ways. It is based on the assumption that it is the degree of emotional security in the relationship that is key to meeting adults' innate needs for being in a reliable, responsive and reciprocal relationship. It attempts to intervene by directly changing the experience of emotional relating in the couple.

Techniques

Emotionally focused marital therapy is a short-term therapy of 8–20 weeks that seeks explicitly to give couples a corrective emotional experience. It focuses on the internal working models of the couple that structure their relating, as these not only give rise to the specifics of the emotional exchanges between them but are themselves generated by these exchanges. An internal working model of greater security in relating allows the couple to experience a wider range of feelings, needs and wishes in relation to each other without leading to a catastrophe. The couple become more resilient and empathic as a result. Anger and distress can be seen as just what they are: feelings that stem from an attachment system being activated, rather than being blown out of all proportion. Emotions are seen as either *primary emotions*, which are the immediate feeling response to something experienced, or as *secondary emotions*, which are the ways in which the primary emotions are responded to, coped with or hidden – an outburst of anger is a secondary emotion having its roots in a primary feeling of loss; giving up and turning away has its roots in despair and loneliness, for example.

The therapy is characterized by a movement between the therapist attending to an emotional experience between the couple, and deliberately structuring and shaping one. It has three main tasks:

- Creating and actively maintaining a positive therapeutic alliance by the use of acceptance and empathy, together with a willingness to demonstrate engagement with the couple through actively validating each partner's experience while seeing it in the context of attachment reactions.
- Seeking out emotional experiences in the sessions – specifically, focusing on instances of anger, fear, surprise, joy, shame and disgust, hurt and anguish – in order to identify the primary feelings behind the secondary feelings. This can lead to a greater understanding in the couple of the way the feelings of each person are affected by the feelings of the other, giving rise to a greater emotional intelligence and the capacity to experience a wider range of feeling. This enables the couple to stay more in touch with each other and not have to resort to dysfunctional coping strategies that leave them distressed and disaffected.
- Using an explicit attachment model to help the couple understand why they are responding to each other in the way that they are, so continuing to normalize their feelings. Then, the therapist will direct the couple to experience a new way of responding to each other when their attachment systems are activated, actively enabling the couple to respond to each other and give voice to their feelings. This deepens their emotional engagement with each other and strengthens their attachment to each other, making them and their relationship more secure.

Indications

- Where the couple want to rebuild the relationship, despite the difficulties between them
- Where the couple have a clear attachment system pattern going on, such as one partner pursuing/attacking and the other withdrawing/avoiding
- Where the couple are not already in the process of separating or divorcing
- Where the couple are able to experience a heightening of difficult emotions between them without recourse to violence.

PSYCHODYNAMIC/ PSYCHOANALYTICAL MARITAL THERAPY

Key texts include Ruszczynski[19] and Clulow.[20]

Characteristics

Psychodynamic and psychoanalytical marital therapy are similar in that both assume the presence of processes operating between the couple that are unconscious to them both but that exert a powerful influence on their cognitions, affects, attributions and overall experience of what a couple relationship is for and like. These unconscious processes are seen as having their roots in the childhood and background of the respective partners, including their conscious and unconscious experience of their parents' couple relationship and their reactions to it. Although the roots of the unconscious processes lie in the past, the couple will be actively engaged in something in the present. The understanding of this takes different forms, according to the theoretical orientation of the therapist: some will focus on the manifestation of internalized representations of the parents – the *internal parental couple* – and the way they seem to encourage or prohibit particular ways of relating; others will focus more on the *state of mind* of the couple, by which is meant the way in which the couple as a couple and as individuals approach their emotional life at any particular moment. This is not so much the nature of any emotion that may be being expressed but rather the inner attitude to it in each of the couple, no matter who is feeling it at that point: is dependency or neediness treated with contempt or sympathy? Are loving feelings cut off prematurely or allowed to flower despite the difficulties? Is anger met with indifference or a struggle for acceptance? And so on.

Key to the psychodynamic/psychoanalytical understanding of the couple relationship is the idea that it is a 'phantasy' relationship – that is, a relationship permeated with unconscious projections on to, and in part accepted by, each other. This means that one partner will manifest emotions, thoughts and behaviours that actually belong to the other partner, forming a complex interlocking system of experience that can be very difficult to unravel. This projective system will be complicated further by the unconscious fit between the couple: what are they trying to achieve in forming a relationship with each other over and above falling in love? Some couples will be attempting to find someone with whom they can develop emotionally, while others will be seeking someone who will protect them from the need to change, in a defensive relationship.

The role of the therapist is to create an environment in which these internal patterns of relating can be seen and experienced 'live' in the room, not only between the couple but also between the couple and the therapist (the *transference*). The therapist is additionally seen as a 'receiver' of the couple's disavowed emotional life. The therapist uses material that obviously belongs to the couple – for example, what they say or how they feel – and compares and contrasts it with their own shifting internal state (the *countertransference*) to form an interpretation as to what might be going on unconsciously in the couple. The idea is that, the more conscious the couple are of what they are doing, and who they really are rather than who they think they are, the greater freedom they have to relate fully with another person.

Techniques

There are regular weekly sessions of 50–60 min, generally on an open-ended basis. The sessions require strict technical handling: informal interactions are kept to a minimum and the sessions are deliberately unstructured with no teaching or guiding. The therapist creates a neutrally expectant space for the couple to use in whatever way they will. Characteristically, the couple will experience this emptiness as though it were full of demands, expectations, prohibitions and punishments, so revealing their unconscious relating.

Attention is paid to everything that happens in the room as of potential meaning for the couple, including asides, jokes, slips of the tongue, and deeply engaged conversation and interactions.

The therapist's personality is used as a tool and as a source of information. Therapists expect to be stirred up by the couple, and their ability to contain this has an impact on the couple.

Interpretations are used as a main instrument of change. Although the therapist will not deliberately create a corrective emotional experience as in emotionally focused therapy, change does not occur without the engagement of both thoughts and feelings, and it is the relationship with the therapist that enables this.

Indications

- Where a couple have a particular interest in the meaning of their relationship – why it is like it is – and want to change it
- Where a couple can make use of symbolism and are not excessively concrete in their thinking
- Where dysfunctional patterns of relating have proved unshiftable through other means, including other therapies, and the couple are prepared to engage in what might be long-term work
- Where one or other of the couple has a narcissistic personality structure.

SYSTEMIC MARITAL THERAPY

Key texts include Weeks and Treat[21] and Jones and Asen.[22]

Characteristics

Systemic marital therapy, like cognitive-behavioural marital therapy, is an overall term that covers a range of different theoretical positions that share common features. Most obviously, there is a focus on a system of interaction and the ways in which the couple act as though responsibility for the system lies with one or other of them. In particular, there may be a focus on the patterns at work in the families of origin of the couple, including a focus on family secrets or on specific behaviours or roles that seem to be repeated through the generations. Some systemic marital therapists also consider the role that the individual has, focusing on the strengths and difficulties (including personal psychopathology) that are brought into the couple system; others see these as more of a manifestation of the action of a wider-arching system, so downplaying the individual.

Systemic therapists are active and assertive, on the basis that changing a destructive system requires greater energy than exists to maintain it. They can take up different roles at different times – guide, teacher, confronter, referee, empathizer – and they may set homework to be done by a couple between sessions. Their aim, however, is to ensure that the couple take more and more responsibility for the quality of their relationship. Attention is paid to the balance of the therapy: the amount of attention paid to each partner, the degree of intensity of confrontation with each, the assumption that both partners are involved in the problem, the equal treatment of both in terms of any individual sessions, and so on.

Systemic therapists assume that any behaviour has a role and a meaning in the system – in effect, that there is a purpose to a behaviour, no matter how reactive it appears. Part of the work of the therapy is to identify why this behaviour has been utilized at this point and to draw the couple's attention to what they are doing and how it has its origins in the different systems at work in the relationship. The couple then have the opportunity to change their actions and so change the system.

Attention is also paid to the use of language by the couple – both at the level of specific content (including the kinds of words chosen) and at the level of process or what the language is meant to do in the couple system. Typically, language patterns are used to manage distance/closeness, to act aggressively or submissively in the relationship, to deal with reactions or responses to the partner, to act defensively to what are perceived as attacks of one kind or another, and to manage levels of intimacy. Attention is also paid to the use of power in the system.

Techniques

Regular 50- or 60-min sessions are held weekly or fortnightly, either open-ended or for a contracted period of time. There may be a reflecting team that observes and comments 'live' on the therapy.

Circular questions such as 'What does he/she do when you are angry?' as opposed to linear questions such as 'How does he/she make you angry?' emphasize the system at work between the couple. Questions such as 'Were your parents angry like this?' emphasize the intergenerational aspect of the couple symptom.

The defensive use of language is addressed, and what it is that is being defended against is looked at. This may involve focusing on the words used and inviting the speaker to say the same thing differently, or it may need to be dealt with by the therapist opening up the feeling behind the words at greater depth, including using comparison and imagery.

Reframing is a key technique in which an intervention is made that describes a process going on between the couple in a way that enables them to change. This is not an attempt to give the couple the truth of what they are doing; instead, it seeks to redefine what is going on in positive terms and in ways that emphasize the system at work between the couple. An example may be when a couple present with one partner suffering from depression; the therapist might indicate how committed that partner is to the relationship as their depression stops them showing angry feelings that they fear their partner would not be able to deal with and so leave. The couple can then be worked with to understand the reciprocal nature of the symptoms of depression and to find a better way of managing feelings in the relationship.

The four different systems at work at any point – the individual, the couple, the families of origin and the social context – are attended to.

Using genograms not only to capture the members of a family but also to explore the feelings they have expressed or avoided can be helpful.

Indications

- When there are clear patterns of relationship stemming from families of origin perceptible in the couple
- Where one partner will need active and effective engagement to join the couple therapy
- Where there are complexities and confusions stemming from multiple sources of input into the couple system (e.g. from social services, schools, other extended family members).

KEY POINTS

- Marital therapy has a supportive and prophylactic role to play in the treatment and management of individual symptoms, in addition to being the treatment of choice in relationship distress.
- Marital therapy is supported by NICE guidelines as a treatment for depression.
- All types of marital therapy recognize the interrelations between communication, behaviour and emotion, though they each emphasize different elements of it.
- Marital therapy is available as short-term, focused treatment and as long-term, exploratory treatment.

REFERENCES

1. Boddington SJA, Lavender A (1995) Treatment models for couples therapy: a review of the outcome literature and the Dodo's verdict. *Sexual and Marital Therapy* **10**: 69–81.
2. Gupta M, Coyne JC, Beach SHR (2003) Couples treatment for major depression: critique of the literature and suggestions for some different directions. *Journal of Family Therapy* **25**: 317–46.
3. Lanman M, Grier F (2003) Evaluating change in couple functioning: a psychoanalytic perspective. *Sexual and Relationship Therapy* **18**: 13–24.
4. Lanman M, Grier F, Evans C (2003) Objectivity in psychoanalytic assessment of couple relationships. *British Journal of Psychiatry* **182**: 255–60.
5. Shmueli A, Clulow C (1997) Marital therapy: definition

and development. *Current Opinion in Psychiatry* **10**: 247–50.

6. Snyder DK, Castellani AM, Whisman MA (2006) Current status and future directions in couple therapy. *Annual Review of Psychology* **57**: 317–44.
7. Denton W, Golden RN, Walsh SR (2003) Depression, marital discord, and couple therapy. *Current Opinion in Psychiatry* **16**: 29–34.
8. Emanuels-Zuurveen L, Emmelkamp PMG (1996) Individual behavioural-cognitive therapy v marital therapy for depression in maritally distressed couples. *British Journal of Psychiatry* **169**: 181–8.
9. Harris TJR, Pistang N, Barker C (2006) Couples' experience of the support process in depression: a phenomenological analysis. *Psychology and Psychotherapy: Theory, Research and Practice* **79**: 1–21.
10. Leff J, Vearnals S, Brewin CR, *et al.* (2000) The London Depression Intervention Trial: randomised controlled trial of antidepressants v. couple therapy in the treatment and maintenance of people with depression living with a partner: clinical outcome and costs. *British Journal of Psychiatry* **177**: 95–100.
11. National Institute for Health and Clinical Excellence (2007) *Depression (Amended): Management of Depression in Primary and Secondary Care.* Clinical guideline 23. London: National Institute for Health and Clinical Excellence.
12. Caldwell BE, Woolley SR, Caldwell CJ (2007) Preliminary estimates for cost-effectiveness of marital therapy. *Journal of Marital and Family Therapy* **33**: 392–406.
13. Snyder DK, Whisman MA (eds) (2003) *Treating Difficult Couples: Helping Clients with Coexisting Mental and Relationship Disorders.* New York: Guilford Press.
14. Baucom DH, Epstein N, LaTaillade J (2002) Cognitive-behavioural couple therapy. In AS Gurman, NS Jacobson (eds) *Clinical Handbook of Couple Therapy.* New York: Guilford Press.
15. Rathus JH, Sanderson WC (1999) *Marital Distress: Cognitive Behavioural Interventions for Couples.* Northvale, NJ: Jason Aronson.
16. Johnson SM (2004) *The Practice of Emotionally Focused Couple Therapy: Creating Connection.* Hove: Brunner-Routledge.
17. Johnson SM (2005) *Becoming an Emotionally Focused Couple Therapist: The Workbook.* Hove: Brunner-Routledge.
18. Bowlby J (1982) *Attachment.* London: Hogarth Press.
19. Ruszczynski S (ed.) (1993) *Psychotherapy with Couples: Theory and Practice at the Tavistock Institute of Marital Studies.* London: Karnac.
20. Clulow C (ed.) (2001) *Adult Attachment and Couple Psychotherapy: The 'Secure Base' in Practice and Research.* London: Brunner/Routledge.
21. Weeks GR, Treat SR (2001) *Couples in Treatment: Techniques and Approaches for Effective Practice.* Philadelphia, PA: Brunner/Routledge.
22. Jones E, Asen E (2000) *Systemic Couple Therapy and Depression.* London: Karnac Books.

Chapter 64

Group therapy

John Gordon and Gabriel Kirtchuk

INTRODUCTION – PSYCHOTHERAPY AND SYSTEM: WHAT THE PSYCHIATRIST NEEDS TO KNOW ABOUT GROUP PSYCOTHERAPY AND GROUP DYNAMICS

Our approach to thinking about groups, emphasized in the subtitle of this chapter, embeds a specific treatment modality in a more comprehensive understanding of group processes.[1] From a biopsychosocial perspective on human development and psychopathology, human beings are group animals – Aristotle's phrase was 'political animals' – through and through. The three major clinically oriented theories of group dynamics – those of Irvin Yalom[2] in the USA and SH Foulkes[3] and WR Bion[4] in the UK – are based on the premise that we are as hardwired through natural selection to interact within groups as we are to breathe air: the group is our natural medium.

The group is essential for survival and protection, originally from external predators and, using a psychodynamic lens, every bit as much from internal predators of the mind, which are frequently externalized in and between groups. The group is also a crucible of identity formation and malformation. Family group cultures and relationships evoke, nurture, facilitate and elaborate the expression of individual potentials, traits and skills on the one hand, and fix, compensate for or further skew immature, maladaptive or pathological responses, patterns and defences on the other. Interactions within school, peer and professional groups continue to shape the development of personality. Our group memberships even influence the extent to which we experience a sense of individuality at all, as well as our ability to be aware of and to cope with our vulnerabilities, pain and anxieties at all phases of the life cycle. Freud viewed the group both as a source of loss of identity (depersonalization) and as a matrix of human creativity.[5] The essence of the group's therapeutic potency derives from this duality of group life, for patients are supported to attend to and understand the reasons for their pathological identities and identifications, which are constantly displayed in the sessions; to relinquish them, usually slowly and painfully (to disinvest from maladaptive ways of experiencing themselves and others); and to create through their interactions with others in the group new capacities for emotional experience, interpersonal sensitivity and relationships.

In a seminar, the authors were discussing how group membership profoundly affects the ways in which individuals feel, think and behave, often out of conscious awareness. Two members of the seminar group, who were trainee psychiatrists from South America, began to talk about 'the bane of our professional life back home'. One described how he had examined a middle-aged woman with a life-threatening condition who had arrived at a large urban hospital from her tribal area some hundreds of miles away. He told his patient that an immediate operation could save her and offered to put her at the top of the list for surgery; otherwise, she would probably die. The woman replied that she must return to her village and consult with her tribe about what to do.

These 'sophisticated' psychiatrists believed that they were merely relating interesting anthropological data from a different, if contemporary, group culture. And it is true that, historically and culturally, enormous variations have existed and continue to exist regarding the degree to which group norms recognize, value, and encourage the differentiation of group members. Individuals as autonomous agents did not inhabit ancient Greece[6] or medieval Europe and emerged only gradually during the Enlightenment; those seventeenth- and eighteenth-century individuals did not view themselves in accordance with our current conception and experience of subjectivity.[7] The authors were able to explore with the seminar members, as we intend to do in this chapter, how an understanding of group dynamics reveals our complex and not always welcome rootedness, as human beings and as professionals, in the ubiquitous play of group forces to which we contribute; and how the potential clinical efficacy of group psychotherapy arises only from this understanding. The unavoidable dilemma, which is intrinsic to the human condition and had been alluded to by our student psychiatrists, was grasped most cogently by Bion:[4]

> One of the problems of group therapy, then, lies in the fact that the group is often used to achieve a sense of vitality by total submergence in the group, or a sense of individual independence by total repudiation of the group, and that part of the individual's mental life, which is being incessantly stimulated and

activated by his group, is his inalienable inheritance as a group animal... The individual is a group animal at war, not simply with the group, but with himself for being a group animal and with those aspects of his personality that constitute his 'groupishness'.

KEY GROUP DYNAMICS

The curriculum of the Royal College of Psychiatrists explicitly and implicitly recognizes the group context of normal and abnormal personality development. There are references, for example, to sociocultural and social psychiatry; to the interactionist approach; to the development and change of attitudes and behaviour, the emergence of visual and auditory perceptions, and the development of self-recognition and personal identity through social interaction; to affiliation, person perception and attribution theory; to social influence, leadership, persuasive communication and obedience in small and large groups; to conformity, polarization and 'groupthink'; to altruism, interpersonal cooperation and social exchange theory; and to the sociology of residential institutions. The Royal College Summary of Areas of Core Medical Knowledge Underpinning Specialist Training in Psychiatry even relates the conceptualization of a 'theory of mind' to interpersonal issues and social behaviour. We would emphasize that the rationale for group psychotherapy rests on the interpersonal basis and manifestations of psychopathology, whatever its ultimate origins. Three group dynamic concepts inherent in the curriculum require further discussion, for they are central to an understanding of the therapeutic action of group psychotherapy and to much of the research in group psychotherapy over the past 30 years: group interaction, group norms and group cohesion.

Group interaction

A group can be defined by the number of interactions between its members. Homans, a sociologist, suggested:

If we say that individuals A, B, C, D, E ... form a group, this will mean that at least the following circumstances hold. Within a period of time, A interacts more with B, C, D, E, ... than he does with M, N, L, O, P, ... whom we choose to consider outsiders or members of other groups. B also interacts more often with A, C, D, E ... than he does with others, and so on for the other members of the group.[8]

Quantity of interaction is very close to intensity of interaction as the emotional significance of group members for one another increases over time. Through the process of interaction, internal differentiations occur with regard to activity, roles, power and status; and the interactions between members are structured accordingly: quantities of sustained interactions become relatively predictable, qualitative patterns of relationship.

Hare studied the process of interaction in small groups (the quantity, sequence and interrelation of acts over time) and found that much human behaviour in groups is directed to solving problems.[9] He highlighted group problems and individual problems, and at each of these levels problem content concerned either tasks or social-emotional issues. The group task is to further the publicly stated aims of the group, the objectives and purposes for which it was formed. In order to succeed, the group members must devise an effective division of labour, but they must also attend to the social-emotional coherence of the group by addressing anxieties, conflicts and special personal relationships that arise in the course of group interaction, which may interfere with or severely jeopardize group survival, let alone realization of the primary task. At the individual level, the task is to achieve those personal goals (to belong, to feel secure, to train, etc.) that led the individual to join the group. Simultaneously, in the social-emotional arena, the individual must manage the strains of membership and self-integration under the impact of multiple interactions.

Most evidently, interpersonal interaction in the psychotherapy group is intimate, intensely emotionally significant and of the utmost importance to group members in terms of their life goals, often literally their life or death. They will be deeply involved at both levels of problem content. The group therapist must also keep in mind the two levels of group problem content. The therapist must structure the group as a goal-directed, focused therapeutic enterprise and contain the inevitable emotional turbulence intrinsic to severe mental illness.

The psychiatrist, even if he or she does not take on the role of group psychotherapist, must be aware of this aspect of group interaction, for psychiatrists are members of groups known as multidisciplinary treatment teams, whether in hospital or community settings. It has been well established that group social-emotional functioning in organizations, in response to intense anxieties posed by the nature of the work, often takes the form of maladaptive defensive behaviour.[10–12] For example, warmly supportive interactions among members of one professional group may be combined with hostile, blaming interactions towards members of another profession (including managers) within the multidisciplinary team. Although such patterns of interaction protect group members from severe tensions, they can divert their efforts away from a clear focus on the vital jobs that need to be done in order to accomplish both group and individual objectives. Psychiatrists' interventions, like those of other colleagues, make up part of a total group response to patients. It is incumbent on the psychiatrists, and perhaps particularly on consultant psychiatrists as highly trained and specialized professionals,[13] to take a leading role in monitoring whether the social-emotional defensive system, a vital ingredient of staff cohesion when it offers mature protection from anxiety, threatens to shift collective work in an anti-task direction.

Group norms

We have mentioned that group interaction sustained over time becomes highly structured and predictable. Task and social-emotional systems must be flexible and adaptable to changing realities, but they need to have a core of stability. Group norms are central to the development of patterned behaviour, which, while sparing individuals from chaos, also determine much that they feel, think and do as group members, both in and out of their awareness. Norms have been studied extensively in the group dynamics and group psychotherapy research literature (see Whiteley and Gordon[1] and Yalom[2] for extended discussions of norms in particular and group dynamics in general).

Mills considers group norms as:

> ... a set of statements about feelings and behaviour. They are cognitive and moral statements which screen, evaluate, prescribe, and proscribe feelings and actions. As statements they are distinct from feelings and from behaviour. They exist in symbolic form in the mind, and are elements of group culture.[14]

Group norms define, explicitly or implicitly, what is appropriate expression, belief and action for individuals in their specific roles as group members in interaction with one another. The normative system offers definitions of deviance, sanctions and how members may legitimately alter the arrangements for social control in the group.

Two classic and very influential studies of group norms stand out from an extensive literature. Sherif demonstrated experimentally the development of group norms when individuals are 'placed in an objectively unstable situation in which all basis of comparison, as far as the external field of stimulation is concerned, is absent'.[15] Individuals were asked to estimate the perceived movement of a point of light in a totally dark room (the autokinetic effect). Alone, each would establish a range of estimations; and within that range, a subjective reference point – the norm – emerged and became fixed over successive trials of 100 judgements. The ranges and norms of individuals varied, but when the individuals were placed together in groups their differing estimates tended to merge. For subjects who faced the experimental condition for the first time not as isolated individuals but in a group, a specific group range and standard were clearly established. Sherif commented that 'every individual need not be aware of the fact that he is being influenced in the group situation, or that he and the other members are converging toward a common norm'.[15]

Asch studied the effects of group (normative) pressure on members' perceptions of an obvious, clearly visible situation.[16] A naive subject placed in a group situation was asked to match the perceived length of a line, drawn on a piece of paper in front of him or her, to one of three other lines drawn on another piece of paper. The experimental condition involved all the other group members, confederates of the experimenter, giving the wrong answer to this extremely simple task at specified times. Asch sought to determine 'the social and personal conditions that induce individuals to resist or to yield to group pressures when the latter are perceived to be *contrary to fact*'.[16]

Although overall 68 per cent of successive estimates were correct and only very few subjects yielded completely in the face of majority group pressure, one-third of erroneous estimates were identical or similar to the (incorrect) majority. Of greater significance from our clinical perspective, however, were the differences among the independent subjects. Only one-quarter were totally independent, while one-third altered their judgements towards the majority norm in 50 per cent or more of the trials. This means that three-quarters of the subjects were affected in some way. Furthermore, not all independents were confidently so. Some maintained their judgement but were emotionally shaken by their deviance from the other group members. Others showed evidence of dissociation, loss of self-esteem or paranoid reactions. Distortions could occur in action (going along with the group majority even while knowing they were wrong); in judgement (the belief that others were probably right despite one's own correct estimate); and, most profoundly, in perception (yielding without knowing that one has been influenced).

The implication of this research is that carefully communicated and consistently applied norms are a pre-eminent therapeutic factor in group psychotherapy. In assessment, pre-group preparation and for the duration of treatment, in every session, the group psychotherapist must reinforce patients' role expectations for productive clinical work and watch for deviations from them. We clarify with prospective patients our recommendations for open and honest communication in the group – about their lives, their reactions to the therapist and to other group members – and underline the primacy of thought and exploration of strong impulses and feelings, rather than immediate resort to action. In particular, we rule out physical violence to others and promote extended working-through of termination in the face of strong temptation towards evasion of mourning. All interactions between group members outside the sessions (if only in the waiting room) should be brought into the group for mutual discussion.

All psychiatrists operate as members of their multidisciplinary work groups; depending on their grade, it is vital that they take responsibility to synchronize the normative system – how professionals ought to behave – both with the reality of the primary tasks of the organization and with the requisite and mature social-emotional relations between group members that enable the work to proceed. Compliance with and submersion in group norms can allow the consequently depersonalized individuals to experience tremendous collective vitality, usually based on scapegoating 'deviant' members or attacking external groups. Psychiatrists can and should be representatives of norms based on reality – the reality of the world outside the hospital and the reality of engagement with the patient.

Group cohesion

Perhaps no other concept in the field of group dynamics has been elaborated so thoroughly, and is so connected with research into the effects of group psychotherapy, as group cohesion (see Yalom[2] for a comprehensive survey of the research literature).[17–19] Group cohesion has been conceptualized as a force, pressure or interpersonal glue that attracts individuals to, and involves and maintains them in, the group. The multiple incentives to join a particular group, whether reflecting a basic need to belong, admiration of the group members, identification with the values, norms or goals of the group, or the status and prestige deemed to flow from group membership, all operate as forces pulling individuals towards and into the group and securing – for as long as they remain salient – allegiance, conformity and commitment.

The 'cohesiveness' of a group is the constellation of such forces at any one time, a resultant of all forces acting on members to stay in the group which takes into account the attractiveness of alternative memberships.[1]

No group can exert power and influence over its members greater than its cohesiveness, for the capacity to influence wanes with the diminution or loss of group attractiveness.

In essence, group cohesiveness refers to the sense of affiliation and belonging shared among group members, the 'we' feeling in the group. In his anthropological study of urban gangs, Whyte demonstrated how deeply dependent the individual's experience of personal identity, esteem and mental health, as well as his perceptions, beliefs and behaviour, are on close patterned relationships with other members of his social group.[20] In the absence of such interactions, due to various interferences with the performance of their accustomed roles, psychosomatic and confusional states affected group members. Their being, just like the South American woman mentioned earlier, was anchored in the group. Such reference groups,[21] those groups of paramount significance to which we belong or to which we aspire to belong (a group in the mind), constantly inform our attitudes and actions even when we are not in immediate contact.

Yalom considers cohesion as the group counterpart to the therapeutic relationship in individual psychotherapy, a key element of therapeutic outcome in all forms of treatment, including – as psychiatrists know – psychopharmacology.[2] In itself, group cohesion is only an essential but not a sufficient factor in bringing about change. However, in conjunction with group norms that promote intense and intimate personal interaction, with an emphasis on open disclosure and a willingness to give spontaneous, frank and respectful feedback to others, a cohesive group provides the safety and containment that enable group members to persevere with their difficult and very painful task.

Psychiatrists will be all too well aware of the organizational complement to group cohesion: the vicissitudes of group morale in health service settings that can so affect the state of mind, ranging from creative collaboration to despair, in which professional tasks are addressed. Whether as clinicians or as clinical managers, a consultant role mandates sustained attention to this aspect of group life.

TRANSITION

Before considering group psychotherapy proper, we offer an example from everyday psychiatric practice of how the group dynamic dimensions just reviewed can affect the psychiatrist's work with patients within the context of the wider professional and hospital systems. A group of junior doctors had been meeting regularly during their rotation with a senior consultant psychiatrist in psychotherapy. The task of the group (a Balint group) was to give the doctors an opportunity to present case material in order to reflect on their interactions with their patients and other staff from a psychodynamic perspective. On this occasion, the consultant arrived to find an apparently random discussion taking place about a recently introduced computerized assessment and selection tool developed to recruit junior doctors.

This new method of job-seeking had confronted doctors with a radical change in the regularized patterns of interaction, expectations (norms) and cohesive primary professional group support for managing an extremely significant career transition. It had been introduced without sufficient communication with the profession, whose leaders had warned of serious problems. Such apprehensions were confirmed, as doctors increasingly found themselves living in uncertainty regarding their futures. They also were concerned about the required online exposure of personal details and were intensely anxious about the severe disruptions to the group patterns of relationship that had enabled them to navigate a difficult stage in their medical training.

The Balint group members were coming to the end of their rotations and were clearly worried about their subsequent employment prospects. The consultant noted that they voiced their anxieties as though they were having a pre-group chat. Soon, one of the psychiatrists began to present a patient. This patient had been in the service for many years, but every time he seemed to his team to be ready for discharge he would act in a manner that would guarantee readmission. The presenting psychiatrist felt frustrated, upset and even angry with herself for feeling so critical towards her patient; she was unable to tolerate or talk to him about his behaviour. She added that the patient had always been in a state of total uncertainty regarding his life. He had experienced no family care and had been in institutions since childhood.

The consultant's intervention linked the psychiatrists' supposedly pre-group anxious preoccupation with their careers to the professional problem in relating to the patient. The patient's terrible history of lack of care and abandonment to institutional processes mirrored these psychiatrists' own current struggle with the effects of losing their accustomed group-based affiliations and patterns on which their professional and (to some extent) personal security depended. Their professional group and system dynamics had been transposed to the treatment setting, where the particular patient repeatedly expressed both the terror of separating from a familiar ward and hospital group and – what the psychiatrists could not put into action – a persistent capacity to control all attempts to make him face an uncertain, even bleak, future. Thinking about the intra- and intergroup interactions in this way supported the members of the Balint group to get more in touch with their own appropriate professional anxieties. They could begin to realize how this discussion of their worries, bringing them in from outside ('pre-group') to centre stage, could provide a model for how to approach the patient and his catastrophic separation anxieties in relation to the ward/treatment group.

GROUP PSYCHOTHERAPY

Just over a century ago, Joseph Hersey Pratt, a physician, conducted 'thought-control clinics' in which he lectured groups of patients with tuberculosis. Through his charismatic leadership, he taught them how to deal with their sputum and attempted to inspire them to live with their illness. Pratt observed the powerful impact of mutual encouragement and learning that inevitably developed among the group members; and with this combination of therapeutic leadership and supportive interpersonal interactions, he had inadvertently stumbled on the basic features of group psychotherapy. Pratt's example gave rise to a number of early, primarily psychoeducational, groups conducted by physicians and psychiatrists with a range of patients, including psychotics.[22] By the late 1920s and 1930s, and particularly during the Second World War,[1] the interest in groups mushroomed, to an extent that the literature – theoretical, clinical and research – became prodigious. A review found that 500–600 articles a year were published on groups in over 400 different sources.[23] Subsequently, the same author estimated that, overall, the group literature consisted of 'approximately 20,000 articles published in hundreds of different journals and thousands of books', while 'literally tens of thousands of psychologists, psychiatrists, social workers, and other mental health practitioners, as well as millions of clients, spend portions of their time in group psychotherapy or group counselling each week'.[24]

Our own review of the more recent literature from the main journals (*International Journal of Group Psychotherapy*, *Group Analysis*, *Group*, *Small Group Behavior*, *Group Dynamics: Theory, Research, and Practice*), covering the period 2001–07 amply confirms Dies' account. In out-patient and in-patient (setting), homogeneous and heterogeneous (patient diagnostic mix), exploratory and structured (therapeutic focus), time-limited and open-ended (duration), peer- and professional-led (leadership role), supportive, psychoeducational, cognitive-behavioural and psychodynamic (theoretical orientation) groups, an unimaginable range of patients are treated (see Montgomery[25] and Knauss[26] for further discussion of these group dimensions). Severely and persistently mentally ill patients; university students with bulimia; residents of nursing homes; gay male survivors of childhood sexual abuse living with human immunodeficiency virus (HIV)/acquired immunodeficiency syndrome (AIDS); patients with fibromyalgia; patients with eating disorders; patients with chronic physical illness; parents; mothers of aggressive children; psychosomatic patients; children with pervasive developmental disorders; homeless people; patients with cancer; traumatized adolescents; patients with bereavement and complicated grief reactions; children with learning disorders; adult survivors of childhood sexual abuse; patients with bipolar disorder; depressed elderly women; patients with post-traumatic stress disorder (PTSD); male spouse abusers; substance abusers; offenders; patients with co-morbidity ... this is only a sample of the types and number of patients treated in group psychotherapy. We will consider separately the indications for group psychotherapy below, but in general, research into group dropout, process and outcome indicates that diagnostic category is no obstacle to referral to a group:

> Thus, the age range and the range of diagnosis would not be considered in itself a problem unless the members were too different to be able to communicate with each other (rather rare, in our experience).[27]

The functioning of psychotherapy groups

The referring psychiatrist, according to the Royal College curriculum, should understand the principles and characteristics of group psychotherapy, and the therapeutic factors in groups, in order to explain this prospective treatment to patients. Our discussion of group dynamics has prepared the ground: group interaction, normative influence and cohesion are central to what happens in psychotherapy groups. Patients who are prepared for and able to participate in these dynamics are likely to derive most benefit from group psychotherapy. To re-emphasize their importance, we briefly consider the clinical theories of group psychotherapy of Yalom,[2] Foulkes[3] and Bion.[4] All reflect the key group dynamic elements, but each theoretical perspective illuminates one of them in a telling way.

From 1970, when the first edition of *The Theory and Practice of Group Psychotherapy* was published, until the (at the time of writing, most recent) fifth edition, Yalom[2] has kept the clinician and researcher in touch with the latest developments in the field. We have relied on his work in this chapter as the most up-to-date and comprehensive handbook for practitioners and referrers. For Yalom, the group is a social microcosm in which interpersonal interaction in the here and now plays the essential role. A patient's capacity to disclose, receive and give personal feedback, and to tolerate the revelation, understanding and reworking of distorted perceptions and interpersonal relationship patterns, indicate the patient's suitability for group treatment, whatever the diagnosis. Sooner or later, the patient will re-enact within the group those maladaptive aspects of his or her personality and symptoms for which he or she has consulted the psychiatrist, and they can be studied in depth as they affect the patient's relationships with other members of the group.

Based on his own and other research, Yalom has elaborated the most significant therapeutic factors. Some factors are inherent in groups, while others pertain to all forms of psychotherapy but take on a particular resonance in the group setting: instillation of hope, universality, imparting information, altruism, the corrective recapitulation of the primary family group, development of socializing techniques, identification/imitative behaviour, interpersonal learning, group cohesiveness, catharsis and existential factors. Of these overlapping and mutually enhancing factors, Yalom distils two vital, group-specific features, each of which potentiates the group as a holding environment (cohesiveness): the group as a here-and-now social microcosm of patients' lives, and the opportunities for therapeutic interventions to derive from member–member, not just therapist–member, interactions.

In the group, hope can come from seeing changes in others with similar problems to one's own, entirely absent in individual forms of treatment. The experience of finding that one is not a unique, irreparably damaged, repulsive or unworthy individual (universality); that, however low one's self-esteem, something one says to another group member is perceived as extremely valuable by the recipient (altruism); that the whole interpersonal configuration of patients' families, through the processes of transference and unconscious role induction, comes alive in the session – these are distinctive group phenomena. Furthermore, in a group, even the non-specific therapeutic factors become socially relevant: imitation of others' self-disclosure, honest, direct feedback, and accurate empathy contribute to a patient's development of social skills. The shared expression of deep feeling (catharsis) and the realization that everyone is to some degree alone, will struggle in life and will die (existential factors) can be especially poignant and meaningful in group psychotherapy, paradoxically helping individuals to overcome states of loneliness and isolation. Yalom's theory highlights how social interaction, connection and integration act as a protective factor and cites 'persuasive evidence that the rate for virtually every major cause of death is significantly higher for the lonely, the single, the divorced, and the widowed'.[2]

Foulkes, the founder of group analysis, propounded a clinical theory that fundamentally located the individual within group relationships, the social matrix. From Foulkes' perspective, there is no such thing as an abstract individual apart from his groups. The concepts of individual and group (society) are totally interrelated; they mutually constitute one another. No other theory so clearly views the individual as contained in and containing (internalizing) the social. Through cultural transmission, group norms are profoundly active inside individuals and make up their identities, patterning the forms of physical, temperamental, emotional and behavioural expression. Although Foulkes fully recognized, depending on the focus of investigation, the conceptual usefulness of distinguishing between a separate 'inside-the-individual' and 'outside-the-individual' (group/society), he suggested that this dichotomous approach could obscure a more complex reality. In this respect, for Foulkes, even the individual mind, inhering in a physical brain, is considered as a reification of mental processes occurring within a wider group network, like neurons interacting within a neural system and being affected by the electrical and chemical properties of the whole.

> This enabled me to say that it is mental processes, not persons, that interact... To do justice to the fact that this mental field of operation very much includes the individual but also transgresses him, I have used the term 'transpersonal processes'. These processes pass through the individual, though each individual elaborates them and contributes to them and modifies them in his own way. Nevertheless, they go through all the individuals – similar to X-rays in the physical sphere.[28]

The most important clinical implication of Foulkes' work is that the aetiology, development and maintenance of an individual's mental health and illness, including psychiatric symptomatology of all kinds, can be understood only by taking account of the group matrix within which wellbeing or psychopathology arises. Only by attention to the X-ray-like group norms, particularly those bearing on the deepest formation of identity, perception of self and others, the range of permissible relationship and feelings, pressures for self-sacrificial loyalty and compliance as opposed to creativity and freedom of thought, can the roots of maladaptive pathology and suffering be identified. This approach has long been accepted in systemic family (group) therapy. In child and family clinics, psychiatrists and other professionals evaluate a child as 'the identified patient', basically an unconsciously constructed (by others and the child) scapegoat whose symptoms play a vital role in securing family homeostasis. Parents, siblings and the child patient all turn out to be invested in keeping the focus away from multiple serious relationship issues and psychopathology of other family members. Treatment characteristically involves supporting others to relinquish their reluctance, often amounting to intense denial of any need, to open up communications within the family network. When this happens, the identified patient is usually freed up from his or her static, painful role, and other members are able to address their problems. The same principle applies fully in group psychotherapy of adults, whose every gesture, symptom and communication can be imbued with meaning when the specific interpersonal context of what seemed before a virtually autistic idiosyncrasy is made evident.

In *Experiences in Groups*, Bion made perhaps the greatest contribution to an understanding of group cohesion by delineating a ubiquitous and powerful type of cohesive group formation that conflicts with the positive cohesion/therapeutic rapport considered so important in group psychotherapy as a necessary condition for successful therapeutic work.[4] Bion's insight, quoted above, is that as group animals we have a built-in capacity to join with others, out of conscious awareness, in ways that undermine more realistic efforts to communicate and to work together. Feelings of vitality, power and even omnipotence can be achieved through such cohesive merger in the group (the depersonalization referred to by Freud[5]), and consequently group members may act in accordance with impulses and emotions that would never be expressed by any one of them as an individual. The group tasks, ultimate objectives and values may be subverted, as more mature forms of thinking and organizing give way to convictions bearing the stamp of reality solely on the basis of the degree of emotion invested in them. As conscious individuals, group members often fear and deny this aspect of their functioning: they are intimidated by their 'groupishness'.[4]

We believe that this form of group cohesion, potentially so destructive of development, can be turned to therapeutic advantage in group psychotherapy. Gordon has pointed to some neglected passages in *Experiences in Groups*, where Bion shows the direction of this positive clinical application.[29] To follow Bion here, the psychiatrist needs to be aware of a particular defence mechanism, projective identification, which is exceedingly prevalent in human relationships, individual and group. Projective identification involves an unconscious phantasy whereby the individual seeks to remove a feared, painful or endangered part of his or her personality or experience. Through 'psychic surgery', an intolerable emotion (grief) or a terrifying impulse (rage) is split off, disowned, from the personality and attributed to (projected into) an object, usually a person in the external world. That person, the recipient of the projected aspect, is identified and perceived as containing the disowned feeling or impulse and will accordingly be treated as, for example, needing consolation or extremely violent and dangerous. In addition to the phantasy of splitting off and projecting, the projector usually exerts real interpersonal pressure on the recipient to elicit feelings and responses in them that mirror the phantasy contents that have been externalized.[30–32]

In the psychotherapy group, Bion showed how members, including the therapist, are constantly and variously recruited by one another into 'playing a part, no matter how difficult to recognize, in somebody else's phantasy ...'.[4] The resulting dramas may, at a more mature level, be re-enactments of family scenes; but the more primitive and enmeshing cohesive configurations reflect the predominance of projective identificatory dispersion of problematic aspects of individuals' identities throughout the group.[33–35] Thus, one patient may be permanently locked into the 'competent' role, another enacts 'anguish', a third 'rage' and yet another 'withdrawal'. Each role or identity represents a fragment of a potentially whole, integrated personality that no patient is yet able to sustain. These configurations – in effect, the ways in which group members attempt to maintain stable, if conflictual, arrays of depersonalized cohesion – can be made the central focus of group exploration, leading to gradual reintegration of personality and concurrent development of realistic empathy in interpersonal relationships. Bion's work demonstrates how, when positive cohesion (the work group) prevails, analysis of the forms of negative cohesion becomes a royal road to therapeutic change.

Indications

On the basis of a considerable corpus of research literature (outcome and dropout studies, in particular) and clinical experience with a huge range of diagnoses and problems, the referring psychiatrist should adopt two approaches to the issue of selection of patients for group psychotherapy: (i) to focus on patient characteristics linked to positive outcome, and (ii) to deselect – to refer everyone except those patients for whom group interaction would be too intolerable or harmful. In order to best apply these perspectives, referrers should be aware of the types of group available in their settings in terms of the multiple dimensions already described (setting, patient mix, therapeutic focus, duration, leadership, theoretical orientation). This requires close collaboration of the psychiatrist with multidisciplinary colleagues and members of his or her own workgroup in order to ascertain whether, for example, even apparently highly unlikely group referrals such as a severely narcissistic patient, a patient with antisocial features, a paranoid personality disorder or a recovering but still hallucinating person with schizophrenia might be able to be placed in a mature, long-term psychodynamic group whose members would be able to contain such seductive, manipulative, aggressive or disturbing patients, who in turn would stimulate the established members to access deeper levels of their maladaptive relationship patterns.

In other words, indication/contraindication inevitably shades into the question of group composition, specifically a matter for the group psychotherapist but which the psychiatrist generally must keep in mind during a consultation. From this perspective, the referring psychiatrist might ask 'Is there a group that can contain this patient and with whose membership and task he or she might identify?' rather than 'Is this patient suitable for group psychotherapy?' Patient variables such as problem complexity, chronicity, functional impairment, coping style, resistance level and degree of distress[36–43] must all be treated as both relevant and relative to the answer the psychiatrist gives to this question.

However, patients with problems in relationships; those who may have failed in individual treatment because of too intense re-enactment of interpersonal pathology with the therapist, whether becoming overintensely intimate or eliciting repeated and intractable negative therapist responses;[44] those who intellectualize excessively and are unaware of their effects on others; those with high psychological mindedness, positive motivation and expectation of treatment;[2] and those with sufficient intelligence and capacity to communicate – or with time to develop this capacity – are all group referrals who could benefit particularly.

Regarding contraindication:

Here is the major guideline: *clients will fail in group therapy if they are unable to participate in the primary task of the group, be it for logistical, intellectual, psychological or interpersonal reasons.*[2]

This *may* include antisocial patients, suicidally depressed patients, and patients with acute situational crises or psychiatric emergencies;[2,44] vulnerable, easily wounded or intensely socially phobic patients;[45] patients with a history of poor attendance in therapy, intimacy problems generalized to extreme personal distrust, excessive use of denial or impulsive behaviour patterns;[24,46] and patients with grave inhibitions in raising or discussing important issues in the presence of others or intolerance of the limited amount of time exclusively devoted to the individual (need to share the therapist).[47] But each of these patient characteristics should be placed in context. If the psychiatrist integrates into the evaluation a survey of previous group memberships experienced by the patient throughout his or her life, the extent to which these features reach an exclusionary threshold for the specific groups at the psychiatrist's disposal should become apparent and can be discussed frankly with the patient.

One of the authors (JG) has for 15 years held two twice-weekly out-patient groups for patients with severe personality disorder. Only one patient out of over 100 referrals, who smoked 30 marijuana joints a day, was rejected, with the recommendation that he first attend to his substance abuse. Although the groups are part of a more comprehensive, hospital-based step-down treatment for personality disorder,[48] group dropout rates within 1 month are considerably lower than the average (8.8%; Yalom gives a rate of 17–57% in a wide range of groups[2]) under conditions in which virtually the only selection criterion is a patient's willingness to try. Nevertheless, clinical outcome and associated major reductions in health service use costs are exemplary for patients in these treatment groups.

CONCLUSION: EVIDENCE-BASED PRACTICE AND PRACTICE-BASED EVIDENCE

Yalom is characteristically upbeat about developments in the research evidence for group psychotherapy over a generation:

Does group therapy help clients? Indeed it does. A persuasive body of outcome research has demonstrated unequivocally that group therapy is a highly effective form of psychotherapy and that it is at least equal to individual psychotherapy in its power to provide meaningful benefit.[2]

In 116 chapter notes, many containing 10 or more individual research studies, Yalom goes a long way to backing his judgement. Although other commentators temper unbridled optimism with concerns about methodological complexities that render any long-term group psychotherapy research extremely daunting[41,49,50] – 'It is questionable whether it is possible on the basis of economic as well as practical and ethical reasons to create study designs for long-term dynamic therapies according to a randomized clinical trial model'[51] – several thorough surveys concur with Yalom's positive evaluation. It is also vital, when evaluating the evidence base, to realize that even randomized controlled trials of psychotherapeutic interventions typically exclude 45–50 per cent of patients.[52]

Lorentzen comments on the over half-century of systematic reviews of the group research literature.[53] From the 1960s, the positive effectiveness of group therapy compared with waiting-list and individual treatments was demonstrated. The development of meta-analysis, using a standardized measure, the effect size, confirmed these positive outcomes, as comparable effects – 0.90 for group and 0.76 for individual psychotherapy – were found. Summing up the period from 1960 to 1990, Lorentzen concluded that group psychotherapy had better outcomes than placebo or waiting list and was equivalent to individual and other psychological interventions. Tschuschke and colleagues confirm effect sizes beyond 1.3 for long-term, out-patient analytical group psychotherapy.[54]

Burlingame and colleagues, agreeing with these positive overall conclusions, also emphasize a consideration that, in the present era of financial constraints and managed healthcare, can only become more and more pertinent: the established cost-effectiveness of group psychotherapy.[55,56] This is both a tremendous advantage and a pitfall of group psychotherapy. MacKenzie, quoting Charles Dickens, called it 'the best of times [and] the worst of times' for group psychotherapy.[57] For although the increasing demand for group treatments should be excellent news, the fact that this development is a result of the primacy of cost-effectiveness over clinical experience – practice-based evidence – and careful evaluation of individual patients' long-term needs may threaten even the most evidence-based practices.

For example, the therapeutic community,[1,48,58–62] based on a rigorous integration of those principles of group dynamics and group psychotherapy highlighted in this chapter, seems to be going the way of many international in-patient psychotherapy settings, whose survival is affected as much by the reality of financial policies as by evidence-based imperatives. However, whatever happens to such exemplars of group dynamic and psychotherapeutic milieu treatment as the Henderson and the Cassel Hospitals, the psychiatrist should continue to view their day-hospital, out-patient and outreach group psychotherapy successors (and any in-patient groups that continue to be provided, especially for severely mentally ill patients) as highly effective and efficient treatment formats. It is now abundantly 'clear that psychotherapy can induce robust changes that are detectable with neuro-imaging'[63] (see also Spence[64]). Such research findings may herald an end to the radical separation of psychiatry and psychotherapy.[65] But beyond the question of treatment outcome, psychiatrists must remain alert to their own inescapable group memberships and the ubiquitous intra- and intergroup dynamics within the hospital or community setting. Whatever the specific mix of clinical interventions deployed, including group psychotherapy, the process and outcome of patients' treatment will depend on this overarching awareness.

KEY POINTS

- Human beings are group animals through and through.
- Group membership crucially affects how we feel, perceive, think and behave.
- All groups have tasks, and interpersonal interaction patterns within groups may facilitate or undermine the achievement of group objectives.
- Groups are characterized by conscious and unconscious norms: rules and sanctions regarding how members should interact.
- Group cohesiveness refers to the sense of affiliation and belonging which members experience.
- The more cohesive the group, the more its members will comply with the group norms.
- Cohesiveness can contribute to effective group development or prevent it, depending on the nature of the norms.
- Symptoms – including psychiatric instability – can arise in individuals from either a too intense compliance with maladaptive group interaction patterns or from a loss of regular group interactions which bolster secure identity.
- Effective psychotherapy groups encourage specific interpersonal interactions based on norms of disclosure, the reception and giving of feedback and the toleration, understanding and reworking of distorted perceptions.
- The theoretical and clinical work of Yalom, Foulkes and Bion are central to the development of group psychotherapy.
- Research in group therapy indicates considerable effectiveness, and selection (i.e. finding a group with which a particular patient can identify) is a crucial consideration.
- Patient variables such as problem complexity, chronicity, functional impairment, coping style, resistance level and degree of distress are relevant and relative to the extent to which a patient can identify with the membership and task of a particular group.
- Group dynamics in general pervade all mental health settings; we live and work in groups so all psychiatrists need to understand them, even if they do not specialize in group psychotherapy.

ACKNOWLEDGEMENT

The authors would like to thank Dr Lakshmiramana Alla, Dr Reshma Inamdar and Dr Himanshu Tyagi, and especially Dr Paul Gilluley, Consultant Forensic Psychiatrist, for their valuable comments on a preliminary draft of this chapter.

REFERENCES

1. Whiteley JS, Gordon J (1979) *Group Approaches in Psychiatry*. London: Routledge & Kegan Paul.
2. Yalom ID, with Leszcz M (2005) *The Theory and Practice of Group Psychotherapy*, 5th edn. New York: Basic Books.
3. Foulkes SH (1964) *Therapeutic Group Analysis*. London: Allen & Unwin.
4. Bion WR (1961) *Experiences in Groups*. London: Tavistock Publications.
5. Freud S (1921) *Group Psychology and the Analysis of the Ego*. London: Hogarth Press and Institute of Psychoanalysis.
6. Dodds ER (1951) *The Greeks and the Irrational*. Berkeley, CA: University of California Press.
7. Elias N (1991) *The Society of Individuals*. London: Basil Blackwell.
8. Homans GC (1992) *The Human Group*. New Brunswick: Transaction Publishers.
9. Hare AP (1962) *Handbook of Small Group Research*. New York: Free Press.
10. Jacques E (1955) Social systems as a defence against persecutory and depressive anxiety. In M Klein, P Heimann, RE Money-Kyrle (eds) *New Directions in Psycho-Analysis*. London: Tavistock Publications.
11. Menzies I (1960) A case-study in the functioning of social systems as a defence against anxiety. *Human Relations* **13**: 95–121. [Reprinted in Menzies I (1988) *Containing Anxiety in Institutions: Selected Essays*, Vol. 1. London: Free Association Press.]
12. Obholzer A, Roberts VZ (1994) *The Unconscious at Work*. London: Routledge & Kegan Paul.
13. Holmes J, Mizen S, Jacobs C (2007) Psychotherapy training for psychiatrists: UK and global perspectives. *International Review of Psychiatry* **19**: 93–100.
14. Mills TM (1962) *The Sociology of Small Groups*. Englewood Cliffs, NJ: Prentice-Hall.
15. Sherif M (1936) *The Psychology of Social Norms*. New York: Harper & Row.
16. Asch SE (1951) Effects of group pressure upon the modification and distortion of judgements. In D Cartwright, A Zander (eds) *Group Dynamics: Research and Theory*, 2nd edn. London: Tavistock Publications.
17. Dion KL (2000) Group cohesion: from 'field of forces' to multidimensional construct. *Group Dynamics: Theory, Research, and Practice* **4**: 7–26.

18. Joyce AS, Piper WE, Ogrodniczuk JS (2007) Therapeutic alliance and cohesion variables as predictors of outcome in short-term group psychotherapy. *International Journal of Group Psychotherapy* **57**: 269–96.
19. Sandahl C (2008) Alliance to the group-as-a-whole as a predictor of outcome in psychodynamic group therapy. *International Journal of Group Psychotherapy* **58**: 163–84.
20. Whyte WF (1943) *Street Corner Society: The Social Structure of an Italian Slum*. Chicago: University of Chicago Press.
21. Newcomb TM (1943) *Personality and Social Change*. New York: Dryden.
22. Ettin MF (1999) *Foundations and Applications of Group Psychotherapy: A Sphere of Influence*. London: Jessica Kingsley Publishers.
23. Dies RR (2001) Commentary on my editorship (1985–1992). *International Journal of Group Psychotherapy* **51**: 161–4.
24. Dies RR (2003) Group psychotherapies. In AS Gurman, SB Messer (eds) *Essential Psychotherapies: Theory and Practice*, 2nd Edn. New York: Guilford Press.
25. Montgomery C (2002) Role of dynamic group therapy in psychiatry. *Advances in Psychiatric Treatment* **8**: 34–41.
26. Knauss W (2005) Group psychotherapy. In GO Gabbard, JS Beck, J Holmes (eds) *Oxford Textbook of Psychiatry*. Oxford: Oxford University Press.
27. Agazarian YM (2005) Destructive forces: cuckoo interrupted. In L Motherwell, JJ Shay (eds) *Complex Dilemmas in Group Therapy: Pathways to Resolution*. New York: Brunner/Routledge.
28. Foulkes SH (1973) The group as matrix of the individual's mental life. In LR Wolberg, EK Schwartz (eds) *Group Therapy 1973: An Overview*. New York: Intercontinental Medical Book Corporation.
29. Gordon J (in press) Some neglected clinical material from Bion's *Experiences in Groups*. In C Mawson (ed) *Bion Today*. London: Routledge and Institute of Psychoanalysis.
30. Klein M (1946) Notes on some schizoid mechanisms. *International Journal of Psychoanalysis* **27**: 99–110. [Reprinted in: Klein M (1975) *The Writings of Melanie Klein*, Vol. 3. London: Hogarth Press.]
31. Ogden TH (1979) On projective identification. *International Journal of Psychoanalysis* **60**: 357–73.
32. Ogden TH (1982) *Projective Identification and Psychotherapeutic Technique*. New York: Jason Aronson.
33. Gordon J, Adebakin D, Jones A (1994) 'The depot group': mutual injection of emotion in community psychiatry. *Group Analysis* **27**: 449–57.
34. Gordon J (1994) Bion's post-*Experiences in Groups* thinking on groups: a clinical example of –K. In VL Schermer, M Pines (eds) *Ring of Fire: Primitive Affects and Object Relations in Group Psychotherapy*. London, York: Routledge & Kegan Paul.
35. Gordon J (1999) Paula Heimann's question and group analysis. *Psychoanalytic Psychotherapy* **13**: 107–16.
36. Piper WE, McCallum M, Joyce AS, *et al.* (2001) Patient personality and time-limited group psychotherapy for complicated grief. *International Journal of Group Psychotherapy* **51**: 525–52.
37. Ogrodniczuk JS, Piper WE, McCallum M, *et al.* (2002) Interpersonal predictors of group therapy outcome for complicated grief. *International Journal of Group Psychotherapy* **52**: 511–35.
38. Lorentzen S, Hoglend P (2002) The change process of a patient in long-term group psychotherapy: measuring and describing the change process. *Group Analysis* **35**: 500–524.
39. Lorentzen S, Hoglend P (2005) Predictors of change after long-term analytic group psychotherapy. *Journal of Clinical Psychology* **61**: 1541–54.
40. Clarkin JF, Levey KN (2004) The influence of client variables on psychotherapy. In MJ Lambert (ed) *Bergin and Garfield's Handbook of Psychotherapy and Behavior Change*, 5th edn. New York: John Wiley & Sons.
41. Beutler LE, Consoli AJ, Lame G (2005) Systematic treatment selection and prescriptive psychotherapy: an integrative approach. In JC Norcross, MR Goldfried (eds) *Handbook of Psychotherapy Integration*, 2nd edn. New York: Oxford University Press.
42. Hannan C, Lambert M, Harmon C, *et al.* (2005) A lab test and algorithms for identifying clients at risk for treatment failure. *Journal of Clinical Psychology* **61**: 1–9.
43. Visintini R, Ubbiali A, Donati D, *et al.* (2007) Referral to group psychotherapy: a retrospective study of patients' personality features associated with clinicians' judgements. *International Journal of Group Psychotherapy* **57**: 515–52.
44. Clarkin JF (2005) Differential therapeutics. In JC Norcross, MR Goldfried (eds) *Handbook of Psychotherapy Integration*, 2nd edn. New York: Oxford University Press.
45. Rutan JS (2005) Treating difficult patients in groups. In L Motherwell, JJ Shay (eds) *Complex Dilemmas in Group Therapy: Pathways to Resolution*. New York: Brunner/Routledge.
46. Dies RR (1993) Research on group psychotherapy: overview and clinical applications. In A Alonso, HI Swiller (eds) *Group Therapy in Clinical Practice*. Washington, DC: American Psychiatric Press.
47. Feldman LB, Feldman S (2005) Integrating therapeutic modalities. In JC Norcross, MR Goldfried (eds) *Handbook of Psychotherapy Integration*, 2nd edn. New York: Oxford University Press.
48. Chiesa M, Fonagy P, Holmes J (2003) When more is less: an exploration of psychoanalytically oriented hospital-based treatment for severe personality disorder. *International Journal of Psychoanalysis* **84**: 637–50.
49. Toseland RW, Siporin M (1986) When to recommend group treatment: a review of the clinical and research literature. *International Journal of Group Psychotherapy* **36**: 171–201.

50. Tschuschke V, Dies RR (1994) Intensive analysis of therapeutic factors and outcome in long-term inpatient groups. *International Journal of Group Psychotherapy* **44**: 185–208.
51. Lorentzen S, Bogwald KP, Hoglend P (2002) Change during and after long-term analytic group psychotherapy. *International Journal of Group Psychotherapy* **52**: 419–29.
52. Westen D, Morrison K Thompson BH (2005) The empirical status of empirically supported psychotherapies: assumptions, findings, and reporting in controlled clinical trials. *Psicoterapia e scienze umane* **39**: 7–90.
53. Lorentzen S (2006) Contemporary challenges for research in group analysis. *Group Analysis* **39**: 321–40.
54. Tschuschke V, Anbeh T, Kiencke P (2007) Evaluations of long-term analytic outpatient group therapies. *Group Analysis* **40**: 140–59.
55. Burlingame GM, MacKenzie KR, Strauss B (2004) Small group treatment: evidence for effectiveness and mechanisms of change. In MJ Lambert (ed) *Bergin and Garfield's Handbook of Psychotherapy and Behavior Change*, 5th edn. New York: John Wiley & Sons.
56. Burlingame GM, Krogel JA (2005) Relative efficacy of individual versus group psychotherapy. *International Journal of Group Psychotherapy* **55**: 607–11.
57. MacKenzie KR (2001) An expectation of radical changes in the future of group psychotherapy. *International Journal of Group Psychotherapy* **51**: 176–80.
58. Main TF (1946) The hospital as a therapeutic institution. *Bulletin of the Menninger Clinic* **10**: 65–70.
59. Main TF (1957) 'The ailment'. *British Journal of Medical Psychology* **30**: 129–45.
60. Jones M (1968) *Social Psychiatry in Practice: The Ideal of the Therapeutic Community.* Harmondsworth: Penguin Books.
61. Hinshelwood RD (1987) *What Happens in Groups: Psychoanalysis, the Individual and the Community.* London: Free Association Books.
62. Norton K (1992) A culture of inquiry: its preservation or loss. *Therapeutic Communities* **13**: 3–25.
63. Etkin A, Pittenger CJ, Kandel ER (2005) Biology in the service of psychotherapy. In JM Oldham, AE Skodol, DS Bender (eds) *The American Psychiatric Publishing Textbook of Personality Disorders.* Arlington, VA: American Psychiatric Publishing.
64. Spence S (2006) All in the mind? The neural correlates of unexplained physical symptoms. *Advances in Psychiatric Treatment* **12**: 349–58.
65. Kandel ER (1998) A new intellectual framework for psychiatry. *American Journal of Psychiatry* **155**: 457–69.

Chapter 65

Cognitive-behavioural therapy

Rebecca Martinez and Chris Williams

INTRODUCTION

After reading this chapter, you will:

- understand the principles and techniques used in cognitive-behavioural therapy (CBT);
- be able to describe behavioural interventions and when they are indicated;
- know when and how to make an appropriate referral for CBT;
- be able to explain to a patient what CBT entails if they are referred for treatment.

CBT is a form of psychotherapy developed by Aaron 'Tim' Beck in the 1960s. In his seminal book *Cognitive Therapy and the Emotional Disorders*, Beck states that psychological problems may result from commonplace processes such as:[1]

- faulty learning;
- making incorrect inferences on the basis of inadequate or incorrect information;
- not distinguishing adequately between imagination and reality;
- thought processes occurring as a result of erroneous premises;
- behaviours that are self-defeating because they are based on unreasonable attitudes.

CBT is characterized by:

- being short-term, problem-focused therapy;
- using step-by-step clear interventions;
- being psychoeducational in nature;
- working by asking effective questions and seeking the right information at the right time;
- a clear underlying model and structure;
- a focus on current problems;
- building on the relationship with the practitioner.

CBT has been researched extensively in a number of different disorders and is recommended for practice by the National Institute for Health and Clinical Excellence (NICE) and Scottish Intercollegiate Guidelines Network (SIGN) guidelines for the following disorders (www.guidance.nice.org.uk/topic/behavioural):

- Anxiety
- Depression
- Panic
- Agoraphobia and other phobias
- Social phobia
- Bulimia
- Obsessive–compulsive disorder (OCD)
- Post-traumatic stress disorder (PTSD).

In addition CBT can be delivered in various self-help formats. These include the following:

- *Written (bibliotherapy) books and workbooks:* currently recommended for use for mild to moderate depression[2] and anxiety.[3]
- *Computerized CBT (CCBT):* the NICE CCBT guidelines[4] recommend the use of CCBT products, with no specific named products suggested. They accept the concept that CCBT has a class effect and that any competently produced package can be effective with support. Such packages include Mood Gym (www.moodgym.anu.edu.au/welcome) and Living Life to the Full (www.livinglifetothefull.com) both free, as well as paid for licenced products such as Beating the Blues (www.beatingtheblues.co.uk) and Fearfighter (www.fearfighter.com).

There is likely to be a significant increase in the delivery of such approaches as part of the English health service emphasis on increasing access to psychological therapies (IAPT) and National Health Service (NHS) Living Life in Scotland where www.livinglifetothefull.com is provided with telephone support from NHS24 staff (the equivalent of NHS Direct in England).

There are no differences in effectiveness between written and computerized self-help approaches, and it is likely that the delivery options for self-help should be based on patient preference.[5]

HOW DOES CBT WORK?

The assessment model based on five key areas provides a clear structure within which to summarize the range of problems and difficulties faced by people.[6] It emphasizes the links between each of the following components:

- Life situation, relationships and practical problems
- Altered thinking
- Altered emotions (also called mood or feelings)
- Altered physical feelings and symptoms
- Altered behaviour or activity levels.

Think of a depressed person with whom you are working at the moment. What do they:

- feel emotionally?
- feel physically?
- say?
- do and not do?

What life situations do they often face?

Use the language they would use and summarize their problems in Figure 65.1.

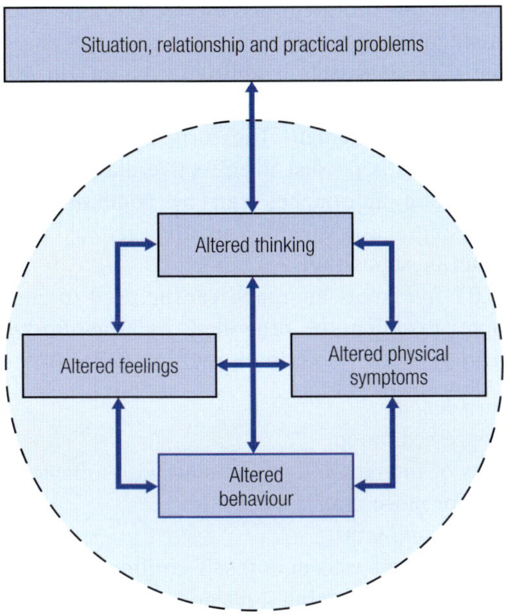

Figure 65.1 Five areas model

Reproduced with permission of Dr Chris Williams (2006) from www.livinglifetothefull.com.

The assessment from a cognitive-behavioural perspective contains all of the elements shown in Figure 65.1, and they form the initial formulation of the patient's difficulties. From a CBT perspective, it is also important to think about how each of the areas interacts with the others and the impact that they may be having in the patient's life. It is useful to think of this five areas assessment as a vicious circle. Problems in any of the areas create and worsen difficulties in the other areas too. This is also a major strength, because it means that making helpful changes in any area is likely to lead to improvement in other areas as well.

CONTENT OF THOUGHTS IN DIFFERENT EMOTIONAL STATES

Experimental research data have confirmed that both the processing styles and the content of thinking vary in different emotional states.[7,8]

Characteristic changes in thinking in depression

Patients with depression are more negative about things when compared with other clinical groups and controls.[9,10] The CBT model proposes the negative cognitive triad:

- Negative view of self
- Negative view of the world
- Negative view of the future.

The following cognitive processes exist in depression:

- Patients with depression have impaired problem-solving skills.
- They take longer to retrieve positive memories and are more readily able to access negative memories.[11] This might explain the common clinical situation when such patients tell you that they have 'done nothing' over recent weeks, despite evidence to the contrary – they are simply remembering the negative and overlooking the things that they have achieved ('negative memory bias').

These thoughts lead to altered behaviour such as reduced activity or unhelpful behaviours such as drinking or cutting to block how they feel.

Characteristic changes in thinking in anxiety disorders

For patients with anxiety disorders (panic disorder, agoraphobia, generalized anxiety, OCD, phobic disorders), the following are common thinking themes:

- Increased perception of danger and threat
- Decreased perception of their own ability to cope with that danger.

Typical thoughts and images include themes of:

- vulnerability;
- loss of control;
- fear of social ridicule;
- physical harm;
- death (e.g. in a panic attack).

In terms of how information is processed, anxious patients are more prone to:

- scan for potential threats;
- have lower thresholds for noticing potential threats.

The result might include the following changes in behaviours:

- Avoidance of anxiety-provoking situations (including people, places and events)
- Start of unhelpful behaviours such as:
  - reassurance-seeking;
  - drinking to excess;
  - misusing sedative medication.

IMPACT OF THOUGHTS ON EMOTIONS

The CBT model emphasizes the reciprocal links between mood state (e.g. anxiety or depression) and altered thinking. Either can affect the other. Thus, adverse changes in mood are associated with extreme and unhelpful thoughts (i.e. thoughts that are more negative or catastrophic). For example, if an individual experiences thoughts such as:

- 'Other people do not like me',
- 'I am inferior to others',
- 'The future is bleak' or
- 'Everything always goes wrong',

then they are likely to feel more anxious or depressed.

Similarly, if mood changes for the worse, then thinking is likely to become more extreme and unhelpful. In this way, a reciprocal relationship is established between extreme thinking and altered mood. Clinically, asking the person 'What went though your mind when you noticed feeling angry/sad/anxious/ashamed?' can help the person to identify upsetting thoughts.

One way of describing such thoughts is negative automatic thoughts. This implies that, during times of low mood, upsetting thoughts pop into the mind more frequently and are harder to dismiss than non-upsetting thoughts. A more user-friendly concept is the idea of 'extreme and unhelpful thoughts'. These are thoughts that make you feel worse, or alter what you do.

What people think can affect what they do

Extreme thoughts may lead individuals to reduce or stop doing activities that previously gave them a sense of pleasure or achievement, or to start doing things that actually worsen how they feel.[6] This establishes a reciprocal relationship between extreme thinking and reduced/avoided activities or unhelpful behaviours.

> I'll never pass the MRCPsych → Give up revising and start watching too much television

Based on this, psychological problems may be tackled by noticing these patterns, correcting misconceptions and learning more helpful attitudes through processes such as reality-testing, introspection and learning. As all of these are cognitive processes, this form of therapy has therefore come to be known as 'cognitive therapy'.

THE CBT FORMULATION (COGNITIVE CONCEPTUALIZATION)

In CBT terms, a formulation is a shared understanding between the therapist or practitioner and the patient about the patient's difficulties, how they came about and what is keeping them going. The formulation acts as a sort of map to guide treatment. CBT is a collaborative form of therapy, which means that the therapist and patient together can discuss and decide on appropriate actions and plans.

CBT can help your patients to make sense of overwhelming problems by breaking them down into smaller parts. This makes it easier to see how they are connected and how they affect your patients. It can also be helpful to see how making changes in one of the five areas can result in improvements in other areas.

Generic CBT skills provide a readily accessible model for patient assessment and management and can usefully inform general clinical skills in everyday practice. CBT can therefore provide an integrated biopsychosocial assessment and management approach.

In the CBT approach, cognitive content or processes, emotional responses and behaviour are all seen as being important for assessment. The form of symptoms is still assessed, as this is needed for effective diagnosis. The CBT and diagnostic approaches can be combined, however, within a single assessment and are seen as compatible rather than in opposition.

The CBT five areas approach can be used to summarize depressive disorder as described by the *International Classification of Diseases*, tenth revision (ICD-10)[12]:

- *Altered mood:*
  - Depressed mood
  - Loss of interest and enjoyment, with anhedonia present for more than 2 weeks
- *Altered thinking:*
  - Reduced self-esteem and self-confidence
  - Thoughts concerning guilt and unworthiness
  - Bleak and pessimistic views of the future
  - Ideas of self-harm
- *Altered physical symptoms:*
  - Diurnal variation of mood
  - Early-morning wakening and disturbed sleep
  - Diminished or increased appetite or weight
  - Loss of libido, fatigue and reduced energy
  - Reduced attention and concentration
  - Constipation
- *Altered behaviour:*
  - Acts of deliberate self-harm or suicide
  - Reduced social activity/work/domestic activities.

A full CBT formulation will contain other elements, as illustrated below, that will help understand how the person has developed these difficulties, what is happening now and what keeps them going (Figure 65.2). Each of the elements of the formulation is explained below.

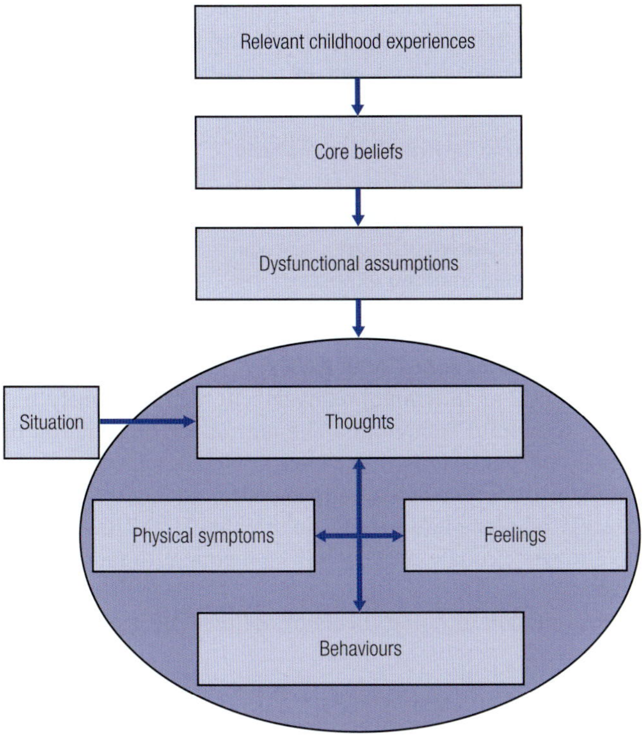

Figure 65.2 Cognitive-behavioural therapy (CBT) formulation

SOME TRADITIONAL CBT DEFINITIONS

- *Relevant childhood data:* aspects of the person's early experience that may have an impact on their current difficulties, beliefs and recurrent patterns of behaviour.
- *Core beliefs:* beliefs and statements that the individual makes about the self or the world. They tend to be global, overgeneralized and absolute, e.g. 'I am useless', 'You can't trust anyone'.
- *Conditional assumptions/dysfunctional assumptions/ beliefs/rules:* these are deeper-seated than automatic thoughts and are 'understandings about how the world works'; they may take the form of 'should' or 'must' statements, or they may be expressed as conditional, in the form 'If ..., then ...', e.g. 'If you don't please everyone, then they will be upset with you', 'I must never complain'.

NEGATIVE AUTOMATIC THOUGHTS AND FORMS OF COGNITIVE BIAS

The cognitive model states that it is our interpretation of a particular situation, rather than the situation itself, that may lead to distress. These interpretations of situations are usually manifested in the form of thoughts, which may be verbal in form or reflect images (black and white, colour, moving, still) or memories.

The term 'automatic thoughts' refers to the stream of consciousness. These thoughts are the overt thoughts that go through a person's mind at a given time.

People experiencing psychological difficulties may distort situations that could otherwise have been conceived as neutral. This is due to certain biases in the thinking patterns, also known as thinking errors or cognitive distortions.

Commonly seen cognitive distortions

(Adapted from Beck.[13])

- *All-or-nothing thinking (back and white thinking):* a situation is viewed under only two categories rather than on a continuum, e.g. 'Unless I do everything right, I am a failure').
- *Catastrophizing:* predicting worse-possible consequences without considering other possible outcomes, e.g. 'If I fail this exam, I will lose my job'.
- *Discounting the positive:* positive experiences or qualities are frequently discounted, e.g. 'I did well in my last exam, but that was just luck'.
- *Emotional reasoning:* thinking that something is true just because it 'feels' true, e.g. 'I feel like such a failure'.
- *Labelling:* giving a global label either to oneself or to others, without considering all the evidence available, e.g. 'I am an idiot'.
- *Magnification/minimization:* a way of manipulating the evidence by magnifying (overly focusing on) the negatives or minimizing (playing down) the positives about a given situation, e.g. 'Anyone can get a good reference'.
- *Selective abstraction:* being unable to see the whole picture, and instead focusing on one particular detail ('mental filter'), e.g. 'That (one) spelling mistake in my essay, means that I am such a bad student'.
- *Mind-reading:* believing that you know what other people are thinking, e.g. 'They think that I can't do anything right'.
- *Overgeneralization:* assuming that, because something has happened once, it will happen again, e.g. 'I can never do anything right'.
- *Personalization:* believing that other people's actions are because of you or something you have done, e.g. 'My colleague didn't stop to talk to me – maybe I have done something wrong'.

FORMULATING A TREATMENT PLAN

The cognitive formulation will help to identify problematic areas in the person's difficulties, which contribute to or help to maintain the problem. Once these areas have been identified, they can become a target for change, and the therapist and patient will use relevant techniques to tackle these difficulties. The areas that may be tackled may be in the cognitive or the behavioural domains – or in other key aspects of the person's life, such as relationships, physically or emotionally (i.e. in any of the five areas).

Cognitive techniques

Cognitive techniques focus on the identification and challenge of negative automatic thoughts. This is done during the encounter with the therapist, which will help to guide the patient through the process.

A technique of dialogue with the patient commonly used in CBT is guided discovery, also known as 'Socratic questioning'. This asks questions to help the person discover or work out the links between their thoughts and how they are and to discover new ways of understanding these.

CBT uses a tool commonly know as the 'thought record' to evaluate and challenge a distressing thought and to help the patient come up with an alternative, more balanced thought (Table 65.1).

It is important for both the patient and the therapist to decide whether to focus on a particular thought, as people have thousands of thoughts in any one day. It is important to work on those thoughts that are associated with situations that have been particularly emotionally charged and upsetting or disruptive for the patient.

Cognitive techniques such as the thought record are commonly used by cognitive-behavioural therapists in a range of disorders. The thought record helps the patient to engage and to become aware of how the cognitive model works in practice.

Behavioural techniques

Behavioural interventions

Behavioural interventions target specific problematic behaviours that are targeted for change.

The initial basis for the development of behavioural techniques was rooted in the theories of operant conditioning. *Operant* conditioning forms an association between behaviour and a consequence. The nature of the consequence will determine whether the behaviour is reinforced or not.

Reduced activity, such as reducing things that used to give a sense of fun, pleasure, achievement, mastery or closeness to others, and unhelpful behaviours, such as drinking to excess, comfort eating, self-cutting, lashing out or withdrawing from others, can continue to affect the individual's mood and energy levels and can maintain the difficulties that they are experiencing.

Using the operant conditioning model, one may understand that individuals who, for example, have a spider phobia would avoid spiders, as in their experience they have learnt the association between spiders and adverse consequences (i.e. symptoms of extreme anxiety). This pattern can be corrected using behavioural techniques.

Unhelpful behaviours can be identified and challenged using a number of behavioural interventions, such as:

- behavioural or functional analysis;
- behavioural activation and activity diaries;
- behavioural experiments;
- systematic desensitization, also called progressive exposure/graded and cue exposure;
- habituation.

Behavioural or functional analysis

Behavioural or functional analysis will help to identify relevant unhelpful behaviours. The aim of the behavioural or functional analysis is to review the details of each of the problem or target behaviours in order to understand the process of precipitation and maintenance, and then to be able to work collaboratively with the patient to tackle these areas.

One method of doing this is to use the ABC approach.[14]

- *A:* antecedents
- *B:* behaviours and beliefs
- *C:* consequences.

When doing this with a patient, it is useful to get the patient to reflect about a recent example and to give as much detail as possible about their understanding of the situation.

Behavioural activation and activity diaries

An *activity diary* may help to assess the types of activity that the patient is currently engaging in and those that they:

- avoid as a result of anxiety;
- have reduced doing, e.g. because of symptoms of depression.

It can also be used to establish the links between certain activities and changes in mood states.

In this way, it is important to collaborate with the patient to establish goals that relate to their activities and those that they are avoiding. Some diaries also allow the person to rate their activities for pleasure, achievement and closeness to others. The activity diary is a useful tool to incorporate activity-scheduling and to monitor regularly the progress that is being made. An example of an activity diary is shown in Table 65.2, and copies of an activity diary and blank five areas assessment sheets can be downloaded free of charge from www.fiveareas.com.

There is a growing evidence base for the use of behavioural activation in depression.[15] The so-called dismantling studies that have examined separately the added benefits of offering cognitive, behavioural or combined cognitive-behavioural approaches suggest that, at least for depression, behavioural activation appears to be as effective as a treatment of depression as offering the full CBT model.[15]

Table 65.1 Thought investigation or thought challenge worksheet

1. Situation/relationship or practical problem when your mood altered	2. Altered emotional and physical feelings	3. What immediate thoughts are present at the time?	4. What unhelpful thinking style(s) occur?	5. Impact of the immediate thought(s)
Think in detail: where am I and what am I doing? Consider: • *The time:* what time of day is it? • *The place:* Where am I? • *The people:* who is present? Who am I with? • *The events:* what has been said? What events happened?	Am I: • Low or sad? Guilty? • Worried, tense, anxious or panicky? • Angry or irritable? • Ashamed or suspicious? (i) State the feelings clearly. Try to be as precise as possible. If more than one feeling occurs, underline the most powerful feeling. (ii) How powerful is this feeling (0–100%)? (iii) Note down any strong physical sensations you notice.	What is going through my mind? How do I see: • Myself? How do others see me? • The current events/situation? • What might happen in the future? • My own body, behaviour or performance? • Any memories or images? (i) State the thought(s) clearly. Try to be as precise as possible. If more than one thought occurs, underline the most powerful thought. (ii) Rate how strongly you believe the most powerful thought at the time (0–100%).	• Bias against myself • Putting a negative slant on things (*negative mental filter*) • Having a gloomy view of the future or jumping to the worst conclusion? • Negative view about how others see me (*mind-reading*) • Bearing all responsibility • Making extreme statements and rules, e.g. using 'must', 'should', 'ought', 'always' and 'never' statements If any of these styles is present, then you have identified an *extreme thought*	(i) What did I do differently? Consider any: • Reduced activity • Unhelpful behaviours (ii) What was the impact on: • Myself? • My view of others? • How I felt? • What I said? • What I did? Overall, was the impact helpful or unhelpful? If there is an unhelpful impact, you have identified an *unhelpful thought*
Situation:	(i) *My feelings:* (ii) *Powerfulness:* 0–100% = (iii) *Physical sensations:*	(i) *My immediate thought(s):* if you have noticed more than one thought, underline the most powerful thought (ii) Rate your belief in the most powerful thought at the time: 0–100% =	*Which unhelpful thinking styles are present?* (state numbers or types)	(i) *What did I do differently?* (ii) *Overall, is it helpful or unhelpful for me to believe the thought?*

Table 65.2 Example: Anne's activity diary

Date and time	Activity (include everything you do)	Duration: how long did you do it for?	Pleasure felt: 0 = no pleasure, 10 = maximum pleasure	How much of an achievement was it, given how you feel? 0 = no sense of achievement, 10 = maximum sense of achievement	How much of a sense of closeness did you feel? 0 = no sense of closeness, 10 = maximum sense of closeness
6–7 a.m.	In bed asleep	7 h	–	–	–
7–8 a.m.	Woke up and listened to the radio	30 min	1	2	5 (favourite DJ)
8–9 a.m.	Got up and had a shower, cleaned my teeth	40 min	3	6	1
9–10 a.m.	Made a coffee	15 min	5	5	0
10–11 a.m.	Watched television	90 min	4	2	2
11–12 p.m.	Watched television	50 min	5	2	2
12–1 p.m.	Friend called by and made them a drink	45 min	7	8	8

Scale: 0 – no pleasure/achievement; 5 – feel okay/reasonable; 10 – maximum pleasure/achievement.

Reproduced by permission of Dr Chris Williams.

Behavioural experiments

Behavioural experiments help patients to collect real-life evidence in order to test out or refute their underlying assumptions and rules. Behavioural experiments can be very effective at producing both emotional and cognitive shifts. The *Oxford Guide to Behavioural Experiments* provides detailed and useful guides to setting up behavioural experiments and tasks in a collaborative manner with clients:[16]

- Practitioners need to present a rationale for conducting the experiment, e.g. that experiments are needed in order to collect solid data regarding central problems and situations.
- The practitioner and patient, collaboratively, are seen as co-investigators, working together to design real-world experiments that test out the validity and utility of dysfunctional cognitions (thoughts, underlying assumptions, and family and cultural rules are amenable to this as well).
- Experiments can take place during a session or set for homework.
- Presenting a rationale, grading tasks and making a task fail-proof can motivate the patient to try it out to see what happens.

When setting up a behavioural experiment, the following steps should be followed:

1. Identify the thought or assumption to be tested – write it down.
2. Brainstorm possible experiments with the patient to come up with activities that will challenge the assumption.
3. If necessary, grade the activities. Start with something easy and make it fail-proof – don't set your patient up for failure.
4. Plan the experiment – specifics, how, when, what, etc.
5. Write down the patient's predictions of the outcome of the experiment ('What do you think will happen?').
6. Carry out the experiment.
7. Record the outcomes.
8. Repeat if necessary, collecting more and more evidence.
9. Analyse the outcomes with the patient.

It is important to keep written records of the experiments. Examples of worksheets on behavioural experiments can be found in the CBT self-help literature and provide a helpful record of the experiment.[17]

Systematic desensitization

This process was described by Wolpe.[18] Initially the patient is taught relaxation techniques, followed by the elaboration of a collaborative hierarchy of feared stimuli with the patient. The patient is encouraged to progress step by step with exposure to each of the stimuli in the hierarchy, starting with those that are predicted to produce lower levels of anxiety, and progressing to those that produce higher levels of anxiety. While they do this, the patient maintains the relaxation, which will *reciprocally inhibit* the fear response.

In reciprocal inhibition, a response that is antagonistic or incompatible to anxiety (e.g. relaxation) is present when the stimulus is presented, and then there is a subsequent reduction of the anxiety response.

Graded and cue exposure (progressive exposure)

Graded exposure is a form of exposure treatment in which the patient and therapist collaboratively create a list or graded hierarchy of feared situations. The patient is exposed to those situations that are predicted to provoke fewer anxiety reactions, until these are mastered. They then gradually work through the hierarchy until the feared stimulus can be faced in its full form. Having a clear step-by-step plan allows progressively more anxiety-provoking situations to be faced and tackled. They key is repeated practice at each step along the way, always then moving on towards the goal. There are no surprises, and always the aim is to push the person forward, but at a pace that they can cope with. This is very different from the flooding approach, in which the patient is exposed to the feared stimulus all at once and is maintained in this situation until the anxiety symptoms decrease. Although effective for some patients, flooding risks the possibility of patient disengagement and anger.

Cue exposure is the exposure of the patient to a 'cue' to a particular stimulus, when the stimuli are paired. This may be encountered in substance abuse, where, for example, a person who may have been previously dependent on alcohol may start to experience cravings or even withdrawal-type symptoms with a stimulus such as the smell of alcohol, which in turn may motivate them to drink alcohol. Cue exposure involves the repeated exposure to such cues so that this extinguishes the response, in this case the craving for alcohol.

Response prevention

Progressive/systematic exposure is especially helpful for phobic anxiety states and obsessive–compulsive symptoms. The person plans how to face up to their fears in a planned, step-by-step way. At the same time, they are encouraged not to leave, run away or try to neutralize the anxiety in unhelpful ways such as using medication, alcohol or distraction. This latter approach is called response prevention. It involves helping the person to recognize the ranges of so-called *safety behaviours* that they use to cope with symptoms and then to plan to slowly drop these behaviours, thereby helping them face their fears more effectively and habituate (get used to) the anxiety, which slowly drops away.

Introducing such behavioural change is also an excellent way of testing out catastrophic fears and building confidence that the very worst does not happen.

Habituation

Habituation is a simple process by which, following repeated exposure to a particular stimulus, the subject stops responding to it. This is also called extinction of the response. So, a particular stimulus that may have provoked an anxiety reaction will stop producing this reaction once the patient has been exposed repeatedly to the stimulus.

DEFINING OUTCOME IN CBT

As CBT is a problem-focused and evidence-based approach, monitoring progress is a central part of the therapy process.

Treatment outcome measures that are commonly used in CBT practice are self-report measures such as the Beck Depression Inventory (BDI)[19] and the Beck Anxiety Inventory (BAI).[20] These can be done weekly just before the start of the session, and they will be used as feedback tools for the patient at review points in the therapy.

Other self-report measures that may be used with the patient are continuum measures for each of the target difficulties, where the patient can rate where they feel they are at. This can help to monitor the patient's progress. Figure 65.3 shows an example.

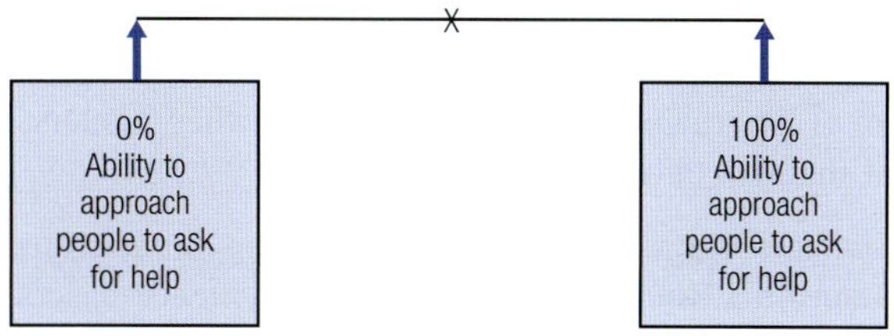

Figure 65.3 Self-report measures: continuum

Readers should be aware of moves to standardize outcome measurement, such as that suggested for the IAPT minimum dataset.

THE EVIDENCE BASE

CBT has been studied for a number of disorders. The evidence base includes randomized controlled trials and meta-analysis of these. The data have been summarized in evidence-based practice guidelines and are recommended for practice by the NICE and SIGN guidelines for the following disorders (www.guidance.nice.org.uk/topic/behavioural):

- Anxiety
- Depression
- Panic
- Agoraphobia and other phobias
- Social phobia
- Bulimia
- OCD
- PTSD.

Selecting and referring patients for CBT

- Consider current evidence-based guidelines.
- The patient prefers to use psychological interventions, either alone or in addition to medication (N.B. the CBT model readily allows the use of medication alongside therapy and may indeed focus on increasing compliance and adherence).
- The target problems for CBT (extreme unhelpful thinking, reduced activity, avoidant or unhelpful behaviours) are present.

- No improvement or only partial improvement has occurred on medication, or the person does not prefer medication.
- Side effects prevent a sufficient dose of medication from being taken over an adequate period.
- Significant psychosocial problems (e.g. relationship problems, difficulties at work, unhelpful behaviours such as self-cutting or alcohol misuse) are present that will not be addressed adequately by medication alone.

EXPLAINING CBT TO THE PATIENT

When a patient is being referred for CBT, as with any other form of treatment, it is important that they understand what this will entail:

- The patient will be required to attend regular sessions for a specified timeframe (although the evidence base suggests that CBT can also be offered equally effectively by telephone).
- The patient will usually meet with a therapist for between 5 and 20 weekly or fortnightly sessions. Each session will be approximately 60 min long.
- At the beginning of each session, the therapist and the patient will establish an agreed agenda of what will be discussed during the session.
- In the first two to four sessions, the therapist will check that the patient can use this sort of treatment and check that the patient feels comfortable with it.
- The patient will be asked to identify goals for the therapy. The patient will decide what they want to deal with in the short, medium and long term.
- Although CBT concentrates on the here and now, the therapist will also ask questions about the patient's past experiences and background, especially to understand how past experiences may still be affecting the patient now.
- The therapy sessions will focus on developing a CBT formulation of the patient's difficulties and will target key unhelpful thoughts and behaviours for intervention.
- Between sessions, the patient will try to put into practice some of the things learned during the therapy sessions. This is done by agreeing with the therapist on a task to complete at home.
- The use of the word 'homework' can be off-putting, so other terms such as 'putting things into action' may be preferred.
- Finally, CBT is increasingly being delivered in all sorts of sizes and shapes – groups, classes, CCBT, written bibliotherapy and more; the so-called 'Low Intensity' methods of delivering CBT.

THE THERAPEUTIC RELATIONSHIP

The CBT model brings three key characteristics seen in evidence-based therapeutic models:

- A model or structure that helps to people understand why they feel as they do
- A focus on problems and symptoms relevant to the patient
- Delivery within a supportive therapeutic relationship.

It is clear that, for any form of psychotherapy, so-called non-specific therapist factors such as warmth, empathy and genuineness contribute the majority of therapeutic effect in a clinical encounter. On top of this, however, the focus and step-by-step structure of CBT have contributed to it having the widest range of NICE recommendations of any of the existing forms of psychotherapy.

CONCLUSION

CBT is a pragmatic, problem-focused therapy that can be used alongside medication and diagnostic approaches. Developed by a medic and founded in empirical research, and yet retaining a strong focus on the individual, it has become the predominant form of psychotherapy offered within the health service today. Increasingly wider and rapid access will occur through routes such as telephone CBT, group-based CBT and the use of CBT self-help alongside the traditional forms of face-to-face CBT. Pragmatically CBT core skills can provide a useful part of the psychiatric armamentarium for everyday clinical use.

FURTHER INFORMATION

www.rcpsych.ac.uk/mentalhealthinformation/therapies/cognitivebehaviouraltherapy.aspx. The Royal College of Psychiatrists produces a helpful guide on its website that may be useful for patients starting a course of CBT treatment.

www.livinglifetothefull.com. Find out about CBT assessment, activity-planning, thought-challenging, relapse prevention and other key CBT techniques. This free CBT life skills site has areas for patients and practitioners.

www.moodgym.anu.edu.au/welcome. A CBT online course that aims to prevent depression. Free and supported by an Australian university.

www.psychiatrycpd.co.uk/learningmodules/anintroductiontocbt.aspx. Paid-for Royal College of Psychiatrist online continuing professional development (CPD) module.

KEY POINTS

- CBT is an evidence-based treatment approach
- Central to effectiveness is working with a clear structure and targeting problems identified through a joint formulation such as the five areas approach
- Translating CBT into accessible language – and helping people make small step by step changes is the key to success
- Psychiatrists can use CBT approaches in clinc sessions by utilising key CBT concepts; targeted cognitive, behavioural and problem solving interventions; or the use of CBT self-help

REFERENCES

1. Beck AT (1976) *Cognitive Therapy and the Emotional Disorders*. New York: Penguin Books.
2. National Institute for Health and Clinical Excellence (2004) *Depression: Management of Depression in Primary and Secondary Care*. Clinical guideline 23. London: National Institute for Health and Clinical Excellence.
3. National Institute for Health and Clinical Excellence (2004) *Anxiety: Management of Anxiety (Panic Disorder, with or without Agoraphobia, and Generalised Anxiety Disorder) in Adults in Primary, Secondary and Community Care*. Clinical guideline 22. London: National Institute for Health and Clinical Excellence.
4. National Institute for Health and Clinical Excellence (2006) *Computerised cognitive behaviour therapy for depression and anxiety*. London: National Institute for Health and Clinical Excellence.
5. Gellatly J, Bower P, Hennessy S, *et al.* (2007) What makes self-help interventions effective in the management of depressive symptoms? Meta-analysis and meta-regression. *Psychological Medicine* **37**: 1217–28.
6. Williams CJ (2006) *Overcoming Depression and Low Mood: A Five Areas Approach*, 2nd edn. London: Hodder Arnold.
7. Williams JMG, Dritschel BH (1988) Emotional disturbance and specificity of autobiographical memory. *Cognition and Emotion* **2**: 221–34.
8. Dalgleish T, Watts FN (1990) Biases of attention and memory in disorders of anxiety and depression. *Clinical Psychology Review* **10**: 589–604.
9. Haaga DA, Dyck MJ, Ernst D (1991) Empirical status of cognitive theory of depression. *Psychological Bulletin* **110**: 215–36.
10. Beck AT, Shaw BF, Rush JA, Emery G (1979) *Cognitive Therapy of Depression*. New York: Guilford Press.
11. Clark DM, Teasdale JD (1982) Diurnal variation in clinical depression and accessibility of memories of positive and negative experiences. *Journal of Abnormal Psychology* **91**: 87–95.
12. World Health Organization (1992) *International Classification of Diseases*, tenth revision. Geneva: World Health Organization.
13. Beck J (1995) *Cognitive Therapy: Basics and Beyond*. New York: Guilford Press.
14. O'Leary KD, Wilson GT (1975) *Behaviour Therapy: Application and Outcome*. Engelwood Cliffs, NJ: Prentice-Hall.
15. Cuijpers P, van Straten A, Warmerdam L (2007) Behavioural activation treatments of depression: a meta-analysis. *Clinical Psychology Review* **27**: 318–26.
16. Bennett-Levy J, Butler G, Fennell M, *et al.* (2004) *Oxford Guide to Behavioural Experiments in Cognitive Therapy*. Oxford: Oxford University Press.
17. Greenberger D, Padesky CA (1995) *Mind over Mood*. New York: Guilford Press.
18. Wolpe J (1958) *Psychotherapy by Reciprocal Inhibition*. Stanford, CA: Stanford University Press.
19. Beck AT, Ward CH, Mendelson M, Mock J, Erbaugh J (1961) An inventory for measuring depression. *Archives of General Psychiatry* **4**: 561–71.
20. Beck AT, Epstein N, Brown G, Steer RA (1988) An inventory for measuring anxiety: psychometric properties. *Journal of Consulting and Clinical Psychology* **56**: 893–7.

Chapter 66

Other individual psychotherapies

Basant K Puri

INTRODUCTION

This chapter primarily describes art therapy and music therapy, which are two of the arts therapies. The arts therapies consist of art therapy, music therapy and dance therapy. (Note that psychodrama is not conventionally considered to be one of the arts therapies.) Although the current body of solid research for creative arts therapies is small compared with that of more traditional medical specialties, the arts therapies are now validating their research through more controlled experimental and descriptive studies.[1] Scientific studies of some of the physical and cerebral effects of music are described in this chapter. At the end of the chapter there is a very brief mention of a few other individual therapies. It should be noted that although the therapies mentioned in this chapter may be used on an individual basis, some of them, such as music therapy, may also often be used in group settings.

ART THERAPY

As David Lomas has pointed out in his foreword to Susan Hogan's history of art therapy, *Healing Arts*, Sigmund Freud, in an essay on Michelangelo's *Moses*, pointed out that the artist's intentions should be capable of being communicated and comprehended in words, which in the case of great works of art might require the application of psychoanalysis; to discover the intentions of the artist, one must be able to *interpret* the artist's work of art.[2]

Classification

Three groups of art therapy have been differentiated:[2,3]

- *Art therapy:* emphasis is placed on the production of the artwork itself, which is not usually interpreted
- *Art psychotherapy:* verbal analysis of the artwork by the therapist takes place; the artwork illustrates the therapeutic relationship or recounts some aspect of the history
- *Analytical art psychotherapy:* draws on the theories of psychoanalysis and emphasizes the transference between client and therapist.

In this chapter, the term 'art therapy' is used as a generic term to refer to all three types.

Techniques

Art therapy may take place on an individual basis, in a small group setting or in an 'open studio' format. The types of artwork that may be produced by the client can involve use of various modalities, including:[2]

- painting;
- collage;
- clay pottery;
- sculpture.

Case vignette

Joy Schaverien has published the paintings shown in Figures 66.1 and 66.2 as part of an instructive case vignette from therapy sessions with a patient named 'Jacqui':[4]

> Jacqui's mother had died suddenly, in her late fifties, when Jacqui was 22. Now Jacqui was in her early fifties but she still felt oppressed by her mother. The internalized mother dominated her every move and denigrated her attempts to work or make relationships ...

Figure 66.1 is of a tree, which she described as showing her chaos, insecurity and depression on one side, and the lively

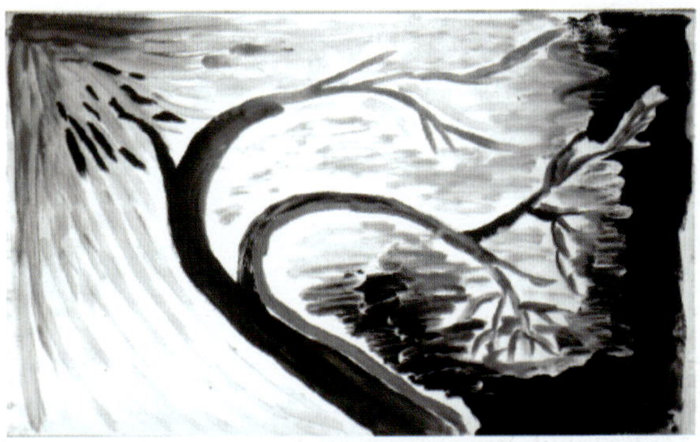

Figure 66.1 Painting of a tree by 'Jacqui', created as part of art therapy
Reproduced from Schaverien.[4]

part of her life on the other. It shows the distorted growth that had emerged as a result of her parental domination and lack of autonomy. The dominating mother had a brother who was 'simple' and who was never really able to function in the world. The family viewed him as rather pathetic and hopeless. At times he was admitted to the local psychiatric hospital for in-patient treatment. Jacqui loved him but her fear of her own vulnerability was at times associated with her uncle and at worst she feared that she was mad. This sense of her own vulnerability, associated with the flaw in her family, emerged as a dark area in many of her paintings.

In a session soon after an insight that connected her fear of madness with her beloved uncle she made Figure 66.2, another painting of a tree. It was an image of growth and she explained how one colour represented the warmth of her feelings for her uncle. The tree had strong roots and branches, but a dark patch, which she felt indicated her relationship to her parents, was like a flaw that ran throughout it.

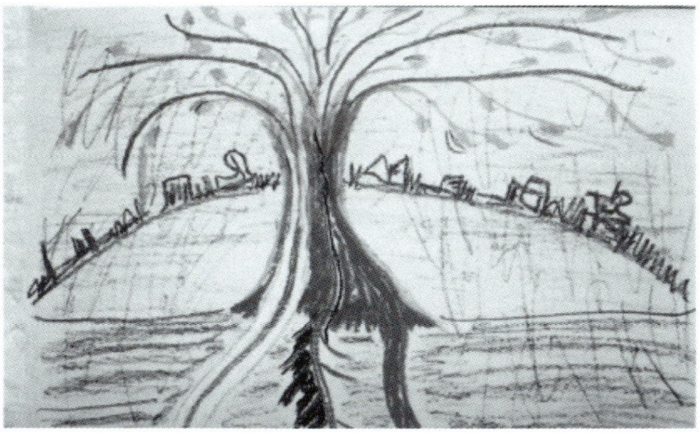

Figure 66.2 Another painting of a tree by 'Jacqui', painted after the one shown in Figure 66.1

Reproduced from Schaverien.[4]

Stages of separation differentiation

Joy Schaverien has identified the following five stages of a separation differentiation that are common in art therapy:[3]

1. *Identification*, which occurs immediately after the creation of the artwork, when there exists a strong connection between the client and his or her artwork.
2. *Familiarization* of the content of the artwork by the client, who begins to become conscious of what it reveals and starts to differentiate its elements.
3. *Acknowledgement* at a conscious level by the client of the implication of his or her artwork; at this stage, discussion with the therapist is possible and interpretations may be received.
4. *Assimilation*, which is the stage of re-integration of the elements of the artwork, which is now owned and the implications of which are now assimilated.
5. *Disposal* of the artwork, which holds powerful affect – before the end of therapy, a conscious decision needs to be made regarding the disposal of the artwork. Will the client take the artwork away with them, or leave it in the art room, or destroy it?

It has been suggested that a transference to the artwork, and the associated transference–countertransference dynamic, may allow art to offer a particular means of psychological transformation in states that may otherwise not be expressible by the client.[5]

Specialized types

There are several variants of art therapy that have been created. For example, the Conversational Model may be applied to art therapy. This model, created by Robert Hobson and Russell Meares, is a developmental model in which what is said and done in therapy is aimed at promoting understanding: a 'conversation', a meeting between two experiencing subjects (an I and a thou), here and now, in such a way that learning can be effective in other relationships.[6] Unconscious traumatic memory may lead to a relative loss of inner speech and intrusion into conventional verbal therapeutic conversation;[7] the client may find it easier, under these circumstances, to express him- or herself by means of artwork.

In image art psychotherapy, free expression, spontaneous expression and thematic drawings are utilized simultaneously. Tokuda has argued that there are image expressions applicable not only to one graphic representation but to a whole series involving the 'drawing–observing–examining–continuing to draw again' process, and somatic self-expression; that these too reflect the preconceptual emotion and total psychosomatic rhythm; and that there exists a process of approaching the true self over the ordinary defences.[8]

Patient groups

A pilot study in 26 patients in a psychosomatic day hospital, involving 16 sessions of art therapy and utilizing standardized rating questionnaires to quantify changes in mood and somatic symptomatology, showed a reduction in somatic symptoms and a tendency to be in a more positive mood during the course of the day treatment.[9] The paintings dealt mainly with the patients' own (current, problematic) issues; the colours chosen for the paintings were particularly important to most patients, and often there was no connection to paintings created during the previous sessions. Subjectively, the patients felt better after the art therapy session. They indicated that they mostly use art therapy as a way to express their problems, and only very few also named other goals of art therapy, such as creativity or relaxation.[9] There is also evidence that art therapy may help to produce a slow partial recovery in patients with chronic somatic symptoms, in whom inability to express emotions is common and is associated with incapacitation and impaired quality of life.[10]

There is preliminary evidence suggesting that art therapy may be helpful to older people with mild to moderate depression,[11] and stronger evidence that it helps to reduce depressive symptoms in prisoners.[12] In a study of 46 seriously delinquent incarcerated male juvenile offenders, Persons examined how art therapy addressed the boys' psychological needs by analysing their self-selected artwork.[13] In descending order of frequency, the eight most frequent need themes were: identity issues; need for security and tranquillity; need for freedom, adventure and fun; need for ideal parental relationships; need for affiliation and affection; erotic and sexual needs; expression of depression, childhood trauma and other psychological problems; and religious or spiritual needs. The juvenile offenders' perceptions of what was most helpful about art therapy, in descending order, were: stress relief and relaxation; reduction of boredom; pride and self-confidence; positive recognition; working through frustration; enjoyment and fun; improvement of ability to concentrate; and the way they were treated.[13]

It has been suggested that art therapy should perhaps be restricted and not applied to patients who are psychotic.[3] A systematic review of art therapy for schizophrenia or schizophrenia-like illnesses has found that randomized studies are indeed possible in this area, but that thus far its benefits or harm in these disorders remain unclear.[14,15]

Art therapy is used to help children with emotional, developmental and behavioural problems.[16] A study of 64 young (age 6–21 years) recipients of renal transplants showed that although art therapy may be of utility in the identification of those who are suffering from depression, it lacks sufficient sensitivity to warrant its use in this population.[17]

A significant improvement in the Hospital Anxiety and Depression Scale (HADS) scores has been reported in patients with cancer receiving chemotherapy who participated in at least four weekly art therapy sessions.[18] Coping resources also improve in women with breast cancer after taking part in art therapy intervention.[19]

In a randomized comparison of a 1-h art therapy session versus watching videos of art therapy in 79 patients with human immunodeficiency virus (HIV) infection, physical symptom mean scores were found to become significantly better for those who participated in art therapy compared with those who viewed the video.[20]

There is preliminary evidence that art therapy may help the speech of children with cerebral palsy, particularly in respect to intelligibility, volume, tempo and control of pauses.[21]

Inter-rater reliability

Eitel and colleagues systematically studied the assessments of 86 raters who evaluated a picture created during an art therapy session. The rating was based on formal (colour, lines, shapes) and contextual criteria. The resulting inter-rater agreement was relatively poor (intraclass correlation coefficient = 0.18–0.52).[22] They also addressed the question of whether raters were able to determine which picture was created at the beginning of the art therapy and which at the end; on the basis of the examination of five sets of pictures, they concluded that the raters were not reliably able to distinguish between the two.[22]

MUSIC THERAPY

Definition

Patients are offered the opportunity to make live music, either improvised or precomposed, with a music therapist who is a trained musician and music therapist, or to listen to music with therapeutic intent.[3]

Techniques

Music therapy may take place on an individual basis or in a group setting. Live music-making may involve:

- tuned and untuned percussion;
- a piano;
- an electric keyboard;
- single-line musical instruments;
- the subject's voice.

Music being listened to may be live or recorded. In the latter case, it may take the form of prerecorded compositions or consist of recordings of music made by the subject.

Cardiovascular, respiratory and mid-cerebral arterial flow velocity effects

Music and musical pauses induce cardiovascular and respiratory changes in the listener. Bernardi and colleagues asked a group of 12 practising musicians and 12 non-musicians to listen, after a 5-min baseline, to a presentation in random order of six different musical styles (first for a 2-min track and then for a 4-min track), with a randomly inserted 2-min pause, in either sequence.[23] Their main findings were as follows: Ventilation, blood pressure and heart rate increased, and mid-cerebral artery flow velocity and baroreflex decreased with faster tempi and simpler rhythmic structures compared with baseline; no habituation effect was observed; the pause reduced heart rate, blood pressure and minute ventilation, even below baseline. An order effect independent of style was evident for mid-cerebral artery flow velocity, indicating a progressive reduction with exposure to music, independent of style. Musicians had greater respiratory sensitivity to the music tempo than did non-musicians.[23] They concluded that music induces an arousal effect, predominantly related to the tempo, with slow or meditative music being able to induce a relaxing effect; relaxation is particularly evident during a pause. Music, especially in trained subjects, may first concentrate attention during faster rhythms, and then induce relaxation during pauses or slower rhythms.[23]

Cerebral changes

Menon and Levitin used functional and effective connectivity analyses to show that listening to music strongly modulates activity in a network of mesolimbic structures involved in reward-processing, including the nucleus accumbens and the ventral tegmental area, as well as the hypothalamus and insula, which are thought to be involved in regulating autonomic and physiological responses to rewarding and emotional stimuli.[24] Responses in the nucleus accumbens and the ventral tegmental area were correlated strongly, pointing to an association between dopamine release and the response of the nucleus accumbens to music.[24] The same group have investigated the neural dynamics of event segmentation in entire musical symphonies under natural listening conditions, by isolating time-dependent sequences of brain responses in a 10-s window surrounding transitions between movements of symphonic works.[25] A strikingly right-lateralized network of brain regions showed peak response during the movement transitions when, paradoxically, there was no physical stimulus. Model-dependent and model-free analysis techniques provided converging evidence for activity in two distinct functional networks at the movement transition: a ventral frontotemporal network associated with detecting salient events, followed in time by a dorsal frontoparietal network associated with maintaining attention and updating working memory. These results provide direct experimental evidence for dissociable and causally linked ventral and dorsal networks during event segmentation of ecologically valid auditory stimuli.[25]

Blood and colleagues carried out a study of emotional responses to pleasant and unpleasant music in subjects who were not professional musicians and who underwent positron-emission tomography (PET) neuroimaging while listening to six versions of a novel melody. As shown in Figure 66.3, they found a significant negative correlation between the degree of dissonance (using major triads as having the least dissonance, and flattened thirteenth triads as the most dissonant) in the melody and the subjective rating of pleasantness.[26] An analysis examining regional cerebral blood flow (rCBF) changes from the PET neuroimaging as a function of increasing dissonance identified significant positive correlations in right parahippocampal gyrus and right precuneus regions, while significant negative correlations, corresponding to increasing consonance, were found in large areas of orbitofrontal cortex bilaterally, medial subcallosal cingulate region (3 mm to the right of

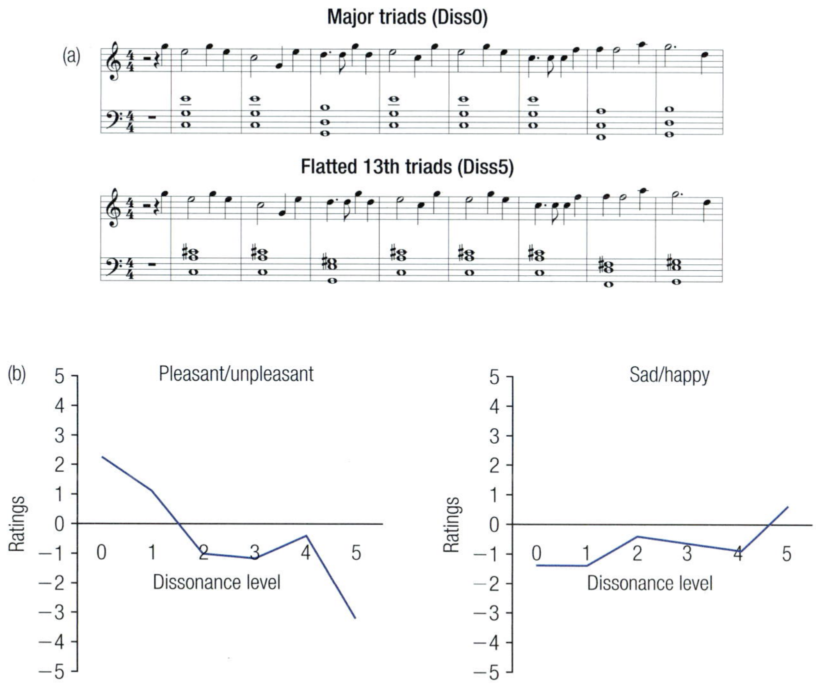

Figure 66.3 Examples of music stimuli and average subject ratings of unpleasant versus pleasant and happy versus sad for each version. (a) Excerpts from the most consonant version (major triads, Diss0) and the most dissonant version (flatted thirteenth triads, Diss5) of music stimuli used in the positron-emission tomography (PET) study (see text). (b) Line graphs demonstrating averaged subject ratings following scans for each of the six versions, Diss0–Diss5. Ratings of very pleasant (+5) versus very unpleasant (−5) demonstrated significant interactions ($P < 0.001$) and a high correlation coefficient ($r = 0.57$) with dissonance level. Ratings of very sad (+5) versus very happy (−5) did not demonstrate significant interactions and had a lower correlation coefficient ($r = 0.33$) with dissonance level

Reproduced from Blood *et al.*[26]

the midline) and right frontal pole.[26] Ratings of increasing unpleasantness correlated, albeit weakly, with rCBF activity in the right parahippocampal gyrus, but in the identical location to that found in the regression with dissonance level; increasing unpleasantness also correlated with activity in the posterior cingulate, whereas ratings of increasing pleasantness correlated with activity in the right orbitofrontal and medial subcallosal cingulate cortex.[26]

Blood and Zatorre went on to use PET to investigate neural correlates of intensely pleasurable responses to music. rCBF changes were measured while subjects listened to music that they selected predictably to elicit the euphoric experience of 'chills' (or 'shivers-down-the-spine'). These were pieces of classical music, such as Rachmaninov's Piano Concerto No. 3 in D Minor, Opus 30, Intermezzo Adagio and Barber's Adagio for Strings. Listening to the chills-inducing musical pieces was associated with increased cardiac rate, electromyographic changes and increased depth of respiration (Figure 66.4).[27] Regression analysis correlating rCBF with increasing chills intensity ratings in the subject-selected and control music conditions identified rCBF increases in the left ventral striatum, dorsomedial midbrain, bilateral insula, right orbitofrontal cortex, thalamus, anterior cingulate cortex, supplementary motor area and bilateral cerebellum, while rCBF decreases with increasing chills intensity were observed in the right amygdala, left hippocampus/amygdala and ventromedial prefrontal cortex, and in widespread, bilateral posterior neocortical regions, particularly in the cuneus/precuneus regions.[27] Subtraction of noise and silent baseline conditions from subject-selected and control music conditions confirmed that activity in the right amygdala, left hippocampus/amygdala and ventromedial prefrontal cortex decreased from baseline during subject-selected music, whereas no cerebral blood flow changes were seen in these structures during control music as compared with the noise and silent baselines.[27] The authors concluded:[27]

> As intensity of these chills increased, cerebral blood flow increases and decreases were observed in brain regions thought to be involved in reward/motivation, emotion, and arousal, including ventral striatum, midbrain, amygdala, orbitofrontal cortex, and ventral medial prefrontal cortex. These brain structures are known to be active in response to other euphoria-inducing stimuli, such as food, sex, and drugs of abuse. This finding links music with biologically relevant, survival-related stimuli via their common recruitment of brain circuitry involved in pleasure and reward.

In 1993, Rauscher and colleagues published a study in which they asked students to listen for 10 min to part of

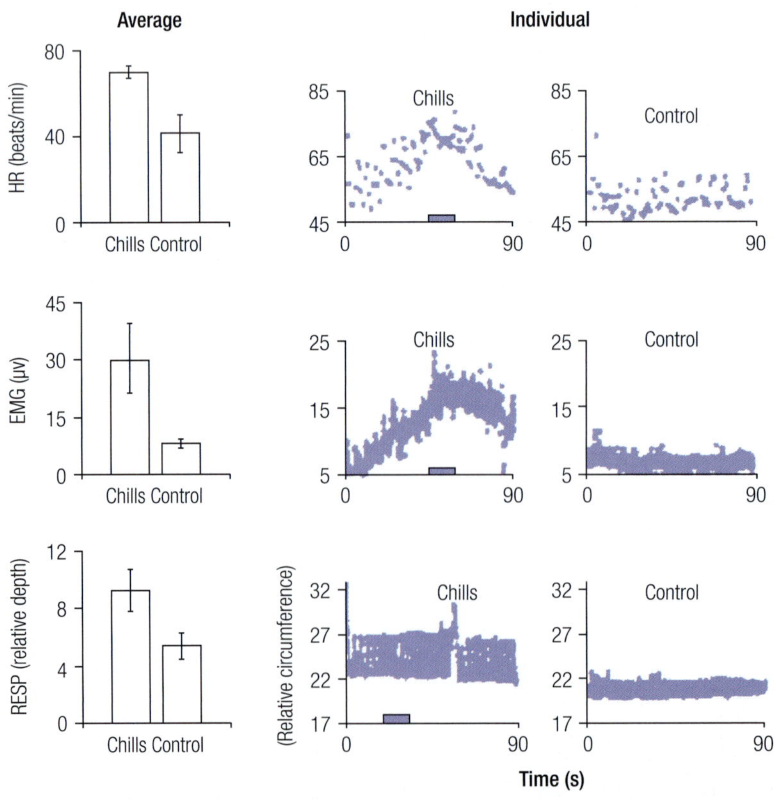

Figure 66.4 Average measurements of heart rate (HR), electromyogram (EMG) and respiration depth (RESP) for subject-selected (chills) and control music conditions, with corresponding examples of individual measurements for each condition over the time course of selected scans (90 s). Error bars indicate standard error for each average. The same subject/scan is shown for individual measurements of HR and EMG (subject 1); a different subject (subject 2) is shown for RESP. Blue bars on the abscissa of graphs in the centre column indicate time periods corresponding to chills. In all three examples, the chills rating was 7 on a scale of 0–10

Reproduced from Blood and Zatorre.[27]

Mozart's Sonata for Two Pianos in D Major, K448, a relaxation tape designed to lower blood pressure or silence, before taking three sets of standard intelligence quotient (IQ) spatial reasoning tasks.[28] Those listening to Mozart's K448 performed significantly better than the other two groups; the mean standard age scores and corresponding spatial IQ scores are shown in Figure 66.5. Pulse rates were measured before and after participation in this experiment, and there was no interaction or main effect for pulse, thereby excluding arousal as a cause for this effect.[28] This effect has come to be known as the Mozart effect and in this original study it was found that enhanced spatial reasoning did not last beyond the 10–15 min during which the subjects were engaged in each spatial task. Subsequently, the Mozart effect has been found to occur in rats:[29]

Rats were exposed in utero plus 60 days post-partum to either complex music (Mozart Sonata (k. 448)), minimalist music (a Philip Glass composition), white noise or silence, and were then tested for five days, three trials per day, in a multiple T-maze. By Day 3, the rats exposed to the Mozart work completed the maze more rapidly and with fewer errors than the rats assigned to the other groups. The difference increased in magnitude through Day 5. This suggests that repeated exposure to complex music induces improved spatial-temporal learning in rats, resembling results found in humans.

Extended exposure to learning and playing music by Mozart and Beethoven has been found to be associated with improved spatiotemporal reasoning that was still present 24 h later in preschool children.[30] With extended exposure, rats have also shown long-term enhancement of maze learning.[31] Furthermore, electroencephalographic studies in humans have shown that the Mozart effect is associated with right frontal and left temporoparietal coherent activity.[32]

Hughes and colleagues carried out an impressive study on the effects of listening to Mozart's K448 on epileptiform activity:[33]

The 'Mozart Effect', using the Piano Sonata in D Major (K.448), was examined in patients with seizures. In 23 of 29 instances significant decreases in epileptiform activity were noted from patients even in coma, with status epilepticus or with periodic lateralized epileptiform discharges (PLEDs). The effect may be immediate or require 40–300 sec to manifest itself. The change in the amount of ictal activity in one patient in coma was from 62% before the music to 21% during Mozart. Amplitudes of these discharges also have often decreased. Examples of PLEDs on both temporal areas are shown in which the effect was only on the left temporal area but in other patients only on the right temporal area. Brain maps during the music showed theta and alpha activity decreased on the central areas, while delta waves increased on the frontal midline area. The basis of this effect is likely that the superorganization of the cerebral cortex with its highly structured radial columns seen throughout both hemispheres may resonate with the superior architecture of Mozart's music.

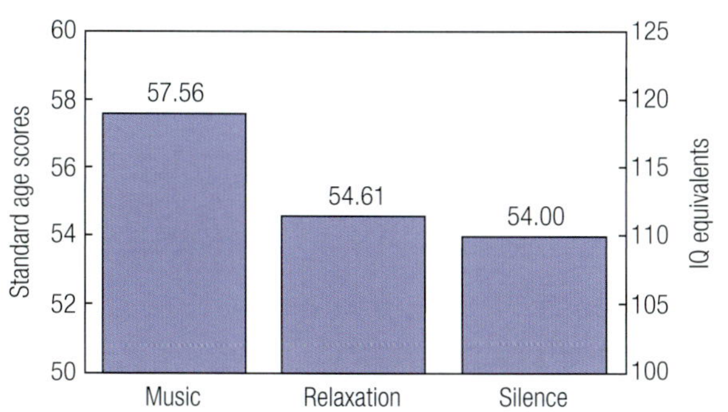

Figure 66.5 Standard age scores and corresponding spatial intelligence quotient (IQ) scores for each of the three listening conditions

Reproduced from Rauscher *et al.*[29]

It is not known how specific the Mozart effect is to his K448 composition. Certainly, there is evidence that the minimalist music of Philip Glass and certain types of pop music do not show beneficial changes in spatial task performance or epileptiform activity. On the other hand, another piece by Mozart, his Piano Concerto No. 23 in A major, K488 has also been found to be associated with improved spatial task performance.[34]

Patient groups

Gold and colleagues have published a systematic review and meta-analysis of the benefits of music therapy for patients with psychiatric disorder. From an initial 166 potentially relevant studies for any mental disorder, they selected 15 studies fulfilling their criteria, which included having a prospective group design. Their findings and conclusions were as follows:[35]

Results showed that music therapy, when added to standard care, has strong and significant effects on global state, general symptoms, negative symptoms, depression, anxiety, functioning, and musical engagement. Significant dose–effect relationships were identified for general, negative, and depressive symptoms, as well as functioning, with explained variance ranging from 73% to 78%. Small effect sizes for these outcomes are achieved after 3 to 10, large effects after 16 to 51 sessions. The findings suggest that music therapy is an effective treatment which helps people with psychotic and non-psychotic severe mental disorders to improve global state, symptoms, and functioning. Slight improvements can be seen with a few therapy sessions, but longer courses or more frequent sessions are needed to achieve more substantial benefits.

The dose–response relationship of music therapy for general symptoms is shown in Figure 66.6, while the dose–response relationships of music therapy for negative symptoms, depressive symptoms and functioning are shown in Figures 66.7, 66.8 and 66.9, respectively.

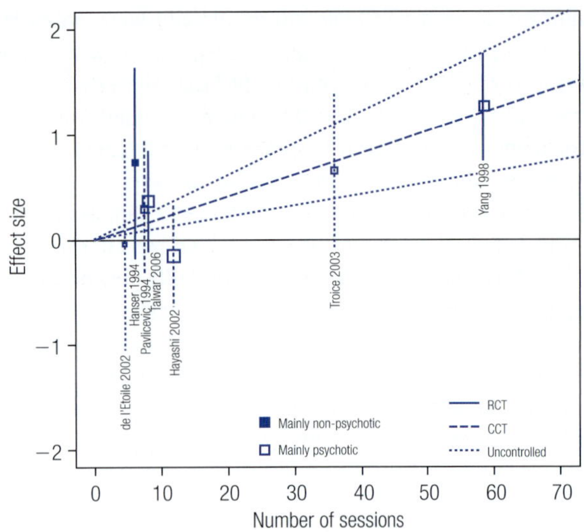

Figure 66.6 Dose–effect relationship of music therapy for general symptoms. Each individual study is plotted at the position indicated by the number of sessions provided and the effect size found in that study. The box symbol for each study is filled white if the majority of participants had a psychotic disorder, and black otherwise. The size of the box represents each study's weight in the analysis. The vertical line added to each individual study indicates the 95% confidence interval (CI) of the observed effect; the line type (solid, dashed, dotted) indicates the strength of the study's design. Finally, the dashed regression line shows the result of a mixed-effects meta-regression analysis, indicating the relationship between the number of sessions provided and the predicted effect size. The 95% CI of the regression is shown by the dotted lines around the regression line

CCT, controlled clinical trial; RCT, randomized controlled trial.

Reproduced from Gold C *et al.*[35]

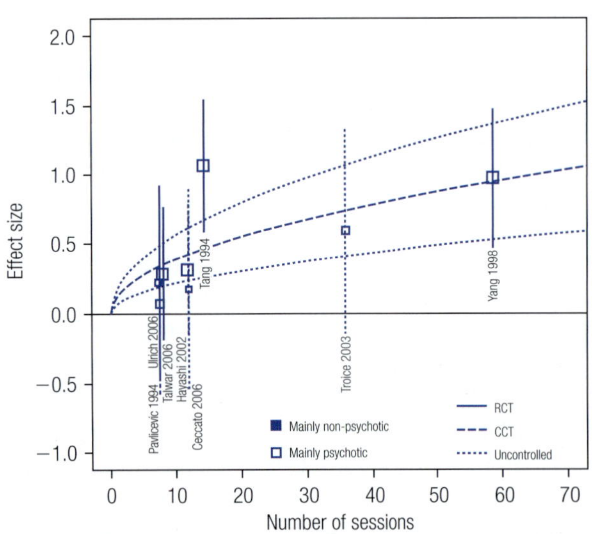

Figure 66.7 Dose–effect relationship of music therapy for negative symptoms. Explanations are as in the legend for Figure 66.9

CCT, controlled clinical trial; RCT, randomized controlled trial.

Reproduced from Gold C *et al.*[35]

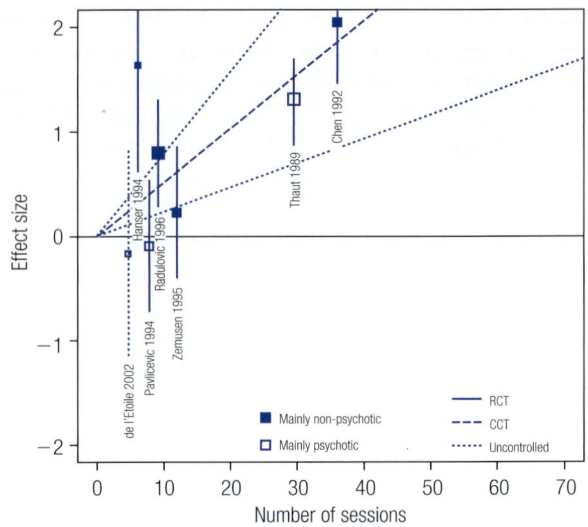

Figure 66.8 Dose–effect relationship of music therapy for depressive symptoms. Explanations are as in the legend for Figure 66.9

CCT, controlled clinical trial; RCT, randomized controlled trial.

Reproduced from Gold C *et al.*[35]

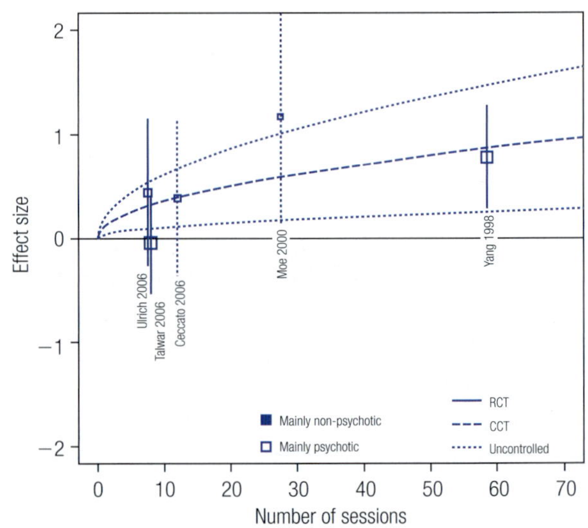

Figure 66.9 Dose–effect relationship of music therapy for functioning. Explanations are as in the legend for Figure 66.9

CCT, controlled clinical trial; RCT, randomized controlled trial.

Reproduced from Gold C *et al.*[35]

OTHER THERAPIES

Table 66.1 gives very brief details of a few selected other therapies. Further details can be found in Windy Dryden's excellent book, *Dryden's Handbook of Individual Therapy*.[36]

Table 66.1 Brief details of other individual psychotherapies

Individual therapy	Founders	Theoretical aspects	Key concepts
Gestalt therapy	Fritz Perls, Laura Perls, Ralph Hefferline, Paul Goodman	Roots in psychoanalysis; includes the notion of dental/oral aggression and Gestalt psychology concepts; process more important than content	Client is encouraged to 'taste' his experience; four 'load-bearing walls' are phenomenological method, dialogical relationship, field-theoretical strategies and experimental freedom
Narrative therapy	Michael White, David Epston	Roots in family therapy and counselling; people ('persons') are complex	Narratives are 'self-stories' (selective memory, multi-stranded and often inconsistent); 're-storying' conceptually to reorient/reposition
Person-centred therapy	Carl Rogers	Emphasizes the internal world of the client, who has lost touch with their 'actualizing tendency'	Therapist's congruence, unconditional positive regard and empathic understanding are required for change to occur
Personal construct therapy	George Kelly	Based on constructive alternativism in which humans act on the world rather than respond to it; behaviour is viewed 'as if' it were an experiment; fundamental postulate – a person's processes are psychologically channelized by the ways in which he or she anticipates events	We view the world via our construing 'goggles'; experience corollary; choice corollary; modulation corollary; cycle of experience; creativity cycle; decision-making cycle; repertory grid technique; laddering; pyramiding; the ABC model; the self-characterization; fixed role therapy

KEY POINTS

- Art therapy and music therapy are two of the arts therapies.
- Types of art therapy include art therapy, art psychotherapy and analytical art psychotherapy.
- Five stages of separation differentiation have been found to be common in art therapy: identification, familiarization, acknowledgement, assimilation and disposal.
- Art therapy may be helpful to patients with depression, somatic symptoms, cancer and cerebral palsy.
- The inter-rater reliability between art therapists is relatively poor.
- Listening to music is associated with cardiovascular, respiratory, cerebral blood flow, emotional and cognitive changes.
- Listening to certain works by Mozart may be associated with improvement in spatial tasks.
- Music therapy, when added to standard care, has strong and significant effects on global state, general symptoms, negative symptoms, depression, anxiety, functioning and musical engagement; significant dose–effect relationships occur in general, negative and depressive symptoms, and in functioning.
- Other psychotherapies that can be used on an individual basis include Gestalt therapy, narrative therapy, person-centred therapy and personal construct therapy.

FURTHER READING

Campbell D (2001) *The Mozart Effect*. London: Hodder & Stoughton.

Dryden W (ed.) (2007) *Dryden's Handbook of Individual Therapy*, 5th edn. London: Sage.

Gabbard GO, Beck JS, Holmes J (eds) (2005) *Oxford Textbook of Psychotherapy*. Oxford: Oxford University Press.

Schaverien J (1991) *The Revealing Image: Analytical Art Psychotherapy in Theory and Practice*. London: Tavistock Routledge.

REFERENCES

1. Pratt RR (2004) Art, dance, and music therapy. *Physical Medicine and Rehabilitation Clinics of North America* 15: 827–41, vi–vii.
2. Hogan S (2000) *Healing Arts: The History of Art Therapy*. London: Jessica Kingsley Publishers.
3. Schaverien J, Odell-Miller H (2005) The art therapies. In GO Gabbard, JS Beck, J Holmes (eds) *Oxford Textbook of Psychotherapy*. Oxford: Oxford University Press.

4. Schaverien J (2005) Art, dreams and active imagination: a post-Jungian approach to transference and the image. *Journal of Analytical Psychology* **50**: 127–53.
5. Schaverien J (1999) Art within analysis: scapegoat, transference and transformation. *Journal of Analytical Psychology* **44**: 479–510.
6. Eisdell N (2005) A conversational model of art therapy. *Psychology and Psychotherapy* **78**: 1–19.
7. Meares R (2004) The conversational model: an outline. *American Journal of Psychotherapy* **58**: 51–66.
8. Tokuda Y (1980) Theory and practice of image art psychotherapy. *Confinia Psychiatrica* **23**: 193–208.
9. Plecity DM, Danner-Weinberger A, Szkura L, Wietersheim JV (2008) [The effects of art therapy on the somatic and emotional situation of the patients: a quantitative and qualitative analysis.] *Psychotherapie, Psychosomatik, Medizinische Psychologie* (in press).
10. Theorell T, Konarski K, Westerlund H, *et al.* (1998) Treatment of patients with chronic somatic symptoms by means of art psychotherapy: a process description. *Psychotherapy and Psychosomatics* **67**: 50–56.
11. McCaffrey R (2007) The effect of healing gardens and art therapy on older adults with mild to moderate depression. *Holistic Nursing Practice* **21**: 79–84.
12. Gussak D (2007) The effectiveness of art therapy in reducing depression in prison populations. *International Journal of Offender Therapy and Comparative Criminology* **51**: 444–60.
13. Persons RW (2008) Art therapy with serious juvenile offenders: a phenomenological analysis. *International Journal of Offender Therapy and Comparative Criminology* (in press).
14. Ruddy R, Milnes D (2003) Art therapy for schizophrenia or schizophrenia-like illnesses. *Cochrane Database of Systematic Reviews* (2): CD003728.
15. Ruddy R, Milnes D (2005) Art therapy for schizophrenia or schizophrenia-like illnesses. *Cochrane Database of Systematic Reviews* (4): CD003728.
16. Waller D (2006) Art therapy for children: how it leads to change. *Clinical Child Psychology and Psychiatry* **11**: 271–82.
17. Wallace J, Yorgin PD, Carolan R, *et al.* (2004) The use of art therapy to detect depression and post-traumatic stress disorder in pediatric and young adult renal transplant recipients. *Pediatric Transplantation* **8**: 52–9.
18. Bar-Sela G, Atid L, Danos S, *et al.* (2007) Art therapy improved depression and influenced fatigue levels in cancer patients on chemotherapy. *Psycho-oncology* **16**: 980–84.
19. Oster I, Svensk AC, Magnusson E, *et al.* (2006) Art therapy improves coping resources: a randomized, controlled study among women with breast cancer. *Palliative and Supportive Care* **4**: 57–64.
20. Rao D, Ņainis N, Williams L, *et al.* (2009) Art therapy for relief of symptoms associated with HIV/AIDS. *AIDS Care* **21**: 64–9.
21. Pachalska M, Franczuk B, Macqueen BD, *et al.* (2001) The impact of art therapy on the intelligibility of speech in children with cerebral palsy. *Ortopedia, Traumatologia, Rehabilitacja* **3**: 508–18.
22. Eitel K, Szkura L, Pokorny D, von Wietersheim J (2008) Do you see what I see? A study about the interrater reliability in art therapy. *Psychotherapy Research* **18**: 216–24.
23. Bernardi L, Porta C, Sleight P (2006) Cardiovascular, cerebrovascular, and respiratory changes induced by different types of music in musicians and non-musicians: the importance of silence. *Heart* **92**: 445–52.
24. Menon V, Levitin DJ (2005) The rewards of music listening: response and physiological connectivity of the mesolimbic system. *Neuroimage* **28**: 175–84.
25. Sridharan D, Levitin DJ, Chafe CH, *et al.* (2007) Neural dynamics of event segmentation in music: converging evidence for dissociable ventral and dorsal networks. *Neuron* **55**: 521–32.
26. Blood AJ, Zatorre RJ, Bermudez P, Evans AC (1999) Emotional responses to pleasant and unpleasant music correlate with activity in paralimbic brain regions. *Nature Neuroscience* **2**: 382–7.
27. Blood AJ, Zatorre RJ (2001) Intensely pleasurable responses to music correlate with activity in brain regions implicated in reward and emotion. Proceedings of the *National Academy of Science, USA* **98**: 11818–23.
28. Rauscher FH, Shaw GL, Ky KN (1993) Music and spatial task performance. *Nature* **365**: 611.
29. Rauscher FH, Robinson KD, Jens JJ (1998) Improved maze learning through early music exposure in rats. *Neurology Research* **20**: 427–32.
30. Rauscher FH, Shaw GL, Levine LJ, *et al.* (1997) Music training causes long-term enhancement of preschool children's spatial-temporal reasoning. *Neurology Research* **19**: 2–8.
31. Aoun P, Jones T, Shaw GL, Bodner M (2005) Long-term enhancement of maze learning in mice via a generalized Mozart effect. *Neurology Research* **27**: 791–6.
32. Sarnthein J, vonStein A, Rappelsberger P, *et al.* (1997) Persistent patterns of brain activity: an EEG coherence study of the positive effect of music on spatial-temporal reasoning. *Neurology Research* **19**: 107–16.
33. Hughes JR, Daaboul Y, Fino JJ, Shaw GL (1998) The 'Mozart effect' on epileptiform activity. *Clinical EEG* **29**: 109–19.
34. Wilson TL, Brown TL (1997) Re-examination of the effect of Mozart's music on spatial task performance. *Journal of Psychology* **131**: 365–70.
35. Gold C, Solli HP, Kruger V, Lie SA (2009) Dose-response relationship in music therapy for people with serious mental disorders: systematic review and meta-analysis. Clinical Psychology Review Apr **29**: 193–207.
36. Dryden W (ed.) (2007) *Dryden's Handbook of Individual Therapy*, 5th edn. London: Sage.

Chapter 67

Therapeutic communities

Kingsley Norton and Fiona Warren

DEFINITIONS

Therapeutic communities (TCs) developed before the psychopharmacological advances of the 1950s and long before the arrival of care in the wider community. Initially, they had represented a psychotherapeutic and sociotherapeutic response to the needs of the huge number of psychosocial casualties generated by the First World War. At that time, TCs were experimental treatments, innovated separately in different institutions. Working at Northfield Hospital, South Birmingham, Tom Main coined the term 'therapeutic community'.[1] For him, the TC was

> ... an attempt to use a hospital not as an organization run by doctors for their greater technical efficiency, but as a community with the immediate aim of full participation of all its members in its daily life and the eventual aim of the re-socialization of the neurotic individual for life in ordinary society.[1]

Main further defined the TC as 'a spontaneous and emotionally structured organisation rather than one which is medically dictated'. He stresses how important it is that

> ... the daily life of the TC [is] related to real tasks, i.e. those which are truly relevant to the needs and aspirations of the small society of the hospital, together with the larger society in which it is set.[1]

For him, it is crucial that patients are viewed as having 'sincere adult roles to play and (are) free to reach for responsibilities and opinions concerning the community of which they are a part'. Main recognizes the central importance of the interaction between patients and the staff – specifically, how the expectations and behaviour of staff exert a profound effect, for good or ill, on patients' treatment outcomes.

TC ideas and practices were extensively developed and deployed, in the UK and North America, by another pioneer, Dr Maxwell Jones. Indeed, the latter was credited by Main with influencing many professionals via his voluminous writings.[2] Working in Surrey, in the UK, at a unit within Belmont Hospital (later named Henderson Hospital), Jones structured the therapeutic day in his TC, giving the community meeting a pre-eminent position and using this forum as the place to sort out the most important and pressing clinical issues that arose.[3] The patients occupied positions of unusual power, for example as enacted through their 'chairing' of some crucial meetings, including the community meeting. When his TC was evaluated over a period of years by a visiting team of social anthropologists, the final report of their research appeared in the form of a book entitled *The Community as Doctor*.[4] The collective, therapeutic essence of the TC is captured by this title.

Subsequently, democratic TCs have been developed, especially along the lines of Henderson Hospital, in many psychiatric subspecialties, including forensic, and in different parts of the world.[5] Therefore, different patient groups and disorders have been treated using Jones' TC approach.[6] In the UK, its application has been deployed most conspicuously in relation to personality disorder (PD).[7] There is a promising and growing evidence base to support the application of this approach to such patients (see below), and recent service developments in the National Health Service (NHS) have seen a resurgence of TCs in community settings.[8] (In this chapter, we concentrate on the 'democratic' TC, as defined by Main and as pioneered in the 1940s, 1950s and beyond by both Main and Jones. We are not concerned here with 'concept' TCs, which have grown up in relation to the treatment of substance misuse, especially in the USA. See also Kennard[6] for a discussion of similarities and differences between these two approaches.)

PRINCIPLES OF TREATMENT

The magnitude of the organizational change in the style and extent of patient–staff collaboration within a ward or unit, which is implied by the TC ideology, requires a radical rethinking of the operation of the multidisciplinary staff team. Importantly, there is a de-emphasis of the staff's technical expertise and the recognition that patients are also 'expert' in the knowledge and experience of their own conditions and disorders. The effect is to flatten the traditional staff hierarchies and to blur the roles that previously were the sole preserve of a particular profession. In practice, this means that nurses and some relatively untrained professionals take on tasks that previously were carried out by more highly trained, including medical, staff.

The democratic TC is exquisitely patient-centred, requiring patients' active involvement in their own and others' treatment, via the preponderance of group-based activities. The therapeutic energy of all who inhabit the environment is needed to carry out its essential activities and functions. In the process, the patients' emotional and interpersonal difficulties, which they might struggle to put into words, are behaviourally manifest, hence potentially easier to recognize and understand. Maladaptive behaviour can be challenged and, with support and encouragement from their peers, patients can learn from one another (as well as from staff) to develop insights and be helped to experiment with other, more effective, more socially acceptable means of coping and expressing themselves.

What appears to make an effective TC is not so much its 'structure' – for example, the presence of community meetings – but the nature of its 'culture'.[2] Main referred to the particular requirement for a TC to provide 'a culture of enquiry ... into personal and interpersonal and intersystem problems and a study of impulses, defences, and relations as these are expressed and arranged socially'. This phrase, reflecting Main's psychoanalytical and systemic orientation, articulates a concern about the TC as a whole and the way in which its constituent human parts need to interrelate.[9] Therefore, an aspiring TC needs to be able to communicate, to disagree (when necessary) and to reach majority decisions with a minimum of hierarchical domination and a maximum of democracy, based on mutual respect for others' viewpoints. Such a culture supports the capacity of a TC subsystem (e.g. patients, as a group) to question directives from its suprasystem (e.g. the staff group). The latter is required to listen to and respond, other than defensively and self-protectively. In this way, an enquiring culture drives the structure, leading to: authentic dialogue among and between staff and patients; conflict identification, based on the empowerment of patients; and collaborative (democratic) management of problematic personal, interpersonal and social situations. This maintains the 'therapeutic' nature of the TC enterprise.

It is within the forum of the community meeting that it is plainest to observe the patient subsystem interacting with that of the staff. The nature and quality of this patient–staff relationship are important signifiers of the health of the TC. A healthy TC's patient subsystem is appropriately empowered, and its staff subsystem is able to relinquish, at least temporarily and thoughtfully, some of the authority invested in it. Internal organization and operation are such as to make use of a range of therapeutic approaches and disciplines, each with its own processes and techniques (e.g. group analytical psychotherapy, art therapy, psychodrama). The TC's hallmark is its successful blending of such individual ingredients, thereby producing a whole that is greater than the sum of its parts.[10]

INDICATIONS FOR REFERRAL AND PREPARATION

TCs have been set up, utilized and, to differing extents, evaluated in disparate settings and with respect to different patient groups, including:

- children and adolescents;
- people with severe and enduring mental illness;
- adults with acute mental health problems;
- people with emerging or established personality disorders;
- offenders;
- people with learning difficulties.[11]

Making judgements about which patients to refer, and when to refer, to TC treatment is dependent on many factors. The referring clinician needs not only to recognize patients who might benefit but also to know about what the treatment entails, so as to prepare the patient to have realistic expectations. As many TCs operate on an in-patient basis, they represent a costly resource. Therefore, most patients who are considered for such specialist treatment will have been marked by failure to improve with less intensive and less costly treatment alternatives. Indeed, such 'failures' might have exacerbated their presenting difficulties and worsened their prognosis. Engaging the patient, while avoiding the raising of falsely high expectations, represents a crucial clinical task. Although insufficient in itself, a reasonably robust therapeutic alliance is needed to support the necessary discussion of the relevant treatments available, enabling the patient to enter the process of referral on an informed basis, with realistic expectations and, optimally, appropriate motivation. As with imparting information to any patient about their possible treatment, much will depend upon the particulars of the case, especially what prior experience and knowledge the patient may already have. Below, we indicate some of the main points of which patients should be made aware in discussions about referral to a TC for treatment. Clearly the language used will need to be tailored to the requirements of the individual patient.

Delegation of traditional power and authority

In a TC, the patients may be struck initially by a difference in the way that patients and staff in a TC relate to each other. This is because the staff offer up to the patients some of the power and authority that are traditionally invested in them by virtue of the role as staff member. However, the relinquishing of authority by staff is not 'all or nothing'. The type and amount of 'power' that is delegated to the patients will vary from TC to TC and within the same TC. In a forensic setting, the range of tasks safely delegated will be narrower than in a non-forensic setting. The degree of the delegation of power to patients will be revealed in the extent to which patients may:

- play a role in selecting new patients for the TC;
- provide some of the response to untoward events that take place in the TC;
- play a part in interpreting rule violation and its consequences;
- exert an influence on continuing memberships of the TC of those who repeatedly break the TC's rules.

Patients need to be aware of this delegated responsibility, not least since it may contradict their previous experiences of being in therapy. This delegation of power contributes to the potential for the patient to have a different experience of themselves and others, including healthcare staff.

Staff–patient collaboration

Many patients (especially patients with antisocial PD) have had unsatisfying interactions or relationships with staff, and their trust in professionals may be low. However, this is not necessarily the case, and the referral to a TC might itself be a marker that the relationship with the referring professional is positive. What should be transmitted to the prospective TC patient, however, is that they should expect an opportunity for genuine empowerment that they might not have encountered previously. There is an expectation, within the TC, that there will be active involvement and a working together with staff, if not from the start, as they become familiar with the treatment model.

Collaboration is thus a potential to be realized, which can only come about as a result of the patient's experience of the TC – that is, via a process that includes mistrusting and testing out (see below).

Rights and responsibilities

Enjoying the privilege of power-sharing comes at a price. There is an expectation on all TC members that their membership is 'active'. This means taking part both in the formal therapy programme, including adhering to the rules (see below), and in the more mundane aspects of the TC's everyday life, including necessary 'domestic' functions, such as washing up, cleaning, ordering and storing food, and creating rotas for escort duties and other support functions. Patients need to engage in therapy sessions (psychotherapy) and also become part of the daily social life of the TC (sociotherapy) in being both a recipient and a provider of therapy. This requirement for them to be part of the whole treatment programme represents a significant challenge. However, there is an expectation that this occurs only gradually, as part of the therapeutic process, and there is much support from their peers, who are struggling, like them, to achieve this.

Rules and rule-breaking

Just as in wider society, from which patients are drawn and to which they will return post-discharge, there are rules in the TC. These mirror (in most instances of open, as opposed to secure, TCs), the mores and laws of the relevant society. Therefore, violence to others and property is proscribed, as is the taking of illicit substances. Other than this, there may be rules governing aspects that ordinarily do not obtain in wider, free society – for example, the proscribing of alcohol (at least the imbibing of it on the TC premises) or the avoidance of sexual contact between patients. What is crucial for a given TC is that its rules are relevant to the TC's membership, neither set too high and outlawing behaviour that cannot voluntarily be curbed, nor set too low, requiring no thought or effort to comply. The optimum is that the patients are under a tolerable degree of stress or anxiety, which enables them also, over time, to reflect on their attitude to rules and authentic belonging to a group. Many habitual rule-breakers exhibit a hypocritical attitude to rules, not relishing others to behave like themselves.

Interaction, exploration and experimentation

During a successful stay in a TC, it is likely that patients will experience and recognize different phases and processes of the therapy, which can be summarized as interaction, exploration and experimentation.[12] In practice, it is difficult for patients to avoid the first – interaction – although some may attempt to do so. There will be a full programme of activities, most of which are group-based, and absences are questioned – part of the culture of enquiry (see above). Exploration relates to this latter aspect, for example to understand the possible meaning of a patient's non-attendance at a therapy session or failure to undertake a practical task, such as doing their share of the communal washing up rota. In this way, the patient's social behaviour (as well as what they might talk about during the therapy sessions) is considered and commented on by their immediate peers and the wider TC, including staff. This provides food for thought; hence, there is scope for the patient to try out new ways of thinking and behaving. Such 'experimentation' can take many forms, and failure is often tolerated by the TC membership, provided that the collective perception is that the member's attempt to reflect and change or adapt is sincere. A patient's successful stay will be marked by involvement in all these phases and processes, including the carrying out of 'failed' experiments. All phases and processes need to be encountered, although the proportion varies according to the patient's requirements. Avoidant patients require more peer support and pressure to interact and experiment, while those with impulse-control problems benefit from peer group reactions and pressure to abstain from their habitual actions and to reflect.[13]

Transition, discharge and aftercare

Leaving a TC can be problematic; therefore, attention is focused on relevant attachment and separation issues from the start of the patient's stay.[14] Those who complete their stay – by no means all who start out – will probably find themselves having become attached to it. For some, it is the first time they will have felt 'at home'.[15] As a consequence, dealing with the leaving process is painful and potentially problematic for all concerned – those remaining as well as those actually departing. TCs vary in how they approach and deal with this crucial phase of the therapeutic journey, although each emphasizes its importance. In many instances, there is an acknowledgement, due to the extent and complexity of the patient's presenting problems, that the patient has not been 'cured' but has made an important start on the road to recovery. Relevant gains often require consolidation, from further out-patient work.

TREATMENT OUTCOME

Studies of the effectiveness of therapeutic community treatment for personality disorder have addressed the key problem domains, from symptomatic change to re-offending, and included studies of cost. Lees and colleagues subjected to meta-analysis 29 studies of TCs, 8 of which were randomized controlled trials (RCTs). They found a summary log odds ratio of −0.512 (95% confidence interval (CI) −0.598 to −0.426), a strong treatment effect.[16] These studies included a range of outcome measures and included both concept and democratic TCs.

In the first study of the effectiveness of the Henderson Hospital therapeutic community, Rapoport's team of researchers classified 64 patients 1 year after their discharge, judging 41 per cent to be 'improved' compared with pretreatment.[17] Subsequent, more rigorous studies have found similar proportions of improvement. Eight months following discharge, 55 per cent of patients improved reliably and 32 per cent improved clinically significantly[18] on the overall measure of neurotic symptoms (Global Severity Index, GSI) of the Symptom Checklist 90 (SCL-90).[19,20] Over 40 per cent of clients who under democratic therapeutic community (DTC) treatment versus 18 per cent of those who were not admitted had improved clinically significantly in symptoms of borderline personality disorder (BPD).[21] In a comparison study with allocation to treatment group on geographical grounds, 80 per cent of clients at the Cassel Hospital had improved clinically significantly on the GSI at around 2 years post-discharge.[22] Importantly, these studies also reported rates of deterioration, which were very small.

Personality-disordered clients are high users of a range of services, from medical through psychiatric to social and criminal justice, and both service usage itself and costs of this have been studied. At Henderson Hospital, early studies of re-admission and reconviction found that at 3 years' post-treatment follow-up, 71 per cent of those patients who stayed in treatment for 9 months or more were neither reconvicted nor re-admitted (*v.* 23% in the not-admitted group, as above); 65 per cent of them remained free of reconvictions and re-admissions at 5 years post-treatment (*v.* 19% in the not-admitted group).[23] An early study of cost-offset showed that post-treatment costs could be as little as 10 per cent of pretreatment costs and offsetting the investment in treatment in just over 2 years.[24–28] Subsequent studies support cost-effectiveness against baseline costs and against general psychiatric service input.[29]

Although there is a demonstrable positive relationship between length of stay in a residential therapeutic community and improvement in symptomatology over the first 3 months,[20] and in symptoms and service usage at 1 year, 3 years and 5 years post-discharge,[21,23] there is some evidence that a shorter period of inpatient treatment, with outpatient follow-up (6 months + 6 months) may be more effective than 12 months of in-patient treatment alone: a significantly larger proportion of patients in the two-stage (39%) than the one-stage (18%) treatment offered at the Cassel Hospital were reliably improved.[22] Research findings suggest that continued improvement may continue beyond the end of treatment.[22,30]

Most of the research on TCs is effectiveness rather than efficacy research – the majority of studies have been naturalistic studies rather than RCTs[31] – although type 1 evidence is also available,[32] suggesting the effectiveness of the TC approach to treating PD. Methodological sophistication has increased as the field of study has developed, and as the rhetoric that funding for services be tied more closely to evidence of effectiveness has been stated more widely.[16] Despite controversy around the appropriateness of the RCT research paradigm for evaluation of a socially complex intervention such as a TC,[33,34] some have been evaluated using RCTs. The principles of good effectiveness research require that robust assessment measures are used to evaluate change in factors that the treatment is designed to change and that these changes are compared with an appropriate alternative condition. Furthermore, it is desirable that assessment is carried out at a suitable point in time *after* the end of treatment. Some guidelines for evaluating treatment for personality disorders exist,[7] and reviews suggest areas in which the evidence base needs to be improved.[35–37] Nonetheless, thus far, the evidence suggests that TCs are an effective approach to reducing both PD features and general symptomatological distress, service usage and costs.

SUMMARY

The development of newer approaches no doubt modified the patient groups who are referred to TCs. However, in spite of having existed in the UK for more than 60 years, TCs remain unusual therapeutic institutions and there remains a place for democratic TCs within the overall treatment armoury. Although there is an evidence base for democratic TCs, part of the preparation and processing of referrals needs to include an assessment of 'fit'. The referring clinician needs not only to undertake a thorough (diagnostic and psychodynamic) assessment of the patient and his or her motivation and treatment needs, but also to impart knowledge of the particular TC to the patient. Without this, there is potentially a mismatch between the service user's capacities and expectations and the service provided, which can be psychologically damaging. It is important that those patients referred understand the nature of the TC's treatment process, in which they would take part, including why they might need to be assessed by the TC before being accepted. Rejection can be traumatic, and this needs to be borne in mind by the referring clinician, being taken into account as part of the preparation of the patient for referral, so as to minimize the risk of iatrogenic harm. Where the fit is good, the therapeutic impact on outcome has been shown to be significantly beneficial.

KEY POINTS

- TCs represent authentic patient-centred psychiatric services.
- TCs have for a long time viewed their patients as 'expert' in their own condition, a view increasingly recognized as important by health systems.
- TCs embody the ethos of patient empowerment, i.e. their involvement in the running of some aspects of hospital organization traditionally the province only of staff.
- TCs function effectively because they are a microcosm of society (in which dysfunction is revealed, leading to insight and experimentation with new coping strategies), and hence what is learned can generalize to life outside.
- TCs are set up to maximize (especially peer group) feedback to the patients so that the effects of their actions or inaction are conveyed clearly and quickly, facilitating insight and learning from such a responsive environment.
- TCs present their patients with the views of other people that challenge their own, even though the 'new' relationships with others are initially mistrusted and therefore (sometimes aggressively) tested for their sincerity and strength.
- TCs require clearly stated and robustly and reliably implemented rules that tolerate degrees of deviance, destructiveness and distress but also set and fairly apply strict limits.
- TCs are relatively long-term treatments, usually more than 6 months, and, although applied to a range of different client groups, cater mostly for patients with personality disorder.
- Preparation for the selection, and also for the joining, processes of the TC, is crucially important as is an assessment of the patient's need for suitable aftercare.
- TCs have a body of research evidence about effectiveness, including health economic benefits.

REFERENCES

1. Main T (1946) The hospital as a therapeutic institution. *Bulletin of the Menninger Clinic* **10**: 66–8.
2. Main TF (1983) The concept of the therapeutic community: its variations and vicissitudes. In M Pines (ed) *The Evolution of Group Analysis*. London: Routledge & Kegan Paul.
3. Jones M (1952) *Social Psychiatry: A Study of Therapeutic Communities*. London: Tavistock Publications.
4. Rapoport R (1960) *The Community as Doctor*. London: Tavistock Publications.
5. Manning N (1989) *The Therapeutic Community Movement: Charisma and Routinization*. London: Routledge & Kegan Paul.
6. Kennard D (1988) *An Introduction to Therapeutic Communities*. London: Karnac Books.
7. Norton K, Dolan B (1995) Assessing change in personality disorder. *Current Opinion in Psychiatry* **8**: 371–5.
8. Crawford M, Rutter D, Price K, *et al.* (2007) *Learning the Lessons: A Multi-Method Evaluation of Dedicated Community-Based Services for Personality Disorder*. London: National Co-ordinating Centre for Service Delivery and Organisation R&D (NCCSDO).
9. Norton K (1992) A culture of enquiry: its preservation or loss. *Therapeutic Communities* **13**: 3–26.
10. Norton K (2003) Henderson Hospital: greater than the sum of its sub-groups. *Group Work* **13**: 65–100.
11. Kennard D (1998) *An Introduction to Therapeutic Communities*, 2nd edn. London: Jessica Kingsley Publishers.
12. Whiteley JS (1986) Sociotherapy and psychotherapy in the treatment of personality disorder: discussion paper. *Journal of the Royal Society of Medicine* **79**: 721–5.
13. Norton K (1992b) Personality disordered individuals: the Henderson Hospital model of treatment. *Criminal Behaviour and Mental Health* **2**: 180–91.
14. Norton KRW (1999) Joining and leaving. In R Haigh, P Campling (eds) *Therapeutic Communities: Past, Present and Future*. London: Jessica Kingsley Publishers.
15. Parker M (1989) Managing separation: the Henderson Hospital leavers' group. *International Journal of Therapeutic Communities* **8**: 21–31.
16. Lees J, Manning N, Rawlings B (2004) A culture of enquiry: research evidence and the therapeutic community. *Psychiatric Quarterly* **75**: 279–94.
17. Rapoport R (1960) Patterns of patient reaction to the unit. In *The Community as Doctor*. London: Tavistock Publications
18. Jacobson NS, Truax P (1991) Clinical significance: a statistical approach to defining meaningful change in psychotherapy research. *Journal of Consulting and Clinical Psychology* **59**: 12–19.
19. Derogatis LR, Rickels K, Rock AF (1976) The SCL-90 and the MMPI: a step in the validation of a new self-report scale. *British Journal of Psychiatry* **128**: 280–89.
20. Dolan BM, Evans CDH, Wilson J (1992) Neurotic symptomatology and length of stay in a therapeutic community. *International Journal of Therapeutic Communities* **13**: 171–7.
21. Dolan B, Warren F, Norton K (1997) Change in border-

line symptoms one year after therapeutic community treatment for severe personality disorder. *British Journal of Psychiatry* **171**: 274–9.

22. Chiesa M, Fonagy P (2003) Psychosocial treatment for severe personality disorder. *British Journal of Psychiatry* **183**: 356–62.
23. Copas JB, O'Brien M, Roberts JC, Whiteley S (1984) Treatment outcome in personality disorder: the effect of social, psychological and behavioural variables. *Personality and Individual Differences* **5**: 565–73.
24. Chiesa M, Iacoponi E, Morris M (1996) Changes in health service utilization by patients with severe personality disorders before and after inpatient psychosocial treatment. *British Journal of Psychotherapy* **12**: 501–12.
25. Davies S, Campling P (2003) Therapeutic community treatment of personality disorder: service use and mortality over 3 years' follow up. *British Journal of Psychiatry* **182**: s24–7.
26. Davies S, Menzies D (2004) Economic evaluations in therapeutic community research. In J Lees, M Manning, D Menzies, *et al.* (eds) *A Culture of Enquiry: Research Evidence and the Therapeutic Community*. London: Jessica Kingsley Publishers.
27. Dolan BM, Warren FM, Menzies D, *et al.* (1996) Cost-offset following specialist treatment of severe personality disorders. *Psychiatric Bulletin* **20**: 413–17.
28. Menzies D, Dolan BM, Norton K (1993) Are short term savings worth long term costs? Funding psychotherapeutic inpatient treatment for personality disorders. *Psychiatric Bulletin* **17**: 517–19.
29. Chiesa M, Fonagy P, Holmes J, *et al.* (2002) Health service use costs by personality disorder following specialist and non-specialist treatment: a comparative study. *Journal of Personality Disorders* **16**: 160–73.
30. Warren F (2004) Outcome of Specialist Therapeutic Community Treatment. PhD thesis. London: St George's Hospital Medical School.
31. Jadad A (1998) *Randomised Controlled Trials*. London: BMJ Books.
32. Khan KS, ter Riet G, Glanville J, *et al.* (eds) (2001) *Undertaking Systematic Reviews of Effectiveness: CRD's Guidelines for Those Carrying Out or Commissioning Reviews*. CRD report no. 4, 2nd edn. York: Centre for Reviews and Dissemination, University of York.
33. Manning N (2004) The gold standard: what are RCTs and where did they come from? In J Lees, N Manning, D Menzies, *et al.* (eds) *A Culture of Enquiry: Research Evidence and the Therapeutic Community*. London: Jessica Kingsley Publishers.
34. Wolff N (2001) Randomised trials of socially complex interventions: promise or peril? *Journal of Health Services Research and Policy* **6**: 123–6.
35. Dolan BM, Coid J (1993) *Psychopathic and Antisocial Personality Disorders: Treatment and Research Issues*. London: Gaskell.
36. Duggan C, Adams C, McCarthy L, *et al.* (2005) *A Systematic Review of the Effectiveness of Pharmacological and Psychological Treatments for those with Personality Disorder*. London: National Programme on Forensic Mental Health.
37. Warren F, Preedy-Fayers K, McGauley G, *et al.* (2003) *Review of Treatments for Severe Personality Disorder*. London: Home Office. www.homeoffice.gov.uk/rds/onlinepubs1.html.

Chapter 68

Effectiveness of psychotherapy

Peter Fonagy

INTRODUCTION

Psychological therapy has been defined as 'an interpersonal process designed to bring about modifications of feelings, cognitions, attitudes and behavior which have proved troublesome to the person who is seeking help from a trained professional'.[1] The psychological therapies are a very diverse set of activities, now including at least seven major classes of approach: (i) psychodynamic psychotherapy, (ii) behavioural and cognitive-behavioural therapy (CBT), (iii) interpersonal psychotherapy, (iv) strategic or systemic psychotherapies, (v) supportive and experiential therapies, (vi) group therapies and (vii) counselling. Each approach provides a model of human behaviour and heuristic foci for interventions.

DETERMINING THE EFFICACY OF TREATMENTS

All psychotherapeutic models provide aetiological formulations, but the evidence base for these is limited. Ideally, as with other medical treatments, the mechanism of therapeutic change entailed in a clinical approach should be understood and tested while simultaneously monitoring the effectiveness of the intervention.[2] The best way to compare these treatments is by randomized controlled trials (RCTs), where variables likely to influence outcome, such as therapist experience and treatment length, are controlled. Studies also increasingly aim to ensure that treatments are carried out in conformity with their theoretical description, for example ensuring that CBT does not include psychodynamic elements and vice versa. To this end, many treatments have been manualized, with the techniques entailed by the therapy pragmatically delineated. Manualization enables reviewers to check whether a treatment was actually delivered in a manner consistent with that advocated by its proponents. There are some limitations to this approach. For example, differences between the groups may occur despite randomization because of small sample sizes. Although the presence of a no-treatment control group would provide an ideal benchmark, it is not ethically viable to withhold treatment in cases other than the very short-term psychotherapies. An increasing number of studies have compared psychosocial interventions with medication or have examined the addition of psychosocial interventions to pharmacological treatment. The criterion used most often to establish the evidence base of a therapeutic approach for a particular condition is the replication of a good-quality RCT with an independent group of investigators testing the same manualized treatment with the same diagnostic group.

Since Hans Eysenck expressed doubts about the overall efficacy of psychotherapy,[3] there have been several meta-analyses of the psychotherapy research literature,[4] as well as narrative reviews,[5] which have examined hundreds of studies measuring the outcome of many forms of therapy. Most studies report a considerable effect size (0.50–0.85) when treatment is contrasted with no treatment, but in most studies other than where a medication arm is used psychotherapy benefits from a placebo effect. The major meta-analyses of therapy outcome have been drawn from rigorously controlled studies (random assignment, careful specification of patient population, use of a treatment manual, raters naive to conditions, statistical power adequate to examine the null hypothesis, and replication by independent investigators).

There is a generally accepted hierarchy of evidence[6] that reflects the degree of certainty with which we can causally attribute observed changes to the treatment under scrutiny. At the top of the hierarchy are RCTs and their aggregation in systematic reviews and meta-analyses. At the second level are controlled trials without randomization and experimental single case designs. At the third level are cohort studies, where groups of patients are allocated to treatments. Ranked below these are case–control studies, where patients with similar outcomes are grouped together and the treatment to which they were exposed is studied retrospectively. At the base of the hierarchy are comparisons across historical times or geographical places, with or without an intervention, alongside the accumulation of professional experience. Finally come descriptive studies.

Although RCTs are at the top of this hierarchy, which is constructed in terms of the clarity of causal inference, RCTs are not without major limitations in the evaluation of psychological therapies. To be proof against chance findings, RCTs require large samples (often over 100 patients per treatment arm in the case of psychotherapies). The comparison of treated and control groups yields the results of the trial. In drug trials the control is uniform (the placebo pill), but in the case of psychological therapies it can be quite variable. Treatment as usual (TAU) in North America is very different from that in Europe or the UK, and this can yield very different results in RCTs of the same treatment conducted in different places, even if that treatment is well manualized. In trials involving two active treatments, assignment to treatment arms is complicated, as patients are likely to have substantial preferences regarding particular styles of psychotherapeutic interventions. (Interventions can, for example, vary in the extent to which they are oriented towards reflection or how directive they are.)

The sheer number of RCTs of psychological therapies presents a challenge for aggregating evidence. Meta-analysis, the arithmetic aggregation of clinical trials, actually entered the medical field via the psychotherapies.[7] The two most commonly used methods of aggregation are averaging *relative risk* (the relative proportion of individuals who no longer meet diagnostic criteria) and the *standardized mean difference* (the difference between treatment and control group means at the end of treatment, divided by the standard deviation of the control group). Both of these statistics can be made more readily applicable by translating them into percentiles indicating the likelihood that a treated client is better off than a control patient or the degree to which the treated client is benefited. These *effect sizes* are stated with 95 per cent confidence intervals (CI). If the confidence interval does not include a null or negative effect, then the results suggest that the treatment is effective. The level of efficacy is indicated by the size of the coefficient, with 0.2 being considered small, 0.5 medium and 0.8 large. Such data aggregation is clearly desirable but, inevitably, there are complications. Aggregation is possible only across a homogeneous set of studies – that is, studies that address the same research question with the same kind of treatment and the same kind of client group, using comparable measures. The sample of studies may not be representative. There appears to be a bias against publishing negative findings. The effect sizes associated with published studies are significantly larger than those of unpublished investigations, both in psychotherapy[8] and in pharmacotherapy.[9] The allegiance of the researcher is also quite a powerful predictor of outcome.[10]

Measuring the outcome of psychotherapy of course depends on finding an appropriate and generally agreed metric for outcome. There can be no doubt that the metrics we mostly use in evaluating psychological therapy are, to a large extent, arbitrary.[11] There are no absolute scales even to measure depression, let alone more subtle constructs such as wellbeing or marital satisfaction. Most measures are 'reactive'. In other words, they interact with the treatment modality, such as measuring the impact of CBT in terms of changes in depressogenic cognitions, which is the primary focus of that type of intervention. Because of this, many have called for the use of biomarkers, such as haemodynamic responses to specific types of stimuli in functional magnetic resonance imaging (fMRI) studies, to assess the effectiveness of psychological therapies.[12]

There are a range of other issues and problems associated with the evaluation of psychotherapies. The range of patients who are willing to participate in an RCT may not be representative, either in terms of ethnicity or in terms of severity or complexity. Follow-ups are rarely long enough to assess accurately whether the impact of the treatment will be lasting. Often authors report significant results on one measure but find no significance on another, and there is no widely accepted method for integrating such disparate observations. Treatments are usually considered in relation to particular disorders, but in reality patients rarely come with a single disorder and in clinical work co-morbidity is the routine rather than the exception. Some disorders are far better researched than others, and some therapies lend themselves more readily to manualization and randomization. The economic impacts of psychotherapies are of enormous concern, but the methodology for calculating economic impact is as yet quite limited.

These limitations have to be borne in mind when treatment guidelines such as those developed by the National Institute for Health and Clinical Excellence (NICE) are implemented. They rely on evidence from controlled studies, thus restricting the range of approaches, are conducted in a clinical context that does not reflect real life, deliberately attempt partially to eliminate factors such as variation in therapist quality from the assessment, and are no better able to answer complex questions concerning outcome than are cohort or case–control studies. Recognizing this, many guidelines development groups take quite a sophisticated approach to addressing the limitations of research-based evidence by adding qualitative methodology to the quantitative. Another difficulty is that guidelines often recommend psychological therapies, but therapists with appropriate specific competencies may not be available. NICE guidelines have tended to recommend CBT as an efficacious treatment for a range of mental health problems, but it should be recognized that CBT is a very broad category and effective practitioners require training to address a number of specific diagnostic conditions. Taking into account these reservations, treatment guidelines have been helpful in improving the quality of care across a number of diagnostic entities.[13]

A GLIMPSE OF THE EVIDENCE BASE

Space does not permit a review of the empirical status of psychotherapy for all mental disorders, but for a comprehensive review see Roth and Fonagy.[5] To illustrate the nature of the evidence base, we will consider only briefly the two most prevalent axis I disorders, anxiety and depression, and the most commonly investigated axis II condition, borderline personality disorder (BPD).

The literature on RCTs clearly identifies behavioural and cognitive-behavioural treatments as highly efficacious in the treatment of anxiety disorders. The best effect sizes have been reported for cognitive therapy for panic disorder (d = 2.9),[14,15] cognitive therapy for post-traumatic stress disorders (d = 1.3–2.2),[16,17] cognitive therapy for social phobia (d = 2.6),[18,19] CBT for generalized anxiety disorder (d = 1.7),[20,21] exposure and response prevention for obsessive–compulsive disorder (d = 1.6),[22,23] and exposure for specific phobias (d = 2.7).[24,25] Many of these studies used unstructured supportive treatment as an attention placebo control.

There are a few RCTs of psychodynamic therapies for anxiety,[26] but there are some notable trials for depression.[27] The National Institute of Mental Health (NIMH) Treatment of Depression Collaborative Research Program is perhaps the most widely cited research programme and set a standard against which other studies could be judged. In this study, patients were randomized to receive one of four interventions: cognitive-behavioural psychotherapy, interpersonal psychotherapy (IPT), imipramine plus clinical management (IMI-CM), or placebo plus clinical management (PLA-CM). Clinical management consisted of a weekly meeting of 20–30 min to discuss medication, side effects and the patient's clinical status. In addition, and where necessary, support, encouragement and direct advice were also offered. On this basis, it is worth noting that both medication conditions contained psychotherapeutic elements. A total of 250 patients, all moderately to severely depressed, were selected for the trial at three research sites; 239 patients actually entered the trial. Patients were assessed before treatment and at 4, 8, 12 and 16 weeks and then followed up at 6, 12 and 18 months. Post-therapy, the general direction of results was similar on all measures and in all samples,[28] with patients who received IMI-CM having the lowest symptomatic scores, those who received PLA-CM the most symptomatic, and the psychotherapies in between and usually closer to IMI-CM. The magnitude of these differences was not large, and pair-wise comparison of treatment conditions revealed no differences between therapies or between therapies and IMI-CM. Patients who received IMI-CM and IPT were significantly more likely to recover than those who had received PLA-CM; a trend toward significance was apparent in the other two patient samples. There were, however, no significant differences between therapies or between therapies and IMI-CM in any patient sample. The lack of significant differences seems attributable to the good performance of PLA-CM (e.g. 62% achieved clinically significant change using the Beck Depression Inventory (BDI) as a measure). For patients with lower levels of depression, PLA-CM (which could be considered a 'minimal support' intervention) was as effective as the active therapies. Relapse was defined as the presence of at least 2 weeks of major depressive disorder (MDD)-level symptoms over the 18-month follow-up period. Only 20 per cent of the original sample and 24 per cent of the patients with follow-up data met the criteria for recovery with no relapse. Of those entering therapies, 24 per cent of patients receiving CBT remained recovered without relapse at 18 months, compared with 23 per cent for IPT, 16 per cent for IMI-CM and 16 per cent for PLA-CM. The findings indicate that few patients recover and remain well with 16 weeks of treatment, and a clear conclusion from this study is that interventions of this length are not sufficient to maintain functioning in the majority of patients.

The studies with the most stringent criteria of methodological rigour indicate the efficacy of interpersonal psychotherapy and CBT. In the single trial that contrasted dynamic-interpersonal therapy and CBT, the two modes of treatment were equivalent in their efficacy. This broad equivalence between outcomes from bona fide therapies is an important finding, suggesting as it does that depression may be responsive to a range of psychotherapeutic techniques. Many large-scale careful studies, such as the Helsinki study, found no difference between therapies with different orientations (e.g. no difference was found between psychodynamic psychotherapy and solution-focused psychotherapy, a systemic psychotherapy[29]). Overall, the generally observed effect size for the psychodynamic treatment for anxiety is hard to estimate, and for depression the outcomes are comparable to CBT, although both types of therapy have only small to medium effects in the long term.[30] In no instance has psychodynamic therapy been shown to be superior to CBT. Most studies compare CBT with drug treatment, and the average effect size across 12 studies (n = 1200) for comparisons with drug treatment indicates that pharmacotherapy is just as effective (effect size = 0.01; 95% CI −0.1, 0.13). In a meta-analysis of short-term psychodynamic psychotherapy, Abbass and colleagues analysed 23 studies of 1431 randomized patients with common mental disorders.[31] These studies covered a range of patient groups, including somatic, anxiety and depressive patients, and patients with social adjustment problems. Moderate effect sizes were obtained in most comparisons, indicating significantly greater improvement in the treatment versus the control groups, which were generally maintained in medium- and long-term follow-up. The findings indicated that short-term dynamic psychotherapy showed modest to moderate gains for a variety of patients, which were mostly sustained. However, there was substantial heterogeneity and variability in treatment delivery and treatment quality, indicating the need for larger studies of higher quality and with specific diagnoses.

For most axis I conditions, various implementations of CBT have the most RCTs, and in general relatively good results are reported. No other therapy has been tested as frequently in trials, but of course we need to remember that the absence of evidence does not imply evidence of the absence of effectiveness.[5] RCTs for personality disorder are less unequivocal in favouring CBT. Some studies of BPD show CBT to be marginal in effectiveness,[32,33] and some even reported slight iatrogenic effects.[34]

Dialectical behavioural therapy (DBT), an outgrowth of CBT that was tailored for BPD, was shown to be highly efficacious in treating suicidality and self-harm in borderline women, but not in treating depression.[35,36] By contrast, a somewhat longer psychodynamic treatment yielded similar effect sizes for para-suicide but also showed improvement for depression and anxiety.[37,38] Head-to-head comparisons have yielded equivocal results. One 3-year treatment trial apparently favoured a version of cognitive therapy over psychodynamic treatment,[39] but another, better controlled trial showed little difference between DBT, psychodynamic therapy and supportive psychotherapy.[40]

RCTs are the gold standard in evidence-based medicine, but the results of these trials are often hard to apply in the context of a medical practice.[41] A major reason for this is that individuals participating in clinical trials will not always resemble the patients that a clinician would see in psychotherapy.[42] It is reasonably clear that in general, 'research therapy' appears more effective than everyday clinical practice.[43] Possible reasons for this include methodological issues, among them the use of focused and structured manualized treatments, careful attention to ensure therapist adherence to protocol, recruitment of participants directly rather than through clinical services, and greater exclusion rates.

COMMON FACTORS IN PSYCHOTHERAPY: SPECIFIC AND NON-SPECIFIC EFFECTS

Psychological treatments work, but by what mechanism? Does it make any difference which method or which theory is the basis for treatment? This issue can be addressed only by conducting comparative trials, in which different forms of treatment are studied head to head.

A number of such studies have been published comparing a wide of range of therapies, including psychodynamic, behavioural, cognitive, interpersonal and client-centred methods. The results are surprisingly consistent: with notable exceptions (e.g. the superiority of CBT over interpersonal therapy for the treatment of obsessive–compulsive disorder and other anxiety disorders), research has failed to show that any one method is more potent than the others. For example, an ambitious comparative trial of transference-focused psychotherapy, DBT and supportive psychotherapy for BPD showed little difference between these three forms of treatment after 1 year of therapy.[40] Over recent decades, psychotherapy research has demonstrated repeatedly that a substantial proportion of the variability in therapeutic outcomes across trials is not explained well by differences between formally defined therapeutic procedures, differences between client groups, or (less well examined) the interaction between these two factors.[44–47] In addition, research has found it hard to show strong correlations between outcome and changes at the level of the mechanism that a particular therapy has postulated as its primary target. For example, in a study of CBT, the extent of focus on 'parental issues' turned out to be positively associated with outcome.[48] In a study of psychodynamic psychotherapy process and outcome, Piper and colleagues found that, in sicker patients with whom the therapeutic alliance is shaky, the use of transference interpretations to deal with problems between therapist and patient made the outcome worse, not better.[49] In another study, a negative association has been reported between the number of transference interpretations and therapy outcome, indicating that the overuse of this technique, frequently regarded by clinicians as essential to therapeutic success, may even be iatrogenic.[50] In fact, it is not so much the differences between procedures that indicate the most effective ingredients of psychological treatments, but the similarities. For, if each therapy is successful in its own way, and if each therapy shares common (or 'non-specific') factors with all others, then success depends on these non-specific factors, which are so-called because we do not know how to specify them.

A methodological review of child psychotherapy treatment studies between 1995 and 2004 found that recent research did not give adequate attention to non-specific therapeutic factors, including the effects of attention, positive regard and therapeutic alliance, as well as the effects of treatment dose, intensity, and actual processes mediating therapeutic change.[51] In an attempt to identify which interventions lead to progress, Orlinksy and colleagues conducted process research on over 50 different variables describing the process of psychotherapy in relation to its outcome.[52] They concluded that 'non-specific' factors are the primary reason behind successful treatment. As a result, they proposed a 'generic model' of psychotherapy, which includes the factors common to all methods, from psychoanalysis to behaviour therapy.[52] It is possible that the common factor uniting therapies is simply that therapists help to make their patients feel hopeful at a time when they are hopeless or demoralized, and that specific theories have little bearing on this matter.[53] Data showing that a good relationship with a therapist is a crucial factor in the outcome of treatment might support this argument.[54,55] The majority of studies in this area find, unsurprisingly, that therapeutic alliance is impacted by the patient's attachment style and quality of object relations,[56–58] although studies also implicate the therapist's attachment security.[59] It is certainly plausible to argue that those with a secure attachment style approach the therapeutic relationship with greater openness and optimism, which might account for the particularly strong associations found in psychotherapy investigations between pretreatment expectancies and the subsequently observed quality of the alliance.[60–63] The paradox is that controlled trials demonstrate repeatedly that the relationship, if not informed by theoretically coherent content, is actually of little therapeutic value.[4,64] It also appears to be the case that the impact of attachment style may be strongest at the initial meeting with the therapist, after which perhaps more subtle processes (arguably still related to attachment) come to determine the alliance.[65] Thus, although all agree that the patient's relationship with the therapist is a key catalyst in psychodynamic treatment, the nature of therapeutic benefit that patients draw from this new relationship seems yet to be resolved.

THERAPIST FACTORS IN THERAPY OUTCOME

Wampold points out that the evidence for common factors highlights the importance of the therapist and his or her skill.[4] The key designs and methods of psychotherapy research peculiarly owe their origins to the common statistical roots that they share with trial methodology in farming, education and medicine.[66] This is understandable, but it is curious that most studies of interventions have tested the effectiveness of therapies without paying very much attention to the role of the therapist.

In Kim and colleagues' analysis of the NIMH Treatment of Depression Collaborative Research Project (TDCRP) dataset, 5–10 per cent of the variance in outcomes was shown to be associated with therapists.[66] In more naturalistic studies, the effects tend to be larger. For example, Okiishi and colleagues examined variations in patient outcomes for 91 therapists treating nearly 2000 patients.[67] The therapists whose patients showed most improvement had an average change rate 10 times greater than the sample's mean rate. This is consistent with other studies using a growth curve approach, where as much as 17 per cent of the variance in rates of patient improvement has appeared to be attributable to the therapist.[68] Very large studies, with datasets of over 5000 patients, consistently report large effects associated with therapists.[69]

Some therapists are better than others, but what contributes to that quality? Beutler and colleagues carefully reviewed studies of the impact of therapist characteristics on outcome.[44,45] The therapist's age, gender and ethnicity appear to have little or no impact on results, and nor are there significant differences in outcome when therapist and client are matched on these variables. Assessment of the impact of therapist personality variables is limited, with some studies attempting post hoc atheoretical analysis, and others a more theory-driven approach, with no consistent or robust findings. There are indications that therapists with better levels of adjustment may have better outcomes, although there is some inconsistency across studies.

Contrary to received wisdom, empirical findings suggest that the therapist's experience does not help to predict outcome. Attempts to show the effects of experience have no conclusive results.[44,70] Wierzbicki and Pekarik's meta-analysis of 125 studies found that there was no correlation between dropout rate and the therapist's experience in years or professional qualifications – although there is some evidence that experience becomes a more important predictor of outcome with patients who are more disturbed.[71]

LONG-TERM PSYCHOTHERAPY

Most psychoanalysts would consider that the aims and methods of short-term once-a-week psychotherapy are not comparable to those of full psychoanalysis. What do we know about the value of intensive and long-term psychodynamic treatment? Here, the evidence base becomes somewhat patchy and we cannot restrict the review to RCTs.

The Boston Psychotherapy Study compared long-term psychoanalytic therapy (two or more times a week) with supportive therapy for clients with schizophrenia in a randomized controlled design.[72] On the whole, clients who received psychoanalytical therapy fared no better than those who received supportive treatment. In the partial-hospital RCT, the psychoanalytical arm of the treatment included therapy groups three times a week as well as individual therapy once or twice a week over an 18-month period.[37,38] A further controlled trial of intensive psychoanalytical treatment of children with chronically poorly controlled diabetes reported significant gains in diabetic control in the treated group, which was maintained at 1 year's follow-up.[73] Experimental single case studies carried out with the same population supported the causal relationship between interpretive work and improvement in diabetic control and physical growth.[74] The work of Chris Heinicke also suggests that sessions four or five times a week may generate more marked improvements in children with specific learning difficulties than a less intensive psychoanalytical intervention.[75]

The Stockholm Outcome of Psychotherapy and Psychoanalysis Project followed 756 people who received national insurance-funded treatment for up to 3 years in psychoanalysis or psychoanalytical psychotherapy.[76–78] The groups were matched on many clinical variables. Analysis four or five times a week had similar outcomes at termination when compared with one to two sessions of psychotherapy per week. During the follow-up period, psychotherapy patients did not change, but those who had had psychoanalysis continued to improve, almost to a point where their scores were indistinguishable from those obtained from a non-clinical Swedish sample.

The German Psychoanalytic Association undertook a major follow-up study ($n = 401$) of psychoanalytical treatments undertaken in that country between 1990 and 1993.[79,80] Between 70 per cent and 80 per cent of the patients achieved (average 6.5 years after the end of treatment) good and stable psychic changes according to the evaluations of the patients, their analysts, independent psychoanalytical and non-psychoanalytical experts, and questionnaires commonly applied in psychotherapy research. The evaluation of mental health costs showed a cost reduction through fewer days of sick leave during the 7 years following the end of long-term psychoanalytical treatments. In the absence of pretreatment measures, it is impossible to estimate the size of the treatment effect.

Another large pre/post study of psychoanalytical treatments examined the clinical records of 763 children who were evaluated and treated at the Anna Freud Centre.[81–84] Children with certain disorders (e.g. depression, autism, conduct disorder) appeared to benefit only marginally from psychoanalysis or psychoanalytical psychotherapy. Interestingly, children with severe emotional disorders (three or more axis I diagnoses) did surprisingly well in psychoanalysis, although they did poorly in psychoanalytical psychotherapy once or twice a week. Younger children derived greatest benefit from intensive treatment. Adolescents appeared not to benefit from the increased frequency of sessions. The importance of the study is perhaps less in demonstrating that psychoanalysis is effective, although some of the effects on very severely disturbed children were quite remarkable, but more in identifying groups for whom the additional effort involved in intensive treatment appeared not to be warranted.

The Research Committee of the International Psychoanalytic Association prepared a comprehensive review of North American and European outcome studies of psychoanalytic treatment.[85] The committee concluded that existing studies failed to unequivocally demonstrate the efficacy of psychoanalysis relative to either alternative treatment or active placebo. Studies showed a range of methodological and design problems, including absence of intent to treat controls, heterogeneous patient groups, lack of random assignments, and failure to use independently administered standardized measures of outcome. Nevertheless, the report, which ran to several hundred pages and briefly describes more than 50 studies, is encouraging to psychoanalysts. A number of studies testing psychoanalysis with state-of-the-art methodology are ongoing and are likely to produce more compelling evidence over the next years. Despite the limitations of the completed studies, evidence across a significant number of pre/post investigations suggests that psychoanalysis appears to be consistently helpful to patients with milder (neurotic) disorders and somewhat less consistently so for patients in other, more severe groups. Across a range of uncontrolled or poorly controlled cohort studies, mostly carried out in Europe, longer, intensive treatments tended to have better outcomes than shorter, non-intensive treatments (demonstration of a dose–effect relationship). The impact of psychoanalysis was apparent beyond symptomatology, in measures of work functioning and reductions in healthcare costs.

CONCLUSIONS

Several conclusions can be drawn from the psychotherapy research literature. First, it appears evident that psychotherapy is effective in treating a wide variety of clinical conditions, with results often equal to those for drug-based treatments. Second, the affinity between patient and therapist (the so-called therapeutic alliance) may be a key factor in effective therapy. Third, although therapist skill is important in establishing this relationship, skill is not dependent upon experience. Fourth, level of functioning and the ability to form a therapeutic alliance are better predictors of outcome than mere diagnosis. Fifth, evidence suggests that common factors and not specific interventions are crucial in therapy. Finally, it appears that most patients benefit from psychotherapy within the first 6 months of treatment, and that long-term therapy has no significant advantage over short-term therapy. However, psychodynamic psychotherapy may be associated with so-called 'sleeper effects', which means that the full benefit of therapy may not be evident until some months after the termination of the trial.

Research into psychotherapy requires further and significant investigation over the coming years, especially enquiry into the nature of therapeutic alliance, as per the evidence for common factors. Further research may provide evidence supporting specific techniques or prove that psychotherapy can be applied more widely than it is at present. Further investigations might also help to determine whether long-term open-ended psychotherapy is consistently effective for the populations for which it is currently prescribed, including chronic depression, severe personality disorder and bipolar disorder.

REFERENCES

1. Strupp HH (1978) Psychotherapy research and practice: an overview. In A Bergin, S Garfield (eds) *Handbook of Psychotherapy and Behavior Change*, 2nd edn. New York: John Wiley & Sons.
2. Kazdin AE (2007) Mediators and mechanisms of change in psychotherapy research. *Annual Review of Clinical Psychology* 3: 1–27.
3. Eysenck HJ (1952) The effects of psychotherapy: an evaluation. *Journal of Consulting Psychology* 16: 319–24.
4. Wampold BE (2001) *The Great Psychotherapy Debate: Models, Methods, and Findings*, Hillsdale, NJ: Lawrence Erlbaum Associates.
5. Roth A, Fonagy P (2005) *What Works for Whom? A Critical Review of Psychotherapy Research*, 2nd edn. New York: Guilford Press.
6. Sheldon TA, Song F, Davey-Smith G (1993) Critical appraisal of the medical literature: how to assess whether health care interventions do more good than

harm. In MF Drummond, A Maynard (eds) *Purchasing and Providing Cost-Effective Health Care*. London: Churchill Livingstone.

7. Smith ML, Glass GV (1977) Meta-analysis of psychotherapy outcome studies. *American Psychologist* **32**: 752–60.
8. Lipsey MW, Wilson DB (1993) The efficacy of psychological, educational, and behavioral treatment: confirmation from meta-analysis. *American Psychologist* **48**: 1181–209.
9. Whittington CJ, Kendall T, Fonagy P, *et al.* (2004) Selective serotonin reuptake inhibitors in childhood depression: systematic review of published versus unpublished data. *Lancet* **363**: 1341–5.
10. Luborsky L, Diguer L, Seligman DA, *et al.* (1999) The researcher's own therapy allegiances: a 'wild card' in comparisons of treatment efficacy. *Clinical Psychology: Science and Practice* **6**: 95–106.
11. Kazdin AE (2005) Evidence-based assessment for children and adolescents: issues in measurement development and clinical application. *Journal of Clinical Child and Adolescent Psychology* **34**: 548–58.
12. Fonagy P (2004) Psychotherapy meets neuroscience: a more focused future for psychotherapy research. *Psychiatric Bulletin* **28**: 357–9.
13. Higgitt A, Fonagy P (2002) Clinical effectiveness. *British Journal of Psychiatry* **181**: 70–7.
14. Clark D, Salkovskis PM, Hackmann A, *et al.* (1994) A comparison of cognitive therapy, applied relaxation and imipramine in the treatment of panic disorder. *British Journal of Psychiatry* **164**: 759–69.
15. Clark DM, Salkovskis PM, Hackmann A, *et al.* (1999) Brief cognitive therapy for panic disorder: a randomized controlled trial. *Journal of Consulting and Clinical Psychology* **67**: 583–9.
16. Ehlers A, Clark D (2003) Early psychological interventions for adult survivors of trauma: a review. *Biological Psychiatry* **53**: 817–26.
17. Ehlers A, Clark DM, Hackmann A, McManus F, Fennell M (2005) Cognitive therapy for post-traumatic stress disorder: development and evaluation. *Behaviour Research and Therapy* **43**: 413–31.
18. Clark DM, Ehlers A, Hackmann A, *et al.* (2006) Cognitive therapy versus exposure and applied relaxation in social phobia: a randomized controlled trial. *Journal of Consulting and Clinical Psychology* **74**: 568–78.
19. Clark DM, Ehlers A, McManus F, *et al.* (2003) Cognitive therapy versus fluoxetine in generalized social phobia: a randomized placebo-controlled trial. *Journal of Consulting and Clinical Psychology* **71**: 1058–67.
20. Ladouceur R, Dugas MJ, Freeston MH, *et al.* (2000) Efficacy of a cognitive-behavioral treatment for generalized anxiety disorder: evaluation in a controlled clinical trial. *Journal of Consulting and Clinical Psychology* **68**: 957–64.
21. Dugas MJ, Ladouceur R, Leger E, *et al.* (2003) Group cognitive-behavioral therapy for generalized anxiety disorder: treatment outcome and long-term follow-up. *Journal of Consulting and Clinical Psychology* **71**: 821–5.
22. McLean PD, Whittal ML, Thordarson DS, *et al.* (2001) Cognitive versus behavior therapy in the group treatment of obsessive-compulsive disorder. *Journal of Consulting and Clinical Psychology* **69**: 205–14.
23. Whittal ML, Thordarson DS, McLean PD (2005) Treatment of obsessive-compulsive disorder: cognitive behavior therapy vs exposure and response prevention. *Behaviour Research and Therapy* **43**: 1559–76.
24. Ost LG, Ferebee I, Furmark T (1997) One-session group therapy of spider phobia: direct versus indirect treatments. *Behaviour Research and Therapy* **35**: 721–32.
25. Ost LG, Alm T, Brandberg M, Breitholtz E (2001) One vs five sessions of exposure and five sessions of cognitive therapy in the treatment of claustrophobia. *Behaviour Research and Therapy* **39**: 167–83.
26. Milrod B, Leon AC, Busch F, *et al.* (2007) A randomized controlled clinical trial of psychoanalytic psychotherapy for panic disorder. *American Journal of Psychiatry* **164**: 265–72.
27. Shapiro DA, Rees A, Barkham M, *et al.* (1995) Effects of treatment duration and severity of depression on the maintenance of gains after cognitive-behavioral and psychodynamic-interpersonal psychotherapy. *Journal of Consulting and Clinical Psychology* **63**: 378–87.
28. Elkin I, Shea MT, Watkins JT, *et al.* (1989) National Institute of Mental Health Treatment of Depression Collaborative Research Program: general effectiveness of treatment. *Archives of General Psychiatry* **46**: 971–82.
29. Knekt P, Lindfors O (eds) (2004) *A Randomized Trial of the Effects of Four Forms of Psychotherapy on Depressive and Anxiety Disorders: Design Methods and Results on the Effectiveness of Short Term Psychodynamic Psychotherapy and Solution Focused Therapy During a 1-Year Follow-Up*. Helsinki: Social Insurance Institution.
30. Leichsenring F, Rabung S, Leibing E (2004) The efficacy of short-term psychodynamic psychotherapy in specific psychiatric disorders: a meta-analysis. *Archives of General Psychiatry* **61**: 1208–16.
31. Abbass A, Hancock J, Henderson J, Kisely S (2006) Short-term psychodynamic psychotherapies for common mental disorders. *Cochrane Database of Systematic Reviews* (4): CD004687.
32. Davidson K, Norrie J, Tyrer P, *et al.* (2006) The effectiveness of cognitive behavior therapy for borderline personality disorder: results from the borderline personality disorder study of cognitive therapy (BOSCOT) trial. *Journal of Personality Disorders* **20**: 450–65.
33. Davidson K, Tyrer P, Gumley A, *et al.* (2006) A randomized controlled trial of cognitive behavior therapy for borderline personality disorder: rationale for trial,

method, and description of sample. *Journal of Personality Disorders* **20**: 431–49.
34. Tyrer P, Tom B, Byford S, *et al.* (2004) Differential effects of manual assisted cognitive behavior therapy in the treatment of recurrent deliberate self-harm and personality disturbance: the POPMACT study. *Journal of Personality Disorders* **18**: 102–16.
35. Linehan MM, Comtois KA, Murray AM, *et al.* (2006) Two-year randomized controlled trial and follow-up of dialectical behavior therapy vs therapy by experts for suicidal behaviors and borderline personality disorder. *Archives of General Psychiatry* **63**: 757–66.
36. Linehan MM, Armstrong HE, Suarez A, Allmon D, Heard H (1991) Cognitive-behavioural treatment of chronically parasuicidal borderline patients. *Archives of General Psychiatry* **48**: 1060–64.
37. Bateman AW, Fonagy P (1999) The effectiveness of partial hospitalization in the treatment of borderline personality disorder: a randomised controlled trial. *American Journal of Psychiatry* **156**: 1563–9.
38. Bateman AW, Fonagy P (2001) Treatment of borderline personality disorder with psychoanalytically oriented partial hospitalization: an 18-month follow-up. *American Journal of Psychiatry* **158**: 36–42.
39. Giesen-Bloo J, van Dyck R, Spinhoven P, *et al.* (2006) Outpatient psychotherapy for borderline personality disorder: randomized trial of schema-focused therapy vs transference-focused psychotherapy. *Archives of General Psychiatry* **63**: 649–58.
40. Clarkin JF, Levy KN, Lenzenweger MF, Kernberg OF (2007) Evaluating three treatments for borderline personality disorder: a multiwave study. *American Journal of Psychiatry* **164**: 922–8.
41. Rothwell PM (2005) External validity of randomised controlled trials: 'to whom do the results of this trial apply?' *Lancet* **365**: 82–93.
42. Westen D, Morrison K (2001) A multidimensional meta-analysis of treatments for depression, panic, and generalized anxiety disorder: an empirical examination of the status of empirically supported therapies. *Journal of Consulting and Clinical Psychology* **69**: 875–99.
43. Weisz JR, Jensen PS (1999) Efficacy and effectiveness of child and adolescent psychotherapy and pharmacotherapy. *Mental Health Services Research* **1**: 125–57.
44. Beutler L, Malik M, Alimohamed S, *et al.* (2004) Therapist variables. In M Lambert (ed.) *Bergin and Garfield's Handbook of Psychotherapy and Behavior Change.* New York: John Wiley & Sons.
45. Beutler LE, Machado PPP, Neufeldt SA (1994) Therapist variables. In AE Bergin, SL Garfield (eds) *Handbook of Psychotherapy and Behavior Change*, 4th edn. New York: John Wiley & Sons.
46. Clarkin JF, Levy KN (2004) The influence of client variables on psychotherapy. In MJ Lambert (ed.) *Bergin & Garfield's Handbook of Psychotherapy and Behavior Change.* New York: John Wiley & Sons.
47. Garfield SL (1994) Research on client variables in psychotherapy. In AE Bergin, SL Garfield (eds) *Handbook of Psychotherapy and Behavior Change*, 4th edn. New York: John Wiley & Sons.
48. Hayes AM, Castonguay LG, Goldfried MR (1996) Effectiveness of targeting the vulnerability factors of depression in cognitive therapy. *Journal of Consulting and Clinical Psychology* **64**: 623–7.
49. Piper WE, Azim HFA, Joyce AS, McCallum M (1991) Transference interpretations, therapeutic alliance, and outcome in short-term individual psychotherapy. *Archives of General Psychiatry* **48**: 946–53.
50. Connolly MB, Crits-Christoph P, Shappell S, *et al.* (1999) Relation of transference interpretations to outcome in the early sessions of brief supportive-expressive psychotherapy. *Psychotherapy Research* **9**: 485–95.
51. Jensen PS, Weersing R, Hoagwood KE, Goldman E (2005) What is the evidence for evidence-based treatments? A hard look at our soft underbelly. *Mental Health Services Research* **7**: 53–74.
52. Orlinksy DE, Ronnestad MH, Willutski U (2004) Fifty years of psychotherapy process-outcome research: continuity and change. In M Lambert (ed.) *Bergin and Garfield's Handbook of Psychotherapy and Behavior Change.* New York: John Wiley & Sons.
53. Frank JD, Frank JB (1991) *Persuasion and Healing.* Baltimore, MD: Johns Hopkins Press.
54. Lambert M (ed) (2004) *Bergin and Garfield's Handbook of Psychotherapy and Behavior Change.* New York: John Wiley & Sons.
55. Luborsky L, Crits-Christoph P, Mintz J, Auerbach A (1988) *Who Will Benefit From Psychotherapy? Predicting Therapeutic Outcomes.* New York: Basic Books.
56. Eames V, Roth A (2000) Patient attachment orientation and the early working alliance: a study of patient and therapist reports of alliance quality and ruptures. *Journal of Psycho-Therapy Research* **10**: 421–34.
57. Hilliard RB, Henry WP, Strupp HH (2000) An interpersonal model of psychotherapy: linking patient and therapist developmental history, therapeutic process, and types of outcome. *Journal of Consulting and Clinical Psychology* **68**: 125–33.
58. Pinsker-Aspen J, Stein M, Hilsenroth M (2007) Clinical utility of early memories as a predictor of early therapeutic alliance. *Psychotherapy: Theory, Research, Practice, Training* **44**: 96–109.
59. Black S, Hardy G, Turpin G, Parry G (2005) Self-reported attachment styles and therapeutic orientation of therapists and their relationship with reported general alliance quality and problems in therapy. *Psychology and Psychotherapy* **78**: 363–77.
60. Meyer B, Pilkonis PA, Krupnick JL, *et al.* (2002) Treatment expectancies, patient alliance, and outcome: further analyses from the National Institute of Mental Health Treatment of Depression Collaborative Research

Program. *Journal of Consulting and Clinical Psychology* **70**: 1051–5.

61. Gaudiano BA, Miller IW (2006) Patients' expectancies, the alliance in pharmacotherapy, and treatment outcomes in bipolar disorder. *Journal of Consulting and Clinical Psychology* **74**: 671–6.
62. Dew SE, Bickman L (2005) Client expectancies about therapy. *Mental Health Services Research* **7**: 21–33.
63. Zuroff DC, Blatt SJ (2006) The therapeutic relationship in the brief treatment of depression: contributions to clinical improvement and enhanced adaptive capacities. *Journal of Consulting and Clinical Psychology* **74**: 130–40.
64. Wampold BE, Minami T, Baskin TW, Callen Tierney S (2002) A meta-(re)analysis of the effects of cognitive therapy versus 'other therapies' for depression. *Journal of Affective Disorders* **68**: 159–65.
65. Goldman G, Anderson T (2007) Quality of object relations and security of attachment as predictors of early therapeutic alliance. *Journal of Counselling Psychology* **54**: 111–17.
66. Kim DM, Wampold BE, Bolt DM (2006) Therapist effects in psychotherapy: a random effects modelling of the NIMH TDCRP data. *Psychotherapy Research* **16**: 161–71.
67. Okiishi J, Lambert MJ, Nielsen L, Ogless BM (2003) Waiting for supershrink: an empirical analysis of therapist effects. *Clinical Psychology and Psychotherapy* **10**: 361–73.
68. Lutz W, Leon SC, Martiniwitch Z, Lyons JS, Stiles WB (2007) Therapist effects in outpatient psychotherapy: a three-level growth curve approach. *Journal of Counselling Psychology* **54**: 32–9.
69. Okiishi JC, Lambert MJ, Eggett D, *et al.* (2006) An analysis of therapist treatment effects: toward providing feedback to individual therapists on their clients' psychotherapy outcome. *Journal of Clinical Psychology* **62**: 1157–72.
70. Propst A, Paris J, Rosberger Z (1994) Do therapist experience, diagnosis and functional level predict outcome in short-term psychotherapy? *Canadian Journal of Psychiatry* **39**: 178–83.
71. Wierzbicki M, Pekarik G (1993) A meta-analysis of psychotherapy dropout. *Professional Psychology: Research and Practice* **24**: 190–95.
72. Stanton AH, Gunderson JG, Knapp PH, *et al.* (1984) Effects of psychotherapy in schizophrenia: I. Design and implementation of a controlled study. *Schizophrenia Bulletin* **10**: 520–63.
73. Moran G, Fonagy P, Kurtz A, Bolton A, Brook C (1991) A controlled study of the psychoanalytic treatment of brittle diabetes. *Journal of the American Academy of Child and Adolescent Psychiatry* **30**: 926–35.
74. Fonagy P, Moran GS (1991) Studies of the efficacy of child psychoanalysis. *Journal of Consulting and Clinical Psychology* **58**: 684–95.
75. Heinicke CM, Ramsey-Klee DM (1986) Outcome of child psychotherapy as a function of frequency of sessions. *Journal of the American Academy of Child Psychiatry* **25**: 247–53.
76. Blomberg J, Lazar A, Sandell R (2001) Outcome of patients in long-term psychoanalytical treatments: first findings of the Stockholm Outcome of Psychotherapy and Psychoanalysis (STOPP) study. *Psychotherapy Research* **11**: 361–82.
77. Grant J, Sandell R (2004) Close family or mere neighbours? Some empirical data on the differences between psychoanalysis and psychotherapy. In P Richardson, H Kächele, C Renlund (eds) *Research on Psychoanalytic Psychotherapy With Adults*. London: Karnac.
78. Sandell R, Blomberg J, Lazar A, *et al.* (2000) Varieties of long-term outcome among patients in psychoanalysis and long-term psychotherapy: a review of findings in the Stockholm outcome of psychoanalysis and psychotherapy project (STOPP). *International Journal of Psychoanalysis* **81**: 921–43.
79. Leuzinger-Bohleber M, Stuhr U, Ruger B, Beutel M (2003) How to study the quality of psychoanalytic treatments and their long-term effects on patients' well-being: a representative, multi-perspective follow-up study. *International Journal of Psychoanalysis* **84**: 263–90.
80. Leuzinger-Bohleber M, Target M (eds) (2002) *The Outcomes of Psychoanalytic Treatment*. London: Whurr.
81. Fonagy P, Target M (1994) The efficacy of psychoanalysis for children with disruptive disorders. *Journal of the American Academy of Child and Adolescent Psychiatry* **33**: 45–55.
82. Fonagy P, Target M (1996) Predictors of outcome in child psychoanalysis: a retrospective study of 763 cases at the Anna Freud Centre. *Journal of the American Psychoanalytic Association* **44**: 27–77.
83. Target M, Fonagy P (1994) The efficacy of psychoanalysis for children with emotional disorders. *Journal of the American Academy of Child and Adolescent Psychiatry* **33**: 361–71.
84. Target M, Fonagy P (1994) The efficacy of psychoanalysis for children: developmental considerations. *Journal of the American Academy of Child and Adolescent Psychiatry* **33**: 1134–44.
85. Fonagy P, Kachele H, Krause R, *et al.* (2002) *An Open Door Review of Outcome Studies in Psychoanalysis*, 2nd edn. London: International Psychoanalytical Association.

PART 6

Clinical specialties

Chapter 69

Addiction psychiatry

Ilana B Crome and Roger Bloor

INTRODUCTION

For the purposes of clinical management of patients it is helpful to distinguish non-dependent substance misuse from dependent use. The criteria for the diagnosis of substance problems for both the *International Classification of Diseases*, 10th revision (ICD-10)[1] and the American Psychiatric Association's *Diagnostic and Statistical Manual of Mental Disorders*, 4th edition (DSM-IV)[2] are outlined and discussed in more detail elsewhere in this chapter.

BASIC PHARMACOLOGY AND EPIDEMIOLOGY OF MISUSED SUBSTANCES

The substances discussed in this chapter may be classified according to their psychopharmacological properties into the following groupings:

- *Sedative-hypnotics (central nervous system (CNS) depressants):*
  - Barbiturates
  - Non-barbiturate hypnotics
  - Ethyl alcohol
  - Benzodiazepines (anxiolytic or anti-anxiety)
- *Narcotic analgesics (opiates):*
  - Opiates
  - Opiate derivatives
  - Synthetic opiates
- *CNS stimulants:*
  - Cocaine
  - Amphetamines
  - Nicotine
  - Caffeine
  - Ecstasy
- *Psychedelics and hallucinogens:*
  - Lysergic acid diethylamide (LSD)
  - Mescaline (peyote cactus)
  - Phencyclidine (PCP; 'angel dust')
- *Cannabis:*
  - delta-9-tetrahydrocannabinol (THC)
- *Inhalants:*
  - Analgesic and anaesthetic gases
  - Glues, solvents and aerosols.

These substances may also be classified according to their mechanistic properties with regard to their binding sites:[3]

- Drugs that bind to G-protein-coupled receptors (GPCRs), e.g. opioids, cannabinoids, γ-hydroxybutyrate (GHB)
- Drugs that interact with ionotropic receptors or ion channels, e.g. nicotine, alcohol, benzodiazepines
- Drugs that target monoamine transporters, e.g. cocaine, amphetamines, methylenedioxymethamphetamine (MDMA, ecstasy).

EPIDEMIOLOGY

Prevalence

The UK has some of the highest levels of substance misuse in Europe. The situation is dynamic, and it has become well recognized that combinations of substances may be misused, including two of the most commonly encountered substances, alcohol and nicotine. Since the early 1990s, despite a fall in overall prevalence from 45 per cent of the adult population in 1974 to 22 per cent in 2006, the prevalence of cigarette-smoking has been higher among 20- to 24-year-olds than in any other age group in Great Britain.[4] In addition, around 25 per cent of the population drink above safe recommended limits of alcohol, with per capita alcohol consumption not only doubling from 1950 to 2000 but also continuing to rise.[5–7] Hospital admissions for conditions related to alcohol consumption doubled in the period 1996–2006, while death rates related to alcohol consumption doubled in the period 1991–2005. Admissions to intensive care units in England and Wales for alcoholic liver disease tripled over the 10-year period from 1996 to 2005.[8]

Alcohol

Alcohol problems comprise 4 per cent of the global burden of disease, and alcohol misuse costs the UK £20 billion per annum. The pattern of alcohol consumption in the UK has shown a dramatic increase since the middle of the twentieth century, and in 2008 the UK had the highest level of alcohol consumption of all European countries. The patterns of consumption in some age groups are of particular concern, with high levels of binge drinking in both males and females in the 16–24 years age group.

UK statistics suggest that 23 per cent of adults drink alcohol at hazardous or harmful levels. This includes 32 per cent of men and 15 per cent of women, equating to approximately 7 million people in England. Over 20 per cent of men and nearly 10 per cent of women are estimated to binge drink. Alcohol dependence is present in 6 per cent of men and 2 per cent of women.[9]

Illicit drugs

Drug misuse costs the UK about £15 billion each year. It is estimated that, of people aged 16–59 years, about 11 million (35%) have used illicit drugs in their lifetime, 3.25 million (10%) have used illicit drugs in the previous year, and 2 million (6%) have used illicit drugs in the previous month. Cannabis is the most likely drug to be used, with 8 per cent of 16- to 59-year-olds reporting use in the previous year. In addition, just over 1 million people aged 16–59 years have used class A drugs in the past year, and the use of class A drugs increased between 1998 and 2007.[10]

There were almost 196 000 people in contact with treatment services in England in 2006–2007, of whom the majority were primary opioid users, with males comprising over 70 per cent of new cases. Estimates derived from a number of sources in the UK suggest that the prevalence of problem drug use is 9.35 per 1000 of the population aged 15–64 years, with a total drug-using population estimated at 360 811.[11] A study of drug use in the younger population of the UK revealed that, among 11- to 15-year-olds, 18 per cent had taken drugs within the past year. The most commonly used drug was cannabis (11%), with 1 per cent reporting the use of heroin and 1 per cent reporting cocaine use.[12] The British Crime Survey 2003/2004 showed that 4 million adults in England and Wales have used a class A drug in their lifetime, with over 1 million having used them in the past year and over 500 000 having used drugs in the past month.[13]

Drug and alcohol problems can present in a variety of settings, including:

- accident and emergency (A&E) units;
- acute hospital settings;
- obstetric and paediatric units;
- mental health wards and clinics.

Prevalence in accident and emergency units

There is an increased risk of traumatic injury among substance users. In a 90-day study, nearly two-thirds of admissions to a trauma centre in the USA were victims of motor vehicle crashes; those who had sustained one traumatic injury were at greatly increased risk of re-injury.[14] In a study of drug and alcohol use in road traffic accident victims in the USA, 59.3 per cent of the sample tested positive for either drugs or alcohol. More patients tested positive for drug use (35.5%) than for alcohol use only (15.8%), while 9.9 per cent tested positive for both. Cannabis and benzodiazepines were the most frequently detected drugs.[14,15]

Screening for drug (or drug and alcohol) use among patients attending emergency or trauma departments in Canada found varying rates of use for a range of different drugs, but overall the studies indicated that about 40 per cent of patients attending these departments were likely to test positive for the use of illicit drugs.[16]

Prevalence in acute general medical settings

In the UK, a study that identified drug use presenting in an acute medical admission unit used both screening questionnaires and the opinion of the admitting doctor to identify drug and alcohol problems.[17] Of the 2988 admissions studied, 609 patients (20%) were found to be misusing drugs or alcohol. The study showed that of the 609 patients with a drug or alcohol problem:

- 437 (72%) had an alcohol problem;
- 116 (19%) were using an illicit drug;
- 56 (9%) were polydrug users.

The most commonly used drug was cannabis.

Prevalence in psychiatric patients

It is well recognized that patients with severe mental illness are especially at risk of substance misuse.[18] Studies of primary care populations in England and Wales have indicated that the co-morbidity rate is increasing by about 10 per cent each year and that co-morbid patients are becoming younger. In studies of patients attending mental health services in the UK, 10 per cent of patients treated by Community Mental Health Teams reported problematic use of illicit drugs and 17 per cent reported alcohol problems in the past year. Of patients attending a community drug and alcohol service, 22 per cent reported a severe mental illness and 46 per cent reported some other form of psychiatric disorder.[19] A study of the prevalence of dual diagnosis in treatment populations in both mental health services and drug treatment services in the UK showed that around 32 per cent of clients in both services were estimated to have dual diagnosis problems. A study in Scotland has shown that problem use of drugs and alcohol is greater in people with schizophrenia than in the general population. More patients than controls reported problem use of drugs in the past year (22 (7%) *v.* 5 (2%)) and at some time before then (50 (20%) *v.* 15 (6%)).[20]

McCann and colleagues report that approximately 50 per cent of adults with attention deficit hyperactivity disorder (ADHD) have a history of psychoactive substance-use disorders.[21] Furthermore, they record that a history of childhood

ADHD has been found in 22–71 per cent of substance-abusing patients. In a sample of patients attending an adult ADHD centre, 33.8 per cent were found to have a positive screen for drug abuse.

A review of the relationship between personality disorder and substance misuse concluded that approximately two-thirds of drug users in treatment have a personality disorder, with antisocial personality disorder being the most common. The review indicated that personality disorder is associated with a range of complications and adverse outcomes in drug users, including psychiatric problems, poor social functioning, dropout from treatment, and increased human immunodeficiency virus (HIV) risk behaviours and infection rates.[22]

Prevalence in patients attending obstetric and paediatric units

Pregnant women and parents are another group to be considered. In Dublin, urine testing of 504 first-visit antenatal patients and a separate sample of 515 post-delivery patients found a prevalence of 2.8 per cent, with the most frequently used drug being cannabis. The authors note that their figures are similar to the results from an earlier study in Birmingham, which found that 2 per cent of women tested positive on their first antenatal visit, but lower than figures reported from studies in the USA in the late 1980s.[23]

Health aspects

Substances impact on every organ system of the body, on the gastrointestinal, cardiovascular, respiratory, musculoskeletal and endocrine systems, and on the CNS. Some problems, such as intoxication, withdrawal, deliberate overdose, injecting accidents, hypothermia and hyperthermia, dehydration, and choking or suffocating may require urgent medical attention; the training of opiate users in the management of these emergencies, including the use of naloxone, may assist the successful reversal of potentially fatal overdoses.[24]

Poor physical health is correlated strongly with poverty and social deprivation, including accidents, dietary neglect, and failure to access primary care. It is not often possible to attribute cause directly, because many of the risk factors for adverse psychosocial consequences and the development of substance misuse are shared. However, once substance misuse is established, further social problems accumulate and persist, so that the removal of the substance alone will not necessarily reduce the social harm.

Substance users are vulnerable to exploitation, especially if they are homeless, mentally ill or have learning difficulties. Unsafe injecting behaviour, high-risk sexual activity, unwanted pregnancy, sexually transmitted infections and accidental overdose compound drug-taking behaviour. Crack cocaine use, common in sex workers, is linked to hepatitis infection and termination of pregnancy.

Furthermore, pregnant teenage substance misusers are at increased risk not only because of their chaotic patterns of use but also due to physical and emotional violence. Substance misuse is associated with early, unplanned or undesired pregnancy and abortion. Since substance use is often accompanied by amenorrhoea, young women may not realize that there is a possibility of pregnancy and may not be aware of their condition until an advanced stage. This can lead to poor antenatal care, with the associated high risks of miscarriage (3% *v.* < 1% in a population attending a specialist drug treatment unit compared with the local maternity population), low birth weight (28% *v.* 9%) and premature babies (20% *v.* 9%).[25]

Substance use, sexual abuse and prostitution have common predisposing factors, including poverty, homelessness, psychiatric illness, and physical and emotional abuse. Cocaine, alcohol and benzodiazepines are commonly used to cope with unmanageable situations. Women involved in prostitution are at risk of sexually transmitted infections, blood-borne viruses and bacterial infections (gonorrhoea, syphilis, chlamydia) that may cause infertility and pelvic disease.

Psychiatric disorders such as depression, anxiety, psychosis, eating disorders and post-traumatic stress disorders are associated with the direct intoxicating effects of acute and chronic substance misuse and withdrawal syndromes, often within a very poor social environment. Treatment of addiction problems in this group must therefore include outreach work, social care, and screening and treatment for sexually acquired infections as part of the spectrum of management. The risk of self-harm and suicide is increased greatly in substance misusers,[26] and strategies to reduce suicide rates necessarily include active management of substance misuse, particularly in high-risk groups such as newly released prisoners.[27]

Mortality

Since 2000, the level of drug problems in the UK has stabilized, but at levels that are the highest in Europe, and there is considerable substance-related mortality.[28] In the UK, 40 000 deaths each year are due to alcohol-related disorders and about 2000 are due to illicit drug use. In Scotland, the standardized mortality ratio (SMR) for Scottish drug users is 12 times as high as that for the general population.[29] In a population of drug users treated in a specialist setting, the SMR was 17 times higher for adult female and male heroin users compared with that of the non-heroin-using population.[30] The mortality of excessive drinkers is at least twice, and that of drug users over 20 times, that of the general population.

Summary

Overall, these studies demonstrate that drug misusers present to a wide range of services, that their problems are not detected, and that failure to recognize their problem may result in inappropriate treatment and recurrence of health issues, since at least one associated factor, the drug misuse, is not being treated effectively. This is why assessment is important.

RESTRICTIONS IMPOSED ON DOCTORS BY THE MISUSE OF DRUGS ACT AND REGULATIONS

The Misuse of Drugs Act (1971) and the Misuse of Drugs Regulations (2001) impose restrictions on the possession and supply of a range of drugs, which apply to everyone, including medical practitioners, unless the practitioner is operating under an exemption within the Regulations.

The Misuse of Drugs Act was designed to control the use of drugs that are viewed as having medical applications. It classifies drugs into three categories (A, B, C) and defines the penalties for production, supply and possession of drugs in these categories. The current UK drug classification system is shown in Table 69.1. It should be noted that cannabis and cannabis resin were reclassified from class B to a class C in 2004, when the Criminal Justice Act (2003) amended the Misuse of Drugs Act. This amendment also increased the maximum penalty for trafficking in class C drugs from 5 years' to 14 years' imprisonment. In 2008 this decision was reversed due to concerns over the increasing prevalence of super-strength strains of the drug and cannabis was reclassified as class B, despite advice to the contrary given by the Advisory Council on the Misuse of Drugs in 2008.[31] Current amendments to the Act are accessible online.[32]

The Misuse of Drugs Regulations (2001)

The Misuse of Drugs Regulations (2001) apply where there are legitimate medical applications for controlled drugs.[33] These Regulations further classify drugs into schedules that reflect the degree of control over possession, use, prescribing and supply. These are summarized in Table 69.2.

Table 69.2 Schedules of the Misuse of Drugs Act

Schedule	Drugs	Comments
1	Cannabis, LSD, opium, psilocin	Can be supplied or possessed only under special licence
2	Amphetamine, cocaine, heroin, methadone, morphine, pethidine, Ritalin®	Available for medical use on prescription; controls on storage and recording of stocks
3	Barbiturates, temazepam, Rohypnol®	Available for medical use on prescription; controls on storage and recording of stocks
4.1	Minor tranquillizers	Illegal to posses without a prescription or to supply
4.2	Anabolic steroids	Can be possessed without a prescription, but illegal to supply
5	Some cough medicines, mild pain killers	Legal to possess, can be bought over the counter, but illegal to supply to another person once purchased

LSD, lysergic acid diethylamide.

Table 69.1 Drug classification under the UK Misuse of Drugs Act (1971)

Class	Example drugs*		Maximum penalty for possession	Maximum penalty for supply
Class A	Cocaine and crack cocaine, ecstasy, heroin, LSD, methadone, methamphetamine, magic mushrooms, any class B drug that is injected	Magistrate's court	6 months + £5000 fine	6 months + £5000 fine
		Crown court	7 years + unlimited fine	Life + unlimited fine
Class B	Amphetamine, barbiturates, codeine	Magistrate's court	3 months + £2500 fine	6 months + £5000 fine
		Crown court	5 years + fine	14 years + fine
Class C	Ketamine, anabolic steroids, minor tranquillizers	Magistrate's court	3 months + £500 fine	3 months + £2000 fine
		Crown court	2 years + fine	14 years + fine

*These are examples and reference should be made to the current amendments to the Act, accessible online.[32]

LSD, lysergic acid diethylamide.

The General Medical Council (GMC) guidance on prescribing reminds doctors that those with full registration may prescribe all medicines, excluding those in Schedule 1 of the Misuse of Drugs Regulations. Doctors who have provisional or limited registration may prescribe medicines in line with the supervisory conditions of their employment. The introduction of a dual system of registration and licence to practise will mean that, in order to prescribe any medication, doctors would have to be both registered with and licensed by the GMC.[34]

Controlled drug prescriptions

Guidance on writing controlled drug prescriptions is available from a number of sources, including the *British National Formulary*.[35]

Notification of drug users

The requirement to notify the Home Office Addicts Register about drug addicts was discontinued in 1997. However, to enable adequate monitoring of data on people presenting with drug problems, doctors and other workers in the addiction field should ensure that they complete the relevant forms for submitting data to the National Drugs Treatment Monitoring System (NDTMS) when a patient starts treatment for drug misuse of any kind. Unlike the Home Office Register, these databases cannot be used as a check on multiple prescribing for drug addicts, because the data are anonymized.[35]

CAUSES, CONSEQUENCES AND RECOGNITION OF HEAVY DRINKING

The concept of 'problem drinking'

Problem drinking incorporates a range of alcohol-related behaviours. The definition of problem drinking has not been standardized; for example, some authors use the term to encompass alcohol dependence, alcohol abuse and hazardous use of alcohol, while others use it to refer to drinking more than the recommended safe level, but short of alcohol dependence.

The use of standardized terms from DSM-IV or ICD-10 avoids such confusion and separates out intoxication from alcohol misuse and alcohol dependence syndrome.

Intoxication

Intoxication is diagnosed in ICD-10 using the following criteria:[1]

A. The following criteria for acute intoxication must be met:

1. There must be clear evidence of recent use of a psychoactive substance (or substances) at sufficiently high dose levels to be consistent with intoxication.
2. There must be symptoms or signs of intoxication compatible with the known actions of the particular substance (or substances), as specified below, and of sufficient severity to produce disturbances in the level of consciousness, cognition, perception, affect, or behaviour that are of clinical importance.
3. The symptoms or signs present cannot be accounted for by a medical disorder unrelated to substance use, and not better accounted for by another mental or behavioural disorder.

B. There must be dysfunctional behaviour, as evidenced by at least one of the following:

1. disinhibition;
2. argumentativeness;
3. aggression;
4. lability of mood;
5. impaired attention;
6. impaired judgement;
7. interference with personal functioning.

C. At least one of the following signs must be present:

1. unsteady gait;
2. difficulty in standing;
3. slurred speech;
4. nystagmus;
5. decreased level of consciousness (e.g. stupor, coma);
6. flushed face;
7. conjunctival injection.

Alcohol abuse or harmful use of alcohol

Alcohol abuse (DSM-IV) or harmful use of alcohol (ICD-10) are diagnosed using the criteria outlined in Tables 69.3 and 69.4.

DSM-IV diagnostic criteria for alcohol abuse

1. A maladaptive pattern of alcohol abuse leading to clinically significant impairment or distress, as manifested by one or more of the following, occurring within a 12-month period:

(a) Recurrent alcohol use resulting in failure to fulfil major role obligations at work, school, or home (e.g. repeated absences or poor work performance related to substance use; substance-related absences, suspensions or expulsions from school; or neglect of children or household).
(b) Recurrent alcohol use in situations in which it is physically hazardous (e.g. driving an automobile or operating a machine).
(c) Recurrent alcohol-related legal problems (e.g. arrests for alcohol-related disorderly conduct).
(d) Continued alcohol use despite persistent or recurrent social or interpersonal problems caused or exacerbated by the effects of the alcohol (e.g. arguments with spouse about consequences of intoxication or physical fights).

2. These symptoms must never have met the criteria for alcohol dependence.[2]

Table 69.3 Criteria for substance abuse (DSM-IV) and harmful use (ICD-10)

DSM-IV	ICD-10
(A) A maladaptive pattern of substance use leading to clinically significant impairment or distress, as manifested by one (or more) of the following occurring within a 12-month period	(A) A pattern of psychoactive substance use that is causing damage to health; the damage may be to physical or mental health
(1) Recurrent substance use resulting in a failure to fulfil major role obligations at work, school, or home	
(2) Recurrent substance abuse in situations that are physically hazardous	
(3) Recurrent substance abuse-related legal problems	
(4) Continued substance abuse despite having persistent or recurrent social or interpersonal problems caused or exacerbated by the effects of the substance	
(B) Has never met the criteria for substance dependence for this class of substance	

DSM-IV, *Diagnostic and Statistical Manual of Mental Disorders*, 4th edition; ICD-10, *International Classification of Diseases*, 10th revision.

ICD-10 diagnostic criteria for harmful use of alcohol

A. There must be clear evidence that the substance use was responsible for (or substantially contributed to) physical or psychological harm, including impaired judgement or dysfunctional behaviour, which may lead to disability or have adverse consequences for interpersonal relationships.

B. The nature of the harm should be clearly identifiable (and specified).

C. The pattern of use has persisted for at least one month or has occurred repeatedly within a 12-month period.

D. The disorder does not meet the criteria for any other mental or behavioural disorder related to the same drug in the same time period (except for acute intoxication).[1]

Components of alcohol dependence syndrome

Alcohol dependence syndrome (ADS) was initially defined as including the following components:[36]

- Subjective awareness of compulsion to drink
- Increased tolerance to alcohol
- Repeated withdrawal symptoms
- Relief or avoidance of withdrawal symptoms by further drinking.

Standardized diagnostic classifications have refined the original concept, and the DSM-IV and ICD-10 classifications are summarized below.

DSM-IV diagnostic criteria for alcohol dependence

A maladaptive pattern of alcohol use, leading to clinically significant impairment or distress, as manifested by three or more of the following seven criteria, occurring at any time in the same 12-month period:

1. Tolerance, as defined by either of the following:

(a) A need for markedly increased amounts of alcohol to achieve intoxication or desired effect.

(b) Markedly diminished effect with continued use of the same amount of alcohol.

2. Withdrawal, as defined by either of the following:

(a) The characteristic withdrawal syndrome for alcohol (refer to DSM-IV for further details).

(b) Alcohol is taken to relieve or avoid withdrawal symptoms.

3. Alcohol is often taken in larger amounts or over a longer period than was intended.
4. There is a persistent desire or there are unsuccessful efforts to cut down or control alcohol use.
5. A great deal of time is spent in activities necessary to obtain alcohol, use alcohol or recover from its effects.
6. Important social, occupational, or recreational activities are given up or reduced because of alcohol use.
7. Alcohol use is continued despite knowledge of having a persistent or recurrent physical or psychological problem that is likely to have been caused or exacerbated by the alcohol (e.g. continued drinking despite recognition that an ulcer was made worse by alcohol consumption).[2]

ICD-10 diagnostic criteria for alcohol dependence

Three or more of the following manifestations should have occurred together for at least 1 month or, if persisting for periods of less than 1 month, should have occurred together repeatedly within a 12-month period:

(1) A strong desire or sense of compulsion to take the substance;

Table 69.4 Criteria for dependence syndrome in *Diagnostic and Statistical Manual of Mental Disorders*, 4th edition (DSM-IV) and *International Classification of Diseases*, 10th revision (ICD-10)

DSM-IV	ICD-10
(A) Diagnosis of dependence should be made if three or more of the following have been experienced or exhibited at any time in the same 12-month period:	(A) Diagnosis of dependence should be made if three or more of the following have been experienced or exhibited at some time during the past year:
(1) Tolerance defined by either need for markedly increased amount of substance to achieve intoxication or desired effect or markedly diminished effect with continued use of the same amount of the substance	(1) A strong desire or sense of compulsion to take the substance
(2) Withdrawal as evidenced by either of the following: • the characteristic withdrawal syndrome for the substance • the same (or closely related) substance is taken to relieve or avoid withdrawal symptoms	(2) Difficulties in controlling substance-taking behaviour in terms of its onset, termination or levels of use
(3) The substance is often taken in larger amounts over a longer period of time than was intended	(3) Physiological withdrawal state when substance use has ceased or been reduced, as evidenced by either of the following: • the characteristic withdrawal syndrome for the substance • use of the same (or closely related) substance with the intention of relieving or avoiding withdrawal symptoms
(4) Persistent desire or repeated unsuccessful efforts to cut down or control substance use	(4) Evidence of tolerance, such that increased doses of the psychoactive substance are required in order to achieve effects originally produced by lower doses
(5) A great deal of time is spent in activities necessary to obtain the substance, use the substance or recover from its effects	(5) Progressive neglect of alternative pleasures or interests because of psychoactive substance use and increased amount of time necessary to obtain or take the substance or to recover from its effects
(6) Important social, occupational, or recreational activities given up or reduced because of substance use	(6) Persisting with substance use despite clear evidence of overly harmful consequences (physical or mental)
(7) Continued substance use despite knowledge of having had a persistent or recurrent physical or psychological problem that was likely to have been caused or exacerbated by the substance	

(2) Impaired capacity to control substance-taking behaviour in terms of its onset, termination, or levels of use, as evidenced by: the substance being often taken in larger amounts or over a longer period than intended; or by a persistent desire or unsuccessful efforts to reduce or control substance use;

(3) A physiological withdrawal state when substance use is reduced or ceased, as evidenced by the characteristic withdrawal syndrome for the substance, or by use of the same (or closely related) substance with the intention of relieving or avoiding withdrawal symptoms;

(4) Evidence of tolerance to the effects of the substance, such that there is a need for significantly increased amounts of the substance to achieve intoxication or the desired effect, or a markedly diminished effect with continued use of the same amount of the substance;

(5) Preoccupation with substance use, as manifested by important alternative pleasures or interests being given up or reduced because of substance use; or a great deal of time being spent in activities necessary to obtain, take, or recover from the effects of the substance;

(6) Persistent substance use despite clear evidence of harmful consequences, as evidenced by continued use when the individual is actually aware, or may be expected to be aware, of the nature and extent of harm.[1]

Physical consequences of alcohol misuse

The physical and metabolic complications of alcohol can affect all systems of the body and may mimic other disease processes.[37] In England and Wales alone, around 28 000 people die prematurely each year from physical diseases, accidents and suicides related to alcohol use.[38]

The physical complications of alcohol use are numerous and are manifested in almost all organs of the body. They relate to the pharmacological effects of alcohol, withdrawal and toxicity, deficiency syndromes as a result of chronic abuse, and secondary effects such as domestic violence and injury resulting from drink-driving offences.

Some studies have demonstrated a protective effect of low levels of alcohol intake for some diseases. However, this possibility needs to be balanced against the clear evidence of harm from excessive or prolonged heavy consumption.

Central nervous system

Any level of blood alcohol concentration will produce some impairment of complex psychomotor skills.[39] Acute intoxication with alcohol may lead to coma or death, resulting from CNS depression leading to respiratory depression and cardiovascular collapse. Intoxicated patients are at increased risk of other traumatic and medical pathologies that may precipitate or be exacerbated by head injury, infection or hypoglycaemia, which must be ruled out or treated appropriately.

Alcohol withdrawal syndrome

Alcohol withdrawal syndrome (AWS) can be classified by severity into three categories:

- Mild alcohol withdrawal occurs less than 24 h after stopping or decreasing alcohol intake and may include tremulousness, anxiety, nausea, vomiting, sweating, hyperreflexia and minor autonomic hyperactivity.
- Moderate alcohol withdrawal is an intermediate position along the continuum, with the hallmark of hallucinosis but an otherwise clear sensorium.
- Severe alcohol withdrawal takes place more than 24 h and up to 5 days after stopping or decreasing alcohol intake. It is characterized by disorientation, agitation, hallucinations and severe autonomic derangement and may be precipitated by a variety of circumstances, including:
    - lack of money to purchase alcohol;
    - acute illness or injury, or postoperatively;
    - nausea and vomiting;
    - a decision to stop drinking.

Seizures, hallucinations and delirium tremens are considered major phenomena. Seizures can occur with any severity level of withdrawal but are normally seen 12–48 h after stopping alcohol.[40] Seizures may also be secondary to intoxication or trauma, or as a toxic effect of alcohol.

Delirium tremens has a mortality of about 5 per cent, the severity generally being related to a previous history of delirium tremens, heavy alcohol consumption and the presence of physical illness. The condition begins 2–3 days after stopping or decreasing alcohol intake and peaks within about a week.[41]

Standardized rating scales for AWS enable objective monitoring and evaluation of interventions. The Clinical Institute Withdrawal Assessment for Alcohol (CIWA-Ar) scale is a short, ten-item scale for clinical measurement of the severity of AWS and can be completed in a few minutes by nursing staff.[42] Points are assigned for categories of symptoms and signs, including sweating, anxiety, tremor, agitation, hallucinations, nausea and vomiting, headache, orientation and impaired consciousness.

Neurological nutritional deficiency syndromes

Nutritional deficiency must be considered in alcohol abusers.[43] The initial presentation may be one of peripheral neuropathy and cardiovascular disorder, such as hypotension or high output cardiac failure (e.g. beriberi), in combination with oral inflammation. This is the result of thiamine deficiency.

The most important presentation of nutritional deficiency is Wernicke–Korsakoff syndrome (WKS), which is a consequence of thiamine deficiency. Wernicke's encephalopathy (WE) and Korsakoff's psychosis (KP) are both part of this syndrome. This is a medical emergency.

Wernicke's encephalopathy is a potentially reversible neurological condition, but untreated it is fatal in 17 per cent of cases, with permanent brain damage occurring in 85 per cent of patients who are managed inappropriately. Postmortem findings indicate that a diagnosis of WE is missed in up to 90 per cent of patients.[44] In its classic form, WE is characterized by the triad of ocular abnormalities, ataxia and a global confusional state; this classic triad is found in only 16 per cent of patients,[45] and the onset of the syndrome may be acute or gradual, evolving over several days.

Korsakoff's psychosis presents as lack of insight, apathy, and anterograde and retrograde amnesia with confabulation. Although originally seen as a distinct syndrome, it is now viewed as part of the progression of WKS and has been shown to share an underlying causation and a common neuropathological basis. Findings from postmortem studies have shown that the most common abnormalities in WKS are in the areas surrounding the cerebral aqueduct and the third and fourth ventricles. The thalamus, mamillary bodies and cerebellum are also affected.[46]

A variety of brain lesions related to alcohol have been defined, including:

- neuronal loss with cerebral dementia;
- alcoholic cerebellar degeneration;
- central pontine myelinolysis;
- Marchiafava–Bignami syndrome.[47]

Liver disease and gastrointestinal disorders

Alcoholic liver disease is a very common cause of morbidity and mortality in the developed world.[48] There is a dose-dependent increase in relative risk for both men and women, with the steepest increase among women.[49] The spectrum of liver disease is not uniform but can be described under three main headings:

- *Alcoholic fatty liver:* this results from the inhibition of oxidation of fatty acids, combined with an increased generation of triglycerides. The early stages produce no changes in liver function tests, other than those related to the direct effect of alcohol on liver function. The condition is asymptomatic and can present with right abdominal pain, nausea and vomiting, which resolve on abstinence. The effects can be reversed within a few weeks of abstinence from alcohol.

- *Alcoholic hepatitis:* this results from chronic alcohol abuse. Alcoholic hepatitis produces liver cell necrosis and inflammation and can raise aspartate aminotransferase (AST), alanine aminotransferase (ALT) and bilirubin levels. AST activity is higher than that of ALT in alcoholic hepatitis and Reye syndrome, in contrast to most types of liver disease, where ALT is higher.[50] The clinical presentation involves jaundice, pyrexia, right abdominal pain, ascites and possible encephalopathy. In patients with poor liver function and a prothrombin time prolonged to a degree that precludes liver biopsy, the prognosis is poor, with a third of patients dying in the acute episode.[51] Severe acute alcoholic hepatitis has a poor outcome with standard supportive management. The reported mortality rate of patients with severe alcoholic hepatitis is 35–46 per cent.[48]
- *Cirrhosis:* this involves a permanent loss of liver cells, which are replaced by fibrosis with loss of the normal liver architecture. Liver function tests may be normal until the process is advanced and diagnosis is confirmed by biopsy. Cirrhosis may be asymptomatic or present with gastrointestinal symptoms, ascites, encephalopathy and oesophageal varices, which may cause haemorrhage. Abstinence and good nutrition are mandatory. Prognosis is poor unless alcohol intake ceases; overall, only 25 per cent of patients with cirrhosis survive 5 years from diagnosis.[51]

Other gastrointestinal consequences of alcohol abuse include acute and chronic pancreatitis, and gastritis and peptic ulcers. Over 70 per cent of cases of chronic pancreatitis are caused by long-term heavy alcohol abuse, which may also result in severe weight loss, diabetes and malabsorption syndrome.

Cancer

Chronic alcohol consumption is a strong risk factor for cancer in the oral cavity, pharynx, hypopharynx, larynx and oesophagus and is also a major aetiological factor in hepatocarcinogenesis. Alcohol increases the risk of cancer of the colorectum and the breast.[52]

Heavy drinkers are more likely to be heavy smokers, and the increased risk from each substance problem appears to be potentiated by the combination. Men who both smoke and drink are nearly 38 times more likely to develop head and neck cancers than men who do neither.[53] The risk of developing cancer of the oesophagus is 50 times greater in heavy drinkers and heavy smokers than in people who abstain.

Cardiovascular disease

The effects of alcohol on the cardiovascular system are well documented and range from the protective effects of light drinking for ischaemic stroke and coronary disease through to the increased risk from heavy drinking for haemorrhagic stroke, cardiomyopathy, hypertension and cardiac arythmias.

Other alcohol-related disorders are detailed in Table 69.5.

WHO USES WHICH DRUGS, AND WHY?

Drug use is affected by age, gender, fashion, availability, regulations and societal values.

Reasons for initiating and continuing drug use

There are a variety of theories used to understand the reasons for initiation and continuation of drug use, which can be classified into three main categories:

- Biological
- Sociological
- Psychological.

Table 69.5 Other alcohol-related disorders

Alcohol-related skeletal muscle disease	Myopathy affects more than 2000 subjects per 100 000 population and, in its chronic form, affects 40–60% of people with alcoholism
Alcohol-related fractures	Common in chronic alcohol misuse. Associated with reduced bone mass and higher incidence of osteoporosis. Poor nutrition and associated smoking habits contribute to the risks of fracture
Fertility	In premenopausal women with alcoholism, there is an increase in the frequency of menstrual disturbances, abortions, miscarriages and infertility. Uncontrolled studies of men with alcoholism have reported that alcohol consumption may affect spermatogenesis and spermiogenesis. Gonadal atrophy, a direct result of toxicity and suppression of the hypothalamic–pituitary axis, is associated with impotence and diminished fertility
Fetal effects	Regular consumption of alcohol during pregnancy may affect the fetus. Abnormalities range from growth retardation to fetal alcohol syndrome. There is no evidence on which to base a recommendation of a safe level of alcohol intake in pregnancy[54]

An alternative classification of theory types has also been proposed, which clusters the majority of current theories into five groups:[55]

- Biological, social or psychological theories
- Theories on the effects of addictive stimuli
- Individual susceptibility theories
- Environmental factor theories
- Recovery and relapse theories.

In reviewing the multiple theories of addiction, West suggested a synthetic theory of addiction, which proposes that addiction is a symptom rather than a unitary disorder and that there are three basic pathologies associated with it:[56]

- A disorder of the motivational systems unrelated to addiction itself
- An abnormality of the motivational system caused by the addictive activity
- Pathological environments that act on normal motivational systems.

This concept has also been suggested in other integrative models, such as those that include a two-component model of availability-proneness.[57,58] These models theorize that drug use occurs when a psychologically prone person is exposed to a high level of drug availability.

Although psychological theories often predominate in the development of interventions for drug addiction, advances in neuroimaging techniques applied to the addiction field could have an increasing impact on available treatments.[59]

Recognizing drug use

A framework for assessing and diagnosing drug problems is provided in the Department of Health's *Drug Misuse and Dependence: UK Guidelines on Clinical Management.*[60] The National Treatment Agency's (NTA) *Care Planning Practice Guide* provides a summary of the characteristics of a selection of tools that can be used for assessment and outcome measurement in a drug treatment setting.[61] The basic principles of the guidelines can be summarized as follows:

- The needs of drug misusers should be assessed in terms of their health, social functioning and criminal involvement.
- A good initial assessment is essential. This may involve a multidisciplinary team.
- Confirmation of drug-taking should be achieved through history, examination and drug testing.
- Any risks to children should be assessed, and child-protection services involved as appropriate.
- Testing for blood-borne infections should be arranged as appropriate.
- A physical and psychological health assessment should be carried out.
- Any ongoing criminal involvement or offences should be determined.
- The drug misuser's expectations and desire to change should be assessed.
- The degree of dependence and need for substitute medication should be assessed.
- Drug testing can help to monitor compliance and treatment outcome.

Taking a drug history

The aim is to elicit as accurately as possible something about past and current drug-taking behaviour and should include the following areas:

- Reason for presentation
- Past and current (past 4 weeks) drug use:
    - Current usage and why patient changed to injecting
    - Supply of needles and syringes
    - Sharing habits, including lending and borrowing injection equipment or paraphernalia
    - Does the patient know how to inject safely?
    - How does the patient clean equipment?
    - How does the patient dispose of used equipment/'works'?
    - Knowledge of HIV/hepatitis B and C issues and transmission
    - Use of condoms
    - Has the patient ever thought of or tried other methods of use?
    - Previous attempts to reduce or stop taking drugs
    - Previous periods of treatment or rehabilitation
- History of injecting and risk of HIV and hepatitis
- Medical history
- Psychiatric history
- Forensic history
- Social history
- Past contact with treatment services
- Drug and alcohol misuse in partner, spouse and other family members
- Impact of drug misuse on other aspects of the patient's life.

Examination

- Assess motivation.
- Assess general health:
    - Signs of drug misuse, e.g. needle track marks, skin abscesses
    - Signs of withdrawal or intoxication
    - Determine the presence of any complications of drug misuse:
        - Viral hepatitis
        - Bacterial endocarditis
        - HIV
        - Tuberculosis
        - Septicaemia
        - Pneumonia
        - Deep vein thrombosis

    - Pulmonary emboli
    - Abscesses
    - Dental disease
- Assess mental health.
- Assess social and family situation.

Investigations

- Full blood screen
- Hepatitis B and C
- HIV
- Urine screening for drugs of abuse at the outset and during prescribing
- Hair analysis (where indicated).

PATTERNS OF USE AND DEPENDENCE ON DIFFERENT DRUGS

Opiates

Effects of intoxication

Heroin may be smoked, injected, or heated on foil and the fumes inhaled. The short-term effects include a rapid onset of euphoria with a sensation of heavy extremities. The user then experiences alternating wakeful and drowsy states. Heroin is a CNS depressant and has effects on reaction times and ability to concentrate.

Diverted pharmaceutical opiates and opioids may be formulated for injection, oral use or as suppositories. Tablets may be crushed and injected. Dependence can develop rapidly, within weeks. Since tolerance also develops rapidly but diminishes quickly after abstinence, relapse can lead to overdose and death. This is also the case for methadone.

Health complications

Repeated use of heroin induces a state of dependency, with a need for increased doses and increased frequency of use. The occurrence of withdrawal symptoms triggers further use to relieve these symptoms. Repeated injections result in collapsed veins, infection of the heart lining, endocarditis, and skin and muscle infections. Sharing of injection equipment also carries a high risk of blood-borne infections such as HIV and hepatitis C. Opiates and opioids depress coughing, breathing and heart rate, dilate blood vessels, reduce bowel activity and produce constipation. Overdose usually occurs in combination with other drugs.

Signs of opiate intoxication

- Apathy
- Sedation
- Disinhibition
- Psychomotor retardation
- Impaired attention
- Impaired judgement
- Interference with personal functioning
- Drowsiness
- Slurred speech
- Pupillary constriction
- Decreased level of consciousness.

Signs of opiate withdrawal

- Craving
- Sneezing, yawning, runny eyes
- Muscle aches, abdominal pains
- Nausea, vomiting, diarrhoea
- Pupillary dilation
- Goose flesh, recurrent chills
- Restless sleep.

Cannabis

Effects of intoxication

Cannabis is either smoked or eaten. Use is accompanied by distorted time perception, impaired coordination and difficulty in thinking. These effects may persist for over 24 h.

Health complications

Cannabis has effects on physical health, with higher rates of lung and heart disease in cannabis users compared with cigarette-smokers. Cannabis use can lead to depression, anxiety and paranoia. Panic attacks are a feature, and there is controversy as to whether cannabis causes an enduring schizophrenia-like psychosis or simply exacerbates it. Memory and learning are affected. Evidence is accumulating of the risk of lung cancer and cancers of the head and neck in cannabis-smokers.

Signs of cannabis intoxication

- Euphoria and disinhibition
- Anxiety and agitation
- Suspiciousness and paranoid ideation
- Impaired reaction time
- Impaired judgement and attention
- Hallucinations with preserved orientation
- Depersonalization and derealization
- Increased appetite
- Dry mouth
- Conjunctival injection
- Tachycardia.

Signs of cannabis withdrawal

- Anxiety
- Irritability
- Tremor
- Sweating
- Muscle aches.

Stimulants – amphetamines, cocaine and ecstasy (MDMA)

Effects of intoxication

The majority of psychostimulants may be used orally, snorted as a powder through the nose, injected or smoked. Psychostimulants produce an intense euphoric state, which may be accompanied by restlessness and agitation, rapid speech rate and increased wakefulness.

Health complications

The use of psychostimulants may precipitate anxiety states, confusion, convulsions and cardiovascular problems. Acute psychotic episodes are a relatively common presentation in mental health settings. The sharing of injection equipment carries the same risks as for heroin use, but the risk is often underestimated in the stimulant-using population. Use of stimulants may lead to exhaustion, depression and weight loss. A paranoid or confusional state may also occur. Hypertension, cardiac arrhythmias, stroke, hepatic and renal damage, and abscesses are the result of heavy use, especially if the drug is injected. Violent and aggressive behaviour may ensue. Snorting cocaine leads to nasal septal perforation and damage to the nasal passages.

Signs of stimulant intoxication

- Euphoria and increased energy
- Hypervigilance
- Repetitive stereotyped behaviours
- Grandiose beliefs and actions
- Paranoid ideation
- Abusiveness, aggression and argumentativeness
- Auditory, tactile and visual hallucinations
- Sweats, chills and muscular weakness
- Nausea or vomiting
- Weight loss
- Pupillary dilation
- Convulsions
- Tachycardia
- Arrhythmias
- Chest pain
- Hypertension
- Agitation.

Signs of stimulant withdrawal

- Lethargy
- Psychomotor retardation or agitation
- Craving
- Increased appetite
- Insomnia or hypersomnia
- Bizarre and unpleasant dreams.

Sedatives – benzodiazepines

Health complications

In the short term, users may experience tiredness, depressed respiration, dizziness and unsteadiness. With other depressants, such as alcohol or opiates, overdose can be fatal. Dependence can develop on low doses, and convulsions occur with withdrawal. Rebound symptoms such as insomnia, anxiety and tension can occur.

Signs of benzodiazepine intoxication

- Euphoria
- Disinhibition
- Lability of mood
- Apathy
- Sedation
- Abusiveness and aggression
- Impaired attention
- Amnesia
- Impaired psychomotor performance
- Unsteady gait
- Slurred speech
- Nystagmus
- Decreased level of consciousness
- Hypothermia.

Signs of benzodiazepine withdrawal

- Confusion and convulsions
- Tremor, postural hypotension
- Nausea and vomiting
- Agitation
- Paranoid ideation
- Tachycardia
- Rebound insomnia and tension.

Sedatives – barbiturates

Barbiturates are classified according to their duration of action:

- Ultra-short-acting
- Short-acting
- Long-acting.

Their effects include relaxation and improved sleep at low levels, but at higher levels they can induce cognitive impairment, lability of mood, and impaired motor behaviour such as slurred speech and slow reaction times.

Signs of barbiturate intoxication

- Apathy
- Sedation
- Abusiveness and aggression
- Impaired attention
- Amnesia
- Impaired psychomotor performance
- Unsteady gait

- Slurred speech
- Nystagmus
- Decreased level of consciousness
- Shallow breathing
- Coma.

Signs of barbiturate withdrawal

Signs of withdrawal can occur up to 20 h after the last dose and include the following:

- Irritability
- Increased heart and respiration rate
- Hallucinations and seizures
- Nightmares
- Insomnia
- Coma
- Death.

Volatile substances

Volatile substances include petrol, acetone, ether and toluene. They may be found in glues, solvents, lighter fluids, spray deodorants and nail-polish removers.

Health complications

The major risks are from the rapid onset of intoxication and method of inhalation. There may be public health and public safety issues where users store large quantities of inflammable solvents in unsafe situations.

Signs of intoxication with volatile substances

- Initial euphoria
- Blurred vision
- Impaired psychomotor function
- Delayed reaction time
- Poor manual dexterity and coordination
- CNS depression
- Respiratory arrest
- Unconsciousness
- Death, due to cardiac arrest.

Signs of withdrawal from volatile substances

There are no withdrawal effects for this category of drug described in DSM-IV. However, after intoxication has worn off, later effects such as headache, stomach ache, conjunctivitis and cough may last for some days.

SPECIFIC POPULATIONS

Adolescents

There is extensive documentation, mainly from cross-sectional studies, of the association of substance misuse and psychiatric disorder in young people. The major diagnostic groups to emerge are affective disorder (bipolar depression, major depression, anxiety, panic, phobias and post-traumatic stress syndrome), personality disorders (conduct, borderline and antisocial) and attention deficit disorders. Learning disability, for example, has not been studied extensively, though clinical experience suggests an association and where assessment and intervention may yield benefits. Moreover, since psychiatric disorders that begin in childhood may continue into adult life, there is an opportunity to intervene early to prevent or reduce conditions complicated by substance misuse, if access to appropriate services is provided. Longitudinal work is vital in order to explore more fully the patterns of co-morbidity and to implement and evaluate the treatment interventions that might contribute to decreasing morbidity and mortality.

Cannabis and psychosis in young people

The possibility of a connection between cannabis use and psychotic symptoms has been the subject of research, and many individual papers have concluded that the connection does, in fact, exist. In a prospective cohort study of cannabis use and its relationship to the development of psychotic symptoms, Henquet and colleagues studied 2437 young people in Europe aged 14–24 years.[62] The study concluded that, at a 4-year follow-up from the baseline, cannabis use has a moderate effect in increasing the risk of psychotic symptoms in young people. This effect was, however, much stronger in young people who showed evidence of a predisposition to psychosis. The study also demonstrated that a predisposition to psychosis at baseline did not predict cannabis use, and the authors concluded that this result could be used to refute the self-medication hypothesis.

A systematic review of general population longitudinal studies was undertaken, which reported the associations between illicit drug use by young people and psychosocial harm.[63] This identified 48 studies, of which only 26 were of a high quality. The review concluded that there were no consistent associations between cannabis use and psychological health problems. Although the evidence did not provide clear support for a causal relationship, it was not robust enough to exclude such a connection, and the authors indicated that better evidence is needed in relation to both cannabis and other illicit substances.

Attention deficit hyperactivity disorder and substance use disorders in adolescents

Longitudinal community studies of children with ADHD have shown that they are at risk for a variety of antisocial activities, which are related mainly to co-morbid drug use.[64] In a longitudinal study in the USA, 158 children aged 4–12 years who had been diagnosed with hyperactivity were followed up for a mean period of 20 years. A matched community control group was followed up over the same time period. Children with co-morbid ADHD and substance use disorders were reported to have a higher severity of drug use and worse treatment outcomes than those with ADHD but no substance use disorder.[65]

Wilens highlighted the lack of evidence on the mechanisms by which untreated ADHD increases the risk of drug or alcohol problems, despite the existence of a considerable body of literature concerning their association.[66] The relationship between early substance use and childhood disorders with externalizing psychopathology such as ADHD, conduct disorder and oppositional defiant disorder has been investigated in a longitudinal community-based study of twins.[67] The results suggested that externalizing psychopathology increases the risks for early initiation of alcohol, nicotine and cannabis use. Progression to regular and more serious use of cannabis by the age of 14 years was reported as having the strongest association with externalizing psychopathology (odds ratio (OR) 3.45). ADHD was the weakest predictor of the three externalizing disorders studied, with conduct disorder being the strongest.

Treating ADHD associated with substance misuse disorders with stimulants has been shown to be effective in treating the hyperactivity disorder but has no effect on the drug or alcohol disorder.[65] The possibility that treating young people with ADHD with stimulants might increase the risk of substance use disorders is a concern for clinicians. A meta-analysis of the literature has been performed to address this concern and concluded that, in fact, such treatment reduces the risk of subsequent drug and alcohol problems.[68]

Anxiety, depression and substance use disorders in adolescents

The relationship between substance use, anxiety and depression in young people is complex, but it reflects many of the general issues that complicate the identification of causal relationships in studies of co-morbidity. A 21-year study of the association between anxiety disorders and substance abuse disorders showed that young people with anxiety disorders are at increased risk of substance use disorders, with ORs between the two disorders in the range of 1.3–3.9.[69] The association is, however, not causal and is dependent on the presence of related confounding factors that are connected with increased risk for anxiety disorder. In constructing the methodology, the authors proposed three possible models: (i) that there would be a common or correlated cause for the disorders; (ii) that self-medication would be confirmed; and (iii) that there would be a causal relationship. The study demonstrated that the first model was the most appropriate.

However, a cross-sectional study that investigated panic attacks, depression and anxiety symptoms, and substance use behaviours during late adolescence demonstrated that 'panickers' were significantly more likely to have ever used sedatives, stimulants, opioids and other drugs, but not tobacco, alcohol, cocaine or hallucinogens.[70] Furthermore, in panickers, substance use and psychological symptoms such as depression and anxiety were related. The authors noted that it was not possible to determine causality, but they did conclude that the relationship between panic attacks and substance use appeared to present before the typical age of onset of substance use and panic disorders. Another study of a clinical sample of adolescents with phobic disorders and substance dependence in Finland showed that adolescents with a phobic disorder were almost five times more likely to develop substance dependence than those without a phobia.[71] Over half of the adolescents had developed substance dependence within 3 years of onset of the phobic disorder. This clearly points to the need to screen, diagnose and treat early on.

A longitudinal study examined the effect of age of first substance use and history of psychiatric disorders on the development of substance use disorder by the age of 16 years.[72] This group reported that the risk of transition to substance use disorder increased with age at onset before age 13 years but began to fall after age 14 years. The findings indicated that early substance use was a major predictor of adolescent substance use disorder, even in the absence of conduct disorder. However, past conduct disorder had a strong additive effect at age 13–15 years; boys with a history of depression were at increased risk of substance use disorder; and anxiety increased the risk of substance use disorder in girls at the age of 16 years.

Pregnant drug users

Pregnancy in a woman who is misusing substances is risky, both for her and the fetus. Pregnant drug users are frequently underweight, anaemic and socially disadvantaged. They are often poor attendees at antenatal clinics, and young users tend to present to maternity services late in their pregnancy. Substance misuse also increases the risk of other conditions, including domestic violence, sexually transmitted diseases, hepatitis B, hepatitis C and HIV. These associated problems can present a significant risk to the pregnant mother and her unborn child, in addition to any effects of the drug use on the growth and maturation of the fetus.[73,74]

Long-term developmental neurocognitive, physical and psychosocial effects resulting from in utero exposure to opioids and other drugs are poorly understood. Moreover, it is increasingly common for substance misusers to take a combination of different drugs at different times during their pregnancy and, because of the complex psychosocial context in which they use substances, research can face serious methodological problems. However, generally, parental substance misuse poses significant risks for children. Child and adolescent mental health services report that a parent's long-standing drug or alcohol misuse is a substantial risk factor for poor mental health in children.[75] Children may also be at high risk of maltreatment, emotional or physical neglect or abuse, family conflict, and inappropriate parental behaviour.[76–78] Children may be exposed to, and involved in, drug-related activities and associated crimes.[79] They are more likely to display behavioural problems,[80] experience social isolation and stigma,[81] misuse substances themselves when older,[82] and develop problem drug use[83] than other children.

Parents with chronic drug addiction spend considerable time and attention on accessing and using drugs, which reduces their emotional and actual availability for their children. Conflicting pressures may be especially acute in economically deprived lone-parent households and where there is little support from relatives or neighbours.[84] In the long term, children of substance-misusing parents may have severe social difficulties, including strong reactions to change, isolation, difficulty in learning to have fun, and estrangement from family and peers.[79] Despite this, substance misusers should not automatically be stereotyped as poor parents.

INTERACTION OF DRUG AND ALCOHOL USE WITH PSYCHIATRIC ILLNESS

Relationship between drug misuse and mental health problems

Research shows that substance use, intoxication, harmful use, withdrawal and dependence (addiction) may lead to or exacerbate psychiatric or psychological symptoms or syndromes.[85] Similarly, psychological morbidity and psychiatric disorders may lead to substance use, harmful use and dependence (addiction). Substance misuse is commonly associated with depression, anxiety and schizophrenia, but eating disorders, post-traumatic stress disorders, ADHD and memory disorders also occur.[86] Alcohol problems, for example, are often seen with bipolar disorders, schizophrenia and personality disorders,[87] while concurrent use of other illicit substances is well recognized in opiate dependence.

Interrelationships in dual diagnosis can be classified as follows:

- A primary psychiatric illness may precipitate or lead to substance use, misuse, harmful use or dependent use, which may also be associated with physical illness and alter social ability.
- Substance use, misuse, harmful use or dependent use may exacerbate a mental or physical health problem, for example painful conditions, and any associated social functioning difficulties.
- Substance use, intoxication, misuse, harmful use or dependent use may lead to psychological symptomatology not amounting to a diagnosis and also to social problems.
- Substance use, misuse, harmful use or dependent use may lead to psychiatric illness, physical illness and social dysfunction.

Co-morbidity

Co-morbidity may present itself in a range of different combinations and permutations, including the following:

- Substance use – even one dose – may lead to psychological symptoms or psychiatric syndromes.
- Harmful use may produce psychiatric symptoms.
- Dependence may produce psychological symptoms.
- Intoxication may produce psychological symptoms.
- Withdrawal from substances may produce psychological symptoms.
- Withdrawal from substances may produce psychiatric syndromes.
- Substance use may exacerbate a pre-existing psychiatric disorder.
- Psychological morbidity not amounting to a disorder may precipitate substance use.
- Primary psychiatric disorder may lead to substance use disorder.
- Primary psychiatric disorder may precipitate substance use disorder, which may in turn lead to psychiatric disorder.[88]

There is a vast body of literature on this topic. However, it must be stated that there are a variety of methodological issues that comprise the comparability of studies, including definitions, criteria for diagnosis, the different healthcare settings and systems in which studies take place, descriptions of combinations of interventions, and changing prevalence. Nonetheless, despite these differences and inherent difficulties, there can be little doubt that these combined disorders now constitute an important component of a psychiatrist's day-to-day workload.

Psychoactive substances have differing psychological effects, including those caused by intoxication and withdrawal. Chronic use, intoxication with depressant drugs and withdrawal from stimulants produce symptoms similar to those seen with depressant drugs, while acute intoxication with stimulants and cannabis may mimic a schizophrenic illness. Withdrawal from depressant drugs may result in symptoms of anxiety, panic and even confusional states. These complex interactions have implications in that not only does drug use interfere with emotional, cognitive and social behaviour, but also the combination of disorders results in poorer treatment compliance and worse outcomes in both the short and the longer term.

An association between drug use and psychiatric conditions has been consistently documented in substance-misusing clinical populations, psychiatric populations, the general population, prison populations and homeless populations. Indeed, in the well-known Epidemiological Catchment Area (ECA) study, drug addiction was associated with a 53.1 per cent lifetime rate of an additional mental disorder.[89]

Furthermore, the interrelationships between physical health, mental health and drug misuse are also well documented. Apart from the direct effects of drugs on general health (see below), there are indirect effects such as dietary neglect, impoverishment, trauma, bereavement and loss. Malnutrition, for instance, may emanate from drug-induced anorexia, malabsorption or economic deprivation. Liver dysfunction, for example as a result of HIV or hepatitis B or C, produces psychological as well as physical problems.

Psychiatric conditions such as anxiety, depression, post-traumatic stress disorder, drug-induced psychosis, schizophrenia, delirium and dementia may lead to, be a consequence of, or coincide with drug misuse. Withdrawal from barbiturates and benzodiazepines leads to delirium, whereas head injuries and serious infections are associated with dementia. The differing mechanisms and types of relationship demand careful history-taking and judicious interpretation. Depression, dementia, delirium and a heightened risk of suicide are probably the problems most commonly faced by clinicians. Of course, some of these conditions are associated with chronic pain and sleep disorders, which may make patients vulnerable and lead to them seeking relief from prescription and non-prescription medications in a non-compliant fashion. Sleep disorders such as insomnia may precipitate an increased alcohol intake and a consequent negative effect on sleep patterns over a prolonged period of excessive intake.

Since there are effective medications and psychosocial interventions available for many psychiatric conditions, correct diagnosis and treatment or referral have tangible benefits.

Another study of mental health centres and substance misuse services in the UK reported that three-quarters of drug service users and 85 per cent of alcohol service users had mental health problems, mostly affective disorders and anxiety disorders. Approximately one-third of the drug treatment population and half of the alcohol treatment population also had multiple morbidity – that is, the co-occurrence of a number of psychiatric disorders or substance misuse disorders.[90] The costs of caring for service users with dual diagnosis are higher than those for single conditions because of the need for greater service use.[91,92] In fact, nearly 40 per cent of drug users had not received help for their mental health problems, and just over 40 per cent of mental health service users reported drug use or hazardous or harmful levels of alcohol use in the past year. These individuals were perceived as being more aggressive and chaotic and less compliant with care plans.[90,93,94]

Drug users attending treatment also tend to carry a heavy burden of additional health problems. These adversely affect their physical and mental health and are accompanied by high rates of unemployment.[95,96] Serious physical illness is an additional co-morbidity and one that is, perhaps, overlooked, underrated and undertreated.[97] Physical problems such as pain, infection, injury and cancer may result from substance misuse and may lead to mental illness. If not treated adequately, these conditions not only add to the patient's suffering but also undermine the treatment provided for substance misuse. As a result, people with multiple conditions often do not access or receive the care they need.

Problems may begin in childhood or adolescence and continue into old age.[5,6,98–103] Child abuse, for example, is known to contribute to the prevalence of co-morbid personality disorder in addiction populations.[104–106] Women who use substances are more likely than a control group to have been exposed to sexual, physical and emotional abuse as children. They are also more likely to experience emotional distress than a control group of women substance misusers who do not have that background.[107,108]

The explanation for differing rates of co-occurring disorders depends on many factors, including the following:

- Differences between or lack of standardization of diagnostic classification systems and diagnostic instruments used for mental disorder and substance use disorders
- The setting in which the condition is studied – for example, a clinical setting is more likely to yield high rates than a general population study
- Services may conceptualize and diagnose the same users differently
- An individual's substance use may fluctuate in type, quantity or frequency
- Time of assessment may influence the result, for example during withdrawal or intoxication
- Mental health presentations may vary, depending on environmental triggers
- Differences between regions in terms of types of presentation and rural or urban communities
- The combination of events that contribute to an individual's life history.

BASICS OF THE BIOLOGICAL, PSYCHOLOGICAL AND SOCIOCULTURAL EXPLANATIONS OF DRUG AND ALCOHOL DEPENDENCE

Substance use and misuse are best viewed through the framework of a multifactorial biopsychosocial model. Age, role, gender, social group and peer pressure, family, community and occupational environment, and overall cultural values and controls on substance use will all act upon substance-taking behaviour.[109]

The biopsychosocial model of addiction is comprehensive and starts from an assumption of multifactorial causality of addiction, including biological, genetic, psychological and sociocultural factors. Within the population of people with alcohol-related problems, this model would propose that there are a series of subpopulations where specific factors may play a more important role in causation than in other groups. The biopsychosocial model may be used to explain the number of cases of coexisting psychiatric and alcohol problems.[110]

The coexistence of psychiatric illness with alcohol dependence is common; for example, the National Institute of Mental Health Epidemiological Catchment Area Program reported that, among people with a mental disorder, the lifetime prevalence of an alcohol disorder was 22 per cent, compared with 13.5 per cent for the total population. Among people with an alcohol disorder, 37 per cent had a co-morbid mental disorder.[85] The self-medication hypothesis suggests that the specific pharmacological properties of addictive substances are used to control the symptoms of psychiatric illness.[111] However, although this view has clinical and empirical support, it has not been supported by consistent research evidence.[112]

A literature review of the use of alcohol to control social anxiety reported that attribution of a self-medicating effect to a substance by the user might not align with the reality of the pharmacological and physiological effects of the substance.[113] For example, the review found support for the fact that individuals with social phobia use alcohol to reduce anxiety, but the evidence that alcohol actually reduced social anxiety was less conclusive.

Attempts to change drinking behaviour can be influenced by a range of factors, including:

- genetic make-up;
- personality;
- sense of control;
- sense of efficacy;
- degree of dependence;
- presence of brain damage;
- psychiatric problems;
- internal and external cues or stimuli;
- financial state;
- values of the treatment programme.

ASSESSMENT AND MANAGEMENT OF DRUG AND ALCOHOL MISUSERS

Guidelines from the British Association of Psychopharmacology (BAP) summarized the evidence base for the pharmacological treatment of substance misuse and co-morbid conditions. The following findings are drawn from this document.[114]

Summary recommendations from the British Association of Psychopharmacology guidelines

Opioids

There is considerable evidence for the use of methadone, buprenorphine and α_2 agonists (clonidine, lofexidine) in the management of withdrawal states. There are differences in choice of medication, depending on the priorities around duration of treatment, adverse effects (bradycardia and hypotension due to α_2-adrenergic agonists) and withdrawal severity. The patient's clinical condition, degree of dependence and preference, and the practitioner's experience, will determine which drug to use.

Similarly, there is an established evidence base for methadone maintenance treatment and, more recently, for buprenorphine. There is inadequate evidence for treatment with naltrexone and injectable opioids, and for using coercive methods.

Stimulants

For stimulant drugs such as cocaine and amphetamine, the guidelines do not recommend the use of dopamine agonists, antidepressants or carbamazepine. Furthermore, there is no clear evidence to support substitute prescription of dexamphetamines. In fact, psychosocial interventions are considered the mainstay of treatment, although the evidence is limited.

Sedatives and hypnotics

The guidelines make recommendations for benzodiazepine dependence, whether the benzodiazepines be used licitly on a prescription or illicitly. In early or mild dependence, minimal interventions such as relaxation or general practitioner (GP) advice are suggested. For more severe dependence, graded discontinuation is advised. For illicit misusers, there is no evidence that continued prescribing is beneficial, apart from to reduce illicit use. The above advice is related to an adult population.

Psychological interventions

The majority of interventions are based on learning theory models, but there is also the recognition that there are non-treatment routes to improvement.[97] Furthermore, information-based approaches such as health education and information are useful in less complex situations. These might include education about harm minimization, immunization and vaccination.

In the addiction literature, the term 'counselling' is used to incorporate brief and intensive interventions, including supportive, directive or motivational counselling, individual, family or group behavioural treatments, and social network behavioural therapy. Counselling may aim to reduce the use of alcohol and drugs, and the associated negative consequences or related problems. The term may encompass assessment, engagement and support, together with the development of therapeutic relationships. The non-judgemental and empathic method of challenging decisions and assumptions in motivational interviewing is included in the gamut of techniques. Important common objectives may include the following:

- *Problem solving:* developing competence in dealing with a specific problem.
- *Acquisition of social skills:* mastery of social and interpersonal skills through assertiveness or anger control.
- *Cognitive change:* modification of irrational beliefs and maladaptive patterns of thought.
- *Behaviour change:* modification of maladaptive behaviour.

- *Systemic change:* introducing change into family systems.

Counselling is a widely used term and is a form of therapy or intervention that includes a wide range of theoretical models. There are many different definitions, each emphasizing specific aspects of the counselling role and processes practised in a multiplicity of settings. Counselling embodies psychodynamics, cognitive-behavioural and person-centred approaches.

There are various treatment options, the choice of which depends on the nature and extent of the problem and the approach that may appear more appropriate and suitable for a particular drug user. The options include:

- non-directive counselling;
- cognitive-behavioural therapy (CBT);
- family dynamics;
- group therapy;
- motivational enhancement.

Non-directive counselling comprises the following components:

The patient determines the content and direction of the counselling and explores conflict and emotions at the time. While allowing empathic reflection, the counsellor does not offer advice and feedback.

A cognitive-behavioural approach assumes that the patient would like to change and analyses the situations that cause drug use, so that these can be altered. Problem-solving techniques, self-monitoring, anger management, relapse prevention, assertiveness training, the acquisition of social skills, and the modification of irrational beliefs or patterns of thought or behaviour are used. Individual, group and family therapies used in the treatment of addiction problems are often based along cognitive-behavioural lines.

Social network behaviour therapy considers the social environment to be important in the development, maintenance and resolution of substance problems. It maximizes positive social support, which is central to the process. The therapist offers advice and feedback and thereby facilitates change in the patient's social world. Behaviour is not interpreted, and engagement with significant others is key in bringing about change and achieving goals.

Family therapy involves attempts to understand and interpret family dynamics in order to change the psychopathology. Substance use is perceived as a symptom of family dysfunction and, therefore, altering the dynamics brings about change in the substance misuse. Family members are viewed as contributory to the problem. Behavioural and psychodynamic techniques may be used in family therapy.

Participation in self-help groups is an important feature of many treatment programmes, in which participants receive support from recovering members who often take members back to the negative consequences of substance misuse. A variant of group therapy is the 12-step approach. Central to the 12-steps philosophy is the idea that recovery from addiction is possible only if the individual recognizes his or her problem and admits that he or she is unable to use substances in moderation. Alcoholics Anonymous and Narcotics Anonymous are examples of groups that use the 12-step philosophy, where drug users have to abstain completely.

Recently, the most influential and popular form of treatment has been a brief or minimal intervention, known as 'motivational interviewing'. This aims to build motivation for change. The focus is on a non-judgemental approach and the patient's concerns about, and choices regarding, future drug use. The treatment thereby elicits strategies from the patient. Motivational enhancement directs the patient to motivation for change by offering empathic feedback and advice and information and selectively reinforces discrepancies that emerge between current behaviour and goals, in order to enhance motivation for change. Significant others play some role in the treatment, but it is not a central role. It is, by and large, a personal therapeutic situation where the individual's motivation is seen as vital. It aims to alter the decisional balance so that the patient directs the process of change.

The key characteristics are best described by the acronym FRAMES:[115]

- Personalized *feedback* or assessment results detailing the target behaviour and associated effects and consequences on the individual
- Emphasizing the individual's personal *responsibility* for change
- Giving *advice* on how to change
- Providing a *menu* of options for change
- Expressing *empathy* through behaviours conveying caring, understanding and warmth
- Emphasizing *self-efficacy* for change and instilling hope that change is not only possible but also within reach.

Evidence is accumulating with regard to the benefits and cost-effectiveness of this type of intervention.[116,117]

Treatment effectiveness

The first relatively long-term, prospective, observational study on outcome in drug misusers in the UK, the National Treatment Outcome Research Study (NTORS), has been under way since 1995.[118] This study follows up 1075 drug misusers in two types of residential service (in-patient and residential units) and two kinds of community service (methadone reduction and methadone maintenance). The age range at baseline was 16–58 years, half of whom were responsible for caring for children.

It is important to note that the specific nature of the treatment modalities provided has not been identified or described in any depth or in detail. Opiates, amphetamines, cocaine, non-prescription benzodiazepines and alcohol have been assessed, and the impact of treatment on psychological health, suicide, mortality and crime has been evaluated. In summary, the study has reported drug use, and injecting and sharing needles, as being reduced. Crime also decreased, with a concurrent improvement in physical and psychological health. However, 20 per cent of the study population continued to use daily, and 40 per cent continued to use once a week. Over a 5-year period, 62 people died, 80 were using two or more illicit drugs and were long-term users, and alcohol use remained at a constantly high level. There was a history of treatment for psychiatric disorder in the 2 years before treatment; in the 3 months before treatment, 30 per cent had suicidal ideation.

NTORS found that over 27 000 acquisitive criminal offences were reported by the cohort examined in the 3 months before starting treatment.[119] Shoplifting was the most common offence. Ten per cent of the sample was responsible for three-quarters of the crimes committed. Frequency of illicit drug use was associated with increased levels of criminal behaviour. Since high-rate offenders were more likely to be regular users of heroin and were three times more likely to have used cocaine regularly, management of this most severely affected group would be important to reduce offending.

At 5 years, 33.3 per cent and 50 per cent of users had achieved abstinence in community and residential services, respectively. However, 20 per cent of users were still using daily. Although 40 per cent used illicit drugs regularly, this had reduced from 66 per cent at intake in the residential services and from 80 per cent in community services. In summary, daily and regular use were found in 20 per cent and 40 per cent, respectively. Likewise, injecting reduced from 60 per cent to 40 per cent, criminal activity halved, and 25 per cent of users were drinking above safe limits. This evidence is encouraging, despite the limitations in the design described above. The study points to some value in the treatment programmes that are being implemented in the UK. This study was on an adult population and so does not include vulnerable groups such as teenagers and older people.

Therefore, despite advances in the effectiveness of pharmacological and psychological treatments for substance misuse, 'it is not clear that these findings will generalise to comorbid major depression and alcohol dependence',[120] as evidence for effective psychological treatment for co-morbidity is still limited.[121] Combined treatments (pharmacological and psychological, or two types of pharmacological treatment) are just beginning to be evaluated in substance-misusing and co-morbid populations. A meta-analysis found that only 14 randomized controlled trials (RCTs) have been carried out in people with both depression and alcoholism.[122] This is surprisingly few trials for two such common conditions. Furthermore, the evidence suggests that, although antidepressants may improve mood, it is not clear that there is a commensurate impact on alcohol consumption. Even 'effective' treatments are not effective for all those who seek help, and not all who need help will seek it.

The most comprehensive review at the time of writing considered both psychological and pharmacological treatments for substance misuse associated with depression, anxiety, schizophrenia, bipolar disorder and severe mental illness.[123] Fifty-nine studies met the standards for inclusion, of which 36 were RCTs. Although there was no clear evidence of superiority of any intervention over the comparison treatment for both psychiatric disorder and substance misuse, and treatments had not been replicated, the review did demonstrate that effective treatments for psychiatric conditions tended to reduce psychiatric symptomatology, and effective treatments for substance misuse tended to reduce substance use. However, the value of integrated treatment was not substantiated.

Despite the fact that there may be more treatment options and services available, these are not as accessible or available as is required, particularly for some especially vulnerable groups. Since both mental health and substance problems may be chronic conditions, treatment cannot be conceptualized or presented as a 'cure', but rather should be considered as support and care that can improve some substance, health and psychosocial outcomes. There is an increasing emphasis on engagement of the service user and carers, on focusing on the community rather than the hospital setting, on continuity, responsiveness and flexibility in care, and on attempting to integrate educational and employment options and accommodation needs, as well as special relationships within the treatment framework. Some of these issues are targeted in models of treatment within the criminal justice system (see below).

DETOXIFICATION PROCEDURES FOR IN-PATIENTS AND OUT-PATIENTS

Opiates

Before embarking on detoxification from opiates, it is advisable to ensure that the patient is fully committed and well informed about the process and is aware of the risk of relapse. Current guidance suggests that the patient should be in a stable supportive social situation or have arrangements in place for this to occur after detoxification. Plans for continuing support should have been finalized.[60]

Guidance on opioid detoxification has been published by the National Institute for Health and Clinical Excellence (NICE),[124] and clinicians should use this as the basis for treatment interventions. In summary, this guidance states the following:

- Methadone or buprenorphine should be offered as a first-line treatment in opioid detoxification, taking into account both the user's preference and the benefit of starting detoxification with the medication that is already being used.

- Lofexidine may be suitable for those who do not wish to use either of the above or who want a more rapid detoxification.
- Clonidine and dihydrocodeine should not be used routinely.
- The treatment should last for up to 4 weeks in a residential setting and up to 12 weeks in a community setting.
- Ultra-rapid and rapid treatment should not be offered routinely, and ultra-rapid detoxification under anaesthesia must not be undertaken.
- In-patient detoxification is suitable for patients with complex needs, such as severe physical or mental health problems and concurrent detoxification for alcohol or other drugs. There must be 24-h medical and nursing support.

The management of detoxification for patients with drug problems within a residential setting is seen in the guidelines as a community-based service unless:

- the user has not responded to a community-based detoxification previously;
- there are significant co-morbid physical or mental health problems;
- the user will need complex detoxification, for example where they will need detoxification from a combination of substances;
- there are particular social problems that are a contraindication to a community-based detoxification.

Although rapid and ultra-rapid detoxification have been the subject of some research, with conflicting results,[125,126] the current guidance is clear that ultra-rapid detoxification under general anaesthesia or heavy sedation carries a high risk of death and must not be offered.

ASSESSMENT AND MANAGEMENT OF NON-SUBSTANCE ADDICTIVE BEHAVIOURS AND RELATED SYNDROMES

The concept of non-substance addictive behaviours has been the focus of much discussion and is currently part of the agenda for the forthcoming revision of the DSM. The application of an addictive behaviour model to activities such as gambling has a long history, although current diagnostic classifications use the concept of an impulse control disorder rather than an addictive model. The advent of the Internet and an exponential increase in access to information and resources has produced the added concept of 'Internet addiction'. The Internet has been described as 'both the means and the object of addiction',[127] and in a wide-ranging review of the concept the authors expressed concern that the proposed development of diagnostic classification based on medical models was premature and lacked an evidence base.[128] Their concern also extended to the use of the concepts in medicolegal cases.

RECOGNITION OF SUBSTANCE MISUSE-RELATED MEDICAL, PSYCHIATRIC AND SOCIAL COMPLICATIONS AND THEIR IMPACT ON PUBLIC HEALTH

Screening and assessment

The aim of screening and assessment measures is to achieve accurate diagnosis and to assist in the development of a relevant management plan. Without rigorous detection, problems will be missed or attributed inappropriately, and the treatment or care response may be inadequate, incorrect or even neglectful as a result. Factors that improve the efficiency of assessment and screening include:

- the experience and environment of the assessment;[129]
- a high index of suspicion;
- a robust assessment process, including taking a thorough history;
- the use of appropriate screening and assessment tools.[5,6]

This is relevant whether the presentation is to social services or to health, mental health or substance misuse services, and it is important to have a clearly defined and agreed approach in a multidisciplinary context,[130] with continual interaction and collaboration across services. The use of a common assessment framework should be seen as standard good practice.[129,131] This will reduce the risk of multiple but similar assessments, which are exhausting and unnecessary,[132] and will ensure a common understanding of terminology, definitions, approaches, interventions and outcome expectations. Any improvement in the user acceptability of assessment processed is to be welcomed, particularly as there is evidence that only half of those who require help ask for it.[133]

There are a range of instruments for the screening and assessment of different substances that can be utilized. These range from standardized tools and medical investigations (blood, urine, hair analysis) through to broader evaluation of factors that may affect the life experience and engagement in treatment of the service user, such as:

- occupational capacity;
- social functioning;
- relationship issues;
- readiness to change;
- motivation for change;
- educational and vocational skill assessment.

Social complications

Substance-related problems can have effects in a range of systems, such as health, education and the criminal justice system. Medication non-compliance, substance abuse and severe mental illness are associated with violence, although violence perpetrated by severely mentally ill people accounts for a small proportion of violent acts in the community.[134–137] Problems associated with dual diagnosis are associated with a poorer prognosis and greater disability. This includes a greater likelihood of medical, psychiatric and social problems that arise as a result of poor compliance with treatment, unplanned discharge, relapse and rehospitalization.[138–140] Self-harm (often by overdose) and eventual suicide also have a strong association, as does early mortality. It is recognized, for example, that service users with dual diagnosis, who constitute 27 per cent of suicides, are treated inadequately.[141–143]

Drug-related violent crime can be divided between violence arising from the effects of the drug, violence associated with the interaction of a psychiatric illness and drug use, violence associated with acquisition of drugs, and violence associated with disputes between drug users, dealers and gangs.[31] There is evidence to suggest that a combination of psychosis and co-morbid use of drugs results in a higher rate and severity of violence than in a population with psychosis and no co-morbid substance use.[144] Reviews of heroin users have also indicated that high rates of aggressive behaviour in this group may be independent of their use of heroin and, rather, related to personality factors that are associated with a risk of heroin dependence.[145] Substance misuse is commonly associated with a range of social problems, such as:

- homelessness;
- economic deprivation;
- unemployment;
- crime and violence;
- victimization;
- family problems;
- childhood abuse.[146–149]

As a result of these complications, co-morbid service users present to a range of services, including:

- primary care;
- secondary care;
- general medical services;
- surgical services;
- mental health services;
- social care services;
- education;
- housing;
- employment services;
- social work (child protection and adult services);
- criminal justice system.[150–153]

It has been noted that the emotional and socioeconomic issues that accompany substance misuse often constitute the major barriers to recovery, both for the individual and for their families.[154]

KEY POINTS

- The UK has among the highest levels of substance misuse in Europe. The situation is dynamic, and it has become well recognized that combinations of substances may be misused, including two of the most commonly encountered licit substances, alcohol and nicotine.
- Drug use is affected by age, gender, geographical location, price, fashion, availability, regulations, and cultural and societal values. There are a variety of theoretical models that are used to explain initiation and continuation of drug use.
- Substance use and misuse are best viewed through the framework of a multifactorial biopsychosocial model. Age, role, gender, social group and peer pressure, the family, community and occupational environment, and overall cultural values and controls on substance use all act upon substance-taking behaviour.
- Substances impact on every organ system of the body, including the gastrointestinal, cardiovascular, respiratory, musculoskeletal and endocrine systems and the CNS.
- It is well recognized that patients with severe mental illness are especially at risk of substance misuse. In studies of patients attending mental health services in the UK, 10 per cent of patients treated by community mental health teams reported problematic use of illicit drugs and 17 per cent reported alcohol problems in the past year.
- Overall, these studies demonstrate that drug misusers present to a wide range of services, that their problems are not detected, and that failure to recognize their problems may result in inappropriate treatment and recurrence of health issues, since at least one associated factor, the drug misuse, is not being treated effectively.
- There is extensive documentation of the association of substance misuse and psychiatric disorder in young people. The major diagnostic groups to emerge are affective disorder (bipolar depression, major depression, anxiety, panic, phobias and post-traumatic stress syndrome), personality disorders (conduct, borderline and antisocial) and attention deficit disorders.
- Pregnancy in a woman who is misusing substances is risky, both for her and the fetus. Pregnant drug users are frequently underweight, anaemic and socially disadvantaged. They are often poor attendees at antenatal clinics, and young users tend to present to maternity services late in their pregnancies.
- Since both mental health and substance problems may be chronic conditions, treatment cannot be conceptualized or presented as a cure but rather should be considered as support and care that can improve some substance, health and psychosocial outcomes.
- Substance-related problems can have effects in a range of systems, including health, education and the criminal justice system. Medication non-compliance, substance abuse and severe mental illness are associated with violence, although violence perpetrated by severely mentally ill people accounts for a small proportion of violent acts in the community.

REFERENCES

1. World Health Organization (1992) *ICD-10 Classification of Mental and Behavioural Disorders*. Geneva: World Health Organization.

2. American Psychiatric Association (1994) *Diagnostic and Statistical Manual of Mental Disorders*, 4th edn. Washington DC: American Psychiatric Association.
3. Lüscher C, Ungless MA (2006) The mechanistic classification of addictive drugs. *PLoS Medicine* **3**: e437.
4. Lader D (2008) *Smoking-Related Behaviour and Attitudes, 2007: A Report Using the National Statistics Omnibus Survey Produced on Behalf of the NHS Information Centre for Health and Social Care*. Newport: Office for National Statistics.
5. British Medical Association (2007) *Fetal Alcohol Spectrum Disorders: A Guide for Healthcare Professionals*. London: British Medical Association.
6. British Medical Association (2008) *Alcohol Misuse: Tackling the UK Epidemic*. London: British Medical Association.
7. Cabinet Office (2004) *Alcohol Harm Reduction Strategy for England*. London: Cabinet Office.
8. Welch C, Harrison D, Short A, Rowan K (2008) The increasing burden of alcoholic liver disease on United Kingdom critical care units: secondary analysis of a high quality clinical database. *Journal of Health Service Research and Policy* **13** (suppl. 2): 40–44.
9. Department of Health (2006) *Models of Care for Alcohol Misusers (MoCAM)*. London: Department of Health.
10. Murphy R, Roe S (2007) *Drug Misuse Declared: Findings From the 2006/07 British Crime Survey – England and Wales*. London: Home Office.
11. National Institute for Health and Clinical Excellence (2007) *Methadone and Buprenorphine for the Management of Opioid Dependence*. Technology appraisal guidance no. 114. London: National Institute for Health and Clinical Excellence.
12. National Centre for Social Research, National Foundation for Educational Research (2006) *Smoking, Drinking and Drug Use Among Young People in England in 2004: Headline Figures*. London: Department of Health.
13. Chivite-Matthews N, Richardson A, O'Shea J (2005) *Drug Misuse Declared: Findings from the 2003/04 British Crime Survey – England and Wales*. London: Home Office.
14. Walsh MJ, Flegel R, Atkins R, *et al.* (2005) Drug and alcohol use among drivers admitted to a level-1 trauma center. *Accident Analysis and Prevention* **37**: 894–901.
15. Walsh JM, Flegel R, Cangianelli LA, *et al.* (2004) Epidemiology of alcohol and other drug use among motor vehicle crash victims admitted to a trauma center. *Traffic Injury Prevention* **5**: 254–60.
16. El-Guebaly N, Armstrong SJ, Hodgins DC (1998) Substance abuse and the emergency room: programmatic implications. *Journal of Addictive Diseases* **17**: 21–40.
17. Canning UP, Kennell-Webb SA, Marshall EJ, *et al.* (1999) Substance misuse in acute general medical admissions. *Quarterly Journal of Medicine* **92**: 319–26.
18. Carey KB, Correia CJ (1998) Severe mental illness and addictions: assessment considerations. *Addictive Behaviour* **23**: 735–48.
19. Trathen B, O'Gara C, Sarkhel A, *et al.* (2007) Co-morbidity and cannabis use in a mental health trust in South East England. *Addictive Behaviour* **32**: 2164–77.
20. McCreadie RG (2002) Use of drugs, alcohol and tobacco by people with schizophrenia: case-control study. *British Journal of Psychiatry* **181**: 321–5.
21. McCann BS, Simpson TL, Ries R, Roy-Byrne P (2000) Reliability and validity of screening instruments for drug and alcohol abuse in adults seeking evaluation for attention-deficit/hyperactivity disorder. *American Journal on Addictions* **9**: 1–9.
22. Seivewright N, Daly C (1997) Personality disorder and drug use: a review. *Drug and Alcohol Review* **16**: 235–50.
23. Bosio P, Keenan E, Gleeson R, *et al.* (1997) The prevalence of chemical substance and alcohol abuse in an obstetric population in Dublin. *Irish Medical Journal* **90**: 149–50.
24. Strang J, Manning V, Mayet S, *et al.* (2008) Overdose training and take-home naloxone for opiate users: prospective cohort study of impact on knowledge and attitudes and subsequent management of overdoses. *Addiction* **103**: 1648–57.
25. Mayet S, Groshkova T, Morgan L, *et al.* (2008) Drugs and pregnancy: outcomes of women engaged with a specialist perinatal outreach addictions service. *Drug and Alcohol Review* **27**: 497–503.
26. Cavanagh JT, Carson AJ, Sharpe M, Lawrie SM (2003) Psychological autopsy studies of suicide: a systematic review. *Psychological Medicine* **33**: 395–405.
27. Farrell M, Marsden J (2008) Acute risk of drug-related death among newly released prisoners in England and Wales. *Addiction* **103**: 251–5.
28. Ghodse H, Oyefeso A, Kilpatrick B (1998) Mortality of drug addicts in the United Kingdom 1967–1993. *International Journal of Epidemiology* **27**: 473–8.
29. Bloor M, Gannon M, Hay G, *et al.* (2008) Contribution of problem drug users' deaths to excess mortality in Scotland: secondary analysis of cohort study. *British Medical Journal* **337**: a478.
30. Hickman M, Carnwath Z, Madden P, *et al.* (2003) Drug-related mortality and fatal overdose risk: pilot cohort study of heroin users recruited from specialist drug treatment sites in London. *Journal of Urban Health* **80**: 274–87.
31. Advisory Council on the Misuse of Drugs (2008) *Cannabis: Classification and Public Health*. London: Home Office.
32. Home Office (2008) *Misuse of Drugs: List of Drugs Currently Controlled Under the Misuse Of Drugs Legislation*. London: Home Office. www.homeoffice.gov.uk/documents/cdlist.pdf.
33. HM Government (2001) *The Misuse of Drugs*

Regulations 2001: Statutory Instrument 2001 – No. 3998. London: The Stationery Office.
34. General Medical Council (2006) *Good Practice in Prescribing Medicines*. London: General Medical Council.
35. Joint Formulary Committee (2008) *British National Formulary 55*. London: British Medical Association and Royal Pharmaceutical Society of Great Britain.
36. Edwards G, Gross MM (1976) Alcohol dependence: provisional description of a clinical syndrome. *British Medical Journal* **1**: 1058–61.
37. Peters TJ (2001) Clinical pathology. In T Stockwell (ed.) *International Handbook of Alcohol Dependence and Problems*. Chichester: John Wiley & Sons.
38. *Drug and Therapeutics Bulletin* (2000) Managing the heavy drinker in primary care. *Drug and Therapeutics Bulletin* **38**: 60–64.
39. Ogden EJ, Moskowitz H (2004) Effects of alcohol and other drugs on driver performance. *Traffic Injury Prevention* **5**: 185–98.
40. Lishman W (1987) *Organic Psychiatry: The Psychological Consequences of Cerebral Disorder*, Oxford: Blackwell Scientific.
41. Chick J (1989) Delirium tremens. *British Medical Journal* **298**: 3–4.
42. Sullivan JT, Sykora K, Schneiderman J, *et al.* (1989) Assessment of alcohol withdrawal: the revised clinical institute withdrawal assessment for alcohol scale (CIWA-Ar). *British Journal of Addiction* **84**: 1353–7.
43. Lishman WA (1990) Alcohol and the brain. *British Journal of Psychiatry* **156**: 635–44.
44. Thomson AD, Cook CC, Touquet R, Henry JA (2002) The Royal College of Physicians report on alcohol: guidelines for managing Wernicke's encephalopathy in the accident and emergency department. *Alcohol and Alcoholism* **37**: 513–21.
45. Harper CG, Giles M, Finlay-Jones R (1986) Clinical signs in the Wernicke–Korsakoff complex: a retrospective analysis of 131 cases diagnosed at necropsy. *Journal of Neurology, Neurosurgery and Psychiatry* **49**: 341–5.
46. Harper C, Dixon G, Sheedy D, Garrick T (2003) Neuropathological alterations in alcoholic brains: studies arising from the New South Wales Tissue Resource Centre. *Progress in Neuropsychopharmacology and Biological Psychiatry* **27**: 951–61.
47. Gabriel S, Grossmann A, Hoppner J, *et al.* (1999) Marchiafava–Bignami syndrome: extrapontine myelinolysis in chronic alcoholism. *Der Nervenarzt* **70**: 349–56.
48. Tome S, Lucey MR (2004) Current management of alcoholic liver disease. *Alimentary Pharmacology and Therapeutics* **19**: 707–14.
49. Becker U, Deis A, Sorensen TI, *et al.* (1996) Prediction of risk of liver disease by alcohol intake, sex, and age: a prospective population study. *Hepatology* **23**: 1025–9.
50. Dufour DR, Lott JA, Nolte FS, *et al.* (2000) Diagnosis and monitoring of hepatic injury: I. performance characteristics of laboratory tests. *Clinical Chemistry* **46**: 2027–49.
51. Finlayson N, Hayes P, Simpson K (2000) Diseases of the liver and biliary system. In NA Boon (ed.) *Davidson's Principles and Practice of Medicine*. London: Churchill Livingstone.
52. Poschl G, Stickel F, Wang XD, Seitz HK (2004) Alcohol and cancer: genetic and nutritional aspects. *Proceedings of the Nutrition Society* **63**: 65–71.
53. Romberger DJ, Grant K (2004) Alcohol consumption and smoking status: the role of smoking cessation. *Biomedicine and Pharmacotherapy* **58**: 77–83.
54. Eustace LW, Kang DH, Coombs D (2003) Fetal alcohol syndrome: a growing concern for health care professionals. *Journal of obstetric, Gynecologic, and Neonatal Nursing* **32**: 215–21.
55. West R (2001) Theories of addiction. *Addiction* **96**: 3–13.
56. West R (2006) *Theory of Addiction*. Oxford: Blackwell.
57. Smart RG (1980) An availability-proneness theory of illicit drug abuse. *NIDA Research Monographs* **30**: 46–9.
58. Barrett ME, Joe GW, Simpson DD (1990) Availability of drugs and psychological proneness in opioid addiction. *Substance Use and Misuse* **25**: 1211–26.
59. Lingford-Hughes AR, Davies SJ, McIver S, *et al.* (2003) Addiction. *British Medical Bulletin* **65**: 209–22.
60. Department of Health (England) and the Devolved Administrations (2007) *Drug Misuse and Dependence: UK Guidelines on Clinical Management*. London: Department of Health.
61. National Treatment Agency (2006) *Care Planning Practice Guide*. London: National Treatment Agency.
62. Henquet C, Krabbendam L, Spauwen J, *et al.* (2005) Prospective cohort study of cannabis use, predisposition for psychosis, and psychotic symptoms in young people. *British Medical Journal* **330**: 11.
63. Macleod J, Oakes R, Copello A, *et al.* (2004) Psychological and social sequelae of cannabis and other illicit drug use by young people: a systematic review of longitudinal, general population studies. *Lancet* **363**: 1579–88.
64. Barkley RA, Fischer M, Smallish L, Fletcher K (2004) Young adult follow-up of hyperactive children: antisocial activities and drug use. *Journal of Child Psychology and Psychiatry* **45**: 195–211.
65. Riggs PD, Hall SK, Mikulich-Gilbertson SK, *et al.* (2004) A randomized controlled trial of pemoline for attention-deficit/hyperactivity disorder in substance-abusing adolescents. *Journal of the American Academy of Child and Adolescent Psychiatry* **43**: 420–29.
66. Wilens TE (2004) Attention-deficit/hyperactivity disorder and the substance use disorders: the nature of the relationship, subtypes at risk, and treatment issues. *Psychiatric Clinics of North America* **27**: 283–301.

67. King SM, Iacono WG, McGue M (2004) Childhood externalizing and internalizing psychopathology in the prediction of early substance use. *Addiction* **99**: 1548–59.
68. Wilens TE, Faraone SV, Biederman J, Gunawardene S (2003) Does stimulant therapy of attention-deficit/hyperactivity disorder beget later substance abuse? A meta-analytic review of the literature. *Pediatrics* **111**: 179–85.
69. Goodwin RD, Fergusson DM, Horwood LJ (2004) Association between anxiety disorders and substance use disorders among young persons: results of a 21-year longitudinal study. *Journal of Psychiatric Research* **38**: 295–304.
70. Valentiner DP, Mounts NS, Deacon BJ (2004) Panic attacks, depression and anxiety symptoms, and substance use behaviors during late adolescence. *Journal of Anxiety Disorders* **18**: 573–85.
71. Ilomaki R, Hakko H, Timonen M, *et al.* (2004) Temporal relationship between the age of onset of phobic disorders and development of substance dependence in adolescent psychiatric patients. *Drug and Alcohol Dependence* **75**: 327–30.
72. Sung M, Erkanli A, Angold A, Costello EJ (2004) Effects of age at first substance use and psychiatric comorbidity on the development of substance use disorders. *Drug and Alcohol Dependence* **75**: 287–99.
73. Scher MS, Richardson GA, Robles N, *et al.* (1998) Effects of prenatal substance exposure: altered maturation of visual evoked potentials. *Pediatric Neurology* **18**: 236–43.
74. Scher MS, Richardson GA, Day NL (2000) Effects of prenatal cocaine/crack and other drug exposure on electroencephalographic sleep studies at birth and one year. *American Academy of Pediatrics* **105**: 39–48.
75. Mountenay J (1998) *Children of Drug Using Parents.* London: National Children's Bureau.
76. Famularo R, Kinscherff R, Fenton T (1992) Parental substance abuse and the nature of child maltreatment. *Child Abuse and Neglect* **16**: 475–83.
77. Wasserman DR, Leventhal JM (1993) Maltreatment of children born to cocaine dependent mothers. *American Journal of Diseases of Children* **147**: 1324–28.
78. Barlow J (1996) *HIV and Children: A Training Manual.* Edinburgh: Children in Scotland.
79. Hogan DM (1998) Annotation: the psychological development and welfare of children of opiate and cocaine users – review and research needs. *Journal of Child Psychology and Psychiatry* **39**: 609–20.
80. Wilens TE, Biederman J, Kiely K, *et al.* (1995) Pilot study of behavioural and emotional disturbances in the high risk children of parents with opioid dependence. *Journal of the American Academy of Child and Adolescent Psychiatry* **34**: 779–85.
81. Kumpfer KL, DeMarsh J (1986) Family environmental and genetic influences on children's future chemical dependence. In S Griswold-Ezekoye (ed.) *Childhood and Chemical Abuse: Prevention and Intervention.* New York: Haworth Press.
82. McIntosh J, Gannon M, McKeganey N, MacDonald F (2003) Exposure to drugs among pre-teenage schoolchildren. *Addiction* **98**: 1615–23.
83. Hoffman JP, Su SS (1998) Parental substance use disorder, mediating variables and adolescent drug use: a non-recursive model. *Addiction* **93**: 1351–64.
84. Rosenbaum M (1979) Difficulties in taking care of business: women addicts as mothers. *American Journal of Drug and Alcohol Abuse* **6**: 431–6.
85. Crome IB (2006) An epidemiological perspective of psychiatric comorbidity and substance misuse: the UK experience/example. In A Baldacchino, J Corkery (eds) *Comorbidity: Perspectives Across Europe.* ECCAS monograph no. 4. London: International Centre for Drug Policy.
86. Bott K, Meyer C, Rumpf H-J, *et al.* (2005) Psychiatric disorders among at-risk consumers of alcohol in the general population. *Journal of Studies on Alcohol* **66**: 246–53.
87. Moran P (2006) Personality and substance use disorders in young adults. *British Journal of Psychiatry* **188**: 374–9.
88. Crome IB, Day E (1999) Substance misuse and dependence: older people deserve better services. *Reviews in Clinical Gerontology* **9**: 327–42.
89. Regier DA, Farmer ME, Rae DS, *et al.* (1990) Comorbidity of mental disorders with alcohol and other drug misuse: results from the Epidemiologic Catchment Area Study. *Journal of the American Medical Association* **264**: 2511–18.
90. Weaver T, Madden P, Charles V, *et al.* (2003) Comorbidity of substance misuse and mental illness in community mental health and substance misuse services. *British Journal of Psychiatry* **183**: 304–13.
91. Hoff RA, Rosenheck RA (1998) Long-term patterns of service use and cost among patients with both psychiatric and substance abuse disorders. *Medical Care* **36**: 843.
92. Hoff RA, Rosenheck RA (1999) The cost of treating substance abuse patients with and without comorbid psychiatric disorders. *Psychiatric Services* **50**: 1309–15.
93. Weaver T, Hart J, Fehler J, *et al.* (2007) *Are Contingency Management Principles Being Implemented in Drug Treatment in England?* London: National Treatment Agency for Substance Misuse.
94. Weaver T, Stimson G, Tyrer P, *et al.* (2004) What are the implications for clinical management and service development of prevalent comorbidity in UK mental health and substance misuse treatment populations? *Drugs: Education, Prevention and Policy* **11**: 329–48.
95. Marsden J, Gossop M, Stewart D (2000) Psychiatric symptoms among clients seeking treatment for drug dependence: intake data from the National Treatment

Outcome Research Study. *British Journal of Psychiatry* **176**: 285–9.

96. Stewart D, Gossop M, Marsden J, Rolfe A (2000) Drug misuse and acquisitive crime among clients recruited to the National Treatment Outcome Research Study (NTORS). *Criminal Behaviour and Mental Health* **14**: S31–6.
97. Crome IB, Ghodse A-H (2007) Drug misuse in medical patients. In E Guthrie (ed.) *Handbook of Liaison Psychiatry*. Cambridge: Cambridge University Press.
98. Advisory Council on the Misuse of Drugs (2006) *Pathways to Problems: Hazardous Use of Tobacco, Alcohol and Other Drugs by Young People in the UK and Its Implications for Policy*. London: Home Office.
99. Boys A, Farrell M, Taylor C, *et al.* (2003) Psychiatric morbidity and substance use in young people aged 13–15 years: results from the Child and Adolescent Survey of Mental Health. *British Journal of Psychiatry* **182**: 509–17.
100. Chiang S-C, Chen S-J, Sun H-J, *et al.* (2006) Heroin use among youths incarcerated for illicit drug use: psychosocial environment, substance use history, psychiatric comorbidity and route of administration. *American Journal on Addictions* **15**: 233–41.
101. Crome IB (2004) Psychiatric comorbidity. In I Crome, AH Ghodse, E Gilvarry, P McArdle (eds) *Young People and Substance Misuse*. London: Gaskell.
102. Crome IB (2004) Comorbidity in young people: perspectives and challenges. *Acta Neuropsychiatrica* **16**: 47–53.
103. Crome IB, Bloor R (2005) Substance misuse and psychiatric comorbidity in adolescents. *Current Opinion in Psychiatry* **18**: 435–9.
104. Bernstein DP, Stein JA, Handelsman L (1998) Predicting personality pathology among adults with substance use disorders: effects of childhood maltreatment. *Addictive Behaviours* **23**: 855–68.
105. Jarvis TJ, Copeland J (1997) Child sexual abuse as a predictor of psychiatric co-morbidity and its implications for drug and alcohol treatment. *Drug and Alcohol Dependence* **49**: 61–9.
106. Kang S-Y, Magura S, Laudet AB, Whitney S (1999) Adverse effects of child abuse victimization among substance-using women in treatment. *Journal of Interpersonal Violence* **14**: 657–70.
107. Booth BM, Curran GM, Han X (2004) Predictors of short-term course of drinking in untreated rural and urban at-risk drinkers: effects of gender, illegal drug use and psychiatric comorbidity. *Journal of Studies on Alcohol* **65**: 63–73.
108. Brady KT, Sinha R (2005) Co-occurring mental and substance use disorders: the neurological effects of chronic stress. *American Journal of Psychiatry* **162**: 1483–93.
109. Crome IB, Bloor RN (2008) Alcohol problems. In R Murray, KS Kendler, P McGuffin, *et al.* (eds) *Essential Psychiatry*. Cambridge: Cambridge University Press.
110. Zimberg S (1993) Introduction and general concepts of dual diagnosis. In E Shollar (ed.) *Dual Diagnosis: Evaluation, Treatment, Training and Program Development*. New York: Plenum.
111. Khantzian EJ (1990) Self-regulation and self-medication factors in alcoholism and the addictions: similarities and differences. *Recent Developments in Alcoholism* **8**: 255–71.
112. Khantzian EJ (1997) The self-medication hypothesis of substance use disorders: a reconsideration and recent applications. *Harvard Review of Psychiatry* **4**: 231–44.
113. Carrigan MH, Randall CL (2003) Self-medication in social phobia: a review of the alcohol literature. *Addictive Behaviour* **28**: 269–84.
114. Lingford-Hughes AR, Welch S, Nutt DJ (2004) Evidence-based guidelines for the pharmacological management of substance misuse, addiction and comorbidity: recommendations. *Journal of Psychopharmacology* **18**: 293–335.
115. Miller WR, Sanchez VC (1993) Motivating young adults for treatment and lifestyle change. In G Howard (ed.) *Issues in Alcohol Use and Misuse by Young Adults*. Notre Dame, IN: University of Notre Dame Press.
116. Dunn C, Deroo L, Rivara FP (2001) The use of brief interventions adapted from motivational interviewing across behavioral domains: a systematic review. *Addiction* **96**: 1725–42.
117. Project MATCH Research Group (1998) Matching alcoholism treatments to client heterogeneity: treatment main effects and matching effects on drinking during treatment. *Journal of Studies on Alcohol* **59**: 631–9.
118. Gossop, M, Marsden J, Stewart D, Kidd T (2003) The National Treatment Outcome Research Study (NTORS): 4–5 year follow-up results. *Addiction* **98**: 291–303.
119. Gossop M, Trakada K, Stewart D, Witton J (2005) Reductions in criminal convictions after addiction treatment: 5-year follow-up. *Drug and Alcohol Dependence* **79**: 295–302.
120. Cornelius JR, Maisto SA, Martin CS, *et al.* (2004) Major depression associated with earlier alcohol relapse in treated teens with AUD. *Addictive Behaviour* **29**: 1035–8.
121. Haddock G, Barrowclough C, Tarrier N, *et al.* (2003) Cognitive-behavioural therapy and motivational intervention for schizophrenia and substance misuse: 18-month outcomes of a randomised controlled trial. *British Journal of Psychiatry* **183**: 418–26.
122. Nunes EV, Levin FR (2004) Treatment of depression in patients with alcohol or other drug dependence: a meta-analysis. *Journal of the American Medical Association* **291**: 1887–96.
123. Tiet QQ, Mausbach B (2007) Treatments for patients with dual diagnosis: a review. *Alcoholism: Clinical and Experimental Research* **31**: 513–36.
124. National Institute for Health and Clinical Excellence (2007) *Drug misuse: Opioid detoxification*. London: National Institute for Health and Clinical Excellence.

125. Krabbe P, Konig J, Heinen N, *et al.* (2003) Rapid detoxification from opioid dependence under general anaesthesia versus standard methadone tapering: abstinence rates and withdrawal distress experiences. *Addiction Biology* **8**: 351–8.
126. Lawental E (2000) Ultra rapid opiate detoxification as compared to 30-day inpatient detoxification program: a retrospective follow-up study. *Journal of Substance Abuse* **11**: 173–81.
127. Shaffer HJ (1996) Understanding the means and objects of addiction: technology, the internet, and gambling. *Journal of Gambling Studies* **12**: 461–9.
128. Warden N, Phillips J, Ogloff J (2004) Internet addiction. *Psychiatry, Psychology and Law* **11**: 280–95.
129. Crome IB, Bloor R, Thom B (2006) Screening for illicit drug use in psychiatric hospitals: whose job is it? *Advances In Psychiatric Treatment* **12**: 375–83.
130. Cohen Z (2006) The single assessment process: an opportunity for collaboration or a threat to the profession of occupational therapy? *British Journal of Occupational Therapy* **66**: 201–8.
131. Advisory Council on the Misuse of Drugs (2003) *Hidden Harm: Responding to the Needs of Children of Problem Drug Users*. London: Home Office.
132. Ogundipe L, Bloor RN (2001) Service innovations: multi-agency standardised assessment schedule as a model of shared-care in managing drug misuse. *Psychiatric Bulletin* **25**: 350–52.
133. McGrath A, Crome P, Crome IB (2005) Substance misuse in the older population. *Postgraduate Medical Journal* **81**: 228–31.
134. Penk WE, Flannery RB, Irvin E (2000) Characteristics of substance abusing persons with schizophrenia: the paradox of the dually diagnosed. *Journal of Addictive Diseases* **19**: 23–30.
135. Scott H, Johnson S, Menezes P, *et al.* (1998) Substance misuse and risk of aggression and offending among the severely mentally ill. *British Journal of Psychiatry* **172**: 345–50.
136. Swanson J, Borum R, Swartz M, Hiday V (1999) Violent behaviour preceding hospitalisation among persons with severe mental illness. *Law and Human Behaviour* **23**: 185–203.
137. Taylor PJ (2004) Mental disorder and crime. *Criminal Behaviour and Mental Health* **14** (suppl. 1): S31–6.
138. Haywood TW, Kravitz HM, Grossman LS, *et al.* (1995) Predicting the 'revolving door' phenomenon among patients with schizophrenic, schizoaffective, and affective disorders. *American Journal of Psychiatry* **152**: 856–61.
139. Swofford C, Kasckow J, Scheller-Gilkey G, Inderbitzin LB (1996) Substance use: a powerful predictor of relapse in schizophrenia. *Schizophrenia Research* **20**: 145–51.
140. Linszen DH, Dingemans PM, Lenior ME (1994) Cannabis abuse and the course of recent-onset schizophrenia. *Archives of General Psychiatry* **51**: 273–9.
141. Appleby L, Shaw J, Kapur N, *et al.* (2006) *Avoidable Deaths: Five Year Report by the National Confidential Inquiry into Suicide and Homicide by People With Mental Illness*. London: National Confidential Inquiry into Suicide and Homicide by People with Mental Illness.
142. Hunt I, Kapur N, Robinson J, *et al.* (2006) Suicide within 12 months of mental health service contact in different age and diagnostic groups: national clinical survey. *British Journal of Psychiatry* **188**: 135–42.
143. Joe S, Neidermeier D (2008) Preventing suicide: a neglected social work research agenda. *British Journal of Social Work* **38**: 507–30.
144. Erkiran M, Özünalan H, Evren C, *et al.* (2006) Substance abuse amplifies the risk for violence in schizophrenia spectrum disorder. *Addictive Behaviour* **31**: 1797–1805.
145. Hoaken PNS, Stewart SH (2003) Drugs of abuse and the elicitation of human aggressive behavior. *Addictive Behaviors* **28**: 1533–54.
146. Johnson AK, Cnaan RA (1995) Social work practice with homeless persons: state of the art. *Research on Social Work Practice* **5**: 340–82.
148. Lewis G. (ed.) (2007) *The Confidential Enquiry into Maternal and Child Health (CEMACH). Saving Mothers' Lives: Reviewing Maternal Deaths to Make Motherhood Safer, 2003–2005*. London: Confidential Enquiry into Maternal and Child Health.
149. Neale J (2004) Gender and illicit drug use. *British Journal of Social Work* **34**: 851–70.
150. Farrell M, Boys A, Bebbington P, *et al.* (2002) Psychosis and drug dependence: results from a national survey of prisoners. *British Journal of Psychiatry* **181**: 393–8.
151. Frisher M, Crome I, Martino O, *et al.* (2009) Epidemiology of co-morbidity in general practice and primary care. In S MacGregor (ed.) *Responding to Drugs Misuse: Research and Policy Priorities in Health and Social Care*. London: Routledge.
152. Holt M, Treloar C, McMillan K, *et al.* (2007) *Barriers and Incentives to Treatment for Illicit Drug Users with Mental Health Comorbidities and Complex Vulnerabilities*. Barton, Australia: Australian Government Department of Health and Ageing.
153. McMurran M (2002) *Expert Paper: Dual Diagnosis of Mental Disorder and Substance Misuse*. London: Department of Health.
154. Baldacchino A, Corkery J (eds) (2006) *Comorbidity: Perspectives Across Europe*. London: International Centre for Drug Policy.

Chapter 70

Child and adolescent psychiatry

Sami Timimi and Kedar Dwivedi

ASSESSMENT OF CHILDREN AND ADOLESCENTS

Assessment is conducted in the context of the developmental level of the child or the adolescent and with the appreciation of multiple perceptions and concerns. Most specialist child and adolescent mental health services (CAMHS) in the UK, after receiving a referral, consider it in a multidisciplinary setting. Often the whole family gets invited, as different family members may have different views, and parents and carers are key to the decision-making process.

The assessment interview should be conducted in a child- and family-friendly environment. Who should be present in the meeting may depend on the purpose of the meeting and the age and wishes of the child. For example, young children usually prefer the presence of one or both parents, while teenagers may wish to have an opportunity to talk on their own. It is essential to establish a good rapport with the young person and their carers. An important aspect of any assessment is an understanding of the young person and their family's strengths, abilities, resilience, coping strategies, and things that are going well.

Assessment interview

The following subheadings act as a useful guide to the areas one should enquire about from parents, the child/adolescent, or both together:

- *Reason for referral:*
  - Presenting complaint
- *Present situation:*
  - Emotional state
  - Cognitive function
  - Sleep
  - Eating
  - Habits of elimination
  - Behaviour
  - Somatic complaints
- *Early developmental history:*
  - Birth and infancy
  - Mother's health during pregnancy
  - Drug treatment, date, place, mode of birth and birth weight
  - Temperament
  - Milestones, e.g. age at sitting, walking, first words, first sentences, bowel and bladder control, acquisition of independence with dressing, crossing the road, eating habits
  - Play
- *Medical history:*
  - Serious medical illnesses and surgery
  - Medication and other treatments
  - Problems with vision or hearing
  - Past psychiatric/psychological problems
- *Family circumstances:*
  - Draw a family tree
  - Who has parental responsibility?
  - Parents' (biological and/or step-parents) history, particularly of medical and psychological problems
  - Siblings' history of medical and psychological problems
  - Parental and other family relationships
  - Other important relationships in extended family
  - Contact arrangements between child and divorced/separated parent if applicable
- *Social circumstances:*
  - Interests, hobbies, structured activities
  - Peer relationships
  - General social functioning
  - Home conditions
  - Family income and financial situation
- *School history:*
  - Behaviour at school
  - Attitude of parents towards school
  - Attitude of child towards school
  - Academic achievement
  - Learning or other academic difficulties
  - Permission to get a school report

  Other agencies involved:
  - Enquire about time, reason and nature of previous contacts
  - Social services
  - Education, including involvement of educational welfare, educational psychologist or emotional behavioural support service (EBSS)
  - Paediatrics
  - Other mental health/counselling services

- Other agencies, including voluntary
- Current legal status
- *Forensic history:*
  - Description of any current or previous offences
  - Convictions
  - Attitudes to offending
  - Contacts with youth justice system
- *Interview with the child:*
  - Use of play materials, drawings, stories, wishes and so on may be helpful with younger children
  - Understanding and perception of the problem
  - Motivation for change
  - Interests and hobbies
  - Friendships
  - Child's ideas on what they would like to achieve therapeutically
  - Child's ideas on how positive change might happen
  - Mental state
- *Interview with the adolescent:*
  - Same as interview with the child, but with further areas for enquiry
  - Substance-misuse history
  - Psychosexual history
  - Identity and self-concept.

Psychometric assessment

Some clinicians supplement the information gained at interview with a variety of psychometric questionnaires (usually given to the parent or teacher of the child). However, this should be done with caution as, apart from questionnaires designed to measure intelligence, such questionnaires have usually been designed for use in epidemiological and other types of research and are thus of questionable clinical utility. Some of the commonly used instruments include the following:

- Child Behavior Checklist (CBCL)[1]
- Conner's Rating Scales – Revised[2]
- Strengths and Difficulties Questionnaire (SDQ)[3]
- Wechsler Intelligence Scale for Children, 3rd edition (WISC-III), for measuring intelligence quotient (IQ).[4]

Assessment of the family and broader context

There are many different schools of family therapy; each has its own approach and attitude towards family assessment:

- *Structural family therapy:* focuses on the structure and power dynamics within a family and examines issues such as generational boundaries, alliances and closeness/distance of family members. The purpose of such assessments is to frame interventions aimed at changing family structure, such as addressing distorted power hierarchies, for example where a child is considered too powerful at home.
- *Systemic therapy:* interested in the dynamics of various systems in which the child is embedded, for example the family, the neighbourhood and the school. The child's problems may be viewed as, at least in part, being a product of dysfunction in the system, or the collective resources in the system are viewed as something that can be harnessed to solve a problem. Thus, treatment may focus little on changing the child and more on changing the dynamic in the system.
- *Strategic family therapy:* interested in the games people play in their relationships and uses this to devise creative and unique strategies, for example 'prescribing' a parent and child who avoid expressing their strong feelings towards each other to practise arguing.
- *Brief solution-focused therapy:* interested in finding out how a young person and his or her family have already solved problems that confronted them. Assessments tend to focus more on what the child and family wish to see change than the presenting problem and its history. Treatment then focuses on goal-setting and using existing problem-solving abilities to find practical ways to achieve these.
- *Narrative therapy:* explores the subjective experience of family members through understanding how each has constructed (individually and together) a set of narratives about themselves, the problem and its relationship to them. Treatment then involves a carefully negotiated process of trying to reshape this narrative away from those aspects that emphasize dysfunction and towards reconnecting with narratives of resilience and coping.

These are just a few of the more well-known schools of family therapy. What this 'family' of therapeutic approaches have in common, though, is scepticism towards narrow medical model approaches that locate dysfunction only in the child. Family therapy has its own rich and varied literature, and familiarity with family therapy approaches is an important part of becoming a competent child and adolescent psychiatrist.

Another area where all mental health clinicians are now expected to have knowledge, skill and capability is that of working with children and families from different cultural backgrounds. Assessments must consider families' cultural beliefs and practices without imposing the values and practices of the dominant Western culture or, conversely, excusing abusive practices as being 'cultural'. Treatment then involves (but is not limited to) utilizing the family's existing beliefs, practices and resources to promote positive change in a culturally congruent manner.[5]

Diagnostic formulation

The place of diagnosis in its narrow sense (i.e. identification by a medical provider of a condition or disease) remains controversial in child and adolescent psychiatry, as practice in this area has changed rapidly in recent years due largely to ideological and cultural changes rather than scientific advances.[6,7] In its broader sense, the term 'diagnosis' refers to a 'critical analysis of the nature of something', and thus a diagnostic formulation avoids the pitfalls of a narrow focus and use of single-word diagnoses. A diagnostic formulation involves a statement about the nature of the presenting problem, identification of risk factors (predisposing/vulnerability, precipitating, maintaining) and protective factors (strengths, resilience, coping) in the child, the family and the broader context, together with relevant aspects of the assessment that will shape the treatment plan (such as those outlined above; see Assessment of the family and broader context).

EFFECTS OF ADULT MENTAL ILLNESS ON CHILDREN

The impact of adult (e.g. a parent's) mental illness or disorder on children is dependent on a variety of factors, such as the nature, severity and duration of the illness, the impact on the adult's functioning, and the degree to which the illness affects the parent–child relationship. Children may experience frequent separations, uncertain relationships, not being looked after properly, having to look after the parent, being upset, frightened or worried about what may happen to that parent, feeling ashamed, or being teased or bullied by other children. Such children are also more likely to experience other environmental factors associated with increased incidence of child psychiatric disorder, such as parental substance misuse, poverty, poor housing and family instability (see Effects of early and continuing experience on later child, adolescent and adult development and functioning, below). About 175 000 young people in the UK are involved in the care of an adult with mental illness.[8]

Effect of depression and other psychiatric symptomatology on parental functioning, and the impact of this on child development and functioning

Neither the *Diagnostic and Statistical Manual of Mental Disorders*, 4th edition (DSM-IV) nor the *International Classification of Diseases*, 10th revision (ICD-10) refers to postnatal mental disorders as formal diagnostic categories; however, mental and behavioural disorders associated with the puerperium are widely recognized in practice and usually start within 6 weeks of birth. Over half of all women feel very emotional in the first week after birth. This is often referred to as the 'baby blues' and usually passes away. In more severe or persistent cases, this can progress to postnatal depression. Postnatal depression usually begins within a month of birth, but it can start as late as 6 months after birth. Generalized anxiety disorder has also been found to be higher in postpartum women than in the general population.[9]

Teenage mothers are more likely than older women to have an insecure attachment and are more likely to experience postnatal depression.[10] Women who have experienced early maternal separation and a low level of maternal care have a higher risk of postnatal depression,[11] as do women who have been abused.[12] The extra burden of caring for a sick baby increases the risk of postnatal depression, as do isolation and lack of social support during or after pregnancy.[13]

Postnatal depression can affect the baby in a variety of ways. In severe cases, it contributes to infant abuse, infanticide and suicidal behaviour.[14] It can affect interpersonal communication, emotional expressiveness and responsiveness to the baby. The mother can become hostile and intrusive, or withdrawn and disengaged, resulting in impairment in mother–infant bonding.[15] Social adversity compounds these effects. Sometimes mothers with postnatal depression experience a distressing lack of maternal feeling, irritability, hostility, aggressive impulses, and pathological ideas about and sometimes outright rejection of the baby.[16] Thus, normal infant development is at risk,[17] and the infant may become fussier, vocalize less, make fewer positive facial expressions, and experience growth problems.[18] Postnatal depression can affect breastfeeding initiation and duration,[19] as there is a complex relationship between maternal identity, breastfeeding and psychological distress.

A variety of parenting practices have been found to be associated with parental depression, including not initiating age-appropriate safety and child development practices, and using more harsh discipline practices for toddlers.[20] Psychiatric effects on children of mothers with maternal postnatal depression include behaviour disturbance, physical ill-health, insecure attachments, depressive symptoms, poor attention,[21] sleep disturbance, eating problems,[22] social problem-solving deficits[23] and poor intellectual development.[24] Male children appear to be more vulnerable than female children.[25] The association between behaviour problems in the child and maternal depressive symptoms has been found to vary according to social support available to the mother and the amount of involvement others have in the care of the child.[26]

Puerperal psychosis

Puerperal psychosis is a more serious condition that usually starts within days or weeks of birth and affects approximately 1 in 500 mothers after birth. There are rapid and extreme changes of mood, withdrawal or overactivity, severe sleeplessness, delusions or unusual experiences. It is more likely if there is a past history or family history of serious mental illness. Puerperal psychosis can manifest as any of the three main psychotic disorders – mania, depression or schizophrenia. It is associated with a higher risk of adverse outcomes for children, including infanticide.[27]

Cultural variations in aetiology and management

The UK government has come to view developing cultural competence in mental health services as a priority.

However, the development of services that have a comprehensive understanding of cultural variations in beliefs and practices and their implication for clinical work remains in its infancy. Greater knowledge and appreciation of cultural diversity also create opportunities for learning about different beliefs, practices and social organizations that can potentially help children and families from a variety of backgrounds.[28]

For example, the prevalence and impact of postpartum depression varies cross-culturally.[29] Although postpartum depression occurs in 10–20 per cent of women in the UK and the USA, it is considered rare in Chinese populations, Fiji and some African populations.[30] Structured social supports after childbirth are described in groups of women with low rates of postpartum depression.[30] In traditional Chinese society, women's bodies are considered weak in the month after childbirth, and the mothers are prohibited from working and visiting. Extra help is brought in: often, the woman's mother or mother-in-law helps with domestic duties, looks after the family and offers advice. Studies in Hong Kong show lower levels of depression at 3 months in women who have this support, although this is dependent to some degree on who offers the support and whether this leads to conflict with the mother.[31]

With regard to psychosis, studies have shown consistently that outcome from schizophrenia is routinely better in developing world settings, a difference that becomes apparent during the initial 2 years of illness.[32] Although extended families can be tyrannical as well as supportive, and most are living in conditions of greater poverty than in developed countries, family involvement, engagement and low criticism appear to be important positive factors contributing to a positive outcome, casting doubt on the stereotype that mental illness is associated with greater stigma in the developing world.[32] It is likely, therefore, that even severe mental illness in a parent may have a less detrimental impact on children in developing countries, particularly where positive family support is available, although this issue has not been investigated adequately.

EFFECTS OF EARLY AND CONTINUING EXPERIENCE ON LATER CHILD, ADOLESCENT AND ADULT DEVELOPMENT AND FUNCTIONING

A substantial body of research has found that rates of emotional and behavioural disturbance in children and young people are associated strongly with environments that create persistent stress for the young person or their family. The most notable of these chronic adversities are poverty, parental psychopathology, parental death, interparental discord, community violence, child maltreatment, entry into the care system (such as foster care) and persistent or chronic medical illness.[33]

One of the most widespread adversities is the experience of parental discord and divorce. The divorce rate varies internationally, with North America and northern Europe having the highest rates globally. Based on annual statistics of marriages and divorce in the USA, it is anticipated that about 50 per cent of first marriages for people under age 45 years may end in divorce.[34] The divorce rate in the UK has been relatively stable for the past couple of decades, at 12–14 divorces per 1000 married couples per year.[35]

Poverty is associated with behaviour problems and poorer cognitive functioning. Parental alcoholism, antisocial behaviour and mental illness (such as schizophrenia and major depression) are associated with slower child development and child psychiatric disorders such as conduct disorder, attention deficit hyperactivity disorder (ADHD) and childhood depression.[33] Many of the risks associated with adversities co-occur (e.g. poverty, parental psychopathology, marital discord), further increasing the loading for the development of emotional and behavioural problems in the offspring.

Long-term implications of early insecure attachment

Attachment theory was first developed by the British psychoanalyst John Bowlby.[36] Attachment theory provides a framework for understanding not only the emotional development of children from birth to adolescence and into adulthood but also the development of a variety of mental health problems and a psychotherapeutic framework for working with children and their caregivers.[37] Attachment refers to an intense emotional relationship between two people that endures over time, with any prolonged separation leading to distress.[38] Development of distress in infancy, and the interpersonal mechanisms by which it can be regulated through attachment relationships, has received significant theoretical consideration. According to attachment theory, early interactions become internalized into an inner working model shaping perceptions, thought and behaviour. A secure attachment helps with the regulation of internal states (e.g. affect, arousal) within an interpersonal context. Adults' representations of their early attachment relationships are believed to predict patterns of parenting and attachment in the next generation (i.e. between them and their offspring).

Three specific patterns of infant–caregiver attachment – secure, insecure–ambivalent and insecure–avoidant – were originally identified based on reactions to the 'strange situation' laboratory task. The 'strange situation' entails observation of infant behaviour during a series of separations and reunions with the caregiver.[39] The original studies using the strange situation with infants found that about 70 per cent of infants demonstrate a secure attachment to their main caregiver, 15 per cent an avoidant (insecure) attachment and 15 per cent an ambivalent (insecure) attachment.[39] Insecure attachment by itself does not mean that the child will necessarily develop psychopathology but leads to an increased vulnerability to psychopathology in the presence of environmental stress.

Many studies demonstrated associations between ambivalent infant attachment and later mental health problems.[40] According to this research, ambivalently attached infants are prone to develop chronic levels of anxiety later in life. This may be due to unpredictable and irregular responsiveness of the caregiver, leading to a fear of separation or abandonment in the infant, which in turn creates a coping strategy centred on chronic vigilance. This may then continue throughout childhood and adulthood and lead to the development of anxiety or behavioural disorders.[41]

There are three broad criticisms aimed at the idea of attachment and its implications of maternal deprivation leading to psychopathology. The first is that Bowlby overstated his case. The studies on which he based his conclusions involved almost complete lack of maternal care, and it was unwarranted to generalize from this that lesser degrees of separation in the first 3 years of life would be damaging. The idea of exclusive care or exclusive attachment to a preferred figure rather than a hierarchy thus places too high an emotional burden on the mother. Second, Bowlby's theory viewed through a historical perspective can be seen as idealizing motherhood and family life after the traumas of the Second World War. Third, Bowlby's theory derives primarily from observations in a nuclear family culture. Thus, it is argued that anthropology has shown that it is normal for childcare to be shared by a stable group of adults, of which maternal care is an important but not exclusive part. Studies attempting to deal with these critiques have provided support for both attachment theory and its critics, for example finding that children who spent their early years in institutions have more emotional and behavioural problems, but also that early loss of the main attachment figure does not necessarily lead to psychopathology that persists into adulthood.[42] However, considerable scepticism remains as to the generalizability of attachment theory, particularly in non-Western and non-nuclear family contexts.[43]

Although attachment insecurity has been found to be a risk factor for later development of psychopathology, its predictive value is poor.[44] However, the more recent proposal for a fourth category of attachment – disorganized attachment – has, some authors argue, increased the potential clinical relevance of attachment theory. Disorganized attachment has been found to have a base rate in low risk families of about 15 per cent but up to 80 per cent in high-risk groups.[45] Disorganized attachment refers to a pattern in which the proximity-seeking behaviour of the infant or child can become disguised, indiscriminate, disorganized and even hostile or violent.[46]

Under the category of 'Disorders of social functioning with onset specific to childhood and adolescence', ICD-10 includes two subcategories that explicitly refer to attachment.[47] 'Reactive attachment disorder of childhood' has an onset before 5 years of age; the clinical features include strongly contradictory or ambivalent social responses that extend across social situations (but may show variability from relationship to relationship), lack of emotional responsiveness, withdrawal reactions, aggressive responses to the child's own or others' distress, and fearful hypervigilance that does not respond to comforting (frozen watchfulness). The clinical features of 'disinhibited attachment disorder of childhood' include attention-seeking and indiscriminately friendly behaviour, poorly modulated social interactions with unfamiliar people and peers, lack of normal tendency to seek comfort from others when distressed, and lack of selectivity in the people from whom comfort is sought. There is often a history of frequent changes in caregivers or institutional upbringing from infancy, resulting in unstable attachment figures during the first 5 years of life.

Short- and long-term effects of other negative life events on development and functioning

Maternal loss

The loss of a parent by death poses a significant developmental challenge on the dependent child. Rates of exposure to parental loss during childhood vary across the world. This affects the meaning attached to parental death and the coping mechanisms that develop to deal with it. For example, in parts of the world where death of a parent is more common, families often have well-developed social networks and extended family support allowing for not only an increase in the availability of other carers to take on childrearing of a youngster well known to them but also the development of more complex identities in carers who may see their own and other extended family members' children as their direct responsibility.

In Western countries, 1.5–4 per cent of children are orphaned of at least one parent during childhood. Studies of Western populations show that disruption of early attachment through death increases the risk of the child developing an attachment disorder, anxiety, depression and other emotional disorders of childhood and adolescence.[48]

Child abuse

The consequences of experiencing abuse depend upon a variety of variables, such as the nature of the abusive act, its frequency, intensity and duration, the relationship between the child and the abuser, the characteristics of the child, others' response to the abuse, and other associated factors. Consequences of abuse include:[49]

- hypothalamic–pituitary axis dysregulation;
- physical harm, including death, life-threatening injuries, long-term physical impairment, or from Munchausen by proxy syndrome, where a parent (about 95% female) feigns, exaggerates or induces illness in the child;
- psychological consequences, such as aggression, anxiety, depression, attachment disorders, post-traumatic stress, substance abuse and psychosis;

- social consequences, such as family disruptions, entering the care system and excessive hospitalization.

The degree of impact of the abuse on the child's life and development is mediated by the degree to which daily functioning is affected and the availability of positive supportive relationships in the child's life. In addition, different types of abuse produce different challenges. For example, sexual abuse can result in a complex interaction between traumatic sexualization, sense of betrayal, sense of powerlessness, guilt, self-blame and self-loathing, behavioural problems, deliberate self-harm, genital/anal injury, sexually transmitted disease, unwanted pregnancy, sexualized behaviour, prostitution, peer relationship problems, educational underachievement, and entry into the care system. In adulthood, such a history can lead to anxiety, depression, self-harm, drug and alcohol abuse, poor sexual functioning, difficulty with maintaining intimate interpersonal relationships, distrust, eating disorders and problems with being a parent.

Child abuse is also discussed below (see Child protection).

Chronic or life-threatening illness

Chronic illness and disability are associated with increased prevalence of psychiatric disorders. Approximately 30–40 per cent of children with a severe paediatric illness also have a co-morbid psychiatric disorder.[50] Illnesses affecting the brain have a stronger association with subsequent and concurrent psychiatric disorders compared with physical illness that does not affect the brain. In Rutter and colleagues' classic Isle of Wight study, rates of psychiatric disorder were 44 per cent among children with structural brain disorders, 29 per cent among children with idiopathic epilepsy, 12 per cent among children with non-cerebral physical disorders and 7 per cent among children free from physical disorders.[51]

CLASSIFICATION AND EPIDEMIOLOGY OF CHILD AND ADOLESCENT PSYCHIATRIC DISORDERS

Classification

The two main systems currently used for classifying child and adolescent psychiatric disorders are ICD-10[47] and DSM-IV.[52] These versions are more similar in their approach to classifying child and adolescent psychiatric disorders than previous versions. Both adopt a multi-axial classification system, although the extent to which this is used in clinical practice is variable.

International Classification of Diseases, 10th revision

ICD-10 is divided into blocks of diagnostic groupings. Blocks F80–F89 (disorders of psychological development) and F90–F98 (behavioural and emotional disorders with onset usually occurring in childhood and adolescence) cover disorders that are specific to childhood and adolescence. A number of disorders placed in other categories can occur in people of almost any age and so can be used for children and adolescents when required. Examples are disorders of eating, sleeping and gender identity. Disorders categorized elsewhere and more commonly found in people over 18 years of age, such as schizophrenia and obsessive-compulsive disorders, can also be used for such presentations in people under 18 years of age.

ICD-10 recommends that clinicians should follow the general rule of recording as many diagnoses as are necessary to cover the clinical picture. When recording more than one diagnosis, ICD-10 advises giving one precedence over the others by specifying it as the main diagnosis and labelling any others as subsidiary or additional diagnoses.

The main ICD-10 categories relevant to child and adolescent psychiatry are as follows:

- *F70–F79 Mental retardation:*
  - F70 Mild mental retardation
  - F71 Moderate mental retardation
  - F72 Severe mental retardation
  - F73 Profound mental retardation
  - F78 Other mental retardation
  - F79 Unspecified mental retardation
- A fourth character may be used to specify the extent of associated behavioural impairment:
  - F7*x*.0 No, or minimal, impairment of behaviour
  - F7*x*.1 Significant impairment of behaviour requiring attention or treatment
  - F7*x*.8 Other impairments of behaviour
  - F7*x*.9 Without mention of impairment of behaviour
- *F80–F89 Disorders of psychological development:*
  - F80 Specific developmental disorders of speech and language
    - F80.0 Specific speech articulation disorder
    - F80.1 Expressive language disorder
    - F80.2 Receptive language disorder
    - F80.3 Acquired aphasia with epilepsy (Landau–Kleffner syndrome)
    - F80.8 Other developmental disorders of speech and language
    - F80.9 Developmental disorder of speech and language, unspecified
  - F81 Specific developmental disorders of scholastic skills
    - F81.0 Specific reading disorder
    - F81.1 Specific spelling disorder
    - F81.2 Specific disorder of arithmetical skills
    - F81.3 Mixed disorder of scholastic skills
    - F81.8 Other developmental disorders of scholastic skills
    - F81.9 Developmental disorder of scholastic skills, unspecified

- F82 Specific developmental disorder of motor function
- F83 Mixed specific developmental disorders
- F84 Pervasive developmental disorders
  - F84.0 Childhood autism
  - F84.1 Atypical autism
  - F84.2 Rett's syndrome
  - F84.3 Other childhood disintegrative disorder
  - F84.4 Overactive disorder associated with mental retardation and stereotyped movements
  - F84.5 Asperger's syndrome
  - F84.8 Other pervasive developmental disorders
  - F84.9 Pervasive developmental disorder, unspecified
- F88 Other disorders of psychological development
- F89 Unspecified disorder of psychological development

- *F90–F98 Behavioural and emotional disorders with onset usually occurring in childhood and adolescence:*
  - F90 Hyperkinetic disorders
    - F90.0 Disturbance of activity and attention
    - F90.1 Hyperkinetic conduct disorder
    - F90.8 Other hyperkinetic disorders
    - F90.9 Hyperkinetic disorder, unspecified
  - F91 Conduct disorders
    - F91.0 Conduct disorder confined to the family context
    - F91.1 Unsocialized conduct disorder
    - F91.2 Socialized conduct disorder
    - F91.3 Oppositional defiant disorder
    - F91.8 Other conduct disorders
    - F91.9 Conduct disorder, unspecified
  - F92 Mixed disorders of conduct and emotions
    - F92.0 Depressive conduct disorder
    - F92.8 Other mixed disorders of conduct and emotions
    - F92.9 Mixed disorder of conduct and emotions, unspecified
  - F93 Emotional disorders with onset specific to childhood
    - F93.0 Separation anxiety disorder of childhood
    - F93.1 Phobic anxiety disorder of childhood
    - F93.2 Social anxiety disorder of childhood
    - F93.3 Sibling rivalry disorder
    - F93.8 Other childhood emotional disorders
    - F93.9 Childhood emotional disorder, unspecified
  - F94 Disorders of social functioning with onset specific to childhood and adolescence
    - F94.0 Elective mutism
    - F94.1 Reactive attachment disorder of childhood
    - F94.2 Disinhibited attachment disorder of childhood
    - F94.8 Other childhood disorders of social functioning
    - F94.9 Childhood disorder of social functioning, unspecified
  - F95 Tic disorders
    - F95.0 Transient tic disorder
    - F95.1 Chronic motor or vocal tic disorder
    - F95.2 Combined vocal and multiple motor tic disorder (de la Tourette's syndrome)
    - F95.8 Other tic disorders
    - F95.9 Tic disorder, unspecified
  - F98 Other behavioural and emotional disorders with onset usually occurring in childhood and adolescence
    - F98.0 Non-organic enuresis
    - F98.1 Non-organic encopresis
    - F98.2 Feeding disorder of infancy and childhood
    - F98.3 Pica of infancy and childhood
    - F98.4 Stereotyped movement disorders
    - F98.5 Stuttering (stammering)
    - F98.6 Cluttering
    - F98.8 Other specified behavioural and emotional disorders with onset usually occurring in childhood and adolescence
    - F98.9 Unspecified behavioural and emotional disorders with onset usually occurring in childhood and adolescence.

Diagnosis of each condition is based on a judgement that the emotions or behaviour being categorized lie outside the usual range found for age and sex of the child/young person and that personal functioning or development is impaired.

ICD-10 employs a multi-axial framework for child and adolescent psychiatric disorders:

- *Axis I:* clinical psychiatric disorders
- *Axis II:* specific disorders of development
- *Axis III:* intellectual level
- *Axis IV:* medical conditions
- *Axis V:* abnormal psychosocial conditions
- *Axis VI:* global social functioning.

Diagnostic and Statistical Manual of Mental Disorders, 4th edition

DSM-IV is a categorical classification system. The categories are 'prototypes', and a patient with a close approximation to the prototype is said to have that disorder. DSM-IV states that there is no assumption that each category of mental disorder is a completely discrete entity with absolute boundaries. Qualifiers are sometimes used, for example mild, moderate or severe forms of a disorder. For nearly half the disorders, symptoms must be sufficient to cause clinically significant distress or impairment in social, occupational or other important areas of functioning.

DSM-IV organizes each psychiatric diagnosis into five levels (axes) relating to different aspects of disorder or disability:

- *Axis I:* clinical disorders, including major mental disorders, and developmental and learning disorders

- *Axis II:* underlying pervasive or personality conditions, and mental retardation
- *Axis III:* medical conditions and physical disorders
- *Axis IV:* psychosocial and environmental factors
- *Axis V:* global assessment of functioning.

Under 'Disorders usually first diagnosed during infancy, childhood or adolescence' the following are found:

- *Mental retardation:*
  - 317 Mild mental retardation
  - 318.0 Moderate mental retardation
  - 318.1 Severe mental retardation
  - 318.2 Profound mental retardation
  - 319 Mental retardation, severity unspecified
- *Learning disorders:*
  - 315.00 Reading disorder
  - 315.1 Mathematics disorder
  - 315.2 Disorder of written expression
  - 315.9 Learning disorder not otherwise specified (NOS)
- *Motor skills disorders:*
  - 315.4 Developmental coordination disorder communication disorders
  - 315.31 Expressive language disorder
  - 315.32 Mixed receptive–expressive language disorder
  - 315.39 Phonological disorder
  - 307.0 Stuttering
  - 307.9 Communication disorder NOS
- *Pervasive developmental disorders:*
  - 299.00 Autistic disorder
  - 299.80 Rett's disorder
  - 299.10 Childhood disintegrative disorder
  - 299.80 Asperger's disorder
  - 299.80 Pervasive developmental disorder NOS
- *Attention-deficit and disruptive behaviour disorders:*
  - ADHD
  - 314.01 Combined subtype
  - 314.01 Predominantly hyperactive–impulsive subtype
  - 314.00 Predominantly inattentive subtype
  - 314.9 Attention-deficit hyperactivity disorder NOS
  - Conduct disorder
  - 312.81 Childhood onset
  - 312.82 Adolescent onset
  - 312.89 Unspecified onset
  - 313.81 Oppositional defiant disorder
  - 312.9 Disruptive behaviour disorder NOS
- *Feeding and eating disorders of infancy or early childhood:*
  - 307.52 Pica
  - 307.53 Rumination disorder
  - 307.59 Feeding disorder of infancy or early childhood
- *Tic disorders:*
  - 307.23 Tourette's disorder
  - 307.22 Chronic motor or vocal tic disorder
  - 307.21 Transient tic disorder
  - 307.20 Tic disorder NOS
- *Elimination disorders:*
  - Encopresis
  - 787.6 Encopresis, with constipation and overflow incontinence
  - 307.7 Encopresis, without constipation and overflow incontinence
  - 307.6 Enuresis (not due to a general medical condition)
- *Other disorders of infancy, childhood, or adolescence:*
  - 309.21 Separation anxiety disorder
  - 313.23 Selective mutism
  - 313.89 Reactive attachment disorder of infancy or early childhood
  - 307.3 Stereotypic movement disorder
  - 313.9 Disorder of infancy, childhood, or adolescence NOS.

Epidemiology

Classic studies

Rutter and colleagues' Isle of Wight study on 10- and 11-year-olds found that:[51]

- 6.8 per cent had a diagnosable psychiatric disorder;
- 4 per cent had a conduct disorder and 2.5 per cent had an emotional disorder;
- the ratio of boys to girls among those with a psychiatric disorder was nearly 2:1;
- 2.5 per cent had an IQ below 70;
- 5.7 per cent of the children had a physical disorder, with higher rates of psychiatric disorder found in those with a physical disorder.

A study with similar methodology in inner London found twice the rate of psychiatric disorders among 10- and 11-year olds than in the Isle of Wight.[53]

Richman and colleagues' study of 3-year-olds in Waltham Forest, London, found that:[54]

- behavioural problems were common, including bedwetting (37%), daytime wetting (17%), poor appetite (17%), regular night-time waking (14%), difficulty settling at night (13%), soiling (13%), strong fears (13%) and overactivity (13%);
- 7 per cent were classed as having moderate to severe behaviour problems;
- prevalence was roughly equal in boys and girls;
- associated factors (with behavioural problems) included speech and language delay, maternal depression, poor parental relationship and psychosocial adversity.

More recent studies

Based on an international literature review,[55] the prevalence of mental disorder in community surveys is reported to be around 20–30 per cent of school-age children, but this figure drops to 12–15 per cent when only moderate to severe (clinically significant) diagnoses are considered.

In a study by the Office for National Statistics of 5- to 15-year-olds, a rate of around 10 per cent for all mental disorders was found.[56] About 5 per cent had a conduct disorder, 4 per cent an emotional disorder and 1 per cent a hyperkinetic disorder. Less common disorders such as autism and eating disorders occurred in about 0.5 per cent. Psychiatric disorders were more common in lone-parent families, reconstituted families, families with more than five children, children of unemployed parents, families in social class V, and families where the parents were social sector tenants.

In the New Zealand child survey, by 11 years of age the prevalence for any psychiatric disorder was found to be approximately 18 per cent.[57] At 15 years of age, approximately 25 per cent of young people met DSM-IV criteria for one of the main mental disorders.[58] At 18 years of age, 45 per cent met criteria for one or more disorder.[59]

These large international variations highlight the difficulties of interpreting the findings due to differing methodologies and variations in the way mental disorders are defined and categorized.

AETIOLOGY OF CHILD PSYCHIATRIC DISORDERS

Knowledge about aetiology is hampered by several factors, including lack of physical or psychological markers for any of the major psychiatric disorders of childhood; differing definitions and categorization; differing interpretations of clinical significance and impairment; cultural relativity and the social construction of diagnostic categories; lack of international studies; differences in meaning attributed to different symptoms by different communities; and the cultural nature of developmental frameworks. One problem is that definitions of disorder rely on definitions of normality; however, cross-disciplinary literature demonstrates that our concepts of childhood, parenting and child development vary enormously cross-culturally and even within Western culture (particularly over time), and thus any system that attempts to impose a universal definition of 'normality' (and thus, by implication, mental disorder) is going to encounter difficulties.[28,43,60]

However, a number of factors that increase the risk for emotional and behavioural problems in children and adolescents have been found and replicated. These factors include poor-quality family relationships, school experiences and community environments, and poor physical health. These factors are also associated with poorer treatment outcomes.[55] These and other potential associations of possible aetiological significance can be subdivided into biological and psychosocial risks.

Biological risks

There is little replicated and undisputed evidence to confirm that common child psychiatric disorders are genetic or related to some form of neurodevelopmental dysfunction or chemical imbalance in the brain. Space does not permit a wider discussion of these complex issues; however, a brief discussion on genetic evidence will give a flavour of the nature of the controversies.

For disorders that child psychiatrists are likely to be asked to assess and manage, hyperkinetic disorders, autism-spectrum disorders (ASD), schizophrenia and anorexia nervosa are the disorders for which evidence for having strong heritability and thus a genetic basis are most frequently claimed. The basis of the evidence comes from familial, twin and adoption studies. All these types of study suffer from numerous methodological problems. Because of the greater methodological problems associated with familial and adoption studies, the main source of information for estimating the relative genetic contribution to heritability comes from twin studies. In twin studies, the difference in the degree to which monozygotic (MZ) twins share a diagnosis compared with dizygotic (DZ) twins forms the basis for estimating the genetic contribution for that particular diagnosis. As MZ twins have all their genes in common whereas DZ twins on average share half their genes, the greater the similarity in MZ than DZ twins, the stronger the genetic contribution. However, for this statement to be true, one has to assume that MZ and DZ twins share the same environment. This is termed the 'equal environment assumption' (EEA). It is accepted that EEA does not hold, as research has demonstrated that being an MZ twin produces psychosocial differences (e.g. MZ twins report more sharing, are more likely to have the same friends, are more likely to be dressed alike, report more identity confusion, and so on, compared with DZ twins). Critics thus contend that twin studies are, as a result, no better than other studies (e.g. family studies) at separating out genetic from environmental factors. Supporters of the twin study method retort that we can still use this method if the violation of EEA is not in the traits or disorder under study. Critics in turn respond by arguing that, when it comes to psychological and behavioural features, it is not possible to speak of 'trait-specific EEA', as psychosocial life does not conform to linear causality, and thus all one needs to prove is that EEA does not hold, and therefore twin studies cannot be used to discover genetic contributions to psychiatric disorders unless a reliable physical marker is found. (For a more detailed overview of these arguments, see the books by Jay Jospeh[61] and Michael Rutter[62]). In addition to these limitations, the lack of identifying consistent genetic linkages to any child psychiatric disorder means that, at present, genetics is of little clinical relevance to the child psychiatrist.

As outlined above (see Chronic or life-threatening illness), physical illnesses, particularly those affecting the brain, increase the risk for co-morbid psychiatric disorders. In addition, children with low IQ and children with specific learning difficulties show increased co-morbid psychiatric disorder (see Mental handicap and developmental disorders, below).

Gender as a risk (with boys being at higher risk of childhood psychiatric disorders, particularly externalizing disorders such as ADHD, conduct disorder and autism) remains a relatively and surprisingly unexplored area. We simply do not know whether the higher rates of diagnosis of these behavioural disorders reflect biological differences or societal attitudes and in what way these two factors interact.[60]

Psychosocial adversity

As outlined above (see Effects of early and continuing experience on later child, adolescent and adult development and functioning, above), a range of adversities, including poverty, parental discord, parental psychopathology, disrupted attachments and violence, are associated with an increased likelihood of developing a psychiatric disorder. In addition, other factors that may increase the likelihood of subsequent psychiatric disorder include environmental factors such as living in an urban setting, poor social networks, going to a school with high rates of behavioural problems, and bullying. Some cross-cultural research finds considerable differences in prevalence rates, with children in politically stable developing countries appearing to have lower rates of child psychiatric disorders;[63,64] however, urbanization and modernization may be associated with an increase in the prevalence of behavioural disorders in these populations.[65]

CHILD PROTECTION

The changing needs of developing children

Concepts of what a child needs at different stages are highly dependent on the model of child development being applied. Our beliefs about what 'normal' child development looks like have continued, and continue, to change over time in Western cultures;[66] in addition, important differences are apparent in different traditions' beliefs and practices about children and their development.[43,67,68] For example, one study found that Indian social work professionals, more than American social work professionals, considered a wider range of adult sexual behaviours and media images to be seriously abusive to children. However, these Indian professionals did not consider physical 'maltreatment' to be as seriously abusive as their American counterparts did.[69] Another example relates to the use of physical punishment on children: Sweden, which has made physical chastisement of children a criminal offence, is often cited as a positive example; however, examination of various morbidity and mortality figures shows Swedish children to be somewhere in the middle of league tables for rich countries.[70] For example, rates of death from child maltreatment in Sweden at 0.6 per 100 000 children are much higher than those in countries that fare best in these tables, namely Spain (0.1/100 000) and Greece and Italy (0.2/100 000), which have not outlawed corporal punishment but which, interestingly, have family-oriented cultures.[71]

The question of how to draw up an ethical framework that provides adequate protection to all children and is able to encompass a proper respect and understanding of this cultural diversity remains an emotive and challenging one. Who has the power and authority to set standards and decide what is acceptable morbidity becomes a loaded issue.[72] Western cultures have a framework that emphasizes rights of the child, and many non-Western cultures also emphasize the responsibilities of the child.[28] Adolescence in many Western cultures is characterized by conflict and the striving for independence, but in many other cultures it is characterized by ambivalence and an exchange of loyalty for protection.[60] There are many other examples of significant cross-cultural differences in the needs of children at different ages, from birth to adulthood. Although it is imperative that every clinician understands, adheres to and explains to families the child protection laws in the country in which they work, every child and family also deserves a competent understanding of this cultural variation in order to properly understand the intentions behind the actions of those in authority towards children, and children towards those in authority.

Types of child abuse and their aetiology, recognition and outcome

Area child protection committees in England and Wales maintain the Child Protection Register and develop procedures and policies for each locality. In England, the estimated rate of children under the age of 18 years registered annually on the Child Protection Register is around 25–30 per 10 000 children. Seventy per cent of registered children are under 10 years of age. Male and female genders are represented equally, but girls account for 60 per cent of those registered for sexual abuse.[73] The categories under which children can be registered are physical abuse, sexual abuse, emotional abuse and neglect.

According to the Department Of Health, in the early to mid-1990s, 1.45 per cent of the 11 million children in England (i.e. 160 000 children) were subject to a child protection enquiry each year. Of these, 15 per cent were placed on the Child Protection Register and 2 per cent were taken into public care.[74]

Physical abuse

Physical abuse includes actual or likely physical injury, or failure to prevent injury or suffering resulting in significant danger or substantial risk of impairment of bodily functions, disfigurement or death. This can include Munchausen by proxy syndrome, which at its most extreme can result in death (e.g. by suffocation or deliberate poisoning). Features such as delay in seeking medical attention, vague and inconsistent accounts of the cause of the injury, and repeated presentations with injuries should raise the suspicion of physical abuse.

Sexual abuse

Sexual abuse refers to involvement of dependent, developmentally immature children and adolescents in sexual activities that they do not truly comprehend, to which they are unable to give informed consent, or that violate the social taboos of family roles. Sexual abuse may involve physical contact, including penetrative or non-penetrative acts and non-contact activities, such as involving children in looking at, or in the production of, pornographic material or watching sexual activities, or encouraging children to behave in sexually inappropriate ways. Some abusers deliberately befriend the victim, 'grooming' them over time towards eventually engaging them in sexual activity. The majority (85–95%) of abusers are male, and the majority of children know their abuser before the abuse starts.

Emotional abuse

Emotional abuse refers to persistent or severe emotional maltreatment or rejection leading to actual or likely severe adverse effects on the behavioural and emotional development of the child. Emotional abuse can involve habitual criticism, humiliation, ridicule, harassment, threat and persistent rejection. Emotional abuse and neglect tend to occur together.

Neglect

Neglect refers to the failure to protect a child from exposure to danger or a lack of attention to daily needs and care to a degree that may result in significant impairment of the child's development or health. Severe neglect is life-threatening and can lead to long-term or severe psychological and physical harm due to the persistent unavailability of parent or guardian. The child is often left alone, and there is non-organic failure to maintain weight and frequent illness and infection because of poor hygiene.

Aetiology

A systemic model proposed by Finkelhor outlines the theories of risk, causation and maintenance of sexual abuse.[75] Prominent factors include:

- motivation to sexually abuse (5–9% of undergraduate males expressed sexual interest in children);
- absence of internal inhibitors (through use of alcohol and drugs, stress, cognitive distortion, e.g. minimization of harmful effects);
- absence of external inhibitors (lack of supervision, availability, access);
- absence of child's resistance by virtue of age, disability, neglect or social isolation.

As children try to adjust, this often results in secrecy, helplessness, entrapment and accommodation, and delayed, unconvincing disclosure and retraction. Thus, sexual abuse, similar to other forms of abuse, has a varied aetiology involving the interaction of several factors.

Interventions and outcome

In the UK, the responsibility for child protection rests primarily with social services. The process leading to intervention by social services starts with someone reporting a concern about possible abuse in a particular child. If the concerns are deemed to warrant further investigation, then a referral to the child protection team takes place. The child protection team then decides whether there is a need for immediate protection (e.g. removing the child from their home and placing them in care) and plans the investigation (which could include interagency discussion, interviewing the child, medical examinations and interviewing members of the family). Other subsequent actions may include convening a child protection conference, developing a protection plan, carrying out a more comprehensive assessment of the child and family, prosecuting the abuser, and referral for therapy. Serious abuse often results in the removal by the courts of parental rights, with parental responsibility then passing to social services.

Once abuse has occurred, there is limited success in treatment. Many children remain in the care system for the rest of their childhood once they have been removed from their family of origin.[73] Thus, prevention acquires a high priority. Prevention can be at different levels:[73]

- *Primary prevention:* involves universal services for the whole population, such as housing, financial support, high-quality childcare, family and child development centres, promoting good parenting practices, and public awareness campaigns.
- *Secondary prevention:* involves targeted services by identifying high-risk populations and offering intervention before abuse and neglect occur, such as targeted home-visiting, school- and hospital-based social services, and targeted therapeutic groups.
- *Tertiary prevention:* involves specialist services for treatment of families where parents and caregivers have already abused their children, such as interdisciplinary services to ensure treatment, care, counselling, management and support, and the use of child-friendly courts.

However, there is no clear evidence of a reduction in abuse associated with any of the above strategies. Therapeutic interventions in relation to the consequences of trauma following abuse may include individual psychotherapy (including eye movement desensitization and reprocessing), group therapy and family therapy.

The potential consequences and outcomes for those who are abused as children are discussed above (see Effects of early and continuing experience on later child, adolescent and adult development and functioning).

INTERACTION BETWEEN PSYCHIATRIC DISORDER AND PHYSICAL ILLNESS

Chronic illness and disability are associated with an increased prevalence of psychiatric disorders. Approximately 30–40 per cent of children with a severe paediatric illness also have a co-morbid psychiatric disorder.[50] Illnesses affecting the brain have a stronger association with subsequent and concurrent psychiatric disorders compared with illnesses that do not affect the brain. In Rutter and colleagues' Isle of Wight study, rates of psychiatric disorder were 44 per cent among children with structural brain disorders, 29 per cent among children with idiopathic epilepsy, 12 per cent among children with non-cerebral physical disorders, and 7 per cent among children free from physical disorders.[51] Many other studies have confirmed this differential prevalence rate.[50]

Although it is important to recognize higher rates of psychiatric disorder in people with physical disorders, it is just as important to recognize that an undiagnosed physical disorder may first present as a psychiatric disorder. Thus, petit mal absences may present as poor concentration, a malabsorption syndrome may first present as hyperactivity, and a variety of endocrine and metabolic disorders may first present as psychosis.

Physical presentation of psychiatric disorder

Physical symptoms often present in the absence of known organic disease. These are often referred to as 'somatization', 'dissociation' or 'conversion' disorders. Many of these conditions involve apparent neurological symptoms, such as convulsions (pseudo-seizures), paralysis or incoordination (dissociative movement disorders). In younger children, headaches and abdominal pain are common presentations often associated with a stressful situation (e.g. difficulties at school). A difficult question facing the clinician is how aggressively to investigate or challenge a child and family with negative findings in the face of anxieties or coping strategies that the child is 'needing' to have the symptom for.

A variety of other psychiatric disorders may first come to the attention of the medical profession via a physical presentation, including eating disorders (e.g. through weight loss, abnormal blood biochemistry, amenorrhoea), depression (through needing treatment for self-harm), hyperactivity and other behavioural disorders (e.g. due to frequent visits to casualty following dangerous and impulsive acts).

COMMON PRESCHOOL PROBLEMS

Prevalence and aetiology

Behavioural problems such as temper tantrums and sleeping and feeding difficulties are very common in preschool children. They are usually considered not as psychiatric disorders but rather as part of normal developmental variation.

Presentation

Behavioural problems such as crying, shouting, aggression, refusal to do what is asked, difficulty settling to sleep, frequent waking during the night, food refusal and faddiness are common. A few problems may be of a more serious nature and require intervention beyond the primary health-care level, such as extreme food refusal or faddiness leading to inadequate dietary intake and failure to thrive.

Treatments

Generally treatment involves reassurance, offering parenting advice, and the use of behavioural management techniques.

Outcome

Although the severity of difficulties will usually decrease during the early school years, it is worth bearing in mind that periods of behavioural problems, including oppositional behaviour, are common throughout childhood and are not usually indicative of a disorder requiring intervention. Research on children's temperament has found that the persistence of early behaviour problems is associated with a mismatch between the child's temperament and their environment, such that even those children who are highly difficult temperamentally can become well adjusted behaviourally if family and social circumstances are supportive.[76]

CONDUCT DISORDER

Prevalence

From the preschool period to middle childhood, there is a decrease in the frequency of temper tantrums and oppositional behaviours. Oppositional problems occur in 5–10 per cent of non-clinical samples.[55] In the Isle of Wight study, Rutter and colleagues found an overall prevalence for conduct disorder of 4.2 per cent among 10- and 11-year-olds.[51] The Ontario Child Health Survey found a rate of 5.5 per cent in 4- to 16-year-olds,[77] while the Christchurch and Dunedin longitudinal study found a rate of 3.4 per cent among 15-year-olds.[78] Little information exists from studies in non-industrialized countries, although available evidence suggests that much lower rates of conduct and other behavioural disorders are found.[63,79] Conduct disorder is more common in boys than girls. Although the majority of studies find that conduct disorders are more common in an urban than a rural setting, some have not found this urban/rural split.

Aetiology

The three most significant associated factors found in the Ontario Child Health Survey were family dysfunction, parental psychopathology and low income (which had a greater effect on children aged 4–11 years than on adolescents).[77] Conduct problems are associated strongly with other disruptive behaviour problems (including ADHD, delinquency and substance misuse), certain internalizing disorders (particularly depression and anxiety), specific developmental disorders, low IQ, family discord, large family size and parental psychopathology.[80]

Presentation

Presentation may be with persistent antisocial behaviour such as fighting, stealing, destruction of property, fire-setting, truancy, cruelty (e.g. to animals), lying and lack of remorse. Conduct disorder can be situation-specific or more pervasive (which is usually more serious). It can also be subdivided into socialized (acts performed along with a peer group) and unsocialized (acts performed alone, which is usually a more serious disorder).

Treatment

With much evidence suggesting an important causal role in the quality of parenting and caregiving, it is not surprising that interventions targeted more towards the parent/carer rather than the young person with the diagnosis are the most common and for which the most evidence for effectiveness is available. Popular parent management training (PMT) programmes include the approaches developed by Patterson and Guillon[81] and the group approach developed by Webster-Stratton.[82] These PMT programmes draw on operant-behavioural and cognitive-behavioural approaches involving developing consistent strategies that reward desired behaviours and ignore or provide negative consequences for undesired behaviours. Approaches that draw on a wider systemic theoretical approach are more popular for use with families of adolescents with conduct disorders. These include functional family therapy,[83] multi-systemic therapy[84] and the seven-steps programme.[85] Other approaches with some supportive evidence include school-based interventions and the use of therapeutic foster care.[80] There is little evidence to support the use of individual therapy (e.g. anger management) on its own or medication on its own.

Outcome

In the classic study by Robins,[86] 45 per cent of children with conduct disorders went on to develop an antisocial personality disorder. Disturbance of conduct is a significant risk factor for substance use.[87] Those individuals who manifest disturbances of conduct earlier in life go on to commit more severe criminal offences.[88] There is a high continuity between failure in school associated with conduct problems and adult unemployment.[55]

HYPERACTIVITY DISORDERS

Prevalence

The American Psychiatric Association estimates the rate of ADHD in school-age children (5–18 years) to be between 3 per cent and 5 per cent.[52] Screening with behavioural questionnaires identifies 10–20 per cent of the population as affected.[89] When more stringent ICD-based criteria are used, about 0.5–2 per cent prevalence rates are found.[90] ADHD occurs much more frequently in males than females, with a ratio of 3–4 : 1 from population-based studies.[91] Lower rates have been reported in studies in some developing countries.[63]

Aetiology

It is often claimed that hyperactivity disorders including ADHD have a primarily genetic basis, albeit through being at the pathological extreme of a normal distribution. However, this claim is contested (see Aetiology of child psychiatric disorders, above). In addition, population twin studies find that symptoms of ADHD share overlapping familial and genetic influences with other neurodevelopmental traits, including reading ability, general cognitive ability, dyspraxia and symptoms of pervasive developmental disorders.[92] ADHD in children and adolescents is also associated with impaired family relationships, higher rates of family conflict, being in foster care, and poverty/lower social class.[93,94]

Presentation

ADHD describes a constellation of poor concentration, hyperactivity and impulsiveness that has been present from an early age. These behaviours must be present in at least two situations (e.g. home and school), associated with impairment of social or academic functioning, present before the age of 7 years and not explained better by another disorder. ICD criteria are more stringent; unlike the DSM, however, the ICD has a category for hyperkinetic conduct disorder, reflecting the common association of hyperactivity with antisocial behaviour. Co-morbidity is high: 30–50 per cent of children with ADHD have co-morbid conduct disorders, 15–75 per cent have a mood disorder, 25 per cent have an anxiety disorder, 40 per cent have oppositional defiant disorder, and 50 per cent have speech or language impairments.[95,96]

Treatment

Recent years have witnessed a phenomenally rapid increase in the use of stimulant medication, usually methylphenidate in its various forms, from short-acting to long-acting preparations. Although effective in reducing ADHD symptoms in the short term, emerging evidence has cast doubt on the long-term effectiveness of stimulants, which, together with increasing concern about risks associated with their use, is likely to result in a more limited role for psychoactive medication in the management of ADHD in coming years.[97] Other treatment approaches include PMT, behavioural therapy, elimination diets and essential fatty acid supplementation.

Outcome

The factors found in childhood to be the most highly predictive of a poor outcome include a family history of ADHD or hyperkinesis, psychosocial adversity and co-morbidity with conduct, mood and anxiety disorders.[98]

SCHOOL-ATTENDANCE PROBLEMS

Prevalence

Non-attendance at school may be the result of truancy (which is often associated with a conduct disorder) or school refusal (which is often associated with an emotional disorder). School refusal affects approximately 1 per cent of school children across the primary and secondary school levels.[99] Truants are more commonly male, whereas school refusal is equally common in boys and girls. There are three main incidence peeks for school refusal: at age 5 years (school entry often associated with separation anxiety), at age 11 years (most common age when transfer from primary to secondary school occurs) and at age 14–16 years.

Aetiology

Truants are associated with having other antisocial symptoms, a family history of antisocial behaviour, academic or learning difficulties, and a large family size. School refusers are associated with having other emotional symptoms, a family history of anxiety, satisfactory to good academic performance, and a smaller family size.[100] In some children, school refusal is associated with a wish to stay at home (e.g. due to concerns about the wellbeing of a parent) rather than a wish to avoid school.

Presentation

In school refusal, there is an inability to go to school or stay in school associated with extreme anxiety. Somatic symptoms may occur that are sometimes fictitious in order to avoid going to school.

Treatment

Problems at school, such as bullying and learning difficulties, need to be dealt with. Treatment then focuses on getting the child back to school as soon as possible. If there is a chronic problem, then a carefully planned graded return involving support from other agencies such as school and education welfare is often required. Little and often is usually better than leaving large gaps between days spent at school. Supplementary interventions for specific problems may also be needed.[101]

Outcome

Prognosis is usually good, particularly in younger children and with successful early intervention.

EMOTIONAL DISORDERS SPECIFIC TO CHILDHOOD

These include anxiety disorders, depression, somatization and conversion disorders.

Prevalence

The Isle of Wight study found a prevalence of 2.5 per cent for emotional disorders in 10- and 11-year-olds.[51] The Dunedin and Christchurch longitudinal studies found a prevalence of anxiety disorders of 7 per cent at age 11 years, with this figure rising to just under 20 per cent by age 18 years.[57] Anxiety disorders are equally frequent in boys and girls until adolescence, after which there is a predominance of girls. Children with separation anxiety disorder (SAD) usually present at a younger age. Although SAD becomes less common as adolescence is approached, generalized anxiety disorder (GAD) then becomes more frequent. Panic disorder is rare before puberty.[102] Post-traumatic stress disorder among at-risk child populations (e.g. who have been exposed to violence or trauma) has been found to have prevalence rates of 3 per cent[103] to 34.5 per cent.[104] Depression is rare in pre-adolescents. Unexplained somatic symptoms are common in children: 2–10 per cent of children experience aches and pains that are mostly unexplained.[105]

Aetiology

As with all child psychiatric disorders, no clear causal pathways have been identified, and aetiology is considered multifactorial. Factors associated include genetics through temperament (early traits of shyness and passivity), parenting style (e.g. high expressed emotion), parental anxiety, traumatic life events and social adversity.[106,107]

Presentation

SAD presents as a preoccupying worry that something may happen to the principal attachment figure or figures or that something may lead to the child being traumatically separated from them. About 75 per cent of children with SAD present with school refusal.[108] Other common associated symptoms include nightmares, social withdrawal and unexplained physical symptoms. Phobic disorders include specific fears (e.g. of animals or the dark), which usually resolve spontaneously, and more generalized fears in older children (e.g. social phobias and school phobias), which may not resolve and can evolve into a GAD.

Treatment

Anxiety disorders are more commonly treated among children in middle- and upper-class families, despite being more common in lower social classes.[55] Treatment is usually with psychosocial therapeutic approaches, including cognitive-behavioural therapy (CBT), family therapy, anxiety management, modelling, in vivo exposure and relaxation training.[109]

Outcome

The outcome depends on several factors, including the presence of co-morbidity and severity. Up to 80 per cent of children with anxiety disorders go into remission during the first year after developing symptoms. Nearly all children with SAD recover; however, some children with GAD who are more severely affected may go on to develop other anxiety disorders that persist into adulthood.[106]

DEPRESSION, OBSESSIVE–COMPULSIVE DISORDER AND SCHIZOPHRENIA IN ADOLESCENCE

Adolescence is generally thought of as the period that extends from the onset of puberty to the attainment of physical maturity (i.e. about 12–20 years). During adolescence, there are rapid biological and psychological changes and a need for intensive readjustment to family, school, work and social life. The multiplicity of changes includes physical, cognitive, social and emotional changes. Factors that contribute to poor adjustment include poor peer relationships, poor family relationships and support, unresolved childhood disorders, low motivation for changing, social disadvantage, family breakdown, brain injury and poor scholastic achievement. Adolescence is essentially a social construction. It is primarily culture rather than biology that decides when adolescence begins and ends, what behaviour is appropriate during this time, when sexual behaviour such as dating and sexual intercourse is accepted, how normal turmoil, unhappiness, rebellion and antisocial behaviour are, how much responsibility young people should be given, and so on.

A widely held view is that from mid-puberty onwards, people in their teens can suffer from psychiatric disorders that are more similar to those seen in adults than in earlier ages.

Depression

Prevalence

Findings in the Oregon Adolescent Depression Project show that the cumulative prevalence of major depressive disorder (MDD) up to age 18 years is 28 per cent (35% for girls, 19% for boys).[110,111] The Dunedin and Christchurch longitudinal studies identified 6.6 per cent of their sample of 15-year-olds as meeting criteria for mood disorder. By age 18 years, this had increased to 22.1 per cent.[57] Depressive disorders are equally frequent in boys and girls until adolescence, after which (from age 14 years) there is a predominance of girls.[112] There is evidence from both clinical studies and population surveys that mild to moderate depressive disorder is becoming more common and beginning earlier.[55] Figures on prevalence are complicated by a rapid change in the way child and adolescent depression has been conceptualized. Before the late 1980s, childhood depression was viewed as very rare, different from adult depression, and not amenable to treatment with antidepressants. A shift in theory, and consequently practice, then took place as influential academics claimed that childhood depression was more common than previously thought (8–20% of children and adolescents), resembled adult depression, and was amenable to treatment with antidepressants (often resulting in antidepressants becoming a first-line treatment).[113]

Aetiology

Important influences include family environment, including depression in parents, marital disharmony, depressive temperament and personality, and chronic adversity.[114] Co-morbidity is the rule rather than the exception and is probably explained by common risk factors, such as family adversity. Anxiety and conduct disorders are the most commonly associated disorders.

Presentation

The diagnostic criteria for depressive disorder in children and adolescents are the same as those for adults. Depressive disorders are partly defined by somewhat arbitrary reference points on a continuum of sadness, lethargy and pessimism.[55] A diagnosis of MDD in children and teenagers requires a minimum 2-week period of pervasive mood change towards sadness or irritability, and loss of interest or pleasure.[52] There needs to be a clear change in functioning, accompanied by impairment in social or other role performance. Diagnosis of major depression also requires the presence of some biological characteristics, such as loss of appetite, insomnia, and reduced energy or libido in adolescents. Children tend to show more anxiety and anger, fewer vegetative symptoms and less verbalization of hopelessness than do adults.

Treatment

Of particular importance is assessment of suicidal risk (which, if significant, is an indication for in-patient treatment). In general, the more severe the symptomatology and the degree of impairment, the more urgent the necessity for early commencement of treatment. There is good evidence to support the use of psychological therapies as the primary treatment modality, including CBT, interpersonal therapy and family therapies.[80,115] Although the use of selective serotonin reuptake inhibitors (SSRIs) for childhood depression became popular during the 1990s and early twenty-first century, following the discovery that drug companies had been manipulating both the data and conclusions most reviews have concluded that SSRIs confer little if any benefit to under-eighteens with depression at the same time as exposing them to small but significant risks, in particular of precipitating suicidal ideation.[116,117] The 2005 National Institute for Health and Clinical Excellence (NICE) guidelines on childhood and adolescent depression recommend only fluoxetine to be used and only if the patient has not responded to psychological approaches after a period of 3 months.[118]

Outcome

Most patients recover within a few months. A small proportion of patients go on to have a more chronic relapsing course, although a larger proportion may experience sub-threshold symptoms. It has been argued that childhood depression is a precursor of adult depression;[119] however, the reliability of this claim has been disputed.[113]

Obsessive–compulsive disorder

Prevalence

Obsessive–compulsive disorder (OCD) is an uncommon condition in childhood, with an overall point prevalence of 0.25 per cent. It is extremely rare in young children, but the point prevalence rises to 0.6 per cent in 13- to 15-year-olds.[120]

Aetiology

Although brain imaging studies in adults and children show evidence of central nervous system abnormalities,[121] successful treatment, including psychological treatment, results in a return to 'normal' morphology and metabolic activity, suggesting that brain imaging abnormalities reflect the effects of an OCD mental state as opposed to its cause. Rates of OCD are about four times greater in relatives of index cases.[122]

Presentation

OCD symptoms fall into four main groups: checking and ruminations, fear of contamination, symmetry and ordering, and hoarding (rare in childhood and adolescence). OCD seems to present at two stages: in the early school years (when boys predominate) and in adolescence (which is more common and when girls predominate).[123]

Treatment

First-line treatment is psychological and involves behavioural techniques such as exposure and response prevention (ERP).[122] Training parents to supervise ERP is used particularly with younger children. Other components that can be added to ERP include cognitive strategies and relaxation. Second-line treatment includes medication, particularly fluoxetine or clomipramine. Medication should be started at a low dose, with careful monitoring, particularly early in treatment, for possible side effects.

Outcome

It has been found that, with treatment, about a third of patients recover, a third continue to have the condition into adulthood, and another third develop other psychiatric disorders.[124]

Schizophrenia

Prevalence

Psychosis is extremely rare before 13 years of age. After age 13 years, the incidence rises rapidly during adolescence, reaching a peak incidence at around 25 years of age. The teenage population prevalence is about 2–3 per 1000.[125] There is a slight excess of males in early-onset psychosis.

Aetiology

Developmental abnormalities, dyspraxia, dyslexia, and speech and language disorders are more common in people who subsequently develop early-onset schizophrenia.[126] A number of conditions that can cause neurological impairment, such as tuberous sclerosis, partial complex seizures and leucodystrophies, are associated with an increased likelihood of developing a psychosis or psychotic symptoms. Together, these suggest a pre-existing neurological vulnerability in at least some patients who subsequently develop a psychosis. Although claims have been made that schizophrenia is a neurological condition associated with a pattern of progressive grey-matter loss, leading (for example) to increase ventricular size, most studies have not controlled properly for the effects of antipsychotics, which also cause atrophy of the brain,[127] and international follow-up studies find a more positive prognosis than previously thought.[32] A growing body of literature has also found a strong association between a history of trauma or abuse in childhood and subsequent psychosis in later life.[128] Thus, schizophrenia is now thought of as a more heterogeneous group of disorders.

Presentation

Schizophrenia is characterized by distortions of thinking and perception, delusions, hallucinations, and disorganized or unusual behaviour. Negative symptoms such as apathy, social withdrawal, poverty of speech and incongruent emotional responses may also be present, but these are rarer in younger patients. In children and adolescents, scholastic ability and self-care may be affected and could be the first signs of a developing psychosis.[55]

Treatment

There is a lack of clear empirical evidence on which to base treatment-planning. However, as child-, adolescent- and adult-onset schizophrenia have many similarities and continuities, using the adult literature has predominated, with treatment strategies being aimed at symptom control, minimizing long-term effects and preventing relapse.[80] In addition to using antipsychotic medication such as risperidone or olanzapine for acutely distressed patients and as a maintenance to prevent relapse, and/or a benzodiazepine such as lorazepam to aid with stabilization of acutely distressed patients, early intervention, psychosocial and psychoeducational approaches have received increasing attention. For example, a broad international, largely user-inspired movement, known as the 'recovery movement', helps patients by focusing on how to manage their lives and regain a sense of 'citizenship' in order to combat the problems of social exclusion, stigma and therapeutic nihilism.

Outcome

Although one study found that 80 per cent of 51 adolescents diagnosed with schizophrenia still had the diagnosis several years later,[129] the majority of studies have found that 50 per cent or more of adolescents diagnosed with schizophrenia are found to have no illness or a different, less severe, diagnosis on follow-up.[125]

ANOREXIA NERVOSA

Prevalence

A median prevalence rate for eating disorders in the 15–20 years age group is estimated at 1.2–1.4 per 1000.[130] This figure relates to young people in the developed Western world; eating disorders are much less common in non-affluent societies. The distribution of childhood-onset anorexia nervosa between social classes seems to be fairly similar to that in adults, with an overrepresentation of higher social classes.[131] The condition is rare at age 12 years but reaches about 1 in 200 girls at age 16 years. There is evidence that both anorexia nervosa and bulimia nervosa are becoming more common and more evenly distributed in social class.[132]

Aetiology

Like most child psychiatric disorders, eating disorders are conceptualized as having multifactorial causation, including biological vulnerability, sociocultural factors and adverse life events. Heritability is high in anorexia but not so with bulimia nervosa. The uneven distribution of eating disorders across populations suggests an important role for prevailing societal attitudes to female body image and size in the context of changing gender roles. Reports of anorexia nervosa in adults and children from African, Asian, Caribbean and Chinese populations suggest that an increasing incidence in these populations is related to exposure to and adoption of Western values.[55]

Presentation

Anorexia nervosa is characterized by self-induced weight loss leading to low weight (typically below 85% expected weight or a body mass index (BMI) of less than 17.5), fear of fatness or weight gain, disturbed body image, and amenorrhoea in postmenarchal females. Bulimia nervosa is characterized by recurrent episodes of binge eating; a preoccupation with eating, often including compulsions to eat; and compensatory behaviours to reduce weight, such as dietary restriction between binges, self-induced vomiting, excessive exercise and laxative abuse. In both conditions, body weight and shape become central to self-evaluation. The disorders occur mainly in females, although 5–10 per cent of cases in adolescents and young adults occur in males. Anorexia nervosa and bulimia nervosa are rare in younger children.[80]

Treatment

Treatment is usually a mixture of psychological therapies, particularly family therapy, together with medical management of physical consequences of low weight and a weight-restoration programme. Typically, a minimum target weight of 95 per cent of expected average body weight is aimed for.[132] In cases of amenorrhoea secondary to weight loss, the return of a regular menstrual cycle is a good indication of a return to a physiologically healthy weight. There is no robust evidence to demonstrate that in-patient treatment achieves better outcomes than out-patient treatment;[133] however, in-patient admission may be preferred in patients who are at a dangerously low weight in order to manage and monitor their physical state in a safe environment.

Outcome

Predictors of good outcome include healthy family functioning and a severe negative life event as precipitant.[134] A long-term follow-up study found that two-thirds of people who had an adolescent eating disorder were free of it 10 years later, although about half had a different psychiatric disorder.[135] Mortality in anorexia nervosa with an age of onset before 18 years is up to 11 per cent, with a mean mortality of 2.16 per cent across studies.[80]

DELIBERATE SELF-HARM IN ADOLESCENCE

Prevalence

In the Western world, suicide is extremely rare before age 14 years, rises rapidly in mid- to late adolescence, and then remains steady until another rise in old age. Suicide increased in males from the 1960s to the 1990s, but then it began to reduce again. It is much more common in boys than girls, occurs mainly in males with a history of aggression, and often occurs when the young person is intoxicated.[136] Surveys show an overall adolescent attempted suicide rate in Western countries of 8–9 per cent, with a rate of 2–3 per cent requiring medical attention.[136] Suicidal ideation is common in teenagers, with rates of about 15–20 per cent.[137]

Aetiology

Self-harm is most strongly predicted by the presence of depressive disorder (in girls) or by a previous suicidal attempt (in boys). Other influences include stress, co-morbid psychiatric disorders (such as depression), family conflict, previous self-harm, a family history of suicide or self harm and perinatal morbidity; sometimes, exposure to knowledge about other actual or fictional suicides can result in mini-epidemics of copycat behaviour.[136]

Presentation

Deliberate self-harm is the most common cause of admission of young people to a general hospital ward and is much more common in females than in males. The most common method is ingestion followed by cutting (although cutting has increased in frequency in recent years). Although pre-planning of a suicide attempt has been considered an indicator of intent, research has shown little correlation between preplanning and successful suicide in youth.[137]

Treatment

Admission to a medical/paediatric unit is often needed for treatment of any physical complications (such as poisoning) or to an adolescent in-patient unit for assessment and treatment of any coexisting psychiatric disorders (such as depression with suicidal ideation). On discharge, the young person and their parents may require advice on staying safe, such as keeping tablets and knives out of reach at home. Further treatment should be arranged to treat any co-morbid psychiatric disorders.

Outcome

The prognostic significance of a suicide attempt ranges from benign to serious, with later completed suicide. This heterogeneity of outcome has made prediction and classification of self-harm problematic. Predictors of recurrence after an attempt include male sex, use of a method other than pills or cutting, persistent suicidal ideas, psychotic symptoms, complications arising from substance abuse or alcohol consumption, a history of previous attempts, and having no adult guardian to supervise them on discharge.[136]

SUBSTANCE MISUSE

Prevalence

It is difficult to give precise prevalence rates, as these vary between countries and within countries over time. In addition, variations in methods of assessment, definition and population studied make comparing the findings of epidemiological studies problematic. However, there appear to be some broad generalizations that can be made from studies on children and adolescents in the past couple of decades in Europe and North America:[138]

- Alcohol and nicotine are the most frequently used substances, closely followed by marijuana, with inhalants (e.g. glue-sniffing), amphetamine, 'downers' (e.g. sleeping pills) and hallucinogens. Cocaine and opiate use is generally rare in under-eighteens, although this may be changing.
- Between one-half and three-quarters of older adolescents have tried an illicit drug.
- 20–40 per cent of those who have used drugs have tried more than one.
- About 1 in 12 of those who take drugs are regular or heavy users.
- Illicit drug use is uncommon in children under the age of 12 years but becomes more frequent during the teenage years.
- Drug use overall is about as common in girls and boys, but there are gender differences in the types of drug used.
- Overall, drug use in young people increased during the 1990s.
- Drug use is more frequent among young people with poor scholastic achievement.

Aetiology

Predisposing factors include environmental factors (e.g. widespread availability of drugs, poverty, parental substance misuse, use of drugs among peers, family conflict, scholastic failure) and individual risk factors (e.g. low self-esteem, persistent behaviour problems, co-morbid psychiatric disorder).[139] Protective factors include easy temperament, good intellectual ability and supportive family and social circumstances.[139]

Presentation

Adolescents who misuse substances differ from adults who do this in a number of ways: they have shorter drug histories, less involvement with certain drugs (particularly opiates), more binge drinking and more polydrug use.[140] ICD-10 uses the following subdivisions for substance misuse:

- *Acute intoxication:* resulting in a disturbed level of consciousness.
- *Harmful use:* a pattern of psychoactive substance use that is causing physical or mental damage to health.
- *Dependence:* a cluster of behavioural, cognitive and physiological phenomena that develop after repeated and regular substance use.
- *Withdrawal state:* a group of symptoms occurring on absolute or relative withdrawal of a substance after persistent use of that substance.

Treatment

Treatment begins with prevention, such as reducing or eliminating exposure and decreasing risk factors.[138] Treatment of people with a substance-misuse problem often includes multi-agency involvement, such as education, child and adolescent mental health services, youth offending, social services, accident and emergency departments, and drug and alcohol services. A variety of individual, educational, family and group approaches, including psychoeducation, motivational interviewing, detox regimes and specific substance-misuse treatment programmes, exist. Physical problems associated with alcohol and drug misuse, such as poor nutrition, overdose, severe intoxication, human immunodeficiency virus (HIV) and hepatitis, also need treatment.

Outcome

The younger people are when they first use drugs, the more likely they are to progress from experimental usage to dependence.[141] Longitudinal studies have shown that considerable risks are associated with substance misuse, especially with respect to suicide, accidental deaths, delinquency, depression and psychosocial dysfunction more broadly.[138]

MENTAL HANDICAP AND DEVELOPMENTAL DISORDERS

Generalized mental handicap

Table 70.1 shows levels of mental handicap based on ICD-10.

Prevalence

The use of an IQ below 70 as the sole criterion would result in prevalence rates of 2–3 per cent, based on a normal distribution curve. However, if some degree of impairment is added as a criterion, then prevalence reduces to about 1 per cent. In the Isle of Wight study, 2.5 per cent of children could be classified as having mental retardation, but about 1.3 per cent had impairments sufficient to require services.[51] In the Aberdeen study of 8- to 10-year-olds, the rate was 2.4 per cent for mental retardation but 0.9 per cent when impairment was added.[142] When compared with the general population, individuals with mental retardation are at much greater risk for having a psychiatric disorder or severe emotional or behavioural dysfunction.[143]

Table 70.1 Levels of mental handicap

Level	IQ range	Approximate mental age in adulthood (years)
Mild	50–70	9–12
Moderate	35–49	6–9
Severe	20–34	3–6
Profound	< 20	< 3

IQ, intelligence quotient.

Aetiology

Historically, researchers have described two groups. One group demonstrates a clear biological cause for their developmental delay; the other has no clear cause and tends to be thought of as part of a continuum in the normal distribution. Although there is not a comprehensive model to explain the increased rate of psychiatric disorder in this population, the following factors are associated with psychopathology in people with mental retardation: atypical motivational styles, increased risk of failure experiences, less differentiated self-concepts, re-enforcement of negative behaviours, poor communication skills, lack of assertiveness skills, peer rejection, compromised social intelligence, family stress, increased rates of seizure disorders, abnormal neurological functioning, and higher than usual risk of genetic anomalies.[144]

Presentation

Diagnosis rests primarily on the use of formal measures of intellectual functioning. However, use of IQ as the sole criterion is problematic, as many people in the mild mental retardation range have no adaptive impairments, cope relatively well with the demands of daily life, and therefore do not come to the attention of professionals. People with accompanying psychopathology often present with emotional or behavioural difficulties, coupled with learning difficulties at school.

Treatment

In addition to diagnosing and treating any accompanying physical disorder (such as epilepsy), treatment for accompanying psychopathology is similar to treatment of people without mental retardation, but with some modifications to take into account the patient's level of functioning and communication. A variety of psychosocial interventions, including behaviour therapy, psychotherapy, systemic interventions and educational interventions, as well as psychopharmacology have been found to be helpful.[144]

Outcome

The majority of people with mild mental retardation go on to live independently and successfully. The more severe the retardation, the greater the likelihood that further support and input from a variety of services will be required.

Specific delays in speech, language and reading

Prevalence

Specific delays in speech and language are common, with an estimated incidence of 3–10 per cent.[145] Estimates of the incidence of specific reading difficulties range between 1 per cent and 9 per cent.[146] Accurate estimates are difficult due to disagreements about cut-off points between 'normal' and delayed.

Aetiology

Most theories on aetiology assume a biological cause for the delay, although this is complicated by what some authors refer to as a 'cult of developmentalism', resulting in an unnecessarily rigid focus on age-specific developmental tasks, which can cause considerable anxiety to parents and educators and introduce competitiveness into child development from a very early age. This makes a more relaxed approach to development, which accepts the different rates at which different individuals develop, much harder to achieve.[60,147]

Presentation

Specific developmental disorders are differentiated from pervasive developmental disorders and general learning difficulties (mental handicap) by having an overall IQ above 70 or a non-verbal IQ above 70 for developmental disorders of speech and language. These children's difficulties are out of line with what is expected for their age and general cognitive difficulties. They include speech and language delays, specific reading difficulties (dyslexia), spelling difficulties (dysgraphia), arithmetic problems (dyscalculia), and problems with motor coordination (dyspraxia). Disorders of speech and language are often associated with a wide range of academic, social, emotional and behavioural problems.[148] Increased prevalence of almost all specific developmental disorders has been found in children presenting with a psychiatric disorder.[149] Most studies find three to four times more boys with specific developmental delays; however, this may be a reflection of coexisting behavioural problems making boys more likely to receive a referral for extra help at school.[150]

Treatment

Treatment is largely educational and includes speech therapy and extra assistance at school, such as an individual education plan or, in more severe cases, a statement of special educational needs.

Outcome

Many children are simply 'late developers' and catch up over time. In a study of 4-year-olds with poor language, most of whom were receiving speech therapy, about half no longer had these difficulties by the time they were 5.5 years old.[151]

Pervasive developmental disorders (including autism and Asperger's syndrome)

Prevalence

A study in preschool children found a rate for ASD of 45.8 per 10 000 children.[152] The National Autistic Society, using an estimated prevalence of 91 per 1000 of the population, estimates that there are around 535 000 people with ASD in the UK and claims that the majority of these may go undiagnosed.[153] ASDs are three to four times more common in males than females.

Aetiology

A specific medical cause is found in only a minority of people with autism, albeit more often in those with pronounced learning problems. Epilepsy occurs more commonly than usual in autism, particularly in people with moderate to severe learning difficulties. Evidence points to genetic factors playing a role in causing ASD, with twin and family studies suggesting an underlying genetic vulnerability to ASD; however, this conclusion has been criticized (see Aetiology of child psychiatric disorders, above). Postmortem and brain scan studies have shown that a number of brain structures may be implicated in autism, although there is no consistent finding or core pathology identified. Severe deprivation (as described in some Romanian orphanages) is also associated with significant developmental delay and autistic patterns of behaviour.[154] Thus, autism is a phenomenological rather than an aetiological diagnosis. It describes a behavioural phenotype that may be arrived at by numerous different aetiological pathways, operating by mechanisms that we do not understand. Furthermore, some authors have pointed out that our changing concept of autism owes more to ideological shifts expanding the notion than to new scientific knowledge.[155,156]

Presentation

Autism is a behaviourally defined disorder, characterized by qualitative impairments in social communication, social interaction and social imagination (the core triad of symptoms), with a restricted range of interests and often stereotyped repetitive behaviours and mannerisms. Sensory hyposensitivities or hypersensitivities to the environment are also common. In DSM-IV, autism is classified as belonging to the pervasive developmental disorders (PDD). There are five subcategories listed under PDD:

- *Autistic disorder.*
- *Asperger's syndrome:* relatively good verbal language, with milder non-verbal language problems, and restricted range of interests and relatedness.
- *PDD-NOS:* non-verbal language and other problems that do not meet the strict criteria for other PDDs.
- *Rett's disorder:* a rare X-linked dominant progressive neurodevelopmental disorder of girls, with poor head growth and microcephaly (prevalence: 1 in 10 000 children). Clinical features include rapid deterioration of behaviour and language, loss of purposeful hand movements, progressive spasticity and ataxia, acquired microcephaly and seizures.
- *Childhood disintegrative disorder:* a rare neurodegenerative disorder (prevalence: 1 in 10 000 children). There is a loss of functioning after 2 years of normal development, with regression of language, social skills, adaptive skills, play, motor skills and continence.

In common practice, Rett's disorder and childhood disintegrative disorder are often considered mainstream medical disorders and are not usually dealt with within services for ASD.

Treatment

Medical examination and investigations are usually required to detect or exclude known organic causes (e.g. hearing problems, tuberous sclerosis), assess neurological deficits, and test for known chromosomal abnormalities such as fragile X syndrome. There are no specific treatments for autism. Treatment for autism is geared largely towards management and support of the associated difficulties that it produces for the individual and their family, with a few requiring multi-agency lifelong integrated care. Behavioural, educational and dietary interventions are used widely. Medications are often used to help families manage behavioural problems, such as aggression, self-injurious behaviour, obsessive–compulsive symptoms and tantrums, which keep the person with ASD from functioning more effectively at home or school. However, the use of medications remains controversial, as there is little evidence to support their producing improved outcomes while exposing children to side effects.[155]

Outcome

Although outcome studies in autism suggest that the disabling features and cognitive style are lifelong, the current fashion for retrospectively diagnosing the great and the good as having had autism (e.g. Einstein, Newton) suggests that at least people some can look forward to exceptionally good outcomes. The fact that IQ levels are the best predictor of future ability to undertake a job and live independently casts doubt on the usefulness of adding autism as a diagnosis for some children.

ENURESIS AND ENCOPRESIS

Enuresis

Prevalence

At the age of 7 years, 15–22 per cent of males and 7–15 per cent of females were found to have nocturnal enuresis. By 18 years, about 1 per cent of males and a lower proportion of females were found to have nocturnal enuresis.[157]

Aetiology

Nocturnal enuresis tends to run in families, as 70 per cent of affected children have a parent or sibling who was late in becoming dry. Nocturnal enuresis is twice as common in MZ than in DZ twins.[158] Other factors may include lack of vasopressin release during sleep or nocturnal insensitivity of renal tubules to vasopressin, incoordination of voiding mechanisms, reduced functional bladder capacity, developmental delay (e.g. late puberty), urinary tract infection or obstruction, and constipation. Environmental factors include stressful life events, social disadvantage, larger family size, teenage pregnancy and mother's smoking.[159]

Presentation

The presentation is characterized by involuntary voiding of urine, by day or night, which is abnormal in relation to the individual's mental age and is not a consequence of a lack of bladder control due to any neurological disorder, to epileptic attacks, or to any structural abnormality of the urinary tract. The condition is generally not diagnosed in children under the age of 5 years or in people with a mental age of less than 4 years.

Treatment

After excluding physical causes, management can include education, a behavioural programme, enuresis alarms, desmopressin and tricyclic antidepressants.[159]

Outcome

Nocturnal enuresis rarely leads to any lasting problems and is not considered an indicator for mental health problems in later life.

Encopresis

Prevalence

Most Western children achieve faecal continence in their second year. Faecal incontinence occurs in about 10 per cent of 3-year-olds, less than 5 per cent of 4-year-olds and 1.5 per cent of 5- to 7-year-olds. At 10–12 years, faecal incontinence occurs in 1.3 per cent of boys and 0.3 per cent of girls.[51] It is very rare after 16 years.

Aetiology

Faecal incontinence may be an abnormal continuation of normal infantile incontinence, be secondary to a medical problem (e.g. constipation, which can in itself be caused by physical or psychological factors), be a monosymptomatic disorder secondary to psychological factors, or be part of a wider psychiatric disorder (e.g. emotional disorder or conduct disorder). Encopresis is also associated with other developmental delays such as enuresis, sensorimotor incoordination, slow language development and learning disability.[159]

Presentation

Presentation is with repeated voluntary or involuntary passage of faeces in places not appropriate for that purpose. The frequency needs to be more than once a month for the diagnosis to be made, and it should not be attributable to a general medical condition.

Treatment

Diagnosis and treatment of organic factors (e.g. constipation) is required. Advice on toilet routine is often used as is appropriate management of any coexisting psychiatric disorder. Particular therapeutic strategies such as externalizing the symptom have also been used successfully.[160]

Outcome

Encopresis usually resolves spontaneously before adolescence. Poor outcomes are associated with developmental disorders, learning difficulties, non-compliance with treatment, disorganized or chaotic family life, and serious social disadvantage.[161]

TIC DISORDERS

Prevalence

Transient tics are commonplace among children, with community surveys indicating that 1–13 per cent of children manifest twitches, tics or other mannerisms at some time, with the highest prevalence being in children aged 7–11 years.[162] Tourette's syndrome is rare, with a prevalence rate of about 4.5 per 10 000 among 16- and 17-year-olds, according to the largest study to date.[163]

Aetiology

The aetiology of tics and Tourette's syndrome remains unknown. Popular aetiological theories for Tourette's syndrome include genetic and perinatal difficulties.[164]

Presentation

Transient tics are characterized by one or more simple motor tics, usually confined to the face or neck, which wax and wane in severity over the course of weeks or months. Tourette's syndrome typically begins in early childhood with bouts of simple motor tics such as eye-blinking or head-jerking. These tics eventually become more persistent and can incorporate virtually any voluntary movement of any portion of the body. Complex motor tics may appear, as may phonic tics such as throat-clearing, grunting, and more complex phonic tics such as coprolalia (excessive and uncontrollable use of foul or obscene language). Tourette's syndrome has a high co-morbidity, particularly with ADHD and OCD.[164]

Treatment

Transient tics resolve spontaneously and thus require no treatment. Tourette's syndrome is treated with supportive psychotherapy and psychoeducation, which is usually sufficient for the majority of patients. Where the child's symptoms are causing significant impairment in day-to-day functioning, other treatments aimed at controlling the involuntary movements may be indicated, including CBT and medication such as haloperidol, sulpiride, risperidone or clonidine.[164]

Outcome

In Tourette's syndrome, the worst severity has been found to occur at about 10 years of age, with about half of those afflicted being virtually symptom-free by 18 years of age.[165]

FAMILY CONFLICT PROBLEMS

Family conflict does not represent a diagnostic category, but it is associated with a wide variety of adverse outcomes. For example, marital conflict is associated with child and adolescent behaviour problems, including aggression and poor social functioning,[166] and has also been found to predict later depressive symptoms, delinquency, alcohol problems,[167] lower levels of closeness to parents, poor self-esteem, and higher levels of distress and violence in the offspring.[168] Assessing the impact of family conflict is complicated by the large cultural variations found in family structure, parenting beliefs and practices, and availability of resources, which thus need to be taken into account in any assessment and treatment.[5] Family therapy approaches (see Aetiology of child psychiatric disorders, above) are the most common therapeutic methods used to try to alleviate family conflict.

CONTINUITIES OF CHILDHOOD PSYCHIATRIC DISORDER INTO ADULT LIFE

The literature on continuities of childhood psychiatric disorder is at an early stage, due to the practical and methodological challenges involved in setting up the type of longitudinal research required. Below is a summary of some of the emerging findings.

Anxiety disorders

Overall, the history of any anxiety disorder in childhood or adolescence is associated with a significant increase in risk for an anxiety disorder occurring in adult life,[169] although the specificity for the same condition recurring is low.[170] A history of a child or adolescent anxiety disorder also increases the risk of substance misuse, poor socialization, depression and educational underachievement; however, the majority of affected children have a good prognosis, being virtually indistinguishable from well controls at follow-up.[171]

Depression

Clinical follow-up studies have shown that adolescent depression is associated with a high risk of depressive relapse extending into the third decade.[172] The risk of recurrence was unaffected by co-morbid diagnoses. Those with depression and conduct disorder also had increased rates of suicide, alcoholism, substance misuse and antisocial personality disorder.[173] The relationship between cause and effect is difficult to establish. For example, poor social adjustment in adults is associated with recurrent adolescent depressive episodes and could be a function of the effects of depression or of persistent adverse social circumstances leading to depression.[174]

Obsessive–compulsive disorder

Unlike anxiety disorders, OCD in childhood, should it recur, tends to recur as OCD. As many as one-half of those with childhood OCD have recurrent episodes into adult life.[175] Other co-morbid disorders such as depression and personality disorders may also arise over time.[124]

Hyperactivity disorders

For many children with a childhood diagnosis of ADHD, outcomes are generally good, with about two-thirds showing no evidence of any mental disorder in adulthood and being gainfully employed.[176] However, compared with 'normal' controls, children with a history of ADHD complete less schooling, hold lower-ranking occupations, have social skills deficits and are more prone to misuse substances.[176]

Conduct disorders

In general, the available evidence suggests a persistence across the life course for childhood-onset conduct disorders, whereas adolescent-onset cases tend to remit in early adulthood in the majority of cases.[177]

Some methodological problems

A number of methodological issues are apparent with longitudinal and other research into long-term outcomes. First, the use of categorical diagnoses for childhood and adult psychiatric disorders based on questionnaires may have only a limited relationship with levels of functioning. Second, high rates of co-morbidity (when the subjects were children and again as adults) makes it difficult to establish the relationship between the childhood and subsequent adult disorder. Third, the studies are unable to differentiate cause and effect (is it the diagnosis or continuing social adversity that may have caused the mental health problems in the first place and that is contributing most to adverse outcomes?). Finally, the studies rarely take into account the possible effects of labelling and any treatment received (e.g. continuing morbidity as a result of toxic side effects of medications taken, and the effect on self-worth together with the psychosocial adversity that arises as a result of becoming a psychiatric patient).[178]

TREATMENT IN CHILD PSYCHIATRY

Child psychiatry sits at the confluence of many different systems of knowledge: medical, psychological, social, paediatric, anthropological, cultural and so on. In addition, child psychiatrists have to become proficient at working not only with children and young people but also with the variety of adults who care for these children and young people. Thus, child psychiatrists need to develop competence in working within a variety of modalities – biological, psychological and social – and in particular need to be able to engage with the young people and also the system of care around them. Familiarity with family and systemic approaches (see Assessment of children and adolescents, above) is therefore important.

In terms of a relationship between methods of treatment and outcome, robust conclusions about specific methods are difficult to establish because of a huge variability in the quality of the research, bias in reporting (e.g. with drug-industry-sponsored trials), inadequate follow-ups and lack of attention to cultural issues.[55,97]

The most marked change in the past couple of decades in the practice of child psychiatry in most Western countries with established child psychiatric services has been the rapid increase in the use of psychopharmacology. In particular, the use of antidepressants for depression, stimulants for ADHD, and antipsychotics such as risperidone for behaviour problems have all taken place against a backdrop of aggressive marketing from the pharmaceutical industry.[97,179] However, we are now aware that the widespread use of SSRI antidepressants in under-eighteens occurred before any data on their safety and efficacy in this age group were available and that the studies, when they did take place, suffered from conflicts of interest, which led to suppression of data.[117] A more objective review of studies using SSRIs in depression leads to the conclusion that SSRIs do not confer significant clinical advantage over placebo and may expose the recipient to unnecessary risks, particular of precipitating suicidal ideation.[116]

Unfortunately, this scenario is not limited to SSRIs. The largest and most influential study on the use of stimulants in ADHD, when it published its findings on the outcome 3 years after the start of the study, found that the advantage seen in patients treated with stimulants compared with those who received behaviour therapy alone had, after 14 months of treatment, been lost; however, patients on medication were now significantly shorter and lighter.[180] This, together with reviews that highlight that we have no evidence to support the contention that treatment with stimulants improves outcome as adults,[181] suggests that, as with SSRIs, it is likely that stimulants have been used too indiscriminately and before robust evidence on their safety and effectiveness was available. This is a problem for child psychopharmacology, particularly as we have limited data on the possible long-term effects of psychiatric drugs on the developing brain and because much of current child psychopharmacology is based on experience and evidence of drugs as they are used in adults, with little robust data on their safety and efficacy in children.[182] As we have discovered with SSRIs, it is likely that we will find different safety and efficacy profiles in under-eighteens, suggesting much greater care needs to be taken in the use of psychotropics in this age group.[183] It is likely, therefore, that in the coming years the use of psychotropics in under-eighteens will be re-evaluated. Predicting from the emerging evidence, this may mean that psychotropics will have a more limited remit than at present, being reserved for patients with more severe impairments and being used in conjunction with non-pharmaceutical approaches as opposed to standalone treatments.

For most of the disorders reviewed in this chapter, there are psychosocial treatments that are grounded solidly in empirical support as standalone treatments. Moreover, the preponderance of available evidence indicates that psychosocial treatments are safer than psychoactive medications. Thus, groups such as the American Psychological Association Working Group on Psychoactive Medications for Children and Adolescents[184] and NICE guidelines on child and adolescent mental health disorders are now recommending that, in the majority of cases, psychosocial interventions should be considered first.

Indications for in-patient and day-patient care

In-patient treatment is indicated when the problems are severe or complex and in the following situations:[185]

- 24-h psychiatric nursing care is required.
- The young person has a rapidly deteriorating condition.
- Out-patient treatment has been unsuccessful.
- There is considerable diagnostic uncertainty.

Day-patient places are a scarce resource, with many units not having provisions for day placements. In those units that do, indications for referral are similar, although the young people referred do not require 24-h nursing care. In-patient units are a mixture of general (the majority) and specialist (e.g. eating disorder, learning difficulty, forensic). The units typically offer a mixture of therapies in addition to the therapeutic milieu and have a hospital school attached to the unit.

DESCRIPTION OF A TYPICAL CHILD PSYCHIATRIC SERVICE

CAMHS are multidisciplinary services with a variety of specialists with training in child and adolescent mental health problems working in them. Different teams have different professionals, depending on national expectations and local factors. Who is in any particular team largely depends on local circumstances (e.g. funding levels, ease of recruitment, availability of any particular professional group, any training or research activities going on there). Different professionals working in CAMHS teams include child and adolescent psychiatrists, clinical psychologists, psychotherapists, family therapists, social workers, specialist nurses, art therapists, occupational therapists and educational psychologists.

CAMHS are organized structurally into four tiers:

- *Tier 1* is aimed at all children and includes all primary healthcare professionals, primary mental health clinicians, teachers, youth workers and welfare officers.
- *Tier 2* is aimed at children at risk of mental health problems and those with mental health problems that require a single professional's input. Professionals working at this level include primary mental health clinicians, child psychiatrists, child psychologists, social workers, paediatricians, educational psychologists, emotional behavioural support workers, specialist nurses and therapists.
- *Tier 3* is aimed at children with recognized psychiatric disorders and includes those that require specialist CAMHS input with a multidisciplinary team working together in a clinic setting.
- *Tier 4* is highly specialist services for children with more severe disorders, including in-patient units.

Other important agencies and institutions that have extensive contact with CAMHS include the following:

- *Paediatrics:* many community (as opposed to hospital) paediatricians run clinics for behavioural disorders, where children with conditions such as ADHD and autism are diagnosed. Referral can come directly from the general practitioner (GP) but also through medical officers (doctors attached to schools). Usually assessments are confined to questions of diagnosis, and treatments tend to revolve around the use of medication and sometimes advice about behavioural strategies. Paediatricians sometimes provide input into a CAMHS team, and members of CAMHS teams (particularly child psychiatrists) sometimes provide input into paediatric teams (e.g. liaison psychiatry on paediatric wards, input into a child development team or centre).

- *Schools:* if the problem is solely or primarily school-based, then the school or education authority has processes and professionals who may get involved. Schools have several services that they can call on to help them with a particular pupil or problem. These include the emotional behavioural support service (EBSS), which helps the school to devise strategies for pupils with emotional or behavioural problems, and educational psychologists, who can assess pupils for learning difficulties and other emotional, behavioural and academic issues. Some schools also employ school counsellors. In addition, all schools and education authorities should have policies and procedures for issues such as bullying. Children in the UK with persistent problems relating to their learning or their behaviour should be given an individual education plan (IEP), which, if the difficulties are severe enough, can lead to an application for a statement of special educational needs. A statement provides pupils with extra input, such as extra teaching, support, mentoring or attendance at a special school such as an emotional behaviour disorder (EBD) school or a mild learning difficulties (MLD) school.
- *Social services:* anyone can request input from social services, but their involvement tends to be around issues such as child protection (see Child protection, above), family support (particularly for families with a disabled child), fostering and adoption, and parenting support and advice.
- *Voluntary:* the voluntary sector includes a variety of organizations that vary from locality to locality. Some may have been set up to support the needs of particular groups (e.g. particular ethnic minority communities; support for children with particular diagnoses such as ADHD; parenting advice groups; counselling for specific events, such as domestic violence, bereavement, victims of abuse) and others are national (e.g. Young Minds, Parentline, National Autistic Society). Thus, each locality has its own specific mixture of local and national groups.
- *Others:* a variety of private therapists are qualified or experienced in working with children and families and run private organizations providing a variety of services for both educational and mental health problems (e.g. services for children with dyslexia, eating disorders, neurodevelopmental disorders, private fostering).

KEY POINTS

- Approaches to assessment and treatment of mental health problems in children and adolescents are characterized by two key features: development and context. Children are changing as they mature physically and psychologically, and so a developmental perspective is necessary. Children are also dependent on adults in a variety of caregiving roles to make decisions on their behalf, and therefore an engagement with the child's context, such as family, school and social services, is necessary for comprehensive assessments and effective interventions.
- Beliefs about what makes up normal or abnormal childhood, child development and child-rearing vary both within and between cultures. Attempts to impose a universal system for defining what should count as abnormal behaviour for a child is therefore problematic. We should be aware that professional beliefs, including those in mainstream child and adolescent psychiatry, are not immune from making this mistake, particularly as no physical or psychological markers accompany the commonly defined disorders. In multicultural societies, high-quality services need to be aware of this in order to engage with services users' perspectives and to develop approaches that make sense to children and families from diverse backgrounds.
- Awareness of child-protection procedures and legal processes for protecting children is vital for any professional working with children. There are four categories of child abuse: sexual abuse, physical abuse, emotional abuse and neglect. Child abuse is associated with a large number of potential adverse consequences for the victim.
- Classification of child psychiatric disorder is taken mainly from the ICD-10, although some categories commonly used in clinical practice (e.g. the diagnosis ADHD) come from the American DSM-IV. In ICD-10, the main groups of diagnoses relevant to children and adolescents' mental health are: mental retardation; disorders of psychological development (which refer mainly to specific learning difficulties and developmental disorders such as autism); and behavioural and emotional disorders with onset usually occurring in childhood and adolescence (which covers disorders that are conceptualized as being specific to childhood and adolescence, such as hyperkinetic disorders, conduct disorders and emotional disorders). In addition, a number of disorders placed in other groupings and that occur more commonly in over-eighteens (e.g. schizophrenia) can also be used for children and adolescents.
- Due to differing approaches to classification and categorization of disorders and differing cut-off points used in research, epidemiological studies have produced figures for the prevalence of child psychiatric disorders that range from about 7 per cent to about 30 per cent of school-aged children.
- As there are no identified physical or psychological markers, clear aetiological pathways have not been found for any child psychiatric disorder. However, research has established a number of associated risk factors, including biological (e.g. being male, having a chronic physical illness – particularly one that affects the nervous system – and low IQ) and psychosocial (e.g. poverty, parental discord, parental psychopathology, disrupted attachments, violence, living in an urban setting, living in a rich country with a high level of social inequality,

poor social networks, going to a school with a high rate of behavioural problems, bullying) ones.

- As child psychiatry sits at the confluence of many different systems of knowledge, competent child psychiatrists need to develop an ability to work in a variety of modalities including biological, psychological and social. In particular, treatment approaches need to engage with the young person's context, such as family and school, where resources to help the young person's mental health problems can often be found. In recent years, child psychiatry has moved towards greater use of psychopharmacology; however, it has now become apparent that much of this change was stimulated more by good marketing than by good science. The place of psychopharmacology is likely to be more limited than recent prescribing trends suggest, as evidence shows that safer alternatives are available and that the drugs that have become more widely used in young people (SSRIs, stimulants, antipsychotics) are associated with risks but no proven long-term benefits

REFERENCES

1. Achenbach TM (1992) *Manual for the Child Behaviour Checklist/2–3 and 1992 Profile.* Burlington, VT: University of Vermont Department of Psychiatry.
2. Conners CK (1997) *Conners' Rating Scales Manual.* North Tonawanda, NY: Multi-Health Systems.
3. Goodman R, Scott S (1999) Comparing the Strengths and difficulties Questionnaire and the Child Behaviour Checklist: is small beautiful? *Journal of Abnormal Child Psychology* **27**: 17–24.
4. Wechsler D (1991) *Manual for the Wechsler Intelligence Scale for Children*, 3rd edn. San Antonio, TX: Psychological Corporation.
5. Dwivedi KN (ed.) (2002) *Meeting the Needs of Ethnic Minority Children.* London: Jessica Kingsley Publishers.
6. Timimi S (2002) *Pathological Child Psychiatry and the Medicalization of Childhood.* London: Brunner/Routledge.
7. Timimi S, Maitra B (eds.) (2006) *Critical Voices in Child and Adolescent Mental Health.* London: Free Association Books.
8. Royal College of Psychiatrists (2006) *Being Seen and Heard: The Needs of Children of Parents with Mental Illness* (DVD). London: Royal College of Psychiatrists.
9. Ross LE, McLean LM (2006) Anxiety disorders during pregnancy and the postpartum period; a systematic review. *Clinical Psychiatry* **67**: 1285–98.
10. Figueiredo B, Bifulco A, Pachecho A, *et al.* (2006) Teenage pregnancy, attachment style, and depression: a comparison of teenage and adult pregnant women in a Portuguese series. *Attachment and Human Development* **8**: 123–38.
11. McLaren L, Kuh D, Hardy R, Mishra G (2007) Postnatal depression and the original mother–child relationship: a prospective cohort study. *Journal of Affective Disorders* **100**: 211–19.
12. Records K, Rice MJ (2005) A comparative study of postpartum depression in abused and non-abused women. *Archives of Psychiatric Nursing* **19**: 281–90.
13. Ueda M, Yamashita H, Yoshida K (2006) Impact of infant health problems on postnatal depression: pilot study to evaluate a health visiting system. *Psychiatry and Clinical Neurosciences* **60**: 182–9.
14. Lee DTS, Chung TKH (2007) Postnatal depression: an update. *Best Practice and Research in Clinical Obstetrics and Gynaecology* **21**: 183–91.
15. Moehler E, Brunner R, Wiebel A, *et al.* (2006) Maternal depressive symptoms in the postnatal period are associated with long-term impairment of mother–child bonding. *Archives of Women's Mental Health* **9**: 273–8.
16. Klier CM (2006) Mother–infant bonding disorders in patients with postnatal depression: the Postpartum Bonding Questionnaire in clinical practice. *Archives of Women's Mental Health* **9**: 289–91.
17. Barr JA (2008) Postpartum depression, delayed maternal adaptation, and mechanical infant caring: a phenomenological hermeneutic study. *International Journal of Nursing Studies* **45**: 362–9.
18. Jung V, Short R, Letourneau N, Andrews D (2007) Interventions with depressed mothers and their infants: modifying interactive behaviours. *Journal of Affective Disorders* **98**: 199–205.
19. Pippins JR, Brawarsky P, Jackson RA, *et al.* (2006) Association of breastfeeding with maternal depressive symptoms. *Journal of Women's Health* **15**: 754–62.
20. McLearn KT, Minkovitz CS, Strobino DM, *et al.* (2006) The timing of maternal depressive symptoms and mothers' parenting practices with young children: implications for pediatric practice. *Pediatrics* **118**: 174–82.
21. Weissman MM, Leckman JF, Merikangas KR, *et al.* (1984) Depression and anxiety disorders in parents and children. *Archives of General Psychiatry* **41**: 845–51.
22. Murray L (1992) The impact of postnatal depression on infant development. *Journal of Child Psychology and Psychiatry* **33**: 543–61.
23. Hay DF, Zahn-Waxler C, Cummings EM, Iannotti RJ (1992) Young children's views about conflict with peers: a comparison of the daughters and sons of depressed and well women. *Journal of Child Psychology and Psychiatry* **33**: 669–83.
24. Sharp D, Hay D, Pawlby S, *et al.* (1995) The impact of postnatal depression on boys' intellectual development. *Journal of Child Psychology and Psychiatry* **36**: 1315–37.
25. Murray L, Kempton C, Woolgar M, Hooper R (1993) Depressed mothers' speech to their infants and its relation to infant gender and cognitive development. *Journal of Child Psychology and Psychiatry* **34**: 1083–101.

26. Lee LC, Halpern CT, Hertz-Picciotto I, *et al.* (2006) Child care and social support modify the association between maternal depressive symptoms and early childhood behaviour problems: a US national study. *Journal of Epidemiology and Community Health* **60**: 305–10.
27. Friedman SH, Hrouda DR, Holden CE, *et al.* (2005) Child murder committed by severely mentally ill mothers: an examination of mothers found not guilty by reason of insanity. *Forensic Science* **50**: 1466–71.
28. Timimi S (2005) Effect of globalisation on children's mental health. *British Medical Journal* **331**: 37–9.
29. McKenzie K, Patel V, Araya R (2004) Learning from low income countries: mental health. *British Medical Journal* **329**: 1138–40.
30. Becker AE, Lee DTS (2002) Indigenous models for attenuation of post partum depression: case studies from Fiji and Hong Kong. In A Cohen, A Kleinman, B Saraceno (eds) *World Mental Health Casebook*. New York: Kluwer.
31. Lee DTS, Yip ASK, Leung TYS, Chung TKH (2004) Ethnoepidemiology of postnatal depression: prospective multivariate study of sociocultural risk factors in a Chinese population in Hong Kong. *British Journal of Psychiatry* **184**: 34–40.
32. Hopper K, Harrison G, Janca A, Sartorius N (eds) (2007) *Recovery from Schizophrenia: An International Perspective: A Report from the WHO Collaborative Project, The International Study Of Schizophrenia*. Oxford: Oxford University Press.
33. Friedman R, Chase-Lonsdale P (2002) Chronic adversities. In M Rutter, E Taylor (eds) *Child and Adolescent Psychiatry*, 4th edn. Oxford: Blackwell.
34. Rose KM, Fields JM (2001) Number, timing, and duration of marriages and divorces: Fall 1996. In *Current Population Reports*. Washington, DC: U.S. Census Bureau.
35. Office for National Statistics (2007) *Divorces*. London: Office for National Statistics. www.statistics.gov.uk/cci/nugget.asp?id=170.
36. Bowlby J (1969) *Attachment and Loss*. New York: Basic Books.
37. Bailham D, Harper PB (2004) Attachment theory and mental health. In KN Dwivedi, PB Harper (eds) *Promoting the Emotional Well-Being of Children and Adolescents and Preventing their Mental Ill Health*. London: Jessica Kingsley Publishers.
38. Loh E, Wragg J (2004) Developmental perspective. In KN Dwivedi, PB Harper (eds) *Promoting the Emotional Well-Being of Children and Adolescents and Preventing their Mental Ill Health*. London: Jessica Kingsley Publishers.
39. Ainsworth M, Blehar M, Waters E, Wall S (1978) *Patterns of Attachment: Assessed in the Strange Situation and at Home*. Hillsdale, NJ: Lawrence Erlbaum Associates.
40. Kobak R, Sudler N, Gamble W (1991) Attachment and depressive symptoms during adolescence: a developmental pathway analysis. *Development and Psychopathology* **3**: 461–74.
41. Cassidy J, Berlin LJ (1994) The insecure/ambivalent pattern of attachment; theory and research. *Child Development* **65**: 971–91.
42. Hodges J, Tizard B (1989) Social and family relationships of ex-institutionalised adolescents. *Journal of Child Psychology and Psychiatry* **30**: 77–97.
43. LeVine RA, New RS (eds) (2008) *Anthropology and Child Development*. Malden, MA: Blackwell.
44. Green J, Goldwyn R (2002) Annotation: attachment disorganization and psychopathology: new findings in attachment research and their potential implications for developmental psychopathology in childhood. *Journal of Child Psychology and Psychiatry* **43**: 835–46.
45. Van IJzendoorn MH, Schuengel C, Bakermans-Kranenberg MJ (1999) Disorganised attachment in early childhood: meta-analysis of precursors, concomitants and sequelae. *Development and Psychopathology* **11**: 225–49.
46. Dwivedi KN (1993) Conceptual frameworks. In KN Dwivedi (ed.) *Group Work with Children and Adolescents*. London: Jessica Kingsley Publishers.
47. World Health Organization (1992) *The ICD-10 Classification of Mental and Behavioural Disorders*. Geneva: World Health Organization.
48. Black D (2002) Bereavement. In M Rutter, E Taylor (eds) *Child and Adolescent Psychiatry*, 4th edn. Oxford: Blackwell.
49. Glaser D (2000) Child abuse and neglect and the brain: a review. *Journal of Child Psychology and Psychiatry* **41**: 97–116.
50. Mrazek D (2002) Psychiatric aspects of somatic diseases. In M Rutter, E Taylor (eds) *Child and Adolescent Psychiatry*, 4th edn. Oxford: Blackwell.
51. Rutter M, Graham P, Yule W (1970) *A Neuropsychiatric Study in Childhood*. London: Heinemann.
52. American Psychiatric Association (1994) *Diagnostic and Statistical Manual of Mental Disorders*, 4th edn. Washington, DC: American Psychiatric Association.
53. Rutter M, Quinton D (1977) Psychiatric disorder: ecological factors and concepts in causation. In H McGurk (ed.) *Ecological Factors in Human Development*. Amsterdam: North-Holland.
54. Richman N, Stevenson J, Graham P (1982) *Preschool to School: A Behavioural Study*. London: Academic Press.
55. Fonagy P, Target M, Cottrell D, Phillips J, Kurtz Z (2002) *What Works For Whom? A Critical Review of Treatments for Children and Adolescents*. New York: Guilford Press.
56. Meltzer H, Gatward R, Goodman R, Ford T (2000) *Mental Health of Children and Adolescents in Great Britain*. London: The Stationery Office.

57. Fergusson D, Horwood J, Lynsky M (1997) Children and adolescents. In PM Ellis, SC Collings (eds) *Mental Health in New Zealand from a Public Health Perspective*. Wellington: Ministry of Health.
58. Fergusson D, Horwood J (2001) The Christchurch Health and Development Study: review of findings on child and adolescent mental health. *Australian and New Zealand Journal of Psychiatry* 35: 287–96.
59. Fergusson D, Poulton R, Horwood J, Miln B, Swain-Campbell N (2003) *Comorbidity and Coincidence in the Christchurch and Dunedin Longitudinal Studies*. Wellington: Ministry of Social Development, Department of Labour and the Treasury.
60. Timimi S (2005) *Naughty Boys: Anti-Social Behaviour, ADHD, and the Role of Culture*. Basingstoke: Palgrave Macmillan.
61. Joseph J (2006) *The Missing Gene: Psychiatry, Heredity, and the Fruitless Search For Genes*. New York: Algora.
62. Rutter M (2006) *Genes and Behaviour*. Oxford: Blackwell.
63. Pillai A, Patel V, Cardozo P, *et al.* (2008) Non-traditional lifestyles and prevalence of mental disorders in adolescents in Goa, India. *British Journal of Psychiatry* 192: 45–51.
64. Cederbald M (1988) Behavioural disorders in children from different cultures. *Acta Psychiatrica Scandinavica* 78: 85–92.
65. Cederbald M, Rahim I (1986) Effects of rapid urbanization on child behaviour and health in a part of Khartoum, Sudan. *Social Science and Medicine* 22: 713–21.
66. Prout A, James A (eds) (1997) *Constructing and Reconstructing Childhood: Contemporary Issues in the Sociological Study of Childhood*. London: Falmer Press.
67. Kakar S (1994) *The Inner World of the Indian Child*. New Delhi: Oxford University Press.
68. Gregg GS (2005) *The Middle East: A Cultural Psychology*. New York: Oxford University Press.
69. Segal U (1992) Child abuse in India: an empirical report on perceptions. *Child Abuse and Neglect* 16: 887–908.
70. Beckett C (2005) The Swedish myth: corporal punishment ban and child death statistics. *British Journal of Social Work* 35: 125–38.
71. UNICEF (2001) *A League Table of Child Deaths By Injury in Rich Nations*. Innocenti report card no. 2. Florence: UNICEF Innocenti Research Centre.
72. Maitra B (1996) Child abuse: a universal diagnostic category? *International Journal of Social Psychiatry* 42: 287–304.
73. Browne K (2002) Child Protection. In M Rutter, E Taylor (eds) *Child and Adolescent Psychiatry*, 4th edn. Oxford: Blackwell.
74. Department of Health (1995) *Child Protection: Messages from Research*. London: HMSO.
75. Finkelhor D (1984) *Child Sexual Abuse*. New York: Free Press.
76. Maziade M (1989) Should adverse temperament matter to the clinician? An empirically based answer. In GA Khonstamm, VE Bates, MK Rothbart (eds) *Temperament in Childhood*. New York: John Wiley & Sons.
77. Offord DR, Boyle MC, Racine YA (1991) The epidemiology of antisocial behaviour in childhood and adolescence. In DJ Pepler, KH Rubin (eds) *The Development and Treatment of Childhood Aggression*. Hillsdale, NJ: Lawrence Erlbaum Associates.
78. Fergusson D, Horwood J, Lynskey M (1993) Prevalence and comorbidity of DSM-III-R diagnoses in a birth cohort of 15 year olds. *Journal of the American Academy of Child and Adolescent Psychiatry* 32: 1127–34.
79. Bird H, Canino G, Rubio-Stipec M (1988) Estimates of the prevalence of childhood maladjustment in a community survey in Puerto Rico: the use of combined measures. *Archives of General Psychiatry* 45: 1120–26.
80. Dunnachie B (2007) *Evidence-based Age-Appropriate Interventions: A Guide for Child and Adolescent Mental Health Services (CAMHS)*. Auckland: The Werry Centre for Child and Adolescent Mental Health Workforce Development.
81. Patterson GR, Guillon ME (1968) *Living With Children: New Methods for Parents and Teachers*. Champaign, IL: Research Press.
82. Webster-Stratton C (1994) Advanced videotape parenting training: a comparison study. *Journal of Consulting and Clinical Psychology* 62: 583–93.
83. Alexander JF, Parsons BV (1982) *Functional Family Therapy*. Monterey, CA: Brooks-Cole.
84. Hengeller SW, Borduin CM (1990) *Family Therapy and Beyond: A Multi-Systemic Approach to Treating the Behaviour Problems of Children and Adolescents*. Pacific Grove, CA: Brooks-Cole.
85. Sells S (2001) *Parenting Your Out of Control Teenager: Seven Steps to Reestablish Authority and Reclaim Love*. New York: St Martin's Press.
86. Robins LN (1996) *Deviant Children Grown Up*. Baltimore, MD: Williams & Wilkins.
87. Loeber R (1988) Natural histories of conduct problems, delinquency, and associated substance use: evidence for developmental progressions. In BB Lahey, AE Kazdin (eds) *Advances in Clinical Child Psychology*, Vol. 11. New York: Plenum Press.
88. Farrington DP (1995) The development of offending and antisocial behaviour from childhood: key findings from the Cambridge study in delinquent development. *Journal of Child Psychology and Psychiatry* 36: 929–64.
89. Walraich ML, Hannah JN, Baumgaertel A, Feurer ID (1998) Examination of DSM-IV criteria for attention deficit/hyperactivity disorder in a country-wide

sample. *Journal of Developmental and Behavioral Pediatrics* **19**: 162–8.

90. Danckaerts M, Taylor E (1995) The epidemiology of childhood hyperactivity. In FC Verhulst, HM Koot (eds) *The Epidemiology of Child and Adolescent Psychiatry.* Oxford: Oxford University Press.
91. Szatmari P, Offord DR, Boyle MH (1989) Ontario child health study: prevalence of attention deficit disorder with hyperactivity. *Journal of Child Psychology and Psychiatry* **30**: 219–30.
92. Willcutt EG, Pennington BF, Olsen RK, *et al.* (2007) Understanding comorbidity: a twin study of reading disability and attention-deficit/hyperactivity disorder. *American Journal of Medical Genetics* **144B**: 709–14.
93. Fletcher KE, Fischer M, Barkley RA, *et al.* (1996) A sequential analysis of the mother–adolescent interactions of ADHD, ADHD/ODD, and normal teenagers during neutral and conflict discussions. *Journal of Abnormal Child Psychology* **24**: 271–97.
94. Green H, McGinnity A, Meltzer H, *et al.* (2005) *Mental Health of Children and Young People in Great Britain.* Basingstoke: Palgrave Macmillan.
95. Biederman J, Newcorn J, Sprich S (1991) Comorbidity of attention deficit hyperactivity disorder with conduct, depressive, anxiety and other disorders. *American Journal of Psychiatry* **148**: 564–77.
96. Jensen PS, Hinshaw SP, Kraemer HC, *et al.* (2001) ADHD comorbidity findings from the MTA study: comparing comorbid sub groups. *Journal of the American Academy of Child and Adolescent Psychiatry* **43**: 792–801.
97. Timimi S (2008) Child psychiatry and its relationship to the pharmaceutical industry: theoretical and practical issues. *Advances in Psychiatric Treatment* **14**: 3–9.
98. Biederman J, Faraone S, Milberger S, *et al.* (1996) Predictors of persistence and remission of ADHD into adolescence: results from a four-year prospective follow-up study. *Journal of the American Academy of Child and Adolescent Psychiatry* **35**: 343–51.
99. Heyne D, King NJ, Tonge BJ, Cooper H (2001) School refusal: epidemiology and management. *Paediatric Drugs* **3**: 719–32.
100. Rutter M, Maughan B, Mortimore P, *et al.* (1982) *Fifteen Thousand Hours: Secondary Schools and Their Effects on Children.* Boston, MA: Harvard University Press.
101. Elliott JG (1999) School refusal: Issues of conceptualisation, assessment and treatment. *Journal of Child Psychology and Psychiatry* **40**: 1001–12.
102. Klein DF, Mannuzza S, Chapman T, Fyer AJ (1992) Child panic revisited. *Journal of the American Academy of Child and Adolescent Psychiatry* **31**: 112–16.
103. Garrison CZ, Bryant ES, Addy CL (1995) Posttraumatic stress disorder in adolescents after Hurricane Andrew. *Journal of the American Academy of Child and Adolescent Psychiatry* **34**: 1193–201.
104. Berman SL, Kurtines WM, Silverman WK, Serafini LT (1996) The impact of exposure to crime and violence on urban youth. *American Journal of Orthopsychiatry* **66**: 329–36.
105. Gerralda E (2003) Somatization and somatoform disorders. In D Skuse (ed.) *Child Psychology and Psychiatry: An Introduction.* Abingdon: Medicine Publishing Company.
106. Fong G, Gerralda E (2003) Anxiety disorders. In D Skuse (ed.) *Child Psychology and Psychiatry: An Introduction.* Abingdon: Medicine Publishing Company.
107. Last CG, Perrin S, Hersen M, Kazdin AE (1992) DSM-III-R anxiety disorders in children: sociodemographic and clinical characteristics. *Journal of the American Academy of Child and Adolescent Psychiatry* **31**: 1070–76.
108. Last CG, Hersen M, Kazdin AE, *et al.* (1992) Comparison of DSM-III separation anxiety and overanxious disorders: demographic characteristics and patterns of comorbidity. *Journal of the American Academy of Child and Adolescent Psychiatry* **26**: 527–31.
109. Dwivedi KN, Varma VP (eds) (1997) *A Handbook of Childhood Anxiety Management.* Aldershot: Arena.
110. Lewinsohn PM, Hops H, Roberts RE, *et al.* (1993) Adolescent psychopathology: I. Prevalence and incidence of depression and other DSM-III-R disorders in high school students. *Journal of Abnormal Psychology* **102**: 133–44.
111. Lewinsohn PM, Rohde P, Klein D, Seeley JR (1999) Natural course of adolescent major depressive disorder: I. Continuity into young adulthood. *Journal of the American Academy of Child and Adolescent Psychiatry* **38**: 56–63.
112. American Academy of Child and Adolescent Psychiatry (1998) Practice parameters for the assessment and treatment of children and adolescent with depressive disorders. *Journal of the American Academy of Child and Adolescent Psychiatry* **37**: 63–83S.
113. Timimi S (2004) Rethinking childhood depression. *British Medical Journal* **329**: 1394–6.
114. Jaffee S, Moffitt T, Caspi A (2002) Early childhood risk factors for juvenile-onset and adult-onset depression. *Archives of General Psychiatry* **59**: 215–22.
115. Dwivedi KN, Varma VP (eds) (1997) *Depression in Children and Adolescents.* London: Whurr.
116. Tsapakis E, Soldani F, Tondo L, Baldessarini R (2008) Efficacy of antidepressants in juvenile depression. *British Journal of Psychiatry* **193**: 10–17.
117. Timimi S (2007) Should young people be given antidepressants? No. *British Medical Journal* **335**: 751.
118. National Institute for Health and Clinical Excellence (2005) *Depression in Children and Young People.* Clinical guideline 28. London: National Institute for Health and Clinical Excellence.

119. Fombonne E, Wostear G, Cooper V, *et al.* (2001) The Maudsley long-term follow-up of child and adolescent depression 2: suicide, criminality and social dysfunction in adulthood. *British Journal of Psychiatry* **179**: 218–23.
120. Heyman I, Fombonne E, Simmons H, *et al.* (2001) Prevalence of obsessive–compulsive disorder in the British nationwide survey of child mental health. *British Journal of Psychiatry* **179**: 324–9.
121. Rosenberg DR, Hanna GL (2000) Genetic and imaging strategies in obsessive–compulsive disorder: potential implications for treatment development. *Biological Psychiatry* **48**: 1210–22.
122. Maskey S (2003) Obsessive–compulsive disorder. In D Skuse (ed.) *Child Psychology and Psychiatry: An Introduction.* Abingdon: Medicine Publishing Company.
123. Swedo SC, Rapoport JL, Leonard HI, Lenane M (1989) Obsessive–compulsive disorder in children and adolescents: clinical phenomenology of 70 consecutive cases. *Archives of General Psychiatry* **46**: 335–41.
124. Wewetzer C, Jans T, Muller B, *et al.* (2001) Long-term outcome and prognosis of obsessive–compulsive disorder with onset in childhood or adolescence. *European Child and Adolescent Psychiatry* **10**: 37–46.
125. Maskey S (2003) Schizophrenia. In D Skuse (ed.) *Child Psychology and Psychiatry: An Introduction.* Abingdon: Medicine Publishing Company.
126. Nicolson R, Lenane M, Singaracharlu S, *et al.* (2000) Pre-morbid speech and language impairments in childhood-onset schizophrenia: association with risk factors. *American Journal of Psychiatry* **157**: 794–800.
127. Moncrieff J (2008) *The Myth of the Chemical Cure.* Basingstoke: Palgrave Macmillan.
128. Read J, Mosher LR, Bentall RP (eds) (2004) *Models of Madness.* Hove: Brunner/Routledge.
129. Hollis C (2000) Adult outcomes of child and adolescent onset schizophrenia: diagnostic stability and predictive validity. *American Journal of Psychiatry* **157**: 1652–9.
130. Fombonne E (1995) Eating disorders: time trends and possible explanatory mechanisms. In M Rutter, D Smith (eds) *Psychosocial Disorders in Young People: Time Trends and their Causes.* Chichester: John Wiley & Sons.
131. Gowers S, Crisp A, Joughin N, Bhat A (1991) Premenarchal anorexia nervosa. *Journal of Child Psychology and Psychiatry* **32**: 515–24.
132. Gowers S (2005) Eating disorders. In S Gowers (ed.) *Seminars in Child and Adolescent Psychiatry.* London: Gaskell.
133. Byford S, Barrett B, Roberts C, *et al.* (2007) Economic evaluation of a randomised controlled trial for anorexia nervosa in adolescents. *British Journal of Psychiatry* **191**: 436–40.
134. North CD, Gowers S, Byram V (1997) Family functioning and life events in the outcome of adolescent anorexia nervosa. *British Journal of Psychiatry* **171**: 545–9.
135. Herpertz-Dahlmann B, Muller B, Herpertz S, *et al.* (2001) Prospective 10 year follow up in adolescent anorexia nervosa: course, outcome, psychiatric morbidity, and psychosocial adaptation. *Journal of Child Psychology and Psychiatry* **42**: 603–12.
136. Shaffer D, Gutstein J (2002) Suicide and attempted suicide. In M Rutter, E Taylor (eds) *Child and Adolescent Psychiatry*, 4th edn. Oxford: Blackwell.
137. Centres for Disease Control (1999) Youth risk behaviour surveillance: United States 1999. *Morbidity and Mortality Weekly Report* **49**: 1–96.
138. Weinberg WA, Harper CR, Brumback RA (2002) Substance use and abuse: epidemiology, pharmacological considerations, identification and suggestions towards management. In M Rutter, E Taylor (eds) *Child and Adolescent Psychiatry*, 4th edn. Oxford: Blackwell.
139. Tsuang MT, Lyons MJ, Meyer JM, *et al.* (1998) Co-occurrence of abuse of different drugs in men: the role of drug specific and shared vulnerabilities. *Archives of General Psychiatry* **55**: 967–72.
140. Lamb C (2005) Substance misuse. In S Gowers (ed.) *Seminars in Child and Adolescent Psychiatry.* London: Gaskell.
141. Fergusson D, Horwood J (1997) Early onset cannabis use and psychosocial adjustment in young adults. *Addiction* **92**: 279–96.
142. Birch HG, Richardson SA, Baird D, *et al.* (1970) *Mental Subnormality in the Community: A Clinical and Epidemiological Study.* Baltimore, MD: Williams & Wilkins.
143. Tong BJ (1999) Psychopathology of children with developmental disorders. In N Bouras (ed.) *Psychiatric and Behavioural Disorders in Developmental Disabilities and Mental Retardation.* Cambridge: Cambridge University Press.
144. Volkmar FR, Dykens E (2002) Mental retardation. In M Rutter, E Taylor (eds) *Child and Adolescent Psychiatry*, 4th edn. Oxford: Blackwell.
145. Nation K (2003) Developmental language disorders. In D Skuse (ed.) *Child Psychology and Psychiatry: An Introduction.* Abingdon: Medicine Publishing Company.
146. Snowling M (2003) Specific learning difficulties. In D Skuse (ed.) *Child Psychology and Psychiatry: An Introduction.* Abingdon: Medicine Publishing Company.
147. Morss JR (1990) *The Biologising of Childhood: Developmental Psychology and the Darwinian Myth.* Hove: Lawrence Erlbaum Associates.
148. Cantwell DP, Baker L (1991) *Psychiatric and Developmental Disorders in Children with Communication Disorders.* Washington, DC: American Psychiatric Press.

149. Cohen NJ, Menna R, Vallance DD, *et al.* (1998) Language, social cognitive processing, and behavioural characteristics of psychiatrically disturbed children with previously identified and unsuspected language impairments. *Journal of Child Psychology and Psychiatry and Allied Disciplines* **39**: 853–64.
150. Shaywitz SE, Escobar MD, Shaywitz BA, *et al.* (1992) Evidence that dyslexia may represent the lower tail of a normal distribution of reading ability. *New England Journal of Medicine* **326**: 145–50.
151. Bishop DVM, Edmundson A (1987) Language-impaired four year olds: distinguishing transient from persistent impairment. *Journal of Speech and Hearing Research* **52**: 156–73.
152. Chakrabarti S, Fombonne E (2001) pervasive developmental disorders in preschool children. *Journal of the American Medical Association* **285**: 3093–9.
153. National Autistic Society (2008) Autism: What is it? www.nas.org.uk/autism.
154. Rutter M, Andersen-Wood L, Beckett C, *et al.* (1999) Quasi-autistic patterns following severe early global privation. *Journal of Child Psychology and Psychiatry and Allied Disciplines* **40**: 537–49.
155. Timimi S (2007) Autism in context. In A Hosen (ed.) *Typical or Atypical Development? Child Psychiatry and Applied Psychology Perspectives.* New York: Edwin Mellen Press.
156. Nadesan M (2005) *Constructing Autism: Unravelling the 'Truth' and Understanding the Social.* London: Routledge.
157. Butler RJ (1998) Annotation: night wetting in children – psychological aspects. *Journal of Child Psychology and Psychiatry* **39**: 453–63.
158. Bakwin H (1971) Enuresis in twins. *American Journal of Diseases of Children* **121**: 225.
159. Clayden G, Taylor E, Loader P, *et al.* (2002) Wetting and soiling in children. In M Rutter, E Taylor (eds) *Child and Adolescent Psychiatry*, 4th edn. Oxford: Blackwell.
160. White M (1989) Pseudoencopresis: from avalanche to victory, from vicious to virtuous circles. In M White (ed.) *Selected Papers.* Adelaide: Dulwich Centre Publications.
161. Levine MD, Bakow H (1976) Children with encopresis: a study of treatment outcome. *Pediatrics* **58**: 845–52.
162. Zohar AH, Apter A, King RA, *et al.* (1998) Epidemiological studies. In JF Leckman, JD Cohen (eds) *Tourette Syndrome, Tics, Obsessions, Compulsions: Developmental Psychopathology and Clinical Care.* New York: John Wiley & Sons.
163. Apter A, Pauls D, Bleich A, *et al.* (1993) An epidemiological study of Gilles de la Tourette syndrome in Israel. *Archives of General Psychiatry* **50**: 734–8.
164. Robertson MM (2003) Tourette syndrome. In D Skuse (ed.) *Child Psychology and Psychiatry: An Introduction.* Abingdon: Medicine Publishing Company.
165. Leckman JF, Zhang H, Vitale A, *et al.* (1998) Course of tic severity in Tourette syndrome: the first two decades. *Pediatrics* **102**: 14–19.
166. Depner CE, Leino EV, Chun A (1992) Interparental conflict and child adjustment: a decade review and meta-analysis. *Family and Conciliation Courts Review* **30**: 323–41.
167. Davies PT, Windle M (1997) Gender specific pathways between maternal depressive symptoms, family discord, and adolescent adjustment. *Developmental Psychology* **33**: 657–68.
168. McNeil C, Amato P (1998) Parents' marital violence: long-term consequences for children. *Journal of Family Issues* **19**: 123–39.
169. Newman DL, Moffitt TE, Caspi A, *et al.* (1996) Psychiatric disorder in a birth cohort of young adults: prevalence, comorbidity, clinical significance, and new case incidence from ages 11 to 21. *Journal of Consulting and Clinical Psychology* **64**: 552–62.
170. Pine DS, Cohen P, Gurley D, *et al.* (1998) The risk for early-adulthood anxiety and depressive disorders in adolescents with anxiety and depressive disorders. *Archives of General Psychiatry* **55**: 56–64.
171. Woodward LJ, Fergusson DM (2001) Life course outcomes of young people with anxiety disorders in adolescence. *Journal of the American Academy of Child and Adolescent Psychiatry* **40**: 1086–93.
172. Fombonne E, Wostear G, Cooper V, *et al.* (2001) The Maudsley long-term follow-up of child and adolescent depression 1: psychiatric outcomes in adulthood. *British Journal of Psychiatry* **179**: 210–17.
173. Fombonne E, Wostear G, Cooper V, *et al.* (2001) The Maudsley long-term follow-up of child and adolescent depression 2: suicide, criminality and social dysfunction in adulthood. *British Journal of Psychiatry* **179**: 218–23.
174. Fergusson DM, Woodward LJ (2002) Mental health, educational, and social role outcomes of adolescents with depression. *Archives of General Psychiatry* **59**: 225–31.
175. March JS, Leonard HL (1996) Obsessive-compulsive disorder in children and adolescents: a review of the past 10 years. *Journal of the American Academy of Child and Adolescent Psychiatry* **35**: 1265–73.
176. Mannuzza S, Klein RG (2000) Long-term prognosis in attention-deficit/hyperactivity disorder. *Child and Adolescent Psychiatric Clinics of North America* **9**: 711–26.
177. Moffitt TE, Caspi A (2001) Childhood predictors differentiate life-course persistent and adolescence-limited antisocial pathways: follow-up at age 26 years. *Developmental Psychopathology* **13**: 355–75.
178. Timimi S (2006) Childhood depression? In S Timimi, B Maitra (eds) *Critical Voices in Child and Adolescent Mental Health.* London: Free Association Books.
179. Sparks JA, Duncan BL (2008) Do no harm: a critical

risk/benefit analysis of child psychotropic medication. *Journal of Family Psychotherapy* **19**: 1–19.

180. Jensen P, Arnold E, Swanson J, *et al.* (2007) 3 year follow-up of the NIMH MTA study. *Journal of the American Academy of Child and Adolescent Psychiatry* **46**: 988–1001.
181. McDonagh MS, Peterson K (2005) *Drug Class Review on Pharmacologic Treatments for ADHD*. Portland, OR: Oregon Health and Science University.
182. Wong IC, Murray ML, Camilleri-Novak D, *et al.* (2004) Increased prescribing trends of paediatric psychotropic medications. *Archives of Disease in Childhood* **89**: 1131–2.
183. Leckman JF, King RA (2007) A developmental perspective on the controversy surrounding the use of SSRIs to treat pediatric depression. *American Journal of Psychiatry* **164**: 1304–6.
184. APA Working Group on Psychoactive Medications for Children and Adolescents (2006) *Report of the Working Group on Psychoactive Medications for Children and Adolescents: Psychopharmacological, Psychosocial, and Combined Interventions for Childhood Disorders – Evidence Base, Contextual Factors, and Future Directions*. Washington, DC: American Psychological Association.
185. Maskey S (2003) In-patient units. In D Skuse (ed.) *Child Psychology and Psychiatry: An Introduction*. Abingdon: Medicine Publishing Company.

Chapter 71

Learning disability psychiatry

Mark Dickinson and Iqbal Singh

INTRODUCTION

There have always been people with learning disability. The effect such a disability will have on an individual will be determined to some extent by the degree of the disability, interacting with family support, opportunities, and the level of sophistication demanded by the society in which they live. It is likely that industrialization and ever-increasing competition have made it progressively more difficult for people with learning disability to fit in and succeed in the UK without help, although the availability and quality of help has improved considerably over the same time.

Current provision for people with learning disability is organized in England on a borough-wide basis (approximate populations of 250 000), with considerable budgets coming from the local authority and the National Health Service (NHS) to offer all kinds of support, in addition to central government funding via channels such as housing benefit. The learning disability budgets of these boroughs are substantial (many tens of millions of pounds annually), of which a small proportion is spent on local specialist health teams.

There has been a revolution in the model of care for people with learning disability in the past 30 years. It has always been the case that the majority of these peoples' needs have been met by families; however, situations inevitably arise requiring the support of statutory services. This may be secondary to difficult behaviour (possibly related to psychiatric illness), the death of parents, a desire to be independent, or other factors.

In the 1960s, and many years before, the standard model of statutory care was institutionalization in one of the giant (1000+ beds) hospitals built by the Victorians and situated on the periphery of large cities and towns. Various legislation since this time, including Better Services for the Mentally Handicapped[1] and Valuing People,[2] along with the effect of scandals relating to standards of care in these institutions and coupled with a more liberal attitude, have resulted in the complete closure of almost all these buildings, with a shift of care into the community.

As a result, people with learning disability who are not living with their parents or family and who require additional support now live in flats, small group homes or small hostels, or with adult carers. Support is available from paid carers, and many organizations have sprung up to provide such support, the level and amount being tailored to the needs of the individual, from a carer visiting on a weekly basis to assist with bills and budgeting, to having 24-h support from two or more carers. Imaginative packages of care are available; for example, an individual with learning disability can continue to live in their family home following the death of their parents, with daily live-in support from a care provider 24 h a day, 7 days a week, the carer sharing the house with the service user. Some of these care packages are extremely expensive, and it remains to be seen whether tax payers and governments will be prepared to continue to fund increasingly expensive options.

Further attempts have been made at social integration, with some success, although it still remains very difficult for a person with a learning disability to hold down a job on the open market, find a partner, get married or have children. It is very uncommon for a person with learning disability to afford, own or use private transport, something hugely valued by people without learning disability. Being slow, particularly in busy places such as cities, meets with very low tolerance, and being different at school may result in bullying. There are opportunities for many interesting day activities and college courses, and some sheltered and voluntary work schemes, but it remains difficult for a person with a learning disability to interact with the rest of society in a meaningful way.

The attitude of society to people with learning disability can be seen as ambivalent. On the one hand, people with Down syndrome may be hugely valued by their families and admired in general through successful national organizations such as the Chicken Shed Theatre Company, while at the same time scientific effort is spent by the same society to perfect prenatal diagnosis of fetuses with the condition so that termination can be offered to parents.

Along with the push towards integration, there has been a similar push for people with learning disability to have full access to the health services available to everyone else. At its most basic level, this means being registered with a general practitioner (GP). It is also required that physicians, surgeons, dentists and other specialist health professionals should be able to successfully treat people with learning disability with expectations as high as those of anyone else, while recognizing that extra input may be required, including issues around increased health need, difficulties in obtaining a history in someone who is non-verbal, performing investigations when the subject does not wish to cooperate, and considering issues such as consent.[3]

There remain limited specialist health services for people with learning disability, in the main organized on a borough-wide basis and usually based in a combined team with social services (forensic, psychotherapeutic and a few other specialist services may be regional). Typically, this specialist health team comprises a small number of psychiatrists (one or two being consultants), a few nurses, occupational therapists, psychologists, speech and language therapists and psychotherapy services (including music, drama and art therapies, and often aimed at people who have limited verbal skills). The complement of a borough-wide health team may be between 10 and 30 individuals, sometimes backed up by a limited number of specialist learning disability psychiatry admission beds (approximately six per district, the private sector providing admission services where none are available locally through the NHS). The age range served is typically 18–65 years, although a few services see children and most services continue to be involved in the care of more elderly people whom they have known for a long time.

Psychiatric illness in people with learning disability is common. Problems of definition make exact figures difficult, but there is probably at least double the prevalence in this group compared with the rest of the population.[4] In addition, the most common behaviour type, challenging behaviour,[5] is largely peculiar to this group. Medicines used by psychiatrists are the same as those used in the general population, although doses prescribed are often smaller due to existing brain damage and sensitivity to side effects. There are many specific syndromes and conditions associated with learning disability, each in turn having its own associations (e.g. Down syndrome and dementia). There is a large amount of epilepsy, probably 50 times the prevalence of that in the non-learning disabled population (rates increasing with greater brain injury and therefore increasing in more severely disabled people). People with learning disability require far more social support and input than non-learning disabled people and may also require extra help with daily living skills, finding employment, communication and many other issues that others take for granted, such as being able to check they are given the correct change at a shop. Research into learning disability is extremely important but is unlikely to be pursued by mainstream services.

The outlook for a person with a learning disability has improved considerably in the past 40 years. A better, longer and more interesting life should be expected, although the goal of real integration with society remains, to some degree, elusive.

DEFINITION

It is important for learning disability services to be able to define who has a learning disability. Other specialist services, for example paediatrics, restrict their activity to their client group, who are easily characterized by age. Whether someone has a learning disability can be far more subjective, and yet it is important to try to make or exclude the diagnosis for various reasons, including the appropriateness of services for the individual, budgeting, and the fact that doubt may cause an individual to be ignored by all services; for example, at the interface between mental health and learning disability, unless a definite diagnosis is made, and in the context of stretched services, both services may choose to assume that the other service is providing help, when in reality neither is.

The three criteria required to make a diagnosis of learning disability are:

- arrested or incomplete development of mind;
- difficulties in adaptive functioning;
- occurring within the developmental period.

The *International Classification of Diseases*, version 10 (ICD-10)[6] and the *Diagnostic and Statistical Manual of Mental Disorders*, 4th edition (DSM-IV)[7] have similar definitions of learning disability, although ICD-10 mentions arrested or incomplete development of mind, which may be deduced from intelligence quotient (IQ) testing.[8,9] DSM-IV specifically mentions such testing, learning disability being suggested by an IQ of 70 or less (two standard deviations from the mean).

Both classifications also stress the importance of problems in adaptive functioning, implying that in certain situations a low IQ may not interfere with the person's ability to be independent in activities of daily living, including washing, cooking and travelling. Finally, both classifications require that the disability occurred during development (in DSM-IV, 'the onset is before 18 years').

IQ measures are certainly important and appear to correlate with various desirable social outcomes; for example, in the USA, higher IQ has been reported to be associated with higher earnings, less chance of imprisonment, lower unemployment and less chance of divorce. These are clearly averages, but they do not necessarily apply to a specific individual. In addition, other factors are important when looking at ultimate performance, for example the ability to concentrate for a prolonged period of time and the amount of determination put towards completing a task. IQ seems to give some sort of indication of the potential an individual has of completing a novel task, but it cannot indicate whether that potential will be used in the real world.

The average IQ of a population is 100, the standard deviation ± 15 points and the standard error 5 points (Figure 71.1). IQ is normally distributed, but with a slight bulge in the lower IQ range. IQ is thought to be inherited through

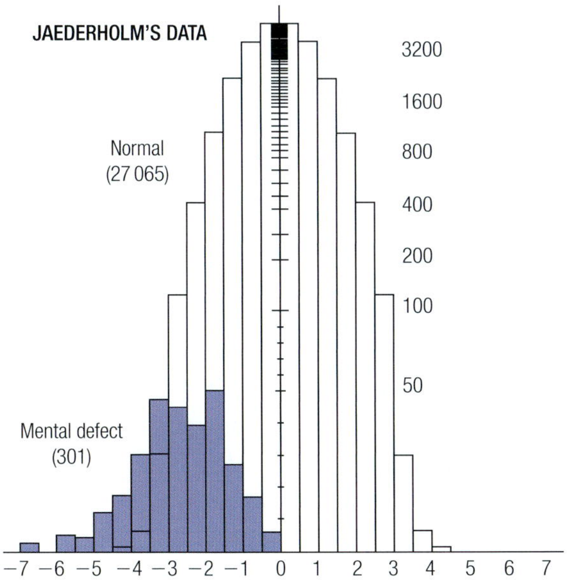

Figure 71.1 Distribution of intelligence quotient (IQ)

multiple genes, in a similar way to height, accounting for the normal distribution. The effect of upbringing on IQ, which may be significant, presumably also operates in a fairly random way and therefore also leads to a normal distribution of scores. The bulge at the lower range is then caused by specific abnormalities, such as Down syndrome and fragile X syndrome.

Ability to socialize is probably as important as IQ when considering the capability of a person to exist in society. In this respect, there has been recent interest in the concept of emotional intelligence.[10]

The population mean IQ score is 100. Two standard deviations from the mean represents approximately 5 per cent of the population and is made up of people with an IQ above 130 and below 70. Therefore, approximately 2.5 per cent of the population has an IQ in the learning disability range. This number is increased by approximately a further tenth (0.25%), representing people with congenital causes for their low IQ (e.g. Down syndrome, fragile X syndrome). On IQ testing, therefore, almost 3 per cent of a population might be expected to have an IQ in the learning disability range. This figure is different from that found in population studies on the prevalence of learning disability, often coming out at about 1 per cent.

The difference may be explained in various ways. Low IQ may not always be associated with problems in adaptive functioning, people with learning disability may not be 'picked up' by services, there may be greater mortality in the low IQ group, and some people with low IQ will not have a learning disability because their problem (e.g. brain injury following a road traffic accident) occurred after the developmental period.

Specialist learning disability services may have a maximum of 1000 patients on their lists in an average borough, representing less than 0.5 per cent of the total population. This low percentage is probably explained by the reasons stated above and the likelihood that many people with an IQ in the learning disability range either look after themselves or are cared for by their families and never come to the attention of specialist services.

Within the learning disability group, further categories are sometimes used, defined to some extent by IQ. 'Mild' learning disability covers approximately 80 per cent of this population and spans an IQ range from 70 to 50. A person with mild learning disability might be expected to have minimal or no physical or sensory problems, to hold down sheltered employment, and to survive with limited support. 'Moderate' learning disability spans an IQ range between 50 and 35 and represents approximately 10 per cent of people with learning disability. These people may be able to help with personal care and travel independently in familiar places, but they require greater levels of support at home. 'Severe' and 'profound' learning disability (IQ ranges 35–20 and 20 or less, respectively) make up the remainder. These people require higher levels of support and may suffer from various physical problems, including epilepsy.[7]

DEVELOPMENT

The human brain develops from ectodermal tissue and, unlike in other species, continues to do so after birth. It reaches its maximum weight at about 10 years of age, with the major growth spurt taking place after birth.[11] There appear to be critical periods of development.[12] Early in pregnancy metabolic upsets or teratogens may produce malformations, while in the mid-trimester neuronal multiplication is at risk. From the last trimester up to 2 years after birth the brain growth spurt takes place, involving glial multiplication, dendritic arborization and synaptogenesis and a high rate of myelination. Poor conditions at any stage may prevent proper brain development, including understimulation. This has been well demonstrated by Hubel and Wiesel,[13] who won the 1981 Nobel Prize for medicine and physiology for their work looking at the critical period for understimulation of cortical neurons in cats. The resulting effect was permanent change of cell function and appearance in the visual cortex.

There are various, somewhat predictable factors associated with problems in brain development, including maternal malnutrition,[14,15] excessive alcohol use[16] and possibly smoking.[17,18] Various drugs taken by the mother may also cause problems for the fetal brain, of which anticonvulsants are particularly important.[19] Exposure to radiation and severe infection may also cause difficulties for the fetus.

Lack of a specific nutrient may result in a specific condition, for example congenital hypothyroidism associated with a lack of iodine. Alternatively, abnormally high levels of a chemical may damage cerebral function, as in phenylketonuria.

There are a number of well-recognized genetic causes of learning disability. These may involve whole chromosomes (and therefore a large number of genes), the most important being Down syndrome. Some learning disability is related to single gene abnormality on the X chromosome (fragile X syndrome[20]). There are also autosomal dominant abnormalities (tuberose sclerosis[21]) and autosomal recessive causes of learning disability (phenylketonuria[22]).

The essentially normally distributed IQ graph suggests multifactorial causes for the majority of people with learning disability, probably caused by the interactions of a number of genes working with various environmental hazards, some of which are listed above. A paper from Brazil describes magnetic resonance imaging (MRI) of 146 children with an IQ of less than 70.[23] Fifty per cent of the scans were reported as normal, while focal thinning at the junction and body of the splenium of the corpus callosum, ventricular asymmetry, periventricular leucomalacia, gliosis and arachnoid cysts were found in the other 50 per cent. Maternal stress and altered blood pressure were the most frequent prenatal findings in the mothers of these children.

A more comprehensive understanding of the genes that appear to be important in the development of learning disability is continually evolving with the identification of autosomal recessive non-syndromic mental retardation genes (ARNSMR).[24] In this context there are even reports of therapeutic interventions in animal models of mental retardation with 'medicines' designed to overcome these gene effects,[25] an example being the work of McBride and colleagues, who demonstrated that synaptic plasticity and courtship behaviour can be restored in a Drosophila model of fragile X syndrome by treatment with metabotropic glutamate receptor antagonist or lithium.[26] For the foreseeable future, however, it is very likely a significant although small proportion of people will be born with learning disability. The most acceptable intervention that may alter this proportion is prenatal care, particularly avoidance of recognized risk factors.

Table 71.1 lists some of the potential causes of learning disability.

Table 71.1 Potential causes of learning disability

Environmental	Consanguineous parents
	Fetal alcohol syndrome
	Anti-epileptics/other drugs taken by the mother in pregnancy
	Prematurity/difficult labour
	Serious infections as an infant, e.g. meningitis
Genetic	Whole gene: Down syndrome
	Autosomal dominant: tuberose sclerosis
	Autosomal recessive: phenylketonuria, mucopolysaccharide disorders (e.g. Sanfilippo syndrome), aspartylglycosaminuria
	Chance mutation/gene deletion: Prader–Willi syndrome

SOCIAL FACTORS

There are many difficulties to be faced by people with learning disability and their parents and carers. Parents may have to come to terms with sadness at the loss of a normally successful child and a real prospect that their son or daughter will never become fully independent. They may also be required to cope with possible burdens of social stigma, self-blame and many practical difficulties in relation to health. These burdens can be overwhelming and may result in a desire to put the child into social care, or they may put sufficient strain on the parents' relationships to precipitate parental separation. None of this is certain, however, and many parents cope superbly, offering an excellent quality of life to their son or daughter. Indeed, recent research has reported lower levels of divorce in families where there is a child with Down syndrome compared with families of children with other birth defects and those of children with no identifiable disability.[27,28]

Schooling may present further difficulties. In the UK, there are many special schools designed for people with learning or physical disabilities. The more recent trend has been to attempt education of people with learning disability in mainstream schools, with additional help. There is considerable controversy around this policy, demonstrated to some degree by looking at the online encyclopaedia Wikipedia. In September 2007, Wikipedia's entry on 'mainstreaming in education' comes with a warning that some statements may be 'disputed, incorrect, unverified, biased or otherwise objectionable'. We suspect this reflects the strongly held but conflicting views of people in relation to this idea. Nevertheless, the article considers advantages and disadvantages of mainstreaming. Possible advantages include increased expectations leading to improved achievements and fostering of better understanding and tolerance. Possible disadvantages are that people with learning disability may feel conspicuous and socially rejected by classmates and may disrupt the learning of their normal intelligence peers through diversion of teacher time and effort to them. Jones, considering the educational needs of people with autistic spectrum disorder, states that 'little rigorous research evidence exists to guide decisions for children with autistic spectrum disorder. This is true for educational practice generally, and for children with other special educational needs.'[29] It seems that, for example, people with Down syndrome may do well in mainstream schools at a very junior level, where their excellent social skills and emotional intelligence will allow integration, but they may require and be happier with transfer to a special school when intellectual demands and expectations increase.

In England the process by which a child with special educational needs receives the additional educational support they need is called 'statementing'. This is an assessment carried out by the local educational authority designed to determine the child's needs in school and what provision will be granted to that child. Possible outcomes include placement in a special school or additional one-to-one support in mainstream classes.

The home environment is very important in determining the later result of an inherited or environmental risk of learning disability, and it is likely that a stimulating home life will improve the IQ score,[30,31] regardless of where the individual is educated. Other factors, including diet, may also be important.

In the middle of the twentieth century, an idea became popular that 'refrigerator parents', particularly mothers, might be causing the devastating condition of autism in their offspring. These parents were thought to be emotionally cut off, cold, and unresponsive to their children, thereby creating an unhappy dull family environment and ultimately causing the social difficulties of their autistic sons and daughters.[32] Such ideas are now discredited. If parents of autistic children appear in any way strange or cut off, then this is much more likely to be due to the stress of caring for a person with autism, although it is recognized that some parents may have autistic traits themselves, which is likely with any partially genetically determined condition.[33,34]

It is becoming increasingly likely that the best treatment for autism, a syndrome with many possible causes and contributory factors, is intensive early intervention with something like social flooding. Children with autism avoid social contact if they can, possibly because of excessive anxiety, and may as a result become progressively cut off from everyone else, exacerbating their difficulties. Intensive social interaction started at as young an age as possible, and aimed at forcing social contact and integration, has been reported to be successful in the treatment of this very disabling condition, although perhaps because of the extremely intensive requirements of the programme (40+ h/week of individual therapy for a period of at least 2 years) it is not widely used or available.[35,36] Bearing in mind the extreme suffering and difficulties faced by people with autism, the lack of successful treatments and the effect it has on their parents and carers, it seems that this social intervention should receive better support than is currently the case.

PSYCHIATRIC DISORDERS IN LEARNING DISABILITY

There is an increased prevalence of psychiatric disorder in people with learning disability compared with the general population. Of crucial importance in making this statement is having some sort of definition of what 'learning disability' means. Professionals with a background in education may describe a person as having a significant or severe learning disability, while a professional from health might describe the same person as having a mild or borderline learning disability. As far as possible we will stick with the definition of learning disability as defined in DSM-IV and starting at an IQ of 70 or below.

Increased rates of psychiatric illness might be expected as a result of the brain damage itself that has caused the learning disability, coupled to a multitude of environmental factors, particularly important being bullying, abuse, loss of opportunities and loss of self-esteem. Difficulty with communication is also very important, causing frustration and anxiety, inability to make one's needs known, and inability to express that one is in pain. Some risk factors for mental illness may, in fact, be lower in people with learning disability compared with the general population, for example drug and alcohol abuse. Fortunately, suicide appears to be relatively rare among adults with learning disability, although suicidal behaviour has been reported to be increased in adolescents.[37]

Much of the information used to make a psychiatric diagnosis comes from what patients actually say. This is particularly important for symptoms relating to more serious psychiatric illness, such as delusional ideas, ideas of reference and hallucinations in schizophrenia. If the person is non-verbal, as may well be the case in severe or profound learning disability, assessment of these symptoms is not possible. In addition, it may be difficult for more able people with mild or moderate learning disability to understand questions related to these symptoms, and there is always the danger of people saying 'yes' because they either do not understand or wish to please.

In this context, the idea of change becomes very important. If, for example, a person who previously attended their day centre, appeared to enjoy it, and had always got up on time and been ready to go is now refusing to get on the morning bus, then something very important has changed. This may be secondary to physical illness or pain. It may be because the person's favourite carer at the day centre has left for another job, or the person now sits next to someone on the bus they do not like, or they are being bullied at the day centre by a new arrival. If, however, factors such as these can be largely excluded, then psychiatric illness is a possible cause of the behaviour change.

Further enquiries may then reveal a previous history of treatment for depression, possibly a positive family history, a more general loss of interest, and some biological changes, for example sleep disturbance plus loss of appetite and uncharacteristic tearfulness. Even in a non-verbal person, it might then be reasonable to consider depression and treatment with antidepressant medication, having first considered issues relating to capacity.

Unfortunately, in practice, it is unusual for the presentation to be so clear-cut. Non-specific behavioural change and difficult behaviour are far more common reasons for psychiatric referral and can be secondary to underlying psychiatric illness. Careful history-taking may elicit auditory hallucinations or delusions of control or reference, suggesting schizophrenia. Paranoid symptoms and catatonia have been reported to be seen more frequently in schizophrenia associated with more severe learning disability.[38,39] Mood disorders are probably relatively common in people with learning disability; rapid-cycling forms and anxiety disorders are also common. Compulsive behaviour may be secondary to an obsessive–compulsive illness or simply a feature of autism.

Biological symptoms are certainly very important in psychiatric diagnosis in learning disability. Weight loss and weight gain should be looked for, along with changes in sleep pattern. Aggression or self-injurious behaviour may sometimes be a symptom of depression, as recognized in the Diagnostic Criteria for Psychiatric Disorders for use with Adults with Learning Disabilities/Mental Retardation (DC-LD).[40] Sleep disturbance can be very important. Sleeping well at night in addition to somnolence during the day may suggest many things, but possibly that the dose of a sedative antipsychotic is too high. Poor sleep and daytime wakefulness may suggest an untreated psychotic process and medicines may be considered or, if already prescribed, the dose reviewed. Otherwise inexplicable changes in behaviour, for example loss of interest in activities or withdrawal, signal the possibility of psychiatric illness.

Table 71.2 summarizes psychiatric assessment in learning disability.

An article looking at the prevalence of psychiatric disorder in learning disability produced some interesting results.[4] First was a perhaps surprisingly low case rate for learning disability in their study population, of 3.3/1000 of the adult population. Of this, perhaps selected, group (who appear from the quoted figures to be less able than a more representative group of people with learning disability), mental ill health was identified in 41 per cent using clinical diagnosis, 35 per cent using DC-LD and 16 per cent using ICD-10 or DSM-IV. Almost all the difference in these rates can be explained by clinical diagnosis and DC-LD rating problem behaviours, which are not recorded by ICD-10 or DSM-IV.

Table 71.2 Psychiatric assessment in learning disability

- History from patient
- Examination
- Corroborative history, from parents, carers, etc.
- Other information, e.g. school reports, past hospital treatment, specialist units
- Investigations, e.g. routine bloods, EEG, head scans
- Specialist psychological testing
- Other specialist assessments, e.g. occupational therapy

EEG, electroencephalogram.

Challenging behaviour

Problem or challenging behaviours are very common in people with learning disability and may cause severe difficulties for the person with the behaviour, their carers and their environment. Perhaps in the general population people with severe challenging behaviour exist but are dealt with by the police and prisons. It seems likely, however, that challenging or problem behaviour is genuinely more common in people with learning disability compared with the general population, probably as a result of factors already mentioned, including bullying, loss of opportunities, difficulty in maintaining self-esteem and difficulties in communication. Another important factor at adolescence and beyond may be the inability of the person with learning disability to achieve independence from their parents and leave home. This coincides with maximum physical strength and can result in very difficult conflicts between children and parents, which in some respects are normal and resolved in the general population by the adolescent leaving home.

Whether challenging behaviour is eventually or helpfully viewed as an illness depends to some degree on whether there are predictable helpful treatments for the condition. Psychiatrists in learning disability are frequently consulted regarding problems of this nature. It is important to look at all possible causative factors when considering such behaviour and possible interventions.

Challenging behaviour is defined by the Challenging Behaviour Foundation (www.thecbf.org.uk) as:

> behaviour which may put themselves or others at risk, or which may prevent the use of ordinary community facilities or a normal home life. The behaviour may be in the form of aggression, self injury, stereotyped behaviour or disruptive and destructive behaviour.

There are a multitude of important considerations to be made during assessment and later when looking at a treatment plan. These include levels of staffing, day activities, social situation, loss and bereavements, physical health, medication side effects and epilepsy. Any of these may be involved in causing or maintaining the challenging behaviour.

At times, however, the challenging behaviour will be secondary to a psychiatric illness, which will require treatment in its own right. Although searching for possible causes and directing interventions at these causes is important, sometimes it may not be possible to significantly alter environmental factors, or none may be found. It may be that the behaviour is present in different environments, for example at the weekend when the child is home with the parents, during the week at the care home, and also at the day centre, suggesting that something relating to the individual is driving, for example, persistent screaming. In such situations, the prescription of medications may be considered, accepting that such prescribing is off-licence. The practice is certainly common in people with learning disability and based on remarkably little evidence.[41] Drugs used include antipsychotics, antidepressants, minor tranquillizers and mood stabilizers.

There have been small studies in the past looking at long-stay hospital populations (no longer particularly relevant, following the closure of these institutions), suggesting that zuclopenthixol and lithium may be helpful in the treatment of challenging behaviour in learning disability.[42,43] A more recent systematic review found only nine randomized controlled trials that could be used for analysis, providing no evidence as to whether antipsychotic medication helps or harms adults with learning disability and challenging behaviour.[44]

The Neuroleptics in Adults with Aggressive Challenging Behaviour and Intellectual Disability (NACHBID) study, organized by Imperial College, was published in 2008.[45] This is a randomized controlled trial looking at the use of risperidone, haloperidol and or placebo in the treatment of aggressive challenging behaviour in people with intellectual disability, examining short- and long-term outcomes of these various prescriptions. The study was faced with major problems in recruitment (86 people entered the research against the planned target of 144), and there may have been some selection bias. The results, however, are quite striking, with no advantage being seen in any of the three treatment groups at 4 weeks. The authors conclude that 'the routine prescription of antipsychotic drugs early in the management of aggressive challenging behaviour, even in low doses, should no longer be regarded as a satisfactory form of care'.[45]

Finally, one paper has reported that it is often possible to reduce antipsychotic medication use in people with learning disability who have been prescribed medication for behavioural problems. One-third of subjects in a mixed group of hospital and community patients were able to come off tablets in this study.[46] Numbers, however, were small and the researchers were not blind to the interventions.

Table 71.3 summarizes the treatments used in learning disability.

Table 71.3 Treatments in learning disability psychiatry

Social	Help with housing, employment and benefits
	Support package to the person's home
	Social outlets, clubs and holidays
	Day activities, e.g. day centres and colleges
Medical	Psychotherapy: supportive, psychodynamic family
	Drug treatments
	Specialist team input: community nurses, occupational therapy, psychology, specialist counselling (art therapy, music therapy), speech therapy (help with communication)
	Referral to other specialists, e.g. neurology

Other psychiatric diagnoses

Other psychiatric diagnoses will be made as in the general population, and similar treatments offered. The problem of diagnosing psychotic illness, particularly in people who are non-verbal, remains, and here reliance will have to be given to changes in behaviour and useful history, for example the presence of a positive family history of psychiatric illness. Symptoms that may be associated with psychotic illness in learning disability include behaviour change, verbal or physical aggression, social withdrawal, speaking to themselves (although this may be a normal habit), and pointing or swiping at things that other people cannot see. It may be that non-verbal forms of assessment are helpful in these situations, for example art or music therapy approaches.

Some assessment schedules are aimed at assisting in making a psychiatric diagnosis in people with learning disability, with well-recognized examples being the psychiatric assessment schedule for adults with developmental disabilities (PAS ADD) and mini-PAS ADD. The mini-PAS ADD can be administered quickly and gives an indication of psychiatric diagnosis in seven possible domains – depression, anxiety and phobias, mania, obsessive–compulsive disorder, psychosis, unspecified disorder (including dementia) and pervasive developmental disorder (autism). Both schedules require formal training before they can be used.[47,48] Other schedules include diagnostic assessment for the severely handicapped (DASH) and psychopathology inventory for mentally retarded adults (PIMRA).[49]

Whether psychological treatments, for example psychotherapy, are suitable for people with learning disability has been the subject of some debate. In the UK, this approach has been pioneered at the Tavistock Clinic in north London, considering issues such as loss, bereavements, sexual abuse and the effect on the individual of having a learning disability.[50]

If drug treatment is prescribed, then starting at a low dose would seem sensible. There are various reasons for this, important ones being the tendency of most psychiatric medicines to lower the seizure threshold, and the possible difficulty of identifying side effects in people with communication problems.

Epilepsy is perhaps 50 times more common in people with learning disability compared with the general population, the greater prevalence being associated with more severe learning disability and obvious brain damage. In this situation, any medicine that lowers the seizure threshold, including all antidepressants and antipsychotics, may precipitate a fit.

Considering side effects, it may be difficult for a person with learning disability to tell a carer that their muscles feel stiff (a possible side effect of antipsychotics), that they have developed a cardiac arrhythmia (a rare but possible side effect of antipsychotics and antidepressants), or that they are unsteady on their feet (possibly related to an anticonvulsant prescription). Remaining vigilant to these consequences of drug use is therefore important, and in this context a gradual introduction of a medicine would seem sensible. Further safety of prescriptions in general will occur if a comprehensive history, examination and investigations are part of the initial assessment process and are given consideration when prescribing a particular drug. In this respect, prescription of these medicines by the patient's GP following specialist advice from the psychiatrist is perhaps the ideal, although not always possible, scenario.

There appear to be some causes of learning disability associated with specific psychiatric diagnoses. It has been reported that approximately 30 per cent of people with velocardiofacial syndrome (deletion of 22q11) will suffer from psychosis;[51] a similar risk seems to be present for people with Prader–Willi syndrome.[52]

SPECIFIC CONDITIONS

There are many different conditions associated with learning disability, some very rare. In this section we look at a few of the more common syndromes – fetal alcohol syndrome, Down syndrome, fragile X syndrome and autism/Asperger's syndrome.

Fetal alcohol syndrome

Fetal alcohol syndrome, as the name suggests, is caused by maternal drinking during pregnancy. It is now often advised that alcohol intake is avoided completely by mothers from conception onwards, although it is also accepted that a mother who has drunk during this period may well have a perfectly healthy baby. It is highly probable that the majority of people reading this chapter were born to mothers who drank alcohol in pregnancy without suffering any obvious untoward consequences.

Fetal alcohol syndrome was first described in 1973, and it may be seen in about 1 in 500 births in the USA. The syndrome can include brain damage, facial deformities, growth defects, heart, lung and kidney defects, hearing and vision problems, and learning disability. There may be microcephaly, with structural abnormalities in various regions of the brain.[53]

Diagnosis is based on the history of excessive alcohol use in pregnancy, along with growth retardation, central nervous system dysfunction or intellectual impairment, and craniofacial abnormalities (microcephaly, narrow receding forehead, flat nasal bridge, epicanthic folds, small palpebral fissures, 'rail track' ears, short upturned nose, smooth philtrum, thin upper lip, micrognathia (Figures 71.2 and 71.3). A clear correlation between the occurrence and severity of neuropsychological problems and the degree of alcohol exposure in utero has been reported.[54] An older study from the *Lancet* reported the 10-year follow-up of 11 children who were the first to be diagnosed with fetal alcohol syndrome. At this time, two of the children were dead, one was lost to follow-up and the remaining eight were described as growth-deficient and dysmorphic. Four of these eight were described as being of borderline intelligence requiring remedial teaching; the other four were described as being severely intellectually handicapped.[55] More recent articles concentrate on the actual neurological problems associated with excessive maternal alcohol use, which include neuronal cell death and abnormal functioning of surviving cells.[56]

The only treatment is avoidance of alcohol during pregnancy, thus preventing fetal exposure to the chemical. Treatment of the established syndrome depends on the needs of the individual, including educational help and residential and occupational assistance to adults.

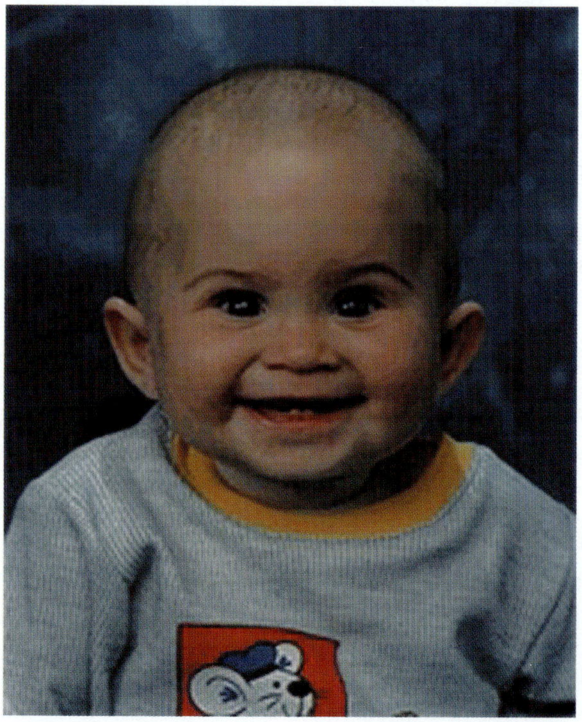

Figure 71.2 Boy with fetal alcohol syndrome, aged 9 months
With thanks to FAS Aware UK.

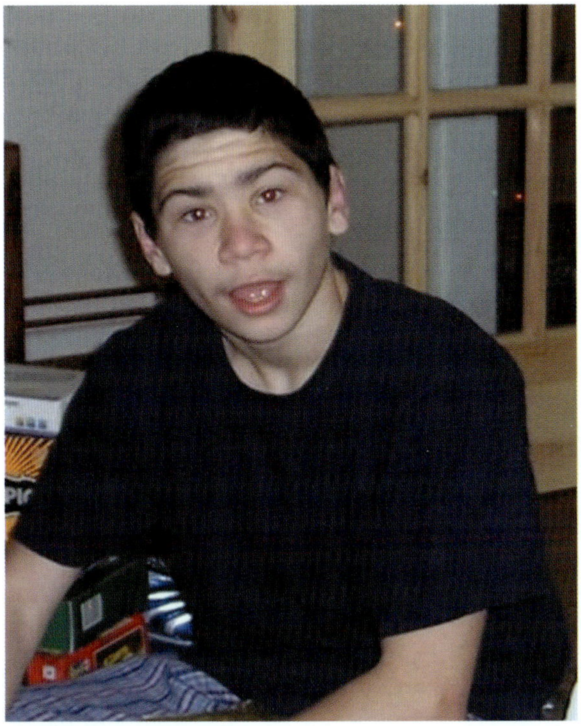

Figure 71.3 Boy with fetal alcohol syndrome, aged 14 years
With thanks to FAS Aware UK.

Similar worries relate to the exposure of the fetus to other toxins during pregnancy, anti-epileptics being an important example.[57]

(For more detailed information, see the website of Foetal Alcohol Syndrome Aware UK at www.fasaware.co.uk.)

Down syndrome

Down syndrome (Figure 71.4) was first described by Langdon Down in 1866. Trisomy 21, the cause of the syndrome, was discovered by Lejeune in 1959.

There is a small risk of the child having Down syndrome in any pregnancy, although the risk increases dramatically with increasing maternal age, rising from about 1 in 1000 in a 20-year-old mother to 40 times this frequency for a 45-year-old mother.[58] Paternal age is probably not important.[59] Prenatal screening, including ultrasound measurements of fetal nuchal translucency and maternal blood tests, is available but not always reliable.[60] Screening may indicate more invasive diagnostic procedures that put the fetus at increased risk, such as amniocentesis. Parents who would not consider termination if their son or daughter has Down syndrome should be advised to avoid having these tests. A couple who already have a child with Down syndrome should have genetic testing if they plan further pregnancies, since relatively rare translocation of chromosome 21 or other genetic abnormalities may increase the risk of them having further children with the syndrome.

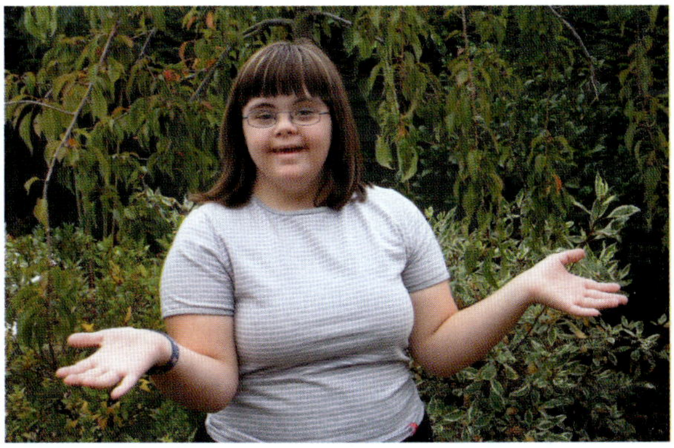

Figure 71.4 Woman with Down syndrome
With thanks to the Down's Syndrome Association.

Life expectancy for people with Down syndrome has improved dramatically over the years. An Australian study describes the follow-up of 1332 people with Down syndrome registered between 1953 and 2000. Average life expectancy was 58.6 years, and the oldest living person in their group was 73 years.[61] This compares to an American study looking at mean life expectancy of all people with learning disability in the USA, showing a dramatic improvement over the same time, and in 1993 an average of 66.2 years.[62] All aspects of medical and surgical care, including cardiac surgery, have been important factors in this success.

Down syndrome is associated with various features, including short stature, a single palmar crease, congenital heart abnormalities and characteristic facial appearance. Most people with Down syndrome also have a significant learning disability.

The various problems faced by people with Down syndrome are ultimately secondary to the additional genetic information coded for on the extra copy of chromosome 21. It is the only trisomy compatible with long-term survival, presumably due to the small size of the chromosome, and it may be secondary to overexpression of some genes with excess production of gene products (e.g. amyloid precursor protein[63]). Other chromosome 21 enzymes may actually be underactive in vivo, for example superoxide dismutase.

Down syndrome is also associated with hypothyroidism, possibly depression and particularly presenile dementia. Unfortunately, the development of dementia is very likely, affecting approximately 50 per cent of people with Down syndrome between the ages of 50 and 60 years, and becoming more common thereafter. It may have a more rapid course than Alzheimer's disease in the general population (although this may be secondary to delay in diagnosis), and it is very commonly associated with the development of swallowing problems, inhalation pneumonia and fits, often presenting as myoclonic jerks.[64] Diagnosis is made by looking at the history of deterioration in the person's skills and abilities, backed up by physical examination and investigations including routine blood tests (thyroid function tests, vitamin B12, folate, lipids), electrocardiogram (ECG), electroencephalogram (EEG) and head scans where possible (scans may well prove too difficult for the patient, as indeed may blood tests). Various rating scales can also be used, some repeated over time and looking for significant deterioration; for example, the Adaptive Behaviour Rating System (ABAS) is carer-rated and looks at all aspects of the person's ability and daily living skills. Other scales can be administered as a single test, for example the Cambridge Examination for Mental Disorders of the Elderly (CAMDEX).[65]

Ball and colleagues have suggested that there may often be a personality change in people with Down syndrome who are about to dement, with 'frontal type' features including reduced empathy, emotional lability, apathy, withdrawal, distractibility, disinhibition and impulsivity.[66]

Treatment of dementia should probably be as in the general population. Social strategies are very important, including, if at all possible, not moving the person from their home. Acetylcholinesterase inhibitors have been used with variable success,[67] with most reports concerning donepezil. Memantine has also been considered.[68]

(For more detailed information, see the website of the Down's Syndrome Association at www.downs-syndrome.org.uk.)

Fragile X syndrome

At a molecular level, fragile X syndrome (Figure 71.5) is caused by an excessive number of CGG (cytosine, guanine, guanine) repeats in a fragment of DNA in the fragile X gene (*FMR1*) on the X chromosome. Normal numbers of copies of the CGG triplet are about 30. There appears to be a 'premutation' stage, with repeats in the range from 55 to 200 seen in male and female carriers.[69] Expansion of the repeat sequence above 200 is known as 'full mutation' and results in hypermethylation at the site of the *FMR1* gene, which in turn leads to underexpression of the fragile X mental retardation protein (FMRP) and the clinical characteristics of the syndrome in males and approximately 50 per cent of affected females. DNA testing is routinely available for fragile X syndrome and can reliably detect not only affected individuals but also carrier males and females.

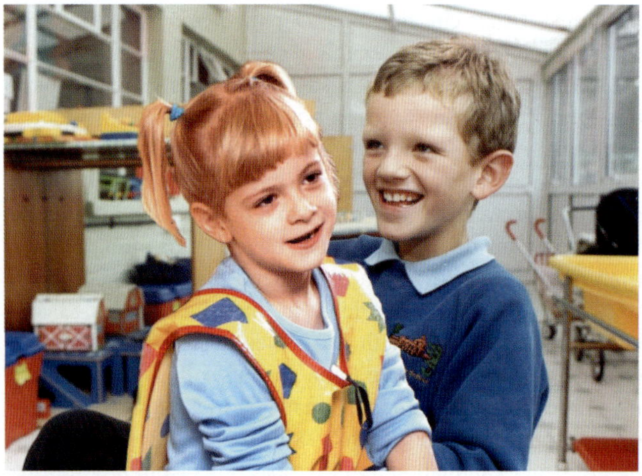

Figure 71.5 Boy and girl with fragile X syndrome
With thanks to the Fragile X Society, UK.

FMRP has been found in most organs, including the brain. In cells it is seen mainly in the cytoplasm, and it may act as an RNA binding/export protein, assisting movement of molecules between the nucleus and the cytoplasm.[70–72]

Fragile X syndrome has been said to be the most common cause of inherited mental handicap,[73] affecting 1 in 4000 males and 1 in 8000 females. It is associated with a wide range of learning disability (from mild to severe in both males and females), attention deficits, hyperactivity (which appears to diminish in adulthood), autism-like features, social phobia, poor eye contact and abnormalities of speech, including repetition, possibly reflecting the effects of physiological arousal caused by hypersensitivity to social and sensory stimuli.[74] Other features include a long thin face and large ears, although these are not seen in all affected people, and large testicles after puberty. There may be a wider connective tissue disorder, with lax joints, flat feet and mitral valve prolapse. Seizures occur in approximately 20 per cent of people with the syndrome, but these usually respond well to anticonvulsants.

There is no specific treatment at present, although recent researchers have suggested that agents acting on γ-aminobutyric acid (GABA) receptors may be helpful in this syndrome.[69,75]

As with all types of learning disability, the main treatment is social, including an educational package designed to meet the needs of the individual, family support and social care where necessary. Genetic counselling should be offered to parents and other family members at risk of producing a child with fragile X syndrome. This may be carried out because there is an existing family member with fragile X syndrome, or in the case of learning disability of unknown cause running in a family, with or without the typical phenotype.

As with other causes of learning disability, there is the possibility, once a diagnosis is known, for parents and families to make contact with other families through relevant support groups, allowing the opportunity of learning from others, sharing experiences, gaining general support and knowing that problems are not faced alone or necessarily unique. (For more detailed information, see the website of the Fragile X Society at www.fragilex.org.uk.)

Early diagnosis is important so that the person can receive appropriate specialist help with education, speech, language and behaviour. Some behavioural disturbance, which may be associated with the syndrome, has been reported to respond to various mainstream 'psychiatric' drugs.[76]

Autism/Asperger's syndrome

This is a fascinating field for researchers and other professionals for various reasons, an important one being that autism seems to represent an illness that affects, in a rather fundamental way, one of the main satisfactions available to most people. Much of the pleasure many of us experience is during interaction with others. For whatever reason, it seems that this shared pleasure is not easily available to people with autism, leading to the main diagnostic criteria of impoverished social interaction, language problems and interest in largely non-social activities, finger-flicking being an example in more severely disabled people and an ability to memorize telephone directories being an example in more able people. Whether there is actually a difference between Asperger's syndrome and autism is uncertain, although we tend to describe people with core symptoms and an associated learning disability (IQ below 70) as having autism, and people with core symptoms and normal intelligence as having Asperger's syndrome.

When autism was originally described by Kanner in 1943, the condition was thought to be rare, with typical autism rates varying between 1.2 and 8.4 in 10 000 children.[77] More recent research has put the figure higher, at 7.1 in 10 000 for typical autism and 20 in 10 000 for autistic spectrum disorder (ASD),[78] the latter usually meaning the presence of autism, pervasive developmental disorder (DSM-IV) or atypical autism (ICD-10). Others have estimated rates as high as 116 in 10 000 for autism and ASD in children.[79]

Autism is defined in DSM-IV by a combination of difficulties in three categories – social interaction, communication and behaviour (restricted, repetitive and stereotyped) – with difficulties in social interaction being particularly important. Onset should be before 3 years of age.[7] Asperger's syndrome has similar criteria, although communication difficulties are not stressed; indeed, clinically significant delays in language should be absent, as should significant delays in cognitive development.

The cause of autism is unknown, although there are many theories. It is far more common in men (male/female ratio: 4 : 1 for autism and 8 : 1 for Asperger's syndrome), which may reflect the fact that men tend to be less verbal and possibly less socially oriented than women and therefore need less of whatever causes autism to express the syndrome. The condition is particularly hard on parents and carers, since the social rewards of loving care (e.g. a smile, hug or thank-you) may be absent or seen only rarely. In addition, the parents and carers have to deal with the difficulties of caring for a child with learning disability and, frequently, behavioural problems, which may be related to lack of empathy. Autism is a very disabling condition. It tends to be lifelong, although it often improves to some extent with age. Worse prognosis has been associated with poor baseline verbal skills. Interestingly, although people with Asperger's syndrome or autism may recognize various difficulties that the syndrome causes them, many also value the unique way in which they are able to perceive the world in general because of their 'problem' and would not wish to lose it.

Multiple investigations have not uncovered much in the way of consistent biological findings. Abnormalities at synapses involving synaptic cleft binding molecules, neuroligin and neurexin, are hypothesized, and large brain sizes have been reported.[80,81] There is an 'androgen theory of autism', proposing that ASD is due in part to elevated fetal testosterone.[82] As with many conditions associated with learning disability, poor conditions during pregnancy and birth may be important, possible risk factors including increasing maternal age, use of medicine during pregnancy and low birth weight.[83] Vaccination as a possible cause of autism achieved much publicity, but this link is no longer accepted.[84] Since autism and autistic traits appear to show a certain amount of genetic inheritance, it is not surprising that genetic theories for autism exist. There is the well-known association between autism and some genetic causes of learning disability, such as fragile X syndrome and phenylketonuria; in addition, very specific genetic abnormalities have been associated with autism, an example being an inversion of the short arm of chromosome 4. This was seen in two brothers both diagnosed with autism, researchers suggesting that GABA transmission may have been impaired as a result of this inversion and possibly underlying the development of the syndrome.[85] Aberrations in brain growth, neuronal patterning and cortical connectivity have been mentioned,[86] and plasma serotonin levels and platelet serotonin binding are consistently found to be raised in the condition, with a negative relationship observed between plasma serotonin levels and speech development.[87] Finally, cerebellar abnormalities have been linked to the syndrome.[88]

It is said that people with autism have difficulties empathizing with other people and cannot put themselves in another person's shoes (sometimes described as 'theory of mind'). This may be through lack of practice following on from social avoidance, or through abnormal brain wiring and connectivity causing abnormal brain function, or both. The 'theory of mind' difficulty may be unique to people with autism, compared with other people with a similar level of intellectual handicap, and may make it hard for them to believe or appreciate others' mental states and experiences. For example, it may be difficult for a person with autism to accept that someone else does not know something. This lack of empathy can make it very difficult to function normally in a social situation and is likely to lead to misunderstandings and suspicion, encouraging further social avoidance. Social avoidance may also be driven by increased levels of anxiety or genuine lack of interest in human interaction. A 'central coherence' theory suggests that people with autism find it difficult to assimilate individual pieces of information into a more coherent ordered whole.[89]

It is widely accepted that treatment should start as early as possible, and generally the degree of success will be related to the early start, intensity and duration. Lovass therapy, for example, has been reported as being successful in significantly improving the functioning of children with autism, although the level of resources required is huge, perhaps 40 h per week of intensive input for at least 2 years.[90] Alternatively, the resources involved in the care of someone with 'untreated' autism are potentially huge, quite apart from the suffering of the patient and carers involved, and it is our belief that much more of this intensive therapy should be available to infants and young children in the UK.

Mainstream psychiatric medications have been used with varying success in autism. Selective serotonin reuptake inhibitors (SSRIs) are sometimes helpful in treating anxiety, depression and obsessionality,[91,92] and small doses of risperidone have been reported to be helpful in children and some adults with the syndrome. Indeed, risperidone is approved for the treatment of irritability associated with autistic disorder in children and adolescents in the USA,[93] and it has nearly achieved a similar licence in the UK.

Highly unsaturated fatty acid supplements have been tried in autism and related conditions, including dyslexia and dyspraxia, apparently with some success.[94] Less mainstream treatments include secretin injections (one review suggests these are ineffective[95]), a casein- and gluten-free diet (a 2004 review concluded that this is an important area for research and that large-scale randomized controlled trials are needed[96]), and many and varied recommendations for various vitamins, trace metals and similar substances,[97] along with avoidance of chemicals such as food colourings and preservatives. It is understandable that such a serious condition with apparently so little in the way of mainstream treatments will attract so many therapeutic suggestions. Providing they are harmless, they may be reasonable and possibly helpful in some people.

Autism is a serious and disabling condition. It seems that there are many possible causes that may lead to a similar presentation. There is probably a significant degree of brain damage at the level of synapses/neuron connectivity, but this damage does not show up on standard brain scans. A certain amount of autism may be normal and helpful in an evolutionary sense, and men seem to be nearer this condition at baseline. Most successful treatment approaches seem to involve considerable mainly social input as early as possible, something that is often not available.

ASSESSMENT IN LEARNING DISABILITY

Making a psychiatric assessment on a person with a learning disability is a similar process to making a psychiatric assessment on anyone else. Initially a detailed history will be taken. This may be from the individual or their carer, or both. The presenting complaint is discussed, along with other standard information, including past medical, surgical and psychiatric history. Family history of psychiatric illness is important and offers clues to diagnosis. Specific questions are asked around developmental history, including any problems during pregnancy or at birth, birth weight and developmental milestones, such as walking alone (usually occurring at about 12 months) and talking (normally some babbling at about 6 months, two-word sentences at 2 years, and longer sentences and incessant talking at 3 years).[98,99] The school attended should be recorded and a note made if this is a special school for people with learning disability, in addition to any examinations entered for or passed. The current social situation should be asked about, including care arrangements and day activities.

A quick test of abilities can be carried out, asking the patient to write a short sentence or their name, read a few lines in a book, and carry out some simple arithmetic. Skills of day-to-day living should also be considered and recorded, including the ability to clean, dress and wash themselves, and the abilities to travel independently, budget and understand money. Employment history is important, including whether the patient has ever been able to work unsupported on the open market (rather unusual for a person with learning disability). Past medical history should be recorded, along with any history of epilepsy and any special investigation results, for example head MRI or EEG. Allergic reactions to drugs or foods should be asked of the carer, since the person with learning disability may not be aware of this potentially important information.

This detailed history will ideally be backed up with a physical examination and various baseline tests, including routine blood tests. Unfortunately, it is not uncommon for a person with learning disability to refuse these investigations, particularly if they do not understand the purpose of the test. Head-scanning all referrals to learning disability psychiatry is probably not practical, although it could be argued that it may be ideal, particularly since MRI scans are probably harmless (which is not necessarily the case with computed tomography (CT) scanning). Apart from helping to exclude organic brain pathology for the presentation, MRI scanning may represent a very useful baseline that can be repeated at a later stage, for example if dementia is suspected in a person with poor verbal skills. An EEG is helpful for patients with diagnosed or suspected epilepsy; it is also better tolerated than scanning and might be ordered when an MRI proves impossible.

Various psychological tests may be helpful. If not already available, an IQ test can prove useful with diagnosis and service provision, particularly for people on the borderline between learning disability and mental health services. The IQ test may demonstrate a difference between verbal and performance skills, which can have a significant effect on day-to-day functioning, or a 'spiky' profile, sometimes seen in autism.

Occupational therapy has many assessment tools to look at daily living skills, including the Adaptive Behaviour Assessment System (ABAS)[100] and Assessment of Motor and Process Skills (AMPS).[101] Speech and language therapy has its own scales and provides dysphagia assessments.

This comprehensive gathering of information can then be

backed up by reports from other services, for example schools, educational psychologists and child and adolescent mental health services, where appropriate. The patient's GP may know the patient and family well and may be the only person with a global knowledge of all the various agencies involved, and therefore the GP is a crucial source of information.

Having completed the assessment, a care plan can be drawn up, which may include referrals to other learning disability specialists, for example family therapy via psychology. If there appears to be an obvious psychiatric illness, appropriate drug treatment may be started.

Sometimes the diagnosis is in doubt or the main problem appears to be challenging behaviour not obviously associated with a psychiatric illness and not responding to initial therapeutic interventions such as psychology or social input. Consideration may then be given to trying a medication as part of a therapeutic trial.[102] This idea is somewhat controversial, but the practice certainly takes place, perhaps justified by the likely possibility that psychiatric illness may present atypically in people with learning disability and that psychiatric drugs may on occasions be helpful in treating behaviour seen largely in people with learning disability (e.g. the use of fluoxetine in the treatment of self-injurious behaviour[103]).

When recommending therapy of this nature, it should be safe, carefully documented, the goals of prescription made clear, reviewed regularly and stopped if proving non-beneficial.

Making a psychiatric diagnosis in a person with learning disability is complicated and challenging and requires considerable effort. A full assessment may direct services towards the most appropriate treatment and therapeutic success.

BEHAVIOURAL PHENOTYPES

Behavioural phenotypes are typical patterns of behaviour that may be associated with certain genetic abnormalities. The concept is potentially helpful, in assisting with diagnosis and helping to explain to parents or carers one factor that may be driving challenging or otherwise difficult behaviour. Equally, however, it should not be given excessive emphasis by assuming that everyone with a certain genetic make-up will behave in a similar way or that because of a particular genetic make-up associated behaviours are unavoidable or untreatable. The behavioural phenotype also describes the typical cognitive abilities associated with a particular genotype.

Some syndromes have been reported to be characterized largely by the behavioural phenotype; for example, Smith–Magenis syndrome (deletion of 17p11.2) is associated with very demanding behaviour, severe temper tantrums, hyperactivity, aggression, self-injurious behaviour, sleeping problems, head-banging and finger-biting.[104]

A behavioural phenotype has been reported in association with Down syndrome, although this is not consistent or inevitable. Being less likely to show maladaptive behaviour than other peers with learning disability has been mentioned,[105] along with strong powers of imitation, a lively sense of humour, obstinacy and amiability. A more recent report suggests the use of and 'over reliance on' social behaviours during cognitively challenging tasks.[106]

Fragile X syndrome has been associated with a behavioural phenotype, including learning disability, autistic features, rapid and disrhythmic speech, anxiety, hand-flapping or hand-biting, shyness and avoidance of eye contact.[107,108]

Prader–Willi syndrome is well known for its association with excessive eating and obesity. It is also associated with learning disability, short stature and neonatal hypotonia, the latter demonstrating the important point that certain behavioural phenotypes may be seen only at specific stages of development. Other behaviours include skin-picking, temper tantrums, compulsive behaviour and mood fluctuations.[109] There may also be differences within the group of people with Prader–Willi syndrome, depending on the genetic subtype. Research has reported that people with the long type I 15q deletion have compulsions around personal cleanliness, and that people with the short type II 15q deletion are more likely to have compulsions around academic areas (e.g. reading and re-reading or counting).[110]

There are many other behaviours associated with genetic causes of learning disability, including self-mutilation following spasticity and choreoathetosis in Lesch–Nyhan syndrome; sleep problems, hyperactivity and non-compliant obsessiveness in tuberose sclerosis; and hyperactivity, anxiety, compulsions, self-injurious behaviour and autistic features in Cornelia de Lange syndrome.[111,112]

Study of behavioural phenotypes with an ever-increasing match to specific biochemical abnormalities may ultimately assist in the development of treatments for these conditions, along with the possibility of a better understanding of the biochemical basis of behaviour in general.

TREATMENTS

Various treatments for psychiatric illness in learning disability have already been mentioned. Biological treatments include all the mainstream psychiatric drugs, such as antipsychotics, antidepressants, mood stabilizers and minor tranquillizers. Electroconvulsive therapy (ECT) is rarely prescribed, although reports exist suggesting efficacy in treatment-resistant mood disorder and psychotic disorder.[113] Clozapine is used more frequently and has been said to be safe, efficacious and tolerated well,[114,115] although, like lithium, clozapine is available only to people who accept regular blood tests.

Attention deficit–hyperactivity disorder (ADHD) is seen in children with learning disability and may respond to psychostimulants such as methylphenidate.[116] This medication may also prove useful in adults. Anti-libidinal drugs, for example cyproterone acetate, are rarely prescribed, but their use has been described in men with learning disability and aberrant sexual behaviour that cannot be managed by educational or behavioural approaches.[117]

Many people with learning disability have epilepsy. For these individuals, consideration needs to be given to the possibility of subclinical seizures causing or complicating a psychiatric presentation in addition to the side effects of the anticonvulsants themselves causing difficulties.

Of the more commonly used anticonvulsants, psychiatric side effects include depression, aggression and activation of psychosis with carbamazepine; aggression and behavioural disturbance with sodium valproate; depression, emotional lability, insomnia, irritability, aggression and psychosis with levetiracetam; confusion and hallucinations with lamotrigine; depression and suicidal ideation with topirimate; and depression, hostility, insomnia, anxiety and hallucinations with gabapentin.[118] Clearly all these side effects, and many others not listed above, are rare, but they should be considered in making a diagnosis.

Vitamin and mineral supplements have been suggested for a number of conditions, including Down syndrome, although there is little evidence that they are helpful. Highly unsaturated fatty acids have been said to be useful in autism and ASD, as have secretin injections and a gluten- and casein-free diet, but again there is little good evidence to recommend these treatments.

Educational approaches are important and early long-term intensive input to children with autism has already been mentioned. Traditionally, psychology will be involved in the behavioural treatment of problem behaviours – various forms of counselling and cognitive-behavioural therapy may be used. Behavioural approaches may look at antecedent, behaviour and consequence (ABC) charts, which might show unintentional reward for challenging behaviour. If, for example, a person with autism and poor communication is feeling socially overwhelmed, they may learn quickly that hitting out will lead to them being removed to their own room and thus avoid the social difficulties. Equally, social reward in the form of social contact may be inadvertently given for unacceptable behaviour, resulting in perpetuation or worsening of the presentation. This may be particularly relevant in unstimulating environments.

Counselling may be verbal or through other mediums such as art or music. In less verbal therapies, patients may be invited to comment on their use of musical instruments or their pictures and drawings and helped in this way to express difficult feelings or thoughts, which may then be therapeutic. The Books Beyond Words series, published by the Royal College of Psychiatrists, offers pictorial representations of various scenarios (epilepsy, bereavement, depression and growing up, among others), allowing shared exploration of a topic, either using words or without the use of language. Cognitive-behaviour therapy has been used with some success in people with learning disability, although it requires a degree of understanding that may be difficult for people with significant intellectual deficit.[119]

Other members of the multidisciplinary team have very important roles to play.

Community nurses will be involved in various activities, including advice around medication, specialist training (e.g. use of rectal diazepam in status epilepticus), monitoring and administering intramuscular injections (contraception and antipsychotics), liaising with GPs, running healthy eating groups, and monitoring and maintaining health action plans in conjunction with GPs.

Social services can assist with benefits, accommodation and day activities. Help is unlikely to be delivered by a social worker, except through duty contact. Instead, an assessment of needs will be followed up by recommendations and, if eligible, the purchase of a care package. This might involve a second agency being contracted to provide care. They may be paid to visit the individual on a daily basis for a few hours to assist with shopping, budgeting, cooking and promoting social contact, this last factor being potentially very important. The current fashion for supported living and supported tenancies has resulted in many people with learning disability now living on their own. When this is coupled with the relatively small realistic peer group available to these people, without sufficient and imaginative support long-term isolation may result in depression and be a significant factor in a psychiatric presentation.

Occupational therapy approaches may assist the individual in finding the confidence to travel independently, seek employment or improve their general abilities in activities of daily living. Success in any of these spheres may well improve self-esteem and reduce depressive feelings. Where problems in communication appear to be important in maintaining anxiety or depression, speech and language therapists may be able to help with aids that allow pictorial representations of spoken words. Books can be produced with photos of various foods, favourite places to visit, rooms (e.g. the toilet, bedroom, bathroom) and pain, among other things. These can then be used by the person with limited vocal communication skills to make their needs known to others.

In conclusion, successful psychiatric treatment of people with learning disability is likely to be multifactorial and involve the input of different professionals, including social services. The prescription of medication will often be an important factor in such treatment.

OFFENDERS WITH LEARNING DISABILITY

It would be very unusual in the UK to find someone in prison who also has a significant learning disability. (IQ has been studied in remand prisoners in Scotland and found to be average although associated with low educational achievement.[120]) This is probably quite right, but what is the response of society to those people who appear to have a significant learning disability and who offend? It might be hoped that people with learning disability will not offend, which may well be the case in respect of crimes such as armed robbery and fraud. However, persistent physical assaults on others, arson and exposure in public certainly occur and require a response. For more extreme and dangerous crimes, a hospital disposal is a possible outcome, while for less serious offences, increased community supervision may be provided, in both instances along with therapeutic endeavours including drug treatment, talking therapies and other treatment options.

The 1983 Mental Health Act describes two grounds for detention under the Act that apply only to people with learning disability, namely mental impairment and severe mental impairment.[121] These are considered, along with mental illness and psychopathic disorder, to constitute 'mental disorder', which may be grounds for involuntary treatment. Both mental impairment and severe mental impairment require that the person has 'arrested or incomplete development of mind', with significant or severe impairment of intelligence and social functioning along with 'abnormally aggressive or seriously irresponsible conduct'.

Thus, a person with a learning disability who has been charged with a crime may be involuntarily detained for hospital treatment on the grounds of mental disorder. This may be after an assault felt to be secondary to a persecutory delusions (a mental illness), or when no obvious mental illness seems to be present, under mental impairment or severe mental impairment, by virtue of the learning disability and behaviour associated with the crime. The Act allows the possibility of providing secure forms of treatment to this group of people as an alternative to prison, usually in a hospital setting.

Since criminal behaviour is not obviously a psychiatric illness, it may be difficult for psychiatrists to treat more persistent offenders, and long admission periods become a possibility. Admissions may take place on general NHS learning disability wards, on forensic units or, more commonly, in private sector provision. Following a crime, 'diversion' of a person with learning disability from the criminal justice system to health and social services may occur at different stages. On many occasions after, for example, an assault on staff by a ward inpatient, the police are not called. If they are called, then it is not uncommon for the police to advise that there is little they can do and for the individual to remain within health and social services provision and treatment. If the alleged offence is more serious, then a hospital disposal under the Mental Health Act (Sections 2 and 3) may be sought, without attempting to charge the individual. If the person is successfully charged with an offence, then an alternative to prison might be the use of a forensic section of the Mental Health Act, for example Section 37, which in the most severe cases could have a Home Office restriction order also applied (Section 41), making ultimate decisions of discharge more complicated and not at the sole discretion of the responsible medical officer.

If a person with an apparent learning disability is to be interviewed by the police, the person should have access to an appropriate adult, whose role is to advise the individual and actively observe the interview process (Police and Criminal Evidence Act, 1984), hopefully safeguarding against issues such as a desire to please, suggestibility and poor understanding, which may result in incorrect and untrue confessions being made.

It may be felt that an apparent offender appearing at court with a learning disability is unfit to plead, meaning that they are unable to put forward a proper defence, challenge a juror, give instructions to their lawyer, and follow the evidence. If this is found to be the case, then a new jury will hear a trial of the facts, a guilty verdict at this stage leading to various possible disposals, including hospital treatment.

Risk assessments have become increasingly part of the remit of psychiatric teams, and attempt to bring some science to the prediction and possibly prevention of undesired future events. In forensic learning disability services, they might, for example, look at the risk of repeated arson.[122]

Recidivism is usually most highly correlated to future risk. Other factors can be important; for example, in a non-learning disabled population, violence and being associated with previous violence were also found to be related to substance abuse, lack of empathy and stress.[123] Risk assessments include personal factors, factors related to the illness, and factors related to the mental state[124] and may be helpful in promoting consideration of issues that might be missed during a normal multidisciplinary case conference. The Historical, Clinical, Risk Management 20 (HCR 20) is one such tool and considers issues such as previous violence, relationship instability, employment problems, insight, attitudes, drug and alcohol use, personal support availability and compliance.[125] Attempts have been made to validate these assessments, and reports exist indicating some success in this respect.[126,127] Other authors have been more critical of their accuracy and usefulness.[128] Even if risk assessments can be made to be more accurate, there remains the difficulty of what should be done when high levels of risk are predicted. Are we prepared to remove a person's freedom for prolonged periods of time based on uncertain assessment tools predicting possible future events? Perhaps their main value is in assisting the research and development of effective treatments for these various undesirable behaviours.

Finally, court reports may be requested at times from psychiatrists working with people with learning disability. Information contained should include some note of the qualifications and experience of the doctor making the report, information made available to the doctor, a full history, the circumstances of the offence, a mental sate assessment, and diagnosis and formulation. Other considerations include fitness to plead, risk assessment and recommendations for disposal.

MENTAL CAPACITY AND CONSENT

Some people with learning disability and their carers are periodically faced with issues around consent. In health, a common example might concern an operation and the consent required of the individual before this can be carried out. (In the UK no one can consent for medical treatment on behalf of another adult.) A person with a severe learning disability will not understand the nature of the operation, the purpose of the operation, the possible risks involved, the risks of doing nothing, and the treatment alternatives (if available), the factors associated with the ability to give valid consent.

If doing nothing is likely to lead to a serious or potentially fatal outcome, then there is not usually any great problem, an example being the surgical treatment of acute bowel perforation. Here, 'consent' may be sought of the nearest relatives or main carers; provided the treatment is in line with what would be considered good medical practice, treatment without proper consent is accepted.

The situation is rather different for procedures that are not life-saving, the most notorious in the learning disability field being sterilization. Almost invariably in situations such as this, involvement of the legal profession and courts will be required.[129]

Lesser situations arise on a daily basis. Blood tests may be requested by a GP. People without learning disability can appreciate the potential value of the test, and know that it will not be particularly painful and that it is very low risk. A person without this understanding will, understandably, actively resist the procedure and may well require restraint if the blood is to be taken. If this is the case, then it is important for the doctor and carers to assess the potential importance of the test. Our feeling is that a blood test would not be justified as a routine check but might be justified where a treatable diagnosable condition is suspected, for example thyroid disorder or diabetes.

Drug treatment may be suggested for a person with a significant learning disability who is unable to understand the possible risks and benefits of the medicine. At times, the ingestion of the drug may be actively resisted. In some situations, this behaviour will be interpreted as refusing consent, and where the necessity of giving the medicine is in doubt the drug may be stopped. This might not be an acceptable outcome if the medicine involved is a powerful anti-epileptic and non-compliance is known to result in multiple seizures or status epilepticus, or the medicine is thyroid replacement treatment with refusal causing life-threatening myxoedema. If the person is felt to have capacity for their refusal, then even life-saving treatment cannot be given; however, in the case of significant learning disability, where capacity is in doubt, treatment may be insisted on, following multidisciplinary discussion and consent from relevant family and carers. Actually delivering this treatment may be easier said than done.

A similar situation occurs on a daily basis in many learning disability homes throughout the UK, where locked doors are used to protect vulnerable individuals from the dangers of the outside world, while at the same time clearly restricting their human rights.

The Mental Capacity Act, 2005, has considered these various issues. Under this Act people are assumed to have capacity for the decisions they make. This can be tested on each individual issue by assessing whether the person is able to understand the information relevant to the decision, is able to retain the information, can use the information in making a decision, and is able to communicate the decision (not necessarily verbally). If the person is felt to lack capacity, then any 'act done or decision made under this Act on behalf of a person who lacks capacity must be done, or made, in his best interests'. It is also noted in the Act that 'a person is not to be treated as unable to make a decision merely because he makes an unwise decision'.[130]

Generally speaking, if it is felt that an individual lacks capacity for a decision, then decisions made on the person's behalf should be documented, in their best interest, in line with current practice, and should follow discussion with family, carers and other involved professionals.

CONCLUSION

Learning disability psychiatry is a fascinating field that touches all aspects of medicine. Forty years ago the majority of statutory care was provided in big institutions geographically removed from the rest of society. Now people with learning disability live in towns and cities with everyone else, with ever-increasing rights and some additional responsibilities. In the vast majority of cases, these changes have improved the quality of life for this group of people.

Providing good healthcare in these changing circumstances has proved challenging, but most GPs now have a list of learning disability patients and are becoming increasingly confident in treating this patient group. In general hospitals liaison work can still be of crucial importance when a patient with a learning disability is admitted for an illness or operation.

When considering behavioural change, physical causes should always be considered. It is important to remember that genuine psychiatric illness may present in atypical ways. Issues around consent, capacity and compliance may all contribute to important challenges in any aspect of treatment. The possibilities for research that could have implications for everyone exist, excellent examples being the association between the additional genetic material in

Down syndrome and presenile dementia, and obesity and Prader–Willi syndrome. There are, however, considerable challenges in carrying out research on people with learning disability, the inability to gain valid consent underlying many of these difficulties.

The role of traditional health services has changed considerably over the past few decades, and social services now head combined learning disability teams. In addition, mainstream medical professionals, particularly GPs but also general psychiatrists, are becoming increasingly involved in learning disability health and psychiatric services. The future of specialist learning disability psychiatry is therefore as a lead profession in the multidisciplinary team. The primary focus will be community work along with advice to other professionals, the development of specialist community teams (challenging behaviour, admission avoidance, autism), research, and an important role in limited admission services and traditional hospital-based care.

REFERENCES

1. Department of Health and Social Security (1971) White Paper. Better Services for the Mentally Handicapped. Cmnd 4683. London: Department of Health and Social Security.
2. Department of Health (2001) White Paper. Valuing People: A New Strategy for Learning Disability for the 21st Century. CM 5086. London: Department of Health.
3. Royal College of General Practitioners (2007) Care of People with Learning Disabilities. Curriculum Statement 14. London: Royal College of General Practitioners.
4. Cooper SA, Smiley E, Morrison J, *et al.* (2007) Mental ill health in adults with intellectual disabilities: prevalence and associated factors. *British Journal of Psychiatry* **190**: 27–35.
5. Emerson E, Kiernan C, Albroz A, *et al.* (2001) The prevalence of challenging behaviours: a total population study. *Research in Developmental Disabilities* **22**: 77–93.
6. Cooper JE, World Health Organization (1994) *Pocket Guide to the ICD-10 Classification of Mental and Behavioural Disorders*. Churchill Livingstone.
7. American Psychiatric Association (1994) *Diagnostic and Statistical Manual of Mental Disorders* 4th edn. Baltimore, MD: American Psychiatric Association.
8. Binet A, Simon T (1916) *The development of intelligence in children*. Baltimore, MD: Williams & Wilkins. [Reprinted 1973, New York: Arno Press.]
9. Wechsler D (1939) *The Measurement of Adult Intelligence*. Baltimore, MD: Williams & Wilkins.
10. Goleman D (1996) *Emotional Intelligence: Why It Can Matter More than IQ*. London: Bloomsbury.
11. Clarke AM, Clarke ADB, Berg J (1985) *Mental Deficiency: The Changing Outlook*, 4th edn. London: Methuen.
12. Hockfield S, Lombroso P (1998) Development of the cerebral cortex: cortical development and experience. *Journal of the American Academy of Child and Adolescent Psychiatry* **37**: 992–3.
13. Hubel DH, Wiesel TN (1970) The period of susceptibility to the physiological effects of unilateral eye closure in kittens. *Journal of Physiology* **206**: 419–36.
14. Yaqoob M, Bashir A, Zaman S, *et al.* (2004) Mild learning disability in children in Lahore, Pakistan: aetiology and risk factors. *Journal of Intellectual Disability Research* **48**: 663–71.
15. Martorell R, Gonzalez Cossio T (1987) Maternal nutrition and birth weight. *Yearbook of Physical Anthropology* **30**: 195–220.
16. Niccols A (2007) Fetal alcohol syndrome and the developing socio emotional brain. *Brain and Cognition* **65**: 135–42
17. Ramsay MC, Reynolds CR (2000) Does smoking by pregnant women influence IQ, birth weight, and developmental disabilities in their infants? A methodological review and multivariate analysis. *Neuropsychological Review* **10**: 1–40.
18. Milberger S, Biederman J, Faraone SV, Chen L, Jones J (1996) Is maternal smoking during pregnancy a risk factor for attention deficit hyperactivity disorder in children? *American Journal of Psychiatry* **153**: 1138–42.
19. Lindhout D, Omtzigt JG (1992) Pregnancy and teratogenicity. *Epilepsia* **33** (suppl. 4): 41–8.
20. Reiss AL, Hall SS (2007) Fragile X syndrome: assessment and treatment implications. *Child and Adolescent Psychiatric Clinics of North America* **16**: 663–75.
21. Schwartz RA, Fernandez G, Kotulska K, Jozwiak S (2007) Tuberose sclerosis complex: advances in diagnosis, genetics, and management. *Journal of the American Academy of Dermatology* **57**: 189–202.
22. Cederbaum S (2002) Phenylketonuria: an update. *Current Opinion in Pediatrics* **14**: 702–6.
23. Da Rocha AF, da Costa Leite C, Rocha FT, *et al.* (2006) Mental retardation: a MRI study of 146 Brazilian children. *Arquivos de Neuro-psiquiatria* **64**: 186–92.
24. Basel Vanagaite L (2007) Genetics of autosomal recessive non syndromic mental retardation: recent advances. *Clinical Genetics* **72**: 167–74.
25. Raymond FL, Tarpey P (2006) The genetics of mental retardation. *Human Molecular Genetics* **15**: R110–16.
26. McBride SM, Choi CH, Wang Y, *et al.* (2005) Pharmacological rescue of synaptic plasticity, courtship behaviour, and mushroom body defects in a Drosophila model of fragile X syndrome. *Neuron* **45**: 753–64.
27. Urbano RC, Hodapp RM (2007) Divorce in families of children with Down syndrome: a population based study. *American Journal of Mental Retardation* **112**: 261–74.
28. Gath A, Gumley D (1986) Family background of children with Down's syndrome and children with a similar degree of mental retardation. *British Journal of Psychiatry* **149**: 161–71.

29. Jones G (2006) Department of Education and Social Skills/Department of Health good practice guidance on the education of children with autistic spectrum disorder. *Child Care, Health and Development* **5**: 543–52.
30. Bradley RH, Whiteside L, Caldwell BM, *et al.* (1993) Maternal IQ, the home environment and child IQ in low birth weight, premature children. *International Journal of Behavioural Development* **16**: 61–74.
31. Bradley RH, Caldwell BM (1984) The relation of infants' home environments to achievement test performance in first grade: a follow up study. *Child Development* **55**: 803–9.
32. Bettelheim B (1967) *The Empty Fortress: Infantile Autism and the Birth of the Self.* New York: Free Press.
33. Spence SJ (2004) The genetics of autism. *Seminars in Pediatric Neurology* **11**: 196–204.
34. Piana H, Fortin C, Noulhiane M, *et al.* (2007) Investigation of the behavioural phenotype of parents of autistic children through the new FAQ self report. *Encephale* **33**: 285–92.
35. Lovaas OI (1987) Behavioural treatment and normal educational and intellectual functioning in young autistic children. *Journal of Consulting and Clinical Psychology* **55**: 3–9.
36. McEachin JJ, Smith T, Lovaas OI (1993) Long term outcome for children with autism who received early intensive behavioural treatment. *American Journal of Mental Retardation* **97**: 359–72, discussion 373–91.
37. Svetaz MV, Ireland M, Blum R (2000) Adolescents with learning disabilities: risk and protective factors associated with emotional well being – findings from the National Longitudinal Study of Adolescent Health. *Journal of Adolescent Health* Nov;**27**: 340–48.
38. Eaton LF, Menolascino FJ (1982) Psychiatric disorders in the mentally retarded: types, problems, and challenges. *American Journal of Psychiatry* **139**: 1297–303.
39. Meadows G, Turner T, Campbell L, *et al.* (1991) Assessing schizophrenia in adults with mental retardation: a comparative study. *British Journal of Psychiatry* **158**: 103–5.
40. Royal College of Psychiatrists (2001) DC-LD. Occasional paper OP48. London: Gaskell.
41. Deb S (2006) Medication for behaviour problems associated with learning disabilities. *Psychiatry* **5**: 368–70.
42. Singh I, Owino WJE (1992) A double blind comparison of zuclopenthixol tablets with placebo in the treatment of mentally handicapped patients with associated behavioural disorders. *Journal of Intellectual Disability Research* **36**: 541–9.
43. Craft M, Ismail IA, Krishnamurti D, *et al.* (1987) Lithium in the treatment of aggression in mentally handicapped patients: a double blind trial. *British Journal of Psychiatry* **150**: 685–9.
44. Brylewski J, Duggan L (2004) Antipsychotic medication for challenging behaviour in people with learning disability. *Cochrane Database Systematic Review* (3): CD000377.
45. Tyrer P, Oliver Africano PC, Ahmed Z, *et al.* (2008) Risperidone, haloperidol, and placebo in the treatment of aggressive challenging behaviour in patients with intellectual disability: a randomised control trial. *Lancet* **371**: 57–63.
46. Ahmed Z, Fraser W, Kerr MP, *et al.* (2000) Reducing antipsychotic medication in people with a learning disability. *British Journal of Psychiatry* **176**: 42–6.
47. Prosser H, Moss S, Costello H, *et al.* (1998) Reliability and validity of the Mini PAS ADD for assessing psychiatric disorders in adults with intellectual disability. *Journal of Intellectual Disability Research* **42**: 264–72.
48. Sturmey P, Newton JT, Cowley A, *et al.* (2005) The PAS ADD checklist: independent replication of its psychometric properties in a community sample. *British Journal of Psychiatry* **186**: 319–23.
49. Balboni G, Battagliese G, Pedrabissi L (2000) The psychopathology inventory for mentally retarded adults: factor structure and comparisons between subjects with or without dual diagnosis. *Research in Developmental Disabilities* **21**: 311–21.
50. Sinason V (1992) *Mental Handicap and the Human Condition: New Approaches from the Tavistock.* London: Free Association Books.
51. Gothelf D, Feinstein C, Thompson T, *et al.* (2007) Risk factors for the emergence of psychotic disorders in adolescents with 22q11.2 deletion syndrome. *American Journal of Psychiatry* **164**: 663–9.
52. Boer H, Holland A, Whittington J, *et al.* (2002) Psychotic illness in people with Prader Willi syndrome due to chromosome 15 maternal uniparental disomy. *Lancet* **359**: 135–6.
53. Niccols A (2007) Fetal alcohol syndrome and the developing socio emotional brain. *Brain and Cognition* **65**: 135–42.
54. Aronson M, Hagberg B (1998) Neuropsychological disorders in children exposed to alcohol during pregnancy: a follow up study of 24 children to alcoholic mothers in Goteborg, Sweden. *Alcoholism, Clinical and Experimental Research* **22**: 321–4.
55. Streissguth AP, Clarren SK, Jones KL (1985) Natural history of the fetal alcohol syndrome: a 10 year follow up of eleven patients. *Lancet* **2**: 85–91.
56. Servais L, Hourez R, Bearzatto B, *et al.* (2007) Purkinje cell dysfunction and alteration of long term synaptic plasticity in fetal alcohol syndrome. *Proceedings of the National Academy of Science USA* **104**: 9858–63.
57. Tomson T, Hiilesmaa V (2007) Epilepsy in pregnancy. *British Medical Journal* **335**: 769–73.
58. Hook EB (1981) Rates of chromosome abnormalities at different maternal ages. *Obstetrics and Gynecology* **58**: 282–5.
59. Roth MP, Feingold J, Baumgarten A, *et al.* (1983)

Reexamination of paternal age effect in Down's syndrome. *Human Genetics* **63**: 149–52.

60. Summers AM, Langlois S, Wyatt P, *et al.* (2007) Prenatal screening for fetal aneuploidy. *Journal of Obstetrics and Gynaecology Canada* **29**: 146–79.
61. Glasson EJ, Sullivan SG, Hussain R, *et al.* (2002) The changing survival profile of people with Down's syndrome: implications for genetic counselling. *Clinical Genetics* **62**: 390–93.
62. Braddock D (1999) Aging and developmental disabilities: demographic and policy issues affecting American families. *Mental Retardation* **37**: 155–61.
63. Mehta PD, Capone G, Jewell A, Freedland RL (2007) Increased amyloid beta protein levels in children and adolescents with Down syndrome. *Journal of the Neurological Sciences* **254**: 22–7.
64. Puri BK, Ho KW, Singh I (2001) Age of seizure onset in adults with Down's syndrome. *International Journal of Clinical Practice* **55**: 442–4.
65. Ball SL, Holland AJ, Huppert FA, *et al.* (2004) The modified CAMDEX informant interview is a valid and reliable tool for use in the diagnosis of dementia in adults with Down's syndrome. *Journal of Intellectual Disability Research* **48**: 611–20.
66. Ball SL, Holland AJ, Hon J, *et al.* (2006) Personality and behaviour changes mark the early stages of Alzheimer's disease in adults with Down's syndrome: findings from a prospective population based study. *International Journal of Geriatric Psychiatry* **21**: 661–73.
67. Prasher VP, Huxley A, Haque MS (2002) A 24 week, double blind, placebo controlled trial of donepezil in patients with Down syndrome and Alzheimer's disease: pilot study. *International Journal of Geriatric Psychiatry* **17**: 270–78.
68. Prasher VP (2004) Review of donepezil, rivastigmine, galantamine and memantine for the treatment of dementia in Alzheimer's disease in adults with Down syndrome: implications for the intellectual disability population. *International Journal of Geriatric Psychiatry* **19**: 509–15.
69. Hagerman RJ, Ono MY, Hagerman PJ (2005) Recent advances in fragile X: a model for autism and neurodegeneration. *Current Opinion in Psychiatry* **18**: 490–96.
70. Bardino B, Mandel JL, Fisch GS (2000) FMR 1 gene and fragile X syndrome. *American Journal of Medical Genetics* **97**: 153–63.
71. Zhang M, Wang Q, Huang Y (2007) Fragile X mental retardation protein FMRP and RNA export factor NXF 2 associate with and destabilize Nxf 1 mRNA in neuronal cells. *Proceedings of the National Academy of Science USA* **104**: 10057–62.
72. Penagarikano O, Mulle JG, Warren ST (2007) The pathophysiology of fragile X syndrome. *Annual Review of Genomics and Human Genetics* **8**: 109–29.
73. Reiss AL, Hall SS (2007) Fragile X syndrome: assessment and treatment implications. *Child and Adolescent Psychiatric Clinics of North America* **16**: 663–75.
74. Belser RC, Sudhalter V (2001) Conversational characteristics of children with fragile X syndrome: repetitive speech. *American Journal of Mental Retardation* **106**: 28–38.
75. D'Hulst C, Kooy RF (2007) The GABAA receptor: a novel target for treatment of fragile X? *Trends in Neuroscience* **30**: 425–31.
76. Berry Kravis E, Potanos K (2004) Psychopharmacology in fragile X syndrome, present and future. *Mental Retardation and Developmental Disabilities Research Reviews* **10**: 42–8.
77. Wing L (1993) The definition and prevalence of Autism: a review. *European Child and Adolescent Psychiatry* **2**: 61–74.
78. Williams JG, Higgins JPT, Brayne CEG (2006) Systematic review of prevalence studies of autistic spectrum disorders. *Archives of Disease in Childhood* **91**: 8–15.
79. Baird G, Simonoff E, Pickles A, *et al.* (2006) Prevalence of disorders of the autistic spectrum in a population cohort of children in South Thames: the Special Needs and Autism Project (SNAP). *Lancet* **368**: 210–15.
80. Garber K (2007) Neuroscience: autism's cause may reside in abnormalities at the synapse. *Science* **317**: 190–91.
81. Hazlett HC, Poe M, Gerig G, *et al.* (2005) Magnetic resonance imaging and head circumference study of brain size in autism: birth through age 2 years. *Archives of General Psychiatry* **62**: 1366–76.
82. Ingudomnukul E, Baron Cohen S, Wheelwright S, Knickmeyer R (2007) Elevated rates of testosterone related disorders in women with autistic spectrum conditions. *Hormones and Behavior* **51**: 597–604.
83. Maimburg RD, Vaeth M (2006) Perinatal risk factors and infantile autism. *Acta Psychiatrica Scandinavica* **114**: 257–64.
84. Taylor B (2006) Vaccines and the changing epidemiology of autism. *Child: Care, Health and Development* **32**: 511–19.
85. Vincent JB, Horike SI, Choufani S, *et al.* (2006) An inversion inv(4)(p12 to p15.3) in autistic siblings implicates the 4p GABA receptor gene cluster. *Journal of Medical Genetics* **43**: 429–34.
86. Pardo CA, Eberhart CG (2007) The neurobiology of autism. *Brain Pathology* **17**: 434–47.
87. Hranilovic D, Bujas Petkovic Z, Vragovic R, *et al.* (2007) Hyperserotonaemia in adults with autistic disorder. *Journal of Autism and Developmental Disorders* **37**:1934–40.
88. Courchesne E, Redcay E, Kennedy DP (2004) The autistic brain: birth through adulthood. *Current Opinion in Neurology* **17**: 489–96.
89. Beaumont R, Newcombe P (2006) Theory of mind and central coherence in adults with high functioning autism or Asperger's syndrome. *Autism* **10**: 365–82.

90. Sallows GO, Graupner TD (2005) Intensive behavioural treatment for children with autism: four year outcome and predictors. *American Journal of Mental Retardation* **110**: 417–38.
91. Moore ML, Eichner SF, Jones JR (2004) Treating functional impairment of autism with selective serotonin reuptake inhibitors. *Annals of Pharmacotherapy* **38**: 1515–19.
92. DeLong GR, Teague LA, McSwain Kamaran M (1998) Effects of fluoxetine treatment in young children with idiopathic autism. *Developmental Medicine and Child Neurology* **40**: 551–62.
93. Scott LJ, Dhillon S (2007) Risperidone: a review of its use in the treatment of irritability associated with autistic disorder in children and adolescents. *Paediatric Drugs* **9**: 343–54.
94. Richardson AJ (2004) Clinical trials of fatty acid treatment in ADHD, dyslexia, dyspraxia and the autistic spectrum. *Prostaglandins, Leukotrienes and Essential Fatty Acids* **70**: 383–90.
95. Williams KW, Wray JJ, Wheeler DM (2005) Intravenous secretin for autistic spectrum disorder. *Cochrane Database Systematic Review* (20): CD003495.
96. Millward C, Ferriter M, Calver S, Connell Jones G (2004) Gluten and caesin free diets for autistic spectrum disorder. *Cochrane Database Systematic Review* (2): CD003498.
97. Kidd PM (2002) Autism, an extreme challenge to integrative medicine: part 2. Medical management. *Alternative Medicine Review* **7**: 472–99.
98. Kaplan HI, Sadock BJ (1990) *Pocket Handbook of Clinical Psychiatry*. Baltimore, MD: Williams & Wilkins.
99. De V Heese H (1992) *The Paediatric Handbook*, 3rd edn. Oxford: Oxford University Press.
100. Harrison P, Oakland T (2000) *Adaptive Behaviour Assessment System*, 2nd edn. New York: The Psychological Corporation.
101. Fisher A (2003) *Assessment of Motor and Process Skills: Development, Standardisation and Administrative Manual*, 5th edn. Fort Collins, CO: Three Star Press.
102. Deb S, Unwin GL (2007) Psychotropic medication for behaviour problems in people with intellectual disability: a review of the current literature. *Current Opinion in Psychiatry* **20**: 461–6.
103. Markowitz PI (1992) Effect of fluoxetine on self injurious behaviour in the developmentally disabled: a preliminary study. *Journal of Clinical Psychopharmacology* **12**: 27–31.
104. Willekens D, De Cock P, Fryns JP (2000) Three young children with Smith Magenis syndrome: their distinct, recognisable behavioural phenotype as the most important clinical symptoms. *Genetic Counselling* **11**: 103–10.
105. Collacott RA, Cooper SA, Branford D, McGrother C (1998) Behaviour phenotype for Down's syndrome. *British Journal of Psychiatry* **172**: 85–9.
106. Fidler DJ (2006) The emergence of a syndrome specific personality profile in young children with Down syndrome. *Down's Syndrome Research and Practice* **10**: 53–60.
107. Turk J (1992) The fragile X syndrome: on the way to a behavioural phenotype. *British Journal of Psychiatry* **160**: 24–35.
108. Einfeld SL, Tonge BJ, Florio T (1994) Behavioural and emotional disturbance in fragile X syndrome *American Journal of Medical Genetics* **51**: 386–91.
109. Holland AJ, Whittington JE, Butler J, *et al.* (2003) Behavioural phenotypes associated with specific genetic disorders: evidence from a population based study of people with Prader Willi syndrome. *Psychological Medicine* **33**: 141–53.
110. Zarcone J, Napolitano D, Peterson C, *et al.* (2007) The relationship between compulsive behaviour and academic achievements across the three genetic subtypes of Prader Willi syndrome. *Journal of Intellectual Disability Research* **51**: 478–87.
111. Fraser W, Kerr M (eds) (2003) *Seminars in the Psychiatry of Learning Disabilities*, 2dn edn. London: Gaskell.
112. Basile E, Villa L, Selicorni A, Molteni M (2007) The behavioural phenotype of Cornelia de Lange syndrome: a study of 56 individuals. *Journal of Intellectual Disability Research* **51**: 671–81.
113. Reinblatt SP, Rifkin A, Freeman J (2004) The efficacy of ECT in adults with mental retardation experiencing psychiatric disorders. *Journal of ECT* **20**: 208–12.
114. Antonacci DJ, de Groot CM (2000) Clozapine treatment in a population of adults with mental retardation. *Journal of Clinical Psychiatry* **61**: 22–5.
115. Thalayasingam S, Alexander RT, Singh I (2004) The use of clozapine in adults with intellectual disability. *Journal of Intellectual Disability Research* **48**: 572–9.
116. Jou R, Handen B, Hardan A (2004) Psychostimulant treatment of adults with mental retardation and attention deficit hyperactivity disorder. *Australasian Psychiatry* **12**: 376–9.
117. Clarke DJ (1989) Antilibidinal drugs and mental retardation: a review. *Medicine, Science and the Law* **29**: 136–46.
118. British Medical Association, Royal Pharmaceutical Society of Great Britain (2006) *British National Formulary*. London: British Medical Association.
119. Haddock K, Jones RS (2006) Practitioner consensus in the use of cognitive behaviour therapy for individuals with learning disability. *Journal of Intellectual Disability* **10**: 221–30.
120. Davidson M, Humphreys MS, Johnstone EC, Owens DG (1995) Prevalence of psychiatric morbidity among remand prisoners in Scotland. *British Journal of Psychiatry* **167**: 545–8.
121. Bluglasss R (1983) *A Guide to the Mental Health Act*. Edinburgh: Churchill Livingstone.

122. Lindsay WR, Hastings RP, Griffiths DM, Hayes SC (2007) Trends and challenges in forensic research on offenders with intellectual disability. *Journal of Intellectual and Developmental Disability* **32**: 55–61.

123. Hartvig P, Alfarnes S, Ostberg B, *et al.* (2006) Brief checklists for assessing violence risk among patients discharged from acute psychiatric facilities: a preliminary study. *Nordic Journal of Psychiatry* **60**: 243–8.

124. Gelder M, Mayou R, Cowen P (2001) *Shorter Oxford Textbook of Psychiatry*. Oxford: Oxford University Press.

125. Webster C (1997) *HCR 20: Assessing the Risk for Violence*, Version 2. Burnaby, Canada: Mental Health, Law, and Policy Institute, Simon Fraser University.

126. Kroner C, Stadtland C, Eidt M, Nedopil N (2007) The validity of the violence risk appraisal guide (VRAG) in predicting criminal recidivism. *Criminal Behaviour and Mental Health* **17**: 89–100.

127. Looman J (2006) Comparison of two risk assessment instruments for sexual offenders. *Sexual Abuse* **18**: 193–206.

128. Edens JF, Buffington Vollum JK, Keilen A, *et al.* (2005) Predictions of future dangerousness in capital murder trials: is it time to 'disinvent the wheel'. *Law and Human Behavior* **29**: 55–86.

129. Knifton C (1998) Non consensual sterilization of the adult with learning disabilities. *British Journal of Nursing* **7**: 1172–6.

130. Alonzi A, Pringle M (2007) Mental Capacity Act 2005 *British Medical Journal* **335**: 898.

Chapter 72

Old-age psychiatry

Boben Benjamin and Alistair Burns

INTRODUCTION

The population of elderly adults is rising in the western world. There will be a significant increase in the total number of people with dementias and functional illnesses in this age group. The psychiatry of old age is likely to become an increasingly important area of specialism over the coming years.

DEMENTIA

Dementia is a clinical syndrome characterized by multiple cognitive deficits. Behavioural, psychological symptoms and neurological difficulties may also be present. The deficits result in impairments in the ability to function at work and socially and to manage activities of daily living. Dementia is an acquired disorder that most commonly develops in late life and does not usually cause impairment in the level of consciousness.

Epidemiology

The number of cases of dementia (all subtypes) in the UK was estimated to be about 700 000 in 2007. This is a prevalence of about 1.1 per cent (1 in 88 of the population). Worldwide, in 2007 nearly 18 million people were thought to have dementia. The prevalence of dementia increases with age, doubling with every 5-year increase across the entire age range, from 30 years to 95 years and over. The number of people with dementia in the UK and the rest of the world is forecast to increase considerably over the next few decades.[1]

Aetiology

The most common cause of dementia in elderly people is Alzheimer's disease (AD), followed by dementia with Lewy bodies (LBD) and Vascular dementia (VaD). Potentially reversible aetiologies include normal-pressure hydrocephalus (NPH), subdural haematoma, metabolic and endocrine causes, and vitamin deficiencies.

The various causes of dementia are listed in Table 72.1.

Table 72.1 Causes of dementia

Cause	Example
Degenerative	Alzheimer's disease, Lewy body disease, frontotemporal dementias, Parkinson's disease, Huntington's disease
Vascular	Single infarct, multi-infarct, diffuse white matter ischaemia
Endocrine	Hypothyroidism, hyperparathyroidism, Cushing's disease, Addison's disease
Metabolic	Hypercalcaemia, uraemia, hepatic encephalopathy
Infectious	Creutzfeldt–Jakob disease, HIV, syphilis
Vitamin deficiency	B12, folate
Toxins	Alcohol, heavy metals
Other	NPH, subdural haematoma, tumours

HIV, human immunodeficiency virus; NPH, normal-pressure hydrocephalus.

Clinical features

A number of cognitive deficits occur in dementia. Memory impairment (amnesia) is a prominent symptom, especially in dementia of the Alzheimer's type. Language difficulties (aphasia) may occur. This may present as a decrease in the quality of speech, and there may be difficulties understanding written and spoken language. In the late stages of dementia, the speech may be incomprehensible or the patient may be mute. Difficulties carrying out coordinated motor tasks are another symptom. This occurs despite intact motor and sensory functions and comprehension of the task (apraxia). Problems such as difficulties with dressing or in using cutlery may be the result. There may be difficulties recognizing objects or familiar people, with no impairment in visual function (agnosia). The ability to plan activities and think abstractly (executive functioning) is often impaired. Executive functioning is particularly impaired in dementia of the frontal lobe type.

Behavioural and psychological symptoms of dementia (BPSD) are common in dementia. Depression occurs frequently. A variety of psychotic symptoms may occur, including paranoid ideation, delusions and hallucinations. Behavioural difficulties such as aggression, wandering, changes in sleep and changes in eating patterns are also common. Changes in personality can be distressing to relatives and are a prominent feature of frontal lobe dementias.

Neurological features may be present early in the course of the disease, depending on the type of dementia. Some common examples are parkinsonism in LBD, focal neurological signs in vascular dementia, and primitive reflexes in the frontotemporal dementias. Rarer dementias may have characteristic neurological features. Myoclonus occurs in Creutzfeldt–Jakob disease and choreathetoid movement in Huntington's disease. All dementias involve a progressive loss of motor function in the end stages.

Dementia causes impairments in all domains of functioning. Difficulties in work may be noticed. Mild degrees of cognitive impairment may impair the individual's ability to perform complex jobs but not less demanding jobs. Social functioning is frequently affected. The person may not remember appointments and may find it hard to remember the names of friends and relatives. With continued deterioration, it may no longer be possible to join friends in activities that are intellectually demanding. The person may lose interest in friends and family as a result of apathy, which is a common symptom of dementia. Neglect of household tasks may become apparent. There is often impairment in the activities of daily living (ADLs). ADLs refer to basic self-care tasks and the skills required to live independently in the community, such as washing, dressing, eating, personal hygiene and toilet activities. A decline in the standard of personal cleanliness may be noticed. Self-neglect of the diet can lead to weight loss. In the late stages of dementia, the ability to eat, use the toilet and dress may become severely affected.

Assessment

The diagnostic process involves identifying a dementia syndrome, determining the likely aetiology, and ruling out other causes of a similar clinical picture.

History

The history is probably the most important component of diagnosing dementia. History must be obtained both from the patient and from appropriate informants, including family members, friends and any professionals involved. Details of cognitive deficits and behavioural and psychological difficulties should be noted. It is essential to note the effect of the cognitive deficits on the patient's functioning. The chronology of the symptoms, including the onset, rate of progression and any fluctuations in the symptoms, is especially important when it comes to elucidating the likely aetiology. A detailed medical history, including risk factors for vascular disease such as diabetes, hyperlipidaemia, hypertension and cardiac arrhythmias, and a history of cigarette use is needed. In addition, an alcohol history and a family history of dementias are also of aetiological significance.

Mental state examination

Mental state examination may reveal inappropriate clothing or reduced hygiene. The patient may be disinhibited or socially inappropriate. There may be signs of depression, such as psychomotor retardation or agitation. Speech in dementia is often fluent, but with a paucity of content. There may be word-finding difficulties and perseveration; as the dementia progresses, speech may get more sparse. In the terminal stages, speech output may be reduced to incomprehensible sounds or mutism. Thought content is often reduced. There may be evidence of psychosis or depression. Hallucinations may be present. Visual hallucinations must raise the suspicion of a delirium or an LBD. Cognitive assessment is a crucial part of the mental state. The patient interview when obtaining the history will give some indication of any cognitive difficulties. However, more formal tests are usually done. The Mini-Mental State Examination (MMSE)[2] and the Abbreviated Mental Test Score (AMTS)[3] are the most commonly used initial screening tests. The patient's level of insight into the cognitive and other symptoms will vary. A degree of awareness may be present. Often, the patient may not be aware of the cognitive difficulties or may minimize their significance.

Physical examination

A complete physical examination must be done. A cardiovascular and neurological examination are of particular importance. An elevated blood pressure or an irregular pulse may have aetiological significance. A neurological examination may show focal neurological deficits, parkinsonism or primitive reflexes. The presence of difficulties in sight or hearing must be noted as these can contribute to cognitive problems.

Investigations

A number of standard blood tests are usually done in order to identify any treatable causes or co-morbid conditions in a dementia. The National Institute for Health and Clinical Excellence (NICE) guidelines in the UK recommend routine haematology, biochemistry including electrolytes, calcium, glucose, kidney and liver function, thyroid function and vitamin B12 and folate levels.[4] Although a syphilis screen was routine in the past, the latest guidelines suggest doing this only if the history or clinical picture is of relevance. A chest X-ray or electrocardiogram (ECG) may be considered, depending on the history. A number of experts recommend doing an ECG routinely before starting cholinesterase inhibitor treatment.

Structural scanning (computed tomography (CT), magnetic resonance imaging (MRI)) is done to exclude pathology, such as a brain tumour, cerebral bleeding or hydrocephalus, which are potentially reversible. Scanning is also helpful in diagnosing the dementia subtype, for example generalized atrophy in AD or evidence of ischaemic changes in vascular dementia. However, specialist interpretation is required, and a number of different pathologies may coexist.

CT screening is the radiological investigation of choice to exclude intracranial lesions, with MRI indicated for a more detailed assessment of cerebral structure.

Single photon emission computed tomography (SPECT) is a functional scan and measures blood flow. It can be of help in differentiating AD and a frontal lobe dementia. Dopamine transporter scans (DATScans) may be helpful in the diagnosis of LBD.

Electroencephalography (EEG) can detect the generalized slowing of brain electrical activity associated with a dementia. The EEG is not used routinely in dementia diagnosis but may help in cases of diagnostic uncertainty. It is certainly useful in Creutzfeldt–Jakob disease or if an associated seizure disorder is suspected.

Rating scales

A number of scales may be used in the assessment and monitoring of dementia. The most commonly used is the MMSE[2]. The MMSE is used as a screening test for dementia and can be helpful in the diagnosis and monitoring of the course of the disease. The test takes about 10 min but will not detect subtle memory difficulties, especially in well-educated people.[5] The MMSE provides measures of orientation, registration (immediate memory), short-term memory (but not long-term memory) and language functioning. A score of 26 or less may indicate significant cognitive impairment. The AMTS is often used in the acute medical setting as a quick screening test for cognitive difficulties; it includes a list of ten items – a score of 6 or less is considered significant. The AMTS is rarely used by psychiatrists, however.

The clock-drawing test is often used, especially in general practice, to screen for dementia.[6] It is easy to administer and is non-threatening. The Alzheimer's Disease Assessment Scale is a more detailed cognitive test commonly used in research.[7] The Clinical Dementia Rating Scale gives an overall severity rating.[8] Neuropsychological symptoms can be monitored using the Neuropsychiatric Inventory (NPI);[9] the NPI also records the distress caused by the symptoms in the carers. Scales for rating ADLs, such as the Bristol Activities of Daily Living Scale,[10] may be used.

Diagnosis

The *Diagnostic and Statistical Manual of Mental Disorders*, 4th edition (DSM-IV) definition of dementia involves multiple cognitive deficits with memory as a required criterion.[11] There should be at least one other cognitive deficit, which must be aphasia, apraxia, agnosia or disturbances in executive functioning. The cognitive deficits must be severe enough to cause significant impairment in social or occupational functioning and must represent a decline from a previous level of functioning.

The *International Classification of Diseases*, 10th revision (ICD-10) requires a decline in memory and thinking sufficient to impair activities of daily living.[12] However, certain dementias such as the frontotemporal lobe type may not have the cognitive deficits required to fulfil the present ICD-10 and DSM-IV criteria in the early stages of the disease.

Some experts feel that the emphasis on memory impairment as an absolute requirement for the diagnosis of a dementia is inappropriate in the non-Alzheimer's dementias.

Differential diagnosis

A number of conditions can mimic dementia and must be considered in the diagnostic process. These include:

- delirium;
- depression;
- drugs;
- normal age-associated memory decline;
- mild cognitive impairment (MCI);
- chronic schizophrenia.

Delirium is usually an acute disturbance (over days) with marked fluctuations in the clinical picture, whereas dementia generally has a relatively stable picture. Cognitive deficits that persist for an extended period (months) suggest a dementia. A LBD may, however, have a similar clinical presentation to a delirium, with fluctuations in the level of consciousness and cognition. People with dementia are at an increased risk of developing a delirium, and the possibility of these two conditions coexisting must be borne in mind.

Depression may present with symptoms similar to those of dementia. However, there are features that are helpful in differentiating between these conditions. In depression the patient may complain of memory loss, whereas in dementia it is often the relatives who notice the patient's memory loss. Affective changes are more common in depression than in dementia. Negative thoughts, including low self-esteem, guilt, hopelessness and thoughts about death, should suggest a depressive disorder. Patients with depression tend to give 'don't know' answers, whereas incorrect answers are more likely in dementia.

A number of drugs can cause symptoms of dementia. Medications with anticholinergic side effects are a particular culprit. A detailed drug history is therefore essential during the assessment process of a dementia.

It is normal for memory to decline with the age. In MCI, there are cognitive difficulties greater than what one would expect to be related to age, but there is no impairment in social and occupational functioning and ADLs, unlike the situation in dementia (see below).

Chronic schizophrenia may be associated with a number of cognitive impairments. However, these are often stable through middle life. The time course of symptoms will help to differentiate this from a dementia. A proportion of patients may show further cognitive decline in old age. Mechanistic explanations may be schizophrenia-related neurodegeneration or a superimposed dementia.[13]

Management

The general principles of dementia management are described here. Specific treatment of issues of the dementia subtypes are described in the relevant sections below.

Dementia management requires a multidisciplinary approach. There may be the need for functional and social support, psychological assistance for both the patient and the carer, and drug treatment. Drug treatment is aimed at cognitive enhancement and the behavioural and psychiatric symptoms.

The needs of the patient and the carer should be assessed when a diagnosis of dementia is made. This may involve a social worker and an occupational therapy assessment. For patients living at home, help may be needed with shopping, cleaning, daytime activities and cooking. Risks at home, such as from fires, intruders and wandering, must be taken into account. Help with the management of financial issues and legal matters (e.g. wills, enduring power of attorney) is often required. If the patient is a, driver the Driver and Vehicle Licensing Agency (DVLA) must be informed. Support for carers, including sit-in services, respite admissions and day-centre placements, is often needed as the dementia progresses.

A number of psychological approaches targeted at the patient and the carer have been shown to be helpful. Reality orientation and verbal or visual cues are used to orient the person to themselves, the time and their environment. Validation therapy focuses on the emotional content of the cognitively impaired person rather than on the factual content.[14] Behavioural analyses using an ABC (antecedent, behaviour, consequence) are helpful in the understanding and management of difficult behaviours. Supportive psychotherapy that uses techniques of reassurance, explanation and education may be beneficial.[15]

Intense individual psychotherapy is often unsuitable in dementia due to the patient's cognitive difficulties. However, some of these techniques may be useful in the early stages of the disease.

Cognition, especially in Alzheimer's dementia, may benefit from the use of the cholinesterase inhibitors or memantine (see Alzheimer's disease, below).

Management of behavioural and psychiatric symptoms of dementia

The first step is to get an accurate assessment of the difficulties from the history and observation. The impact on both the patient and the carer should be noted. Standardized rating scales such as the NPI may be used. A behavioural analysis as described above should be considered.

When drug treatment is considered for agitation and psychosis, antipsychotics are often used. These have been shown to be effective, but there are a number of adverse effects, including increased mortality, risk of strokes, falls and drowsiness, worsening cognitive decline and parkinsonism. There is evidence that the cholinesterase inhibitors are effective in the treatment of agitation and psychosis, and these are increasingly being used as alternatives to antipsychotics. Although the current evidence base is limited, clomethiazole or anti-epileptics are sometimes considered. Antidepressants should be considered for depression. In the UK, Kings College in collaboration with the Alzheimer's Society is conducting a study looking at the effectiveness of the antidepressants setraline and mirtazapine in people with dementia and depression. The study is being carried out at a number of centres nationally and was still in progress at the time of writing (http://www.iop.kcl.ac.uk/projects/?id=10179). The judicious use of hypnotics for insomnia and the use of benzodiazepines for agitation may be options in some cases. The risk of falls and drug dependence must be borne in mind.

Non-pharmacological treatments for agitation, including aromatherapy[16] and bright-light therapy,[17] have some evidence of efficacy.

Mild cognitive impairment

MCI refers to a state of cognitive difficulties beyond that of normal age associated decline but not sufficient to meet the criteria for a dementia. Although MCI may involve any cognitive domain, memory impairment is most commonly involved. People with MCI progress to AD at a greater rate than would be expected for healthy individuals of the same age.

There are no consensus criteria for MCI. However, the following criteria formalized by Peterson and colleagues are frequently used:[18]

- Cognitive complaint, usually memory
- Normal general cognitive function (i.e. cognitive screening test) in normal range for age (e.g. MMSE)
- 1.5 standard deviations (SD) below age-appropriate norms on memory tests or memory component of other cognitive tests (tests determined by clinician's judgement)
- ADLs not affected significantly
- Not meeting DSM dementia criteria (i.e. impairments not sufficient to impair professional and social activities).

Vascular cognitive impairment is MCI related to a vascular cause; however, the term is also used in the literature as an umbrella term to cover the entire range of cognitive impairment due to vascular causes, ranging from vascular MCI to vascular dementia. There is some evidence that cholinesterase inhibitors have symptomatic benefit in MCI, but it is unclear whether cognitive decline is prevented by their use.[19]

Alzheimer's disease

Alzheimer's disease was first described by Alois Alzheimer in 1907. It is the most common type of dementia, accounting for 50–70 per cent of cases. The number of people in the UK with AD in 2007 was estimated at 417 000.[1] One in eight people over the age of 65 years has AD, and nearly half of people over the age of 85 years have AD.

Clinical features

The onset of the disease is insidious. Memory loss is the characteristic early symptom of AD. Although memory for recent events is lost first, as the disease progresses long-term memory is affected as well. Disorientation to time is common, and the patient may get lost in unfamiliar places. In the early stages of the disease, the standards of self-care may deteriorate. Language is commonly affected early in the disease. Word-finding difficulty (nominal dysphasia) is the most common language difficulty. Patients may describe the function of an object without being able to recall the name – for example, saying 'a thing you write with' instead of 'pen'. Fluent dysphasia – fluent speech but with a paucity of understandable content – is the second most common language problem. The other cognitive, behavioural and psychiatric features of dementia as described above also develop. Impairment of judgement is an important symptom that may put the patient at risk and cause concern to their family.

Pathophysiology

A characteristic feature of the brain of a person with AD is generalized atrophy of the cerebral hemispheres, in particular the medial temporal lobes, hippocampus and amygdala. The microscopic hallmark is the extracellular neuritic plaque and the intracellular neurofibrillary tangle. The plaques are composed of an amyloid core surrounded by neuritic processes. The amyloid core consists primarily of a small peptide known as Aβ, which is derived from the larger amyloid precursor protein (APP).

Neurofibrillary tangles are intracellular structures associated with hyperphosphorylated tau. The neurochemical basis of AD is thought to be a cholinergic deficit, and this forms the basis of the cholinergic hypothesis of AD. Other neurotransmitters such as γ-aminobutyric acid (GABA) may also be involved.

Diagnosis

The gold standard for the diagnosis of AD is the National Institute of Neurological and Communicative Disorders and Stroke (NINCDS)–Alzheimer's Disease and Related Disorders Association (ADRDA) criteria (Box 72.1).

Box 72.1 NINCDS-ADRDA criteria for Alzheimer's disease (summarized)

1. Probable Alzheimer's disease: Dementia defined by deficits in two or more cognitive domains (including memory) with a progressive course. There should be no disturbance of consciousness and no other systemic disease that could explain the deficits.
2. Possible Alzheimer's disease: A dementia syndrome with an aberrant course or a second disease that could cause the deficits.
3. Definite Alzheimer's disease: Probable Alzheimer's disease together with histopathological evidence.

Source: McKhann G, Drachman D, Folstein M, et al. (1984) Clinical diagnosis of Alzheimer's disease: report of the NINCDS-ADRDA Work Group under the auspices of Department of Health and Human Services Task Force on Alzheimer's Disease. *Neurology* **34(7):** 939–44.

Management

Drug treatment has been available for AD since the 1990s. The drugs used are the cholinesterase inhibitors and memantine. There are currently three cholinesterase inhibitors licensed for the treatment of mild to moderate AD in the UK – donepezil, galantamine and rivastigmine. Memantine is licensed for the treatment of severe AD. Of these, donepezil is the most widely prescribed.[20] These medications inhibit the enzyme acetylcholinesterase, which results in an increase in the amount of acetylcholine available for neurotransmission. Memantine blocks glutamate-mediated cell damage by binding to the *N*-methyl-D-aspartate (NMDA) receptors.

Cholinesterase inhibitors have been shown to slow down the rate of cognitive and functional decline. They are also beneficial in the treatment of neuropsychiatric symptoms and behavioural difficulties. Studies have shown that caregivers of patients on treatment may have reduced emotional distress. The benefits may last up to 3 years.[21] In severe dementia, behavioural rather than cognitive benefits tend to be the goal. Memantine has similar benefits to the cholinesterase inhibitors. The most common side effects of the cholinesterase inhibitors are gastrointestinal – nausea, vomiting and anorexia. Caution in the case of a history of cardiac and respiratory disease, peptic ulcer disease or gastrointestinal bleeding is advisable. Memantine tends to be tolerated better.

In the UK, NICE introduced controversial guidelines in 2006 recommending that the cholinesterase inhibitors should be used only in moderate dementia. NICE does not recommend the use of memantine.[4] These decisions were based on cost–benefit analyses and have been challenged. A subsequent court case resulted in NICE having to have a more inclusive definition of moderate dementia and has had to make it explicit that it would be based on the judgement of the clinician.

Prognosis

AD is a progressive disease and the life expectancy is shortened. A figure of 8 years is often quoted. There is however considerable variation in between individuals and people may survive between 5 and 20 years after the onset of symptoms. The cause of death is often a medical condition such as a chest infection.

Vascular dementia

Vascular dementia occurs as a result of impairment in the vascular supply of the brain. This impairment can have many causes, but atherosclerotic changes are the most common. Vascular dementia is the third most common type of dementia after AD and LBD.

Clinical features

The classical history for vascular dementia described in textbooks is acute or subacute cognitive impairment after an acute neurological event, with a stepwise progression. However, the onset may be more gradual, especially if it is due to lacunar infarcts or white matter ischaemia. There may be neurological signs such as hemiparesis, sensory change, dysphasia or visual disturbances. Mood disturbances, including mood lability, depression and anxiety, are more common than in AD and may predate the cognitive impairments, especially if the onset is gradual. Headache, dizziness, tinnitus, syncope and other non-specific features may be early features that present before the cognitive or neuropsychiatric complaints. Neuropsychological testing in vascular dementia typically shows patchy deficits, whereas AD shows global impairment with memory difficulties prominent early in the disease.

Diagnosis

There are a number of criteria used in the diagnosis of vascular dementia. Hachinski and colleagues devised a list of criteria in the 1970s to differentiate vascular dementia and AD (Box 72.2).[22] Based on the number of criteria present, a score below 4 was said to be AD and a score of 7 or above a vascular dementia. Patients scoring between 4 and 7 were thought to have a mixed picture. These criteria are rarely used nowadays because they do not take into account neuroradiological findings and are not as useful if the vascular dementia has a more gradual onset.

The DSM-IV criteria include focal neurological signs and symptoms or laboratory evidence of cerebrovascular disease (radiological evidence) that are judged to be aetiologically related to the dementia. This is sensitive but not very specific for vascular dementia. The National Institute of Neurological Disorders and Stroke (NINDS)–Association Internationale pour la Recherché et l'Enseignement en Neurosciences (AIREN) criteria are the most specific of all the available criteria and are used most commonly in research.[23] These criteria provide three levels of certainty: definite, probable and possible (Box 72.3).

Pathology

There may be a number of different types of pathological change. Large single infarctions can affect the cerebral cortex and underlying white matter, usually in watershed areas (parts of the brain at the ends of the distribution areas of the cerebral arteries). Multiple cortical infarcts can occur. There may be lacunar infarcts (deep small infarcts < 1.5 cm in diameter). White-matter changes (leucoariosis), best seen on MRI as areas of hyperintensity, are believed to be caused by ischaemia as a result of small-vessel disease and are increasingly recognized as a cause of dementia, especially if the changes are in the periventricular area. If the white-matter changes are diffuse and widespread, then the resulting dementia is termed 'Binswanger's disease'. There may be a combination of the various pathologies.

Box 72.2 Modified Hachinski score

Score < 4: suggests a primary dementia e.g. Alzheimer's disease
Score 4–7: indeterminate
Score > 7: suggests a vascular dementia.

	Feature	Score
1.	Abrupt onset of symptoms	2
2.	Stepwise deterioration	1
3.	Fluctuating course	2
4.	Nocturnal confusion	1
5.	Personality relatively preserved	1
6.	Depression	1
7.	Somatic complaints	1
8.	Emotional lability	1
9.	History or presence of hypertension	1
10.	History of stroke	2
11.	Evidence of co-existing atherosclerosis	1
12.	Focal neurological symptoms	2
13.	Focal neurological signs	2

Source: Hachinski VC, Iliff LD, Zilkha E, et al. (1975) Cerebral blood flow in dementia. *Archives of Neurology* **32:** 632–7.

Box 72.3 NINDS – AIREN criteria for vascular dementia (summarized)

1. Probable vascular dementia: Dementia defined by a decline in memory and two or more other cognitive domains. There should be focal neurological signs consistent with a stroke and evidence of cerebrovascular disease by brain imaging. The dementia should arise within 3 months of the stroke or there should be an abrupt decline in cognitive functioning or a fluctuating, stepwise course.
2. Possible vascular dementia: Dementia with focal neurological signs in the absence of brain imaging studies.
3. Definite vascular dementia: Probable vascular dementia together with histopathological evidence.

Source: Román GC, Tatemichi TK, Erkinjuntti T, et al. (1993) Vascular dementia: Diagnostic criteria for research studies. Report of the NINDS-AIREN International Workshop. *Neurology* **43:** 250.

Management

There is no treatment currently available to reverse the brain damage caused by cerebrovascular discasc. Thc management of vascular dementia involves monitoring and treating the risk factors in an attempt to reduce the risk of further deterioration. This includes administering antiplatelet drugs and controlling major vascular risk factors (e.g. hypertension, hypercholesterolaemia, smoking, diabetes mellitus). There is some evidence that the drug pentoxifylline, which increases blood flow, improves cognition in vascular dementia.[24] There is evidence that treatment with cholinesterase inhibitors may be of benefit; however, these drugs are not currently approved for this indication in the UK or the USA.

Prognosis

The course is extremely variable. The underlying vascular risk factors may lead to a stroke or a myocardial infarction; this may result in a pneumonia leading to death.

Dementia with Lewy bodies

Dementia with Lewy bodies and dementia in Parkinson's disease are often described as distinct entities determined by the relationship between the onset of motor symptoms and dementia. However, it is unclear whether they are the same or different disorders.

Epidemiology

Although older textbooks state that vascular dementia follows AD in prevalence, many experts now believe that LBD is the second most common type of dementia.[25] The prevalence in the community is between 0.1 per cent and 5 per cent. LBD accounts for about 22 per cent of all cases of dementia.[26–28] LBD is more common in men than in women.

Clinical features

The age of onset is 50–83 years. Fluctuations in the cognitive performance are a characteristic feature. Alterations in the level of consciousness and visual hallucinations may occur, as in delirium.[29] The visual hallucinations tend to be complex and are often of people or animals. The complexity of the visual hallucinations is thought to decrease with the progression of the dementia. Hallucinations may also occur in other modalities, and delusions may be present. Symptoms of depression are common: studies show its presence in between one-third and one-half of patients.[29,30] Parkinsonism is present in up to 70 per cent of patients. Recurrent falls and syncope are common. Neuroleptic sensitivity may occur in a third of cases and may involve worsening parkinsonism, impaired consciousness and autonomic disturbances.[31] Sleep disturbances are an important feature in LBD and include rapid-eye-movement sleep behaviour disorder (RBD), excessive daytime sleepiness, insomnia, sleep apnoea and restless legs syndrome.[32,33]

The differentiation from AD can be difficult in practice; however, patients with LBD tend to have more visuospatial impairment and less memory impairment in the early stages than patients with AD. Thus, memory changes on the MMSE may be more prominent with AD, whereas difficulties in clock-drawing or figure-copying may be more indicative of LBD.[34]

Box 72.4 International Consensus Consortium Criteria for dementia with Lewy bodies

1. Progressive cognitive decline of sufficient magnitude to interfere with normal social or occupational function. Prominent or persistent memory impairment may not necessarily occur in the early stages but is usually evident with progression. Deficits on tests of attention and frontal-subcortical skills and visuospatial ability may be especially prominent.
2. Two of the following are required for a diagnosis of probable dementia with Lewy bodies:
   - Fluctuating cognition with pronounced variations in attention and alertness
   - Recurrent visual hallucinations which are typically well formed and detailed
   - Spontaneous motor features of Parkinsonism.
3. Features supportive of the diagnosis are:
   - Repeated falls
   - Syncope or transient loss of consciousness
   - Neuroleptic sensitivity
   - Systematized delusions.
   - Hallucinations in other modalities

Source: reference 35

Diagnostic criteria

The consensus criteria by McKeith and colleagues are shown in Box 72.4.[35]

Pathology

Lewy bodies are intracytoplasmic inclusion bodies and are found in LBD and Parkinson's disease. They consist of abnormally phosphorylated neurofilament proteins aggregated with ubiquitin and alpha synuclein. The Lewy bodies are present in the brainstem or limbic areas, or they may have a diffuse distribution. Alzheimer's-type plaques are present in a similar density and distribution to that seen in Alzheimer's disease, but neurofibrillary tangles are less common.[36] Evidence suggests that the clinical presentation is driven by AD pathology and not Lewy body distribution.[37]

Management

The treatment of hallucinations and delusions is challenging in LBD because of the symptom severity, the patient's sensitivity to treatment and the high stress levels of the patient's carers. If the symptoms are mild, no medication treatment may be needed. Cholinesterase inhibitors are often used as first-line treatment for troublesome symptoms.[4] A multicentre trial has shown behavioural and cognitive benefits when rivastigmine is used in LBD. At the time of writing, rivastigmine was the only one of the cholinesterase inhibitors licensed for the treatment of dementia in Parkinson's disease and so it is often used for LBD. A more recent trial has shown that all three currently available cholinesterase inhibitors – rivastigmine, galantamine and donepezil – are of benefit, in terms of both neuropsychiatric symptoms and cognition.[38] Cholinesterase inhibitors may worsen tremor; however, this worsening is usually very mild and not too troublesome clinically. Cholinesterase inhibitors are not routinely prescribed solely for the cognitive difficulties seen in LBD, unlike in AD. There is evidence of cognitive benefit, but the slowing of cognitive decline is harder to establish in LBD and has not been adequately demonstrated. The early symptomatology of LBD tends to be dominated by behavioural and psychiatric issues.

Antipsychotics can be effective for the treatment of psychosis in DLB, but there is a risk of neuroleptic sensitivity with both typical and atypical antipsychotics.[39] There are also other risks associated with the use of antipsychotics in dementia, including increased mortality and cognitive decline. If an antipsychotic is considered, atypical antipsychotics, particularly quetiapine, may be preferred. A study by Roger and colleagues showed that quetiapine did not worsen parkinsonism;[40] however, other studies have not shown this. The NICE guidelines for dementia in the UK allow severe behavioural symptoms in LBD to be treated with antipsychotics, but they advocate monitoring for worsening parkinsonism and acute physical deterioration.

There is no evidence to suggest that depression should be treated any differently from usual. RBD may be treated with clonazepam.[41] Other treatments include antidepressants and melatonin.

Parkinsonism may sometimes be helped with medications such as levodopa. However, there is the risk of worsening confusion and psychotic symptoms, and the effect on the movement disorder is probably less than that in Parkinson's disease.[42]

Prognosis

The rate of progress in LBD is similar to that of AD, although some authors believe that the course is shorter in LBD.[43,44] The functional impairment may be greater and quality of life may be more impaired than in AD.[45]

Frontotemporal dementia

Frontotemporal dementia (FTD) is a group of disorders that primarily affect the frontal and temporal lobes of the brain.

Epidemiology

Frontotemporal dementia is the second commonest cause of early onset dementia (<65 years) after AD. Although some studies had suggested that FTD occurred more frequently in men than in women, the most recent evidence shows an equal prevalence in both sexes.[46,47,48]

Pathology

There are three types of histopathological finding in FTD. The first type, which is the most common, shows neuronal loss, spongiform change and minimal gliosis. The second type (Pick type) includes argentophilic inclusions, with neuronal loss and abundant gliosis. The third type involves either of the first two patterns plus evidence of motor neuron disease in the anterior horn cells of the brainstem and spinal cord.[49,50]

Clinical features

The clinical features include personality changes, behavioural changes, language problems and, as the disease progresses, neurological signs. Memory and other cognitive functions tend to be affected less severely in the early stages of the disease.

A key feature is a decline in social conduct. This might include socially inappropriate behaviours such as stealing, sexually inappropriate behaviour, disinhibition and tactlessness. The patient may become apathetic, with a loss of drive, or may be overactive. There may be decreased emotional expression than was the case premorbidly. A lack of awareness of the behavioural problems and the difficulties they cause commonly occurs.

Compulsive or repetitive behaviour such as foot-tapping, collecting things or hand-washing is another feature. An increase in appetite and a preference for sweet foods, leading to weight gain, is a symptom. Loss of speech and language, and various verbal stereotypies, may be present. There may be a decreased response to painful stimuli.

As the disease progresses, parkinsonian symptoms may develop.

There are two related disorders with similar histological characteristics.[51] The clinical presentation depends on the topography of the disease and not on the pathology. Semantic dementia involves the temporal lobes bilaterally and results in a loss of ability to understand the meaning of words and objects. Progressive non-fluent aphasia is associated with the Sylvian fissure in the left hemisphere and involves language difficulties.[52]

Diagnostic criteria

The Lund Manchester criteria are given in Box 72.5.

Investigations

Although the history is the most important component in the diagnosis, neuropsychological testing including frontal lobe tests may be of benefit. The tests may often be normal. CT or MRI scanning may reveal frontotemporal lobe shrinkage. SPECT scanning may be helpful in differentiating this disorder from AD. The EEG is usually normal.

Box 72.5 Lund–Manchester criteria for frontotemporal dementia

The Lund–Manchester diagnostic criteria for frontotemporal dementia require all of the following core components to be present:

1. Insidious onset and gradual progression
2. Early decline in social interpersonal conduct
3. Early impairment in regulation of personal conduct
4. Early emotional blunting
5. Early loss of insight.

Supportive diagnostic features include:

A. Behavioural disorder:
   - decline in personal hygiene and grooming;
   - mental rigidity and inflexibility;
   - distractibility and impersistence;
   - hyperorality and dietary change;
   - utilization behaviour.

B. Speech and language: altered speech output (aspontaneity and economy of speech, press of speech), stereotypy of speech, echolalia, perseveration, mutism.

C. Physical signs: primitive reflexes, incontinence, akinesia, rigidity, tremor, low/labile blood pressure.

D. Investigations:
   - neuropsychology: impaired frontal lobe tests; no amnesia or perceptual deficits;
   - EEG: normal on conventional EEG despite clinically-evident dementia;
   - brain imaging: predominant frontal and/or anterior temporal abnormality.

Source: reference 50

Management

A multidisciplinary approach involving the family and other caregivers is needed in view of the frequent difficulties in managing these patients. The patients are relatively young and physically well, can demonstrate a number of behavioural difficulties and have limited insight.

There is currently no treatment that helps to prevent the progression of FTD. Symptomatic drug treatment for the behavioural problems may be considered. Antipsychotics may be of benefit for aggression and if there any psychotic features. Selective serotonin reuptake inhibitors (SSRIs) have been shown to be of benefit for compulsions, disinhibition and overeating.[53] Caregivers may need assistance from support groups and planned respite admission; 24-h care may be needed.

Prognosis

The disease progresses over 2–10 years before resulting in death.

Mixed dementias

AD pathology often coexists with vascular pathology, and this is sometimes referred to as 'mixed dementia'. Although both DSM-IV and ICD-10 include a category of mixed dementia, there are no consensus criteria. 'Pure' AD or vascular dementia may not be as common as previously thought. About 40 per cent of patients in the community with dementia have been found to have mixed pathology.[54] The diagnosis during life may be based on clinical and imaging factors. In clinical practice, the results of neuroimaging are probably the most common reason for changing an initial clinical diagnosis of AD to that of a mixed dementia.[55] Treatment involves cholinesterase inhibitors or memantine and the management of vascular risk factors.[56]

DELIRIUM

Delirium, or acute confusional state, is a state of cerebral dysfunction. It usually has an acute onset and fluctuates over the course of the day. It is characterized by a disturbance of consciousness, which manifests as impaired attention. The patient's attention wanders and they may be distracted by irrelevant stimuli. There are cognitive difficulties, particularly with short-term memory, and disorientation to time or place. Speech may be rambling and incoherent. Perceptual disturbances including distortions, illusions and hallucinations, especially in the visual mode, are common. The patient may be overactive and restless, or lethargic and drowsy; sleep patterns are frequently affected. Mood may be one of perplexity, euphoria or apathy and may shift rapidly and unpredictably.

Delirium is a medical emergency and has a high mortality and morbidity rate in elderly people. In elderly patients, delirium is associated with increased length of hospital stay and a higher rate of entry into nursing homes. Risk factors for delirium include cognitive and sensory impairment, use of restraints, malnutrition, the use of more than three medications, bladder catheterization, and increasing number of iatrogenic events.[57] Common precipitants for delirium in elderly patients include infections, constipation, medications and electrolyte abnormalities. Delirium is common after surgery.

As for younger people, the treatment involves identifying the cause and offering supportive measures.

LATE-ONSET SCHIZOPHRENIA

The classification of schizophrenic illnesses starting late in life has been contentious. A number of different terminologies and cut-off age limits have been used in the literature. The term 'late paraphrenia' was used by some authors to describe paranoid delusions and hallucinations in older people. Other authors prefer the term 'late-onset schizophrenia' (LOS) because of a number of similarities to early-onset disease. The DSM-IV and ICD-10 classifications do not include a separate category for late-onset psychotic illnesses; however, schizophrenia may be diagnosed at any age.

The Late Onset Schizophrenia Group, which comprised 17 international representatives of basic science and clinical schizophrenia research and academic and clinical geriatric psychiatry centres, issued a consensus statement in 2000 that divided schizophrenia into three groups based on age. The early-onset group is said to have an age of onset below 40 years, the late-onset group between ages 40 years and 60 years, and the very late schizophrenia-like group at an age above 60 years.[58]

Epidemiology

The epidemiology for new-onset schizophrenia has not been established clearly; however, the proportion of patients with schizophrenia whose illness first emerged after the age of 40 years was estimated to be 23.5 per cent in one study.[59] An incidence rate of 12.6 per 100 000 population per year has been calculated using the age of onset of 45 years. The 1-year prevalence rate of schizophrenia in individuals aged 45–64 years was shown to be 0.6 per cent.[60] The prevalence of schizophrenia in older adults in the community is less than 0.5 per cent.[61,62] The risk for females is higher than that for males in late life.

Clinical features

LOS is frequently characterized by persecutory delusions, which may relate to the patient's neighbours. Partition delusions – usually relating to some material or radiation passing through the patient's walls or ceilings from a neighbour's house – may occur in two-thirds of patients with very-late-onset schizophrenia-like illness. Auditory hallucinations are the second most common psychotic symptom. The auditory hallucinations may range from a hum to those of a Schneiderian first-rank symptom nature. Visual, tactile and olfactory hallucinations are not uncommon. Thought disorder, negative symptoms and catatonia are rare, especially after the age of 60 years.

Aetiology

Structural imaging is similar to that of early-onset cases, with higher ventricular to brain ratio versus age-matched controls and focal abnormalities such as reduction in the volume of the left temporal lobe.[63]

Some studies reported an increase in infarcts or white-matter hyperintensities in very-late-onset cases.[64] However, when patients with focal neurological abnormalities and dementia were excluded, there was no demonstrable excess of these changes.[65]

It is possible that an increase in the number of D4 receptors plays a role in the development of LOS.

There are often lifelong paranoid and schizoid traits in people who develop LOS. However, there is probably less psychosocial, educational and occupational dysfunction than in people with early-onset disease.[66]

There is an association between sensory deficits, especially deafness and visual impairment, and late-life schizophrenia. However, causation has not been established.

Management

Elderly patients who develop schizophrenic symptoms frequently have poor insight into their experiences. Often they manage in the community for long periods until their behaviour becomes a significant risk to themselves or others, when they are brought to the attention of the mental health team. They may resist investigations and treatment. Many will agree to take medications for symptomatic relief while not accepting the medical opinion regarding the diagnosis.

Antipsychotic agents continue to be the first-line treatment for late-onset psychosis, despite the lack of robust randomized clinical trials in this population. Clinical experience, however, suggests that these drugs are of benefit. It is important to select patients appropriately and to carefully weigh the benefits and risks when initiating these agents. Dosages of one-quarter to one-half of those used in early-onset cases are often sufficient. Elderly people starting antipsychotics are at an increased risk of having side effects compared with working-age adults. The risk of developing tardive dyskinesia may be three to five times greater in elderly patients than in younger adults.[67] Psychosocial interventions may be helpful in helping the patient and their family to cope with the symptoms. There is very little published evidence on specific psychotherapies in schizophrenia with first onset in old age.

Prognosis

Fully developed symptoms rarely go away completely; however, their intensity and the disruption they cause will fluctuate over time. One small study suggested a link with AD.[68] However, other evidence indicates that patients with very-late-schizophrenia-like disorder present with stable cognitive and everyday functioning, compared with chronically institutionalized elderly patients with schizophrenia.[69]

Older people with chronic schizophrenia

People who have had a diagnosis of schizophrenia from an early age and have grown old with the disease are sometimes referred to as 'graduates', especially in the UK literature. This term has been used since the early 1970s and predominantly describes people with schizophrenia; however, other enduring mental illnesses such as mood disorders are also included. People are thought of as 'graduating' from services designed for the needs of adults of working age to those designed for older people.

Epidemiology

The number of older people with chronic schizophrenia is not known. This is due partly to the variety of settings in which these individuals are now based. It is estimated that people who develop schizophrenia before the age of 45 years, and who age with it, represent about 85 per cent of all people with schizophrenia.[70] In the UK, the number of elderly people with chronic psychoses in the 1980s was estimated at around 30 per 100 000 of the population.[71]

Clinical issues

Older people with chronic schizophrenia have complex mental and physical health difficulties and social needs.[72] Hallucinations and delusions tend to become less severe with time, but negative symptoms tend to worsen. Some studies have shown evidence of continued cognitive decline in elderly people with chronic schizophrenia.[73] Cognitive deficits are associated with poor social and community functioning.[74]

Elderly people with chronic schizophrenia may be at risk of having unrecognized physical health problems and poor management of illnesses. This may be for a number of reasons, including poor insight and poor medication compliance.[75] The rates of cardiovascular diseases and diabetes in people with schizophrenia have been reported to be increased above those in people without the disease.[76]

Elderly people with chronic schizophrenia tend to have varying degrees of social impairment, but their general coping skills may improve.[75] Social impairment is associated with impaired cognition, negative symptoms and parkinsonism.[77] There may also be issues of stigma due to the long history of mental health difficulties and the side effects of antipsychotic medications.

Management

Elderly people with chronic schizophrenia are managed by adult, old-age or rehabilitation psychiatry. The Royal College of Psychiatrists in the UK produced a report in 2002 to highlight the needs of 'graduates'. This report recommended that health and social services identify these needs and draw up individual care plans to meet these needs, taking into account the available resources.[78]

Older people with schizophrenia may be on high doses of medications started when they were young. With the pharmacokinetic and pharmacodynamic changes of the ageing process, lower doses may be more suitable in older people. Cognitive-behavioural therapy (CBT) has been shown to be helpful in treating persistent symptoms in younger patients.[79] In older people, a cognitive-behavioural approach may also be of benefit, particularly for improving social functioning.[80] Social care needs may be complex and should be addressed on an individual basis.

AFFECTIVE DISORDERS IN ELDERLY PEOPLE

Depression

Epidemiology

Depression is the most common psychiatric illness in elderly people.[81] The prevalence of major and minor depression in elderly people living in the community is 10–15 per cent. About 2 per cent of these people meet the criteria for a major depressive disorder. A number of people have subthreshold depression – symptoms of depression that do not fulfil the standard criteria for a depressive disorder but that still cause suffering and are treatable.[82]

Clinical presentation

It may be more appropriate to think of depression as a spectrum ranging from subthreshold symptoms to a major depressive disorder. Sticking rigidly to the categories in ICD-10 and DSM-IV may be less appropriate in elderly people, due to the variety of clinical presentations.

The diagnostic criteria for depression do not take age into account; however, there may be some differences in presentation in elderly people compared with in younger adults. Low mood or sadness may not be reported in elderly people, while anxiety, feelings of not being able to cope, and irritability may be more frequent. Memory may be impaired and can present with a dementia-like picture. Somatic and hypochondriacal symptoms may occur in elderly people, making the differentiation from physical disorders difficult. Depression may present with behavioural changes such as refusing care, aggression and new-onset alcohol dependence. Physical symptoms such as low energy, anorexia and weight loss may be difficult to interpret due to co-morbid physical disorders.[83]

There is evidence for a subtype of depression (vascular depression) that arises primarily in later life and is associated with cerebrovascular disease. Distinct clinical features may include reduced depressive ideation (e.g. guilt), greater cognitive impairment, particularly including executive functioning, and psychomotor retardation. An association has been reported between deep white-matter changes, especially in the frontal lobe and basal ganglia, and depression on MRI scanning. These changes may reflect small-vessel ischaemia. The concept of vascular depression is not without its critiques, however, and there are no consensus criteria at present.[84]

Management

Antidepressants are effective in elderly people, with tricyclic antidepressants and SSRIs having equal efficacy in this age group.[85] The altered pharmacokinetics and pharmacodynamics of elderly people make it essential to use antidepressants with caution. The SSRIs are often preferred because of the anticholinergic side effects of tricyclic antidepressants. The SSRIs are also safer in an overdose.

However, there is an increased risk of gastrointestinal bleeding with SSRIs: it is advisable to use caution if there is a history of gastrointestinal bleeding or if the patient is on aspirin or non-steroidal anti-inflammatory drugs (NSAIDs), and concomitant use of a proton-pump inhibitor may be an option worth considering in some cases. There is also the risk of hyponatraemia in elderly people as a result of the syndrome of inappropriate antidiuretic hormone secretion (SIADH), particularly with the SSRIs; monitoring of serum electrolytes is therefore advisable. Venlafaxine and mirtazapine have also been shown to be effective in elderly people.[86,87] Medical co-morbidity is associated with a decreased tolerability of, and a poorer response to, antidepressants

Electroconvulsive therapy (ECT) is a safe and effective treatment in major depression in old age, with a recovery rate of 70–80 per cent of patients.[87] ECT is generally used for severe depression when other treatment options have failed and when there is a threat to life from poor dietary intake or suicidal ideation. There is evidence that it is particularly effective in psychotic depression.[84] The current NICE guidelines recommend ECT only for short-term treatment and not for maintenance treatment. Patients should have ongoing cognitive checks due to the risk of post-ECT memory impairment.[88]

CBT is increasingly used in the treatment of mild and moderate depression and is recommended by NICE in the UK. CBT is at least as good for treating depression in older people as it is for younger adults.[89]

Interpersonal therapy is effective in preventing relapse.[90] Cognitive therapy may, however, be better than interpersonal therapy in more severe depression.[91] Cognitive analytical therapy may be considered particularly if unresolved issues from the patient's past form a significant part of the clinical picture.[92] In more severe depression, a combination of psychotherapy and medications may be the most effective option.

Prognosis

The recovery rates of depression in elderly people are lower than those in younger adults.[93] If confounders such as physical illness are taken into account, the rates in late life are little different from those in midlife, but relapse rates appear higher.[94] A number of patients develop chronic symptoms.[95]

Late-life depression may increase the risk of mortality. A study in 2008 showed that increasing depression severity corresponds to a greater mortality risk, with elderly men on antidepressants being at a particularly high risk.[96] The risk was thought not to be pharmacological but to be related to the depression. The mortality is due in part to cardiac causes.

Bipolar affective disorder

Although bipolar affective disorder is relatively uncommon in elderly people, it can be a diagnostic and management challenge. Mania in older people can either be in the context of a patient with a previous diagnosis of a bipolar disorder or have its first onset in old age.

Epidemiology

The prevalence of mania in the community decreases with age, from 1.4 per cent in younger adults to 0.1 per cent in people over 65 years.[97] However, first admission rates increase with age, perhaps relating to an increased need for inpatient treatment.[98] Twelve per cent of all affective disorders treated on specialized geriatric psychiatry units are due to mania.[99]

Clinical presentation

The clinical features of older people with mania are similar to those seen in younger adults with mania. The former may have a less severe form of the illness and less sexual preoccupation.[100,101] A late-onset mania is more likely to be associated with organic mental illness, although one study showed that overall there was only a slight increase in the association with organic pathology in late-onset versus early-onset bipolar disorder.[102]

Management

A thorough physical examination and appropriate investigations have to be carried out in late-onset mania in order to rule out an organic cause. Neuroleptics, lithium and anticonvulsants are used as for younger people, but in lower doses and at a slower titration. Social and psychological support is important to consider.

Prognosis

Although not supported by all studies, there may be a poorer prognosis in elderly people with bipolar affective disorder compared with those with unipolar depression. A risk of increased risk of mortality was found in the former by Shulman and colleagues.[103] Late-life bipolar disorders are associated with cognitive impairments.[104] It is unclear whether there is an increased risk of dementia.

ANXIETY DISORDERS

Epidemiology

The prevalence of anxiety disorders has been estimated at 1–10 per cent of the elderly population.[105] Up to one in seven adults may have appreciable levels of anxiety if life-disrupting subsyndromal anxiety is included.[106] There is an excess of females for most disorders. The prevalence and incidence tend to fall with age.

Clinical presentation

The full range of anxiety disorders seen in younger people may occur in elderly people. A relatively common type of phobia in elderly people called 'space phobia' has been described. This involves a fear of falling in open spaces and may lead to confinement at home.[107]

Abnormal illness behaviour, including somatization and hypochondriasis, may develop. In the majority of patients, these behaviours have their onset in early life. First presentations in old age are usually secondary to depression or an anxiety disorder. Obsessional disorders rarely appear for the first time in old age. The possibility of focal or generalized organic causes must be considered.

Assessment

Detection of anxiety symptoms in elderly people is complicated by a number of factors, including physical illnesses, multiple medications, the difficulty of differentiating anxiety from depression, and the tendency of some older adults to resist psychiatric evaluation.[108] The anxiety may be dismissed by health professionals as being 'understandable' given the life situation.

Symptoms starting for the first time in elderly patients require thorough investigation. Due to the range and overlap of anxiety symptoms and co-morbidity with medical illnesses, some authors have suggested that a dimensional rather than a categorical approach may be more useful in the evaluation of these symptoms.[109]

Management

Medication treatment is as for younger people. However, the side effects of medications and the effects of ageing need to be taken into account. Antidepressants may be considered, especially if there are symptoms of depression. SSRIs are usually the preferred choice, but the risks of gastrointestinal bleeding and hyponatraemia must be borne in mind. Short-term use of benzodiazepines for relief from troublesome symptoms may be an option. The possibility of dependence, memory impairment, risks of falls and delirium in elderly people should be taken into consideration.

Psychological therapies have been shown to be of benefit in treating anxiety disorders in younger adults. Trials in older people are also supportive of the use of psychological approaches. Research conducted to date suggests that CBT produces significant improvement in anxiety symptoms among elderly patients. However, there is some concern that CBT does not benefit elderly patients with anxiety as much as it does younger patients with anxiety. Methods of augmenting or supplementing CBT are being developed to make it more suitable for older adults.[110]

Smit and colleagues identified risk factors for developing anxiety in late life, which include depression, two or more chronic illnesses, poor sense of mastery, poor self-rated health and low educational level. The authors suggested that this may offer opportunities for prevention.[111]

LEGAL ISSUES

Mental capacity

Mental capacity refers to a person's ability to make a decision regarding an action. This is of particular relevance in old-age psychiatry and is often an issue when making decisions regarding medical treatment, place of residence, finances and care arrangements.

Mental Capacity Act

The Mental Capacity Act 2005 came into force in England and Wales in October 2007. It is a statutory framework that enables decision-making on behalf of adults aged 16 years and over who lack capacity to make decisions on their own behalf.

The Act sets out a clear test for a person who lacks capacity. This involves the inability to:

- understand the information relevant to the decision;
- retain that information;
- use or weigh that information as part of the process of making the decision; or
- communicate the decision.

The test of capacity is decision-specific, for example a decision regarding a particular treatment, and is not a global characteristic of the person concerned. People are presumed to have capacity unless it is proved otherwise. The Act also states that the ability of a person to make a decision must be maximized before a conclusion about the lack of capacity can be made; this might include writing things down or using a translator. People are allowed to make 'unwise' decisions.

When a person lacks capacity, decisions must be taken based on the person's best interests. The Act provides a checklist for determining best interests; these include taking into account the person's past and present wishes (in particular, any relevant written statements made by the person when capacity was present), the person's beliefs and values, and the views of anyone involved in the care of the person and any donee of a lasting power of attorney.

The Act has introduced a number of new powers and bodies. The Lasting Powers of Attorney (LPA) allows individuals to appoint another person (an attorney) to look after their property and financial affairs and to make health and personal welfare decisions when they lack the capacity to make these decisions themselves in the future. The attorney(s) can use the LPA only after it has been registered with the Office of the Public Guardian. The Act creates a new Court of Protection, which is ultimately responsible for the proper functioning of the legislation. Independent mental capacity advocates (IMCAs) have been introduced by the Act. The role of the IMCAs is to assist incapacitated adults who do not have anyone else to help them in the decision-making process for serious medical treatment or place of residence.[112]

Living wills and advance directives (decisions)

Any person with capacity has the right to accept or refuse medical treatment. Living wills are statements made about accepting or refusing medical treatment at a future date when capacity is not present. Living wills are not legally binding but should be taken into account when treatment is being considered in an incapacitated person. Advance directives are a type of living will concerned specifically with decisions made in advance about the refusal of treatment when it is being considered and capacity is not present. Advance directives have a legal basis in the Mental Capacity Act and must be respected; however, there are circumstances when an advance directive might not be acted upon, such as when the person has acted in a manner inconsistent with the decision (e.g. a change of religious faith) or an unanticipated change in circumstances (e.g. treatment advances that change the prognosis of the condition).[112]

Testamentary capacity

This refers to the ability of a person to make a will. The criteria for testamentary capacity are based on the case of Banks versus Goodfellow (1870) and involve the following. The person making a will (testator) must:

- understand the nature of a will;
- have knowledge of the nature and extent of their assets;
- be able to recall and understand the claims of potential heirs;
- be free of delusions or hallucinations that influence their testamentary decisions.

Understanding the nature of a will refers to understanding that the will deals with the distribution of the testator's property to the named person or people after the testator's death.

The testator need not have a detailed knowledge of their property, but they do need to have a reasonable idea of what their property constitutes. A psychiatrist may be asked to assess a person's testamentary capacity in difficult cases. They may also be asked to give evidence if the will is contested after the testator's death on issues of capacity and undue influence.

Driving

Driving is a complex activity and requires the integration of perception, motor function and cognition. Ageing is associated with slower cognitive functioning and reduced musculoskeletal strength and flexibility. There is a slight increase in the crash risk in people over 70 years (the highest risk is in males aged 16–24 years). Practical steps to continue safe driving include driving for shorter periods, taking frequent breaks, driving during only daylight hours, and maintaining longer stopping distances.

In the UK, the DVLA is responsible for issuing driving licences. The law governing the issue of driving licences is contained in the Road Traffic Act 1988 and the Motor Vehicles (Driving Licences) Regulations 1999. Age is not a bar to having a UK licence. However, at the age of 70 years, the DVLA requires confirmation that there is no medical disability; thereafter, the licence is reviewed every 3 years.

A diagnosis of a dementia has consequences for driving. As the disease progresses, the ability to drive is usually lost. Over the course of the disease, evidence suggests that the risk of a crash is increased significantly. As a general rule, however, the risk seems to remain acceptably low for up to 3 years after the onset of dementia, by which time most patients have stopped driving.[113]

The DVLA acknowledges that it is extremely difficult to assess the driving ability in people with dementia and that the presentations and rates of progression are variable. In early dementia, when sufficient skills are retained and progression is slow, a licence for group 1 vehicles (cars, motorcycles) may be issued, subject to annual review. A formal driving assessment may be necessary. The licence for group 2 vehicles (vehicles over 3.5 tonnes, including lorries and buses) will be revoked on the basis of a diagnosis of a dementia in view of the increased risks relating to the size of the vehicle and the time spent in occupational driving.

Notifying the DVLA of a medical condition that affects driving is the responsibility of the licence holder. It is the duty of the doctor to inform patients of this responsibility. Failure to notify the DVLA is a criminal offence. There is also a duty to inform the insurance company. The DVLA may require a medical report and a driving assessment.

The General Medical Council (GMC) advises doctors that, in some circumstances, it may be necessary for them to break confidentiality and contact the DVLA if the patient continues to drive when they may not be fit to do so.

The psychological and practical negative consequences of revoking a licence must be borne in mind. It is an independent risk factor for entry into a nursing home.[114]

OLD-AGE PSYCHIATRY SERVICES

Older people have often been overlooked when it comes to the planning of services. As the population ages and the number of older people with mental illnesses rises, it is important that planned and funded services exist to address the need. The cut-off age for entry into services is usually 65 years. There have been discussions as to whether separate services should exist for elderly people, since this has implications of ageism. However, older people do have unique requirements, such as physical co-morbidity, increased incidence of cognitive difficulties and frailty. A continued separate service with the required expertise is probably the most useful way of addressing the needs of these people.

Community mental health teams

Mental health services in the UK are provided through specialist community mental health teams (CMHT). The role of the team is to provide assessment and treatment of the mental health of older people with complex needs. The team consists of members from a variety of professional backgrounds who work in a concerted manner. The National Service Framework for Older People in the UK recommended that the core members of the team should include a consultant psychogeriatrician, community mental health nurses, a clinical psychologist, a social worker and an occupational therapist.[115] There should be referral arrangements with other professionals, including physiotherapists, speech and language therapists and dieticians.

The role of the community nurse may include monitoring the mental health of the patients and providing advice and support to the carers. The nurse can alert the general practitioner (GP) or psychiatrist if the patient's condition worsens and needs further medical input. Nurses in the UK have the opportunity to become supplementary prescribers and can do this as part of an agreed care plan.

Psychologists play a vital role in neuropsychological assessments of people with cognitive impairments. Specific psychological treatment may also be offered, depending on the local arrangements.

Occupational therapists are needed to assess patients' skills for independent living; this is particularly relevant in dementia. They may help in setting up adjustments to the patient's home in order to enable the patient to continue to function well in that environment.

A CMHT social worker helps in coordinating care arrangements in the community and in organizing 24-h residential or nursing placements. An approved mental health worker (most often a social worker with specialized training) in the UK also has the role of assessing the needs of people being considered for detention under the Mental Health Act.

Day hospitals

Day hospitals form an important part of the psychiatric services for older people in the UK, with more than 90 per cent of teams in the UK having access to places.[116] However, a number of Mental Health Trusts have recently been reviewing the need for Day Hospital access.

The roles and benefits of day hospitals include the following:

- Assessment of patients to help with diagnostic clarification and for observation of behavioural difficulties in dementia
- May be an alternative to more expensive in-patient admission in some cases
- May help in the transition from in-patient settings to the community and reduce the length of in-patient admission
- Rehabilitation of patients with dementia
- Psychotherapeutic interventions for behavioural difficulties
- Respite for carers
- Longer-term support for those with relapsing illness or poor response to treatment.

Day hospitals are distinct from day centres.

In-patient care

Elderly people frequently have considerable physical health needs and may be frail. They are best managed in wards for older people and not together with working-age adults.[117] In-patient settings around the UK vary as to whether they have separate units for people with organic and functional disorders or whether such patients are admitted together. This may depend on local resources and practicalities such as the number of patients. Patients with dementia may have a number of behavioural difficulties, and it is advantageous to manage them separately, as this will require specific staff expertise and ward environment. Old-age psychiatric units are best located in or close to general hospitals, where there is access to geriatric or general medical expertise and laboratory and radiological resources.

Memory clinics

Memory clinics are specialized clinics that aim to diagnose and treat people with memory problems. The staff must consist of a psychiatrist, nurses and a neuropsychologist. The role of the doctor is to help with the diagnosis of dementia and to assess co-morbid psychiatric and medical conditions, which may contribute to the memory problems. Some memory clinic teams are nurse-led. The nurses may be involved in the initial diagnostic process and help in the monitoring of treatment. A psychologist must carry out comprehensive cognitive assessments, especially in cases of diagnostic difficulty. The clinic may advise the patient and their carers on issues to do with driving and social care. Longer-term issues such as financial arrangements, living wills and advance directives may also be addressed. There is evidence to suggest that memory clinics provide better-quality assessment, care-planning and follow-up than do traditional old-age psychiatry home assessment visits for people with memory disorders.[118]

Liaison service

There is a very high prevalence of mental health disorder among older people within the general hospital setting. Delirium in elderly people is common, with a prevalence of up to 20 per cent on medical wards and even higher in surgical wards.[119] Dementia is found in up to 30 per cent of elderly in-patients.[120] The rates of depression vary between studies but may be as high as 40 per cent.[121] These illnesses are often underdiagnosed and undertreated, with resulting increased morbidity.

Despite this, liaison psychiatry for older people is generally a poorly resourced part of the psychiatric service. In the UK, the service is generally on an ad hoc consultation basis, usually by a psychiatrist. A liaison model may be more suitable. One option is to have a multidisciplinary team, including psychiatrists, social workers, occupational therapists, psychologists and psychiatric nurses. In addition to helping with the diagnosis and management of mental illness, the role of the team would be to provide training to the general hospital staff. The liaison model would facilitate easier access to psychiatric advice, help with ongoing management difficulties and may help to improve clinical outcomes.[122]

KEY POINTS

- Dementia is a clinical syndrome of a number of cognitive deficits along with behavioural, psychological and neurological symptoms; it causes significant morbidity in older people and has an impact on the patient's family, health and social services, and the economics of a country. The prevalence is expected to increase considerably over the next few decades.
- The commonest cause of dementia is Alzheimer's disease. Early memory loss is a characteristic feature of Alzheimer's disease; however all cognitive domains are affected over time. A cholinergic deficit is thought to be an important cause of the symptomatology, and treatment with acetylcholinesterases such as Aricept can slow down the course of the disease.
- The second most common cause of dementia is Lewy body disease. Marked fluctuations in cognition and level of consciousness, parkinsonism, visual hallucinations and neuroleptic sensitivity frequently occur. Lewy body disease may cause more severe functional impairment than Alzheimer's disease. Treatment of the visual hallucinations can be problematic; cholinesterase inhibitors are a useful option.
- Vascular dementia has a variety of presentations, ranging from the classical stepwise progression to a slow and gradual course. Neurological symptoms and psychological symptoms are commoner than in Alzheimer's disease, and the cognitive deficits are patchier with early memory loss being a less prominent symptom. There is no specific treatment; however the vascular risk factors need to be monitored closely to reduce the risk of further brain damage. Vascular dementia may coexist with Alzheimer's disease.
- Frontotemporal dementia is common in people under the age of 65. Behavioural and personality changes are the presenting symptoms. There is no treatment at present which affects the course of the disease.
- A delirium is an acute confusional state with fluctuations in consciousness and perceptual disturbances. It may coexist with a dementia and requires urgent medical attention.
- Cases of schizophrenia in old age may refer to those with chronic disease – 'graduates' – who have aged, or to those whose first episode of illness starts late in life. There are differences in symptoms, with the latter having less thought disorder and reduced treatment requirements.
- Depression is the most common mental illness in older adults and there are a greater variety of presentations than in younger people. Memory may be impaired and it is a differential diagnosis when a dementia is suspected. Antidepressants are effective; however lower doses are used in view of the altered pharmacokinetics and risk of side effects in older people.
- The assessment of mental capacity is important when it comes to deciding on treatment, competence to manage financial affairs and writing wills. The Mental Capacity Act in England and Wales provides a statutory basis for this.
- Services for older adults with mental health problems vary across the UK; however they are usually based primarily in the community and have a multidisciplinary team approach.

REFERENCES

1. Dementia UK (2007) *A Report into the Prevalence and Cost of Dementia Prepared by the Personal Social Services Research Unit at the London School of Economics and the Institute of Psychiatry at King's College London for the Alzheimer's Society*. London: Alzheimer's Society.
2. Folstein MF, Folstein SE, McHugh PR (1975) 'Mini-mental state': a practical method for grading the cognitive state of patients for the clinician. *Journal of Psychiatric Research* **12**: 189–98.
3. Hodkinson HM (1972) Evaluation of a mental test score for assessment of mental impairment in the elderly. *Age and Ageing* **1**: 233–8.
4. National Institute of Health and Clinical Excellence. (2006) *CG 42 Dementia: Supporting people with dementia and their carers in health and social care*. London: National Institute of Health and Clinical Excellence.
5. Small GW (2002) What we need to know about age related memory loss. *British Medical Journal* **324**: 1502–5.
6. Sunderland T, Hill JL, Mellow AM, *et al.* (1989) Clock drawing in Alzheimer's disease: a novel measure of dementia severity. *Journal of the American Geriatric Society* **37**: 725–9.
7. Rosen WG, Mohs RC, Davis KL (1984). A new rating scale for Alzheimer's disease. *American Journal of Psychiatry* **141**: 1356–64.
8. Morris JC (1993) The Clinical Dementia Rating (CDR): current version and scoring rules. *Neurology* **43**: 2412–4.
9. Cummings JL, Mega M, Gray K, *et al.* (1994). The Neuropsychiatric Inventory: comprehensive assessment of psychopathology in dementia. *Neurology* **44**: 2308–14.
10. Bucks RS, Ashworth DL, Wilcock GK, Siegfried K (1996) Assessment of activities of daily living in dementia: development of the Bristol Activities of Daily Living Scale. *Age Ageing* **25**: 113–20.

11. American Psychiatric Association (2000) *Diagnostic and Statistical Manual of Mental Disorders*. Washington, DC: American Psychiatric Association.
12. World Health Organization (1992) *International Classification of Diseases*. Geneva: World Health Organization.
13. O'Donnell F (2007) Cognitive impairment in schizophrenia: a life span perspective. *American Journal of Alzheimer's Disease and Other Dementias* **22**: 398–405.
14. Jones GMM (1997) A review of Feil's validation method for communicating with and caring for dementia sufferers. *Current Opinion in Psychiatry* **10**: 326–32.
15. Junaid O, Hegde S (2007) Supportive therapy in dementia. *Advances in Psychiatric Treatment* **13**: 17–23.
16. Ballard CG, O'Brien J, Reichelt K, Perry E (2002) Aromatherapy as a safe and effective treatment for the management of agitation in severe dementia: the results of a double blind, placebo controlled trial. *Journal of Clinical Psychiatry* **63**: 553–8.
17. Lyketsos C, Veiel LL, Baker A, Steele C (1999) A randomised controlled trial of bright light therapy for agitated behaviours in dementia patients residing in long-term care. *International Journal of Geriatric Psychiatry* **14**: 520–25.
18. Peterson RC, Doody R, Kurz A, *et al.* (2001) Current concepts in mild cognitive impairment. *Archives of Neurology* **58**: 1985–92.
19. Salloway S, Ferris S, Kluger A, *et al.* (2004) Efficacy of donepezil in mild cognitive impairment: a randomized placebo-controlled trial. *Neurology* **63**: 651–7.
20. Benjamin B, Burns A (2007) Donepezil for Alzheimer's disease. *Expert Review of Neurotherapeutics* **7**: 1243–9.
21. Burns A, Gauthier S, Perdomo C (2007) Efficacy and safety of donepezil over 3 years: an open-label, multicentre study in patients with Alzheimer's disease. *International Journal of Geriatric Psychiatry* **22**: 806–12.
22. Hachinski VC, Ibiff LD, Zilhka E, *et al.* (1975) Cerebral blood flow in dementia. *Archives of Neurology* **32**: 632–7.
23. Roman GC, Tatemichi TK, Erkinjuntti T, *et al.* (1993) Vascular dementia: diagnostic criteria for research studies: report of the NINDS-AIREN International Workshop. *Neurology* **43**: 250–60.
24. European Pentoxifylline Multi-Infarct Dementia Study (1996) *European Neurology* **36**: 315–21.
25. National Institute of Neurological Disorders and Stroke (2009) *NINDS Dementia with Lewy Bodies Information Page*. www.ninds.nih.gov/disorders/dementiawithlewybodies.
26. Yamada T, Hattori H, Miura A, Tanabe M, Yamori Y (2001) Prevalence of Alzheimer's disease, vascular dementia and dementia with Lewy bodies in a Japanese population. *Psychiatry and Clinical Neurosciences* **55**: 21–25.
27. Rahkonen T, Eloniemi-Sulkava U, Rissanen S, *et al.* (2003) Dementia with Lewy bodies according to the consensus criteria in a general population aged 75 years or older. *Journal of Neurology, Neurosurgery and Psychiatry* **74**: 720–24.
28. McKeith I, Mintzer J, Aarsland D, *et al.* (2004) Dementia with Lewy bodies. *Lancet Neurology* **3**: 19–28.
29. Byrne EJ, Lennox G, Lowe J, Godwin-Austen RB (1989) Diffuse Lewy body disease: clinical features in 15 cases. *Journal of Neurology, Neurosurgery and Psychiatry* **52**: 709–17.
30. Aarsland D, Ballard C, Larsen JP, McKeith I (2001) A comparative study of psychiatric symptoms in dementia with Lewy bodies and Parkinson's disease with and without dementia. *International Journal of Geriatric Psychiatry* **16(5)**: 528–36.
31. McKeith IG (2002) Dementia with Lewy bodies. *The British Journal of Psychiatry* **180**: 144–7.
32. Schenck CH, Bundlie SR, Mahowald MW (2003) REM behavior disorder (RBD): delayed emergence of parkinsonism and/or dementia in 65% of older men initially diagnosed with idiopathic RBD, and an analysis of the minimum & maximum tonic and/or phasic electromyographic abnormalities found during REM sleep. *Sleep* **26(Suppl)**: 0794.M.
33. Boeve B, Silber M, Ferman T, *et al.* (2001) Association of REM sleep behavior disorder and neurodegenerative disease may reflect an underlying synucleinopathy. *Movement Disorder* **16**: 622–30.
34. Ballard CG, Ayre G, O'Brien J, *et al.* (1999) Simple standardised neuropsychological assessments aid in the differential diagnosis of dementia with Lewy bodies from Alzheimer's disease and vascular dementia. *Dementia and Geriatric Cognitive Disorders* **10**: 104–8.
35. McKeith IG, Galasko D, Kosaka K, *et al.* (1996) Consensus guidelines for the clinical and pathologic diagnosis of dementia with Lewy bodies (DLB): report of the consortium on DLB international workshop. *Neurology* **47**:1113–24.
36. Weiner MF (1999) Dementia associated with Lewy bodies: dilemmas and directions. *Archives of Neurology* **56**: 1441–2.
37. Weisman D, Cho M, Taylor C, *et al.* (2007) In dementia with Lewy bodies, Braak stage determines phenotype, not Lewy body distribution. *Neurology* **69**: 356–9.
38. Bhasin M, Rowan E, Edwards K, McKeith I (2007) Cholinesterase inhibitors in dementia with Lewy bodies: a comparative analysis. *International Journal of Geriatric Psychiatry* **22**: 890–95.
39. McKeith IG (2002) Dementia with Lewy bodies. *The British Journal of Psychiatry* **180**: 144–7
40. Kurlan R, Cummings J, Raman R, Thal L, for the Alzheimer's Disease Cooperative Study Group (2007) Quetiapine for agitation or psychosis in patients with dementia and parkinsonism. *Neurology* **68**: 1356–63.
41. Gagnon J-F, Postuma RB, Montplaisir J (2006) Update

on the pharmacology of REM sleep behavior disorder. *Neurology* **67**: 742–747.

42. Mosimann UP, McKeith IG (2003) Dementia with Lewy bodies: diagnosis and treatment. *Swiss Medical Weekly* **133**: 131–42.
43. Ballard C, O'Brien J, Morris CM, *et al.* (2001) The progression of cognitive impairment in dementia with Lewy bodies, vascular dementia and Alzheimer's disease. *International Journal of Geriatric Psychiatry* **16**: 499–503.
44. Walker Z, Allen RL, Shergill S, Mullan E, Katona CL (2000) Three years survival in patients with a clinical diagnosis of dementia with Lewy bodies. *International Journal of Geriatric Psychiatry* **15**: 267–73.
45. Ratnavalli E, Brayne C, Dawson K, Hodges JR (2002) The prevalence of frontotemporal dementia. *Neurology* **58**: 1615–21.
46. Mercy L, Hodges JR, Dawson K, *et al.* (2008) Incidence of early-onset dementias in Cambridgeshire, United Kingdom. *Neurology* **71(19)**: 1496–9.
47. Ratnavalli E, Brayne C, Dawson K, Hodges JR (2002) The prevalence of frontotemporal dementia. *Neurology* **58**: 1615–21.
48. Rosso SM, Kaat LD, Baks T, *et al.* (2003) Frontotemporal dementia in The Netherlands: patient characteristics and prevalence estimates from a population-based study. *Brain* **126**: 2016–22.
49. Snowden JS, Neary D, Mann DMA (1996) *Frontotemporal Lobar Degeneration: Frontotemporal Dementia, Progressive Aphasia, Semantic Dementia.* New York: Churchill Livingstone.
50. Neary D, Snowden JS, Gustafson L, *et al.* (1998) Frontotemporal lobar degeneration. A consensus on clinical diagnostic criteria. *Neurology* **51**: 1546–54.
51. Snowden JS, Neary D, Mann DM (2002) Frontotemporal dementia. *British Journal of Psychiatry* **180**: 140–43.
52. Swartz JR, Miller BL, Lesser IM, *et al.* (1997) Frontotemporal dementia: treatment response to serotonin selective reuptake inhibitors. *Journal of Clinical Psychiatry* **58**: 212–16.
53. Jellinger K, Attems J (2007) Neuropathological evaluation of mixed dementia. *Journal of the Neurological Sciences* **257**: 80–87.
54. Rockwood K, Macknight C, Wentzel C, *et al.* (2000) The diagnosis of 'mixed' dementia in the Consortium for the Investigation of Vascular Impairment of Cognition (CIVIC). *Annals of the New York Academy of Sciences* **903**: 522–8.
55. Langa KM, Foster NL, Larson EB (2004) Mixed dementia: emerging concepts and therapeutic implications. *Journal of the American Medical Association* **292**: 2901–8.
56. Inouye SK, Viscoli CM, Horowitz RI, Hurst LD, Tinetti ME (1993) A predictive model for delirium in hospitalised elderly medical patients based on admission characteristics. *Annals of Internal Medicine* **119**: 474–81.
57. Carlson LA, Gottfries CG, Winblad B, Robertsson B (1999) Delirium in the elderly: Epidemiological, pathogenetic, diagnostic and treatment aspects. 3rd Symposium on Aging and Aging Disorders, Stockholm, September 3-4, 1998. *Dementia and Geriatric Cognitive Disorders* **10**: 393–400.
58. Howard R, Rabins PV, Seeman MV, Jeste DV, International Late-Onset Schizophrenia Group (2000) Late-onset schizophrenia and very-late-onset schizophrenia-like psychosis: an international consensus. *American Journal of Psychiatry* **157**: 172–8.
59. Harris MJ, Jeste DV (1988) Late-onset schizophrenia: an overview. *Schizophrenia Bulletin* **14**: 39–45.
60. Keith SJ, Regier DA, Rae DS (1991) Schizophrenic disorders. In LN Robins, DA Regier (eds) *Psychiatric Disorders in America: The Epidemiologic Catchment Area Study.* New York: Free Press.
61. Copeland JRM, Dewey ME, Scott A, *et al.* (1998) Schizophrenia and delusional disorder in older age: community prevalence, incidence, comorbidity and outcome. *Schizophrenia Bulletin* **24**: 153–61.
62. Castle DJ, Murray RM (1993) The epidemiology of late-onset schizophrenia. *Schizophrenia Bulletin* **19**: 691–700.
63. Naguib M, Levy R (1987) Late paraphrenia: neuropsychological impairment and structural brain abnormalities on computed tomography. *International Journal of Geriatric Psychiatry* **2**: 83–90.
64. Breitner J, Husain M, Krishnan K, Figiel G, Boyko O (1990) Cerebral white matter disease in late-onset paranoid psychosis. *Biological Psychiatry* **28**: 266–74.
65. Howard R, Cox T, Almeida O, *et al.* (1995) White matter abnormalities in the brains of patients with late paraphrenia and the normal community living elderly. *Biological Psychiatry* **38**: 86–91.
66. Jeste DV, Harris MJ, Krull A, *et al.* (1995) Clinical and neuropsychological characteristics of patients with late-onset schizophrenia. *American Journal of Psychiatry* **152**: 722–30.
67. Woerner MG, Alvir JMJ, Saltz BL, Lieberman JA, Kane JM (1998) Prospective study of tardive dyskinesia in the elderly: rates and risk factors. *American Journal of Psychiatry* **155**: 1521–8.
68. Brodaty H, Sachdev P, Koschera A, Monk D, Cullen B (2003) Long-term outcome of late-onset schizophrenia: 5-year follow-up study. *British Journal of Psychiatry* **183**: 213–19.
69. Mazeh D, Zemishlani C, Aizenberg D, Barak Y (2005) Patients with very-late-onset schizophrenia-like psychosis: a follow-up study. *American Journal of Geriatric Psychiatry* **13**: 417–19.
70. Harris A, Jeste D (1998) Late-onset schizophrenia: an overview. *Schizophrenia Bulletin* **14**: 39–55.
71. Royal College of Psychiatrists (2002) *Caring for People who Enter Old Age with Enduring or Relapsing Mental*

Illness ('Graduates'). Council Report CR110 October 2002. London: Royal College of Psychiatrists. www.rcpsych.ac.uk/files/pdfversion/cr110.pdf

72. Karim S, Overshott R, Burns A (2005) Older people with chronic schizophrenia. *Aging and Mental Health* **9**: 315–24.
73. O'Donnell BF (2007) Cognitive impairment in schizophrenia: a life span perspective. *American Journal of Alzheimer's Disease and Other Dementias* **22**: 398–405.
74. Green MF (1996) What are the functional consequences of neurocognitive deficits in schizophrenia? *American Journal of Psychiatry* **153**: 321–30.
75. Cohen CI, Cohen GD, Blank K, *et al.* (2000) Schizophrenia and older adults: an overview – directions for research and policy. *American Journal of Geriatric Psychiatry* **8**: 19–28.
76. Baldwin JA (1979) Schizophrenia and physical disease. *Psychological Medicine* **9**: 611–18.
77. Bozikas VP, Kosmidis MH, Kafantari A, *et al.* (2006) Community dysfunction in schizophrenia: rate-limiting factors. *Progress in Neuro-Psychopharmacology and Biological Psychiatry* **30**: 463–70.
78. Jolley D, Nick K, Holloway F (2004) Older people with long-standing mental illness: the graduates. *Advances in Psychiatric Treatment* **10**: 27–34.
79. Turkington D, Sensky T, Scott J, *et al.* (2008) A randomized controlled trial of cognitive-behavior therapy for persistent symptoms in schizophrenia: a five-year follow-up. *Research* **98**: 1–7.
80. Granholm E, McQuaid JR, McClure FS, *et al.* (2007) Randomized controlled trial of cognitive behavioral social skills training for older people with schizophrenia: 12-month follow-up. *Journal of Clinical Psychiatry* **68**: 730–37.
81. Beekman AT, Copeland JR, Prince MJ (1999) Review of community prevalence of depression in later life. *British Journal of Psychiatry* **174**: 307–11.
82. Age Concern (2007) *Mental Health Services Letting Down Older People*. www.ageconcern.org.uk/AgeConcern/pr_mental_health_inquiry.asp.
83. Evans M, Mottram P (2000) Diagnosis of depression in elderly patients. *Advances in Psychiatric Treatment* **6**: 49–56.
84. Baldwin RC, O'Brien J (2002) Vascular basis of late-onset depressive disorder. *British Journal of Psychiatry* **180**: 157–60.
85. Mottram P, Wilson K, Strobl J (2006) Antidepressants for depressed elderly. *Cochrane Database of Systematic Reviews* (1): CD003491.
86. Ibor JJ, Carrasco JL, Prieto R, García-Calvo C, Ceres Study Group (2007) Effectiveness and safety of venlafaxine extended release in elderly depressed patients. *Archives of Gerontology and Geriatrics* **46**: 317–26.
87. Nelson JC, Hollander SB, Betzel J, *et al.* (2006) Mirtazapine orally disintegrating tablets in depressed nursing home residents 85 years of age and older. *International Journal of Geriatric Psychiatry* **21**: 898–901.
88. Institute of Clinical Excellence (2003) Guidance on the use of electroconvulsive therapy. Technology Appraisal 59, April 2003. London: National Institute of Clinical Excellence.
89. Walker DA, Clarke M (2001) Cognitive behavioural psychotherapy: a comparison between younger and older adults in two inner city mental health teams. *Aging and Mental Health* **5**: 197–9.
90. Reynolds CF, III, Miller MD, Pasternak RE, *et al.* (1999) Treatment of bereavement-related major depressive episodes in later life: a controlled study of acute and continuation treatment with nortriptyline and interpersonal psychotherapy. *American Journal of Psychiatry* **156**: 202–8.
91. Luty SE, Carter JD, McKenzie JM, *et al.* (2007) Randomised controlled trial of interpersonal psychotherapy and cognitive-behavioural therapy for depression. *British Journal of Psychiatry* **190**: 496–502.
92. Hepple J, Sutton L (2004) *Cognitive Analytic Therapy and Later life: A New Perspective on Old Age*. Philadelphia, PA: Brunner/Routledge.
93. Tuma TA (2000) Outcome of hospital-treated depression at 4.5 years: an elderly and a younger adult cohort compared. *British Journal of Psychiatry* **176**: 224–8.
94. Mitchell AJ, Subramaniam H (2005) Prognosis of depression in old age compared to middle age: a systematic review of comparative studies. *American Journal of Psychiatry* **162**: 1588–1601.
95. Cole MG, Bellavance F (1997) The prognosis of depression in old age. *American Journal of Geriatric Psychiatry* **5**: 4–14.
96. Ryan J, Carriere I, Ritchie K, *et al.* (2008) Late-life depression and mortality: influence of gender and antidepressant use. *British Journal of Psychiatry* **192**: 12–18.
97. Weissman MM, Leaf PJ, Tichler GL (1988) Affective disorders in five United States communities. *Psychological Medicine* **18**: 141–53.
98. Eagles JM, Whalley LJ (1985) Ageing and affective disorders: the age at first onset of affective disorders in Scotland, 1969–1978. *British Journal of Psychiatry* **147**: 180–87.
99. Shulman K (1993) Mania in the elderly. *International Review of Psychiatry* **5**: 445–53.
100. Young RC, Kiosses D, Heo M, *et al.* (2007) Age and ratings of manic psychopathology. *Bipolar Disorders* **9**: 301–4.
101. Broadhead J, Jacoby R (1990) Mania in old age: a first prospective study. *International Journal of Geriatric Psychiatry* **5**: 215–22.
102. Almeida OP, Stephen F (2002) Bipolar disorder: similarities and differences between patients with illness

onset before and after 65 years of age. *International Psychogeriatrics* **14**: 311–22.

103. Shulman K, Tohen M, Satlin A, *et al.* (1992) Mania compared with unipolar depression in old age. *American Journal of Psychiatry* **149**: 341–5.
104. Gildengers AG, Butters MA, Seligman K, *et al.* (2004) Cognitive functioning in late-life bipolar disorder. *American Journal of Psychiatry* **161**: 736–8.
105. Eastwood R, Cobin S (1985) Epidemiology of mental health disorders in old age. *Recent Advances in Psychogeriatrics* **1**: 17–33.
106. Cohen CI, Magai C, Yaffee R, Walcott-Brown L (2006) The prevalence of anxiety and associated factors in a multiracial sample of older adult. *Psychiatric Services* **57**: 1719–25.
107. Marks I (1981) Space 'phobia': a pseudo-agoraphobic syndrome. *Journal of Neurology, Neurosurgery and Psychiatry* **44**: 387–90.
108. Lauderdale SA, Sheikh JI (2003) Anxiety disorders in older adults. *Clinics in Geriatric Medicine* **19**(4): 721–41.
109. Krasucki C, Howard R, Mann A (1998) The relationship between anxiety disorders and age. *International Journal of Geriatric Psychiatry* **13**: 79–99.
110. Gorenstein EE, Papp LA (2007) Cognitive-behavioral therapy for anxiety in the elderly. *Current Psychiatry Reports* **9**: 20–25.
111. Smit F, Comijs H, Schoevers R, *et al.* (2007) Target groups for the prevention of late-life anxiety. *British Journal of Psychiatry* **190**: 428–34.
112. Department of Constitutional Affairs (2005) Mental Capacity Act 2005: Summary. www.dh.gov.uk/assetRoot/04/10/85/96/04108596.pdf.
113. Breen DA, Breen DP, Moore JW, Breen PA, O'Neill D (2007) Driving and dementia. *British Medical Journal* **334**: 1365–9.
114. Zuin D, Ortiz H, Boromai D, Lopez LZ (2002) Motor vehicle crashes and abnormal driving behaviours in participants with dementia in Mendoza, Argentina. *European Journal of Neurology* **9**: 29–34.
115. Department of Health (2001) National Service Framework for Older People. London: Department of Health.
116. Royal College of Psychiatrists (2001) *Faculty of the Psychiatry of Old Age. Old Age Psychiatric Day Hospital Survey,* April 2001. London: Royal College of Psychiatrists. http://www.rcpsych.ac.uk/pdf/DH%20survey.pdf
117. Draper B (1994) The elderly admitted to a general hospital psychiatry ward. *Australian and New Zealand Journal of Psychiatry* **28**: 288–97.
118. Royal College of Psychiatrists (2002) Memory clinics complement traditional approaches to management of memory disorders. London: Royal College of Psychiatrists. www.rcpsych.ac.uk/pressparliament/pressreleasearchive/pr297.aspx.
119. Rockwood K (1989) Acute confusion in elderly medical patients. *Journal of the American Geriatrics Society* **37**: 150–54.
120. Pitt B (1991) The mentally disordered old person in the general hospital ward. In FK Judd, GD Burrows, DR Lipsitt (eds) *Studies on General Hospital Psychiatry.* Amsterdam: Elsevier.
121. Pitt B (1991) Depression in the general hospital setting. *International Journal of Geriatric Psychiatry* **6**: 363–70.
122. Strain JJ, Lyons JS, Hammer JS, *et al.* (1991) Cost offset from a psychiatric consultation: liaison intervention with elderly hip fracture patients. *American Journal of Psychiatry* **148**: 1044–9.

Chapter 73

Rehabilitation psychiatry

Frank Holloway and Sridevi Kalidindi

WHAT IS REHABILITATION PSYCHIATRY?

The development of rehabilitation psychiatry

Rehabilitation psychiatrists in the UK date the origins of their trade to the opening in 1796 of the Retreat in York by the Quaker merchant William Tuke. This institution pioneered what came to be known as 'moral treatment' for, as Tuke described the client group, 'people deprived of their reason'. The Retreat offered humane care in an environment that resembled a family, with a strong emphasis on encouraging people to be active and to take responsibility for themselves, while at the same time managing risk. The Retreat became the model for the Asylum, in the early nineteenth century a cutting-edge and evidence-based technology for promoting the recovery of people experiencing episodes of what we now term 'severe mental illness'. Discharge rates from the early asylums were impressive, although by the latter part of the nineteenth century the asylums had entered their 'long sleep', losing their initial impetus for recovery and discharge.

The best asylums always retained some focus on recovery. Organized aftercare for people discharged from a mental hospital dates back to the foundation of the Mental After Care Association in 1869 'to facilitate the readmission of the poor friendless convalescent from Lunatic Asylums into social life'.[1] The potential importance of work as a stimulus to rehabilitation (as opposed to something necessary for the economical running of the asylum) was recognized in the UK in the 1930s and became a major theme in the 1950s and 1960s, with the development of industrial therapy workshops both for in-patients and for people who had been discharged from hospital.

Throughout the Western world the large mental hospitals have been closing, to be replaced by systems of community care: mental hospital bed numbers peaked in the UK and the USA in 1954. An 'open door' movement both literally opened the previously locked doors within the mental hospital and metaphorically led to hospitals admitting and discharging many more people. During this process, the term 'rehabilitation' became synonymous with 'resettlement' – in other words, discharging long-stay patients from hospital. Careful evaluation of hospital closure programmes, notably in the large-scale Team for the Assessment of Psychiatric Services (TAPS) study into the closure of Friern Hospital in North London, led by Julian Leff, has confirmed that people do well with adequate support, even if discharged after decades of living in a hospital.[2]

In the USA, psychiatric rehabilitation is seen as having emerged in the 1970s as a consequence of deinstitutionalization, the large-scale, rapid closure of state mental hospitals that occurred in the 1960s and 1970s. This challenged community mental health services to address the needs of people with severe mental illnesses. The challenge was not generally taken up with enthusiasm, and as a consequence specialist psychosocial rehabilitation services emerged.[3] The situation was different in the UK, where deinstitutionalization was a slower process and the evolving community mental health services always focused on those most in need. In the UK psychiatric rehabilitation has continued to serve a small minority of people with the most severe illnesses, most commonly schizophrenia, who required longer-term hospital treatment and intensive community support.[4]

Social inclusion

People with severe mental illness are among the most marginalized members of our society, commonly experiencing poverty, educational failure, unemployment, lack of access to leisure and recreation, and poor housing. On average, their social networks are smaller and less reciprocal compared with the general population, and in relationships they are more likely to give than to take. They are less likely to be married or cohabiting than their peers. They are more likely to be the victims of crime than the general population, and they are more likely to end up in prison having committed a crime. Severe mental illness is associated with increased physical morbidity and consequent decreased life expectancy. Mental illness carries with it a burden of stigma and discrimination that no longer applies to physical illness or disability. The experience of someone with a mental illness is therefore commonly, although not inevitably, one of social exclusion.[5] The corollary of exclusion is inclusion, and a major aim of contemporary mental health services is to foster social inclusion.

Recovery

Contemporary mental health policy emphasizes the importance of 'recovery' within mental health services. The term 'recovery' has additional meanings to the ordinary concept of becoming free of symptoms and disability, although the starting point for the movement was the observation that the inevitability of continuing disability inherent in the Kraepelinian concept of schizophrenia was wrong:[6] a substantial proportion of people who have psychotic episodes do get better.

Equally salient is the concept of recovery while living with a mental illness, or, as Patricia Deegan put it, 'recovery as a journey of the heart'.[7] Here, the focus is on user-defined outcomes, quality of life, empowerment, the installation of hope, facilitating self-management and helping people to find personal meaning in life.[8]. A narrative approach – listening to people's stories of living with and recovering from severe mental illness – informs the contemporary recovery movement (Box 73.1).[9] The aim of recovery-oriented services is to enable people to 'live well despite any limitations caused by the disability or illness'.[10]

Understanding mental illness

According to the vulnerability–stress–coping–competence model,[11] biological vulnerabilities (which can themselves be the result of environmental factors) predispose to mental illness and interact with multiple factors, which include psychosocial stressors and the social environment, to determine outcome.

Interventions can:

- alleviate predisposing factors;
- mitigate triggering and maintaining factors;
- improve coping skills;
- increase personal resilience in the face of adversity.

Box 73.1 Recovery: key issues from the patient's perspective

THINGS THAT HELP RECOVERY

- Hope
- Involvement in meaningful activities
- Experiencing illness as only one aspect of oneself (rather than being defined by the illness)
- Managing the symptoms and impairments associated with the illness
- Experiencing successes and pleasure
- Opportunities for reciprocity – giving back to others
- Feeling part of a broader community.

THINGS THAT HINDER RECOVERY

- Being the object of stigma and discrimination
- Experiencing repeated failure and loss
- Losing control of one's life and key decisions
- The constriction of possibilities, expectations and roles open to the person
- Being confined to a passive 'patient role', where the person has nothing to offer others
- Pessimistic and paternalistic attitudes from staff and carers
- Institutional culture in services
- Lack of activity and structure in daily life.

Institutionalization

In his powerful book *Asylums*, the sociologist Erving Goffman described the phenomenon of institutionalization.[12] He described the ways in which the behaviours of patients could be understood as a response to the bureaucratic and dehumanizing processes of the mental hospital. A sociologically informed study by John Wing (a psychiatrist) and George Brown (a sociologist) on patients with schizophrenia living in three mental hospitals in England carefully teased out the effect of the social environment of the wards on the patients.[13] They showed that the negative symptoms that patients demonstrated were related, in part, to the impoverishment of the wards and in particular to the amount of time patients were left doing nothing at all.

Understanding disability

The concepts of social inclusion and recovery are fashionable. Less fashionable are concepts relating to the disabilities that are associated with severe mental illness. According to John Wing, the effects of mental illness on an individual are can be understood in terms of the following:[14]

- *Impairments:* the direct effects of illness, e.g. positive and negative symptoms, cognitive impairment, lack of drive and motivation.
- *Disabilities:* the difficulties the person experiences in carrying out day-to-day tasks.
- *Social handicaps:* the effects of impairments and disabilities on performing social roles and living a good life.
- *Personal reactions to illness:* the person's responses to the illness experience, and that of their immediate social network.
- *Stigma and discrimination:* the effects of societal views towards mental illness.

Impairments, disabilities and handicaps are influenced by psychological and social factors, which include the person's reaction to the illness experience, the stigma associated with mental illness, and other aspects of the social environment.

These concepts lie behind the definition of rehabilitation adopted by the World Health Organization, 'reducing the impact of disabling and handicapping conditions and enabling disabled people to achieve social integration'.[15]

There are two elements to this definition:

- It is an active process for the individual in acquiring attitudes and skills that allow the person to overcome the effects of an illness or disorder.
- It can involve changing the environment in order to decrease the impact of illness at both the individual and the societal level.

Psychiatric rehabilitation: a contemporary definition

A whole system approach to recovery from mental ill health which maximizes an individual's quality of life and social inclusion by encouraging their skills, promoting independence and autonomy in order to give them hope for the future and which leads to successful community living through appropriate support.[4]

This is an inclusive and person-centred definition. It focuses both on a desired end – successful community living – and on the aims that people have for themselves. These aims tend to include both everyday concerns, such as improving one's financial situation, social relationships and physical health, and improving cognitive capacities and symptoms, particularly symptoms of depression and anxiety.[16] The quality of life literature confirms that people experiencing severe mental illness are concerned about the same issues as the general population, such as housing, finances, relationships, safety, health and occupation, although people living impoverished lives tend to lower their expectations and aspirations. The core skills of the rehabilitation practitioner are to encourage people who may lack motivation and have often lost hope to identify achievable goals for change and then support them in achieving these goals.

What's different about rehabilitation psychiatry?

Rehabilitation psychiatry is now recognized as a specialty in its own right, becoming one of the faculties of the Royal College of Psychiatrists in 2004. It differs from traditional psychiatric practice in a number of ways (Box 73.2). The rehabilitation psychiatrist's primary focus is on functioning and quality of life. However, the rehabilitation psychiatrist will always be seeking optimal management of symptoms for a patient group that has, by definition, responded poorly to standard treatments.[17] Given that all forms of mental disorder affect functioning and result in social exclusion, rehabilitation skills and attitudes are clearly relevant to all psychiatrists.

Box 73.2 What's different about psychiatric rehabilitation?

- Focus on function rather than symptoms
- Focus on strengths rather than weaknesses
- Focus on the person's goals
- Time to take stock of the patient as a person
- Opportunity to replace despair with hope
- Opportunity to offer a different experience of mental health services for the patient and their carers
- Requirement to take the long view – developing a strategic approach.

ASSESSMENT

People who come to a rehabilitation service need to be assessed in a responsive and adaptable fashion, as they may not be able to tolerate a more formal approach. The assessment process needs to be truly person-centred if it is to be effective, and it should as far as possible be a collaboration between the service user, carers and staff members. The focus should be on the strengths of the individual, without ignoring or glossing over areas that require support. A good starting point is to get the person to tell their life story, putting the illness and its treatment as far as possible to one side. This should be supplemented by a through review of available case records, which will document the person's 'illness career'.

Thorough assessment of needs is core to the process of rehabilitation. People who come under the remit of rehabilitation services often have needs that have previously not been properly recognized or met, for example co-morbid mental disorders. Unrecognized or unmet needs can often lead to recurrent hospital admissions, further decline in function and a loss of hope for all concerned. In-depth assessment requires a multidisciplinary approach and should be a continuing process. Key assessment domains are discussed below.

Mental health

Assessment of mental (ill-)health should include an accurate primary diagnosis and identification of co-morbidities. A thorough understanding of past and current symptomatology is required. Co-morbidity may include substance misuse/dependence, personality disorder, learning disability, mood and anxiety disorder, and autism-spectrum disorder. It is important to have a clear understanding of the user's perception of their illness. Assessment will lead to a treatment plan that works towards symptom control and risk reduction and encourages self-management.

Physical health

Severe mental illness is associated with markedly increased physical morbidity. Risk of ill-health is exacerbated by social exclusion, poverty and underactivity. There is an increased prevalence of obesity, smoking is common with all the associated increases in physical health problems, and the metabolic abnormalities that can arise with psychotropic medication may lead to cardiovascular risk factors such as hyperlipidaemia, glucose intolerance or frank diabetes mellitus. Service users can be particularly reluctant to engage in screening programmes such as cervical smears. Rehabilitation services will work closely with primary healthcare in addressing these issues.

Family and personal relationships

Forming and maintaining relationships is core to quality of life and as such any existing relationships should be supported. There are often conflicts and unresolved issues that may impact negatively on both the service user and significant others, and these should be identified.

The lack of meaningful relationships in a user's life can also be starkly apparent; support towards positive change in this area is possible.

Daytime activities

How we spend our days impacts hugely on our mood and self-esteem. Finding out what the user is able to engage in regularly can be used as a starting point to set goals for future activities. Gross underactivity is an indication of severe social impairment.

Housing

The person's current housing situation, with an indication of whether there are any issues in this setting, should be clarified. A full accommodation history with the support received in each placement, and any clear reasons for a breakdown of a placement, should be explored. This can aid planning for future placement and support requirements.

Occupation and education, including functional skills

Activities of daily living such as self-care, care of the user's living space, and ability to shop, cook, launder, use public transport safely and manage finances should be looked at in depth so that a plan for support and work towards improvement in any relevant areas can be formulated.

Finances and welfare benefits

How much money is received in benefits or otherwise, and how the user manages their money, is an important practical concern. In cases where there are serious concerns about an inability to self-manage funds – for example, running up large debts, falling into arrears with rent, or running out of money for food and essential items before the next amount of money arrives – appointeeship may be considered. Another suitable adult such as a relative or the local social services can take on this responsibility to support the user and ensure all bills and expenses are dealt with and then pass on the remainder of the funds to the user at agreed regular time intervals. Budgeting skills can be an area for support to work towards, whenever possible, a return to independent management by the user.

Risk issues

Risk assessment is part of standard psychiatric practice. It is important to consider risks around self-neglect, vulnerability, fire-setting and other challenging behaviours that are more common in this population. By identifying and appropriately managing the risks they present, the user can be supported to take positive risks. When considering placement, adequate support and contingency plans can be put into place, thus maximizing the likelihood that the placement will be a successful one.

Many users will have a forensic history: this should be seen in context. Is the offending secondary to times of deterioration in mental health, linked to substance misuse, or simply criminality in its own right? Some understanding of the context within which risk behaviours occurred will enable the service user and the team to move forwards and the current risks to be assessed and managed appropriately, alongside other agencies when appropriate, such as the probation service and the local police-led multi-agency public protection arrangements (MAPPA).

Substance misuse

It is important to identify co-morbid substance misuse, which is common, and to develop an understanding of the user's recognition of this as an issue and willingness (or otherwise) to address it. (The issues surrounding dual diagnosis for rehabilitation services are very complex and not amenable to simple solutions,[18] but the fact of co-morbid substance misuse cannot be a reason for exclusion from contemporary rehabilitation services.)

Medication, including side effects

Many users who come to rehabilitation services continue to experience positive and negative psychotic symptoms, depression, anxiety and obsessional symptoms, despite vigorous pharmacological management. A full review should be undertaken of the user's illness history, including their medication history, noting which medication was prescribed, at which dose and for what period of time, and the compliance of the user with it (including blood levels of medication where available). Periods of relative stability and best function should be correlated with medication regimes at the time, as well as social factors. It is important to hear the user's and their carers' views on which regimes may have worked best, or not, for them in the past, and to take side effects seriously. One should ensure that the diagnosis is correct, that co-morbidity has been accounted for, and that other primary diagnoses such as organic mental disorder have not been missed.

Early warning signs, relapse indicators and contingency plans

Discussion of past episodes of acute illness can tap into the user's and carers' current understanding of the illness and their coping strategies. A discussion with the user of what they have and have not found a helpful response from services also can be enlightening.

Assessment should also include a number of other areas. The psychological approach of the individual incorporates information about their early life experiences, triggers for relapse, core beliefs, coping strategies, emotional and behavioural consequences of the illness, relapse indicators and support networks. *Cognitive function*, particularly memory and executive functioning, is often severely impaired in the rehabilitation client group and can be a specific target for rehabilitation interventions.[19] Unfortunately formal cognitive assessment is uncommon in current clinical practice. Were it to be assessed routinely, then treatment and management plans could be informed by an understanding of any specific deficits that the individual experienced. Structured assessment of quality of life may be revealing: this will include consideration of the person's religious, spiritual and cultural needs. These issues are often neglected, and addressing them can lead to both a greater understanding of the person and reconnection with potentially powerful sources of social support, for example through faith communities. Identification of recovery factors enables an understanding of the individual's motivation for self-management, goals, roles, strengths and illness understanding.

Carers' assessment

Most National Health Service (NHS) mental health trusts have a standardized format for assessing and making a care plan around the needs ot the patient's carers. The role of carer can impose a huge burden on individuals and families, and the importance of supporting carers cannot be overemphasized. When carers do not receive adequate support, the result may be their disengagement from the user because of an inability to cope, which is clearly an enormous potential loss for the user. Rehabilitation services may need to rebuild shattered relationships between the service user and their carers.

Assessment tools

A standardized approach to assessment is important to ensure an adequate assessment in these complex individuals. There are many tools that can be used in routine clinical practice,[20] a number of which deserve specific mention. The Camberwell Assessment of Need – Clinical Version covers 22 life domains and can incorporate the views of the assessor, user and carer.[21] It identifies serious need and also incorporates the view of the user as to what they would find useful support. The Social Functioning Questionnaire is composed of five eight-item scales that assess a person's level of competence in an area of social functioning.[22] The areas are self-care, domestic skills, community skills, social skills and responsibility. The Health of the Nation Outcome Scale is a summary outcome measure that focuses mainly on symptoms.[23] The Manchester Short Assessment of Quality of Life provides a useful brief assessment of quality of life in a number of domains.[24]

Symptom questionnaires for psychotic, mood or anxiety symptoms also can be used, tailored to each individual's needs. These instruments can be used at the beginning of a user's time with the service, and then at relevant intervals, but they should certainly be rated again at the end of a period of intervention and treatment – for example, at the end of a stay on a rehabilitation unit. This can provide evidence of outcomes as a result of specific interventions and overall change from receiving rehabilitation.

Other important outcomes to measure include whether the user moves on to a more or less independent living situation following time in receipt of rehabilitation services, and the number and length of admissions to an acute hospital setting before and after rehabilitation. Improvements to social networks can also be measured.

Formulation

An overall formulation of the user once these assessments are complete can provide insight into why the individual is in the current situation at this point in time and can be used to forge a way forward collaboratively with them and their carers.

INTERVENTIONS

Pharmacological treatments

It is beyond the scope of this chapter to discuss in detail issues of pharmacological management in the rehabilitation population, many of whom have treatment-resistant psychosis. Clozapine is the drug of choice in this situation. Its use is described at length in the *Maudsley Prescribing Guidelines*.[25] The key to successful use of clozapine is management of its many side effects.[17] Augmentation strategies can be adopted when clozapine, along with psychological and social interventions, fails to provide adequate symptom control. If clozapine cannot be tolerated, adherence is a major problem or symptomatic improvement is not adequate after a good trial other regimes may be tried.[17] When prescribing in this situation, where the evidence base is limited, it is wise to seek a second opinion wherever possible and certainly to employ routine outcome measures.

Psychological treatments

A wide range of psychological interventions have been shown to be effective in the treatment of psychotic illnesses. These include cognitive-behavioural therapy (CBT) and family therapy,[26–28] cognitive remediation therapy[19,29] behavioural therapy based on operant conditioning paradigms[30,31] and psychoeducation.[32] Psychodynamic understanding can also be useful in complex cases, particularly for the staff team in helping them to understand the patient and their reactions to him or her.[33]

The psychoeducational component of treatment should incorporate collaborative and wherever possible user-led plans of how to stay well by, for example, using the Wellness Recovery Action Plan, which is described below.[34] The trick here is to work out with the user an agreed treatment plan that enables the user to work towards their goals more effectively.

Skills training

People referred to rehabilitation services tend to have deficits in functional and social skills. A key task of rehabilitation practitioners is to help the user to improve these skills. Formal, manualized social skills training is much favoured in the USA.[35] A meta-analytical review of controlled trials showed no clear evidence of efficacy in terms of relapse rate, social functioning, quality of life or treatment adherence.[36] The problem appears to be with the generalization of skills outside the artificial treatment setting. In vivo interaction with staff (primarily occupational therapists, nurses and support time and recovery (STR) workers, whose role is described in more detail below) and peers is likely to be more effective than artificial programmes, and that is what good rehabilitation services offer.

Rehabilitation services also provide environments that have positive expectations on service users in terms of interpersonal behaviour and functioning. The Three Hospitals Study demonstrated the powerful effect that the social environment has on the functioning of people with schizophrenia.[13] Encouraging people to structure their time is particularly important in maintaining social functioning, an insight that was well understood by the pioneers of the Asylum 200 years ago.

RECOVERY AND REHABILITATION IN THE COMMUNITY

The aim of rehabilitation is for people experiencing severe mental illness to live successful and fulfilled lives. This requires a range of therapeutic interventions that have already been described and a set of supporting services – hence the need for a whole-system approach.[4]

In England, mental health services are coordinated under the overarching umbrella of the Care Programme Approach (CPA).[37] Its central principles are quite simple:

- Assessment of health and social care needs, including housing and employment (described in some detail above)
- Assessment of risk issues, including risks to self and others
- Development of a written care plan to address needs and risks
- Identification of contingency, crisis and relapse plans
- Regular review of the plan by all those involved in the plan
- Identification of a care coordinator who brings people together
- Full involvement of the service user and carers in care-planning
- Interprofessional collaboration and cooperation.

These principles are fully consistent with rehabilitation practice. However, there is a clear potential tension between the essentially user-defined concept of 'recovery as a journey of the heart' and the necessarily reductive and professionally led process of elaborating a CPA care plan within a formal meeting. Self-management strategies have an important potential role here, and the Wellness Recovery Action Plan is an influential and popular tool.[34] This involves the service user identifying actions, thoughts and behaviours that are associated with staying well and then developing a written plan of action, warning signs and a crisis plan: crucially, the process is patient-led rather than professionally driven.

Community support services

Most people in the UK living with severe and disabling mental illness are treated by their general practitioner (GP) or a community mental health team (CMHT). Their community support will come from family, friends, informal agencies such as places of worship, and, for those in contact with a CMHT, a package of care overseen by the care coordinator under the CPA.

In England, mental health services employ STR workers, who are:

> people who come from different walks of life with different backgrounds including volunteers and existing and former service users ... to help service users to have an ordinary life assisting them with their everyday, practical needs in whatever setting they find themselves to facilitate recovery.[38]

This includes, for example, helping people to manage their finances and address their housing needs. The STR role is intended to complement that of the care coordinator and is oriented towards rehabilitation and recovery.

Stein and Test published a landmark controlled study into what became known as 'assertive community treatment' (ACT).[39] ACT is a form of intensive community support designed specifically to help people at risk of admission because of their severe mental illness to live successfully outside hospital. The service was designed around what they felt to be the requirements for successful community tenure (Box 73.3). These requirements reflect concern with the individual's basic needs (including treatment needs) but also attention to the person's motivation, morale and social environment. The ACT model emphasizes staff offering support in vivo, in the person's own environment, in contrast to standard care in the USA, which remains clinic-based.

Box 73.3 Requirements for community tenure of people at risk of hospital admission

- *Material resources:* e.g. food, shelter, clothing, medical care
- *Coping skills:* e.g. budgeting, cooking, using public transport in vivo
- *Motivation:* e.g. systems of support to help people cope with stress
- *Freedom from dependent relationships:* aiming to break the cycle of dependency
- *Support and education of community members:* to help community members to interact appropriately with the patient
- *Assertive support system:* to preclude the tendency to drop out of care.

Adapted from Stein and Test.[39]

ACT, or assertive outreach (AO), as it is known in the UK, has become the standard method of supporting people who disengage from treatment and are recurrently admitted to hospital. Success in maintaining people in the community seems to be related to adherence to a specific service model that involves a team-based approach to care and in vivo treatment.[40] ACT has been significantly less effective in UK studies than in those carried out in the USA, but undoubtedly AO teams can keep marginalized patients in contact with services more successfully than can generic CMHTs. This may be because of the recovery-oriented practices that successful AO teams adopt, which foster engagement with the treatment team.[40]

Early intervention in psychosis (EIP) teams provide intensive community support to people who newly present with psychotic illnesses. EIP teams follow the principles of ACT, but in addition provide phase-specific interventions that are age-appropriate and take into account the needs of patients and carers who are new to the mental health system. EIP is an extremely promising approach, although to date the proposition that EIP improves long-term outcomes is unproven.[41]

All mental health services in England are required to provide AO and EIP services. The community rehabilitation team (CRT), designed to offer intensive community support to a minority of patients with the most severe disabilities, predates this requirement.[4] Increasingly, specialist CRTs focus on working with individuals placed in high-support residential and nursing care.

Work, daycare and education

Work plays an important part in most people's lives. This goes beyond the obvious financial rewards to include opportunities for social relationships and offering meaning and structure to daily life. Being unemployed has very well-documented bad effects on both physical and mental health. Work is a powerful aid to social inclusion and the majority of people with mental illness want to be occupied and to work.[42] However, the employment prospects of people with schizophrenia in the UK have worsened markedly over the past 50 years,[43] and until recently interest in providing work opportunities for people with a mental illness had been waning.

There are a wide range of work options for people with a mental illness (Box 73.4). By far the most preferable is remaining in employment following the onset of the illness, something that EIP services prioritize, or rapid return to the workforce following an episode of illness. Some people lack basic skills and will benefit from re-entry into education before seeking employment. For others, a period of voluntary work acts as a stepping stone into open employment. The welfare benefits system is very complex and can act as a disincentive to people to seek a return to work, although part-time employment can be undertaken without loss of benefit if it is an element of a rehabilitation programme.

Box 73.4 Work options for people with a mental illness

- Maintaining pre-illness employment
- Voluntary work
- Sheltered employment
- Prevocational training
- Clubhouse Model
- Social firms
- Supported employment
- Service user employment programmes
- Mainstream employment.

Work assessment, sheltered employment, prevocational training and supported employment are provided by specialist agencies. The influential Clubhouse Model brings these elements together in a service that is user-run, offers a welcoming and supportive environment for people with a severe mental illness, and provides good employment outcomes for service users.[44] Social firms are businesses designed to support paid employment for people with disabilities who work alongside non-disabled colleagues. The current research evidence favours programmes that offer supported employment ('place and train') over elaborate prevocational training schemes ('train and place').[45]

Mental health services are increasingly developing specific employment programmes for people who have a mental illness, with the aim of recruiting current and former service users to work as paid members of staff, on the grounds that they have a particular and valuable perspective to offer.

Not everyone wants or can achieve paid employment. Many find voluntary work both rewarding in itself and a potentially valuable stepping stone into open employment. Daycare may provide similar psychological benefits to work. Informal projects that offer a drop-in function may offer a safe place for people to go to. Projects may specifically promote people's creative skills or engage them in sporting activities that encourage active lifestyles. Further education may give people life skills that they lack and offers an excellent venue for developing social skills in a mainstream environment.

Housing

Most people with severe mental illness live in their own homes or with family members. A minority live in one of the many forms of supported housing that are available (Table 73.1).[46,47] These include family placement schemes (where the person lives with a paid carer), supported lodging schemes (where a carer oversees the person but does not live with them), housing with peripatetic support (which can be in individual units or in shared housing – what used to be called 'group homes') and staffed housing.

There is an extremely wide range of staffed housing available, from services that have a few hours a day of support worker time, through services that provide a member of staff available on a sleep-in basis at night to 24-h staffed units, which offer residential and nursing care. Most forms of supported housing rely on staff who do not have professional qualifications, although nursing homes are required to have minimum numbers of nursing staff. Supported housing can be oriented towards 'rehabilitation' in the sense of helping the person to become more independent or merely offer a form of continuing care, which, at its worst, can foster institutionalization and undermine people's autonomy and practical skills. Some services specialize in particular client groups, for example forensic patients or people with co-morbid learning disability and mental illness.

A key skill in rehabilitation practice is to identify the appropriate form of housing for an individual given their current level of functioning and the clinical problems that they present. Placement is no easy task and requires complex negotiations between the patient, their carers, potential care providers and funding authorities. Once the person is placed, the CRT may work with the individual and their

Table 73.1 Classification of residential services (costs of care generally increase down the list)

Facility	Description
Community care	
Independent living	Own house, flat, bedsit
Independent living with support	Domiciliary support (e.g. from home care team) or sheltered housing project with in situ support
Living with family/supported lodgings	May involve considerable support from informal or paid carers
Group home/shared housing/supported housing	Shared accommodation with varying levels of support
Staffed housing	Daily contact with staff team
Residential care home/registered nursing home	24-h staff cover (night-waking) – both may offer rehabilitation or long-term care
Hospital care	
Acute ward	Short stay
Rehabilitation unit	Medium stay – may be open or locked
Continuing care unit	Long stay
Intensive care unit	Locked short stay
Low secure unit	Locked long stay
Medium secure unit	Locked, with significant perimeter security
Special hospital	Locked, with high security

Adapted from Ramsay and Holloway.[46]

placement provider to ensure that realistic rehabilitation and recovery goals are being pursued.

Funding for housing and supports to live independently comes from a range of sources: people's earned income or savings, housing benefit, 'supporting people' monies (a funding stream developed to encourage vulnerable people from a range of client groups to live as independently as possible), social services authorities and health authorities.

Current policy is aimed at decreasing the numbers of people living in residential care and nursing homes in favour of packages of care that allow people to live in their own homes. These packages may provide practical support with tasks of daily living and prompts to take medication. The policy reflects the aims and aspirations of service users, who, unless they have been living in the system for many years, rarely opt for some form of communal living, whatever their assessed disabilities.

Limits of community care

Experience of the hospital closure programme, notably the TAPS study, has confirmed that even former long-stay inpatients can live successfully in ordinary housing with the support of non-professional care staff,[48] although a minority require initial placement in specialized hospital-based facilities.[49] Contemporary rehabilitation in-patient services aim to work intensively with people for a year or less before discharging them to independent living (relatively uncommon) or some form of supported or staffed housing, although a small proportion have to move on to continuing care units.[4]

A small group of patients exhibit 'challenging behaviours'. No generally agreed service model has yet emerged in the era of deinstitutionalization for this patient group, which is diagnostically heterogeneous but characterized by non-compliance with treatment, absconding, violence, disturbance at night and bizarre behaviour.[50] Some of these patients will improve after intensive rehabilitation and active pharmacological management over a period of years.[49] When behavioural disturbance, risk or offending behaviour is extreme, patients may be treated in a special hospital or medium secure unit, although the latter were not designed or resourced to provide long-term care. More recently, long-term low secure units have opened to provide continuing, institutionally based care and treatment for people who present with challenging behaviours.[31]

A significant proportion of people requiring longer-term high-support care cannot be cared for locally and are placed as out-of-area treatments (OATs). Until recently very little was known about the numbers and characteristics of OATs: however, the client group is known to be very heterogeneous, with, in general, little systematic attempt being made by the placing services to review the users' needs and to facilitate return to their local area.[51] Good-quality local mental health services follow up OATs very carefully and are constantly seeking to help people to return to life in community settings.

REHABILITATION: ETHICAL ASPECTS

Coercion versus empowerment

Mental health services are often experienced as coercive. When the individual's views of what is and is not acceptable differ too greatly from the treatment team conflict and coercion can result. The simple process of supporting a user's rehabilitation may be seen as coercive, for example taking control over someone's financial affairs or strongly prompting them to attend to their activities of daily living.

Empowering people to manage their own illness as far as possible rather than fostering a paternal approach to care produces rewards for the individual and the team supporting them. Putting the user at the centre of the care and involving them and their carers in a meaningful and informed way is the best approach to achieving empowerment. Access to advocacy can support this, and advance directives can be useful. The service user agrees at a time when they have capacity what they would and would not find useful or agree to should their condition deteriorate. Jointly formulated crisis plans may lead to a decrease in compulsory admissions.[52]

There does come a point when, usually for reasons of risk to self or others or in the face of marked self-neglect, the locus of control passes to the mental health staff supporting the user, who will need to act in the best interests of the user and others. This can clearly be perceived as coercive. It is important that decision-making and control are handed back as soon as is practicable. Actions by staff and lay carers need to be undertaken in the light of relevant legislation – in England and Wales, the Mental Health Act and the Mental Capacity Act – which requires decisions surrounding treatment and care to be taken in the best interests of the patient or service user.

Confidentiality

Confidentiality and joint working is another contentious area. There is guidance about confidentiality from regulatory bodies such as the General Medical Council (GMC), but this can be difficult to reconcile at times with day-to-day practice. For example, there is the need to share information with the criminal justice system for the purposes of public protection or in the best interests of the patient when they may not have consented to such information-sharing (the GMC test for this being extremely high). CPA policies may state that information must be shared between relevant others – both professionals and carers. What approach should be taken when service users emphatically do not wish information about their care to be shared with carers from whom they may nonetheless derive a great deal of support and who may be at risk? How can carers support a care plan of which they have no knowledge? These are extremely sensitive issues for which there is no easy answer.

Acknowledging ethical dilemmas

Ethical issues need to be recognized and debated at team and service level, taking into account the legislative framework, advice from professional codes of conduct and the growing ethical literature. In this way, an appropriate way forward may be found for each individual.

SERVICE DEVELOPMENT AND EVALUATION IN REHABILITATION

Successful practice in rehabilitation requires a whole-system approach, which implies working with multiple actors and agencies (e.g. the patient, lay and paid carers, the care team, independent sector providers, funders of care packages, commissioners of services). Given that there is a stark gap between what is available and what we believe to be the ideal provision, the effective rehabilitation psychiatrist will inevitably become involved in service development. This requires complex managerial skills that can only be acquired in practice, albeit supplemented by relevant courses and texts (e.g. Bhugra *et al.*[53]). Useful practical experiences include working closely with voluntary-sector organizations, including joining management committees, and helping to develop business plans for service innovations.

Promoting service development rests on three core issues: What is the need? What is the policy? What is the potential funding? Currently, funding streams for service development rely on responding to policy initiatives or identifying activities that will lead to immediate cost savings (e.g. by decreasing expenditure on residential care by improving the available community support). Rehabilitation psychiatrists require advanced skills in population needs assessment. This demands a grasp of epidemiological principles (relating to the incidence and prevalence of disabling severe mental illnesses) and the ability to undertake or support local evaluation of the needs for high-support care.

Evaluation of rehabilitation services is challenging. Seven stages of evaluation in a rehabilitation service have been identified (Table 73.2).[54] There are complexities surrounding the desired outcomes of rehabilitation (e.g. bed use, costs, personal satisfaction, symptomatology, social functioning) and the definitions of the interventions provided by rehabilitation services. In comparison with other countries the hospital closure programme in the UK was well evaluated, providing data that remain relevant to contemporary rehabilitation services.[2] Locally, rehabilitation services should audit their activities by measuring patient outcomes, patient and carer views of services, lengths of in-patient stay and other service use data, and the overall costs, which is where any evaluation programme should start.[54]

Table 73.2 Stages of evaluation in a rehabilitation service

Stage of evaluation	Tasks to be completed
1 Feasibility and acceptability	Simple audit studies
2 Enquiry	Qualitative and observational studies
3 Outcome	Follow-up of cohorts
4 Intervention dissection	Exploratory trials (case–control and randomized)
5 Confirmation of efficacy in practice	Large randomized controlled trial
6 Audit of standards	Constant monitoring
7 International dissemination	Policy and promotion

Adapted from Tyrer.[54]

SPECIALIST REHABILITATION SERVICES

Forensic rehabilitation

As the large mental hospitals closed and the traditional high secure hospitals (e.g. Broadmoor) downsized, in-patient provision for offender-patients in medium secure and low secure units expanded very rapidly. A new specialism of Forensic Rehabilitation, devoted to reintegrating offender-patients with significant social disabilities into the community, was born.[55] Balancing ongoing risk management with rehabilitation and reintegration into the community lies at the core of Forensic Rehabilitation. The recognition that for each user there may be a level of support that to go below would be unsafe is an important part of the management of forensic patients. It is also key not to forget risk at any time, however long the user may have been stable. Long-term support and monitoring are vital, particularly in less supported placements, as the re-emergence of risk may occur at any time as destabilizing factors come into play for the user, such as substance misuse and relapse of psychosis.

The forensic population tends to be complex, with the majority being co-morbid for any or all of the following: low intellectual function, substance misuse, personality disorder and physical problems. For effective management, this co-morbidity must be identified and addressed appropriately.[55]

Rehabilitation and learning disability

Service users who have both significant learning disability and co-morbid mental illness with rehabilitation needs are often not cared for at a local level. They are commonly placed in very costly OAT settings within the independent sector, which may offer continuing care rather than rehabilitation.

The key points for assessment, treatment and management of this group of individuals are that a flexible, user-centred approach needs to be adopted.[56] A highly skilled staff group with expertise in the concepts of learning disability, rehabilitation, care-planning and the ability to liaise across relevant services and with the service user's family and carers with adequate resources is also central to success. The strengths of the individual should be recognized and sufficient onus placed on quality of life.

Impairments, disabilities, handicaps and stigma need to be taken into account, and where possible the root causes of behavioural problems need to be identified and addressed. This can prove challenging in service users who have limited ability to communicate. Adequate risk assessment can also prove to be a challenge, and this in turn impacts on the user's management and progress. If triggers for risk behaviour cannot be identified or communicated, then the individual may remain in a more restrictive setting for extended periods of time.

Acquired brain injury

The common causes of brain injury include anoxia, hypoglycaemia, trauma, subarachnoid haemorrhage, infectious causes such as meningitis, and alcohol use.[57] The main psychiatric symptoms that develop are psychosis, depression, anxiety disorders and aggression. Aggression has a number of causes, for example being secondary to disinhibition as a consequence of frontal lobe damage, seizure activity or psychotic symptoms. Assessing the underlying cause is essential if aggression is to be treated appropriately and effectively.

Pre-existing psychiatric conditions may have given rise to the head injury, for example following a suicide attempt or as a result of risky behaviour in a patient with attention deficit hyperactivity disorder (ADHD). Patients with both a severe mental illness and an acquired brain injury are most likely to present to psychiatric rehabilitation services because of the increased likelihood of them developing a chronic disability.[58]

It is important to have an understanding of the type and severity of the head injury in order to provide appropriate input for each individual.[58] Care must be taken with treatment of psychiatric symptoms post-head injury because, although the symptoms can generally be treated using the relevant medication for a particular diagnosis (e.g. antipsychotics for psychosis, antidepressants for depression), some caveats exist. Anticholinergic side effects of medication can worsen confusion in this patient group. Generally there is an increased sensitivity to side effects. Starting at a low dose initially with gradual increases and avoiding drugs that may have central nervous system side effects is advisable.

When the brain injury is severe and obvious rehabilitation is undertaken in a neuropsychiatric brain injury unit, with the possibility of move-on to a community-based service. The rehabilitation programme is dictated by each individual's pattern of enduring disability: the keys to success are detailed understanding of the cognitive deficits and the elaboration of an individualized and highly structured programme.

For patients with moderate to severe impairments, cognitive rehabilitation focuses on improving independence in specific areas of function, such as being able to cook a simple meal and goal-planning. Staff, who will often be clinical psychologists or occupational therapists, provide an individualized programme of activities to address the person's needs that is undertaken in a graduated and carefully evaluated manner. Memory impairment may be assisted by the use of electronic devices such as a watch with an alarm that sounds at times when medication must be taken.

Behaviour modification is another useful intervention that can reinforce wanted behaviour and reduce unwanted behaviour. A functional analysis of unwanted behaviour should be carried out before formulating the plan in order to understand the triggers and potential gains from such behaviour (a similar approach to that adopted in the management of challenging behaviours in psychiatric rehabilitation settings[31]). A consistent approach is imperative for all staff involved in a person's care in order for behaviour modification to be implemented successfully.

THE FUTURE OF REHABILITATION AND RECOVERY IN PSYCHIATRIC PRACTICE

Potential users of rehabilitation and recovery services are characterised not only by particular diagnostic labels (notably schizophrenia) and the consequent stigma, but also by multiple indices of social exclusion: they tend to be poor, socially isolated, inadequately housed, unemployed and at risk of victimisation.[59]

The UK currently has no clear government policy relating to specialist recovery and rehabilitation services. Given that potential users are those with a mental illness who are in most need, are most socially excluded and take up a large proportion of the currently available resources (e.g. through recurrent acute hospital admissions, long-term daycare, residential care and high-cost placements[60]), this is a puzzling anomaly. The Rehabilitation and Social Psychiatry Faculty of the Royal College of Psychiatrists has sought to remedy this policy gap,[61] and the Irish College of Psychiatrists has published detailed guidance on establishing rehabilitation and recovery services.[62]

In addition to the elaboration of a coherent policy for recovery and rehabilitation services, there are a number of areas where further development is clearly required. Of prime importance is for services to move towards a more user-led pattern of care, with a much greater emphasis on a truly collaborative approach between staff, user and carers than currently occurs in many care settings. Supporting users to make informed choices both empowers them and will, in the long term, lead to better outcomes. In many services, this will require a change in culture.

We need to take much more seriously the positive impact on people of returning to meaningful activity: this includes improving opportunities for work and education. Effective reintegration of people who are experiencing severe mental illness also requires efforts to tackle the barriers that perpetuate stigma and discrimination and is an ongoing but important part of the task of rehabilitation services in collaboration with users. Enabling a devalued group to participate on equal terms can reduce prejudice.[63]

Traditionally there were barriers to accessing recovery and rehabilitation services for people with a history of offending, who were experiencing co-morbid substance misuse, or who had functional disabilities occurring in the context of a personality disorder. These barriers will fall. As an example, a significant minority of people with severe personality disorders are found in expensive placements. By developing local strategies for joint working with specialist psychotherapy services, these individuals can be supported in moving to progressively less dependent settings.

There is an increasing need for rehabilitation services to prove their worth by ensuring that the work they undertake is measured appropriately and reported to commissioners. This requires services to embrace routine measurement of patient outcomes, including feedback from users and carers, together with regular reviews of the service that ensure that treatment and care are evidence-based and that provision is relevant to the needs of the local population, responsive and of a high quality.

KEY POINTS

- Rehabilitation and recovery concepts and attitudes are relevant to all areas of psychiatric practice.
- The assessment process must be thorough and identify all areas of need, as this patient group often experiences unidentified and unmet needs.
- Rehabilitation focuses on the individual's skills and abilities as well as on symptoms and disabilities.
- Many rehabilitation clients suffer from treatment-resistant psychoses for which evidence-based treatment is available.
- There is a focus on the working alliance between patients/service users and carers.
- Rehabilitation services have as explicit aims fostering hope, social inclusion and individual recovery in the face of continuing illness and disability.
- The Royal College of Psychiatrists Faculty of Rehabilitation and Social Psychiatry has developed a reading list for trainees (see www.rcpsych.ac.uk).

REFERENCES

1. Bennett DH (1983) The historical development of rehabilitation services. In FN Watts, DH Bennett (eds) *Theory and Practice of Psychiatric Rehabilitation.* Chichester: John Wiley & Sons.
2. Holloway F (2004) Reprovision for the long-stay patient. *Psychiatry* **3**: 5–9.
3. Pratt CW, Gill KG, Barrett NM, Roberts MM (2007) *Psychiatric Rehabilitation.* Burlington, MA: Academic Press.
4. Killaspy H, Harden C, Holloway F, King M (2005) What do mental health rehabilitation services do and what are they for? A national survey in England. *Journal of Mental Health* **14**: 157–66.
5. Office of the Deputy Prime Minister (2004) *Mental Health and Social Exclusion.* London: Office of the Deputy Prime Minister.
6. Warner R (2003) *Recovery from Schizophrenia: Psychiatry and Political Economy*, 3rd edn. London: Routledge.
7. Deegan P (1996) Recovery as a journey of the heart. *Psychiatric Rehabilitation Journal* **19**: 91–7.
8. Roberts G, Wolfson P (2006) New directions in rehabilitation: learning from the recovery movement. In G Roberts, S Davenport, F Holloway, T Tattan (eds) *Enabling Recovery: Principles and Practice of Psychiatric Rehabilitation.* London: Gaskell.
9. Davidson L (2003) *Living Outside Mental Illness: Qualitative Studies of Recovery in Schizophrenia.* New York: New York University Press.
10. Care Standards Improvement Partnership (2007) *A Common Purpose: Recovery in Future Mental Health Services.* Leeds: Care Standards Improvement Partnership.
11. Anthony WA, Liberman RP (1986) The practice of psychiatric rehabilitation: historical, conceptual and research base. *Schizophrenia Bulletin* **12**: 542–59.
12. Goffman E (1961) *Asylums: Essays on the Social Situation of Mental Patients and Other Inmates.* Edison, NJ: Transaction Publishers.
13. Wing JK, Brown G (1970) *Institutionalism and Schizophrenia.* Cambridge: Cambridge University Press.
14. Wing JK (1993) Social consequences of severe mental illness. In D Bhugra, J Leff (eds) *Social Psychiatry.* Oxford: Blackwell.
15. World Health Organization (1980) *International Classification of Impairment, Disabilities and Handicaps: A Manual of Classification Relating to the Consequences of Disease.* Geneva: World Health Organization.

16. Lecomte T, Wallace CJ, Perreault M, *et al.* (2005) Consumers' goals in psychiatric rehabilitation and their concordance with existing services. *Psychiatric Services* **56**: 209–11.
17. Sweeting M (2006) Management of medication when treatment is failing. In G Roberts, S Davenport, F Holloway, T Tattan (eds) *Enabling Recovery: Principles and Practice of Psychiatric Rehabilitation.* London: Gaskell.
18. Corrigan PW, Mueser KT, Bond GR, Drake RE, Solomon P (2008) *Principles and Practice of Psychiatric Rehabilitation: An Empirical Approach.* New York: Guilford Press.
19. Wykes T (2006) Cognitive rehabilitation. In G Roberts, S Davenport, F Holloway, T Tattan (eds) *Enabling Recovery: Principles and Practice of Psychiatric Rehabilitation.* London: Gaskell.
20. Kemp L, Tattan T (2006) Rating scales. In G Roberts, S Davenport, F Holloway, T Tattan (eds) *Enabling Recovery: Principles and Practice of Psychiatric Rehabilitation.* London: Gaskell.
21. Slade M, Thornicroft G, Loftus L, Phelan M, Wykes T (1999) *CAN: Camberwell Assessment of Need – A Comprehensive Needs Assessment Tool for People with Severe Mental Illness.* London: Gaskell.
22. Clifford P, Morris I (1983) *The Social Functioning Questionnaire.* London: Research and Development for Psychiatry.
23. Wing J, Curtis R, Beevor AS (1996) *Health of the Nation Outcome Scales (HoNOS).* London: Royal College of Psychiatrists Research Unit.
24. Priebe S, Huxley P, Knight S, *et al.* (1999) Application and results of the Manchester Short Assessment of Quality of Life (MANSA). *International Journal of Social Psychiatry* **45**: 7–12.
25. Taylor D, Paton C, Kerwin R (2007) *The Maudsley 2007–2008 Prescribing Guidelines*, 9th edn. London: Taylor & Francis.
26. Pilling S, Bebbington P, Kuipers E, *et al.* (2002) Psychological treatments in schizophrenia: meta-analysis of family interventions and cognitive behaviour therapy. *Psychological Medicine* **32**: 763–82.
27. Fadden G (2006) Family interventions. In G Roberts, S Davenport, F Holloway, T Tattan (eds) *Enabling Recovery: Principles and Practice of Psychiatric Rehabilitation.* London: Gaskell.
28. Turkington D, Arjundas R (2006) Cognitive-behavioural therapy. In G Roberts, S Davenport, F Holloway, T Tattan (eds) *Enabling Recovery: Principles and Practice of Psychiatric Rehabilitation.* London: Gaskell.
29. Kurtz MM, Moberg PJ, Gur RC, *et al.* (2001) Approaches to cognitive remediation of neuropsychological deficits in schizophrenia: a review and meta-analysis. *Neuropsychology Review* **11**: 197–210.
30. Davies W (1993) *The RAID Programme for Challenging Behaviour.* Leicester: Association for Psychological Therapies.
31. Beer D (2006) Managing challenging behaviours. In G Roberts, S Davenport, F Holloway, T Tattan (eds) *Enabling Recovery: Principles and Practice of Psychiatric Rehabilitation.* London: Gaskell.
32. McGorry P (2005) Royal Australian and New Zealand College of Psychiatrists clinical practice guidelines for the treatment of schizophrenia and related disorders. *Australian and New Zealand Journal of Psychiatry* **39**: 1–30.
33. Davenport S (2006) Psychodynamic considerations in rehabilitation. In G Roberts, S Davenport, F Holloway, T Tattan (eds) *Enabling Recovery: Principles and Practice of Psychiatric Rehabilitation.* London: Gaskell.
34. Copeland ME (2002) Overview of WRAP: wellness recovery action plan. *Mental Health Recovery Newsletter* **3**: 1–9.
35. Corrigan PW, Mueser KT, Bond GR, Drake E, Solomon P (2006) *Principles and Practice of Psychiatric Rehabilitation: An Empirical Approach.* New York: Guilford Press.
36. Pilling S, Bebbington P, Kuipers E, *et al.* (2002) Psychological treatments in schizophrenia: II. Meta-analyses of randomized controlled trials of social skills training and cognitive remediation. *Psychological Medicine* **32**: 783–91.
37. Kingdon D, Amanullah S (2005) The care programme approach: relapsing or recovering? *Advances in Psychiatric Treatment* **11**: 325–9.
38. Department of Health (2003) *Mental Health Policy Implementation Guide: Support Time and Recovery (STR) Workers.* London: Department of Health.
39. Stein LI, Test MA (1980) Alternative to mental hospital treatment: I. Conceptual model, treatment program, and clinical evaluation. *Archives of General Psychiatry* **37**: 392–7.
40. Killaspy H (2007) Assertive community treatment in psychiatry. *British Medical Journal* **335**: 311–12.
41. Marshall M, Rathbone J (2004) Early intervention for psychosis. Cochrane Database of Systematic Reviews (2): CD004718.
42. Boardman J, Robinson B (2006) Working to recovery: meaningful occupation and vocational rehabilitation. In G Roberts, S Davenport, F Holloway, T Tattan (eds) *Enabling Recovery: Principles and Practice of Psychiatric Rehabilitation.* London: Gaskell.
43. Marwaha S, Johnson S (2004) Schizophrenia and employment: a review. *Social Psychiatry and Psychiatric Epidemiology* **39**: 337–49.
44. Macias C, Rodican CF, Hargreaves WA, *et al.* (2006) Supported employment outcomes of a randomized controlled trial of ACT and clubhouse models. *Psychiatric Services* **57**: 1406–15.
45. Crowther RE, Marshall M, Bond GR, Huxley P (2001) Helping people with severe mental illness to obtain work: systematic review. *British Medical Journal* **322**: 204–8.

46. Ramsay R, Holloway F (2007) Mental health services. In G Stein, G Wilkinson (eds) *General Psychiatry: College Seminars in Psychiatry*, 2nd edn. London: Gaskell.
47. MacPherson R, Shepherd G, Edwards T (2004) Supported accommodation for people with severe mental illness: a review. *Advances in Psychiatric Treatment* **10**: 180–88.
48. Leff J, Treiman N (2000) Long-stay patients discharged from hospitals. *British Journal of Psychiatry* **176**: 319–23.
49. Trieman N, Leff J (2002) Long term outcome of long-stay psychiatric inpatients considered unsuitable to live in the community TAPS project 44. *British Journal of Psychiatry* **181**: 428–32.
50. Holloway F, Wykes T, Petch E, Lewis-Cole K (1999) The new long stay in an inner city service: a tale of two cohorts. *International Journal of Social Psychiatry* **45**: 93–102.
51. Ryan T, Hatfield B, Sharma I, Simpson V, McIntyre A (2007) A census study of independent mental health sector usage across seven strategic health authorities. *Journal of Mental Health* **16**: 243–53.
52. Henderson C, Flood C, Leese M, *et al.* (2004) Effect of joint crisis plans on use of compulsion in psychiatric treatment: single blind RCT. *British Medical Journal* **329**: 136–8.
53. Bhugra D, Bell S, Burns A (2007) *Management for Psychiatrists*, 3rd edn. London: Royal College of Psychiatrists Publications.
54. Tyrer P (2006) Evaluation of rehabilitation services. In G Roberts, S Davenport, F Holloway, T Tattan (eds) *Enabling Recovery: Principles and Practice of Psychiatric Rehabilitation*. London: Gaskell.
55. Davies S, Abbott P (2006) Forensic rehabilitation. In G Roberts, S Davenport, F Holloway, T Tattan (eds) *Enabling Recovery: Principles and Practice of Psychiatric Rehabilitation*. London: Gaskell.
56. Simpson N (2006) Psychiatric rehabilitation for people with learning disability. In G Roberts, S Davenport, F Holloway, T Tattan (eds) *Enabling Recovery: Principles and Practice of Psychiatric Rehabilitation*. London: Gaskell.
57. Teasdale GM (1995) Head injury. *Journal of Neurology, Neurosurgery and Psychiatry* **58**: 526–39.
58. Allin M, Fleminger S (2006) Acquired brain injury. In G Roberts, S Davenport, F Holloway, T Tattan (eds) *Enabling Recovery: Principles and Practice of Psychiatric Rehabilitation*. London: Gaskell.
59. Davenport S, Holloway F, Roberts G, Tattan T (2006) Rehabilitation and recovery in the 21st century. In G Roberts, S Davenport, F Holloway, T Tattan (eds) *Enabling Recovery: Principles and Practice of Psychiatric Rehabilitation*. London: Gaskell.
60. Holloway F (2006) Resource allocation. *Psychiatry* **6**: 72–5.
61. Executive Committee, Faculty of Rehabilitation and Social Psychiatry, Royal College of Psychiatrists (2005) *The Forgotten Need for Rehabilitation in Contemporary Mental Health Services*. www.rcpsych.ac.uk/pdf/frankholloway_oct05.pdf.
62. Irish College of Psychiatrists (2007) *How to Set Up Rehabilitation and Recovery Services in Ireland: Guide for Consultants in Rehabilitation Psychiatry Produced by the Faculty of Rehabilitation and Social Psychiatry, Irish College of Psychiatrists*. Occasional paper OP64.
63. Hewstone M (2003) Intergroup contact: panacea for prejudice? *Psychologist* **16**: 352–5.

PART 7

Mental health service provision

Chapter 74

Management of psychiatric services

Hameen Markar and Borislav Iankov

INTRODUCTION

We live in times of great scientific and medical inventions. Psychiatry has undergone one of the most dynamic developments over the past 50 years. The fast-developing pharmaceutical industry has armoured us with a range of effective psychotropic medication, which has greatly affected the way our services are now organized. In recent years, we have seen specialist community mental health teams established across the country, offering home treatment, early intervention and intensive support for people with complex needs. The National Service Framework (NSF) for Mental Health, published in 1999, is a strategic document for the development of adult mental health services in the National Health Service (NHS).[1] The NHS Plan, which followed the NSF in July 2000, promotes new models of care and contains key targets and core standards for the health and social care sectors, based on the NSF.[2] This ambitious and far-reaching plan requires strong clinical leadership and managerial skills for its successful implementation.

Doctors constantly strive to improve services and have learned to adjust to service changes. As front-line clinicians, we are best placed to understand and deal with intricate clinical issues and help organize and develop services that will suit our patients.

Clinical involvement in such innovative service developments is crucial, but this can only be achieved in a meaningful and constructive manner if clinicians have a good understanding of the issues involved in such service change. Service change and development is linked closely with service improvement, but our training, which is largely clinical, hardly deals with the complexities involved in effecting such changes.

Our aim in this chapter is to provide an overview of the intricate logistics of organizing, leading and developing a new psychiatric service or change of service while ensuring the delivery of a high standard of care.

Staff members are sometimes resistant to change. This may be due to several reasons, such as a lack of understanding of the issues involved, feeling threatened because of the changes, or a fundamental disagreement with the proposal. Such resistance may also present in different forms, ranging from open hostility and refusal to cooperate to indifference and covert sabotage. Management of these issues can be both difficult and sensitive and requires considerable skill, understanding and maturity. As clinicians, we receive no training in any of these core management skills.

We discuss various aspects of management, including communication, difficult colleagues, resistance and the principles of project management.

EFFECTIVE MEDICAL MANAGEMENT

Who is an effective medical manager? What are the specifications required to be an effective medical manager? The job is unique, in that it requires an excellent grasp of not only clinical but also managerial issues. The need to work effectively with both managers and clinicians, without compromising credibility, honesty and transparency, is not an easy task and requires good management skills. The key attributes necessary to be an effective medical manager can be conveniently listed under two main headings: personal characteristics and core skills.

Personal characteristics

The medical manager leads, plans, organizes, completes and evaluates. Effective leadership requires as a minimum good skilful management of multidisciplinary teams. To achieve this, one needs to have the respect of the team members. Respect is earned and never automatic by virtue of one's position. To gain respect, the leader must work tirelessly and demonstrate competency to lead the team in an appropriate and constructive manner that encourages collaboration and maximum team cooperation. Unlike multidisciplinary clinical teams, where clinical knowledge is usually the central focus, service development and project teams have a wider remit with not only clinical but also financial and political dimensions. A good medical manager is flexible and remains receptive to the views and opinions of other team members, who may not have a clinical background. Clearly, the leader of such a team has the knowledge and interpersonal skills to gain the trust and confidence of others within the team. Individual differences may exist within team members, borne out of certain beliefs and convictions, and these should be recognized and acknowledged. A medical leader should not be seen as driving a medical model, giving no consideration to the disparate views of other professionals in the team. Instead, the leader should be open, honest, fair and transparent and should adopt an inclusive approach. These are the essential ingredients to gain trust, credibility and, above all, respect.

When working with colleagues, one could come across the difficult ones, ranging from the aggressive and manipulative to the incompetent. An accomplished leader will have clear strategies to diagnose and manage such diverse personalities and get the best out of them. Similarly, when team functioning is affected, it is necessary to identify the possible causes and to take early remedial action. The common causes of team dysfunction include poor leadership, lack of role clarity and perceived inequalities.

Probity and integrity are of paramount importance, not only in one's personal life but also in one's professional dealings. These are linked closely but not exclusively with financial and commercial issues and include matters such as ethical provision of information, writing reports, giving evidence and dealing with pharmaceutical companies and other commercial organizations.

A good leader is able to devise good plans that are achievable and takes into account the diverse views and opinions of others. The best of plans could go wrong and, therefore, one must have subsidiary plans to deal with such eventualities. All plans must have clear and unambiguous objectives, with a well-defined pathway to reach the endpoint. Both the endpoint and the pathway may require change, depending on circumstances, and a competent leader will adjust accordingly.

No plan will be successful if it is not linked to conscientious and meticulous organization. This involves attention to detail, careful coordination and accurate analysis with methodical administration.

A leader must be a completer, and no amount of planning or organization would help if one does not have the skills and qualities necessary to complete. A medical leader should relentlessly pursue the aims and objectives outlined in the service change, showing great courage and resilience in the face of repeated obstacles and resistance. This is possible only if the change is driven by a firm belief and conviction that such change is necessary for the benefit of all users of the service, staff and the organization.

Once implementation is complete, attention moves to consolidation and evaluation of the change, first to determine the effectiveness, both clinical and financial, of the change, and second to replicate such change in other appropriate clinical settings.

Core skills

Leadership and management require not only personality characteristics but also a number of core skills, explained in the sections below.

Communication skills

Communication skills are central to effective leadership and require the highest priority. Faulty and ineffective communication is the root cause of many problems within teams. Change and communication are inextricably linked, and an effective medical leader requires excellent communication skills, including the ability to listen, assimilate and synthesize information, consider the range of views expressed, and communicate in a clear, precise and unambiguous manner. Communication is a two-way process – top-down and vice versa – with a beginning but no end. Middle managers are a useful source for developing good communication with front-line staff and must be utilized fully throughout the process. Honesty, appropriate challenges and clarity are the hallmarks of good communication.

Chairing meetings

This requires specific skill and experience that one would expect in effective leadership. A quality chairperson commands the respect of the team, is able to adhere to time limits, has control of the meeting, is unfailingly courteous and listens to all views expressed. The chair of a committee can have personal opinions, but these must not be allowed to dominate the meeting. A good chair will encourage others to express their views, allocate adequate time for debate on different issues, lead the group towards decisive action and, above all, maintain a good sense of humour at all times.

Setting clear objectives

In any form of service change, it is important to define the aims and objectives as clearly as possible. In a health organization, the objectives are usually driven by health or financial priorities. Aims must be clear, precise, achievable and preferably measurable against established targets. In service development, it is often necessary to differentiate between immediate objectives and outcome measures. Thus, for example, in the development of a home treatment service, the immediate aim is to establish the service in both structural and functional terms (see below). However, the outcome measures and targets are different and will be in relation to user satisfaction, reduced hospital admissions, and so on.

Developing a project plan

Once the objectives have been defined clearly, the next step is to develop a project plan that outlines the actions and activities necessary towards implementation. At the outset, a project team should be constituted. This will consist of staff with varying skills and different professional backgrounds, who are capable and motivated and also share a firm belief in the need for change. The project plan will consist of a series of operational measures that are set out in chronological order, with one activity leading to another, until eventually the endpoint is reached. The leader will delegate authority and responsibility to individual members of the project committee, for each of the action points, which may be divided into several components, if necessary.

Delegating

Appropriate delegation demands a good understanding of the knowledge, skills and ability of each individual in the team. Every individual will have some special aptitude or talent, and a good clinical leader will mobilize and channel such skills effectively. Past performance is often a useful guide in such situations.

Timescales

Good project management involves establishing achievable timescales, with a defined completion date for each activity. This should take into account both expected and unexpected events such as annual leave and sick leave, the competency of the individuals, and resource and capacity issues. The timescales must be realistic and, to some extent, flexible.

Resistance

No project runs entirely to plan. In the process of implementation, one often encounters obstacles and difficulties. These may arise from external or internal sources. The cardinal rule is to be one step ahead and to anticipate such issues. At the very outset, it is necessary to have some understanding of the possible sources of resistance within the service and, as far as possible, to take action to deal with them. Unexpected complications could also arise that may hinder progress. In all such situations, a good clinical leader will retain the support, loyalty and cooperation of the team, so that working together such issues are overcome and dealt with appropriately. It is the responsibility of the leader to encourage, facilitate, persevere and respond adequately, ensuring at all times that morale is maintained and the project remains on course. Feedback to project members must be realistic, positive and encouraging.

IMPLEMENTATION OF A SERVICE CHANGE

Having discussed the personality and core characteristics of an effective medical manager, the rest of this chapter deals with the process involved in effecting a service change.

Setting the scene

What is the proposed change? This can vary from a minor change in existing clinical practice to more significant and substantial changes in the development and delivery of a new service.

Is the change really necessary? This is not an easy question to answer, particularly when changes are imposed from the department or the strategic health authority. In such cases, it is good practice to carefully assess the issues involved and, if necessary, to seek clarification from higher authorities.

It may be necessary to research the proposal, taking into consideration the current practice, including its strengths and weaknesses; the likely benefits from the change, which may be clinical, organizational or financial; the effects on staff and service users; the impact on other clinical services; and the views of the stakeholders, including voluntary organizations, and if available, the experience of other organizations that have implemented such change. Careful consideration and wide-ranging discussions and consultations may be necessary before a final decision is made regarding the need for change. This is a critical decision that requires considerable thought, since it will form the basis for all other actions. It is vital that the person leading the change should be convinced firmly of the need for such change.

The next step is formation of a project team. Careful consideration must be given to the composition of the project team, in terms of numbers, professional representation and the skill mix required.

Action plan

Once the project team is in place, a project plan including operational action points and dates for future meetings should be developed. This will form the working document for the future.

The action plan is essentially a pathway that leads to the implementation of the project. This will have, as outlined above, several action points, some of which may be broken down into several components. The action plan also defines responsibility and specific timescales.

Implementation

This is the hub of the service change. This process can take from a few weeks to several months, depending on the proposed change. The implementation of the action plan can be considered under two broad components:

- *Structure:* what is the structure of a service? This comprises the buildings and service facilities that are necessary. Depending on the nature of the proposed service, accessibility to users and carers, soundproof interview rooms, conference rooms, storage space and security are some of the provisions that need consideration. Structure must also deal with staff composition, skill mix and staff members' professional needs such as computers, telephones, fax machines, and the general working environment.
- *Function:* The functional component relates to the development of appropriate operational policies and guide-

lines. This will vary from one service to another, taking into account the roles of different professional groups, job descriptions and service requirements.

The functional part of the service has to be developed carefully and built around the agreed aims and objectives of the service. The operational policy, the job descriptions of the different professionals, guidelines on staff training, and clinical/managerial supervision are important components that must relate to the aims and objectives of the service. This is not an easy task, and it is essential that, throughout this phase, one remains focused on the key objectives.

Both structural and functional changes will require wide-ranging discussion with all members of the project team, as well as stakeholders from within and outside the organization. Effective communication processes must be established across different staff groups, community teams, in-patient services, medical staff committee, staff unions, general practitioners (GPs), commissioners and other stakeholders. Throughout the entire process, it is essential to monitor the financial impact and to ensure that the project remains within the allocated budget. The potential for further development of the project and possible expansion into future markets, both locally and outside the region, must be borne in mind.

At this stage, the project team may wish to break down the action plan into manageable components, with appropriate delegation and agreed timescales, based on skill and expertise.

The implementation phase, which includes structural and functional development, is the body of the service change and will take a considerable amount of time and effort. It is during this stage of project management that resistance will emerge. Such resistance can take many forms, ranging from passive expressions of discontent to open hostility, anger and even sabotage. Different forms of resistance need to be handled differently, based on the probable cause. Throughout this process, and despite the numerous distractions, the project team has to maintain focus and a grip on the task at hand. Tact, patience and diplomacy are useful, as is emotion in some situations, but these must never lead to poor judgement or indecisiveness.

Consolidation and review

Once a service is established and fully operational, it must be accepted and embedded within the organization. Staff and users who are involved with the service need to recognize its value and benefits as well as its deficiencies. This will facilitate regular reviews and changes within the service in order to meet the varying demands of the users and the organization. The establishment of a new service is not the end but rather the beginning of further changes, which will be driven by surveys, audits and other outcome measures.

Evaluation of a new service is a continuous process and has different dimensions, which may be clinical, financial or operational. More often than not, it is a combination of all three. The central role of the customer is paramount throughout the process of evaluation. The customer is the service user, who is not only the patient but also others such as the carers, community and in-patient teams, professionals, outside stakeholders and commissioners.

CONCLUSION

Service development and delivery will continue to remain at the forefront of NHS reforms for many future years. If such change and development are to have meaningful clinical engagement, it is necessary for clinicians to provide strong, effective clinical leadership. In this chapter, we have outlined the main personal characteristics and core skills that are needed for such a role. Essentially, these are the qualities of leadership, which make one credible, trustworthy and dependable. Individuals who are genuinely interested in medical management acquire these features over a period of time through experience, training and apprenticeship. A young doctor requires multiple skills along clinical, academic, research and management lines. Irrespective of one's main interest, knowledge of the basic principles of medical management is essential for the delivery of a good-quality service.

The second part of this chapter deals with the processes involved in implementing a major service change. This is about higher-level medical management and will be beneficial mainly to those who aspire to develop a career in management. However, all clinicians, both medical and non-medical, would benefit from a knowledge of the fundamentals involved in the process of implementing a service change.

KEY POINTS

- The health service is changing and evolving constantly. It is crucial that there is strong clinical involvement and engagement with such changes.
- The medical manager leads, plans, organizes, completes and evaluates.
- The personal characteristics of an effective medical manager include sound knowledge, interpersonal and communication skills, flexibility, adaptability and transparency, fairness and credibility.
- The core skills of a medical manager include an ability to communicate effectively, chair meetings, set clear objectives, delegate and deal with resistance.
- The process involved in effecting a service change includes development of a project plan, identification of a project team, establishing realistic timescales, implementation, consolidation and review.
- The implementation can be considered under two broad components – structure and function.

- In the consolidation phase, the new service must be accepted and embedded within the organization.
- The evaluation phase has different dimensions, which may be clinical, financial or operational.

REFERENCES

1. Department of Health (1999) *National Service Framework for Mental Health: Modern Standards and Service Models*. London: Department of Health.
2. Department of Health (2000) *The NHS Plan: A Plan for Investment – a Plan for Reform*. London: Department of Health.

FURTHER READING

Bhugra D, Bell S, Burns A (2007) *Management for Psychiatrists*, 3rd edn. London: Royal College of Psychiatrists.

NHS Modernisation Agency (2003) *NHS Leadership Qualities Framework*. London: NHS Institute for Innovation and Improvement. www.nhsleadershipqualities.nhs.uk.

Reynolds A, Thornicroft G (1999) *Managing Mental Health Services*. Buckingham: Open University Press.

Chapter 75

Advice to special medical services

Geoffrey Lloyd

INTRODUCTION

Psychiatric problems are commonplace throughout clinical medicine.[1] It follows that no clinical service in secondary or tertiary care hospitals can function adequately without access to psychiatric advice on diagnosis and management, although the frequency with which this advice is sought varies across the specialties. In recognition of this need, liaison psychiatry has developed as a subspecialty within psychiatry, and many hospital trusts now have established liaison psychiatry services. The number of consultant posts has expanded from a small base in the 1980s,[2] but not as rapidly as the Royal College of Psychiatrists has recommended.[3] Clinical expansion has been accompanied by increased professional recognition,[4] liaison psychiatry now having faculty status within the College.

Following the purchaser/provider separation introduced into the UK National Health Service (NHS), the commissioning of secondary care is in the hands of primary care trusts. Services in acute general hospitals are commissioned according to the perceived needs of the community that the hospital serves. The provision of psychiatric services to special medical services is complicated by the fact that mental health services are commissioned separately and are provided by distinct mental health trusts. Liaison psychiatry services are usually managed by mental health trusts, even though the patients that these services treat are fundamentally looked after by acute hospital trusts. There needs to be close collaboration between commissioners, acute trusts and mental health trusts if good psychiatric care is to be delivered within general hospitals.

But the provision of services is extremely variable within the UK. This chapter reviews the need for services and makes recommendations for their development. Whenever possible, reference is made to recommendations from official bodies such as medical royal colleges, the Department of Health and the National Institute for Health and Clinical Excellence (NICE), bearing in mind that these recommendations aspire to a standard of clinical practice that is seldom, if ever, achieved.

Joint reports from the Royal College of Physicians (RCP)[5] and the Royal College of Psychiatrists (RCPsych)[6] have drawn attention to the high prevalence of psychiatric problems in emergency departments and acute wards and have called for an expansion of services so that a liaison psychiatry service is established in every general hospital. These recommendations have been echoed by a report from the Academy of Medical Royal Colleges,[7] which has pointed out that there has been no incentive to commission or develop services as they are not a priority for mental health or acute trusts. The Academy's report emphasized that there is an urgent need to develop national standards that inform the commissioning services, thus ensuring that patients in need receive prompt assessment and management by appropriately trained professionals. The guiding principles of an ideal service were as follows:

- The quality of care given to people with mental health problems should be the same as the care given to people with physical health problems.
- The quality of care should be the same, regardless of the patient's racial, religious or cultural background.
- Particular attention should be given to people with learning difficulties.
- Emergency department staff should be trained to carry out initial mental health and risk assessments.
- Emergency departments should receive timely support from mental health services, led and coordinated by liaison psychiatry teams.
- Patients in acute hospitals should have similar access to the opinion of a consultant psychiatrist as they would to a consultant in physical health problems.
- There should be good referral pathways and communications with primary care.

There should be access to more specialized services for children and older people and a brief intervention service for patients with alcohol-related problems. Rapid access to effective interpreting services must also be available.

EMERGENCY DEPARTMENT

The emergency department holds a key position at the interface between acute medical and mental health services. The prevalence of psychiatric illness is high among attendees, and in many trusts the emergency department is the agreed place of safety for patients to be assessed if they have been detained by the police under the Mental Health Act. This arrangement is advantageous in that it allows physical and psychiatric examination to be conducted in the same place, but the emergency department does not often provide a suitably calm environment for a detailed mental state assessment. It is important that the place of safety for a particular catchment area is agreed by clinicians and managers from acute and mental health trusts and by the local police service.

The profile of patients attending with psychiatric problems has been described in several studies. Salkovskis *et al.* showed that approximately one-third of attendees at an emergency department had scores on a self-report questionnaire indicative of psychiatric disorder.[8] Many patients have deliberately harmed themselves by drug overdose or injury, and there is a high prevalence of drug and alcohol problems. Attendance outside normal working hours is common, this factor probably contributing to many patients leaving the department before being assessed adequately. Up to a third of patients attending inner-city hospitals live outside the catchment area of the local mental health service. For patients in many districts, the emergency department is a major point of entry to the mental health service.[9] A survey in Manchester found that 16 per cent of patients newly admitted to the mental health service made their first contact via the emergency department.[10]

The Department of Health has advised that in England and Wales no patient should wait in the emergency department for more than 4 h from the time of arrival to the time of admission, transfer or discharge. This target time cannot always be achieved, and patients with psychiatric problems form a high proportion of those whose stay exceeds the 4-h target. Delays occur due to lack of available staff, particularly approved doctors and social workers, and difficulties in finding beds for patients who need admission.

Psychiatric services to emergency departments vary widely with regard to their configuration and available clinical staff. Problems of contacting psychiatric staff are particularly common where the mental health trust has no presence in the acute hospital and where no liaison psychiatry service has been developed. These deficiencies need to be addressed, and a joint report from the Royal College of Psychiatrists and the British Association for Accident and Emergency Medicine has made several recommendations to improve the standard of psychiatric care:[11]

- Local policies should be agreed on the management of common clinical problems.
- There should be agreement on the responsibility for managing children, adolescents and older people.
- Rapid access to patient information (e.g. databases, care plans) should be available.
- Staff should be aware of customs and beliefs of patients from ethnic minorities. Access to interpreters should be available.
- Emergency department personnel should have knowledge of mental health issues sufficient to make an initial assessment. Mental health training needs to be part of the education of emergency department staff.
- A consultant psychiatrist needs to be identified as the senior member of mental health staff responsible for liaising with the emergency department.
- The first point of contact from the mental health service may be with an experienced mental health nurse or a junior doctor.
- There should be locally agreed standards regarding attendance times of mental health staff. Suggested times for first-line attendance were 30 min from being called in urban areas and 90 min in rural areas. For an approved doctor's attendance, the times were 60 min in urban areas and 120 min in rural areas.
- There should be unambiguous arrangements regarding the attendance of social workers in emergency departments.
- Interview rooms should allow for privacy but should also include standard safety features.
- Staff should be trained in safety techniques.

These recommendations are most likely to be achieved if there is a 24-h liaison service to the emergency department; the case for such a service is particularly strong for inner-city departments.[12]

Deliberate self-harm

Deliberate self-harm (DSH) is such a common problem that it warrants special consideration. It was the only area of liaison psychiatry discussed in the National Service Framework (NSF) for mental health in England.[13] It has been estimated that there are over 150 000 admissions annually to hospitals in the UK following DSH. Most of these come through the emergency department and are initially assessed there or in adjacent observation wards, sometimes known as clinical decision units. Although evidence for its effectiveness is not convincing, it is generally agreed that all patients should undergo a specialist psychosocial assessment. There is an increasing trend for this to be carried out by a suitably trained mental health nurse, preferably someone who is a member of a liaison psychiatry team. The topics to be covered in the assessment are well-established:

- Events leading up to DSH
- Suicidal intent at the time of the episode
- Current and ongoing psychosocial difficulties
- History of previous psychiatric treatment
- Previous episodes of DSH
- Family and personal history
- Personality traits
- Misuse of alcohol and other drugs
- Evidence of current mental illness
- Current suicidal intent

- Coping strategies and external support
- Patient's willingness to engage in aftercare.

It is essential for the nurse or doctor who completes this assessment to have good rapport with community mental health teams so that appropriate aftercare can be arranged. In some cases the general practitioner (GP) will be the most suitable person to provide further treatment, but in any case the GP should be informed of the episode of DSH as soon as possible. Unfortunately, the evidence base for the effectiveness of treatment to prevent repetition is very weak.[14] Most services aim to identify people at high risk of repetition and to focus treatment on this group. These people have usually developed a severe depressive illness or schizophrenia or have evidence of a borderline personality disorder. Medication will be appropriate for those with an identifiable illness; psychotherapy is more suitable for personality disorders.

Some patients refuse to cooperate with psychiatric assessment or may refuse treatment for the physical complications of the self-harm. In such circumstances it is important for emergency department and mental health staff to be familiar with the concept of mental capacity and to be able to assess whether or not the patient lacks capacity to make decisions concerning refusal of treatment. It is unlikely that the Mental Capacity Act can be used in acute decision-making. If there are grounds for believing the patient lacks capacity, common law can be applied to detain the patient in the department and to administer whatever medical treatment is thought to be in the patient's best interest. If a patient is detained under common law, arrangement should be made for an urgent psychiatric evaluation by an approved doctor and social worker to determine whether hospital admission under the Mental Health Act is required. Non-psychiatric staff in the emergency department need to know their responsibilities under common law with regard to detaining and treating a patient who lacks capacity.

Royal College of Psychiatrists guidelines recommend that all patients over the age of 65 years who harm themselves should be referred to an old-age psychiatry team.[15] The prevalence of psychiatric illness is high in this age group, as is the risk of subsequent suicide. Similarly, children and adolescents should be referred to a child and adolescent service.[16] It is usually appropriate to admit children to a paediatric ward following an episode of DSH so that a full evaluation of the family background can be undertaken.

MEDICAL DEPARTMENTS

The high prevalence of psychiatric illness among medical patients is due to several factors, which often interact with one another:

- Pre-existing psychiatric illness contributing to development of physical illness
- Psychological reaction to physical illness, e.g. anxiety, depression, acute psychosis
- Organic effects of illness on mental function, e.g. delirium, dementia
- Influence of medically prescribed drugs on mental function and behaviour
- Medically unexplained symptoms that mask underlying psychiatric illness
- Alcohol and drug misuse.

Psychiatric illness adds to the distress experienced by medically ill patients and complicates their management. Almost certainly it prolongs their hospital admission. Most in-patient referrals to liaison psychiatry services come from medical specialties, particularly neurology, oncology and gastroenterology. Much depends on the ability of medical and nursing staff to identify their patients' psychiatric problems. Psychiatrists have a responsibility to educate these professionals by enhancing their communication skills and their psychiatric diagnostic acumen. They should indicate which patients are most likely to benefit from psychiatric referral and treatment. The choice of psychotropic drug, if required, has to be made with attention to side effects complicating the medical condition and to interactions with drugs already prescribed. Protocols are required to advise on the general management and pharmacological treatment of acutely disturbed patients.

Patients who attend hospital frequently but whose symptoms cannot be explained adequately in terms of physical pathology constitute a troublesome group who use up considerable resources in terms of medical time and expensive investigations. Many have an underlying psychiatric disorder, most often a depressive illness, anxiety disorder or panic attacks. Referral for psychiatric assessment should be encouraged at an early stage if the presenting symptoms do not conform to a recognized pattern of illness or if routine investigations prove to be negative. Psychiatric treatment is more likely to be effective if it can be started before a pattern of chronic invalidism is established.

Psychiatric input may be required by specific units that wish direct access to a particular psychiatrist.[17] Such arrangements work well but must not be allowed to develop at the expense of other departments of the hospital. Funding must be arranged to allow clinical sessions to be devoted to whichever specialty requires them. Examples where special links have been developed include pain clinics, palliative care services and neurology. Indeed, some psychiatrists have specialized in providing a service solely to neurology patients, and a subspecialty of neuropsychiatry has emerged.

Alcohol misuse

Increasing consumption of alcohol, particularly among young adults, is responsible for a growth in alcohol-related medical admissions and in mortality related to alcohol, for example from cirrhosis.[18] The prevalence of problem drinkers among medical in-patients varies from one hospital to another and between medical specialties. However, among male in-patients, prevalence rates of 25 per cent have often been reported. Alcohol-related problems are also common in emergency departments.[19]

Different degrees of problem drinking have been described. Harmful drinking is defined as drinking that has led to demonstrable physical damage or dependence. Hazardous drinking describes a level of consumption that increases the risk of harm. It is equivalent to 'at risk' drinking and is usually defined as an average daily consumption of over 5 units of alcohol for men and 2.5 units for women. Conditions that are directly related to alcohol include alcoholic liver disease, acute alcoholic poisoning and withdrawal fits. In other conditions alcohol is a contributory factor; these include hypertension, cardiac arrhythmias, self-poisoning, fractures, tuberculosis and various types of cancer. Detection of harmful and hazardous drinking is essential if further harm is to be prevented. Clinicians must be able to take a drinking history, with particular reference to the quantity of consumption, usually expressed in units of alcohol per week, the pattern of drinking, evidence of dependence and alcohol-related harm. Laboratory tests are useful corroborators of high consumption. They are sometimes the first indicators of problem drinking. Various questionnaires are also available as screening instruments. A report from the RCP recommended that hospitals should develop a defined strategy for managing patients with alcohol problems.[20] This strategy should include:

- screening for early detection of harmful and hazardous drinkers;
- early assessment of severity of dependence;
- protocols for pharmacological treatment of detoxification;
- good links with liaison psychiatry or specialist alcohol service for management of patients with complex withdrawal;
- assessment of need for referral to specialist service;
- brief intervention for coincidental hazardous drinkers;
- provision of general staff education and support;
- good links with the GP after the patient's discharge;
- occupational policy for alcohol for all hospital healthcare workers.

With regard to staffing implications, the report advised that senior members of the medical and nursing staff should be identified to act as a focus for the alcohol strategy and to provide support for junior staff. A senior psychiatrist with an interest in alcohol misuse should act as a link between the acute hospital and mental health trusts, and one or more dedicated alcohol health workers should be employed to coordinate strategies, provide brief intervention (in the form of counselling) and have sufficient knowledge of local services to refer on for more specialized treatment.

Drug misuse

Similar comments apply to drug misuse. Although not as prevalent as alcohol misuse, drug-related problems can create substantial difficulties in clinical management. A survey by Canning *et al.* found that, of the 6 per cent of medical in-patients identified as dependent on illicit drugs, the great majority were taking cannabis.[21] In most cases cannabis causes few problems in medical management; acute psychotic reactions can occur but are uncommon. More difficult problems are associated with opiates, ecstasy, amphetamines and sedatives. Hospital trusts need to develop protocols for the management of patients with acute intoxication and withdrawal states. Pregnant users need to be encouraged to withdraw from drugs in early pregnancy. Withdrawal is best undertaken as an in-patient. It should be conducted gradually to avoid precipitating premature labour and causing fetal distress. Few acute hospitals need a specialized drug treatment service, but there is much to be said for incorporating this responsibility into the work of the alcohol treatment service.

Sexual dysfunction

A decision needs to be taken on whether to establish a sexual dysfunction service to help people with sexual problems attending medical, surgical and gynaecological clinics. Some trusts in the UK have special sexual dysfunction clinics; others employ sexual counsellors attached specifically to one service, usually gynaecology. Much depends on the identified need and the ability to persuade commissioners to fund the service. If a clinic of this nature is established, then it will almost inevitably attract referrals from GPs.

SURGICAL DEPARTMENTS

Surgeons refer fewer patients for psychiatric assessment than do their physician colleagues. In general surgical practice, most referrals request help in the management of postoperative delirium. Advice on managing behavioural problems following head injury is sometimes requested by neurosurgeons and orthopaedic surgeons. More chronic psychological problems occur in the aftermath of major surgery such as mastectomy for breast cancer, colectomy followed by colostomy for bowel disease, and limb amputation for trauma, malignancy or vascular disease. Disfigurement from trauma, malignancy and burns is also a major source of distress. Depression is a well-recognized problem and results from body-image disturbance and its effects on morale and relationships. Surgical departments now employ clinical nurse specialists to help patients adjust to postoperative problems. Breast-care and stoma nurses acquire considerable expertise in providing emotional and practical support. Close links between nurse specialists and liaison departments should be encouraged and can be facilitated by regular clinical meetings.

Victims of road traffic accidents, assault and other forms of trauma are at risk of developing post-traumatic stress disorder during the weeks following the trauma and should be asked about relevant symptoms at follow-up appointments.

Preoperative psychiatric assessment may be requested if there is doubt about a patient's capacity to consent to surgery. Although in principle all registered doctors are entitled to make a judgement concerning capacity, in practice surgeons may prefer the opinion of a psychiatrist, especially where there is evidence of previous psychiatric illness affecting judgement. Preoperative assessment is also requested for some patients who seek plastic surgery for cosmetic reasons, a rapidly growing population in the USA and the UK. The most frequent operations requested are breast enlargement or reduction, rhinoplasty and pinnaplasty. Cosmetic surgery is generally contraindicated in three groups of conditions:[22]

- Mania, schizophrenia and severe depression, when judgement about the effects of surgery is likely to be impaired
- Eating disorders, when abdominoplasty is desired as a weight-reduction procedure
- Body dysmorphic disorder, which is characterized by a preoccupation with an imagined defect in appearance or excessive concern with a slight physical abnormality. The underlying concern is often unchanged or made worse by surgery.[23]

It is important that the surgeon asks screening questions at the initial consultation to uncover an underlying psychiatric disorder and seeks specialist advice if there is any doubt about the indication for surgery. Very rarely, a patient may request amputation of a perfectly healthy digit or limb. This is a manifestation of a condition known as amputee identity disorder. The outcome of surgery and the long-term prognosis of this condition are unknown.

MATERNITY SERVICES

The association between childbirth and psychiatric illness is well established. Postnatal depression develops in 10–15 per cent of women in the months following childbirth. A more serious psychotic disorder occurs in two women for every 1000 live births. Predisposing factors include a previous or family history of psychiatric illness and a complicated delivery. There is also some evidence that pregnancy itself is a vulnerable period as far as psychological symptoms are concerned. Women with pre-existing psychiatric illness may be at risk of an exacerbation of symptoms, not least because many women stop psychotropic medication abruptly once they discover they are pregnant. For these reasons, attention has been given to providing better care for women during the antenatal and postnatal periods.

The NICE guidelines recommend the establishment of a network of perinatal mental health services managed by a coordinating board of healthcare professionals, commissioners, managers, service users and carers.[24] There should be a multidisciplinary perinatal service in each district; in areas of high morbidity, these services may be provided by a separate specialist perinatal mental health team. Each network should have access to a designated specialist inpatient service, providing facilities for the admission of mothers and babies, but a decision for joint admission must be taken only after a very careful appraisal of risk to the baby. Admission is usually needed for managing the small number of women who develop a postnatal psychosis or who have a poorly controlled pre-existing psychotic illness.

Identification of vulnerable women begins at the time of the first antenatal booking appointment by asking screening questions concerning past or previous mental illness, previous treatment by a psychiatrist and a family history of mental illness. Specific questions should also be asked about current or previous use of illicit drugs. A midwife is well placed to conduct this screening. Some clinics like to supplement this with self-report questionnaires. A written care plan should be developed for women at risk. If a possible mental health problem is identified, further assessment should be considered according to the severity of symptoms. When severe mental illness is suspected, referral should be made to a mental health service, including, if available, a specialist perinatal mental health service. Similar screening questions should be used to detect mental illness at the postnatal visit.

NICE guidelines recommend a stepped care approach to the treatment of postnatal depression. Much of this involves psychological therapy, and so it is important for a range of treatments to be accessible. Self-help strategies, non-directive counselling, brief cognitive-behaviour therapy and interpersonal psychotherapy all have their place for mild to moderate depression. Antidepressant medication is recommended only if psychological therapy is not available, is declined or does not work.[25]

PLANNING FOR MAJOR DISASTERS

Every acute hospital has (or should have) a coordinated plan for dealing with unexpected major disasters such as train and plane crashes and the effects of terrorist activity. Most of the planning deals with the medical and surgical management of serious physical injuries, but in recent years many hospital plans have included advice for dealing with the psychosocial effects of disasters. Liaison psychiatrists should be involved closely with the development and implementation of these plans. Bisson *et al.* have provided useful advice.[26] Planning for a psychosocial response should be a multidisciplinary exercise. It should be sufficiently flexible to cope with a range of situations and be capable of immediate response. A core multidisciplinary team should be identified, roles defined and a team leader appointed.

In the immediate aftermath of a major incident, psychosocial care should comprise giving basic emotional and practical support. Universal counselling is not recommended. Survivors can be offered the opportunity to discuss their experiences and feelings if they wish to do so but must not be forced to do so. This support is most appropriately given by non-mental health professionals. Mental health staff should be available to deal with the small proportion of survivors who develop acute anxiety states or psychoses. For the majority, verbal advice and written information should be given about the normal emotional response to disasters, with emphasis on the fact that emotional symptoms tend to resolve within a few weeks. Using alcohol and drugs as a method of coping should be discouraged. If symptoms do not resolve within a few weeks, victims should be encouraged to consult their GP, a special telephone helpline or some other identified local resource. Counselling or cognitive-behaviour therapy might be suitable at that stage. For patients admitted to hospital, the team should maintain contact with ward staff to help identify patients who may be developing persistent problems such as post-traumatic stress disorder or depression and to provide intervention accordingly.

ESTABLISHING A SERVICE

Where no specific liaison psychiatry service exists, it will be necessary to make a case for its establishment if the recommendations of the Academy of Medical Royal Colleges are to be fulfilled. This will involve persuading commissioners to fund an adequately staffed service and to agree its managerial arrangement. Psychiatrists may have to undertake some fairly basic educational work in this regard. Although physicians and surgeons are becoming increasingly aware of psychological factors in their clinical practice, commissioners may have little knowledge of liaison psychiatry and the diagnostic and therapeutic skills it has to offer. The NSF for mental health had little to say about liaison psychiatry, but the Scottish Executive specifically acknowledged the evidence supporting the effectiveness of liaison psychiatry and made a commitment to develop it further.[27] Subsequent publications such as the NHS Cancer Plan[28] and the NSF for older people[29] have stressed the importance of access to psychological care and psychiatric services. Reference should also be made to government targets such as the waiting time initiative and the reduction of the national suicide rate. The effectiveness of treatment needs to be emphasized. Psychological therapies are of proven benefit in the treatment of functional somatic conditions,[30] and behavioural interventions are recognized as effective in the management of chronic physical illness.[31] Psychotropic drugs have an established role in the treatment of co-morbid mental illnesses, but their use often has to be modified in order to avoid drug interactions and dangerous side effects.

Estimating the demand

A helpful guide has been provided by Morris, based on her own experience of establishing a service at Hull Royal Infirmary.[32] It is important to be familiar with research that demonstrates the high prevalence of psychiatric illness, but only a fraction of these patients will require a specialist opinion. Some idea of the likely demand can be gleaned partly by examining patterns of referral to a psychiatrist (if data exist) before developing a new service. However, this is likely to underestimate the demand because experience shows that a specific service is almost certain to increase the rate of referrals once it is established and accepted as part of the acute hospital.[33] More useful information can be obtained by looking at reported referral rates from other hospitals of a similar size and nature. Teaching hospitals tend to report higher rates than district general hospitals, as do hospitals with tertiary services such as neurology, oncology and transplantation.

Service profile

It is essential for liaison psychiatry to be located within the general hospital that it serves. This enables the service to be accepted as an integral part of the hospital and facilitates a prompt response to urgent referrals. It also helps to reduce the stigma that is still attached to psychiatry and psychiatric hospitals. The presence of the service can be enhanced if its clinicians participate in aspects of the hospital's management and contribute to postgraduate teaching of nurses and junior doctors. Presenting cases at medical grand rounds further raises the profile.

Ideally, referrals should be accepted from all departments of the hospital, regardless of where the patient lives. Clinicians from other specialties often find it exasperating to be told a referral cannot be made to a particular psychiatrist because the patient does not reside at an appropriate address. This is clearly a denial of choice. There should also be agreement as to whether out-patients can be seen and whether referrals can be accepted from GPs as well as from hospital consultants. Some liaison psychiatrists have developed special skills in managing chronic somatizers who are often frequent attendees at GP surgeries, medical out-patient clinics and emergency departments and who make considerable demands on medical time and expensive investigations. Chronic fatigue is another condition for which expertise has been developed and for which patients could be referred by GPs.

If patients are seen in an out-patient clinic, they usually prefer this to be located on the same site as the clinics they attend for other medical reasons. It follows that adequate clinic rooms should be provided together with office space for clinical and secretarial staff. Data must be collected and stored to enable audit and clinical research to be conducted.

However, if referrals are accepted from all specialties, the commissioning must reflect this demand on the liaison service, which must be funded correspondingly. It should be clear what age groups the service covers. Children and adolescents (up to the age of 16 years) should be seen by a specialist child and adolescent team. Some services accept referrals of all adults aged 16 years and over, but where there is a well-developed old-age service this team may accept responsibility for adults over 65 years of age. This responsibility needs to be clarified and agreed with commissioners.

The level of staffing is difficult to define. It is likely that a liaison service will start with relatively few staff but will expand as it becomes established and demand increases. It is important that there should be an appropriate range of clinical skills within the team The joint report from the RCP and RCPsych estimated that, for an acute hospital of approximately 600 beds serving a population of 250 000, the team should comprise:

- one full-time consultant liaison psychiatrist;
- one trainee psychiatrist;
- five liaison nurses;
- one or two health psychologists/clinical psychologists;
- one secretary.

A teaching hospital, serving an inner-city population with several tertiary specialist centres requires a larger service with at least two full-time consultant liaison psychiatrists. Most services operate predominantly on a consultation basis, patients being seen following a specific request by the referring team. The referral process should be uncomplicated and the response timely. During periods of heavy workload, the liaison service must be flexible and give priority to urgent referrals. There should be good channels of communication with medical, nursing and other professionals within the general hospital and with community psychiatric teams. A liaison, as opposed to a consultation, model should be developed with certain medical units if there is demand. Closer links can be forged through regular multidisciplinary meetings, which help to improve the detection and management of psychological problems; some psychiatrists seek referrals proactively in this manner.

The newly appointed consultant in liaison psychiatry is at some risk of professional isolation, given that most of the groundwork in establishing the service will involve working with clinicians and managers who are not concerned directly with mental health issues and persuading commissioners who may be sceptical about what liaison psychiatry has to offer. Psychiatric colleagues may be working elsewhere in mental health units or community clinics. Links with psychiatrists must be retained and developed by attendance at postgraduate case-conferences, lectures and committee meetings. Soon after appointment, the consultant should approach a mentor who is familiar with the acute hospital and nature of the clinical work. The mentor should agree to provide regular support and advice, thereby helping to alleviate the obstacles and frustrations that are inevitably experienced.

Training

Experience of managing mental health problems within a general hospital is a valuable part of training for junior psychiatrists. It is essential for those who wish to consider a career as a liaison psychiatrist. Each psychiatry training scheme should have at least one junior liaison training post and opportunities for further specialized experience towards the end of training, at which stage scope for research should also be available. Posts in liaison psychiatry should also be available during the first or second foundation years. The consultant's job plan must recognize the training role so that adequate time is available for weekly supervision.

Funding and management

The joint RCP and RCPsych report advocated that a liaison service should be funded from within the acute trust's budget and also managed within the acute trust, given that the patients treated are primarily the responsibility of staff employed by the acute trust. The more recent report from the Academy of Medical Royal Colleges also recommended that the liaison service should be commissioned via the acute trust. Local primary care trusts should therefore fund the acute trust accordingly. There must also be recognition of the demands made by patients attending the acute hospital from outside the immediate catchment area. Tertiary referral patients, for example to neurology and oncology, have many psychological needs and make demands on the liaison service. Funding for tertiary care must provide for this clinical activity.

SUMMARY

The establishment of a liaison psychiatry service should be achieved in all acute general hospitals. It is warranted by the high prevalence of mental health problems and supported by medical royal colleges and official government documents. Commissioners must be actively engaged in providing this service through the acute trust.

REFERENCES

1. Yates WR (2002) Epidemiology of psychiatric disorders in medically ill patients. In MG Wise, JR Rundell (eds) *Textbook of Consultation-Liaison Psychiatry*, 2nd edn. Washington, DC: American Psychiatric Publishing.
2. Mayou R, Lloyd G (1985) A survey of liaison psychiatry

in the United Kingdom and Eire. *Bulletin of the Royal College of Psychiatrists* **9**: 214–17.

3. Swift G, Guthrie E (2003) Liaison psychiatry continues to expand: developing services in the British Isles. *Psychiatric Bulletin* **27**: 339–41.
4. Lloyd GG (2001) Origins of a section: liaison psychiatry in the College. *Psychiatric Bulletin* **25**: 313–15.
5. Royal College of Physicians and Royal College of Psychiatrists (1995) *The Psychological Care of Medical Patients: Recognition of Need and Service Provision*. London: Royal College of Physicians and Royal College of Psychiatrists.
6. Royal College of Physicians and Royal College of Psychiatrists (2003) *The Psychological Care of Medical Patients: A Practical Guide*. London: Royal College of Physicians and Royal College of Psychiatrists.
7. Academy of Medical Royal Colleges (2008) *Managing Urgent Mental Health Needs in the Acute Trust*. London: Academy of Medical Royal Colleges.
8. Salkovskis P, Storer D, Atha C, *et al.* (1990) Psychiatric morbidity in an accident and emergency department. *British Journal of Psychiatry* **156**: 483–7.
9. Johnson S, Thornicroft G (1995) Emergency psychiatric services in England and Wales. *British Medical Journal* **311**: 287–8.
10. Gater R, Goldberg D (1991) Pathways to psychiatric care in south Manchester. *British Journal of Psychiatry* **159**: 90–96.
11. Royal College of Psychiatrists and British Association for Accident and Emergency Medicine (2004) Psychiatric Services to Accident and Emergency Departments. Council report 118. London: Royal College of Psychiatrists.
12. Hodgkiss A (2007) The emergency department. In GG Lloyd, E Guthrie (eds) *Handbook of Liaison Psychiatry*. Cambridge: Cambridge University Press.
13. Department of Health (1999) National Service Framework for Mental Health. London: Department of Health.
14. National Collaborating Centre for Mental Health (2004) *Self-Harm: The Short-Term Physical and Psychological Management and Secondary Prevention of Self-Harm in Primary and Secondary Care*. Leicester and London: British Psychological Society and Royal College of Psychiatrists.
15. Royal College of Psychiatrists (2004) Assessment Following Self-Harm in Adults. Council report 122. London: Royal College of Psychiatrists.
16. Royal College of Psychiatrists (1998) Managing Deliberate Self-Harm in Young People. Council report 64. London: Royal College of Psychiatrists.
17. Peveler R, Feldman E, Friedman T (2000) *Liaison Psychiatry: Planning Services for Specialist Settings*. London: Gaskell.
18. Leon DA, McCambridge J (2006) Liver cirrhosis rates in Britain from 1950 to 2002: an analysis of routine data. *Lancet* **367**: 52–6.
19. Pirmohamed M, Brown C, Owens L, *et al.* (2000) The burden of alcohol misuse on an inner-city general hospital. *Quarterly Journal of Medicine* **93**: 291–5.
20. Royal College of Physicians (2001) *Alcohol: Can the NHS Afford it? Recommendations for a Coherent Alcohol Strategy for Hospitals*. London: Royal College of Physicians.
21. Canning UP, Kennell-Webb SA, Marshall EJ, Wessely S, Peters TJ (1999) Substance misuse in acute general medical admissions. *Quarterly Journal of Medicine* **92**: 319–26.
22. Veale D (2007) Cosmetic procedures. In GG Lloyd, E Guthrie (eds) *Handbook of Liaison Psychiatry*. Cambridge: Cambridge University Press.
23. Phillips KA, Grant J, Siniscalchi J, *et al.* (2001) Surgical and non-surgical medical treatments for patients with body dysmorphic disorder. *Psychosomatics* **42**: 504–10.
24. National Institute for Health and Clinical Excellence (2007) *Antenatal and Postnatal Mental Health: The NICE Guideline on Clinical Management and Service Guideline*. London: National Institute for Health and Clinical Excellence.
25. Musters C, McDonald E, Jones I (2008) Management of postnatal depression. *British Medical Journal* **337**: 399–403.
26. Bisson JI, Bolton J, Mackway-Jones K, Guthrie E (2007) Major disaster planning. In GG Lloyd, E Guthrie (eds) *Handbook of Liaison Psychiatry*. Cambridge: Cambridge University Press.
27. Scottish Executive Health Department (2000) *Our National Health: A Plan for Action, a Plan for Change*. Edinburgh: The Stationery Office.
28. Department of Health (2002) *The NHS Cancer Plan*. London: Department of Health.
29. Department of Health (2001) *A National Service Framework for Older People*. London: Department of Health.
30. Kroenke K, Swindle R (2000) Cognitive behaviour therapy for somatisation and symptoms syndromes: a critical review of controlled trials. *Psychotherapy and Psychosomatics* **69**: 205–15.
31. Von Korff M, Tiemens B (2000) Individualised stepped care of chronic illness. *Western Journal of Medicine* **172**: 133–7.
32. Morris S (2007) Establishing a service. In GG Lloyd, E Guthrie (eds) *Handbook of Liaison Psychiatry*. Cambridge: Cambridge University Press.
33. Brown A, Cooper AF (1987) The impact of a liaison psychiatry service on patterns of referrals in a general hospital. *British Journal of Psychiatry* **150**: 83–7.

PART 8

Legal and ethical aspects of psychiatry

Chapter 76

Forensic psychiatry

Ian Treasaden

INTRODUCTION

Forensic psychiatry is the application of psychiatric knowledge to issues related to the courts and law. The principal work of forensic psychiatrists is the assessment of and preparation of psychiatric reports for the court on mentally abnormal offenders and their treatment. In practice, however, nearly all general psychiatrists will have to undertake such work on their own patients from time to time. In addition, forensic psychiatrists are also asked to provide advice on the management of aggressive and other severely behaviourally disturbed patients, who may not have been formally charged with offences or reached the courts, for example very aggressive in-patients in ordinary psychiatric hospitals.

Forensic psychiatrists in the UK are most often based in secure psychiatric hospitals such as medium secure units or special hospitals, for example Broadmoor in the UK, but they frequently undertake work in prisons to provide reports for the courts on people on remand in prison awaiting trial and to advise the prison medical service on the psychiatric management of particular inmates. Forensic psychiatrists have characteristically undertaken specialist forensic psychiatry training and are not formally legally trained. However, they are often more familiar than most lawyers with the legal issues surrounding the field of mentally abnormal offenders.

The term 'forensic' comes from the Roman forum, where offenders were tried. The Romans took the view that the 'mad' were punished enough by their madness and should not be additionally punished (*satis furore punitor*). The Bethlem Hospital in London, from where the term bedlam originated, was given cash from the early nineteenth century to take mentally disordered offenders, but due to the resulting stigma associated with such patients, which persists today, they were eventually placed in a new facility, the State Criminal Lunatic Asylum, which opened in 1863, following the Criminal Lunatics Asylums Act of 1860, and which was later renamed Broadmoor Hospital, the first of the special hospitals.

Special hospitals

In the UK, as constituted under the National Health Service Act of 1977 (Section 4), special hospitals are for individuals subject to detention who also require treatment under conditions of special (i.e. maximum) security on account of their 'violent, dangerous or criminal propensities'. Such patients are considered an immediate and grave danger to others, either to the public or to staff and patients in hospital. The level of security in special hospitals is equivalent to that of a category B prison in terms of preventing a patient escaping, but not in terms of preventing people breaking in to obtain an individual's release, as in category A prisons.

The three special hospitals in England are Broadmoor Hospital in Berkshire, Rampton Hospital in Nottinghamshire, and Ashworth Hospital in Liverpool. Rampton Hospital provides for all English female special hospital cases and is the national special hospital for those with learning disability and those with hearing problems. Rampton and Broadmoor hospitals also have dangerous and severe personality disorder (DSPD) units. These hospitals have the advantage of having large sites facilitating greater freedom and therapeutic activities compared with less secure units.

Most admissions to special hospitals in the UK come via the courts. Some patients are transferred from ordinary psychiatric hospitals, where they have behaved dangerously, but may not have been formally charged with offences. Others are transferred during custodial sentences from prison. Women are admitted at least five times less frequently than men[1] and are more likely to be civilly detained, have personality disorder and be suicidal.[2]

Special hospitals and their equivalents throughout the world have in the past been frequently criticized concerning their physical conditions, repressive regimes and the maltreatment of patients by staff. They have often tended to develop in isolation from the developments in practice in ordinary psychiatric facilities. A number of official inquiries have commented on the abuse of patients in such facilities, which have arisen due to the combination of poorly trained staff and a difficult to manage patient population, among other factors. In the UK, the Fallon Inquiry in 1999 severely criticized the lack of control in a special unit for people with personality disorder in Ashworth Special Hospital.[3] Such hospitals have been described as being in a 'no-win situation', being criticized for keeping patients in too long, or letting the wrong ones out who, on occasions, may kill or otherwise behave dangerously again, often many years later. However, the latter may have more to do with the patients' subsequent situation or their psychiatric follow-up than with decisions made by the special hospitals. It can be difficult, in any case, to assess whether a patient will be dangerous in the community while he or she is still in a secure, single-sex ward without access to, for instance, alcohol, drugs or potential victims. The risk of re-offending is, however, long-term.[4] Nonetheless, such hospitals clearly fulfil a need in many countries, with the demand for admissions often exceeding capacity. Of relevance is Penrose's law, which was based on a 1936 study of different European countries and states that a higher national homicide rate correlates with a lower national number of psychiatric hospital beds.

Medium secure units

These were set up in England on a regional basis (hence, the previous term 'regional secure units') following the 1975 Butler[4a] and the 1974 Glancy[4b] reports in response to an unmet need for secure care. This arose from the open-door policy since the early 1950s of ordinary psychiatric hospitals, overcrowding in special hospitals, and increasing numbers of mentally abnormal offenders in prisons needing in-patient psychiatric treatment. Mentally abnormal offenders were sent by the courts to ordinary psychiatric hospitals after conviction; they would then abscond and re-offend, but not so dangerously as to require special hospital admission. They would end up in prison again, and the vicious cycle of admission and re-offending continued.

Medium secure units were set up for people whose severely disruptive or dangerous behaviour requires psychiatric treatment in conditions of medium security – that is, more than that available in ordinary hospitals but less than that in special hospitals – and who also have a prospect of responding to care within about 18 months.[5] However, provisions for longer-stay patients in medium secure units have also now been developed. Many patients have committed dangerous offences such as homicide, rape or arson. The majority have severe (psychotic) mental illness, mainly schizophrenia. Aggressive psychopaths are not considered suitable for such units, as there is no definite evidence that they are amenable to treatment in such conditions within the original maximum recommended duration of admission. Severely mentally handicapped people are also excluded, as they can generally be managed within locked units of hospitals for mentally handicapped people.

In general, patients admitted to medium secure units are detained under the 1983 Mental Health Act. The largest number, at least 40 per cent, come via the courts, having dangerously offended. Most, up to 90 per cent, are male, but more recently women's enhanced medium secure (WEMS) units have been developed – the term 'enhanced' referring to the therapeutic input rather than the level of security. Such units have allowed chronic behaviourally disturbed females to be transferred out of special hospitals.

Over a third of patients have been transferred to medium secure units from special hospitals as a graded step in their rehabilitation to conditions of less security and, ultimately, the community. Some patients are admitted from prison, either while on remand awaiting trial or after becoming mentally ill during a custodial sentence. Others are transferred from ordinary psychiatric hospital facilities. Most patients admitted to medium secure units are either discharged to the community, often to supervised hostels, or transferred to ordinary psychiatric facilities. A few require transfer to a special hospital.

The National Adolescent Forensic Network in the UK has developed medium secure units (five in number to date) for 12- to 18-year-olds with severe mental illness who have committed serious offences.

The number of places available in specialized secure psychiatric facilities is limited compared with the large number of mentally abnormal offenders. Thus, most mentally abnormal offenders continue to be dealt with by ordinary psychiatric hospitals as either in- or out-patients.

Low secure units often admit, under locked conditions, chronic behaviourally disturbed, sometimes violent, patients who have offended less seriously. *Locked psychiatric intensive care units* are usually for acute mentally ill individuals who are violent, destructive or suicidal, and length of admission is usually short (less than 2 months).

Community forensic psychiatry

Forensic psychiatry services have historically been institutionally based and for mentally disordered individuals who present a substantial or persistent risk to others. However, increasingly specific forensic psychiatry out-patient services are being developed,[6] which should offer specialist skills not available to non-forensic teams, such as anger-management and specific brief treatments. These services may be either parallel to those of adult general psychiatry services or integrated with them,[7,8] and they have had a duty to cooperate with multi-agency public protection arrangements (MAPPAs) since 2003.[9]

CRIME AND PSYCHIATRY

Psychological motives for crime can be found in nearly all offenders, and this has led to psychiatric and, in particular, psychoanalytical interest since the time of Freud. The problem has been that this has not led to successful psychological treatments for offenders in general. Crime is now increasingly seen as a sociological phenomenon, better explained by sociological theories than by individual psychological theories. Psychiatric explanations for an offence, although providing understanding of the offender, do not necessarily provide an excuse for, or remove legal responsibility from, the offender, although this is often perceived by the public to be the case. Psychiatrists are trained to detect the presence or absence of psychiatric disorder; they are not especially equipped to assess a defendant's responsibility for his or her actions, which is a legal concept. It is a philosophical question as to whether an individual in fact has complete free will: our response to events is due to the combination of our genes, previous experience and the current stresses in our life. There is also a contrast between the legal system's attempt to clarify whether an individual offender is either 'mad', and therefore in need of psychiatric treatment, or 'bad', and therefore in need of punishment, and the often multifactorial psychiatric explanations of behaviour. Offending is not a characteristic symptom of any mental disorder, and an offender's behaviour may arise from a combination of mental illness, premorbid personality difficulties and background.

The courts are, in general, sympathetic to offers of psychiatric treatment as an alternative to other sentences, particularly custodial sentences, which are generally known to be ineffective, although guaranteeing that an individual will not offend for the period of sentence. Occasionally the court can be dismissive of psychiatric evidence, especially as this may be perceived as being based largely on the history obtained from the individual (e.g. whether or not the individual says they hear voices).

A psychiatric assessment is particularly likely to be requested if there is no apparent motive for an offence, if the offender is female rather than male, and in cases of sexual offending. Even where the psychiatrist does not consider that an individual has a specific mental disorder or is amenable to psychiatric treatment, the court may be assisted in sentencing by the psychological understanding provided by a psychiatric assessment.

For instance, although a theft may appear to be committed for financial gain, it will rarely be the entire explanation, and other motivations, such as excitement, may be important. People with personality difficulties, for example, may be unable to sustain relationships or work and may find life generally unrewarding and meaningless; they may obtain 'kicks' not only from alcohol and drug abuse but also from the excitement of offending. One reason burglars may urinate in the homes they enter is such excitement, sometimes compounded by alcohol abuse, which itself may have given them the courage to offend. Such behaviour may also be an act of defilement. Burglars may also find it exciting to creep around while the owners are at home and asleep and, on occasions, the excitement generated may lead to a serious offence such as rape. At a deeper unconscious psychological level, offenders may, for instance, be standing up to their parents or stealing to obtain symbolic affection.

Aspects of criminology

Crime is socially determined and varies between societies and over time. In the past in the UK, both suicide and certain homosexual acts were illegal; hence, the saying that 'the major cause of crime is the law'. Studies indicate that almost everyone commits a crime at some time in their life. There is thus a less clear cut-off between offenders and non-offenders than is generally assumed. Most crime goes undetected, and crime statistics may merely reflect changes in detection rates, or a reduced tolerance of the public to a particular behaviour, or increased police recording of offending, rather than, for instance, a real increase in crime. Increasing police numbers is thus likely to increase the number of offences detected and recorded. Currently about 60 per cent of offending in the UK is related to motor vehicles. The British Crime Survey[10] collects information independently from the police and suggests that nearly twice as much crime may be committed (over 10 million crimes per year) than is reported to the police (about 5 million crimes).[11] The best deterrent appears to be the certainty of arrest rather than, for instance, the severity of punishment.

Although certain categories of crime may have increased over the past 25 years, it is likely that the public's perception that we live in a less law-abiding society than formerly is misplaced. The term 'hooligan' may originate from the name of an Irish gang leader in Victorian London involved in what would now be termed 'mugging'. Even in the early twentieth century in the UK, public-house brawls were common and sometimes observed by several hundred individuals at a time as entertainment. Industrial and political violence were also more common in the early part of the twentieth century than at present.

The peak age of offending in the UK is 14 years for girls and 17–18 years for boys (Figure 76.1). Studies in inner London have shown that up to one in five boys there have at least one conviction by the age of 21 years. Half the indictable crimes (more serious and eligible for trial by jury) are committed by people under the age of 21 years, and 30 per cent of males have been convicted of such an offence by the age of 30 years. Crime in general decreases with age as personality matures, except for a small peak for women aged 40–50 years, around the menopause. With the falling numbers of people aged 14–15 years in the UK (i.e. the peak age of committing crime), there has been a corresponding fall in the rates of certain offences.

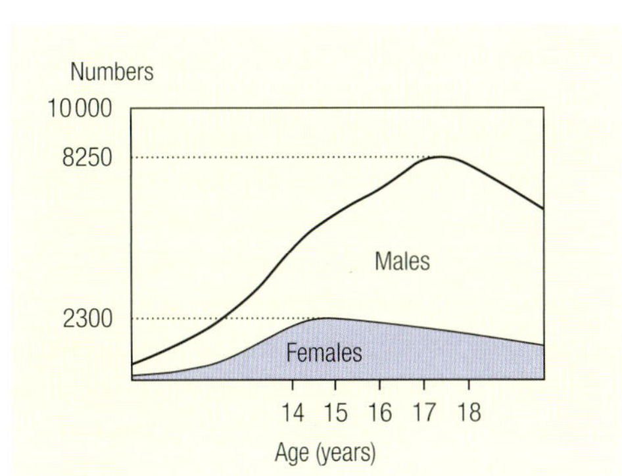

Figure 76.1 People found guilty or cautioned for indictable offences in England and Wales

Sexual differences in offending rates

In the UK, convicted males outnumber females by five to one, although this preponderance is only half of what it was 25 years ago. The excess may be due, among other factors, to the strength of males in general for repetitive violence (females tend to commit only isolated offences of violence), opportunity at work (e.g. fraud, although this is an area where females are also increasingly being convicted), the psychology of the male as 'breadwinner', and females being generally more conforming in behaviour. A female offender generally comes from a more damaged background and is otherwise more psychologically and behaviourally disturbed than a male who has committed the same offence. This in turn is reflected in the fact that females in prison tend to be more behaviourally and psychiatrically disturbed than their male counterparts. Females are also reported less frequently for crimes, particularly by male police officers, and yet are up to three times more likely to go to prison for their first offence than males in the UK.

In the past it was argued that the female equivalent to male delinquency was promiscuity, but evidence suggests that delinquent males are equally likely to be promiscuous. Some offences are, by definition, more common in women (e.g. those related to prostitution). Economic motives are commonly given as a rationalization for prostitution, although prostitutes as a group show an excess of mental disorder, self-harm, alcohol or drug abuse, physical disorders, personality disorders and bisexuality.

Premenstrual tension and crime

There is evidence that women are more likely to offend, be violent in an institution or harm themselves premenstrually than at other times during the menstrual cycle. Indeed, some women have successfully used premenstrual tension as a defence to a charge of homicide.[12,13] It is most likely, however, that premenstrual tension is only an exacerbating factor in such individuals, and it does not imply that women in general are overall 'less responsible' at that time of the month.

JUVENILE DELINQUENCY

Delinquency is defined as law-breaking behaviour. Juvenile delinquency usually means such behaviour committed by 10- to 21-year-olds. The majority of boys under the age of 17 years may commit a delinquent act. Up to one in five males in London have a conviction by the age of 21 years, and half of all indictable crimes (the more serious offences eligible for trial by jury) are committed by individuals under the age of 21 years.[14] Five males are convicted for every one female. Recidivism (chronic offending) is associated with an earlier age at first offence and with both loss of life experience and institutionalization due to repeated custodial sentences.

Aetiology

This is multifactorial and is not associated with an established psychiatric disorder. Some such individuals do have a personality disorder, but opportunity may be more important. For those with personality disorder, the aetiology of their offending is likely to be that of their personality disorder. There is evidence that adult criminality may have an inherited genetic predisposition, especially for acquisitive crime, but this is not definitely so for juvenile delinquency.

Sociological theories include delinquent subcultures and associated peer pressure, differential association[15] and social protest theories[16] of the 'have-nots'. Differences in juvenile delinquency rates have also been related to residence in large towns and even particular bad schools. There is also evidence of labelling effects: those labelled as delinquent by conviction in court are more likely to continue with such behaviour than if they are not apprehended and convicted.

Individual developmental factors

Studies of children with conduct disorder show that 28 per cent grow up to be psychopathic adults, compared with 4 per cent of those with neurotic disorder and 2 per cent of controls.[17] The factors summarized in Figure 76.2, if present, are associated with the development of delinquency.

If three of these five factors are present, then there is a 40 per cent chance of the individual showing delinquent behaviour during adolescence. Also, if troublesomeness at school is noted, then there is a 50 per cent chance of later showing delinquent behaviour.

Prevention and management

Many of the factors associated with juvenile delinquency are present before birth. It might therefore be countered, for instance, by reducing family size, increasing family income

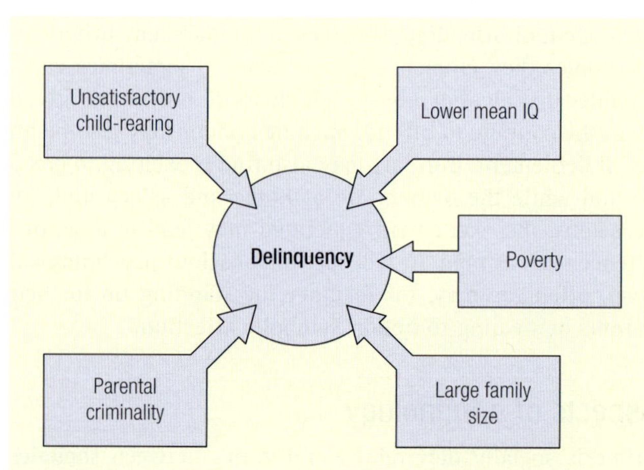

Figure 76.2 Factors associated with the development of delinquency
IQ, intelligence quotient.

to counter poverty, and countering low intelligence by special attention and remedial education. Individual counselling to improve self-esteem and counter feelings of resentment may help suitable individuals, particularly those who are of high intelligence and show good motivation, but a paternalistic, strict regime tends to be more helpful than a psychodynamically based regime for people who are immature and of low intelligence.

Box 76.1

DUNEDIN MULTI-DISCIPLINARY HEALTH & DEVELOPMENT STUDY 32-YEAR FOLLOW-UP OF BIRTH COHORT OF 1000 NEW ZEALANDERS (MOFFITT)

(A) LIFE COURSE PERSISTENT OFFENDERS

- Rare – small numbers but responsible for half crime rate
- Neuro-development problems ↓
- Temperament difficulties ← Disrupted attachments ↓
- Disruptive behaviour ← Ineffective discipline ↓
- Social learning poor ← Delinquent peer influences, truanting, etc. ↓
- Personality disorder, particular antisocial personality disorder (15–25%) ↓
- Serious violence
- Victimization of partners and children
- Poor physical, sexual and psychiatric health (especially depression)
- Substance dependence (opiates) and alcoholism
- More traumatic injuries

Management

- Requires early childhood interventions in family but as chronic cumulative condition requires lifelong interventions.

(B) ADOLESCENT LIMITED OFFENDERS

- Common
- Good neuro-development and also social and academic skills
- Maturation gap in period 15–25 years
- Extrovert, sensation seeking, risk taking
- Prognosis better if good partner and job
- Requires individual treatment, e.g., cognitive-behavioural skills training, during teen years to counteract delinquent peer influence. (Group treatments facilitate deviant peer networks)
- Parent management training and education

Juvenile delinquency may be ameliorated by a good relationship with one parent or, in its absence, a counsellor, by improved emotional harmony in the home and a good experience in school, together with a good peer group.[18] Successful employment and a good relationship/marriage also improve the prognosis with regard to adult criminality.

Prognosis

By 19 years of age, half will have stopped their delinquent behaviour. The half who will continue are more likely to be abusing alcohol and drugs, and to gamble, to smoke and to be more sexually promiscuous. Delinquency in teenagers is also associated with criminality in adult life. The best predictor of future criminality remains the extent of previous delinquency, although offending usually ceases in the early twenties.

More recently, a 32-year follow-up of a birth cohort of 1000 New Zealanders has differentiated, apart from adult onset offenders and discontinuous offenders, life-course-persistent offenders and adolescence limited offenders and the implications for treatment (Box 76.1).[19,20]

MENTALLY ABNORMAL OFFENDERS

It has been variously estimated that 1–3 per cent of all offenders and up to one-third of those in prison have a mental abnormality. Other estimates are even higher. Most of these people have personality disorder/psychopathy or alcohol and drug dependency. Nevertheless, there is an over-representation in prison of people with learning disabilities, and people with both functional and organic mental illnesses. Imprisonment may precipitate mental illness. In the UK, men outnumber women in prison by 30 to 1, but female prisoners have more mental and physical disorders.

Mentally abnormal offenders have usually committed petty and minor offences. In fact, it is not certain that mentally disordered people break the law more often than non-mentally disordered people. Both mental illness and law-breaking are common. Up to 40 per cent of ordinary psychiatric hospital admissions may follow threatened or actual aggression, but in most of these cases it is usually considered pointless for such individuals to be charged with their offences. When assessing offenders, it is important to bear in mind that they may become mentally ill before or after an offence, due to being in custody or to fear of the likely consequences of their offending.

After committing an offence, a mentally abnormal individual may be arrested and detained in hospital under the civil provisions of a country's mental health legislation, be cautioned by police or be charged. An individual must normally be charged within 3 days of arrest in the UK. If charged, the individual may be remanded on bail or in custody (e.g. in prison) until the court case is heard.

Box 76.2 Forensic psychiatric assessment

- Full history and mental state of patient, including fantasies and impulses to offend
- Objective account of offence, e.g. from arresting police officer or from statements (depositions) in Crown Court cases
- Objective accounts of past offences, if any, e.g. obtain list of previous convictions
- Additional information gathering, e.g. interviews with informants (e.g. relatives), reading a social enquiry report from a probation officer (if prepared)
- Review of previous psychiatric records, e.g. to ascertain relationship of mental disorder to previous behaviour and response to psychiatric treatment and need for security.

Forensic psychiatric assessments

Referrals to psychiatrists may be made by the court itself, the probation service or defence solicitors. Custom in England and Wales is that all individuals charged with murder have reports prepared on them by two psychiatrists.

Psychiatrists are expected to assess whether an individual is fit to plead and stand trial, whether mental disorder is present, the individual's level of mental responsibility, and detainability under the relevant Mental Health Act (e.g. Sections 37 and 41 of the Mental Health Act 1983 in England and Wales), and to arrange any treatment recommended, on either an in- or out-patient basis as required. Psychiatrists are also expected to give an opinion (make a risk assessment) as to the degree of dangerousness of an offender, as far as they are able.

Areas to be considered in a forensic psychiatric assessment are shown in Box 76.2.

To rely solely on an offender's account may lead to an underestimate of the severity of the circumstances of the offence. For example, a paranoid psychotic patient may complain of being threatened by a victim of his violence when in fact the victim plausibly states that the offence was unprovoked. Also with incomplete information about previous convictions, a psychiatrist runs the risk of being discredited in court.

Box 76.3 outlines the areas to be covered in a clinical forensic psychiatric risk assessment and management plan.

Multifactorial nature of offending

When assessing an offender, it is important to bear in mind that no psychiatric disorder is specifically characterized by

Box 76.3 Clinical risk assessment and risk management planning

The aim is to get an understanding of the risk from a detailed historical longitudinal overview, obtaining information not only from the patient, who may minimize his or her past history, but also from informants. Ideally it should not be a one-off single interview assessment.

Reconstruct in detail what happened at the time of the offence or behaviour causing concern.

Independent information from statements of victims or witnesses or police records should be obtained where available. Do not rely on what the offender tells you or the legal offence category – for example, arson may be of a wastepaper bin in a busy ward or with intent to kill. Possession of an offensive weapon may have been prelude to homicide.

Offence = offender × victim × circumstances/environment

Risk factors associated with violence to be sought in a forensic assessment have been usefully summarized and are detailed later in this chapter.

Consider also protective factors:
Practical risk assessment (history × mental state × environment) can be supplemented by standardized instruments of risk, including actuarial risk instruments based on static risk factors, such as the Violence Risk Appraisal Guide (VRAG), and dynamic risk instruments, such as the Historical, Clinical, Risk-20 (HCR-20) based on factors that can change or be managed, for example symptoms of mental illness and non-compliance.

In conclusion:

- Aim to answer how serious the risk is (i.e. its nature and magnitude): is it specific or general, conditional or unconditional, immediate, long-term or volatile? Have the individuals or situational risk factors changed? Who might be at risk?
- From such a risk assessment, a risk-management plan should be developed to modify the risk factors and specify response triggers. This should ideally be agreed with the individual. Is there a need for more frequent follow-up appointments, an urgent care programme approach meeting or admission to hospital, detention under the Mental Health Act, physical security, observation or medication? If the optimum plan cannot be undertaken, then reasons for this should be documented and a back-up plan specified.
- Risk assessments and risk-management plans should be communicated to others on a 'need to know' basis. On occasions, patient confidentiality will need to be breached if there is immediate grave danger to others. The police can often do little unless there is a specific threat to an individual, whereupon they may warn or charge the subject. Very careful consideration needs to be given before informing potential victims to avoid their unnecessary anxiety. Their safety is often best ensured by management of those at risk.

offending, and it is important to see an offence as being due to a combination of the offender, the victim and the situation/environment.

The offender

For those with a psychiatric disorder, being young and male increases the chance of committing an offence. Overall, chronically mentally ill people are more likely to commit offences than those who are acutely ill. People whose mental illness has relapsed and who are not compliant with treatment are also more likely to commit offences. The motivation for crime may be the same as for those who are not mentally ill (e.g. as a reaction to rejection), but also it may be due to delusions or hallucinations, or as a result of a deterioration in social functioning and personality due to mental illness, so that such individuals are more impulsive and have a lower stress tolerance (e.g. in schizophrenia or depressive disorder).

People with paranoid schizophrenia may develop isolated paranoid delusions about particular individuals, which may go unrecognized, and they may otherwise appear to function adequately in daily life. They may plan attacks and are more effective in their execution compared with individuals with other types of schizophrenia. Specific parts of the body, e.g. the eyes, are more likely to be attacked by such patients.

The victim

This is most commonly a family member with whom the individual is in close proximity. This is true for victims of both mentally disordered people and 'normal' individuals. Most conflicts in any case occur within the family. Although it is important not to overrate the role of the victim, the victim can unintentionally provoke an offence, especially if they are physically or mentally ill themselves or have been abusing alcohol or drugs. The victim may also not appreciate the degree of stress that a potential assailant is under. Battered children are more likely to be temperamentally more difficult to manage.

The circumstances

These may also be important, for example in a pub, where victim and offender have both abused alcohol. Mentally ill individuals will tend to commit offences of criminal damage against public rather than private property, and in situations where they are likely to be apprehended. The availability of weapons is also important.

Outcomes of sentencing

Box 76.4 shows the outcomes of sentencing. In England and Wales, an individual charged with an imprisonable offence may be detained in a psychiatric hospital under Section 37 of the Mental Health Act 1983 (a 6-month renewable treatment order). A Section 41 Restriction Order may be added by a Crown Court. This requires Ministry of Justice authorization for leave, transfer or conditional or

Box 76.4 Outcome of sentencing of mentally abnormal offenders

- The law takes its course, e.g. a fine, prison
- Conditional or absolute discharge, possibly with voluntary psychiatric treatment
- Probation order, with or without condition of psychiatric treatment (e.g. Community Rehabilitation Order in England and Wales)
- Detention under the Mental Health Act (e.g. under Section 37, with or without a Section 41 Restriction Order under the Mental Health Act 1983 of England and Wales).

absolute discharge of the individual from hospital – that is, it removes the final decision from the patient's consultant psychiatrist and responsible clinician. The order is made 'to protect the public from serious harm' and allows for conditional discharge subject to conditions such as place of residence and compliance with psychiatric treatment.

Under English law, a shoplifter with depression would be found guilty but might be placed on a community rehabilitation (previously, probation) order with a condition of psychiatric out-patient treatment.[21] An individual with schizophrenia who smashed shop windows would be found guilty of criminal damage and might then be admitted to a psychiatric hospital under a hospital order (e.g. Section 37 of the Mental Health Act 1983 in England and Wales). See Figure 76.3 for an indication of the prevelance of community rehabilitation orders.

In countries other than the UK, mentally abnormal offenders are not considered legally guilty; they thus do not have a conviction recorded against them and are merely ordered to be detained in hospital for treatment. Under UK law, alcohol and drug dependence are not grounds for detention under the Mental Health Act, although again this does not always pertain in other countries.

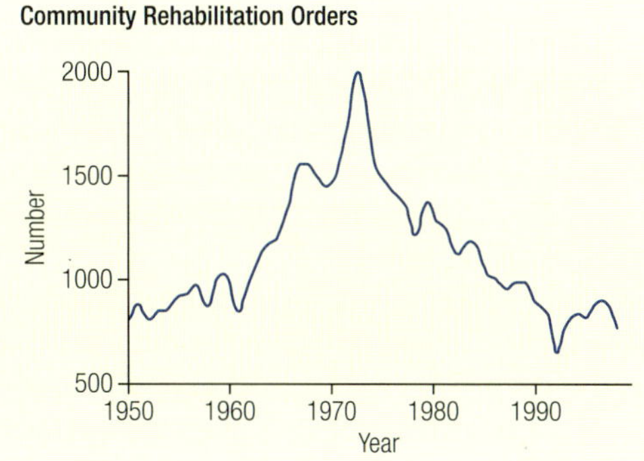

Figure 76.3 Community rehabilitation orders. Reproduced with permission from ref. 21

The courts

Doctors, whatever their specialty, are likely to have to attend court at some time in their career, if only to give evidence to a coroner's court or regarding personal injury cases.

Over 98 per cent of all criminal prosecutions in England and Wales are dealt with by magistrates' courts. Three magistrates usually preside. A juvenile court is composed of a special panel of three magistrates, one of whom is usually a woman. It deals with offences committed by children and young people. In these courts, the defendant's name must not be disclosed by newspapers and other media without the court's permission.

The UK system of law is adversarial. If called to give evidence, for example by the defendant's legal advisors, then a witness will initially undergo examination-in-chief by them, followed by cross-examination, in this case by the prosecution, and then a re-examination. It is important as a doctor not to overstate one's professional views. One should indicate clearly the limits of opinion and in what areas one cannot comment.

In most cases it will be sufficient for a psychiatrist to give an opinion to the court in a report. Oral evidence is usually requested only when there is a dispute regarding the medical evidence, such as in cases of homicide where a disputed psychiatric defence has been put forward (such as diminished responsibility) in order to reduce the charge from murder to manslaughter, or where oral evidence is legally required, for example in supporting an individual being made subject to restrictions under Section 41 of the Mental Health Act 1983 of England and Wales.

ASSOCIATION OF PARTICULAR MENTAL DISORDERS WITH OFFENDING

Offending is not a primary characteristic of any mental disorder. When considering an offence, it is important to consider not only the offender but also the victim and the circumstances.

Organic mental disorders

The onset of minor offending such as shoplifting, minor sex offences and fraud at a late age may be due to dementia (e.g. Alzheimer's disease) owing to its reduction of intellectual functioning, judgement and normal inhibitions in social behaviour. Elderly people in general often show coarsening of their personality characteristics and disinhibition with increasing age.

Brain damage from head injury, even in the absence of significant cognitive impairment, may produce a profound alteration in personality, resulting in excessive aggression, for example to a partner, who may then find it impossible to continue to live with the individual. Brain damage also reduces alcohol tolerance, which in turn may predispose to further head injuries.

Huntington's disease may present in the early stages with psychopathic behaviour.[22]

The association of epilepsy with offending is discussed in detail later.

Schizophrenia and delusional disorders

Most individuals with schizophrenia do not commit criminal offences, but overall schizophrenia is overrepresented among offenders, particularly compared with affective psychoses. Most convictions are for minor offences and are secondary to the associated deterioration in the individual's personality and social functioning, rather than arising from delusions and hallucinations. Schizophrenia, especially paranoid schizophrenia, can, on occasions, lead to dangerous offending and may result in planned assaults, including homicide, without apparent motive.

Antisocial behaviour is occasionally seen in the prodromal phase of schizophrenia, when the clinical picture may be referred to as 'pseudo-psychopathic schizophrenia'. Schizophrenia may otherwise distort the perceptions, judgement and voluntary control of actions. Matricide (the killing of one's mother) is frequently, but not invariably, associated with schizophrenia.

Morbid delusional sexual jealousy (Othello's syndrome) does not infrequently lead to severe aggression towards, and the killing of, a sexual partner about whom delusions of sexual infidelity are held. This is discussed in detail later.

Querulous paranoia (litigious paranoia or morbid querulousness) leads to a profound sense of being wronged and a desire to seek redress through the courts.[23]

Mood (affective) disorders

Overall, people with mood disorders are underrepresented in forensic psychiatric populations. Depressive disorder is more generally associated with the risk of suicide, but it is an occasion associated with homicide, for example the 'altruistic' homicide of a family where the individual feels that the family may be better off out of this 'wicked' world. Homicides associated with depressive disorder are more likely to occur in the morning and usually involve family members. As will be discussed later, up to one-third of individuals suspected of committing homicide commit suicide, with up to one-half trying, although this predominantly reflects the psychological difficulty of living with having committed such an offence. Shoplifting may also be associated with depression, particularly in middle-aged females of previously good record who may shoplift as a cry for help to bring attention to their mental state.

Hypomania or manic episodes are often associated with disinhibited behaviour, irritability, intolerance and increased sexual drive. This may lead to convictions for breach of the peace, road-traffic offences, impulsive violence and sexual offending such as rape. Such patients spend money excessively, often due to their belief that they will soon make this up, but it can also lead to fraud.

Disorders of adult personality

These are common among offenders, but there is no clear cut-off between psychiatrically 'normal' individuals who offend and individuals with personality disorder. Some individuals are given a diagnosis of personality disorder on the basis of the circular argument that they have a personality disorder because they have offended. However, it is possible to contrast psychopathic offending, which is impulsive and unplanned, with more organized planned criminality with co-defendants. People with personality disorder who offend have frequently abused alcohol or drugs, or are dependent on them, and often have chronic neurotic and stress-related disorders as well.

Learning disabilities (mental retardation)

People with learning disabilities are three to four times overrepresented among offenders and even higher among violent offenders.[24] This may be because they lack understanding of the nature of their behaviour and its legal consequences, they are more suggestible and they are easier to catch. Learning disabilities may also lead to feelings of frustration, which in turn may lead to violence and even homicide. Also, in panic or frustration, such people may commit arson or sexual offences that relate to their difficulty initiating and sustaining interpersonal and sexual relationships.

CRIMINAL RESPONSIBILITY

Criminal responsibility is a legal concept and begins at 7 years in the Republic of Ireland; 8 years of age in Scotland but at 10 years of age in England and Wales and Northern Ireland. Individuals can commit serious offences before this age, but in the UK they will not be held legally responsible (*doli incapax*) and cannot be convicted, although they may be placed on a social services care order and held in a secure children's home. After the age of 10 years in England and Wales, an individual is considered legally responsible for his or her actions, unless they were due to:

- a mistake;
- an accident;
- duress;
- necessity, e.g. self-defence;
- responsibility being affected by mental disorder.

It is questionable how good psychiatrists are in judging responsibility as opposed to diagnosing mental disorder.

Some offences require specific guilty intent (*mens rea*) as well as an unlawful act (*actus rea*), for example murder, rape and arson (i.e. specific intent). Other offences do not require proof of guilty intent, for example motoring offences (i.e. basic or non-specific intent). Certain mental states interfere with the patient's intention (*mens rea*) and may be defences in law to the *actus rea*.

Insanity has always been regarded as a defence in English law. A judge in King Alfred's time was hung for having ordered the hanging of an insane man. By the early eighteenth century, for insanity to be a defence in law it had to be such as to cause the subject to be like a 'wild beast' – devoid of all reason and memory. However, in 1780 a soldier was acquitted of murder because he was found to be suffering from a delusion about the victim as a result of insanity.

Following an offence, an individual may be detained under a civil section of the Mental Health Act 1983 (e.g. Sections 2, 3, 4, 136), or cautioned by the police, or charged. If charged, the individual may be remanded on bail or in custody (e.g. in prison) until the court case.

Mental abnormality as a defence in court

In most cases, the alleged offender stands his or her trial. If the defendant is found guilty or pleads guilty, he or she then presents the medical evidence in mitigation to alter the sentencing of the court; for example, instead of a custodial sentence, the individual may be placed on a community rehabilitation (old probation) order with or without a condition of in- or out-patient psychiatric treatment or be detained in hospital under Sections 37 and 41 of the Mental Health Act 1983. In countries other than the UK, mentally abnormal offenders are not legally convicted.

In certain uncommon cases the offender offers evidence of their mental disturbance, either:

- to excuse their being tried (not fit to plead); or
- to agree to having done the act but not to have been fully responsible at the time (insane or diminished responsibility or automatism or infanticide).

In these cases, the psychiatric evidence is presented as part of the arguments to the court and is heard before conviction.

Criminal Procedure (Insanity and Unfitness to Plead) Act 1991

Unfit to plead

A mentally disordered offender may plead that he or she is unfit to plead (under 'disability' in relation to trial). This refers to the time of trial.

The defendant would have to prove, using medical evidence, in a Crown Court hearing, that he or she was not fit to do at least one of the following (based on the original test used in 1836 in R *v*. Pritchard):

- Instruct counsel ('so as to make a proper defence')
- Appreciate the significance of pleading
- Challenge a juror
- Examine a witness
- Understand and follow the evidence of court procedure.

The defendant does not have to be fit to give evidence him- or herself.

If raised by the judge or the prosecution, this must be proved beyond reasonable doubt, but if raised by the defence, this only has to be proved on the balance of probabilities. This is a very rare plea and is likely to be successful only in cases such as severe mental impairment or for patients who are extremely paranoid, for example about the court or their legal representatives. In psychotic patients, unfitness to plead is significantly related to thought disorder and delusional thinking.[25] Physical illness, such as pneumonia, may also result in unfitness to plead and stand trial.

If the individual is found unfit to plead, a decision for a Crown Court judge since the Domestic, Violence, Crime and Victims Act 2004 (see Appendix i), then there is a provision for a trial of the facts. If the individual is found unfit to plead, then this results in discretionary sentencing, including detention in hospital, a guardianship order, a supervision and treatment order or absolute discharge.

Historically, the concept originates from dealing with deaf-mute people. In medieval times, defendants were pressed under weights to give a plea, without which they could not be convicted or executed or their property given to the Exchequer – hence, the phrase 'press for an answer'.

In Scotland, individuals are found unfit to plead more commonly, including in cases where in England they would be convicted and detained under a Section 37 hospital order. Fitness to plead is also often a major issue in the USA, where the term 'competency' is used.

In England and Wales, as an alternative to finding the individual unfit to plead, Section 37(3) of the Mental Health Act 1983 can be used, including in a magistrate's court, for detention without conviction, or the individual can be remanded to hospital for treatment (e.g. Section 36) in order to get the individual well enough to be fit to plead.

Not guilty by reason of insanity ('special verdict') (insanity defence) (McNaughton Rules)

Historically, this defence arose from the case of McNaughton in 1843. McNaughton, believing himself to be poisoned by Whigs, attempted to shoot the prime minister, Robert Peel, missed (or misidentified), and shot and killed Peel's secretary. Because McNaughton was deluded and insane, he was acquitted, but this caused a great deal of argument, including from Queen Victoria ('Insane he may be, but not guilty he is not'), and the law lords were asked to issue guidance for the courts in response to five questions. Their guidance is known as the 'McNaughton Rules'.[26]

In this defence, the offender is arguing that he or she is not guilty (not deserving of punishment) by reason of his or her insanity. It has to be proven to a court, on the balance of probabilities, that at the time of the offence the offender laboured under such defect of reason that he or she met the McNaughton Rules – that is:

- that by reason of such defect from disease of the mind, the individual did not know the nature or quality of his or her act (this means the physical nature of the act); or
- the individual did not know that what he or she was doing was wrong (forbidden by law).
- If an individual was suffering from a delusion, then his or her actions would be judged by their relationship to the delusion – that is, if the individual believed their life to be immediately threatened, then they would be justified in striking out, but not otherwise.

Technically, this plea may be put forward for any offence, but in practice it is usually put forward only for murder and other serious offences. In fact, such a plea is rare.

Evidence from two or more medical practitioners, one approved under Section 12 of the Mental Health Act 1983, is required before the return of the verdict 'not guilty by reason of insanity'. Such a verdict implies lack of intent. However, legally a psychiatrist can only give evidence regarding an individual's capacity to form intent (a legal concept), not the fact of intent at the time of the offence.

Under the Criminal Procedure Act 1991, if found not guilty by reason of insanity, then the judge has freedom to decide on the sentencing and disposal of the defendant (discretionary sentencing), including detention in hospital under forensic treatment orders of the Mental Health Act 1983.

- A psychiatrist does a retrospective mental state examination for the time of the offence when assessing whether the individual is not guilty by reason of insanity (McNaughton Rules).
- In the McNaughton Rules, the legal concept 'disease of mind' is used. (In diminished responsibility, the legal concept 'abnormality of mind' is used.)
- From case law, 'mind' refers to reason, memory and understanding. 'Disease' can be organic or functional, permanent or temporary, treatable or not treatable, is 'internal' (R *v.* Quick) or 'manifests in violence and is prone to recur' (Bratty *v.* AG for N Ireland 1961). It can also include epilepsy (R *v.* Sullivan, 1984).

Criticism of the McNaughton Rules and diminished responsibility

The McNaughton Rules are now almost obsolescent. Points against them are include the following:

- 'Hardly anybody is "mad" enough to fit the rules' (Lord Bramwell). Even McNaughton would not have been.
- The rules assumes a doctrine that mind is made up of separate independent compartments, of which cognition is most important (a Victorian view).
- The rules are too unfair, as abnormal mental states do not fit into rigid categories.
- The rules ignore the importance of emotional disturbance and failure of will, when cognition is normal.

Homicide by mentally disordered offenders in England and Wales

Definition

Homicide is the killing of another human being. It is not necessarily unlawful.

Epidemiology

There have been around 500–600 homicides each year in England and Wales in the first decade of the twenty-first century.[27] These figures include for 2003 the 172 victims of Dr Harold Shipman, an English general practitioner (GP) who killed many of his elderly patients. Around a third of all homicide victims are female (half killed by their partners). This compares with around 16 000 externally caused deaths each year (of these, half are suicides, others misadventure, accidents, etc.).

Of note is that in England and Wales between 1996 and 1999, the three highest at-risk occupational groups of being homicide victims were security staff (25 victims), medical staff (24 victims) and social workers (14 victims).[28]

Legal classification in England and Wales

Homicide may be lawful or unlawful.

Lawful homicide

Lawful homicide may be:

- justifiable, e.g. on behalf of the state, such as actions taken by people in the army or the police force;
- excusable, e.g. a pure accident or an honest or reasonable mistake.

Unlawful homicide

Unlawful homicide is defined in England and Wales as the unlawful killing of any reasonable creature in being and under the Queen's (or King's) peace. Types of unlawful homicide include:

- murder;
- manslaughter;
- child destruction;
- genocide;
- causing death by dangerous driving;
- suicide pacts;
- infanticide.

Clinical categories of homicide

Parricide, the killing of near-relatives, is disproportionately committed by males in late adolescence[29] and includes patricide (killing of one's father), matricide (killing of one's mother, which in the UK is more common than patricide[30] and tends to be committed by people with schizophrenia,[31] perhaps reflecting the psychological difficulty of normally doing so), uxoricide (killing of one's wife) and filicide (the killing of one's child).

Serial killing involves killing individuals over time, spree killings involve killing individuals in different locations during one episode, and mass killing involves killing multiple individuals at the same time and in the same location.

Murder

Murder is an offence at common, as opposed to statute (Parliament-passed) law in England and Wales. It is defined as an unlawful killing with malice aforethought. Malice aforethought requires an intention to kill or to cause grievous bodily harm. Murder, like any other crime requiring proof of intent, involves proof of a subjective state of mind on the part of the accused. The *actus reus* of murder consists of both of the following:

- An unlawful act
- The act causes the death of another human being.

Murder results in a mandatory life custodial sentence in England and Wales. On average, 11.5 years is served in prison, and then the prisoner is released on life licence. A few murderers do serve life.

Manslaughter

Manslaughter may be categorized into three groups:

- Voluntary manslaughter
- Involuntary manslaughter
- Corporate liability.

The third of these will not be considered further here.

Voluntary manslaughter

There are cases of homicide in which the defendant would be guilty of murder if it were not for the availability of one of the following partial defences: diminished responsibility, provocation, killing in pursuance of a suicide pact.

Diminished responsibility (Section 2 Homicide Act 1957)

As a reaction against the fact that mentally disordered people who had killed were still being hanged, given the then mandatory death sentence for murder (abolished in the UK in 1965), despite other defences, such as not guilty by reason of insanity (the McNaughton Rules), a movement was created to bring in a defence of diminished responsibility – that is, the responsibility of the offender is not totally absent because of mental abnormality but is only partially impaired; therefore, the offender would be found guilty but the sentence modified. This was made law in the Homicide Act 1957 and applies only to a charge of murder. The murder charge is reduced to manslaughter on the grounds of diminished responsibility.

Under the 1957 Homicide Act (Section 2), as a defence against the charge (only) of murder, the offender may plead that at the time of the offence, he or she had diminished responsibility. The offender has to show that at the time:

> where a person kills ... he shall not be convicted of murder if he was suffering from such abnormality of mind, whether arising from a condition of arrested or retarded development of mind or any inherent causes or induced by disease or injury, as substantially impaired his mental responsibility for his acts.

'Abnormality of mind' is left to the defendant (or his or her medical advisors) to define and is not synonymous with mental disorder as defined in the Mental Health Act 1983. It has been ruled in the Court of Appeal, in the case of R *v.* Byrne (1960), regarding the defence that 'abnormality of mind' would have affected at the time of the offence the individual's perception, judgement (between right and wrong, between good and bad), or the voluntary control of (capacity to control, a legal concept) his or her actions.

Thus, abnormality of mind is:

> A state of mind so different from that of the ordinary human beings that the reasonable man, earlier defined as 'a man with a normal mind', would term it abnormal. It appears to us to be wide enough to cover the mind's activities in all its aspects, not only the perception of physical acts and matters, and the ability to form a rational judgement as to whether the act was right or wrong, but also the ability to exercise will power to control physical acts in accordance with that rational judgement (R *v.* Byrne 1960).

The authoritative interpretation of the term 'abnormality of mind' was given by Lord Parker (R *v.* Byrne 1960) as follows:

> Whether the accused was at the time of killing suffering from 'any abnormality of mind' in the broad sense in which we have indicated above is a question for the jury. On this question medical evidence is, no doubt, important, but the jury are entitled to take into consideration all the evidence including the acts or statements of the accused and his demeanour. They are not bound to accept the medical evidence, if there is other material before them which, in their good judgement, conflicts with it and outweighs it. The aetiology of the abnormality of mind (namely, whether it arose from a condition of arrested or retarded development of mind or any inherent causes or was induced by disease or injury) does, however, seem to be a matter to be determined on expert evidence ...

'Substantially' is also undefined and is left to the jury to decide, although the doctors may give their opinions.

> Substantial does not meant total... At the other end [it] does not mean minimal or trivial. It is something in between. (R *v.* Lloyd 1996).

The effect of a successful plea of diminished responsibility is to reduce the charge from murder to manslaughter. The verdict 'unties the judge's hands'. Murder carries a statutory sentence of life imprisonment, but the court is free to make any sentence at all with regard to manslaughter, including a hospital or community rehabilitation (probation) order or, indeed, a life prison sentence, in which case research has shown that such individuals may spend longer in custody than those convicted of murder.[32] This may reflect concern that although abnormality of mind was identified in these cases of diminished responsibility, no ameliorating treatment is undertaken, for example in hospital, if the individual received a life prison sentence.

In addition to a report supporting the plea of diminished responsibility, the psychiatrist may also, if appropriate, wish to arrange for the appropriate hospital treatment and offer the appropriate Mental Health Act 1983 section (detention) recommendations to the court to help them with their sentencing (e.g. sections 37 and 41 of that act).

The diminished responsibility defence has been used where a defence of insanity would have no hope of success. Examples include:

- mercy killing;
- when the subject kills his or her spouse in a state of reactive depression;
- individuals who kill in jealous frenzies;
- individuals who are subject to an 'irresistible impulse' to kill (cited more often in the USA);
- subjects who kill and who are 'deranged' by psychopathic disorder.

The diminished responsibility defence has largely replaced the insanity defence in England and Wales for individuals charged with murder.

The most important points in favour of diminished responsibility are that:

- it allows for an overall assessment of the person;
- it allows more flexible sentencing.

Against diminished responsibility are the following points:

- There is a problem of balancing the concept of responsibility with 'determinism', e.g. does a greater propensity to lose one's temper imply less responsibility?
- It assumes that a distinction can be made between psychopathy and 'wickedness' in terms of moral or criminal responsibility.
- Does diminished responsibility mean less power to resist temptation? If so, should the irresponsible be punished less than the responsible?
- Does an irresponsible act in a normally responsible person indicate a greater aberration of mind than irresponsible behaviour in an irresponsible person?
- If a person is found to have diminished responsibility, then it may mean that the court will return such a person to society faster than a responsible offender.

Provocation (Section 3 Homicide Act 1957)

Provocation is the sudden or temporary loss of control under provocation that might make a 'normal' person kill. Whether this occurred is for the jury to decide, although a psychiatrist's opinion may be requested. More recently, psychiatric evidence about the propensity of individuals with certain vulnerable personalities or conditions, such as learning disability, to be provoked has been accepted as admissible.

Following criticism that this defence is used inappropriately by individuals who kill after losing their temper, and that it is not sufficiently tailored to those who kill out of fear of serious violence, for example those subject to prolonged domestic violence (as illustrated in the case of R *v.* Ahulwalia, 1992), the Ministry of Justice has proposed that this defence should be replaced with a new partial defence for people who (i) kill in response to fear of serious violence or (ii) have a justified sense of being seriously wronged.[33]

Killing in pursuance of a suicide pact (which the offender has to prove) (Section 4 Homicide Act 1957)

A suicide pact is defined as being a common agreement between two or more people, having for its object the death of all of them, whether or not each is to take his or her own life.

Involuntary manslaughter

Involuntary manslaughter refers to cases of homicide without malice aforethought. It can take several forms, including the following:

- An unlawful and dangerous act: 'constructive manslaughter' – the *actus reus* consists of an unlawful act that is dangerous and causes death.
- Gross negligence: the *actus reus* consists of a breach of a duty of care that the accused owes to the victim, with the result that the breach leads to the victim's death.

Infanticide

Under the Infanticide Acts 1922 and 1938 (Section 1), infanticide is defined as having occurred when a woman by any wilful act caused the death of her child under the age of 12 months, but at the time of the act or omission the balance of her mind was 'disturbed by reason of her not being fully recovered from the effect of giving birth to the child or the effect of lactation consequent upon the birth of the child'. This is technically an offence rather than a defence.

The grounds for this plea, as an alternative to murder, are less stringent than those for diminished responsibility (i.e. there is no need to prove abnormality of mind); nor does it require proof of a mental disorder, for example mental illness. It is the policy of the Director of Public Prosecution and the Crown Prosecution Service to use this plea for such mothers. It does not apply to adopted children or to any child other than the youngest (otherwise a manslaughter plea has to be used), as it is possible to give birth on two occasions within 1 year.

When this plea was introduced, many such mothers had acute organic confusional puerperal psychoses. Nowadays, infanticide is rather an historical anachronism; only about one in six of such mothers have functional puerperal psychoses, the remainder being not dissimilar from those who batter their children. A conviction for infanticide usually results in a sentence of a community rehabilitation (probation) order, often with a condition of psychiatric treatment (out- or in-patient).

Amnesia

Some 40–50 per cent of people charged with homicide claim amnesia for the actual act.

Amnesia is not in itself a defence, but the underlying condition may be – for example, a post-traumatic state, epileptic fit or acute psychosis. In the 1959 Podola Appeal case in England and Wales (Podola's amnesia was, in fact, not genuine), it was ruled that even if amnesia is genuine, it is no bar to trial.

Amnesia may be feigned by lying or caused by:

- hysterical amnesia (denial);
- failure of memory registration owing to overarousal (comparable to 'exam phobia');
- alcohol;
- other psychoactive drugs;
- head injury.

Drugs and alcohol

It has always been considered in England and Wales that a person is fully responsible for their actions if they knowingly used drugs or alcohol (voluntary intoxication). It is assumed that everyone knows that drunkenness is associated with aggressive and irresponsible behaviour and therefore one is responsible for not becoming drunk. The same rule applies to drug abuse. This would not apply if an individual were 'slipped' drugs or alcohol or if their doctor did not inform them of the side effects and interactions (e.g. with alcohol) of prescribed medication.

Successful defences have been based on:

- being so drunk as to be incapable of forming intent in offences requiring specific intent;
- developing a mental illness, e.g. psychosis, as a result of the ingestion of a drug or alcohol (as in delirium tremens);
- where the use of a drug, which might be legitimate, produces a mental state abnormality that could not have been anticipated by the subject, e.g. hypoglycaemia after the use of insulin.

Thus, overall, successful defences following consumption of alcohol or drugs are based on either (i) involuntary intoxication or (ii) if intoxicated voluntarily, lack of specific intent where offences, such as murder, require this.

Automatism

Automatism is a rare plea generally restricted (although not entirely) to cases of homicide. The defendant pleads that at the time of the offence their behaviour was automatic (no *mens rea*). The law uses this term to mean a state almost near unconsciousness. It refers to unconscious, involuntary, non-purposeful acts where the mind is not conscious of what the body is doing. There is a separation between the will and the act, or the mind and the act – 'Mind does not go with what is being done' (Bratty *v*. AG for N Ireland, 1963).

This is an extremely rare plea and has been successfully pleaded, particularly in cases of homicide, for offences occurring during hypoglycaemic attacks, sleepwalking or sleep, for example fighting tigers and snakes in dreams (theoretically this should be during night terrors in slow-wave sleep, as in dreams one should be paralysed in rapid eye movement (REM) sleep, but it has been argued that such offences may occur as an individual wakes from a dream). Such must be the degree of automatism that there is no capacity to form any intent to kill or any capacity to control actions.

In certain cases, such as offending while sleepwalking, individuals have walked free from the court on the understanding that they always lock their bedroom door.

Where a defence of *sane automatism* is put forward, the subject hopes to receive a total acquittal. However, the law has become aware that some automatism states are really the result, in the legal sense, of a disease of the mind, such as epilepsy, which may recur, and therefore in such cases the jury may be invited to consider that the defence of automatism should be regarded as evidence of insanity (insane automatism) and to return the special verdict – that is, not guilty by reason of insanity – which would allow for discretionary sentencing, including detention in hospital.

Although historically sleepwalking and night terrors have been accepted as automatisms and led to acquittal, case law now differentiates sane automatism due to external causes (extrinsic factors), such as hypoglycaemia due to insulin use, from insane automatism due to disease of the mind caused by mental illness or brain disease (intrinsic factors), such as diabetes mellitus, epilepsy and even hysterical dissociative fugue states, where the special verdict (not guilty by reason of insanity) should be returned.

Pathological intoxication (as defined in the tenth revision of the *International Classification of Diseases*; ICD-10) is sudden onset of aggression and often violent behaviour, not typical of an individual when sober, very soon after drinking amounts of alcohol (only) that would not produce intoxication in most people.[34]

Mute defendants

Rarely, one may be asked to help the court decide whether an individual who appears to be mute (i.e. with no speech at all) is being mute 'by malice or a visitation of God'. If mute 'by malice', then the case proceeds with a not guilty plea entered on the defendant's behalf. If 'by visitation of God', for example if the defendant is deaf and dumb, then the question of fitness to plead arises, with a view to disposal under the Criminal Procedure (Insanity and Unfitness to Plead) Act 1991.

MENTALLY DISORDERED OFFENDERS INVOLVED WITH THE POLICE AND COURTS IN ENGLAND AND WALES

Following an offence, an individual may be admitted informally to a psychiatric hospital, compulsorily detained under civil sections of the Mental Health Act 1983 (e.g. Section 2, 3, 4, 136), be cautioned by the police, which the individual has to voluntarily accept, or be charged. If charged, the individual may be remanded on bail or in custody (e.g. prison) until the court case. The police may also check whether the person is an absconding detained patient and return him or her to hospital under Section 18 or Section 138.

Under the Police and Criminal Evidence Act 1984 (PACE), there is a code of practice that covers detention, treatment and questioning of people by police officers. If the individual is suspected by a police officer to be mentally disordered, then an 'Appropriate Adult' must be informed and asked to come to the police station. This should ideally be an individual trained or experienced in dealing with mentally disordered people rather than an unqualified relative. An Appropriate Adult should be present while the individual is told their rights and can advise the person being interviewed, observe the fairness of the interview and facilitate communication with the interviewee. They may also require the presence of a lawyer.

If a decision is taken by the police to prosecute, the case is passed to the Crown Prosecution Service, which will also consider the public interest and likely adverse effects of prosecution of a mentally disordered individual.

Police and court liaison

Terminology

- *Diversion or early diversion:* this is the transfer to the healthcare system of a mentally disordered individual in police custody or at first court hearing.
- *Diversion or police or court diversion schemes:* specific psychiatric services provided to the police or courts, usually to a magistrate's court (where 98 per cent of offenders are tried). Such services reduce the time on remand in custody for mentally ill individuals but may not affect the long-term risk of offending.[34a,34b,34c] However, it is unlikely that serious offenders, such as those charged with murder, will be suitable for such diversion.

Psychiatric issues relevant to police and court liaison include:

- Evidence of mental disorder
- Need for out- or in-patient psychiatric treatment
- Urgency if in-patient psychiatric treatment required
- Nature of alleged offence and risk to others
- Fitness to remain in police custody
- Fitness to be interviewed by police
- Fitness to plead if individual is to appear in court.

Remember that the technical legal offence may not reflect the actual risk. For example, arson may be of a wastepaper bin in front of others on a busy hospital ward or committed with intent to endanger the lives of others in a tower block. Similarly, possession of an offensive weapon may have been with a view to seriously harming others.

Fitness to remain in police custody

- There is no legal definition.
- An individual may be unfit to remain in police custody due to physical illness or psychiatric disorder.
- Serious and immediate risk to an individual's health will usually make the individual unfit to remain in police custody. Detention under a civil section of the Mental Health Act 1983 may then be indicated.

Fitness to be interviewed by police

- There is no legal definition.
- The individual should be able to understand the police caution after it has been explained.
- Full orientation to time, place and person is required.
- Fitness may be questioned if the individual is likely to give answers due to their mental disorder that may be wrongly interpreted by the court.
- If the individual is fit to be interviewed but has a history of mental disorder, then an Appropriate Adult should be present. Such individuals can be provided by Appropriate Adult schemes.

False confessions (after Gudjonnson 1993)[35]

Three types of false confession have been described:

- *Voluntary:* e.g. due to depression or morbid guilt.
- *Coerced-compliant:* due to being pressurized during the interrogation. Individuals often retract such false confessions after interrogation.
- *Coerced-internalized:* the individual becomes confused by interrogation and comes to believe the false story. This is seen particularly in people with learning disability.

In cases of possible suggestibility and false confessions:

- assess the individual's intellectual level;
- use the Gudjonnson Suggestibility Scale.

Procedure before trial

The presumption is always in favour of remanding an individual on bail rather than in custody. Bail could include a condition of residence in a psychiatric hospital, although the individual would be an informal patient there unless detained under the Mental Health Act 1983.

Where the individual might otherwise be remanded to prison, the Mental Health Act 1983 allows for the following:

Section 35 – remand to hospital for report

This order can be made under Subsection (3) (i) 'if the court is satisfied on the written or oral evidence of a registered medical practitioner that there is reason to suspect the accused person is suffering from mental disorder'; and (ii) 'the court is of the opinion that it would be impractical for a report on his mental condition to be made if he were remanded on bail'.

A hospital bed must be available within 7 days. If awaiting a bed, the accused must be kept in a 'place of safety', e.g. a 'police station, prison or remand centre or any hospital the managers of which are willing temporarily to receive him' (Section 55(1)). The remand period is for a maximum of 28 days, although it is renewable for further periods of 28 days, without the necessity of the patient attending court, up to a maximum of 12 weeks. Part IV provisions on consent to treatment do not apply, and so the individual cannot be treated without their consent, except in an emergency under common law. Some psychiatrists therefore additionally detain such individuals under Section 3 when they wish to treat them without their consent; the code of practice states that this may be considered if there is a delay in getting to court. The use of Section 36 might, however, then be more appropriate.

Section 36 – remand to hospital for treatment

This may be used only by the Crown Court and is an alternative to remand to custody. It can apply to individuals waiting for trial or sentence. It requires the written or oral evidence of two doctors that the individual is 'suffering from a mental disorder of a nature or degree which makes it appropriate for him to be detained in hospital for treatment'. It cannot be used for people charged with murder. The remand is for a maximum of 28 days, although this may be renewed for further periods of 28 days, without the necessity of the patient attending court, up to a maximum of 12 weeks. Part IV provisions of consent to treatment apply. A hospital bed must be available within 7 days and the individual must meanwhile be kept in a 'place of safety' (Section 55(1)). Problems arise if the individual has to wait for more than the maximum 12 weeks of the order to appear in the Crown Court. In these circumstances, detention under a civil section or the use of Section 48 may be required.

Section 48 – remand to hospital of other prisoners (including those on remand in custody)

This section gives the Justice Secretary powers to direct the transfer to hospital of a person waiting for trial or sentence and who has been remanded in custody. It also applies to individuals detained under the Immigration Act 1971 and civil prisoners. The Justice Secretary requires two medical reports, which do not need to specify the availability of a bed at a particular hospital, stating that the individual has a mental disorder of a nature or degree that makes it appropriate for him or her to be detained in hospital for medical treatment and that he or she is in urgent need of such treatment. The period of detention is variable and can continue to the time of sentence. This order has increasingly been used to divert severely mentally ill (psychotic) offenders from custody to hospital, even when the need may not be 'urgent'. It has the advantage that it does not require a court hearing to impose the order. On occasions, e.g. when an acutely mentally ill offender has appeared in court, such an individual may only nominally be remanded to a named custodial facility and, by arrangement with the Ministry of

Justice, is transferred directly to hospital without being placed in custody.

Unfit to plead (Criminal Procedure (Insanity and Unfitness to Plead) Act 1991)

This was described earlier.

Mental disorder as a defence

As described previously, such defences include the following:

- Not guilty by reason of insanity (McNaughton Rules)
- Diminished responsibility: Section 2 of the Homicide Act 1957
- Infanticide Act 1938.

Sentencing

The following options for sentencing were made available under the Mental Health Act 1983.

Hospital order – Section 37 of the Mental Health Act 1983

This may be made by the Crown Court or a magistrate's court, the latter being able to make such an order without conviction under Section 37(3) as long as the court is satisfied that the individual committed the act or omission in question. The individual has to be charged with an imprisonable offence rather than simply any offence. For this sentence to be made, a hospital bed must be available within 28 days, beginning from the date of the order. The patient, meanwhile, must be kept in a 'place of safety' (Section 55(1)). The availability of a bed within 28 days and the evidence of two registered medical practitioners, one approved under Section 12 of the Mental Health Act 1983, are essential before the court can impose such an order.

Interim hospital order – Section 38 of the Mental Health Act 1983

If it is uncertain that a full Section 37 hospital order is appropriate, then this can be tested out by making an interim order. It can be made for up to 12 weeks in the first instance and then renewed by the court for periods of up to 28 days at a time, to a maximum of 1 year. The patient does not have to attend court in person when the order is renewed. This order is also useful for psychiatrists who are uncertain whether the individual's mental disorder is going to be amenable to psychiatric treatment, for example in cases of personality disorder. If, in the end, a Section 37 hospital order is not considered appropriate, then the court can use its discretion to otherwise sentence the individual, including to prison.

Restriction order – Section 41 of the Mental Health Act 1983

Section 41(1) states:

> ... where a hospital order is made in respect of an offender by the Crown Court, and it appears to the court, having regard to the nature of the offence, the antecedents of the offender and the risk of him committing further offences if set at large, that it is necessary for the protection of the public from serious harm so to do, the court may, subject to the provisions of this section, further order the offender shall be subject to special restrictions set out in the section, without limit of time; and the order under this section shall be known as a 'Restriction Order'.

That the order is made 'without limit of time' reflects the therapeutic uncertainty of how quickly an individual will progress. One of the two doctors recommending Section 37 must attend court to give evidence, but it is for the court to decide whether a Section 41 restriction order should be imposed. The main restrictions are that the patient can only be absolutely or conditionally discharged, given leave of absence, or transferred to another hospital with the approval of the Justice Secretary. A restriction order therefore is an added safeguard, so that the decision to, for example, discharge, is not left to the responsible clinician alone.

If conditionally discharged, compulsory aftercare, which will involve statutory supervision by either a social worker or probation officer and usually a psychiatrist, is required. The main advantage of this order for professionals is that it facilitates the long-term management of mentally abnormal serious offenders by specifying the conditions of their discharge, for example their place of residence, such as a supervised care home or hostel, and compliance with psychiatric treatment, including medication, upon threat of recall to hospital. If recalled, the individual is subject to a mandatory mental health review tribunal hearing within the first 6 months.

Guardianship order – Section 37 of the Mental Health Act 1983

The grounds are as for a Section 37 hospital order. It is used rarely. A proposed guardian must agree to it. If the patient absconds from a place where they are required to live, then they may be recaptured and returned there. There are, however, no effective sanctions for a patient refusing to cooperate with psychiatric treatment, for example with medication treatment, although attendance to see a psychiatrist can be enforced. It was hoped in the 1975 Butler Report that this order might be increasingly used, but many social services departments are reluctant to use this order for mentally abnormal offenders, although again it can facilitate the management of a mentally abnormal offender in the community.

Hospital and limitation directions – Section 45A of the Mental Health Act 1983

This was brought in by the Crime (Sentences) Act 1997 (on 1 October 1997). It is referred to as the 'hybrid order', as it is a prison sentence accompanied by hospital and limitation (equivalent to a restriction order) directions. It is available only to the crown court and, currently, only for people with psychopathic disorder alone. Written or oral evidence from two doctors is required, and the treatability test applies.

Psychiatric community rehabilitation (old probation) orders

These can be made in any court for any offence other than one with a fixed penalty, such as murder which carries a mandatory life prison sentence, but they do require conviction. Supervision by a probation officer is for a specified period between 6 months and 3 years. In cases where there is a condition of psychiatric treatment, the court will require evidence from a doctor approved under Section 12 of the Mental Health Act 1983. Conditions may include that the subject receives treatment as an in-patient or in a nursing home or as an out-patient at a specified hospital or place from or under the direction of a named doctor. The court must explain the requirements of the order to the offender and obtain the offender's consent. If the individual subsequently refuses to cooperate with psychiatric treatment, then the doctor can only report this to the supervising probation officer, who may take proceedings on these grounds for breach of the probation order. Detention in hospital under the civil provisions of the Mental Health Act 1983 is an alternative, if appropriate, in such circumstances.

After sentencing

Transfer direction from prison – Section 47 of the Mental Health Act 1983

This allows the Justice Secretary to order the transfer of a sentenced prisoner following conviction if he or she has a mental disorder. The patient is subject to consent to treatment provisions. This order can continue until the earliest date of release, whereupon a notional Section 37 hospital order automatically follows without the need for further completion of legally required medical recommendation reports. Commonly, a restriction direction is also made under Section 49, which has the same effect as a restriction order under Section 41. Such individuals can be returned to prison to complete a sentence before their earliest date of release, for example if they recover from their mental illness or they no longer require in-patient treatment. The two groups of individuals most frequently transferred from prison on this order are those who develop mental illness during a prison sentence and those where the mental illness was missed at the time of sentence.

Transfer of individuals kept in custody during Her Majesty's Pleasure – Section 46 of the Mental Health Act 1983

This also covers members of the armed forces. It has the same effect as a hospital order with restrictions without limit of time.

PSYCHIATRIC EXPERT EVIDENCE AND PSYCHIATRIC COURT REPORTING

The areas of psychiatric expert evidence and psychiatric court reporting are summarized in Boxes 76.5 and 76.6.

Table 76.1 details forensic treatment orders under the Mental Health Act 1983. Box 76.7 shows the Mentally Disordered Offenders and the Crime Sentences Act 1997.

Box 76.5 Psychiatric expert evidence

- Fitness to plead
- Mental responsibility, e.g. not guilty by reason of insanity, diminished responsibility
- Mental disorder, e.g. mental illness, learning disability, personality disorder
- Is the client treatable?
- Have arrangements been made for such treatment, e.g. community rehabilitation order with condition of out-patient treatment, or in-patient treatment under Section 37 of the Mental Health Act 1983?
- Is the client dangerous? e.g. Section 41 Mental Health Act 1983, placement in a special hospital
- Suggestions about non-psychiatric management, e.g. community rehabilitation order, supervised hostel.

Problem areas in police/court liaison and reporting

A plea of not guilty

If the individual is pleading not guilty or is undecided upon their plea but you think the individual was mentally ill at the time of the offence, it is best to say, for example, 'for the time of the offence, Mr X showed symptoms of mental illness such as …' This avoids having to comment on likely guilt before a plea is entered.

Explaining the relationship of mental illness to offending

An offence may have arisen directly from paranoid or passivity delusions due to mental illness or indirectly due to a deterioration in personality and social functioning, for instance in schizophrenia. There may be no relationship between the offence and the mental disorder. The offence and legal consequences may precipitate a mental illness, for example depression.

Personality disorder

If you do not think the individual's personality difficulties are amenable to specific in-patient psychiatric treatment, then say so and add the words 'In the absence of mental illness I do not consider him detainable under the Mental Health Act'.

Box 76.6 Court reporting

A report may be requested:

- by a court (magistrate's, crown or higher), usually through the probation service. Written authorization by the court must be given;
- by the defence solicitors, in which case the patient's written permission is required before giving a report to the solicitor, which remains the solicitor's and client's to use or not in court.

Information required for a report includes:

- information about the charge;
- a social enquiry report from a probation officer;
- a list of previous convictions;
- previous medical hospital records;
- previous reports (social and medical);
- depositions where available, e.g. Crown Court, but not magistrates' cases.

The history will be taken from the patient and, if possible, a relative or friend.

The client should ideally be examined fully physically.

Questions that the court or solicitor will be particularly interested in include the following:

- Does he or she have a mental disorder?
- Is it susceptible to or requiring specific treatment?
- Can arrangements be made for such treatment, e.g. hospital, out-patient?
- Is the client dangerous?
- Have you any suggestions as to the client's management, apart from the psychiatric aspects?

After interview and examination of other reports, etc., one can valuably discuss the case again with the probation officer or others, such as other psychiatrists involved in the case:

- Discuss particularly your findings and compare them with other professionals' observations, which may reveal gross discrepancies.
- Discussion may reveal unexpected channels for disposal or unforeseen difficulties.

The general principles of the written report are as follows:

- It should be in clear English, and technical terms should be avoided if possible. If such terms are used, an explanation of them should be given, e.g. paranoid (persecutory) delusions (false beliefs), auditory and visual hallucinations (voices and visions).
- Use the report to help the court reach the most appropriate disposal for the patient.
- The report is a recommendation to the court. The court may have other psychiatric opinions that oppose yours and may itself be unconvinced by your opinion. Thus, the onus is on you to provide the evidence in the report for your opinion.
- The onus is also on the reporting doctor to make all the necessary medical arrangements for the disposal and management of the patient.
- Be accurate, complete and brief. The court is extremely busy and will resent a turgid, overwritten medical report. For magistrates' courts, which may deal with dozens of cases a day, around two pages may suffice; even then, only the opinion may be read.

People use different forms for their report, but the following is suggested. Paragraph numbers and headings can be used for clarity and are valued by the legal profession:

- *Para 1 – Introduction:* inform the court of when and where the patient was seen, and at whose request, what information was available, who the informants were, and sometimes what information was not available. State the current offence(s) for which the patient is charged and its date, and the plea if known, i.e. guilty or not guilty.
- *Para 2 – Past medical history:* inform the court of this and of the result of medical examination, e.g. 'Physical examination revealed no abnormality'.
- *Para 3 – Family history:* report the important, relevant points, including family history, or not, of psychiatric disorder and criminality.
- *Para 4 – Personal history:* report the important points of the patient's physical development (e.g. birth, milestones), early development (e.g. bed-wetting (enuresis)), schooling (e.g. truancy) and occupational history (e.g. difficulties with a job, sackings, difficulty sustaining employment, difficulties with colleagues or supervisors at work).
- *Para 5 – Sexual history:* be reasonably discreet. The report may be read in open court.
- *Para 6 – Previous personality:* report details of personality in terms of social interaction, emotions and habits, e.g. drinking, gambling, drugs.
- *Para 7 – Past forensic history:* technically, past convictions should not be admissible before conviction, but they are admissible when the report is to assist sentencing. In practice, often only one psychiatric report is prepared for both trial and sentencing.
- *Para 8 – Past psychiatric history:* report dates, diagnosis, relevant details and relationship of mental disorder and treatment to offending.
- *Para 9 – Circumstances surrounding index offence(s):* report the circumstances leading to current offence(s) and the defendant's state of mind at the time of the offence, sticking to the phenomena reported, e.g. 'for the time of the offence, the patient gives a history of tearfulness, loss of hope, poor sleeping... These are symptoms of a depressive mental illness'.

– *Para 10 – Interview:* report the result of the interview, e.g. 'the patient showed/did not show evidence of mental illness'. Then give a brief outline of the evidence, e.g. 'the patient muttered and looked around the room as though hearing voices (auditory hallucinations)', or list the symptoms and say, for example, 'these are symptoms of the severe mental illness of schizophrenia'.

Information in Paragraphs 1–10 should be factual, verifiable and ideally agreed by all, even if others' opinions differ from your own.

– *Para 11 – Opinion:* the final paragraph should express your opinion. The court will be interested particularly in your opinion regarding the following:
  - Is the individual fit to plead and stand trial?
  - Does the individual have a mental disorder as defined in the Mental Health Act 1983?
  - Where appropriate, comment on issues of responsibility, e.g. not guilty by reason of insanity or diminished responsibility in cases of homicide.
  - If so, can arrangements be made for the patient's treatment (sort this out if you can)? Make suggestions to the court about which disposal would be appropriate, e.g. Section 37 hospital order with or without a Section 41 restriction order, or out-patient psychiatric treatment as a condition of a Community Rehabilitation Order (formerly known as a probation order).

For example – a case of a mentally abnormal offender with diminished responsibility in the case of a homicide:

This man is fit to plead and stand trial.

In my opinion he suffers from a mental disorder as defined in the Mental Health Act 1983, the severe mental illness of schizophrenia, characterized by delusions (false beliefs) of passivity (being externally controlled) and paranoid (persecutory) content and auditory hallucinations (voices) talking about him in a derogatory way in the third person.

In my opinion, at the time of the alleged offence of murder, Mr X was suffering from an abnormality of mind, due to the severe mental illness of paranoid schizophrenia, affecting his perception, judgement and voluntary control of his actions, as substantially impaired his responsibility for his acts.

I consider he would benefit from treatment in a psychiatric hospital. I have made arrangements for a bed to be reserved for him at X Hospital under Section 37 of the Mental Health Act 1983 if the court considers that this would be appropriate.

I recommend, if the court so agrees, that he additionally be made subject to restrictions under Section 41 of the Mental Health Act 1983 to protect the public from serious harm and to facilitate his long-term psychiatric management, including by specifying the conditions of his discharge from hospital, e.g. of residence, and compliance with out-patient treatment, and by providing the ability to recall him to hospital should his mental state or behaviour deteriorate or he otherwise gives rise to concern.

As an alternative:

In my opinion this man does not suffer from mental disorder and is not detainable in hospital under the Mental Health Act 1983. He has an immature personality and requires considerable support and would benefit from group psychotherapy as an out-patient. If the court is prepared to consider an alternative to a custodial sentence in this case, I would recommend that, subject to the probation service's agreement, he be made subject to the direction of a probation order with a condition that he attend an out-patient group under my direction at X Mental Health Unit.

Comment on any mitigating circumstances, e.g. marital or work stress, and on the prognosis.

Express any doubts you may have as to the likelihood of benefit from or risks associated with treatment in the person's case.

If you have no psychiatric recommendation, say so: for example, 'I have no psychiatric recommendation to make in this case'.

Finally, if essential information is lacking, or if time is not sufficient to make the necessary arrangements for a hospital bed, then do not hesitate to state your findings to date, state what you would like to do, and ask for a further period of remand.

Psychiatric and psychological treatment can be offered after the law has taken its course when the individual is free to take it up, or as a condition of a community rehabilitation (previously probation) order.

Substance misuse

In general it may be best to allow the law to take its course and to offer treatment or help on a voluntary basis only when the individual is free to take this up, except where specific drug rehabilitation residential placements are recommended as a condition of, for instance, a community rehabilitation order, to which, however, the patient must agree. In general, the recommendation is usually that the individual must stop abusing alcohol or drugs, and that this is something that the individual must primarily decide to do, although the ability or will of the individual to do so may be in doubt, but the individual may additionally be helped by services in doing so.

Table 76.1 Forensic treatment orders for mentally abnormal offenders

	Grounds	Made by	Medical recommendation	Maximum duration	Eligibility for appeal to mental health review tribunal
Section 35 – Remand to hospital for report	Mental disorder	Magistrate's or Crown Court	Any doctor	28 days; renewable at 28-day intervals; maximum 12 weeks	
Section 36 – Remand to hospital for treatment	Mental disorder (not if charged with murder)	Crown Court	Two doctors: one approved under Section 12	28 days; renewable at 28-day intervals; maximum 12 weeks	
Section 37 – Hospital and guardianship orders (Section 37(3) without conviction)	Mental disorder – accused or convicted of an imprisonable offence	Magistrate's or Crown Court	Two doctors: one approved under Section 12	6 months; renewable for further 6 months and then annually	During second 6 months; then every year; mandatory every 3 years
Section 41 – Restriction order	Added to Section 37 – to protect public from serious harm	Crown Court	Oral evidence from one doctor	Usually without limit of time; effect – leave, transfer or discharge only with consent from Justice Secretary	As Section 37
Section 38 – Interim hospital order	Mental disorder – for trial of treatment	Magistrate's or Crown Court	Two doctors: one approved under Section 12	12 weeks; renewable at 28-day intervals; maximum 12 months	None
Section 47 – Transfer of sentenced prisoner to hospital	Mental disorder	Justice Secretary	Two doctors: one approved under Section 12	Until earliest date of release (EDR) from sentence	Once in the first 6 months; then once in the next 6 months; thereafter, once a year
Section 48 – Urgent transfer to hospital of remand prisoner	Mental disorder	Justice Secretary	Two doctors: one approved under Section 12	Until date of trial or sentence	Once in the first 6 months; then once in the next 6 months; thereafter, once a year
Section 49 – Restriction direction	Added to Section 47 or Section 48	Justice Secretary		Until end of Section 47 or 48; effect – leave, transfer or discharge only with consent of Justice Secretary	As for Sections 47 and 48 to which applied

Box 76.7 Mentally disordered offenders and the Crime (Sentences) Act 1997

- *Mandatory life sentence* for second 'serious offence' (attempted murder, manslaughter, rape, attempted rape) unless exceptional circumstances (which do not include mental disorder alone)
- *Hospital direction and limitation direction* (equivalent to restriction order) for psychopathic disorder only; if patient benefits, can stay entire sentence in hospital
- *Transfers to hospital:*
  - Court and Justice Secretary can specify unit
  - Justice Secretary's consent required for transfer of restricted patients between hospitals, even if in same trust
  - Section 47 transfer now allowed to mental nursing home
- *Interim hospital orders:*
  - Maximum duration extended to 1 year (from 6 months)
  - Can use before a hospital direction.

Individuals citing hearing a 'voice' telling them to commit an offence where a mental illness is not suspected

Note the absence of other characteristic symptoms of severe mental illness, such as of schizophrenia. Such isolated voices may reflect only pseudo-hallucinations, which are usually perceived as in the mind rather than external space, occur in individuals with severe personality disorder under stress, or may be due to substance abuse.

History of mild head injury or mild learning disability

Such a history does not necessarily imply that the condition is of a degree that would adversely affect the individual's ability to otherwise normally sustain him- or herself adequately in the community and be responsible for their acts. Frequent problems occur in people with borderline learning disability who are not suitable for learning disability services, although the courts and social services look to the medical profession to manage them in spite of the 'normal' intelligence level. Their offending is usually due to personality difficulties.

PSYCHODYNAMIC AND EPIDEMIOLOGICAL ASPECTS OF HOMICIDE

Homicide followed by suicide

This outcome, which precludes a criminal trial, occurred in around 7 per cent of such offences between 1966 and 2004 in England and Wales.[36] The rates of homicide followed by suicide have probably been higher in England and Wales in the past, with estimates of up to a half attempting suicide and a third succeeding in the 1960s, at a time when most homicides were domestic, with an overrepresentation of female offenders and child victims[37] and thus perhaps more psychologically difficult to cope with the consequences.

Psychodynamic aspects

Most individuals who have killed do not regard themselves as typical murderers, and many resent the implications of the word 'manslaughter'. Nevertheless, although murderous thoughts can be normal, acting on them is not. Homicide can be seen as preventing something even more psychologically worse for the individual. After committing homicide, some individuals, due to psychological defence mechanisms, may appear callously indifferent, idolize the victim, or claim amnesia as the act is too painful to think or talk about.[38]

In terms of prevention, the Jason Mitchell Inquiry in the UK argued that all psychiatric in-patient units that include offenders with disturbed personalities should have access to specialist psychodynamic expertise to provide a psychodynamic formulation of the case.[39]

Trends in homicide rates due to mental disorder in England and Wales

Using the legal classifications of homicide described in this chapter, Large and colleagues have shown that, in England and Wales, the annual number of homicides due to mental disorder rose from fewer than 50 in 1957 to more than 100 in the 1970s but has now returned to the earlier low levels while other homicides have continued to rise.[36] The initial rise in homicide by mentally disordered people was attributed to the same factors responsible for the increase in other homicides, such as substance misuse and increased availability of weapons, and the subsequent decline to the improved awareness of, services for and treatment of mental disorder.

These findings contradict those of Coid, who argued that the rate of homicide by mentally ill people is related to the prevalence of mental illness, which itself is fairly constant in all countries – that is, in countries with high homicide rates, this is due to high numbers of non-mentally ill offenders, their violence being related to criminal activities, drug-dealing and subcultural and economic factors, and, as a consequence, these countries with high homicide rates had a lower proportion of mentally ill homicide offenders.[40]

There is thus no evidence of increasing rates of homicide by mentally ill people in England and Wales (this is also supported by Bennett[41] and Taylor and Gunn[42]) in spite of this being the media and public perception, which in turn probably reflects only increasing awareness. Homicides by mentally ill people have a negligible effect on public safety in England and Wales compared with other factors, such as road-traffic accidents.

VIOLENCE AND MENTAL ILLNESS

Violence has multifactorial causes and is a biopsychosocial environmental phenomenon. All behaviour has a biochemical basis. Although biochemical abnormalities can cause psychological symptoms, including aggression, there is also increasing evidence that psychological events, such as severe abuse in childhood and severe psychological trauma in adulthood, may cause neurobiological abnormalities, for example in serotonin (5-hydroxytryptamine, 5-HT) metabolism in adults, which in turn is associated with aggression, which is usually inhibited by serotonin.[43] Models of violence are shown in Table 76.2. No model can adequately explain all violence and different models may be best for different situations.

Aggression, using the biological definition, is intraspecific fighting. Normal aggression is seen in all members of a species, but pathological aggression or violence is excessive in degree or arises from mental disorder. Almost all forms of mental disorder can be associated with aggression and violence (Table 76.3), although anyone can become violent. There has been a debate about whether aggression is an instinct – that is, genetically determined but called out by

Table 76.2 Models of and factors in violence

Biological factors	Fight or flight response Males and young people more violent Testosterone levels Reduced serotonin levels in brain
Alcohol, drugs	50% violent offences follow alcohol abuse in UK Disinhibition
Psychological models	
Instrumental aggression	Learn to achieve ends by violence
Cognitive model	Look at world aggressively
Behavioural model	Inconsistent, erratic parental punishment
Social learning	Peer pressure/modelling
Status	Status of being violent
Psychodynamic models	
Freudian	Primary drive due to frustration; later, primary drive libido, aggression secondary drive
Kleinian	Annihilation anxiety
Kohut	Secondary to developmental insults or deprivations
Object relation school (Winnicott)	Creative of another
Attachment theory	Aggression in insecurely attached infant, e.g. deprived or abused, relates to others with hostility
Family factors	Physical abuse as child Parental discord and violence Parental irritability, usually due to depression
Social models	Subcultural norm, e.g. Hell's Angels, pub brawls Sporting, political and industrial violence Relative poverty and inequality Comparative anthropology, e.g. Mead's studies
Environmental factors	Avoidance of frustration by well-structured and staffed milieu and non-provocative regime

Table 76.3 Violence and psychiatric disorder

Non-psychiatric causes (social and economic)	Criminal, e.g. drug-dealing
	Cultural, e.g. subcultures
Psychiatric causes	Violence or threats of violence in 40% pre-admission to psychiatric units Schizophrenia – paranoid and non-paranoid Mania, hypomania, also depression Alcohol abuse/withdrawal Drug abuse/withdrawal, e.g. hallucinogens, PCP, benzodiazepine withdrawal Organic mental disorder and brain damage, epilepsy (especially TLE), dementia Personality disorder, particularly antisocial, impulsive and borderline Learning disability Child and adolescent behaviour disorders Post-traumatic stress disorder Dissociative states
Intrafamilial	Spousal abuse Child abuse Elder abuse

PCP, phencyclidine; TLE, temporal lobe epilepsy.

the environment – or learned. Probably there is a normal inborn assertiveness, with aggression being secondary to early developmental deprivation and insults or mental disorder, rather than a primary drive.

Karl Lorenz has noted that a personal bond and individual friendship is found only in animals with highly developed intraspecific aggression.[44] In fact, the more aggressive the particular animal or species, the firmer is the bond. Real intimacy thus may occur only when individuals share real aggressive and good feelings.

Aggression often follows frustration and threat, for example in a person with low self-esteem, and increasing tension. Aggression may be displaced from the original object on to a symbolic representation of it, for example arson, or anger towards the mother displaced on to women in general. Aggression can also be a social phenomenon, for example in altruistic aggression and war.

Violence is action while dangerousness is a potential and a matter of opinion. The term 'risk' is now used increasingly in professional practice in preference to 'dangerousness'. Risk is, ideally, a matter of statistical fact. It emphasizes a continuum of levels of risk, varying not only with the individual but also with the context. It may change over time and, in principle, should be based on objective assessment. Dangerousness tends to imply an all-or-none phenomenon and a static characteristic of an individual. However, risk assessment is less important than risk management, although risk management does not imply risk elimination.

Risk factors include dispositional factors (e.g. demographic factors), historical factors (including past violence), constitutional factors (including stress and social support) and clinical factors (including diagnoses, symptoms and substance abuse). Risk may change rapidly over time.

In the past, factors associated with violence were said to be the same, regardless of whether the offender was mentally ill – that is, personality disorder, impulsivity, anger, violent family background and substance abuse.[45] However, since 1992, studies have shown that having a diagnosis of mental illness is associated weakly with violence due to a subgroup with specific types of symptoms such as paranoid (persecutory) delusions (false beliefs) and delusions of passivity (being under external control). It is thus certain symptoms, and not particular psychiatric diagnoses alone, that are associated with violence. Nevertheless, the risk of violence is still better predicted by being a young male than by having a diagnosis of schizophrenia.[46]

Psychiatrists are better than chance or laypeople in predicting violence and better still at assessing situations where there is no risk; however, they tend to underestimate the risk of violence in females.[47] Professionals also underestimate the high background base rates of violence in the community in general; for example, up to 40 per cent of males in a London sample had been seriously violent by the age of 32 years.[48] The majority of violence never results in criminal charges. This also applies to in-patients who are violent, where formal charges may often be seen as serving little purpose if the patient is to remain in hospital.

Among individuals with mental illness, affective disorders are underrepresented in forensic psychiatric facilities. Violence is, however, increased in people with schizophrenia,[49] especially those who have drifted out of treatment, and in young males with acute schizophrenia compared with those with chronic schizophrenia. Violence may arise directly from positive symptoms of mental illness, such as delusions (false beliefs) and hallucinations (e.g. voices). Mental illness, especially schizophrenia, may, however, lead indirectly to violence through associated deterioration in social functioning and personality, so that such individuals become more antisocial and impulsive and develop a lower tolerance to stress. This may lead to disputes in court in England and Wales about the disposal of such individuals with few or no positive psychotic symptoms who have killed, with such individuals sometimes being given, wrongly, an additional diagnosis of personality disorder to explain their violence. A mentally ill individual may also behave violently for 'normal' emotional reasons, such as fear and anger, and then experience accompanying corresponding psychotic symptoms, such as hallucinations of aggressive content. Violence, law involvement and imprisonment may precipitate mental illness.

For a mentally ill person, the key issue is whether the individual has a delusion of a content on which he or she might act dangerously, for example of persecution or infidelity, but even then not all morbidly jealous individuals, for instance, assault their partner. Twenty per cent of people presenting to hospital with their first episode of schizophrenia have threatened the lives of others, but among these patients half have already been ill for a year.[50] Overall, however, it is unusual for a person with schizophrenia to present for the first time with serious violence including homicide. One established period of higher risk is within a few months of discharge from hospital.[51] People with both schizophrenia and substance abuse have higher rates of violence than those with substance abuse alone, who in turn have higher rates than those with schizophrenia alone.[46]

Research has generally shown, but not universally,[52] a consistent association between violence and delusions, particularly of threat/control override content, for example persecutory delusions, passivity delusions and thought insertion.[53] These findings are in keeping with social psychology theory that violence in general is associated with the individual feeling under threat or losing control of his or her situation.

Based particularly on the work of Steadman and Monahan's group in the USA (the McArthur Foundation Violence Risk Assessment Study),[54] the Royal College of Psychiatrists for the UK and Ireland in 1996, in its booklet *Assessment and Clinical Management of Risk of Harm to Other People*, detailed 'warning signs' of which professionals should be aware.[55] These were:

- beliefs of persecution or control by external forces;
- previous violence or suicide attempts;
- social restlessness;
- poor compliance with medication or treatment;
- substance abuse;
- hostility, suspiciousness and anger;
- threats.

Psychiatric patients tend to peak for violent offending at a later age than the general population. It is important to be aware that the oft-quoted 'best predictor of future behaviour is past behaviour' (after Kvaraceus[56]) is based on non-psychiatric populations and, in any case, accounts for only 5 per cent of the variance.[54] A history of previous violence is required for this to be relevant in any case. Among severely (psychotic) mentally ill people, delusions of threat/control override appear to be better predictors than past behaviour.

Among all individuals, including mentally ill people, a history of expressed threats (as opposed to generalized anger), substance misuse and personal deprivation or abuse are associated with violence. Indeed, it has been suggested that homicide rates in general may be reduced in the UK by coordinated multi-agency responses and more policy and educational initiatives targeted specifically to counter domestic violence, child abuse, alcohol abuse and the carrying of knives and other weapons.[28]

Law-breaking behaviour in general, and violence in particular, usually decreases when the basic needs of an individual are met. For instance, an individual with schizophrenia who kills may have a characteristic history of not only poor compliance with medication, leading to relapse of his or her mental illness, but also of being in a situation of social isolation and poor home conditions. Some individuals may even offend to remove themselves from their situation in the community to the security of prison or hospital. The risk of self-harm or suicide is, however, greater for people with schizophrenia, even if they have before behaved seriously violently, than is homicide or serious harm to others.

In summary, although no mental illness is characterized by serious violence, including homicide, the existing evidence suggests that there is a link between mental illness and violence. Mental illness is a risk factor, but not a large one, and the risk is increased by substance abuse[56a].

Developments in brain scanning may elucidate this area further. Our research group has found evidence, using 31-phosphorus magnetic resonance spectroscopy (MRS), of increased cerebral metabolism in male patients with schizophrenia who have dangerously offended, including by homicide.[57] In a structural magnetic resonance imaging (MRI) voxel-based morphometry study, evidence of reduced grey-matter volume bilaterally in Brodmann areas 39 and 40 and the cerebellum was found in people with schizophrenia who had violently offended, including by homicide, compared with matched individuals with schizophrenia who had not so offended (Figure 76.4).[58] A strong connection has been hypothesized between the supramarginal region corresponding to Brodmann area 39/40 and Broca's area, which may correspond largely to the arcuate fasciculus, with the connectional pattern of the language regions of this model fitting the network of parietotemporal–prefrontal connections that participate in working memory. This points to the possibility of an abnormality in neural circuits involved in verbal working memory in this group of patients.[58]

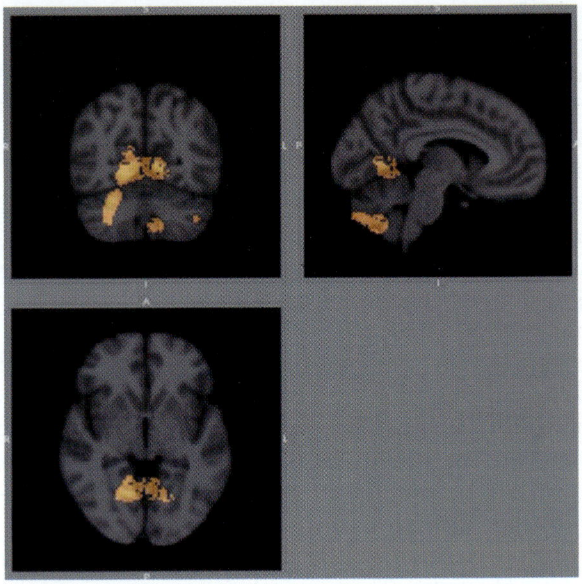

Figure 76.4 Results of a voxel-based morphometry study of male patients with schizophrenia who had seriously dangerously offended compared with male patients with schizophrenia who had not violently offended. The *P*-value map, showing significant clusters, corrected for multiple comparisons overlaid on a standard template (MNI152), demonstrates reduced grey-matter volume bilaterally in Brodmann areas 39 and 40 and in the cerebellum. Reproduced from Puri *et al.*[57]

These results, and additional findings relating to lipid peroxidation, may be consistent with increased cerebral oxidative stress in patients with schizophrenia who have seriously and dangerously offended.[59]

Avoidable deaths: the national confidential inquiry into suicide and homicide by people with mental illness, University of Manchester, England

This inquiry for England and Wales was set up in 1996 to collect detailed clinical information on homicides and suicides by individuals in contact with mental health services.[60,61]

Shaw and colleagues, using data from this inquiry over a 5-year period from April 1999 to December 2003, identified 249 such cases of homicide from a total of 2670 homicides – that is, 9 per cent of all homicides.[62] This equated to 52 patient homicides a year. There was no evidence of a rise in homicides, including stranger homicides, by mentally ill people. The typical perpetrator of stranger homicides in England and Wales is a young male who has been drinking alcohol or abusing drugs.[63]

People with schizophrenia were responsible for 30 patient homicides a year. Half were current or recent patients, but one-third had no previous contact with services.

People with personality disorder and a history of current or previous contact with psychiatric services were responsible for ten cases per year.

Rates of mental disorder in all perpetrators of homicide were as follows:

- *Lifetime mental disorder:* 30%
- *Schizophrenia (lifetime):* 5%
- *Contact with mental health services:* 18%
- *Contact within past 12 months:* 9%
- *Mental illness at time of offence:* 10%
- *Convicted of manslaughter on grounds of diminished responsibility (Section 2 Homicide Act 1957):* 4%
- *Hospital order:* 6%.

Fourteen per cent of homicides (7 per year) were considered 'most preventable' due to service failures, for example lack of adequate supervision or poor compliance.

The resulting recommendations included the following:

- *Ensure high-risk patients receive enhanced care-planning, backed up by peer review:* lack of this was considered the cause of 53 per cent of the most preventable homicides.
- *Respond robustly when a care plan breaks down:* lack of response was considered to have caused 18 per cent of the most preventable homicides. Twenty-five per cent of patient homicides were preceded by non-compliance.
- *Develop services for dual-diagnosis patients:* 36 per cent of homicide cases had dual diagnoses, i.e. mental disorder and substance abuse.

A review of homicides by patients with severe mental illness was also conducted by Maden, who looked at 25 cases from the National Confidential Inquiry into Homicides by psychiatric patients between 1995 and 2007.[64] Maden emphasized the value of structured clinical assessment of violence risk, especially using the Historical Clinical Risk-20 (HCR-20).[65] The HCR-20 includes 20 items of historical (H) factors (which reflect long-term risk), clinical (C) factors (which reflect current risk) and risk-management (R) factors. It thus covers both dynamic and actuarial risk factors. It can be used as an enquiry guide and a prompt rather than a numerical rating scale. The cases reviewed by Maden resembled forensic psychiatric service cases with high H item scores, but most were under general psychiatric services at the time.

Lack of patient compliance and compulsory treatment in the community were seen by Maden as the major issues. The Mental Health Act 2007 for England and Wales has now introduced increased powers to treat patients compulsorily in the community. Risk assessment alone however was deemed insufficient without adequate risk management.

A dual diagnosis with drug and alcohol misuse was present in 23 of 25 cases reviewed by Maden. Intoxication at the time of the homicide offence was very frequent. Abstinence was therefore recommended as a condition of discharge from hospital. The need for setting limits and early intervention was highlighted. Clinicians should be clear where to draw a line for intervention. Maden also made the point that diagnosis is only one factor in the assessment of the risk of violence. Drug-induced psychosis is just as dangerous as schizophrenia. The importance of involving carers was also emphasized, as they are most at risk.

However, risk management does not equate to risk elimination, and some violence, including homicides, by mentally disordered people is probably inevitable.

Inquiries into homicides by psychiatric patients

Such inquiries have been mandatory in England and Wales since 1994,[66] following a critical and widely reported inquiry into the killing in 1992 of Jonathan Zito by Christopher Clunis, who had chronic schizophrenia.[67] Such inquiries have emphasized failures in care due to poor communication between professionals and agencies, downgrading of previous violence, failure to recognize and manage social restlessness and escalating problems, lack of contact of subjects with consultant psychiatrists, rigid catchment area practice, lack of resources (e.g. acute beds, trained staff), failure to use the Mental Health Act appropriately to detain for reasons of health before violence occurs, and lack of carer involvement, although the latter may raise issues of patient confidentiality. Non-compliance with treatment in the community has perhaps been the most common major factor characterizing these cases. However, even Hippocrates noted that patients tend not to take their prescribed treatments. Also, there can be no real 'supervision' in the community in the sense of continual observation.

Overall, such inquiries have highlighted not the limitations of risk assessment, as real as these are, but failure to communicate or manage known risk. Improving community psychiatric care may thus be more useful in reducing the risk of violence than attempts at perfecting risk-assessment instruments. Certainly, the use of standardized structured risk-assessment instruments would not alone prevent most homicides by psychiatric patients.

Government responses to inquiry findings

The political pressure of 'something must be done' led to the following:

- Care-programme approach (CPA)[68]
- Supervision registers[69]
- Guidance on Discharge of Mentally Disordered People[69]
- Mental Health (Patients in the Community) Act 1995 (supervised discharge order)

- Community treatment order under the Mental Health Act 2007.

The usefulness of the above measures remains open to question. The CPA is a process rather than a treatment; individuals may be unable or unwilling to comply, and their families may or may not wish to be involved. On the positive side, the CPA is a needs-led multidisciplinary approach to developing a care plan, which has to be monitored and should always include a risk assessment. Drawbacks to its implementation include lack of resources, large caseloads, increase in time required for meetings and documentation, and it leading to defensive practice.

These government responses also occured against a background of a general decline in psychiatric hospital beds (from 152 000 in 1954 to 53 700 in 1993). Those psychiatric patients who have been violent in the community, however, tend not to be those who might previously have been on long-stay wards. However, if one closes 100 long-term hospital beds, there is an additional need for about 10 new acute beds in order to cope with resulting revolving-door admissions, and this can lead to a lack of acute beds for the emergency admission of violent patients. Increasing the number of hospital beds alone is not the whole solution, as there is also a need for other measures such as short-term crisis community facilities. Although inquiries emphasize the need for direct face-to-face contact between professionals and the patient, an average inner-city caseload for a social worker is 20 and for a consultant psychiatrist 450–500, with 300 new patients a year – and yet CPA arrangements are technically required for all patients and a legal duty of care applies to any patient to whom a professional talks. Funding has also not been related to epidemiology, for example in urban areas where there is an excess of schizophrenia due to social drift and where drug abuse and a younger population are also more evident, and there has otherwise been increased identification of cases, including via court and prison-diversion schemes. One response by clinicians has been to increase the rates of detention under the Mental Health Act 1983, which has been most pronounced for Section 3 and for mental illness. Although there has been no significant change in the number of Section 37 hospital orders, there has been an increase in Section 41 restriction orders. Another response has been the development of assertive outreach programmes.

Proactive measures to manage violence include adequate training of community mental health terms and the development of protocols for potential violent scenarios in hospital and in the community, for example for home visits. Risk assessment should also lead to the identification of warning signs indicating early signs of relapse or increased risk. The importance of communication between the GP, hospital and social services, housing, police and probation is paramount. Clearly, the better a patient is known, the more likely the accuracy of the risk assessment. If there is doubt about the safety of continued community care of an individual prone to violence, admission should be considered.

The Royal College of Psychiatrists has produced clinical practice guidelines for the management of imminent violence.[70] This covers ward design and organization, the need for adequate space, comfort and privacy, the anticipation and prevention of violence, including by fostering open communication with patients, anticipating risk and avoiding confrontation in a crisis, training for staff to recognize warning signs of violence and to self-monitor verbal and nonverbal behaviour, and training in the appropriate use of medication. However, the guidelines acknowledge the lack of funding available for training, the shortage of qualified staff, and the levels of stress currently reported among those who work in the mental health field and deal with violence.

HABIT AND IMPULSE-CONTROL DISORDERS AND RELATED OFFENCES INCLUDING ARSON & SHOPLIFTING

Impulse-control disorders are disorders in which the person acts on an impulse that is potentially harmful and that he or she fails to resist. The impulses are usually perceived as pleasurable (egosyntonic). There is an increasing sense of wishing to commit the act, with a sense of pleasure occurring once the act has been committed. These disorders have also been conceptualized as non-substance-related addictions. They do not represent personality disorders. They are described in the fourth edition of the American Psychiatric Association's *Diagnostic and Statistical Manual of Mental Disorders* (text revision; DSM-IV-TR) as 'impulse-control disorders'[71] and in the World Health Organization's (WHO) ICD-10 as 'habit and impulse disorders'.[34]

In DSM-IV-TR, their essential features include the following:

- There is a failure to resist an impulse, drive or temptation to perform an act that is harmful to the person or to others.
- For most disorders, the individual feels an increasing sense of tension or arousal before committing the act and then experiences pleasure, gratification or relief at the time of committing the act.
- Following the act, there may or may not be regret, self-reproach or guilt.

Included are the conditions of pathological gambling, pyromania, kleptomania, trichotillomania and intermittent explosive disorder.

The ICD-10 has a similar definition for this group of disorders (Table 76.4), but it also includes intermittent explosive (behaviour) disorder. The ICD-10 points out that these disorders have no clear rational motivation.

Pathological gambling, pyromania and intermittent explosive (behaviour) disorder are more common in men,

Table 76.4 ICD-10 habit and impulse disorders

Pathological gambling	Persistently repeated gambling that continues and often increases despite social consequences
Pathological fire-setting (pyromania)	Repeated fire-setting without any obvious motive; intense interest in watching fires burn
	Feelings of increasing tension before the act and intense excitement immediately after it
Pathological stealing (kleptomania)	Repeated failure to resist impulses to steal objects that are not required for personal use or monetary gain
	Objects may be discarded, given away or hoarded
	Increasing sense of tension before and a sense of gratification during and immediately after the act
Trichotillomania	Noticeable hair loss due to a recurrent failure to resist impulses to pull out hair
	Hair-pulling usually preceded by mounting tension and followed by sense of relief or gratification (responds to behaviour therapy and SSRI antidepressants)
Intermittent explosive (behaviour) disorder	

ICD-10, *International Classification of Diseases*, 10th edition; SSRI, selective serotonin reuptake inhibitor.

while kleptomania and trichotillomania are more common in women. There is an absence of epidemiological studies of the prevalence of these disorders, but rates among psychiatric in-patients may be higher than in the general population. Using the Minnesota Impulsive Disorders Interview,[72] Grant and colleagues found the following rates, mainly co-morbid with depression, among in-patients:[73]

- *Kleptomania:* 8%
- *Pathological gambling:* 7%
- *Intermittent explosive (behaviour) disorder:* 6.4%
- *Trichotillomania:* 3.4%.

Overall, such impulse-control disorders are probably underdiagnosed.

Other disorders, such as pathological buying (oniomania or shopaholism), characterized by buying items that are not needed and often storing them unopened, and workaholism, have also been considered to be impulse-control disorders but are not classified as such in DSM-IV-TR or ICD-10. Such behaviours may be motivated by a need for compensation or as a substitute for something missing in life or as a depressive equivalent.

Impulse-control disorders may lead to offending either directly, for instance in pyromania, or indirectly, for instance for financial gain in a pathological gambler. Individuals who commit crimes due to such a disorder have, however, usually been deemed legally culpable for their actions, even though their propensity is psychiatrically considered to be irresistible. It has been argued, however, that this may be a legal injustice, as such individuals clinically apparently have little or no control over their actions.

The interface between impulse-control disorders and offending raises philosophical questions, including questions about the nature of free will and whether all behaviours are determined by the effects of genes, environment and background. Are people with impulse-control disorders less responsible for their behaviour, and should they therefore be punished less than people of normal responsibility? Even if impulse-control disorders have a biological basis, in clinical practice the aim is, however, to encourage the patient to take responsibility for his or her actions.

History

During the eighteenth century, the concept of 'monomania with propensity' developed, referring to the fact that apparently insane, incomprehensible actions did not always appear to be the result of delusional thinking. This and subsequent historical developments have been discussed by Gibbens and Prins, who cite the following historical landmarks:[74]

- Philippe Pinel (1745–1826), in the eighteenth century, referred to 'mania without delirium' as being a disease of the willpower.
- Esquirol referred in 1885 to instinctive monomanias, including homicide, fire-setting and alcoholism – that is, respectively, homicidal monomania, pyromania and dipsomania, where the individual acts 'without passion or motive but only under involuntary instinctive impulse'.
- Referring to some cases of theft and homicide, Rush in 1810 described them as an illness of the moral willpower and equated this illness with the involuntary movements of convulsions.
- Mathey coined the term 'kleptomania' (theft) to add to the list of other manias, including dipsomania and pyromania.

As noted by Topp,[75] it was a Frenchman, Marc, in 1833 who first used the term 'kleptomania' when describing a number of wealthy individuals who carried out bizarre, worthless thefts in which they had little intrinsic interest and to which they confessed spontaneously when challenged.

Subsequently, it has been considered that instinctive monomanias such as kleptomania are very rare and, indeed, it has been questioned whether they, in fact, exist. Terms such as 'pyromania' and 'kleptomania' have indeed tended to be increasingly discarded. Neustatter doubted whether kleptomania existed as an entity, but, if it did, he suggested that it was part of a psychopathic personality that gives way to impulses.[76]

Differentiation from obsessive–compulsive disorder

An important differentiation in this area is between compulsions and impulses. Compulsions, as seen in obsessive–compulsive disorder, are characterized by non-situational preoccupation with subjective compulsion, despite conscious resistance, such preoccupations being thoughts (ruminations or obsessions) or acts (rituals or compulsions). Where there is poor impulse control, impulses are poorly resisted, and this is much more common than compulsions. In the case of obsessive–compulsive disorder, patients in general do not act on their ruminations, unlike people with poor impulse control. The key difference between impulse-control disorders and obsessive–compulsive disorder is that although both may lead to relief of anxiety and tension, in obsessive–compulsive disorder the thought of carrying out the act must not in itself be pleasurable – that is, the thought must be egodystonic.

Pathological gambling

This is defined in ICD-10 as persistently repeated gambling that continues and often increases despite social consequences. Gambling involves risking something of value, not necessarily money, in a game or other uncertain event, with the aim of achieving greater value. There is a range of gambling behaviours, from the culturally normal to hazardous, professional, problematic and pathological gambling. In contrast to professional gamblers, who may carefully plan their gambling and base it on information in order to decrease the risk, pathological gamblers will myopically gamble despite repeated and heavy losses, resulting in adverse family and social consequences and financial ruin, to which they appear hyposensitive. Four phases may be distinguished: winning, losing, desperation and eventual giving up. Problems do not arise from the gambling itself but from the consequences, as seen in alcoholism. Indeed, pathological gambling shows features characteristic of an addiction, with loss of control, extremes of emotions reflecting autonomic nervous system changes, and withdrawal phenomena when not gambling.

DSM-IV-TR defines the essential feature of pathological gambling as a chronic and progressive failure to resist impulses to gamble, with behaviour leading to much damage to personal and family life. Evidence suggests this to be a valid and reliable diagnosis.[77] Efforts to control, resist or stop gambling generally fail, and the behaviour has been equated to an addiction, with withdrawal symptoms of irritability and restlessness if the person is unable to gamble, and an escalation in the size and frequency of bets or other stakes in order to achieve a desired level of excitement. Such individuals tend to respond to repeated losses by gambling further to 'chase' their losses, in spite of increasing debts, marital breakdown and law involvement. They anticipate losses, as shown in functional magnetic resonance imaging (fMRI) studies (reduced activity in the ventromedial prefrontal cortex), even while their appetite for gambling and their impulsivity increase, and they will continue gambling until they have lost their available resources. Psychodynamically, they appear unconsciously to aim to lose their money. They tend to focus on their winnings, disavow or deny their losses, lack the courage to own up to losses, and gamble more to break even. This is a pattern also seen in stock-market 'rogue traders'.

Pathological gambling may also lead to disturbances in eating, sleeping and sexual relationships, and to difficulties in sustaining employment. Lying to and relying financially on friends is also characteristic. Some gamblers steal in order to finance their habit, and pathological gambling may come to light only following a court case regarding an acquisitive offence such as theft, fraud or embezzlement.

Some individuals present following an overdose or self-harm, which occurs in 10 per cent of pathological gamblers, or with depression. Suicide occurs in 2 per cent of attenders at Gamblers Anonymous (Gam-Anon). Legg-England and Gotestam[78] and Raylu and Oei[79] have reviewed pathological gambling in detail.

Epidemiology

Gambling itself is common, with estimates of prevalence around 40 per cent of the British population and 60 per cent of the US population.[80] Even these figures may now be underestimates, given the current availability of national television and other lotteries. Wardle and colleagues found the prevalence of gambling in the UK to be 68 per cent, but 48 per cent when the UK national lottery was excluded.[81] Gambling is said to be more common among Chinese people and less common among Scandinavian people. It is more common in men, people with a past history of psychiatric disorder and criminals. Problem gamblers cause themselves or others to suffer. It is possible to lose control and bankrupt oneself through gambling in just one day. Pathological gambling is associated with tolerance and withdrawal phenomena and has been found to have a prevalence of 0.25 per cent in Australia[82] and 0.77 per cent in the USA. Shaffer and Korn reviewed 120 studies and suggested a lifetime rate of 1.6 per cent, a figure not dissimilar to that for schizophrenia.[83] Wardle and colleagues in the UK estimated that 0.5–0.6 per cent of the population were problem gamblers.[81] The Royal College of Psychiatrists in the UK in 1977 described around 10 per cent of prisoners as pathological gamblers.

Pathological gambling is certainly more obvious but probably also more common among people, especially men, who indulge in horse- and dog-racing, in which losses soon become apparent. Female pathological gamblers, on the other hand, have been reported to be more likely to make use of specialized helplines.[84] In the UK, it is said that women prefer bingo, which may lead to less pathological gambling and in which losses tend to be smaller.

Aetiology

The predominant motivation for pathological gambling is the sense of thrill and pleasure at the risk-taking, as reflected in changes of heart rate demonstrated during gambling. Winning produces euphoria, said to be comparable to the effects of amphetamines, and helps individuals to switch from negative internal mood states, including despondency and loneliness. Dostoyevsky, in his autobiographical novel *The Gambler*, described the reward of a sense of power obtained from gambling. Freud, commenting on this, considered that Dostoyevsky did his best writing after a big loss from gambling as he was then freed from unconscious guilt feelings concerning patricidal urges that inhibited his creativity.[85] Gambling has also been described as serving to gratify oedipal wishes, for example wishing to defeat a tyrannical father or to woo a mother.[86,87] Moran cited social pressures, early exposure to gambling, and a father who gambled or drank alcohol as aetiological factors among male gamblers, while having an alcoholic spouse who was often absent was characteristic more of women who gamble.[80] Gambling increases with the number of gamblers in one's social network, being initially a social activity, but when pathological it is usually undertaken alone.

Learning theory has suggested that the pattern of intermittent (variable ratio) reinforcement, the most potent schedule for conditioning, particularly applies to gambling, where repeated losses with frequent near-misses are combined with occasional random wins with immediate payouts. The prospect of small but immediate rewards is preferred to higher but delayed rewards. Evidence of psychological dependence may become manifest by the appearance of what can be considered withdrawal symptoms and craving following the stopping of such activity.

Biological factors may also be important.[88] The orbitofrontal cortex and anterior cingulate gyrus are involved in reward mechanisms. Potenza and colleagues undertook an fMRI study of pathological gamblers, which showed, compared with controls, decreased activation of the orbitofrontal cortex, basal ganglia and thalamus, which have been linked to impulsivity and disinhibition.[89]

Pathological gambling has been suggested to be associated with low central serotonin levels, as seen in other impulse-control disorders, and low central dopamine activity, as seen in other addiction disorders. Serotonin is involved in mood and impulse control, and dopamine in reward, pleasure and motivation. Of note is the increasingly recognized phenomenon of individuals with Parkinson's disease, who have low levels of the neurotransmitter dopamine, presenting for treatment of gambling after having been treated with pro-dopaminergic agents such as L-dopa.[90] Noradrenaline (norepinephrine), which is involved in arousal and excitement, and opioids, involved in urges and pleasure, may also be important.

Co-morbidity

Although pathological gambling often arises in the absence of other psychiatric disorders, personality disorder, especially antisocial, narcissistic and borderline types, and depression may also be present. The presence of personality disorder will, however, explain only part of the excess of impulsivity. Hypomanic or manic episodes of bipolar disorder, which may be associated with general overspending and grandiose beliefs about one's wealth and ability to make money, including the ability to counter losses, may also lead to excessive gambling. Problem gambling is associated with attention deficit hyperactivity disorder (ADHD), delinquency and recidivist offenders, and is especially high among young offenders.

Risk factors

These include being male, being over 45 years of age, cigarette-smoking, alcohol abuse, low income, having debts, being a foreign national, having a depressive disorder, flat affect, having the metabolic syndrome, and sleep difficulties in females. A history of previous treatment for gambling is an important risk factor.

Assessment

This should include eliciting when gambling started and when it became regular, who introduced the individual to gambling or encouraged the individual to gamble, the circle of gambling friends, and the history of escalation in patterns of gambling. Is gambling increased when the individual is despondent or after alcohol consumption?

The onset and presence of symptoms of pathological gambling should be noted, for example inability to stop despite debts, withdrawal symptoms such as restlessness and irritability when not gambling, chasing losses, and raising stakes for the thrill.

The motivation to change should also be assessed. Stages of change include the following:

1. Precontemplation, when the need to change is recognized.
2. Contemplation, when the problem is acknowledged and the individual is willing to change.
3. Action taken to change.
4. Maintenance to sustain control of or abstinence from gambling.

Screening instruments such as the South Oaks Gambling Screen (SOGS)[91] can be useful, especially in screening populations at risk (a score of 3–5 out of 10 indicates problem gambling, while a score over 5 indicates pathological gambling). The SOGS may produce excessive false-positives compared with the National Opinion Research Center DSM Screen for Gambling Problems (NODS)[92], which was developed as a population-based telephone screening tool to identify gambling problems according to DSM-IV criteria.[93] Stinchfield found that the SOGS demonstrated good to excellent classification accuracy in his large gambling treatment sample, but it had poorer accuracy in the general population sample, with a 50 per cent false-positive rate; the SOGS overestimated the number of pathological gamblers in the general population compared with DSM-IV diagnostic criteria.[94]

A further tool is the Canadian Problem Gambling Severity Index,[95] which contains 9 items of the 30-item Canadian Problem Gambling Inventory (CPGI).

Management

Health promotion to populations at risk as identified by screening to counter excessive gambling before problems develop is ideal. However, pathological gambling may not always follow a chronic and persisting course. Slutske reported that among individuals with a lifetime history of pathological gambling, 36–39 per cent did not experience any gambling-related problems in the past year, even though only 7–12 per cent had ever sought either formal treatment or attended meetings of Gamblers Anonymous.[96] About one-third of the individuals with pathological gambling disorder in her study of two nationally representative US samples were characterized by natural recovery.

Co-morbid psychiatric disorders should be excluded or treated, for example depression. As with other addictive behaviours, selective serotonin reuptake inhibitor (SSRI) antidepressants at high doses have been recommended,[97] as has the opioid antagonist naltrexone. The selective noradrenergic reuptake inhibitor (SNRI) venlafaxine, the 5-HT^{1A} partial agonist buspirone, the stimulant cognitive enhancer modafinil, and the psychostimulant methylphenidate have all been used.

Cognitive-behavioural therapy (CBT), which concentrates on reducing the preoccupation with gambling and can involve motivational interviewing and risk- and harm-reduction strategies, has been used successfully and has also been combined with a 12-step group programme.[98] There is no real evidence for the efficacy of psychodynamic psychotherapy or aversive behavioural therapy in this disorder. Dickerson described 22 uncontrolled studies offering a variety of management approaches, including most forms of psychotherapy.[99] Support and counselling for the family, which can include brief focal marital counselling, may also be required.

Help is often sought only as a result of the consequences of gambling, such as debt, deteriorating marital and other relationships, and law involvement, rather than as a result of a primary desire to stop gambling itself. Most gamblers cannot contemplate complete abstinence, although some may consider as a reasonable goal stopping gambling for a number of months, with a view to continuing controlled gambling thereafter.

One approach is for the family income to be paid into an account over which only the gambler's partner has control.[80] Gamblers Anonymous adopts the approach used by Alcoholics Anonymous and may be more helpful than standard traditional psychiatric approaches. For relatives, Gamblers Anon is available for mutual support, akin to Al-Anon for relatives of people with alcoholism. Local citizens' advice bureaux and money advisory services may assist with resulting financial difficulties.

Few pathological gamblers will consider a goal of total abstinence. In spite of management approaches, the prognosis is generally considered poor, although 10 per cent stop spontaneously and progression and chronicity are not inevitable. Relapse rates after treatment vary from two-thirds to 70 per cent. Duration of the disorder and neurocognitive measures of disinhibition and decision-making are powerful predictors of relapse in pathological gambling.[100]

As the ease of availability of gambling increases, so does the risk of developing pathological gambling. For example, legislation controlling casinos and countering society's hedonistic attitudes to, for instance, national lotteries and so on may be important in prevention, although a study by Bondolfi and colleagues in Switzerland showed no increase in pathological gambling following an increase in the opening of casinos.[101]

Pathological fire-setting (pyromania)

ICD-10 defines pathological fire-setting as repeated fire-setting without any obvious motive. There is an intense interest in watching fires burn and feelings of increasing tension before the act and intense excitement immediately after it.

In DSM-IV-TR, it is referred to as pyromania and also classified as an impulse disorder. There is deliberate and purposeful fire-setting on more than one occasion. Tension or affective arousal is present before the act. There is intense pleasure, gratification or relief when setting fires or when witnessing or participating in their aftermath. Such individuals, also referred to as 'firebugs', are fascinated with, curious about and attracted to fire.

This group of fire-setters includes those who are described as having an irresistible impulse and a repeated urge to set fires, which they do not fully understand and about which they are often inarticulate. They are often isolated and inadequate people who set a number of fires impulsively and who may escalate the seriousness of their fire-setting. This group also overlaps with people who set fires for tension or depression reduction – that is, as an anxiolytic or antidepressive act. Such individuals discover that fire-setting relieves feelings of despondency or tension. An analogy can be made with the calming effect that normal individuals report when observing and sitting in front of a glowing open fire.

In the past, fire-setting by men was considered to be frequently associated with direct sexual arousal by such an act – that is, the use of fire as a fetish – and there was considerable psychodynamic interest in the symbolism of fire, for example flames of passion, burning desire, blazing rows and so on. Freud described the glow of fires as reflecting sexual excitement and the motion of flames as symbolic of the phallus in action.[102] However, although a number of fire-setters may indeed obtain a sense of excitement from their actions, those who are specifically sexually aroused and who may even masturbate after setting fires are rare.

Pathological fire-setters are a subset of those who tend to set more fires and to whom the fire is a thing of interest in itself. Individuals have a fascination with fire and hence the arson appears outwardly motiveless. There may also be an associated fascination with fire engines and calling out the fire service. The making of false telephone calls to the emergency services can result in a charge of 'wasting electricity' in the UK.

Other clinical features include evidence of advanced preparation and indifference to the consequences of fire-setting to property or life.

It is rare in children but more common in male adolescents, particularly those with poor social skills and learning difficulties.

The offence of arson

Arson is the offence associated with fire-setting and is the unlawful and malicious (wilful) destruction of or damage to property by setting a fire. Legally, the more serious charge is arson with intent to endanger life or being reckless as to whether life was endangered. Owing to problems of detection, only 5 per cent of cases of arson end in successful prosecution in the UK. In the UK, one in eight schools is subject to arson each year.

If an individual is charged with arson, it is important to reconstruct in detail what happened at the time of the offence, for example reading witness statements related to the case and not simply depending on the actual legal offence category. For instance, arson may be the setting fire to a wastepaper bin in a busy hospital ward in front of observing staff and fellow patients, or an impulsive or planned serious fire, in circumstances unlikely to be detected, with intent to kill. Of psychodynamic note is the fact that fire almost uniquely can make things disappear, including evidence. Historically, one reason individuals were burned at the stake was to avoid the spilling of blood.

Epidemiology

Approximately 40 per cent of all serious fires in the UK are started deliberately. Six per cent of fires in the UK are recorded as arson. Arson is responsible for 1 per cent of all serious crimes in the UK. However, as the evidence is often burned, only about a quarter of arson offences result in conviction. The peak age for arson is 17 years for men and 45 years for women. Eighty per cent of people convicted of arson are men. There is increased incidence of arson among people with learning disabilities and people with alcohol dependence syndrome. Fifty per cent of cases of arson follow alcohol abuse, especially binge drinking of alcohol.

Clinical classification

Numerous attempts have been made to classify arson clinically, for example by Puri and colleagues.[103]

There is no typical arsonist. Psychiatric difficulties are common, but the most common diagnoses are personality disorder and substance abuse, in up to two-thirds of cases, with about 8 per cent of arsonists having a psychosis. Pure pyromania appears rare (1%) among convicted arsonists.[104]

A classification based on these studies is as follows:

Fire as a means to an end (motivated)

Individuals who set few fires include the following:

- *Psychosis, such as schizophrenia:* such individuals may set fires to, for instance, burn out the devil or evil, or in response to hallucinatory voices.
- *Displaced revenge, anger or jealousy:* rather than overt direct aggression against an individual, aggression may be displaced into setting fire to that individual's property. For instance, an employee who is told off by the boss, may, rather than retaliate directly, physically or aggressively, return after business hours to set fire to the boss's property. This is the most common reason (in almost 50% of cases) found by psychiatrists among arsonists referred to them.
- *Cover-up of other crimes, e.g. homicide:* modern forensic science, however, usually overcomes such attempts at a cover-up.
- *For insurance:* this has become increasingly common in recent years, e.g. setting a chip-pan fire to finance the redecoration of a kitchen.
- *Political motivation:* e.g. to further their rise to power, Nazi storm troopers set fire to the Reichstag in 1932 in Berlin.
- *Adolescent gangs:* individuals are generally more likely to be disinhibited and behave antisocially in a group than when alone. This group is associated with a low rate of recidivism, except among gang leaders.

Individuals who set more fires include the following:

- *Desire to be powerful or a hero:* members of this group often have an inadequate personality. Their low self-esteem is bolstered by the sense of power they feel at the results of their having set fires, e.g. the panic and the emergency services with flashing lights rushing to the scene. Sometimes this is combined with a desire to be a hero, so that after setting a fire the individual may rush

into the premises and rescue pets or elderly or infirm people. On occasions, they are caught owing to being seen repeatedly or even photographed, for instance in a local newspaper, at the scenes of the fires.
- *To earn money:* this occurs when part-time firemen on call-out rates set a fire. It is a particular problem in rural areas and in some countries such as France. Some individuals may be drawn to the fire service because of their fascination with fire, and psychodynamic associations have been made regarding the phallic symbolism of hoses. Anthropologists and evolutionists have suggested that females may have been impressed by the ability of males to put fires out by urinating.
- *As a cry for help:* to bring attention to a distressed emotional state.

Fire as a thing of interest

This includes pathological fire-setting (pyromania).

Differential diagnosis of pyromania

This includes conduct, adjustment, affective and psychotic disorders.

Co-morbidity of pyromania

This may include substance misuse, past history of sexual or physical abuse, and personality disorder, especially antisocial personality disorder. High rates of previous sexual abuse in women who set fires have been described frequently in clinical practice.

Assessment of arsonists

Assessment depends not only on a careful, detailed history and mental state examination but also on the gathering and study of objective information such as witness statements related to the case. It is important to determine the presence or absence of psychiatric abnormality, especially at the time of the offence, and its relationship with the offence itself. It is important to determine whether there is a history of previous fire-setting and to examine precipitants.

It should be noted that *suicide by fire* is particularly associated with schizophrenia, perhaps explaining the choice of this most painful means of suicide. Historically, it has been described in the early nineteenth century among Hindu widows in India (*suttee*) and among monks protesting in Vietnam during the twentieth-century Vietnam War.

Management

This should clearly address any underlying or co-morbid psychiatric disorders. For example, psychological intervention with CBT may be helpful, particularly in cases of pyromania.

The potential dangers of fire-raising must always be borne in mind. The view of the fire service is that a large fire is merely a small fire not brought under control.

In cases where an individual is charged with arson, the courts will be particularly concerned with the protection of the public. The courts are likely to be unwilling in serious cases of arson to consider out-patient care or placement in an open psychiatric ward. Ordinary psychiatric hospitals are also inevitably reluctant to admit patients who have set fires, so if hospital treatment is required it is frequently undertaken under conditions of medium or maximum security. In the absence of a psychiatric disposal, the courts usually impose a custodial sentence. In England and Wales, under the Criminal Damage Act 1971, a maximum sentence of life imprisonment can be imposed for arson (Section 1) or arson endangering life (Section 2).

Prognosis

Further offences of arson are increasingly likely if there has been a history of previous arson and if the offender continues to have an irresistible impulse to set fires or to relieve tension or obtain pleasure or sexual excitement from such fire-setting. Increased risk of further fire-setting is seen in individuals with psychosis, learning disability or dementia. However, in an individual case, it may be difficult to tell whether that individual will re-offend. The risk of further serious offending after a period in prison or hospital is low; however, the risk of re-offending may not be apparent in the short term but only on longer follow-up. For example, Soothill and Pope found a 4 per cent recidivism rate over a 20-year period,[105] and Sapsford and colleagues reported a recidivism rate over time of 2–20 per cent.[106]

Pathological stealing (kleptomania)

In ICD-10, pathological stealing is defined as repeated failure to resist impulses to steal objects that are not required for personal use or monetary gain. Objects may be discarded, given away or hoarded. The person may even later offer to pay for items stolen. An increasing sense of tension before and a sense of gratification during and immediately after the act are seen.

Epidemiology

Kleptomania is usually seen in women of a mean age of 36 years, with a mean duration of illness of 16 years (often after an onset in childhood).[107]

The term 'kleptomania' comes from the Greek for 'stealing madness'. The disorder is generally said to be rare, with fewer than 5 per cent of arrested shoplifters giving a history consistent with kleptomania.[71] However, such individuals rarely seek psychiatric help and often avoid detection, so that estimates of the prevalence of kleptomania have been variable – even up to a quarter of all shoplifters. Up to a quarter of people with bulimia nervosa are said also to meet the diagnostic criteria for kleptomania. Kleptomania is certainly more prevalent in females than males, unlike other impulse-control disorders such as intermittent explosive disorder and pyromania, where males predominate. Onset is around 20 years of age, but diagnosis is usually made one or two decades later. The individuals concerned are typically married. Males may be underrepresented because they are more likely to receive custodial sentences precluding re-offending in the community during periods of imprisonment.

Clinical features

Stealing is perpetrated without much planning and without the assistance of others. The objects taken are not needed for personal use or for their monetary value and may be given away, discarded or returned surreptitiously, or kept and hidden. The individual invariably has enough money to pay for the stolen objects, but the theft is not committed to express anger or vengeance. Typically, when diagnosed, such individuals have appeared in court several times, feel guilt or remorse, but have not sought psychiatric treatment. There is often a history of a number of years of chronic dysphoric mood, and of the display of signs of depression and anxiety. Individuals' relationships and marriages are often unhappy. There is frequently a history of sexual difficulties and dysfunction and a past history of a turbulent childhood. Individuals often show poor impulse control generally and evidence of personality disorder, but the stealing is not primarily the result of conduct disorder or antisocial personality disorder. They share similarities, therefore, with people who have a past history of childhood sexual abuse.

Differential diagnosis

In ordinary shoplifting, the act is usually well planned, although it may be impulsive, but it is motivated by need or monetary gain and the objects taken are for the individual's use or to be used for financial gain. Some individuals who shoplift may attempt upon arrest to simulate kleptomania; they are then referred to as 'malingering'.

Shoplifting may also occur in conduct disorder, antisocial personality disorder, depression, hypomanic or manic episodes, schizophrenia and organic mental disorders, but in such circumstances the act is related to the primary diagnosis.

Co-morbidity

This includes eating disorders and substance-abuse disorders. Kleptomania may be precipitated by major stressors such as life events. Depression is common, and bipolar disorder may not be infrequent.[108]

Aetiology

There is no definite evidence of a specific genetic or inherited predisposition, although a biological basis has been suspected; for example, Grant and colleagues found decreased white-matter integrity in the inferior frontal brain regions in women with kleptomania.[109]

Kleptomania has been viewed as a variant of depressive disorder. People with kleptomania often have depressive symptoms, and the thieving itself may produce a stimulating excitement that has an antidepressive effect. Kleptomania has also been viewed as a variant of obsessive–compulsive disorder, but only about half of people with kleptomania experience with stealing the relief of tension characteristic of that disorder, and in obsessive–compulsive disorder there is not typically the sense of gratification seen in kleptomania.

Psychodynamic theories

Psychodynamic theories of kleptomania have included the following (Figure 76.5):

- *Loss substitution*, in which kleptomania provides symbolic compensation for threatened or actual loss[110]

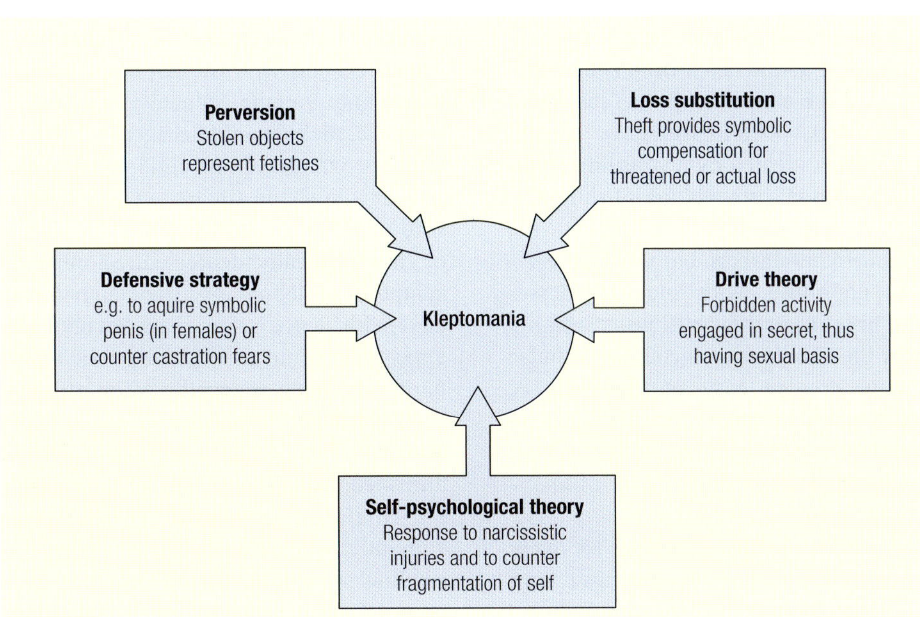

Figure 76.5 Psychodynamic theories of kleptomania

- *Drive theory*, which considers kleptomania in terms of a forbidden activity, engaged in secret and thus having a sexual basis
- *Perversion*, in which stolen objects represent fetishes as described by Fenichel
- *Defensive strategy* used by females, e.g. to acquire a symbolic penis to counter castration fears
- *Self-psychological theory*, in which kleptomania is seen as a response to narcissistic injuries and a means to counter fragmentation of self.

Management

In keeping with the view that kleptomania may be an equivalent of depressive or obsessive–compulsive disorder, kleptomaniac individuals often respond well to antidepressant medication, especially SSRIs such as fluoxetine. CBT has also been found to be effective.[111] Psychotherapeutic approaches, including family therapy, have also been reported. A self-imposed ban on shopping may, however, be required where treatment fails.

Prognosis

The condition tends to be chronic but waxes and wanes.

The offence of shoplifting

The technical offence is theft from shops, an offence that, as with all offences of theft, requires the intent permanently to deprive, as well as the act, in order for the offence to be proved in court. Intent would clearly be indicated if an individual were seen to be hiding an object in their coat and to be looking around to make sure they were not being observed. In absent-minded shoplifting, there would, in theory, be no intention to deprive.

Epidemiology

In the UK, about 5 per cent of all shoppers shoplift.[112] However, up to 50 per cent of goods taken from shops may be taken by the staff of those shops, as is the case with many thefts from businesses. Sociologists have viewed shoplifting as a social disorder created by a consumer society and precipitated by the visual provocation of shop displays. Open shelves increase sales and reduce the requirement for staff, as in supermarkets, but they are associated with increased shoplifting, with such businesses having to take this into account in their business planning. Some items are left near the checkout to encourage impulse buying but, in addition, provide easy but inexpensive objects to be shoplifted. Objects are often taken suddenly on impulse and are of trivial value or useless. Some individuals appear to regard shoplifting as an accepted perk of shopping and may pay for other items.

Until the early 1970s, most shoplifters in the UK were women, who then undertook more of the shopping than now, and 15 per cent showed evidence of psychiatric disorder. Ninety per cent did not re-offend after conviction.[74] However, the majority of shoplifters in the UK are now male and aged 10–18 years, as reflected in signs on shops limiting the number of children allowed in at one time. Males are now more likely than females to have previous convictions. The incidence of psychiatric disorder has been reduced to about 5 per cent, and it is questionable now whether shoplifting deserves more psychiatric attention than other thefts (90% of all offences are acquisitive). The previous predominance of female offenders coincided with the view that female offenders in general tended to be psychiatrically disordered, which may explain the tendency of courts to request psychiatric reports more often in shoplifting offences than in other, male-dominated offences.

Classification

Shoplifters have been subject to lay and legal stereotyping as needy, greedy or seedy. Bluglass distinguished three groups of shoplifters: professional, amateur and associated with psychiatric disorder.[113] Building on Bluglass's work, a more detailed classification is as follows:

Shoplifting for simple gain, plus excitement with or without associated marked antisocial attitudes

The principal motivation is excitement. Such individuals are responsible for a significant proportion of shoplifting in large cities. Individuals often feel less constrained by another country's laws when abroad. This category also includes organized gangs and people with chaotic lives who steal impulsively and commit other offences. They may come from antisocial families and be subject to relative poverty. Such shoplifting may be associated with resentment and feelings of bitterness associated with other individuals' lifestyle.

Shoplifting associated with psychiatric disturbance

The most common association in this group has historically been with depression in people of previous law-abiding personality. A study in Montreal found that 1 per cent of 1649 shoplifters had depression or bipolar disorder.[114] People in this group may include isolated younger women with children, but also include middle-aged women isolated from their families, who have lost children, who have experienced the loss of a husband (including loss owing to his career) and who may have significant physical complaints or ill-health or be chronically depressed. Shoplifting may be an early symptom of depression. The depression may also be associated with acute losses. Law involvement, including court appearances and associated publicity, can precipitate self-harm or suicide, especially when offenders are depressed.

In cases of shoplifting and depression, the motivation may arise from feelings of guilt or a desire to be caught and punished, may be a cry for help, or may represent an act of self-comfort or a treat. Other dynamics include secondary gain in newly poor people to 'keep up appearances' and stealing something for oneself that is not purchased with money from parents or a partner. In married female offenders, there may particularly be sexual difficulties or rejection and marital problems. Shoplifting may be an act of revenge on a partner to induce shame or punishment. For instance, it may result in the female having to be accompanied by her male partner when shopping in future or alternatively in the male partner having to undertake the shopping from which the woman can then opt out. For such individuals, a prison sentence may at one level be a relief from their marital or family situation.

Other psychiatric disorders associated with shoplifting include anorexia and bulimia nervosa, which may reflect both hunger for food and impulsivity, and early dementia, which is associated with disinhibited behaviour, lower resistance to temptation, poor judgement and late-onset offending. Shoplifting may also occur on occasion in association with other psychotic mental illnesses, alcoholism and learning disability.

Absent-minded shoplifting

This implies no intent permanently to deprive and, if successfully argued in court, a not guilty verdict will result. Such shoplifting may result from undue preoccupation, distractions or harassment, for example caused by the shopper's own accompanying children. Other causes cited include claustrophobia in shops and various medical or psychiatric drugs that impair concentration or cause confusion. It is the prescribing doctor's responsibility to warn of such side effects from medication. Although a defence based on medication side effects, including the effects of benzodiazepines, is not infrequently put forward in court by shoplifters, in reality it is rarely a primary cause.

Shoplifting in children

This peaks around age 14–15 years, with boys being predominant. Boys steal sweets and books, while girls tend to steal cosmetics and clothes. The items stolen are usually of little value. The most common group is 'normal' children stealing for excitement. However, child shoplifting may also occur due to subcultural standards or as an expression of emotional disturbance, for example as an act of defiance against parents, as a cry for help, or in association with feelings of depression, worthlessness and guilt.

Assessment

An examination of the history and mental state of the individual should elucidate the motives and detect any evidence of formal psychiatric disorder. The motive may often initially appear obscure, with useless objects or objects of trivial value taken suddenly on impulse, sometimes as a treat or arising from concealed resentment. Alcohol or drug abuse is often associated with shoplifting. Additional information should be obtained if possible, for example from the arresting police officer. It is often useful to discuss the case with the probation officer if one has been requested by the court to prepare a social enquiry report, which should also be read. It is essential to establish whether there is a history of previous convictions for shoplifting and any past psychiatric history and its relationship to offending.

Management

If it is argued on psychiatric grounds that there was no intent to shoplift and the patient pleads this successfully, then a finding of not guilty will result. However, individuals are often deterred from such a defence, for example a defence involving absent-minded shoplifting, as it will often require a number of court appearances and considerable legal expense to plead this successfully, and it may well involve local publicity.

Where the court accepts that intent permanently to deprive was present, the individual is legally convicted of theft. If the individual does have a psychiatric disorder, including kleptomania, requiring treatment, then psychiatric evidence may be used in mitigation with a view to altering the sentence; for example, a psychiatric recommendation of out-patient psychiatric treatment may be made as part of a community rehabilitation (the old probation) order.

Trichotillomania

This is a habit and impulse disorder characterized by noticeable hair loss resulting from recurrent failure to resist impulses to pull out the hair. Hair-pulling is usually preceded by mounting tension and followed by a sense of relief or gratification. It is not itself directly associated with criminality, although it can be associated with personality disorder, which in turn may be associated with offending. It has been well reviewed by Walsh and McDougall.[115]

Intermittent explosive (behaviour) disorder or episodic dyscontrol syndrome

Intermittent explosive (behaviour) disorder is included in ICD-10 under habit and impulse disorders, while intermittent explosive disorder is included in DSM-IV-TR under impulse-control disorders, and is characterized by episodes of sudden unprovoked violence. Onset is in adolescence, and males outnumber females in a ratio of four to one. It was originally conceptualized as a form of limbic epilepsy, but this has not been borne out. The syndrome may, however, be associated with soft neurological signs and temporal lobe electroencephalogram (EEG) abnormalities, and it may be helped by anticonvulsants such as carbamazepine and sodium valproate. These are also mood stabilizers, and lithium and SSRI antidepressants may also help, suggesting a link to mood (affective) disorder. This disorder, in fact, usually occurs in people with a severe, often explosive personality disorder with a propensity under stress to intemperate outbursts of anger and impulsive violence when frustrated, which equates to the emotionally unstable impulsive-type personality disorder of ICD-10 and falls within the antisocial personality disorder of DSM-IV-TR. It is of note that half of persistently aggressive offenders in general are said to have an abnormal EEG record, often an immature record (persistence of excess posterior slow-wave activity), characteristic of people with psychopathic disorder and not diagnostic of epilepsy.

Conclusions

Impulse-control disorders are a disparate group of conditions with different characteristics and epidemiologies. Whether the urges and impulses and resulting criminality are irresistible is open to question. Perhaps no impulse is irresistible, if an individual is motivated to try hard enough to resist. Certainly in practice, impulse-control disorders appear to be controllable at times but uncontrollable at others, when momentary excitement leading an individual to act on the impulse appears to overwhelm control. A disordered function of control may better describe the situation than an irresistible impulse. Indeed, the impulse to act is often combined with a desire not to act.

The conditions included in habit and impulse-control disorders do not reveal an identical psychopathology. Pathological gambling is a more complex condition, requiring attention to the whole person, than an impulse-control disorder such as trichotillomania. A pathological gambler shows features akin to substance addiction, with characteristic histories of escalation from use, abuse, and then addiction with tolerance and withdrawal symptoms, with gambling becoming the centre of the person's life, unlike the situation in pyromania or trichotillomania.

Impulse-control disorders are at least as prevalent as schizophrenia, but the research interest in such disorders and the evidence base for treatments are limited. Current treatments demonstrated to be effective include CBT and SSRIs. Other treatments for impulsivity with a weaker evidence base include SNRIs, anticonvulsants, stimulants such as methylphenidate, and the cognitive enhancer modafinil. Other approaches being considered and researched include biofeedback, repetitive transcranial magnetic stimulation, deep-brain stimulation and stereotactic neurosurgery.

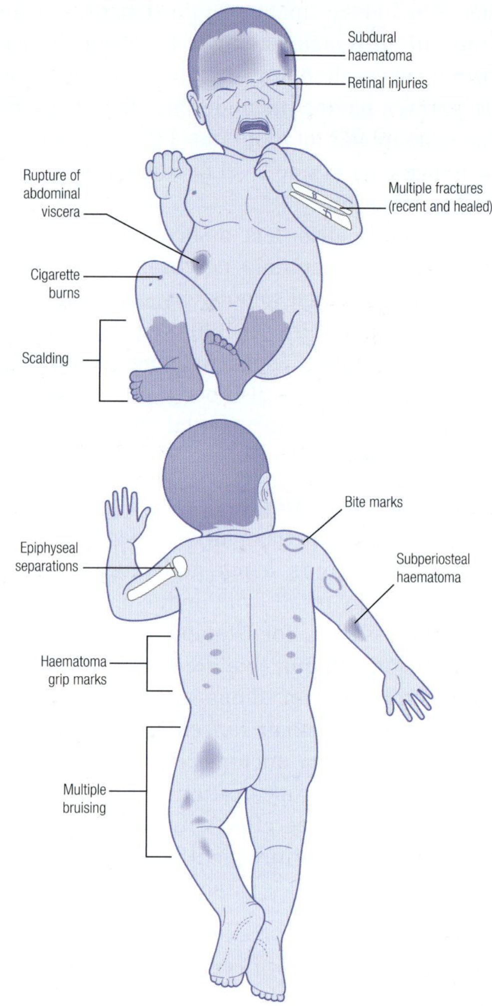

Figure 76.6 Possible clinical features of non-accidental injury in children

NON-ACCIDENTAL INJURY OF CHILDREN

The term 'non-accidental injury of children' has replaced the term 'baby battering', coined by Kempe and Kempe in 1961 as an emotive term to highlight the problem.[116]

Characteristic features of different members of the families in which non-accidental injury of children occurs are as follows:

- *Children:*
  - Usually under 3 years of age
  - Failure to thrive
  - Persistent crying
  - Multiple injuries in time and space
  - Delay in reporting and contradictory histories of injuries.
- *Parents:*
  - Often abused themselves and unhappy children
  - From lower social class families
  - Isolated and no support
  - Marital disharmony
  - Unwanted pregnancy
  - No contraception.
- *Mother:*
  - Often teenager, unmarried, neurotic or with a learning disability
  - Expects love from child
  - Not infrequently taking diazepam.
- *Father:*
  - In about half the cases, not the biological father
  - Two-thirds not married
  - Often has a personality disorder
  - Criminal in two-thirds of cases; one in three has a conviction for violence
  - Beats wife in one-quarter of cases
  - Competes with the child, whom he rejects, for his partner's attention.

Possible clinical features of non-accidental injury in children are shown in Figure 76.6.

The incidence of psychosis in parents is low but may be higher in severely abused cases. In the UK there are 80 child murders a year, 60 of whom are killed by their parents and 10 by strangers.

Note that filicide is the killing of one's son or daughter.

Management

Early recognition of children at risk is paramount for people working in baby clinics and general practice. It depends on high professional awareness, including from health visitors and from people working in nursery facilities and schools. Child protection registers are held by local authorities, which must also be able and prepared to undertake rapid emergency action (e.g. an emergency protection order). Around 32 000 children are at present on at-risk registers in the UK. Multidisciplinary case conferences, with the designation of key workers, are essential in the management of such families. Specific family and marital therapy may be necessary to improve the family and marital situation and to counter unrealistic expectations and consequent feelings of resentment about the child.

Homicide of infants and children

Of children killed under 1 year of age, 60 per cent are killed by their mother. On occasions, a mother will kill her child to spite a partner or spouse (*Medea syndrome* or *complex*).

NEONATAL HOMICIDE

There are about 20 cases per year in England and Wales of neonatal homicide, most within 1 day of life and committed by the mother. The mothers are typically of previous good behaviour but from chaotic or dysfunctional homes. They are isolated, as reflected in their taking pregnancies to term without telling others. They may deny their pregnancy, attributing nausea to something eaten and the kicks from the baby as due to wind. Their denial, combined with psychological splitting and tendency to concealment, may result in the mother making no noise during labour. The precipitant to homicide may be the baby's first cry or a desire to kill the baby at birth before the 'beginning of life'. Alternatively, the baby may be abandoned, whereupon it may be difficult to decide whether this was with intent to kill or not.

CHILD ABDUCTION

The relevant law in England and Wales is the Child Abduction Act 1984. There are three main groups:

- Abduction by parents, usually in custody disputes
- Abduction of older children, usually by a man with a sexual motive[117]
- Baby-stealing, the least common group, usually carried out by women.

In the UK, in the nineteenth century children were stolen in order to obtain their clothes. When females steal babies, in general the babies are well cared for and usually quickly recovered.

Categories of baby-stealing

These include the following:[118]

- *Comforting offences*: e.g. people with learning disability who steal a baby to play with or for comfort
- *Manipulative offences:* the motive may be an attempt to influence the woman's partner in an insecure relationship by presenting the baby to him and pretending the child is his, e.g. following a miscarriage of a pregnancy by him or threatened desertion
- *Psychotic offences:* motivated by delusional ideas, e.g. that the child is a Messiah.

SPOUSE ABUSE AND INTIMATE PARTNER VIOLENCE

The term 'spouse abuse' has replaced the term 'wife battering'. Historically in England and Wales, in the sixteenth century a male was not allowed to beat his wife after 10 p.m. In the eighteenth century, the 'rule of thumb' applied, as a result of which a male was not legally allowed to beat his wife with a stick or implement wider than a thumb. Under the Matrimonial Causes Act 1878, a husband was allowed a free hand with his wife to the extent that he could forcibly return his wife to their home.

The true incidence of such abuse is obscured by the hidden nature of the behaviour and problems in definition, for example over the degree of violence. This category accounts in England and Wales for 16 per cent of all violent crimes and results in two homicides of females a week; 40 per cent of these are killed in the bedroom or kitchen. The abuse is often associated with psychological abuse and behaviour linked to excessive jealousy and control of money. In the USA it has been estimated that in 25–30 per cent of marriages, one partner will push, shove or grab the other at some point. Punches and kicks occur in 13 per cent of marriages, and beating up or using a weapon occurs in 5 per cent of marriages. Surveys show that although women attack their husbands at a not substantially lesser frequency, such attacks are much less violent and usually defensive.

Male abusers are often inarticulate and demanding and find violence empowering. Typologies include men with a frequent loss of temper and men who undertake cold deliberate assaults, as well as overcontrolled individuals who eventually 'snap' under stress. Jealousy within the relationship is a factor noted in two-thirds of cases. Half of offenders have been exposed to domestic violence as a child. Fifty per cent of assaults follow alcohol abuse. Being a male abuser has also been associated with gambling, unemployment and a criminal record. Offenders are often remorseful following their violence but this does not prevent repetition. Women may be trapped in violent marriages economically, due to a lack of alternative housing, because of feelings of responsibility for their children, or by learned helplessness. A graphic account of spouse abuse has been given by Pizzey.[119]

Battered woman syndrome

This has been described as being characterized by:

- depression;
- loss of self-esteem;
- post-traumatic stress disorder;
- substance abuse;
- suicidality;
- physical health problems
- sexual problems.

Intimate partner abuse affects mainly women. If intimate partner abuse is suspected, it can be difficult to persuade the female victim to admit that she has been physically and mentally abused. A Canadian screening randomized trial found that women prefer self-completed questionnaire approaches to face-to-face questioning.[120] Assessment of the victim must be carried out with great sensitivity. Check that the victim is not suicidal or depressed, that she is not abusing alcohol or drugs and that she does not have an anxiety disorder.

Management

Management can be difficult, particularly if the victim denies the abuse and insists on returning to the abusive partner. If there is a high risk of the abuse continuing, social services may need to be involved and the police may need to be informed. If the risk is lower, and the victim and her partner agree, then marital therapy may be arranged.

Voluntary refuges are now widely available. Anger management techniques can be applied to offenders. A non-molestation injunction can also be sought, including with attached power of arrest. A new multidisciplinary case conference management approach (MARAC) has been developed in the UK.

ELDER ABUSE

Estimates of up to 500 000 older people being abused a day in the UK have been made. Elder abuse includes violence, neglect and emotional abuse of elderly relatives, often surviving widowed elderly mothers. The term 'elder abuse' replaces the term 'granny bashing'.[121] The offender is often a son or daughter (50% aged ≥60 years) of the victim and lives with the victim. The British prevalence rate is 1.5–5.6 per cent. Abused elders are no more physically or mentally infirm than non-abused elders.

The abuser may be otherwise under stress from marital or financial problems, be depressed, have a history of substance misuse or a personal history of abuse themselves, and be unable to cope with the added stress of looking after the victim, who may be emotionally and economically dependent. Unresolved emotional conflict is often present.

There is often a history of families being reluctant to take over the care of elder relatives but being put under pressure to do so. Occasionally, elder abuse arises due to an equally aged spouse having to cope with or care for the victim. Emotional conflict may be present between the abuser and the abused. Unqualified staff in poorly managed nursing homes may also abuse elderly people.

Victim vulnerability factors, such as disability, dementia or paranoid illness, may be present.

Non-accidental injury of children, spouse- and elder-abuse, reflect the fact that most violence is in the family, where individuals are most physically and emotionally close to others.

SPECIAL SYNDROMES

Morbid jealousy (Othello syndrome)

Delusions of infidelity about a sexual partner can lead an individual to examine, for example, the partner's underwear and sexual organs, in an attempt to find proof of unfaithfulness, and, on occasions, attempt to extract confessions by violence. It not infrequently leads to severe aggression towards, and the killing of, the sexual partner about whom the delusions are held. The condition occurs in males over six times more commonly than in females (c.f. erotomania, which is more frequent in females). It usually commences in the forties, after about 10 years of the relationship, and is present for about 4 years before presentation. It is responsible for 12 per cent of homicides due to mental illness.[122]

Aetiology

Evolutionary theories suggest that males may be predisposed to sexual jealousy as they cannot know whether it is their sperm that results in a pregnancy. Ten per cent of male birds look after offspring that are not biologically their own.

Morbid jealousy is associated with alcoholism, schizophrenia and delusional disorder. Morbid jealousy may be a forerunner of a later schizophrenic illness, this manifesting only after serious violence. It is also associated with impotence in males. Psychodynamic theories postulate that the suspicious attitudes may be a projection of the individual's own desires for infidelity on to the victim-partner or a more internally acceptable, conscious manifestation of repressed homosexuality. Morbid jealousy is often associated with low self-esteem, with resulting feelings of insecurity that the partner may not really love him and may wish to leave him for someone else.

Management

This is often difficult due to lack of insight of the subject and the sexual partner's belief that they can overcome the subject's unjustifiable beliefs. Underlying psychiatric conditions should be treated adequately, for example stopping alcohol abuse. Antipsychotic medication may help if compliance can be obtained. Separation of the couple may be the only answer. There is a risk of recurrence in future relationships: an example is the case of Iliffe, who killed four wives in spite of having spent periods in Broadmoor Hospital. It is best to work with a co-therapist, such as a social worker, who remains involved with the partner (e.g. advising her of refuges), while the psychiatrist concentrates on the patient.

Other terms

Rivalry is where two individuals are in competition for the same object. There is no aggression to the object.

Envy is where one individual desires someone or something that belongs to another person. Aggression is to the competitor or the self, but not to the object.

Jealousy is where there are fantasies of losing the object to a rival. Aggression is directed not to the rival but to the object, for example the partner. Historically and across cultures, the main cause of female homicide is male jealousy.

Jealousy can be normal or excessive. Sometimes even in the absence of delusions it may still be termed morbid – that is, for neurotic, obsessional, as well as delusional reasons – including being secondary to an affective disorder. It also arises in paranoid personalities. The boundary between normal and pathological jealousy may be indistinct. However, psychotic jealousy often responds better than neurotic jealousy to treatment.

Delusional jealousy can develop even when the partner has, in fact, been unfaithful. The way the delusional belief develops may be more important diagnostically than the pure content of the belief.

Erotomania (de Clérambault's syndrome)

This is a delusional disorder that another person, often unobtainable and of higher social status, loves the patient (usually female) intensely. It may be primary or secondary due to a paranoid or affective disorder. It is usually associated with paranoid psychosis or schizophrenia rather than being a pure monodelusional disorder. Only some people with this disorder cause disruptive antisocial behaviour (e.g. making phone calls, writing letters, following the victim), but repeated rebuttals may lead to hatred and dangerous behaviour. Gilles de la Tourette, who gave his name to Tourette's syndrome, was killed by an erotomanic patient. Dangerousness is increased if there is a history of multiple delusional objects in the past and a premorbid antisocial personality.[123] De Clérambault, after whom the syndrome was named, shot himself while dressed in a toga and was found by Lacan, the French psychotherapist.

Stalking

This is the wilful, malicious and repeated following and harassing of another person that threatens his or her safety. Eighty per cent of victims are female. Typologies of the stalker include the following:[124]

- *The rejected stalker who acts through a mixture of revenge and desire for reconciliation:* as a group, these people tend to be more assaultative but more likely to respond to judicial sanctions.
- *Intimacy-seeking:* these individuals include deluded patients. Such individuals may stalk famous people and mental health professionals.
- *Incompetent stalker/suitor:* such individuals lack social skills and may be intellectually limited.
- *Resentful stalkers:* these individuals often intend to cause fear.
- *Predatory stalkers:* these individuals are rare but may have fantasies about or have intent to commit sexual assaults.

There may also be false victims, including those deluded that they are being stalked. Post-traumatic stress disorder occurs in over a third of victims. Fifty per cent of stalkers threaten violence, three-quarters of whom are not subsequently violent or destructive of property. The risk of violence is increased if there are prior convictions or substance misuse. Stalking offences are now covered by the Protection from Harassment Act 1997 in England and Wales (an injunction combined with a criminal sentence), but prevention, when possible, may be most effective.

Munchausen syndrome (hospital addiction syndrome)

Originally described by Dr Richard Asher in the *Lancet* in 1951 and named after Baron Karl von Munchausen, Raspe's 1785 fictious French cavalry officer who lied harmlessly about his military exploits, this is the intentional production or feigning of illness to bring about repeated hospital admissions, investigations and operations.[125] It is a factitious disorder, consciously produced. Symptoms simulated are suggestive of severe physical illness and deceive medical staff. Men appear to be affected more commonly than women. The patient's history is plausible but overdramatic. Self-inflicted injuries, including simulating symptoms in a bizarre way, for example by swallowing needles, are seen. Abdominal symptoms are most common. Pathological lying (pseudologia fantasica) is often present. Variants include presenting with psychiatric complaints, including a false history of bereavement. When feigning comes to light, such individuals abscond from hospital. They frequently change their name and the hospitals they approach. To fund their wandering, they may commit theft and create disturbances.

Note: people in prison suspected of feigning mental illness are usually found on follow-up to have been genuinely mentally ill.

Munchausen's syndrome by proxy

In this, physical symptoms are intentionally produced in others, for instance by a mother in her child. The perpetrator frequently has nursing experience. The chosen method of producing symptoms is often by poisoning or suffocation. The term was coined by Meadow.[126,127] In one-third of cases, there is a history of fictitious illness in the mother. The father is usually emotionally, if not physically, absent, while the perpetrator appears superficially an exemplary mother. In the past, cameras installed on children's wards unknown to the mother (now questioned legally and ethically) revealed mothers suffocating or otherwise harming their children in the nurses' absence. It is rare for the mother to confess, due to feelings of shame and humiliation and low self-esteem, which in turn may lead to prolonged legal disputes about allegations.

SPECIFIC GROUPS OF MENTALLY DISORDERED OFFENDERS

Ethnic minorities

Afro-Caribbean people, but not Asian people, are overrepresented in the psychiatric and criminal justice systems. The reasons for this are controversial. Studies have shown an excess of Afro-Caribbean people, particularly British-born young men, admitted with a diagnosis of schizophrenia. The rates in their countries of origin are, however, not raised, making genetic factors unlikely to be the cause. Admissions of Afro-Caribbean people are more likely following contact with the police and social services, and following detention under the Mental Health Act 1983, in particular, under forensic Part III sections (25 times greater).[128–130] They are also overrepresented in special hospitals, medium secure units and locked wards. Twenty per cent of patients in special hospitals are Afro-Caribbean, but very few of these have had a Mental Health Act 1983 pre-2007 legal diagnosis of psychopathic disorder. Afro-Caribbean people are also overrepresented among those arrested, are more likely to be remanded into custody and are overrepresented in the prison population (5% in the general population compared with 11% of men and 25% of women in the prison population, according to Home Office figures). There is also an excess of women normally resident in West Africa serving sentences in England and Wales for drug smuggling. Afro-Caribbean people are also more likely to be the victims of murder.

Reasons suggested for such overrepresentation of Afro-Caribbean people include sociodemographic factors, such as overrepresentation among young people, unemployed people, lower social classes and socially deprived people, which in turn is associated with higher rates of offending,[131] differences in referral (non-Afro-Caribbean people are admitted via GPs and at an earlier stage than Afro-Caribbean people, who tend to be referred by the courts, the police and probation officers and for whom white psychiatric services may carry more stigma, leading to a later presentation), and overrepresentation among remand prisoners, leading to an increase in identification of mental illness ('differential filter theory'). In London Afro-Caribbean people represent one-fifth of the population but two-fifths of those detained. The statistics are not explained by drug abuse, higher rates of mental illness in the country of origin, differential migration or the stress of migration. Other factors postulated for the differences include the stress of prejudice and cultural acculturation of second-generation immigrants, higher rates of post-traumatic stress disorder due to being subject to violence in countries of origin, relative lack of father figures and peer group pressures. There is some evidence for stereotyping Afro-Caribbean people as taller and of bigger build and as more violent when mentally ill,[132] but not for systematic discrimination by psychiatrists (as opposed to the courts or the police); however, the institutional racism of psychiatric services was raised in an inquiry into the circumstances of the death of an Afro-Caribbean man, David Bennett, who died after being restrained in a medium secure unit.[132a]

Substance misuse and crime

Association of crime with substance misuse may be due to:

- altered mental states due to drug intoxication, withdrawal or long-term consequences, e.g. organic mental disorder;
- acquisitive offences to finance substance misuse;
- technical offences under the Misuse of Drugs legislation.

Crimes requiring specific intent, such as murder, wounding with intent, theft and burglary (in contrast to those requiring basic intent, such as manslaughter, assault and unlawful wounding), can be 'negatived' by intoxication.

Drug and alcohol abuse usually has disinhibiting effects on behaviour, impairs judgement and is associated with violence. Alcohol abuse, including acute intoxication, is present in up to one-half of individuals at the time they commit offences of violence in the UK.

Alcohol dependence syndrome is associated with an eight times higher rate of convictions for criminal offences, including especially motoring, drunkenness and acquisitive offences. There may be a history of alcohol abuse for 3

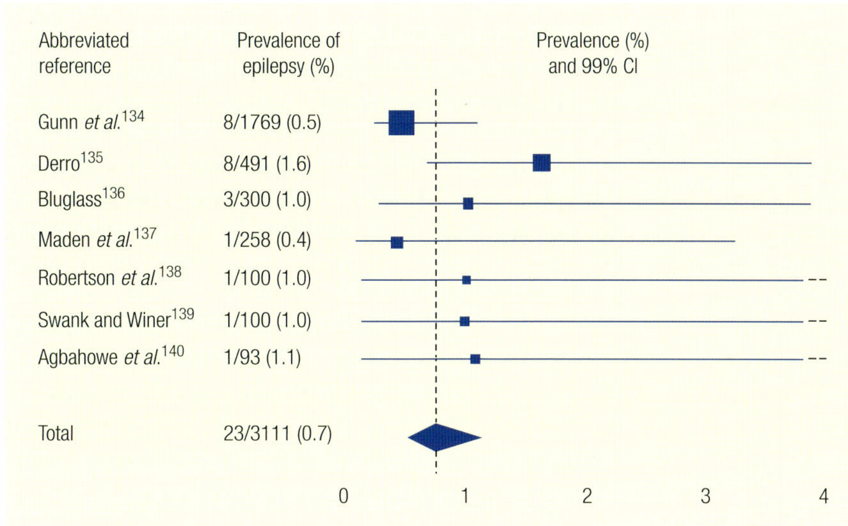

Figure 76.7 Prevalence of epilepsy in the prisoners found in seven surveys. CI, confidence interval.

years before initial offence, within 3 years of which the individual is often dependent on alcohol.

About half of people with a drug dependence syndrome have convictions before they become dependent.

Glue-sniffers may be charged with breach of the peace or depositing rubbish, such as crisp bags from which they have inhaled glue and which are then dropped when the individual becomes intoxicated. In non-mentally ill people, cannabis may be the only drug that has anti-aggressive properties.

Epilepsy

The prevalence of epilepsy in prisons in England and Wales was noted in the 1970s to be two to four times that in the general population (7.2 per 1000 compared with 4.2 per 1000).[132b] However, a more recent study in 2002 has shown a prevalence of 1 per cent in prison, which is equivalent to that in the community (Figure 76.7).[133] Individuals with epilepsy are no more likely than other prisoners to be serving a custodial sentence for a violent offence. Violence associated with epilepsy is, in fact, rare.[141] Ictal phenomena, including automatism, do not account for this overrepresentation. Alternative explanations include:

- underlying organic mental disorder being responsible for both epilepsy and offending;
- development of epilepsy adversely affecting an individual's self-esteem and resulting in social rejection, which in turn leads to antisocial behaviour;
- adverse social circumstances leading to both epilepsy and antisocial behaviour, e.g. being a 'battered baby';
- a tendency to be impulsive and antisocial, leading to offending and brain injuries and thus post-traumatic epilepsy.

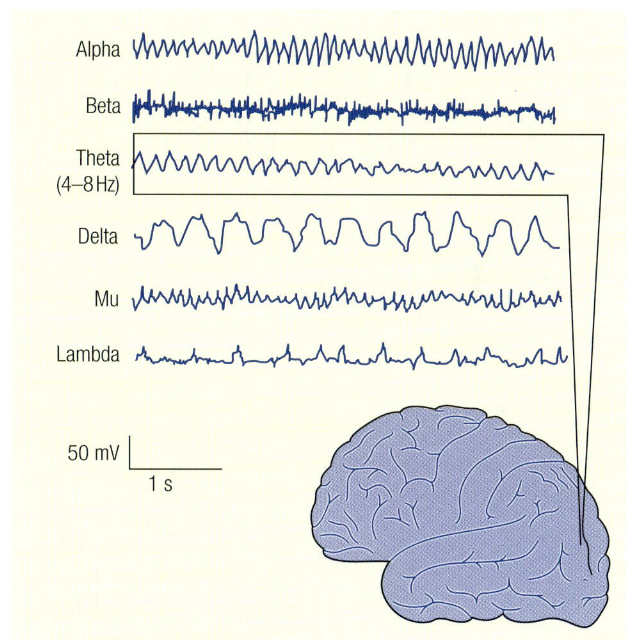

Figure 76.8 Electroencephalogram (EEG) study showing posterior slow (theta) waves in a psychopath

If linked, the most likely relationship between epilepsy and imprisonment is that such individuals show the same biosocial disadvantages.[132]

The association between aggressive behaviour and temporal lobe epilepsy has been reported widely. There is some evidence for amygdaloid foci, but psychosocial factors are also important. As a generalization, however, neurologists say that without a history of a fit, epilepsy is unlikely to be a cause of aggression.

Half of persistently aggressive offenders are said to have an abnormal EEG, often an immature record (persistence of excess posterior slow-wave theta activity), characteristic of individuals with psychopathic disorder and not diagnostic of epilepsy (Figure 76.8).

Episodic dyscontrol syndrome (intermittent explosive (behaviour) disorder) is characterized by episodes of sudden, unprovoked violence. It was originally conceptualized as limbic epilepsy, which has not been borne out. However, the syndrome may be associated with soft neurological signs and temporal lobe EEG abnormalities and may be helped by anticonvulsants such as carbamazepine. It usually occurs in people with a severe, often explosive personality disorder. However, as already noted, half of persistently aggressive offenders have an abnormal EEG.

Deaf people

One in ten referrals to the three main specialist psychiatric units for deaf people in England (in Birmingham, London and Manchester) come from the police, courts or solicitors. The majority have committed minor or acquisitive offences, but there is a high proportion of those charged with sexual offences, reflecting a lower threshold for referral rather than a disproportionate number of deaf individuals committing sexual offences. Deaf offenders are more likely to be found unfit to plead.[142] Grubin found 7 deaf people in his series of 295 cases unfit to plead. Rampton Special Hospital in England provides a maximum secure unit for the deaf.

PERSONALITY DISORDER

Personality disorder is an extreme persistent variation from the normal (statistical) range of one or more personality attributes (traits), causing the individual, their family or society to suffer.

Personality = character (acquired) + temperament (hereditary or congenital)

The history of the term psychopathic personality disorder

During the nineteenth century, it was recognized that there was a group of individuals who had neither mental illness nor mental retardation but who showed abnormally aggressive, antisocial, seriously irresponsible or inadequate behaviour from an early age, with which society felt impelled to deal. In 1801, Pinel, the humanitarian psychiatrist who first unlocked the chains from patients in the French psychiatric hospital Bicêtre, coined the term '*manie sans délire*' to describe this group of patients. Not all the patients he described appeared to be what we would nowadays call psychopathic. A typical case, however, was that of a man, spoiled by a weak mother, who killed any animal who 'offended' him. He was found to be intellectually normal and was able to run his own estate, but he had thrown a woman who was abusive to him down a well.

In 1835, the psychiatrist and anthropologist Pritchard coined the term 'moral insanity' for this group of patients, the term 'moral' at that time meaning psychological more than ethical. His cases also included individuals with bipolar disorder (manic-depressive psychosis). In 1891 Koch used the term 'psychopathic inferiority', in 1909 Kraepelin the term 'psychopathic traits', and in 1927 Schneider the term 'psychopathic personalities'. In 1930, the term 'sociopathy' was used by Partridge in the USA, which indicated and emphasized the social malfunctioning of such patients. The term 'psychopathy' originally included all personality disorders, which still applies on the European continent. The term became restricted in the USA to antisocial personality disordered people and was imported to the UK with that meaning by Henderson in 1939. He distinguished three kinds of psychopathic personality:

- Predominantly aggressive people
- Predominantly inadequate people (e.g. pathological liars or those who show pseudologia phantastica, swindlers and con artists – who are themselves the most easily conned)
- Creative psychopaths, who have high ability combined with their severe personality disorder, such as Lawrence of Arabia and the Renaissance sculptor Cellini.

Table 76.5 Historical nomenclature

Manie sans delire	Pinel, 1801
Moral insanity	Prichard, 1835
Moral imbecile (from early age)	Royal Commission for Care and Control of Feeble-Minded, 1904
Moral insanity (acquired)	
Psychopathic inferiority	Koch, 1891
Psychopathic traits	Kraepelin, 1909
Psychopathic personalities	Schneider, 1927
Sociopathy	Partridge, 1930
Character neurosis	Alexander
Psychopathy:	Henderson, 1930
(a) Predominantly aggressive	
(b) Predominantly inadequate	
(c) Predominantly creative	
ICD-9: antisocial, explosive, asthenic, paranoid	
DSM-III: antisocial, borderline	
ICD-10: dissocial, emotionally unstable, impulsive and borderline types, dependent, paranoid	
DSM-IV: antisocial, borderline, histrionic, narcissistic	

The term 'psychopathic disorder' was incorporated into the English Mental Health Act in 1959, and in the 1983 Mental Health Act it was defined as a persistent disorder or disability of mind (whether or not including impairment of intelligence) that results in abnormally aggressive or seriously irresponsible conduct on the part of the patient. As a legal diagnosis it was used to detain people suffering from all clinical personality disorders. However, to detain an individual on such grounds, it had to be stated that the condition was treatable. There is no legal diagnosis of psychopathic disorder in the mental health legislation of Scotland or Northern Ireland.

In England and Wales, following the amendment of the Mental Health Act 1983 by the Mental Health Act 2007, the term psychopathic disorder was removed and subsumed under a single definition of mental disorder.

The equivalent of the clinical diagnosis of psychopathic disorder in DSM-IV-TR is antisocial personality disorder, and in ICD-10 it is dissocial personality disorder, although some psychopathic individuals are best described by the category 'emotionally unstable personality disorder, impulsive type'. The term 'psychopath' is also used clinically in a pejorative sense to describe unreliable, uncooperative and often difficult male patients. The definition of psychopathy has also been used in a circular fashion – antisocial behaviour is presumed to be due to psychopathy, and yet psychopathy is presumed present from the behaviour. Table 76.5 summarizes the historical nomenclature.

Table 76.6 Clinical features of psychopathic disorder

	Clinical feature
Classically	Affectionless Impulsive
As a result	Egocentric and lacks empathy Lacking in shame, totally guiltless, no regret No ability to profit from experience, including punishment No life plan, lacks normal drive or motivation Viciousness Unable to sustain emotional relationships, but may present as initially articulate and charming
Other features	Very low anxiety/tension Breathtaking escapades Autonomic nervous system abnormalities, with slower conditioning Rarely seeks assistance Untreatable in pure form
Negative features	Lack of psychosis Lack of intellectual deficit Lacks criminal motive

Table 76.7 Cleckley's differentiation of primary and secondary psychopaths

Primary	Secondary (neurotic)
Very low anxiety/tension	High anxiety/tension
Totally guiltless	Hidden guilt
No regret	Hidden regret
Breathtaking escapades	Banal escapades
Behaviour not understandable in terms of family dynamics	Behaviour understandable in terms of family dynamics
Apparent intelligence	Low self-esteem
Articulate (charming) qualities	
ANS abnormalities and slower conditioning	
Does not seek assistance, e.g. guiltless prisoner	Seeks assistance, e.g. tense, aggressive
Not treatable	Better prognosis

ANS, autonomic nervous system.

Psychopathy

This is a term used:

- as a Mental Health Act 1983 definition, prior to its amendment by the Mental Health Act 2007, allowing detention (of abnormally aggressive and seriously irresponsible patients);
- for antisocial or all personality disorders;
- as a term of abuse for uncooperative, usually male patients.

Characteristics of clinical psychopathy include affectionlessness, impulsivity, seeking immediate gratification, lack of guilt and failure to learn by experience and punishment. There is an association with XYY syndrome.

The classic features of psychopathic personality are shown in Table 76.6.

Cleckley usefully differentiated primary from secondary psychopaths (Table 76.7).[143] As classically described, a primary psychopath would rarely seek assistance from a clinician and is most likely to be found within the penal system. Secondary psychopaths, however, are described with higher levels of anxiety or tension, hidden guilt and regret, and low self-esteem. They may impulsively harm themselves under stress, seek assistance from psychiatric services and have a better prognosis. Contrary to popular belief, psychopaths do not make good soldiers, as they are too impulsive and do not work cooperatively, although they can on occasion undertake breathtaking and heroic acts. The general characteristic of psychopaths – the seeking of immediate gratification of needs – may result in sexual offending.

Management of antisocial personality disorders and psychopathy

In the antisocial group of personality disorders, it may be difficult to engage the patient in treatment. Low stress tolerance may lead the patient to make insistent demands for treatment, including for drugs, and for instant results from such treatment, upon threat of self-harm or harm to others. Patients may often stop treatment themselves, unless they are forced to receive it while detained in hospital or are encouraged to do so during a custodial sentence to speed release. They may do best with younger therapists, whom they perceive as being less authoritarian. However, such patients often lack motivation for treatment.

Group therapy is usually preferable to individual psychotherapy. This may be undertaken within a therapeutic community, where the patient lives with other patients and staff and where the consequences of antisocial behaviour are immediately apparent, which contrasts with the delayed punishment for such behaviour given by the legal system. In therapeutic communities, there is open communication and shared examination of problems between patients and staff in a democratic and communal environment, with regular feedback (reality confrontation) given to individuals about their behaviour. This allows social learning to take place. People with severely handicapped personalities may, however, be unable to tolerate the stress of such a regime and may act out, and they may benefit from a more paternalistic authoritarian approach. Therapeutic community treatment can be effective,[143a,143b] as was offered at the Henderson Hospital in Surrey, UK, where research showed subsequent decreases in levels of hospitalization and criminality and also cost-savings in subsequent care, and, for those non-mentally ill personality disordered individuals who are serving a custodial sentence, at both Grendon Underwood and Wormwood Scrubs prisons in England. The Henderson Hospital Unit and HMP Wormwood Scrubs units have now closed.

Among people with borderline personality disorder, interpersonal group therapy and dialectical behaviour therapy have been shown to be effective, the latter reducing parasuicidal behaviour.

Depression, suicidal impulses and general impulsivity and aggression may be countered by low-dose antipsychotic medication, in either oral or depot injection form. The latter helps to overcome the usually poor compliance with oral drug treatment in this group of patients. However, as such treatment is usually required on a long-term basis, there is a risk of tardive dyskinesia. Levels of serotonin in the brain have been shown to be low in the brain of impulsive, self-harming and aggressive personalities, and thus antidepressants, especially the newer serotonin reuptake inhibitors, may also be of benefit, as may lithium carbonate, which also raises serotonin levels, because of its anti-aggressive and mood-stabilizing properties. The anticonvulsant carbamazepine is regarded as a stabilizer of the limbic system and is promoted as a treatment for 'dyscontrol syndrome'. Benzodiazepines should be avoided, as they may release paradoxical aggression.

Aggressive psychopaths are generally not admitted to medium secure units in England and Wales. Those with a legal diagnosis of psychopathic disorder may be detained in special hospitals such as Broadmoor, where treatment may do little more than keep such individuals out of the community, free from drugs and alcohol, and away from potential victims during the years of their greatest risk to others, while their personality matures naturally with age. The more recent DSPD units are described below.

People with antisocial personality disorder or psychopathy tend to improve naturally with age and maturation. Normal individuals become less emotional and impulsive and more cautious and careful with age. Individuals with psychopathy are most destructive in their early life and tend to 'burn out' after age 30–35 years, becoming less antisocial, although family difficulties, such as violence to their partner or children, alcohol and drug abuse, and depression and self-blame may persist. There is also a higher incidence of death by violence and suicide. It may also increase the vulnerability and adversely affect the course and treatment of co-morbid mental illness, such as depression and episodes of paranoid psychosis.

The Psychopathy Checklist – revised (PCL-R)

This was devised by Hare and is used to measure the presence and level of psychopathy. It has been proven to be a good predictor of risk. A short version (PCL-SV) can be used in non-forensic populations.

The Psychopathy Checklist has two factors:

- *Personality traits:*
  - Superficial
  - Grandiose
  - Manipulative
  - Lacks remorse
  - Lacks empathy
  - Does not accept responsibility
- *Deviancy of social behaviour:*
  - Impulsive
  - Poor behavioural controls
  - Lacks goals
  - Irresponsible
  - Adolescent antisocial behaviour
  - Adult antisocial behaviour.

Only one-third of people with antisocial personality disorder reach the checklist criteria for psychopathy on this scale. Scores on the deviancy of social behaviour factor may vary between cultures, e.g. low in Scotland compared with the USA.

Neuroimaging findings

Subjects with high PCL-R scores have been found to have reduced prefrontal grey-matter volumes and reduced autonomic arousal to social stressors.[144] Functional hypoactivation of the amygdala[145] and evidence of dysfunction of the orbitofrontal cortex, which receives projections from the amygdala, have also been found in psychopathy. Amygdala-empathy impairments have been seen as resulting in the callous unemotional traits of psychopathy in the Integrated Emotion System Theory of Blair.[146]

Evidence for treatability

Psychopathic disorder has been removed as a legal category in the Mental Health Act 1983 by the amended Mental Health Act 2007 and incorporated in the category of 'mental disorder'. The Treatability Test – that is, such treatment is likely to alleviate or prevent a deterioration – was also removed from the Mental Health Act 1983 by the Mental Health Act 2007. The new criterion is that treatment is available that is appropriate to the patient – that is, it must have the purpose of improving the patient's condition or preventing deterioration.

One important argument for treating psychopathic disorder is that it may lead to the next generation of people with personality disorder.

Dolan and Coid wrote in 1993 that there is 'no convincing evidence psychopaths can or cannot be treated'.[147] Much the same could be said today. Indeed, there is some evidence that insight-oriented programmes may increase the psychopathic individual's ability to manipulate and deceive and thus increase the risk.[148]

To summarize, there is evidence for treatability for the following:

- Dialectical behaviour therapy for borderline personality disorder
- Cognitive skills programme:
  - Enhanced thinking skills (UK)
  - Reasoning and rehabilitation (R + R) (USA)
- Drug treatment.

Possible mechanisms for the effectiveness of drugs in personality disorder are suggested in Table 76.8.

Evidence for treatability has also been shown in the following facilities:

Table 76.8 Possible mechanisms for the effectiveness of drugs in personality disorder

Symptom	System	Treatment
Affective instability	Adrenergic, cholinergic	Lithium, carbamazepine
Transient psychotic symptoms and over sensitivity	Dopaminergic	Low dose neuroleptics
Impulsive aggressive behaviour	Serotonergic	SSRIs, lithium, carbamazepine

SSRI, selective serotonin reuptake inhibitor.

- *In prison:* HMP Grendon Underwood near Aylesbury, Buckinghamshire, was purpose-built for treatment by group therapy of offenders with psychopathic personality disorder who are already serving a prison sentence with at least 1 year to serve. Remaining at HMP Grendon is voluntary. Referral is by the prison medical service itself. Psychiatrists in court reports and judges in court can recommend placement at HMP Grendon but cannot order such a placement. Gunn and colleagues[148a] showed that self-image, attitudes to staff and behaviour improved in Grendon compared with controls in other prisons. However, the beneficial effect of the prison regime is counteracted by the environment to which the prisoner returns on release – that is, factors in the community after release are just as important in the ultimate outcome. Thus, overall the regime does not significantly affect re-conviction rates for serious offences, but it may do so in terms of the overall number of offences.
- *In hospitals:* Henderson Hospital in Sutton (now closed) was famous for the development under Maxwell Jones of a therapeutic community approach. This unit treated people with psychopathic disorder on an open unit within the National Health Service (NHS). It did best with articulate, intelligent, younger psychopaths without too much violence. The patient had to be resilient enough to withstand this approach and not act out excessively. Those who previously received standard inpatient psychiatric care did less well, probably because this encourages dependency and discourages taking responsibility for oneself. Claims made for beneficial effects included cost-effectiveness through saving from future in-patient psychiatric hospital admissions and prison sentences.
- In the Netherlands, offenders with severe personality disorder can be detained in special forensic psychiatric institutions, Ter Beschikking Stelling (TBS) hospitals, for treatment and rehabilitation into society after having served their prison sentence.[149] A sustained fall in recidivism rates has been reported.[150]

An early forerunner of these special therapeutic communities was the Van Der Hoeven Clinic, Utrecht. This famous secure unit is run as a therapeutic community treating young adult psychopathic offenders by group psychotherapy in combination with an education, rehabilitation and resocialization programme.

The Butler Committee recommendations for psychopaths were that for aggressive psychopaths the law should take its course, e.g. imprisonment, inadequate psychopaths should be placed in hostels with social service care, and people with intervening mental illness hospitalized.

Dangerous and severe personality disorder (DSPD) units have been established in Broadmoor and Rampton special hospitals, and at HMP Whitemoor and HMP Frankland. Their establishment was controversial,[151] but they are now in place.[152] The criterion for admission is that there must be more than a 50 per cent risk of committing a serious offence due to a severe personality disorder.

PRISON PSYCHIATRY

Psychiatrists may be requested to assess prisoners:

- to provide court reports;
- to provide assessments on management and advice, including for sentenced prisoners, at the request of prison medical officers;
- for statutory purposes, such as preparing reports for the parole board.

To visit a prisoner, arrangements need to be made with the healthcare wing of the prison. Psychiatrists may need security clearance. Assessments have to fit in with prison routine, which allows only 2–3 h in the morning or the afternoon to see a patient, and the psychiatrist will usually need to wait for prison staff escorts upon arrival.

Issues relevant to psychiatric care in prison include the following:

- Prevention of offending and imprisonment by psychiatric care in the community
- Police station/court diversion schemes
- Screening should be undertaken on reception of inmates to prison (three-quarters of psychiatric cases may be missed due to inadequate screening[153])
- Measures to counter suicide risk (highest in first 2 months, especially among young people on remand, who are not necessarily formally mentally ill)
- Return to psychiatric hospital care under the relevant sections of the Mental Health Act 1983 while on remand, by means of court sentence or during custodial sentence
- Substance misuse/detox services – abstinence may result in a medical emergency due to withdrawal; there are also high mortality rates in cases of substance misuse upon release from prison due to loss of tolerance
- Sex offender treatment programmes (SOTPs)
- Special therapeutic community units for sentenced prisoners with personality disorder, e.g. at HMP Grendon in England
- DSPD units at HMP Whitemoor and HMP Franklin.

The Mental Health Act 1983 does not apply in prison, but medical treatment can be administered in good faith under common law in prison where there is lack of capacity to consent and in the best interests of the individual, for example to prevent immediate serious risk to others or self.

The aim is that healthcare in prison should ensure an equivalence of services to NHS care outside,[154] with 24-h psychiatric care/in-reach for remanded and sentenced prisoners, on both medical wings and ordinary locations, provided by local general or forensic mental health services.

The National Offender Management Service (NOMS) has been established to manage offenders across the criminal justice system.[155] Healthcare services in prison have been devolved to the NHS.[156]

Suicide risk in prison

Suicide risk in prison is nine times higher than in the community. Risk is highest in the first 2 months in custody. Formal mental illness may be absent.

At-risk groups include:

- people on remand;
- young people;
- people with a history of substance misuse;
- people with a history of violent offences.

Other factors, such as anxiety about the consequences of future court hearings, bullying, isolation and poor conditions in prison, may also be relevant.

Assessment is often compounded by the limited information available in prison. Attempts should be made to gather a background history, including from psychiatric services previously involved in the care of the individual.

Prediction remains difficult. Suicide remains the most common cause of death in prisons and is most commonly by hanging. An assessment, care in custody and teamwork (ACCT) approach has been developed for suicide/self-harm risk assessment based on case management, individualized care-planning and multidisciplinary teamwork.[157]

Although the prevalence of mental disorder in prison populations is high, with perhaps the majority suffering from mental disorder, albeit mainly personality disorder (40–60%) or substance misuse, and with major depression in 10–12 per cent and psychotic illness in around 4 per cent,[158] the criterion for transfer to hospital under the Mental Health Act is that the individual requires detention for in-patient psychiatric treatment, not simply that the individual might benefit from psychiatric or psychological help, including in prison. However, shortage of low-, medium- and maximum-secure beds leads to mentally ill prisoners remaining in custody for lengthy periods.[159] The Bradley Report (2009) has recommended that individuals in prison in need of hospitalization should be transferred within 14 days, as well as other recommendations regarding early intervention, diversion and the development of joint criminal justice mental health teams.[159a]

A useful guide when assessing offenders with regard to their need for psychiatric treatment is not to focus alone on the offence but to assess the need for in- or out-patient treatment as if one were seeing the individual as a new outpatient case.

Psychiatry and prisons

The UK has a daily population of over 80 000 prisoners, with about 130 000 people received each year. There are about 20 male prisoners to 1 female prisoner. Weekly updates on the prison population are available at www.hmprisonservice.gov.uk. This equates to about 1 in 15 children experiencing a parent in prison at some point, or about 25 000 at any one time.

Penrose's Law described an inverse relationship between the number of psychiatric in-patients and prisoners in a country. The UK has a greater proportion of both compared with the rest of Europe, except for prisoners in Turkey. However, it is true that as the UK's psychiatric hospital population has decreased, so the prison population has risen. The USA, which has 5 per cent of the world's population, has 25 per cent of the world's prisoners (around 2 million), perhaps due largely to policies of zero tolerance to drug-related crime (60% of people in prison are there because of this). One in three of New York's male African-Americans has been in prison or on parole.

Prisons in England and Wales may be:

- *local*, such as HMP Brixton and HMP Wandsworth, which are closed and for people on remand, awaiting trial or sentence, or for convicted prisoners serving less than 2 years, and serve local courts; or
- *training prisons*, which may be open, such as HMP Ford, or closed, such as the high-security HMP Belmarsh or HMP Long Lartin, for prisoners serving more than 2 years. Some are dispersal prisons for high security risk prisoners, e.g. HMP Wormwood Scrubs.

London's local prison for women is HMP Holloway. Female training prisons include HMP Styal and HMP Cookham Wood. HMP Durham provides a unit for women requiring special security. HMP Holloway and HMP Styal contain mother-and-baby units. Female prisoners have higher rates of learning disability, personality disorder, neurosis and substance misuse.[137,160–162]

All prisoners are classified on security considerations, from category A prisoners, who are considered to require maximum security and are subject to many restrictions, down to category D prisoners, who are suitable for open conditions.

Young offender institutions (HMYOI) take people aged 15–21 years requiring custody, for example HMYOI Feltham, near London.

Although custodial sentences prevent re-offending during such sentences and are increasing in length in the UK, 60 per cent of prisoners re-offend within 2 years.

Prevalence of psychiatric disorder in prison

Psychiatric symptoms are common in the first 2 months of imprisonment. Between one-third and one-half of prisoners may have an ICD-10 diagnosable psychiatric disorder, but personality disorder and substance misuse are the most common diagnoses. There is an excess of psychoses among prisoners on remand for psychiatric reports, but among sentenced prisoners, the prevalence of psychosis is not raised.

The number of elderly (age ≥60 years) people in prison in the UK increased three-fold between 1988 and 1998, to 1.7 per cent of the population. In more than half of such cases, psychiatric disorder is present, with personality disorder and depression (about 30% often undetected or under-treated) being the most common diagnoses.[163]

The Mental Health Act 1983 does not apply in prison, but treatment can be given in urgent circumstances in 'good faith' under common law.

Other examples of special units in prisons

The special unit at Barlinnie Maximum Security Prison in Scotland was developed for psychopaths who had been very violent, for example killing within a prison setting, and who were destructive within the ordinary prison regime. The unit was run as a small therapeutic community with emphasis on developing the inmates' creative talents, as described in the memoirs of Jimmy Boyle. Admission to this special unit was voluntary.

Herstedvester Prison in Denmark was a forerunner of the prisons attempting to treat psychopaths. Based on therapeutic community principles, it relied heavily on the effect of an indeterminate sentence to motivate prisoners, which is no longer in place. It also used castration for sex offenders. However, follow-up studies showed that 3 years after release, the re-offending rate had returned to that of prisoners from a control group prison.

VICTIMOLOGY

Forensic psychiatry has been defined as 'the prevention, amelioration and treatment of victimisation which is associated with mental disease'[164] – that is, victims of specific offences, or mentally disordered offenders who themselves are the victims of childhood abuse or mental ill-health, or of their own offending behaviour and secondary victimization because of it. Forensic, as opposed to other subspecialties of, psychiatry expertise in this area has been questioned. The victims of childhood abuse and neglect develop an excess of psychological sequelae, including post-traumatic stress disorder, and may become offenders in later life – the abused becoming the abuser ('identification with the aggressor'). A study of 1000 male offenders found that those with post-traumatic stress disorder were five times more likely to have committed acts of serious violence.[165]

MENTAL HEALTH LEGISLATION IN THE UK, WITH SPECIAL REFERENCE TO THE MENTAL HEALTH ACT 1983 OF ENGLAND AND WALES

In the UK there are different legal systems in Scotland, Northern Ireland, the Isle of Man and the Channel Islands to those in England and Wales, although they have developed in parallel. UK mental health legislation covers more than the compulsory detention of patients, although it is this that is usually concentrated on in descriptions of the Acts. In general, compulsory hospitalization depends not only on a diagnosis of mental disorder within the meaning of the Act in question, but also on its necessity for the patient's health or safety or for the protection of others.

Mental Health Act of England and Wales 1983

The Mental Health Act 1983, which replaced the Mental Health Act 1959, remains the basis of current mental health law in England and Wales, but it was amended substantially by the Mental Health Act 2007.

Mental Health Act 2007: an Act to amend the Mental Health Act 1983

The purpose of the Mental Health Act 2007 was to bring mental health legislation into line with service provision, to strengthen patient safeguards and to tackle human rights incompatibilities. Most provisions came into force on 3 November 2008. The Deprivation of Liberty provisions amending the Mental Capacity Act 2005 came into force in April 2009. Age-appropriate services provisions come into force in April 2010.

Definition of mental disorder

The previous four categories of mental disorder are replaced by one: mental disorder. Mental disorder means any disorder or disability of the mind. Exclusions for dependence on alcohol or drugs are retained. If a patient has a learning disability, however, this must also be associated with abnormally aggressive or seriously irresponsible conduct if long-term sections (orders) are used.

Detention criteria

These are that the individual should have a mental disorder of a nature or degree necessary for the patient's health or safety or for the protection of others. Appropriate treatment must be available for longer-term sections. The previous treatability test is removed.

Medical treatment

A new definition includes a broader range of treatments and applies to manifestations of the disorder rather than only the disorder itself. The phrase 'under medical supervision' has been removed.

The term 'appropriate treatment' means treatment that is appropriate in the person's case, taking account of the nature and degree of mental disorder or other circumstances of the case.

Professional roles

The role of approved social worker (ASW) is replaced by approved mental health professional (AMHP). This role is open not only to social workers but also to nurses, occupational therapists and psychologists. AMHPs are approved by the local social services authority, which also provides training for this role.

The term 'responsible medical officer' (RMO) is replaced by 'responsible clinician' (RC), who may also be a psychologist.

Renewing detention

This is no longer solely the task of the RC. Another professional person concerned with the patient must agree that the renewal conditions are met.

Nearest relative

A patient now has the right to make an application to displace their nearest relative, who may also be displaced by a county court when there are reasonable grounds to do so. This overcomes the risk of the technical nearest relative being an abuser of the patient. Nearest relative also now includes civil partners.

Supervised community treatment (SCT)

Supervised community treatment (SCT) replaces supervised discharge and is now also referred to as a community treatment order (CTO). This allows the patient to be under 'compulsion' in the community. However, before such an order can be made, the patient must have been detained in hospital (Sections 3, 37, 47). The order is made by the RC and AMHP. It is renewable after 6 months, and then a further 6 months, and then annually. However, this order does not allow forcible treatment outside hospital. The RC can recall a patient for up to 72 h. The RC and AMHP, if agreed, can revoke a CTO, which re-starts the previous order for its full duration – e.g. a further full Section 3. Section 17 leave is still available, but the RC must consider a CTO if leave is greater than 7 days and document the reasons for this.

Mental health review tribunals (MHRTs)

Time is reduced before a case has to be referred to the mental health review tribunal (MHRT). An annual referral is required for people under age 18 years.

Age-appropriate services

From April 2010, hospital managers must consult child and adolescent mental health service (CAMHS) specialists when detaining people under 18 years of age and ensure that such individuals are admitted to a suitable environment. Since January 2008, parental authority is no longer sufficient to allow admission of 16- or 17-year-olds as informal patients. The Mental Health Act 1983 must be used. There are also more safeguards for the use of electroconvulsive therapy (ECT) for such individuals.

Advocacy

There is a new role for the independent mental health advocate (IMHA), for which formal training is now required. Hospital managers must ensure that advocacy services are available. Advocates have the right to meet with patients in private, to meet with professionals and to access health records with the patient's consent.

Consent to treatment, including for electroconvulsive therapy

For medication, arrangements are largely unchanged (Table 76.9). However, for patients being treated under an SCT, the patient's consent is required, as is a Second Opinion Appointed Doctor (SOAD) by the Secretary of State for Health (in practice the Care Quality Commission) within a month. If the patient lacks the capacity to consent, others can authorize.

No ECT can be administered, except in an emergency, if a

Table 76.9 Consent to treatment under Mental Health Act 1983*

Type of treatment	Informal	Compulsory
Urgent treatment	No consent	No consent
Irreversible, hazardous or non-established treatments, e.g. psychosurgery (e.g. leucotomy), hormone implants (for sex offenders), surgical operations (e.g. castration)	Consent and second opinion	Consent and second opinion
Section 58	Consent	Consent or second opinion
Psychiatric drugs, ECT		Consent and second opinion

Consent to treatment should be informed and voluntary (implies mental illness, e.g. dementia, does not affect judgement).
For first 3 months of treatment, a detained patient's consent is not required for Section 58 medicines but is for ECT.
Patients can withdraw voluntary consent at any time.
ECT, electroconvulsive therapy.

Table 76.10 Civil treatment orders under the Mental Health Act 1983

Civil treatment order under Mental Health Act 1983	Grounds	Application by	Medical recommendations	Maximum duration	Eligibility for appeal to MHRT
Section 2 – Admission for assessment	Mental disorder	Nearest relative or approved mental health practitioner	Two doctors (one approved under Section 12)	28 days	Within 14 days
Section 3 – Admission for treatment	Mental disorder	Nearest relative or approved mental health practitioner	Two doctors (one approved under Section 12)	6 months	Within first 6 months; if renewed, within second 6 months, then every year; mandatory every 3 years
Section 4 – Emergency admission for assessment	Mental disorder (urgent necessity)	Nearest relative or approved mental health practitioner	Any doctor	72 h	————
Section 5(2) – Urgent detention of voluntary in-patient	Danger to self or others		Doctor in charge of patient's care	72 h	————
Section 5(4) – Nurse's holding power of voluntary in-patient	Mental disorder (danger to self, health or others)	Registered mental nurse or registered nurse for mental handicap	None	6 h	————
Section 136 – Admission by police	Mental disorder	Police officer	Allows patient in public place to be removed to 'place of safety'	72 h	————
Section 135	Mental disorder	Magistrate	Allows power of entry to home and removal of patient to place of safety	72 h	————

MHRT, mental health review tribunal.

patient has capacity and refuses. Patients under age 18 years must have consent and SOAD authorization. No ECT may be administered, unless in an emergency, if a patient lacks capacity but has a valid advance decision (AD) refusing ECT or has an attorney who refuses ECT.

Provisions for mentally abnormal offenders

The new definition of mental disorder is wider-ranging, resulting in Sections 48, 36 and 45A now being applicable to patients with all forms of mental disorder. Restriction orders must be indefinite, not time-limited as was possible previously. There are new provisions for sharing certain information with victims, extending this beyond the Domestic Violence, Crimes and Victims Act 2004.

Revised code of practice

This sets out five guiding principles of purpose to inform decisions under the Act – least restrictive alternative, respect, participation and effectiveness, efficiency and equity.

Mental health review tribunals

These are independent bodies consisting of a doctor, lawyer and layperson whose responsibility is to consider the justification for continued compulsion under the 1983 Mental Health Act. The chair of the MHRT is a lawyer, and in the case of restricted patients is a judge.

Patients are allowed legal aid to assist in representation, for example private psychiatric reports can be commissioned.

The MHRT can order discharge or delayed discharge, and recommend (not order) transfer to another hospital or leave of absence. It can also order discharge or conditional discharge (i.e. with conditions such as place of residence) or a deferred conditional discharge (pending the conditions being in place) of a Section 41 restricted patient.

Table 76.10 shows the eligibility for hearings for civil orders. That for forensic orders is shown in Table 76.3.

Patients on a 72-h detention order have no MHRT rights but can appeal against detention to hospital managers.

The Care Quality Commission

This body now incorporates the Mental Health Act Commission (MHAC; Section 121 of the Mental Health Act 1983) and the Social Services Inspectorate. It is an independent body of about 100 part-time members (doctors, nurses, psychologists, social workers, lawyers and laypeople) appointed by the Secretary of State for health. It, as did the MHAC, provides approved doctors to give second opinions on consent to treatment. It receives, reviews and scrutinizes detention documents and exercises a general protective function for all detained patients. It regularly visits psychiatric hospitals to interview detained patients and makes sure that their complaints are being properly handled. It also visits special hospitals monthly and other psychiatric units once or twice a year.

It is responsible for the code of practice (Section 118) on detention, treatment of all psychiatric patients (informal or detained) and consent to treatment, for the guidance of clinical and administrative staff in psychiatric hospitals and social workers.

Court of Protection

Originally empowered by Section 94 of the Mental Health Act 1983, but made a new body under the Mental Capacity Act 2005, this is for the protection and management of the property of mentally disordered patients. Medical evidence that any form of mental disorder renders a person incapable of managing his or her property and affairs can be put to a judge in the special court of protection. If the judge is satisfied, he or she may then appoint a receiver to act on behalf of the patient, keep the patient's accounts and manage the patient's affairs. The receiver may be a relative or friend of the patient, a solicitor, a bank trustee or an official solicitor of the supreme court. The patient and their affairs may be checked from time to time by medical and legal visitors appointed by the Lord Chancellor.

Medical visitors must have special knowledge and experience of mental disorder.

The Court of Protection is used especially for dementing patients, but also for people with other mental disorders, such as mania and schizophrenia. In practice, many acutely ill psychiatric patients upon admission are unable to manage their property, but rapid treatment response makes this rather ponderous procedure of the Court of Protection unnecessary.

Patients' rights under the Mental Health Act 1983

On admission, detained patients must be advised of their legal status, their rights to appeal to an MHRT, their rights in respect of consent to treatment, those who have authority to discharge them, and the Care Quality Commission.

Correspondence to and from informal patients cannot be interfered with. Correspondence from detained patients in ordinary psychiatric hospitals can be withheld only if the person to whom the correspondence is addressed has asked for that to happen. Special hospitals can withhold correspondence to and from patients, except about staff and to solicitors and members of Parliament (MPs) or the sovereign. (In the latter case, correspondence can be sent free of charge as it is the sovereign's mail.) Patients in any psychiatric hospital must be informed if their correspondence is withheld.

Informal inpatients have voting rights.

Health and social services have a duty to provide aftercare for detained patients when they leave hospital (Section 117).

Mental Health (Scotland) Act 2003

Section 328 defines mental disorder as any mental illness, personality disorder or learning disability. Sexual orientation, sexual deviancy, transsexualism, transvestism and dependency on or use of alcohol or drugs are excluded from this definition. Under the Act, provisions exist for an RMO, an Approved Medical Practitioner (AMP) (Section 22), a Mental Health Officer (MHO) (in practice a social worker), designated Medical Practitioners (DMPs), Mental Welfare Commission and Mental Health Tribunal. All patients have a right to advocacy (Section 259). Advanced statements are possible under Sections 275 and 276.

Part 5 of the Act details emergency detention orders, Part 6 details short-term admission orders and Part 7 community treatment orders for hospital or community.

Mental Health Act (Northern Ireland) Order 1986

Mental illness is defined in the Act as a state of mind that affects a person's thinking, perceiving, emotion or judgement, to the extent that they require care or medical treatment in their own interests or in the interests of other people. Medical treatment is defined as including nursing and also care and treatment under medical supervision.

There are definitions in the Act for mental handicap, severe mental handicap and severe mental impairment. To be placed in the severe mental handicap category, there must be associated 'abnormally aggressive or seriously irresponsible conduct'.

It is stated that no person should be treated as having a mental disorder by reason of only a personality disorder, promiscuity or other immoral conduct, sexual deviancy or dependence on alcohol and drugs.

Part II of the Order allows compulsory admission for assessment for up to 14 days before being admitted for treatment. For the purposes of application for detention in Northern Ireland, the nearest relative can be someone living in the Republic of Ireland or the UK. Temporary holding powers are available for voluntary patients already in hospital, as with the English and Welsh, and Scottish Acts. These holding powers are for 6 h by a professionally registered charge nurse and 48 h by a doctor on the staff of a hospital concerned, which also includes a general hospital.

If the patient is not well enough to become a voluntary patient or to be discharged before the end of the 14-day assessment period, they may in the first instance be detained for up to 6 months if they are diagnosed as having mental illness or severe mental impairment and they remain at high risk of serious physical harm to themselves or others. The period of detention is renewable for a further 6 months and then annually, subject to approval, following an examination by a doctor from another hospital appointed by the Mental Health Commission.

Provisions for consent to treatment and guardianship are similar to those set out in the English Act.

Provisions exist similar to those in the 1983 English Act for individuals involved in criminal proceedings; for example, the courts have the power to remand for examination or treatment, and interim hospital orders are also available. Hospital orders may be made regardless of the apparent availability of places, unlike in the rest of the UK, and a court may also impose a restriction order on the patient's discharge. In all hospital order cases, psychiatrists are expected to give oral evidence in the court.

Individuals detained for 2 years are automatically referred to an MHRT.

The Mental Health Commission, unlike the English equivalent, covers voluntary patients, people in guardianship and people in residential accommodation or, indeed, anybody with a mental disorder. Where it receives complaints, it has the power to hold a formal inquiry in order to establish the facts.

At any one time, Northern Ireland has fewer than ten patients in Britain's mainland maximum security hospitals. Northern Ireland has no maximum security hospital itself.

Also of note – therapeutic abortion is allowed in Northern Ireland only where there is undoubted grave risk to the continuing physical or mental health of the pregnant woman. This leads to women crossing from Northern Ireland to the British mainland each year to have abortions.

MENTAL HEALTH LEGISLATION IN THE REPUBLIC OF IRELAND

The Central Mental Hospital Dundrum, which opened in 1850, is the only security hospital in the country. It accepts many prison transfers (remand and sentenced) and also the majority of people found 'guilty but insane' and people judged 'unfit to plead'.

The Mental Treatment Act 1945 remained the main mental health legislation in Eire until recently.

Mental Health Act 2001

This replaces the Mental Treatment Act 1945 and the Acts passed in 1953, 1961 and 1981. However, its implementation has been gradual. Section 4 details the principles underlying the Act, including the best interests of the person but with due regard to the interests of others who may be at serious harm.

Definition of mental disorder

Section 3 defines mental disorder as 'mental illness, severe dementia or significant intellectual impairment'. Compulsory detention should be as a result of (i) mental disorder causing immediate and serious harm to the patient or to other people; or (ii) because of the severity of the mental disorder, the judgement of the person is so impaired that, if the patient is not admitted to an approved centre, would lead to a serious deterioration; or (iii) because detention in an approved centre is likely to benefit or alleviate the condition.

Table 76.11 Comparison of urgent civil detention under mental health legislation in the UK and the Republic of Ireland

	Legislation	Out-patient	In-patient
England and Wales	Mental Health Act 1983	Section 2 or 3 should be used rather than Section 4	Section 5(2) immediately or Sections 2 or 3
Scotland	Mental Health (Care and Treatment) (Scotland) Act 2003	Part 5 if arranging; Part 6 would involve undesirable delay	Part 5 if arranging; Part 6 would involve undesirable delay
Northern Ireland	Mental Health (Northern Ireland) Order 1986	a. 4	a. 7(2) may be detained under a. 4
Republic of Ireland	Mental Health Act 2001	Sections 9 and 10	Section 2

Table 76.12 Comparison of legal provisions for mentally disordered offenders in the UK and the Republic of Ireland

	England & Wales	Scotland	Northern Ireland	Republic of Ireland
	Mental Health Act 1983	Mental Health (Care and Treatment) Scotland Act 2003	Mental Health (Northern Ireland) Order 1986	Mental Health Act 2001
Police				
Detention of mentally disordered person found in public place	Section 136	Section 297	a130	Section 12
Detention of mentally disordered person in private premises	Section 135	Section 293	a129	Section 12
Pre-trial		Criminal Procedure (Scotland) Act 1995		
Remand to hospital for assessment	Section 35	Section 52B–J	a42	–
Remand to hospital for assessment	Section 36	Section 52K–S	a43	–
Transfer of untried prisoner to hospital	Section 48	Section 52K–S	a54	–
Trial				
Criteria for fitness to plead	*R v Prichard* 1836	*HMA v Wilson Stewart v HMA* 1942	*R v Prichard*	*R v Prichard* (Section 3 CL(I)B2002)
Procedure relating to a finding of unfitness to plead	Sections 2–3 and sch 1–2 CP(IUP) A1991	Sections 54–57 CP(S)A 1995	a49 and 50A	Lunacy (Ireland) Act 1821, Juries Act 1976
Criteria for insanity at the time of the offence	*McNaughten Rules* 1843	*HMA v Kidd* 1960	CJ(NI)A 1966	*Doyle v Wicklow County Council* 1974
Procedure relating to a finding of insanity at the time of the offence	Sections 1&3 and sch 1–2 CP(IUP)A 1991	Sections 54 and 57	a50 and 50A CJ(NI)O 1996	Trial of Lunatics Act 1883
Criteria for diminished responsibility	Section 2 Homicide Act 1957	*Galbraith v HMA* 2001 Culpable Homocide	CJ(NI)O 1996	

Table 76.12 *Continued*

	England & Wales	Scotland	Northern Ireland	Republic of Ireland
	Mental Health Act 1983	Criminal Procedures (Scotland) Act 1995	Mental Health (Northern Ireland) Order 1986	Mental Health Act 2001
Post-conviction but pre-sentence				
Remand to hospital for assessment	Section 35	Section 52B–J Section 200	a42	–
Remand to hospital for treatment	Section 36	Section 52K–S	a43	–
Interim hospital/compulsion order	Section 38	Section 53	–	–
Transfer of untried prisoner to hospital	Section 48	Section 52B–J Section 52K–S	a54	Previous legislation applies
Sentence				
Compulsory treatment in hospital under MHA	Section 37	Section 57A	a44	–
Restriction order	Section 41	Section 59	a47	–
Hybrid order (hospital disposal with prison sentence)	Section 45A–B	Section 59A	–	–
Compulsory treatment in community under MHA	–	Section 57A	–	–
Guardianship	Section 37	Section 58(1A)	a44	–
Intervention order for incapable adult	–	Section 60B	–	–
Psychiatric probation order	sch 2 (p5) Powers of Criminal Courts (Sentencing) Act 2000	Section 230	sch 1 (p4) CJ(NI)O 1996	–
Post-sentence		Mental Health (Care and Treatment) Scotland Act 2003		
Transfer of sentenced prisoners to hospital	Section 47	Section 136	a53	Previous legislation applies
Restriction direction for transferred prisoner	Section 49	All	a55	–

Mental illness means a state of mind affecting thinking, perceiving, emotion or judgement. Significant intellectual disability means a state of arrested or incomplete development of mind, including significant impairment of intelligence and social functioning and abnormally aggressive or seriously irresponsible conduct.

Other official terms

Approved centres include in-patient facilities, hospitals and other facilities registered with the Mental Health Commission (MHC). There are Review Tribunals and an Inspector of Mental Health Services who is a consultant psychiatrist appointed by the MHC.

Important sections of the Mental Health Act 2001

These include the following:

- Application for involuntary admission (Section 9)
- Medical assessment (Section 10)
- Power of the Garda to detain and apply for involuntary admission (Section 12)
- Removal to an approved centre (Section 13)
- Admission to an approved centre (Sections 14 and 15).

Part 4 of the Act concerns consent to treatment for patients subject to compulsion.

COMPARISON OF UK AND REPUBLIC OF IRELAND LEGISLATION

Table 76.11 compares civil detention under mental health legislation in the UK and the Republic of Ireland. Table 76.12 compares the legal provisions for mentally disordered offenders in the UK and the Republic of Ireland.

MENTAL HEALTH LEGISLATION IN CANADA

The courts are under provincial jurisdiction. The ten provinces and two territories also have a court of appeal. The highest court, the Supreme Court of Canada, is situated in Ottawa, the national capital. There is a criminal code that covers mentally abnormal offenders, but their management varies between provinces due to their respective mental health legislations. The criminal code does, however, allow a trial judge to remand an offender for psychiatric assessment, and the court of appeal has similar provision.

There are two maximum-security hospitals in Canada, the Mental Health Centre at Penetanguishene, Ontario, and the Institut Philip Pinel in Montreal.

The maximum-security hospital at the Oak Ridge Division of the Mental Health Centre at Penetanguishene has around 200 patients. The majority are warrants of the lieutenant governor patients, having been found not guilty by reason of insanity, or involuntary patients under the Ontario Mental Health Act 1980. Patients who have been stabilized are referred to long-term medium security units. When fit for rehabilitation in the community, such patients may be referred to a university based forensic service, such as the Clarke Institute of Psychiatry in Toronto.

The Metropolitan Toronto Forensic Service (METFORS) is well known for its provision of psychiatric services to the courts and prisons. METFORS has a brief assessment unit and otherwise undertakes standard forensic psychiatric pre-trial assessments and treatments. In Ottawa there is a well-developed clinic for the treatment of and research into sexual offenders, and it has a close relationship with the probation service.

With the provinces and territories having differing mental health legislation, definitions of mental disorder vary between them. The criteria for involuntary civil committal are wide in all the provinces, except Ontario, where objective evidence of potential dangerousness to self or others is required. Provinces other than Ontario have less stringent admission criteria regarding general health, welfare and safety. Most provinces require certification by two physicians before involuntary admission of a patient to a psychiatric facility. Periods of detention vary with the various mental health acts of the provinces. Most provinces have provision for police officers to take a person for a psychiatric examination and for judges to order that an individual charged with a criminal offence be examined, admitted and treated in a psychiatric facility.

Regarding consent to treatment, an incompetent involuntarily detained patient has the right to refuse all forms of psychiatric treatment in Nova Scotia and Ontario. If found incompetent, consent from the nearest relative is required; in the absence of the nearest relative, review board procedures exist to hear the case and issue treatment orders.

There is considerable variability in the roles and powers of the mental health tribunals of the various provinces and territories of Canada. People found not guilty by reason of insanity or found unfit to proceed with a trial and who are made subject to conditions of a warrant of the lieutenant governor of the province of Ontario are reviewed by an advisory board, appointed by the lieutenant governor in council on at least one occasion every 12 months.

There are provisions under sections of the Criminal Code of Canada to remand a mentally abnormal offender for a psychiatric assessment for fitness to proceed with trial, if that individual is mentally ill or the balance of the individual's mind is disturbed. The period of assessment is up to 30 days. If the person is deemed not fit to plead or stand trial, then a trial of fitness is ordered. If the person is found unfit, then the court orders that the person be kept in custody until the pleasure of the lieutenant governor of the province is known. Similarly, if found not guilty by reason of insanity, the individual is also made subject to the terms of the lieutenant governor's warrant and kept in a place of custody. Custody is nearly always a psychiatric facility with either maximum or medium security.

If the offence committed is minor, then a probation order with a condition of psychiatric treatment may be ordered. Some correctional institutions have programmes for psychiatric treatment. If a prisoner becomes mentally ill while serving a sentence, there are provisions in the criminal code to transfer the patient to a psychiatric facility for treatment.

MENTAL HEALTH LEGISLATION IN THE USA

Most aspects of mental health law are delegated to the various states, so that they can enact legislation to suit local needs. Mental health legislation in the USA has been shaped by social and political forces and case law. The emphasis has always been on the least restrictive treatment. Involuntary psychiatric treatment has been considered in many ways out of keeping with the US constitution and philosophy of upholding the individual's rights of freedom, speech and behaviour.

In the past 30 years, there has been a trend away from detention (certification) on grounds of need for treatment and towards increasing patients' rights and restricting involuntary treatment. This, together with a desire to reduce the number of in-patients and the cost of their care, has led to the general adoption as a criterion for detention a standard of future or potential dangerousness to the patient or others, rather than grave disability, for reasons of health alone or the patient's need for treatment. Emergency hospitalization can be initiated without prior judicial approval, but subsequent commitment needs to be ordered by a judge.

Involuntary patients have the right to refuse medication. Medication to control dangerous patients in an emergency has been sanctioned if the need to prevent violence outweighs the possibility of harm to the patient and all less restrictive alternatives have been ruled out. If the patient is not dangerous, then in many states the only way to enforce medication is to have the patient declared incompetent, whereupon treatment conditions can be made, often on the basis of what the patient would have decided were he or she competent to do so rather than what might be in the patient's best interests.

In keeping with the idea of the least restrictive treatment, orders allowing out-patient committal to psychiatric treatment have emerged in nearly all states. This assists the large number of patients who have been discharged from hospital in the USA and who are clearly incapable of coping with the outside world and meeting their basic needs. Such community commitment orders have been legally challenged on the grounds that if an individual is well enough to live outside an institution, then it is hard to justify such a restriction of their constitutional liberty. American states are divided widely on this issue. Some have developed a new lower threshold for involuntary out-patient care.

The ruling in the case of Tarasoff *v.* Regents of University of California in 1974–76 (a duty to warn in 1974 modified to a duty to protect in 1976) has led many American psychotherapists to acknowledge that patient confidentiality can be violated, in view of the court's assertion that 'protected privilege ends where community peril begins'.

MENTAL HEALTH LEGISLATION IN AUSTRALIA AND NEW ZEALAND

Each of the six states of Australia and its territories has its own separate mental health act and its own judicial system. Australian law is derived from, but is not identical to, the common law of England. Australian and UK mental health services and laws are, however, similar. Much Australian psychiatric care is privately based, with state provision concentrating on patients with severe (psychotic) mental illness. Mental health legislation in Australia has been under constant review over recent years, with new acts drafted and frequent amendments made to earlier acts. The Mental Health Act 1986 of the State of Victoria introduced a community treatment order. This Act, together with the Mental Health Act 1990 of New South Wales, had a significant influence on the development of legislation throughout Australia.

New Zealand has one Mental Health Act, which also has provisions for the compulsory treatment of patients in the community.

KEY POINTS

- Most mentally abnormal offenders are dealt with by ordinary psychiatric hospital facilities as out- or in-patients.
- Special hospitals treat people with mental disorder who are considered to be an immediate and grave danger to the public if they were to abscond, and who cannot be managed under conditions of medium security.
- Medium secure units in England and Wales provide psychiatric treatment under conditions of medium security, greater than ordinary hospitals but less than special hospitals.

- Juvenile delinquency (law-breaking behaviour) is associated with low normal intelligence, large family size, poverty, unsatisfactory child-rearing, parental criminality and troublesomeness at school.
- Up to one in five boys in London may have a conviction by the age of 21 years, and half of indictable crimes are committed by under-21-year-olds.
- Schizophrenia is associated mostly with minor offending secondary to deterioration in personality and social functioning, rather than with serious or dangerous offences or offences arising directly from delusions or hallucinations.
- Depressive disorder is underrepresented among offenders but is associated with homicide and shoplifting.
- Morbid delusional sexual jealousy is associated with repetitive and serious violence to the individual's partner.

- In the UK, most mentally abnormal offenders stand trial. If found guilty, they are convicted, but medical evidence is given in mitigation to alter the sentencing of the court, e.g. a hospital treatment order may be recommended instead of a custodial sentence.
- Some offences require specific guilty intent (*mens rea*) as well as an unlawful act (*actus rea*), e.g. murder, rape, arson. Other offences do not require proof of guilty intent, e.g. motoring offences (i.e. on the basis of non-specific intent).
- Fitness to plead refers to the time of the trial, not of the offence.
- Not guilty by reason of insanity (the special verdict) refers to the time of the offence. The grounds (McNaughten Rules) are that, by reason of such defect of the mind, the subject did not know the nature or quality of the act, or did not know that what he or she was doing was wrong (forbidden by law).
- Diminished responsibility (Homicide Act 1957) is only a defence to a charge of murder that carries a mandatory life sentence. It refers to

the time of the offence and is on the grounds of the presence of abnormality of mind ... which substantially impaired mental responsibility for the act. It results in a reduction of the charge to manslaughter, which allows discretionary sentencing, including a hospital order.
- Infanticide is the unlawful killing of a child of under 1 year of age by the child's mother at a time when the balance of her mind was disturbed due to giving birth or from lactation.
- In general an individual is regarded as legally fully responsible if he or she knowingly took, or was voluntarily intoxicated with, drugs or alcohol unless offence requies specific intent which may be 'negatived' by intoxication.
- Amnesia itself is not a legal defence, although the underlying condition may be. Amnesia may reflect lying, hysterical denial, overarousal preventing registration, alcohol or drug intoxication, or head injury.

- Risk varies not only with the individual but also with the context and over time; it is not a static characteristic, as it is implied by the now less often used term 'dangerousness'.
- Risk of dangerous behaviour is increased by the presence of substance misuse, the availability and use of weapons, morbid jealousy and the sadistic murderer syndrome.
- Short-term prediction is better than that for the longer term.
- Past behaviour is the best predictor of risk for non-mentally ill people, but for mentally ill people positive psychotic symptoms, such as paranoid delusions and delusions of passivity, are better predictors.
- When risk is identified, a risk-management plan should be developed, but this may not result in risk elimination.

- Most shoplifting offenders are now male. The peak age of offending is 10–18 years.
- About 5 per cent of shoplifters have a formal psychiatric disorder.
- Shoplifting may be an early symptom of depressive disorder or dementia.
- Pathological stealing (kleptomania) is an impulse-control disorder characterized by recurrent failure to resist impulses to steal objects not needed for personal use or monetary gain. It is present in only a minority of shoplifters.

- Arson is unlawfully or maliciously (wilfully) destroying or damaging property by setting fire.
- A more serious charge is arson with intent to endanger life.
- Arson may be motivated for psychotic reasons, or by displaced revenge, anger or jealousy.
- Alternatively, arson may be due to fire being a thing of interest to the fire-setter, as in the impulse disorder pathological fire-setting (pyromania).

- Abused children are usually under 3 years of age and present with multiple injuries in time and space.
- Delay in reporting and contradictory histories of injuries are often given by the parents.
- Abusive parents have often been abused themselves as children.
- High professional awareness is required to allow early recognition.
- Multidisciplinary case conferences are essential for management, and placement of the child on a local authority child protection register may be required.
- In the assessment of violence:
  - Ask informants about a history of violence.
  - Request previous summaries, e.g. of in-patient care, and past psychiatric and probation reports.
  - Document above and otherwise keep and use proper records.
  - Make plans to manage the risk, and document this.
  - Be particularly cautious in cases where treatment is refused, reduced or withheld.

REFERENCES

1. Jamieson E, Butwell M, Taylor P, Leese M (2000) Trends in special (high security) hospitals: 1. Referrals and admissions. *British Journal of Psychiatry* **176**: 253–9.
2. Taylor PJ, Leese M, Williams D, *et al.* (1998) Mental disorder and violence: a special (high security) hospital study. *British Journal of Psychiatry* **172**: 218–26.
3. Fallon P, Blueglass R, Edwards B, Daniels G (1999) *Report of the Committee of Inquiry into the Personality Disorder Unit, Ashworth Special Hospital.* London: The Stationery Office.
4. Bucanan A (1998) Criminal conviction after discharge from special (high security) hospital: incidence in the first ten years. *British Journal of Psychiatry* **172**: 472–6.

4a. Home Office and Department of Health (1975) *Report of Committee of Mentally Abnormal Offenders (Butler Committee).* CMMD 6244. London: HMSO.

4b. Department of Health and Social Secuirty (1974) *Revised Report of the Working Party on Security in NHS Psychiatric Hospitals (Glancy Report).* London: DHSS.

5. Treasaden IH (1985) Current practice in medium secure units. In L Gostin (ed.) *Secure Provision: A Review of the Special Services for the Mentally Ill and the Mentally Handicapped in England and Wales.* London: Tavistock Publications.
6. Judge J, Harty M, Fahy T (2004) Survey of community forensic psychiatry services in England and Wales. *Journal of Forensic Psychiatry and Psychology* **15**: 244–57.
7. Snowden P, McKenna J, Jasper A (1999) Management of conditionally discharged patients and others who present similar risks to the community: Integrated or parallel? *Journal of Forensic Psychiatry and Psychology* **110**: 583–96.
8. Mohan R, Slade M, Fahy TA (2004) Clinical characteristics of community forensic mental health services. *Psychiatric Services* **55**: 1294–8.

9. Royal College of Psychiatrists (2006) *Psychiatrists and Multi-Agency Public Protection Arrangements: Guidelines on Representation, Participation, Confidentiality and Information Exchange*. London: Royal College of Psychiatrists
10. Office for National Statistics (2008) About National Statistics and ONS. www.statistics.gov.uk/SSD/surveys/british_crime_survey.asp.
11. Home Office (2009) Crime in England and Wales 2007/2008. www.homeoffice.gov.uk/rds/crimeew0708.html.
12. Brahms D (1981) Premenstrual syndrome: a disease of the mind? *Lancet* **II**: 1238–40.
13. Brahms D (1982) Rejection of the premenstrual syndrome as a defence in English Law. *Lancet* **I**: 1134–5.
14. West DJ, Farrington DP (1977) *The Delinquent Way of Life*. London: Heinemann Educational.
15. Sutherland EH (1942) Development of the theory. In K Schuessler (ed.) *Edwin H. Sutherland on Analyzing Crime*. Chicago, IL: University of Chicago Press.
16. Merton RK (1957) *Social Theory and Social Structure*, revised edn. Glencoe, IL: Free Press.
17. Robbins LN (1966) *Deviant Children Grown Up: A Sociological and Psychiatric Study of Sociopathic Personality*. Baltimore, MD: Williams & Wilkins.
18. Rutter M (1978) Family, area and school influences in the genesis of conduct disorders. In L Hersov, M Berger, D Schaffer (eds) *Aggression and Antisocial Behaviour in Childhood and Adolescence*. Oxford: Pergamon.
19. Moffitt TE, Caspi A (2001) Childhood predictors differentiate life-course persistent and adolescence limited antisocial pathways among males and females. *Development Psychopathology* **13**: 355–79.
20. Moffitt TE, Caspi A, Harrington H, Milne BJ (2002) Males on the persistent and adolescent antisocial pathways: follow-up at age 26. *Developmental Psychopathology* **14**: 179–207.
21. Clarke T, Kemey-Herbert J and Humphrey SM (2002) Community rehabilitation orders with additional requirements of psychiatric treatment. *Advances in Psychiatric Treatment* **8**: 281–90.
22. Oliver JE (1970) Huntington's chorea in Northamptonshire. *British Journal of Psychiatry* **116**: 241–53.
23. Rowlands MW (1988) Psychiatric and legal aspects of persistent litigation. *British Journal of Psychiatry* **153**: 317–23.
24. Hodgins S (1992) Mental disorder, intellectual deficiency, and crime: evidence from a birth cohort. *Archives of General Psychiatry* **49**: 476–83.
25. James DV, Duffield G, Blizard R, Hamilton LW (2001) Fitness to plead: a prospective study of the inter-relationships between expert opinion, legal criteria and specific symptomatology. *Psychological Medicine* **31**: 139–50.
26. Memon R (2006) Legal theory and case law defining the insanity defence in English and Welsh law. *Journal of Forensic Psychiatry and Psychology* **17**: 230–52.
27. Coleman K, Hird C, Povey D (2005) *Violent Crime Overview, Homicide and Gun Crime 2004/5*, 2nd edn. London: Home Office.
28. Brookman F, Maguire M (2003) *Reducing Homicide: Summary of a Review of the Possibilities*. RDS occasional paper no. 84. London: Home Office.
29. Shon PCH, Targonski JR (2003) Declining trends in US parricides 1976–1998: testing the Freudian assumptions. *International Journal of Law and Psychiatry* **26**: 387–402.
30. Green CM (1981) Matricide by sons. *Medicine, Science and the Law* **21**: 207–14.
31. Gillies H (1965) Murder in the West of Scotland. *British Medical Journal* **111**: 1087–94.
32. Dell S (1984) *Murder into Manslaughter: The Diminished Responsibility Defence in Practice*. Oxford: Oxford University Press.
33. Ministry of Justice (2008) *Murder, Manslaughter and Infanticide: Proposal for Reform of the Law*. Consultation paper CP19/08. London: Home Office.
34. World Health Organization (1992) *International Classification of Diseases and Related Health Problems*, 10th revision. Geneva: World Health Organization.
34a. Joseph P, Potter M (1993) I Diversion from custody – psychiatric assessment at the magistrate's court. *British Journal of Psychiatry* **162**: 325–30.
34b. Joseph P, Potter M (1993) II Effect on hospital and prison responses. *British Journal of Psychiatry* **162**: 330–34.
34c. James D (1999) Court diversion at 10 years: can it work, does it work and has it a future? *Journal of Forensic Psychiatry* **10**: 507–24.
35. Gudjonnson GH (1993) *The Psychology of Interrogation, Confessions and Testimony*. Chichester: Lodey.
36. Large M, Smith G, Swinson N, Shaw J, Neeson O (2008) Homicide due to mental disorder in England and Wales over 50 years. *British Journal of Psychiatry* **193**: 130–37.
37. West DJ (1965) *Murder Followed by Suicide*. London: Macmillan.
38. Treasaden I (2003) Assessment of violence in medium secure units. In R Doctor (ed.) *Dangerous Patients: A Psychodynamic Approach to Risk Assessment and Management*. London: Karnac Books.
39. Bloom-Cooper L, Grounds A, Guinan P, Parker A, Taylor M (1996) *The Case of Jason Mitchell: Report of the Independent Panel of Enquiry*. London: Gerald Duckworth & Co.
40. Coid J (1983) The epidemiology of abnormal homicide and murder followed by suicide. *Psychological Medicine* **13**: 855–60.
41. Bennett D (1996) Homicide, inquiries and scapegoating. *Psychiatric Bulletin* 20, 298–300.

42. Taylor PJ, Gunn J (1999) Homicides by people with mental illness: myth and reality. *British Journal of Psychiatry* **174**: 9–14.
43. Linnoila VM, Virkkunen M (1992) Aggression, suicidality and serotonin. *Journal of Clinical Psychiatry* **53** (suppl.): 46–51.
44. Lorenz K (1966) *On Aggression*. New York: Harcourt.
45. Monohan J (1981) *Predicting Violent Behaviour: An Assessment of Clinical Techniques*. Beverly Hills, CA: Sage.
46. Swanson JW, Holzer CE, 3rd, Ganju VK, Jono RT (1990) Violence and psychiatric disorder in the community: evidence from epidemiologic catchment area survey. *Hospitals and Community Psychiatry* **41**: 761–70.
47. Lidz CW, Mulvey EP, Gardner W (1993) The accuracy of predictions of violence to others. *Journal of the American Medical Association* **269**: 1007–11.
48. Farrington DP (1995) The Twelfth Jack Tizard Memorial Lecture: the development of offending and antisocial behaviour from childhood – key findings from the Cambridge Study in Delinquent Development. *Journal of Child Psychology and Psychiatry and Allied Disciplines* **36**: 929–64.
49. Mullen PE (2006) Schizophrenia and violence: from correlations to preventative strategies. *Advances in Psychiatric Treatment* **12**: 239–48.
50. Humphreys MS, Johnstone EC, MacMillan JF, Taylor PJ (1992) Dangerous behaviour preceding first admissions for schizophrenia. *British Journal of Psychiatry* **161**: 501–05.
51. Taylor PJ (1993) Schizophrenia and crime: distinctive patterns in association. In S Hodgins (ed.) *Crime and Mental Disorder*. Beverly Hills, CA: Sage.
52. Applebaum PS, Robbins PC Monahan J (2000) Violence and delusions: data from the MacArthur Violence Risk Assessment Study. *American Journal of Psychiatry* **157**: 566–72.
53. Link BG, Stueve A (1994) Psychotic symptoms and violent/illegal behaviour of mental patients compared to community controls. In J Monahan, HJ Steadman (eds) *Violence in Mental Disorder: Developments in Risk Assessment*. Chicago, IL: University of Chicago Press.
54. Steadman HJ, Mulvey EP, Monahan J, *et al.* (1998) Violence by people discharged from acute psychiatric inpatient facilities and others in the same neighbourhoods. *Archives of General Psychiatry* **55**: 393–401.
55. Royal College of Psychiatrists Special Working Party on Clinical Assessment and Management of Risk (1996) *Assessment and Clinical Management of Risk and Harm to Other People*. Council report CR53. London: Royal College of Psychiatrists.
56. Kvaraceus W (1966) *Dangerous Youth*. Columbus, OH: Columbus Press.
56a. Fazel S, Långström N, Hjern A, Grann M, Lichtenstein P (2009) Schizophrenia, substance abuse, and violent crime. *Journal of the American Medical Association* **301**: 2016–23.
57. Puri BK, Counsell SJ, Hamilton G, *et al.* (2004) Cerebral metabolism in male patients with schizophrenia who have seriously and dangerously offended: a 31P magnetic resonance spectroscopy study. *Prostaglandins, Leukotrienes and Essential Fatty Acids* **70**: 409–11.
58. Puri BK, Counsell SJ, Saeed N, *et al.* (2008) Regional grey matter volumetric changes in forensic schizophrenia patients: an MRI study comparing the brain structure of patients who have seriously and violently offended with that of patients who have not. *BMC Psychiatry* **8** (suppl. 1): S6.
59. Treasaden IH, Puri BK (2008) Cerebral spectroscopic and oxidative stress studies in patients with schizophrenia who have dangerously violently offended. *BMC Psychiatry* **8** (suppl. 1): S7.
60. Appleby L, Shaw J, Amos T, *et al.* (1999) *Safer Services: Report of the National Confidential Inquiry into Suicide and Homicide by People with Mental Illness*. London: The Stationery Office.
61. Appleby L, Shaw J, Sherratt J, *et al.* (2001) *Safety First: Report of the National Confidential Inquiry into Suicide and Homicide by People with Mental Illness*. London: The Stationery Office.
62. Shaw J, Hunt IM, Flynn S, *et al.* (2006) Rates of mental disorder in people convicted of homicide: a national clinical survey. *British Journal of Psychiatry* **188**: 143–7.
63. Shaw J, Amos T, Hunt IM, *et al.* (2004) Mental illness in people who kill strangers: longitudinal study and national clinical survey. *British Medical Journal* **328**: 734–7.
64. Maden A (2007) *Treating Violence: A Guide to Risk Management in Mental Health*. Oxford: Oxford University Press.
65. Webster CD, Douglas KS, Eaves D, Hart SD (1997) *HCR-20: Assessing Risk of Violence*, version 2. Vancouver: Mental Health, Law and Policy Institute, Simon Fraser University.
66. Department of Health (1994) *Guidance on the Discharge of Mentally Disordered People and their Continuity of Care in the Community*. HSG (94) 27. London: NHS Executive.
67. Ritchie J, Dick D Lingham R (1994) *The Report of the Inquiry into the Care and Treatment of Christopher Clunis*. London: HMSO.
68. Department of Health (1990) *The Care Programme Approach for People with a Mental Illness Referred to the Specialist Psychiatric Services*. London: HMSO.
69. NHS Management Executive (1994) *Introduction of Supervision Registers for Mentally-Ill People from 1 April 1994*. Leeds: NHSME.
70. Royal College of Psychiatrists (1998) *Clinical Practice*

Guidelines For The Management Of Imminent Violence. London: Royal College of Psychiatrists.
71. American Psychiatric Association (2000) *Diagnostic and Statistical Manual of Mental Disorders*, 4th edn, text revision. Washington, DC: American Psychiatric Association.
72. Christenson GA, Faber RJ, de Zwaan M, *et al.* (1994) Compulsive buying: descriptive characteristics and psychiatric comorbidity. *Journal of Clinical Psychiatry* **55**: 5–11.
73. Grant JE, Levine L, Kim D, Potenza MN (2005) Impulse control disorders in adult psychiatric inpatients. *American Journal of Psychiatry* **162**: 2184–8.
74. Gibbens TCN, Prins J (1962). *Shoplifting*. London: Institute for the Study and Treatment of Delinquency.
75. Topp DO (1973) Fire as a symbol and weapon of death. *Medicine, Science and the Law* **13**: 79–86.
76. Neustatter WL (1953) *Psychological Disorder and Crime*. London: Christopher Johnson.
77. Stinchfield R (2003) Reliability, validity and classification accuracy of a measure of DSM-IV diagnostic criteria for pathological gambling. *American Journal of Psychiatry* **160**: 180–82.
78. Legg-England S, Gotestam KG (1991) The nature and treatment of excessive gambling. *Acta Psychiatrica Scandinavica* **84**: 113–20.
79. Raylu N, Oei TP (2002) Pathological gambling: a comprehensive review. *Clinical Psychology Review* **22**: 1009–61.
80. Moran E (1983) Gambling. In GFM Russell, LA Hersov (eds) *Handbook of Psychiatry 4: The Neuroses and Personality Disorders*. Cambridge: Cambridge University Press.
81. Wardle H, Sproston K, Orford J, *et al.* (2007) *British Gambling Prevalence Survey 2007*. London: National Centre for Social Research.
82. Dickerson MG (1988) The prevalence of excessive and pathological gambling in Australia. *Journal of Gambling Behaviour* **4**: 125–51.
83. Shaffer HJ, Korn DA (2002) Gambling and related mental disorders: a public health analysis. *Annual Review of Public Health* **23**: 171–212.
84. Potenza MN, Steinberg MA, McLaughlin SD, *et al.* (2001) Gender-related differences in the characteristics of problem gamblers using a gambling helpline. *American Journal of Psychiatry* **158**: 1500–505.
85. Freud S (1928) Dostoyevsky and parricide. In J Strachey (ed.) *The Complete Works of Sigmund Freud*. London: Hogarth Press.
86. Frosch WA, Frosch JP, Frosch J (1985). The impulse disorders. In R Michels, JO Cavenar (eds) *Psychiatry*, vol. 1. Philadelphia, PA: J.B. Lippincott.
87. Greenson R (1947) On gambling. *American Imago* **4**: 61.
88. Sharpe L (2002) A reformulated cognitive-behavioural model of problem gambling: a biopsychosocial perspective. *Clinical Psychology Review* **22**: 1–22.
89. Potenza MN, Leung HC, Blumberg HP, *et al.* (2003) An fMRI Stroop task study of ventromedial prefrontal cortical function in pathological gamblers. *American Journal of Psychiatry* **160**: 1990–94.
90. Driver-Dunkley E, Samanta J, Stacy M (2003) Pathological gambling associated with dopamine agonist therapy in Parkinson's disease. *Neurology* **61**: 422–3.
91. Lesieur H, Blume S (1987) The South Oaks Gambling Screen (SOGS): a new instrument for the identification of pathological gamblers. *American Journal of Psychiatry* **144**: 1184–8.
92. Gerstein D, Murphy S, Toce M, *et al.* (1999) *Gambling Impact and Behavior Study: Report to the National Gambling Impact Study Commission*. Chicago, IL: National Opinion Research Center.
93. Hodgins DC (2004) Using the NORC DSM screen for gambling problems as an outcome measure for pathological gambling: psychometric evaluation. *Addictive Behaviors* **29**: 1685–90.
94. Stinchfield R (2002) Reliability, validity, and classification accuracy of the South Oaks Gambling Screen (SOGS). *Addictive Behaviors* **27**: 1–19.
95. Ferris J Wynne H (2001) *The Canadian Problem Gambling Index: Final Report*. Ottawa: Canadian Centre on Substance Abuse.
96. Slutske WS (2006) Natural recovery and treatment-seeking in pathological gambling: results of two US national surveys. *American Journal of Psychiatry*, **163**: 297–302.
97. Grant JE, Kim SW (2002) Effectiveness of pharmacotherapy for pathological gambling: a chart review. *Annals of Clinical Psychiatry* **14**: 155–61.
98. Petry NM, Roll JM (2001) A behavioral approach to understanding and treating pathological gambling. *Seminars in Clinical Neuropsychiatry* **6**: 177–83.
99. Dickerson MG (1989) Gambling: dependence without a drug. *International Review of Psychiatry* **1**: 157–72.
100. Goudriaan AE, Oosterlaan J, De Beurs E, Van Den Brinic W (2008) The role of self-reported impulsivity and reward sensitivity versus neurocognitive measures of disinhibition and decision-making in the prediction of relapse in pathological gamblers. *Pathological Medicine* **38**: 41–50.
101. Bondolfi G, Jermann F, Ferroero F, *et al.* (2008) Prevalence of pathological gambling in Switzerland after the opening of casinos and the introduction of new preventative legislation. *Acta Psychiatrica Scandinavica* **117**: 236–9.
102. Freud S (1932) The acquisition of power over fire. *International Journal of Psycho-Analysis* **13**: 405–10.
103. Puri BK, Baxter R, Cordess CC (1995). Characteristics of firesetters: a study and proposed multiaxial psychiatric classification. *British Journal of Psychiatry* **166**: 393–6.

104. Ritchie EC, Huff TG (1999) Psychiatric aspects of arsonists. *Journal of Forensic Science* **44**: 733–40.
105. Soothill K, Pope PJ (1973) Arson: a twenty-year cohort study. *Medicine, Science and the Law* **13**: 127–38.
106. Sapsford RJ, Banks C, Smith DD (1978) Arsonists in prison. *Medicine, Science and the Law* **13**: 247–54.
107. McElroy ES, Pope HJ, Jr, Hudson N (1991) Kleptomania: a report of 20 cases. *American Journal of Psychiatry* **148**: 652–7.
108. Lejoyeux M, Arbarataz M, McLoughlin M, Adès J (2002) Impulse control disorders and depression. *Journal of Nervous and Mental Diseases* **190**: 310–14.
109. Grant JE, Correia S, Brennan-Krohn T (2006) White matter integrity in kleptomania: a pilot study. *Psychiatric Research* **147**: 233–7.
110. Cupchik W, Atcheson JD (1983) An occasional crime of the moral majority. *Bulletin of the American Academy of Psychiatry and the Law* **11**: 343–52.
111. Gudjonsson GH (1990) Psychological and psychiatric aspects of shoplifting. *Medicine, Science and the Law* **30**: 45–51.
112. Buckle A, Farrington DP (1984) An observational study of shoplifting. *British Journal of Criminology* **24**: 63–73.
113. Bluglass R (1990) Shoplifting. In R Bluglass, P Bowden (eds) *Principles and Practice of Forensic Psychiatry*. Edinburgh: Churchill Livingstone.
114. Lamontagne Y, Carpentier N, Hetu C, Lacerte-Lamontagne C (1994) Shoplifting and mental illness. *Canadian Journal of Psychiatry* **39**: 300–302.
115. Walsh KH, McDougall CJ (2001) Tricotillomania: presentation, etiology, diagnosis and therapy. *American Journal of Clinical Dermatology* **2**: 327–33.
116. Kempe CH, Kempe RS (1978) *Child Abuse*. London: Fontana.
117. D'Orban PT, Haydn-Smith P (1985) Men who steal children. *British Medical Journal* **290**: 1784.
118. D'Orban PT (1976) Child stealing: a typology of female offenders. *British Journal of Criminology* **16**: 275–81.
119. Pizzey E (1974) *Scream Quietly or the Neighbours Will Hear*. London: Penguin.
120. MacMillan HL, Wathen N, Jamieson E, *et al.* (2006) Approaches to screening for intimate partner violence in healthcare settings: a randomised trial. *Journal of the American Medical Association* **296**: 530–36.
121. Renvoize J (1978) *Web of Violence*. London: Routledge & Kegan Paul.
122. Mowat RR (1966) *Morbid Jealousy and Murder*. London: Tavistock Publications.
123. Menzies RP, Federoff JP, Green CM, Isaacson K (1995) Prediction of dangerous behaviour in male erotomania. *British Journal of Psychiatry* **166**: 529–36.
124. Mullen PE, Pathe M, Purcell R (2000) *Stalkers and Their Victims*. Cambridge: Cambridge University Press.
125. Bursten B (1965) On Munchausen's syndrome. *Archives of General Psychiatry* **13**: 261.
126. Meadow R (1982) Munchausen's syndrome by proxy. *Archives of Disease in Childhood* **57**: 92–8.
127. Meadow R (1989) Munchausen's syndrome by proxy. *British Medical Journal* **299**: 248–50.
128. Jones G, Berry M (1986) Regional secure units: the emerging picture. In G Edwards (ed.) *Current Issues in Clinical Psychology IV*. London: Plenum.
129. McGovern D, Cope R (1987) The compulsory detention of males of different ethnic groups with special reference to offender patients. *British Journal of Psychiatry* **150**: 505–12.
130. Cope R, Ndegwa D (1990) Ethnic differences in admission to a regional secure unit. *Journal of Forensic Psychiatry* **1**: 365–78.
131. Fitzgerald M (1993) *Ethnic Minorities and the Criminal Justice System*. Royal Commission on Criminal Justice research study 20. London: HMSO.
132. Lipsedge M (1994) Dangerous stereotypes. *Journal of Forensic Psychiatry* **5**: 14–19.
132a. Norfolk, Suffolk and Cambridgeshire Strategic Health Authority (2003) *Independent Inquiry into the Death of David Bennett: An Independent Inquiry Set Up under HSG(94)27*. Cambridge: Norfolk, Suffolk and Cambridgeshire Strategic Health Authority.
132b. Gunn J (1977) *Epileptics in Prison*. London: Academic Press.
133. Fazel S, Vassos E, Danesh J (2002) Prevalence of epilepsy in prisoners: a systematic review. *British Medical Journal* **324**: 1495.
134. Gunn J, Maden A, Swinton M (1991) Treatment needs of prisoners with psychiatric disorders. *British Medical Journal* **303**: 338–41.
135. Derro R (1978) Admission health evaluation of inmates of a city-county workhouse. *Minnesota Medicine* **61**: 333–7.
136. Bluglass R (1966) A psychiatric study of scottish convicted prisoners. University dissertation. St Andrews: University of St Andrews.
137. Maden A, Swinton M, Gunn J (1994) Psychiatric disorder in women serving a prison sentence. *British Journal of Psychiatry* **164**: 44–54.
138. Robertson R, Bankier R, Schwartz L (1987) The female offender: a Canadian study. *Canadian Journal of Psychiatry* **32**: 749–55.
139. Swank G, Winer D (1976) Occurrence of psychiatric disorder in a country jail population. *American Journal of Psychiatry* **133**: 1331–3.
140. Agbahowe S, Ohaeri J, Ogunlesi A, Osahon R (1998) Prevalence of psychiatric morbidity among convicted inmates in a Nigerian prison community. *East African Medical Journal* **75**: 19–26.
141. Hindler CG (1989) Epilepsy and violence. *British Journal of Psychiatry* **155**: 246–9.
142. Grubin DH (1991) Unfit to plead in England and Wales

1976–1988: a survey. *British Journal of Psychiatry* **158**: 540–48.

143. Cleckley H (1982) *The Mask of Sanity*. St Louis, IL: Mosby.

143a. Lees J, Manning N, Rawling B (1999) *Therapeutic Community Effectiveness: A Systematic International Review of Therapeutic Community Treatment of People with Personality Disorders and Mentally Disordered Offenders. CRD Report 17*. NHS Centre for Reviews and Dissemination. York: University of York.

143b. Warren F, Preedy-Fayers IC McGauley G (2003) *Review of Treatment for Severe Personality Disorders*. Home Office. On-line report 30/03. London: Home Office.

143c. Linehan MM (1993) *Cognitive-Behavioural Treatment of Borderline Personality Disorder*. New York: Guilford Press.

143d. Lineham MM (1993) *Skills Training Manual for Treatment of Borderline Personality Disorder*. New York: Guilford Press.

144. Raine A, Lencz T, Bihrle S, *et al.* (2000) Reduced prefrontal grey matter volume and reduced autonomic activity in antisocial personality disorder. *Archives of General Psychiatry* **57**: 119–27.

145. Kiehl KA, Smith AM, Mendrek A, *et al.* (2004) Temporal lobe abnormalities in semantic processing by criminal psychopaths as revealed by functional magnetic resonance imaging. *Psychiatry Research* **130**: 297–12.

146. Blair RJ (2005) Applying a cognitive neuroscience perspective to the disorder of psychopathy. *Developmental Psychopathology* **17**: 865–91.

147. Dolan B, Coid J (1993) *Psychopathic and Antisocial Personality Disorders: Treatment and Research Issues*. London: Gaskell.

148. Losel F (1998) Treatment and management of psychopaths. In DJ Cooke, AE Forth, RD Hare (eds) *Psychopathy: Theory, Research and Implications for Society*. Dordrecht: Kluwer.

148a. Gunn J, Robertson G (1982) An evaluation of Grendon Prison. In J Gunn, DP Farrington (eds) *Abnormal Offenders, Delinquency and the Criminal Justice System*. Chichester: John Wiley.

149. TBS (1991) *A Special Measure within the Criminal Code*. Leiden: Zorn Publishing.

150. WODC (2006) *Outpatient Supervision Programs for Forensic Psychiatric Patients after an Intramural Punishmentor Measure: a Systematic Review*. The Hague: Ministerie van Justitie: Buiten Behandeling.

151. Treasaden IH, Weller M (2004) An update on managing dangerous people with severe personality disorder: 'the Human Timebombs'. *Medico-Legal Journal* **72**: 105–10.

152. Madden A (2007) Dangerous and severe personality disorder: antecedants and origins. *British Journal of Psychiatry* **190**: S8–11.

153. Birmingham L, Mason D, Grubin D (1998) A follow-up study of mentally disordered men remanded to prison. *Criminal Behaviour and Mental Health* **8**, 202–13.

154. Department of Health (2001) *Changing the Outlook: A Strategy for Developing and Modernising Mental Health Services in Prisons*. London: Department of Health.

155. National Offender Management Service (2006) *The NOMS Offender Management Model*. London: Home Office.

156. Department of Health (2007) *National Partnership Agreement between the Department of Health and the Home Office for the Accountability and Commissioning of Health Services for Prisoners in Public Sector Prisons in England*. London: Department of Health.

157. HM Prison Service (2005) *Safer Custody Group: The ACCT Approach – Caring for People At Risk in Prison*. London: HM Prison Service.

158. Fazel S, Danesh J (2002) Serious mental disorder in 23 000 prisoners: a systematic review of 62 surveys. *Lancet* **359**: 545–50.

159. Birmingham L (2004) Mental disorder and prisons. *Psychiatric Bulletin* **28**: 393–7.

159a. Bradley KJC (2009) *The Bradley Report. Review of People with Mental Health Problems or Learning Disabilities in the Criminal Justice System*. London: Department of Health.

160. Maden A, Taylor CJA, Brooke D, Gunn J (1995) Mental disorder in remand prisoners. London: Institute of Psychiatry.

161. Singleton N, Meltzer H, Gateward R, Coid J, Deasy D (1998) *Psychiatric Morbidity Among Prisoners in England and Wales: The Report of a Survey Carried Out in 1997 by the Social Survey Division of the Office of National Statistics on Behalf of the Department of Health*. London: The Stationery Office.

162. O'Brien M, Mortimer L, Singleton N, Meltzer H, Goodman R (2003) Psychiatric morbidity among women prisoners in England and Wales. *International Review of Psychiatry* **15**: 153–7.

163. Fazel S, Hope T, O'Donnell I, Jacoby R (2001) Hidden psychiatric morbidity in elderly prisoners. *British Journal of Psychiatry* **179**: 535–9.

164. Gunn J, Taylor P (1993) *Forensic Psychiatry: Clinical, Legal and Ethical Issues*. London: Butterworth Heinemann.

165. Collins J, Bailey S (1990) Traumatic stress disorder and violent behaviour. *Journal of Traumatic Stress* **3**: 203–20.

Chapter 77

Legal aspects of psychiatric care, with particular reference to England and Wales

Ian Treasaden

INTRODUCTION

Psychiatry and the law are connected. The law must protect not only the patient but also society, and this raises the problem of individual liberty of the patient (the autonomy of the patient, e.g. concerning consent) versus, among other matters, the compulsory treatment of patients against their wishes (the duty of care of the doctor, e.g. to avoid negligence) – that is, the dilemma between the compulsory care and treatment of mentally disordered people and their rights. This balance has varied through history and varies between countries.

Law

Law is the body of rules sanctioned formally by parliament and the courts and administered by legal fora. It is important to distinguish psychiatric terms and diagnosis, such as schizophrenia, from legal concepts, such as not only particular crimes but also legal diagnostic categories, for example abnormality of mind, giving rise to diminished responsibility, and mental disorder. For instance, the legal concept of psychopathic disorder used in the Mental Health Act 1983 before it was amended by the Mental Health Act 2007 did not equate to the clinical diagnosis of psychopathy. Morality also does not equate with legality, and vice versa.

Legal sources

Common law arises out of common customs developed by judicial court decisions. This results in the law continuously evolving through precedents and exceptions established in court.

Statute law arises from Acts of Parliament. Statute law trumps and sits upon common law.

Equity refers to the principles of justice in cases not covered by statute or common law.

Legal fields

In *criminal law*, the state initiates proceedings on behalf of society against an individual where Parliament and other courts have defined an activity as a crime. It includes the offences of murder and manslaughter on grounds of diminished responsibility.

Civil law relates to citizens' rights and civil wrongs and involves one individual against another as regards any matter defined by parliament or the courts as civil, including the Mental Health Act 1983.

The law courts (legal fora)

Criminal courts

Criminal courts include the following:

- *Magistrates' courts* deal with over 98 per cent of all criminal prosecutions in England and Wales – hence, the usefulness of psychiatric magistrate court division schemes. They try cases 'summarily' – that is without a jury
- *Crown Courts* include the Central Criminal Court (the Old Bailey). They are for more serious indictable offences, where cases are tried by a jury
- *Appeal Courts (criminal division)* e.g. the Courts of Justice in the Strand
- The Supreme Court of the UK, which replaced the House of Lords (Judicial Committee) in 2009.

The UK system of law is adversarial (in contrast to many European inquisitorial systems, which are based on the Napoleonic Code). If called to give evidence, for example by the defendant's legal advisors, then a witness will initially undergo an examination-in-chief by the legal advisors, followed by cross-examination, in this case by the prosecution, and then a re-examination. It is important for doctors not to overstate their professional views and for them to indicate clearly the limits of their opinion and in what areas they cannot comment. In most cases, a psychiatrist is able to give his or her opinion to the court in a report. Oral evidence is usually required only where there is dispute regarding medical evidence, for example over diminished responsibility, or where oral evidence is legally required, for example in supporting an individual being made subject to restrictions under Section 41 of the Mental Health Act 1983 in England and Wales.

A magistrate should be addressed as 'your worship', a judge in a Crown Court as 'your honour' and a High Court judge as 'my lord'. Barristers address a judge as 'my lud', a fellow barrister as 'my learned friend' and a solicitor as 'my friend'.

Civil courts

Civil cases are dealt with mainly by County Courts, although a few matters are heard in magistrates' courts, for example domestic cases such as maintenance payments. More serious cases are heard in the High Court, including the Courts of Justice in the Strand in London. In County Courts and High Courts, the case is usually heard before a single judge and only rarely in front of a jury, for example in cases of defamation The single judge when sitting without a jury will therefore decide on both the facts and the law.

The High Court is divided as follows:

- The Queen's Bench Division, which deals with most cases such as contracts and damage
- The Chancery Division, which deals with financial matters, company law, tax, trusts and wills
- The Family Division, which deals with adoption, divorce and wardship.

There is also an Appeal Court.

The Supreme Court of the UK, which replaced the House of Lords in 2009 as the final UK civil court, considers appeals on grounds of points of law only.

In civil courts the plaintiff seeks 'remedy' to alleged injuries such as damage, including psychiatric damage. Damages are to compensate, not punish – hence, damages will be greater for brain damage than for death. Nominal damages may be awarded, for example if a bad reputation is not damaged further by libel or slander. The Criminal Compensation Board is a civil court. Most civil cases are settled before they come to court or at the court before a hearing. The defendant will pay the costs if he or she pursues a case to a court hearing and is not awarded a sum greater than a settlement offered before the court hearing.

Appeals can be made to the European Court of Justice on points of European Law and on questions of citizens' rights.

Civil psychiatric court reports

Psychiatrists are usually placed under greater scrutiny in civil than criminal cases, and their evidence is more often discredited. It is often prudent to refer to accepted classifications such as the tenth revision of the *International Classification of Diseases* (ICD-10), e.g. severe, moderate or mild depressive episode, and the fourth edition of the *Diagnostic and Statistical Manual of Mental Disorders* (DSM-IV), although the court will take note of a psychiatrist's experience if a case is atypical. The prognosis in civil cases is usually very important with regard to damages.

Juvenile courts

These deal with juvenile criminal and care/residence order proceedings.

A juvenile court is composed of a special panel of three magistrates, one of whom is usually a woman. The defendant's name must not be disclosed by newspapers or other media without the court's permission.

Coroners' courts

Coroners should be called 'sir' when being addressed. If a coroner 'invites' you to attend, then attendance is mandatory. It is the court most often attended by the medical profession. Under Rule 22, the verdict must not be framed in a way to determine civil liability.

Mental health review tribunals

These tribunals are quasi-judicial courts. Their decisions can be appealed against at the High Court Queen's Bench Division, and subsequently in courts above.

Note the difference in burden of proof between criminal courts (beyond reasonable doubt) and civil courts (on the balance of probabilities). For example, an individual may be found not guilty of criminal paedophile offences but may have his children removed from him by a civil court.

PSYCHIATRIC OPINIONS IN CIVIL LAW (CIVIL CAPACITY)

The burden of proof in such matters is on the balance of probabilities.

Issues of mental fitness

Contracts

Contracts require free full consent. If an individual is of unsound mind (not equivalent to being detained under the Mental Health Act 1983) at the time of making a contract, then that contract is regarded as void. However, 'mentally incapable' people are bound by contracts unless the other party or parties to the contract knew or should have known of the individual's incapacity. Under employment law an individual can be dismissed only for behavioural effects of mental disorder, not for mental disorder itself.

Testamentary capacity

This is the ability to make a valid will. To do this in the UK, individuals must be over the age of 18 years and not be of 'unsound mind'.

This becomes an issue either at the time the individual

makes a will, where a solicitor may ask for medical, including psychiatric, advice, or after the individual's death. Accurately assessing the capacity of a person to make a will would prevent the current high levels of litigation in this area.[1]

If a patient decides to make a will, then they may ask the doctor attending them to witness the will, particularly if the patient is seriously ill. Doctors should be aware they will be regarded in law as not acting as mere lay witnesses. If a doctor does agree to witness the will, then he or she is said to have 'attested the will', which implies that the doctor considers the patient to be of 'sound disposing mind and memory'. This is most often undertaken by a general medical practitioner rather than a psychiatrist. If the will is subsequently contested, the doctor may be required to appear in court to give evidence about the patient's mental state at the time the patient made the will.

Although not specifically defined in law, to have a 'sound disposing mind' by custom (based on Banks *v.* Goodfellow (1870)), the individual must:

- know the nature and extent of his property, although not necessarily the details;
- know all people and their names having a claim on his bounty, and the relative strength of their claim (e.g. bearing on the distribution between people);
- have no morbid state of mind that might distort his or her natural feelings and influence his or decisions;
- have the ability to realize the nature of a will and its consequences;
- be able to express him- or herself clearly and without ambiguity.

The presence of mental disorder, such as mild dementia, does not necessarily affect testamentary capacity, although if the will is complex it may do so. Testamentary capacity, however, may be severely affected if the individual has paranoid delusions about an individual who would normally be considered to have a claim on his or her property. The 1826 case of Dew *v.* Clark established, however, that even if one was deluded (in this case, believing he was being pursued by evil spirits), this did not necessarily preclude an individual from having testamentary capacity.

If an individual dies having left a will, then they die 'testate' and a grant of probate enables the executor or trustee to administer the will. Wills must be in writing, except if on 'actual military service'. Wills must be made without force, fear, fraud and undue influence. A person making a will is a testator or testatrix. The similarity of such words to testes is not by chance. The ancient Romans swore oaths by placing their fingers on the testes. The relevant law is the Administration of Estates Act 1982.

Marriage

Marriage is a contract, so that if an individual has a mental disorder at the time so as not to appreciate the nature of the contract, then that contract is 'voidable' (not void). Lack of valid (competent) consent is rare, as most mentally disordered individuals appreciate the nature of marriage.

A marriage may be annulled if:

- one partner has a mental disorder at the time of the marriage so as not to appreciate the nature of the contract;
- one partner did not disclose that he or she had epilepsy or a communicable venereal disease;
- either party was under 16 years of age at the time of marriage;
- pregnancy by another male at the time of marriage was not disclosed;
- there was non-consummation (no intromission of the penis);
- one of the partners was forced to agree to the marriage under duress.

Marriage continues until challenged successfully in the courts by one of the parties, resulting in the marriage being deemed 'voidable'.

Legal capacity to marry is different from the legal capacity to have sexual relations.

Apart from an inability to give valid competent consent, an individual may be deemed, even if he or she can give valid consent, as unable to marry due to '*unfitness for marriage*' – that is, having a mental disorder in terms of the definition of the Mental Health Act 1983, resulting in an incapacity to carry out the ordinary duties of marriage (not just be 'difficult to live with'). For a marriage to be 'voidable' on such grounds, the individual must be incapable of living in a married state or carrying out the ordinary duties of marriage. Psychiatric grounds must be substantial. A registrar will only rarely refuse to marry on the basis of unfitness for marriage but will more commonly do so on the basis of incapacity to consent. Any person, including a doctor, may enter a 'caviat' pre-marriage with a superintendent registrar, who must then investigate it.

Sexual relationships between in-patients

Article 8 of the European Convention on Human Rights secures the right of all to respect for private and family life, which is taken to include sexual relationships between patients.

In practice, competent detained in-patients are not precluded from marriage, but secure hospitals, such as special hospitals in the UK (e.g. Broadmoor Hospital), have, on the basis of need for rules governing in-patients, successfully resisted to date the right of such in-patients to have provisions made for sexual relations between them.

The United Nations (UN) Declaration of Rights of Mentally Retarded Persons (1971) gives the right of mentally disabled people to live with their own family. It does not specifically refer to sexual relations, but it is taken to imply this.

It is illegal for male staff to have a sexual relationship with a patient, a male guardian with a subject of a guardianship order, and anyone with a patient with 'severe mental handicap' in the UK.

Divorce

This is covered by the Matrimonial Causes Act 1973. Mental disorder may affect the capacity to consent to divorce. Non-consensual divorce is achievable only on the basis of behaviour as specified in the Matrimonial Causes Act. Thus, mental disorder is the basis for divorce only when it results in the relevant legal behaviour – that is, adultery, unreasonable behaviour (which replaced the term 'cruelty'), desertion and living apart for more than 2 years if the respondent consents or for 5 years without consent (irretrievable breakdown). 'Quickie' divorces are based on filing affidavits, in contrast to divorces defended in court. Mental disorder most often leads to divorce by causing an irretrievable breakdown in marriage due to unreasonable behaviour.

Issues relating to the children of marriage following divorce are governed by 'supremacy of the interest of the child'. Separation/divorce usually results in residence, which replaced the term 'custody', of the children with the mother, unless, for example, mental disorder, among other factors, 'affects her capacity to love and care for the child'. Contact has replaced the term 'access', and the Child Support Agency has taken over many of the past roles of lawyers contesting financial issues related to childcare in court.

A Care Order (Children and Young Persons Act 1989) is taken out where a parent, or the parents, cannot safely care for the child – that is, on grounds of actual, or risk of, serious harm and this is attributable to care. Objective, especially current, behavioural evidence carries more weight than predicted behaviour in court.

Tort

This is a civil wrong to a person, a reputation or the estate of an individual, for example libel, slander, fraud, trespass, negligence or breach of copyright. Mentally disordered individuals are considered incapable of committing a tort unless the disorder does not preclude them understanding the nature or probable consequences of their acts. Defamation, which covers slander (spoken) and libel (written, but also includes spoken words on television, film or video), is not eligible for legal aid and is heard and adjudicated (e.g. amount of damages) by a jury – hence, the occasional huge damages in such cases awarded by a jury. Defences include 'justification', 'fair comment' and 'mere vulgar abuse'.

Mentally disordered people as witnesses

Mentally disordered individuals may give evidence in court or make a written statement, but it is for the magistrates or the judge to determine whether they are fit to do so and can understand the nature and obligation of the oath. To this end, medical evidence may be called for and the jury will have to consider how much weight to attach to the witness's evidence.

Certificate or report of sanity

This may be required for the purposes of a mental health review tribunal, when making a will, when signing legal documents or to rescind receivership.

Always read carefully and consider with great care any document given to you to sign, because of the risk of legal or professional General Medical Council (GMC) proceedings if you don't.

Power of attorney and enduring power of attorney

These remain legally valid if set up before the Mental Capacity Act 2005, which introduced the lasting power of attorney.

A power of attorney is a means whereby one person (the donor) gives legal authority to another person (the attorney or donee) to manage the donor's affairs.

An ordinary power of attorney is automatically revoked by law when the donor loses his or her mental capacity to manage and administer his or her own property and affairs, and accordingly the attorney's authority to act under the power then ceases.

Unlike an ordinary power of attorney, an *enduring power of attorney* (EPA; introduced in 1986 after the Enduring Powers of Attorney Act 1985) may continue in force after the donor has lost his or her mental capacity to manage and administer his or her financial affairs, provided it has been registered with the Public Trust Office.

Guardianship may be useful to help someone over age 16 years having difficulty with looking after themselves.

An *appointee* is someone authorized by the Department of Social Security in England and Wales to receive and administer benefits on behalf of someone else.

An *advocate* has no formal legal status.

Mental Capacity Act 2005 of England and Wales

The main provisions of this Act are as follows:

- *Designated decision-makers for people who lack capacity:*
  - Lasting power of attorney (LPA) – these are like EPAs but can make health and welfare decisions
  - Court appointed deputies – these replace receivership in the Court of Protection. They can make decisions on welfare, healthcare and financial matters, but they cannot refuse consent to life-sustaining treatment.
- *Two new public bodies:*
  - A new Court of Protection
  - A new Public Guardian will:
    - register LPAs and deputies;
    - supervise deputies;
    - be scrutinized by a Public Guardian Board.
- *Three provisions to protect vulnerable people:*
  - Independent mental capacity advocate (IMCA)
  - Advance decisions to refuse treatment, including, if expressly stated, 'even if life is at risk'
  - New criminal offence of ill-treatment or neglect of a person who lacks capacity.

Introduction into law

- IMCAs became available on 1 April 2007.
- The code of practice and the criminal offence of ill-treatment and wilful neglect became law in April 2007.
- From October 2007, all other elements of legislation, including the new Court of Protection, Public Guardian and Office of the Public Guardian, became operational.
- Deprivation of liberty safeguards (MCA DOLs) became law in April 2009.

Scope of the Act: exclusions under Section 27

No decision on the following is to be made on behalf of a person:

- Consent to marriage, civil partnership or sexual relations
- Consent to divorce/dissolution of a civil partnership on the basis of 2 years' separation
- Consent to a child being placed for adoption or making of an adoption order
- Discharging parental responsibilities in matters not relating to a child's property
- Consent under the Human Fertilisation and Embryology Act 1990.

Treatment of detained patients under the Mental Health Act 1983 is separate from the Mental Capacity Act. Mental Health Act 1983 consent to treatment provisions apply.

Capacity

A person may lack capacity:

- at the material time;
- if he or she is unable to make a decision for him- or herself in relation to the matter;
- because of an impairment of, or a disturbance in the functioning of, the mind or brain (Section 2).

It does not matter whether the impairment or disturbance is permanent or temporary.

Impairment or disturbance

The impairment or disturbance may occur in a wide range of situations ... people who are affected by ... alcohol or drug misuse ... delirium ... following head injury ... mental illness ... dementia ... learning disabilities ... long-term effects of brain damage ... grave physical conditions producing confusion, drowsiness or loss of consciousness including as a result of treatment [from the Code of Practice].

Able to make a decision?

Under Section 3, individuals should be able to :

- understand information relevant to the decision, including potential consequences of different decisions;
- retain that information for long enough to make a decision – not permanently;
- use that information to make a decision;
- communicate the decision, including by gesture or sign language.

A surprising or unwise decision does not of itself indicate lack of capacity.

Statutory principles

Under Section 1(1):

- everyone is assumed to have capacity, unless shown otherwise;
- no one is to be treated as unable to make a decision unless all practicable steps to assist have failed;
- a person is not to be treated as lacking capacity only because he or she makes an 'unwise' decision;
- any act or decision on behalf someone who lacks capacity must be done in his or her best interests;
- before any act, there must be consideration of whether the objective can be as well achieved in a less restrictive way.

Section 4: best interests

One must consider all the relevant circumstances, in particular the following:

- Involve the person if possible in any decision
- Other wishes/beliefs, made with capacity, or values that indicate preference
- Anyone already nominated, or any carers, etc., e.g. lasting power of attorney or court appointed deputy
- Likely to regain capacity? If so, when?
- Not to seek the subject's death where the decision relates to life-sustaining treatment; consider whether is in the best interests of the person concerned. ('Life-sustaining treatment' is treatment that the provider clinician considers necessary to sustain life.)

Section 4(a): a reasonable belief

There is sufficient compliance with the best interests requirement if (having complied with the requirements of Section 4) the person making the determination reasonably believes that what he or she does or decides is in the best interests of the person concerned.

New process for making decisions

- Advance decision (AD)
- Lasting power of attorney donee (LPA)
- Section 5
- Court of Protection or court appointed deputy (CAD).

Advance decisions (Section 24)

An AD is a decision made by an adult with capacity that if:

- at a later time a specified treatment is proposed to be carried out by a person providing health care; *and*
- at that time he or she lacks capacity to consent to that treatment,

then the specified treatment is not to be carried out or continued.

An AD is not necessarily binding if the following tests are met:

- *Capacity test:* if the person still has capacity to consent to the treatment proposed

- *Validity test:* if the person withdrew the AD at any time when able to do so, or has done anything clearly inconsistent with the AD
- *Applicability test:*
  - Not the treatment specified in the AD
  - Any specified circumstances are absent
  - Reasonable grounds for believing that important unforeseen circumstances exist, not anticipated at the time of the AD
- *Life-sustaining threshold:* an AD is not applicable to life-sustaining treatment unless it is verified by a statement to the effect that it is to apply to that treatment even if life is at risk, and the decision is in writing, signed and witnessed.

Lasting power of attorney (Section 9)

An LPA is a power under which the donor confers on a donee or donees authority to make decisions about:

- his or personal welfare or specific aspects thereof; and
- his or her property and affairs or specified aspects thereof.

This includes authority to make such decisions in circumstances where the donor no longer has capacity.

The authority conferred by an LPA is subject to:

- any conditions or restrictions specified in the document;
- the provisions of the Mental Capacity Act and, in particular, Section 1 (Principles) and Section 4 (Best Interests).

Section 5: liability for care or treatment

Where the Section 5 conditions are satisfied, someone who does an act 'in connection' with an incapacitated person's care or treatment will incur legal liability only if the act would have been unlawful if it was done with consent; as an example, negligent acts are not protected.

Section 5 conditions are as follows:

- The act is 'in connection with' care or treatment.
- The person doing it takes reasonable steps to establish whether the subject has capacity.
- The person reasonably believes that the subject lacks capacity.
- The person reasonably believes that the act is in the subject's best interests.
- If restraint is used, then the person reasonably believes that it is necessary to do the act in order to prevent harm to the subject *and* that the act is a proportionate response to the likelihood of the subject's suffering harm and the seriousness of that harm.

Restraint is the use, or threat of use, of force to achieve an outcome, or restriction of liberty of movement, whether or not resisted.

The Court of Protection and its elements

The Court is assisted by:

- the Public Guardian;
- the deputies;
- the Court of Protection visitors.

Section 16 powers of the court: where a matter concerns personal welfare or property and affairs, and a person lacks capacity in relation to it, then the court may decide the matter or appoint a deputy (CAD) to make decisions about where to live, contact with others and medical treatment

Powers of the court over property and affairs include:

- managing, buying and selling property;
- trade, profession, business and partnership matters;
- contracts and debts;
- wills and trust powers;
- legal proceedings.

Advocacy and Independent Advocacy Service (Section 35)

The appropriate authority must arrange for IMCAs to be available to support people to whom decisions proposed under Sections 37, 38 and 39 relate:

- *Section 37:* serious medical treatment
- *Section 38*: accommodation provision by National Health Service (NHS)
- *Section 39:* provision of accommodation by local authority.

Exceptions include where there is:

- a person nominated by the subject (in whatever manner) to be consulted in matters affecting his interests; or
- a donee of an LPA created by the subject;or
- a deputy appointed by the court (CAD) for the subject; or
- a donee of an EPA created by the subject under earlier legislation.

In such circumstances, the duty to consult an IMCA in relation to decisions under Sections 37–39 does not apply.

Deprivation of liberty safeguards

The Mental Health Act 2007 updated existing mental health legislation and was used as a vehicle for introducing the deprivation of liberty safeguards into the Mental Capacity Act 2005. The new safeguards provide a framework for the lawful deprivation of liberty of people who lack capacity to consent to arrangements made for their care or treatment in either a hospital or care home, and who need to be deprived of liberty in their own best interests in order to protect them from harm.

The Mental Capacity Act 2005 Deprivation of Liberty Safeguards (MCA DOLS) are a response to a European Court of Human Rights (ECtHR) judgment in October 2004 in the Bournewood case of HL *v.* UK. The court found that a man with autism and a learning disability, who lacked the capacity to decide about his residence and medical treatment, and who had been admitted informally to Bournewood Hospital, was unlawfully deprived of his liberty in breach of Article 5 of the European Convention on Human Rights (ECHR).

The MCA DOLS remedy to the breach of the ECHR is perceived as a major step towards better protecting the rights of vulnerable individuals in hospitals and care homes. They will make a big difference to the people in care who have no or only limited choice about their life. However, there is no doubt that implementing the safeguards will be challenging for care homes, primary care trusts (PCTs) and NHS trusts.

In the main, the people covered by the safeguards will be those with severe learning disabilities, older people with one of a range of dementias, and people with neurological conditions such as brain injury. The safeguards apply only to those people not covered by the Mental Health Act 1983.

The safeguards apply to people in hospitals, including independent hospitals, and care homes registered under the Care Standards Act 2000, whether they have been placed there by a PCT or a local authority or through private arrangements.

The MCA DOLS apply to people in hospitals and care homes who meet all of the following criteria. The person must:

- be aged 18 years or over;
- have a mental disorder such as dementia or a learning disability;
- lack capacity to consent to arrangements made for their treatment or care;

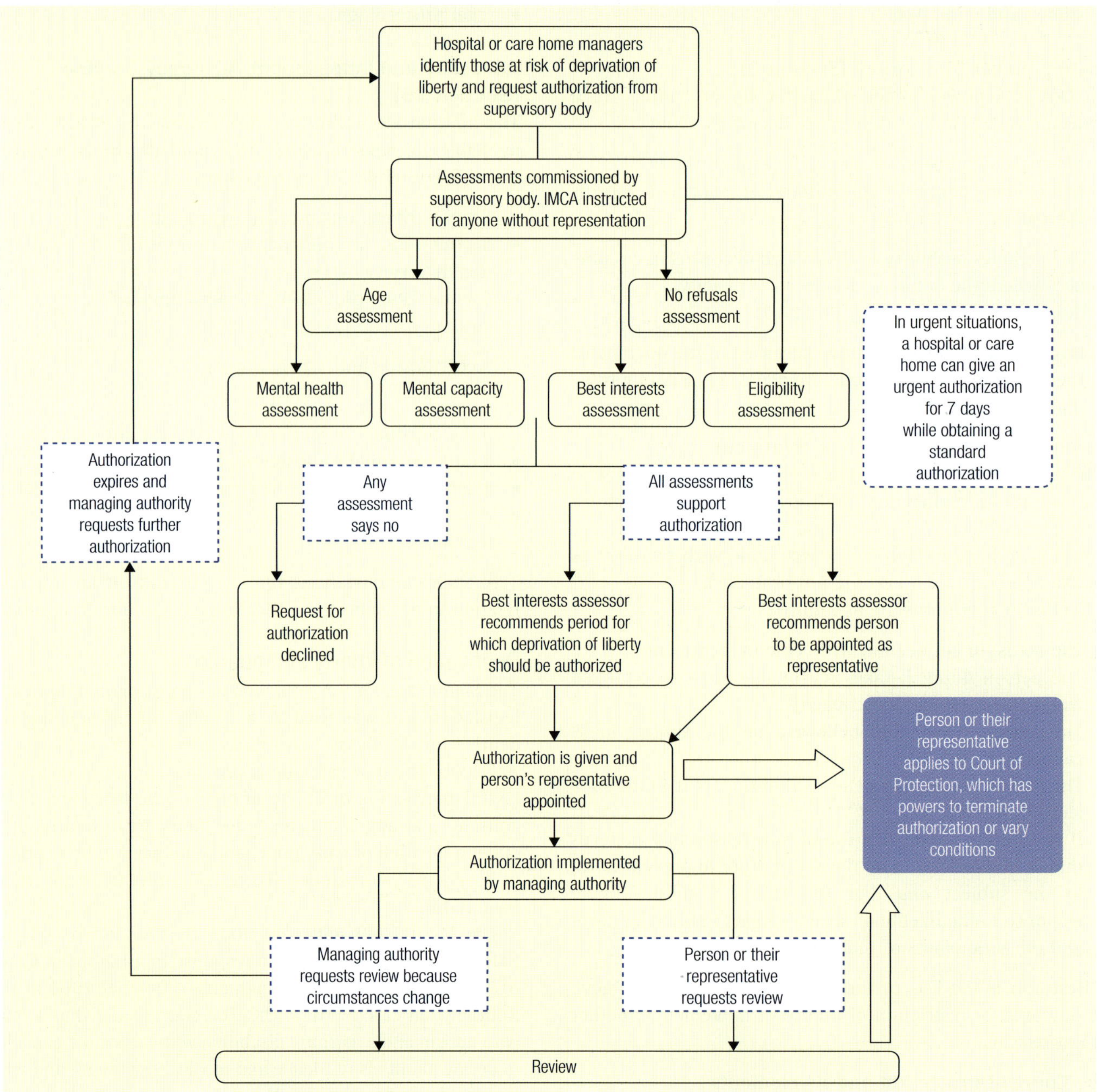

Figure 77.1 Overview of the deprivation of liberty safeguards process

Reproduced from Briefing 175: Mental Capacity Act 2005 Deprivation of Liberty Safeguards. NHS Confederation March 2009. London: NHS Confederation Publications.

- need to have their liberty taken away in their own best interests in order to protect them from harm.

Figure 77.1 gives an overview of the deprivation of liberty of safeguards process.

ISSUES OF PSYCHIATRIC DAMAGE

Normal ordinary emotional reactions such as grief are not eligible for compensation, but 'psychiatric damage' (legal term 'nervous shock') is. Issues regarding psychiatric damage have arisen in cases of post-concussional syndrome, accident and compensation neurosis, malingering, victims of torture, pathological grief and, since 1989, post-traumatic stress disorder, following the sinking in the English Channel of the ferry *Herald of Free Enterprise*. The vulnerability of the complainant is not relevant (e.g. an 'eggshell skull' is no defence) and the defendant must take the plaintiff as they find him or her. Dissociative (conversion) disorders constitute psychiatric damage, but malingering does not, although in practice there is a spectrum between these conditions and it is thus important to assess the degree of unconscious production of symptoms. In general, symptoms persist longer, the longer it takes to settle a case, regardless of whether there are issues of compensation or not.

Cases arising from the Hillsborough football stadium fire in Sheffield, England in 1988 led to rulings that symptoms are eligible for compensation if they result from the individual being directly subjected to the trauma, from seeing in real life a close (first-degree) but not a distant (e.g. nephew, fiancé) relative being killed, from seeing the killing of a close relative broadcast on television, and from hearing about this from a third person such as a police officer. Symptoms attributed to news about those not related, for example learned from the radio or from watching a recording of the disaster on a television programme, did not lead to compensation. In fact, police officers attending the scene were compensated before these cases were heard.

For psychiatric damage an individual must have a psychiatric illness. Psychiatric damage can be:

- secondary to physical sequelae, e.g. after loss of a limb;
- primarily psychological;
- psychological but secondary, such as witnessing the fate of another person, e.g. a lecturer having a heart attack.

A psychiatrist must define the mental disorder and give a prognosis, which is very important in cases of damage. The court then puts a 'tariff tag' on the disorder and prognosis.

Psychiatric negligence (a tort)

There are three elements:

- *A duty of care to a 'neighbour' (with whom the defendant has a natural relationship):* this applies to the NHS in the UK. If an individual is under private care, then he or she can also sue for breach of contract
- *Breach of duty of care:* this includes technical and advice errors
- *Damage to other party results:* i.e. foreseeable and would not have happened anyway.

The onus of proof is on the plaintiff to prove that a breach of duty of care caused damage.

An individual is usually judged by the standards of his or her professional peers or by a professional standard. Costs may result from nervous shock, cost of care and loss of work.

The following are some common causes of psychiatric negligence in order of frequency, according to UK medical defence societies:

- *Suicide or attempted suicide (50%):* this is due to failure of assessment or management. Proper care should have been present. If suicide is not prevented, then the presence of good operational suicide policies, documentation of suicide risk and management plans to counter it in the medical records, and the informing of all relevant staff, such as nursing staff, of the suicide risk will be defences.
- *Negligent use of drugs (30%):* this arises from the wrong drug being prescribed, the patient not being monitored properly or not being warned properly, or no proper consent procedure being followed. This arises particularly where drug toxicity results. For example, with lithium:
  - Delays in laboratory telling doctor result
  - Failure to check patient's thyroid and renal functioning
  - Failure to monitor blood levels
  - Most due to use of diuretics.
- *Misdiagnosis:* especially failure to diagnose organic disorders.

Other causes include homicide by a patient, sexual misconduct of a doctor, breach of confidentiality and lack of supervision (advice, instruction, monitoring and control), for example by a consultant of a trainee. In practice, a doctor should never have a relationship with even an ex-patient.

Cases are scrutinized to see whether 'reasonable care' compared with that of professional peers was present – that is, that the clinician used reasonable clinical judgement to weigh up the risks of illness, treated or untreated, and the risks of treatments or also alternative treatments and their risks.

An error of judgement or mistake becomes negligent if an individual did not exercise reasonable care.[2] Psychiatrists as a specialty consult medical defence associations frequently but are not among the medical specialties at high risk of litigation.

Negligence cases arise from:

- the dereliction of duty directly causing damage to plaintiff (the '4Ds' of US law);

- a bad outcome plus bad feelings, e.g. guilt, rage, grief, surprise.

It remains likely that, in spite of the current litigious culture, psychiatry is no different from other medical specialties in that, for every case of negligence brought, many more meritorious cases are not.

Medical records

If a risk is identified and documented, then it is incumbent on the psychiatrist to manage that risk and to record a management plan, for example to tell staff of the risk. The importance of good medical records is rightly emphasized as a way of countering litigation – 'if it's not recorded, it didn't occur'. However, psychiatrists will often have the opportunity to expand on their written records, for example if cross-examined in court. Merely recording the patient as saying that he or she is 'not homicidal' or 'not suicidal' in the records would not prevent successful litigation if other evidence suggested otherwise; for example, a suicidal patient may deny being at risk of suicide but clearly be at risk of committing suicide on the basis of admitted symptoms of severe depression. NHS medical continuation sheets have letters and numbers at the base of the page, which give some indication of the age of the sheet, and this can sometimes reveal when entries are made inappropriately after an adverse event.

LEGAL PRINCIPLES UNDERLYING MENTAL HEALTH LAW

In Western countries, mental health law originates from the efforts by the state in the early nineteenth century to protect the public from violent acts of 'mad' people. Subsequently, laws developed to protect vulnerable mentally ill individuals from their own neglect or self-harm and from abuse or exploitation by others.

Political ideology has influenced psychiatric services, even in the past 50 years; for example, in the Soviet Union, a diagnosis of 'slow schizophrenia' was used to detain political dissidents,[3] and in Italy 'Law No. 10' sought to close mental hospitals.

International declarations and principles relevant to the involuntary admission and treatment of mentally ill people include the following:

- *The European Convention for the Protection of Human Rights and Fundamental Freedoms (1953)*
- *United Nations Principles for the Protection of Persons with Mental Illness and for the Improvement of Mental Health Care (1991)*, and its international covenant on civil and political rights.

Cases brought by individuals against their governments at the Court of Human Rights in Strasbourg led to the committee of ministers of the Council of Europe enunciating further principles – Recommendations for the Legal Protection of Persons Suffering from Mental Disorders Placed as Involuntary Patients (1983).

Internationally approved principles include the following:

- Detention can only be by procedure defined in law.
- The individual or their representative must be informed of a decision to detain and the reasons for it.
- There should be a review of decisions to detain by an independent body, including independent from the state
- The individual has a right of appeal against detention.
- Mental disorder should not include social non-conformity alone.
- Mental disorder should be of sufficient severity to justify the initial deprivation of liberty and the continuation of detention.
- Detention should be reviewed at regular intervals.
- Circumstances and facilities of detention should be approved by law for that purpose, and such premises should be inspected regularly by an independent body.

Other issues highlighted have included the need for a legal framework to cover the following:

- Consent to treatment by detained patients
- Validity of detaining those for whom no effective treatment or resources exist
- Compulsory treatment in the community.

The World Health Organization (WHO) in 2003 described general principles for the development of mental health legislation.[4] These include the following:

- The 'least restrictive alternative' principle applies.
- If institutional treatment is required, then voluntary admission should be encouraged, with involuntary care being used only in exceptional circumstances.
- Information gathered should be treated as confidential.
- Free and informed consent to treatment should be available. Treatment without consent should be undertaken only in exceptional circumstances, for example involuntary patients lacking capacity to consent and where treatment is required to improve mental health or prevent deterioration in mental health or prevent risk of harm to self or others.
- The rights of involuntary patients are protected by rights of appeal against involuntary care and the ability to obtain a second opinion.
- Legislation should state explicitly the circumstances under which involuntary admission should be considered.
- Provision should be made for automatic independent review of involuntary admission or treatment.
- Guardians should be appointed for people not capable of making decisions.
- Involuntary treatment in the community should be considered.

Legislation may also lay down the framework for delivery of psychiatric services nationally, for example statutory requirements on local health authorities to provide services. Legislation alone generally does not improve services without corresponding funding. Legal safeguards should not be unworkable or exceedingly expensive and divert funding from services, and procedures should not be excessively detailed and impractical.

Deprivation of liberty is a major matter for any citizen, and such a human rights issue remains the most important issue in mental health legislation.

THE OVERLAP OF LEGAL AND ETHICAL CONSIDERATIONS IN PSYCHIATRY

Ethics

Ethics is a branch of philosophy. It is the science of the philosophy of morals. Ethics is concerned with which actions are right, which ends are good, whether the rightness of actions is inferable from the consequences, and whether the virtuousness of motives is inferred from the rightness of actions; for example, is it less bad to shoplift from a supermarket than from a corner shop, or for a person who repeatedly loses his temper to kill compared with one of previously good character who does so?

The word 'ethics' originates from the Greek *ethos* (nature, disposition) and the word 'morals' from the Latin *moris*, the generic form of *mos* (custom). Although the two words are often used synonymously, ethics is the science of the philosophy of morals, and morals is the practice or enactment of ethics. (Latin terms usually refer to real everyday matters, while Greek terms refer to an idealized theoretical understanding). Thus, ethics involves the analysis of universal principles on which decisions are made, while morals regulate day-to-day judgement and refer to particular actions and beliefs. The law is silent on many matters. Theoretically, morals should override political and legal requirements. The term 'moral' is, however, also tainted by association with immorality and sexual misconduct.

The interest in ethical aspects of psychiatry has increased rapidly in the past 20 years, especially concerning the rights of patients, particularly in their dealings with psychiatrists and particularly in the USA. This concern led directly to the Code of Practice being established as prescribed in the Mental Health Act 1983 of England and Wales.

Ethics may assist where there is uncertainty and assist in obtaining the best-quality judgements. It can help to distinguish facts from values and in elucidating roles and duties. Law may follow ethics, or ethics may follow law.

The four principles of ethical medical practice are:[5,6]

- *Autonomy:* respecting the patient's wishes.
- *Beneficence:* doing good.
- *Non-maleficence:* avoiding doing harm.
- *Justice:* fairness in the provision of care.

In practice, these principles often conflict and a balance has to be drawn. In medical ethics there is often a central conflict between the autonomy of the patient (e.g. concerning consent) and the duty of care of a doctor (e.g. negligence). Ethical dilemmas cannot therefore usually be solved by an algorithm.

Expert psychiatric reports

The Royal College of Psychiatrists states that expert psychiatric reports should be prepared only by a consultant psychiatrist or a trainee under a consultant psychiatrist's supervision – so, for example, not a prison medical officer. Reports should be independent, regardless of whether the psychiatrist has been instructed by the Crown Prosecution Service or a defence solicitor. The individual should be informed and warned that an interview to provide a court or similar report is not a normal medical interview, is not confidential, and may be used in sentencing and sent even if the subject does not cooperate. This is sometimes referred to as 'a contract of confidentiality'. However, the British Medical Association (BMA) states that doctors may properly refuse to examine subjects who do not wish to be examined. Problems arise if a psychiatrist is asked to compile a court report on a patient that the psychiatrist knew previously. The BMA advises doctors to make clear to the patient their two roles. It may be necessary to detail in the report only what took place in the interview for the report and not to refer, if the patient does not agree, to the past psychiatric history, and then to state explicitly that this is what has been done. Alternatively, it may be necessary to override the patient's wishes and to reveal the past psychiatric history, not only for reasons of public interest but also in the patient's own interest. It is important to distinguish findings, which should be objective and, ideally, agreed by all, from opinion. If reports are requested by a solicitor, then it is the solicitor's decision as to whether to use or make available the psychiatrist's report.

Judicial guidance for expert reports is shown in Box 77.1.

Ethics of predicting dangerousness

For a psychiatrist, ethical dilemmas may arise when recommending a Section 41 restriction order under the Mental Health Act 1983 of England and Wales in the case of a mentally disordered offender ('to protect the public from serious harm'), in Mental Health Review Tribunals, and, in the USA, in relation to the death penalty if an offender is a 'continuing threat to society'. Issues include the inaccuracy of prediction, the traditional medical ethic against the death

Box 77.1

JUDICIAL GUIDANCE ON EXPERT REPORTS

There have been a number of cases before the Court of Appeal in which expert evidence has been considered. Within the judgments the Court has provided judicial guidance on the content and presentation of expert reports.

In *R v Harris, Rock, Cherry and Faulder* [2005] EWCA Crim 1980, the Court stated:

(i) Expert evidence presented to the court should be and be seen to be the independent product of the expert, uninfluenced as to form or content by the exigencies of litigation.
(ii) An expert witness should provide independent assistance to the court by way of objective unbiased opinion in relation to matters within his expertise. An expert witness… should never assume the role of advocate.
(iii) An expert witness should state the facts or assumptions on which his opinion is based. He should not omit to consider material facts which detract from his concluded opinions.
(iv) An expert should make it clear when a particular question or issue falls outside his expertise.
(v) If an expert's opinion is not properly researched because he considers that insufficient data is available, then this must be stated with an indication that the opinion is no more than a provisional one.
(vi) If after exchange of reports, an expert witness changes his view on material matters, such change of view should be communicated to the other side without delay and when appropriate to the court.

In *R v Bowman* [2006] EWCA Crim 417, the Court went on to say that any such expert report must include:

(i) Details of the expert's academic and professional qualifications, experience and accreditation relevant to the opinions expressed in the report and the range and extent of the expertise and any limitations upon the expertise.
(ii) A statement setting out the substance of all the instructions received (whether written or oral), questions upon which an opinion is sought, the materials provided and considered, and the documents, statements, evidence, information or assumptions which are material to the opinions expressed or upon which those opinions are based.
(iii) Information relating to who has carried out measurements, examinations, tests, etc. and the methodology used, and whether or not such measurements etc. were carried out under the expert's supervision.
(iv) Where there is a range of opinion in the matters dealt with in the report, a summary of the range of opinion and the reasons for the opinion should be given. In this connection any material facts or matters which detract from the expert's opinion and any points which should fairly be made against any opinion expressed should be set out.
(v) Relevant extracts of literature or any other material which might assist the court.
(vi) A statement to the effect that the expert has complied with his/her duty to the court to provide independent assistance by way of objective unbiased opinion in relation to matters within his or her expertise and an acknowledgement that the expert will inform all parties and where appropriate the court in the event that his/her opinion changes on any material issues.
(vii) Where on an exchange of experts' reports matters arise which require a further or supplemental report the above guidelines should, of course, be complied with.

penalty, and that if a psychiatrist does not offer treatment but states that the patient is dangerous, this may result in prolonged detention in prison (e.g. people convicted of manslaughter rather than murder in England and Wales, on grounds of diminished responsibility, but who are not offered hospital treatment and who receive a life sentence, serve longer in prison than people convicted of murder[7]).

Ethics of assessing responsibility

Responsibility is a legal concept. It is questionable whether psychiatrists, who can make a valid diagnosis of mental disorder, can accurately assess responsibility, for example for reasons of diminished responsibility to reduce the charge from murder to manslaughter in homicide cases in England and Wales. Courts, however, may use psychiatric evidence in mitigating sentencing.

Ethics of detaining patients

Patients may have a right to be treated even against their will. In some countries and in certain states of the USA, it is more difficult to detain patients compared with the UK.

Ethics of consent

It is assumed, unless contested, that every adult has the right and the capacity (legal concept) (competence) to decide whether or not he or she will accept medical treatment, even if refusal risks permanent injury to health or premature death.[8]

In England and Wales it is illegal to treat without consent, except in an emergency in good faith or under the Mental Health Act 1983 Part IV. Legally if a patient is 'medically touched' without consent, this constitutes battery.

Consent should be informed and voluntary, which implies that mental disorder such as dementia does not affect judgement. In practice, a lower threshold for capacity is adopted for patients who consent to treatment compared with those who refuse. Refusal is not the same as lack of capacity to consent. It is important to never threaten to impose treatment if a patient refuses, and always to ensure that a patient is not simply consenting for a 'quiet life'. A distinction is to be made between coercion and a patient's acceptance of the reality of his or her situation.

Valid ethical consent requires competence and information, resulting in understanding. Understanding and voluntariness can then result in an affirmative decision.[9]

Regarding consent being based on sufficient information, to date the standard applied to this in the UK has been predominantly profession-based – that is, giving the level of information that is normally given by the profession in that medical situation based on the duty of care. The alternative standard is patient-based – that is, the level of information necessary in order to allow a patient to operate his or her autonomy. Information should refer to alternative treatments and advice about substantial or unusual risks. No or very little information given may result in the professional being liable to a charge of battery. Inadequate information may result in a doctor being held liable to a charge of negligence (breach of duty of care). 'Informed consent' is a US term and is not specifically enshrined in UK law.

A decision about consent may vary over time, and different messages may be given by the patient in different modalities.

A consent form is only evidence as to consent and does not amount to fact of consent.

The UK standard for sufficient information for valid consent is now closer to the US law – the *objective prudent patient test* (what a reasonable patient should be told) rather than the *reasonable doctor medical test* (profession-based) – due mainly to changing GMC guidelines.

Relevant case law from England and Wales includes the following:

- *Sidaway* v. *Board of Governors of Bethlem Royal and Maudsley Hospital (1985):* the majority of the five Law Lords supported the doctor-based standard of not telling of the 1 per cent risk of damage to spinal cord, after a neurosurgical procedure on the cervical vertebrae. However, the judgment suggested that if doctors were lax in informing patients, then the courts may intervene.
- *Bolam* v. *Friern Hospital Management Committee (1957):* the 'Bolam test' – a doctor is required to exercise the ordinary skills of a competent practitioner in the field (profession-based standard).
- *Maynard* v. *West Midlands RHA (1985* ***1*** *All ER 635):* even if the body of medical opinion cited is a minority, this may still be defendable.
- *Bolitho* v. *Hackney Health Authority (1997 All ER 771):* in order to avoid negligence, even if following a 'responsible body' of medical opinion, a doctor needs to convince the court that the amount of information given or omitted can be defended.

Courts are reluctant to put a percentage figure on risk of which a patient should be warned, as the individual significance of injury to the individual is also important. Always put a note of warnings given to the patient in the notes and in a letter to the patient's general practitioner (GP) (not the consent form).

Individuals under the age of 16 years can give valid consent if there is sufficient understanding. Parental consent is valid for individuals aged 16–18 years who do not understand.

Consent in English law for adults (aged ≥18 years) and minors

The following apply to competent adult patients:

- The patient may refuse any, including life-saving, treatment (otherwise battery).
- The patient should be given information about the nature of the procedure, any serious side effects, the likely benefits and alternatives (otherwise negligence).

For incompetent adult patients, the following principles apply:

- The doctor should act in the best interests of the patient.
- The patient's relatives and friends cannot give or withhold consent (they can only assent), but they may be sources of information regarding best interests.

For minors, the following points apply:

- A person under 18 years of age should not be allowed to come to serious harm on the grounds of the minor or the parents refusing consent to necessary and urgent treatment.
- Patients aged 16–17 years are presumed by statute to have the capacity to give consent, unless the contrary is shown.
- A child under age 16 years who does have capacity ('Gillick competent' in common law[10,11]) can give consent, but if the child refuses treatment consent can be overridden by the people with parental responsibility or a court.
- Courts are unlikely to consider that people aged 13 years or under have capacity.
- For children who are not Gillick competent, the people with parental responsibility give consent but have a legal obligation to act in the child's best interests.

Although psychiatric disorders can affect a patient's judgement and therefore capacity to consent, this can also occur in medical disorders, albeit less often.

The House of Lords has ruled that doctors have a common law duty (justification of necessity) to act in the best possible interests of the patient, for example if the patient is physically ill and not competent (e.g. unconscious) or if the patient is permanently unable to consent (e.g. due to severe learning disability) to treatments not covered by the Mental Health Act 1983.

Patients detained under the Mental Health Act 1983 may be able to give free valid consent to treatment, providing they are not complying simply to get out of hospital. The patient should know the nature and consequences of the proposed treatment, the consequences of not having the treatment, and the risks of the treatment.

Although some doctors argue that it would be negligent in the case of patients not consenting if one did not test for medical conditions suspected (i.e. duty of care), this is not accepted legally. Undertaking a human immunodeficiency virus (HIV)/acquired immunodeficiency syndrome (AIDS) test without the patient knowing the nature of such a test, and its personal and social implications, constitutes assault, even if the patient consented to give blood for unspecified or other tests.

Exceptions to usual requirements for consent

- *Implied consent:*
  - By fact of consultation
  - Patient's consent unavailable, but reasonable person would consent, e.g. unconscious patient after overdose
- *Necessity:*
  - Some level of patient incompetence and serious harm or death likely to occur
  - Doctor owes duty of care
- *Emergency:* to prevent serious harm to patient or other
- *Post-suicide attempt:* can reverse effects of suicide attempt (anachronism, as suicide was previously a crime), but can not stop a suicidal patient from leaving hospital if not detainable under the Mental Health Act 1983
- *Detention under Mental Health Act 1983.*

Capacity and competency

Capacity is a legal concept. Competency is clinical concept but is occasionally used legally. The terms mean the ability to know and understand the nature and consequences of legal proceedings, including for medical purposes.

Assessment of capacity

This is required in many branches of medicine, including psychiatry, for example:

- *Old-age psychiatry:*
  - Testamentary capacity
  - Power of attorney
  - Social care, e.g. sheltered home
- *Forensic psychiatry:* fitness to plead and stand trial
- *Liaison psychiatry:*
  - Treatment refusal
  - Leaving hospital without medical consent.

Capacity may vary over time, for example in delirium.

Legal principles relating to capacity

- An imprudent decision is not itself grounds for incapacity (analyse the way decision was made, not the decision itself).
- Capacity is function-specific, not global.
- Standard of proof is on the balance of probabilities.
- There are three stages of assessing capacity (Re C [1994] All ER 819):
  - Comprehension and retention of relevant information
  - Ability to believe information (e.g. no delusion interfering)
  - Weigh information and make decision.

Approaches to making decisions for incompetent patients

- Best interests
- Proxy
- Advance directive (living will)
- Substituted judgements (e.g. if patient became competent, what treatment would he or she choose?).

The final three of these are available in the Mental Capacity Act 2005.

British Medical Association and Law Society guidelines (1994) on assessing capacity

- Can the patient understand the nature and purpose of the procedure or treatment and why it is being proposed?
- Does the patient understand the principle benefits and risks, the alternatives, and the risks and consequences of not being treated?
- Capacity does not depend on detainability under the Mental Health Act 1983.
- Take into account the patient's anxiety, language problems and cultural and educational background.
- There is no relation to clinical reality, e.g. severity of illness if treatment is refused.

The MB test for capacity (1997) (needle phobia)

- Comprehend and retain information.
- Weigh information in balance and reach decision.

Patient attempts suicide and then refuses treatment in accident and emergency department

Theoretically, if competent, such a patient can refuse treatment. However, medical defence organizations in the UK comment that competence can always be questioned if an individual has harmed him- or herself, and so it is defendable to intervene. The common law justification of 'necessity' allows reasonable interventions, including medical treatments, reasonable to the circumstances, where the competence of the individual is unknown.

Case law propositions on medical treatment

Lord Donaldson MR in Re T (critically ill young woman) (adult refusal of medical treatment) (1994) 4 All ER 649 CA

Incapacity may be due to the following:

- Long-term mental incapacity or retarded development
- Temporary factors:
  - Unconsciousness
  - Confusion
  - Fatigue
  - Shock
  - Pain.

NB: in the case of MB (1997), with needle phobia, panic, indecisiveness and irritability were ruled not to be factors causing incapacity.

Capacity may be reduced, not removed (i.e. could be taught, not simply assessed). The patient's decision must be independent (e.g. from relatives and religious advisors).

Thorpe J, in Re C Adult Refusal of Medical Treatment (1994) 1 All ER 819

Refusal of treatment can be a declaration never to consent or never in some future circumstances, for example to electroconvulsive therapy (ECT) (equivalent to 'living will').

Advance directives are now legal under the Mental Capacity Act 2005; for example, the individual may state that, if mental illness relapses again, he or she wants no haloperidol, only risperidone, antipsychotic medication.

Consent obtained by coercion or duress invalid

Freeman *v.* Home Office (1983) All ER 589

Freeman claimed that his relationship as a prisoner with the prison doctor prevented valid consent due to his role in influencing disciplinary procedures. Issue was of covert, as opposed to overt, coercion instead of voluntary consent. The case was lost by Freeman.

Barbara *v.* Home Office (1984)

Barbara was injected in prison against his will. The case was won by Barbara.

Too much information may preclude patient making valid judgement

This was stated by Lord Templeman in Sidaway *v.* Board of Governors of Bethlem Royal and Maudsley Hospital (1985).

Medical treatment for mental disorder under Part IV of Mental Health Act 1983

Section 63

Consent is not required for medical treatments that do not fall within Section 57 or 58, for example nasogastric feeding of detained patient with borderline personality disorder refusing to eat ruled by Court of Appeal within scope of Section 63 (B *v.* Croydon Health Authority (1995) (1 All ER 683).

Section 145

Medical treatment includes nursing and also includes care, habilitation, and rehabilitation under medical supervision.

Wall J, in Thameside and Glossop Acute Services Trust *v.* UCH (1996) 1 FLR 792

Induction of labour and possible Caesarean section of a 41-year-old 38-week-pregnant woman with schizophrenia was ruled treatment within scope of Section 63. The woman consented to induction, but medical staff feared that she would change her mind. The decision was obtained on grounds (i) to prevent deterioration in the patient's mental state, (ii) that a live baby would promote the patient's health and (iii) that antipsychotic medication was contraindicated during pregnancy. However, the real issue is competence. Such decisions are often made in a rush, with the patient in labour and taking analgesics, so that 'not competent' is accepted. Also such cases are often heard in court often ex-parte with no representation of the individual (which does not prevent liability). Note that the Court of Appeal ruled in 1988 that a fetus is not a person with legal rights.

Re C (adult refusal of medical treatment) (1994)

C's gangrene was ruled not likely to affect his mental condition. C was a patient at Broadmoor Hospital and was deluded that he was a great doctor. He insisted on no amputation in the future and, in fact, he recovered.

Confidentiality

The BMA and the Royal College of Psychiatrists[12] state that the ideal ethical position is that doctors must protect any information acquired in the course of a doctor–patient relationship. The GMC accepts that this is not an absolute position and that doctors can reveal such information if there is an immediate grave risk to the patient or others ('risk of death or serious harm').[13] In other circumstances, a doctor should not reveal information until forced to do so, for example by a court order.[14]

The general duty regarding confidentiality is covered in guidelines e.g. from the GMC. Exceptions to confidentiality include the following:

- Court order
- Statute – by law for legal proceedings (all have strict narrow criteria for information that can be divulged):
  - Misuse of Drugs Law: notification of addicts
  - Road Traffic Act 1988: identification of drivers in road traffic accidents
  - Police and Criminal Evidence Act 1984
  - Preventing terrorism
- Warrant
- Data Protection Act 1984 (for computer-stored clinical data)
- Venereal Diseases Regulations 1974 (applies to health authority employees)

- Human Fertilisation and Embryology Act 1990 and amendment of 1992.

Disclosure is allowed in the following circumstances:

- In the public interest
- With consent
- Without identification.

In the UK, a patient or their lawyer can easily gain access to their medical records under the following regulations:

- Supreme Court Act 1981 (personal injury claims)
- Access to Medical Records Act 1988 (reports)
- Access to Health Records Act 1990 (from 1 November 1990).

Issues regarding confidentiality to third parties may also arise. Confidentiality is compromised by accessibility of information by multi-disciplinary professionals, such as the following:

- Advocates
- Case workers
- Care assistants/carers
- Social workers who share information with child agencies
- Key workers

Psychiatrists are asked to share information with police, probation officers, including for victim liaison, and for Multi-Agency Public Protection Arrangements (MAPPAs). Always bear in mind the importance of the 'need to know' principle and note that people in old age or with learning difficulties pose special problems.

Incapacity to drive a motor vehicle

In the UK, the patient should be advised that if he or she does not inform the Driver Vehicle Licensing Authority (DVLA) about a relevant condition, then the doctor is obliged to do so. The only absolutely prescribed psychiatric disability is severe mental handicap. For lesser degrees of mental handicap, in order to be able to drive the individual would need to demonstrate adequate functional ability at the wheel. In the USA, the American Psychiatric Association takes the view that there should be no expectation that a psychiatrist can accurately assess capacity to drive a motor vehicle.

Consent to disclose

This is considered reasonable if the patient realizes the nature and consequences. It is also considered reasonable by the BMA and GMC for a doctor to share information with other people who are concerned professionally in assisting with or collaborating in the patient's clinical care (viewed as 'implicit consent').

Information to relatives and carers

In general, this requires the patient's consent. It may be ethical to give information to relatives and carers if it is considered undesirable to tell a patient the full implications of their disorder or the patient is incapable of consent. However, the Royal College of Psychiatrists states that 'families [are] not on a par with outsiders'.

Information required by due legal process

This includes information required by statute, for example notifiable infectious diseases, and by court order. A patient is not 'privileged' in UK law, as in some other countries – that is, the patient is not protected from disclosure without his or her consent in all circumstances. If the doctor refuses a court order to disclose, then the doctor is in contempt of court.

Although it is a fundamental principle of administration of justice that legal professional privilege with clients is absolute (this includes lawyer–doctor communications about a client), this does not apply to the doctor–patient relationship. The court respects this private relationship, but the relationship may be outweighed by public interest, legal process or the safety of others. In this respect, the doctor–patient relationship is comparable to that of a journalist and their sources, or a priest and a penitent.

Duty to society

In the UK, this can override the duty to maintain patient confidentiality. In the case of W *v.* Dr H Egdell (Court of Appeal 8.11.89), a psychiatrist revealed a patient's dangerousness to the then assistant medical director at Ashworth Hospital, knowing that it was likely that this information would be conveyed to the Home Office, although the psychiatrist's mental health review tribunal report regarding this was not submitted to the tribunal by the instructing solicitors. The psychiatrist's actions were upheld in court.

A similar ruling was made in the case of R *v.* Crozier (1990). Crozier attempted to murder his sister. Dr Wright said that Crozier was sane. Crozier was about to be sentenced to prison when a defence psychiatrist, Dr D McDonald, arrived late and gave his report, indicating mental illness, to the prosecution, as a result of which Crozier was detained under Sections 37 and 41 of the Mental Health Act 1983 against his wishes.

The ideal is to try to persuade the patient to give consent, but otherwise the patient must be advised that absolute confidentiality, for example regarding crimes, cannot be given. If a doctor does reveal information without a patient's consent, then the doctor will need to be able to justify this to the GMC, which takes a very hard line on this issue. Breach of confidentiality can lead to a charge of serious professional misconduct.

In the Tarasoff case in the USA, it became evident to a psychotherapist that his patient, Mr Podder, at the University of California at Berkeley was dangerous. The therapist consulted colleagues and subsequently recommended the patient's detention in hospital. However, the campus police involved in the detention process released Podder, as he appeared rational and said that he would stay away from his potential victim, Tatiana Tarasoff, who had rejected his efforts to continue a courtship. Podder realized that his psychotherapist must have talked to the police, and he broke off treatment. Two months later, in 1969, he shot, stabbed and killed Tarasoff after he had returned from a holiday. Relatives of Tarasoff sued the therapist and the campus police, complaining that they should have warned of the danger (Tarasoff *v.* Regents of University of California). This was initially dismissed and then upheld at the California Supreme Court, which initially ruled in 1974 that there was a duty to warn Tarasoff. This was later modified in 1976 to place a duty on the therapist to use reasonable care, for example to hospitalize (interpreted as a duty to protect). From this case comes the phrase 'Protective privilege ends where community peril begins'. Similar rulings were later given in other states of the USA, but they have not resulted in the expected increased litigation and have not been made law in the UK. Associated problems include distinguishing real from false threats, and the effect on the patient's willingness to confide in a therapist. This case reflects the ethical conflict of having to balance patient confidentiality against breaching it and negligence to third parties.

Medical research

It may be justifiable to disclose information without a patient's consent if approved by an ethics committee (e.g. case note studies), but some people question this. A detained patient may not be incompetent to give consent, but there should be no suggestion that participation in research should lead to an earlier release. If the patient, however, is incompetent to give consent, then there is no legal basis for proceeding with research, but in practice, both before and since the Mental Capacity Act 2005, it has been considered ethical to do so if the patient does not resist inclusion in the study, if the relatives are informed and give agreement (assent; although this carries no legal authority as relatives cannot give consent for a patient), and if the patient is considered likely to have consented if he or she had had the capacity. Case history reports are usually disguised to avoid identification, but increasingly, especially among psychotherapists, patients' consent is being obtained. The World Medical Association's Declaration of Helsinki is the established guidance for the ethics of clinical trials on human subjects.[15]

Information for Mental Health Review Tribunals

By law, responsible doctors must submit psychiatric reports with or without the patient's consent, and the patient's medical records will be made available with or without the patient's consent to the Mental Health Review Tribunal, usually to the medical member but not exclusively so. Solicitors for patients now expect to be free to examine the medical records for themselves, if the patient consents to this. A copy of the mental health review tribunal psychiatric report is given to the patient unless the doctor states that it will result in serious harm, including to third parties. Reasons must be given for this to the tribunal. It is therefore good practice to discuss one's opinion with the patient before he or she receives the report.

Disclosure of information in other situations

No consent is required for information to be given for hospital managers' hearings, and managers are not obliged to request to see the records of the patient. Ministry of Justice reports on Section 41 and other restricted patients have not usually had, nor require, the patient's consent, but it is good practice usually to explain what the Ministry of Justice has been told. The Care Quality Commission (previously Mental Health Act Commission), including its non-medical members, can examine records without a detained patient's consent, and its medical representatives can similarly do so when considering second opinions regarding consent to treatment.

Ethics of control of detained patients

There are rights for staff to restrain or impose treatment on psychiatric patients under common law (to prevent a criminal act, to save life or to prevent serious harm, e.g. when the patient is unconscious) and under the Mental Health Act 1983. Staff are protected under Section 139 of the Mental Health Act 1983, so that patients cannot undertake civil proceedings against staff without leave of the High Court unless there is a prima facie case (e.g. of bad faith or treatment undertaken without reasonable care) or undertake criminal proceedings without leave of the Director of Public Prosecutions.

Physical restraint may include a spectrum from instruction to time out to seclusion. It is important for all staff to follow agreed policies and, in England and Wales, the Code of Practice of the Mental Health Act 1983.

If treatment with clozapine is to be imposed without consent under the Mental Health Act 1983, venepuncture can be undertaken without the patient's consent (Mental Health Act Commission Practice Note No. 1 June 1993). However, one cannot make a patient swallow tablets.

A duty of care of a doctor may be shared by his or her team. The BMA highlights, however, that a doctor is responsible for the continuing care of a patient until care is handed on to another doctor.

Ethics of working with prisoners and other detained people

These ethics have been addressed in the United Nations Declaration in 1981, the World Medical Association 1975 Declaration of Tokyo and the World Psychiatric Association 1983 Declaration of Hawaii, as well as the Royal College of Psychiatrists ethical guidelines specifically concerning psychiatric care in prison (1992).

Declaration of Hawaii

As approved by the General Assembly of the World Psychiatric Association in Vienna, on 10 July 1983:

No procedure shall be performed nor treatment given against or independent of a patient's own will, unless because of mental illness, the patient cannot form a judgement as to what is in his or her own best interest and without which treatment serious impairment is likely to occur to the patient or others.

Ethics of medical care in prison

Particular issues for prisoners are that they cannot choose their doctor and their medical care may be less than desirable. However, prisons are not hospitals. There may be a conflict of interest between the duty of care for the patient and a responsibility to the institution, although it is clear that the doctor's first responsibility is to the patient and not to the institution. The BMA states that doctors should not be associated with any punishment damaging to health. This may be an issue in prison adjudications of misconduct and fitness for punishment. The doctor may, however, be able to justify their involvement on the basis that their findings may excuse the patient or help in mitigation due to the patient being sick. Administering drugs in prison in general requires the patient's consent and is not covered by the Mental Health Act 1983. If the prisoner does not consent, then the prisoner may not be treated or secluded, except to save life, to restrain violence or to prevent an irretrievable deterioration in the prisoner's health.

Ethics of punishment

Punishment may be justified on grounds of revenge, deterrence, reform or the protection of others. Punishment may be on the basis that an individual has free will and thus punishment for his or actions is justified in terms of retribution or 'just deserts'. The utilitarian view (the greatest good for the greatest number) may justify punishment for reasons of deterrence on the basis that offenders choose to offend. However, although the death penalty for parking offences may stop such offending, such an argument is not usually taken to this extreme.

Doctors and torture

The European Convention of Human Rights Article 3 states that no one should be subjected to 'inhuman and degrading treatment or punishment'. Inspectors from the Convention make unannounced visits to facilities in countries that are signatories and where people are detained and bring any deficiencies in practice to the notice of those in authority. If no action is taken, the inspectors will publish their findings.

Human Rights Act 1998

This incorporated the European Convention on Human Rights to UK law with full effect from October 2000. Articles relevant to mental health care include the following:

- *Article 2:* right to life.
- *Article 3:* inhuman treatment.
- *Article 5:* right to liberty.
- *Article 5 (1):* protects patients' autonomy – no one is to be detained, except in specified cases as prescribed by law.
- *Article 5 (1)e:* concerns lawful detention of people only if reliably shown to be of 'unsound mind', which equates to, but is not referred to as, incapacity.
- *Article 5 (4):* guarantees the right to a speedy court review of a person's detention.
- *Article 6:* right to a fair trial.
- *Article 8:* right to privacy, including private and family life and correspondence.

Ethics of allocation of resources

Traditional medical ethics, such as the Hippocratic Oath, in which doctors tell each other how to behave but emphasize that their patient should always come first, may provide little help with issues of allocation of resources to other patients.

There is no single ethical solution to the problem of allocating resources. Psychiatrists need to balance legal, practical and ethical issues.[16] For instance, resources could be preferentially allocated to the following:

- *The youngest:* because they are the most productive and have the longest life (on the basis of utilitarianism and welfare maximization).
- *The kindest:* on the basis of just deserts.
- *The most in need:* on the basis of Marxist theory and 'justice'.
- *By chance:* on the basis of lottery.

Quality-adjusted life years (QALYS) may be one way forward in trying to balance the demands of, for example, the need for heart transplants against treatment for depression. The dilemma is in trying to meet the overall population's welfare and other needs (e.g. education) compared with an individual patient's needs. We are conditioned from childhood, and by society and our own psychological needs, to provide a single answer to a dilemma and, indeed, this is often valued, as in business. However, rarely are there single 'right' answers, although there are wrong ones. To balance competing needs, society needs a sense of proportion and to this end will argue about what is right repetitively. Doctors must act as advocates for their own patients, but they must also accept that decisions may be taken by others, such as managers and government, on the basis of cost–benefit.

Multidisciplinary working

A professional may be guided by his or own personal ethics but may also be governed by a code of ethics of his or her profession, which may conflict with that of other professions, for example the insistence of social services of breaking confidentiality where there is any risk to children. This is against a background of society itself becoming increasingly litigious. Professionals are often left in a dilemma – for example, it may be negligent not to restrain a psychiatric patient, but to do so risks being accused of battery and false imprisonment. General principles are often much easier to discuss and resolve than individual clinical cases. Beware the risk of 'freedom always wearing the trousers' in arguments.

The 'wise doctor principle' is being replaced by the 'wise patient principle'. Paternalism in doctors is being replaced by an adult relationship between the doctor and patient.

Ethics of genetic screening

Ethical debate often proceeds on the basis of either assumptions about what the patient wants or what doctors care about; for example, it was previously widely assumed in the case of genetic screening for Huntington's disease that it would be harmful to the patient if the tests were positive, and thus such testing would be unethical (the principle of non-maleficence). Clinical experience has shown this to be not infrequently untrue.

Euthanasia

Treatment for depression rarely alters the attitude of patients considering euthanasia, which is often settled, considered, rational and fixed.

Methods of ethical reasoning

Most ethical dilemmas in psychiatry and, indeed, medicine, are due to one of the following issues:

- Consent
- Autonomy
- Rationality
- Confidentiality.

Principles

This approach offers a top-down approach to tackling ethical problems – that is, from a general theory to particular cases, for example the 'four principle' perspective:

- *Autonomy:* respecting the patient's wishes.
- *Beneficence:* doing good.
- *Non-maleficence:* avoiding doing harm.
- *Justice:* fairness in the provision of care.

These principles, however, may conflict in individual cases; for example, respecting the patient's wishes (autonomy) to have a detailed explanation of his or her condition may be at the expense of time spent with other patients (unjust). Autonomy may include the patient asking the doctor to decide for him or her.

Paradigms (casuistry – case-based reasoning)

This offers a bottom-up approach, starting from cases, and emphasizes two questions:

- What changes to the case would make it clearer what to do?
- What related situations would be less problematic ethically?

For example, in thinking about how to manage risk of death in an individual with mild learning disability pathologically water-drinking, if one alters the scenario, for example to an overdose, then the ethical issues become clearer.

The advantages of this approach include the real life case method and its offering practical solutions. It is, however, professionally centred and can be biased by prejudices.

Perspectives

This approach is based on the practical skill of the capacity to view problems not only from professionals' perspective but also from the perspective of the patient, the patient's relatives and other members of the multidisciplinary team. It is thus patient- and knowledge-centred, but it may have the disadvantage of relativism.

Ethical theories

These may be:

- *Substantive:* concerned with establishing particular ethical conclusions:
  - Deontological (rule-based): these theories emphasize rights, duties and responsibilities, regardless of consequences, e.g. Kant's 'categorical imperatives'.[17]
  - Consequentialist (teleology): these theories emphasize the importance of evaluating the consequences of actions, e.g. utilitarianism.[18]

For example, on confidentiality, consequentialist reasoning emphasizes the consequences if the patient cannot trust their doctor, while deontological reasoning emphasizes the patient's right to privacy. Similarly, in a case where one conjoined twin must die in order to allow the other to live, otherwise both will die, or in the oft-quoted example of a certain number of men being in a boat with provisions for one fewer than that number, deontologists would say that one should not kill while consequentialists would emphasize the need for the greatest good.

- *Virtue ethics:* rather than making binding, often rather negative, rules and duties, virtue ethics emphasizes changing people's attitudes to embrace the virtues, e.g. compassion, trustworthiness, integrity, conscientiousness and good relationships.
- *Analytical:* concerned with the meaning of value terms and general logical form of ethical argument.

Ethics, guidelines and clinical practice

A summary of the issues to be considered in ethical dilemmas is shown in Table 77.1. Ethical or moral conflict is

Table 77.1 Issues to be considered in ethical and legal dilemmas

Defining the problem	What are the clinical problems or key clinical features? What are the ethical or legal issues raised? What are the conflicts and dilemmas?
Who is involved?	Patient, others
Differences in value systems, perspectives and religious beliefs	What are the perspectives of the patient, the partner and family? What are the relevant psychological and social aspects?
Myths and misunderstandings	What is the empirical evidence relevant to decision-making in this case?
What ethical principles are involved?	Autonomy, consent, beneficence, non-maleficence, confidentiality, justice, fairness, truth, integrity, etc.
Are ethical principles in conflict?	
Can they be resolved?	What are the strengths and weaknesses of these arguments?
Should one take priority?	
Short- and long-term consequences	
Professional guidance	
Legal guidance	
Research ethics, if relevant	
Precedent	
Involving other parties	Which colleagues do you suggest involving? Who else could you involve? What use have you made of the network of services and resources available?
Multidisciplinary team views and agreement	
Integrating information and analysis – an holistic management plan	How did you propose to move forward? How do you explain this proposal in terms of your ethics/legal assessment and the available information/evidence?

central to human life. Some moral philosophers argue that conflict is mere appearance and can be resolved by moral homework. This does not reflect real life, however. Aristotle argued that we should test our ethical convictions against ordinary experiences. Bertrand Russell argued that philosophy teaches one to live with uncertainty rather than to answer uncertainty. General principles can be set down as guidelines, but there will always be exceptions. However, a doctor will always need to be able to justify any divergence from accepted guidelines. Doctors, especially psychiatrists, have to make a lot of difficult decisions quickly, with often incomplete information against the background of heavy workloads and understaffed and under-resourced services and a litigious climate, with medical treatments often not resulting in cure.

KEY POINTS

- Psychiatric (and medical) negligence has three main elements:
  - Duty of care to a 'neighbour'
  - Breach of duty of care
  - Damage to other party results.
- Other elements include the following:
  - Behaviour below the standard required by law
  - Reasonably foreseeable damage
  - Actual casual connection
  - Bolam principal: if care is in keeping with a body of recognized opinion, then it is usually defendable, but courts act as a safety net and may disagree.

- Consent requires:
  - Information (knowing) to either profession- or patient-based standard
  - Competency
  - Voluntariness.
- Competence + information ⟶ understanding.
- Understanding + voluntariness ⟶ decision.
- Competence is not an absolute quality and is no longer considered global.
- Competence is not statutorily defined.
- Competence depends on the patient's functioning (e.g. intelligence level) and the nature of the treatment (e.g. complexity of issue): it is action-specific.
- An incompetent patient is incapable of giving valid consent (capacity is a legal concept).
- The Mental Health Act 1983 states that competence means 'knowing the nature, purpose and likely effects of treatment'.
- Treatment without consent is battery. Harm is presumed and does not have to be proven.
- Detention without consent is false imprisonment.
- Consent by proxy (assent) is not legal (c.f. surrogacy in the USA).
- The general duty regarding confidentiality is covered in guidelines e.g. from the GMC.
- Exceptions to confidentiality include the following:
  - Court order
  - Statute – by law for legal proceedings (all have strict narrow criteria for information that can be divulged):
    - Misuse of Drugs Law: notification of addicts
    - Road Traffic Act 1988: identification of drivers in road traffic accidents
    - Police and Criminal Evidence Act 1984
    - Preventing terrorism
  - Warrant
  - Data Protection Act 1984 (for computer-stored clinical data)
  - Venereal Diseases Regulations 1974 (applies to health authority employees)
  - Human Fertilisation and Embryology Act 1990 and amendment of 1992.
- Disclosure is allowed in the following circumstances:
  - In the public interest
  - With consent
  - Without identification.
- In the UK, a patient or their lawyer can gain access to their medical records under the following regulations:
  - Supreme Court Act 1981 (personal injury claims)
  - Access to Medical Records Act 1988 (reports)
  - Access to Health Records Act 1990 (from 1 November 1990).

REFERENCES

1. Jacoby R, Steer P (2007) How to assess capacity to make a will. *British Medical Journal* **335**: 155–7.
2. Olojugba C, Darwiche F (2006) Clinical negligence. *British Medical Journal* (7570 suppl.): **129**.
3. Bloch S, Reddaway P (1977) *Russian Political Hospitals: The Abuse of Psychiatry in the Soviet Union*. London: Gollanz.
4. World Health Organization (2003) *Mental Health Legislation and Human rights*. Geneva: World Health Organization.
5. Beauchamp TL, Childress J F (1994) *Principles of Biomedical Ethics*, 4th edn. New York: Oxford University Press.
6. Gillon R (1986) *Philosophical Medical Ethics*. Chichester: John Wiley & Sons.
7. Dell S (1984) *Murder into Manslaughter: The Diminished Responsibility Defence in Practice*. Oxford: Oxford University Press.
8. General Medical Council (2006) *Consent: In Good Medical Practice*, 4th edn. London: General Medical Council.
9. Lidz CW, Meisel A, Zerutavel E, *et al.* (1984) *Informed Consent*. London: Guilford Press.
10. Gillick *v.* West Norfolk and Wisbeach Area Health Authority [1986] AC 112.
11. Department of Health and Welsh Office (1999) *Mental Health Act 1983: Code of Practice*. London: The Stationery Office.
12. Royal College of Psychiatrists (2009) *Good Psychiatric Practice*. College report CR154. London: Royal College of Psychiatrists.
13. General Medical Council (2004) *Confidentiality: Protecting and Providing Information*. London: General Medical Council.
14. Hagger L (2005) Patient confidentiality. *BMJ Careers* **330** (suppl.): 258.
15. General Assembly of the World Medical Association (1964) Declaration of Helsinki. Adopted by the General Assembly of the World Medical Association at Helsinki, Finland.
16. Sabin JE, Daniels N (1999) Ethical issues in mental health resource allocation. In: S Block, P Chodoff, SA Green (eds) *Psychiatric Ethics*, 3rd edn. Oxford: Oxford University Press.
17. Kant I (1959) *Foundations of Metaphysics and Morals*, transl. L White Beck. Indianapolis, IN: Bobbs-Merrill Co.
18. Mill JS (1861 [1998]) *Utilitarianism*. New York: Oxford University Press.

Chapter 78

Ethics and law

Gwen Adshead

INTRODUCTION

There is no specific ethics and law section in most curricula for psychiatric trainees. However, if the curriculum and the clinical competencies for psychiatric practice are read carefully, then it will be clear that ethical awareness and the capacity to reason thoughtfully about ethical dilemmas are essential requirements of good psychiatric practice. Arguably, ethical theory and reasoning are central to all aspects of the psychiatric curriculum, because good psychiatric practice is about relationships and ethical theory deals with how we should act towards others. All psychiatrists need ethical competence if they are to be competent in their clinical care of patients, their work with colleagues and their own personal probity.

A useful way to think about this is to complement evidence-based medicine (EBM) with values-based medicine (VBM).[1] Certainly, we need facts in order to make decisions, and those facts need to be based on good-quality evidence. But a values-based approach emphasizes two things: first, how many difficult dilemmas in medicine (and especially psychiatry) arise because of different perspectives on values; and second, how an awareness of our value perspectives can help us to make the best-quality ethical decisions possible.

CASE 1 PRIVACY AND CONFIDENTIALITY

Mrs Jenkins is referred by her general practitioner (GP) because she seems depressed and withdrawn. Her husband comes with her and wants to come into the interview room with her. He insists that she cannot talk to you without him, saying, 'She needs me, doctor'. What do you do?

The first point to note about this story is its ordinariness. Ethical dilemmas occur daily in psychiatry – sometimes more than once a day. It is therefore easy for psychiatrists to mistake the ethical for the clinical. The dilemma here is that it is ethically and clinically desirable to see Mrs Jenkins on her own. Ethically, she has a claim to privacy, and you have a duty to keep what she says confidential. Clinically, it is essential to speak to Mrs Jenkins on her own, because otherwise you will not be able to find out whether Mr Jenkins is the problem. It will also be clinically relevant if she really is unable to talk to you without him present. However, it is also going to be clinically relevant to interview Mr Jenkins at some point. Ethically, respect for her includes respect for his viewpoint (which does not mean agreement, necessarily); further, he may really be the best person to represent Mrs Jenkins' viewpoint.

The second point to note is that ethical dilemmas in clinical practice have to be resolved; they cannot be avoided. You will have to answer Mr Jenkins' request one way or the other. The purpose of taking time to think and read about ethics in psychiatry is to try to learn to make the best-quality decisions you can. Sometimes this will mean taking time to think and talk with other colleagues; discussions with others, especially from other disciplines, are often very helpful.

Third, whatever you decide to do about Mrs Jenkins, you need good-quality communication skills to do it. You may decide that you need to talk to Mrs Jenkins alone, even if it is just to get her consent to her husband joining you. Or you may decide to let Mr Jenkins into the room to get his account of what has been happening, and then ask him if he minds stepping outside so you can talk to his wife alone. However you decide to play it, you need to be able to quickly establish a rapport with two people – one of whom is possibly severely depressed, and the other of whom is anxious or angry or both. The therapeutic relationship is crucially important in psychiatric ethics.

In relation to ethics, therefore, the important skills that every psychiatrist needs to have are as follows:

- *Awareness of the distinction between an ethical dilemma and a clinical dilemma:* the language of ethical dilemmas often involves the words 'should' and 'ought'. You *can* see Mrs Jenkins with her husband, but *ought* you to?
- *Awareness of the ways that one can analyse an ethical dilemma using different theories of ethics:* you already have skills in ethical reasoning. The purpose of the training is to improve those skills.

- *Awareness of the different perspectives and value systems that you will meet in your professional practice:* your values, beliefs and attitudes influence how you make ethical decisions and how you decide what the right thing is to do. However, your values, beliefs and attitudes may conflict with those of the patient or your colleagues.
- *Awareness of the role of the law in regulating relationships between people, and responding to ethical dilemmas:* the law is secondary to ethics conceptually; it offers a public and social structure for resolving ethical dilemmas. For this reason, it is often helpful to look at what the legal response to a dilemma might be. But legal is not necessarily the same as ethical, as a quick reflection on the Nazi and apartheid race laws makes clear.
- *Good enough communication skills to facilitate discussion of views and values by everyone involved in ethical decision-making.*

ETHICS AND THE CLINICAL CARE OF PATIENTS

It is (we hope) obvious that it is ethically unjustifiable to give a patient poor clinical care. We think that it is wrong because:

- patients have an expectation that they will be cared for by a doctor when they are made vulnerable by illness or disability;
- you have acquired a duty towards the vulnerable because of your training as a doctor and a psychiatrist. As your knowledge grows, so too do your ethical duties;
- mental disorder makes people especially vulnerable, both in terms of asking for help and in terms of being exploited by others, including healthcare professionals.

CASE 2 BEST INTERESTS AND THE DUTY OF CARE

You are trying to manage Janie according to the best practice guidelines for borderline personality disorder (BPD), which means that you do not admit her except in crisis. She has just been discharged this morning after a lengthy admission; she returns at 11 p.m. the same night, begging to be admitted again. She says that she feels really suicidal and can't cope outside.

Ethics is the study of how we 'should' treat people. During the psychiatric training, you will learn how to treat people's mental distress, using a variety of interventions. Ethical dilemmas arise when you know that you *can* take a course of action; but *should* you? In this case, you can admit Janie: but should you?

A traditional ethical analysis might go like this. You have a duty of care to Janie that arises from your professional identity as a doctor. The ethical aspects of that duty are sometimes summarized as:

- a duty to respect the patient's autonomy, i.e. respect the judgements they make for themselves, based on good-quality information;
- a duty to do the best for the patient's welfare;
- a duty not to harm the patient;
- a duty to act justly and fairly.

These principles form the basis of a theory of ethics based on duties of doctors. There are also ordinary ethical principles of being a citizen, including generally telling the truth and respecting the law. Within psychiatry, we might also want to add the duty to do what we can in order to support and enhance autonomy, given that so many of our patients may lack it or have a fluctuating capacity to be autonomous. We have a duty to assess capacity in order to make autonomous decisions carefully. We also have particular duties to act justly and fairly because many psychiatric patients are vulnerable to exploitation in ways that general medical patients are not.

In this case, we could argue that there is a duty to respect Janie's request for care. In terms of her welfare, she will be safe in hospital, and especially safe from self-harm. There also does not seem to be any failure to respect justice or act fairly if she is admitted. So, from the duty point of view, one could argue that admitting her is the right thing.

But another ethical theory states that the consequences of one's actions matter most in deciding what is right. If you do admit her, then you are undermining the therapeutic relationship that she agreed with her team. There is an evidence base for treatment of BPD that suggests that long-term admissions are not helpful. You may actually do her a harm in the long run if you admit her.

At this point, clinicians sometimes ask what the law says on these matters. Mental health legislation gives you the power to detain someone if you feel that they need treatment for a mental disorder and are refusing it. You have no legal duty to admit Janie, however, just because she asks you to.

Two other theories of medical ethics are especially relevant in psychiatry: virtue ethics and the ethics of care and values-based practice. *Virtue ethics* sets out what a good psychiatrist is and then invites you to act likewise. In this case, the virtuous psychiatrist has regard both to Janie's immediate need for relief from anxiety and to her longer-term needs to learn not only how to manage her negative affects but also how to believe that she can. The *ethics of care* places most importance on the relationship with Janie and would suggest that you have a duty to use the therapeutic relationship to relieve her anxiety and her distress, which need not include admitting her. It might mean that you spend 2 h talking to her, helping her to manage her immediate distress.

CASE 3 ETHICS AND WORKING WITH COLLEAGUES

You are asked to go out and assess the mental state of a man at home. When you get there, you find he has barricaded himself inside his room and is crying. His mother is crying too. Everyone is very distressed, and the community psychiatric nurse (CPN), who knows the family well, says, 'You must arrange for him to be sectioned straight away.' However, you know that the patient is doing well in his sheltered work placement and that an in-patient admission may lead to the loss of this work. When you put this to the CPN, she is angry and says that you are dismissing her opinion because she is 'just a nurse'. What is the right thing to do?

Most patient care in psychiatry is delivered by teams of professionals, which reflects the diversity of needs of most psychiatric services users. The role of the psychiatrist has changed from a traditional medical one of making diagnostic and therapeutic decisions, and asking others to carry them out (as might be done by a surgeon), into one in which the different mental health professionals engage with different aspects of the patient's life. The consultant psychiatrist then acts as a coordinator of information and intelligence about the patient, making sure that no sources of information are overlooked. Although in legal terms the psychiatrist will be responsible for patients (especially any that are admitted under the Mental Health Act), in clinical terms other professionals may take the lead on care coordination.

There are two aspects to this scenario that involve ethical reflection, and they are subtly different. The first aspect is the difference in value perspective between you and the nurse. She is clearly responding to the patient's immediate distress, and she sees it as her ethical duty to relieve that distress. She may also be thinking about a duty to the patient's mother, whereas you may be thinking primarily about the patient's needs, both long- and short-term. Exploring the differences in your perspective will make it easier for you to come to some resolution.

However, the second aspect relates to the values that are put on to professional status. We have professional duties to respect the different contributions that different healthcare professionals make to patient care. Culturally, doctors are often depicted as being the dominant decision-makers in medicine, but in reality the care of very sick patients is always a matter of teamwork, and the clinical care can be compromised if professionals do not work together closely and respectfully. Ethically competent doctors ensure, through good communication skills and discussions about differences in professional opinion, that they are seen to be respectful of their co-workers.

CASE 4 PERSONAL PROBITY

Janie, the patient in Case 2, has made good progress and has been discharged form the clinic. A year later, you meet her at a social event organized by a friend of yours. You and Janie get on well, and she suggests that you meet up again for a drink the following week. When you meet, she confides in you that she had a sexual relationship with one of the other junior doctors that she met in the hospital.

This is a case that raises issues about professional boundaries in psychiatric practice. The 'boundary' here refers to the line between our professional identity (those verbal and non-verbal behaviours that mark us as professional) and our personal identity (again, those verbal and non-verbal behaviours that make us who we are personally). In theory, there is a strict boundary between the professional and the personal; when that boundary is crossed, we call it a 'boundary crossing' or, in serious cases, a 'boundary violation'.[2]

Meeting an ex-patient at a party is a boundary crossing; this is an overlap between your personal and professional identities. It needs to be handled thoughtfully so that both parties' confidences are respected. It is debateable whether psychiatric patients can ever have relationships with their doctors that do not have some professional aspect to them; some would argue that it is not wise to have a drink with Janie, although it is legal and does not undermine any of the ethical duties described above. However, boundary crossings often lead to boundary violations,[3] where there is complete collapse between personal and professional functions; such violations are usually harmful to the patient. Having a sexual relationship with a patient, as this colleague seems to have done, is always harmful to the patient and often to the doctor involved as well.

In these cases, it is essential to get good advice from a trusted senior colleague before any action is taken. There is no legal duty to report this allegation, but the General Medical Council (GMC) takes the view that doctors should always disclose when they have concerns about other doctors' practices that may cause harm to patients. The ethical justification for disclosure is the prevention of harm to future patients. However, such situations are always personally delicate and potentially distressing for all concerned; it is vital to take the time that you need to discuss any future course of action.

Such cases also bring up the issue of confidentiality or, more properly, the general ethical duty to keep patient information private and to not disclose without express consent. If the patient consents to disclosure, then all is well; in this case, you might say to Janie that you would like to discuss her disclosure with a senior colleague, and if she agrees that is fine. If she disagrees, then this means that your duty to protect Janie's confidences, and your professional duty to report concerns about others doctors, are in direct conflict.

Respect for confidentiality is not the same as secrecy, and there are justifications for breaching confidentiality; for example, Section 30 Annex B of the National Health Service (NHS) code of confidentiality for all staff states that staff are permitted to breach confidentiality in the '*detection, investigation and punishment* of violent crime' (author's italics).[4] However, it might be hard to argue that Janie's experience constitutes violent crime. If, however, Janie were alleging that she had been raped, then there is clear justification for disclosing her allegations to a senior colleague, even in the face of Janie's flat refusal. There is justification to do so; it is still open to you whether to disclose or not. This might be a case where overriding Janie's refusal is the lesser of two evils.

LAW AND PSYCHIATRY

The law is the codification of a social consensus and is a mixture of statutes (which are debated and made law by Parliament) and case law, which is decided by argument in different types of court. Laws change as social circumstances change, and so what was lawful 200 years ago may not be lawful now. In theory, at least, law should follow ethics, and not the other way round: it may be lawful for you to take some form of action, but it may not be ethically right.

It is not possible to describe all the law with which a psychiatrist should be familiar in a short textbook such as this. What I will set out here are the general areas of law that psychiatrists need to know about, and the types of law in which they may be involved.

Civil and criminal law

There is a crucial distinction between the civil law and the criminal law, namely that they regulate different kinds of social relationship. The criminal law deals with antisocial behaviour: it specifies what shall be a criminal offence and what the penalties are for breaking the law. Criminal offences are those that are antisocial and harmful and result in social condemnation and exclusion. Criminal law determines guilt and innocence; the criminal courts are where magistrates and juries determine whether someone is responsible for a crime and what their punishment should be. Not all social rule-breaking is criminal (traffic and parking offences are a good example), but criminal activity is defined in terms of law-breaking, which is usually defined by legal statutes.

In contrast, civil law matters are about different kinds of problem in social relationships. It starts from the premise that relationships give rise to duties, and if that duty is breached then one party can claim that they have been wronged by the other. Civil law includes medical negligence, family law, contract law, and the law on capacity to make decisions. Psychiatrists need to be familiar with the Capacity Act, which in ethical terms reflects the principle of respect for autonomy. However, the capacity to exercise autonomy may be compromised in different ways and by different illnesses (not all mental); the Act sets out how doctors should behave in relation to patients whose autonomy is impaired.

Psychiatrists may find themselves advising different kinds of court in different ways. Medicolegal work is a specific psychiatric competency, and no junior doctor should attempt it without proper supervision and advice, especially where it involves giving expert testimony in the criminal or family courts. The two most important things to know before getting involved in any medicolegal work are (i) what sort of psychiatric question is being asked, and why, and (ii) whether you are the right person to answer it. If there is no psychiatric question – or there is, but you are not the right person to answer it – then you are entitled to tell any lawyer that you refuse to be involved.

Mental health law

Mental health law is a particular branch of civil law that addresses the problems of citizens who have mental illnesses. Since Roman times, it has been recognized that people with mental illnesses may need special protection because they are mentally vulnerable; it has also been recognized that a small minority pose a risk to the public. Most countries have specific mental health legislation, which is set out in some from of legal statute and then regulated and reviewed by subsequent case law. In England and Wales, Jones's *Mental Health Act Manual* is an invaluable guide.[5]

Specific legislation is needed because it is generally harmful to detain people against their will, and it is ethically unjustifiable to do harm to others unless there is a strong justification in terms of either the consequences or justice. Psychiatric practice often involves assessing and treating people who either cannot consent or who are refusing for mad reasons, and so there needs to be legislation to protect vulnerable patients. There also needs to be a legal mechanism to protect the public from the tiny minority of patients who may pose a risk of harm to others but for whom the criminal law is inappropriate.

Much of the debate in the past 20 years between psychiatrists, lawyers and the government has been about the extent to which mental health law should be primarily about protecting the public or primarily about protecting the vulnerable patient. At present, psychiatry seems to be in a highly risk-averse mode, where the protection of the public is seen as a primary duty. It has not always been so in psychiatry, and it is to be hoped that this mode will change in the future.

CONCLUSION

Our professional competencies are acquired through training and experience. Our professional ethical identity, however, is made up of our professional values and attitudes. It begins with the MRCPsych training, but it continues to deepen and grow; we never stop learning how to be 'good' psychiatrists. Note that we do not have to be perfect; we only have to be (as a famous paediatrician once said), 'good enough'. We will inevitably sometimes make mistakes, and mature people learn from those mistakes. The ethical aspect of psychiatry is what makes it fascinating; paying close attention to ethical tensions in the work, and honing ethical reasoning skills, will make the job rich, human and enjoyable for years to come. At least, I have found it so.

KEY POINTS

- Ethics is the study of how we ought to treat people.
- Competence in ethical reasoning is essential for psychiatric practice.
- What is legally permissible is not necessarily ethically justifiable.
- In difficult situations, get advice and spend time in discussion: don't let anxiety rush you.
- Good communication skills make ethical discussions easier.
- Good-quality ethical reasoning involves considering all perspectives, especially the ones you disagree with.
- A good outcome does not justify treating people badly: what is good clinically may not be ethically justifiable.

FURTHER READING

Adshead G (2008) In D Bhugra, O Howes (eds) *Handbook for Psychiatric Trainees*. London: Royal College of Psychiatrists.

Bloch S, Green S (2009) *Psychiatric Ethics*, 4th edn. Oxford: Oxford University Press.

Robertson M, Waller G (2007) Overview of psychiatric ethics: 1. Professional ethics and psychiatry. *Australasian Psychiatry* **15**: 201–6.

Royal College of Psychiatrists (2001) *Good Psychiatric Practice*. London: Royal College of Psychiatrists.

Royal College of Psychiatrists (2006) *Good Psychiatric Practice: Confidentiality and Information Management*. College report CR 133. London: Royal College of Psychiatrists.

REFERENCES

1. Woodbridge K, Fulford KWM (2004) *Whose Values? A Workbook for Values Based Practice*. London: Sainsbury Centre for Mental Health.
2. Gutheil T, Gabbard G (1993) The concept of boundaries in clinical practice: theoretical and risk management dimensions. *American Journal of Psychiatry* **150**: 188–96.
3. Sarkar SP (2004) Boundary violations and sexual exploitation in psychiatry and psychotherapy: a review. *Advances in Psychiatric Treatment* **10**: 312–20.
4. Department of Health (2003) *Confidentiality: NHS Code of Practice*. London: Department of Health.
5. Jones RM (2005) *Mental Health Act Manual*, 9th edn. London: Sweet & Maxwell.

Chapter 79

Risk assessment

Anthony Maden

INTRODUCTION

Violence risk assessment has assumed increasing importance in mental health services over the past two or three decades. Of the many pressures that have led to a greater emphasis on risk, most are not specific to mental health but reflect wider cultural changes. Society as a whole has become more risk-averse. Popular concern about crime and violence borders on hysteria, despite evidence that the frequency of many offences has fallen.

It is tempting to dismiss the increased concern with violence risk as a further example of the health and safety fascism that demands children wear protective goggles to play conkers. It is tempting, but it is also wrong; the other side of the story is that the past 30 years have seen massive improvements in attitudes towards vulnerable people in general and towards victims in particular.

From being virtually ignored, victims have become a central concern of the criminal justice system. Once the rights of victims are acknowledged, the inevitable next step is a greater emphasis on protection and prevention. Specific examples include the greater consideration we now give to victims of rape and other sexual offences, and our willingness to confront the realities of child physical and sexual abuse, much of it perpetrated by carers and authority figures. At the same time, there has been an expansion of offending behaviour programmes aimed at reducing rates of sexual re-offending.

So, although some psychiatrists dismiss violence risk management as interference by the nanny state, a stronger case can be made that is an aspect of progress towards a more civilized society. Concern for vulnerable people implies a desire to take all reasonable steps to minimize victimization.

THE ETHICS OF RISK ASSESSMENT

One source of professional resistance to violence risk assessment derives from concern that it is unethical. Concern with violence risk has been portrayed as stigmatizing to patients and therefore inconsistent with the caring role of a health professional. We need to confront this attitude head-on. Training in risk assessment is pointless if mental health professionals are reluctant to use it because they see it as a dark art that is essentially anti-patient. Fortunately, there is plenty of evidence to show that good risk management is an essential part of medical care. It is part of a doctor's duty of care to manage violence risk competently, as the following sections illustrate.

Risk versus safety

Opponents assume that risk assessment attaches negative labels and leads to detention or other adverse consequences. This assumption has no basis. The aim of risk assessment is to distinguish different levels of risk and to inform decisions about resource allocation. The process would be pointless if it labelled all patients as high-risk. Any effective risk-assessment system discriminates between different levels and types of risk and ought to lead to low ratings more often than it leads to high.

Safety is the other side of the risk coin. There can be no ethical objection to describing a patient or, more accurately, a management plan as 'safe'. On the contrary, it is unethical to deny patients an assessment that would identify them as low-risk simply because the same assessment would identify a (smaller) number of patients as high-risk. Most doctors would have no qualms about an assessment that suggests a patient can be treated safely in a particular setting; once that principle is accepted, there is no basis on which to argue against the same assessment just because the outcome for another patient is an indication of higher risk.

The inevitability of decisions about risk

Mental health professionals routinely take decisions that depend on estimates or 'guesstimates' of safety and risk. We take those decisions in a climate of intense scrutiny, where there are often accusations of institutional racism relating to the detention of patients from ethnic minorities. These difficult decisions are not going to go away. We cannot avoid risk assessment and management; the question is how well we are going to do it. The best course of action is to make the decisions, and the ethical dilemmas, explicit.

We can then deal with them transparently so our decisions can be questioned and challenged.

Conflicts in values

It is helpful to make explicit the conflict of values inherent in violence risk management. On the one hand, we place great value on respect for patient autonomy and minimize medical interference in their lives. On the other hand, we value the right of the public to live safely and free from the fear and threat of violence.

This conflict of values is real and we cannot avoid it by emphasizing only one side of the equation, whether it is the rights of patients or those of wider society. Instead, we need to find defensible and transparent means of negotiating that conflict. The process of violence risk assessment and management can help us to find a path through the minefield. It allows acknowledgment of the conflict, and it encourages openness about the compromises we make in order to negotiate a way through the dilemma.

Third-party risk in medicine

Finally, we need to bear in mind the wider context of medical practice. Since medicine now deals with chronic diseases where the aim is management rather than curative intervention, risk management is a core function of most branches of healthcare. The specialist in hypertension aims through treatment to minimize the risk of complications such as myocardial infarction and stroke. The specialist in diabetes aims through treatment to minimize a wealth of complications, including eye disease, renal failure and peripheral vascular disease. In this sense, violence risk management falls within the mainstream of medical practice.

Yet violence risk management in mental health is different because it sometimes involves compulsory treatment, which is, of course, rare in other fields of medicine. Psychiatry is exceptional because of the extent to which it deals with third-party risk, which is rare in most areas of medicine. Once we accept the proposition that some patients with mental disorders and without proper treatment will not only suffer harm but also inflict serious harm on others, we take on obligations rarely faced by medical professionals in other specialties.

Psychiatry is not quite unique in this respect, and there are some examples of third-party risk in physical medicine. They include the control of infectious diseases, restrictions on driving motor vehicles in people who are impaired by visual problems or epilepsy, and medical involvement in childcare proceedings when a mother is unfit through disease to look after her children. In all of these cases, the doctor is required to balance the rights of the patient against the rights of others, whether they are specific individuals or the general public.

Although the examples are hard to find, the principle of management in these cases is absolutely clear. There is a low threshold for intervening and restricting patients' lives when disease involves risk to others. Society has a low tolerance for any risk to third parties that may be associated with diseases and their medical treatment. It is psychiatry's misfortune that it deals routinely with third-party risks that are exceptional in other branches of medicine, but the principles are the same.

Common ground

Although there is sometimes a true conflict between the rights of the patient and the rights of the public, there is a lot of common ground. One of the most depressing things about the debate over the 2007 revision of the Mental Health Act 1983 was the tendency of the Bill's opponents to present patients as an enlightened and embattled minority besieged by a hostile and ill-informed public.

In reality, patients are members of the public too. Mental illness is common and can affect anyone. Patients are more likely to be victims of violence rather than its perpetrators, and so there is a common interest in reducing the prevalence of violence.

The other sense in which there is common ground is that an act of serious violence has profound negative consequences for the perpetrator as well as the victim. The perpetrator is likely to spend a long time in custody, even if the setting is a secure hospital rather than a prison. The perpetrator will have to come to terms with having caused serious injury to another person, often a loved one, and suicide is not uncommon. The perpetrator may have to live with lifelong restrictions on his or her freedom. The violent act may split up a marriage or cause a rift within a family.

These dire consequences for the perpetrator amount to one of the most negative of all negative outcomes in mental illness. Leaving aside concern for potential victims, doctors have an ethical duty to take reasonable steps to reduce the chances of such a disastrous complication of serious mental illness.

Summary

A proper concern with the safe management of violence risk is not in any sense anti-patient. Risk management is an essential part of medical care, and the failure to manage violence risk properly can have devastating consequences for other people, for the patient, and for the public image of mental health.

THE ASSOCIATION BETWEEN MENTAL DISORDER AND VIOLENCE

Having dealt with the ethical aspects of violence risk management, it is appropriate to consider briefly the underlying science before moving on to the practicalities of managing risk.

One reason for the slow adoption of violence risk assessment in psychiatry is that, until recently, doctors were taught that violence was of little or no importance in mental illness. As recently as the late 1980s, the orthodox teaching within mental health was that there was no statistical association between mental illness and violence. Until then, most studies had methodological flaws that obscured the true picture. Only in 1990, with the emergence of large-scale epidemiological community studies, did it become apparent that there was a significant association. For example, Swanson and colleagues found self-reported violence during the past 12 months in 2 per cent of community respondents without a psychiatric diagnosis but in 8 per cent of community respondents with a diagnosis of schizophrenia.[1]

The epidemiology of violence and mental disorder is now supported by a vast literature, and a review is beyond the scope of this chapter. It has been shown consistently that a diagnosis of schizophrenia is statistically associated with an increased risk of violence.[2] The association with violence is even stronger for diagnoses such as substance misuse and antisocial personality disorder.

Apparent contrary findings, which show no statistical association between schizophrenia and violence, usually arise because the control group includes diagnoses such as personality disorder that carry an even higher risk. The true picture is summed up well in a paper by Shaw and colleagues, which showed a probability of schizophrenia of 5 per cent in men remanded on a charge of homicide compared with approximately 1 per cent in the general population.[3]

The implication of these findings is inescapable. Once it has been demonstrated that some common mental disorders are associated at the population level with a significant increase in the risk of violence, their management becomes part of the core business of mental health services.

APPROACHES TO RISK ASSESSMENT AND MANAGEMENT

Underlying principles

The awakening of interest in violence risk assessment has brought with it a range of methods, techniques and instruments. They can be helpful, but they can also be misleading; in order to use them sensibly, it is essential to be aware of their underlying assumptions and limitations. There is also a tendency for the debate to focus on which method or tool is 'best'. The concept is meaningless unless we are clear about what we should expect from risk assessment. The underlying principles are helpful here because they show how much the various instruments have in common, and they help us to have realistic expectations of what they can do.

The past is the best guide to the future

The old clichés are the best, and it is impossible to overstate the value of this ancient one. It applies well beyond mental health and is the basis of aphorisms about learning from history, lest we be compelled to repeat it.

Critics point out that, if the cliché is taken at face value, then creativity could not exist and there would truly be nothing new under the sun. There would be no surprises. This criticism is valid but not fatal to a proper use of history. The future is similar to the past often enough to make it foolish in the extreme to ignore history. Also, surprises often come because somebody does something different; one of the things services can do differently is to improve treatment.

It is because of this principle that the management of violence risk begins with a careful description of the internal and external factors associated with previous violence. We hope to identify factors that we can change in order to influence the risk of future violence.

It is worth noting also that the principle of consistency is the basis of all science. Many scientific laws can be reduced to the formula: when x and y apply, z will follow. In most cases also, the scientific law originated from historical observations that, whenever x and y were observed together, z tended to follow. The next step is prediction based on a series of observations, which allows us to say how likely it is that z follows given that x and y are both present.

For our purposes, z is violence, or a particular type of violence. Risk assessment is the process of identifying the variables (internal and external) associated with previous violence and making predictions about the likely circumstances in which violence will recur.

Psychiatry is not physics. We will never have the luxury of precise formulae to link violence to its antecedents. The practical problem is that mental health services have to contend with variables a through to w as well as x, y and z. Nevertheless, the principle is sound. We should not neglect x and y just because there are other factors that we cannot influence.

There are fewer than 20 common indicators of risk

On the other hand, psychiatry has more of a scientific basis than we sometimes admit. Most management of violence risk deals with a surprisingly limited range of variables. They include non-compliance with medication, relapse, lack of insight, intoxication and psychopathy. The Historical Clinical Risk 20 (HCR-20) is so-called, rather than HCR-2000, for a reason: namely, that 20 variables cover most general indicators of violence risk.[4] The Violence Risk Appraisal Guide (VRAG) has 12 items, as does the Hare Psychopathy Checklist: Screening Version (PCL-SV),[5] whereas the full Hare Psychopathy Checklist Revised (PCL-R) has 20.[6]

Standardized measures of risk in sex offending also tend to concentrate on a small number of variables, including psychopathy, non-sexual offending, victims unknown to the perpetrator, paraphilias, male victims, and inability to establish stable relationships. Of course, it would be ridiculous to suggest that such a small amount of information is all you need to know about a case, but the fact remains that a handful of variables tell us a great deal about the background risk of violence.

In summary, a small number of variables can account for much of the variance in the risk of re-offending. There is often overlap between the items used in different standardized measures. Once the basic list of variables is covered, little added value results from extending the list. Other, more idiosyncratic risk factors are best included as part of the overall clinical formulation rather than trying to develop a standardized measure that includes everything.

Violence risk is multidimensional

Violence risk is not like height and weight: it cannot be reduced to a score on a single dimension or number. Instead, it needs to be measured in a way that includes qualitative and descriptive factors.

The various facets of violence risk include nature, severity, immediacy and likely victims. A probability can be attached to any one of these dimensions. For example, a man with morbid jealousy may be very likely to attack his partner, moderately likely to attack a member of her family, and unlikely to attack a member of the general public. A predatory sexual offender may present a high risk of sexual assault to women but a low risk of violence to other groups of people.

The other difference from height and weight is that violence risk is not simply an inherent property of the individual. It depends also on external circumstances and contingencies, which make the description even more complicated. The use of alcohol and drugs increases most violence risks and, it may be more or less likely in the individual patient. Non-compliance with medication is one of the most important risk factors associated with violence in schizophrenia, so a patient on effective medication may present very different risks from the same patient when untreated.

A comprehensive assessment is therefore a detailed description, taking into account the history, present state and likely future conditions, and including an account of factors likely to increase and decrease risk. It is relative rather than absolute, and attempts to reduce risk to a number or percentage are misleading.

As a result, the quality of a risk assessment cannot be judged simply by its predictive ability. Testing of predictions lends itself readily to statistical analysis, but it should never be seen as the whole story. The true test of a risk assessment is the extent to which it aids treatment by improving risk management – which is much more difficult to measure but also much more important and useful than prediction.

If this sounds impossibly complicated, then we can take comfort from the fact that clinicians routinely juggle multi-faceted risks. We are used to trading different dimensions off against each other. We decide almost automatically that a significant risk of minor physical assault can be tolerated and defended, whereas we have a very low tolerance when dealing with life-threatening assaults or potential risk to vulnerable groups such as children. The formal process of violence risk management simply makes these considerations more explicit and transparent – and therefore more defensible.

Individual consistency helps clinical prediction

Doctors have an advantage over physicists because doctors are concerned in clinical practice with risk prediction in the individual patient rather than in all patients or in the average patient. So, a rule about the relationship between delusions and violence may be impossible to formulate in a general sense for all patients, but a specific patient whose delusions have been associated with violence in the past will probably exhibit violence when deluded in the future. The greater accuracy is possible because, in scientific terms, many of the variables associated with the individual patient are controlled; they remain constant over time.

For this reason, statistical studies may understate the extent to which we can predict violence in association with mental illness. As a general rule, a patient who has been violent during a previous psychotic episode should be assumed to be likely to behave violently during a future episode, all other things being equal.

The main priority is to prevent repetition

It is much more difficult to foresee a first act of violence than it is to predict a repetition. Although this fact is rarely stated explicitly, it is implicit in any risk-management tool that relies on history. It follows from the first principle – that the past is the best guide to the future: when there is no history, it is difficult to say much about the likely future.

The same principle shapes expectations and criticisms of mental health services. The most critical homicide inquiries condemn failure to manage a patient who has already behaved violently, rather than failure to predict a first act of serious violence. In this sense, the attitude of the public is consistent with the science. One can understand and sympathize with professionals when a serious act of violence comes out of the blue, but there is less sympathy when there has been previous violence in similar circumstances. The more serious the previous violence, and the greater its similarity to the present act, the less any failing will be understood or tolerated.

This principle is also a powerful response to those who oppose risk management as 'locking up people who have not done anything'. If a risk-management system works properly, then it should give priority to those cases in which

there has been previous violence. It is almost impossible for any patient to be rated as presenting a high risk of violence without a history of violence.

Psychopathy is a risk factor for violence

Many risk-assessment instruments incorporate items related directly or indirectly to psychopathy because psychopathy has consistently shown a positive association with violence risk. One can accept this association without necessarily accepting psychopathy as a diagnostic entity. For example, features such as lack of empathy and callous unconcern for others are likely to increase violence risk, whether they derive from schizophrenia, autism or a personality disorder. It may also be the case that the value of such a measure derives from a careful recording of the range and extent of previous antisocial behaviour rather than the diagnosis of any underlying personality disorder.

An elevated psychopathy score increases violence risk, irrespective of other diagnoses, but the reverse is not true. It is a serious mistake to assume that the absence of features of psychopathy necessarily means a low risk of violence, and this mistake is made most easily when dealing with mental illness. Schizophrenia and other serious mental illness can result in a high risk of violence, even in the absence of all other historical indicators of violence risk. Hence, standardized instruments that rely heavily on indicators of psychopathy can be misleading in mentally ill people.

THREE APPROACHES TO RISK ASSESSMENT

Having set out some principles of violence risk assessment, we turn to attempts to apply them in clinical practice. The three approaches considered here are unstructured clinical assessment, actuarial or standardized assessment, and structured clinical assessment. The evidence strongly favours a structured clinical approach, so the other two approaches are given only brief consideration. See Maden[7] for a more detailed discussion.

Unstructured clinical assessment

As the title suggests, there are no rules other than the basic rules of good clinical practice. Until recently, this was probably the most common method of assessing violence risk in the UK. It has the virtue of being used widely and flexible. It can be adapted endlessly to fit any clinical case.

The disadvantage is that there is wide variation in individual practice, and standards vary widely according to the skill and experience of the practitioner. It is also difficult to challenge the opinion or to communicate the basis of the assessment to others. These are serious criticisms in an era when mental health services are often criticized for apparent discriminatory practice. A more structured approach to assessment could be justified solely on the grounds that it helps to reduce discriminatory practice, even if it made no other contribution to improving risk management.

Actuarial or standardized risk assessment

This term is derived from the insurance industry, in which a small number of facts are gathered and then combined according to a strict formula in order to estimate the level of risk associated with life insurance. Actuarial risk assessment lies at the opposite end of the spectrum from the unstructured clinical method. There are fixed rules about the data that must be gathered, and about the way in which data are used to arrive at an assessment of violence risk.

The link with the insurance industry is a key to both the strengths and the weaknesses of this method. The strengths are that it is systematic, eliminates variation between individual practitioners and excludes clinical judgement. Statistical evaluation shows that such methods are reliably better than chance in predicting violence.

Of course, such statistical evaluations are done on populations rather than individuals. The insurance industry requires only that its methods work for populations and has no interest in individual prediction. By contrast, clinical risk management deals with individuals. When dealing with individual patients, the inflexibility of the actuarial method becomes a major drawback. For example, an individual may have a single, idiosyncratic problem (e.g. morbid jealousy) that leads to a high risk of violence. In the absence of other generic risk factors, an actuarial assessment would be misleading, with potentially disastrous consequences.

VRAG is one of the most widely used actuarial scales.[8] Its authors won notoriety by claiming it could and should supplant clinical estimation of risk. The scale was developed on 600 adult male patients followed up after release from a high-security hospital in Ontario, Canada, with violent re-offending as the outcome measure. From a mass of data, 12 items were found to predict re-offending (Box 79.1).

The claimed strength of actuarial instruments such as the VRAG is that they express risk in simple percentage terms. Put in 12 variables and the VRAG gives a risk of violent re-offending between, for example, 10 per cent and 20 per cent. Such precision would be wonderful if it were valid but, as we have seen above, violence risk is multifaceted and cannot be reduced to a single number.

A further problem is that the percentages are derived from groups and cannot be applied directly to an individual patient. We gain some useful information from knowing that an individual patient closely resembles a group with a particular risk of re-offending, but it is misleading to assume that all members of the group will behave in the same way. Idiosyncratic features and events may lead to a very different outcome. A simplistic example is the high-risk offender who is incapacitated by a broken leg or a serious physical illness; the VRAG score does not change, but the actual risk may be very different.

Box 79.1 The 12 items of the Violence Risk Appraisal Guide

- PCL-R score
- Problems at junior school
- Personality disorder
- Alcohol abuse
- Separated from parents before age 16 years
- Failure on prior conditional release
- History of non-violent offending
- Never married
- Schizophrenia*
- Extent of victim injury*
- Age*
- Female victim*

*Negative correlation with risk of violence.

Total scores on the instrument have been divided into nine bins, along a spectrum of violence risk. Each bin has an attached probability of violence, expressed in percentage terms and relating to a 7-year timeframe.

Incidentally, none of this matters in large groups, where the oddities cancel each other out. Actuarial measures such as the VRAG are useful and valid for commissioners and planners who may wish to compare services or allocate resources, but the clinician dealing with individuals needs to be more cautious in interpreting scores.

The other problem of the actuarial approach is that it is relevant only for patient groups very similar to the group on which it was developed. One of the oddities of the VRAG is the negative effect on risk of a diagnosis of schizophrenia. This anomaly arises because the personality-disordered patients in the original study group presented even higher risks. The research literature would not support the downgrading of risk because the diagnosis is schizophrenia.

Structured clinical assessment of violence risk

The structured clinical method represents a compromise between actuarial or standardized assessment on the one hand and the unstructured clinical method on the other (Box 79.2). A structured clinical assessment requires the collection of a certain amount of standard data about the individual (the small number of standard variables mentioned above), but there is flexibility in the use of additional data and in the way data are used to draw conclusions. In the example given above, morbid jealousy would simply be included as an additional variable, and the shrewd clinician would give it appropriate weight in the risk assessment, unconstrained by any of the rules that apply in actuarial assessments.

The best-known example of structured clinical risk assessment is the HCR-20. The HCR-20 requires the collection of 20 data items: ten items are historical and refer to the past; five items are clinical and relate to present state; and five risk-management items relate to the future (Box 79.3).

Each of the 20 items is scored as definitely present (2), probably or partially present (1) or absent (0). The definitions for each item are described by Webster and colleagues,[4] and they are a major part of training in the use of the HCR-20. They are intended to be not operational but ostensional – that is, they provide only examples of the

Box 79.2 Structured clinical management of violence risk

- *Step 1:* Collection of data from records, patient interview and informants.
- *Step 2:* Standardized assessment of static and dynamic risk factors.
- *Step 3:* Consideration of idiosyncratic risk factors.
- *Step 4:* Description of violence risks, including nature, likely victims, and factors increasing and decreasing the risk.
- *Step 5:* Description of plans to address the risks, including contingency plans.
- *Step 6:* Assign priorities.

Box 79.3 The 20 items of the Historical Clinical Risk 20 (HCR-20)

HISTORICAL ITEMS

- *H1:* previous violence
- *H2:* young age at first violent incident
- *H3:* relationship instability
- *H4:* employment problems
- *H5:* substance use problems
- *H6:* major mental illness
- *H7:* psychopathy
- *H8:* early maladjustment
- *H9:* personality disorder
- *H10:* prior supervision failure.

CLINICAL ITEMS

- *C1:* lack of insight
- *C2:* negative attitudes
- *C3:* active symptoms of major mental illness
- *C4:* impulsivity
- *C5:* unresponsive to treatment.

RISK-MANAGEMENT ITEMS

- *R1:* plans lack feasibility
- *R2:* exposure to destabilizers
- *R3:* lack of personal support
- *R4:* non-compliance with remediation attempts
- *R5:* stress.

type of behaviour that should receive a particular rating. Other examples are always possible. Therefore, the rating requires judgement and the exercise of discretion.

With the basic data in place, the clinician is then required to add any idiosyncratic variables and to make an assessment of risks. There is complete freedom to interpret the data as seems appropriate in the individual case.

So far, the method appears to be no more than a flexible form of standardized risk assessment, with allowance for the exercise of clinical discretion. But there is one further stage to the HCR-20 that turns it from a risk-assessment instrument into a tool for risk management. The second stage of the HCR-20 is to formulate feared scenarios of violence based on the available data. For each scenario, the assessor is required to describe factors that will increase or decrease the risk, leading to the formulation of interventions and the assignment of priority to the case.

The three steps to developing a risk management plan in the HCR-20 are:

1 Description of feared scenarios of violence.
2 Development of a risk-management strategy.
3 Prioritization of the case and arrangements for review.

The task may seem daunting because the number of scenarios is potentially infinite. In practice, the same scenarios and situations recur frequently – sometimes in a way that is embarrassing to mental health services because we fail to deal with them adequately.

Examples of common scenarios include the following:

- A patient stabilized on depot changes to oral medication, engages in covert non-compliance and then relapses.
- A non-compliant patient relapses, takes drugs and then assaults a family member, friend or fellow hostel resident.
- A male patient assaults his partner when he is unwell, because of his jealousy or her infidelity.
- A decrease in monitoring or support (e.g. discharge or transfer from hostel to the community) leads to non-compliance or drug-taking, relapse and violence.

The familiar themes of non-compliance, relapse and intoxication occur repeatedly. Common warning signs of an increased violence risk in mentally ill patients include relapse and non-compliance, from which case-management strategies follow automatically. Victim safety planning is often forgotten, but it is well known that relations and carers are disproportionately likely to be the victims of violence by mentally ill patients.

Protective factors tend also to be neglected, but they should be part of any risk-management plan.

STRENGTHS AND WEAKNESSES OF THE HCR-20

The HCR-20 and other structured clinical methods have become popular because they help clinicians without telling them what to do. They inform and can improve clinical judgement without attempting to substitute for it. The clinical team makes the final decisions.

This strength of the HCR-20 is potentially also its main weakness. Clinicians may feel disappointed that the final decisions and judgements remain with them. Unfortunately, there is no escape from this reality. Violence risk management involves making choices in a complicated situation in which conflicting values have to be balanced against each other and there is a range of possible right answers rather than a single one. It is unrealistic to expect any standard formula to come up with the 'right' answer, because the single right answer does not exist.

The structured clinical method goes beyond assessment into risk management. Violence is not a neutral occurrence. It is always a bad outcome. Good assessment automatically implies management aimed at avoiding the negative outcome.

A potential source of error in the HCR-20 is to add up the scores and use it as an actuarial instrument. In fact, this practice may be adopted as a way of measuring the predictive validity of the HCR-20's items; it is difficult to think of any other way of measuring its predictive abilities.

Statistical evaluations of this type have value, and they suggest that the HCR-20 is comparable to actuarial measures of violence risk. We can derive comfort from that finding – the HCR-20 has indeed chosen 20 of the right variables – while also bearing in mind that it does not reflect best clinical use of the HCR-20.

It is interesting to reflect on how the HCR-20 can be better evaluated. It allows for idiosyncratic variables that, by definition, apply only to the individual patient and so cannot be included in statistical analysis. It also allows for the use of discretion, and so a high score need not imply a clinical judgement of high risk.

The point of the HCR-20 is to formulate a good risk management plan rather than to make a precise prediction. It is against that standard that it should be judged. In other words, it is judged against the standards of clinical practice, and not by the standard (predictive accuracy) of the fortune-teller or the actuary. The problem is that we do not have good ways of measuring standards of clinical practice; the task of the profession is to develop them rather than to allow ourselves to be judged by inappropriate statistical measures.

Meanwhile, the HCR-20 and other structured clinical approaches fit easily into the care programme approach (CPA), which is based on planning for the future and includes regular reviews. The HCR-20's three strands relating to past, present and future are ideally suited to the CPA framework.

RISK-SHARING AND OWNERSHIP

Accurate prediction is never possible in the individual, and we can never eliminate violence risk entirely. Therefore, we have to confront the problem of dealing with uncertainty, and we have to manage negative outcomes. It is inevitable that things will go wrong sometimes, and preparation for a bad outcome is part of risk management.

The first step is to clarify one's responsibilities. Risk assessment and management can be considered as a three-stage process that addresses the following questions:[9]

- *What are the risks associated with treatment of this mental disorder?* Mental health professionals should be able to give a reasonable answer, whether the issue concerns general risks or a specific patient. Professional expertise is relevant.
- *How can the risks be reduced?* Again, professional expertise is relevant, and so this is a reasonable question to address to mental health professionals. We may not be able to implement the measures concerned, but we can give an opinion on the likely effects of particular interventions or non-interventions.
- *Are the residual risks acceptable?* Unlike the previous two questions, the answer to this is to be found not in professional expertise but in moral, social or philosophical considerations. As it is not a technical question, mental health professionals have no claim to special expertise. There are also risks for the profession because, if we take on this responsibility, then we are held to account when things go wrong.

These considerations may seem abstract, but they underpin measures such as the restricted hospital order. Mental health services give their opinions on the risks and the effects of treatment, but the decision on discharge, which is effectively a consideration of whether the risk is acceptable, rests with the Ministry of Justice or with a tribunal.

Similar considerations should apply when dealing with risk in other contexts. At the lowest level, it is essential to involve relations and carers in decisions. The views of other members of the multidisciplinary team should always be sought. When dealing with mentally disordered offenders, there may be joint working with the probation service or the involvement of a multi-agency public protection panel. The common theme is a wider sharing of risks.

It is wrong to dismiss this approach as defensive practice. Once the issues involved go beyond technical questions, the quality of decision-making is improved by the involvement of other perspectives.

THE SECOND OPINION

Risk assessments are rarely right or wrong in categorical terms, but they vary in quality. Similarly, there is usually room for discretion in the way risks are managed. The final arbiter is almost always a matter of clinical judgement. The preceding section stressed the importance of multidisciplinary and multi-agency approaches as a way of sharing risks and improving the quality of decision-making.

In particularly difficult cases, the best course of action is to seek a second opinion. Greater use should be made of forensic services in this respect. There may be no expectation that the service will take over the patient or suggest anything new, but the endorsement of current treatment can be invaluable. When there is no absolute right or wrong answer, it is reassuring to know you have the support of others. After all, a homicide inquiry is nothing more than a second opinion delivered with the benefit of hindsight; it is far better to have the benefit of all that wisdom before the event rather than after it.

KEY POINTS

- Violence risk assessment always requires a detailed history of previous violence and the circumstances in which it occurred.
- Violence risk is multidimensional, and so a comprehensive assessment can never be reduced to a number or percentage on a single measure.
- Structured risk assessment enhances but can never replace clinical judgement.
- The best risk assessments are relative rather than absolute. They facilitate risk management by describing factors that will increase or decrease risk.
- Clinical and non-clinical factors contribute to violence risk. Multi-agency working allows better management and appropriate sharing of risk.
- Decisions on the acceptability of risk are social and political rather than medical. High-risk cases often involve courts and tribunals. Clinicians should take all reasonable steps to involve relatives and carers.
- Violence risk can never be eliminated, and so comprehensive risk management includes planning for a negative outcome.
- There are few absolutes in risk management. There is usually a spectrum of reasonable decisions rather than a single right answer. In doubtful and high-risk cases, the best protection is a second opinion.

REFERENCES

1. Swanson JW, Holzer CE, Ganju VK, Jonjo RT (1990) Violence and psychiatric disorder in the community: evidence from the epidemiologic catchment area surveys. *Hospital and Community Psychiatry* **41**: 761–70.
2. Mullen PE (2006) Schizophrenia and violence: from correlations to preventative strategies. *Advances in Psychiatric Treatment* **12**: 239–48.
3. Shaw J, Hunt IM, Flynn S, *et al.* (2006) Rates of mental disorder in people convicted of homicide: a national clinical survey. *British Journal of Psychiatry* **188**: 143–7.
4. Webster CD, Douglas KS, Eaves D, Hart SD (1997) *HCR-20: Assessing Risk for Violence, Version 2.* Vancouver: Mental Health, Law and Policy Institute, Simon Fraser University.

5. Hart S, Cox D, Hare R (1995) *The Hare Psychopathy Checklist: Screening Version.* Toronto: Multi-Health Systems.
6. Hare RD (1991) *The Psychopathy Checklist Revised.* Toronto: Multi-Health Systems.
7. Maden A (2007) *Treating Violence: A Guide to Risk Management in Mental Health.* Oxford: Oxford University Press.
8. Quinsey VL, Harris GT, Rice ME, Cormier CA (1998) *Violent Risk Appraisal Guide.* Washington: American Psychological Association.
9. Maden A (2005) Violence risk assessment: the question is not whether to do it but how. *Psychiatric Bulletin* 29: 121–2.

APPENDIX I

Domestic Violence, Crime and Victims Act 2004

Provisions for unfitness to plead and insanity

1. Judge rather than jury will determine fitness to plead.
2. Secretary of State loses role in deciding whether defendant is admitted to hospital. Now a matter for Court.
3. Court can no longer order psychiatric hospital admission without medical evidence that justifies detention on grounds of mental state.
4. New range of disposals.
   (a) S. 37 Mental Health Act 1983 with or without a Restriction Order under S. 41.
   (Also S. 38 Interim Hospital Order).
   N.B: Court can now require a hospital to admit.
   (b) Supervision Order for physical and/or mental disorder, but not as inpatient without consent.
   (c) Absolute Discharge.

   Extension of Victim Contact Scheme to victims of Mentally Disordered Offenders.

   Includes offenders:
   - Transferred from prison to hospital.
   - Subject to Hospital Orders with Restriction Orders.

Index

Note: *vs* denotes differential diagnosis or comparisons.
Abbreviations used in index subentries: ADHD – attention deficit hyperactivity disorder, CFS – chronic fatigue syndrome, ECS – electroconvulsive shock, ECT – electroconvulsive therapy, HPA – hypothalamic–pituitary–adrenal, MCS – multiple chemical sensitivity, ME – myalgic encephalomyelitis, OCD – obsessive–compulsive disorder, MS – transcranial magnetic stimulation